Veterinary Cytology

Veterinary Cytology

Leslie C. Sharkey, DVM, PhD, Diplomate ACVP (Clinical Pathology)
Professor
Department of Clinical Sciences
Cummings School of Veterinary Medicine
Tufts University
North Grafton, MA, USA

M. Judith Radin, DVM, PhD, Diplomate ACVP (Clinical Pathology)
Professor Emerita
Department of Veterinary Biosciences
College of Veterinary Medicine
The Ohio State University
Columbus, OH, USA

Davis Seelig, DVM, PhD, Diplomate ACVP (Clinical Pathology)
Associate Professor
Department of Veterinary Clinical Sciences
College of Veterinary Medicine
University of Minnesota
St. Paul, MN, USA

WILEY Blackwell

This edition first published 2021

Registered Office
John Wiley & Sons, Inc., 111 River Street, Hoboken, NJ 07030, USA

Editorial Office
111 River Street, Hoboken, NJ 07030, USA

For details of our global editorial offices, customer services, and more information about Wiley products visit us at www.wiley.com.

Wiley also publishes its books in a variety of electronic formats and by print-on-demand. Some content that appears in standard print versions of this book may not be available in other formats.

Library of Congress Cataloging-in-Publication Data
Names: Sharkey, Leslie C., editor. | Radin, M. Judith, editor. | Seelig, Davis, editor.
Title: Veterinary cytology / [edited by] Leslie C. Sharkey, M. Judith Radin, Davis Seelig.
Description: Hoboken, NJ : Wiley-Blackwell, 2021. | Includes bibliographical references and index.
Identifiers: LCCN 2019047670 (print) | LCCN 2019047671 (ebook) | ISBN 9781119125709 (cloth) | ISBN 9781119125723 (adobe pdf) | ISBN 9781119125716 (epub)
Subjects: MESH: Animal Diseases–diagnosis | Cytodiagnosis–veterinary | Animal Diseases–pathology | Cytological Techniques–methods | Pathology, Veterinary–methods | Pets
Classification: LCC SF757.25 (print) | LCC SF757.25 (ebook) | NLM SF 757.25 | DDC 636.089/1–dc23
LC record available at https://lccn.loc.gov/2019047670
LC ebook record available at https://lccn.loc.gov/2019047671

Cover Design: Wiley
Cover Images: Microscopic view of animal cell Photo credit – Judith Radin, Brown cat with closed eyes Photo credit – Sandra Diaz, Black and white image of veterinary cytology Photo Credit – Charlotte Hollinger

Set in 9.5/12.5pt STIXTwoText by SPi Global, Pondicherry, India

SKY10096026_011325

Contents

Preface

From its conception, this text was developed to be an evidence-based complement to the range of excellent, albeit species-restricted, published cytology atlases. Although rich in figures, this text is not intended to be a comprehensive atlas, but rather a more traditional textbook in which the editors and an international team of esteemed authors pull together an expansive and enlarging body of veterinary cytology literature. In the spirit of comparative medicine and pathology, we sought to represent as complete a range of species as possible, although there are a few omissions that we hope to address in future editions. A second goal of the text was to introduce, often through coauthorship, perspective from the clinicians with whom we work so closely. We feel this approach adds depth, context, and a new and unique dimension to the presentation and interpretation of the cytology material.

The book contains 66 chapters divided into 16 parts. The first two parts are technique focused, while the subsequent 11 parts are organ/tissue based. The content in these chapters predominantly reflects what is known about the canine, feline, and equine species, in which the cytology literature is most robust. This content is followed by parts on non-traditional species, including exotic companion mammals, rabbits, cattle, camelids, non-human primates, reptiles and birds, amphibians, fish, invertebrates, and sheep and goats. The last part highlights some unique features of the applications of cytology in industry settings.

Finally, this text sought to be evidence based and up to date. However, due to the inevitable delays in the production of a project of this magnitude, new material was undoubtedly published during the editorial process, and some material was no doubt omitted. Regardless, we hope that this text will provide a robust basis for the study of veterinary cytology, including identification of gaps in knowledge that will set the stage for future research. We hope it will be a valuable resource for the veterinary community.

Acknowledgments

We would like to express our sincere appreciation to all those that contributed chapters and images to this book. This has been both a challenging and rewarding experience that we could not have accomplished without you. We would like to thank the clinical pathologists and those from other veterinary disciplines that partnered together to enhance the depth of expertise and critical assessment of their material.

As pathologists, we depend heavily on our laboratory personnel for support, ideas, keeping things organized, finding archived material, and a sense of humor when dealing with us. For this, we want to express our gratitude to the hardworking residents and laboratory staff at The Ohio State University, Cummings School of Veterinary Medicine at Tufts University, and the University of Minnesota.

On a personal note:

I would like to express profound appreciation for the love, patience, and support of my children during this project and all the ones that preceded it.

Leslie C. Sharkey

I would like to thank my family for their love, support, and putting up with me during this process.

M. Judith Radin

I would like to thank my clinical pathologist colleagues and resident trainees at the University of Minnesota and my mentors at Colorado State University.

Davis Seelig

List of Contributors

Editors

M. Judith Radin, DVM, PhD, Diplomate ACVP (Clinical Pathology)
Professor Emerita
Department of Veterinary Biosciences
College of Veterinary Medicine
The Ohio State University
Columbus, OH, USA

Davis Seelig, DVM, PhD, Diplomate ACVP (Clinical Pathology)
Associate Professor
Department of Veterinary Clinical Sciences
College of Veterinary Medicine
University of Minnesota
St. Paul, MN, USA

Leslie C. Sharkey, DVM, PhD, Diplomate ACVP (Clinical Pathology)
Department of Clinical Sciences
Cummings School of Veterinary Medicine
Tufts University
North Grafton, MA, USA

Contributors

Laura Adhikari, MD
Director of Cytopathology
Department of Pathology
University of Oklahoma Health Sciences Center
Oklahoma City, OK, USA

Irina Amorim, DVM, PhD
Assistant Professor
Department of Pathology and Molecular Immunology
Institute of Biomedical Sciences Abel Salazar (ICBAS)
University of Porto
Porto, Portugal

Kari L. Anderson, DVM, Diplomate ACVR
Professor of Medical Imaging
Department of Veterinary Clinical Sciences
College of Veterinary Medicine
University of Minnesota
Minneapolis, MN, USA

Luca Aresu, DVM, PhD
Department of Veterinary Sciences
Università degli Studi di Torino
Turin, Italy

Anne C. Avery, VMD, PhD
Associate Professor
Department of Microbiology, Immunology and Pathology
College of Veterinary Medicine and Biomedical Sciences
Colorado State University
Fort Collins, CO, USA

Paul R. Avery, VMD, PhD, Diplomate ACVP
Department of Microbiology, Immunology and Pathology
Colorado State University
Fort Collins, CO, USA

Kirstin F. Barnhart, DVM, Diplomate ACVP, PhD
Abbvie, Inc.
Associate Director, Clinical Pathology
Senior Pathologist
North Chicago, IL, USA

Janet Beeler-Marfisi
Assistant Professor
Department of Pathobiology
University of Guelph
Guelph, Ontario, Canada

Catherine J. Benson, DVM, Diplomate ACVP (Clinical and Anatomic)
Specialist Veterinary Pathologist
IDEXX Laboratories
East Brisbane, QLD, Australia

Walter Bertazzolo, DVM, ECVCP Diplomate
Clinical Laboratory
Ospedale Veterinario Città di Pavia
Laboratorio di Analisi Veterinarie LaVallonea
Alessano, Italy

Joseph J. Bertone, DVM, MS, Diplomate ACVIM (Large Animal)
Professor, Equine Medicine
College of Veterinary Medicine
Western University of Health Sciences
Pomona, CA, USA

Dorothee Bienzle, DVM, PhD, Diplomate ACVP
Professor and Canada Research Chair in Veterinary Pathology
Department of Pathobiology
University of Guelph
Guelph, Ontario,
Canada

Ugo Bonfanti, Med. Vet. ECVCP Diplomate
Veterinary Laboratory La Vallonéa,
Passirana di Rho, MI, Italy

Jennifer L. Brazzell, DVM, MVetSc, MRCVS, Diplomate ACVP (Clinical and Anatomic)
Veterinary Pathologist
Marshfield Labs
Marshfield, WI, USA

Matthew Breen, PhD, CBiol, FRSB
Oscar J. Fletcher Distinguished Professor of
Comparative Oncology Genetics
Department of Molecular Biomedical Sciences
College of Veterinary Medicine
North Carolina State University
Raleigh, NC, USA

Jeff Bryan, DVM, PhD, Diplomate ACVIM
Department of Veterinary Medicine and Surgery
University of Missouri College of Veterinary Medicine
Columbia, MO, USA

Erin N. Burton, DVM, MS, Diplomate ACVP
Department of Veterinary and Biomedical Sciences
College of Veterinary Medicine
University of Minnesota
St. Paul, MN, USA

Jenna H. Burton, DVM, MS, Diplomate ACVIM (Oncology)
Assistant Professor of Clinical Oncology
Department of Surgical and Radiological Sciences
School of Veterinary Medicine
University of California
Davis, CA, USA

Shelley Burton, DVM, MSc, Diplomate ACVP (Clinical Pathology)
Professor of Clinical Pathology
Department of Pathology and Microbiology
Atlantic Veterinary College
University of Prince Edward Island
Charlottetown, Prince Edward Island, Canada

Christopher K. Cebra, VMD, MA, MS, Diplomate ACVIM-LA
The Pfefferkorn and Wendorf Professor
of Camelid Medicine
Oregon State University College of Veterinary Medicine
Corvallis, OR, USA

Joan Ripley Coates, BS, DVM, MS, Diplomate ACVIM (Neurology)
Professor of Veterinary Neurology and Neurosurgery
Department of Veterinary Medicine and Surgery
Neurology & Neurosurgery Service Leader
Veterinary Health Center (Small Animal Hospital)
University of Missouri
Columbia, MO, USA

Stefano Comazzi, DVM, PhD, Diplomate ECVCP
Department of Veterinary Medicine and Public Health
University of Milan
Milan, Italy

Francisco de Oliveira Conrado, DVM, MSc, Diplomate ACVP (Clinical)
Assistant Professor
Department of Biomedical Sciences
Cummings School of Veterinary Medicine
Tufts University
North Grafton, MA, USA

Michelle Cora, DVM, Diplomate ACVP, Veterinary Medical Officer/NTP Clinical Pathologist
National Toxicology Program
National Institute of Environmental Health Sciences
Research Triangle Park, NC, USA

Etienne Côté, DVM, Diplomate ACVIM (Cardiology, Small Animal Internal Medicine)
Associate Professor
3M National Teaching Fellow
Department of Companion Animals
Atlantic Veterinary College
University of Prince Edward Island
Charlottetown, Prince Edward Island, Canada

Sarah Crain, DVM, MS, Diplomate ACVIM
Cummings School of Veterinary Medicine at Tufts University
Department of Clinical Sciences
North Grafton, MA, USA

Alice Defarges Bichot, DVM, MSc, Diplomate ACVIM (Small Animals)
Assistant Professor in Small Animal Internal Medicine
Department of Clinical Studies
Ontario Veterinary College
University of Guelph
Guelph, Ontario, Canada

Sharon M. Dial, DVM, PhD, Diplomate ACVP
Director
Arizona Veterinary Diagnostic Laboratory
University of Arizona
Tucson, AZ, USA

Sandra Diaz, DVM, MS, Diplomate ACVD
Assistant Professor
Department of Veterinary Clinical Sciences
College of Veterinary Medicine
The Ohio State University
Columbus, OH, USA

Olivier Dossin, DVM, PhD, Diplomate ECVIM-CA (Internal Medicine)
Associate Professor
Small Animal Internal Medicine
INP – Ecole Vétérinaire
Université Fédérale Toulouse Midi Pyrénées
Toulouse, France

Jean-Yves Douet, DVM, PhD, Diplomate ESV (Ophthalmology)
Associate Professor in Veterinary and Comparative Ophthalmology
Département des Sciences Cliniques
INP-Ecole Nationale Vétérinaire
Toulouse, France

Jill Schappa Faustich, DVM, Diplomate ACVP
Clinical Instructor
Department of Veterinary Clinical Sciences
University of Minnesota Veterinary Medical Center
St. Paul, MN, USA

Eric J. Fish, DVM, PhD, Diplomate ACVP (Clinical)
Clinical Pathologist II
IDEXX Laboratories, Inc.
Westbrook, ME, USA

Thomas Gibson, BSc, BEd, DVM, DVSc, Diplomate ACVS (Small Animal)
Associate Professor, Small Animal Surgery
Department of Clinical Studies
Ontario Veterinary College
University of Guelph
Guelph, Ontario, Canada

Jennifer Graham, DVM, Diplomate ABVP (Avian/Exotic Companion Mammal), Diplomate ACZM
Associate Professor of Zoological Companion Animal Medicine
Department of Clinical Sciences
Cummings School of Veterinary Medicine
Tufts University
North Grafton, MA, USA

Fanny Granat, DVM, PhD, ECVCP Diplomate
Consultant in Clinical Pathology
LAPVSO Laboratory
Toulouse, France

Angela Gwynn, MEd, DVM, Diplomate ACVP (Clinical Pathology)
Clinical Pathology Resident
Department of Veterinary Sciences
University of Minnesota
St. Paul, MN, USA

Daniel Heinrich, DVM, Diplomate ACVP (Clinical)
Clinical Pathology Resident
University of Minnesota Veterinary Medical Center
St. Paul, MN, USA

Sally E. Henderson, DVM, PhD, Diplomate ACVP (Clinical Pathology)
Veterinary Clinical Pathologist
IDEXX Laboratories, Inc.
Worthington, OH, US

Michala de Linde Henriksen, DVM, PhD, Diplomate ACVO
Assistant Professor, Comparative Ophthalmology
Department of Clinical Sciences
College of Veterinary Medicine and Biomedical Sciences
Colorado State University
Fort Collins, CO, USA

Natalie Hoepp, DVM, MS, Diplomate ACVP
Medical Director
Scopio Labs
Philadelphia, PA, USA

Charlotte Hollinger, VMD, MS, Diplomate ACVP (Clinical and Anatomic)
Associate Pathologist
Wildlife Conservation Society
Zoological Health Program
Bronx, NY, USA

Emma Hooijberg, BVSc (pret), CertGP(SAP), Diplomate ECVCP
Senior Lecturer, Veterinary Clinical Pathology
Department of Companion Animal Clinical Studies
Faculty of Veterinary Science
University of Pretoria
Pretoria, South Africa

K. Lisa Hulme-Moir, BVSc (Dist), PhD
Gribbles Veterinary Ltd.
Auckland, New Zealand

Thomas Jenei, DVM, Diplomate ACVS
Assistant Clinical Professor
Department of Veterinary Clinical Sciences
Tufts Cummings School of Veterinary Medicine
North Grafton, MA, USA

Courtney Johnson, BS, DVM
Veterinary Clinical Pathology Resident
Department of Veterinary Clinical Sciences
University of Minnesota
St Paul, MN, USA

John Keating, DVM, Diplomate ACVP
Director of Pathology
CBSET, Inc.
Lexington, MA, USA

William C. Kisseberth, DVM, PhD, Diplomate ACVIM (Oncology)
Associate Professor
Department of Veterinary Clinical Sciences
College of Veterinary Medicine
Ohio State University
Columbus, OH, USA

Joyce S. Knoll, VMD, PhD, Diplomate ACVP (Clinical Pathology)
Associate Professor and Chair
Department of Biomedical Sciences
Cummings School of Veterinary Medicine
North Grafton, MA, USA

Sandra Nogueira Koch, DVM, MS, Diplomate ACVD
Associate Professor, Dermatology
Veterinary Clinical Sciences
Veterinary College
University of Minnesota
St. Paul, MN, USA

Judith Koenig, Mag Vet Med, Dr. Med Vet, DVSc, Diplomate ACVS, Diplomate ECVS, Diplomate ACVSMR
Associate Professor, Large Animal Surgery & Equine Medicine and Rehabilitation
Department of Clinical Studies
Ontario Veterinary College
University of Guelph
Guelph, Ontario, Canada

Paula M. Krimer, DVM, DVSc, Diplomate ACVP
Athens Veterinary Diagnostic Laboratory and Department of Pathology
University of Georgia
Athens, Georgia

Mary Anna Labato, DVM, Diplomate ACVIM (SAIM)
Clinical Professor
Section Head Small Animal Medicine
Department of Clinical Sciences
Cummings School of Veterinary Medicine
North Grafton, MA, USA

Jessica Lawrence, DVM, Diplomate ACVIM (Oncology), Diplomate ACVR (Radiation Oncology), MRCVS
Senior Lecturer & Head of Oncology
University of Edinburgh
The Royal (Dick) School of Veterinary Studies
Easter Bush Campus
Midlothian, United Kingdom

Sarah E. Leavell, DVM
Post-Doctoral Fellow
Department of Microbiology, Immunology, and Pathology
College of Veterinary Medicine and Biomedical Sciences
Colorado State University
Fort Collins, CO, USA

Christine C. Lim, DVM, Diplomate ACVO
Assistant Professor of Ophthalmology
College of Veterinary Medicine
University of Minnesota
St. Paul, MN, USA

Cheryl London, DVM, PhD, Diplomate ACVIM (Oncology)
Professor
Department of Veterinary Biosciences
The Ohio State University
Columbus, OH, USA

Susan Lowum, MS, DVM, Diplomate ABVP (Canine and Feline Practice)
Assistant Professor, Primary Care
Veterinary Clinical Science Department
College of Veterinary Medicine
University of Minnesota
St. Paul, MN, USA

Catriona Lyle, BVM&S, MSc, Diplomate ECEIM
Senior Lecturer in Equine Medicine
Department of Companion Animal Clinical Studies
Faculty of Veterinary Science
University of Pretoria
Pretoria, South Africa

Scott Madill, BVSc, DVSc, Diplomate, American College of Theriogenologists
Assistant Professor and Associate Medical Director
Department of Veterinary Population Medicine
College of Veterinary Medicine
University of Minnesota
St. Paul, MN, USA

Carlo Masserdotti, DVM, Dipl ECVCP, Spec Bioch Clin IAT
Anatomic and Clinical Pathologist
Idexx Laboratories
Italy

Camille A. McAloney, DVM
Department of Veterinary Biosciences
College of Veterinary Medicine
The Ohio State University
Columbus, OH, USA

Meredeth Crandall McEntire, DVM, MS, Diplomate ACVP (Clinical Pathology)
Clinical Pathologist
Pet Emergency Clinic & Referral Center
Spokane, WA, USA

Melissa Dawn Meachem, DVM, MVetSc, Diplomate ACVP (Clinical Pathology)
Clinical Associate
Department of Veterinary Pathology
Western College of Veterinary Medicine
University of Saskatchewan
Saskatoon, Saskatchewan, Canada

Helen Michael
Comparative Pathology Fellow
Center for Cancer Research, National Cancer Institute
Bethesda, MD, USA

Doris M. Miller, DVM, PhD, Diplomate ACVP
Associate Director of State Government Relations
Professor
Athens and Tifton Veterinary
Diagnostic Labs
College of Veterinary Medicine
University of Georgia
Athens, GA, USA

Laurie Millward, DVM, MS, Diplomate ACVP
Assistant Professor- Clinical
Department of Veterinary Clinical Sciences
College of Veterinary Medicine
The Ohio State University
Columbus, OH, USA

Elspeth Milne, BVM&S, PhD, Diplomate ECVCP, FRCPath, FHEA, FRCVS
Head of Veterinary Pathology
Royal (Dick) School of Veterinary Studies
The University of Edinburgh
Easter Bush Campus
Midlothian, United Kingdom

Julia Bettina Montgomery, Med Vet, PhD, Diplomate ACVIM (Large Animal)
Assistant Professor
Department of Large Animal Clinical Sciences
Western College of Veterinary Medicine
University of Saskatchewan
Saskatoon, Saskatchewan, Canada

Alisa L. Newton, VMD, Diplomate ACVP
Head, Aquatic Health
Wildlife Conservation Society
Zoological Health Program
New York Aquarium
Brooklyn, NY, USA

Jed Overmann, DVM, Diplomate ACVP
Assistant Professor, Clinical Pathology
Department of Veterinary Clinical Sciences
University of Minnesota
St. Paul, MN, USA

Liron Pantanowitz, MD
Director, Division of Anatomic Pathology
A. James French Professor of Pathology
Department of Pathology & Clinical Labs
University of Michigan
Ann Arbor, MI, USA

Reema T. Patel, DVM, Diplomate ACVP
Clinical Pathologist
Antech Diagnostics
Annapolis, MD, USA

Helene Pendl, Dr. Med. Vet.
Pendl Lab
Diagnostic Microscopy
Hematology, Cytology, and Histopathology in Birds and Reptiles
Switzerland

Allan P. Pessier, DVM, Diplomate ACVP
Clinical Associate Professor
Washington Animal Disease Diagnostic Laboratory
Department of Veterinary Microbiology and Pathology
College of Veterinary Medicine
Washington State University
Pullman, WA, USA

Cesar Piedra-Mora, DVM
Anatomic Pathology Resident
Department of Biomedical Sciences
Cummings School of Veterinary Medicine
Tufts University
North Grafton, MA, USA

Florence Poitout-Belissent, DVM, Diplomate ACVP, Diplomate ECVCP
Scientific Director Clinical Pathology
Charles River Laboratories, Inc.
Montreal, Quebec, Canada

Heather L. Priest, DVM, Diplomate ACVP
Clinical Pathologist II
Charles River Laboratories
Reno, NV, USA

Nicholas A. Robinson, BVSc (Hons), PhD, MACVSc, Diplomate ACVP
Associate Professor
Department of Biomedical Sciences
Cummings School of Veterinary Medicine
Tufts University
North Grafton, MA, USA

Margaret V. Root Kustritz
Assistant Dean of Education and Professor, Theriogenology
Department of Veterinary Clinical Sciences
University of Minnesota
St. Paul, MN, USA

Kelly S. Santangelo, DVM, PhD, Diplomate ACVP
Assistant Professor, Clinical Pathology Section
Department of Microbiology, Immunology, and Pathology
College of Veterinary Medicine and Biomedical Sciences
Colorado State University
Fort Collins, CO, USA

Deanna M.W. Schaefer, DVM, MS, MT(ASCP), Diplomate ACVP
Assistant Professor of Veterinary Clinical Pathology
Department of Biomedical and Diagnostic Sciences
University of Tennessee
Knoxville, TN, USA

Jodi A. Scholz, DVM, Diplomate ACLAM
Assistant Professor
Department of Comparative Medicine
Rochester, MN, USA

Diana Schwartz, DVM
Resident, Clinical Pathology
Department of Pathology, Microbiology and Immunology
School of Veterinary Medicine
University of California Davis
Davis, CA, USA

Cleverson D. Souza, DVM, MSc, PhD, Diplomate ACVP
Department of Veterinary Clinical Sciences
College of Veterinary Medicine
Washington State University
Pullman, WA, USA

Wendy S. Sprague, DVM, PhD
Sprague Medical and Scientific Communications, LLC
Fort Collins, CO, USA

Nicole I. Stacy, DVM, Dr. Med. Vet, Diplomate ACVP
Aquatic, Amphibian, and Reptile Pathology
Department of Comparative, Diagnostic and Population Medicine
College of Veterinary Medicine
University of Florida
Gainesville, FL, USA

Jennifer D. Steinberg, DVM, Diplomate ACVP (Clinical)
Senior Clinical Pathologist
Lacuna Diagnostics
Baltimore, MD, USA

Kevin S. Stepaniuk, DVM, FAVD, Diplomate AVDC
Columbia River Veterinary Specialists
Vancouver, WA, USA

Mark A. Suckow, DVM, Diplomate ACLAM
Associate Vice President for Research
Attending Veterinarian
Professor, Department of Biomedical Engineering
University of Kentucky
Lexington, KY, USA

Marian Taulescu, DVM, MSc, PhD, Diplomate ECVP
Associate Professor
Department of Veterinary Pathology
Faculty of Veterinary Medicine Cluj-Napoca
Cluj-Napoca, Romania

Mary Anna Thrall, DVM, MS, Diplomate ACVP
Professor
Department of Biomedical Sciences
Ross University School of Veterinary Medicine
Basseterre, St Kitts, West Indies

Julie Tomlinson, DVM, Diplomate ACVP
Clinical Pathologist
Lacuna Diagnostics
Auckland, New Zealand

Susan J. Tornquist, DVM, MS, PhD, Diplomate ACVP
College of Veterinary Medicine
Oregon State University
Corvallis, OR, USA

Cathy Trumel, DVM, PhD, ECVCP Diplomate
Professor of Veterinary Clinical Pathology
Université de Toulouse
Toulouse, France

Harold Tvedten, DVM, PhD
Clinical Veterinarian
University Animal Hospital
Swedish University of Agricultural Sciences
Uppsala, Sweden

Linda M. Vap, DVM, Diplomate ACVP (Clinical Pathology)
Associate Professor
Department of Microbiology, Immunology and Pathology
College of Veterinary Medicine
Colorado State University
Fort Collins, CO, USA

Karen M. Vernau, DVM, MAS, Diplomate ACVIM (Neurology)
Professor of Neurology/Neurosurgery
Department of Surgical and Radiological Sciences
School of Veterinary Medicine
University of California, Davis
Davis, CA, USA

William Vernau, BSc, BVMS, DVSc, PhD, Diplomate ACVP
Professor of Clinical Pathology
Director of Clinical Laboratories
Department of Pathology, Microbiology and Immunology
School of Veterinary Medicine
University of California, Davis
Davis, CA, USA

Koranda A. Walsh, VMD, Diplomate ACVIM (SAIM), Diplomate ACVP (Clinical Pathology)
Assistant Professor of Clinical Pathobiology
University of Pennsylvania
Philadelphia, PA, USA

Jillian Zientek Walz, DVM, Diplomate ACVIM (Oncology)
Resident in Small Animal Oncology
Department of Veterinary Clinical Sciences
College of Veterinary Medicine
University of Minnesota, St. Paul, MN, USA

Robert Washabau, VMD, PhD, Diplomate ACVIM
Professor
University of Minnesota
Department of Clinical Sciences
St. Paul, MN, USA

Kyle Lauren Webb, DVM, Diplomate ACVP (Clinical)
Clinical Pathologist
ANTECH Diagnostics
Orlando, FL, USA

Amy L. Weeden, DVM, Diplomate ACVP (Clinical)
Diagnostic Clinical Pathologist
Gribbles Veterinary
Auckland, New Zealand

Nicole M. Weinstein, DVM, Diplomate ACVP
Associate Professor
Department of Pathobiology
University of Pennsylvania
Philadelphia, PA, USA

Maxey L. Wellman, DVM, MS, PhD, Diplomate ACVP (Clinical Pathology)
Professor
Department of Veterinary Biosciences
College of Veterinary Medicine
The Ohio State University
Columbus, OH, USA

Peter M. Wencel, DVM
Al Aseefa Falcon Clinic
Dubai, United Arab Emirates

Marlyn S. Whitney, DVM, PhD, Diplomate ACVP (Clinical Pathology)
Associate Clinical Professor
Department of Veterinary Pathobiology
Veterinary Medical Diagnostic Laboratory
College of Veterinary Medicine
University of Missouri
Columbia, MO, USA

Charles E. Wiedmeyer, DVM, PhD, Diplomate ACVP
Associate Professor
Department of Veterinary Pathobiology
College of Veterinary Medicine
University of Missouri
Columbia, MO, USA

Angela Wilcox, BVSc, MS, Diplomate ACVP, Diplomate ABT
Senior Clinical Pathologist
Charles River Laboratories, Inc.
Reno, NV, USA

Carrie A. Wood, DVM, Diplomate ACVIM (Oncology)
Clinical Instructor, Harrington Oncology
Cummings School of Veterinary Medicine
Tufts University
North Grafton, MA, USA

R. Darren Wood, DVM, DVSc, Diplomate ACVP (Clinical Pathology)
Associate Professor
Department of Pathobiology
Ontario Veterinary College
University of Guelph
Guelph, Ontario, Canada

List of Abbreviations

α-SMA	α-smooth muscle actin
ABK	acute bullous keratopathy
ACM1	muscarinic acetylcholine receptor M1
ACTH	adrenocorticotropic hormone
AGID	agarose gel immunodiffusion
AgNOR	argyrophilic nucleolar organizer regions
AHS	airway hypersensitivity
AI	antibody index
ALP	alkaline phosphatase
AMH	anti-Müllerian hormone
ANAE	alpha naphthyl acetate esterase
ANBE	alpha naphthyl butyrate esterase
AO	atlanto-occipital space
APOT	amyloid-producing odontogenic tumors
APUD	amine precursor uptake and decarboxylation
AQ	albumin quotient
AR	antigen retrieval
ASA	anti-sperm antibodies
ASCUS	atypical cells of undetermined significance
AST	aspartate aminotransferase
ASVCP	American Society for Veterinary Clinical Pathology
AV	artificial vagina
BAC	bacterial artificial chromosome
BAL	bronchoalveolar lavage
BALF	bronchoalveolar lavage fluid
BBB	blood–brain barrier
BCG	bromocresol green
BCR	breakpoint cluster region
Bd	*Batrachochytrium dendrobatidis*
BFG	blood-to-fluid glucose
BLV	bovine leukemia virus/bovine leukosis virus
BPH	benign prostatic hyperplasia
BPV	bovine papillomavirus
BPV-DNA	bovine papillomavirus DNA
Bsal	*Batrachochytrium salamandrivorans*
BSE	breeding soundness examination
CAA	canine acanthomatous ameloblastoma
CAEV	caprine arthritis-encephalitis virus
CANARA	canine androgen receptor assay
CAP	College of American Pathologists
CASA	computer-assisted sperm analysis
CAV	canine adenovirus
CB	cell block
CBC	complete blood count
CB-MSCs	umbilical cord blood-derived mesenchymal stromal cells
CC	calcinosis circumscripta
CCLR	cranial cruciate ligament rupture
CD	cluster of differentiation
CDV	canine distemper virus
CD25	cluster of differentiation 25 (interleukin-2 receptor subunit)
CEH	cystic endometrial hyperplasia
cerb	C-erbB-2 oncoprotein
CFA	*Canis familiaris* autosome (dog chromosome)
CGH	comparative genomic hybridization
CHF	congestive heart failure
CHOP	cyclophosphamide, doxorubicin, vincristine, prednisone
CHV	canine herpesvirus-1
CI	confidence interval
CK	cytokeratins
CKD	chronic kidney disease
c-KIT	tyrosine protein kinase kit or CD117
CK7	cytokeratin 7
CLs	corpora lutea
CLE	cutaneous lupus erythematosus
CLIA '88	Clinical Laboratory Improvement Amendments of 1988
CM	cerebellomedullary cistern
CMG-3G5	cell membrane ganglioside recognized by the antibody 3G5
CML	chronic myelogenous leukemia
CNS	central nervous system
COPD	chronic obstructive pulmonary disease
CPDD	calcium pyrophosphate deposition disease
cPLI	pancreas-specific lipase immunoreactivity
CPSE	canine prostate specific esterase
CQI	continuous quality improvement

CSF	cerebrospinal fluid
CT	computed tomography
CTMC	connective mast cells
cTn-I	cardiac troponin I
CV	coefficient of variation
DAPI	4′,6-diamidino-2-phenylindole
DART	developmental and reproductive toxicology
DCX	doublecortin
ddPCR	droplet digital polymerase chain reaction
DHB	Birt–Hogg–Dube gene
DIC	differential interference contrast
DLBCL	diffuse large B cell lymphoma
DRE	digital rectal exam
DTM	dermatophyte test medium
EATL	enteropathy associated T-cell lymphoma
EBC	evidence-based cytology
EBL	enzootic bovine leukosis
EBM	evidence-based medicine
ECM	extracellular matrix
EDTA	ethylenediaminetetraacetic acid
EEE	eastern equine encephalitis
EGC	eosinophilic granuloma complex
EGFR	epidermal growth factor receptor
EHV	equine herpes virus
EHV-1	equine herpes virus-1
EIPH	exercise-induced pulmonary hemorrhage
ELISA	enzyme-linked immunosorbent assay
EMEA	European Agency for Evaluation of Medicinal Products
EMH	extramedullary hematopoiesis
EN	eosin-nigrosin
ENTV	enzootic nasal tumor virus
EPM	equine protozoal myeloencephalitis
ER	estrogen receptor
ERU	equine recurrent uveitis
FAS	fibrosarcoma
FCoV	feline coronavirus
FDA	US Food and Drug Administration
FFH	focal fibrous hyperplasia
FFPE	formalin fixed paraffin embedded
FH	fibrohistiocytic nodule
FHV	feline herpesvirus
FIC	feline idiopathic cystitis
FIMCT	feline intestinal mast cell tumors
FIOT	feline inductive odontogenic tumors
FIP	feline infectious peritonitis
FISH	fluorescence *in situ* hybridization
FL	follicular lymphoma
FNA	fine-needle aspirate
FNAB	fine-needle aspiration biopsy
FNCB	fine-needle capillary biopsy
FROMS	feline restrictive myofibroblastic sarcoma
FSA	fibrosarcoma
FSH	follicle stimulating hormone
FURTD	feline upper respiratory tract disease
FVH1	feline herpesvirus 1
G	gauge
GATA-4	transcription factor GATA-4
GBM	glioblastoma multiforme
GC	germinal center
GCT	granular cell tumor
GFAP	glial fibrillary acidic protein
GIST	gastrointestinal stromal tumors
GIT	gastrointestinal tract
GME	granulomatous meningoencephalomyelitis
GMS	Gomori methenamine silver
GnRH	gonadotropin releasing hormone
GP	gastric polyps
GST α	glutathione S-transferase α
H&E	hematoxylin and eosin
HBME-1	Hector Battifora mesothelial epitope-1
HCC	hepatocellular carcinoma
HEP	hemangiopericytoma
HER-2	human epidermal growth factor receptor 2
HG	HistoGel™
HHS	hemophagocytic histiocytic sarcoma
HIER	heat-induced epitope retrieval
HLL	Hodgkin-like lymphoma
HMB-45	human melanoma black monoclonal antibody against melanosomal glycoprotein gp100 (Pmel17)
HPF	high powered field, 400× magnification
HPV	human papillomavirus
HRP	horseradish peroxidase
HS	histiocytic sarcoma
HSA	*Homo sapiens* autosome (human chromosome)
HSL	hepatosplenic lymphoma
HUMARA	human androgen receptor assay
IAD	inflammatory airway disease
IB	inclusion body
IBD	inflammatory bowel disease in Chapters 9 and 32
IBD	inclusion body disease in Chapter 61
ICC	immunocytochemistry
ICIB	intracytoplasmic inclusion bodies
ICP	intracranial pressure
ICT	interstitial cell tumor (Leydig tumor)
IFAT	indirect fluorescent antibody test
Ig	immunoglobulin
IGCNU	intratubular germ cell neoplasia of undifferentiated origin
IGF	insulin-like growth factor
IGFBP2	insulin-like growth factor binding protein 2
IgG	immunoglobulin G
IGR	immunoglobulin receptor

IHC	immunohistochemistry
IL	interleukin
IL-8	interleukin-8
IM	intramuscular
IMMK	immune-mediated keratitis
IMPA	immune-mediated polyarthritis
INIB	intranuclear inclusion bodies
IR-LPP	immunomodulatory-responsive lymphocytic-plasmacytic pododermatitis
ITC	isolated tumor cells
IVDH	intervertebral disc herniation
KCS	keratoconjunctivitis sicca
Ki67	nonhistone protein found in the nucleus of proliferating cells
KIT	gene that encodes c-Kit
KPI	karyopyknotic index
L : E	lymphocyte to epithelial ratio
LBC	liquid-based cytology
LBL	lymphoblastic lymphoma
LC3	microtubule-associated protein light chain 3
LDH	lactate dehydrogenase
LDIF	leukocyte differential count
LE	lupus erythematosus
LGL	large granular lymphocyte
LH	luteinizing hormone
LINE	long interspersed nuclear element
LIS	laboratory information system
LPS	lipopolysaccharide
LRT	lower respiratory tract
LS	lumbosacral cistern
LYVE-1	lymphatic vessel endothelial receptor-1
mAbs	monoclonal antibodies
MALT	mucosa-associated lymphoid tissue
MAP-2	microtubule-associated protein-2
MART-1	melanoma-associated antigen recognized by T cells
MCE	multiple cartilaginous exostosis
MCL	mantle cell lymphoma
MCP-1	monocyte chemoattractant protein
MCT	mast cell tumors
MEED	multisystemic eosinophilic epitheliotrophic disease
melan-A	melanoma antigen recognized by T cells 1 or MART-1
MHLW	Japan's Ministry of Health, Labor and Welfare
MiTF	melanoma-associated transcription factor
MMC	mucosal mast cells
MMP	matrix metalloproteinase
MPNST	malignant peripheral nerve sheath tumors
MPO	myeloperoxidase
MPS	mononuclear-phagocytic system
MRD	myeloma-related disorders
MRI	magnetic resonance imaging
MST	median survival time
MUM1/IRF4	multiple myeloma oncogene 1/interferon regulatory factor 4
MUO	meningoencephalomyelitis of unknown origin
MZL	marginal zone lymphoma
N:C	nuclear to cytoplasmic ratio
NALT	nasal-associated lymphoid tissue
NBT/BCIP	nitro blue tetrazolium chloride/5-bromo-4-chloro-3-indolyl phosphate
NE	necrotizing encephalitis
NETs	neutrophil extracellular traps
NGFR	nerve growth factor receptor
NHP	nonhuman primate
NLE	necrotizing leukoencephalitis
NMB	new methylene blue
NME	necrotizing meningoencephalitis
NPV	negative predictive value
NSE	neuron-specific enolase
NT-proBNP	N-terminal pro-B-type natriuretic peptide test
NZW	New Zealand white
OA	osteoarthritis
OCD	osteochondritis dissecans
OIF	oil immersion field with 1000× magnification
Olig2	oligodendrocyte transcription factor 2
OSA	osteosarcoma
pAbs	polyclonal antibodies
PAGE	polyacrylamide gel electrophoresis
PALs	periarterial lymphatic sheaths
Pap	Papanicolaou
PAP	prostatic acid phosphatase
PARR	polymerase chain reaction for antigen receptor rearrangement
PAS	periodic acid-Schiff
PAS-D	periodic acid-Schiff after diastase
PBS	phosphate-buffered saline
PCNA	proliferating cell nuclear antigen
PCR	polymerase chain reaction
PCV	packed cell volume
PDGFRα	platelet derived growth factor alpha receptor
PECAM	platelet endothelial cell adhesion molecule
PEH	pseudo-placentational endometrial hyperplasia
PF	pemphigus foliaceus
PGP 9.5	member of the ubiquitin hydrolase protein family
PH	portal hypertension
PHP	primary hyperparathyroidism
PI	propidium iodide
PIN	prostatic intraepithelial neoplasia

PLAP	placental alkaline phosphatase
PMNs	polymorphonuclear cells or neutrophils
PMRCT	primitive malignant round cell tumor
PNET	primitive neuroectodermal tumor
PNL2	anti-melanoma antibody against a fixative resistant melanocyte associated antigen
PNST	peripheral nerve sheath tumors
POC	point-of-care
POF	peripheral odontogenic fibroma
PPV	positive predictive value
PR	progesterone receptor
PROT	CSF protein concentration
PROX-1	prospero-related homeobox gene
PRP	platelet-rich plasma
PSA	prostate-specific antigen
PTAH	phosphotungstic acid-hematoxylin
PTCL-NOS	peripheral T-cell lymphoma not otherwise specified
PTH	parathyroid hormone
PTHrp	parathyroid hormone-related protein
PWT	perivascular wall tumor
QA	quality assurance
QC	quality control
RAO	recurrent airway obstruction
RBC	red blood cells
RCC	red cell count
REAL	Revised European-American Classification of Lymphoid Neoplasms
RI	reference interval
ROSE	rapid on-site sample evaluation
rRNA	ribosomal ribonucleic acid
RSAT	rapid slide agglutination test
S-100	a calcium binding protein
SAA	serum amyloid A
SARA	subacute rumen acidosis
SCC	squamous cell carcinoma in Chapters 20, 21, 30, 31, 40, 56, and 65
SCC	somatic cell count in Chapter 58
SCF	stem cell factor
SCID	severe combined immunodeficiency
SCSA	sperm chromatin structure assay
SCT	Sertoli cell tumor
SD	standard deviation
SE	standard error
SES	subsurface epithelial structures
SFT	Society for Theriogenology
SFV	Shope fibroma virus
SG	specific gravity
SHC	sterile hemorrhagic cystitis
SIL	squamous intraepithelial lesion
SIPS	subinvolution of placental sites
SIV	simian immunodeficiency virus
SLE	systemic lupus erythematosus
SOA	sino-orbital aspergillosis
SOP	standard operating procedure
SOX9	sex-determining region Y box9 gene
SPA	surfactant protein A
SRMA	steroid responsive meningitis arteritis
STP	Society of Toxicologic Pathology
Strep. zoo.	*Streptococcus equi* subspecies *zooepidemicus*
T4	thyroxine
TAT	turnaround time
TCB	transcervical biopsy
TCC	transitional cell carcinomas
TCR	T-cell receptor
TJC	The Joint Commission
TLR	Toll-like receptor
TNFα	tumor necrosis factor alpha
TNCC	total nucleated cell count
TOTW	transoral tracheal wash
TP	total protein
TPS	The Paris System
TQM	total quality management
TRM	transrectal massage
TRP	tyrosinase-related protein
TSH	thyroid stimulating hormone
TTF	thyroid transcription factor
TTF1	thyroid transcription factor 1
TTW	transtracheal wash
TVT	transmissible venereal tumor
TZL	T zone lymphoma
UC	urothelial carcinoma
UP III	uroplakin III
URT	upper respiratory tract
US	ultrasound
USG	urine specific gravity
VEE	Venezuelan equine encephalitis
VEGF	vascular endothelial growth factor
VEGF-R	vascular endothelial growth factor receptor
VLA-QAP™	Veterinary Laboratory Quality Assurance Program
vWF	von Willebrand factor
WB	Western blot
WBC	white blood cell (leukocyte)
WDL	well-differentiated liposarcomas
WF	Working Formulation
WHO	World Health Organization
WNV	West Nile virus
WT-1	Wilms' tumor antigen
XCIP	X-chromosome inactivation profiling
ZVL	zoonotic visceral leishmaniasis

Part I

Basic Cytology Techniques

1

Sample Collection

Kari L. Anderson, Angela Gwynn, Carrie A. Wood, and Leslie C. Sharkey

Introduction

One of the most appealing features about diagnostic cytology is its capacity to provide a timely, inexpensive, and minimally invasive diagnosis. However, the acquisition of a diagnostic quality sample can be strewn with pitfalls contributing to pre-analytical error that can heavily influence the ability to obtain an accurate diagnosis. Understanding and preventing these sources of error will help avoid the frustration of a nondiagnostic sample or diagnostic error. Screening of sample quality is also discussed in Chapter 5; however, briefly, to be diagnostic, a cytology sample should be representative of the lesion, cellular enough to obtain a diagnosis, relatively free of contaminants (e.g. lubricant, gel, bacteria, blood, etc.), appropriately prepared to allow for the interpretation of cellular material, and sufficiently stained (see Chapter 2 for more detail). Four of these five criteria fall under the process of sample acquisition. As such, recognizing the importance of sample acquisition is particularly relevant for clinicians that are submitting their samples to reference laboratories. Based on tissue and lesion type, some samples will have a higher probability of yielding a diagnostic quality slide, and variations in acquisition and preparation methods are required to maximize obtaining diagnostic samples.[1] The specifics of sample collection for particular species or tissues are addressed in those chapters, and Chapter 50 describes the laboratory analysis of fluid samples in detail.

Methods of Sample Collection

There are a number of technical approaches that can be used in the collection of samples for cytologic analysis. The choice of a particular method should be driven primarily by the features of the lesion, the sampled tissue, and the clinical suspicion.[2]

Sampling Superficial or Subcutaneous Masses

Fine-needle aspiration (FNA) is a relatively simple noninvasive technique used to obtain tissue samples. Samples are generally considered to be sensitive with good agreement between cytology and histopathology results for many lesion types.[3,4] Although the procedure is well recognized, there is variability in recommended techniques.[5] Regardless, aspiration is typically performed without clipping or sterile preparation of the site; however, the area should be free of gross contamination. Necrotic or overtly infected areas should also be avoided as these generally yield samples that may not be reflective of the underlying process.

The term aspiration often refers to the application of negative pressure with a syringe attached to a needle. Fine needle is sometimes reserved for needles 20 G or smaller.[6,7] Another option is the capillary, core, or fenestration technique, which can also be referred to as "needle-off" since a syringe is not attached when the needle is introduced into the tissue. This technique was first described in human medicine in 1986 but has been a commonly recognized sampling method in veterinary medicine for many years.[8] Three to four short, rapid redirections are used to obtain the sample; the bevel of the needle cuts through the mass and directs the sample into the inner diameter of the needle. Redirecting the needle into multiple planes significantly increases tissue yield as opposed to unidirectional core sampling.[9] The needle is then attached to an air-filled syringe for expulsion of the sample. Avoiding suction can minimize hemodilution of the sample, and less material is lost to coating the inside of the syringe.

Capillary sampling can be superior in areas where blood contamination can negatively impact sample acquisition, which is more important in highly vascular areas such as the spleen, but can be relevant for hemorrhagic lesions of the skin and subcutaneous tissue as well.[8] Lymph nodes are often aspirated using the capillary technique.[3,5] Because lymphoid cells are prone to rupture, capillary sampling can

Veterinary Cytology, First Edition. Edited by Leslie C. Sharkey, M. Judith Radin, and Davis Seelig.

improve the diagnostic yield. When the needle is inserted, the tip of a finger is positioned to cover the end of the needle hub. This prevents sample leakage from the end of the needle as it is withdrawn. Alternatively, a syringe can be attached to the end of the needle in the capillary method but without suction. The attached syringe provides negative pressure as the needle is withdrawn. Attaching the syringe can aid in manipulating the needle in difficult-to-reach areas or for operators with mobility or dexterity limitations. Sampling complications for superficial structures are typically minimal, but can include hemorrhage, particularly for vascular lesions or if there is a coagulopathy.

Sample Collection Using Advanced Imaging

Indications

Sampling structures that are not superficially accessible or cannot be palpated and stabilized manually can be challenging. Additionally, some lesions will have regions of necrosis or cavitation, which, if sampled, will not reflect the underlying disease process (i.e. "geographic misdiagnosis"). Percutaneous image-guided sampling with FNA, fine-needle biopsy, or tissue-core biopsy can guide precise needle placement and facilitate procurement of samples from deeper lesions in an efficient, effective, and relatively safe manner. Additionally, with image guidance, samples can be obtained from regions of viable tissue suspected to represent the true underlying disease process.[10,11] Image guidance allows the operator to avoid other important structures and minimize risk of laceration of major blood vessels or inadvertent puncture of adjacent organs.[12,13] Image-guided sampling can be more efficient and safe than other methods and result in more positive diagnostic samples, with follow-up imaging assessment for post-biopsy complications possible.[13–15]

Imaging Modalities

Ultrasound (US), fluoroscopy, computed tomography (CT), and magnetic resonance imaging (MRI) have all been described as means to directly visualize and guide sampling of lesions in veterinary patients.[10,13,15–23] The choice of modality depends upon availability of equipment, location of lesion, and preference and experience of the sampler.[10] Each modality has unique advantages and limitations for use during image-guided sampling.[10,16,23] For example, while fluoroscopy provides real-time guidance and can be utilized to sample lesions deep within the lung or bone, staff are exposed to radiation; the internal structure of the lesion cannot be visualized; and it is more challenging to accurately differentiate lesions from adjacent vital structures.[10] Cross-sectional imaging modalities (US, CT, and MRI) have mostly replaced fluoroscopy for percutaneous biopsy because of greater contrast resolution, better visualization of needle placement, and greater overall ability to procure diagnostic samples. CT provides improved tissue evaluation and provides unobstructed visualization of needle pathway and target but generally does not allow real-time guidance, resulting in blind needle passage and in longer procedure times with possible geographic misses.[1,15,16] Compared with CT, MRI has superior soft tissue resolution, lacks beam-hardening artifacts from nearby bone, and involves no radiation exposure, but image-guided sampling with MRI necessitates specialized non-ferromagnetic equipment.[10,11] CT and MRI are generally less available, are more costly, and often require deep sedation or general anesthesia; therefore they are often reserved for lesions that are difficult to biopsy with US guidance.[10,16,23] US-guided sampling is readily accessible, portable, cost effective, and rapid; affords continuous, real-time monitoring of needle insertion; and involves no radiation exposure.[12,13,15] For US-guided fine-needle biopsy, the patient often needs no or minimal sedation. The major limitation to US-guided sampling is inability to identify an acoustic window, such as when overlying gas or bone prevents identification of the lesion.[10]

Materials Required

In general, materials required for image-guided sampling, beyond the imaging equipment, are simple and similar to those needed for non-image-guided sample collection. In our practice, a small gauge (e.g. 22 G) hypodermic (1.5 in.) or spinal (3.5 in.) needle coupled to a 6 cc syringe with either aspiration (FNA) or non-aspiration techniques are employed based on radiologist preference. In some instances, an extension set is attached to the needle and syringe for gentle suction, particularly in the case of sample collection from fluid-filled or more technically challenging structures. Additional materials may be required depending upon the modality used. For example, a localizer method (localizing needles or grid) can be placed on the patient during CT-guided sampling.[16] A needle guidance system can be utilized while procuring samples in order to target very deep, small lesions.[16–18,24,25] A discussion of technique for image guidance with each modality is beyond the scope of this chapter, and the reader is referred to other sources.[10,11,16–18,20–23,26,27]

Complications

A complete discussion of the potential complications per modality is beyond the scope of this chapter. Potential complications depend upon operator experience, sampling needle size, and the location and nature of lesions sampled. Potential complications include pain, fever, hemorrhage, intraparenchymal hematoma, hematuria, peritonitis, pneumothorax, epistaxis, hemoptysis, seizures, spread of infection, tumor seeding, and death.[12,16,17,21,28–34] Complications occurring during image-guided sampling will depend upon the location of the lesion but are reported to be low for fine-needle and tissue-core biopsy with higher risk for bleeding during tissue-core biopsy in the presence of thrombocytopenia.[13,14,35–39] Bleeding at the site is the most commonly reported complication of sampling abdominal structures, but is often minor and self-limiting.[12,40] The risk of hemorrhage is reported to be 0–16.9% in the veterinary literature, with higher risk associated with renal biopsy.[12,13,40–42] A review of FNA utilizing image guidance (fluoroscopy, scintigraphy, CT, and ultrasonography) in over 11 000 human patients demonstrated low risk for any type of complication with a mortality rate of 0.008%, major complication rate of 0.05%, and other complications at a rate of 0.49%.[28] Pneumothorax has been the most commonly reported complication of sampling thoracic structures, especially when aerated lung is penetrated. Typically only a small volume of air is identified and no intervention is necessary.[21,32] Imaging can be repeated after the sampling procedure to assess for any immediate or delayed complications from the procedure.

Sample Preparation and Staining

Once an aspiration sample is obtained, it is transferred to a slide. It is helpful to lay out several clean glass sides before the aspiration procedure. Some slides may retain glass or dust debris, which can significantly interfere with creation of a monolayer of cells on the slide surface. If the slides are not pre-cleaned, wiping with lens paper or a Kimwipe® can significantly improve outcomes. Care should be taken to minimize handling of slides to avoid contamination with keratinocytes. A 10–12 mL syringe can be used with 6–8 mL of air in the syringe to transfer fenestration and capillary samples to glass slides. The syringe with the air is attached to the needle with the sample, and the air should be gently expelled from the syringe to allow a single drop of material to be placed on each slide. Control is important at this step; if excessive amounts of material are placed on the slide, an excessively thick preparation may result. Thick preparations are very difficult to evaluate as they do not stain well, individual cells may not be visible, and excessive pressure may be needed to create the slide increasing the risk of cell rupture (Figure 1.1).[5]

Several methods have been described for preparing slides, but no significant case–control studies have been performed to validate various techniques. Individual outcomes, operator preference, and prior instruction will generally dictate the method. When preparing a slide, any technique creating multiple small droplets should be avoided. Droplets will dry quickly, resulting in excessive thick smears. Many veterinary oncologists use squash preparation when preparing slides. The goal of the slide preparation is to create a monolayer of intact cells that will stain readily and for optimal cytomorphology. To create a squash preparation, two slides are placed at right angles to each other centered over the sample drop on the slide. As the slide is applied, the sample will begin to slowly spread under the slide. When the sample begins to spread, the top slide is gently drawn to the bottom of the other slide to smear the material in a uniform layer on the glass surfaces. It is recommended that the two slides be held in the air while this is done and not placed on a hard surface to avoid excessive downward pressure. This method is not as well suited to liquid specimens, and there is a risk for thick smears if too little pressure is applied or for nondiagnostic ruptured cells if excessive pressure is applied.[5]

The blood smear technique is more appropriate for serous or fluid samples. This method is similar to blood smear preparation. To begin, a clean slide is placed on a stable, hard surface; a drop of the sample is deposited at one end of the slide; and a second slide is directed a third of the way into the sample at a 45° angle. The angled or spreader slide is then quickly drawn down to the bottom of the first slide using gentle pressure to create the feathered edge. A modified method is to combine the squash prep and blood smear techniques and use a 90° rotated flat slide to smear the fluid sample. This is sometimes referred to as a line technique.

Once a slide is created, it must be allowed to dry for one to two minutes at a minimum. Direct heat application especially with an open flame is not recommended because of uneven distribution of heat, cell deformation, and risk for injury. When the slides are dried, a representative slide should be stained and evaluated for adequate cellularity. Diff-Quik is a modified Romanowsky stain readily available in most practice settings. It is generally considered to be a reliable stain for screening smears and most diagnostic applications. Some mast cell granules may not stain with Diff-Quik (Chapter 13), and the lipid contained in lipoma cells is dissolved by the alcohol fixative in step 1 of the staining process.[43,44] Dipping rather than passive immersion is recommended to enhance stain uptake and reduce the time for stain to set.[45] Additional detail on staining is presented in Chapter 2. It is essential that a slide be evaluated for adequate cellularity and quality prior to lab submission. In a UK study, lack of cellularity was the most common reason for a sample to be rejected as nondiagnostic.[1] Screening can also help confirm successful sampling of the target tissue. For example, aspiration of salivary tissue can inadvertently occur during attempts to aspirate

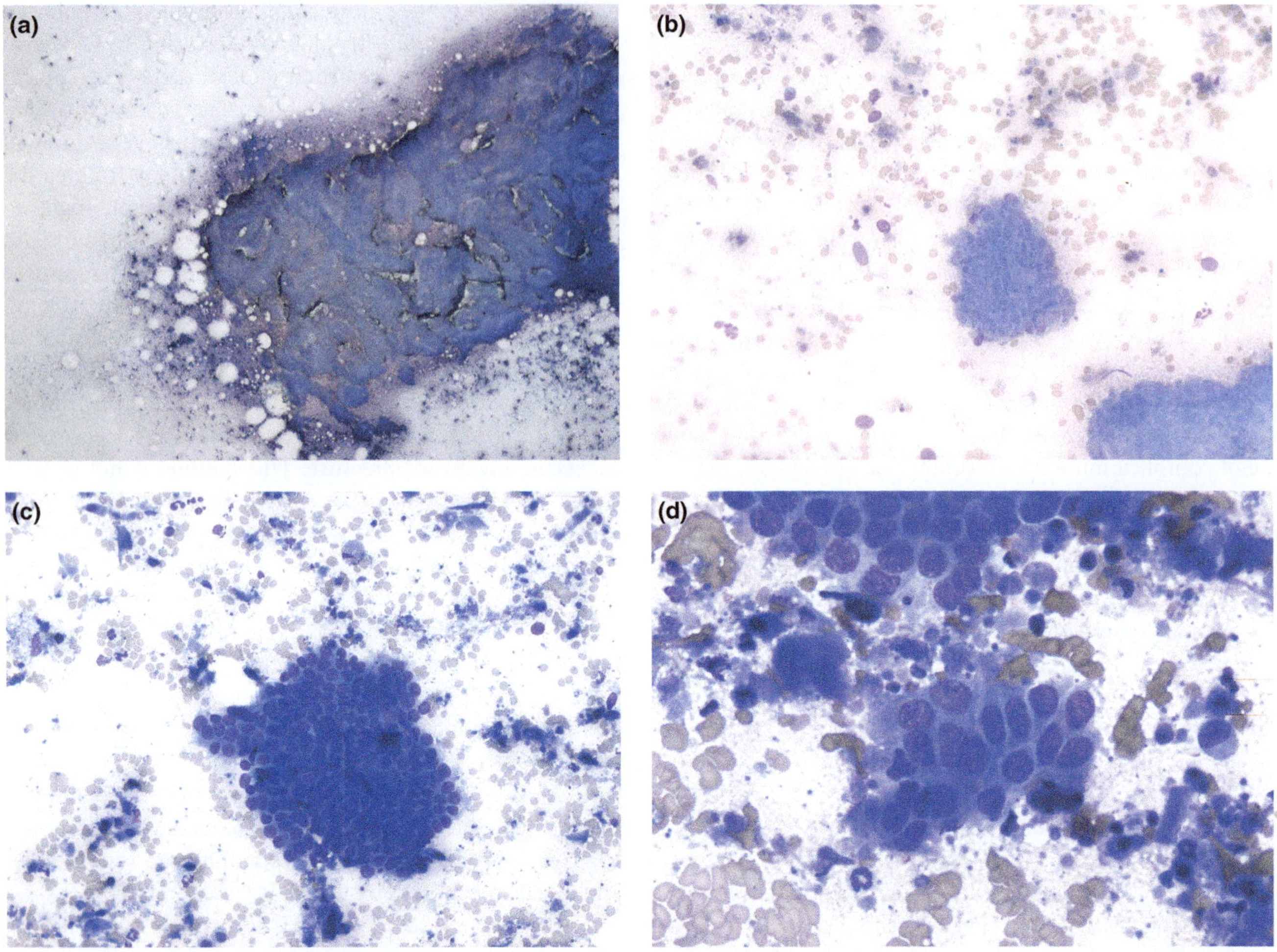

Figure 1.1 Cytology smears from a subcutaneous mass on the ventral abdominal midline from an adult dog with a history of removal of a colonic adenocarcinoma. Multiple smears were submitted and there was regional variation in the thickness of the smears. (a) A region of the smear demonstrating clusters of cells that are too thick to stain (Wright Giemsa, 200×). (b) A region of the smear that was understained, but thin enough that repeat staining might improve cytologic detail (Wright Giemsa, 200×). (c and d) Thinner, better stained areas with good cytologic detail (Wright Giemsa, 200× and 500×, respectively). A cytologic diagnosis of metastatic carcinoma due to seeding of the laparotomy incision site was made.

the mandibular lymph nodes. All slides, including those pre-stained, should be submitted for evaluation. Smear quality and content can vary and impact the diagnosis, so submission of multiple smears optimizes the diagnostic process (Figures 1.1 and 1.2). Cytology slides should never be submitted in the same shipping container as a formalin sample. Formalin is known to destroy the cells on the slide and render them nondiagnostic (Figure 1.3).

Diagnostic Yield

Maximizing diagnostic yield can require use of multiple collection methods. The recovery rate (or the rate of collecting diagnostic quality samples) is also dependent upon the experience of the sampler and the nature of the lesion.[8,46–49] Interestingly, reporting the diagnostic recovery rate is not emphasized in veterinary medicine, although it is reported in some studies.[3,37,50–53] Recovery rate should be noted by clinicians in evaluating the appropriateness of cytology as a diagnostic tool in individual cases. Absence of nucleated cells, poor cell preservation, and cell disruption are cited as causes of nondiagnostic samples.[54,55] Many studies of the diagnostic value of cytology focus on the agreement between cytologic and histologic diagnoses. Often, correlations are performed using only diagnostic cytology samples, which can minimize the impact of difficulties obtaining diagnostic specimens. In studies that choose to report the number of nondiagnostic samples as part of their findings, the diagnostic accuracy of cytology

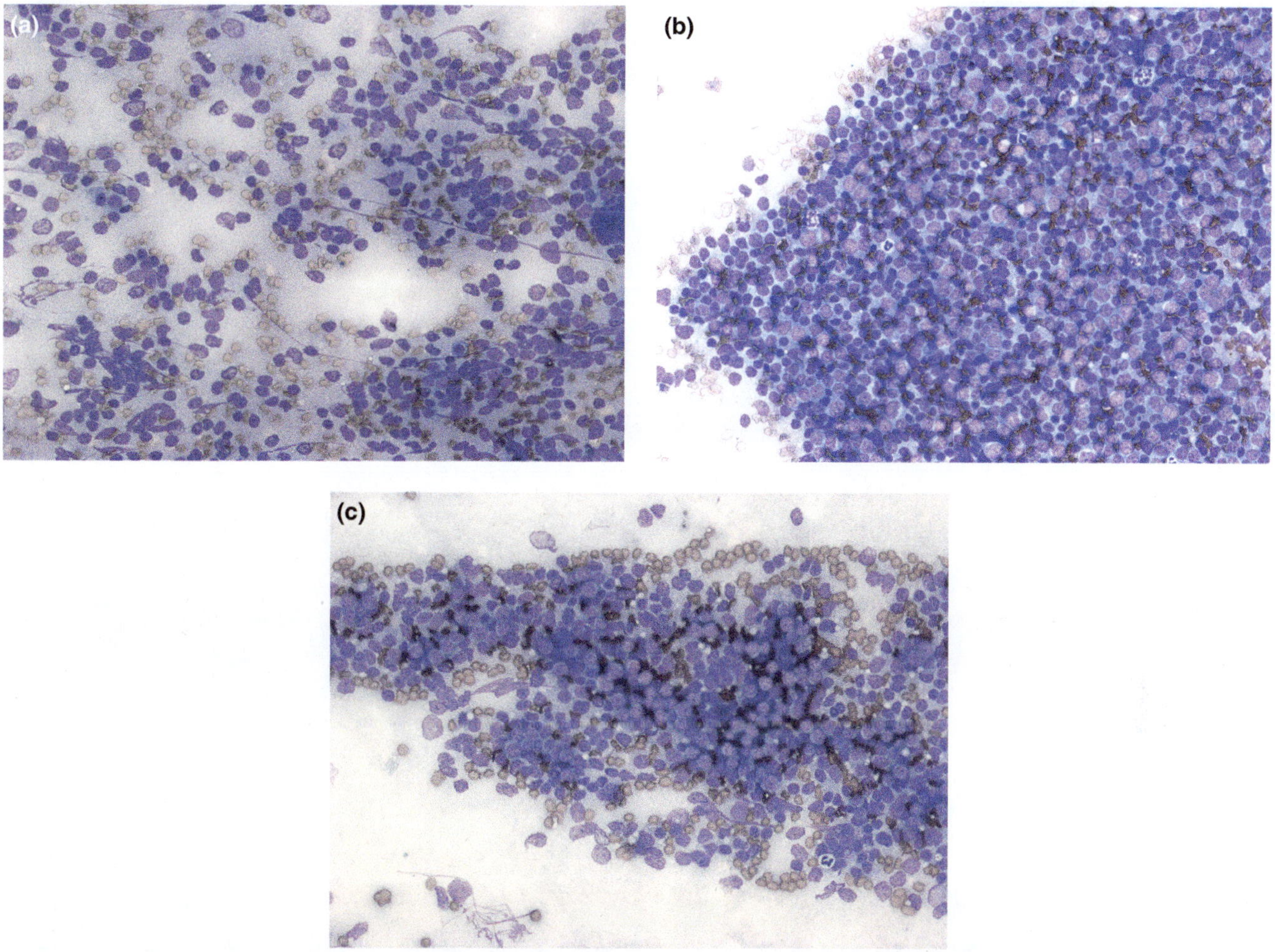

Figure 1.2 Prescapular lymph node aspirate from an adult dog. (a) Broken cells that cannot be interpreted are present in several of the smears. (b) Other areas of the smear were composed of predominantly intact well-stained cells. The population was heterogeneous and included many small cells as well as intermediate and some large cells. Occasional mitotic figures and non-degenerate neutrophils were observed. (c) Some regions contained moderate numbers of broken cells, and intact cells were predominantly a uniform population of medium lymphocytes (Wright Giemsa, 200×).

tends to be lower.[56] Studies in human medicine report that up to 32% of aspirates obtained by clinicians were considered unsatisfactory. More specifically in one study, half of these patients either had to repeat the procedure or undergo additional diagnostic testing.[46] Definitive diagnosis was obtained in 61% of human abdominal FNA cases with the first needle pass, with a further increase of 21% with the second FNA attempt using a new needle, 8% with the third FNA attempt, and 6% with the fourth FNA attempt.[57]

Implications of Nondiagnostic Samples

Nondiagnostic or low cellularity samples are frustrating for clinicians and cytopathologists; however, interpreting inadequate samples is not recommended. Sample quality can affect the diagnostic accuracy, with low quality samples risking being reported as either a false negative or a false positive. Although this seems intuitively obvious and is often alluded to in studies of veterinary cytology, the impact is rarely quantitatively assessed. One study of bone cytology in dogs revealed that cellularity significantly affected rates of cytologic-to-histopathologic correlation with high, moderate, and poor cellularity samples having concordant primary process in 88, 77, and 47% of cases, respectively.[58] This study highlights the potential harm that may result from forcing a cytologic interpretation on substandard samples. Unfortunately, in many cases, the slides are not examined prior to submission, making it difficult, if not impossible, for the clinician to know if a high-quality sample has been obtained. In a study of veterinary

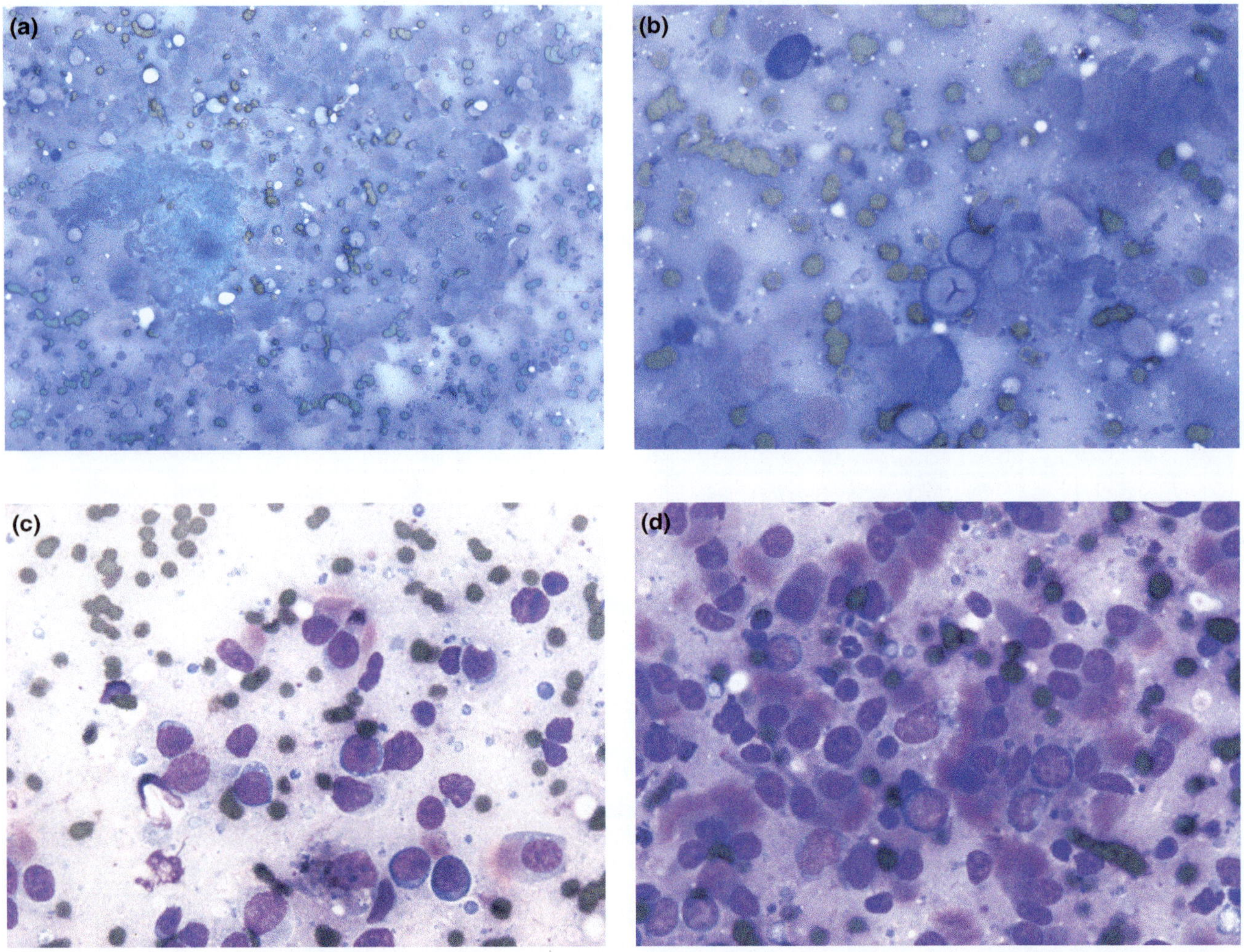

Figure 1.3 Nasal flush cytology from an adult cat. Smears were submitted in the same container with a histology sample in a container of formalin. (a and b) Smears that were unstained prior to submission and exposed to formalin fumes. Staining is inadequate and smears cannot be interpret (Wright Giemsa, 200× and 400×, respectively). (c and d) Smears pre-stained prior to submission were unaffected and revealed numerous mature ciliated columnar respiratory epithelial cells and a population of medium to large atypical lymphocytes, suggesting a potential diagnosis of lymphoma (Diff-Quik, 200× and 400×, respectively). The histologic diagnosis was intermediate cell lymphoma.

practitioners in the United Kingdom, the majority of samples submitted (51%) were not evaluated prior to submission. Of those samples submitted, 19% were classified as low cellularity. Low cellularity may not always reflect poor sampling techniques as many of these samples were classified as a "suspect lipoma" but were of insufficient quality to allow for any diagnostic interpretation.[1]

Conclusion

Aspiration is a skill that any practitioner can gain proficiency with repeated use. By avoiding the pitfalls of inadequate sampling, excessive cell damage, or thick samples in slide preparations, the diagnostic utility of cytology can be implemented to its fullest for both specialist and general practitioners.

References

1 Skeldon, N. and Dewhurst, E. (2009). The perceived and actual diagnostic utility of veterinary cytological samples. *J Small Anim Pract* 50: 180–185.

2 MacNeill, A.L. (2011). Cytology of canine and feline cutaneous and subcutaneous lesions and lymph nodes. *Top Companion Anim Med* 26: 77–85.

3 Ghisleni, G., Roccabianca, P., Ceruti, R. et al. (2006). Correlation between fine-needle aspiration cytology and histopathology in the evaluation of cutaneous and subcutaneous masses from dogs and cats. *Vet Clin Pathol* 35: 24–30.

4 Sontas, B.H., Yuzbasioglu Ozturk, G., Toydemir, T.F. et al. (2012). Fine-needle aspiration biopsy of canine mammary gland tumours: a comparison between cytology and histopathology. *Reprod Domest Anim* 47: 125–130.

5 Liffman, R. and Courtman, N. (2017). Fine needle aspiration of abdominal organs: a review of current recommendations for achieving a diagnostic sample. *J Small Anim Pract* 58: 599–609.

6 Laprais, A. and Olivry, T. (2017). Is CCNU (lomustine) valuable for treatment of cutaneous epitheliotropic lymphoma in dogs? A critically appraised topic. *BMC Vet Res* 13: 61.

7 Wypij, J.M. (2011). Getting to the point: indications for fine-needle aspiration of internal organs and bone. *Top Companion Anim Med* 26: 77–85.

8 Leblanc, C.J., Head, L.L., and Fry, M.M. (2009). Comparison of aspiration and nonaspiration techniques for obtaining cytologic samples from the canine and feline spleen. *Vet Clin Pathol* 38: 242–246.

9 Titoria, P., Siva, T.M., and Malik, T. (2010). An assessment of fine-needle sampling techniques. *Ann R Coll Surg Engl* 92: 429–431.

10 Finn-Bodner, S.T. and Hathcock, J.T. (1993). Image-guided percutaneous needle biopsy: ultrasound, computed tomography and magnetic resonance imaging. *Semin Vet Med Surg (Small Anim)* 8: 258–278.

11 Vignoli, M., Ohlerth, S., Rossi, F. et al. (2004). Computed tomography-guided fine-needle aspiration and tissue-core biopsy of bone lesions in small animals. *Vet Radiol Ultrasound* 45: 125–130.

12 Leveille, R., Partington, B.P., Biller, D.S., and Miyabayashi, T. (1993). Complications after ultrasound-guided biopsy of abdominal structures in dogs and cats: 246 cases (1984–1991). *J Am Vet Med Assoc* 203: 413–415.

13 Barr, F. (1995). Percutaneous biopsy of abdominal organs under ultrasound guidance. *J Small Anim Pract* 36: 105–113.

14 Schwerk, W.B. and Schmitz-Moormann, P. (1981). Ultrasonically guided fine-needle biopsies in neoplastic liver disease: cytohistologic diagnoses and echo pattern of lesions. *Cancer* 48: 1469–1477.

15 Britt, T., Clifford, C., Barger, A. et al. (2007). Diagnosing appendicular osteosarcoma with ultrasound-guided fine-needle aspiration: 36 cases. *J Small Anim Pract* 48: 145–150.

16 Tidwell, A.S. and Johnson, K.L. (1994). Computed tomography-guided percutaneous biopsy in the dog and cat: description of technique and preliminary evaluation in 14 patients. *Vet Radiol Ultrasound* 35: 445–456.

17 Koblik, P.D., LeCouteur, R.A., Higgins, R.J. et al. (1999). CT-guided brain biopsy using a modified Pelorus Mark III stereotactic system: experience with 50 dogs. *Vet Radiol Ultrasound* 40: 434–440.

18 Chen, A.V., Wininger, F.A., Frey, S. et al. (2012). Description and validation of a magnetic resonance imaging-guided stereotactic brain biopsy device in the dog. *Vet Radiol Ultrasound* 53: 150–156.

19 Penninck, D.G., Crystal, M.A., Matz, M.E., and Pearson, S.H. (1993). The technique of percutaneous ultrasound guided fine-needle aspiration biopsy and automated microcore biopsy in small animal gastrointestinal diseases. *Vet Radiol Ultrasound* 34: 433–436.

20 Penninck, D.G. and Finn-Bodner, S.T. (1998). Updates in interventional ultrasonography. *Vet Clin North Am Small Anim Pract* 28: 1017–1040.

21 McMillan, M.C., Kleine, L.J., and Carpenter, J.L. (1988). Fluoroscopically guided percutaneous fine-needle aspiration biopsy of thoracic lesions in dogs and cats. *Vet Radiol* 29: 194–197.

22 Fischer, A., Mahaffey, M.B., and Oliver, J.E. (1997). Fluoroscopically guided percutaneous disk aspiration in 10 dogs with diskospondylitis. *J Vet Intern Med* 11: 284–287.

23 Vignoli, M. and Saunders, J.H. (2011). Image-guided interventional procedures in the dog and cat. *Vet J* 187: 297–303.

24 Troxel, M.T. and Vite, C.H. (2008). CT-guided stereotactic brain biopsy using the Kopf stereotactic system. *Vet Radiol Ultrasound* 49: 438–443.

25 Taylor, A.R., Cohen, N.D., Fletcher, S. et al. (2013). Application and machine accuracy of a new frameless computed tomography-guided stereotactic brain biopsy system in dogs. *Vet Radiol Ultrasound* 54: 332–342.

26 Menard, M. and Papageorges, M. (1995). Ultrasound corner technique for ultrasound-guided fine needle biopsies. *Vet Radiol Ultrasound* 36: 137–138.

27 Tidwell, A.S. and Johnson, K.L. (1994). Computed tomography-guided percutaneous biopsy: criteria for accurate needle tip identification. *Vet Radiol Ultrasound* 35: 440–444.

28 Livraghi, T., Damascelli, B., Lombardi, C., and Spagnoli, I. (1983). Risk in fine-needle abdominal biopsy. *J Clin Ultrasound* 11: 77–81.

29 Smith, E.H. (1984). The hazards of fine-needle aspiration biopsy. *Ultrasound Med Biol* 10: 629–634.

30 Hager, D.A., Nyland, T.G., and Fisher, P. (1985). Ultrasound-guided biopsy of the canine liver, kidney, and prostate. *Vet Radiol* 26: 82–88.

31 Nyland, T.G., Wallack, S.T., and Wisner, E.R. (2002). Needle-tract implantation following us-guided fine-needle aspiration biopsy of transitional cell carcinoma of the bladder, urethra, and prostate. *Vet Radiol Ultrasound* 43: 50–53.

32 Zekas, L.J., Crawford, J.T., and O'Brien, R.T. (2005). Computed tomography-guided fine-needle aspirate and tissue-core biopsy of intrathoracic lesions in thirty dogs and cats. *Vet Radiol Ultrasound* 46: 200–204.

33 Proot, S.J. and Rothuizen, J. (2006). High complication rate of an automatic Tru-Cut biopsy gun device for liver biopsy in cats. *J Vet Intern Med* 20: 1327–1333.

34 Warren-Smith, C.M., Roe, K., de la Puerta, B. et al. (2011). Pulmonary adenocarcinoma seeding along a fine needle aspiration tract in a dog. *Vet Rec* 169: 181.

35 Crystal, M.A., Penninck, D.G., Matz, M.E. et al. (1993). Use of ultrasound-guided fine-needle aspiration biopsy and automated core biopsy for the diagnosis of gastrointestinal diseases in small animals. *Vet Radiol Ultrasound* 34: 438–444.

36 de Rycke, L.M., van Bree, H.J., and Simoens, P.J. (1999). Ultrasound-guided tissue-core biopsy of liver, spleen and kidney in normal dogs. *Vet Radiol Ultrasound* 40: 294–299.

37 Cordner, A.P., Sharkey, L.C., Armstrong, P.J., and KD, M.A. (2015). Cytologic findings and diagnostic yield in 92 dogs undergoing fine-needle aspiration of the pancreas. *J Vet Diagn Invest* 27: 236–240.

38 Crabtree, A.C., Spangler, E., Beard, D., and Smith, A. (2010). Diagnostic accuracy of gray-scale ultrasonography for the detection of hepatic and splenic lymphoma in dogs. *Vet Radiol Ultrasound* 51: 661–664.

39 Reichle, J.K. and Wisner, E.R. (2000). Non-cardiac thoracic ultrasound in 75 feline and canine patients. *Vet Radiol Ultrasound* 41: 154–162.

40 Vaden, S.L., Levine, J.F., Lees, G.E. et al. (2005). Renal biopsy: a retrospective study of methods and complications in 283 dogs and 65 cats. *J Vet Intern Med* 19: 794–801.

41 Stefanello, D., Valenti, P., Faverzani, S. et al. (2009). Ultrasound-guided cytology of spleen and liver: a prognostic tool in canine cutaneous mast cell tumor. *J Vet Intern Med* 23: 1051–1057.

42 Watson, A.T., Penninck, D., Knoll, J.S. et al. (2011). Safety and correlation of test results of combined ultrasound-guided fine-needle aspiration and needle core biopsy of the canine spleen. *Vet Radiol Ultrasound* 52: 317–322.

43 Sabattini, S., Renzi, A., Marconato, L. et al. (2018). Comparison between May-Grünwald-Giemsa and rapid cytological stains in fine-needle aspirates of canine mast cell tumour: diagnostic and prognostic implications. *Vet Comp Oncol* 16 (4): 511–517.

44 Jackson, D.E., Selting, K.A., Spoor, M.S. et al. (2013). Evaluation of fixation time using Diff-Quik for staining of canine mast cell tumor aspirates. *Vet Clin Pathol* 42: 99–102.

45 Jorundsson, E., Lumsden, J.H., and Jacobs, R.M. (1999). Rapid staining techniques in cytopathology: a review and comparison of modified protocols for hematoxylin and eosin, Papanicolaou and Romanowsky stains. *Vet Clin Pathol* 28: 100–108.

46 Carson, H.J., Saint Martin, G.A., Castelli, M.J., and Gattuso, P. (1995). Unsatisfactory aspirates from fine-needle aspiration biopsies: a review. *Diagn Cytopathol* 12: 280–284.

47 Feoli, F., Paesmans, M., and Van Eeckhout, P. (2008). Fine needle aspiration cytology of the breast. Impact of experience on accuracy, using standardized cytologic criteria. *Acta Cytol* 52: 145–151.

48 Welch, R.A., Salem-Elgharib, S., Wiktor, A.E. et al. (2006). Operator experience and sample quality in genetic amniocentesis. *Am J Obstet Gynecol* 194: 189–191.

49 Petrone, M.C. and Arcidiacono, P.G. (2014). Basic technique in endoscopic ultrasound-guided fine needle aspiration for solid lesions: how many passes? *Endosc Ultrasound* 3: 22–27.

50 Bonfanti, U., Bertazzolo, W., Gracis, M. et al. (2015). Diagnostic value of cytological analysis of tumors and tumor-like lesions of the oral cavity in dogs and cats: a prospective study on 114 cases. *Vet J* 205: 322–327.

51 Crain, S.K., Sharkey, L.C., Cordner, A.P. et al. (2015). Safety of ultrasound-guided fine-needle aspiration of the feline pancreas: a case-control study. *J Fel Med Surg* 17: 858–863.

52 McAloney, C.A., Sharkey, L.C., Feeney, D.A. et al. (2018). Evaluation of the diagnostic utility of cytologic examination of renal fine-needle aspirates from dogs and the use of ultrasonographic features to inform cytologic diagnosis. *J Am Vet Med Assoc* 252: 1247–1256.

53 McAloney, C.A., Sharkey, L.C., Feeney, D.A., and Seelig, D.M. (2018). Diagnostic utility of renal fine-needle aspirate cytology and ultrasound in the cat. *J Fel Med Surg* 20: 544–553.

54 Amores-Fuster, I., Cripps, P., Graham, P. et al. (2015). The diagnostic utility of lymph node cytology samples in dogs and cats. *J Small Anim Pract* 56: 125–129.

55 Zachar, E.K., Burgess, H.J., and Wobeser, B.K. (2016). Fine-needle aspiration in the diagnosis of equine skin disease and the epidemiology of equine skin cytology

submissions in a western Canadian diagnostic laboratory. *Can Vet J* 57: 629–634.

56 Cohen, M., Bohling, M.W., Wright, J.C. et al. (2003). Evaluation of sensitivity and specificity of cytologic examination: 269 cases (1999–2000). *J Am Vet Med Assoc* 222: 964–967.

57 Dähnert, W.F., Hoagland, M.H., Hamper, U.M. et al. (1992). Fine-needle aspiration biopsy of abdominal lesions: diagnostic yield for different needle tip configurations. *Radiology* 185: 236–268.

58 Berzina, I., Sharkey, L.C., Matise, I., and Kramek, B. (2008). Correlation between cytologic and histopathologic diagnoses of bone lesions in dogs: a study of the diagnostic accuracy of bone cytology. *Vet Clin Pathol* 37: 332–338.

2

Routine Stains and Automated Stainers

Harold Tvedten

Introduction to Routine Cytology Stains

This chapter assumes that sample collection has resulted in adequately cellular and representative slides that contain intact cells of good morphological quality (Chapter 1). Samples should be thin enough to stain uniformly and should lack background material. The choice of stains for a given practice or laboratory will vary according to the variety and volume of samples to be analyzed and the diagnoses to be made. Most laboratories also perform hematology and urinalysis; therefore, it is an advantage to have stains that have multiple uses. Some laboratories include bacteriology and mycology analysis that may require specialized stains (Chapter 3).

Traditional Romanowsky-Type Stains

Most veterinary cytologists use a Romanowsky-type stain as their primary stain. While human cytologists currently use mainly the Papanicolaou stain, Romanowsky-type stains were originally chosen by cytopathology pioneers because of their hematopathologic roots.[1,2] Romanowsky-type stains provide unique information that cause it to be recommended even in human medicine as a complement to Papanicolaou staining.[1] Romanowsky-type stains use various combinations of red and blue dyes, methanol, and phosphate buffers.[3] The red dye (eosin) is an anionic dye that binds to alkaline substances (e.g. hemoglobin and other proteins) and stains them reddish-orange (i.e. eosinophilic). The blue dyes, including azure B and azure A, are cationic (basic) dyes originating from demethylation breakdown products of methylene blue. They are in the thiazine family and bind to acidic structures (e.g. DNA and RNA) to color them blue (basophilic).[4] The two most commonly used red and blue dyes are eosin Y and azure B, respectively, although there are alternatives, such as xanthene and thiazine. In the final reaction, the dyes together produce the "Romanowsky effect" that is a polychromic purple hue to the nuclear chromatin, certain cytoplasmic structures (e.g. neutrophil granules), and background material. If the Romanowsky effect is not observed, this usually indicates a technical failure (see section "Disadvantages of Romanowsky-Type Stains"). On Romanowsky-stained slides, colors are described as *basophilic* (blue), *eosinophilic* (orange-red), and *neutrophilic* (no color). Additional descriptors include *amphophilic*, which means a tissue that stains with both acidic and basic dyes, and *metachromatic*, which indicates the color produced is different than the original color of the dye (e.g. purple-colored mast cell granules stained by blue dyes).

It is important to note that there is no one "standard" Romanowsky-type stain. Pathologists such as Dmitri Romanowsky, Paul Ehrlich, William Leishman, James Wright, Gustav Giemsa, and others needed practical stains for microscopy and made various modifications and improvements that allow more consistent staining of smears. Staining methods are named after these men, for example, Giemsa, May-Grunwald-Giemsa, and Wright stain. In Europe these stains are generally termed a Giemsa-type stain, and in the United States they are usually called a Wright-type stain. The use of just one name such as "Giemsa" or "Wright" falsely suggests that the various methods are the same. There are a number of method-specific modifications to these stains including various methods of dye preparation, staining time, and pH requirements.

Advantages of Romanowsky-Type Stains

Romanowsky-type stains provide excellent cytoplasmic detail, including the differential staining of cytoplasmic granules, vacuoles, and other cytoplasmic structures.[1] As cytoplasmic granule, staining is used for the identification of certain neoplasms (e.g. thyroid, large granular lymphocytes,

Veterinary Cytology, First Edition. Edited by Leslie C. Sharkey, M. Judith Radin, and Davis Seelig.

mast cells) and for the classification of leukocytes, Romanowsky-type stains are useful in the interpretation of both neoplasia and inflammation. Plasma cells, with their mRNA-rich dark blue cytoplasm and their mRNA-poor pale blue Gogi zone, are readily identified with a Romanowsky-type stain. Romanowsky-type stains are also optimal in the detection of microorganisms as bacteria and fungi. *Mycobacterium* spp. can be identified by their negative staining (clear rods seen against a blue background; Figure 11.3).

In addition to its useful staining properties, the air-dried fixation approach used for Romanowsky-type stains results in greater spreading of cells on the glass slide than the wet (alcohol) fixation needed for Papanicolaou staining.[1] This cell spreading amplifies nuclear and size differences and allows for interpretation of relative size comparisons such as nuclear to cytoplasmic ratios. With Romanowsky-type stains, the background material in the sample is differentially stained, thus allowing identification of protein, necrosis, and other materials such as collagen, elastin, cartilage, osteoid, amyloid, fat droplets, or glycogen-rich material.[1] Although evaluation of nuclear chromatin and nucleolar detail is adequate with Romanowsky-type stains, stains discussed later outperform Romanowsky-type stains for evaluation of nuclear detail especially with thicker smears and tissue fragments. In addition to their microscopic advantages, Romanowsky-type stains are practical, quick, and readily applied to nearly all types of diagnostic samples. Finally, the long history of Romanowsky-stained samples in veterinary pathology has resulted in decades of published diagnostic material that can be used for years to come.

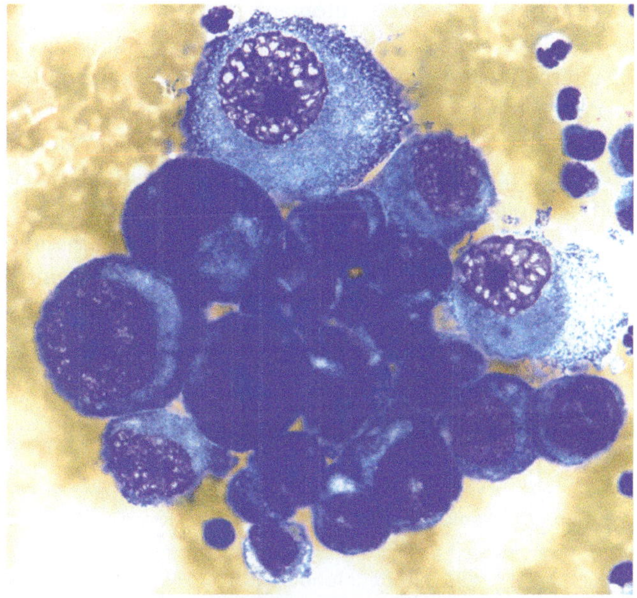

Figure 2.1 Abdominal fluid from a dog. As Romanowsky-type stains are not semitransparent, the thicker areas often stain too dark to allow for robust examination of nuclear and cytoplasmic detail. Note that the cells in the center are too darkly stained to evaluate, whereas cells at the edge lay flat enough to show better morphological detail (May-Grunwald-Giemsa, 1000×).

Disadvantages of Romanowsky-Type Stains

Romanowsky-type stains are not semitransparent, and thus thicker tissue particles or material can be troublesome to interpret. This can hinder the diagnosis of neoplasia because such a diagnosis is greatly aided by evaluating the architectural relationship among cells in thicker particles. However, these thicker tissue fragments and thicker areas of the smear usually stain too darkly using a Romanowsky-type stain (Figure 2.1).[5] In addition, Romanowsky-type stains do not illustrate sharp chromatin detail in nuclei and nucleoli. As such, heterochromatin granules and nucleoli are less distinct with Romanowsky staining than with Papanicolaou or new methylene blue (NMB) stains. This can be a disadvantage in the identification of malignant cells.

Technical Aspects of Romanowsky-Type Stains

There are a number of variables that influence the final staining intensity when using a Romanowsky-type stain, including the ratio of azure B to eosin Y, the duration of staining, the pH of the solutions and buffers, the age of the slide, and the purity of the stains.[3,6] Proteins can have a net positive or negative charge (zwitterion) based on the pH of the environment they are in; thus the same protein can bind a given dye differently according to the pH of the stain and appear more acidophilic or basophilic as a result. Generally, the purple nuclear color of the Romanowsky effect is greatest at neutral to slightly alkaline pH (7–8) and decreases with increasing acidity.[3] If the pH is too high, erythrocytes can appear blue-green.[3,5] Duration of staining also affects final staining intensity as the purple nuclear color is more intense with longer staining times.

The author uses a May-Grunwald-Giemsa stain first optimized for use with a CellaVision hematology instrument (CellaVision, Lund, Sweden).[7] The same stain is currently used for our hematological and cytological specimens (Table 2.1). The stock solutions are a mixture of azure A, azure B, methylene violet, methylene blue, and eosin Y dissolved in a mixture of methanol and glycerol. The working solutions are diluted with water or an aqueous buffer and are stable for a period of hours (one working day).

Rapid Romanowsky-Type Stains

Rapid versions of Romanowsky-type stains are commonly used in veterinary pathology and can result in complete slide staining within 3–5 minutes as compared with

20–30 minutes for many automatic stainers. These rapid stains offer a simple, inexpensive, and good quality staining alternative for small clinics and laboratories. Examples of rapid Romanowsky-type stains are Diff-Quik (Dade Behring Inc., Deerfield, IL, USA) and Hemacolor (Merck KGaA, Darmstadt, Germany). These rapid methods have modified red and blue dyes that mimic the classical Romanowsky-type stain, but in contrast to the methanol-based classical Romanowsky-type stains, these quick stains are usually aqueous based.[8] However, these quick stains usually have a post drying methanol fixation step as their first step, which improves the differential staining of heterochromatin and euchromatin. Additionally, Diff-Quik adds triarylmethane dye to the methanol fixative in the first solution and includes sodium azide and a pH buffer with the red dye solution (xanthene) to prevent microbial contamination. Hemacolor is advertised as a two minute quick variation of the Pappenheim stain but has staining appearance of a Romanowsky stain and is designed for blood smears. Hemacolor has a similar three-solution system like Diff-Quik with a methanol fixing solution, one red (eosin) and one blue (azure) staining solution.

Table 2.1 May-Grunwald-Giemsa (MGG) method used with a Molek automated stainer.[a]

Position #	Solution	Reaction time
1	MGG stock solution[b]	5 minutes
2	Buffer solution[c]	5 dips
3	Giemsa working solution[d]	10 minutes
4	Buffer solution	5 dips
5	Deionized water	5 dips

[a] The Molek stainer (Molek Medical Equipment, Enskede, Sweden) is an automated dip-type stainer with some agitation.
[b] May-Grunwald-Giemsa stock solution (Merck HX 935559 eosin-methylene blue solution modified for microscopy; contains methanol; Merck K GaA, Darmstadt, Germany).
[c] Buffer stock solution 7.2 is made from buffer tables (Merck K GaA TP937068806, Darmstadt, Germany).
[d] Dilute 1 part Giemsa stain stock solution (Merck HX807294 azur-eosin-methylene blue solution for microscopy; contains methanol; Merck K GaA, Darmstadt, Germany) with 19 parts of buffer solution (stable for 8 hours).

Rapid Romanowsky-type stains are often used in practices with small volumes of samples and involve hand dipping slides in and out of three solutions (fixative, red stain, and blue stain) in separate Coplin jars. Dipping instead of passive immersion may reduce the time needed in each solution. Additional or less red or blue color can be obtained by more or fewer dips in the different colored dyes. Across the aqueous methods, instability of the various dyes has prevented standardization of any one quick methodology.[3] Aqueous Romanowsky-type stains, including the quick stains, offer both advantages and disadvantages. One disadvantage is that these methods may fail to stain granules of mast cells, basophils, and large granular lymphocytes, which is in contrast to methanol-based methods (Figures 2.2, 2.3, and 13.3).[4] However, there can be differences between laboratories even when similar stains are used. For example, using an automated stainer (Hematek 3000, Siemens, Tarrytown, NY, USA), the author's laboratory consistently failed to detect mast cell granules despite using a methanol-based stain (Figure 2.2). One advantage of the aqueous stains is that the viral inclusions of canine distemper stain more distinctly than the classical methanol-based stains.[8]

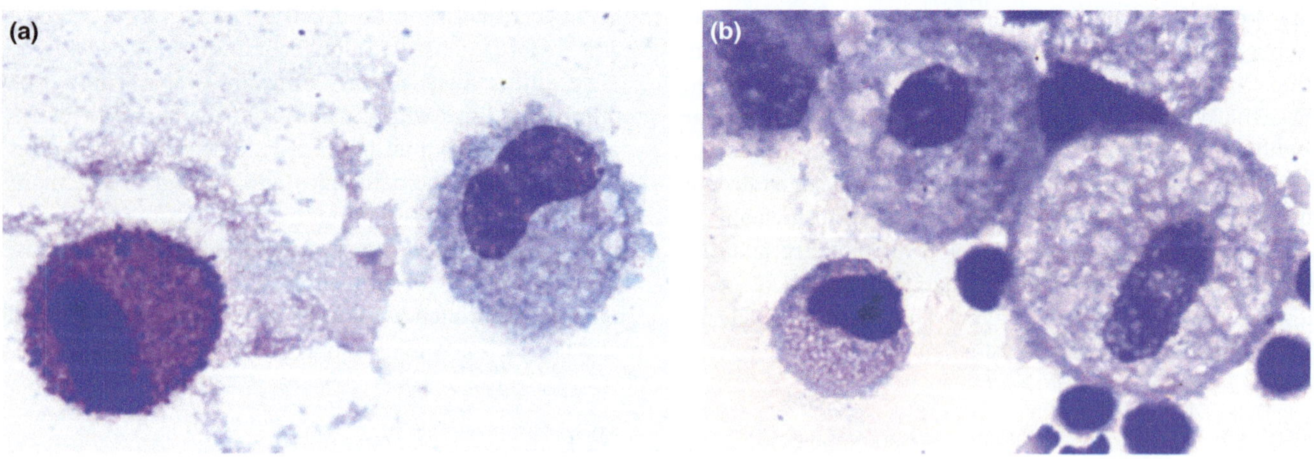

Figure 2.2 Bronchoalveolar lavage from a horse. (a) Note the robust staining of mast cell granules in the sample stained with May-Grunwald-Giemsa (1000×) as compared with (b) weaker staining using the Hematek "modified Wright's stain" (Siemens, Tarrytown, NY, USA) (1000×).

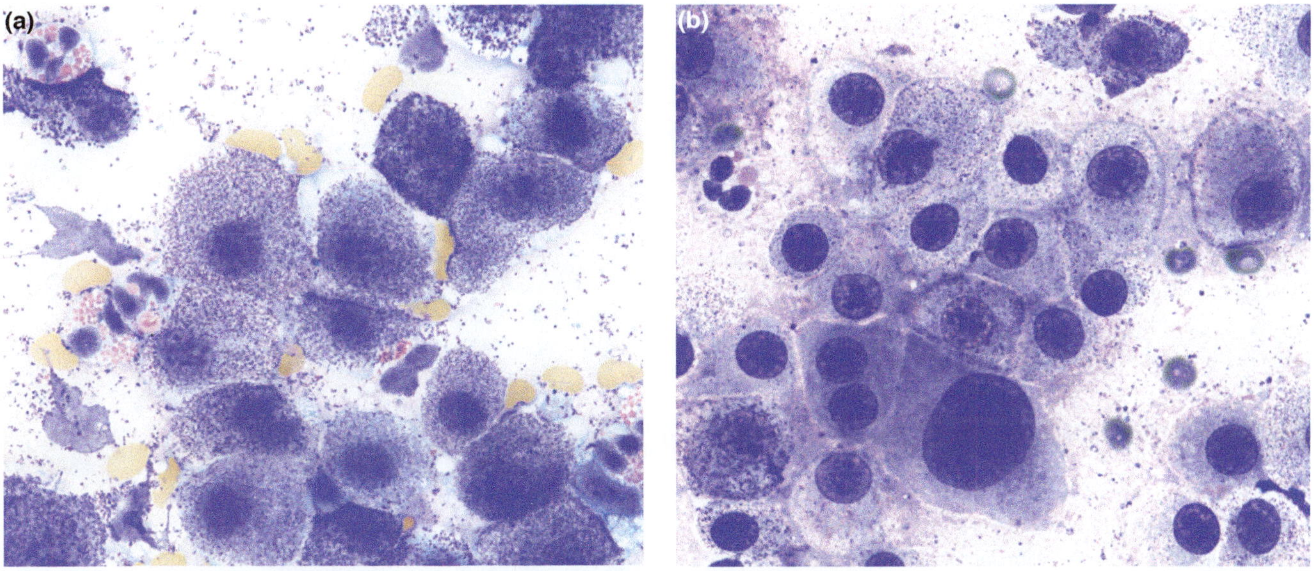

Figure 2.3 Skin mass from a dog. (a) Notice the more prominent mast cell and eosinophil granules when stained with the methanolic May-Grunwald-Giemsa stain (1000×) as compared with (b), which was stained with an aqueous quick stain. Notably, the chromatin detail was superior in the quick stain (Diff-Quik, 1000×).

Papanicolaou Stain

The Papanicolaou stain (Pap stain) is commonly used in human cytopathology for cervical cancer screening and other cytological diagnoses. The most commonly cited advantage of the Papanicolaou stain is its ability to highlight nuclear detail. The hematoxylin used in the Pap stain has a high affinity for heterochromatin, which is the inactive form of DNA and stains as granules, but has a lower affinity for euchromatin, which is actively replicating DNA. As blast cells and malignant cells often have high levels of DNA activity, their "immature nuclei" will appear more "open" and lighter staining. Using the Pap stain, these changes in nuclear chromatin detail and distribution and changes in shape and size of nucleoli can be used to evaluate risk of malignancy.[5] For example, an irregular pattern of parachromatin clearing, which describes the pattern of unstained euchromatin in relation to well-stained heterochromatin, can be used to suggest malignancy.

In contrast to the air-dried smears used for Romanowsky staining, Papanicolaou staining requires immediate "wet fixation" in 95% ethanol for 30 minutes or alternative fixation methods (e.g. 100% methanol, 95% denatured alcohol, 80% propanol, and 80% isopropanol). Rehydration of air-dried smears with physiological saline within 30 minutes of collection still allows the use of a Pap stain on air-dried slides.[5] The original, and still routinely used, Pap stain method has five dyes including hematoxylin and eosin (H&E). The inclusion of H&E made the Pap stain attractive to histopathologists accustomed to evaluating similarly stained tissue sections. One additional advantage of the Pap stain is its ability to detect cytoplasmic keratinization due to the inclusion of an orange G dye, which makes it particularly useful in the evaluation of cervical or squamous cell neoplasia in women. Lastly, the Pap stain is a semitransparent stain that allows for the evaluation of thicker tissue fragments.

There are a number of limitations to the use of the Pap stain in veterinary cytopathology, chief of which is that most veterinary cytologists are not trained in its interpretation. Another disadvantage of the original Pap stain was that it took 30 or more minutes to perform. However, ultra-fast Pap stains that take two to three minutes are available. Jörundsson et al. described how to perform these quick Pap stains and compared results with Romanowsky-type-stained smears.[5] They described how air-dried smears made at the time of collection could be rehydrated (within 30 minutes of collection) for later Pap staining. Based on their results, they recommended that all smears be air-dried and that one or more slides, including the thinnest preparations, but not all slides, be stained with a Romanowsky-type stain. After preliminary evaluation of the Romanowsky-type-stained smear, it would be decided whether it is necessary to perform a Pap. This approach has not been adopted by most veterinary cytologists, and further published work using the Pap stain in veterinary cytopathology is sparse. Roszel et al. promoted a similar Sano's stain for cytology, but that has not become popular.[9]

New Methylene Blue Stain

NMB is a technically simple stain that has the advantages of being rapid, semitransparent (which allows for the evaluation of thicker tissue fragments), and useful in illustrating chromatin and nucleolar detail. NMB is a monochromic blue stain that also stains bacteria and fungi. No alcohol is used and therefore fat droplets and cholesterol crystals are visible.[8] NMB can also be used to evaluate urine sediment and detect peripheral blood reticulocytes and as a counterstain for other stains such as fat stains (Sudan or Oil red O). This combination can be used to confirm that clear intracellular vacuoles in hepatocytes or macrophages contain lipid. Disadvantages of NMB include its lack of staining of cytoplasmic structures (e.g. hemoglobin and eosinophil granules), the need to evaluate slides immediately, and that no permanent smear is available for later review. To optimize NMB staining, a large coverslip (20 × 50 mm) should be used to draw a drop of NMB over the cells while avoiding air bubbles.

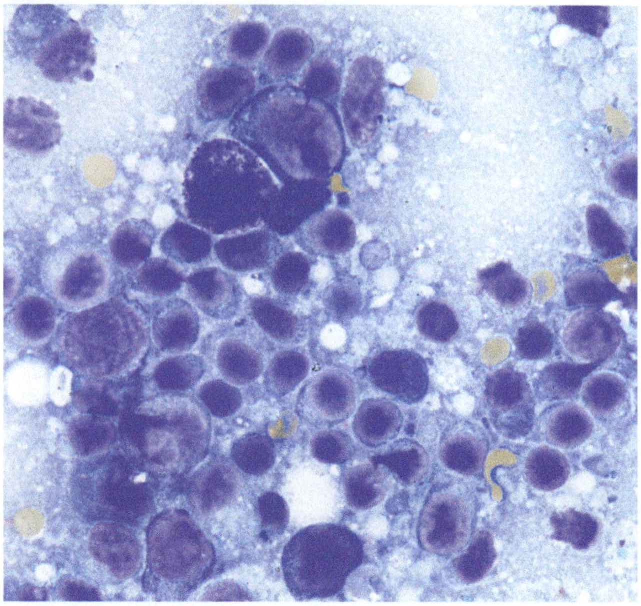

Figure 2.4 Lymph node from a dog. Inadequate drying of material can cause darkly stained central areas in nuclei that resemble a large nucleolus. The artifact can falsely suggest a predominance of lymphoblasts and perhaps malignant lymphoma instead of being primarily small lymphocytes in this reactive lymph node (Diff-Quik, 1000×).

Fixation

The most common method of fixation in veterinary cytology is air drying. Slides should be dried at room to body temperature, and the drying can be aided by waving them in the air. Heating or flaming should be avoided as both methods damage cells. While drying can cause artifacts such as nuclear distortion and vacuolization, there is less loss of cells from air-dried slides as compared with those that are wet fixed. These artifacts tend to occur if drying is delayed or insufficient; thus smears should be very thin to speed the drying process.[5] When using Romanowsky-type stains, inadequate drying can cause dark blue central nuclear artifacts that resemble large nucleoli (Figure 2.4).[5] If necessary, air-dried smears can be rehydrated for Pap staining by dipping smears in 0.9% NaCl for 30 seconds.[5] For best effect, rehydration should be performed within 30 minutes of making the smear. Notably, rehydration can lyse erythrocytes and may give a cleaner background than air-dried slides.

Stain Contamination

The contamination of stains with organisms or cells can cause an incorrect diagnosis. As such, cytologists need to be diligent in evaluating samples for potential contamination. Contamination may be suspected when (i) yeast, bacteria, or cellular exudate is noted on the back side of the slide or on parts of the slide away from the area of the smear that appears to contain the patient's true sample, (ii) organisms are seen in greater than expected numbers, (iii) organisms are found in unexpected sites (e.g. CSF, peripheral blood, or lipoma aspirates), or (iv) neutrophils in an area of the smear appear more darkly stained and shrunken compared with other neutrophils in areas, more likely representing the sample. In addition to infectious organisms, tumor cells can float off the correct slide and fasten to an incorrect slide.

Stain contamination can result from any source, but ear swabs (particularly those with abundant yeast or bacterial exudate) are a common offender. To mitigate the risk of contamination, ear swabs and other smears that appear thick or "flaky" should be stained using dedicated staining solutions or stained at the end of the day (when fresh stain is prepared in the morning). In addition, stains should be filtered often (e.g. every morning in practices with high volumes of cytology samples or during the day if contamination is suspected). In practices with only a few cytological specimens, filtering or changing stains can be done more infrequently (e.g. weekly or when contamination is suspected). Filtering of stains can be performed with a funnel and filter paper or with a Millipore-type syringe filter (0.2–0.5 μm pore size) that can remove bacteria as well as larger fungi. However it is important to note that filtering may not successfully remove contamination; therefore, stain replacement is recommended whenever contamination is suspected.

References

1 Krafts, K.P. and Pambuccian, S.E. (2011). Romanowsky staining in cytopathology: history, advantages and limitations. *Biotech Histochem* 86: 82–93.

2 Söderström, N. (1966). *Fine-Needle Aspiration Biopsy: Used as a Direct Adjunct in Clinical Diagnostic Work*. New York: Grune & Stratton.

3 Horobin, R.W. (2011). How Romanowsky stains work and why they remain valuable: including a proposed universal Romanowsky staining mechanism and a rational troubleshooting scheme. *Biotech Histochem* 86: 36–51.

4 Allison, R.W. and Velguth, K.E. (2010). Appearance of granulated cells in blood films stained by automated aqueous versus methanolic Romanowsky methods. *Vet Clin Pathol* 39: 99–104.

5 Jorundsson, E., Lumsden, J.H., and Jacobs, R.M. (1999). Rapid staining techniques in cytopathology: a review and comparison of modified protocols for hematoxylin and eosin, Papanicolaou and Romanowsky stains. *Vet Clin Pathol* 28: 100–108.

6 Dunning, K. and Safo, A.O. (2011). The ultimate Wright-Giemsa stain: 60 years in the making. *Biotech Histochem* 86: 69–75.

7 Tvedten, H.W. and Lilliehook, I.E. (2011). Canine differential leukocyte counting with the CellaVision DM96Vision, Sysmex XT-2000iV, and Advia 2120 hematology analyzers and a manual method. *Vet Clin Pathol* 40: 324–339.

8 Raskin, R. and Meyer, D.J. (2016). *Canine and Feline Cytology: A Color Atlas and Interpretation Guide*, 3e. St. Louis, MO: Elsevier.

9 Roszel, J.F., MacVean, D.W., and Monlux, A.W. (1978). Use of cytology for tumor diagnosis in private veterinary practice. *J Am Vet Med Assoc* 173: 1011–1014.

3

Microbiologic Review of Cytology Samples

Erin N. Burton, Sharon M. Dial, and Leslie C. Sharkey

Introduction

A primary indication for cytologic examination of lesions is to evaluate samples for the presence of microorganisms and to assess potential pathogenicity. The sensitivity and specificity of cytology for the breadth of organisms in various tissues is not always established; however, for many, microscopic identification is considered strong evidence of the presence of an agent (high specificity), particularly if there is concurrent inflammation, while the absence is harder to interpret (variable sensitivity). The presence of an appropriate inflammatory cell population can be suggestive for microbial organisms and may guide additional diagnostic testing when cytologic evaluation is negative. A variety of organisms can be present as environmental contaminants and commensal species. Potential pathogenicity is interpreted in light of knowledge of commensal organisms in a particular sample (i.e. Chapter 30), understanding of the collection environment and technique, other evidence of sample contamination, the concurrent presence of inflammation, and if organisms are intracellular or extracellular. This chapter will provide a general overview of major organism types, with a focus on dogs, cats, and horses, and will reference images throughout the text in addition to the figures specifically associated with this chapter. The reader is directed to tissue- and species-specific chapters for more detailed information since an encyclopedic review of organisms is beyond the scope of this chapter. While a loose phylogenetic approach is used, frequent reclassification of organisms, often based on genotype, means that classification does not always correspond to microscopic appearance and may change with time. Some of the species chapters are particularly rich in infectious agents, including Chapters 60, 61, and 63 that feature unusual organisms specific to primates, avian and reptile species, and fish that will not be emphasized in this chapter.

Bacterial Cytological Evaluation

While culture is often considered, the reference standard for the detection of bacterial infection, cytologic evaluation is an important complementary technique. Preliminary assessment of smears, especially with Gram stain, provides valuable information to guide initial treatment, especially in the context of increasing concerns about antimicrobial resistance.[1] In many instances, cytologic evaluation provides additional context for culture data (Figure 3.1). In people and animals, cytology is used to help distinguish colonization from true infection, to identify a predominant organism in tissues when cultures grow several species, or to identify fastidious or slow growing organisms that may grow poorly and not be represented in culture results.[1–3] Quantitation in some tissues such as the ear and skin (Chapters 11 and 17) can facilitate interpretation. Cytology can be particularly important if there is the potential for false-positive results associated with culture growth due to sample contamination, or poor recovery of organisms associated with pre-analytical factors, including prolonged transport or other delays in processing[4]. The sensitivity of both cytology and culture can be negatively impacted by previous antimicrobial therapy, so when possible, samples should be acquired prior to initiation of treatment, or at a minimum, the treatment history should be included in the clinical information submitted to the laboratory.[1]

Evaluation of a cytology specimen for bacterial pathogens begins with assessment of smear quality. Very low cellularity suggests the potential for an inadequate culture sample, while the absence of inflammatory cells, the presence of debris, squamous epithelial cells with or without epicellular bacteria, or numerous extracellular bacteria of mixed morphology could be consistent with contamination of the sample that might yield growth of bacteria of uncertain pathological significance (Figure 50.8). Evidence of oropharyngeal contamination of respiratory samples

Veterinary Cytology, First Edition. Edited by Leslie C. Sharkey, M. Judith Radin, and Davis Seelig.

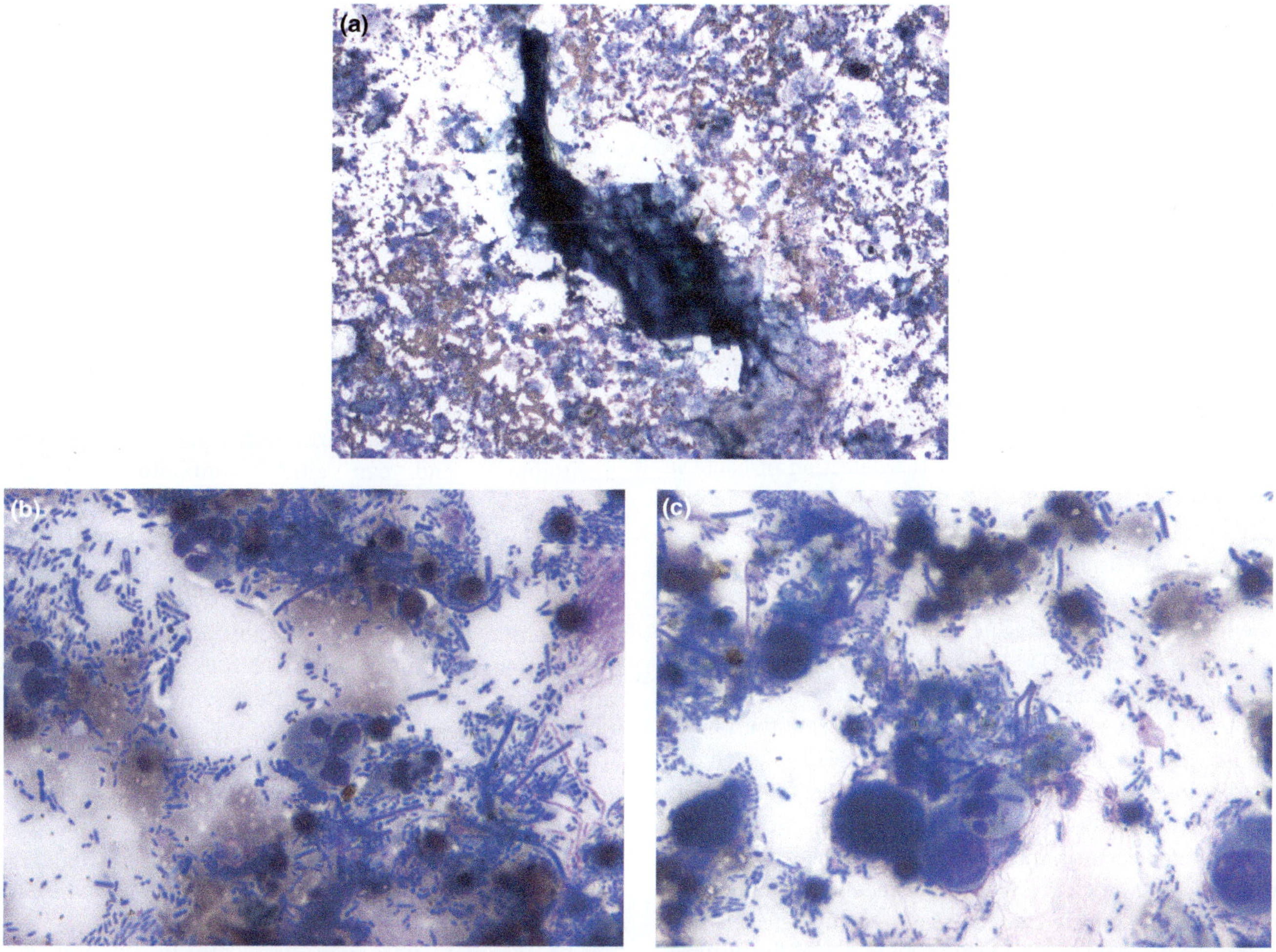

Figure 3.1 An adult Irish Draught gelding presented for a history of colic. Abdominal fluid was submitted for analysis, which revealed a total protein concentration of <2.0 g/dL and 1000 cells/μL. (a) Microscopy revealed numerous heterogeneous extracellular bacteria and plant material consistent with enterocentesis or acute gastrointestinal rupture (Wright Giemsa stain, 100×). (b and c) Closer inspection revealed neutrophils with intracellular bacteria, more suggestive for acute rupture; however, enterocentesis with *in vitro* phagocytosis of organisms could not be fully excluded cytologically (Wright Giemsa stain, 1000×). Due to declining clinical condition, the horse was euthanized, and necropsy was consistent with a septic peritonitis due to rupture.

(numerous extracellular bacteria of mixed morphology, squamous epithelial cells, and/or *Simonsiella* sp.) should call into question the value of culture results, and repeat collection should be considered (Chapters 25 and 26).

Cytology samples assessed to be of acceptable cellularity and free of artifacts that compromise interpretation should be characterized in terms of the relative presence of different inflammatory cells, as well as their morphologic characteristics, especially degenerate vs. non-degenerate neutrophils. The morphology of all bacteria should be described, including rod or coccoid shape, size (small, large, pleomorphic), patterns of association (i.e. diplococci, chaining, formation of mats), the presence of capsules or spores, and intra- or extracellular localization (Figures 17.2, 19.3, 20.11, 21.9, 25.7, 25.12, 31.4, 33.3, 33.5, 39.2, 39.8, 50.7, 53.2, 53.3, 55.5, 57.1, 58.2, 58.7, 59.5, 60.1, 60.5, 60.7, 60.8, 60.19, 60.22, and 61.1, for example). Ideally, Gram staining should be performed, keeping in mind that Gram-positive organisms can appear variably Gram-positive or Gram-negative if they are degenerating, which can be associated with death or antimicrobial use. These factors can also impact morphology. Organisms such as *Actinomyces* and *Nocardia* spp. typically appear as thin, chaining beaded rods using Wright Giemsa stain and can be variable in their Gram staining characteristics and are often highlighted better using acid-fast techniques (Figure 58.7). They are fastidious in culture and may be missed, so cytologic identification can be clinically useful, especially since they are an important consideration in antimicrobial choice. Mycobacteria rarely take up typical stains and appear as negatively staining rod-shaped intra- or extracellular structures. Acid-fast staining is recommended for confirmation, and these organisms require special culture techniques and grow slowly (often many months) (Figures 11.3, 58.8, and 61.19).

Best practices in the interpretation of cytologic identification of bacteria can depend on the clinical context. For urine, bacterial culture remains the reference standard; however, timely appropriate treatment can be facilitated by cytologic evaluation of urine specimens.[5–7] Studies show the presence or absence of neutrophils is not a good indicator of infection in all cases, cytologic examination of modified Wright-stained urine preparations had a sensitivity of 83% and a specificity of 99% for the detection of bacteria compared with culture, while the use of Gram stain can further improve sensitivity (Chapter 39).

In cases of suspected pyoderma, cytology is valuable to distinguish overgrowth from pathogenicity and to quantitate the relative numbers and likely clinical significance of organisms (Chapter 11).[3] In lip fold or commissure dermatitis, a combination of clinical signs and neutrophils in cytology samples correlated better with disease than numbers of organisms alone.[8] Likewise, a study of infected dog bite wounds used clinical and cytologic indicators of infection (>85% neutrophils, degenerate change in neutrophils, intracellular bacteria) rather than culture because culture results could not distinguish between a contaminated wound and an infected wound.[9] In this study, infected bites were significantly more likely to have a positive culture; however, of 83 wounds considered to be noninfected, 66 cultured positive. Thus, reliance on bacterial culture results in the absence of other clinicopathologic findings supportive of infection could result in overtreatment.

In canine bacterial keratitis, in-house cytologic evaluation and culture results correlated in 70% of 71 cases, while 14 cases had negative cytology with a positive culture and 7 dogs had identification of leukocytes and/or bacteria on cytology but a negative culture (Chapter 19).[10] Bacteria were found cytologically in 20–30% of canine and feline bile samples, typically associated with inflammation in the cat, but only in 1/6 of the canine cases. Cytology was minimally more sensitive than culture (24 vs. 21%) for the detection of organisms.[11] In contrast, a retrospective study of 34 cases of suspected canine septic arthritis found synovial fluid culture to be relatively insensitive for the detection of bacteria (44%) compared with cytology, suggesting an important role for cytology in the evaluation of this disease.[12] These studies illustrate the need for specific evaluation of the role of cytology and bacterial culture to determine best practices for the diagnosis of bacterial pathogenesis in different conditions.

Fungal Cytological Examination

Fungal disease presents in myriad forms and mimics many other diseases. Thus, evaluation of cytological and histological preparations is often the initial method of diagnosis. The morphology of specific fungal agents can be sufficient for definitive diagnosis except for the opportunistic saprophytic species. For certain agents such as dimorphic fungi, geographic location, or travel history can support the diagnosis. Many fungi are commonly identified in cytological preparations such as fine-needle aspirates, body cavity fluids, cerebrospinal fluid, impression smears, fecal smears, urine sediments, and skin scrapings. As with bacteria, fungal structures can be present in the environment and can either contaminate samples (Figure 26.3) or in some cases can be commensal or nonpathogenic, so interpretation in the cytologic and clinical context is necessary.

Pyogranulomatous inflammation with or without an eosinophilic component is the most common inflammatory response to fungal infection. Most fungal infections are chronic, resulting in the presence of variable numbers of macrophages, neutrophils, small lymphocytes, and well-differentiated to reactive fibrocytes in the cytological preparations. Less commonly, primarily histiocytic (granulomatous) inflammation with giant cells is seen with minimal numbers of neutrophils. Both fibrocytes and large epithelioid macrophages can exhibit pleomorphism with moderate to marked anisokaryosis, anisocytosis, and prominent nucleoli. Dermatophytes, *Pythium insidiosum*, *Lagenidium* spp., and *Cryptococcus* spp. are the organisms most commonly associated with a significant eosinophilic component. In some cryptococcal lesions, inflammation may be absent.

Routine Wright Giemsa stains will adequately stain most fungal agents. However, many of the saprophytic fungal agents often fail to stain in routine preparation and appear as negatively stained linear elements. In addition, Wright Giemsa stains can obscure identification of dematiaceous fungi. Evaluation of an unstained preparation can often reveal the pigmented fungi. Small fungal organisms like *Pneumocystis carinii* can be difficult to identify on Wright Giemsa stains due to size and light staining (Figures 25.13 and 60.9). To assist in identification of poorly staining or small organisms, air-dried cytological preparations can be stained using special stains more often used for histopathology. The two most commonly used stains are the Gomori methenamine silver (GMS) and the periodic acid-Schiff (PAS). The advantage for both the GMS and PAS stain is the increased sensitivity for identification of fungal agents that are small or fail to stain adequately with Wright Giemsa stain. The primary disadvantage is that these stains are not available as in-house stains, requiring submission of slides to a diagnostic laboratory to increase sensitivity for cytologic detection.

Fungal organisms can be divided morphologically into three broad categories: dimorphic fungi, mycelial fungi, and yeast. Dimorphic fungal agents, *Blastomyces dermatitidis*, *Histoplasma capsulatum*, *Coccidioides* spp., and yeast predominant organisms such as *Cryptococcus* spp., *Sporothrix schenckii*, and *Candida* sp. present with typical morphologic characteristics that can allow determination of species. In contrast, the mycelial fungi, which are often opportunistic and saprophytic, are more difficult to classify microscopically. In most cases, a differential list for these organisms can be provided based on width and uniformity of the hyphae, septation, pigmentation, and presence and type of spores, but culture is required for definitive classification.

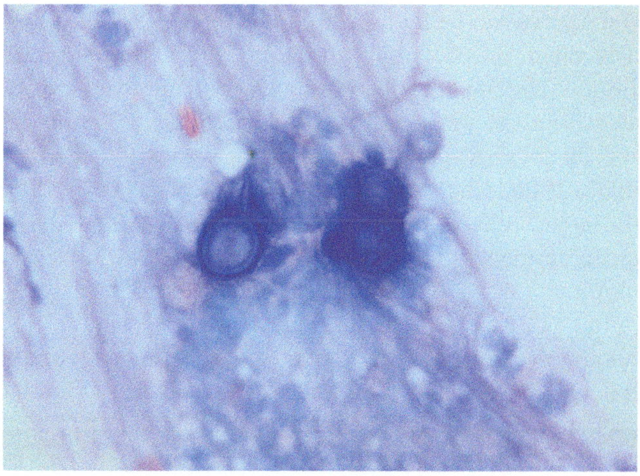

Figure 3.2 Skin aspirates with a single and a budding *Blastomyces dermatitidis* yeast forms (Wright Giemsa stain, 1000×).

Dimorphic Fungi

The dimorphic fungi (*Coccidioides* spp., *B. dermatitidis*, *H. capsulatum*, *Cryptococcus* spp., and *S. schenckii* complex) have distinct morphology within tissues and grow in mycelial form in culture at room temperature. *Cryptococcus* spp. is somewhat of an exception because it grows in yeast form in tissue and traditional culture; the mycelial form is only propagated using specialized culture parameters. Rarely, dimorphic fungi form mycelia in tissues usually with higher oxygen tension.[12–15] These organisms usually result in systemic infections, resulting in the identification of the organisms in multiple sites. Having a good understanding of the specific characteristics of each of these fungal agents is essential for making a cytological diagnosis.

Blastomyces dermatitidis

B. dermatitidis in cytological preparations has a thick cell wall and broad-based budding (Figure 3.2). These yeast organisms are 5–20 μm in size. These organisms can be confused with small spherule of *Coccidioides* spp. The organism often collapses with the capsule forming distinct folds (Figures 3.2, 25.10, and 39.11). Cytological diagnosis is most common from consolidated lung and enlarged lymph nodes. Like *Coccidioides* spp., *B. dermatitidis* is a cause of fungal osteomyelitis.[16] Historically, *B. dermatitidis* is the dimorphic fungus most commonly associated with uveitis.[17] *H. capsulatum*, *Cryptococcus* spp., and *Coccidioides* spp. are less commonly reported in association with the uveal tract. Aspirates of the anterior and posterior chambers may provide a diagnosis when the ocular exam suggests granulomatous lesions within the uveal tissues (Chapter 19).

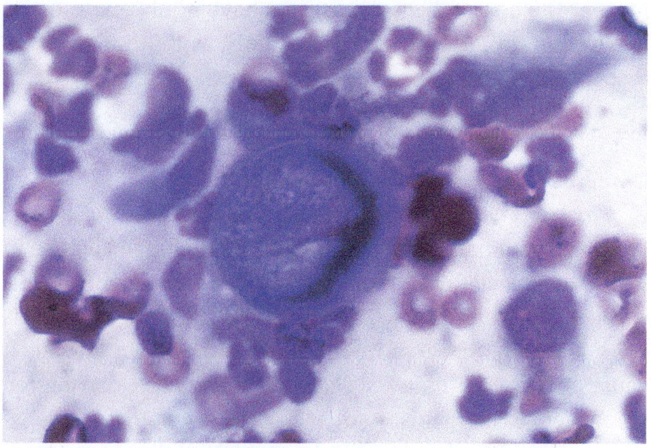

Figure 3.3 Bone aspirates with a single *Coccidioides* sp. spherule and concurrent inflammation (Wright Giemsa stain, 1000×).

Coccidioides spp.

The genus *Coccidioides* has two species with distinct genotypes but identical phenotypes, *Coccidioides immitis* and *Coccidioides posadasii*. Dogs are most commonly affected; however, infection has been reported in many mammalian and reptilian species. Feline cases are increasingly being identified as awareness of the disease in this species is improving.[18] The organisms in tissue are characterized by a spherical structure (spherule) with a distinct thick cell wall that undergoes internal septation with the production of a large number of endospores (endosporulation) (Figures 3.3 and 59.2). When mature, the spherule ruptures and releases the endospore that can then be phagocytized and spread to other locations. The spherules stain deeply basophilic with Wright Giemsa stain and can collapse forming prominent folds. Endosporulation is difficult to appreciate cytologically unless the spherule is ruptured. Rarely, intracytoplasmic endospores can be found within macrophages. The spherules range in size from 10–120 μm and endospores are 1–2 μm. The smaller spherules can be difficult to differentiated from the yeast form of *B. dermatitidis*. *Coccidioides* spp. do not show budding as would be seen with *B. dermatitidis*. If budding is absent, diagnosis depends on finding the larger spherules, evidence of endosporulation, and history of residence or travel in an endemic area. The increased movement of people and their pets often confounds separation of these two diseases by regions of endemicity. Aspirates of internal and cutaneous/subcutaneous mass lesions, consolidated lung fields, lymph nodes, lytic and proliferative bone lesions, and pleural, abdominal, and pericardial effusions are the most common preparations in which spherules are found. It is important to remember that granulomas containing spherules have been found in all organ systems in affected animals in endemic areas. While central nervous system involvement is not uncommon in the dog and cat, organisms have not been reported in cerebral spinal fluid samples. Rarely, aspirates of masses associated with the spinal meninges have revealed pyogranulomatous inflammation with spherules.

Cryptococcus spp.

Cryptococcus neoformans var. *neoformans* and *C. neoformans* var. *gattii* both have been identified to cause fungal disease in veterinary species. The two species cannot be reliably differentiated cytologically.[19] *C. neoformans* var. *neoformans* is considered the most common fungal pathogen in the cat. It causes disease in many species and should be considered whenever yeast organisms are identified in cytological preparations. The organism is a 4–7 μm yeast with thin-based budding and a thick nonstaining capsule (Figures 24.4, 39.11, and 48.1). In most preparations, background cellular and protein staining usually outlines the capsule without any special staining such as India ink. However, preparations with minimal inflammation or insufficient protein background such as cerebral spinal fluid can make identification of the capsule difficult. In these cases, India ink may be helpful. *C. neoformans* var. *gattii* is a reportable disease in Washington and Oregon. The Center for Disease Control encourages reporting of all culture-confirmed cases regardless of state of origin for the case.[20] The organisms are most commonly identified in aspirate preparations from the upper respiratory tract including mass lesions overlying the nasal planum and sinuses. *Cryptococcus* spp. are the most commonly reported fungal agents in cerebral spinal fluid.

Histoplasma capsulatum

H. capsulatum organisms are characterized as 2–3 μm yeast forms that usually have a thin pseudocapsule (Figure 3.4). The organisms are both intracellular and extracellular in most preparations. Organisms are most often found within macrophages but can be seen in neutrophils. As with *Coccidioides* spp. and *B. dermatitidis*, the primary infection is respiratory with systemic extension. As a result, consolidated lung lesions are common sites for diagnosis of histoplasmosis with liver, spleen, and lymph nodes commonly involved with systemic disease. *H. capsulatum* is the dimorphic fungus most commonly associated with the gastrointestinal tract with the organism found on rectal scrapings. Less commonly, *H. capsulatum* can be found in aspirates of cortical bone lesions, within joint fluid and cerebral spinal fluid, and in blood films and bone marrow preparations.[21–23]

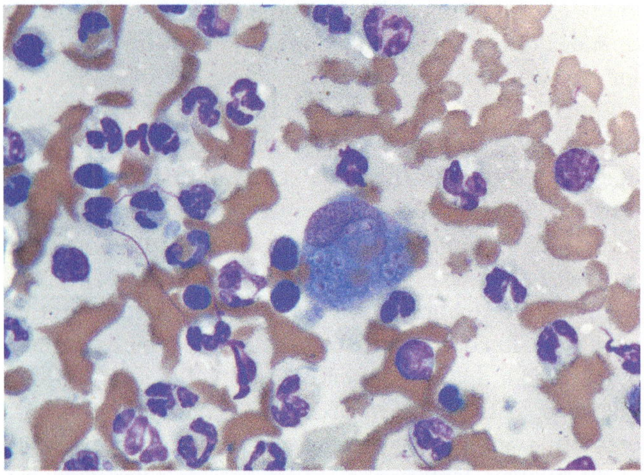

Figure 3.4 Aspirates from dermal lesions on the face of an adult Siamese cat. Several small *Histoplasma capsulatum* yeasts are within a single macrophage (Wright Giemsa stain, 1000×).

Sporothrix schenckii Complex

The *S. schenckii* species complex consists of six species, two of which are most common in veterinary medicine, *S. schenckii* and *Sporothrix brasiliensis*.[24,25] The yeast form is found in tissues and cytological preparations and is an ovoid to fusiform (cigar-shaped) pleomorphic yeast with thin-based budding. Multiple buds can be seen on a single parent yeast.[26] The organisms are 2 μm in width with variable lengths. Occasionally, mycelial forms are seen in both histological and cytological preparations.[27] In most affected animals, only a small number of organisms are usually seen in diagnostic samples. Cats are an exception; numerous pleomorphic yeast organisms can be found both within macrophages and free in the background of feline cytological preparations.[28] When organisms are infrequent, the distinct fusiform morphology may not be evident, making it difficult to differentiate *Sporothrix* species from *H. capsulatum* and *Candida* spp. Most infections are cutaneous and result from implantation of environmental forms of the fungus into tissues. Disseminated disease with multiple cutaneous lesions with or without lymph node involvement is common in the cat and can be seen in dogs. Systemic infection with involvement of visceral organs such as the liver or lungs is uncommon but has been reported in feline cases due to *S. brasiliensis*.[27] Sporotrichosis is a zoonotic disease with well-documented animal to animal and animal to human transmission. Unlike *Cryptococcus gattii*, sporotrichosis is not currently reportable in the United States.

Mycelial Fungi

There are numerous saprophytic mycelial fungi that are opportunistic pathogens in veterinary species, while others such as dermatophytes are more zoophilic. Dermatophytosis is an important skin disease in dogs and cats with zoonotic potential that will be presented in greater detail in Chapter 11. Of the saprophytic organisms, *Aspergillus* spp. is often singled out as a separate entity with specific site propensities, including the nasal cavity and vertebra in the dog (Figure 25.8). Other examples include *Fusarium* spp. However, for cytologic evaluation, it is not useful to distinguish the saprophytic fungi because they cannot be reliably identified based on morphology in cytological or histological preparations.[29] It is most appropriate to provide a cytological diagnosis of saprophytic fungal infection with a differential list of possible species for the mycelial morphology found in the preparations. This approach has been recommended for the histological diagnosis of fungal disease as well. The mycelial fungi can be grouped based on their morphologic characteristics including, pigmentation, presence and number of septae, and type of branching. In addition, the presence of unusual features such as chlamydospores, conidiospores, and crystal formation can all be used to provide a differential list of possible fungal species based on cytology or histopathology. Figures illustrating examples in various tissues include 21.10, 25.8, 39.10, and 61.21.

Yeast

The most common yeast infections are *Malassezia* spp. (covered in greater depth in Chapter 11, Figure 17.2) and *Candida* spp., which can be a commensal organism with the potential for overgrowth and pathogenicity in immunocompromised animals and with disruption of normal microbiota with antimicrobial therapy (Figures 39.9 and 52.6). Systemic spread and mycelial growth are reported but very rare in animals.[30] *Candida* spp. organisms are typically oval, 3–8 μm in diameter, and often with a thin halo. They can occur intra- or extracellularly and can be characterized by narrow-based budding as well as the formation of germ tubes, pseudohyphae, or true hyphae that can be seen in cytology samples.[31]

Miscellaneous Organisms

Pythium insidiosum

P. insidiosum is an oomycete that primarily affects horses, dogs, and humans with a small number of cases in other mammalian species.[32] The organism was originally thought to be a zygomycete due to the broad pauci-septate hyphal form seen in tissues. The hyphae range from 3 to 12 μm in diameter, are sparsely septate and hyaline, and form 90° branches. Infection occurs following exposure to motile zoospores in water.[33] In most species, the organism usually causes cutaneous tumorlike growths, often on the distal limbs. Gastrointestinal disease is the most common manifestation of the disease in dogs (Figure 31.5). Primary pulmonary and cutaneous disease in the dog is also reported.[34,35] Systemic disease can be seen with extension of lesions to the pancreas, mesenteric lymph nodes, liver, and eye. The organism is associated with arteritis as well.[32] Historically, the disease is regionally limited to tropical, subtropical, and temperate environments. However, cases have been reported outside in the Southeastern United States suggesting expansion of its environmental niche.[36] As with other organisms that form hyphae, *Pythium* sp. cannot be specifically identified on histological sections or cytology. Their hyphae are indistinguishable from *Zygomycetes* such as *Mucor*, *Conidiobolus*, and *Basidiobolus*. Differentiation requires either culture, immunohistochemical stains, or molecular methods to confirm the species. The organisms do not stain well in cytological or histological preparations. Grocott's methenamine silver is considered superior to periodic acid-Schiff stain for demonstration of the organism in both cytological and histological preparations. Eosinophilic inflammation is a common inflammatory response to this organism. Because the organism is often in small numbers within lesions, the disease should be considered when the clinical, cytological, or histological findings are suggestive of infection in the endemic regions.

Prototheca spp.

Prototheca spp. are achlorophyllous algae closely related to *Chlorella* sp. While infection with *Prototheca* spp. organisms is not common, it is well documented in veterinary species.[37] It is most often reported in dogs and rarely in cats. *Prototheca* spp. is a well-documented cause of mastitis in ruminants (Figure 58.9) and a cause of rhinitis in the horse.[38,39] *Prototheca zopfii* is the most common species identified in dogs.[40] *Prototheca wickerhamii* is the predominant species identified in cats with only one report of *P. zopfii*.[41] Infection by the algae is most common in immunosuppressed individuals although it is considered a primary pathogen that can infect immunocompetent individuals. The most common lesion in cats is cutaneous, while visceral disease is most common in dogs. The disease can disseminate to involve the intestine, kidney, liver, heart, eyes, and brain. Primary protothecal meningitis has been reported with no evidence of disease outside of the central nervous system. In cytological preparations the organisms are 3–30 µm round to oval sporangia with internal compartmentalization and formation of sporangiospores. The sporangiospores are separated by thick walls that are contiguous with the outside wall of the sporangia.[42] The inflammatory response is pyogranulomatous with or without an eosinophilic component. Organisms are usually in low to moderate numbers in cytological preparations. The organisms are readily stained with Wright Giemsa stain precluding the need for additional stains.

Rhinosporidium seeberi

Originally thought to be a protozoal organism similar to *Coccidia*, then considered a fungus, *R. seeberi* is a unique infectious agent that is currently considered a member of the order *Dermocystida* (DRIP clade).[43] These organisms are not fungi but show morphology similar to *Coccidioides* spp. The organisms that share this classification are primarily fish pathogens. Infection due to *R. seeberi* is limited to reports of upper respiratory tract and conjunctiva.[44] The disease is most commonly reported in the horse with sporadic cases in the dog (Figure 24.5) and other species. Granulomatous rhinitis and, rarely, laryngitis are the usual presentations. The lesions are often polypoid.[45] Within the inflammatory lesion, the organism forms large sporangia that contain endospores. Immature early forms contain a single nucleus with central nucleolus that range in size from 60 to 500 µm with a thick eosinophilic wall.[43] As the sporangia matures 1–2 µm endospores are formed. In cytological preparations, the endospores are often deeply basophilic with no internal structure. Occasionally, a ruptured sporangium is seen associated with myriad endospores. The organisms are usually associated with significant pyogranulomatous inflammation.

Protozoal Cytological Examination

Detection of parasites cytologically can be difficult and frustrating because the site of greatest pathology or tissue injury does not always correlate well with the life cycle and subsequently organism detection. Thus, some background knowledge of how clinical signs correlate with the life cycle is needed for optimal sample selection and diagnostic successes.

Apicomplexan Protozoans

Toxoplasma, *Neospora*, and *Sarcocystis* spp. are intracellular apicomplexan protozoan parasites that can infect virtually all mammals. In domestic animals, specifically dogs and cats, these infections are generally associated with neurologic manifestations. In cattle, neosporosis is a common cause of abortion and economic losses.[46] Merozoites or tachyzoites are most notably seen on cerebrospinal fluid but also cutaneous, mammary, and respiratory cytological evaluations. In the central nervous system, neutrophilic pleocytosis is often observed with low number of merozoites or tachyzoites seen intracellular and/or extracellular. Tachyzoites and merozoites can be observed clustered or individualized, ovoid to banana shape, 1–7 µm in length with pale blue cytoplasm and an eccentrically placed, round to ovoid nucleus. These three protozoans are difficult to distinguish using morphology alone; thus serology and/or molecular diagnostics are often necessary for a definitive diagnosis.[47,48]

Leishmaniasis

Leishmania spp. are protozoan parasites transmitted by sandflies and divided into three broad categories based on clinical manifestation; cutaneous, mucocutaneous, and visceral leishmaniasis. While leishmaniasis is considered a primarily foreign animal disease in the United States, several autochthonous cases are reported each year. *Leishmania mexicana*, a cutaneous leishmaniasis, infecting both dogs and cats is considered endemic to Texas with the Southern Plains Woodrat being the primary sylvatic reservoir.[49] *Leishmania infantum*, a zoonotic visceral leishmaniasis (ZVL), is reported in the United States, and dogs are considered to be the primary domestic reservoir.[50] While sandflies are also considered the primary means of transmission, there is evidence that vertical transmission can also be a primary means of transmission. In the United States, there has been an increased incidence of ZVL within the Foxhound population in regions of the country that lack the biological vector. Fine-needle aspirates or impression smears of the lesions reveal a pyogranulomatous to granulomatous inflammation with small lymphocytes, plasma cells, and multinucleated giant cells also usually present. Amastigotes are found within parasitophorus vacuoles or free in the background. The amastigotes are ovoid to round, 1.5–2 µm × 2.5–5.0 µm with pale blue to color less cytoplasm that contains an eccentrically placed small ovoid to round, red to light purple nucleus (Figure 19.5). Perpendicular to the nucleus, a single kinetoplast that is bar shape and deep purple is noted. The kinetoplast tends to be located between the nucleus and the edge of the organism that contains the greatest amount of cytoplasm.

It is an important morphological feature as it can help distinguish leishmaniasis from other infectious etiologies such as, *H. capsulatum* and *S. schenckii*.

Cytauxzoonosis

Cytauxzoon felis is a tick borne hemoprotozoan parasite of cats with swift and severe clinical course, which left untreated has almost a 100% mortality.[51] Infected cats initially present with nonspecific clinical signs including depression, anorexia, fever, lymphadenomegaly, and malaise, making diagnosis challenging. Veterinarians have traditionally relied on identification of erythrocyte piroplasms on blood film examination for definitive diagnosis[50]. Advanced molecular techniques, such as polymerase chain reactions, are known to be more sensitive but are more expensive than cytologic diagnostics and require days to complete.[52] Because the entire course of disease is typically less than five days from initial clinical signs to death, any delay in diagnosis is likely to result in mortality.[53] Blood smear evaluation has both biological and technical limitations. Biologically, at the onset of clinical illness, the parasite is usually still in the tissue phase of development (i.e. schizogenous phase) and has not entered the intraerythrocytic phase.[54] It is the intraerythrocytic piroplasm phase that is detected on blood smear evaluation. Therefore, cats may present for clinical care prior to the appearance of piroplasms in the peripheral blood. It has been estimated that piroplasms may not be evident in circulation at onset of disease in up to 50% of infected cats.[55] Parasitemia alone cannot differentiate between active disease and persistently infected. There is evidence that identification of schizont-laden macrophages in liver, splenic, and lymph node cytology may be an additional option for the diagnosis of cytauxzoonosis as these cats are traditionally present during the tissue stage of disease that is hallmarked by widespread vascular parasite thrombi in visceral organs. Schizont-laden macrophages should not be present in the visceral organs of cats that are persistently infected and may aid in diagnosing active disease. Schizont-laden macrophages are round varying from >15 to 75 µm in diameter. The nucleus of the macrophage is eccentrically placed, pale pink, and ballooned with a single macronucleus. Within the cytoplasm, numerous, small, round to comma shape, (1–2 µm) purple merozoites can be observed (Figure 3.5).

Intestinal Parasites

By far, one of the most common samples submitted for parasite screening is feces. Intestinal parasites consist of the majority of pathogenic veterinary endoparasites. Please refer to Chapter 33 for dry mount fecal cytology; however, an extensive description of parasitical examination of feces is beyond the scope of this text. Dry mount fecal cytology can be useful for identification of parasitic ova and cysts while simultaneously evaluating the bacterial composition; however, motile forms (trophozoites) of certain protozoans such as *Giardia* spp., *Trichomonads,* or amoebae, and motile bacteria, such as *Campylobacter* spp., are easier to evaluate using a wet mount preparation.[56] It is imperative that samples be collected and prepared within five minutes of fecal loop extraction or defecation as the motile protozoan parasites degrade rapidly when exposed to the external environment. Commonly, Lugol's iodine or lactophenol cotton blue is added to the wet mount preparation to enhance visualization of both trophozoites and/or the internal structures of cyst/ova for further identification. Unfortunately, these stains, specifically iodine, result in rapid death of motile forms of protozoans; thus it is recommended to review unstained and stained wet mount concurrently or sequentially to increase the sensitivity of detection.[56]

Miscellaneous Parasites Diagnosed Cytologically

An exhaustive list of parasites that can be diagnosed cytologically is beyond the scope of this chapter. Specific examples are described in other chapters and include respiratory tissues (Chapters 24 and 25, Figure 25.14), the urinary system (Chapters 37, and 39, Figure 39.12), and hepatobiliary (Chapters 34 and 37, Figure 37.4) in small animals and a wider range in exotic species (Chapters 61 and 63).

Dracunculus spp. larvae and adult females are nematodes that can be found in the subcutaneous tissue, usually the distal extremities, of various domestic species and wildlife.[57,58] Common clinical presentation for dracunculiasis includes a non-healing wound in a distal extremity with a previous history of access to freshwater with copepods and/or frogs, which can overlap with the geographic, clinical, and cytologic features of some oomycete infections, most commonly *Lagenidium* and *Pythium* spp. These lesions are generally localized to the distal extremities; as the adult male and female worms mate in the retroperitoneal space or various connective tissues, then the female migrates to the subcutaneous tissue of distal extremities. In the subcutaneous tissues, female produces various toxins that result in blistering of the skin and an inflammatory reaction (eosinophilic to neutrophilic) that eventually results in a small pore in the skin. Upon contact with water, the female will extrude a portion of her body from the wound releasing larvae into the water. In cases where dracunculiasis is suspected, caution should be taken before attempting fine-needle aspiration of the wound. Damaging the adult female during aspiration may result in anaphylaxis in the patient. On cytological evaluation, larvae stages are

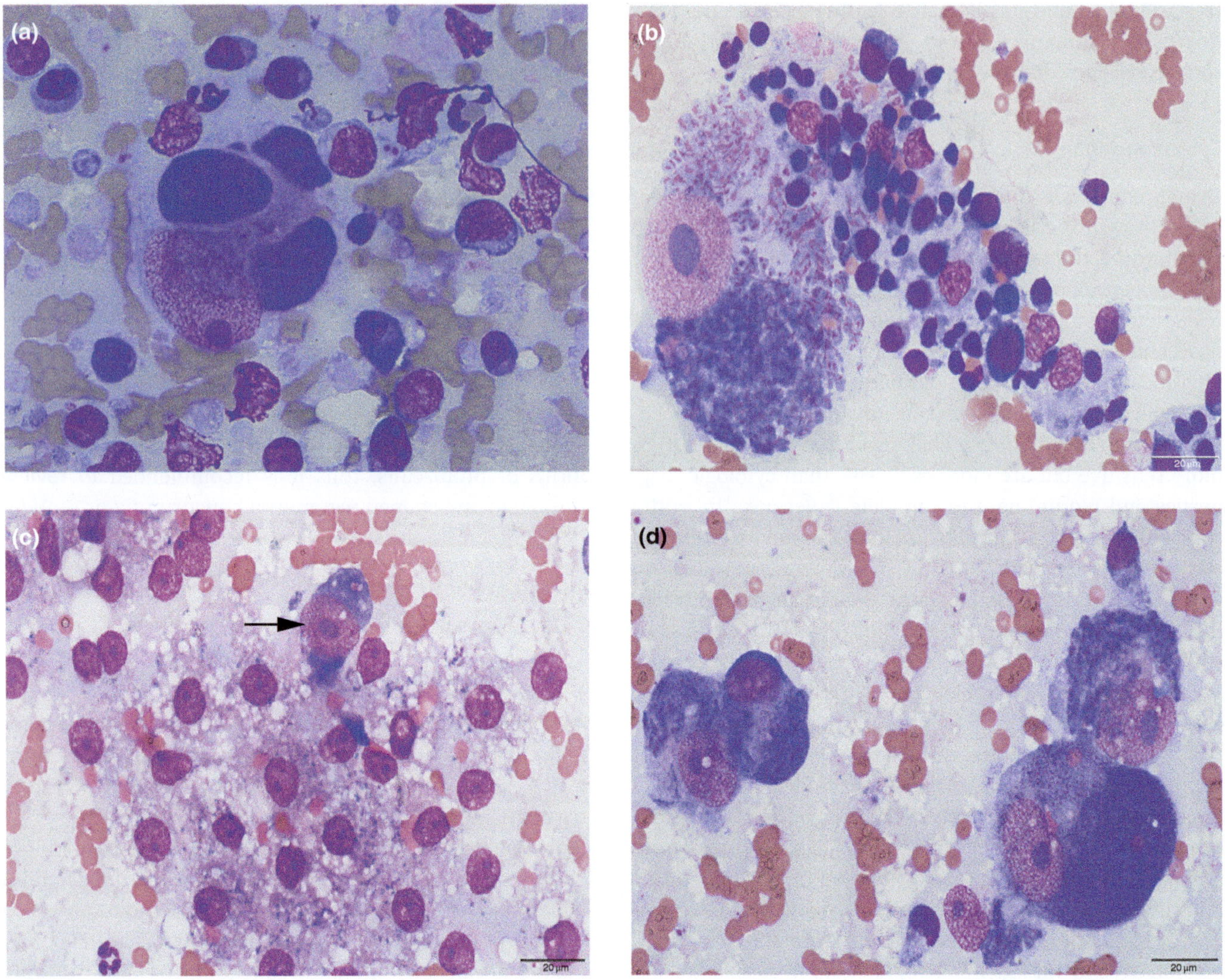

Figure 3.5 (a) Splenic aspirates with a single schizont-laden macrophages containing numerous *Cytauxzoon felis* merozoites (1–2 µm) (Wright Giemsa stain, 600×). (b) Splenic aspirates from a 2.5-year-old, neutered male, domestic shorthair cat presented for a two-day history of inappetence and lethargy. The spleen was enlarged and coarsely heterogeneous on ultrasound. A large, partially lysed schizont-laden macrophage is seen associated with a heterogeneous lymphoid population (Wright Giemsa stain, 1000×). (c and d) Fine-needle aspirate from the enlarged hypoechoic liver of the same cat. (c) A cluster of mildly atypical hepatocytes exhibiting moderate distinct vacuolization (lipid accumulation) is seen surrounding a schizont-laden macrophage containing several *C. felis* organisms (arrow). (d) Several schizont-laden macrophages containing numerous *C. felis* organisms in various stages of maturation (Wright Giemsa stain, 1000×. *Source:* Images (b–d) courtesy of Francisco Conrado).

identified. The larvae are approximately 600 × 40 µm, pale blue to colorless with many horizontal striations (cuticle), have a curved anterior end and a long-tapered tail (Figure 3.6). These larvae are observed closely associated with inflammatory cells highlighting their morphologic features.[58] In the United States, *Dracunculus insignis* and *Dracunculus medinensis* are the most common species in dogs and wildlife; however, molecular diagnostics are needed for specific diagnosis as the larvae cannot be differentiated using cytology alone.[57,58]

Setaria spp. adult nematodes are generally found in the peritoneal cavities of equids and domestic and wild ruminants. After sexual reproduction, larvae are released into the abdominal cavity of the host, migrate to the peripheral blood, are ingested by a mosquito, and ultimately continue the life cycle.[59] While *Setaria* microfilariae are most commonly described in the peripheral blood, migration of the larvae to the central nervous system, resulting in an eosinophilic pleocytosis, and eyes have been reported in cattle and horses and skin in horses.[60–63] In the peripheral

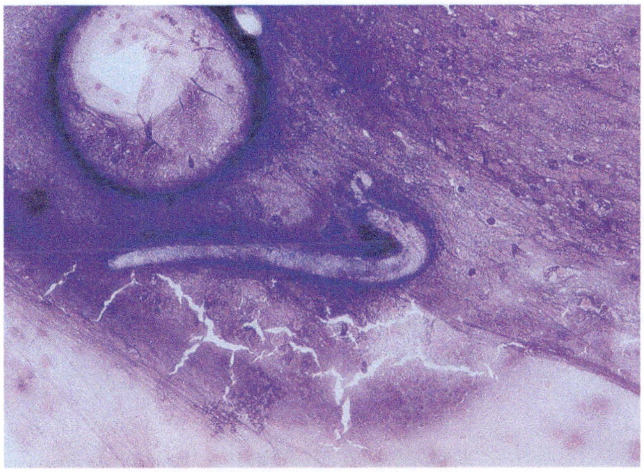

Figure 3.6 *Dracunculus* larva (L1) in a cutaneous lesion on the distal limb of a dog. A single serpentine larva with characteristic cuticle with horizontal striation, curved anterior end, and tapered tail against pink cellular debris and inflammatory cells (Wright Giemsa stain, 200×).

blood, the microfilariae are approximately 268–285 µm long with a sheath and basophilic internal structures; however, these same features would be observed on other cytological specimens.[63]

Ectoparasites

Many ectoparasites are diagnosed by gross examination, and a comprehensive review is beyond the scope of this chapter. However, cytologic examination of ear smears and dermatologic samples from small animal species and a range of exotic species is routinely performed to screen for small mites. In dogs and cats, the most common entities are demodicosis, sarcoptic mange (Chapter 11), and ear mites such as *Otodectes cynotis*. Additional examples are described in the species-specific chapters.

Conclusion

Cytology is capable of assisting in the identification of a wide range of microbiologic agents, as well as refining the interpretation of potential pathogenicity. There are limitations to the role of cytology, which can sometimes lack sensitivity in the identification of organisms. Utilization of a wider range of staining options can facilitate visualization of some organisms. In addition, additional complementary testing may be required to more specifically identify at the genus and species level.

References

1. Thys, J.P., Jacobs, F., and Byl, B. (1994). Microbiological specimen collection in the emergency room. *Eur J Emerg Med* 1: 47–53.
2. Woods, G.L. and Walker, D.H. (1996). Detection of infection or infectious agents by use of cytologic and histologic stains. *Clin Microbiol Rev* 9: 382–404.
3. Beco, L., Guaguère, E., Lorente Méndez, C. et al. (2013). Suggested guidelines for using systemic antimicrobials in bacterial skin infections (1): diagnosis based on clinical presentation, cytology and culture. *Vet Rec* 172: 72–78.
4. Wilson, M.L. (1996). General principles of specimen collection and transport. *Clin Infect Dis* 22: 766–777.
5. Swenson, C.L., Boisvert, A.M., Gibbons-Burgener, S.N., and Kruger, J.M. (2011). Evaluation of modified Wright-staining of dried urinary sediment as a method for accurate detection of bacteriuria in cats. *Vet Clin Pathol* 40: 256–264.
6. Way, L.I., Sullivan, L.A., Johnson, V., and Morley, P.S. (2013). Comparison of routine urinalysis and urine Gram stain for detection of bacteriuria in dogs. *J Vet Emerg Crit Care* 23: 23–28.
7. O'Neil, E., Horney, B., Burton, S. et al. (2013). Comparison of wet-mount, Wright-Giemsa and Gram-stained urine sediment for predicting bacteriuria in dogs and cats. *Can Vet J* 54: 1061–1066.
8. Doelle, M., Loeffler, A., Wolf, K. et al. (2016). Clinical features, cytology and bacterial culture results in dogs with and without cheilitis and comparison of three sampling techniques. *Vet Dermatol* 27: 140–147.
9. Meyers, B., Schoeman, J.P., Goddard, A., and Picard, J. (2008). The bacteriology and antimicrobial susceptibility of infected and non-infected dog bite wounds: fifty cases. *Vet Microbiol* 127: 360–368.
10. Hindley, K.E., Groth, A.D., King, M. et al. (2016). Bacterial isolates, antimicrobial susceptibility, and clinical characteristics of bacterial keratitis in dogs presenting to referral practice in Australia. *Vet Ophthalmol* 19: 418–426.
11. Peters, L.M., Glanemann, B., Garden, O.A., and Szladovits, B. (2016). Cytological findings of 140 bile samples from dogs and cats and associated clinical pathological data. *J Vet Intern Med* 30: 123–131.
12. Scharf, V.F., Lewis, S.T., Wellehan, J.F. et al. (2015). Retrospective evaluation of the efficacy of isolating bacteria from synovial fluid in dogs with suspected septic arthritis. *Aust Vet J* 93: 200–203.
13. Kaufmann, A.F., Kaplan, W., and Kraft, D.E. (1979). Filamentous forms of Ajellomyces (blastomyces) dermatitidis in a dog. *Vet Pathol* 16: 271–273.

14 Schuetz, A.N., Pisapia, D., Yan, J., and Hoda, R.S. (2012). An atypical morphologic presentation of *Coccidioides* spp. in fine-needle aspiration of lung. *Diagn Cytopathol* 40: 163–167.

15 Tonelli, A.R., Khalife, W.T., Cao, M., and Young, V.B. (2008). Spherules, hyphae, and air-crescent sign. *Am J Med Sci* 335: 504–506.

16 Roberts, R.E. (1979). Osteomyelitis associated with disseminated blastomycosis in nine dogs. *Vet Radiol* 20: 124–134.

17 Kern, T. (1995). Canine uveitis. In: *Kirk's Current Veterinary Therapy XII* (ed. J.D. Bonagura), 1248–1253. Philadelphia, PA: W.B. Saunders.

18 Graupmann-Kuzma, A., Valentine, B.A., Shubitz, L.F. et al. (2008). Coccidioidomycosis in dogs and cats: a review. *J Am Anim Hosp Assoc* 44: 226–235.

19 Chang, Y.C., Khanal Lamichhane, A., Bradley, J. et al. (2015). Differences between *Cryptococcus neoformans* and *Cryptococcus gattii* in the molecular mechanisms governing utilization of D-amino acids as the sole nitrogen source. *PLoS One* 10: e0131865.

20 CDC (2015). *C. gatti* Infection Statistics. https://www.cdc.gov/fungal/diseases/cryptococcosis-gattii/statistics.html (accessed 17 July 2018).

21 Meadows, R.L., MacWilliams, P.S., Dzata, G., and Delauche, A.J. (1992). Diagnosis of histoplasmosis in a dog by cytologic examination of CSF. *Vet Clin Pathol* 21: 122–125.

22 Prater, M.R., Ruiz De Gopegui, R., Burdette, K. et al. (1999). Bone marrow aspirate from a cat with cutaneous lesions. *Vet Clin Pathol* 28: 52.

23 Huss, B.T., Collier, L.L., Collins, B.K., and Pittman, L.L. (1994). Polyarthropathy and chorioretinitis with retinal detachment in a dog with systemic histoplasmosis. *J Am Anim Hosp Assoc* 30: 217–224.

24 Pohlman, L.M., Bagladi-Swanson, M.S., and Torres-Irizarry, M.S. (2014). Pathology in practice. Disseminated pyogranulomatous inflammation with intralesional Sporothrix organisms in a cat. *J Am Vet Med Assoc* 245: 187–189.

25 López-Romero, E., Reyes-Montes, M.R., Pérez-Torres, A. et al. (2011). *Sporothrix schenckii* complex and sporotrichosis, an emerging health problem. *Future Microbiol* 6: 85–102.

26 Barros, M.B., de Almeida Paes, R., and Schubach, A.O. (2011). *Sporothrix schenckii* and Sporotrichosis. *Clin Microbiol Rev* 24: 633–654.

27 Gremião, I.D., Menezes, R.C., Schubach, T.M. et al. (2015). Feline sporotrichosis: epidemiological and clinical aspects. *Med Mycol* 53: 15–21.

28 Bernstein, J.A., Cook, H.E., Gill, A.F. et al. (2007). Cytologic diagnosis of generalized cutaneous sporotrichosis in a hunting hound. *Vet Clin Pathol* 36: 94–96.

29 Guarner, J. and Brandt, M.E. (2011). Histopathologic diagnosis of fungal infections in the 21st century. *Clin Microbiol Rev* 24: 247–280.

30 Willems, N., Houwers, D.J., Schlotter, Y.M. et al. (2017). Disseminated candidiasis in a young, previously healthy, dog and review of literature. *Mycopathologia* 182: 591–596.

31 Bradford, K., Meinkoth, J., McKeirnen, K., and Love, B. (2013). Candida peritonitis in dogs: report of 5 cases. *Vet Clin Pathol* 42: 227–233.

32 Gaastra, W., Lipman, L.J., De Cock, A.W. et al. (2010). *Pythium insidiosum*: an overview. *Vet Microbiol* 146: 1–16.

33 Schurko, A.M., Mendoza, L., Lévesque, C.A. et al. (2003). A molecular phylogeny of *Pythium insidiosum*. *Mycol Res* 107: 537–544.

34 Grooters, A.M. (2003). Pythiosis, lagenidiosis, and zygomycosis in small animals. *Vet Clin North Am Small Anim Pract* 33: 695–720, v.

35 Kepler, D., Cole, R., Lee-Fowler, T. et al. (2019). Pulmonary pythiosis in a canine patient. *Vet Radiol Ultrasound* 60 (2): E20–E23.

36 Oldenhoff, W., Grooters, A., Pinkerton, M.E. et al. (2014). Cutaneous pythiosis in two dogs from Wisconsin, USA. *Vet Dermatol* 25: 52–54.

37 Hollingsworth, S.R. (2000). Canine protothecosis. *Vet Clin North Am Small Anim Pract* 30: 1091–1101.

38 Kurumisawa, T., Kano, R., Nakamura, Y. et al. (2018). Is bovine protothecal mastitis related to persistent infection in intestine? *J Vet Med Sci* 80: 950–952.

39 Schöniger, S., Roschanski, N., Rösler, U. et al. (2016). Prototheca species and *Pithomyces chartarum* as causative agents of rhinitis and/or sinusitis in horses. *J Comp Pathol* 155: 121–125.

40 Shank, A.M., Dubielzig, R.D., and Teixeira, L.B. (2015). Canine ocular protothecosis: a review of 14 cases. *Vet Ophthalmol* 18: 437–442.

41 Huth, N., Wenkel, R.F., Roschanski, N. et al. (2015). *Prototheca zopfii* Genotype 2-induced nasal dermatitis in a cat. *J Comp Pathol* 152: 287–290.

42 Greene, C.E., Rakich, P.M., and Latimer, K.S. (2006). Protothecosis. In: *Infectious Diseases of the Dog and Cat*, 3e (ed. C.E. Greene). St. Louis, MO: Elsevier.

43 Fredricks, D.N., Jolley, J.A., Lepp, P.W. et al. (2000). *Rhinosporidium seeberi*: a human pathogen from a novel group of aquatic protistan parasites. *Emerg Infect Dis* 6: 273–282.

44 Burgess, H.J., Lockerbie, B.P., Czerwinski, S., and Scott, M. (2012). Equine laryngeal rhinosporidiosis in western Canada. *J Vet Diagn Invest* 24: 777–780.

45 Meier, W.A., Meinkoth, J.H., Brunker, J. et al. (2006). Cytologic identification of immature endospores in a dog with rhinosporidiosis. *Vet Clin Pathol* 35: 348–352.

46 Marugan-Hernandez, V. (2017). *Neospora caninum* and bovine neosporosis: current vaccine research. *J Comp Pathol* 157: 193–200.

47 Dubey, J.P., Barr, B.C., Barta, J.R. et al. (2002). Redescription of *Neospora caninum* and its differentiation from related coccidia. *Int J Parasitol* 32: 929–946.

48 Bisby, T.M., Holman, P.J., Pitoc, G.A. et al. (2010). *Sarcocystis* sp. encephalomyelitis in a cat. *Vet Clin Pathol* 39: 105–112.

49 Esch, K.J. and Petersen, C.A. (2013). Transmission and epidemiology of zoonotic protozoal diseases of companion animals. *Clin Microbiol Rev* 26: 58–85.

50 Boggiatto, P.M., Gibson-Corley, K.N., Metz, K. et al. (2011). Transplacental transmission of *Leishmania infantum* as a means for continued disease incidence in North America. *PLoS Negl Trop Dis* 5: e1019.

51 Meinkoth, J., Kocan, A.A., Whitworth, L. et al. (2000). Cats surviving natural infection with *Cytauxzoon felis*: 18 cases (1997–1998). *J Vet Intern Med* 14: 521–525.

52 Birkenheuer, A.J., Marr, H., Alleman, A.R. et al. (2006). Development and evaluation of a PCR assay for the detection of *Cytauxzoon felis* DNA in feline blood samples. *Vet Parasitol* 137: 144–149.

53 Cohn, L.A. and Birkenheuer, A.J. (2012). Cytauxzoonosis. In: *Infectious Diseases of the Dog and Cat* (ed. C.E. Greene), 764–771. St. Louis, MO: Elsevier.

54 Meinkoth, J.H. and Kocan, A.A. (2005). *Feline cytauxzoonosis. Vet Clin North Am Sm Anim Pract* 35: 89–101, vi.

55 Ferris, D.H. (1979). A progress report on the status of a new disease of American cats: cytauxzoonosis. *Comp Immunol Microbiol Infect Dis* 1: 269–276.

56 Broussard, J.D. (2003). Optimal fecal assessment. *Clin Tech Small Anim Pract* 18: 218–230.

57 Cleveland, C.A., Garrett, K.B., Cozad, R.A. et al. (2018). The wild world of Guinea Worms: a review of the genus. *Int J Parasitol Parasites Wildl* 7: 289–300.

58 Bulla, C. and Thomas, J.S. (2009). What is your diagnosis? Subcutaneous mass fluid from a febrile dog. *Vet Clin Pathol* 38: 403–405.

59 Tung, K.C., Cheng, F.P., Lai, C.H. et al. (2004). Demonstration of vector competence of *Culex quinquefasciatus* (Diptera: Culicidae) for *Setaria digitata*. *Vet Parasitol* 123: 279–284.

60 Tung, K.C., Lai, C.H., Ooi, H.K. et al. (2003). Cerebrospinal setariosis with *Setaria marshalli* and *Setaria digitata* infection in cattle. *J Vet Med Sci* 65: 977–983.

61 Shin, S.S., Cho, K.O., and Wee, S.H. (2002). Ocular infection of cattle with *Setaria digitata*. *J Vet Med Sci* 64: 7–10.

62 Shin, J., Ahn, K.S., Suh, G.H. et al. (2017). First blindness cases of horses infected with *Setaria Digitata* (Nematoda: Filarioidea) in the Republic of Korea. *Korean J Parasitol* 55: 667–671.

63 Zanzani, S., Piseddu, E., Barelli, A., and Manfredi, M.T. (2014). What is your diagnosis? CBC and blood film from an Italian thoroughbred gelding. *Microfilaremia Vet Clin Pathol* 43: 609–610.

4

Evidence-Based Cytology

Laura Adhikari

What Is Evidence-Based Medicine?

Healthcare providers are entrusted with the task of easing the pain and suffering of their patients. Most who chose to pursue a career in healthcare welcome this charge with open arms and view it as a privilege. However, the goal is not just to provide any care, but, in modern medicine, it is to provide the *best and most efficient care*. Healthcare providers are acutely aware of the dynamic nature of their profession and are consistently striving for deeper knowledge and understanding of physiology and care delivery and, thus, constantly seeking process improvement to provide this best and efficient care. One important way to do so is by adopting an evidence-based approach. This approach, which is termed evidence-based medicine (EBM), is an intentional, judicious, and rational perspective on the practice of medicine that is guided by modern and best evidence. As physicians strive to provide quality and effective care within the most current realm of available knowledge, their practice becomes much more than just healing, but it morphs into *sustainable* healing backed by evidence without overusing resources. The practice of EBM can be informed by an array of methods, ranging from exchanging ideas with fellow care providers to combing through journals and electronic databases. However, it is important to keep in mind that some resources are more credible than others.

History of Evidence-Based Medicine

In the mid to late twentieth century, the focus on healthcare and its delivery shifted from traditional practice and expert witnesses to a new approach based on research and evidence. The establishments of Cochrane collaboration based on the works of Archie Cochrane and clinical learning strategy developed by McMaster Medical School in England in 1970s paved the way, so to speak, for evidence-based care.[1] The driving forces behind the implementation of evidence-based practice are the need for highest quality care, role expansion, focus on cost containment, and the demand for improved healthcare delivery. In the United States, there was a significant focus on improvement in healthcare delivery during the 1970s, which sparked considerable interest in research and evidence-based care.[2] This momentum led to the establishment of the National Institute of Health to make clinical decisions. During that time, physicians learned to recognize the variation in the patient population based on their beliefs, socioeconomic status, values, and goals. At the same time, physicians also began to appreciate different areas of expertise among care providers. Often, those important aspects were disconnected that led to a patient not getting expert care because a care provider failed to pay attention to the patient variation. For example, in fee-for-service systems, such as veterinary medicine, these social aspects can have a huge impact on the application of new clinical practice if only a small population of owners can afford to pay for the care regardless of its effectiveness. In addition, if care providers are to prescribe treatment options that contradict with the patient's cultural or societal beliefs, the patient is less likely to follow the treatment plan. Thus care options have to be tailored based on the entire patient.

In its modern form, EBM (or evidence-based practice) seeks to bridge the gap between the diverse expertise of care providers and their patients using the best research evidence so as to maximize patient care. The motivation behind this process is to address questions such as: "What have others done in similar situations?" "What was the outcome?" "What evidence do we have that has led us to believe that our interventions will be fruitful?" Specifically, the approach is defined as "the conscientious, explicit, and judicious use of current best evidence in making decisions about the care of individual patients".[3] These questions are the cornerstones of EBM, which is, in essence, a process of utilizing research evidence to guide clinical practice. EBM

Veterinary Cytology, First Edition. Edited by Leslie C. Sharkey, M. Judith Radin, and Davis Seelig.

has evolved clinical practice over time, and the current standards of practice are built upon the foundation and principles of EBM.

Defining Evidence-Based Cytology

As is the case with EBM, evidence-based cytology (EBC) can be best defined by its goal, which is to generate "a reproducible, high quality and clinically relevant test result in the field of cytology."[4] This test result, which traditionally represents the final diagnosis, should, if developed in an EBC-based system, best explain the available diagnostic findings when those findings are evaluated through the most appropriate diagnostic algorithm(s).[5] It is the design and refinement of these diagnostic algorithms that form the foundation of EBC. The components of an EBC-based diagnostic algorithm include (i) objective evidence from well-designed, peer-reviewed studies, (ii) transparent rationale linking the evidence to the diagnostic algorithm (i.e. should be easily understood by those using the algorithm), and (iii) periodic updating. From a practical perspective, EBC should seek to determine (i) the reliability by which a particular morphologic feature can be identified and (ii) the relevance of that (and other) morphologic feature(s) on the clinical progression of a particular patient population.[4]

Notably, the incorporation of evidence-based guidelines into cytology does not seek to eliminate pathologist experience (e.g. anecdotal evidence) as a component of the diagnostic algorithm but rather seeks to determine how that experience can be weighted to achieve the most accurate final diagnosis. The remainder of this chapter will focus on the role, including types and origin, of evidence in EBC and how that evidence can be identified.

Examples of Evidence-Based Cytology

In cytology, the gold standard remains in the histopathology. The level of certainty in any diagnosis is grounded in the experience and training of the practitioner and, when available, their use and understanding of published guidelines. In the practice of cytology, there have been several areas including thyroid, uterine cervix, pancreas, urine, and salivary gland, in which these guidelines have been written. The publishing of guidelines can be attained in many different ways. In infancy, some guidelines are opinion based in which a single researcher or a group publishes an experience with any given tissue. These guidelines become refined when more data is available for review, which then becomes consensus based. Over time, additional experiences and epidemiological studies are collected to refine, modify, or correct prior recommended guidelines by a group of individuals considered to be experts in their field. For example, sample adequacy for thyroid cytology was first proposed by Goellner et al. in 1987 with an institutional experience guided by the retrospective review of 6300 biopsies.[6] This initial work was modified by subsequent publications from Sidawy et al.[7] and Baloch et al.[8] and ultimately resulted in the development of *The Bethesda System for Reporting Thyroid Cytopathology* in 2009.[9]

Diagnostic Reproducibility

As noted above, a key component of EBC is professional self-assessment. Namely, pathologists must be aware of how reliable they (and their profession) are at all facets of their discipline. This includes the identification of specific morphologic features (e.g. mitotic figures, infectious agents, or criteria of malignancy) and how those features are used to generate a specific diagnosis. If a particular feature cannot be reliably identified or a particular diagnostic interpretation cannot be reliably made by a group of pathologists, then its utility is significantly limited. This self-assessment also extends to the final diagnosis. That is, how reliable are pathologists at the assigning the same diagnosis to a particular set of samples? What is the reproducibility of a particular diagnosis when applied to a representative set of samples by a representative group of pathologists? The answer to these questions is addressed by intra- and interobserver variability studies. While this approach is common, it is important to note that these studies have shortcomings. As well stated by Fleming in a 1996 editorial, many interobserver variation studies involve "small numbers of pathologists...usually devoting unusual attention to the material examined. This implies that the observer variation in the general community is likely to be significantly worse...."[10]

In veterinary cytopathology, there are small numbers of studies that address the issue of diagnostic reproducibility. Across reproducibility studies, the degree of agreement is commonly presented as a kappa score or kappa statistic. In this approach, an agreement is presented as a quantitative and qualitative value and can range from −1 to +1, where 0 represents the degree of agreement that occurs from random chance only and +1 represents perfect agreement. Although there is no standardized score for the interpretation of the kappa value, one recent publication on the use of kappa in healthcare suggests the following: 0–0.20 (no agreement), 0.21–0.39 (minimal), 0.40–0.59 (weak), 0.60–0.79 (moderate), 0.80–0.90 (strong), and >0.90 (almost perfect).[11] In a study examining the accuracy of cytology in differentiating adrenal cortical tumors from adrenal medulla tumors in dogs and cats, Bertazzolo et al. report a high degree of agreement (kappa = 0.95) between four cytopathologists with varying levels of diagnostic training and experience, including three board-certified clinical pathologists and one resident in clinical pathology.[12] In a second study, Perazzi et al. report fair to perfect interobserver agreement between two cytopathologists across nine descriptive categories in the cytologic assessment of canine superficial ocular samples.[13] Finally, in the evaluation of canine splenic fine-needle aspiration samples, LeBlanc et al., report partial to complete agreement (not using a kappa score) in the evaluation of the quality of canine splenic cytology samples between two cytopathologists.[14]

The Evidence in Evidence-Based Cytology

Levels of Evidence in EBC

The clinical observations from an experienced pathologist handed down to an apprentice represent one form of evidence-based practice. However, although valuable, these observations (i.e. anecdotal evidence) are rarely ever published and may or may not withstand the scrutiny of peer criticism and can ultimately lead to patient harm. That is why the use of literature and its application can help improve patient outcomes when applied to everyday practice. In the literature, there is a hierarchy of EBM in which study designs can propose a more solid foundation of clinical evidence. Case reports followed by case series help introduce new ideas and interesting findings to the general practice that can be further investigated by retrospective reviews to include a larger population of patients. These studies are often limited due to unforeseen bias created by the author(s) in patient selection and outcome. Ideally, evidence-based physicians are guided by a larger meta-analysis of the available clinical literature. However, one must also realize that the best evidence may never be sufficient to replace clinical decision making. Rather, the incorporation of an individual clinical patient into a general model of the disease (whether it is diagnosis or treatment of the disease) defines the "art" of medicine.[5] As a clinical decision maker, it is important to weigh benefits, risks, resources, and patient values when choosing a treatment modality.

Identification of Evidence in EBC

Seeking evidence, although a relatively simple quest, could become an exhausting exercise. While the inclination is to comb through textbooks in search of answers, they often fall short in today's ever-evolving scientific landscape (i.e. the publication lag).[15–17] At the same time, the online landscape is littered with information that one must become cautious in blindly accepting. Therefore, it is crucial to carefully scrutinize the resources while looking for the major aspects of credible sources. For the purpose of the rest of the chapter, the author will refer to the internet-based publications. For instance, when performing an evidence-based search, the publishing website is one of the first clues as to whether or not the material is trustworthy. Nonprofit, government, and well-acclaimed scientific websites are considered superior over other. Organizations such as Cochrane review, National Institute of Health and Human Services, and Centers for Medicare and Medicare Services are some of the reliable sources where credible information can be obtained. Among research publications, peer-reviewed publications undergo additional scrutiny by experts and are desirable. Research studies that have undergone Institutional Review Board (IRB) approval process are usually preferred to others. It is essential to venture beyond the textbooks and look at real-life examples including case studies, quality research publications, and systematic reviews along with expert consult before making a decision.

Identification of Credible Sources

Finding a reliable source can be an exhausting endeavor. The first step in finding an answer is to identify a problem and formulate a concise and logical question. Robust scientific databases include, but are not limited to, PubMed, Cochrane Database of Systematic Reviews, Academic Search Complete, Update, and Google Scholar. All of these databases are constantly monitored and are committed to publishing credible researches. Most of these databases are free and can be accessed via hospital, library, and other educational institutions' networks. The third step is to conduct a search of most recent publications on the desired topic with desired limiters such as peer-reviewed articles to capture the most up-to-date publications. A similar approach can be employed to conduct a search on government websites. Finally, once the research publications are retrieved, it is essential to scrutinize them for validity, conflict of interest, adaptability, and transferability.

Vetting the Evidence

As noted above, the Internet is flooded with a whole host of "research publications" that makes sifting through each and every one of them to isolate the credible publications impossible. Determining the essential components of a proper paper is one of the easiest ways to identify them besides reading the entire paper. The components of a proper paper include relevance, a thorough literature review, a properly formulated research question, fitting scientific methodology, appropriate sample size, valid statistical analysis, internal as well as external validity, transferability, credible authors, and full disclosure of any conflict of interest.

Relevance refers to the theoretical as well as the practical need for the research. A relevant research study must either add to the existing body of knowledge or expand its applications to enhance the quality of care. A complete literature review is the backbone of an investigation. Redundant research without a clear appreciation for existing knowledge and applications rarely advances the field in which that research is conducted. Hence, every proper paper must include a succinct overview of what is currently known and how the research adds to the growing body of knowledge. Scientific methodology defines the logical progression of how the research was carried out. It includes the IRB approval process, participant recruitment process, sample collection, and data collection process. Ideally, the study should contain a sufficient number of samples that have been collected to avoid statistical errors and add to its validity. The research data must be thoroughly scrutinized using proper scientific analysis. Different types of data require different modes of statistical analysis to analyze them appropriately. The author encourages the readers to refer to statistical analysis textbooks to familiarize themselves with the various options for statistical analysis. Sound methodology and well-suited scientific analysis enhance the validity of a proper paper.

Finally, the research must be transferable. That is, the results must be applied to the relevant discipline. Transferability goes farther than reproducibility. Reproducibility, although a critical component of proper research, applies to be able to reproduce the results while following a similar research methodology. Reproducibility alone may or may not necessarily enhance its application. Hence, the findings of a proper paper must be transferable and applicable to its relevant audience. The researches must possess adequate knowledge to be able to transfer to others and contribute to the discipline. The authors must, also, disclose any existing or potential conflict of interest in the paper. It is part of the ethical standard that is held high in the scientific community. Once a proper research is conducted and a paper to, it should be presented to the scientific community for due scrutiny.

Application of Evidence in EBC

One of the key components of EBC is that its adoption is transparent. That is, the users of an EBC-based diagnostic algorithm should have access to the material(s) used in its crafting. This approach allows for continued scrutiny of the algorithm and its incremental improvement. To this end, the construction of an evidence archive, preferably Internet based, is another important aspect of providing EBC. Such a database should allow users to quickly isolate relevant findings and encourages constant assessment of the algorithm. We must become critical thinkers not only to appreciate the research but also to appraise it and discover the ways to incorporate the research findings in our practice.

Final Outcome

Following the identification and appraisal of credible research, the building of an accessible database, we need to create a set of guidelines. It is referred to as the best practice guidelines. Best practice guidelines originate from the most current body of knowledge, based on sound research findings, and are accepted by the authorities in the field as standards. These guidelines are designed to help steer the decision-making process. Best practice guidelines, although a valuable tool, is not free of limitations. The readers must realize that these are guidelines and each situation must be examined individually in order to make the appropriate decision, similar to the story presented above. These guidelines are not absolute and should not be viewed as the end all and be all. On the contrary, these are guidelines that any reasonable clinician would accept as a logical way to make a decision.

References

1 Stavrou, A., Challoumas, D., and Dimitrakakis, G. (2014). Archibald Cochrane (1909-1988): the father of evidence-based medicine. *Interact Cardiovasc Thorac Surg* 18: 121–124.

2 Guyatt, G.H., Sackett, D.L., and Cook, D.J. (1993). Users' guides to the medical literature. II. How to use an article about therapy or prevention. A. Are the results of the study valid? Evidence-Based Medicine Working Group. *JAMA* 270: 2598–2601.

3 Sackett, D.L., Rosenberg, W.M., Gray, J.A. et al. (1996). Evidence based medicine: what it is and what it isn't. *BMJ* 312: 71–72.

4 Dey, P. (2007). Time for evidence-based cytology. *Cytojournal* 4: 1.

5 Costa, J. (2007). Reflections about evidence-based pathology. *Int J Surg Pathol* 15: 230–232.

6 Goellner, J.R., Gharib, H., Grant, C.S., and Johnson, D.A. (1987). Fine needle aspiration cytology of the thyroid, 1980 to 1986. *Acta Cytol* 31: 587–590.

7 Sidawy, M.K., Del Vecchio, D.M., and Knoll, S.M. (1997). Fine-needle aspiration of thyroid nodules: correlation between cytology and histology and evaluation of discrepant cases. *Cancer* 81: 253–259.

8 Baloch, Z.W., Fleisher, S., LiVolsi, V.A., and Gupta, P.K. (2002). Diagnosis of "follicular neoplasm": a gray zone in thyroid fine-needle aspiration cytology. *Diagn Cytopathol* 26: 41–44.

9 Cibas, E.S. and Ali, S.Z. (2009). NCITFSotS Conference. The Bethesda System for reporting thyroid cytopathology. *Am J Clin Pathol* 132: 658–665.

10 Fleming, K.A. (1996). Evidence-based pathology. *J Pathol* 179: 127–128.

11 McHugh, M.L. (2012). Interrater reliability: the kappa statistic. *Biochem Med (Zagreb)* 22: 276–282.

12 Bertazzolo, W., Didier, M., Gelain, M.E. et al. (2014). Accuracy of cytology in distinguishing adrenocortical tumors from pheochromocytoma in companion animals. *Vet Clin Pathol* 43: 453–459.

13 Perazzi, A., Bonsembiante, F., Gelain, M.E. et al. (2017). Cytology of the healthy canine and feline ocular surface: comparison between cytobrush and impression technique. *Vet Clin Pathol* 46: 164–171.

14 Leblanc, C.J., Head, L.L., and Fry, M.M. (2009). Comparison of aspiration and nonaspiration techniques for obtaining cytologic samples from the canine and feline spleen. *Vet Clin Pathol* 38: 242–246.

15 Booth, A. (1999). Mapping the evidence base of pathology. *J Pathol* 188: 344–350.

16 McAlister, F.A., Straus, S.E., Guyatt, G.H., and Haynes, R.B. (2000). Users' guides to the medical literature: XX. Integrating research evidence with the care of the individual patient. Evidence-Based Medicine Working Group. *JAMA* 283: 2829–2836.

17 Friedland, D. (2014). Evidence-based medicine: a framework for emotional regulation, intuition, and conscious engagement. *Glob Adv Health Med* 3: 3–4.

5

General Approach to Diagnostic Cytology

Jed Overmann

Assessment of Sample Adequacy and Quality

Regardless of sample type, there are some general components involved in assessment of the sample and arriving at a diagnosis or interpretation.[1,2] The first step in evaluating cytologic specimens is to assess sample adequacy and quality. Although the specific features will vary across diagnoses, a diagnostically adequate sample will contain a sufficient number of intact and well-stained cells that represent the underlying process. The assessment of adequacy is typically subjective and initially seeks to characterize if sufficient sample (most often intact cells) is present for interpretation. A more quantitative approach to assessing sample adequacy and quality and its effect on diagnosis has been described as in the case of endoscopic sampling of the gastrointestinal tract in dogs and cats.[3] For cytopathologists working in referral hospitals or academic institutions, the timely assessment of sample adequacy may be unique and offer opportunities for resampling. In these settings, the cytopathologist may be located near where sampling is taking place (e.g. especially image-assisted sampling). This approach toward the immediate assessment of the diagnostic adequacy of a cytology sample is known as ROSE (rapid on-site evaluation). ROSE has been evaluated in human medicine across a variety of tissues and lesions in terms of its economic impacts and effects on sample adequacy and has repeatedly been shown to increase the diagnostic adequacy rate regardless of sampling site.[4–7] The diagnostic utility and financial effects of implementing ROSE in veterinary medicine have yet to be described.

The failure to obtain a diagnostic quality sample can result from the inadvertent aspiration of elements that are not representative of the mass. As such, it is important to consider the gross and/or imaging appearance of a lesion when determining sample adequacy. For example, large tumors can have areas of inflammation, necrosis, fibrosis, or cyst formation, and limited sampling can result in an incomplete or misleading interpretation. For lesions that are large, and especially those with a heterogeneous appearance, sampling from multiple areas of the lesion is ideal. Further information on the best practices of sample collection is available in Chapter 1. Irrespective of the approach, a diagnostic cytopathology report should contain some description of overall quality or cellularity.

Cytologic Interpretation

Once a sample is determined to be of diagnostic quality, the initial approach is to characterize the findings as normal or a combination of one or more of the following categories: hyperplasia, inflammation, neoplasia (benign vs. malignant), or other (e.g. hemorrhage, necrosis, etc.). Familiarity with normal findings for a given tissue is essential in recognizing pathologic or physiologic alterations.

Hyperplasia

Hyperplasia is defined by the enlargement of an organ or tissue by an increased number of otherwise normal cells. Hyperplastic tissue consists of cells that microscopically resemble those from normal tissue. Samples from hyperplastic tissues can be of increased cellularity and can also display minor cytomorphologic changes. For example, mild cytomorphologic alterations, including variation in cytoplasmic volume and cytoplasmic staining properties, have been described for benign prostatic hyperplasia in dogs, conjunctival hyperplasia in cats, and goiterous thyroid nodules in people.[1,2,8]. Establishing a cytologic interpretation of hyperplasia is aided by physical exam or imaging results demonstrating a mass, nodular lesion, or symmetrical tissue enlargement. However, because of the morphologic overlap between them, cytologically

Veterinary Cytology, First Edition. Edited by Leslie C. Sharkey, M. Judith Radin, and Davis Seelig.

distinguishing hyperplastic tissue from a well-differentiated neoplastic process can be difficult in some instances (e.g. differentiating a hyperplastic liver nodule from a well-differentiated hepatocellular tumor).[9,10] Owing to these difficulties, the provision of a complete patient history including imaging findings is needed to prioritize otherwise morphologically similar cytologic differentials.

Inflammation

Inflammatory processes are categorized based on the predominant cell type or types. This allows for prioritization of an underlying process if one is not clearly evident. Inflammatory processes are typically categorized as neutrophilic, eosinophilic, pyogranulomatous or mixed, granulomatous, and lymphocytic/lymphoplasmacytic. It is noteworthy that, with rare exceptions, there are no defined numerical thresholds for the morphologic characterization of inflammatory processes.

Neutrophilic Inflammation

Neutrophilic inflammation, which is cytologically defined according to tissue-specific guidelines, can result from a number of etiologies such as bacterial, fungal, or protozoal infection, autoimmune disease, and neoplasia. To provide some etiologic insights, neutrophils in cytologic specimens are assessed for morphologic changes and described as non-degenerate or degenerate. Non-degenerate neutrophils appear similar to peripheral blood neutrophils. In contrast, degenerate neutrophils have swollen, pale-staining nuclei (termed karyolysis). Degenerate neutrophils are described to be the result of a toxic local environment that is commonly due to bacterial infection (especially Gram-negative endotoxin-producing organisms). Karyolysis is the result of failure of the cell to maintain water balance in addition to the direct action of endonucleases. While identification of large numbers of degenerate neutrophils suggests the possibility of a septic process (most often bacteria), it should be noted that degenerate neutrophils can be present in non-septic lesions and non-degenerate neutrophils can predominate in some septic lesions. Condensed, dark-staining nuclei (pyknosis) with fragmentation of the nuclear material (karyorrhexis) also can be seen in neutrophils from inflammatory lesions. Condensation of nuclear material along with vacuolization of cytoplasm are morphologic features of apoptotic neutrophils.[11] Functionally, apoptosis of neutrophils prevents the release of damaging neutrophil contents and promotes removal of these cells by macrophages, whereas necrosis of neutrophils can compound local inflammation and tissue damage.

Eosinophilic Inflammation

Primary considerations for eosinophilic inflammation include allergic or hypersensitivity reactions, parasitism, paraneoplastic syndromes (especially mast cell tumor), idiopathic eosinophilic conditions, and some fungal infections. While eosinophils can be the predominant inflammatory cell in some of these lesions, eosinophilic inflammation should be considered when >10% eosinophils are present. Eosinophils are generally identified by their characteristic granules on Romanowsky-type stains, though eosinophils with nonstaining granules (i.e. "vacuolated" or gray eosinophils) have been described in Greyhounds, other sighthounds, and occasional Golden Retrievers.[12,13]

Histiocytic Inflammation

Histiocytic or macrophagic inflammation and granulomatous inflammation are characterized cytologically by a predominance of macrophages. While the number of macrophages needed to diagnose this pattern of inflammation is not fully defined, additional cytologic features (regardless of numbers) can be used to support this diagnosis. Macrophages can be variably vacuolated and contain phagocytosed debris or organisms. In the case of granulomatous inflammation, epithelioid macrophages (i.e. macrophages with often polygonal cell borders and/or found in "epithelial-like" aggregates) and/or multinucleate forms may be evident. Macrophages can predominate in fungal infections, foreign body responses, *Mycobacterium* spp. infections, and inflammation associated with calcinosis circumscripta, cellulitis, or panniculitis (Chapters 3, 11, and 12).

Mixed or Pyogranulomatous Inflammation

Mixed or pyogranulomatous inflammation is characterized by significant numbers of both macrophages and neutrophils with smaller numbers of lymphocytes and plasma cells. Causes of pyogranulomatous inflammation include fungal infections, foreign body responses, *Mycobacterium* spp. infections, *Actinomyces* or *Nocardia* spp. infections, or chronic tissue trauma/inflammation. With either pyogranulomatous or histiocytic inflammatory lesions, additional staining such as Gram stain or acid-fast stain could be considered to help ensure small numbers of organisms are not missed during evaluation.

Lymphocytic and Lymphoplasmacytic Inflammation

Lymphocytic and lymphoplasmacytic (or mononuclear) inflammation can result from many immune reactions (e.g. vaccine reactions, lymphocytic inflammation associated with canine histiocytoma), allergic disease, and some viral infections. Lymphocytes and plasma cells can also be seen along with a variety of other inflammatory cell types in chronic inflammatory lesions. As there may be significant concern for a lymphoid neoplasm in samples demonstrating notable lymphocytic inflammation, further diagnostic assessment may be indicated (Chapter 27).

Neoplasia

When neoplasia is cytologically suspected, sample characteristics and cytomorphologic features can often allow placement of the tumor type into one of four general categories: round cell tumor, epithelial tumor, mesenchymal cell tumor, and naked nuclei tumor. Melanoma is often considered separately as it can mimic characteristics of multiple categories. General characteristics of the four major categories are summarized in Table 5.1. While this scheme helps to narrow interpretation, identification of a specific tumor type (e.g. mast cell tumor, sebaceous adenoma, etc.), when possible, is ideal. The reliability of this approach was demonstrated in a cytology/histopathology correlation study of cutaneous and subcutaneous masses from dogs and cats. In this study, cytology correctly categorized 175 out of 175 true positive cytologic diagnoses of neoplasia as mesenchymal tumor, round cell tumor, epithelial tumor, or melanoma.[14] In this same study, cytologic diagnosis of a specific tumor type (e.g. mast cell tumor, squamous cell carcinoma, hemangiopericytoma) was most likely with round cell tumors compared with epithelial or mesenchymal cell tumors. Exceptions to this approach certainly exist. For example, certain epithelial tumors such as squamous cell carcinomas can have relatively little cell cohesion and clustering, some carcinomas such as renal carcinoma or nasal adenocarcinoma can have a "round cell tumor" appearance, and some aspirates from mesenchymal cell tumors can be very cellular.

Criteria of Malignancy

Once a diagnosis of neoplasia is established, assessment for cytologic criteria of malignancy is performed to differentiate benign versus malignant tumors. A summary of some of the general cytologic criteria of malignancy is presented in Table 5.2. This assessment must be performed with knowledge of the known cytologic profile of the tumor type under consideration. While the characterization of criteria of malignancy is typically subjective, computer-assisted evaluation of some of these features (e.g. computer-assisted nuclear morphometry of canine mammary gland tumors) has been described for some types of

Table 5.2 General cytologic criteria of malignancy.

Hypercellularity
Anisocytosis
Macrocytosis
Anisokaryosis
Irregular nuclear fragments
Abnormal multinucleation
Nuclear molding
Large, multiple, or irregularly shaped prominent nucleoli
Abnormal or variable nuclear to cytoplasmic ratios
Increased mitotic figures (especially when atypical)

Table 5.1 General cytologic characteristics of the major categories of tumors.

Round cell tumors	Epithelial tumors
High cellularity Discrete cells Intact, well-defined cell margins Round nuclei **Examples:** lymphoma, histiocytoma, transmissible venereal tumor, plasmacytoma, mast cell tumor	High cellularity Evidence of clustering or cellular cohesion Visible cell junctions Intact, well-defined cell margins Round to oval nuclei Evidence of glandular origin (e.g. acinar structures, secretory material) **Examples:** sebaceous adenoma, perianal adenoma, squamous cell carcinoma, hepatocellular carcinoma
Mesenchymal cell tumors	**Naked nuclei tumors**
Lower cellularity Individualized or in aggregates Spindloid to plump cells with less distinct cell margins Round to oval nuclei Extracellular matrix **Examples:** fibrosarcoma, hemangiosarcoma, osteosarcoma	High cellularity Disrupted cellular margins Many free nuclei on ruptured cytoplasmic contents Sometimes small numbers of intact round to polygonal cells Round nuclei **Examples:** insulinoma, chemodectoma, carcinoids, anal sac adenocarcinoma

neoplasia.[15] Nuclear and nucleolar changes tend to be stronger cytologic criteria of malignancy, and the presence of multiple criteria also increases suspicion of malignancy. As previously stated, the interpretive thresholds for criteria of malignancy are variable based on the tissue of origin or suspected tumor type. For example, canine transitional cell carcinomas (Chapter 38) generally have marked and multiple cytologic criteria of malignancy, whereas canine thyroid adenocarcinomas (Chapter 45), and many neuroendocrine malignancies, often have relatively mild criteria of malignancy.

For some types of neoplasia, cytologic features beyond the general criteria of malignancy may be useful for interpretation. For example, hepatocyte dissociation, acinar or palisading hepatocyte arrangements, and the presence of naked nuclei and capillaries were described in well-differentiated canine hepatocellular carcinomas.[9] Assessment of criteria of malignancy is ultimately done with the goal of providing the clinician with accurate information regarding the prognosis and potential behavior of a neoplastic process. This is clearly illustrated in the recent efforts to identify criteria that may be useful in the cytologic grading of canine mast cell tumors.[16,17]

Hemorrhage, Cystic Fluid, and Necrosis

Other processes that can be identified cytologically are hemorrhage, cystic fluid, and necrosis. Hemorrhage can result from a number of causes including trauma, inflammation, neoplasia, and coagulopathies. The cytologic appearance of hemorrhagic lesions can vary with time course. In peracute hemorrhage, RBCs may predominate with minimal erythrophagocytosis and lack of RBC breakdown products. However, it is important to note that *in vitro* erythrophagocytosis by macrophages can begin within minutes, though this process may take longer within some hemorrhagic lesions.[18] Degradation of heme from phagocytosed RBCs within macrophages results in release of iron and formation of hemosiderin. Hemosiderin can be seen within macrophages or extracellularly, and the color can vary from blue to black (most common), but can be yellow, gold, or green on Wright Giemsa-stained samples.[19] Prussian blue stain can be used to confirm iron content and help differentiate hemosiderin from other dark pigments, including bile and lipofuscin. Studies from animals and humans have shown the first appearance of hemosiderin at 33 hours to 7 days following clinical or experimental hemorrhage.[20–22] Hematoidin crystals can also be seen in areas of previous hemorrhage. Hematoidin is a crystalline, golden-amber material that forms in areas of low oxygen tension as a heme breakdown product after removal of iron from the heme molecule. Hematoidin often appears as a rhomboid shaped crystal, but can also be seen in needlelike forms.[19] Further information on the cytologic appearance of hemorrhage is available in Chapters 50 and 52.

Cystic fluid most often consists of a low cellularity, proteinaceous appearing (i.e. pale blue/pink-staining and sometimes bubbly background) sample. Foamy macrophages often predominate, and minimal evidence of hemorrhage can also be seen in some lesions. Fluid-filled cystic structure can be associated with benign and malignant lesions. Necrosis is most often recognized cytologically as amorphous basophilic debris/material. Necrosis of cells and tissue can be associated with a variety of processes including tissue trauma, inflammation, and benign and malignant tumors.

References

1 Raskin, R. and Meyer, D.J. (2016). *Canine and Feline Cytology: A Color Atlas and Interpretation Guide*, 3e. St. Louis, MO: Elsevier.

2 Cowell, R.L. and Valenciano, A.C. (2014). *Cowell and Tyler's Diagnostic Cytology and Hematology of the Dog and Cat*, 4e. St. Louis, MO: Elsevier.

3 Jergens, A.E., Andreasen, C.B., Hagemoser, W.A. et al. (1998). Cytologic examination of exfoliative specimens obtained during endoscopy for diagnosis of gastrointestinal tract disease in dogs and cats. *J Am Vet Med Assoc* 213: 1755–1759.

4 Nasuti, J.F., Gupta, P.K., and Baloch, Z.W. (2002). Diagnostic value and cost-effectiveness of on-site evaluation of fine-needle aspiration specimens: review of 5,688 cases. *Diagn Cytopathol* 27: 1–4.

5 Burgess, C., Dias, L., Maughan, E., and Moorthy, R. (2013). Neck lump clinics: is on-site assessment of fine needle aspirate diagnostic adequacy cost-effective? *J Laryngol Otol* 127: 1122–1126.

6 Witt, B.L. and Schmidt, R.L. (2013). Rapid onsite evaluation improves the adequacy of fine-needle aspiration for thyroid lesions: a systematic review and meta-analysis. *Thyroid* 23: 428–435.

7 Iglesias-Garcia, J., Larino-Noia, J., Abdulkader, I., and Domínguez-Muñoz, J.E. (2014). Rapid on-site evaluation of endoscopic-ultrasound-guided fine-needle aspiration

diagnosis of pancreatic masses. *World J Gastroenterol* 20: 9451–9457.

8 Layfield, L.J., Wax, T., and Jones, C. (2003). Cytologic distinction of goiterous nodules from morphologically normal thyroid: analyses of cytomorphologic features. *Cancer* 99: 217–222.

9 Masserdotti, C. and Drigo, M. (2012). Retrospective study of cytologic features of well-differentiated hepatocellular carcinoma in dogs. *Vet Clin Pathol* 41: 382–390.

10 Roth, L. (2001). Comparison of liver cytology and biopsy diagnoses in dogs and cats: 56 cases. *Vet Clin Pathol* 30: 35–38.

11 Quinn, M.T., Deleo, F., and Bokoch, G.M. (2007). *Neutrophil Methods and Protocols*. Totowa, NJ: Humana Press.

12 Iazbik, M.C. and Couto, C.G. (2005). Morphologic characterization of specific granules in Greyhound eosinophils. *Vet Clin Pathol* 34: 140–143.

13 Giori, L., Gironi, S., Scarpa, P. et al. (2011). Grey eosinophils in sighthounds: frequency in 3 breeds and comparison of eosinophil counts determined manually and with 2 hematology analyzers. *Vet Clin Pathol* 40: 475–483.

14 Ghisleni, G., Roccabianca, P., Ceruti, R. et al. (2006). Correlation between fine-needle aspiration cytology and histopathology in the evaluation of cutaneous and subcutaneous masses from dogs and cats. *Vet Clin Pathol* 35: 24–30.

15 Simeonov, R. and Simeonova, G. (2007). Computerized cytomorphometric analysis of nuclear area, nuclear perimeter and mean nuclear diameter in spontaneous canine mammary gland tumours. *Vet Res Commun* 31: 553–558.

16 Camus, M.S., Priest, H.L., Koehler, J.W. et al. (2016). Cytologic criteria for mast cell tumor grading in dogs with evaluation of clinical outcome. *Vet Pathol* 53: 1117–1123.

17 Scarpa, F., Sabattini, S., and Bettini, G. (2016). Cytological grading of canine cutaneous mast cell tumours. *Vet Comp Oncol* 14: 245–251.

18 Gemsa, C., Woo, C.H., Fudenberg, H.H., and Schmid, R. (1973). Erythrocyte catabolism by macrophages in vitro. The effect of hydrocortisone on erythrophagocytosis and on the induction of heme oxygenase. *J Clin Invest* 52: 812–822.

19 Radakovich, L.B. and Olver, C.S. (2017). Pigments: iron and friends. *Vet Clin North Am Small Anim Pract* 47: 17–29.

20 Sherman, J.M., Winnie, G., Thomassen, M.J. et al. (1984). Time course of hemosiderin production and clearance by human pulmonary macrophages. *Chest* 86: 409–411.

21 Epstein, C.E., Elidemir, O., Colasurdo, G.N., and Fan, L.L. (2001). Time course of hemosiderin production by alveolar macrophages in a murine model. *Chest* 120: 2013–2020.

22 Cao, S., Zheng, M., Hua, Y. et al. (2016). Hematoma changes during clot resolution after experimental intracerebral hemorrhage. *Stroke* 47: 1626–1631.

Part II

Quality Control and Special Laboratory Techniques

6

Quality Assurance in Cytology

Liron Pantanowitz

Introduction

It is important to acknowledge that all cytology tests have inherent limitations. Hence, even in the hands of an excellent veterinary pathologist, one may encounter a false-negative or false-positive cytology result. False-negative results may occur due to sampling error (e.g. lesional cells were not collected) or laboratory error (e.g. abnormal cells were missed during screening or misinterpreted as benign/reactive). An ongoing quality management program designed to monitor and evaluate the overall quality of the cytology laboratory testing process can help prevent, detect, reduce, and correct such deficiencies, ideally as quickly as possible.[1,2] The primary reason for employing a quality assurance (QA) program is to improve patient care. Another reason may include regulatory compliance. In the United States, the Clinical Laboratory Improvement Amendments of 1988 (CLIA '88) are federally mandated standards that serve as the foundation of quality programs in cytology laboratories performing testing on human samples. To obtain a CLIA certificate, a human cytology laboratory must be accredited and inspected by The Joint Commission (TJC) or the College of American Pathologists (CAP). CLIA '88 established such quality measures as rescreening, cytologic–histologic correlation, daily workload limits, and proficiency testing. Although similar federal mandates do not govern veterinary diagnostic pathology, the approach toward laboratory best practices are not unique to any one species.

In cytology, the test process includes everything from the time a specimen is collected from a patient (e.g. fine-needle aspiration) until the final report is delivered. Quality control (QC) is concerned largely with the technical quality of products (e.g. cytology slides) to make sure that they meet specified quality criteria. QA focuses more on outcome (i.e. patient care) and involves a global assessment of the entire testing process. Total quality management (TQM), or continuous quality improvement (CQI), evaluates the testing process with the intent of continuously improving all its aspects.[3] TQM requires focused data collection, measurement of performance, introduction of improvements, and, if necessary, implementation of corrective actions if the laboratory falls below an approved standard.

Additional components of a successful TQM program can include (i) participation in an accreditation program and interlaboratory comparisons, (ii) establishing indicators of quality with relevant thresholds (i.e. benchmarks), (iii) developing procedure/policy manuals for the laboratory, (iv) documenting and maintaining records of QC/QA activity, (v) engaging in peer review of difficult or borderline cases, (vi) undertaking quality audit projects, and (vii) continuing education of staff who work in the cytology laboratory. To maintain quality during the testing process, it may be necessary that all screening take place within an appropriately certified laboratory facility or an approved referral laboratory.

To perform QA activities, laboratories often need access to electronic data, typically extracted from a laboratory information system (LIS), and the capacity to analyze these data. The LIS can be leveraged to monitor the overall test process, including the pre-analytic (e.g. specimen collection), analytic (e.g. screening and diagnostic performance), and post-analytic (e.g. cytology reports) phases. Ideally, quality metrics need to be universally applicable for a variety of practice settings. The adoption of QA procedures in routine daily practice of human cytology laboratories has proven to be pivotal in their success, most notably for the Pap test that is used to screen for cervical cancer.[4–7]

While the practice of veterinary cytology may be similar in many regards to its human counterpart, there are notable differences (e.g. the patients, diseases encountered, and reimbursement models). Moreover, the workflow of cases differs between the two disciplines. Whereas typically only pathologists review cytopathology specimens in veterinary laboratories, in human cytology laboratories most cases are first screened by cytotechnologists before being forwarded

Veterinary Cytology, First Edition. Edited by Leslie C. Sharkey, M. Judith Radin, and Davis Seelig.

to a cytopathologist for final interpretation and reporting. In veterinary medicine there is also no correlate for cancer monitoring, such as occurs with the Pap smear. Nevertheless, employing a QA program in veterinary laboratories is still necessary to assure that cytology testing is performed in a safe environment and that all animals from which cytology samples are obtained receive high quality diagnoses and therefore good care. The aim of this chapter is to review the QA measures utilized in laboratories involved in performing cytology tests on humans so that, if appropriate, they can be extrapolated to veterinary practice in order to prevent and control potential errors and to benefit veterinary patients.

Quality Indicators

QA metrics can be used to monitor each phase of the cytology laboratory test cycle.[8] Specific metrics include those applied to the pre-analytic phase (e.g. evaluation of rejected and unsatisfactory specimens, the rate of mislabeled specimens, and delays in transportation), the analytic phase (e.g. cytopreparation problems, diagnosis verification, the rates of amended reports, and the re-biopsy rate), and the post-analytic phase (e.g. turnaround time [TAT], transcription errors on reports, and client satisfaction). TAT is often measured. TAT reflects the time from which a specimen is received in the laboratory to the time the final report is issued. The concept of TAT is crucial in veterinary medicine. In academic centers, same-day cytology TAT is almost a universal expectation, and it is not unusual for veterinarians to check in on their patient's result within an hour of sample submission. Clearly, timely results are important, especially in emergent cases. However, it is equally important to remember that "speed kills" because rushing through the testing process to meet clinician demand can sometimes result in missing important features or failing to thoroughly evaluate all diagnostic possibilities. One way to address this is to offer a verbal preliminary impression with a warning that the final diagnosis may differ after a more thorough evaluation of the case.

To assess diagnostic proficiency, laboratories can also monitor the frequency of their various diagnostic categories. Occasionally, rendering a definitive primary interpretation (e.g. negative or positive for malignancy) or a specific diagnosis (e.g. mast cell tumor) may not be possible, especially if there is only limited sample available, artifact, or obscuring material such as blood is present and/or performing ancillary studies is not possible. Such cases may instead be reported as being "atypical" or only "suspicious" for a lesion. It may be valuable to monitor the "atypical" rate for the entire laboratory, as well as for individuals relative to each other and to the laboratory average. For Pap tests in women, human cytology laboratories monitor various ratios such as the "atypical cells of undetermined significance (ASCUS)/squamous intraepithelial lesion (SIL)" ratio and "ASCUS/human papilloma virus (HPV)" positivity rates.[9,10] These ratios serve as better benchmarks than certain individual diagnostic rates, as they often take into account the prevalence of disease in high-risk populations.

A variety of other QA processes can be adopted. These include proficiency testing and interlaboratory comparisons. Participating in peer interlaboratory programs, for both technical and interpretive components of the testing process, allows a laboratory to compare its performance to peer laboratories.[11] For Pap tests in humans, several well-established external QA programs are available around the world.[12] Some laboratories also randomly seed known abnormal cases into their routine workload, which is intended to increase screening concentration and identify those screeners with unsatisfactory performance. The Veterinary Laboratory Quality Assurance Program (VLA-QAP™, provided by the Atlantic Veterinary College, University of Prince Edward Island) is an external QA program that facilitates interlaboratory proficiency testing. This program offers testing the areas of bacteriology, chemistry, toxicology, cytology, endocrinology, hematology, histopathology, parasitology, serology, therapeutic drug monitoring, and urinalysis.

Rescreening

In human cytology laboratories, additional quality indicators of diagnostic accuracy include rescreening measures. Rescreening is the reevaluation of negative Pap tests either in real time (i.e. prospective rescreening) or using archived case material (i.e. retrospective rescreening). While this may not apply to veterinary laboratories, rescreening of Pap tests is mandated by CLIA in the United States. This includes prospective and retrospective rescreening of selected cases. Rescreening is most useful for detecting screening errors, as opposed to diagnostic errors. Prospective rescreening involves the reexamination of 10% of negatively interpreted Pap tests screened by cytotechnologists (not pathologists) prior to reporting. These cases are selected randomly or by including high-risk women based on preestablished criteria (e.g. women with a known history of a prior lesion). This allows errors in diagnosis to be corrected before a final report is issued. CLIA regulations in the United States also mandate a retrospective review of all archived negative Pap tests for the last five years (so-called 5-year look-back) from women with a new Pap test interpretation of a high-grade squamous intraepithelial lesion or cancer. If a significant discrepancy is found that could impact current patient care, the clinician is notified and an amended report is issued. By uncovering previously missed lesions, rescreening provides educational feedback to cytologists. In a scenario with applicability to veterinary clinical pathology, some human cytology laboratories have applied rescreening measures to nongynecologic cases in which selected cases get assigned to a second QA cytopathologist for review. This prospective peer review mechanism helps to prevent diagnostic errors and allows for corrective action prior to reporting. Not surprisingly, there is a greater likelihood of detecting an abnormality with higher rescreening intensity. However, rescreening adds to workload and thus may be challenging to undertake in large cytology laboratories involved in screening a high volume of cases with limited staff.

Cytologic–Histologic Correlation

Histologic outcome is a commonly used gold standard against which cytologic interpretations are measured. However, it is not uncommon to find cases in which the histologic diagnosis is incorrect. Monitoring cytologic–histologic correlation results is one way to flag discrepancies. Infrequently, reevaluating all case material in light of a patient's clinical findings or outcome may warrant revising a diagnosis. Some contributing causes of both incorrect cytologic and histologic diagnoses include sample bias or incorrect interpretation (e.g. well-differentiated malignancies interpreted as potential hyperplastic processes or overinterpretation of reactive conditions as neoplasia). In human cytology laboratories, cytologic–histologic correlation is conducted for both gynecologic (i.e. Pap test and cervical biopsy) and nongynecologic cases. These correlations can be performed in real time (ideal, if feasible) and/or retrospectively (e.g. three or six monthly). When identified, diagnostic discrepancies can be reviewed by the pathologist responsible for diagnosing a current tissue biopsy, by the pathologist who made the original cytology interpretation, at weekly consensus conferences, or independently by different pathologists. Nevertheless, if significant disparities exist, they need to be resolved, and, if needed, diagnostic practices may need to be altered. In addition to the direct impact on patient care, this exercise also serves as the basis for developing and refining cytologic diagnostic criteria.

Workload Limits

Some laboratories have a reputation for being "sweatshops" that generate low-quality cytology reads. Such laboratories attempt to lower costs by assigning large numbers of cases to pathologists. They may even offer financial incentives to read additional slides. One mechanism to prevent this from happening, and improve diagnostic quality, is to limit the number of cases any one individual can review. In the United States, an important component of a QA program for cytology laboratories that handle human specimens includes provisions for establishing and monitoring the maximum workload (described in terms of slides per hour) for individual cytotechnologists. Indeed, US federal law requires that cytotechnologists document the number of slides they screen within each 24 hour period and the number of hours they spend screening slides each day. This includes gynecologic and nongynecologic cases, as well as slides rescreened for QC purposes. For this purpose, a cellular fine-needle aspirate smear that covers more than half of the slide counts as a full slide. Slides counted as half slides include cytocentrifuge specimens (e.g. cytospins), liquid-based slides (e.g. ThinPrep), and cell block sections. Guidelines for human laboratories prohibit manually screening more than 100 conventional Pap smear slides per day. This applies not only to cytotechnologists but also to pathologists who perform primary screening. The maximum of 100 slides/24 hours is not intended as a performance target, but rather as an absolute maximum allowed by law. Higher limits are permissible when screening Pap tests that have been imaged and screened by computer systems, since the cytotechnologist reviews a smaller surface area microscopically. Available data indicate that lower screening rates are associated with higher screening sensitivities.[13,14] For this reason, evidence-based recommendations published in 2013 by the American Society of Cytopathology task force proposed that the average cytotechnologist workload should not exceed 70 slides/day for Pap tests subject to image-assisted screening.[15] The LIS can be leveraged to keep track of these metrics and, if needed, can lock out individuals once their case limits have been reached.

Miscellaneous Performance Measures

Cytology laboratories can utilize various other objective measures of an individual's "diagnostic competency." For example, screening skills can be evaluated by monitoring an individual's abnormal rate (abnormal cases/total cases) and false-negative cases. Such interpretive skills can be compared with laboratory statistics (e.g. cytotechnologist–cytopathologist discrepancy log for cases submitted to pathologists for review), as well as tracking performance on proficiency tests. Rates below the average imply that errors may be occurring (e.g. abnormal cases are being missed).

Conclusion

Several factors can affect the overall quality of a cytology diagnosis including sampling, screening, and misinterpretation. In the cytology laboratory a continuous quality management plan is therefore essential to avoid erroneous results. Achieving a high level of quality requires QA monitors to be systematically implemented for all phases of the testing process. Establishing and maintaining a sound quality management plan requires considerable time, effort, and dedicated staff. However, commitment to such a continuous program is important to instill confidence in the clients of a cytology laboratory and to ensure optimal patient care.

References

1 Frable, W.J. (2007). Error reduction and risk management in cytopathology. *Semin Diagn Pathol* 24: 77–88.

2 Cibas, E.S. (2014). Laboratory management. In: *Cytology: Diagnostic Principles and Clinical Correlates*, 4e (eds. E.S. Cibas and B.S. Ducatman), 519–546. Philadelphia, PA: Elsevier.

3 Idowu, M.O. and Nakhleh, R. (2011). Quality assurance in anatomic pathology. In: *Laboratory Administration for Pathologists* (eds. E.A. Wagar, R.E. Horowitz and G.E. Seigal), 137–150. Northfield, IL: CAP Press.

4 Mody, D.R., Davey, D.D., Branca, M. et al. (2000). Quality assurance and risk reduction guidelines. *Acta Cytol* 44: 496–507.

5 Miller, A.B. (2002). Quality assurance in screening strategies. *Virus Res* 89: 295–299.

6 Tworek, J.A., Henry, M.R., Blond, B., and Jones, B.A. (2013). College of American Pathologists gynecologic cytopathology quality consensus conference on good laboratory practices in gynecologic cytology: background, rationale, and organization. *Arch Pathol Lab Med* 137: 158–163.

7 Branca, M. and Longatto-Filho, A. (2015). Recommendations on quality control and quality assurance in cervical cytology. *Acta Cytol* 59: 361–369.

8 Clary, K.M., Davey, D.D., Naryshkin, S. et al. (2013). The role of monitoring interpretive rates, concordance between cytotechnologist and pathologist interpretations prior to sign-out, and turn-around-time in gynecologic quality assurance: findings from the College of American Pathologists gynecologic cytopathology quality consensus conference. Working group 1. *Arch Pathol Lab Med* 137: 164–174.

9 Cibas, E.S., Zou, K.H., Crum, C.P., and Kuo, F. (2008). Using the rate of positive high-risk HPV test results for ASCUS together with the ASCUS/SIL ratio in evaluating the performance of cytopathologists. *Am J Clin Pathol* 129: 97–101.

10 Renshaw, A., Deschene, M., and Auger, M. (2009). ASC/SIL ratio for cytotechnologists. A surrogate marker of screening sensitivity. *Am J Clin Pathol* 131: 776–778.

11 Eversole, G.M., Moriarty, A.T., Schwartz, M.R. et al. (2010). Practices of participants in the College of American Pathologists interlaboratory comparison program in cervicovaginal cytology. *Arch Pathol Lab Med* 134: 331–335.

12 Shield, P.W., Frost, F., Finnimore, J.L. et al. (2017). External quality assurance in nongynecologic cytology: The Australasian experience. *Cancer Cytopathol* 125: 349–361.

13 Elsheikh, T.M., Kirkpatrick, J.L., Cooper, M.K. et al. (2010). Increasing cytotechnologist workload above 100 slides per day using the ThinPrep Imaging System leads to significant reductions in screening accuracy. *Cancer Cytopathol* 118: 75–82.

14 Levi, A.W., Galullo, P., Gordy, K. et al. (2012). Increasing cytotechnologist workload above 100 slides per day using BD FocalPoint GS Imaging System negatively affects screening performance. *Am J Clin Pathol* 138: 811–815.

15 Elsheikh, T.M., Austin, R.M., Chieng, D.F. et al. (2013). American Society of Cytopathology workload recommendations for automated Pap test screening: developed by the productivity and quality assurance in the era of automated screening task force. *Diagn Cytopathol* 41: 174–178.

7

Special Staining Techniques: Application and Quality Assurance

Kelly S. Santangelo, Deanna M.W. Schaefer, Sarah E. Leavell, and Heather L. Priest

Immunocytochemical Staining

General Principles of Immunocytochemistry

Immunocytochemistry (ICC) involves the detection of specific antigens of interest in cytologic samples. As a diagnostic tool, it is typically performed on cell populations prepared as direct smears, cytospins, cell blocks, cytoscraped cell blocks, or impression smears from biopsies.[1–10] When employed in research, monolayer and suspension cultures are additional ICC options.[11] This is in contrast to immunohistochemistry (IHC), which is typically performed on formalin-fixed paraffin-embedded or frozen tissue sections. While ICC and IHC share many methodological similarities, there are important differences between the two techniques that will be highlighted below, including fixation options, storage considerations, and controls.[12]

Antibody and Antigen Interactions

ICC utilizes antibodies that target antigens characteristic of certain cells or infectious agents. Antibodies, or immunoglobulins (Ig), are "Y" shaped and consist of two identical light chains and two identical heavy chains (Figure 7.1). The most commonly used Ig for ICC is IgG, with IgM used less frequently.[13,14] Use of nontraditional antibody options, such as recombinant single-chain variable fragments[15] and single-domain antibodies,[16] may become routine, but the focus of this section will remain on the more typical antibody construct.

Polyclonal Antibodies Polyclonal antibodies (pAbs) are produced by immunizing an animal, most often a rabbit, with purified antigen.[14] The resultant antiserum is collected and includes several different antibodies to the target protein (i.e. polyclonal). Polyclonal antisera have a higher affinity and broader reactivity than monoclonal antibodies (mAbs) but lower specificity.[17] Hence, pAbs are more likely to bind to multiple epitopes of the target antigen, but there is a greater likelihood of cross-reactivity with similar epitopes in nontarget proteins, leading to false-positive results. In addition, variations in antibody titer and quality can fluctuate from lot to lot, depending on the animal(s) immunized.[18]

Monoclonal Antibodies mAbs are produced by immunizing an animal, typically a mouse, with purified antigen.[19] Specific antibody-producing B lymphocytes are then harvested from the spleen and fused with mouse myeloma cells, which create immortal hybrid cells that produce Igs specific for a single epitope. These cells form hybridomas that are screened for specificity and maintained long term. Advantages of mAbs over pAbs include higher specificity and reduced background reactivity.[12] The higher specificity of mAbs does not eliminate the possibility of cross-reactivity with other antigens due to either shared epitopes or epitopes resulting from protein cross-linking during fixation.

Advantages and Challenges

When properly executed, ICC can be a valuable tool with several advantages compared with IHC and, in certain cases, flow cytometry. As ICC is rooted in cytology, it allows for simultaneous assessment of cell morphology and organization with immunostaining. The shorter turnaround time of ICC offers the opportunity for near-bedside results, which can allow for timely (pre- and intra-procedure) diagnoses, same-day treatment planning, and rapid resampling.[20–23] Additionally, certain antibodies, such as some T-lymphocyte and histiocytic markers, are only effective in cytologic preparations and not in formalin-fixed tissue.[24] Lastly, other advantages of ICC include those intrinsic to traditional fine-needle aspiration cytology, including minimally invasive sampling, limited anesthetic risk, and diminished patient discomfort. The primary challenges of ICC, as well as potential solutions, are provided in Table 7.1. Briefly, the most daunting disadvantages include pre-analytical

Veterinary Cytology, First Edition. Edited by Leslie C. Sharkey, M. Judith Radin, and Davis Seelig.

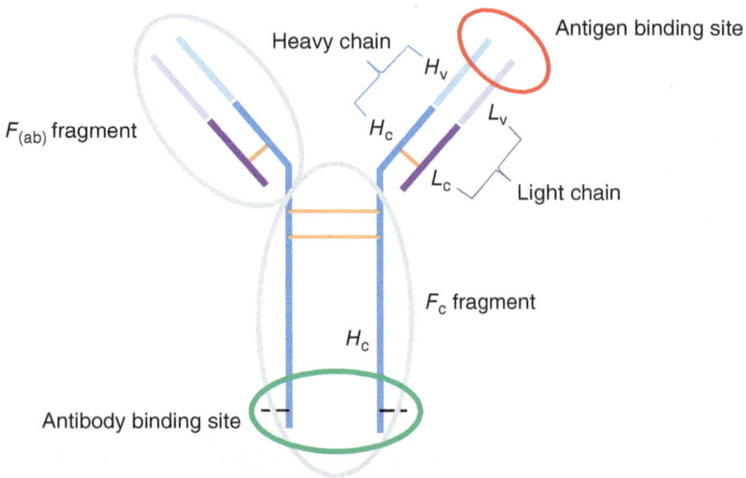

Figure 7.1 The classic structure of an immunoglobulin showing the constant fragment (F_c) and the antigen binding fragment (F_{ab}). The structure can further be broken into heavy and light chains, with constant (H_c, L_c) and variable regions (H_v, L_v). The variable regions of the heavy and light chains allow for a multitude of antigen binding abilities. The structural, constant heavy chain on the Fc portion provides for antibody binding and helps define the isotype of the immunoglobulin.

Table 7.1 The primary challenges of ICC and potential solutions.

Challenge	Potential solutions
Difficulty in obtaining an adequate number of diagnostic smears for a full ICC panel	Ship samples in transport media to allow for cytospin preparations, liquid-based cytology, and/or cell block techniques Divide smears into multiple sections using a barrier pen
Inability to assess smear quality prior to ICC staining	Evaluate unstained smears with the light decreased and condenser lowered on the microscope to enhance contrast Utilize phase-contrast microscopy
Lack of easy access to appropriate control samples	Maintain communication with necropsy service to allow collection of fresh tissues Utilize cell lines with known expression of antigens of interest
Possibility for excess background immunoreactivity in ruptured, necrotic, or poorly preserved samples	Validate optimal antibody titer Utilize negative assay controls If provided in fluid media, wash sample with neutral buffer/solution
Shortage of standardized protocols and ICC/IHC comparison studies to validate techniques	Promote communication among diagnostic labs Request that groups provide adequate information when publishing results

ICC, immunocytochemistry; IHC, immunohistochemistry.

variations in sample quality, inadequate sample to complete a full ICC panel, and a shortage of published protocols for groups wanting to include ICC in their laboratories.[5,12,25]

Overview and Protocol

ICC testing can be separated into three phases: (i) the pre-analytical phase, which constitutes sample collection through slide storage; (ii) the analytical phase, which focuses on methods employed for optimal visual localization of the target; and (iii) the post-analytical phase, which encompasses interpretation and reporting of results. While this summary of ICC is based upon the available literature, it is important to note that each phase needs to be optimized for each antigen–antibody combination.[14]

Pre-analytical Phase

Sample Collection and Transport In veterinary medicine, ICC samples are typically smears of fine-needle aspirates or biopsies or cytospin preparations of cavity, cyst, or joint fluids.[25] The advantages and disadvantages of each are presented in Table 7.2. As with routine cytology, the quantity and quality of cells will dictate the diagnostic utility of ICC. High numbers of ruptured, necrotic, or

Table 7.2 Advantages and disadvantages of select methods for ICC sample preparation.

Method	Advantages	Disadvantages
Direct smears	Can use slides that were initially obtained Most cost-effective option	Inability to reduce background artifact present on smears Limited slide numbers may preclude evaluation of complete ICC panels Excessively thick samples can result in both false-positive and false-negative results
Cytospin preparations	Useful with samples that have limited starting material Best preservation of cell morphology Complete ICC panels may be possible Ability to wash and concentrate samples, potentially minimizing background artifact	Extra cost, time, and equipment required
Cell block methods	Samples and controls can be handled similarly to IHC Complete ICC panels may be possible Materials are easily stored	Extra cost, time, and equipment required As samples are fixed, use of certain antibodies may be precluded

ICC, immunocytochemistry; IHC, immunohistochemistry.

poorly preserved cells will not only preclude sufficient antibody–antigen interactions but may also result in high amounts of background.[3,5]

The application of ICC in veterinary medicine is often hindered by the submission of insufficient number of diagnostic quality slides. A number of alternate sample processing techniques, including cytospin, ThinPrep, and cell block techniques (Chapter 8), offer a potential solution to this hurdle.[5,24] In these techniques, non-fluid samples (i.e. tissue aspirates) are collected into transport media and shipped to diagnostic laboratories for slide or block preparation. Examples of such media are provided in Table 7.3. In addition to preserving cellular architecture, these techniques offer the ability to concentrate low cellular samples, the option to simultaneously fix samples, and the capacity to remove substances (protein, carbohydrate, or lipid) that may cause undesired background.

Table 7.3 Select examples of noncommercial collection/transport media for cytology and ICC.

Contents of media	Comments/notes
2 mL of stock solution (normal saline, 5% acetone, and 1% BSA) in a 5 mL EDTA tube[24]	
Solution of 10% acetone and 5% BSA in saline[24]	Recommended when shipping will be delayed by one to three days
1 mL of normal saline and 40 µL of 22% BSA in a 3 mL EDTA tube[23]	Utilize when samples are stained within 24 hours of collection
1 mL of saline with 0.1 mL of serum from the patient or same species in a red top tube (authors' experience)	As would be done for flow cytometry samples

BSA, bovine serum albumin; EDTA, ethylenediaminetetraacetic acid; ICC, immunocytochemistry.

Fixation Fixation of samples for ICC is often needed to prevent autolysis and stabilize cellular materials.[12,14] Unfortunately, no single fixative is perfect. Common fixatives for ICC and their caveats are presented in Table 7.4. Acetone pre-cooled to 4 °C and applied for at least one minute is the most common choice, as it reportedly provides the most consistent results.[24,26] Of note, acetone solubilizes cell membranes, leading to diffusion of small peptides out of cells and potential false-negative results.[12] Alternately, fixation with formalin offers some advantages over acetone, including superior preservation of cellular morphology, long-term retention of antigenicity, and more firm adhesion of cells to the slide.[24,27] Notably, formalin fixation may be necessary for use with some antigens, particularly nuclear antigens.[3] However, antigen retrieval (AR) (see section "Antigen Retrieval") may be needed with formalin fixation, and some antigens, such as estrogen or progesterone receptors, may be rendered completely inactive.[12] If utilizing multiplex ICC, selection of an appropriate fixative that will preserve all target epitopes, particularly when combining cell surface and cytoplasmic antigens, is a critical consideration. In addition to fixation choice, the selection of an appropriate slide is an important consideration in preparing samples for ICC. Generally, charged, silanized, or poly-L-lysine-coated slides provide excellent sample retention regardless of the fixative used.[12]

Storage Depending on the antigen of interest, the diagnostic utility of unfixed air-dried samples varies from one to two weeks at room temperature.[3,28] While this can be prolonged with refrigeration,[29] even acetone-fixed slides

Table 7.4 Common fixatives for ICC and their caveats, if documented.

Fixative	Comments/notes
100% acetone (4 °C)	Solubilizes cell membranes, leading to possible diffusion of small peptides out of cells (possible false-negative results) Charged or pretreated slides are recommended to avoid loss of cells during protocol
4–10% formalin	Preferred fixative for nuclear antigens
Alcohol fixatives, such as 95% ethanol, 1 : 1 mixture of methanol–absolute ethanol, 100% methanol (chilled to −20 °C), absolute alcohol, propylene glycol in alcohol	Antigens such as S-100 protein, Hep Par 1, and GCDFP-15 are leached by alcohol fixatives (false-negative results)
0.1% formal saline	
0.4–4% paraformaldehyde	

GCDFP-15, gross cystic disease fluid protein 15, a marker of mammary carcinoma; Hep Par 1, hepatocyte paraffin 1 recognizes mitochondrial antigen of hepatocytes; ICC, immunocytochemistry.

can lose their antigenicity after three to four months at 4 °C.[24] Some laboratories fix cytologic samples for ICC with methanol and cover with 3% polyethylene glycol for long-term storage.[30] When kept at −70 °C, cells can retain their immunogenicity for a year or more.[3,31] Although global recommendations are not possible, it is generally recommended that samples archived for future ICC studies be refrigerated, frozen, and/or fixed.

Use of Previously Stained Slides Chromogenic ICC can be performed on currently and previously stained, decolorized smears stained with Romanowsky-type or Papanicolaou stains.[32–36] Notably, the same slide can be sequentially stained with multiple antibodies if the first test is negative. However, cell loss, disruption, and antigenic degradation from repeated exposure to graded alcohols can cause inadequate results.[12] In cases with limited slides, single samples can be divided into multiple zones, or the smear can be divided using tissue transfer techniques.[33] If this latter technique is utilized, non-adhesive-treated slides should be used. Previously stained slides are subject to auto-fluorescence, making them unsuitable for fluorescent ICC.

Analytical Phase

General Methodology Specific ICC techniques are dictated by (i) the location of the epitope of interest (membrane versus nuclear versus cytoplasmic), (ii) the type of fixation, (iii) whether AR is necessary, (iv) whether direct or indirect methods are employed, and (v) whether chromogenic versus fluorescent detection is utilized. A typical indirect chromogenic ICC protocol with AR is provided (Table 7.5).

Table 7.5 Example of a chromogenic ICC protocol for an intracellular target epitope, including optional antigen retrieval.

1) Ensure that slides, preferably charged or pretreated, are fully air-dried.
2) Briefly rinse 1X with PBS.
3) Fix cells for recommended length of time.
4) Antigen retrieval (optional step): Perform HIER with preheated buffer for suggested length of time.
5) Wash slides 3X with PBS.
6) Permeabilize samples with diluted detergent. (Note: Acetone-fixed and some methanol-fixed slides do not require additional permeabilization. This step will not be required for membrane antigens.)
7) Wash slides 3X with PBS.
8) Block endogenous enzyme activity.
9) Wash slides 3X with PBS.
10) Perform nonspecific antibody binding blocking step.
11) Wash slides 3X with PBS.
12) Incubate with primary antibody.
13) Wash slides 3X with PBS.
14) Incubate with secondary antibody.
15) Utilize detection reagents to visualize the immunoreaction.
16) Counterstain.
17) Coverslip.

HIER, heat-induced epitope retrieval; ICC, immunocytochemistry; PBS, phosphate-buffered saline.

Manual Versus Automated ICC While it requires more attention than automated staining, manual staining permits the division of a single slide into multiple areas with a barrier pen, as well as more conservative use of reagents.[37] For a diagnostic service with a large number of submissions, an automated stainer is recommended. Should an automated stainer be used, it is important that the staining system be sufficiently flexible so as to accommodate antibodies and reagents from a variety of sources.

Detection Systems In order to visualize the ICC reaction, one of the reaction reagents, typically either the primary, secondary, or tertiary antibody, must be labeled with a reporter molecule. Typical labels include fluorescent compounds, metals, or enzymes such as peroxidase, alkaline phosphatase (ALP), and glucose oxidase.[12] Generally, as the visualization of fluorescent and metal labels requires specialized microscopes, enzyme-based detection systems, which produce a colored precipitate that can be visualized with light microscopy, are preferred. The optimal detection system maximizes sensitivity with a high signal to noise ratio, optimizes reproducibility, and can be performed as efficiently as possible. Importantly, the selected system must be compatible with the species of interest, as methods that perform well with human cells may not be adequate with animal samples.

Direct Methods

Direct detection of antibody–antigen complexes is a one-step process that uses a primary antibody directly conjugated to reporter molecules (Figure 7.2). This method is the most time-efficient option but often lacks satisfactory sensitivity for detection of many antigens relevant to diagnostic cytology.[14]

Indirect Methods

Two-step (or indirect) ICC protocols allow for more sensitive antigen detection (Figure 7.2). In this approach, a secondary antibody, which is conjugated to a reporter molecule, is directed against the primary antibody.[14] This technique is superior to direct ICC because the unlabeled primary antibody retains full avidity to the epitope, resulting in stronger binding, and the higher number of labels per molecule of primary antibody allows for increased reaction sensitivity.[12] A variety of commercial kits are available that work well in veterinary species, including newer systems that directly link the reporter molecule to the secondary antibody in a proprietary polymer. This eliminates a step in the technical process while maintaining or improving the sensitivity and specificity of the reaction.[38]

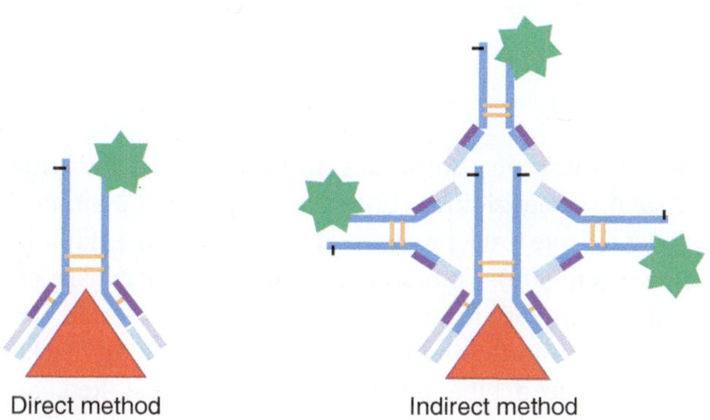

Figure 7.2 A comparison of direct and indirect methods of ICC. The direct ICC method uses an antibody that has been directly conjugated to a fluorescent molecule or a chromogen detection substrate. The indirect method uses a primary antibody to directly bind to the antigen, followed by a secondary anti-primary antibody that is conjugated to a fluorescent molecule or a chromogen detection substrate. Signal can be amplified with indirect methods, as multiple secondary antibodies can bind to the primary.

Multiplex ICC

Multiple immunolabeling (Figure 7.3) is utilized to simultaneously localize different antigens on the same sample and can be performed with either direct or indirect methods. In the case of the former, antibodies raised in the same species can be used. For indirect methods, primary antibodies raised in differing species are typically selected for simultaneous labeling, with secondary antibodies then targeted toward the individual species utilized. The availability of various enzymes, chromogens, and fluorescent molecules makes this technique feasible. False-positive labeling due to cross-reactivity among different components of the reaction is a concern that can be overcome with careful planning and use of multiple controls. Selecting an adequate set of substrates for multiplex ICC can also be difficult, particularly when antigen co-localization causes mixing of chromogenic color reactions. The use of semiquantitative multispectral analysis and alternative labels, such as quantum dots, have made high-throughput biomarker quantification and dual labeling more accurate and less burdensome.[39,40]

Controls The inclusion of both positive and negative controls with each clinical sample is vital for proper interpretation of ICC. Positive controls should be samples in which immunostaining is expected, and negative controls are samples in which immunostaining is not expected. Negative controls are commonly either negative antibody controls or negative sample controls. Examples of the former include incubation of case samples with one of the following: (i) buffer only (i.e. antibody omission), (ii) buffer with an isotype-matched Ig, or (iii) buffer with an unrelated mAb.[25,41] The latter consists of a sample in which the epitope of interest is not expressed. Controls should be prepared and processed using the same methods as the test case. A common mistake is to use improper control specimens, such as formalin-fixed paraffin-embedded sections, to interpret ICCs.[5] As maintaining a bank of control slides is challenging, potential options include the use of cell lines and postmortem samples.[24]

Antigen Retrieval Fixation, particularly with formalin and other cross-linking agents, can alter the three-dimensional structure of target proteins, rendering epitopes undetectable by specified antibodies. In such situations, depending upon the specific antigen–antibody interaction, AR may be needed.[24] The most common AR used for ICC is heat-induced epitope retrieval (HIER), with enzyme-induced

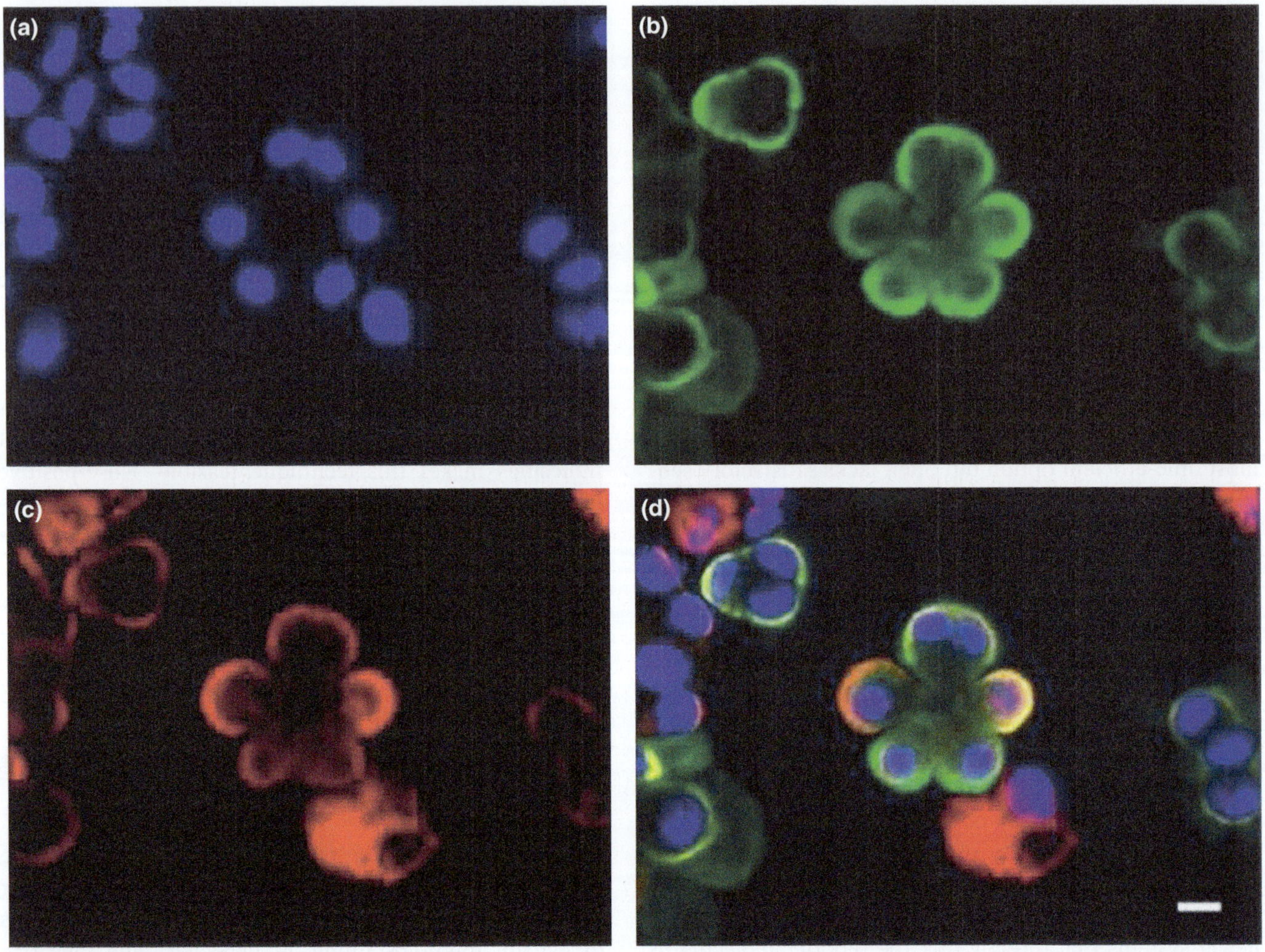

Figure 7.3 Multiplex immunofluorescent ICC image of vimentin-only macrophages and neutrophils adjacent to dual-cytokeratin- and vimentin-positive mesothelial cells. The quadrants are divided to show each fluorescent stain individually and combined. (a) DAPI imparts blue nuclear staining. (b) Cytokeratin (AE1/AE3 + 8/18) positivity of mesothelial cells is shown as green. (c) Vimentin (SP20) positivity of all three cell types appears red. (d) An overlay of the three antibodies demonstrates dual cytokeratin and vimentin positivity of the mesothelial cells (bar = 10 μm).

epitope retrieval used less often.[4] In veterinary medicine, HIER using a citrate buffer of pH 6.0 has been successful in detecting nuclear antigens on ethanol or formalin-fixed smears.[3,12,42] Few cytoplasmic or membrane antigens require AR, although it has been reported to enhance immunopositivity[43] and has been used to decolorize stained slides.[35] While AR enhances ICC, it can also increase background staining.[12] Owing to the wide range of fixation techniques and the uniqueness of each antigen–antibody interaction, standardization of AR is difficult and should be optimized for each ICC protocol.

Chromogen and Counterstaining Options In chromogenic ICC, a colored precipitate is formed from the reaction of an enzyme, typically horseradish peroxidase (HRP) or ALP, with a substrate. Substrates utilized for HRP include 3,3′-diaminobenzidine (brown precipitate), 3-amino-9-ethylcarbazole (red precipitate), and 4-chloro-1-naphthol (blue precipitate). Common substrates for ALP consist of a combination of nitro blue tetrazolium chloride and 5-bromo-4-chloro-3-indolyl phosphate (NBT/BCIP, black to purple to deep blue precipitate), Vulcan Fast Red, and Vector Black. While enzymes and/or chromogens utilized in single antibody reactions can be dictated by personal preference, multiplex chromogenic ICC requires selecting compatible color combinations. When multiplexing, a chromogenic approach is more successful when distinguishing different cell types rather than attempting to co-localize epitopes within one cell type.[39] For the latter, immunofluorescent techniques are preferred. The counterstain in ICC should allow assessment of cell morphology but differ in hue from the chosen chromogen.[12] Available counterstains include hematoxylin, methyl green, and nuclear fast red.[44] However, counterstaining may not be recommended in ICC protocols, such as when staining for nuclear antigens.[14] In fluorescent ICC, a nuclear stain, such as 4′,6-diamidino-2-phenylindole (DAPI), is useful.

Post-analytical Phase

Interpretation and Reporting ICC is not a stand-alone diagnostic and should be performed in concert with routine cytology and interpreted with knowledge of other related clinicopathologic data.[12,25] Interpretation also requires appropriate positive and negative controls. As there is no single threshold that defines a positive ICC result, each laboratory should quantify the number of positive cells or infectious organisms, the intensity of staining, and the cellular location of the staining (nuclear versus cytoplasmic versus membranous).[12] The interpretation should also provide the reader with an assessment of confidence in the results based on personal experiences and/or (ideally) peer-reviewed literature. Guidelines for the publication of ICC data are available.[25]

Caveats and Pitfalls

Incorrect Results

As with any diagnostic test, erroneous ICC results can be classified as either false positives or false negatives. Common causes of false positivity include (i) inadequate or inappropriate fixation for the antigen of interest, (ii) insufficient blocking, (iii) high background labeling with pAbs, (iv) interpretation of immunoreactivity in the incorrect cell of interest, (v) spurious staining of phagocytized cells, or (iv) reagent trapping in clusters or layers of cells.[3,5,12] False positivity also can result from antigen cross-reactivity, which is defined as inappropriate but specific binding of a pAb to a cell type in which the antigen of interest is not expressed. Evaluation of cross-reactivity in the diagnostic setting is dictated by whether the antibody is targeting an infectious agent or a cell marker.[12,45] For antibodies against pathogens, it is particularly important that the antibody be tested against other organisms that are morphologically similar.[12] Antibodies against microorganisms have also been reported to cross-react with cellular organelles.[12] While cross-reactivity of an antibody does not preclude its usage in ICC, the appropriate interpretation requires this is acknowledged and reported.[12] For neoplastic markers, antibodies to specific cell types or components should be evaluated more extensively to prevent the possibility of false-positive results.[46] False-negative results can be associated with improper fixation, insufficient antibody concentrations, inadequate AR, or cell damage during slide preparation.[3,5] It can be particularly challenging to interpret ICC performed on inflamed or necrotic samples, and in these situations, negative controls are critical.

Species Cross-Reactivity

It should not be assumed that antigen detection is consistent among species, as identical antibody clones can differ drastically in reactivity.[47] For instance, melan-A has been reported to label melanocytes in many species, but not horses.[48] It is advisable to optimize ICC tests for each new species, which can be directed by literature searches and/or consultations with antibody manufacturers.

Quality Assurance and Quality Control

Assay Optimization and Standardization

Standardization refers to optimization of an ICC protocol, including incubation time, incubation temperature, antibody dilutions, AR approach, controls, buffers, and detection systems.[3,12] The goal of standardization is the production of reproducible and consistent results, even with different reagents and protocols, and is particularly important as many veterinary diagnostic laboratories vary their approach toward ICC.[12,45]

Assay Validation

Once an assay has been developed, optimized, and standardized, it is then validated to confirm the accuracy of the test within the intended species. Validation begins with evaluation of the analytical characteristics of a test, including sensitivity, specificity, repeatability, and reproducibility.[12] In addition to confirming antibody specificity, validation examines other variables that can affect the immunoreaction, including pre-analytical and analytical variables.[3] Optimally, ICC assays should be validated by comparing results among laboratories using similar techniques and using a diagnostic "gold standard," such as IHC. As robust validation can be difficult to achieve given the small number of veterinary laboratories performing ICC, published data may be used to assist with test validation.[49]

Diagnostic Applications

ICC has a variety of diagnostic applications, including lymphoma immunophenotyping, neoplastic cell lineage assignment or identification, identification of infectious agents, and prognostication of neoplastic lesions. The following section includes a diagnostic approach to integrating ICC into a diagnostic plan and a summary of useful veterinary antibodies. A list of many of these antibodies is also provided in Table 7.6.

Table 7.6 Summary of selected antibodies used in immunocytochemistry as reported in the veterinary literature.

	Antibody	Target cells
Lymphoid	CD3	T cells
	CD4	T helper cells, canine neutrophils, activated macrophages/monocytes
	CD8	Cytotoxic T cells
	CD20	B cells
	CD79a	B cells
Histiocytic	CD1a	Dendritic cells, thymocytes
	CD1c	Dendritic cells, thymocytes, subset of B cells
	CD11b	Macrophages and subset of dermal interstitial dendritic cells, granulocytes, monocytes
	CD11c	Granulocytes, monocytes, and dendritic cells (Langerhans cells and interstitial dendritic cells)
	CD11d	Macrophages of splenic red pulp and bone marrow, T cells
	CD18	All leukocytes, low levels on lymphocytes
	CD90	Dermal interstitial dendritic cells, T cells, thymocytes, monocytes
	CD204	Tissue-resident macrophages
	E-cadherin	Langerhans cells
	Lysozyme	Granulocytes, monocytes, macrophages
	MHCII	Dendritic cells and macrophages
Epithelial	Broad-spectrum CK	All epithelial cells
	CK7	Glandular and transitional epithelial cells
	CK20	Gastric and intestinal epithelial cells
	Uroplakin III	Urothelial cells
Mesenchymal	Vimentin	Mesenchymal cells
	Desmin	Cells of muscle origin, canine mesothelial cells
	von Willebrand factor	Endothelial cells, megakaryocytes, platelets
Melanoma	Melan-A	Melanocytes
	S-100	Variety of cell types including melanocytes
Infectious agents	Feline coronavirus	
	Bovine respiratory syncytial virus	
	Chlamydophila	
Prognostic markers	Ki67	Proliferating cells
	c-kit/CD117	Mast cells, stem cells

Diagnostic Approach to Using Immunocytochemistry

ICC results can only be interpreted with appropriate clinical and cytologic differential diagnoses. From this list of cytologic differential diagnoses, an ICC diagnostic plan using the most appropriate panel of antibodies should be used with the intention of confirming one diagnosis and refuting other(s). It is important to note that such antibody panels will vary from case to case (depending upon the cytologic differential diagnoses) and, if possible, should contain both discriminatory and redundant antibodies. Specific approaches are outlined in the sections that follow. However, this approach can be challenging and costly as it requires multiple diagnostic quality samples and multiple antibodies. As such, one of the common ICC mistakes is requesting too few immunostains, thereby creating bias toward the favored diagnosis.[5] Lastly, it is important to note that there is no "magic" antibody that can differentiate reactive and neoplastic lesions and between benign and malignant neoplasms. As such, a cytologic diagnosis is absolutely required. Figure 7.4 outlines a simple diagnostic

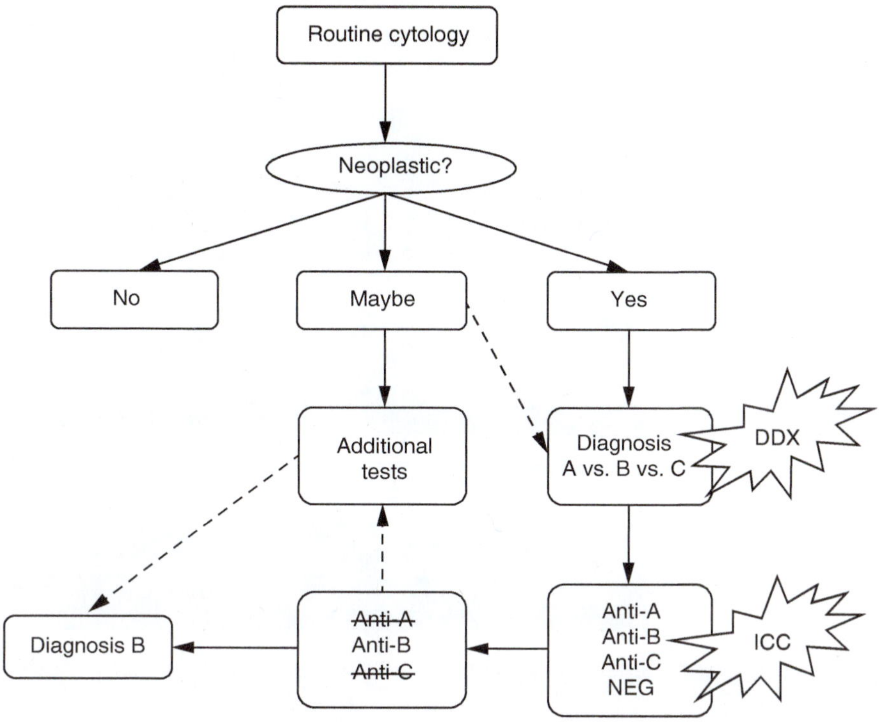

Figure 7.4 Algorithm for the application of immunocytochemistry (ICC) in the diagnosis of veterinary neoplasia. When cytomorphology is compatible with a neoplastic process, a list of differential diagnoses (DDX) is determined, designated above by A, B, and C. A panel of antibodies directed against antigens expected to be expressed in each of these possible diagnoses (anti-A, anti-B, and anti-C) are applied along with a negative control (NEG). Diagnosis B is made when expression for the expected antigen in diagnosis B is found and no expression is observed for the antigens expected in diagnoses A and C. Immunocytochemistry in cases when a diagnosis of neoplasia is uncertain can aid in assignment of cellular lineage, but additional tests are often needed to confirm a neoplastic process (represented by dashed lines).

algorithm for the application of ICC in veterinary cancer diagnosis. Sufficient slides are required to follow this approach, but this can be achieved using some of the techniques detailed in Table 7.1.

Immunophenotyping of Lymphoma

Based on a recent survey of veterinary oncologists and clinical pathologists, the most common application of ICC is the immunophenotyping of lymphoma.[25] Differentiating between T- and B-cell tumors is of prognostic importance, with T-cell neoplasms having a broad spectrum of clinical courses, and may eventually have treatment implications as subtype-specific therapies are developed, including antibody-based treatment of B-cell lymphoma.[50,51] Multiplex immunofluorescence lymphoma ICC has been described, thus allowing for the immunophenotyping of T- and B-cell markers on a single smear.[52] Excellent correlation between ICC and IHC has been shown in several publications.[20,21,53] Most laboratories and publications report CD3 as a T-cell marker and CD79a, CD20, and PAX5 as B-cell markers in canine, feline, and equine specimens.[21,25,54–59] ICC can also detect T-cell subsets using CD4 and CD8 antibodies.[60] Figure 7.5 illustrates the use of the ICC in the phenotyping of a B-cell lymphoma. Co-expression of T- and B-cell markers in lymphoma has been reported and demonstrates the importance of multiple antibodies and the need for additional diagnostic testing in these cases, such as PCR for antigen receptor rearrangements.[56]

Neoplastic Cell Lineage Identification

ICC can be used to characterize cell lineage in cases where routine cytology does not allow for a definitive diagnosis. Table 7.6 lists many of the antibodies that have been published to be effective in veterinary ICC, including the identification of cells of histiocytic, epithelial, or mesenchymal origin.

Histiocytic Tumors Histiocytes are a family of bone marrow-derived phagocytic cells whose membership includes macrophages and various dendritic cell subsets.[61] As the cytomorphology of neoplastic histiocytic cells can overlap with other cells, including those of hematopoietic, mesenchymal, or epithelial origin, ICC may be useful in differentiating histiocytic neoplasms from lymphoma, carcinoma, and sarcoma.[62] Using ICC, histiocytic

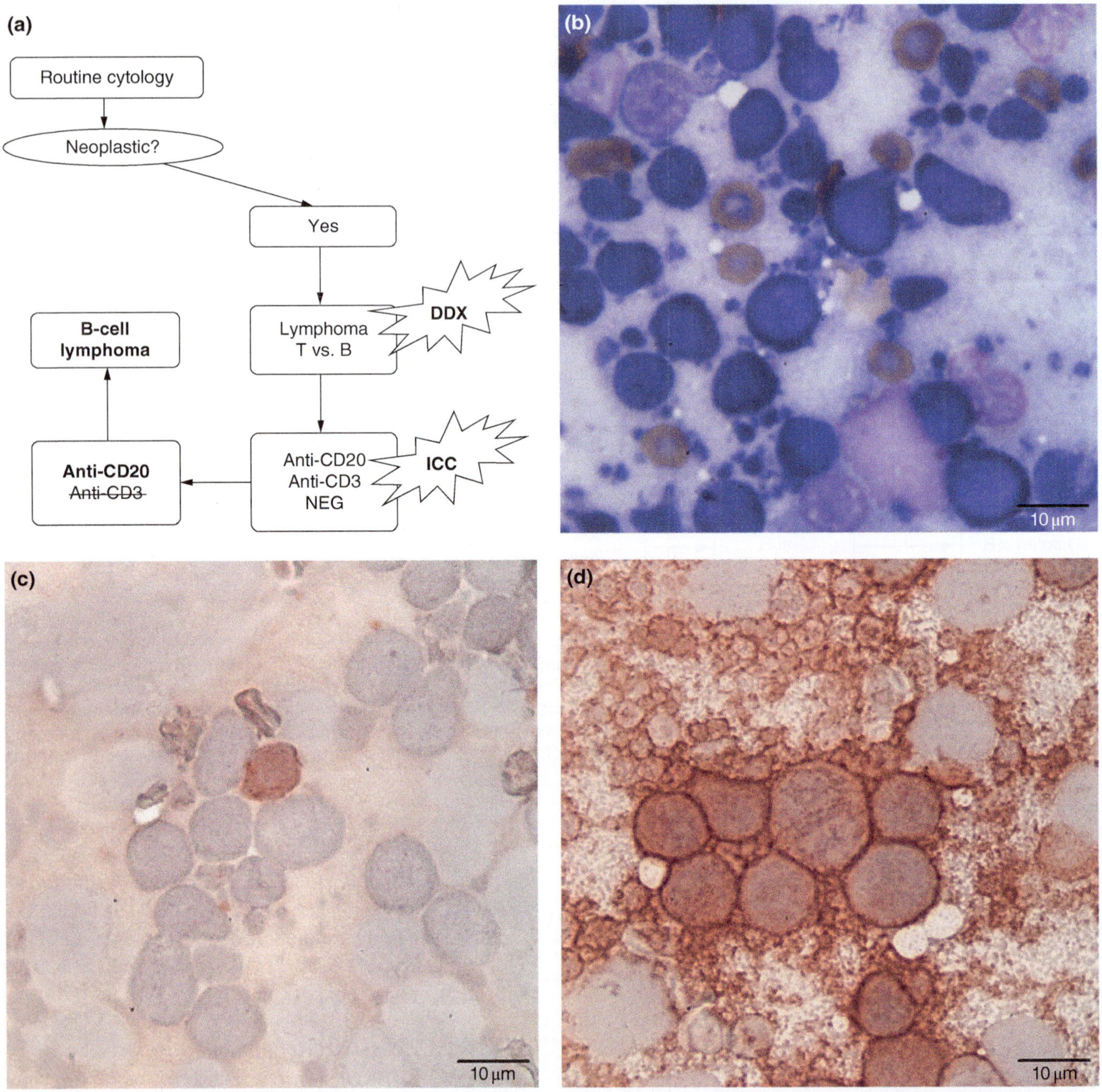

Figure 7.5 (a) Diagnostic algorithm in the immunophenotyping of a case of lymphoma using a canine lymph node aspirate. (b) Large neoplastic lymphocytes predominate consistent with a diagnosis of lymphoma (Wright's, 1000×). (c) No expression of CD3 is detected in the large neoplastic cells. A single small residual lymphocyte exhibits strong cytoplasmic immunoexpression of CD3 (Dako, A 0452, 1000×). (d) Strong cytoplasmic immunoexpression of CD20 in the neoplastic cells and in the background due to cell rupture (Thermo Fisher, RB 9013-PO, 1000×). Positive and negative controls stained as expected (not shown).

neoplasms can be identified, and potentially subclassified, using antibodies directed against a variety of surface antigens (Table 7.6).[61] Several reports describe using ICC to facilitate the diagnosis of histiocytic neoplasia in the cerebrospinal fluid or peripheral blood, thus demonstrating the advantage of ICC in the diagnosis of lesions not easily accessible for biopsy.[63–68] Although histiocytic neoplasms are less common in cats, ICC has also been applied to feline samples using antibodies directed against CD1a, CD1c, CD11b, and CD18.[69]

Epithelial Tumors Assignment of an epithelial origin to a cell of uncertain lineage is accomplished using antibodies directed against cytokeratins (CK). Anti-CK antibodies can have either broad-spectrum specificity, such as the pancytokeratin clone EA1/AE3, or they may be directed against single, more tissue-specific CK. The latter allows for further characterization of the origin of epithelial cells, such as anti-CK7 and anti-CK20 antibodies. ICC studies using AE1/AE3 in canine tissues have reported strong immunoexpression in epithelial cells,[9,59,70–75] and Figure 7.6 demonstrates immunoreactivity in feline tissues using a multiplex immunofluorescent ICC. Moreover, expected immunoexpression patterns using tissue-specific CK have been reported in canine tissues,[70] suggesting that these antibodies may be useful in the subclassification of epithelial tumors. As some carcinomas can display co-expression of CK and vimentin (which is traditionally considered a marker of mesenchymal origin),[72,74,76] it is important to stress the importance of panels of antibodies rather than just one. The importance of antibody panels in providing the most accurate lineage assignment is demonstrated by a report describing a joint metastasis of a transitional cell carcinoma in a dog, in which immunoexpression of uroplakin III further refined an ambiguous neoplasm demonstrating co-expression of CK and vimentin.[72]

ICC has also been used for the characterization of metastatic carcinoma in canine lymph node impression smears,[71] in peripheral blood and bone marrow smears,[77,78] and in canine and feline bone marrow using cell block cytology.[9] In lymph node smears, the authors demonstrated a higher sensitivity of ICC using clone AE1/AE3 as compared with routine cytology to detect metastasis[71] as has been described in human studies.[79,80]

Mesenchymal Tumors Antibodies against vimentin, which is considered a pan-mesenchymal marker, as well as tissue/cell-specific antibodies have been successfully used in canine ICC for the diagnosis of mesenchymal neoplasia.[31,81,82] As shown in Figure 7.6, this antibody can also be used in feline tissues. Further subtyping of canine mesenchymal tumors into either muscle or endothelial origin using antibodies directed against desmin[31,82] and von Willebrand factor,[31] respectively, has been reported.

Melanoma Given its lack of characteristic melanin pigment and an often high degree of cellular atypia, which may mimic many malignant neoplasms, ICC can be particularly useful in the diagnosis of amelanotic melanoma. Specific antibodies would include a melanocytic marker, vimentin, a broad-spectrum CK, and possibly others. Melan-A[31,83,84] and S-100[31,83] have both been used in ICC for the detection of canine melanocytic cells. Melan-A has been shown to be a more specific marker with only weak expression in squamous cell carcinoma and

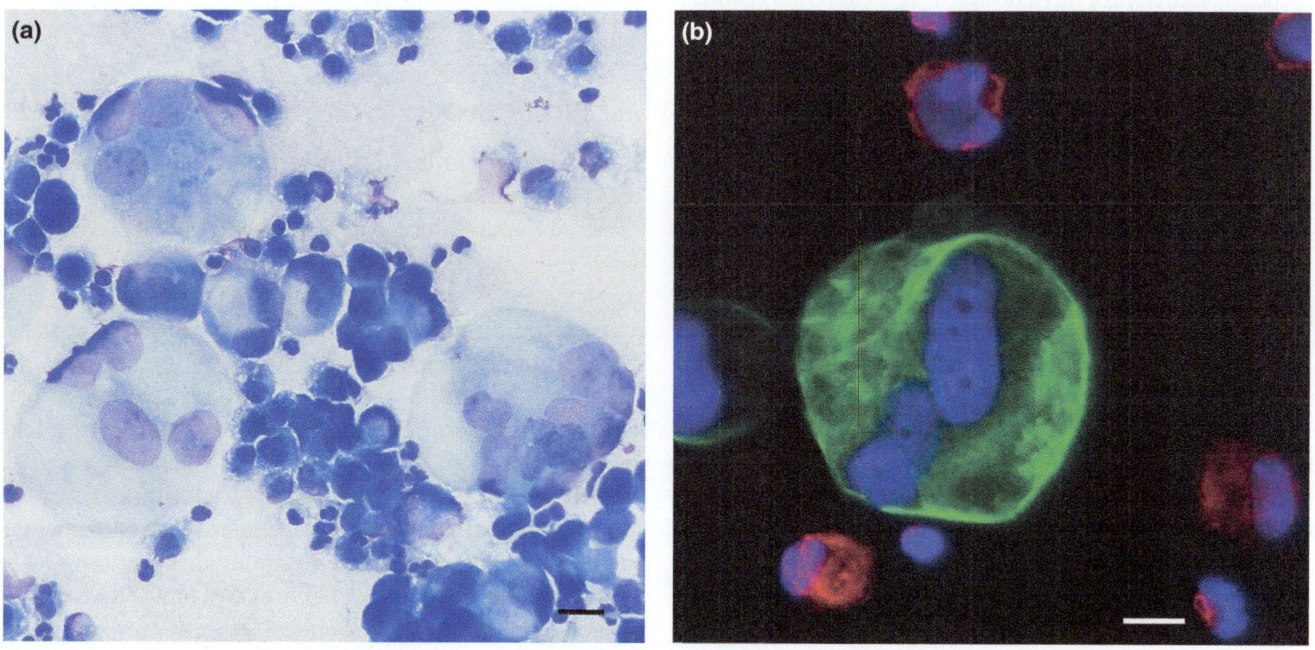

Figure 7.6 Thoracic fluid samples from a cat. (a) Note the large, atypical, multinucleated cells within this fluid sample (Wright's stain, 500×, bar = 10 μm). (b) Multiplex immunofluorescent ICC of same sample fluid, which confirms the presence of cytokeratin-only (green) positive cells admixed with vimentin-positive (red) inflammatory cells. DAPI imparts blue nuclear staining. These findings are consistent with a diagnosis of carcinoma (630×, bar = 10 μm).

normal canine testicular cells, whereas S-100 showed positive reactions in several different tissues and tumor types.[83] An ICC panel using antibodies directed against melan-A, CK, and vimentin was shown to have perfect agreement with histopathology and IHC in the diagnoses of 38 cases of canine oral amelanotic melanomas.[84] However, a case report of a single S-100-positive, melan-A-negative melanoma in the dog has been reported, and, as such, staining for both markers may be worthwhile.[31]

Mesothelioma The light microscopic diagnosis of canine mesothelioma is, in part, difficult due to the cytomorphologic overlap of neoplastic mesothelial cells with the neoplastic cells from many other tumor types, including carcinomas and sarcomas, and the lack of a mesothelial cell-specific antibody. While panels of antibodies are reported to aid in the diagnosis of human mesothelioma,[85] many of these antibodies have not been validated in a veterinary setting. Studies in canine tissues have shown positive immunoexpression of CK, vimentin, and desmin in normal and reactive mesothelial cells, whereas neoplastic mesothelial cells demonstrate only CK and vimentin positivity.[74] This profile may be helpful in the diagnosis of mesothelioma, although additional confirmatory studies are needed.[31,74]

Identification of Infectious Agents

While non-antibody-based cytochemistry can aid in the detection of certain infectious agents, this approach tends to lack specificity for any one agent. ICC for feline coronavirus (FCoV) in cats with feline infectious peritonitis (FIP) is the most well-studied scenario. Using a direct immunofluorescent approach, intramacrophagic detection of FCoV was detected with 100% sensitive and 71.4% specificity in cats with FIP.[86] This sensitivity was considerably lower when an immunoperoxidase technique was used on liver and kidney aspirates from FIP-positive cats (11 and 31%, respectively).[87] The ICC detection of *Chlamydophila* spp. within the peripheral blood heterophils of a red-tailed hawk[88] and of bovine respiratory syncytial virus within mononuclear cells in transtracheal wash fluid from an infected calf has been reported.[89]

Other Applications of Immunocytochemistry

ICC of the proliferation marker Ki-67 has been performed on canine mammary tumor[90] and lymph node[58] samples to assess its potential as a prognostic marker as well as on canine liver lesions to assess its potential to differentiate between neoplastic and nonneoplastic lesions.[91] Immunocytochemical detection of CD117 (*c-kit*) in canine mast cell tumors has been performed, and a report demonstrates (i) that the patterns of staining reported on IHC samples (i.e. membrane associated, paranuclear, and diffuse) can be identified in cytologic specimens, (ii) that low-grade mast cell tumors predominantly demonstrate a membrane-associated pattern, and (iii) that a diffuse staining pattern was restricted to high-grade tumors.[92] Future studies on the application of ICC are needed to provide additional information on the diagnostic value of these techniques.

Cytochemical Staining

General Principles

In cytochemistry, stainable components on a slide (cells or extracellular material) interact with a stain to cause a detectable color change.[93] Staining intensity and selectivity for specific tissue components is related to the affinity of tissue components for the stain and staining duration.[93] Stain affinity depends on the nature of the interaction of the stain with the tissue, including electrostatic, hydrogen, and covalent bonding, or hydrophobic effects[93] and with other elements of the staining system, including solvents. Staining duration is also important as different tissue compartments show differential staining profiles according to their respective duration of stain exposure.[93] As with ICC, there are a number of potential technical pitfalls associated with cytochemistry that may result in inappropriate results, including inadequate stain purity, stain degradation, or errors in staining procedure. As such, appropriate positive and negative controls should be included with every set of stained slides.[93]

Indications and Applications

Cytochemistry further characterizes cellular or extracellular components, beyond which can be assessed with a traditional Romanowsky-type stain (Table 7.7). As fewer steps and reagents are required, cytochemistry is generally cheaper, faster, simpler, and less labor intensive than ICC. As cytochemical reagents are generally subject to less species specificity than the antibodies in ICC, cytochemistry is often quite useful in veterinary diagnostic pathology, particularly in the examination of nontraditional species. Like any adjunctive staining approach, cytochemistry occupies a niche within the overall diagnostic algorithm and is best suited to identify cells or extracellular material for which appropriate species-validated immunodiagnostics (ICC or flow cytometry) are not available or cost prohibitive and for which appropriate cytochemical reagents are available. Specific diagnostic applications of cytochemistry in veterinary medicine include (i) lineage determination of hematopoietic cells, (ii) detection and characterization of infectious agents, or (iii) identification of cellular and

Table 7.7 Summary of histochemical and cytochemical stains.

	Cytochemical stain	Cell/substance detected	Positive color	Background color
Infectious agents	Gram stain[a]	Gram-positive bacteria, some fungal elements	Purple	Pink
	Gram stain[a]	Gram-negative bacteria	Pink	Pink
	Ziehl–Neelsen[a]	*Mycobacterium*, *Cryptosporidium*, ±*Nocardia*	Pink or red	Blue or green
	Kinyoun	*Mycobacterium*, *Cryptosporidium*, ±*Nocardia*	Pink or red	Blue or green
	Fite-Faraco	*Mycobacterium*, *Cryptosporidium*, ±*Nocardia*	Pink or red	Blue or green
	Gimenez	*Chlamydia*, *Helicobacter*, *Acanthamoeba*	Red or magenta	Blue or blue-green
	Macchiavello	Chlamydia, *Helicobacter*, *Acanthamoeba*	Red or magenta	Blue or blue-green
	Warthin–Starry	Spirochetes and other curved bacteria, *Clostridium piliforme*	Dark brown to black	Yellow to gold
	Modified Steiner	Spirochetes and other curved bacteria, *C. piliforme*	Dark brown to black	Yellow to gold
	Grocott methenamine silver[a]	Fungal hyphae, yeast, *Pneumocystis* cysts	Black	Light green
Minerals and pigments	Perls' Prussian blue[a]	Ferric iron	Blue	Pink to red
	Rubeanic acid	Copper	Greenish black	Pale red
	Rhodanine	Copper	Orange-red to red	Blue-green
	Alizarin red S	Calcium salt deposits	Orange-red	Green
	von Kossa	Large calcium salt deposits	Black or brown-black	Red
	Hall's (Fouchet's)	Bile	Green to blue-green	Yellow (muscle) to red (collagen)
	Masson-Fontana[a]	Melanin, some lipofuscin, some neuroendocrine cells (chromaffin and argentaffin cells)	Black	Red
	Schmorl's reaction	Melanin, some lipofuscin, some neuroendocrine cells (chromaffin and argentaffin cells)	Blue	Red
Lipids	Oil red O	Fat	Bright red	Blue
Collagenic and reticular connective tissue	Masson trichrome	Collagen	Blue	Red cytoplasm, blue-black nuclei
	Reticulin silver impregnation	Reticulin	Black	Depends on counterstain, often pink or red

(*Continued*)

Table 7.7 (Continued)

	Cytochemical stain	Cell/substance detected	Positive color	Background color
Carbohydrates, mucins, and glycoproteins	Periodic acid-Schiff[a]	A wide variety of carbohydrates and mucin	Magenta	Nuclei are blue
	Periodic acid-Schiff with diastase	A wide variety of carbohydrates and mucin, *except* glycogen	Magenta	Nuclei are blue
	Alcian blue[a]	Acid mucins, acid proteoglycans	Blue	Red
	Toluidine blue	Mast cell granules, acid mucins, cartilage	Red-purple	Blue
	Mucicarmine	Acid mucins (particular epithelial origin), mucinous bile, chordoma cells, *Cryptococcus* capsules	Deep red	Black nuclei, other tissue elements are yellow
Other intracellular and extracellular constituents	Alkaline phosphatase[a]	Osteosarcoma, some leukemias, and other tumors, various normal tissues (e.g. osteoblasts, hepatocytes, intestinal epithelial cells, kidney, placenta, some leukocytes)	Black or brown-black by NBT/BCIP method (blue by some methods)	Light red and blue (light Romanowsky-type counterstaining)
	Nonspecific esterases	Histiocytic cells, monocytic cells, megakaryocytes, T lymphocytes	Red to brown	Depends on counterstain
	Phosphotungstic acid–hematoxylin	Fibrin, striated muscle, the cytoplasmic granules in granular lymphocytes and oncocytoma cells	Blue or blue-black	Orange to red
	Congo red[a]	Amyloid	Red by standard bright-field microscopy; apple green birefringence with polarized light	Blue
	Luxol fast blue	Myelin	Blue	Pink-violet

[a] These stains have been validated for use on slides previously stained with Romanowsky stains.[33,94,95]
NBT/BCIP, nitro blue tetrazolium chloride/5-bromo-4-chloro-3-indolyl phosphate.

extracellular constituents. Additionally, unless stated otherwise, all the stains listed below can be performed in histologic as well as cytologic samples.

Sample Collection and Submission

Cytochemistry is often performed on unstained cytology slides, including tissue aspirates, impression smears, body cavity fluid smears, or blood smears. However, a number of cytochemical stains have been validated for use on previously stained stains, usually after destaining with a microwave method or with acid alcohol.[33,94,95]

Specific Cytochemical Stains

Hematopoietic Cells

Cytochemistry performed on blood and bone marrow smears can help assign lineage to normal and neoplastic hematopoietic cells, including leukocyte subsets across domestic and non-domestic.[96–106] However, owing to concerns regarding interpretation, quantification, and reproducibility, this approach has nearly entirely been replaced (when possible) by antibody-based analysis (e.g. flow cytometry and ICC). As such, only the nonspecific esterases are presented below. For more specific information, the reader is referred to veterinary hematology references.[96–106]

Nonspecific Esterases Esterase enzymes are present in a wide variety of tissues. Two of these, alpha naphthyl acetate esterase (ANAE) and alpha naphthyl butyrate esterase (ANBE), can be detected cytochemically and may be useful in veterinary diagnostic pathology. By adjusting the pH, temperature, and reaction time, esterase cytochemical staining can be made somewhat specific for detection of monocytes, histiocytic cells, megakaryocytes, and T lymphocytes.[96] ANBE is considered more specific for monocytic and histiocytic cells than ANAE, but ANAE may be more sensitive.[96] Sodium fluoride treatment can be used to increase specificity of the ANAE reaction. Monocytic, histiocytic, and megakaryocytic cells have negative or weakened staining with ANAE after sodium fluoride treatment, while T lymphocytes will remain positive. Sodium fluoride treatment is not commonly used with ANBE staining.[96] Nonspecific esterase cytochemistry has been used in veterinary medicine to help classify types of acute leukemia and to aid in the diagnosis of histiocytic neoplasia.[96,107–109]

Minerals and Pigments

Perls' Prussian Blue The Prussian blue stain is used to detect iron in cells and tissues. It is most commonly used on bone marrow samples to estimate iron stores; on blood and/or bone marrow samples to assess for siderocytes, sideroblasts, or sideroleukocytes; on liver samples to evaluate for hemochromatosis; and on other tissues to detect hemosiderin-laden macrophages (often indicating previous hemorrhage).[110–118] Tissue sections are acidified with dilute hydrochloric acid and treated with potassium ferrocyanide, which reacts with ferric iron to form a blue product, ferric ferrocyanide, also known as Prussian blue (Figure 7.7).[119]

Rubeanic Acid, Rhodanine The two most common staining techniques for histologic or cytologic detection of copper are rubeanic acid and rhodanine. Both techniques have been used in evaluation of liver samples of various species on both tissue sections and cytology slides (Figure 7.8).[116,119–123]

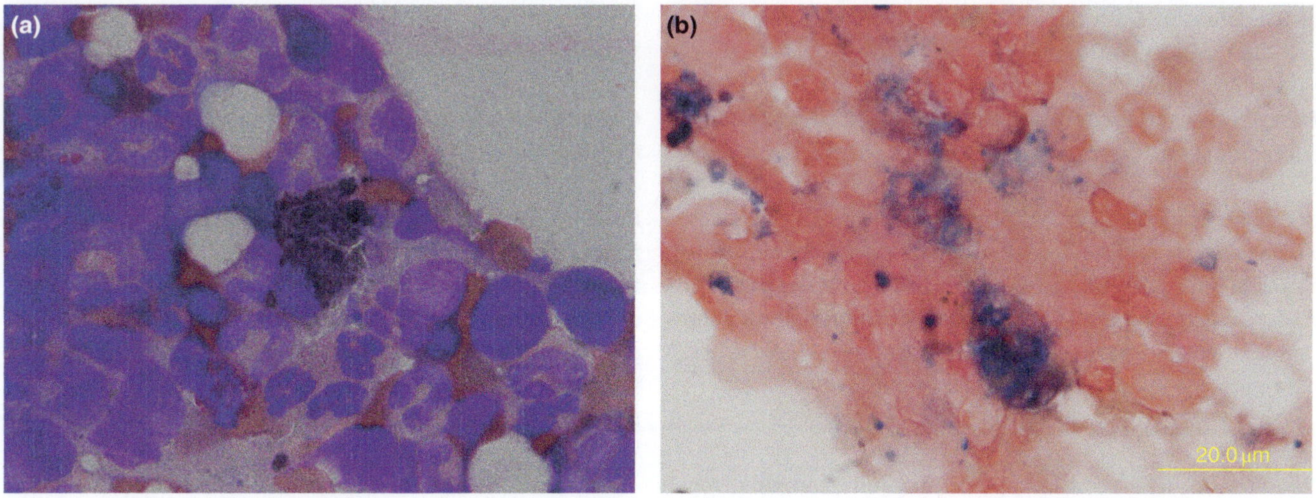

Figure 7.7 Bone marrow from a dog. (a) Macrophages contain a black pigment when stained with a routine Romanowsky-type stain (Wright's, 100×). (b) Note the positive blue staining within macrophages, confirming the presence of iron (Prussian blue, 100×).

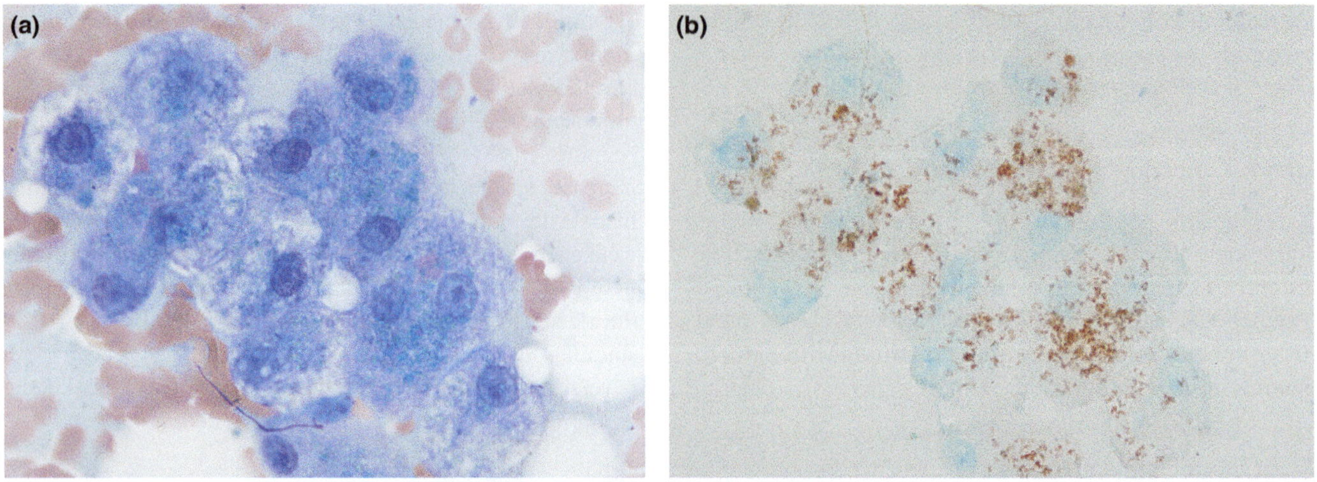

Figure 7.8 Liver aspirate from a dog. (a) Hepatocytes contain small, turquoise-colored granules (Wright's, 100×). (b) The orange/brown positive staining of the granules is compatible with copper (rhodanine, 100×).

Alizarin Red S, von Kossa Free ionic calcium cannot be demonstrated by special stains, but alizarin red S and von Kossa can be used to detect a variety of calcium salts (e.g. calcium phosphate, calcium carbonate, and calcium oxalate) in cytology and histology slides.[119,124] Diagnostically, alizarin red S or von Kossa can be useful to document tissue necrosis, dystrophic mineralization, calcinosis circumscripta, calcium oxalate nephrosis, and osteosarcoma.[124–130] Neither stain is completely specific for calcium, but alizarin red S is considered to be more specific than von Kossa, especially when performed at a pH of 4.2.[119] It also has the advantage over von Kossa of being able to detect smaller deposits of calcium.[119]

Hall's (Fouchet's) Hall's stain is a bile stain suitable for both histology and cytology samples and can be used to differentiate bile from other similarly colored pigments (e.g. hemosiderin or lipofuscin).[119,131,132]

Masson-Fontana, Schmorl's Reaction The Masson-Fontana and Schmorl's stains are two stains that exploit melanin's capacity to reduce silver or acid ferricyanide, thus producing a detectable color change. In veterinary medicine, the Masson-Fontana stain is more commonly used than the Schmorl's reaction, and it is most commonly used for diagnosis of melanocytic tumors.[94,133–136] However, it is important to note that neither staining method is specific for melanin and other pigments (e.g. lipofuscin) may also stain positively.[118,119,137]

Lipids

Oil Red O The routine processing of samples for histopathology extracts lipids from tissue sections, thus rendering them undetectable in traditional formalin-fixed paraffin-embedded sections.[93] However, the use of unfixed cytology samples that are not treated with lipid solvents (including alcohols) resolves this problem. Oil red O is a lipid stain used that can be used in the diagnosis of lipid-producing tumors, including liposarcoma, and lipid accumulations in nonneoplastic tissues such as the liver or peritoneal fluid.[138–144]

Collagenic and Reticular Connective Tissue

Masson Trichrome and Reticulin Silver Impregnation Masson trichrome is a common histochemical stain used to detect coarse collagen fibers, usually to assess for fibrosis or to support the diagnosis of a collagen-producing tumor.[145–148] Reticulin stains, including Gomori's and Gordon and Sweets' methods, stain reticular fibers, which are fine, argyrophilic forms of collagen often seen in myelofibrosis.[143,149–152] The use of these connective tissue stains has not been well published, likely because of the poorly exfoliative nature of collagen.[153]

Carbohydrates, Mucins, and Glycoproteins

Periodic Acid-Schiff The periodic acid-Schiff (PAS) stain detects a wide variety of carbohydrate-containing substances, including mucin, glycogen, basement membranes, many fungi capsules or cell walls, acanthamoeba, thyroid colloid, zymogen granules, Russell bodies, granular cell tumors, and oncocytomas.[55,94,154–169] To confirm the presence of glycogen versus other carbohydrates, PAS can be combined with pre-staining diastase treatment, which will digest glycogen into smaller sugar units that are subsequently washed out of the section.[155]

Alcian Blue The alcian blue stain binds to cationic groups in certain tissue components, particularly mucins and proteoglycans. In veterinary medicine, alcian blue positivity is reported in a number of neoplasms, including chondrosarcoma, myxoma, myxosarcoma, other myxoid mesenchymal tumors (e.g. myxoid liposarcoma and myxoid leiomyosarcoma), chordoma, various mucin-producing epithelial tumors, and mast cell tumors.[170–181] Alcian blue has also been used in diagnosis of some nonneoplastic conditions, including gelatinous bone marrow transformation, mucinous bile peritonitis, and primary secretory otitis media.[131,182,183]

Toluidine Blue Toluidine blue staining is a metachromatic method (i.e. the color of the dye when bound to tissue is different than the color of the original dye) that is most often used to highlight mast cell granules, acid mucins, and cartilage (Figure 7.9).[155,184] Although toluidine blue staining is reported in many of the same conditions in which alcian blue staining is positive, it is most commonly used in the diagnosis of mast cell neoplasia.[172,181,185–188] Additionally, toluidine blue has been used to quantify mast cell numbers in canine liver and equine bronchoalveolar lavage cytology samples.[189,190]

Mucicarmine Mucicarmine stains acidic mucins of epithelial origin and has been used to aid a diagnosis of adenoma or adenocarcinoma.[155,177,180,191,192] Mucicarmine will also stain the extracellular mucin in peritoneal fluid from dogs with mucinous bile peritonitis, the non-vacuolated portions of cytoplasm from chordoma cells, and the capsule of *Cryptococcus* spp. yeast.[131,176,193,194]

Other Intracellular and Extracellular Constituents

Alkaline Phosphatase The ALPs are a group of enzymes expressed in many tissues, including liver, bone, kidney, intestine, and placenta, and leukocytes.[195] The cytochemical detection of ALP is most commonly performed through incubation with a NBT/BCIP toluidine salt followed by counterstaining in a modified Romanowsky stain.[196] Diagnostically, ALP cytochemistry is most frequently used to refine a cytologic diagnosis of sarcoma to the more specific diagnosis of osteosarcoma (Figure 7.10). The technique is reported to be quite sensitive (88–100%) and specific (89–94%) when compared with histopathology.[95,196] It is important to note that ALP does not distinguish neoplastic from nonneoplastic bone lesions.[197] Moreover, limited studies have reported ALP positivity in non-osteosarcoma mesenchymal tumors, including two of nine melanomas, two of five chrondosarcomas, one of four gastrointestinal stromal tumors, one of three anaplastic sarcomas, a multilobular tumor of bone, and a collision tumor that included a histiocytic sarcoma and a bronchoalveolar carcinoma.[95,196,197] In addition to mesenchymal tumors, acute myelomonocytic and monocytic leukemia in dogs are reportedly strongly positive for ALP, and acute T-lymphoid leukemias may be weakly positive.[97] Lastly, ALP positivity is reported on tissue sections in some reproductive tumors, either by IHC[198–200] or by Gomori metal salt histochemistry; however, these findings have not be confirmed using traditional cytochemical approaches.[201]

Phosphotungstic Acid–Hematoxylin (Mallory's) The phosphotungstic acid–hematoxylin (PTAH) stain is applied more frequently to tissue sections than cytology slides and is commonly used to identify fibrin, striated muscle, rhabdomyomas, and rhabdomyosarcomas.[149,202–205] Other PTAH-positive tumors and tissue components include

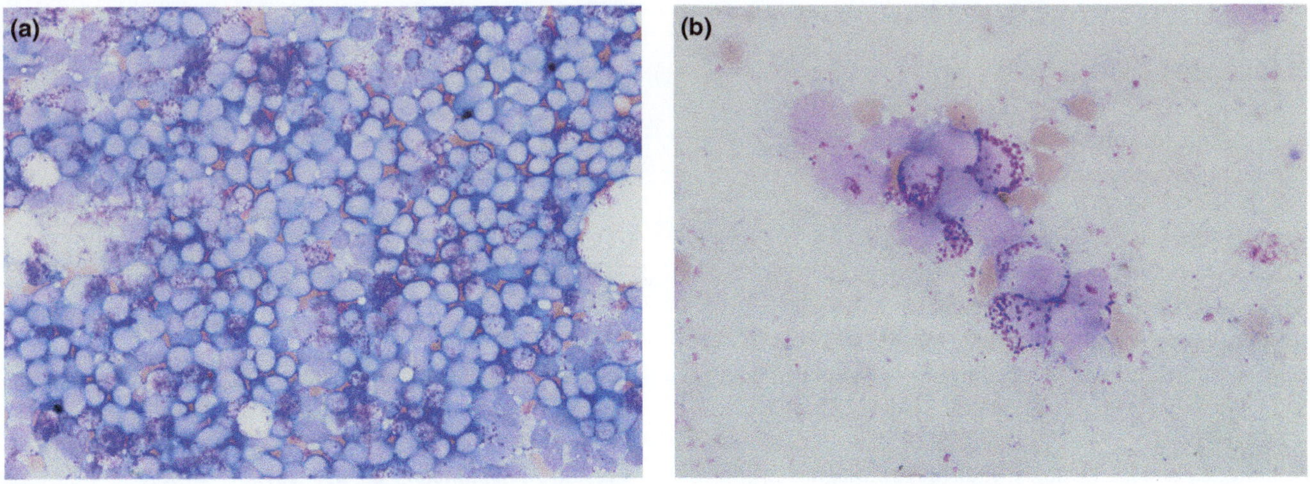

Figure 7.9 Lymph node from a dog with large granular lymphoid leukemia. (a) A methanolic Romanowsky-type stain detects the metachromatic granules in the neoplastic large granular lymphocytes. These granules did not stain with Diff-Quik (not shown) (Wright's, 100×). (b) Toluidine blue highlights the large granules in these cells (1000×. *Source:* Images courtesy of Samantha Evans).

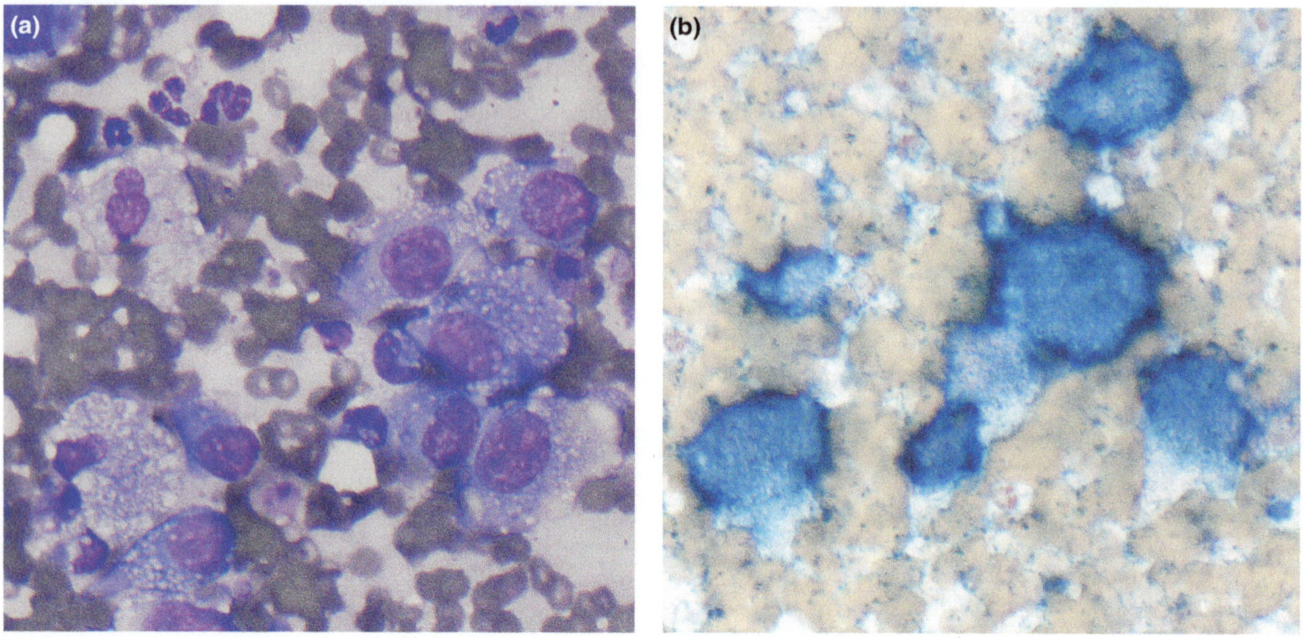

Figure 7.10 Rib mass from a dog. (a) Differential diagnoses for the neoplastic mesenchymal cells included osteosarcoma and histiocytic sarcoma (Wright's, 500×). (b) Positive staining for alkaline phosphatase within the cytoplasm was consistent with a diagnosis of osteosarcoma (500×). These cells did not stain with alpha naphthyl butyrate esterase (not shown).

oncocytoma cell cytoplasmic granules and some granular lymphocyte cytoplasmic granules.[168,206–208]

Congo Red Congo red is a flattened dye molecule that intercalates into the β-pleated sheets of amyloid, which are polypeptides that principally accumulate in extracellular spaces.[140,209–218] This interaction results in bright green birefringence under polarized light.[209] Congo red can be used on tissue sections and on cytology samples, although birefringence is best seen in tissues that are 5–10 μm thick, so thickly prepared cytology slides are recommended for Congo red staining.[140,210–215,217,218] A tissue transfer technique for performing Congo red staining on a portion of the material from a previously stained cytology slide has been described.[33]

Luxol Fast Blue Luxol fast blue is used on nervous system tissue to detect myelin.[219] It has been used to demonstrate myelin-like material on a cerebrospinal fluid cytology sample from a dog.[220]

References

1 Chivukula, M. and Dabbs, D. (2011). Immunocytochemistry. In: *Diagnostic Immunohistochemistry*, 3e (ed. D.J. Dabbs). Philadelphia, PA: W.B. Saunders.

2 Dupré, M.P. and Courtade-Saidi, M. (2012). Immunocytochemistry as an adjunct to diagnostic cytology. *Ann Pathol* 32: e47–e51, 433–437.

3 Skoog, L. and Tani, E. (2011). Immunocytochemistry: an indispensable technique in routine cytology. *Cytopathology* 22: 215–229.

4 Zhang, Z., Zhao, L., Guo, H. et al. (2012). Diagnostic significance of immunocytochemistry on fine needle aspiration biopsies processed by thin-layer cytology. *Diagn Cytopathol* 40: 1071–1076.

5 Fowler, L.J. and Lachar, W.A. (2008). Application of immunohistochemistry to cytology. *Arch Pathol Lab Med* 132: 373–383.

6 Gong, Y., Sun, X., Michael, C.W. et al. (2003). Immunocytochemistry of serous effusion specimens: a comparison of ThinPrep vs cell block. *Diagn Cytopathol* 28: 1–5.

7 Kirbis, I.S., Maxwell, P., Fležar, M.S. et al. (2011). External quality control for immunocytochemistry on cytology samples: a review of UK NEQAS ICC (cytology module) results. *Cytopathology* 22: 230–237.

8 Roh, M.H., Schmidt, L., Placido, J. et al. (2012). The application and diagnostic utility of immunocytochemistry on direct smears in the diagnosis of pulmonary

adenocarcinoma and squamous cell carcinoma. *Diagn Cytopathol* 40: 949–955.

9 Taylor, B.E., Leibman, N.F., Luong, R. et al. (2013). Detection of carcinoma micrometastases in bone marrow of dogs and cats using conventional and cell block cytology. *Vet Clin Pathol* 42: 85–91.

10 Varsegi, G.M. and Shidham, V. (2009). Cell block preparation from cytology specimen with predominance of individually scattered cells. *J Vis Exp* (29): e1316.

11 Bratthauer, G.L. (2010). Processing of tissue culture cells. *Methods Mol Biol* 588: 85–92.

12 Ramos-Vara, J.A. and Miller, M.A. (2014). When tissue antigens and antibodies get along. *Vet Pathol* 51: 42–87.

13 Burry, R.W. (2011). Controls for immunocytochemistry: an update. *J Histochem Cytochem* 59: 6–12.

14 Ramos-Vara, J.A. (2005). Technical aspects of immunohistochemistry. *Vet Pathol* 42: 405–426.

15 Nezlin, R. (2016). Use of aptamers in immunoassays. *Mol Immunol* 70: 149–154.

16 de Marco, A. (2013). Perspectives offered by single-domain antibodies in clinical diagnostic of pediatric tumors. *Curr Med Chem* 20: 2188–2194.

17 Hayat, M. (2002). *Microscopy, Immunohistochemistry, and Antigen Retrieval Methods: For Light and Electron Microscopy*, 1e. New York, NY: Kluwer Academic/Plenum Publishers.

18 Nelson, P.N., Reynolds, G.M., Waldron, E.E. et al. (2000). Monoclonal antibodies. *Mol Pathol* 53: 111–117.

19 Köhler, G. and Milstein, C. (1976). Derivation of specific antibody-producing tissue culture and tumor lines by cell fusion. *Eur J Immunol* 6: 511–519.

20 Fisher, D.J., Naydan, D., Werner, L.L., and Moore, P.F. (1995). Immunophenotyping lymphomas in dogs: a comparison of results from fine needle aspirate and needle biopsy samples. *Vet Clin Pathol* 24: 118–123.

21 Sapierzyński, R. (2010). Practical aspects of immunocytochemistry in canine lymphomas. *Pol J Vet Sci* 13: 661–668.

22 Caniatti, M., Roccabianca, P., Scanziani, E. et al. (1996). Canine lymphoma: immunocytochemical analysis of fine-needle aspiration biopsy. *Vet Pathol* 33: 204–212.

23 Aulbach, A.D., Swenson, C.L., and Kiupel, M. (2010). Optimized processing of fine-needle lymph node biopsies for automated immunostaining. *J Vet Diagn Invest* 22: 383–388.

24 Valli, V., Peters, E., Williams, C. et al. (2009). Optimizing methods in immunocytochemistry: one laboratory's experience. *Vet Clin Pathol* 38: 261–269.

25 Priest, H.L., Hume, K.R., Killick, D. et al. (2017). The use, publication and future directions of immunocytochemistry in veterinary medicine: a consensus of the Oncology-Pathology Working Group. *Vet Comp Oncol* 15: 868–880.

26 Dabbs, D.J. and Wang, X. (1998). Immunocytochemistry on cytologic specimens of limited quantity. *Diagn Cytopathol* 18: 166–169.

27 Ikeda, K., Tate, G., Suzuki, T., and Mitsuya, T. (2011). Comparison of immunocytochemical sensitivity between formalin-fixed and alcohol-fixed specimens reveals the diagnostic value of alcohol-fixed cytocentrifuged preparations in malignant effusion cytology. *Am J Clin Pathol* 136: 934–942.

28 Atkinson, B. (2004). *Atlas of Diagnostic Cytopathology*, 2e. Philadelphia, PA: W.B. Saunders.

29 Fetsch, P.A. and Abati, A. (2010). The clinical immunohistochemistry laboratory: regulations and troubleshooting guidelines. *Methods Mol Biol* 588: 399–412.

30 Venkatraman, L., Catherwood, M.A., Patterson, A. et al. (2006). Role of polymerase chain reaction and immunocytochemistry in the cytological assessment of lymphoid proliferations. *J Clin Pathol* 59: 1160–1165.

31 Höinghaus, R., Hewicker-Trautwein, M., and Mischke, R. (2008). Immunocytochemical differentiation of canine mesenchymal tumors in cytologic imprint preparations. *Vet Clin Pathol* 37: 104–111.

32 Miller, R. and Kubier, P. (2002). Immunohistochemistry on cytologic specimens and previously stained slides (when no paraffin block is available). *J Histotechnol* 25: 251–257.

33 Stone, B.M. and Gan, D. (2014). Application of the tissue transfer technique in veterinary cytopathology. *Vet Clin Pathol* 43: 295–302.

34 Naito, Y., Okabe, Y., Kawahara, A. et al. (2012). Guide to diagnosing primary pancreatic lymphoma, B-cell type: immunocytochemistry improves the diagnostic accuracy of endoscopic ultrasonography-guided fine needle aspiration cytology. *Diagn Cytopathol* 40: 732–736.

35 Abendroth, C.S. and Dabbs, D.J. (1995). Immunocytochemical staining of unstained versus previously stained cytologic preparations. *Acta Cytol* 39: 379–386.

36 Shtilbans, V., Szporn, A.H., Wu, M., and Burstein, D.E. (2005). p63 immunostaining in destained bronchoscopic cytological specimens. *Diagn Cytopathol* 32: 198–203.

37 Koss, L. and Melamed, M. (2006). *Diagnostic Cytology and Its Histopathologic Bases*, 5e. Philadelphia, PA: Lippincott Williams & Wilkins.

38 Ramos-Vara, J.A. and Miller, M.A. (2006). Comparison of two polymer-based immunohistochemical detection systems: ENVISION+? and ImmPRESS? *J Microsc* 224: 135–139.

39 van der Loos, C.M. (2008). Multiple immunoenzyme staining: methods and visualizations for the observation with spectral imaging. *J Histochem Cytochem* 56: 313–328.

40 Jin, Z. and Hildebrandt, N. (2012). Semiconductor quantum dots for in vitro diagnostics and cellular imaging. *Trends Biotechnol* 30: 394–403.

41 Dabbs, D. (2014). *Diagnostic Immunohistochemistry: Theranostic and Genomic Applications*, 4e. Philadelphia, PA: Elsevier/Saunders.

42 Suthipintawong, C., Leong, A.S., Chan, K.W., and Vinyuvat, S. (1997). Immunostaining of estrogen receptor, progesterone receptor, MIB1 antigen, and c-erbB-2 oncoprotein in cytologic specimens: a simplified method with formalin fixation. *Diagn Cytopathol* 17: 127–133.

43 Denda, T., Kamoshida, S., Kawamura, J. et al. (2012). Optimal antigen retrieval for ethanol-fixed cytologic smears. *Cancer Cytopathol* 120: 167–176.

44 van Hecke, D. (2002). Routine immunohistochemical staining today: choices to make, challenges to take. *J Histotechnol* 25: 45–54.

45 Ramos-Vara, J.A., Kiupel, M., Baszler, T. et al. (2008). Suggested guidelines for immunohistochemical techniques in veterinary diagnostic laboratories. *J Vet Diagn Invest* 20: 393–413.

46 Ramos-Vara, J.A. and Miller, M.A. (2007). Immunohistochemical detection of protein gene product 9.5 (PGP 9.5) in canine epitheliotropic T-cell lymphoma (mycosis fungoides). *Vet Pathol* 44: 74–79.

47 Ramos-Vara, J.A., Miller, M.A., Johnson, G.C. et al. (2002). Melan A and S100 protein immunohistochemistry in feline melanomas: 48 cases. *Vet Pathol* 39: 127–132.

48 Ramos-Vara, J.A., Frank, C.B., DuSold, D., and Miller, M.A. (2014). Immunohistochemical expression of melanocytic antigen PNL2, Melan A, S100, and PGP 9.5 in equine melanocytic neoplasms. *Vet Pathol* 51: 161–166.

49 Raskin, R. and Meyer, D. (2016). *Canine and Feline Cytology: A Color Atlas and Interpretation Guide*, 3e. St. Louis, MO: Elsevier.

50 Jain, S., Aresu, L., Comazzi, S. et al. (2016). The development of a recombinant scFv monoclonal antibody targeting canine CD20 for use in comparative medicine. *PLoS One* 11: e0148366.

51 Rue, S.M., Eckelman, B.P., Efe, J.A. et al. (2015). Identification of a candidate therapeutic antibody for treatment of canine B-cell lymphoma. *Vet Immunol Immunopathol* 164: 148–159.

52 Sawa, M., Yabuki, A., Setoguchi, A., and Yamato, O. (2015). Development and application of multiple immunofluorescence staining for diagnostic cytology of canine and feline lymphoma. *Vet Clin Pathol* 44: 580–585.

53 Vail, D.M., Kravis, L.D., Kisseberth, W.C. et al. (1997). Application of rapid CD3 immunophenotype analysis and argyrophilic nucleolar organizer region (AgNOR) frequency to fine needle aspirate specimens from dogs with lymphoma. *Vet Clin Pathol* 26: 66–69.

54 Sapierzyński, R., Dolka, I., and Fabisiak, M. (2012). High agreement of routine cytopathology and immunocytochemistry in canine lymphomas. *Pol J Vet Sci* 15: 247–252.

55 Kol, A., Christopher, M.M., Skorupski, K.A. et al. (2013). B-cell lymphoma with plasmacytoid differentiation, atypical cytoplasmic inclusions, and secondary leukemia in a dog. *Vet Clin Pathol* 42: 40–46.

56 Granum, L., Gorman, E., Ruaux, C., and Vernau, W. (2015). Biphenotypic B-cell lymphoma in 2 cats. *Vet Clin Pathol* 44: 320–325.

57 Cian, F., Tyner, G., Martini, V. et al. (2013). Leukemic small cell lymphoma or chronic lymphocytic leukemia in a horse. *Vet Clin Pathol* 42: 301–306.

58 Bauer, N.B., Zervos, D., and Moritz, A. (2007). Argyrophilic nucleolar organizing regions and Ki67 equally reflect proliferation in fine needle aspirates of normal, hyperplastic, inflamed, and neoplastic canine lymph nodes (n = 101). *J Vet Intern Med* 21: 928–935.

59 Wallace, K.A., Goldschmidt, M.H., and Patel, R.T. (2015). Converting fluid-based cytologic specimens to histologic specimens for immunohistochemistry. *Vet Clin Pathol* 44: 303–309.

60 Turinelli, V., Marchal, T., Ponce, F. et al. (2005). Aggressive large granular lymphocyte lymphomas in five dogs: a clinical cytohistolgoical and immunological study. *Comp Clin Path* 13: 109–118.

61 Moore, P.F. (2014). A review of histiocytic diseases of dogs and cats. *Vet Pathol* 51: 167–184.

62 Sapierzyński, R., Jagielski, D., Dolka, I., and Jagielski, D. (2012). Cytopathological diagnosis of visceral histiocytic sarcoma in five dogs. *Pol J Vet Sci* 15: 751–758.

63 Tzipory, L., Vernau, K.M., Sturges, B.K. et al. (2009). Antemortem diagnosis of localized central nervous system histiocytic sarcoma in 2 dogs. *J Vet Intern Med* 23: 369–374.

64 Zimmerman, K., Almy, F., Carter, L. et al. (2006). Cerebrospinal fluid from a 10-year-old dog with a single seizure episode. *Vet Clin Pathol* 35: 127–131.

65 Stowe, D.M., Escobar, C., and Neel, J.A. (2012). What is your diagnosis? Cerebrospinal fluid from a dog. *Vet Clin Pathol* 41: 429–430.

66 Cluzel, C., Aboulmali, A.A., Dugas, S. et al. (2016). Diffuse leptomeningeal histiocytic sarcoma in the cerebrospinal fluid of 2 dogs. *Vet Clin Pathol* 45: 184–190.

67 Allison, R.W., Brunker, J.D., Breshears, M.A. et al. (2008). Dendritic cell leukemia in a Golden Retriever. *Vet Clin Pathol* 37: 190–197.

68 Rossi, S., Gelain, M.E., and Comazzi, S. (2009). Disseminated histiocytic sarcoma with peripheral blood involvement in a Bernese Mountain dog. *Vet Clin Pathol* 38: 126–130.

69 Pinto da Cunha, N., Ghisleni, G., Scarampella, F. et al. (2014). Cytologic and immunocytochemical characterization of feline progressive histiocytosis. *Vet Clin Pathol* 43: 428–436.

70 Höinghaus, R., Hewicker-Trautwein, M., and Mischke, R. (2007). Immunocytochemical differentiation of neoplastic and hyperplastic canine epithelial lesions in cytologic imprint preparations. *Vet J* 173: 79–90.

71 Höinghaus, R., von Wasielewski, R., Hewicker-Trautwein, M. et al. (2007). Immunocytological detection of lymph node metastases in dogs with malignant epithelial tumours. *J Comp Pathol* 137: 1–8.

72 Colledge, S.L., Raskin, R.E., Messick, J.B. et al. (2013). Multiple joint metastasis of a transitional cell carcinoma in a dog. *Vet Clin Pathol* 42: 216–220.

73 Sprague, W. and Thrall, M.A. (2001). Recurrent skin mass from the digit of a dog. *Vet Clin Pathol* 30: 189–192.

74 Przeździecki, R. and Sapierzyński, R. (2014). Using of immunocytochemistry in differential diagnosis of neoplasms of serosal cavities in dogs. *Pol J Vet Sci* 17: 149–159.

75 Sawa, M., Yabuki, A., Miyoshi, N. et al. (2012). A simple and rapid immunocytochemical technique for detection of cytokeratin, vimentin, and S-100 protein in veterinary diagnostic cytology. *Res Vet Sci* 93: 1341–1345.

76 Grieco, V., Patton, V., Romussi, S., and Finazzi, M. (2003). Cytokeratin and vimentin expression in normal and neoplastic canine prostate. *J Comp Pathol* 129: 78–84.

77 Piane, L., Sayag, D., Lermuzeaux, J. et al. (2014). What is your diagnosis? Abnormal cells on a blood smear from a dog. *Vet Clin Pathol* 43: 461–462.

78 Mischke, R., Höinghaus, R., Lütkefels, E. et al. (2003). Immunocytological confirmation of bone marrow metastases in a dog with cholangiocarcinoma. *J Small Anim Pract* 44: 411–414.

79 Munakata, S., Aihara, T., Morino, H., and Takatsuka, Y. (2003). Application of immunofluorescence for intraoperative evaluation of sentinel lymph nodes in patients with breast carcinoma. *Cancer* 98: 1562–1568.

80 Salem, A.A., Douglas-Jones, A.G., Sweetland, H.M. et al. (2002). Evaluation of axillary lymph nodes using touch imprint cytology and immunohistochemistry. *Br J Surg* 89: 1386–1389.

81 Andreasen, C.B., Mahaffey, E.A., and Duncan, J.R. (1988). Intermediate filament staining in the cytologic and histologic diagnosis of canine skin and soft tissue tumors. *Vet Pathol* 25: 343–349.

82 Avallone, G., Pinto da Cunha, N., Palmieri, C. et al. (2010). Subcutaneous embryonal rhabdomyosarcoma in a dog: cytologic, immunocytochemical, histologic, and ultrastructural features. *Vet Clin Pathol* 39: 499–504.

83 Höinghaus, R., Mischke, R., and Hewicker-Trautwein, M. (2002). Use of immunocytochemical techniques in canine melanoma. *J Vet Med A Physiol Pathol Clin Med* 49: 198–202.

84 Przeździecki, R., Czopowicz, M., and Sapierzyński, R. (2015). Accuracy of routine cytology and immunocytochemistry in preoperative diagnosis of oral amelanotic melanomas in dogs. *Vet Clin Pathol* 44: 597–604.

85 Hasteh, F., Lin, G.Y., Weidner, N., and Michael, C.W. (2010). The use of immunohistochemistry to distinguish reactive mesothelial cells from malignant mesothelioma in cytologic effusions. *Cancer Cytopathol* 118: 90–96.

86 Headley, S.A., Voltarelli, D., de Oliveira, V.H.S. et al. (2015). Association of *Histophilus somni* with spontaneous abortions in dairy cattle herds from Brazil. *Trop Anim Health Prod* 47: 403–413.

87 Giordano, A., Paltrinieri, S., Bertazzolo, W. et al. (2005). Sensitivity of Tru-cut and fine needle aspiration biopsies of liver and kidney for diagnosis of feline infectious peritonitis. *Vet Clin Pathol* 34: 368–374.

88 Johns, J.L., Luff, J.A., Shooshtari, M.P. et al. (2009). What is your diagnosis? Blood smear from an injured red-tailed hawk. *Vet Clin Pathol* 38: 247–252.

89 Brazzell, J.L., Kaese, H.J., and Borjesson, D.L. (2006). Bold fusion: transtracheal wash from a Jersey calf. *Vet Clin Pathol* 35: 247–249.

90 Zuccari, D.A.P.C., Santana, A.E., Cury, P.M., and Cordeiro, J.A. (2004). Immunocytochemical study of Ki-67 as a prognostic marker in canine mammary neoplasia. *Vet Clin Pathol* 33: 23–28.

91 Neumann, S. and Kaup, F.-J. (2005). Usefulness of Ki-67 proliferation marker in the cytologic identification of liver tumors in dogs. *Vet Clin Pathol* 34: 132–136.

92 Sailasuta, A., Ketpun, D., Piyaviriyakul, P. et al. (2014). The relevance of CD117 immunocytochemistry staining patterns to mutational exon-11 in c-kit detected by PCR from fine-needle aspirated canine mast cell tumor cells. *Vet Med Int* 2014: 1–8.

93 Horobin, R. (2013). How histological stains work. In: *Bancroft's Theory and Practice of Histological Techniques* (eds. S.K. Suvarna, C. Layton and J.D. Bancroft). London: Churchill, Livingstone, Elsevier.

94 Marcos, R., Santos, M., Santos, N. et al. (2009). Use of destained cytology slides for the application of routine special stains. *Vet Clin Pathol* 38: 94–102.

95 Ryseff, J.K. and Bohn, A.A. (2012). Detection of alkaline phosphatase in canine cells previously stained with Wright-Giemsa and its utility in differentiating osteosarcoma from other mesenchymal tumors. *Vet Clin Pathol* 41: 391–395.

96 Raskin, R. (2010). Cytochemical staining. In: *Schalm's Veterinary Hematology*, 6e (eds. D.J. Weiss and K.J. Wardrop), 391–395. Ames, IA: Wiley-Blackwell.

97 Stokol, T., Schaefer, D.M., Shuman, M. et al. (2015). Alkaline phosphatase is a useful cytochemical marker for the diagnosis of acute myelomonocytic and monocytic leukemia in the dog. *Vet Clin Pathol* 44: 79–93.

98 Bezjian, M., Diep, A.N., de Matos, R., and Schaefer, D. (2013). Chinese Box turtle (*Cuora flavomarginata*) with lymphoid leukemia characterized by immunohistochemical and cytochemical phenotyping. *Vet Clin Pathol* 42: 368–376.

99 Silverstone, A., Garner, M.M., Wojcieszyn, J.W. et al. (2007). Acute lymphoblastic leukemia in a diamondback terrapin, *Malaclemys terrapin*. *J Herpetol Med Surg* 17: 92–99.

100 Modiano, J.F., Smith, R., Wojcieszyn, J. et al. (1998). The use of cytochemistry, immunophenotyping, flow cytometry, and in vitro differentiation to determine the ontogeny of a canine monoblastic leukemia. *Vet Clin Pathol* 27: 40–49.

101 Woolford, L., Wong, A., Sneath, H.L. et al. (2015). Hematology of dugongs (*Dugong dugon*) in southern Queensland. *Vet Clin Pathol* 44: 530–541.

102 Salakij, C., Salakij, J., Prihirunkit, K. et al. (2014). Quantitative and qualitative morphologic, cytochemical, and ultrastructural characteristics of blood cells in captive Asian water monitors. *Vet Clin Pathol* 43: 538–546.

103 Bricker, N.K., Raskin, R.E., and Densmore, C.L. (2012). Cytochemical and immunocytochemical characterization of blood cells and immunohistochemical analysis of spleen cells from 2 species of frog, *Rana (Aquarana) catesbeiana* and *Xenopus laevis*. *Vet Clin Pathol* 41: 353–361.

104 Clark, P. and Swenson, C.L. (1999). Cytochemical staining characteristics of leukocytes of the common brushtail possum (*Trichosurus vulpecula*). *Aust Vet J* 77: 605–606.

105 Work, T.M., Raskin, R.E., Balazs, G.H., and Whittaker, S.D. (1998). Morphologic and cytochemical characteristics of blood cells from Hawaiian green turtles. *Am J Vet Res* 59: 1252–1257.

106 Alleman, A.R., Jacobson, E.R., and Raskin, R.E. (1992). Morphologic and cytochemical characteristics of blood cells from the desert tortoise (*Gopherus agassizii*). *Am J Vet Res* 53: 1645–1651.

107 Wong, V.M., Snyman, H.N., Ackerley, C., and Bienzle, D. (2012). Primary nasal histiocytic sarcoma of macrophage-myeloid cell type in a cat. *J Comp Pathol* 147: 209–213.

108 Lester, G.D., Alleman, A.R., Raskin, R.E., and Mays, M.B. (1993). Malignant histiocytosis in an Arabian filly. *Equine Vet J* 25: 471–473.

109 Wellman, M.L., Krakowka, S., Jacobs, R.M., and Kociba, G.J. (1988). A macrophage-monocyte cell line from a dog with malignant histiocytosis. *In Vitro Cell Dev Biol* 24: 223–229.

110 Gale, E., Torrance, J., and Bothwell, T. (1963). The quantitative estimation of total iron stores in human bone marrow. *J Clin Invest* 42: 1076–1082.

111 Phiri, K.S., Calis, J.C.J., Kachala, D. et al. (2009). Improved method for assessing iron stores in the bone marrow. *J Clin Pathol* 62: 685–689.

112 Harvey, J.W. (ed.) (2009). Evaluation of erythrocytes. In: *Veterinary Hematology: A Diagnostic Guide and Color Atlas*, 49–121. St. Louis, MO: Elsevier-Saunders.

113 Gaunt, S.O. and Baker, D.C. (1986). Hemosiderin in leukocytes of dogs with immune-mediated hemolytic anemia. *Vet Clin Pathol* 15: 8–10.

114 Mete, A., Hendriks, H.G., Klaren, P.H.M. et al. (2003). Iron metabolism in mynah birds (*Gracula religiosa*) resembles human hereditary haemochromatosis. *Avian Pathol* 32: 625–632.

115 Sprague, W.S., Hackett, T.B., Johnson, J.S., and Swardson-Olver, C.J. (2003). Hemochromatosis secondary to repeated blood transfusions in a dog. *Vet Pathol* 40: 334–337.

116 Whittemore, J.C., Newkirk, K.M., Reel, D.M., and Reed, A. (2012). Hepatic copper and iron accumulation and histologic findings in 104 feline liver biopsies. *J Vet Diagn Invest* 24: 656–661.

117 Doucet, M.Y. and Viel, L. (2002). Alveolar macrophage graded hemosiderin score from bronchoalveolar lavage in horses with exercise-induced pulmonary hemorrhage and controls. *J Vet Intern Med* 16: 281–286.

118 Barger, A. and Riensche, M. (2009). What is your diagnosis? Hemorrhagic effusion in a dog. *Vet Clin Pathol* 38: 529–531.

119 Orchard, G. (2013). Pigments and minerals. In: *Bancroft's Theory and Practice of Histological Techniques*, 7e (eds. S.K. Suvarna, C. Layton and J.D. Bancroft), 239–270. London: Churchill, Livingstone, Elsevier.

120 Johnson, G.F., Gilbertson, S.R., Goldfischer, S. et al. (1984). Cytochemical detection of inherited copper toxicosis of Bedlington terriers. *Vet Pathol* 21: 57–60.

121 Ramirez, C.J., Kim, D.Y., Hanks, B.C., and Evans, T.J. (2013). Copper toxicosis in New Zealand White rabbits (*Oryctolagus cuniculus*). *Vet Pathol* 50: 1135–1138.

122 Moore, A.R., Coffey, E., and Hamar, D. (2016). Diagnostic accuracy of Wright-Giemsa and rhodanine stain protocols for detection and semi-quantitative grading of copper in canine liver aspirates. *Vet Clin Pathol* 45: 689–697.

123 Teske, E., Brinkhuis, B.G., Bode, P. et al. (1992). Cytological detection of copper for the diagnosis of inherited copper toxicosis in Bedlington terriers. *Vet Rec* 131: 30–32.

124 Marcos, R., Santos, M., Oliveira, J. et al. (2006). Cytochemical detection of calcium in a case of calcinosis circumscripta in a dog. *Vet Clin Pathol* 35: 239–242.
125 Radi, Z.A. and Sato, K. (2010). Bilateral dystrophic calcinosis circumscripta in a cynomolgus macaque (*Macaca fascicularis*). *Toxicol Pathol* 38: 637–641.
126 Nguyen, F., Cherel, Y., Guigand, L. et al. (2002). Muscle lesions associated with dystrophin deficiency in neonatal Golden Retriever puppies. *J Comp Pathol* 126: 100–108.
127 Valentine, B.A., Cooper, B.J., Cummings, J.F., and de Lahunta, A. (1990). Canine X-linked muscular dystrophy: morphologic lesions. *J Neurol Sci* 97: 1–23.
128 Speight, K.N., Boardman, W., Breed, W.G. et al. (2013). Pathological features of oxalate nephrosis in a population of koalas (*Phascolarctos cinereus*) in south Australia. *Vet Pathol* 50: 299–307.
129 Chae, I.H., Kwon, H.J., Kim, E.-K. et al. (2016). Value of additional von Kossa staining in thyroid nodules with echogenic spots on ultrasound. *Pathol Res Pract* 212: 415–420.
130 Ringenberg, M.A., Neitzel, L.E., and Zachary, J.F. (2000). Meningeal osteosarcoma in a dog. *Vet Pathol* 37: 653–655.
131 Owens, S.D., Gossett, R., McElhaney, M.R. et al. (2003). Three cases of canine bile peritonitis with mucinous material in abdominal fluid as the prominent cytologic finding. *Vet Clin Pathol* 32: 114–120.
132 Merchant, S.H., Haghir, S., and Gordon, G.B. (2000). Granulomatous peritonitis after laparoscopic cholecystectomy mimicking pelvic endometriosis. *Obstet Gynecol* 96: 830–831.
133 Stern, A.W. and Lamm, C.G. (2009). Malignant melanoma of the subcutaneous tissues in an Umbrella Cockatoo (*Cacatua alba*). *J Avian Med Surg* 23: 303–306.
134 Vala, H., Pópulo, H., Mesquita, J.R. et al. (2012). Melanocytic tumour in a black sheep never exposed to ultraviolet radiation. *J Comp Pathol* 146: 160–164.
135 Schulman, F.Y., Lipscomb, T.P., and Atkin, T.J. (2005). Canine cutaneous clear cell adnexal carcinoma: histopathology, immunohistochemistry, and biologic behavior of 26 cases. *J Vet Diagn Invest* 17: 403–411.
136 Gregory, C.R., Harmon, B.G., Latimer, K.S. et al. (1997). Malignant chromatophoroma in a canebrake rattlesnake (*Crotalus horridus atricaudatus*). *J Zoo Wildl Med* 28: 198–203.
137 Barbosa, A.J., Castro, L.P., Margarida, A., and Nogueira, M.F. (1984). A simple and economical modification of the Masson-Fontana method for staining melanin granules and enterochromaffin cells. *Stain Technol* 59: 193–196.
138 Masserdotti, C., Bonfanti, U., De Lorenzi, D., and Ottolini, N. (2006). Use of Oil Red O stain in the cytologic diagnosis of canine liposarcoma. *Vet Clin Pathol* 35: 37–41.
139 Choi, U.S., Seo, K.W., Oh, S.-Y. et al. (2005). Intra-abdominal mass aspirate from a cat in heat. *Vet Clin Pathol* 34: 275–277.
140 Tei, M., Uchida, K., Chambers, J.K. et al. (2012). Mammary lipid-rich carcinoma with extensive amyloid deposition in a dog. *J Vet Med Sci* 74: 809–811.
141 Dobromylskyj, M.J., Copas, V., Durham, A. et al. (2011). Disseminated lipid-rich peritoneal mesothelioma in a horse. *J Vet Diagn Invest* 23: 615–618.
142 Hunt, G.B., Luff, J.A., Daniel, L., and Van den Bergh, R. (2013). Evaluation of hepatic steatosis in dogs with congenital portosystemic shunts using Oil Red O staining. *Vet Pathol* 50: 1109–1115.
143 Trott, K.A., Giannitti, F., Rimoldi, G. et al. (2014). Fatty liver hemorrhagic syndrome in the backyard chicken. *Vet Pathol* 51: 787–795.
144 Brown, J.S., Johnson, M.C., Sims, W.P. et al. (2011). Oil Red O-positive lipid in peritoneal fluid from a horse with a rectal tear. *Vet Clin Pathol* 40: 265–269.
145 Yhee, J.-Y., Yu, C.-H., Kim, J.-H., and Sur, J.H. (2008). Effects of T lymphocytes, interleukin-1, and interleukin-6 on renal fibrosis in canine end-stage renal disease. *J Vet Diagn Invest* 20: 585–592.
146 Sánchez-Lara, A.C., Elliott, J., Syme, H.M. et al. (2015). Feline chronic kidney disease is associated with upregulation of transglutaminase 2: a collagen cross-linking enzyme. *Vet Pathol* 52: 513–523.
147 Teredesai, A. and Wohrmann, T. (2005). Metastasizing seminal vesicle adenocarcinoma in a Wistar rat. *J Vet Med Ser A* 52: 131–134.
148 Mete, A., Woods, L., Famini, D., and Anderson, M. (2012). Disseminated pleomorphic myofibrosarcoma in a grizzly bear (*Ursus arctos horribilis*). *J Comp Pathol* 147: 376–380.
149 Bancroft, J. and Layton, C. (2013). Connective and mesenchymal tissues with their stains. In: *Bancroft's Theory and Practice of Histological Techniques*, 7e, 187–214. London: Churchill, Livingstone, Elsevier.
150 Blue, J.T. (1988). Myelofibrosis in cats with myelodysplastic syndrome and acute myelogenous leukemia. *Vet Pathol* 25: 154–160.
151 Thiele, J., Kvasnicka, H.M., Facchetti, F. et al. (2005). European consensus on grading bone marrow fibrosis and assessment of cellularity. *Haematologica* 90: 1128–1132.
152 Karttunen, T., Alavaikko, M., Apaja-Sarkkinen, M., and Autio-Harmainen, H. (1988). An immunohistochemical study of laminin, type-IV collagen and type-III pN-

collagen with relation to reticular fibres in Hodgkin's disease. *Int J cancer* 41: 52–58.

153 Yang, G.C.H., Yang, G.-Y., and Tao, L.-C. (2003). Cytologic features and histologic correlations of microacinar and microtrabecular types of well-differentiated hepatocellular carcinoma in fine-needle aspiration biopsy. *Cancer* 102: 27–33.

154 Grossniklaus, H.E., Waring, G.O., Akor, C. et al. (2003). Evaluation of hematoxylin and eosin and special stains for the detection of acanthamoeba keratitis in penetrating keratoplasties. *Am J Ophthalmol* 136: 520–526.

155 Layton, C. and Bancroft, J. (2013). Carbohydrates. In: *Bancroft's Theory and Practice of Histological Techniques*, 7e (eds. S.K. Suvarna, C. Layton and J.D. Bancroft), 157–171. London: Churchill, Livingstone, Elsevier.

156 Kumar, R. and Dey, P. (2016). Fine-needle aspiration cytology of non-neoplastic adrenal pathology. *Diagn Cytopathol* 44: 472–476.

157 McCue, M.E., Armién, A.G., Lucio, M. et al. (2009). Comparative skeletal muscle histopathologic and ultrastructural features in two forms of polysaccharide storage myopathy in horses. *Vet Pathol* 46: 1281–1291.

158 Bisby, T.M., Pratt, S.M., Kent Fenton, R. et al. (2009). What is your diagnosis? Perifemoral mass in a cow. *Vet Clin Pathol* 38: 343–347.

159 Benoit-Biancamano, M.-O., Morin, M., and Langlois, I. (2005). Histopathologic lesions of diabetes mellitus in a domestic ferret. *Can Vet J* 46: 895–897.

160 Langohr, I.M. and Tanabe, M. (2005). Idiopathic complex polysaccharide storage disease in an abyssinian cat. *Vet Pathol* 42: 502–506.

161 Kanehara, T., Matsui, N., Murakami, M. et al. (2016). B-cell lymphoma with Mott cell differentiation in a cat. *Vet Clin Pathol* 45: 356–360.

162 Stacy, N.I., Nabity, M.B., Hackendahl, N. et al. (2009). B-cell lymphoma with Mott cell differentiation in two young adult dogs. *Vet Clin Pathol* 38: 113–120.

163 Kodama, A., Sakai, H., Kobayashi, K. et al. (2008). B-cell intestinal lymphoma with Mott cell differentiation in a 1-year-old miniature Dachshund. *Vet Clin Pathol* 37: 409–415.

164 Patnaik, A.K. (1993). Histologic and immunohistochemical studies of granular cell tumors in seven dogs, three cats, one horse, and one bird. *Vet Pathol* 30: 176–185.

165 Campos, C.B., Nunes, F.C., Gamba, C.O. et al. (2015). Canine low-grade intra-orbital myxosarcoma: case report. *Vet Ophthalmol* 18: 251–253.

166 Brown, C.A., Elliott, J., Schmiedt, C.W., and Brown, S.A. (2016). Chronic kidney disease in aged cats: clinical features, morphology, and proposed pathogeneses. *Vet Pathol* 53: 309–326.

167 Quigley, K.A., Jackson, M.L., and Haines, D.M. (2001). Hyperlipasemia in 6 dogs with pancreatic or hepatic neoplasia: evidence for tumor lipase production. *Vet Clin Pathol* 30: 114–120.

168 Doughty, R.W., Brockman, D., Neiger, R., and McKinney, L. (2006). Nasal oncocytoma in a domestic shorthair cat. *Vet Pathol* 43: 751–754.

169 Buergelt, C.D. and Adjiri-Awere, A. (2000). Bilateral renal oncocytoma in a Greyhound dog. *Vet Pathol* 37: 188–192.

170 Akkoc, A., Ozyigit, M.O., and Cangul, I.T. (2007). Valvular cardiac myxoma in a dog. *J Vet Med Ser A* 54: 356–358.

171 Khachatryan, A.R., Wills, T.B., and Potter, K.A. (2009). What is your diagnosis? Vertebral mass in a dog. *Vet Clin Pathol* 38: 257–260.

172 Chikata, S., Nakamura, S., Katayama, R. et al. (2006). Primary chondrosarcoma in the liver of a dog. *Vet Pathol* 43: 1033–1036.

173 Forlani, A., Roccabianca, P., Palmieri, C. et al. (2015). Pathological characterization of primary splenic myxoid liposarcomas in three dogs. *Vet Q* 35: 181–184.

174 Boyd, S.P., Taugner, F.M., Serrano, S. et al. (2005). Matrix "blues": clue to a cranial thoracic mass in a dog. *Vet Clin Pathol* 34: 271–274.

175 Labelle, P. and Holmberg, B.J. (2010). Ocular myxoid leiomyosarcoma in a cat. *Vet Ophthalmol* 13: 58–62.

176 Yui, T., Ohmachi, T., Matsuda, K. et al. (2015). Histochemical and immunohistochemical characterization of chordoma in ferrets. *J Vet Med Sci* 77: 467–473.

177 Brunetti, B., Sarli, G., Marcato, P.S., and Benazzi, C. Histochemical and immunohistochemical characterization of canine mammary mucinous carcinoma. *J Comp Pathol* 129: 131–136.

178 Sakai, H., Murakami, M., Mishima, H. et al. (2012). Cytologically atypical anal sac adenocarcinoma in a dog. *Vet Clin Pathol* 41: 291–294.

179 Monteiro, L.N., Salgado, B.S., Grandi, F. et al. (2011). Ovarian mucinous cystadenoma in a gray brocket deer (*Mazama gouazoupira*). *J Vet Diagn Invest* 23: 589–592.

180 Radi, Z.A., Miller, D.L., and Hines, M.E. (2004). Rete testis mucinous adenocarcinoma in a dog. *Vet Pathol* 41: 75–78.

181 Simoes, J.P.C. and Schoning, P. (1994). Canine mast cell tumors: a comparison of staining techniques. *J Vet Diagn Invest* 6: 458–465.

182 Beeler-Marfisi, J., Gallastegui Menoyo, A., Beck, A. et al. (2011). Gelatinous marrow transformation and hematopoietic atrophy in a miniature horse stallion. *Vet Pathol* 48: 451–455.

183 Weinstein, N.M., Boes, K.M., Mauldin, E., and Rossmeisl, J. (2016). What is your diagnosis? Middle ear material from a dog. *Vet Clin Pathol* 45: 195–196.

184 Sridharan, G. and Shankar, A.A. (2012). Toluidine blue: a review of its chemistry and clinical utility. *J Oral Maxillofac Pathol* 16: 251–255.

185 Martínez, J., Martínez, V., Grau-Roma, L. et al. (2011). Multiple cutaneous mast cell tumors in a pig. *J Vet Diagn Invest* 23: 1222–1225.

186 Millward, L.M., Hamberg, A., Mathews, J. et al. (2010). Multicentric mast cell tumors in a horse. *Vet Clin Pathol* 39: 365–370.

187 Makino, T., Utsunomiya, T., Kamino, Y. et al. (2002). Nerve sheath myxoma of the tongue in a child. *Int J Oral Maxillofac Surg* 31: 451–454.

188 Kindblom, L.G. and Angervall, L. (1975). Histochemical characterization of mucosubstances in bone and soft tissue-tumors. *Cancer* 36: 985–994.

189 Masserdotti, C. (2013). Proportion of mast cells in normal canine hepatic cytologic specimens: comparison of 2 staining methods. *Vet Clin Pathol* 42: 522–525.

190 Leclere, M., Desnoyers, M., Beauchamp, G., and Lavoie, J.P. Comparison of four staining methods for detection of mast cells in equine bronchoalveolar lavage fluid. *J Vet Intern Med* 20: 377–381.

191 Loynachan, A.T., Bryant, U.K., and Williams, N.M. (2008). Renal mucus gland cystadenomas in a horse. *J Vet Diagn Invest* 20: 520–522.

192 Corapi, W.V., Rodrigues, A., and Lawhorn, D.B. (2011). Mucinous adenocarcinoma and T-cell lymphoma in the small intestine of 2 Vietnamese potbellied pigs (*Sus scrofa*). *Vet Pathol* 48: 1004–1007.

193 Headley, S.A., Di Santis, G.W., de Alcântara, B.K. et al. (2015). *Cryptococcus gattii*-induced infections in dogs from southern Brazil. *Mycopathologia* 180: 265–275.

194 Mandrioli, L., Bettini, G., Marcato, P.S. et al. (2002). Central nervous system cryptococcoma in a cat. *J Vet Med A Physiol Pathol Clin Med* 49: 526–530.

195 Fernandez, N.J. and Kidney, B.A. (2007). Alkaline phosphatase: beyond the liver. *Vet Clin Pathol* 36: 223–233.

196 Barger, A., Graca, R., Bailey, K. et al. (2005). Use of alkaline phosphatase staining to differentiate canine osteosarcoma from other vimentin-positive tumors. *Vet Pathol* 42: 161–165.

197 Britt, T., Clifford, C., Barger, A. et al. (2007). Diagnosing appendicular osteosarcoma with ultrasound-guided fine-needle aspiration: 36 cases. *J Small Anim Pract* 48: 145–150.

198 Yu, C.-H., Hwang, D.-N., Yhee, J.-Y. et al. (2009). Comparative immunohistochemical characterization of canine seminomas and Sertoli cell tumors. *J Vet Sci* 10: 1–7.

199 Banco, B., Giudice, C., Ghisleni, G. et al. (2015). Immunohistochemical study of mixed germ cell sex cord stromal tumours in 13 canine testes. *J Comp Pathol* 152: 182–187.

200 Park, J., Goo, M., Hong, I. et al. (2009). Immunohistochemistry diagnosis of an ovarian dysgerminoma in one bitch. *Reprod Domest Anim* 44: 855–858.

201 Chandra, A.M., Woodard, J.C., and Merritt, A.M. (1998). Dysgerminoma in an Arabian filly. *Vet Pathol* 35: 308–311.

202 Cotovio, M., Monreal, L., Armengou, L. et al. (2008). Fibrin deposits and organ failure in newborn foals with severe septicemia. *J Vet Intern Med* 22: 1403–1410.

203 Cesarini, C., Cotovio, M., Ríos, J. et al. (2016). Association between necropsy evidence of disseminated intravascular coagulation and hemostatic variables before death in horses with colic. *J Vet Intern Med* 30: 269–275.

204 Dunbar, M.D., Ginn, P., Winter, M. et al. (2012). Laryngeal rhabdomyoma in a dog. *Vet Clin Pathol* 41: 590–593.

205 Chapman, S., Nabity, M., and Calise, D. (2008). What is your diagnosis? Lingual mass in a dog. *Vet Clin Pathol* 37: 133–139.

206 You, M.-H., Kim, Y.-B., Woo, G.-H. et al. (2011). Nasopharyngeal oncocytoma in a cat. *J Vet Diagn Invest* 23: 391–394.

207 Herraez, P., Berridge, B., Marsh, P. et al. (2001). Small intestine large granular lymphoma in a horse. *Vet Pathol* 38: 223–226.

208 Pohlman, L.M., Higginbotham, M.L., Welles, E.G., and Johnson, C.M. (2009). Immunophenotypic and histologic classification of 50 cases of feline gastrointestinal lymphoma. *Vet Pathol* 46: 259–268.

209 Gilbertson, J. and Hunt, T. (2013). Amyloid. In: *Bancroft's Theory and Practice of Histological Techniques*, 7e (eds. S.K. Suvarna, C. Layton and J.D. Bancroft), 271–290. London: Churchill, Livingstone, Elsevier.

210 Paltrinieri, S., Sironi, G., Giori, L. et al. (2015). Changes in serum and urine SAA concentrations and qualitative and quantitative proteinuria in Abyssinian cats with familial amyloidosis: a five-year longitudinal study (2009–2014). *J Vet Intern Med* 29: 505–512.

211 Segev, G., Cowgill, L.D., Jessen, S. et al. (2012). Renal amyloidosis in dogs: a retrospective study of 91 cases with comparison of the disease between Shar-Pei and non-Shar-Pei dogs. *J Vet Intern Med* 26: 259–268.

212 Flatland, B., Moore, R.R., Wolf, C.M. et al. (2007). Liver aspirate from a Shar Pei dog. *Vet Clin Pathol* 36: 105–108.

213 Kim, D.Y., Taylor, H.W., Eades, S.C., and Cho, D.Y. (2005). Systemic AL amyloidosis associated with multiple myeloma in a horse. *Vet Pathol* 42: 81–84.

214 Burrough, E.R., Myers, R.K., Hostetter, S.J. et al. (2012). Amyloid deposition in 2 feline thymomas. *Vet Pathol* 49: 616–620.

215 Bock, P., Hach, V., and Baumgärtner, W. (2011). Oral masses in two cats. *Vet Pathol* 48: 906–910.

216 Vite, C.H. and Head, E. (2014). Aging in the canine and feline brain. *Vet Clin North Am Small Anim Pract* 44: 1113–1129.

217 Elitok, O.M., Elitok, B., and Unver, O. (2008). Renal amyloidosis in cattle with inflammatory diseases. *J Vet Intern Med* 22: 450–455.

218 Zini, E., Lunardi, F., Zanetti, R. et al. (2016). Endocrine pancreas in cats with diabetes mellitus. *Vet Pathol* 53: 136–144.

219 Highley, J. and Sullivan, N. (2013). Techniques in neuropathology. In: *Bancroft's Theory and Practice of Histological Techniques*, 7e (eds. S.K. Suvarna, C. Layton and J.D. Bancroft), 353–380. London: Churchill, Livingstone, Elsevier.

220 Bauer, N.B., Bassett, H., O'Neill, E.J., and Acke, E. (2006). Cerebrospinal fluid from a 6-year-old dog with severe neck pain. *Vet Clin Pathol* 35: 123–125.

8

Cell Block Preparation Techniques and Applications in Veterinary Medicine

Koranda A. Walsh and Reema T. Patel

Introduction

The cell block (CB) is a sample processing technique in which a routine cytology sample, including fine-needle aspiration (FNA) and fluid samples, is concentrated to create a "button" of cells that is then processed as a histopathologic sample. The CB provides an adjunctive method to cytologic slides of tissue needle aspirates, cavitary effusions, and liquid-based cytology (LBC). With LBC, a sample is collected, and rather than being placed on a slide, it is transferred to transport medium and later processed for placement onto a slide. The traditional CB technique was first described more than a century ago in 1896 using collodion (nitrocellulose) bag methods, but it did not gain widespread use in human medicine until 1947.[1,2] While its usage in veterinary medicine is only sporadically described in the veterinary literature, there have been multiple publications since 2012, suggesting that this old technique may have a new niche in modern diagnostic veterinary clinical pathology.

Advantages and Disadvantages of the Cell Block

By the nature in which samples are collected and processed, the CB technique merges the best parts of routine FNA cytology with histopathology. Accordingly, one of the chief benefits of the CB is that it provides some residual tissue architecture on samples that were collected with minimal invasiveness. By preserving this architecture, CB preparations have been shown to improve the detection of malignant populations in effusions, detect nodal metastasis, and subclassify certain types of lymphoma.[3–5] In addition, as CB samples are processed similarly to routine tissue biopsy specimens, the CB technique generates archivable material suitable for ancillary tests such as immunocytochemistry (ICC), immunohistochemistry (IHC), *in situ* hybridization tests, cytogenetics, and polymerase chain reaction.[6–9] Lastly, as one of the initial steps in the processing of samples for CB is centrifugation, this approach will concentrate low cellularity samples and may improve diagnostic yield. Similar to its advantages, the disadvantages of CB represent the shortcomings of the two techniques it combines. This includes the shortcomings of routine FNA cytology, including potentially low cellularity samples and processing steps that can affect ancillary tests (e.g. alcohol fixation hinders some IHC). The shortcomings of traditional biopsy shared with CB methods include increased cost, prolonged processing time, and, in some cases, the need for specialized equipment.

In general, CB samples are especially useful when biopsy tissue is not available. In human medicine, CBs are often prepared as a standard practice, especially on fluid specimens.

The Cell Block in Diagnostic Veterinary Pathology

There are few publications that have examined the diagnostic utility of the CB in veterinary diagnostic pathology. While there are differences in sample processing techniques, the CB has been shown to be useful in the evaluation of lymphoid tissue, in the detection of bone marrow carcinoma metastasis, in the detection of carcinoma in fluid samples, and in the diagnosis of infectious agents (leishmaniasis, fungal osteomyelitis).[10–17]

Preparation Techniques

There are a wide variety of CB preparation protocols that combine the basic steps of (i) cellular concentration, (ii) sample fixation, and (iii) paraffin embedding for processing

Veterinary Cytology, First Edition. Edited by Leslie C. Sharkey, M. Judith Radin, and Davis Seelig.

as a histopathologic specimen. Variations in the technique are found in the method of cell concentration, fixation method and medium, and materials used for embedding cells. Although many techniques have not been documented in veterinary medicine, it is worth mentioning them since further investigation of these techniques could be explored by the veterinary community.

Cell Tube Blocks

In this technique, the sample is placed in a plain microhematocrit tube with one opening occluded by clay.[16] The authors recommended using Jovi clay (Jovi Plastilina, Rubi, Spain), a xylene-resistant modeling clay, rather than Giotto clay (Giotto Pongo, Fila Hispania, Barcelona, Spain) as Giotto clay tended to dissolve during formalin fixation.[16] If the sample is of low cellularity, it can be initially concentrated by centrifugation (2000 g for 5 minutes) prior to adding the sediment to the microhematocrit tube. To increase sample recovery, the microhematocrit tube is filled approximately three quarters full. A small volume of air is added by rocking the tube into a parallel position, and approximately 10 μL of Percoll or Ficoll is then added. This creates a bubble between the sample and the Percoll or Ficoll. The tube is sealed with clay and centrifuged for 5 minutes at 14 500 g. After centrifugation, the tube is scored near the liquid–air interface and broken. The cellular portion of the sample, including the surrounding capillary tube, is placed into 10% buffered formalin for 24 hours. The sample is then extruded from the capillary tube using one end of a paper clip and embedded horizontally into the paraffin block. Horizontal embedding provides that each section will contain all layers of cells, from red blood cells to nucleated cells. Sections are amenable to special and IHC stains, and a single block yields approximately 100 sections of 5 μm thickness.[16] The advantages of this technique include easy access to sample processing materials and the separation of nucleated cells from red blood cells in blood-contaminated samples.

Needle Rinse Method

In this method, the needle used for sample collection is sequentially rinsed with 20–30 mL of normal saline, special medium (e.g. Roswell Park Memorial Institute medium [RPMI]), formalin, paraformaldehyde, or ethanol, followed by centrifugation.[18,19] Rinsing with balanced saline prior to fixation may provide flexibility for ancillary tests.[20] Alternatively, the contents of the needle can be rinsed with 4% buffered paraformaldehyde, which offered better results for ICC than the originally proposed 7.5% buffered formalin.[21,22] Subsequent steps as exemplified by Zito et al. are well described.[21] After rinsing from the needle, cells are pelleted in a 10 mL soft, plastic, tapered centrifuge tube for 10 minutes at 1000 rpm [*sic*]. The supernatant is decanted and 70% ethyl alcohol is added to the sediment. The sediment is resuspended by agitation and centrifuged again for 10 minutes at 1000 rpm [*sic*]. This step is repeated once more before a final decantation and removal of the sediment via a spatula. The sediment is then wrapped in lens paper, placed in a tissue cassette, and embedded in paraffin after a short processing in xylene. The major disadvantages to this method are the potential loss of specimen and the potential negative effects on IHC that can occur with ethyl alcohol fixation.

Tissue Clot Methods

There are two well-characterized tissue clot approaches. In the first, the material in the needle lumen is allowed to clot.[19] It is then pushed out of the needle with a syringe or wire stylet and collected on filter paper in a tight circular motion to build up a cone. This cone is then allowed to dry slightly to ensure that the coagulum is congealed. The coagulum is then gently wrapped in tissue paper and transferred to formalin and processed as a histologic sample.[19]

The second approach is best documented for effusion samples but can also be applied to FNA samples collected into normal saline after needle rinsing. In both cases, the cell suspension is centrifuged and the supernatant is removed. The sample is resuspended in 0.1 mL of pooled, room temperature plasma followed by the addition of 0.2 mL of reconstituted, room temperature thrombin and quickly mixed well.[23–25] If after five minutes, no clot forms, an additional 0.2 mL of thrombin can be added.[25] The clot is then slid onto a piece of filter paper and wrapped within it. Finally, the pellet is fixed in 10% buffered formalin and embedded in paraffin. Notably, cell-free thrombin (e.g. Simplastin Excel S, bioMerieux, Durham, NC, USA) is recommended as reagents prepared from rabbit lung or brain can contain epithelial cells that may cause erroneous interpretations.[26] Some authors point out that plasma or thromboplastin can result in possible cross-reactions with non-patient human proteins during staining and recommend the use of other media to stabilize the pellet.[27,28]

Cell Block Embedding Materials

There are a variety of materials that can be used as matrices for embedding concentrated cells, including agar, HistoGel™ (HG), gelatin albumin, collodion bags, pregelatinized starch, sodium alginate, gelatin foam, polyvinyl alcohol foam, and acetone-melted paraffin.[11,15,17,29–38] An embedding material provides physical support to the concentrated sample (pellet or sediment) prior to paraffin embedding. With low cellularity samples, the collodion bag or Shidham's method have been recommended (see sections "HistoGel™ with Shidham's Method" and "Collodion Cell Bag Method"). Commonly used materials are described below.

Agarose Gel Method

Following conventional FNA, the sample is expelled into a 0.6 mL Eppendorf tube containing 70% ethanol and is centrifuged (2817 g for 10 minutes).[11] The supernatant is decanted, 2% liquid agarose gel is added, and the sample is centrifuged again (2817 g for 10 minutes). The pellet is then paraffin embedded and processed as a routine histologic specimen. This method has been cited in veterinary medicine primarily for preservation of architectural patterns but also as an example of the use of CBs for ancillary testing (cytochemical, ICC, molecular, and proteomic analysis).[11]

HistoGel™ Method

HG (Thermo Fisher Scientific, Inc., Waltham, MA, USA) is an inert aqueous processing gel that can be used on unfixed or formalin-fixed tissues. The mixture of sample and HG is embedded in paraffin, providing a double-embedding process. In veterinary medicine, HG has been used to prepare friable tissue biopsies, biopsies that require specific orientation, highly cellular fluids, urine sediment, peripheral blood, and bone marrow samples.[2,39] In these reports, samples retain excellent cell morphology, some architectural integrity, and immunoreactivity for cytokeratin, vimentin, glial fibrillary acidic protein, and muscle-specific actin. The advantage of HG is that it uses a readily available medium and requires no specialized equipment or processing once the tissue is embedded. However, its usefulness in poorly cellular fluids is uncertain, and for such samples, an alternate approach is advised (see sections "HistoGel™ with Shidham's Method" and "The Rapid and Cellient™ Methods").

HistoGel™ with Shidham's Method

This technique is a modification of the standard HG approach and is used to process low cellularity samples, in particular samples with individually scattered cells or small groups of cells.[32] This procedure has been optimized for liquid-based, low cellularity, human cervicovaginal specimens. However, it is also applicable to nongynecologic specimens including effusions, FNAs, brushings, and cyst contents. This method compensates for low cellularity samples by creating a pellet that can be more efficiently sectioned by the histotechnician. Specific modifications include concentrating cells parallel to the plane of sectioning and marking the level in the paraffin where the cells are concentrated such that the histotechnician does not cut too shallow or too deep relative to the cells. In contrast to the traditional HG technique, this modified version does require specialized equipment, including flat-bottom glass tubes and a swiveling centrifuge. A video of the process is provided at www.jove.com/video/1316.

Collodion Cell Bag Method

Collodion cell bags are made by coating the inside of a 10–15 mL test tube with a nitrocellulose-based film.[40] Once the bag material lining the inside of the tube has hardened, a sample fixed with either 95% alcohol or 10% formalin is added. The sample is centrifuged at 3000 rpm [*sic*] for 10 minutes, and the supernatant is discarded. The bag containing the sediment is gently extracted from the tube, twisted closed above the sediment, and excess bag material cut off. The bag is whisked through a 1% alcohol solution of eosin to more easily identify the cell pellet and then processed as a histologic specimen.[40]

Gelatin-Foam Method

Gelatin-foam CBs have been utilized in both human and veterinary medicine.[41] For this technique, the sample is placed into a 1.5 mL conical tube, centrifuged, and the resultant cell sediment retained. An approximately 4×4×2 mm piece of gelatin foam is then placed on top of the sediment, prodded to encourage absorption, and incubated for 30 minutes to allow for full absorption into the foam. To "seal" the cells into the foam and to dislodge the foam from the tube, methanol is then poured over the gel foam for 30 seconds. It is notable that CBs have been prepared without methanol with good results (Koranda Walsh, personal communication). After discarding the methanol, the foam is fixed for at least six hours in 10% buffered formalin. The gelatin foam is then processed as a normal histology specimen.[41]

Commercially Available Cell Block Kits

Thermo Scientific Shandon Cytoblock™ Method

This all-in-one kit (Thermo Fisher Scientific, Inc., Waltham, MA, USA) facilitates preparation of paraffin-embedded blocks from cell suspensions, cell aggregates, and tissue fragments.[42] Notably, the reagents in the kit are incompatible with traditional buffered formalin or any phosphate-containing fixative. Either an unbuffered formal saline or the Thermo Scientific Shandon Formal-Fixx™ (Thermo Fisher Scientific, Inc., Waltham, MA, USA) must be used. In contrast to the methods described above, specimens prepared using the Cytoblock™ kit are fixed prior to processing.

The Rapid and Cellient™ Methods

The Rapid CB method (UMass Memorial Medical Center, Worcester, MA, USA), a method later developed into the Cellient™ method (Hologic Corporation, Marlborough, MA, USA), was designed for samples with low cellularity.[43–45] Rapid CBs involve trapping cellular material on a polycarbonate filter with 12 µm pores that is positioned below a modified cassette.[45] The collected sample passes through an opening in the cassette and is gathered onto the filter. Absolute alcohol, xylene, and molten paraffin flow through the sample after which a column of wax is added, cooled, and hardened. This leaves a disc of cells on the undersurface of the cassette.[44] The cassette is then dropped into a biopsy mold and remelted for 15 minutes.

The Cellient™ method is an automated version of the Rapid CB.[43] In this approach, samples are centrifuged, fixed in a methanol-based fixative (ThinPrep PreservCyt®, Hologic Corporation, Marlborough, MA, USA), and concentrated using vacuum-assisted filtration. The Cellient™ processor loads the sample onto a cassette and embeds the sample in paraffin. Similar diagnostic performance was reported in a study comparing traditionally prepared CBs (method not specified) and Cellient™ CBs.[45]

Fixation Method and Material

There are many different fixation methods available and each can have a different effect on IHC and molecular tests. In general, as CB samples can be considered modified versions of traditional histopathology specimens, protocols for their preparation can often be extrapolated from studies on formalin-fixed paraffin-embedded tissues. However, modifications may be needed.

Formalin

Owing to its widespread availability and the lack of a need for special equipment or reagents, formalin (alone or in mixtures with ethanol) is a commonly used fixative. However, disadvantages of formalin include poorer cytologic detail and possible impediments to DNA extraction.[20,46] As with traditional histopathology specimens, changes in fixation time can have anticipated interferences, e.g. increased fixation time can decrease the sensitivity for detection of certain antigens. For molecular testing, formalin can cause DNA fragmentation/denaturation, poor yield for RNA and false positives, and sequencing artifacts.[20,46]

Alcohol

Several of the commercial CB preparation kits (e.g. Cellient™, ThinPrep® Liquid Based Cytology [Hologic Corporation, Marlborough, MA, USA], and BD SurePath™ liquid-based Pap test [BD, Franklin Lakes, NJ, USA]) utilize alcohol-based fixation (e.g. methanol, ethanol, or isopropanol). Alcohol fixation generally provides good cytological perseveration aside from cell shrinkage and holes within cells and provides superior nucleic acid quality.[20,46] However, there are generally fewer published IHC protocols as compared with ones designed for formalin-fixed specimens.

Microwave

Although microwave fixation provides satisfactory histologic detail and excellent quality genomic DNA, there is little available literature about the known effects of microwave fixation on immunostaining.[20]

Conclusions

CBs require longer turnaround time than FNAs and not all specimens will have sufficient cellularity or volume for this technique. The additional cost and the excess material that is required to obtain a good quality cellular pellet may limit routine use of CBs. However, CBs provide distinct advantages as far as providing histology-like specimens and additional available material for ancillary testing. These advantages make it likely that more veterinary laboratories will institute them as part of routine practice.

References

1 Bahrenberg, L. (1896). On the diagnostic results of the microscopical examination of the ascitic fluid in two cases of carcinoma involving the peritoneum. *Clevel Med Gaz* 11: 274–278.

2 Chapman, C. and Whalen, E. (1947). The examination of serous fluids by cell block technique. *N Engl J Med* 237: 215–220.

3 Koksal, D., Demirag, F., Bayiz, H. et al. (2013). The cell block method increases the diagnostic yield in exudative pleural effusions accompanying lung cancer. *Turkish J Pathol* 29: 165–170.

4 Engohan-Aloghe, C., Hottat, N., and Noël, J.-C. (2009). Accuracy of lymph nodes cell block preparation according

to ultrasound features in preoperative staging of breast cancer. *Diagn Cytopathol* 38: 5–8.

5 Salomao, M., Remotti, H., Allendorf, J.D. et al. (2014). Fine-needle aspirations of pancreatic serous cystadenomas: improving diagnostic yield with cell blocks and α-inhibin immunohistochemistry. *Cancer Cytopathol* 122: 33–39.

6 Keyhani-Rofahga, S., O'Toole, R., and Leming, M. (1984). The role of cell block in fine-needle aspiration cytology. *Acta Cytol* 28: 630–631.

7 Fetsch, P.A., Simsir, A., Brosky, K., and Abati, A. (2002). Comparison of three commonly used cytologic preparations in effusion immunocytochemistry. *Diagn Cytopathol* 26: 61–66.

8 Billah, S., Stewart, J., Staerkel, G. et al. (2011). EGFR and KRAS mutations in lung carcinoma. *Cancer Cytopathol* 119: 111–117.

9 Young, N.A., Naryshkin, S., and Katz, S.M. (1993). Diagnostic value of electron microscopy on paraffin-embedded cytologic material. *Diagn Cytopathol* 9: 282–290.

10 Taylor, B.E., Leibman, N.F., Luong, R. et al. (2013). Detection of carcinoma micrometastases in bone marrow of dogs and cats using conventional and cell block cytology. *Vet Clin Pathol* 42: 85–91.

11 Zanoni, D.S., Grandi, F., and Rocha, N.S. (2012). Use of the agarose cell block technique in veterinary diagnostic cytopathology: an "old and forgotten" method. *Vet Clin Pathol* 41: 307–308.

12 Fernandes, N.C.C.A., Guerra, J.M., Réssio, R.A. et al. (2016). Liquid-based cytology and cell block immunocytochemistry in veterinary medicine: comparison with standard cytology for the evaluation of canine lymphoid samples. *Vet Comp Oncol* 14: 107–116.

13 Zanoni, D., Grandi, F., Cagnini, D. et al. (2012). Agarose cell block technique as a complementary method in the diagnosis of fungal osteomyelitis in a dog. *Open Vet J* 2: 19–22.

14 Menezes, R.C., Madeira, M.F., Ferreira, L.C. et al. (2016). Cell-block immunohistochemistry of bone marrow aspirates: a novel tool to improve the diagnosis of Leishmania infection in dogs. *J Comp Pathol* 154: 157–160.

15 Wallace, K.A., Goldschmidt, M.H., and Patel, R.T. (2015). Converting fluid-based cytologic specimens to histologic specimens for immunohistochemistry. *Vet Clin Pathol* 44: 303–309.

16 Marcos, R., Santos, M., Marrinhas, C., and Caniatti, M. (2017). Cell tube block: a new technique to produce cell blocks from fluid cytology samples. *Vet Clin Pathol* 46: 195–201.

17 Joiner, K.S. and Spangler, E.A. (2012). Evaluation of HistoGel™-embedded specimens for use in veterinary diagnostic pathology. *J Vet Diagn Invest* 24: 710–715.

18 Chandra, A., Cross, P., Denton, K. et al. (2009). The BSCC Code of Practice: exfoliative cytopathology (excluding gynaecological cytopathology). *Cytopathology* 20: 211–223.

19 Yung, R.C.W., Otell, S., Illei, P. et al. (2012). Improvement of cellularity on cell block preparations using the so-called tissue coagulum clot method during endobronchial ultrasound-guided transbronchial fine-needle aspiration. *Cancer Cytopathol* 120: 185–195.

20 Jain, D., Mathur, S.R., and Iyer, V.K. (2014). Cell blocks in cytopathology: a review of preparative methods, utility in diagnosis and role in ancillary studies. *Cytopathology* 25: 356–371.

21 Zito, F.A., Gadaleta, C.D., Salvatore, C. et al. (1995). A modified cell block technique for fine needle aspiration cytology. *Acta Cytol* 39: 93–99.

22 Kung, I.T., Yuen, R.W., and Chan, J.K. (1989). Optimal formalin fixation and processing schedule of cell blocks from fine needle aspirates. *Pathology* 21: 143–145.

23 Kulkarni, M.B., Desai, S.B., Ajit, D., and Chinoy, R.F. (2009). Utility of the thromboplastin-plasma cell-block technique for fine-needle aspiration and serous effusions. *Diagn Cytopathol* 37: 86–90.

24 Karnauchow, P.N. and Bonin, R.E. (1982). "Cell-block" technique for fine needle aspiration biopsy. *J Clin Pathol* 35: 688.

25 Castro-Villabón, D., Avello, Y., Ruiz, N., and Rodriguez-Urrego, P.A. (2014). Implementation of routine thromboplastin-plasma cell block technique in the evaluation of non-gynecologic specimens: a methodologic comparison with conventional cytology. *J Microsc Ultrastruct* 2: 177–181.

26 Henwood, A.F. and Charlton, A. (2014). Extraneous epithelial cells from thromboplastin in cell blocks. *Cytopathology* 25: 412–413.

27 Heyderman, E. and Brown, B.E. (1986). Preparation of fine needle aspirates for immunocytochemical studies. *Lancet* 328: 520–521.

28 Kaneko, C., Kobayashi, T.K., Hasegawa, K. et al. (2010). A cell-block preparation using glucomannan extracted from *Amorphophallus konjac*. *Diagn Cytopathol* 38: 652–656.

29 Munfus-McCray, D., Harada, S., Adams, C. et al. (2011). EGFR and KRAS mutations in metastatic lung adenocarcinomas. *Hum Pathol* 42: 1447–1453.

30 Mohamed, S., Yasufuku, K., Nakajima, T. et al. (2008). Analysis of cell cycle-related proteins in mediastinal lymph nodes of patients with N2-NSCLC obtained by

EBUS-TBNA: relevance to chemotherapy response. *Thorax* 63: 642–647.

31 Kerstens, H.M.J., Robben, J.C.M., Poddighe, P.J. et al. (2000). AgarCyto: a novel cell-processing method for multiple molecular diagnostic analyses of the uterine cervix. *J Histochem Cytochem* 48: 709–718.

32 Varsegi, G.M. and Shidham, V. (2009). Cell block preparation from cytology specimen with predominance of individually scattered cells. *J Vis Exp* (29): e1316.

33 Koss, L. (1979). *Diagnostic Cytology and Its Histopathologic Bases*, 3e. Philadelphia: JB Lippincott.

34 Fahey, C. and Bedrossian, U.K. (1993). Collodion bag: a cell block technique for enhanced cell collection. *Lab Med* 24: 94–96.

35 He, Q.-L., Zhu, Y.-Z., Zheng, G.-J. et al. (2012). A new convenient technique for making cell blocks. *Cell Tissue Res* 350: 395–400.

36 Noda, Y., Fujita, N., Kobayashi, G. et al. (2010). Diagnostic efficacy of the cell block method in comparison with smear cytology of tissue samples obtained by endoscopic ultrasound-guided fine-needle aspiration. *J Gastroenterol* 45: 868–875.

37 Mayall, F.G. (2012). An FNA cytology foam core device for making cell blocks. *J Clin Pathol* 65: 959–961.

38 Krogerus, L.A. and Andersson, L.C. (1988). A simple method for the preparation of paraffin-embedded cell blocks from fine needle aspirates, effusions and brushings. *Acta Cytol* 32: 585–587.

39 Craig, F., Soma, L., Melan, M. et al. (2008). MUM1/IRF4 expression in the circulating compartment of chronic lymphocytic leukemia. *Leuk Lymphoma* 49: 273–280.

40 Bussolati, G. (1982). A celloidin bag for the histological preparation of cytologic material. *J Clin Pathol* 35: 574–576.

41 Mayall, F.G. and Wood, I. (2011). Gelatin foam cell blocks made from cytology fluid specimens. *J Clin Pathol* 64: 818–819.

42 Khan, S., Omar, T., and Michelow, P. (2012). Effectiveness of the cell block technique in diagnostic cytopathology. *J Cytol* 29: 177–182.

43 Akalin, A., Lu, D., Woda, B. et al. (2008). Rapid cell blocks improve accuracy of breast FNAs beyond that provided by conventional cell blocks regardless of immediate adequacy evaluation. *Diagn Cytopathol* 36: 523–529.

44 Istvanic, S., Fischer, A.H., Banner, B.F. et al. (2007). Cell blocks of breast FNAs frequently allow diagnosis of invasion or histological classification of proliferative changes. *Diagn Cytopathol* 35: 263–269.

45 Fischer, A., Vartanian, H., Hanc, B. et al. (2006). Efficient technique for making paraffin-embedded "rapid cell blocks" in 12 minutes. *Mod Pathol* 19: 57.

46 Srinivasan, M., Sedmak, D., and Jewell, S. (2002). Effect of fixatives and tissue processing on the content and integrity of nucleic acids. *Am J Pathol* 161: 1961–1971.

9

Molecular Clonality Testing

Davis Seelig and Anne C. Avery

Role of Clonality Analysis

At its most basic level, clonality testing seeks to determine whether a cellular population is derived from a single clone. In the context of diagnostic medicine, the assignment of a clonal origin to a group of cells strongly implicates a neoplastic origin to that group of cells.[1] As such, the detection of clonality can be used, when interpreted in the context of clinical and other laboratory data, as an indicator of neoplasia. However, as will be discussed below, it is important to recognize that monoclonality is not equivalent to neoplasia nor does the lack of monoclonality exclude neoplasia. The chapter will focus on clonality testing for hematopoietic malignancies, including lymphoid and non-lymphoid neoplasms. The former will entirely emphasize PCR-based testing through evaluation of the antigen receptor genes that will, for the sake of brevity, be abbreviated as PARR. It is important to note that the term PARR is used only in veterinary medicine and is not applied to the human lymphoid clonality assay. The latter will review X-chromosome inactivation profiling (XCIP). In addition to providing a review of the molecular underpinnings, methods, and clinical applicability of clonality testing, this chapter will also address its quality assurance aspects.

Lymphoid Clonality Testing

Molecular Basis of Lymphoid Clonality Testing

The technical aspects of the PARR assay have been well described. In brief, the assay exploits the unique antigen receptor genes (the T-cell receptor, TCR, and immunoglobulin receptor IgR genes) for the detection of either a polyclonal (i.e. reactive) or monoclonal (i.e. neoplastic) process. During their development and maturation, both B and T cells undergo somatic DNA rearrangement of their antigen receptor V, D, and J genes to produce cell-specific immunoglobulin and T-cell receptors (IGR and TCR), respectively. The end result of these normal rearrangements is the formation of genes that are, on a cell-to-cell basis, unique in both length and sequence. With continued maturation, the sequence of the antigen receptor genes is locked in both B and T cells and passed along to all subsequent cellular progeny. Given that the neoplastic transformation of a lymphoid cell occurs *after* this process of antigen receptor rearrangement, the relative heterogeneity of this gene sequence can be used as a surrogate marker of a monoclonal or polyclonal lymphocyte population.

In response to an inflammatory stimulus, lymphocytes mount a diverse reaction to a spectrum of antigens that results in the activation and proliferation of lymphocytes that are heterogeneous with regard to their receptor genes (i.e. a polyclonal expansion). In contrast, a neoplastic population can be characterized by the uncontrolled proliferation of a single lymphocyte with a single receptor gene (i.e. a monoclonal expansion). The PARR assay exploits this difference. In a lymphocyte-rich sample, a monoclonal expansion is highly suggestive of lymphoid neoplasia, whereas a polyclonal expansion is more consistent with a reactive lymphoid process. Clonality testing is most useful in face of biologically ambiguous lymphocyte population (i.e. a neoplastic vs. an inflammatory population) as an adjunctive immunophenotyping tool (in concert with immunohistochemistry (IHC) and/or flow cytometry) and in determining if two neoplasms are clonally related. However, as will be reviewed in the remaining sections, there are a number of important diagnostic considerations to the interpretation of PARR testing, including sampling considerations, its unique terminology, and the transparency of interpretation guidelines.[2]

Veterinary Cytology, First Edition. Edited by Leslie C. Sharkey, M. Judith Radin, and Davis Seelig.

Diagnostic Aspects of Lymphoid Clonality Testing

Sampling Considerations

PARR testing is primarily performed on genomic DNA isolated from cells in which a neoplastic process is suspected. In clinical practice, PARR has successfully detected clonal lymphoid populations in fresh solid tissue aspirates, peripheral blood, body cavity fluids, cerebrospinal fluid, stained or unstained cytology samples, aqueous humor, and urine.[3] This includes recently collected samples, samples from previously stained slides, and archived samples. Increasingly, there are reports of successful utilization of formalin-fixed, paraffin-embedded (FFPE) samples in lymphoid clonality assays.[4] This includes of the successful application of PARR to FFPE lymph node and intestinal and mediastinal mass samples.[5–9] However, as the quality and integrity of DNA extracted from formalin fixation can impart a number of confounding artifacts, including background smearing, decreased DNA yield, and fragmented DNA, it is important that laboratories report their diagnostic performance to the end user.[5,10] Such reporting should include the diagnostic performance in both unfixed and FFPE samples. While all potential variables have yet to be investigated, the quality of the extracted DNA is at least inversely proportional to storage time with older samples, demonstrating more abnormalities than more recently collected samples.[5] According to published canine and feline reports, the yield of adequately quality DNA from veterinary FFPE samples varies from 60 to 100%.[5–9] One review article recommends that DNA yield and purity be evaluated by spectrophotometry with an input goal of 100 ng per 50 μL reaction; however this suggestion is not based upon published veterinary data.[2]

Analytical Aspects of Lymphoid Clonality Testing

Following PCR amplification, samples must be evaluated for the presence of either a monoclonal or polygonal gene product. Historically, this analysis was performed using polyacrylamide gel electrophoresis (PAGE). The nature of the PCR products will vary depending on the primer pairs used, but typically one or two discreet peaks would be seen in the immunoglobulin clonality assay, and two to multiple peaks with the TCR gamma PCR assay. However, owing to concerns regarding diagnostic resolution and the identification of either small or closely spaced PCR products, gel electrophoresis is increasingly being replaced by capillary electrophoresis.[11] To date, there is no published consensus in the detection of either a monoclonal or polyclonal expansion using capillary electrophoresis. However, general guidelines define a monoclonal population as a single peak that is 2–3× the height of any background peaks, whereas a polyclonal population is described to consist of numerous small peaks distributed over the size range of the primer set in a Gaussian or Gaussian-like distribution.[5,12,13] Importantly, the criteria used by laboratories performing PARR testing should be both objective and reported. Capillary electrophoresis is performed on a wide range of instruments with variable resolving capacity.

Outside of these two diagnostic categories, laboratories may report samples as having an oligoclonal profile, which is characterized by multiple peaks and may indicate either a neoplastic (i.e. monoclonal) or reactive/nondiagnostic sample depending upon the diagnostic criteria established by the performing laboratory.[2] It is important to note that more than one peak can be seen in neoplastic populations. In addition, the term pseudoclonal may be used to describe samples containing one or more discrete peaks that are nonneoplastic in origin but may resemble a monoclonal process.[14] Pseudoclonality is reported in samples containing insufficient DNA (i.e. hypocellular samples).[2] As is the case with mono- and polyclonality, the criteria used to define oligo- and pseudoclonality are not well established in the veterinary literature and should be reported by the laboratory performing the assay.

Diagnostic Accuracy of Lymphoid Clonality Assays

The sensitivity and specificity of the PARR assay will be reviewed below. While these data are important in the assessment of the diagnostic performance of the assay (and should be reported by laboratories performing the test), the results of clonality assays, like any diagnostic testing, should be considered in conjunction with the other diagnostic and clinical information available to the veterinarian or pathologist. Although not currently offered by most laboratories that perform clonality testing, an assessment of sensitivity and specificity is a reasonable expectation of clinicians submitting this testing. Clinicians submitting samples for clonality testing should provide the laboratory with cytology/histology results and clinical information. Samples from non-lymphoid sites or low cellularity samples may have a greater propensity for giving pseudoclonal results, and performing the samples in replicate is not a guarantee that this will not happen. Although the clonality assay should be interpreted objectively, knowing what information the clinician is seeking is important in assessing the results.

Diagnostic Sensitivity of the Clonality Assay

Including the original publication, the published sensitivity of PARR for the detection of either B- or T-cell neoplasms in canine samples ranges from 63 to 100%, with sensitivity seeming to increase with modification of PCR primer sets.[15–18] In the cat, the published sensitivity of PARR using FFPE samples ranges from 65 to 87%.[19–21] The sensitivity of the clonality assay is primarily influenced by two factors, namely, (i) the recognition spectrum of the primers used in the assay and (ii) the number of clonal (neoplastic) cells within a sample. As successful detection of a clonal population requires the binding of primers to the appropriate gene regions, unique variations of those genes (including polymorphisms or mutations) that do not result in primer binding may cause a false-negative result. One example of this is somatic hypermutation, which describes the failure of the assay primers to bind as a result of normal mutations within the antigen receptors of B cells. It is also reported that "dilution" of the tumor cell population by large numbers of inflammatory cells (i.e. a polyclonal background) can result in the number of tumor cells falling below the detection limit of the assay and a polyclonal test result despite the presence of a neoplastic process.[4] Based upon dilution studies, clonal rearrangements can be detected when 0.1–10% (or 1 tumor cell in 100 normal cells) of the DNA was derived from neoplastic cells.[11,15]

Diagnostic Specificity of Clonality Testing

The published specificity of PARR in canine tissues ranges from 94 to 98%, whereas in the cat the specificity is reported to be 95%.[13,20–22] Known false-positive PARR results describe nonneoplastic monoclonal lymphoid expansions (i.e. benign clonal lymphoid proliferations) and PARR+, non-lymphoid neoplasms. Benign clonal lymphoid expansions are reported in canine and feline inflammatory bowel disease (IBD), *Ehrlichia* sp. infection, and canine thymoma.[6,9,15,23,24] Also, positive PARR test results are reported in non-lymphoid neoplasms, including 64% (16/25) cases of canine acute myeloid leukemia.[25] However it is important to note that the performance of the PARR assay, including sensitivity and specificity, continues to evolve as the methodologies of the test (including primers) are revised. As such, current interpretative guidelines (including the existence of benign clonal expansions) are likely to change.

Lymphoid Clonality in Intestinal Tissues

Owing to the unique confounding factors to PARR testing, in the impact of background lymphoid inflammation, it is important to note that there may be tissue- and disease-specific interpretation guidelines. This is best highlighted by the role of PARR in the discrimination between IBD and lymphoma using intestinal samples. There are four studies that report the accuracy of PARR the detection of monoclonal lymphocytes in dogs with intestinal lymphoma. Across the four studies, the sensitivity ranges from 67 to 88%, and the specificity is reported as 100%.[4,26–28] In the cat, the sensitivity of PARR for the diagnosis of intestinal lymphoma (generally as compared with histology ± IHC) ranges from 50 to 91%, with the lowest value reported in B-cell neoplasms.[5,7,29,30] Similar to the dog, the specificity of PARR in the diagnosis of feline intestinal lymphoma is 90–100%.[6,29,30] However, as will be highlighted below, the current approach in the diagnosis of feline intestinal lymphoma is imperfect (particularly when relying upon histology and IHC as a "gold" standard), and diagnostic method comparison studies (including those assessing the diagnostic performance of PARR) should be interpreted with caution.

In a study of 77 feline intestinal biopsies, 52 of which were classified as inflammatory and 25 as T-cell lymphoma (according to histopathology and IHC), a monoclonal population could be found in 38 cases. When using survival as the determining outcome data, cats with a clonality-based diagnosis of lymphoma had a 2.8 times higher risk of an enteropathy-related death than cases diagnosed by cytology, histology, or IHC.[6] Based on their results, the authors suggest that the sensitivity of histology and IHC for the diagnosis of feline intestinal lymphoma is low to moderate (38 and 64%, respectively) and that clonality assessment should be added in a stepwise fashion.[6] Similarly, in a series of 63 cats with clinical signs of enteric disease, the addition of PARR on FFPE tissues resulted in the reclassification of eight cases, namely, five cases originally diagnosed as IBD were changed to T-cell lymphoma and two cases originally diagnosed as T-cell lymphoma were changed to IBD.[31]

Lineage Assignment of Hematopoietic Neoplasms

In addition to assessing clonality, the PARR assay also provides immunophenotyping data. In light of concerns regarding cross-lineage rearrangement (i.e. the rearrangement of T-cell loci by B cells or of B-cell loci by T cells), there are suggestions that PARR should not be used as tool for neoplastic cell lineage assignment. However, there are important caveats to this literature, including (i) a lack of reported objective criteria for the defining of clonality, (ii) a lack of clinical follow-up (to rule out the existence of multiple neoplasms), and (iii) the known occurrence of coincident B- and T-cell lymphoma (particularly indolent T-zone lymphoma in dogs with B-cell lymphoma), which may overestimate impact of true cross-lineage rearrangements.[16,32]

It is important to note that while B- and T-cell immunophenotyping is certainly an important step in the process of lymphoma subtyping, when used in isolation it may provide potentially misleading prognostic information provided by simple B- or T-cell immunophenotyping (in which biologically indolent forms of lymphoma may be lumped with more aggressive forms of the disease).[16,32] In one study comparing the immunophenotyping results of 62 cases of canine nodal lymphoma, the percent agreement between PARR and IHC was 70% and between PARR and flow cytometry was 63%.[33] Also, in cases of acute leukemia in which the lineage of the neoplastic cell may not be evident on microscopy alone, the results of clonality testing may erroneously assign a lymphoid origin to a myeloid neoplasm as 64% of cases of a canine acute myeloid leukemia demonstrate clonally rearranged lymphocyte receptor genes.[25] In feline lymphoma, the use of PARR as a lineage assignment tool is similarly not recommended with reported sensitivities (as compared with IHC) of 25 and 89% (for T-cell and B-cell neoplasms) and specificities of 100 and 75% (for T- and B-cell neoplasms).[34]

PARR Testing in the Horse

In the horse, PARR has been used to support the diagnosis of T-cell-rich B-cell lymphoma, diffuse large B-cell lymphoma, and five equine cases of B-cell neoplasia characterized by monoclonal gammopathy, peripheral blood involvement, and tissue infiltration by small- to medium-sized cells.[35–37]

Non-lymphoid Clonality Testing

Non-lymphoid cells lack well-characterized and cell lineage-specific DNA sequences that can be probed for clonality. As such, detecting clonality in these lineages requires an alternate approach. This approach, known as X-chromosome inactivation profiling, exploits the normal process of X-chromosome inactivation. In female animals, one copy of the X chromosome (of either maternal or paternal origin) undergoes random inactivation by methylation. As a result of this inactivation, there is an approximately 1 : 1 ratio between transcriptionally active paternally and maternally derived X-chromosome genes in normal tissue. In contrast, clonal cells from a neoplasm demonstrate a uniform pattern of X-chromosome inactivation and a skewed ratio between maternally and paternally derived X chromosomes. As such, the detection of a skewed (or nonrandom) XCIP is indicative of a clonal origin to a cell population.[38,39]

In female animals, X-chromosome inactivation can be measured using the androgen receptor gene. This gene contains repeated DNA elements (CAG repeats), the number of which varies within a population. If an animal is heterozygous for the number of repeats, it is possible to determine if the same X chromosome is inactivated in all the cells in a particular sample. Methylated genes resist the action of restriction enzymes. Thus in an animal with clonally expanded cells, digestion of DNA with specific restriction enzymes will eliminate one of the alleles, leaving a single allele for detection by PCR. In a reactive process, where only half of the X alleles from each source (maternal and paternal) are methylated, restriction enzyme digestion would not eliminate either gene, and both could be detected using a PCR assay. In humans this assay is referred to as the human androgen receptor assay (HUMARA), and in the dog at least one group has denoted it the canine androgen receptor assay (CANARA).[40] At the time of preparation of this chapter, there is limited published data on the applicability of XCIP to veterinary samples. In the dog, it is been successfully used to document the clonality of lymphoma, chronic myelogenous leukemia, acute myelogenous leukemia, and histiocytoma.[38,40] In the cat, XCIP has been successfully applied to three mammary gland adenocarcinoma cell lines and multiple primary tumor samples, including those from cases of myelodysplastic syndrome, pulmonary carcinoma, ceruminous carcinoma, lymphoma, fibrosarcoma, and leiomyosarcoma.[41]

Quality Assurance and Clonality Testing

Similar to traditional microscopy-based diagnostics, clonality testing would also benefit from interlaboratory standardization of sample analysis and interpretation guidelines.[2,42] To that end, future studies should include the simultaneous analysis of matched samples with known biologic outcomes to determine the best performing assay. Furthermore, it is recommended that laboratories performing clonality analysis provide an assessment of the sensitivity and specificity of their assay, including reports of both false-positive and false-negative result percentages.[11]

References

1 Swerdlow, S.H. (2003). Genetic and molecular genetic studies in the diagnosis of atypical lymphoid hyperplasias versus lymphoma. *Hum Pathol* 34: 346–351.

2 Keller, S.M., Vernau, W., and Moore, P.F. (2016). Clonality testing in veterinary medicine: a review with diagnostic guidelines. *Vet Pathol* 53: 711–725.

3 Pate, D.O., Gilger, B.C., Suter, S.E., and Clode, A.B. (2011). Diagnosis of intraocular lymphosarcoma in a dog by use of a polymerase chain reaction assay for antigen receptor rearrangement. *J Am Vet Med Assoc* 238: 625–630.

4 Fukushima, K., Ohno, K., Koshino-Goto, Y. et al. (2009). Sensitivity for the detection of a clonally rearranged antigen receptor gene in endoscopically obtained biopsy specimens from canine alimentary lymphoma. *J Vet Med Sci* 71: 1673–1676.

5 Gress, V., Wolfesberger, B., Fuchs-Baumgartinger, A. et al. (2016). Characterization of the T-cell receptor gamma chain gene rearrangements as an adjunct tool in the diagnosis of T-cell lymphomas in the gastrointestinal tract of cats. *Res Vet Sci* 107: 261–266.

6 Sabattini, S., Bottero, E., Turba, M.E. et al. (2016). Differentiating feline inflammatory bowel disease from alimentary lymphoma in duodenal endoscopic biopsies. *J Small Anim Pract* 57: 396–401.

7 Moore, P.F., Rodriguez-Bertos, A., and Kass, P.H. (2012). Feline gastrointestinal lymphoma: mucosal architecture, immunophenotype, and molecular clonality. *Vet Pathol* 49: 658–668.

8 Kaneko, N., Tanimoto, T., Morimoto, M. et al. (2009). Use of formalin-fixed paraffin-embedded tissue and single-strand conformation polymorphism analysis for polymerase chain reaction of antigen receptor rearrangements in dogs. *J Vet Med Sci* 71: 535–538.

9 Vessieres, F., Rasotto, R., Peters, I. et al. (2018). Assessment of lymphoid molecular clonality in canine thymoma. *J Comp Pathol* 158: 66–70.

10 Lenze, D., Müller, H.-H., and Hummel, M. (2012). Considerations for the use of formalin-fixed and paraffin-embedded tissue specimens for clonality analysis. *J Hematopathol* 5: 27–34.

11 Avery, A.C. (2012). Molecular diagnostics of hematologic malignancies in small animals. *Vet Clin North Am Small Anim Pract* 42: 97–110.

12 Keller, S.M. and Moore, P.F. (2012). A novel clonality assay for the assessment of canine T cell proliferations. *Vet Immunol Immunopathol* 145: 410–419.

13 Waugh, E.M., Gallagher, A., Haining, H. et al. (2016). Optimisation and validation of a PCR for antigen receptor rearrangement (PARR) assay to detect clonality in canine lymphoid malignancies. *Vet Immunol Immunopathol* 182: 115–124.

14 Boer, A., Tirumalae, R., Bresch, M., and Falk, T.M. (2008). Pseudoclonality in cutaneous pseudolymphomas: a pitfall in interpretation of rearrangement studies. *Br J Dermatol* 159: 394–402.

15 Burnett, R.C., Vernau, W., Modiano, J.F. et al. (2003). Diagnosis of canine lymphoid neoplasia using clonal rearrangements of antigen receptor genes. *Vet Pathol* 40: 32–41.

16 Valli, V.E., Vernau, W., de Lorimier, L.P. et al. (2006). Canine indolent nodular lymphoma. *Vet Pathol* 43: 241–256.

17 Chaubert, P., Baur Chaubert, A.S., Sattler, U. et al. (2010). Improved polymerase chain reaction-based method to detect early-stage epitheliotropic T-cell lymphoma (mycosis fungoides) in formalin-fixed, paraffin-embedded skin biopsy specimens of the dog. *J Vet Diagn Invest* 22: 20–29.

18 Gentilini, F., Calzolari, C., Turba, M.E. et al. (2009). GeneScanning analysis of Ig/TCR gene rearrangements to detect clonality in canine lymphomas. *Vet Immunol Immunopathol* 127: 47–56.

19 Roccabianca, P., Avallone, G., Rodriguez, A. et al. (2016). Cutaneous lymphoma at injection sites: pathological, immunophenotypical, and molecular characterization in 17 cats. *Vet Pathol* 53: 823–832.

20 Mochizuki, H., Nakamura, K., Sato, H. et al. (2011). Multiplex PCR and Genescan analysis to detect immunoglobulin heavy chain gene rearrangement in feline B-cell neoplasms. *Vet Immunol Immunopathol* 143: 38–45.

21 Mochizuki, H., Nakamura, K., Sato, H. et al. (2012). GeneScan analysis to detect clonality of T-cell receptor gamma gene rearrangement in feline lymphoid neoplasms. *Vet Immunol Immunopathol* 145: 402–409.

22 Avery, A. (2009). Molecular diagnostics of hematologic malignancies. *Top Companion Anim Med* 24: 144–150.

23 Olivero, D., Turba, M.E., and Gentilini, F. (2011). Reduced diversity of immunoglobulin and T-cell receptor gene rearrangements in chronic inflammatory gastrointestinal diseases in dogs. *Vet Immunol Immunopathol* 144: 337–345.

24 Qurollo, B.A., Davenport, A.C., Sherbert, B.M. et al. (2013). Infection with Panola Mountain *Ehrlichia* sp. in a dog with atypical lymphocytes and clonal T-cell expansion. *J Vet Intern Med* 27: 1251–1255.

25 Stokol, T., Nickerson, G.A., Shuman, M., and Belcher, N. (2017). Dogs with acute myeloid leukemia have clonal rearrangements in T and B cell receptors. *Front Vet Sci* 4: 76.

26 Couto, K.M., Moore, P.F., Zwingenberger, A.L. et al. (2018). Clinical characteristics and outcome in dogs with small cell T-cell intestinal lymphoma. *Vet Comp Oncol* 16: 337–343.

27 Ohmura, S., Leipig, M., Schopper, I. et al. (2017). Detection of monoclonality in intestinal lymphoma with polymerase chain reaction for antigen receptor gene rearrangement analysis to differentiate from enteritis in dogs. *Vet Comp Oncol* 15: 194–207.

28 Carrasco, V., Rodriguez-Bertos, A., Rodriguez-Franco, F. et al. (2015). Distinguishing intestinal lymphoma from inflammatory bowel disease in canine duodenal endoscopic biopsy samples. *Vet Pathol* 52: 668–675.

29 Hammer, S.E., Groiss, S., Fuchs-Baumgartinger, A. et al. (2015). Sensitivity and specificity of the PCR-based lymphocyte clonality assay (PARR) for the diagnosis of B- and T-cell lymphoma in cats. *Vet Clin Pathol* 44: E15–E16.

30 Moore, P.F., Woo, J.C., Vernau, W. et al. (2005). Characterization of feline T cell receptor gamma (TCRG) variable region genes for the molecular diagnosis of feline intestinal T cell lymphoma. *Vet Immunol Immunopathol* 106: 167–178.

31 Kiupel, M., Smedley, R.C., Pfent, C. et al. (2011). Diagnostic algorithm to differentiate lymphoma from inflammation in feline small intestinal biopsy samples. *Vet Pathol* 48: 212–222.

32 Weiss, A.T., Klopfleisch, R., and Gruber, A.D. (2011). T-cell receptor gamma chain variable and joining region genes of subgroup 1 are clonally rearranged in feline B- and T-cell lymphoma. *J Comp Pathol* 144: 123–134.

33 Thalheim, L., Williams, L.E., Borst, L.B. et al. (2013). Lymphoma immunophenotype of dogs determined by immunohistochemistry, flow cytometry, and polymerase chain reaction for antigen receptor rearrangements. *J Vet Intern Med* 27: 1509–1516.

34 Sato, H., Fujino, Y., Uchida, K. et al. (2011). Comparison between immunohistochemistry and genetic clonality analysis for cellular lineage determination in feline lymphomas. *J Vet Med Sci* 73: 945–947.

35 Badial, P.R., Tallmadge, R.L., Miller, S. et al. (2015). Applied protein and molecular techniques for characterization of B cell neoplasms in horses. *Clin Vaccine Immunol* 22: 1133–1145.

36 Collar, E.M., Parker, J.E., Gorman, E.M. et al. (2019). PCR for antigen receptor rearrangement (PARR) clonality testing in a horse with a solitary retropharyngeal lymphoma. *Equine Vet Educ* 31 (8): 413–418.

37 Meichner, K., Kraszeski, B.H., Durrant, J.R. et al. (2017). Extreme lymphocytosis with myelomonocytic morphology in a horse with diffuse large B-cell lymphoma. *Vet Clin Pathol* 46: 64–71.

38 Mochizuki, H., Goto-Koshino, Y., Takahashi, M. et al. (2015). Demonstration of the cell clonality in canine hematopoietic tumors by X-chromosome inactivation pattern analysis. *Vet Pathol* 52: 61–69.

39 Chen, G.L. and Prchal, J.T. (2007). X-linked clonality testing: interpretation and limitations. *Blood* 110: 1411–1419.

40 Delcour, N.M., Klopfleisch, R., Gruber, A.D. et al. (2013). Canine cutaneous histiocytomas are clonal lesions as defined by X-linked clonality testing. *J Comp Pathol* 149: 192–198.

41 Mochizuki, H., Goto-Koshino, Y., Takahashi, M. et al. (2012). X-chromosome inactivation pattern analysis for the assessment of cell clonality in cats. *Vet Pathol* 49: 963–970.

42 Langerak, A.W. (2016). Toward standardization of clonality testing in veterinary medicine. *Vet Pathol* 53: 705–706.

10

Cytogenetics

Matthew Breen

Introduction to Cytogenetics

Somatic alterations to the constitutional genome of cells represent key biological markers for diagnosis and prognosis of numerous human cancers, as well as for monitoring residual disease during therapy. Alterations to genome architecture take many forms, and, in general, the development of tumors is associated with an accumulation of a series of genome changes. By the time cancer patients present with disease, their cancers may be at various stages, and while some alterations are easily detected in routine clinical specimens, others are more challenging. At one end of the spectrum are changes to single nucleotides and small (few base pairs) deletions/duplications/insertions of DNA, each of which may alter a critical amino acid sequence and hence function of the gene product. At the other end of the spectrum are larger structural and numerical changes that can take the form of partial to whole chromosome copy number changes. Such changes can alter the karyotypic architecture of the genome and thus be visible as chromosome aberrations under a light microscope, while others are more subtle, requiring visualization with the aid of targeted fluorescence *in situ* hybridization (FISH) reagents. Alterations to the structure of chromosomes (e.g. translocations, inversions, insertions) may lead to deregulation of transcription of gene expression and even to chimeric transcripts that could drive malignant transformation.

In human medicine, the use of conventional metaphase-based cytogenetics for the analysis of large numerical and structural changes to the genome in cancer cells has been ongoing for almost 50 years. Since the discovery of the Philadelphia chromosome in 1960 as the first visible genetic abnormality associated with cancer,[1] the use of cytogenetics has identified chromosome aberrations in over 69 551 human neoplasms (as of October 2019), representing 75 different types of cancer (see http://cgap.nci.nih.gov/Chromosomes/Mitelman). This approach has been very fruitful for aiding the localization of cancer-associated genes and has identified over 22 000 gene fusions, many of which have aided selection of the most appropriate therapeutic approaches for patients and subsequent monitoring for recurrent disease.

Cytogenetics has contributed enormously to developing improvements in the clinical management of patients. Patients with cytogenetic signatures indicative of a poor prognosis may be directed to receive more aggressive treatments to improve the probability of positive outcomes, while those with signatures associated with a good prognosis may be spared unnecessary treatment. The World Health Organization recognizes that genetic abnormalities offer some of the most reliable criteria for the classification of tumors and has stressed the importance of further research into this area. Here we will briefly review the techniques of molecular cytogenetics and provide examples of recent findings in veterinary oncology that demonstrate the potential implications for diagnosis and prognosis in animal patients.

Animal Cytogenetics: The Basics of Nomenclature

The DNA of all animals is packaged into chromosomes, nature's biological filing cabinets. For historical reasons, the structure of chromosomes is described by their visual appearance through a light microscope, with nomenclature making reference to the size of the chromosome and location of the centromere. As a cell progresses through mitosis, it passes through metaphase and it is this stage of division that the chromosomes are evident as discrete structures (Figure 10.1) Chromosomes with a centromere located at the end are described as either telocentric or acrocentric. When there are two clearly distinguishable arms on either side of the centromere, such chromosomes

Veterinary Cytology, First Edition. Edited by Leslie C. Sharkey, M. Judith Radin, and Davis Seelig.

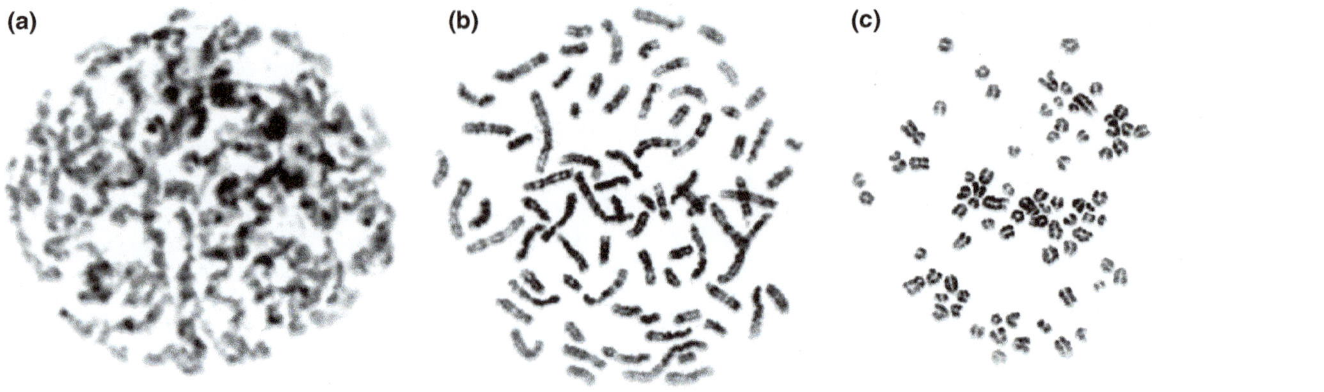

Figure 10.1 To visualize chromosome through a microscope requires that the dividing cell be in the metaphase stage of mitosis. Depending on the needs of the cytogeneticists, chromosome condensation increases as the cell passes through (a) prometaphase, (b) mid-metaphase, or (c) late metaphase. Conventional cytogenetic approaches require the chromosome to be in early to mid-metaphase, while molecular approaches can accommodate the use of cells in any stage of mitosis.

are referred to as either metacentric, where the centromere is located approximately in the middle and the two arms are of comparable size, or submetacentric, where the non-central location of the centromere produces arms of different size. In the case of bi-armed chromosomes, the visibly shorter of the two arms is referred to as the "p arm," and the longer arm as the "q arm" (Figure 10.2). For all species, it is first important to determine the number and visual appearance of the chromosomes in the "healthy" cell nucleus. As such, each chromosome of a species is assigned a specific number or letter. Though there have been some inconsistencies in how this has been done, animal chromosomes have generally been numbered from the largest to smallest autosomes, with the two sex chromosomes (X and Y) placed at the end. An example of the karyotype for the domestic dog is shown in Figure 10.3.

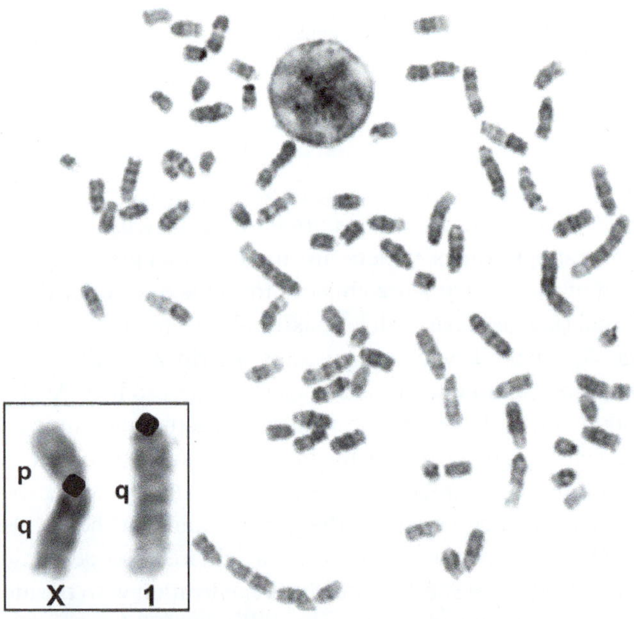

Figure 10.2 Mid-metaphase preparation showing the 78 chromosomes of the domestic dog. Each chromosome has a centromere, and the position of the centromere dictates the nomenclature of the chromosome. Inset shows enlarged and correctly oriented dog chromosome CFA X and CFA 1 with black circles overlaying the location of the centromere. Chromosomes with two clearly distinguishable arms on either side of the centromere, such as for CFA X, are referred to as bi-armed. In this case, the shorter of the two arms is referred to as the p arm, and the longer as the q arm. When the centromere is located at one end of the chromosome, such as for CFA 1, there is a single chromosome arm (referred to as the q arm), and these are reported as acrocentric/telocentric.

Chromosome Aberrations

The "normal" karyotypes of companion animals have been well studied and documented. Deviations from normal are reported as aberrations, which may be numerical or structural, or both. Numerical changes result from a net gain or loss of genetic material, whereas structural changes are due to altered DNA organization. In either case changes may be simple or complex. An abnormal chromosome with an intact centromere is termed derivative chromosome, and the number used to identify the structure is determined by the origin of the centromere. For example, an aberrant chromosome that results from an inversion of the distal end of dog chromosome 5 would be referred to as derivative chromosome 5, and a translocation of a segment of chromosome 7 onto the distal end of chromosome 20 would be derivative chromosome 20. An example of the presence of extensive rearrangements of the karyotype of the domestic dog is shown in Figure 10.4. The challenge for cytogenetics is to be able to identify which segments of the genome are contributing to the derivative chromosomes.

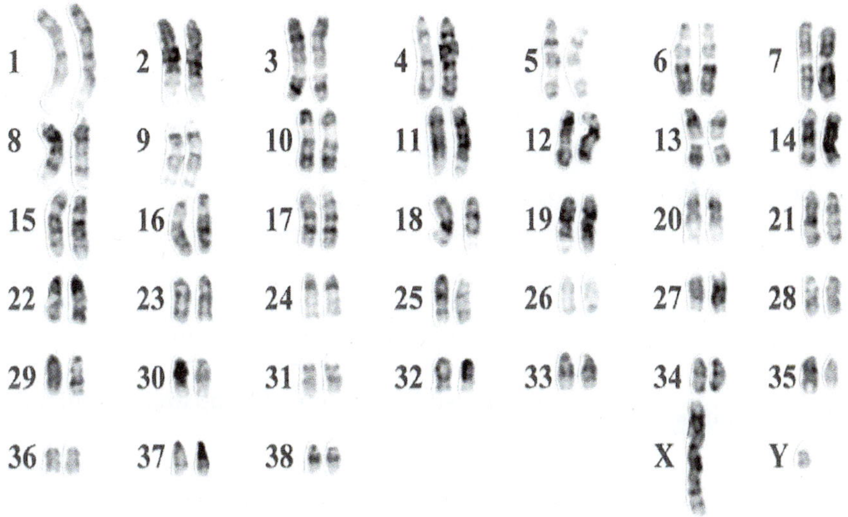

Figure 10.3 DAPI-banded karyotype of the chromosomes of the domestic dog. All autosomes are acrocentric, and the two sex chromosomes are submetacentric.

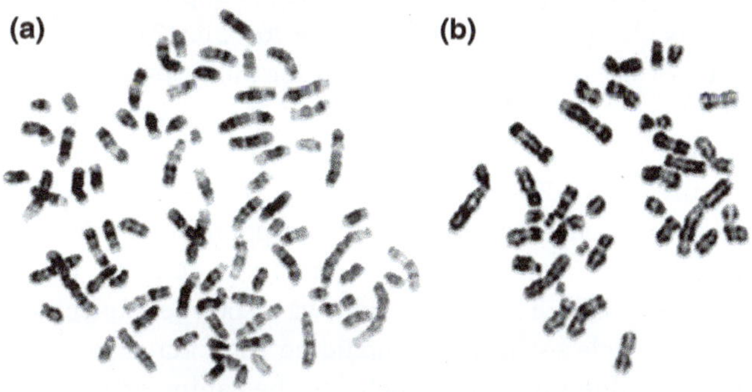

Figure 10.4 The extent of cytogenetic aberrations can be extensive in a cancer cell. (a) DAPI-banded metaphase preparation from a healthy male dog (2n = 78, XY). (b) DAPI-banded metaphase preparation of a cell from a canine osteosarcoma biopsy. The cell has 36 chromosomes, most of which are bi-armed, the result of centric fusions. The high complexity of the rearrangements makes it impossible to identify which segments of the canine genome are associated with each derivative chromosome. Indeed, looking at this metaphase spread without prior knowledge of its origins, one would not even consider it was from a dog.

In this example, the extent of structural rearrangement renders it virtually impossible (using chromosome banding patterns alone) to identify which centromere is associated with each derivative chromosomes, and so such chromosomes cannot be readily identified.

Simple Numerical Changes

If an aberration is the result of an addition/gain or deletion/loss of a whole chromosome (i.e. a change in the total number of chromosomes), the term aneuploidy is used. If the aberration involves gain or loss of a piece of a chromosome that is visible through a microscope, such changes are referred to as segmental aneuploidy. When such changes are submicroscopic, these are referred to as cryptic or focal aberrations. For diploid organisms, such as companion animals, an increase in the number of copies of a genomic region above $n = 2$ could be any number, whereas deletions can only be either a single copy ($n = 1$) or a complete loss ($n = 0$).

Complex Numerical Changes

If an aberration involves the presence of multiple copies (generally five or more copies) of the same region of the genome, the term amplification is used. Amplifications can be subtle, with perhaps 5–8 copies of a genomic region, or can involve 30, 40, and even more than 50 copies of a specific genomic region.

Simple Structural Changes

Structural alterations to single chromosomes can take several forms and are described by the type of change. For example, if a segment of a chromosome breaks from the rest of the chromosome, rotates 180°, and reattaches to the same chromosome, the aberration is referred to as an inversion. Such inversions can occur at the end of a chromosome and include an entire chromosome arm or just a segment within the body of a chromosome. If the inversion includes the centromere, the aberration is termed a pericentric inversion, while if it does not involve reorientation of the centromere, it is termed a paracentric inversion.

Complex Structural Changes

Structural alterations can also involve more than one chromosome, for example, when a piece of one chromosome is transferred to another. This is referred to as a translocation, and if the event involves an exchange of chromosomal material between two chromosomes, the aberration is referred to as a reciprocal translocation.

Impact and Role of Cytogenetic Changes

Either numerical or structural chromosomal changes can result in major cellular consequences, including the formation of novel gene sequences and controlling elements that can alter gene regulation and/or generate new gene products. From a diagnostic perspective, many human cancer subtypes are so strongly associated with a unique cytogenetic abnormality that the detection of such an abnormality is considered pathognomonic for that cancer, or cancer subtype. While the generation of new gene products resulting from cytogenetic abnormalities may drive certain malignancies, such products may also be novel therapeutic targets and might allow for early targeted therapy. The pairing of diagnosis and treatment such that the detection of a characteristic mutation might result in a specific treatment is referred to as companion diagnostics, where the presence of an event not only diagnoses a disease but also indicates an appropriate means to effectively treat that disease. Studies have also identified correlations between the presence of key cytogenetic events in a tumor cell population and the clinical outcome of the patient receiving a particular therapy. Chromosome aberrations may thus be considered of prognostic value, providing clinicians with added information to aid determination of the most appropriate therapy and likely survival times.[2]

Cytogenetics of Animal Cancers

The routine use of cytogenetics in human medicine has to date not been broadly mirrored in veterinary medicine. This is due to a combination of factors including a paucity of baseline information on the nature of cytogenetic changes apparent in animals, a lack of suitable reagents to interrogate veterinary species for disease-specific cytogenetic changes, a lack of information about the clinical relevance of any cytogenetic changes, few skilled individuals to perform such studies, and of course financial constraints. Of the key veterinary species studied by cytogenetics, the domestic dog has received the most attention, and so this species will be used to highlight progress and what can be achieved.

Canine Cancer Cytogenetics, Past, Present, and Future

A History of the Development of Diagnostic Canine Cytogenetics

To achieve consistency in chromosome description, the canine cytogenetics community established a Committee for the Standardization of the Karyotype of the Domestic Dog in the early 1990s. This committee was able to reach a consensus on the identification of dog chromosomes 1–21 (*Canis familiaris* autosome or CFA 1-21) and concluded that a complete standardized karyotype would require the use of molecular cytogenetic reagents.[3] In parallel, Langford et al. generated a panel of whole chromosome paint probes for FISH analysis of the dog.[4] FISH is a direct approach that allows visualization of genomic organization in individual cell nuclei and, notably, is considered the "gold standard" for many diagnostic assays in human oncology. The use of FISH led to the development of a consensus chromosome nomenclature for CFA 21–38, and a numbering system was proposed for all chromosomes of the dog[3,5,6] that was later endorsed by the International Society of Animal Genetics Dog Map workshop in 2000 (Figure 10.3). The introduction of multicolor FISH in canine cytogenetics provided new opportunities to expedite the physical mapping of numerous genomic clones (Figure 10.5). This approach was soon enhanced by genome-wide techniques, including the microarray.[7] The initial canine microarray included the canine orthologues of 31 human cancer genes and provided an opportunity for a first-pass screen of large copy number aberrations in canine cells. Subsequently, the usage of a canine comparative genomic hybridization (CGH) array, which was constructed with 2122 canine bacterial artificial chromosome (BAC) clones from the CHORI-82 canine BAC library,[8] allowed the identification of recurrent DNA copy number aberrations in a variety of canine cancers, including osteosarcoma, brain tumors, transmissible venereal tumors, and histiocytic malignancies.[9–12] The release of a high quality domestic dog genome in 2005[13] facilitated the creation of a genome-wide CGH canine microarray comprising over 170 000 oligonucleotide probes spaced at ~13 kb intervals, which has been used to characterize numerous canine cancer specimens representing canine lymphoma, osteosarcoma, hemangiosarcoma, melanoma, mast cell tumor, leukemia, and urothelial carcinoma.[14–21]

A common theme in all these studies is the ability to identify cancer, and occasionally tumor subtype-specific, DNA copy number changes. This work affirms the potential of cytogenetics to provide both diagnostic and prognostic information in canine cancer patients. Notably, the

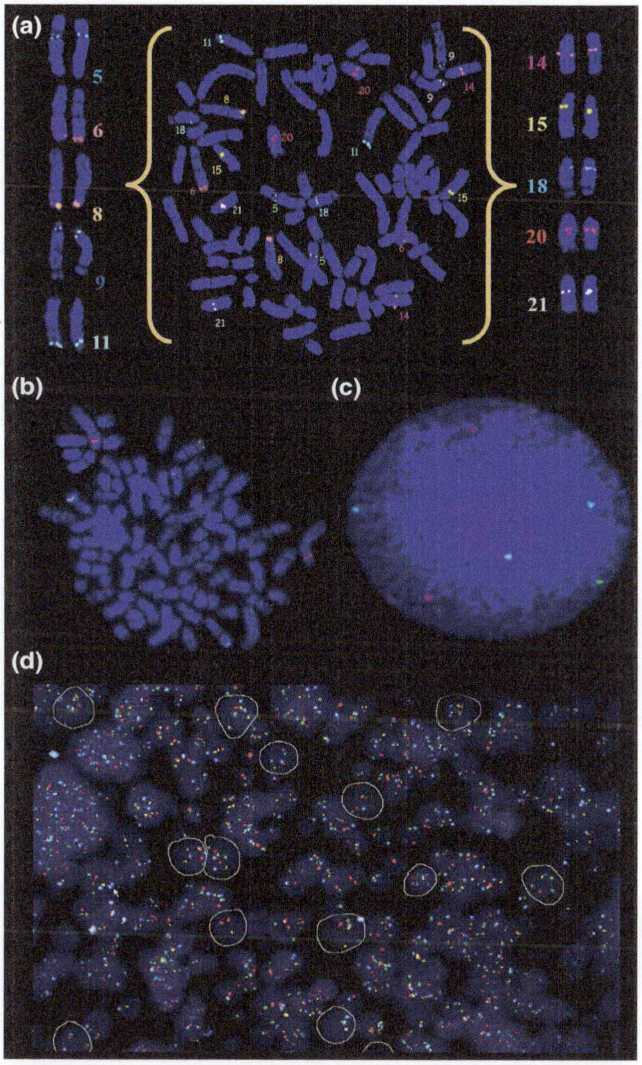

Figure 10.5 Applications of molecular cytogenetics. (a) Single-locus FISH probes can be used individually or, as is the case here, labeled with multiple fluorophores to permit their use in combinations as a means to identify numerous chromosomes simultaneously in metaphase spreads from healthy individuals. (b) Multicolor FISH can be used to determine the copy number of select regions in individual metaphase spreads and (c) interphase nuclei from cancer cells. In this example, in both the metaphase spread and interphase nucleus, the green, red, and aqua probes are visible as $n = 1$, $n = 2$, and $n = 3$ copies, respectively, indicating monosomy of the green locus and trisomy of the aqua locus. (d) To increase throughput, populations of cells can be imaged simultaneously and sophisticated software used to identify discrete nuclei from which multiple probe enumeration or association is automatically determined.

cytogenetic testing approaches that have emerged from these studies may be performed using the same cytological preparations that are presented to the clinical pathologist daily for evaluation, including a blood smear, a fine-needle aspirate of a suspected lesion, a touch preparation of an excised tissue mass, and even a urine cytospin. Specific clinical examples include the identification of a *BCR-ABL* translocation in canine leukemia (the Raleigh chromosome), the assessment of a key cytogenetic signature to detect cells shed from a canine urothelial carcinoma in a free-catch urine specimen, the prediction of the disease-free interval in canine lymphomas treated with cyclophosphamide, doxorubicin, vincristine, and prednisolone (CHOP)-based chemotherapy, and the enumeration of genome regions to differentiate canine histiocytic malignancies from other round cell neoplasms.

Molecular Cytogenetics in Canine Oncology: The Here and Now

Canine Leukemia: The Raleigh Chromosome

The first chromosome aberration to be associated with a specific cancer in people was the Philadelphia chromosome, named after the city in which it was identified.[1] The Philadelphia chromosome is observed in patients with chronic myelogenous leukemia (CML) and results from a translocation event between chromosomes 9 and 22 that brings together the c-*abl* oncogene at *Homo sapiens* autosome (HSA) 9q34 and the breakpoint cluster region (BCR), located at HSA 22q11, to form a derivative human chromosome 22.[22] The juxtaposition of *BCR* and *ABL* has been reported in over 95% of CML patients and is now considered a hallmark feature of this disease.[23] The co-localization of these two genomic regions results in the production of a fusion protein that elevates tyrosine kinase activity, thus enhancing cellular proliferation. The therapeutic significance of this discovery was realized with the identification that imatinib mesylate (Gleevec®, Novartis Pharmaceuticals, Basel, Switzerland) was an antagonist to this fusion protein and thus able to prevent blast crisis.[23–25] In the years following the approval of Gleevec, it was reported that almost two thirds of Philadelphia chromosome-positive CML patients showed a cytogenetic response and almost 90% were free of disease progression.[26,27] Evaluation of cells for the presence of cytogenetic response remains an important surrogate marker of survival in human CML patients.[28,29]

In veterinary species, CML is a rare disease that is largely diagnosed by exclusion and is considered to have a poor prognosis.[30–33] A cytogenetic study of canine CML showed that affected dogs also may present with a functional active BCR-ABL translocation.[33] This study resulted in the first molecular cytogenetic test for a clinically significant genomic alteration in a veterinary cancer and has since been used to identify the presence of the Raleigh chromosome in a further 30 dogs with possible CML (Breen, personal communication). The identification of a functional

BCR-ABL translocation suggests that treatment with Gleevec or other tyrosine kinase inhibitors may be an option for therapy of canine CML. It should be noted that the presence of the Raleigh chromosome should not be interpreted as the dog having CML. Rather, it should be taken as the dog having a BCR-ABL translocation and thus is a candidate for tyrosine kinase therapy. Dogs with a BCR-ABL translocation have been evaluated further during treatment,[34–36] and as more cases are associated with clinical follow-up, we will learn more about the significance of this cytogenetic aberration in canine leukemia.

Canine Urothelial (Transitional Cell) Carcinoma

Canine transitional cell carcinomas (TCC), now referred to as urothelial carcinoma (UC), is estimated to represent ~1–2% of all canine cancers (Chapter 38).[37] Published studies have suggested that over 20 000 cases of canine UC/TCC are diagnosed in the United States each year. However, with an estimated 6 000 000 cancer diagnoses in the United States, a 1–2% incidence would equate to 60 000–120 000 new cases each year, and so published suggestions may be grossly underestimated. UC/TCC can affect the bladder, urethra, and kidneys of male and female dogs and the prostate of males. UC/TCC is most often detected in the trigone of the bladder and can cause partial or complete obstruction of urine entering the bladder from the ureters or prevent urine voiding.[38] At the time of diagnosis, approximately 20% of cases of canine UC/TCC have detectable metastases, with approximately 50% having metastases detected at necropsy.[39] The diagnosis of canine UC/TCC may be delayed as its signs overlap with more common urinary tract disorders (e.g. polyps, stones, or infection), including stranguria, pollakiuria, periuria, dysuria, hematuria, and bacteriuria. During this delay, the underlying UC/TCC may develop into a more advanced, larger, and more invasive neoplasm with a greater likelihood of metastasizing. Once treatment is initiated, most dogs die within the first year of treatment.

The noninvasive diagnosis of canine UC/TCC can be challenging. The routine cytological examination of urine is often inconclusive, and the bladder tumor antigen test offers less than ideal specificity (see Chapter 38). While high-resolution ultrasound can identify small urinary bladder masses, it may miss lesions in the urethra and cannot determine their biologic behavior. The gold standard for the diagnosis of UC/TCC is histologic assessment of a biopsy specimen; however, there may be reluctance to perform an invasive procedure, and there are concerns about cross seeding the cancer when using cystocentesis or surgery.[40,41]

Genome-wide DNA copy number profiling of confirmed canine UC/TCC biopsy specimens identified recurrent aneuploidy of several regions, including gain of a region of dog chromosome CFA 13 in 97% of cases.[18] The same aberration has been found in several other canine cancers,[9,14–17,20,42,43] suggesting that a gain of CFA 13 is an indicator of neoplasia, but is not specific to one cancer type. In addition, copy number gain of CFA 36 was detected in 84% of canine UC/TCC, and the loss of one or both copies of CFA 19 was detected in 77% of these cases.[18] The presence of all three aberrations was detected in 68% of cases of canine UC/TCC and comprises a cytogenetic signature not detected in hundreds of cases of non-UC/TCC cancers. A gain of CFA 13 and CFA 36 offers an odds ratio of 422 in the diagnosis of canine UC/TCC (i.e. a dog with cells containing both aberrations is 422 times more likely to have a UC/TCC than not). To leverage this finding, a multicolor FISH assay designed to detect this unique cytogenetic signature has evaluated urine cytology specimens from hundreds of suspected cases of canine UC/TCC. Thus far, the sensitivity and specify of this assay for the detection of this signature is greater than 99%. When translated to droplet digital polymerase chain reaction (ddPCR), which is more cost effective and higher throughput than traditional FISH, malignant (i.e. UC/TCC) urinary bladder samples could be separated from nonmalignant samples with a 100% sensitivity and specificity when using biopsy specimens and with 67% sensitivity and 100% specificity when using patient-matched urine.[44] The findings show that while FISH analysis remains the gold standard for individual cells, ddPCR offers higher-throughput, lower-cost detection of aneuploidy in cell populations.

In parallel to the identification of this characteristic cytogenetic signature, it was demonstrated that 85% of canine UC/TCC cases harbor a single base mutation in exon 15 of the canine *BRAF* gene.[45,46] This mutation produces a single amino acid change in the *BRAF* protein (valine to glutamic acid or V595E), leading to increased kinase activity, enhanced proliferation, and ultimately tumorigenesis. The absence of this mutation in nonneoplastic bladder tissues, including inflammatory bladder tissue and polyps, led to the development of a rapid and highly sensitive assay using cells shed into the urine.[45] To date, this assay appears to be unaffected by bacteriuria or hematuria and provides a highly effective means to detect the presence of malignant UC/TCC cells in conventional free-catch urine specimens. This noninvasive assay is the first liquid biopsy for the detection of a canine cancer and has been commercialized as the CADET® *BRAF* Mutation Detection Assay (Sentinel Biomedical, Raleigh, NC, USA) with 85% sensitivity and over 99% specificity. The use of ddPCR to further assess the DNA copy number of three key regions of the genome (described above) has been shown detect over two thirds of the 15% of canine UC/TCC cases with expected clinical signs that are not associated with the BRAF mutation. This assay has been commercialized as CADET® *BRAF*-PLUS (Sentinel Biomedical, Raleigh, NC, USA). In combination, the use of CADET® *BRAF* and *BRAF*-PLUS on several thousand cases of canine UC/TCC and controls offers over a combined overall sensitivity of greater than 95% to detect the presence of a canine UC/TCC in a free-catch urine specimen (Breen et al., personal communication).

Canine Lymphoma Prognosis

Canine lymphoma is estimated to affect in excess of 250 000 pet dogs each year in the United States and is one of the most commonly diagnosed canine cancers. While many dogs with lymphoma respond to multi-agent chemotherapy and enter remission, the duration of that remission is highly variable, and there is a lack of reliable means to predict its duration. Recent cytogenetic studies of canine lymphoma have identified a series of DNA copy number changes, some of which are generalized between subtypes and some of which are restricted to one subtype.[20,42] In a recent study, select recurrent DNA copy number changes have been significantly associated with duration of first remission in canine lymphoma treated with either single agent doxorubicin or multi-agent CHOP therapy (Breen et al., in preparation). These data have been used to develop a cytogenetic assay in which regions of the canine genome are evaluated in from lymph node samples and may be used to predict duration of remission in dogs treated with either single agent doxorubicin or multi-agent CHOP therapy.

Histiocytic Malignancies

Histiocytic malignancies are neoplasms derived primarily from the dendritic cells of the skin and visceral organs (Chapter 28). They typically have a very poor prognosis and are considered generally unresponsive to current therapeutic options. Across all dog breeds, histiocytic malignancies are rare, but they do have an overabundance in several purebred dogs, including the Bernese Mountain Dog, Flat-coated Retriever, Golden Retriever, and Rottweiler.[9,47,48] Current testing approaches in the diagnosis of histiocytic neoplasia, including histology and immunohistochemistry, are time consuming and may not be readily accessible. Genome-wide DNA copy number profiling of canine histiocytic malignancies and lymphomas across a range of breeds identified regions of the canine genome that are aberrant in one of these two cancers but not the other. While deletions of dog chromosomes 2, 16, and 31 are frequent aberrations detected in histiocytic neoplasms,[9,49] these deletions have not been reported in several other round cell neoplasms, including lymphoma and soft tissue plasma cell tumors. In fact, dog chromosome 31 is one of the more frequently detected gains in copy number in canine lymphoma.[20] Using these features, a cytogenetic assay was developed to simultaneously assess the mean copy number status of regions of dog chromosomes 2, 16, and 31. The assay has over 97% specificity and over 97% sensitivity to distinguish between histiocytic neoplasia and lymphoma.[50] The use of this cytogenetic assay should add value to the diagnostic toolbox by providing a complementary approach to help differentiate challenging histiocytic malignancies from other round cell cancers.

Conclusion

In summary, the development of sophisticated, well-characterized, molecular cytogenetic reagents for veterinary species provides new opportunities in veterinary oncology. It is likely that, as in human medicine, cytogenetic screening of cancers in our pets could become common practice in veterinary oncology, with assays offering new ways to aid diagnosis, direct therapy, and even offer insights into prognosis.

References

1 Nowell, P.C. and Hungerford, D.A. (1960). A minute chromosome in human chronic granulocytic leukemia. *Science* 132: 1497.

2 Oudejans, J.J., van Wieringen, W.N., Smeets, S.J. et al. (2009). Identification of genes putatively involved in the pathogenesis of diffuse large B-cell lymphomas by integrative genomics. *Genes Chrom Cancer* 48: 250–260.

3 Switonski, M., Reimann, N., Bosma, A.A. et al. (1996). Report on the progress of standardization of the G-banded canine (*Canis familiaris*) karyotype. Committee for the Standardized Karyotype of the Dog (*Canis familiaris*). *Chrom Res* 4: 306–309.

4 Langford, C.F., Fischer, P.E., Binns, M.M. et al. (1996). Chromosome-specific paints from a high-resolution flow karyotype of the dog. *Chrom Res* 4: 115–123.

5 Breen, M., Reimann, N., Bosma, A.A. et al. (1998). Standardization of the chromosome nos. 22–38 of the dog (*Canis familiaris*) with the use of chromosome painting

probes. *Proceedings of the 13th European Colloquium on Cytogenetics of Domestic Animals*, Budapest (1–6 June 1998).

6 Breen, M., Bullerdiek, J., and Langford, C.F. (1999). The DAPI banded karyotype of the domestic dog (*Canis familiaris*) generated using chromosome-specific paint probes. *Chrom Res* 7: 401–406.

7 Thomas, R., Duke, S.E., Bloom, S.K. et al. (2007). A cytogenetically characterized, genome-anchored 10-Mb BAC set and CGH array for the domestic dog. *J Hered* 98: 474–484.

8 Thomas, R., Duke, S.E., Karlsson, E.K. et al. (2008). A genome assembly-integrated dog 1 Mb BAC microarray: a cytogenetic resource for canine cancer studies and comparative genomic analysis. *Cytogenet Genome Res* 122: 110–121.

9 Hedan, B., Thomas, R., Motsinger-Reif, A. et al. (2011). Molecular cytogenetic characterization of canine histiocytic sarcoma: a spontaneous model for human histiocytic cancer identifies deletion of tumor suppressor genes and highlights influence of genetic background on tumor behavior. *BMC Cancer* 11: 201.

10 Thomas, R., Duke, S.E., Wang, H.J. et al. (2009). 'Putting our heads together': insights into genomic conservation between human and canine intracranial tumors. *J Neurooncol* 94: 333–349.

11 Thomas, R., Rebbeck, C., Leroi, A.M. et al. (2009). Extensive conservation of genomic imbalances in canine transmissible venereal tumors (CTVT) detected by microarray-based CGH analysis. *Chrom Res* 17: 927–934.

12 Thomas, R., Wang, H.J., Tsai, P.C. et al. (2009). Influence of genetic background on tumor karyotypes: evidence for breed-associated cytogenetic aberrations in canine appendicular osteosarcoma. *Chrom Res* 17: 365–377.

13 Lindblad-Toh, K., Wade, C.M., Mikkelsen, T.S. et al. (2005). Genome sequence, comparative analysis and haplotype structure of the domestic dog. *Nature* 438: 803–819.

14 Angstadt, A.Y., Motsinger-Reif, A., Thomas, R. et al. (2011). Characterization of canine osteosarcoma by array comparative genomic hybridization and RT-qPCR: signatures of genomic imbalance in canine osteosarcoma parallel the human counterpart. *Genes Chrom Cancer* 50: 859–874.

15 Angstadt, A.Y., Thayanithy, V., Subramanian, S. et al. (2012). A genome-wide approach to comparative oncology: high-resolution oligonucleotide aCGH of canine and human osteosarcoma pinpoints shared microaberrations. *Cancer Gen* 205: 572–587.

16 Poorman, K., Borst, L., Moroff, S. et al. (2014). Comparative cytogenetic characterization of primary canine elanocytic lesions using array CGH and fluorescence in situ hybridization. *Chrom Res* 23: 171–186.

17 Roode, S., Rotroff, R., Avery, A. et al. (2015). Genome-wide assessment of recurrent genomic imbalances in canine leukemia identifies evolutionarily conserved regions for subtype differentiation. *Chrom Res* 23: 681–708.

18 Shapiro, S.G., Raghunath, S., Williams, C. et al. (2015). Canine urothelial carcinoma: genomically aberrant and comparatively relevant. *Chrom Res* 23: 311–331.

19 Thomas, R., Borst, L., Rotroff, D. et al. (2014). Genomic profiling reveals extensive heterogeneity in somatic DNA copy number aberrations of canine hemangiosarcoma. *Chrom Res* 22: 305–319.

20 Thomas, R., Seiser, E.L., Motsinger-Reif, A. et al. (2011). Refining tumor-associated aneuploidy through 'genomic recoding' of recurrent DNA copy number aberrations in 150 canine non-Hodgkin lymphomas. *Leuk Lymphoma* 52: 1321–1335.

21 Mochizuki, H., Thomas, R., Moroff, S., and Breen, M. (2017). Genomic profiling of canine mast cell tumors identifies DNA copy number aberrations associated with KIT mutations and high histological grade. *Chrom Res* 25: 129–143.

22 Rowley, J.D. (1973). Letter: A new consistent chromosomal abnormality in chronic myelogenous leukaemia identified by quinacrine fluorescence and Giemsa staining. *Nature* 243: 290–293.

23 Kurzrock, R., Kantarjian, H.M., Druker, B.J., and Talpaz, M. (2003). Philadelphia chromosome-positive leukemias: from basic mechanisms to molecular therapeutics. *Ann Intern Med* 138: 819–830.

24 Mauro, M.J. and Druker, B.J. (2001). Chronic myelogenous leukemia. *Curr Opin Oncol* 13: 3–7.

25 Mauro, M.J., O'Dwyer, M.E., and Druker, B.J. (2001). ST1571, a tyrosine kinase inhibitor for the treatment of chronic myelogenous leukemia: validating the promise of molecularly targeted therapy. *Cancer Chemother Pharmacol* 48 (Suppl 1): S77–S78.

26 Kantarjian, H.M. and Talpaz, M. (2001). Imatinib mesylate: clinical results in Philadelphia chromosome-positive leukemias. *Semin Oncol* 28: 9–18.

27 Hernandez-Boluda, J.C. and Cervantes, F. (2002). Imatinib mesylate (Gleevec, Glivec): a new therapy for chronic myeloid leukemia and other malignancies. *Drugs Today (Barc)* 38: 601–613.

28 Deininger, M.W. (2003). Cytogenetic studies in patients on imatinib. *Semin Hematol* 40: 50–55.

29 Rosti, G., Testoni, N., Martinelli, G., and Baccarani, M. (2003). The cytogenetic response as a surrogate marker of survival. *Semin Hematol* 40: 56–61.

30 Tarrant, J.M., Stokol, T., Blue, J.T. et al. (2001). Diagnosis of chronic myelogenous leukemia in a dog using morphologic, cytochemical, and flow cytometric techniques. *Vet Clin Pathol* 30: 19–24.

31 Leifer, C.E., Matus, R.E., Patnaik, A.K., and EG, M.E. (1983). Chronic myelogenous leukemia in the dog. *J Am Vet Med Assoc* 183: 686–689.

32 Pollet, L., Van Hove, W., and Mattheeuws, D. (1978). Blastic crisis in chronic myelogenous leukaemia in a dog. *J Small Anim Pract* 19: 469–475.

33 Breen, M. and Modiano, J.F. (2008). Evolutionarily conserved cytogenetic changes in hematological malignancies of dogs and humans: man and his best friend share more than companionship. *Chrom Res* 16: 145–154.

34 Perez, M.L., Culver, S., Owen, J.L. et al. (2013). Partial cytogenetic response with toceranib and prednisone treatment in a young dog with chronic monocytic leukemia. *Anticancer Drugs* 24: 1098–1103.

35 Culver, S., Ito, D., Borst, L. et al. (2013). Molecular characterization of canine BCR-ABL-positive chronic myelomonocytic leukemia before and after chemotherapy. *Vet Clin Pathol* 42: 314–322.

36 Figueiredo, J.F., Culver, S., Behling-Kelly, E. et al. (2012). Acute myeloblastic leukemia with associated BCR-ABL translocation in a dog. *Vet Clin Pathol* 41: 362–368.

37 Knapp, D. and McMillan, S. (2013). Tumors of the urinary system. In: *Withrow and MacEwen's Small Animal Clinical Oncology* (eds. S.J. Withrow, R. Page and D.M. Vail), 572–582. St. Louis, MO: Elsevier Saunders.

38 Knapp, D.W., Glickman, N.W., Denicola, D.B. et al. (2000). Naturally-occurring canine transitional cell carcinoma of the urinary bladder A relevant model of human invasive bladder cancer. *Urol Oncol* 5: 47–59.

39 Patrick, D., Fitzgerald, S., Sesterhenn, A. et al. (2006). Classification of canine urinary bladder urothelial tumours based on the World Health Organization/International Society of Urological Pathology consensus classification. *J Comp Pathol* 135: 190–199.

40 Nyland, T.G., Wallack, S.T., and Wisner, E.R. (2002). Needle-tract implantation following us-guided fine-needle aspiration biopsy of transitional cell carcinoma of the bladder, urethra, and prostate. *Vet Radiol Ultrasound* 43: 50–53.

41 Higuchi, T., Burcham, G.N., Childress, M.O. et al. (2013). Characterization and treatment of transitional cell carcinoma of the abdominal wall in dogs: 24 cases (1985–2010). *J Am Vet Med Assoc* 242: 499–506.

42 Thomas, R., Smith, K.C., Ostrander, E.A. et al. (2003). Chromosome aberrations in canine multicentric lymphomas detected with comparative genomic hybridisation and a panel of single locus probes. *Brit J Cancer* 89: 1530–1537.

43 Thomas, R., Valli, V.E., Ellis, P. et al. (2009). Microarray-based cytogenetic profiling reveals recurrent and subtype-associated genomic copy number aberrations in feline sarcomas. *Chrom Res* 17: 987–1000.

44 Mochizuki, H., Shapiro, S.G., and Breen, M. (2016). Detection of copy number imbalance in canine urothelial carcinoma with droplet digital polymerase chain reaction. *Vet Pathol* 53: 764–772.

45 Mochizuki, H., Shapiro, S.G., and Breen, M. (2015). Detection of BRAF mutation in urine DNA as a molecular diagnostic for canine urothelial and prostatic carcinoma. *PLoS One* 10: e0144170.

46 Mochizuki, H., Kennedy, K., Shapiro, S.G., and Breen, M. (2015). BRAF mutations in canine cancers. *PLoS One* 10: e0129534.

47 Affolter, V.K. and Moore, P.F. (2002). Localized and disseminated histiocytic sarcoma of dendritic cell origin in dogs. *Vet Pathol* 39: 74–83.

48 Moore, P.F. (2014). A review of histiocytic diseases of dogs and cats. *Vet Pathol* 51: 167–184.

49 Kennedy, K., Thomas, R., and Breen, M. (2016). Canine histiocytic malignancies: challenges and opportunities. *Vet Sci* 3: 2–12.

50 Kennedy, K., Thomas, R., Durrant, J. et al. (2019). DNA copy number and targeted transcriptional analysis of canine histiocytic malignancies identifies diagnostic signatures and highlights disruption of spindle assembly complex. *Chrom Res* 27(3): 179–202.

Part III

Skin and Subcutis

11

Inflammatory Diseases of the Skin

Sandra Diaz and M. Judith Radin

Introduction

Inflammatory skin conditions vary widely and include infection, hypersensitivity reactions, and autoimmune diseases. Grossly, inflammatory lesions can manifest as papules, pustules, crusts, scaling, plaques, erosions, ulcers, and draining tracts. Depending on the etiology and chronicity of the conditions, lesions can be localized or widespread. It is not unusual for primary dermatologic conditions to be complicated by secondary bacterial infection as the normal skin barriers are broken down. Evaluation of skin conditions requires a minimum dermatologic database. Commonly performed diagnostic procedures that comprise this database include cytology, skin scrapings, trichograms, Wood's lamp evaluation, bacterial and fungal cultures, and skin biopsy.

Sampling Techniques

Skin Scrapings

Skin scraping is an essential tool in the diagnosis of most skin conditions as it allows identification of parasites. It is relatively simple and easy to perform. An area is selected based on the suspected condition (e.g. ear margins in a suspect case of scabies) while avoiding traumatized skin (excoriations, erosions, ulcerations). To perform the scraping, a surgical microspatula or #10 scalpel blade is used, and multiple sites are sampled. If follicular mites are suspected (*Demodex canis, Demodex injai, Demodex cati*), the skin is firmly squeezed and released, followed by a deep scraping until capillary bleeding is observed. For superficial mites that live on the stratum corneum (*Sarcoptes scabiei, Cheyletiella* spp., *Demodex gatoi, Otodectes cynotis*), superficial scrapings can be performed, and there is no need for capillary bleeding. Applying mineral oil on the skin and blade facilitates sample collection. All collected material (scales and crusts) is transferred to a microscope slide with mineral oil and covered with a coverslip. Slides are examined using the 4× or 10× objective with the condenser lowered to increase contrast.

Acetate Tape Impression with Skin Squeezing

This method has been recently described as an alternative to deep skin scrapings for the identification of demodex mites and was found to be very sensitive.[1] For acetate tape impressions, a 10cm piece of clear tape (Scotch 3M®, Maplewood, MN, USA) is placed on the selected lesion, and the skin is squeezed. The tape strip is removed, fixed on a microscope slide without staining, and examined with a light microscope using the 10× objective immediately after collection.

Flea Comb

Collecting a sample utilizing a flea comb aids in the diagnosis of flea allergy. It also allows identification of other surface ectoparasites such as *Cheyletiella* spp., *D. gatoi*, and lice. Hairs and scales are collected with the comb, transferred to a microscope slide with mineral oil, and covered with a coverslip. Samples are examined with the 4× or 10× objective with the condenser down to increase contrast. The presence of fleas, mites, eggs, and fecal pellets is recorded.

Trichography

Hair examination allows the identification of surface ectoparasites. It also helps in the diagnosis of dermatophytosis by visualization of hyphae and spores, confirmation of pruritus-traumatized hair, identification of roots in anagen and telogen, follicular dysplasias, and visualization

Veterinary Cytology, First Edition. Edited by Leslie C. Sharkey, M. Judith Radin, and Davis Seelig.

of follicular demodex mites. Hair plucking has good sensitivity (85.1%) when compared with deep skin scrapings for the identification of demodex mites, and it may be easier to perform than deep skin scrapings in difficult-to-reach areas (e.g. paws) or in uncooperative patients.[2] However, a negative sample does not rule out the presence of mites.

Hairs are collected by firmly grasping a small group of hairs with the fingertips or a hemostat and plucking them in a fast motion following the direction of the hair growth. The epilated hairs are placed in the same orientation on a microscope slide with mineral oil and covered with a coverslip. The hair shaft is examined from tip to root using the 4× or 10× objective with the condenser lowered to increase contrast.

Cytologic Examination

Cytological examination is a very useful diagnostic tool and is performed in almost every patient with skin lesions at initial presentation. It allows the diagnosis of common infectious conditions, such as superficial pyoderma, *Malassezia* infections, and otitis externa, as well as less common dermatoses such as neoplasms and autoimmune skin diseases. The technique varies depending on the type and location of the lesion.

Impression Smear

Impression smears are used to collect samples (i) from the surface of exudative lesions; (ii) after opening a pustule, vesicle, or papule (Figure 11.1a); or (iii) after removing a crust. The slide is gently pressed against the surface of the lesion so the cells can adhere to the slide without being altered (Figure 11.1b). The slide is air-dried and stained with a quick stain such as Diff-Quik® or a Romanowsky stain. The sample is first examined at low magnification (4× and 10× objectives) to identify areas of interest, followed by examination at higher magnification (50× or 100× immersion oil objective).

Adhesive Tape Preparation

Clear adhesive tape can be used to collect samples from lesions that are dry, oily, or difficult to reach with a microscope slide, e.g. interdigital spaces. To stain the tape following collection of material, the first and second steps of Diff-Quik® are omitted, and the tape is dipped in the third step stain (thiazine dye), rinsed, and let dry (Figure 11.2). A strip of immersion oil is placed on a glass slide, and the tape is placed on top so that the tape acts as a coverslip. Alternatively, the tape can be placed directly on a drop of the third step dye on the slide. The slide is examined with the 100× oil objective to identify *Malassezia* spp. and bacteria. Unstained adhesive tape can be used to identify superficial mites using the 4× or 10× objectives with the condenser down to increase contrast.

Cotton Swabs

Swabs are used to collect samples from ear canals, draining tracts, nail fold, and moist skin lesions (Figure 11.1c). The swab is gently rolled over the lesion or placed in the ear canal. It is then pressed against the microscope slide, allowed to dry, and routinely stained and examined as for impression smears. Cotton swabs can also be used to collect samples to identify ear mites (*O. cynotis*). After introducing the swab in the ear canal and retrieving the sample, the collected material is mixed with mineral oil on a microscope slide and covered with a coverslip. The slide is examined with the 4× or 10× objective with the condenser down to increase contrast.

Microspatula, #10 Scalpel Blade, Toothpick

A microspatula or #10 scalpel blade can aid in sample collection for surface cytology (Figure 11.1d). In addition, a microspatula or a toothpick can be used when collecting samples from difficult-to-reach places, like the nail fold. After gently scraping the surface of the affected skin, the instrument is firmly pressed against the microscope slide. The slide is then routinely stained and examined as for impression smears. A recent review comparing the use of tape preparations, direct impression smears, and toothpicks to identify bacteria, yeast, and inflammatory cells from the nail folds found a higher number of organisms present in the samples collected by toothpick.[3]

Fine-Needle Aspiration

Fine-needle aspiration (FNA) is used to collect samples from nodules, tumors, plaques, and abscesses. Typically, a 20–22 G needle and a 6–12 mL syringe are used for skin lesions. The methods for aspiration and slide preparation are described in Chapter 1. Smears are usually made by the squash method and stained with a Romanowsky stain or quick stain. Stained slides are first examined with a low power objective (4× and 10×) to identify areas of interest, followed by examination with an oil immersion (50× and 100×) objective.

Wood's Lamp

A Wood's lamp is an ultraviolet light with a wavelength of 253.7 nm, filtered through a cobalt or nickel filter. It is used for the diagnosis of dermatophytosis. The primary dermatophyte of veterinary importance that produces fluorescence is *Microsporum canis*. The characteristic "apple green" fluorescence observed on *M. canis*-infected hair

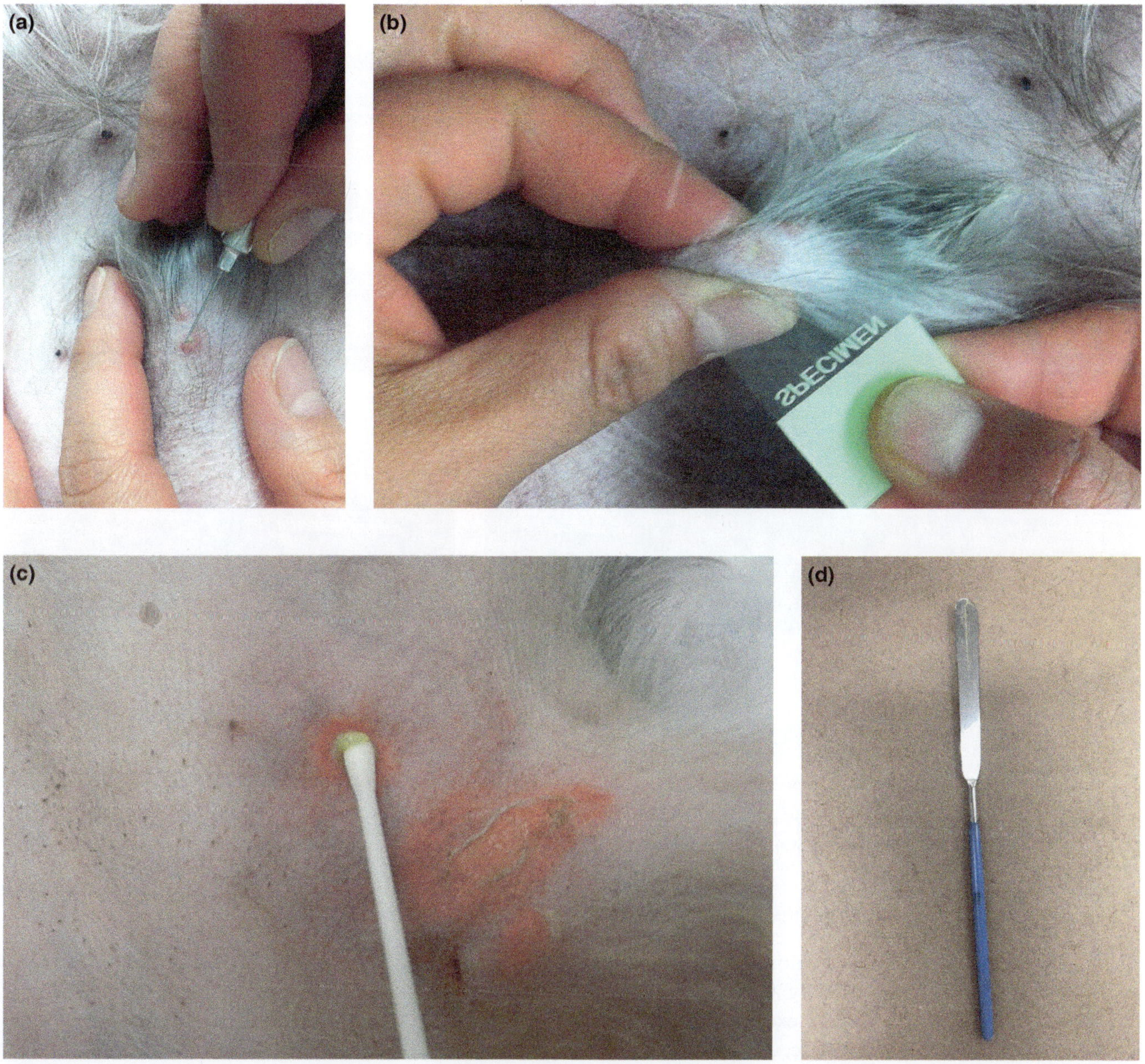

Figure 11.1 Common methods for obtaining cytologic samples of skin lesions. (a) Opening a pustule with a needle prior to making an impression smear. (b) Impression smear of a pustule. (c) A cotton swab can be used to collect samples from draining tracts, nail folds, moist skin lesions, and ear canals. (d) A microspatula is used to obtain samples by scraping.

shafts is due to pteridine, a water-soluble chemical metabolite located within the cortex or medulla of the hair; therefore, fluorescence should be seen in individual hairs. Scales and crusts do not fluoresce. False negatives can be observed, and it is anecdotally reported that only approximately 50% of *M. canis* isolates fluoresce. A recent review stated that in untreated cats, positive fluorescence varied from 91 to 100%, while fluorescence varied from 39 to 53% in animals that were previously treated.[4] False positives can be seen with keratin, soaps, petroleum jelly, and some bacteria (*Pseudomonas* spp., *Corynebacterium* spp.); however, in these cases, the fluorescence is not apple green.

Fungal Culture

Fungal culture is usually considered the gold standard for the diagnosis of dermatophytosis; however, in a recent consensus paper, no one test was identified as a "gold standard."[4] False-negative and false-positive culture results can occur. A recent study comparing real-time polymerase

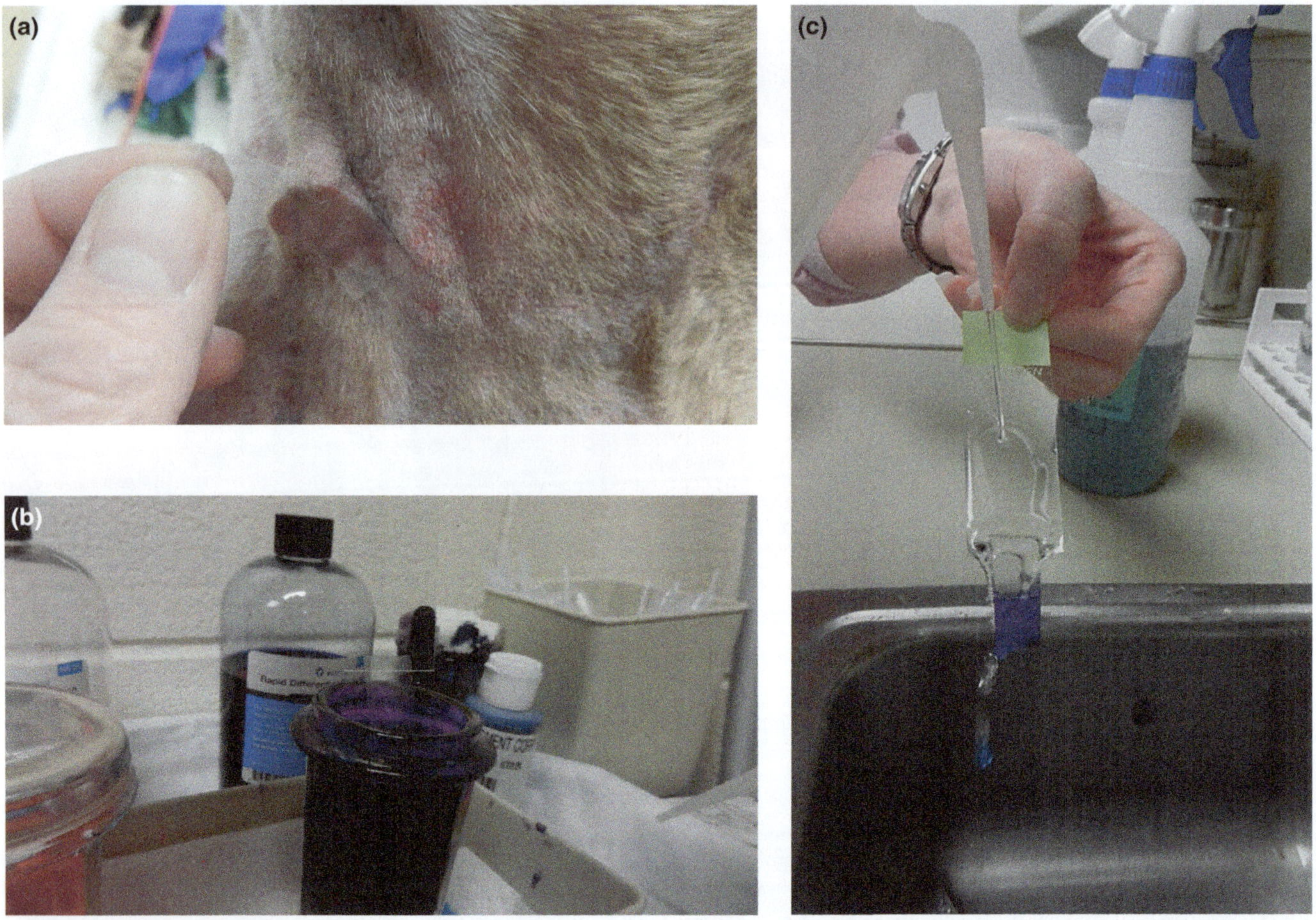

Figure 11.2 The tape method for collecting samples. (a) Tape is applied to the lesion. (b) The tape is stained using only the third step (thiazine dye) of the Diff-Quik stain. (c) Staining is followed by rinsing with water and applying the tape over immersion oil on a microscope slide.

chain reaction (PCR) with fungal culture for the diagnosis of *M. canis* reported 100% sensitivity and specificity, with the advantage of rapid diagnosis or exclusion of dermatophytosis.[5] A positive PCR test can occur with active infection but also with fomite carriage or nonviable fungal organisms from a successfully treated infection.[4] A false-negative test can occur because of sampling technique or the presence of pathogens other than *M. canis*.[4]

Dermatophyte test medium (DTM) agar is used to selectively culture for dermatophytes. DTM contains Sabouraud's dextrose agar, cycloheximide (antifungal), gentamicin (antibacterial), chlortetracycline (antibacterial), and phenol red (a pH indicator). Sample collection can be performed with the help of a Wood's lamp to identify infected hairs or from the periphery of a lesion, making sure to include damaged hairs, scales, and crusts. If the condition involves deep lesions (e.g. kerions, dermatophytic pseudomycetomas), a tissue sample should be collected for culture.[6] When nodules or plaques are to be cultured, the surface of the skin is disinfected, and a biopsy aseptically collected. The tissue is then placed in a sterile container. The laboratory should be consulted about transport media, but generally culturettes with transport media are adequate. A three-week incubation period is usually recommended; however, a recent retrospective study suggested that two weeks can be sufficient. In this study, *M. canis* isolates were recovered within 14 days from 98.2% of pretreatment samples and 96.5% of samples from cats receiving treatment.[7]

Punch Biopsy

Histopathology is required for the diagnosis of some skin diseases such as neoplasia, immune-mediated diseases, dermatomyositis, sebaceous adenitis, zinc responsive dermatosis, and follicular dysplasias. It also assists in the diagnosis of parasitic disease, bacterial infection, fungal infection, sterile dermatoses, and paraneoplastic syndromes. A biopsy is indicated when (i) the history and clinical examination suggest a disease that needs to be confirmed by histopathology, (ii) the clinical approach has not given a diagnosis, (iii) the condition has been refractory to appropriate treatment for a previous diagnosis, (iv) a disease that requires prolonged treatment potentially associated with serious side effects needs to be confirmed (e.g. immune-mediated diseases), and (v) nodules, vesicles, and/or ulcers are present.[8] The type of lesions to be sampled will depend on the clinical presentation. Primary lesions are ideally sampled, but are not always present. If no primary lesions are present, secondary lesions representing different stages of evolution can be sampled. For example, in pemphigus foliaceus (PF), the primary lesion is a pustule; if absent, an intact, adhered crust can be sampled. If there are variable lesions present, collecting a sample of each type increases the chances of a diagnosis.

Most samples can be collected with a 6 mm punch biopsy, but punches as large as 8 mm can be used. When collecting samples from sensitive places like the nose and the paw pads, a 4 mm punch can be used. To perform the biopsy, the lesion to be sampled is selected, and the hair gently clipped if needed, taking care to avoid touching the skin surface. The periphery of the lesion is marked with a permanent marker and infiltrated with 2% lidocaine. "Normal" skin is not included, except when collecting a sample from an ulcer or scar, in which case the junction of lesional and normal skin is included. The punch biopsy is slightly pressed against the skin and rotated in a clockwise motion to penetrate the full thickness of the skin. The punch is then removed to expose the sample that is usually adhered to the subcutaneous tissue. To collect the sample, the subcutaneous fat is cut carefully with iris scissors, and small forceps can be used to support the subcutaneous tissue. Care should be taken to not damage the sample with the forceps, which can create artifacts. Excess blood is removed by gently blotting the sample with a piece of gauze. The biopsy is then placed in 10% formalin. The incision can be closed with suture or staples. If small nodules that can be completely excised or deep lesions (e.g. panniculitis) are present, elliptical wedge biopsies are recommended.

Infectious Agents

Infection of the skin can occur when there is disruption of the cutaneous barrier through trauma, wounds (surgical or otherwise), parasites, allergy, immunosuppression, endocrine disease, or environmental conditions (e.g. heat and humidity). Lesions vary and include papules, pustules, nodules, crusting lesions, alopecia, ulcers, draining tracts, and granulomatous nodules.[9] Inflammatory response patterns range from neutrophilic (typical with most bacteria) to granulomatous to pyogranulomatous (often seen with fungal agents). Lesions can have an eosinophilic component, depending on the infectious agent and if allergies are contributing to disease development.

Bacteria

Cytology is useful in detecting bacteria in cutaneous samples and for evaluation of inflammatory patterns and efficacy of antimicrobial therapy (see Chapter 3 for discussion of correlation of cytology and culture for bacterial and fungal organisms).[10–14] Fewer than 2 cocci and less than 2 rods per 1000× oil immersion field (OIF) are expected on normal canine skin.[15] Distinguishing active bacterial infection from surface colonization requires the presence of both neutrophils and phagocytosis of bacteria on cytology.[12,13] In one study, impression smear cytology had a diagnostic sensitivity of 93% in distinguishing dogs with superficial pyoderma from normal dogs when criteria for infection included the presence of neutrophils, intracellular (phagocytized) bacteria, and either >2 or >5 extracellular cocci or rods/OIF.[16] Tape, impression smear, and swab methods are all able to detect inflammation and bacteria. Tape and impression smear methods outperformed the swab method in experimentally defined conditions.[17]

Increased numbers of extracellular bacteria can indicate a pathologic skin condition. Using the tape method, bacterial overgrowth syndrome in dogs is suggested when five or more extracellular bacteria are seen in an OIF.[14,18] While affected dogs had the highest numbers of bacteria in areas with cutaneous lesions, extracellular bacterial numbers were higher even in those areas without obvious lesions when compared with skin of normal dogs.[18] Bacterial counts were shown to decrease in response to antibiotic therapy but still not decline to numbers as low as on the skin of healthy dogs.

Active infection (pyoderma, folliculitis, furunculosis) is typically characterized by degenerate neutrophils. Isolates from cutaneous lesions are frequently bacteria that are found on healthy skin as part of the normal microflora and may represent opportunistic infections. Staphylococcal species, especially *Staphylococcus pseudintermedius*, are cultured most often from canine superficial and deep pyoderma.[14] Similarly, *Staphylococcus* spp. are commonly isolated from the cat and horse.[19–21] Rod-shaped bacteria are less commonly isolated from skin infections and include *Proteus* spp., *Pseudomonas aeruginosa*, and *Escherichia coli* in dogs and cats, *Rhodococcus equi* in cats, and *Corynebacterium* in horses.[14,22–25] *Dermatophilus congolensis* is a common isolate in horses with higher prevalence in tropical climates or in the autumn and winter in temperate climates.[26,27] Diagnosis of *D. congolensis* is based on the presence of typical lesions and demonstration of the characteristic "railroad track" pattern of bacterial cocci by impression cytology from crusts (Figure 58.2).[26,27] Because bacteria can be scarce, especially with chronic lesions, newer tests such as real-time quantitative PCR are being evaluated.[27,28]

The inflammatory pattern observed with actinomycosis, nocardiosis, and mycobacterial infections is pyogranulomatous dermatitis and panniculitis. *Actinomyces* and *Nocardia* spp. appear as filamentous bacteria on cytology. Cutaneous infection with *Mycobacterium* spp. can be diagnosed by cytology in cats and dogs.[29,30] FNAs are characterized by mixed inflammation with predominantly macrophages and occasional multinucleated giant cells.[31–35] Variable numbers of neutrophils, lymphocytes, plasma cells, and fibroblasts are seen. Because of their lipid cell wall, the bacilli do not stain with Romanowsky-type stains (Figure 11.3). Consequently, mycobacteria appear as negatively-stained, clear, thin, rod-shaped spaces within macrophages and giant cells and free in the background. *Mycobacteria* spp. are acid-fast and will stain red with a modified acid-fast stain (e.g. Ziehl–Neelsen).

Malassezia

Malassezia spp. are commonly found on the skin of healthy dogs and cats (see Figure 17.2a).[36] Anatomic location and sampling technique can influence the ability to detect organisms on the skin, with the tape method showing some advantages.[37,38] In a control group of healthy cats, <2 yeast/OIF were found in 7/18 cats and usually in only one anatomic site.[39] In one study, *Malassezia* spp. were found on swab smears prepared from the nail fold in 61% of 46 cats, and the presence of yeast correlated with brown greasy material in the nail folds.[40] Likewise, normal skin of dogs typically yields <2 yeast/OIF with higher populations around the mouth and chin.[37,41] Basset Hounds and Devon Rex cats appear to harbor higher numbers of yeast on normal appearing skin compared with other breeds.[41,42] In horses, *Malassezia* is most commonly found in intertriginous areas such as the groin, intermammary area, and prepuce where numbers of yeast may exceed 10/OIF.[43–45] Other cutaneous areas usually exhibit <2 yeast/OIF.

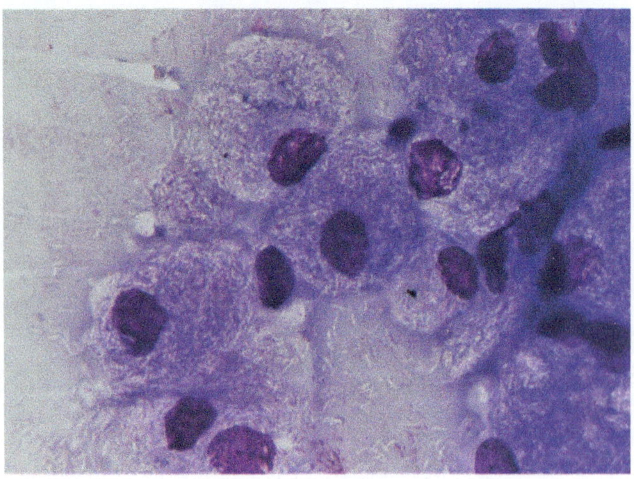

Figure 11.3 Aspirate of a skin mass from a cat with feline leprosy. Numerous nonstaining rods compatible with *Mycobacterium* spp. are observed within the cytoplasm of the macrophages and free in the background (Wright's, 1000×).

Overgrowth of *Malassezia* spp. associated with dermatitis in cats is suggested when >2 yeast/OIF are found in at least two separate anatomic locations when sampled by the tape method.[39] Diagnosis of *Malassezia* dermatitis in dogs is based on finding 3–5 or more yeast/OIF using tape samples.[37,41] Fewer numbers may be significant if the dog has developed a hypersensitivity to the yeast. *Malassezia* dermatitis is uncommon in the horse.[9,26,46]

Dermatophytes

Dermatophytosis is common in dogs, cats, and horses. Lesions are variable and can be minimal to more severe, characterized by alopecia, folliculitis, granuloma, and kerion formation. Diagnostic techniques were reviewed in a recent consensus paper, and no single test was identified as a "gold standard."[4] Hair examination and cytology including skin scrapes, impression smears, and FNA are useful diagnostic aids.[47,48] In one study of dogs with kerions, spores and hyphae were detectable in 15/39 dogs using impression smears and FNAs.[48] On cytology, spores (arthroconidia) are 2–5 μm in diameter, round, and basophilic and sometimes have a clear halo (Figure 11.4).[47,49,50] Hyphae are 2–3 μm in diameter and septate and exhibit variable staining.[47,49] Organisms can be seen in association with squamous epithelial cells, keratin, and hair. Cellularity is consistent with pyogranulomatous inflammation, including neutrophils, lymphocytes, plasma cells, macrophages, multinucleated giant cells, eosinophils, and fibroblasts.[9,47,49,51,52] Acantholytic keratinocytes can be seen in some cases of dermatophytosis, especially *Trichophyton* spp.[50,53,54] Culture and speciation of the dermatophyte involved helps to guide prevention.

Demodex

Demodex mites are normal inhabitants of the skin that occupy the hair follicles and sebaceous glands. The cause

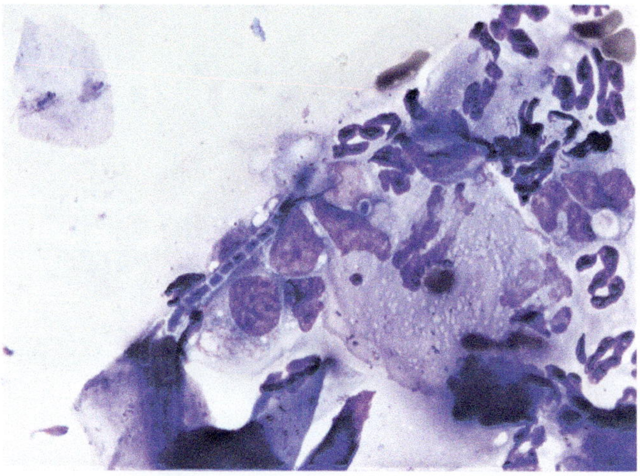

Figure 11.4 Cytology from the pinna of an 8-year-old dog with crusting and alopecia. Septate fungal hyphae and spores are admixed with keratin, neutrophils, and macrophages. *Trichophyton* sp. was cultured from hair samples (Diff-Quik, 1000×).

of generalized demodicosis appears to be related to genetic predisposition in the juvenile form and immunosuppression secondary to endocrinopathy, neoplasia, drugs, or other infections in the adult-onset form.[55] Deep skin scrapes are most commonly used to detect *Demodex* (Figure 11.5), and finding more than one mite is considered suggestive for clinical disease.[56,57] Tape preparations can be used to demonstrate mites, especially with generalized demodicosis due to the large number of mites that come to the surface of the skin.[1,2,57,58] Several studies suggested that tape with skin squeezing is of similar or better sensitivity as deep skin scrapes.[1,58] Trichograms are not as diagnostically sensitive as scraping or tape methods. Trichograms examining 50–100 hairs will detect mites in about 50–80% of cases.[2,55,56] Multiple stages including adults, immature mites, and eggs can be seen. Exudate cytology from expression of pustules can help determine if there is secondary pyoderma and may be of similar sensitivity as deep skin scrapes.[2] Degenerate neutrophils with intracellular bacteria, usually *Staphylococcus* spp., are found in association with the mites (Figure 11.5).

Sarcoptic Mange

Scabies, caused by *S. scabiei*, is a pruritic, contagious disease that primarily affects dogs, cats, and horses. Because the mites are not host specific, human owners can be infected. Deep skin scraping of crusted papules or in heavily scaled areas is frequently used to demonstrate mites, ova, and feces (scybala) (Figure 11.6). However, a negative scrape does not exclude infection as scraping may detect mites in only 20% of cases.[59] One study suggested that the tape method may be more sensitive than deep skin scrapes at finding sarcoptes mites.[58]

Other Agents

Protozoal and other fungal agents are detectable by cytology. For images and descriptions, see Chapter 3. For canine papilloma virus, see Chapter 12. Feline herpes virus 1 is discussed in section "Eosinophilic Dermatitides."

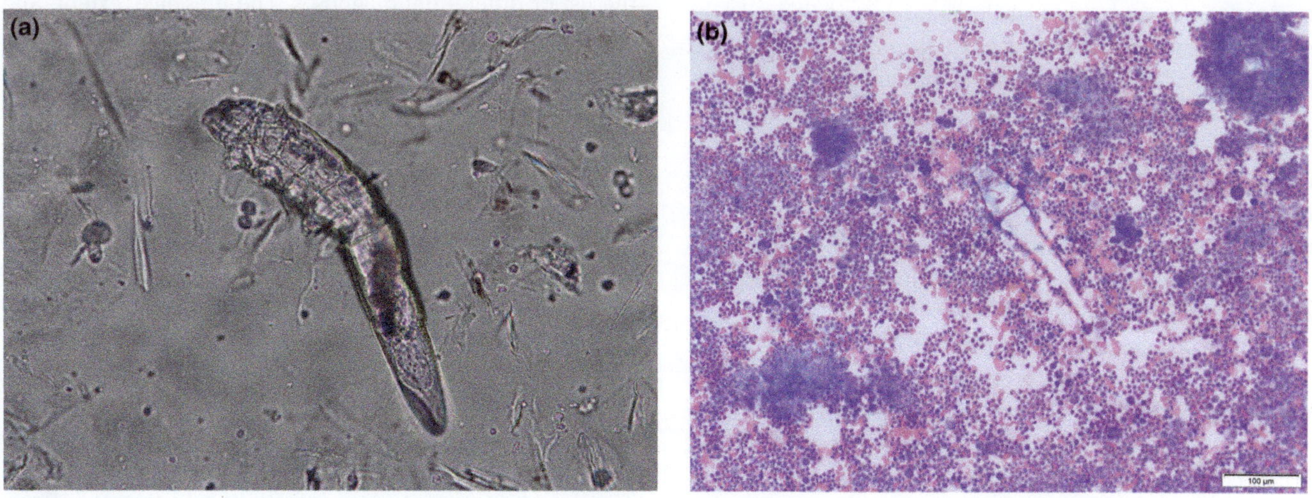

Figure 11.5 (a) Demodex mite and keratin flakes obtained by skin scraping (unstained, in mineral oil). (b) Demodex mite (center) with numerous neutrophils in the background, compatible with a secondary pyoderma (Wright's stain. *Source:* Image courtesy of Erin Burton).

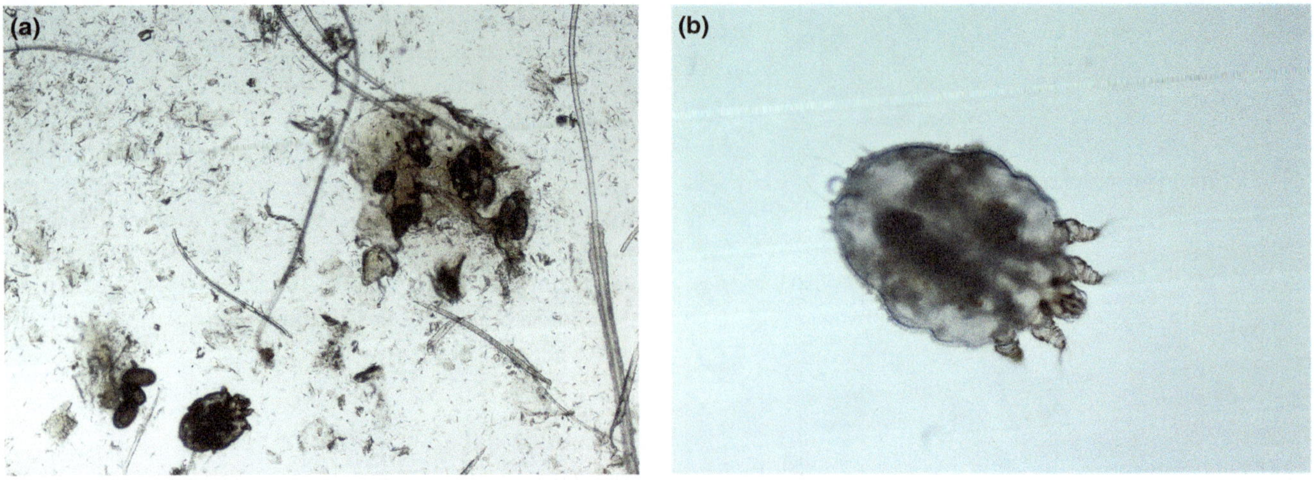

Figure 11.6 (a) Scabies mite and eggs obtained by skin scraping (unstained, in mineral oil.) (b) Scabies mite (unstained, in mineral oil, 400×).

Hypersensitivity and Autoimmune Skin Diseases

Fleabite Hypersensitivity

Fleabite hypersensitivity is a common hypersensitivity reaction to flea saliva antigens. Clinically, the lesions consist of erythematous and crusted papules, erythema, and, in most cases, severe pruritus. In dogs, fleabite affects the lumbosacral area, caudal aspect of hind limbs, and tail base. In chronic cases, clinical signs may become more generalized. In cats, unlike dogs, the distribution of the clinical signs and type of lesions is more variable. Cats with hypersensitivity reactions usually present with one of the following patterns: miliary dermatitis, self-induced alopecia, eosinophilic granuloma complex (EGC), or head and neck pruritus. Other insects and mites also can cause papular dermatitis. In addition, in the cat, hypersensitivity reactions to environmental and/or food allergens can have a similar clinical presentation.

The diagnosis of fleabite hypersensitivity is based on the clinical response to strict flea control. Intradermal testing can be used to support the diagnosis, but a negative result does not exclude fleabite hypersensitivity.[60] Although cytology of the papules is not diagnostic for fleabite hypersensitivity, it will allow the clinician to exclude the presence of a bacterial folliculitis and help to confirm the suspicion of fleabite hypersensitivity. Samples for cytologic evaluation can be collected from an erythematous papule by impression smear after carefully opening the surface with a 25 g needle or a scalpel blade or after gently removing the small crusts covering the papules. Skin cytology will reveal variable number of eosinophils, intermixed with neutrophils and small numbers of mast cells.[61–64] Lymphocytes, macrophages, and plasma cells predominate in chronic cases.[64]

Feline Miliary Dermatitis

Feline miliary dermatitis is characterized clinically by numerous, small, localized or generalized erythematous and crusted papules. It is the most common feline problem in small animal dermatology. The list of differential diagnoses for miliary dermatitis is lengthy and includes allergies (fleabite hypersensitivity, atopic dermatitis, and/or adverse food reactions), parasitic diseases (*Cheyletiella*, *Notoedres*, *Otodectes*, and *D. gatoi*), infectious conditions (bacterial and fungal), immune-mediated diseases such as PF, and dietary imbalances like essential fatty acid and biotin deficiencies.[65] In addition, urticaria pigmentosa-like disease has been reported in Sphynx and Devon Rex cats in which the papules are generalized with a linear configuration.[66,67] A detailed history will often provide information that helps to narrow the list of differential diagnoses. The presence, extent, and severity of pruritus, the occurrence of skin lesions in animals or people in contact with the patient, seasonality, and response to previous medications are especially helpful.

Initial evaluation includes collecting skin scrapings to look for mites and skin cytology to characterize the inflammatory infiltrate and identify the presence of secondary infections (bacterial and yeast). Since dermatophytosis is an important differential diagnosis for military dermatitis, direct examination of the hair shafts for presence of spores and hyphae is done, and, if negative, a fungal culture is indicated.

If skin scrapings are negative, treatment trials are recommended to exclude the presence of external parasites. If there is secondary bacterial or yeast infection, it is recommended to treat them before pursuing further diagnoses. The presence of secondary infections will trigger inflammation; therefore, diagnostic cytology and histopathologic findings may be masked.

As with flea hypersensitivity, samples are collected after gently removing the small crust covering the erythematous papules. After removing the crust, an impression smear of the "opened" papule can be made. Samples will show a variable number of eosinophils and neutrophils, and in more chronic cases, lymphocytes and macrophages can also be present.[50,68] Rarely, basophils are seen.[50] Secondary pyoderma with neutrophils and bacteria can complicate cytologic diagnosis.[68] Acantholytic epithelial cells are not expected with miliary dermatitis.[69]

Pemphigus Foliaceus

PF is an autoantibody-mediated skin disease that has been documented in dogs, cats, horses, goats, sheep, and a cow.[70] PF is the most common autoimmune skin disease in dogs. The major autoantigen targeted in people is desmoglein-1; however, it has been recently demonstrated that the major antigen in dogs is desmocollin-1, with desmoglein-1 being only a minor antigen in this species.[71] Desmogleins and desmocollins are cadherins, transmembrane glycoproteins that form part of the desmosomes. Alteration of these components of the cell adhesion junctions results in the separation of the keratinocytes, known as "acantholysis," the hallmark of PF. The lesions are found in the superficial spinous and granular layers of the epidermis. Acantholysis results in formation of vesicles, which are quickly infiltrated by neutrophils, forming pustules.

The primary lesions seen in cases of canine PF are pustules (Figure 11.7a). As the pustules are superficial and fragile, only the resultant crusts are observed in most cases. Consequently, the most common clinical sign in dogs and

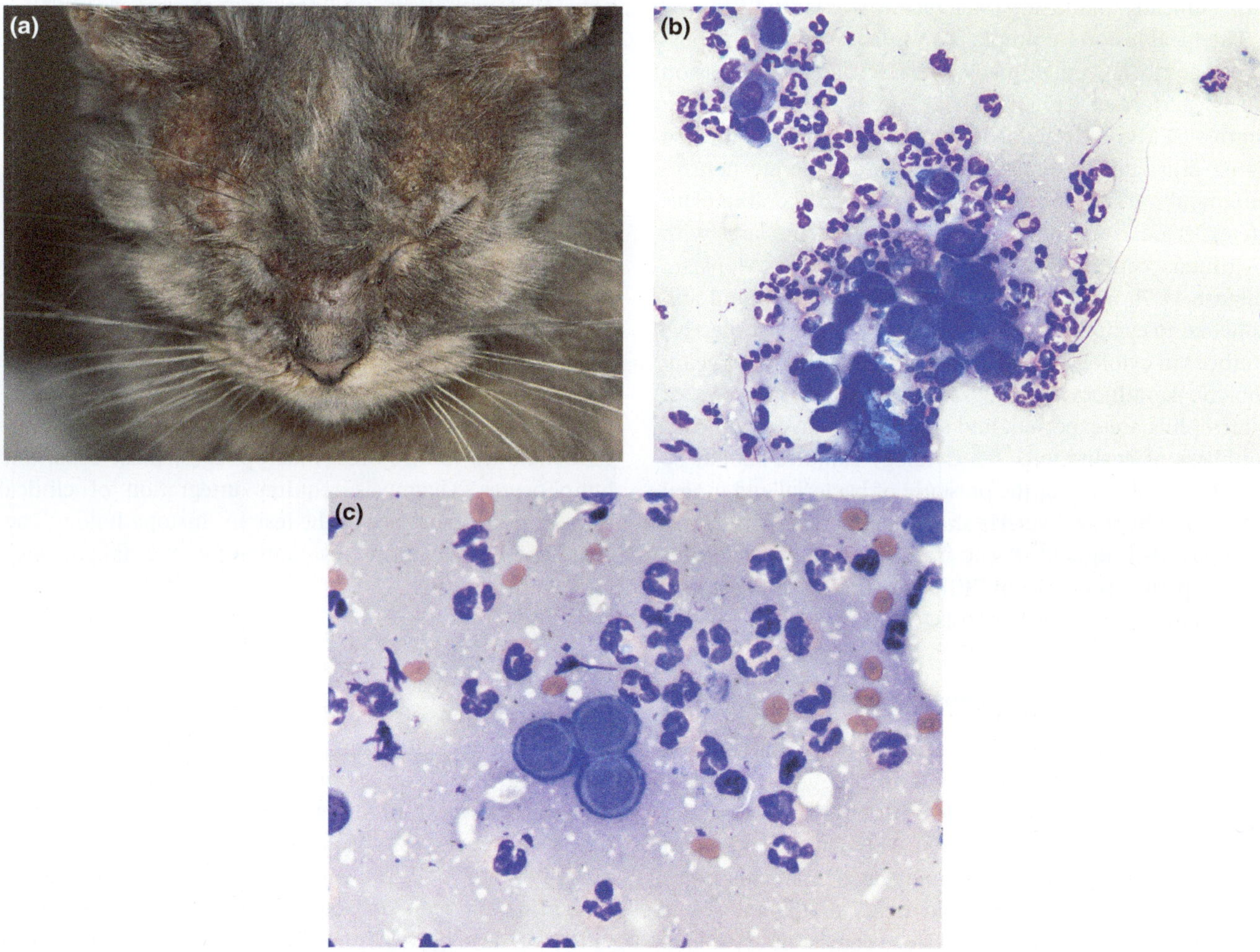

Figure 11.7 (a) A cat with pemphigus foliaceus. (b) Acantholytic epithelial cells and neutrophils from the muzzle of a cat with pemphigus foliaceus. Some of the acantholytic cells have deeply basophilic cytoplasm that obscures the nucleus (Wright's, 500×). (c) Acantholytic cells from the cat exhibit a round nucleus and deeply basophilic cytoplasm (Wright's, 1000×).

cats with PF is crusting, followed by pustules and alopecia. In horses, edema and crusts have been identified as the most common lesions.[72] While lesions in some cases of canine and feline PF have a generalized distribution, lesions are often seen in the inner pinnae, dorsal muzzle, trunk, paw pads, and periocular region. In cats, a recent retrospective study indicated the pinnae, head, and face to be commonly affected.[73] Periareolar skin and nail beds are also often involved in cats. In horses, the most commonly affected areas include the face, trunk, neck, and extremities.[72,74] Other areas involved are the coronary band, mane, prepuce, and dorsum. Mucous membranes are rarely affected.

Important clinical differential diagnoses for canine PF are bacterial folliculitis and dermatophytosis; therefore, bacterial and fungal cultures are indicated to exclude these conditions. Some *Staphylococcus* spp. produce exfoliative toxins that can cause significant acantholysis.[75] Superficial pustular dermatophytosis caused by *Trichophyton* spp. can look clinically and histopathologically similar to PF.[53]

The ideal lesion to sample is an intact pustule. The pustule is gently lanced with a 25 g needle, and an impression smear performed (Figure 11.1a and b). Alternatively, a sample can be collected from underneath a newly formed moist crust. On cytology, many non-degenerate neutrophils and variable number of acantholytic keratinocytes are expected.[76,77] Acantholytic keratinocytes are large with a round central nuclei and dark blue cytoplasm (Figure 11.7b and c). These cells can often be found still attached to each other, forming clusters. In a retrospective study, skin cytology samples showed the presence of acantholytic keratinocytes in 37/48 dogs.[76] High numbers of neutrophils are expected, and some cases have significant numbers of eosinophils.[76,78] Cytology samples should be carefully evaluated for the presence of bacterial and fungal spores and hyphae. Bacteria should not be seen if the sampled pustule is intact.[77] Because acantholytic keratinocytes are not pathognomonic for PF, histopathology must be performed to confirm the diagnosis.[79]

Cutaneous Lupus Erythematosus

Canine cutaneous lupus erythematosus (CLE) variants are diverse. A recent publication proposes a new classification for CLE in the dog that includes subacute CLE (vesicular CLE) and chronic CLE (exfoliative CLE, facial/generalized discoid lupus erythematosus, and mucocutaneous lupus erythematosus).[80] Facial discoid lupus erythematosus is the most common form. Skin lesions consist of erythema, depigmentation, and scaling that progress to erosions and ulceration. Differential diagnoses include mucocutaneous pyoderma, pemphigus complex, cutaneous drug reaction, erythema multiforme, cutaneous lymphoma, uveodermatologic syndrome, squamous cell carcinoma, solar dermatitis, and deep fungal infections.

Sample collection from erosive to ulcerative lesions is difficult. To identify secondary infections, an impression smear can be performed from superficial lesions. When collecting a sample from a deeper ulcer, a scalpel blade can be used to gently scrape the edge of the ulcer and place the sample onto a microscope slide. Findings must be interpreted carefully since blood and environmental contaminants can be present. The visualization of intracellular bacteria helps to identify the presence of mucocutaneous or deep pyoderma. However, in cases of deep pyoderma, the absence of organisms does not exclude infection. Therefore, a tissue sample should then be submitted for bacterial culture if an infection is suspected.

Ulcerative lesions rarely provide diagnostic samples since they are highly contaminated. As with most ulcerative diseases, CLE can be only diagnosed by histopathology. Histopathology findings are characterized by a lichenoid, cell-rich, lymphocytic interface dermatitis with basal keratinocyte vacuolar degeneration, apoptosis, loss of basal cells, and basement membrane thickening.[9,80]

Eosinophilic Dermatitides

Eosinophilic inflammation in the skin often results from a hypersensitivity reaction to foreign material, environmental allergens, flea and insect bites, parasites, some infectious agents, drugs, and food.[81] While cytology of these conditions typically has an eosinophilic component, eosinophils often are one part of a mixed inflammatory picture that includes neutrophils, macrophages, mast cells, and lymphocytes. Diagnosis requires integration of clinical signs, gross appearance of the lesions, histopathology, bacterial and fungal culture, evaluation for external parasites, and allergy testing.

Eosinophilic Granuloma Complex of Cats

EGC of cats consists of indolent or rodent ulcers, eosinophilic plaques, and eosinophilic granulomas. An individual cat can exhibit one or multiple of these lesions. EGC is a manifestation of an allergic reaction and is observed in cats with hypersensitivity to a variety of allergens (fleas, mosquito bite, food, and environmental factors) and atopic dermatitis.[82–85] Genetic factors possibly modulate susceptibility for development of EGC.[86,87] Feline herpesvirus 1 (FHV1) has been found in eosinophilic granulomas in cats.[88] Diagnosis of EGC is aided by the appearance of gross lesions, cytology, and histology. FNA, tapes, and skin scrapes help exclude other etiologic agents and conditions such as neoplasia. Peripheral eosinophilia is common with eosinophilic plaque but less common with indolent ulcer and eosinophilic granuloma.[81]

Cytology of EGC is characterized by numerous eosinophils with variable numbers of neutrophils and macrophages (Figure 11.8).[83,89] Cytology is useful in determining if there is secondary bacterial infection, as evidenced by the presence of degenerate neutrophils with phagocytized bacteria.[83,84,89] Secondary infection with *Staphylococcus* spp. is common. In one study, all cats with eosinophilic plaque or indolent ulcer had cytologic evidence of bacterial infection with cocci most commonly observed.[89] Secondary yeast infection, commonly *Malassezia* spp., also can be detected by cytology.[84] Histologic lesions vary, depending on chronicity of the lesion and if ulceration and secondary infection occur. Common histologic characteristics include diffuse dermal infiltrates of eosinophils with variable numbers of neutrophils, macrophages, lymphocytes, and mast cells.[9,81,90] Flame figures, consisting of collagen fibers surrounded by degenerating and degranulating eosinophils, are observed within the inflammation. With chronic lesions, particularly indolent ulcers, inflammation tends to be more lymphocytic with fibrosis,[9] and cytology would be expected to reflect this.

Feline Herpesvirus 1 (FHV1)

FHV1 infection can result in an ulcerative dermatitis primarily involving the nose, muzzle, and eyelids but can occur elsewhere on the body.[91,92] These lesions usually occur in the absence of respiratory signs or conjunctivitis, although cats can have a previous history of respiratory infection. Histologically, there is ulcerating and necrotizing dermatitis and folliculitis that is characterized by eosinophilic and neutrophilic inflammation.[91] Flame figures can be seen. Intranuclear viral inclusions can be difficult to detect, and infection may need to be confirmed by PCR or immunohistochemistry.[88,93,94] There are no reports of finding viral inclusions on cytologic preparations.

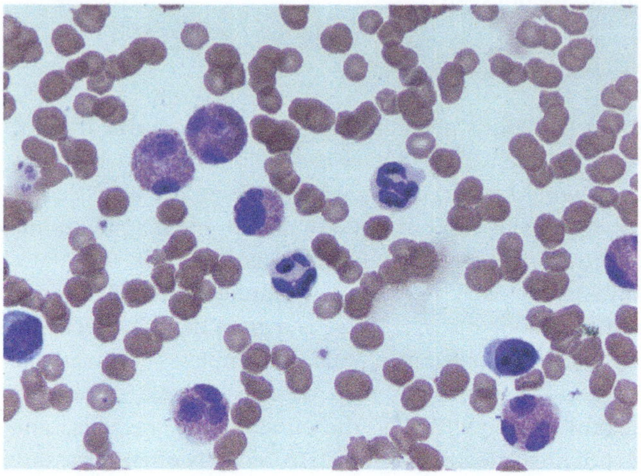

Figure 11.8 Aspirate of an eosinophilic plaque from a 12-year-old spayed female domestic short-haired cat. Eosinophils, non-degenerate neutrophils, and occasional small lymphocytes are present (Wright–Giemsa, 1000×).

Canine Eosinophilic Granuloma

Eosinophilic granuloma is rare in the dog. It is most commonly reported in Siberian Huskies and Cavalier King Charles Spaniels but occurs in other purebred and mixed breed dogs.[95–101] It is more common in young dogs, <3 years of age. Some dogs have a peripheral eosinophilia. The etiology is assumed to be a hypersensitivity reaction as cases often respond to immunomodulatory therapy. Gross lesions appear as papules, plaques, and nodules with ulceration and secondary bacterial infection possible. While most frequently reported in the oral cavity, lesions can occur in the skin and in the ear.[95,96,98–104]

Smears taken by impression, FNA, or scraping consist of eosinophils, neutrophils, and macrophages with fewer numbers of lymphocytes, plasma cells, and mesenchymal cells (Figure 11.9).[95,98,104] One report failed to demonstrate eosinophils in FNAs, and specimens only contained macrophages and degenerate neutrophils with occasional

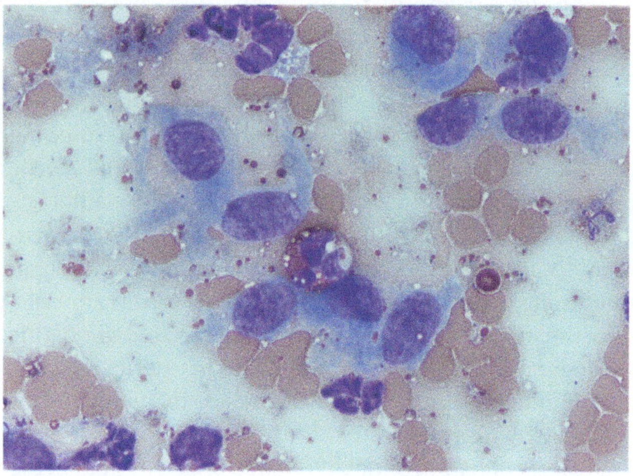

Figure 11.9 Aspirate of a sublingual eosinophilic granuloma from a 4-year-old female Siberian Husky. Both the breed and location are typical for eosinophilic granuloma in the dog. In addition to intact eosinophils, eosinophil granules are scattered in the background. Spindle-shaped cells compatible with reactive fibroblasts exhibit some atypia with mild anisokaryosis and anisocytosis, stippled chromatin, and multiple prominent nucleoli (Wright–Giemsa, 1000×).

intracellular cocci.[100] On histology, eosinophilic and granulomatous or pyogranulomatous inflammation is seen in the dermis.[9] Numbers of multinucleated giant cells, lymphocytes, and plasma cells vary.[98]

Equine Eosinophilic Granuloma

Eosinophilic granuloma constitutes 3.5–3.9% of nodular and proliferative cutaneous lesions in horses.[105–108] As in other species, eosinophilic granulomas in the horse are thought to be a hypersensitivity reaction to a variety of stimuli, including insect bites, trauma, injection site reactions, atopy, food allergy, or embedded hair.[109] Granulomas that develop in response to *Habronema* larvae can appear similar. Because equine mast cell tumors can have a nodular appearance with a marked eosinophilic infiltrate, distinguishing an eosinophilic granuloma from mast cell tumor based on cytology is problematic and often requires histopathology.[110]

Multisystemic eosinophilic epitheliotropic disease is a rare condition in the horse characterized by eosinophilic and lymphoplasmacytic inflammation of the skin and multiple internal organs including the liver, intestine, bile ducts, mesenteric lymph nodes, pancreatic duct, salivary glands, and kidney.[111,112]

Panniculitis

Panniculitis is inflammation of the subcutaneous adipose tissue and has been associated with infectious or noninfectious etiologies in dogs, cats, and horses.[113–116] Panniculitis manifests as single or multiple nodules that can be painful and sometimes accompanied by systemic clinical signs such as fever, anorexia, and lethargy.[114,117] Nodules can be soft or firm, be ulcerated or have draining tracts. Distinction between infectious causes and sterile panniculitis is based on culture, cytology, histopathology, and special stains for organisms. Causes of sterile panniculitis include trauma, injection reactions, vasculopathies, pancreatitis, immune-mediated disease, neoplasia, nutritional deficiencies, metabolic disease, and idiopathic in dogs and cats.[113,114,117–121] Idiopathic sterile nodular panniculitis also is described in horses, including a case associated with pancreatitis.[115,116,122,123]

Cytology of panniculitides is characterized by lipid in the background and within foamy macrophages.[114,115,118–121] Numbers of neutrophils, lymphocytes, plasma cells, and eosinophils are variable. Reactive mesenchymal cells and necrotic debris can be present. Cytology is reported to be inconsistent with histology.[119,120] Distinguishing panniculitis from neoplasia can be problematic using cytology, especially when mesenchymal cells are present. In one study, FNA of firm nodules consisted of predominantly mesenchymal cells that exhibited atypia and criteria of malignancy that raised suspicion of neoplasia.[119] Histologic findings in these cases were of pyogranulomatous inflammation with varying degrees of fibrosis and no evidence of neoplasia.

Cytology is useful in detecting a variety of infectious agents associated with panniculitis. Documented reports where organisms were observed on FNA include *Mycobacteria* spp.,[34,124] *Nocardia* spp.,[125] *Toxoplasma gondii*,[126–128] *Sporothrix schenckii*,[129] and *Dirofilaria repens*.[130]

Pododermatitis

Plasma Cell Pododermatitis of Cats

Plasma cell pododermatitis is characterized by swelling and erythema of multiple foot pads and often involves all four feet.[131–136] Lesions can progress to ulceration with secondary infection and proliferation of granulation tissue. Several reports describe swelling over the bridge of the nose with similar plasmacytic infiltrates.[137,138] Cats often exhibit polyclonal hypergammaglobulinemia and variable leukocytosis.[131–133,137,139] FNA of lesions are described as poorly cellular with variable numbers of plasma cells, neutrophils, lymphocytes, mast cells, and fibroblasts.[133,137,138] Histology is needed to confirm the diagnosis. Histologic lesions are characterized by superficial and deep dermatitis with perivascular infiltrates of plasma cells, including Mott cells, and lesser numbers of lymphocytes.[131–136,140] Suppurative to pyogranulomatous inflammation is associated with ulceration and granulation tissue. Notably, eosinophils are not seen.

Canine Pododermatitis

Pedal folliculitis and furunculosis is common in the dog and can involve the dorsal and palmar/plantar surfaces, interdigital spaces, and nail folds. There are a myriad of etiologies that cause pododermatitis in the dog, including infectious/parasitic agents such as demodex, dermatophytes and bacteria, allergy, immune-mediated disease, and metabolic disease. There is a great deal of overlap in the clinical appearance, and a complete dermatologic workup is necessary.[141,142] As described above, cytology is helpful in characterizing the inflammatory response and identifying infectious agents. Histology is often necessary for a definitive diagnosis.

Immunomodulatory-responsive lymphocytic–plasmacytic pododermatitis (IR-LPP) is a chronic dermatitis of unknown etiology, and diagnosis is by exclusion of other etiologies and by characteristic histologic lesions. IR-LPP is characterized by erythema, pruritus, alopecia, and thickening of the skin of the dorsal and palmar/plantar surfaces of the feet of dogs.[143,144] Ulceration, serosanguinous discharge, and draining tracts vary over the course of the disease. On cytology, cellularity is low to moderate with lymphocytes and plasma cells and variable numbers of other inflammatory cells.[143] Histologic lesions are characterized by perivascular infiltrates of lymphocytes and plasma cells extending from the superficial to deep dermis.[143,144] Neutrophilic to mixed inflammation is variably seen. A moderate increase in mast cells and occasional eosinophils are described. Epidermal lesions include hyperplasia, hyperkeratosis, and spongiosis.

Conclusion

Cytology is useful for characterizing the type of inflammatory response and the detection of infectious agents and parasites. Histopathology is often needed for a definitive diagnosis, especially with autoimmune diseases such as PF and CLE. For both cytology and histology, identification and sampling of the primary lesion improves the likelihood of correctly identifying the cause of the dermatologic condition.

References

1 Pereira, A.V., Pereira, S.A., Gremiao, I.D. et al. (2012). Comparison of acetate tape impression with squeezing versus skin scraping for the diagnosis of canine demodicosis. *Aust Vet J* 90: 448–450.

2 Saridomichelakis, M.N., Koutinas, A.F., Farmaki, R. et al. (2007). Relative sensitivity of hair pluckings and exudate microscopy for the diagnosis of canine demodicosis. *Vet Dermatol* 18: 138–141.

3 Lo, K.L. and Rosenkrantz, W.S. (2016). Evaluation of cytology collection techniques and prevalence of *Malassezia* yeast and bacteria in claw folds of normal and allergic dogs. *Vet Dermatol* 27: 279-e67.

4 Moriello, K.A., Coyner, K., Paterson, S., and Mignon, B. (2017). Diagnosis and treatment of dermatophytosis in dogs and cats: Clinical Consensus Guidelines of the World Association for Veterinary Dermatology. *Vet Dermatol* 28: 266-e68.

5 Brillowska-Dabrowska, A., Michalek, E., Saunte, D.M. et al. (2013). PCR test for *Microsporum canis* identification. *Med Mycol* 51: 576–579.

6 Cornegliani, L., Persico, P., and Colombo, S. (2009). Canine nodular dermatophytosis (kerion): 23 cases. *Vet Dermatol* 20: 185–190.

7 Stuntebeck, R., Moriello, K.A., and Verbrugge, M. (2018). Evaluation of incubation time for *Microsporum canis* dermatophyte cultures. *J Feline Med Surg* 20: 997–1000.

8 Linder, K.E. (2001). Skin biopsy site selection in small animal dermatology with an introduction to histologic pattern-analysis of inflammatory skin lesions. *Clin Tech Small Anim Pract* 16: 207–213.

9 Mauldin, E. and Peters-Kennedy, J. (2016). Integumentary system. In: Jubb, Kennedy, and Palmer's Pathology of Domestic Animals, 6e (ed. M.G. Maxie), 509–736. St. Louis, MO: Elsevier.

10 Wildermuth, B.E., Griffin, C.E., and Rosenkrantz, W.S. (2006). Feline pyoderma therapy. *Clin Tech Small Anim Pract* 21: 150–156.

11 Marsella, R. and Akucewich, L. (2007). Investigation on the clinical efficacy and tolerability of a 0.4% topical stannous fluoride preparation (MedEquine Gel) for the treatment of bacterial skin infections in horses: a prospective, randomized, double-blinded, placebo-controlled clinical trial. *Vet Dermatol* 18: 444–450.

12 Yu, H.W. and Vogelnest, L.J. (2012). Feline superficial pyoderma: a retrospective study of 52 cases (2001–2011). *Vet Dermatol* 23: 448-e86.

13 Bajwa, J. (2017). Cutaneous cytology and the dermatology patient. *Can Vet J* 58: 625–627.

14 Loeffler, A. and Lloyd, D.H. (2018). What has changed in canine pyoderma? A narrative review. *Vet J* 235: 73–82.

15 Colombo, S. (1997). Quantitative evaluation of cutaneous bacteria in normal dogs and dogs with pyoderma by cytological evaluation. Doctoral thesis. Faculty of Veterinary Medicine, Milan, Italy.

16 Udenberg, T.J., Griffin, C.E., Rosenkrantz, W.S. et al. (2014). Reproducibility of a quantitative cutaneous cytological technique. *Vet Dermatol* 25: 435-e67.

17 Doelle, M., Loeffler, A., Wolf, K. et al. (2016). Clinical features, cytology and bacterial culture results in dogs with and without cheilitis and comparison of three sampling techniques. *Vet Dermatol* 27: 140-e37.

18 Pin, D., Carlotti, D.N., Jasmin, P. et al. (2006). Prospective study of bacterial overgrowth syndrome in eight dogs. *Vet Rec* 158: 437–441.

19 Medleau, L. and Blue, J.L. (1988). Frequency and antimicrobial susceptibility of *Staphylococcus* spp isolated from feline skin lesions. *J Am Vet Med Assoc* 193: 1080–1081.

20 Chiers, K., Decostere, A., Devriese, L.A., and Haesebrouck, F. (2003). Bacteriological and mycological findings, and in vitro antibiotic sensitivity of pathogenic staphylococci in equine skin infections. *Vet Rec* 152: 138–141.

21 Abraham, J.L., Morris, D.O., Griffeth, G.C. et al. (2007). Surveillance of healthy cats and cats with inflammatory skin disease for colonization of the skin by methicillin-resistant coagulase-positive staphylococci and *Staphylococcus schleiferi* ssp. schleiferi. *Vet Dermatol* 18: 252–259.

22 Zink, M.C., Yager, J.A., and Smart, N.L. (1986). *Corynebacterium equi* infections in horses, 1958–1984: a review of 131 cases. *Can Vet J* 27: 213–217.

23 Aleman, M., Spier, S.J., Wilson, W.D., and Doherr, M. (1996). *Corynebacterium pseudotuberculosis* infection in horses: 538 cases (1982–1993). *J Am Vet Med Assoc* 209: 804–809.

24 Heffner, K.A., White, S.D., Frevert, C.W., and Jakowski, R. (1988). *Corynebacterium folliculitis* in a horse. *J Am Vet Med Assoc* 193: 89–90.

25 Fairley, R.A. and Fairley, N.M. (1999). *Rhodococcus equi* infection of cats. *Vet Dermatol* 10: 43–46.

26 White, S.D. (2005). Equine bacterial and fungal diseases: a diagnostic and therapeutic update. *Clin Tech Equine Pract* 4: 302–310.

27 Awad, W., Nadre-Elwgoud, M., and El-Sayed, A. (2008). Diagnosis and treatment of bovine, ovine and equine dermatophilosis. *J Appl Sci Res* 4: 367–374.

28 Frank, L.A., Kania, S.A., and Weyant, E. (2016). RT-qPCR for the diagnosis of dermatophilosis in horses. *Vet Dermatol* 27: 431-e112.

29 Malik, R., Smits, B., Reppas, G. et al. (2013). Ulcerated and nonulcerated nontuberculous cutaneous mycobacterial granulomas in cats and dogs. *Vet Dermatol* 24: 146-53.e32-3.

30 Gunn-Moore, D.A. (2014). Feline mycobacterial infections. *Vet J* 201: 230–238.

31 Charles, J., Martin, P., Wigney, D.I. et al. (1999). Cytology and histopathology of canine leproid granuloma syndrome. *Aust Vet J* 77: 799–803.

32 Malik, R., Hughes, M.S., James, G. et al. (2002). Feline leprosy: two different clinical syndromes. *J Feline Med Surg* 4: 43–59.

33 Foley, J.E., Borjesson, D., Gross, T.L. et al. (2002). Clinical, microscopic, and molecular aspects of canine leproid granuloma in the United States. *Vet Pathol* 39: 234–239.

34 Malik, R., Shaw, S.E., Griffin, C. et al. (2004). Infections of the subcutis and skin of dogs caused by rapidly growing mycobacteria. *J Small Anim Pract* 45: 485–494.

35 Torii, E., Reppas, G., Krockenberger, M.B. et al. (2016). Autochthonous feline leprosy caused by *Mycobacterium* sp. strain Tarwin affecting a cat from the Central Coast of New South Wales. *Aust Vet J* 94: 285–289.

36 Chen, T.A. and Hill, P.B. (2005). The biology of *Malassezia* organisms and their ability to induce immune responses and skin disease. *Vet Dermatol* 16: 4–26.

37 Kennis, R.A., Rosser, E.J. Jr., Olivier, N.B., and Walker, R.W. (1996). Quantity and distribution of *Malassezia* organisms on the skin of clinically normal dogs. *J Am Vet Med Assoc* 208: 1048–1051.

38 Omodo-Eluk, A.J., Baker, K.P., and Fuller, H. (2003). Comparison of two sampling techniques for the detection of *Malassezia* pachydermatis on the skin of dogs with chronic dermatitis. *Vet J* 165: 119–124.

39 Ordeix, L., Galeotti, F., Scarampella, F. et al. (2007). *Malassezia* spp. overgrowth in allergic cats. *Vet Dermatol* 18: 316–323.

40 Colombo, S., Nardoni, S., Cornegliani, L., and Mancianti, F. (2007). Prevalence of *Malassezia* spp. yeasts in feline nail folds: a cytological and mycological study. *Vet Dermatol* 18: 278–283.

41 Bensignor, E., Jankowski, F., Seewald, W. et al. (2002). Comparison of two sampling techniques to assess quantity and distribution of *Malassezia* yeasts on the skin of Basset Hounds. *Vet Dermatol* 13: 237–241.

42 Ahman, S., Perrins, N., and Bond, R. (2007). Carriage of *Malassezia* spp. yeasts in healthy and seborrhoeic Devon Rex cats. *Med Mycol* 45: 449–455.

43 Nell, A., James, S.A., Bond, C.J. et al. (2002). Identification and distribution of a novel *Malassezia* species yeast on normal equine skin. *Vet Rec* 150: 395–398.

44 White, S.D., Vandenabeele, S.I., Drazenovich, N.L., and Foley, J.E. (2006). *Malassezia* species isolated from the intermammary and preputial fossa areas of horses. *J Vet Intern Med* 20: 395–398.

45 Shokri, H. (2016). Occurrence and distribution of *Malassezia* species on skin and external ear canal of horses. *Mycoses* 59: 28–33.

46 Kim, D.Y., Johnson, P.J., and Senter, D. (2011). Severe bilaterally symmetrical alopecia in a horse. *Vet Pathol* 48: 1216–1220.

47 Mendelsohn, C., Rosenkrantz, W., and Griffin, C.E. (2006). Practical cytology for inflammatory skin diseases. *Clin Tech Small Anim Pract* 21: 117–127.

48 Albanese, F. and Caruso, C. (2007). Dermatophytic kerion: etiology, clinical aspects, diagnosis and therapy in 39 dogs. *Vet Dermatol* 21: 9–18.

49 Zimmerman, K., Feldman, B., Robertson, J. et al. (2003). Dermal mass aspirate from a Persian cat. *Vet Clin Pathol* 32: 213–217.

50 Albanese, F. (ed.) (2017). Cytology of canine and feline non-neoplastic skin diseases. In: Canine and Feline Skin Cytology, 77–290. Cham, Switzerland: Springer.
51 Abramo, F., Vercelli, A., and Mancianti, F. (2001). Two cases of dermatophytic pseudomycetoma in the dog: an immunohistochemical study. *Vet Dermatol* 12: 203–207.
52 Van Rooij, P., Declercq, J., and Beguin, H. (2012). Canine dermatophytosis caused by *Trichophyton rubrum*: an example of man-to-dog transmission. *Mycoses* 55: e15–e17.
53 Peters, J., Scott, D.W., Erb, H.N., and Miller, W.H. Jr. (2007). Comparative analysis of canine dermatophytosis and superficial pemphigus for the prevalence of dermatophytes and acantholytic keratinocytes: a histopathological and clinical retrospective study. *Vet Dermatol* 18: 234–240.
54 Scott, D.W. (1994). Marked acantholysis associated with dermatophytosis due to *Trichophyton equinum* in two horses. *Vet Dermatol* 5: 105–110.
55 Mueller, R.S. (2004). Treatment protocols for demodicosis: an evidence-based review. *Vet Dermatol* 15: 75–89.
56 Rosychuk, R.A.W. (2010). Canine and feline demodicosis: what's new. *Proceedings of the North American Veterinary Conference on Small Animal and Exotics*, Orlando, FL (16–20 January 2010), 445–447.
57 Mueller, R.S., Bensignor, E., Ferrer, L. et al. (2012). Treatment of demodicosis in dogs: 2011 clinical practice guidelines. *Vet Dermatol* 23: 86–96, e20-e21.
58 Pereira, D.T., Castro, L.J.M., Centenaro, V.B. et al. (2015). Skin impression with acetate tape in *Demodex canis* and *Scarcoptes scabiei* var. vulpes diagnosis. *Arq Bras Med Vet Zootec* 67: 49–54.
59 Curtis, C. (2012). Canine sarcoptic mange (sarcoptic acariasis, canine scabies). *Companion Animal* 17: 32–36.
60 Laffort-Dassot, C., Carlotti, D.N., Pin, D., and Jasmin, P. (2004). Diagnosis of flea allergy dermatitis: comparison of intradermal testing with flea allergens and a FcepsilonRI alpha-based IgE assay in response to flea control. *Vet Dermatol* 15: 321–330.
61 Gross, T.L. and Halliwell, R.E. (1985). Lesions of experimental flea bite hypersensitivity in the dog. *Vet Pathol* 22: 78–81.
62 Raskin, R.E. (2016). Skin and subcutaneous tissues. In: Canine and Feline Cytology: A Color Atlas and Interpretation Guide, 3e (eds. R.E. Raskin and D.J. Meyer), 36. St. Louis, MO: Elsevier.
63 Sood, N.K., Mekkib, B., Singla, L.D., and Gupta, K. (2012). Cytopathology of parasitic dermatitis in dogs. *J Parasit Dis* 36: 73–77.
64 Nesbitt, G.H. and Schmitz, J.A. (1978). Fleabite allergic dermatitis: a review and survey of 330 cases. *J Am Vet Med Assoc* 173: 282–288.
65 Marcella, R. (2013). Hypersensitivity disorders. In: Muller and Kirk's Small Animal Dermatology, 7e (eds. W.H. Miller Jr., C.E. Griffin and K.L. Campbell), 412. St. Louis, MO: Elsevier/Mosby.
66 Vitale, C.B., Ihrke, P.J., Olivry, T. et al. (1996). Feline urticaria pigmentosa in three related Sphinx cats. *Vet Dermatol* 7: 227–233.
67 Noli, C., Colombo, S., Abramo, F., and Scarampella, F. (2004). Papular eosinophilic/mastocytic dermatitis (feline urticaria pigmentosa) in Devon Rex cats: a distinct disease entity or a histopathological reaction pattern? *Vet Dermatol* 15: 253–259.
68 Bell, A.G., Chard, W.G., Grayson, J.L., and James, M.P. (1995). Eosinophilic papulocrustous dermatitis (miliary dermatitis) and eosinophilic inflammatory bowel disease in two cats. *N Z Vet J* 43: 153–157.
69 Jackson, A. and Foster, A. (2006). Management of feline miliary dermatitis: a clinical update. *In Pract* 28: 147–151.
70 Olivry, T. (2018). Auto-immune skin diseases in animals: time to reclassify and review after 40 years. *BMC Vet Res* 14: 157.
71 Bizikova, P., Dean, G.A., Hashimoto, T., and Olivry, T. (2012). Cloning and establishment of canine desmocollin-1 as a major autoantigen in canine pemphigus foliaceus. *Vet Immunol Immunopathol* 149: 197–207.
72 Vandenabeele, S.I., White, S.D., Affolter, V.K. et al. (2004). Pemphigus foliaceus in the horse: a retrospective study of 20 cases. *Vet Dermatol* 15: 381–388.
73 Jordan, T., Affolter, V., Outerbridge, C. et al. (2018). Clinicopathological findings and clinical outcomes in 49 cases of feline pemphigus foliaceus examined in northern California, USA (1987–2017). *Vet Dermatol* 29: 277.
74 Zabel, S., Mueller, R.S., Fieseler, K.V. et al. (2005). Review of 15 cases of pemphigus foliaceus in horses and a survey of the literature. *Vet Rec* 157: 505–509.
75 Amagai, M., Matsuyoshi, N., Wang, Z.H. et al. (2000). Toxin in bullous impetigo and staphylococcal scalded-skin syndrome targets desmoglein 1. *Nat Med* 6: 1275–1277.
76 Mueller, R.S., Krebs, I., Power, H.T., and Fieseler, K.V. (2006). Pemphigus foliaceus in 91 dogs. *J Am Anim Hosp Assoc* 42: 189–196.
77 Rosenkrantz, W. (2013). Immune-mediated dermatoses. *Vet Clin North Am Equine Pract* 29: 607–613.
78 Vaughan, D.F., Clay Hodgin, E., Hosgood, G.L., and Bernstein, J.A. (2010). Clinical and histopathological features of pemphigus foliaceus with and without

eosinophilic infiltrates: a retrospective evaluation of 40 dogs. *Vet Dermatol* 21: 166–174.

79 Olivry, T. and Linder, K.E. (2009). Dermatoses affecting desmosomes in animals: a mechanistic review of acantholytic blistering skin diseases. *Vet Dermatol* 20: 313–326.

80 Olivry, T., Linder, K.E., and Banovic, F. (2018). Cutaneous lupus erythematosus in dogs: a comprehensive review. *BMC Vet Res* 14: 132.

81 Bloom, P.B. (2006). Canine and feline eosinophilic skin diseases. *Vet Clin North Am Small Anim Pract* 36: 141–160, vii.

82 Hobi, S., Linek, M., Marignac, G. et al. (2011). Clinical characteristics and causes of pruritus in cats: a multicentre study on feline hypersensitivity-associated dermatoses. *Vet Dermatol* 22: 406–413.

83 Buckley, L. and Nuttall, T. (2012). Feline eosinophilic granuloma complex(ities): some clinical clarification. *J Feline Med Surg* 14: 471–481.

84 Scott, D.W. and Miller, W.H. Jr. (2013). Feline atopic dermatitis: a retrospective study of 194 cases (1988–2003). *Jpn J Vet Dermatol* 19: 135–147.

85 Ravens, P.A., Xu, B.J., and Vogelnest, L.J. (2014). Feline atopic dermatitis: a retrospective study of 45 cases (2001–2012). *Vet Dermatol* 25: 95–102, e27–e28.

86 Colombini, S., Hodgin, E.C., Foil, C.S. et al. (2001). Induction of feline flea allergy dermatitis and the incidence and histopathological characteristics of concurrent indolent lip ulcers. *Vet Dermatol* 12: 155–161.

87 Leistra, W.H., van Oost, B.A., and Willemse, T. (2005). Non-pruritic granuloma in Norwegian forest cats. *Vet Rec* 156: 575–577.

88 Lee, M., Bosward, K.L., and Norris, J.M. (2010). Immunohistological evaluation of feline herpesvirus-1 infection in feline eosinophilic dermatoses or stomatitis. *J Feline Med Surg* 12: 72–79.

89 Wildermuth, B.E., Griffin, C.E., and Rosenkrantz, W.S. (2012). Response of feline eosinophilic plaques and lip ulcers to amoxicillin trihydrate-clavulanate potassium therapy: a randomized, double-blind placebo-controlled prospective study. *Vet Dermatol* 23: 118, e24–e25.

90 Fondati, A., Fondevila, D., and Ferrer, L. (2001). Histopathological study of feline eosinophilic dermatoses. *Vet Dermatol* 12: 333–338.

91 Hargis, A.M., Ginn, P.E., Mansell, J.E.K.L., and Garber, R.L. (1999). Ulcerative facial and nasal dermatitis and stomatitis in cats associated with feline herpesvirus 1. *Vet Dermatol* 10: 267–274.

92 Gaskell, R., Dawson, S., Radford, A., and Thiry, E. (2007). Feline herpesvirus. *Vet Res* 38: 337–354.

93 Hargis, A.M. and Ginn, P.E. (1999). Feline herpesvirus 1-associated facial and nasal dermatitis and stomatitis in domestic cats. *Vet Clin North Am Small Anim Pract* 29: 1281–1290.

94 Suchy, A., Bauder, B., Gelbmann, W. et al. (2000). Diagnosis of feline herpesvirus infection by immunohistochemistry, polymerase chain reaction, and in situ hybridization. *J Vet Diagn Invest* 12: 186–191.

95 Madewell, B.R., Stannard, A.A., Pulley, L.T., and Nelson, V.G. (1980). Oral eosinophilic granuloma in Siberian husky dogs. *J Am Vet Med Assoc* 177: 701–703.

96 Potter, K.A., Tucker, R.D., and Carpenter, J.L. (1980). Oral eosinophilic granuloma of Siberian huskies. *J Am Anim Hosp Assoc* 16: 595–600.

97 Turnwald, G.H., Hoskins, J.D., and Taylor, H.W. (1981). Cutaneous eosinophilic granuloma in a labrador retriever. *J Am Vet Med Assoc* 179: 799–801.

98 Bredal, W.P., Gunnes, G., Vollset, I., and Ulstein, T.L. (1996). Oral eosinophilic granuloma in three cavalier King Charles spaniels. *J Small Anim Pract* 37: 499–504.

99 Tellado, M.N., Michinski, S.D., Olaiz, N. et al. (2014). Canine oral eosinophilic granuloma treated with electrochemotherapy. *Case Rep Vet Med* 2014: 519197.

100 Knight, E.C. and Shipstone, M.A. (2016). Canine eosinophilic granuloma of the digits treated with prednisolone and chlorambucil. *Vet Dermatol* 27: 446-e119.

101 Kussmann, I., Zimmermann, O., and Herder, V. (2017). Eosinophilic granuloma in a Pug dog. *Kleintierpraxis* 62: 744–747.

102 Curiel, J.M.A., Kraus, K.H., Brown, T.P., and Chastain, C.B. (1988). Eosinophilic granuloma of the nasal skin in a dog. *J Am Vet Med Assoc* 193: 566–567.

103 Poulet, F.M., Valentine, B.A., and Scott, D.W. (1991). Focal proliferative eosinophilic dermatitis of the external ear canal in four dogs. *Vet Pathol* 28: 171–173.

104 Vercelli, A., Cornegliani, L., and Portigliotti, L. (2005). Eyelid eosinophilic granuloma in a Siberian husky. *J Small Anim Pract* 46: 31–33.

105 Pascoe, R.R. and Summers, P.M. (1981). Clinical survey of tumours and tumour-like lesions in horses in south east Queensland. *Equine Vet J* 13: 235–239.

106 Scott, D.W. and Miller, W.H. (eds.) (2011). Miscellaneous skin diseases. In: Equine Dermatology, 2e, 436–467. St Louis, MO: Elsevier Saunders.

107 Valentine, B.A. (2005). Equine cutaneous non-neoplastic nodular and proliferative lesions in the Pacific Northwest. *Vet Dermatol* 16: 425–428.

108 Souza, T.M., Brum, J.S., Fighera, R.A. et al. (2011). Prevalence of equine skin tumors diagnosed at the Laboratory of Veterinary Pathology of the Federal University Santa Maria, Rio Grande do Sul, Brazil. *Pesqui Vet Bras* 31: 379–382.

109 Slovis, N.M., Watson, J.L., Affolter, V.K., and Stannard, A.A. (1999). Injection site eosinophilic granulomas and collagenolysis in 3 horses. *J Vet Intern Med* 13: 606–612.

110 Millward, L.M., Hamberg, A., Mathews, J. et al. (2010). Multicentric mast cell tumors in a horse. *Vet Clin Pathol* 39: 365–370.

111 Nimmo Wilkie, J.S., Yager, J.A., Nation, P.N. et al. (1985). Chronic eosinophilic dermatitis: a manifestation of a multisystemic, eosinophilic, epitheliotropic disease in five horses. *Vet Pathol* 22: 297–305.

112 Bosseler, L., Verryken, K., Bauwens, C. et al. (2013). Equine multisystemic eosinophilic epitheliotropic disease: a case report and review of literature. *N Z Vet J* 61: 177–182.

113 Shanley, K.J. and Miller, W.H. (1985). Panniculitis in the dog: a report of five cases. *J Am Anim Hosp Assoc* 21: 545–550.

114 Scott, D.W. and Anderson, W.I. (1988). Panniculitis in dogs and cats: a retrospective analysis of 78 cases. *J Am Anim Hosp Assoc* 24: 551–559.

115 Karcher, L.F., Scott, D.W., Paradis, M., and Anderson, W.I. (1990). Sterile nodular panniculitis in five horses. *J Am Vet Med Assoc* 196: 1823–1826.

116 Waitt, L.H., Cebra, C.K., Tornquist, S.J., and Löhr, C.V. (2006). Panniculitis in a horse with peripancreatitis and pancreatic fibrosis. *J Vet Diagn Invest* 18: 405–408.

117 Contreary, C.L., Outerbridge, C.A., Affolter, V.K. et al. (2015). Canine sterile nodular panniculitis: a retrospective study of 39 dogs. *Vet Dermatol* 26: 451–458, e104–e105.

118 Dal-Bó, Í.S., Macedo, A.S., Gottlieb, J. et al. (2012). Traumatic panniculitis in a dog. *Acta Sci Vet* 40: 1090.

119 Kim, H.J., Kang, M.H., Kim, J.H. et al. (2011). Sterile panniculitis in dogs: new diagnostic findings and alternative treatments. *Vet Dermatol* 22: 352–359.

120 O'Kell, A.L., Inteeworn, N., Diaz, S.F. et al. (2010). Canine sterile nodular panniculitis: a retrospective study of 14 cases. *J Vet Intern Med* 24: 278–284.

121 Yamagishi, C., Momoi, Y., Kobayashi, T. et al. (2007). A retrospective study and gene analysis of canine sterile panniculitis. *J Vet Med Sci* 69: 915–924.

122 Dagleish, M.P., De Jaham, C., Suprenan, S., and Scudamore, C.L. (2000). Serum alpha-1-proteinase inhibitor concentration in 2 Quarter Horse foals with idiopathic pyogranulomatous panniculitis. *Equine Vet J* 32: 449–452.

123 Menzies-Gow, N.J., Patterson-Kane, J.C., and McGowan, C.M. (2002). Chronic nodular panniculitis in a three-year-old mare. *Vet Rec* 151: 416–419.

124 Bezerra, B.M.O., Lopes, C.E.B., Matos, M.G. et al. (2018). Cytologic diagnosis of feline cutaneous mycobacteriosis in Fortaleza (Ceará) – case report. *Rev Bras Hig Sanid Anim* 12: 87–91.

125 Malik, R., Krockenberger, M.B., O'Brien, C.R. et al. (2006). Nocardia infections in cats: a retrospective multi-institutional study of 17 cases. *Aust Vet J* 84: 235–245.

126 Anfray, P., Bonetti, C., Fabbrini, F. et al. (2005). Feline cutaneous toxoplasmosis: a case report. *Vet Dermatol* 16: 131–136.

127 Hoffmann, A.R., Cadieu, J., Kiupel, M. et al. (2012). Cutaneous toxoplasmosis in two dogs. *J Vet Diagn Invest* 24: 636–640.

128 Oliveira, T.S., Turchetti, A.P., Barbosa, F.B.S. et al. (2014). Cutaneous toxoplasmosis in an immunosuppressed dog. *Arq Bras Med Vet Zootec* 66: 797–800.

129 Bernstein, J.A., Cook, H.E., Gill, A.F. et al. (2007). Cytologic diagnosis of generalized cutaneous sporotrichosis in a hunting hound. *Vet Clin Pathol* 36: 94–96.

130 Albanese, F., Abramo, F., Braglia, C. et al. (2013). Nodular lesions due to infestation by *Dirofilaria repens* in dogs from Italy. *Vet Dermatol* 24: 255-e56.

131 Gruffydd-Jones, T., Orr, C.M., and Lucke, V.M. (1980). Food pad swelling and ulceration in cats: a report of five cases. *J Small Anim Pract* 21: 381–389.

132 Medleau, L., Kaswan, R.L., Lorenz, M.D., and Mansell, J. (1982). Ulcerative pododermatitis in a cat: immunofluorescent findings and response to chrysotherapy. *J Am Anim Hosp Assoc* 18: 449–451.

133 Taylor, J.E. and Schmeitzel, L.P. (1990). Plasma cell pododermatitis with chronic footpad hemorrhage in two cats. *J Am Vet Med Assoc* 197: 375–377.

134 Drolet, R. and Bernard, J. (1984). Plasma cell pododermatitis in a cat. *Can Vet J* 25: 448–449.

135 Dias Pereira, P. and Faustino, A.M. (2003). Feline plasma cell pododermatitis: a study of 8 cases. *Vet Dermatol* 14: 333–337.

136 Guaguere, E., Prelaud, P., Degorce-Rubiales, F. et al. (2004). Feline plasma cell pododermatitis: a retrospective study of 26 cases. *Vet Dermatol* 15 (Suppl. 1): 27.

137 Declercq, J. and Man, M. (2002). Swelling of the nose in three cats with plasmacytic pododermatitis. *Vlaams Diergeneeskd Tijdschr* 71: 277–281.

138 Declercq, J. and De Bosschere, H. (2010). Nasal swelling due to plasma cell infiltrate in a cat without plasma cell pododermatitis. *Vet Dermatol* 21: 412–414.

139 Scarampella, F. and Ordiex, L. (2004). Doxycycline therapy in 10 cases of feline plasma cell pododermatitis: clinical, haematological and serological evaluations. *Vet Dermatol* 15 (Suppl. 1): 27.

140 Bettenay, S.V., Mueller, R.S., Dow, K., and Friend, S. (2003). Prospective study of the treatment of feline plasmacytic pododermatitis with doxycycline. *Vet Rec* 152: 564–566.

141 Duclos, D. (2013). Canine pododermatitis. *Vet Clin North Am Small Anim Pract* 43: 57–87.

142 Gortel, K. (2013). Recognizing pyoderma: more difficult than it may seem. *Vet Clin North Am Small Anim Pract* 43: 1–18.

143 Breathnach, R.M., Baker, K.P., Quinn, P.J. et al. (2005). Clinical, immunological and histopathological findings in a subpopulation of dogs with pododermatitis. *Vet Dermatol* 16: 364–372.

144 Breathnach, R.M., Fanning, S., Mulcahy, G. et al. (2008). Canine pododermatitis and idiopathic disease. *Vet J* 176: 146–157.

12

Dermal and Subcutaneous Masses

Jennifer L. Brazzell, Daniel Heinrich, and Jillian Zientek Walz

Introduction

Skin tumors represent a third and a quarter of all tumors in the dog and cat, respectively.[1] Cutaneous lesion cytology can be particularly instrumental in differentiating neoplastic from non-neoplastic lesions, with a reported sensitivity of 89% and specificity of 98–100%.[2,3] In veterinary species, diagnostic cytology of cutaneous lesions is reported to agree with histologic diagnosis in 66% of cases. However, when insufficient (nondiagnostic) samples are excluded, this agreement increases to 70–90%.[3,4] Rates of insufficient sampling range from 11 to 17%.[3,4] The disparity in diagnostic accuracy when considering adequate to insufficient samples underscores the importance of conscientious sampling technique. Sampling error, preparation error, or lesion characteristics can lead to samples with insufficient cellularity, excessive blood contamination, pervasive sample thickness, or ubiquitous cell rupture. Additionally, concurrent processes associated with the lesion such as ulceration, infection, inflammation, and/or widespread necrosis can result in samples that are nonrepresentative or difficult to interpret (Figure 12.1). That being said, with adequate sampling, correlation between fine-needle aspiration (FNA) and histopathology of canine skin and adnexal tumors has been reported to be as high as 86%.[5]

Sample Collection

The reader is directed to Chapters 1 and 11 for a thorough discussion of sample collection and preparation techniques. Additionally, a number of high-quality review articles contain detailed suggestions for collection and preparation of cytology samples in veterinary species.[6,7]

There are certain situations where obtaining a representative sample may be difficult such as sampling of fluid-filled, vascular, or ulcerated masses. When sampling fluid-filled masses, an effort should be made to aspirate both the fluid contents of the mass as well as the wall of the mass. The non-aspirate (fenestration) technique is often more useful for very vascular lesions where aspiration causes significant hemodilution of the sample. Care should be taken to sample distant from or deep to any sites of ulceration to avoid confounding collection of necrotic and/or inflamed tissue. Similarly, one should avoid superficial impression smears or skin scrapes of the ulcerated portion of a mass since skin scrapings and impression smears will primarily exfoliate the secondary superficial inflammation and infection and rarely will the primary pathology be represented. Evidence of necrosis and inflammation should be noted in the diagnostic report but considered carefully in the interpretation of the sample since these are often secondary lesions and not the primary pathology.

When faced with interpretation of suboptimally collected or prepared samples, the cytologist may also employ certain techniques to maximize information recovery. Evaluation of the feathered edge of highly blood contaminated samples often reveals the greatest density of lesion-associated cells. Similarly, the edges of excessively thick samples often contain regions of diagnostic quality (i.e. a monolayer of adequately stained cells).

Complications associated with sample collection for cutaneous and subcutaneous lesion cytology have not been evaluated in veterinary species but are considered minimal. In the authors' experience, common complications of cutaneous lesion cytology include mild discomfort or pain on aspiration and mild hemorrhage and/or bruising. Rare complications include moderate hemorrhage; aggravation of lesions such as edema and pruritus associated with mast cell degranulation; or post-aspiration swelling, edema, or infection.

Veterinary Cytology, First Edition. Edited by Leslie C. Sharkey, M. Judith Radin, and Davis Seelig.

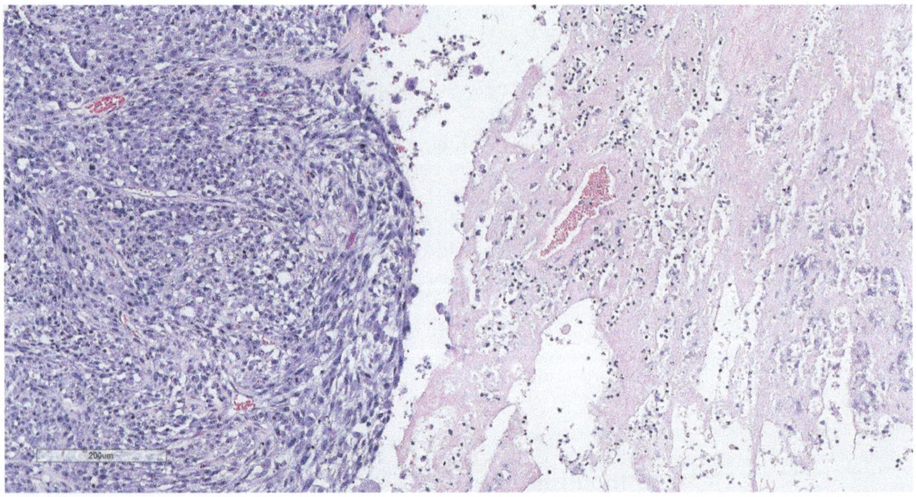

Figure 12.1 Histology of a canine soft tissue sarcoma with a necrotic center depicting the potential for sampling bias during FNA. Aspiration of the non-necrotic malignancy (left side of image) would yield a population of spindle cells, while aspiration of the necrotic and inflamed center of the malignancy (right side of image) would yield proteinaceous fluid, necrotic debris, and a mixed inflammatory infiltrate (hematoxylin and eosin, 200×).

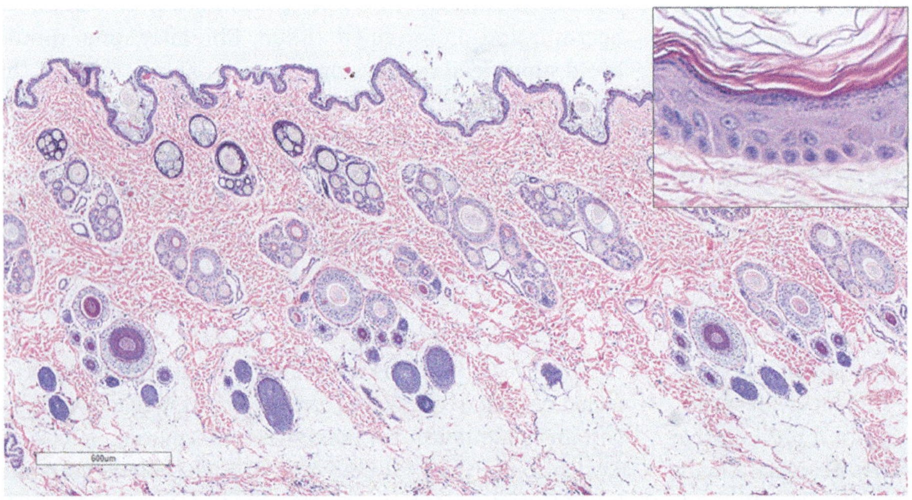

Figure 12.2 Histology of canine skin demonstrating the epidermis, dermis, and subcutis. Cross sections of pilosebaceous units are found in the dermis and superficial subcutis (hematoxylin and eosin, 100×). Inset. Magnification of the epidermis demonstrating the four layers of the epidermis, which are from deep to superficial, the basal layer (stratum basale), spinous layer (stratum spinosum), granular layer (stratum granulosum), and cornified layer (stratum corneum) (hematoxylin and eosin, 400×).

Histologic Architecture of the Skin

Skin is composed of the epidermis, dermis, and subcutis (hypodermis) (Figure 12.2). The epidermis consists of four layers, which are, from deep to superficial, the basal layer (stratum basale), spinous layer (stratum spinosum), granular layer (stratum granulosum), and cornified layer (stratum corneum) (Figure 12.2 inset). The cuboidal basal keratinocytes mature through all layers of the epidermis until they are exfoliated from the skin surface as flattened, polygonal, anucleate, keratinized superficial squamous cells. The dermis lies deep to the epidermis and consists primarily of collagen fibers with few interspersed elastic fibers. The dermis contains hair follicles, adnexal structures (apocrine, sebaceous, and in some anatomic locations eccrine glands), smooth muscle bands, blood and lymphatic vessels, and nerves. The subcutis, composed primarily of adipose tissue, lies deep to the dermis. Hair follicles may extend into the subcutis depending on the phase of the hair cycle. The hair follicle is divided into three segments that are associated with three different types of keratinization, proceeding from superficial to deep. The upper/infundibulum segment extends from the epidermal surface to the entrance of the sebaceous gland duct, exhibits epidermal or squamous keratinization, and yields anucleate squamous cells. The middle/isthmus segment extends from sebaceous gland duct to the insertion of the arrector pili muscle, exhibits trichilemmal keratinization, and yields amorphous eosinophilic keratin. The lower/inferior segment extends from the insertion of the arrector pili muscle to the hair follicle bulb, exhibits matrical keratinization, and yields anucleate cells with a central empty zone known as "ghost cells."[8,9]

Epithelium-Derived Masses Diagnosed by Cytology

Epithelium-derived masses represent a large majority of cutaneous and subcutaneous masses in dogs, cats, and horses – approximately a quarter to a third of all canine, feline, and equine cutaneous tumors.[10–13] A survey of canine and feline skin masses in central Italy found that follicular tumors and tumor-like lesions (follicular and dermoid cysts, dilated pore and focal adnexal dysplasia) accounted for approximately 10 and 8% of all skin tumors in dogs and cats, respectively, with the majority of true tumors in dogs and cats diagnosed as trichoblastomas.[14] Note however that most feline trichoblastomas have been reclassified as apocrine ductular adenomas since that publication.[15]

Epithelial tumors tend to exfoliate well with FNA. Cytologic features of epithelial tumors include cells in clusters, sheets, and rafts with intercellular junctions that may display a pavement, honeycomb, acinar, palisade, papillary, or trabecular structure.[16–18] General characteristics of a benign tumor include a uniform population of cells cytologically similar to those of normal tissue, while those of a malignant tumor include a pleomorphic cell population displaying anisocytosis, anisokaryosis, and increased nuclear to cytoplasm (N:C) ratios with the exception being in those cell populations where a high N:C ratio is expected such as basilar epithelial cells and lymphocytes.[16,18,19] Inflammation within and adjacent to and/or trauma and irritation of non-neoplastic or benign neoplastic lesions can result in significant cellular dysplasia that can be misinterpreted as malignant change. Interpretation of cellular atypia in inflamed lesions should therefore be made with caution. Limited studies have been performed utilizing nuclear morphometry on cytologic and histologic specimens to attempt to differentiate benign from malignant epithelial lesions with limited success.[20,21] Therefore, a cytologic diagnosis of malignancy should always be correlated with signalment and history and should be confirmed histologically prior to definitive diagnosis and prognostication.

Histologically, epithelial masses are categorized based on their histogenesis and predominant morphological component and are subcategorized as hyperplastic, cystic, benign neoplastic, or malignant neoplastic lesions (Table 12.1).[8,15,22] The histologic appearance of the many types of epithelium-derived masses is well-documented;[8,15,22] however, the cytologic appearance of the same lesions is poorly documented. In addition, the cytologic appearance of many epithelium-derived cysts and masses overlap, and therefore, the use of generic cytologic morphologic diagnoses such as "basilar epithelial neoplasm"[23] or "keratin-containing mass/cyst" – a term preferred by one author (JLB) – may be more appropriate and should be considered in lieu of specific cytologic morphologic diagnoses such as "trichoblastoma."

Basilar Epithelial Neoplasms

The term "basilar epithelial neoplasm" is a catch-all diagnosis denoting a heterogeneous group of histologically distinct epidermal, hair follicle, and adnexal (sweat or sebaceous gland) skin tumors with basal cell characteristics that have similar cytologic appearance.[18,24,25] Included in this group of neoplasms are true tumors of the undifferentiated basal cell layer of the epidermis (basal cell epithelioma, basal cell carcinoma), follicular tumors (trichoblastomas or pilomatricomas), sebaceous/modified sebaceous tumors (sebaceous epitheliomas), and apocrine tumors (apocrine ductular adenomas).

Most basilar epithelial neoplasms exfoliate variably sized cohesive clusters; palisading rows; or papillary formations of uniform, small, round to cuboidal or rarely spindled cells, often with poorly defined borders. Cells exhibit high N:C ratios and contain scant, lightly basophilic cytoplasm that may contain melanin pigment; small round or ovoid nuclei; clumped chromatin; and indistinct nucleoli (Figure 12.3a). The occurrence of other cell populations and cellular constituents such as variable numbers of background keratin bars and flakes, superficial nucleate and anucleate squamous cells, fibrocytes, and inflammatory cells can complicate the interpretation.[23,26] Due to variable histogenesis and architecture of basilar epithelial neoplasms, the characteristic clusters of basilar epithelial cells may not exfoliate upon FNA. For example, trichoblastomas have numerous morphologic variants including ribbon, trabecular, spindle, and granular cell variants.[8,15] Trabecular-type trichoblastomas have been described as exfoliating elongated cells with cigar-shaped nuclei

Table 12.1 Histological classification of epithelial tumors, cysts, hamartomas, and tumor-like lesions.

Undifferentiated basal cell epithelial tumors	Basal cell epithelioma Basal cell carcinoma
Epidermal tumors	Viral papilloma (exophytic or inverted) Subungual keratoacanthoma Actinic or solar keratosis Multicentric squamous cell carcinoma (bowenoid in situ carcinoma) Squamous cell carcinoma Basosquamous carcinoma

Follicular adnexal tumors[a]	Upper/infundibulum
	  Infundibular keratinizing acanthoma
	Middle/isthmus
	  Tricholemmoma
	Lower/inferior
	  Trichoblastoma
	  Trichoepithelioma
	  Malignant trichoepithelioma (a.k.a. metrical carcinoma)
	  Pilomatricoma
	  Malignant pilomatricoma

Adnexal tumors of sebaceous and modified sebaceous glands	Sebaceous adenoma Sebaceous ductal adenoma Sebaceous epithelioma Sebaceous carcinoma Meibomian adenoma Meibomian ductal adenoma Meibomian epithelioma Meibomian carcinoma Circumanal/perianal gland adenoma Circumanal/perianal gland epithelioma Circumanal/perianal gland carcinoma Apocrine gland Eccrine gland
Adnexal tumors of apocrine glands	Apocrine secretory adenoma/cystadenoma Complex and mixed apocrine adenoma Apocrine secretory adenocarcinoma Complex and mixed apocrine secretory adenocarcinoma Apocrine ductular adenoma Apocrine ductular carcinoma Anal sac (apocrine gland) adenoma Anal sac (apocrine gland) adenocarcinoma
Adnexal tumors of eccrine glands	Eccrine adenoma Eccrine carcinoma
Undifferentiated adnexal tumors	Clear cell adnexal carcinoma

Cysts	Follicular cyst[a]
	  Infundibular (epidermal inclusion cyst)
	  Isthmus (tricholemmal)
	  Matrical
	  Panfollicular/hybrid
	Dilated pore
	Dermoid cyst
	Sebaceous duct cyst
	Apocrine cyst
	Ciliated cyst
	Subungual epithelial inclusion cyst

Table 12.1 (Continued)

Hyperplastic, hamartomatous, and other tumor-like masses	Epidermal hamartoma (pigmented epidermal nevus)
	Follicular hamartoma
	Sebaceous hamartoma
	Apocrine hamartoma
	Fibroadnexal hamartoma/dysplasia
	Trichofolliculoma
	Pressure point comedones
	Cutaneous horn
	Pawpad keratoma (pawpad corn, callus)
	Squamous papilloma
	Warty dyskeratoma
	Sebaceous, meibomian, circumanal gland hyperplasia

[a] Follicular tumors and cysts are subcategorized based on the portion of the hair follicle from which they arise. From superficial to deep, upper/infundibulum includes epidermal surface to duct of the sebaceous gland; middle/isthmus includes the duct of the sebaceous gland to the insertion of arrector pili muscle; lower/inferior includes the insertion of arrector pili muscle to the hair follicle bulb.[8]

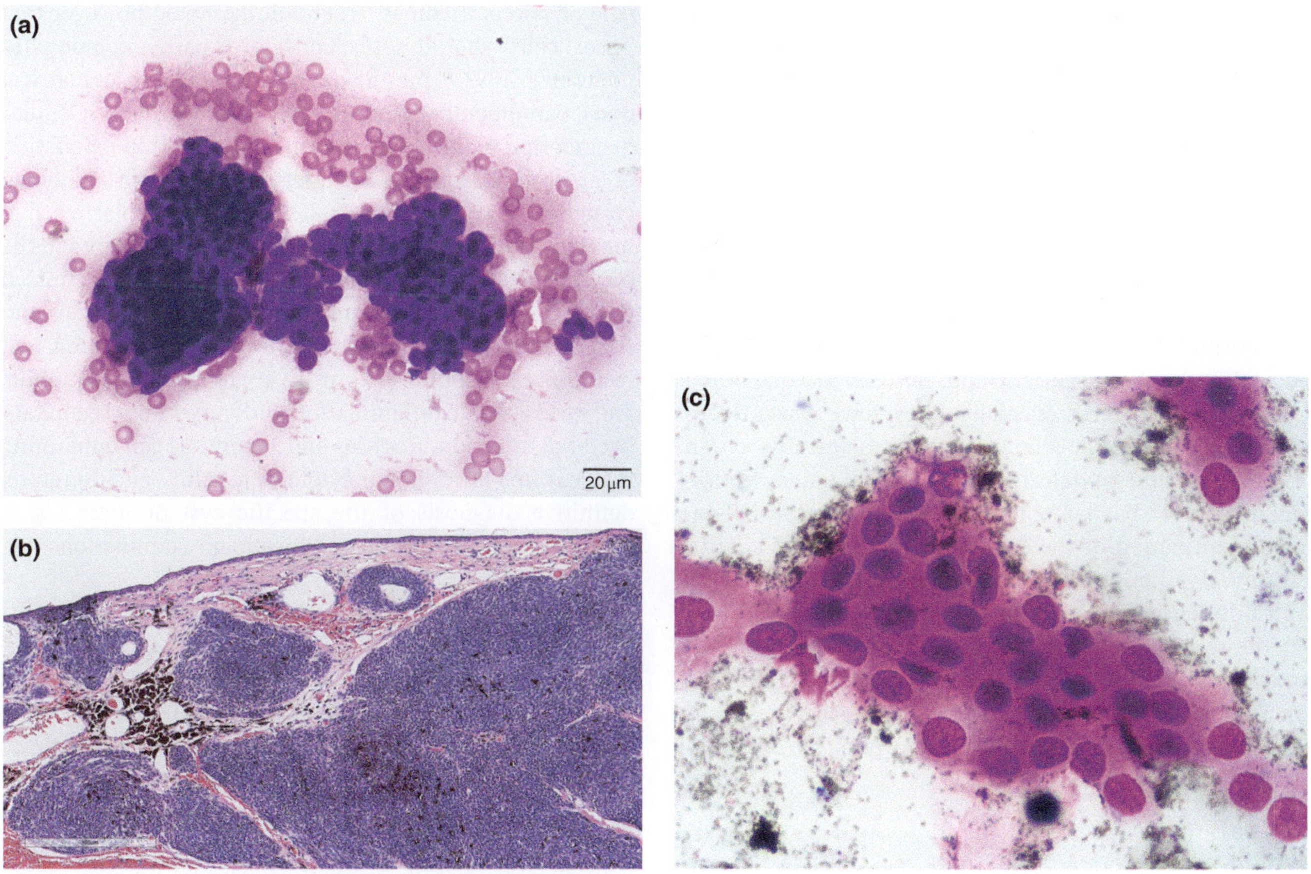

Figure 12.3 (a) FNA of a feline basilar epithelial neoplasm displaying a uniform population of basilar epithelial cells that have exfoliated in small clusters (Wright–Giemsa, 500×). (b) Histology of feline pigmented apocrine ductular adenoma displaying a uniform population of pigmented basilar epithelial cells with high N:C ratios (hematoxylin and eosin, 200×). (c) FNA of a canine basilar epithelial neoplasm displaying a raft of uniform, pigmented, cuboidal to polygonal epithelial cells. Numerous melanin granules are noted in the background (Wright–Giemsa, 100×).

arranged individually and in cohesive aggregates associated with eosinophilic fibrillar extracellular material.[27] The presence of eosinophilic fibrillar extracellular material and spindled cells can be characteristic of trichoblastomas and permit a more specific cytologic diagnosis.[28] The concurrent presence of keratinized squamous cells and sebaceous cells, with or without spindle cells, can be more suggestive of aspiration of a fibroadnexal hamartoma.[28] Granular cell trichoblastomas exfoliate many individualized medium-to-large, round-to-polygonal cells dispersed in linear streams in a light purple background.[29] Additionally, cystic variants of basilar epithelial neoplasms, which are common in cats, may only exfoliate the amorphous keratinized debris from the cystic cavity if the wall of the lesion is not aspirated.[30] Some basilar epithelial neoplasms, particularly solid-cystic apocrine ductular adenomas in cats, may be pigmented (Figure 12.3b). Aspiration of these pigmented masses may exfoliate pigmented keratinized debris and/or pigmented basilar epithelial cells that should not be misinterpreted as aspiration of a melanocytic neoplasm (Figure 12.3c). Therefore, definitive diagnosis of the exact histogenesis of basilar epithelial neoplasms requires surgical excision and histologic analysis of the lesion.[23]

The majority of basilar epithelial tumors are benign, but malignant variants do occur, and malignancy may be suggested by cytologic observation of cellular pleomorphism. Cytologic examination of a malignant pilomatricoma revealed round to cuboidal, basaloid cells arranged individually and in loosely cohesive clusters displaying pleomorphism, anisocytosis, anisokaryosis, prominent nucleoli, rare binucleation, and mitoses.[31] That being said, nuclear criteria of malignancy have been documented in cytologic specimens from histologically benign lesions.[26] Definitive determination of benignancy versus malignancy of basilar epithelial tumors requires histologic examination of the entire tumor as there is significant overlap between normal, hyperplastic, benign, and well-differentiated malignant basal epithelial cells. Therefore, surgical removal of these basilar epithelial neoplasms and submission for histopathologic analysis should be recommended, particularly if the mass has recently grown in size, changed in morphology, or is otherwise clinically indicated.

Keratin- and Squamous Cell-Containing Masses

There are a number of cutaneous epithelial masses that are composed largely of cystic centers that exfoliate primarily keratinized debris or anucleate superficial squamous cells (Figure 12.4a). Keratin and squamous cell-containing masses include true cysts such as follicular cysts, dermoid cysts, and subungual inclusion cysts; follicular tumors such as infundibular keratinizing acanthomas, trichoepitheliomas, and pilomatricomas; subungual keratoacanthomas; and a variety of hyperplastic/hamartomatous/tumor-like lesions such as fibroadnexal hamartomas and warty dyskeratomas. Cysts in dogs, cats, and horses may be congenital or acquired (typically secondary to repeated trauma) and can be single or multiple.[32–34] Grossly, contents of these cysts and masses are often described as off-white and caseous or chalky.[6] Aspirates from keratin- and squamous cell-containing lesions exhibit few cells (primarily keratinocytes that are anucleate or contain karyolytic nuclei) with abundant keratinized debris.[18,23–25] Keratinized debris is basophilic and can exfoliate as angular keratin bars or amorphous debris (Figure 12.4b–d). Squamous "ghost cells" are characterized as a polygonal basophilic anucleate squamous cells with a central unstained zone corresponding to the site previously occupied by the nucleus. Ghost cells, with or without concurrent exfoliation of basilar epithelial cells, can be a cytologic characteristic of pilomatricomas.[9] It should be noted however that "ghost cells" should not be considered pathognomonic for pilomatricomas as they also can be aspirated from matrical cysts, panfollicular cysts, and trichoepitheliomas.[9] Cellular degradation within cystic lesions may result in exfoliation of large, clear, rectangular cholesterol crystals with notched corners (Figure 12.4c and d). If the cyst or neoplasm is pigmented, few to many melanin granules can be found in the background or within squamous cells and keratinized debris (Figure 12.3c). Trauma and rupture of keratin- and squamous cell-containing mass lesions are common and result in neutrophilic (Figure 12.4c) to mixed neutrophilic and macrophagic inflammation with or without secondary bacterial infection. Keratin- and squamous cell-containing masses often have similar cytologic features, and therefore, definitive diagnosis of the specific cyst or mass lesion requires surgical excision and histologic examination.

Superficial Squamous Cell Masses

Superficial squamous cell masses arising from the epidermis include viral and nonviral (idiopathic) papillomas and squamous cell carcinomas. Superficial squamous cell masses are typically exophytic and originate in the epidermis and dermis but if invasive, as in the case of squamous cell carcinoma, may extend into the subcutis. In contrast, lesions that may mimic squamous cell masses (including follicular cysts and tumors) may bulge on the skin surface but originate in the dermis and subcutis. Occasionally, squamous cell carcinomas will emanate from areas of ductular squamous metaplasia within glandular tissues such as the mammary gland or circumanal gland,[35,36] in which case they may present as a primarily dermal or subcutaneous mass.

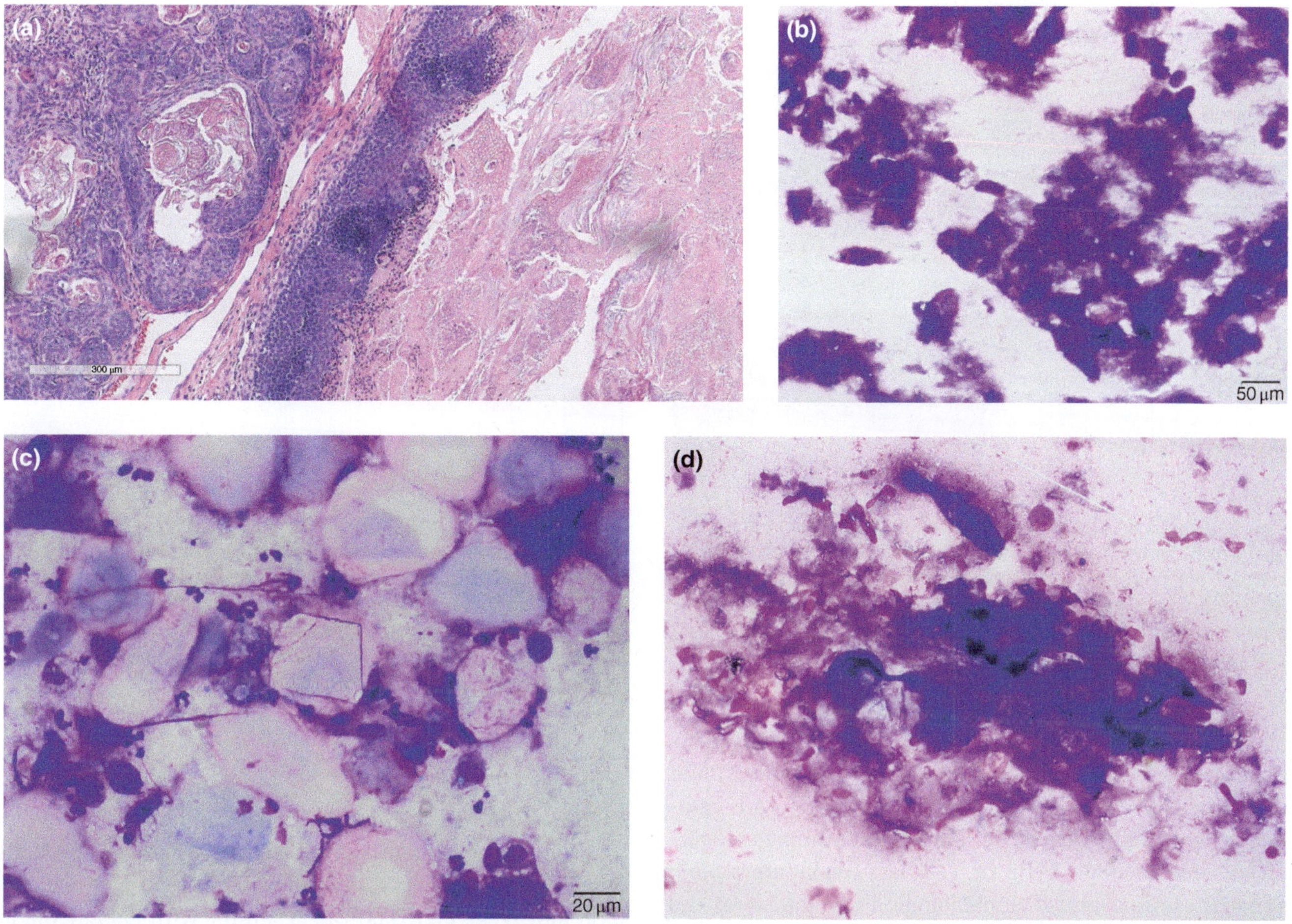

Figure 12.4 (a) Histology of a canine pilomatricoma. If the cystic center on the right was aspirated, ghost cells and keratinized debris would exfoliate. If the solid portion of the mass on the left was aspirated, basilar epithelial cells would exfoliate (hematoxylin and eosin, 200×). FNAs of canine keratin-containing masses illustrating how these types of masses are cytologically variable. (b) Exfoliated amorphous basophilic keratinized debris (Wright–Giemsa, 200×). (c) Superficial nucleate and anucleate squamous cells. Note the central, clear, cholesterol crystal. Low numbers of degenerate neutrophils are also present (Wright–Giemsa, 400×). (d) A combination of amorphous keratinized debris, keratin flakes, and keratin bars. A cholesterol crystal is at the bottom right (Wright–Giemsa, 200×).

Papillomas

Viral papillomas have exophytic and endophytic (inverted) variants, are due to infection with various canine and feline papillomaviruses, and display viral cytopathic effects cytologically and histologically.[8,15,37–39] Idiopathic squamous papillomas are considered by most to be a tumor-like, hyperplastic or dysplastic lesion that is not virally induced and not a true neoplasm.[8,15] Scrapings or aspirates of viral papillomas exfoliate a unique population of large, polygonal to fusiform cells with lightly basophilic and foamy to eosinophilic and granular cytoplasm, round eccentric nuclei, and clumped chromatin[39] (Figure 12.5). These cells, which may be referred to as koilocyte-like cells, are presumed to represent hypertrophied keratinocytes that have undergone degeneration and dysplasia.[39] The cytologic appearance of the fusiform-shaped cells may overlap with that of mesenchymal cells in which case immunocytochemistry using a broad-spectrum cytokeratin can be used to confirm their epithelial origin.[39] Scrapings or aspirates of idiopathic squamous papillomas exfoliate primarily uniform, mature flattened, keratinized squamous epithelial cells with fewer intermediate and basal squamous epithelial cells.[16,39,40] Intermediate and basal squamous epithelial cells are smaller and rounder and have increased cytoplasmic basophilia and slightly increased N:C ratios than mature superficial squamous cells, which are angular and contain light blue keratinized cytoplasm and small dense, often pyknotic nuclei. Although koilocyte-like cells are not

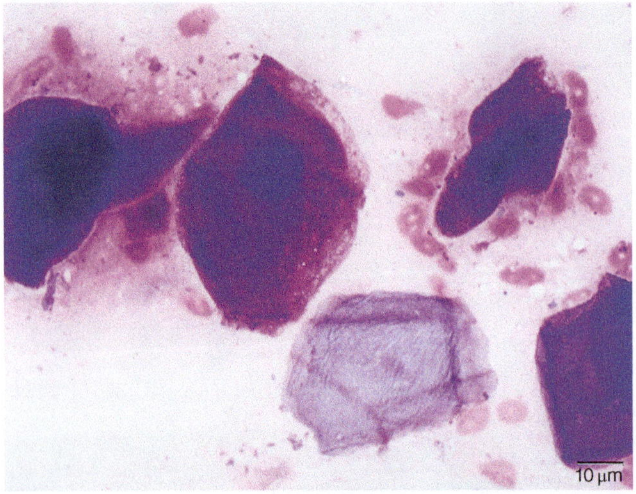

Figure 12.5 FNA of a canine viral papilloma demonstrating a fusiform hypertrophied squamous epithelial cell (center) with atypical eosinophilic cytoplasmic granularity presumed to represent viral cytopathic effect. Contrast this cell to the typical blue cytoplasm of the anucleate squamous cell (bottom) (Wright–Giemsa, 1000×).

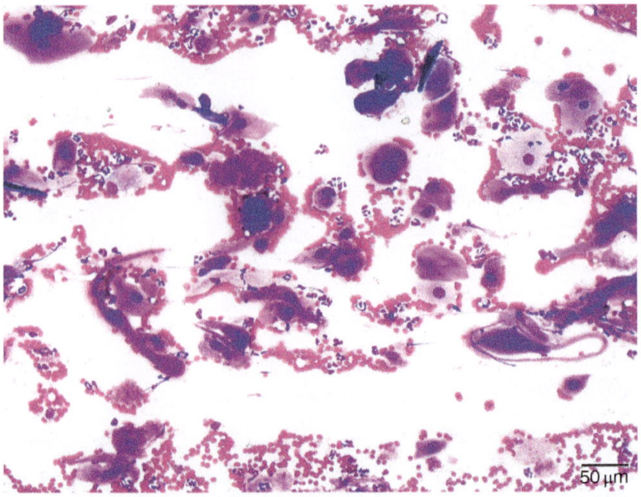

Figure 12.6 FNA of a feline squamous cell carcinoma. Malignant squamous cells exhibit numerous criteria of malignancy including anisocytosis, anisokaryosis, multinucleation, prominent nucleoli, aberrant "tadpole" shape, and nuclear to cytoplasmic asynchronous maturation. Neoplastic cells are admixed with lipid, peripheral blood, and neutrophilic inflammation (Wright–Giemsa, 400×).

observed in non-viral squamous papillomas, mild dysplastic changes such as mild anisocytosis, anisokaryosis, and increased N:C ratios may be observed if the lesion is traumatized and/or inflamed.[16,18] If increased numbers of basilar or intermediate cells or cellular atypia are noted, surgical excision and histopathologic examination of the mass should be considered to rule out a well-differentiated squamous cell carcinoma.

Squamous Cell Carcinoma

Squamous cell carcinomas can be induced by exposure to ultraviolet light and/or by papillomavirus infection.[37,41,42] The cytologic appearance is variable, depending on the degree of tumor differentiation. Squamous cells aspirated from squamous cell carcinomas exfoliate singly or in sheets and are variably mature. Less mature basilar cells are smaller and rounder, have higher N:C ratios, and contain a small amount of more deeply basophilic cytoplasm, while more mature superficial cells are angular and contain abundant characteristic, light blue, keratinized cytoplasm.[43,44] Occasionally, neoplastic cells from squamous cell carcinomas may demonstrate asynchronous nuclear to cytoplasmic maturation as a criterion of malignancy. Microscopically, this is evident in cells demonstrating mature cytoplasmic characteristics (i.e. angular margins with keratinized, light blue to pink cytoplasm) with retained (i.e. immature) large, round nuclei. Other features often identified in squamous cell carcinomas include emperipolesis, teardrop- or tadpole-shaped squamous cells, and perinuclear punctate vacuoles (assumed to represent colorless and atypical keratohyalin granules) (Figure 12.6). Occasionally, if the squamous neoplasm is poorly differentiated, the squamous origin of the cells may not be evident cytologically. In such cases, consideration may be given to staining a sample with Papanicolaou stain. The cytoplasm of squamous cells stained with a Papanicolaou stain is orangeophilic and indicative of keratinization and squamous differentiation.[43,45] Squamous cell carcinomas are frequently inflamed, and variably degenerate neutrophils will exfoliate alongside the neoplastic cells. Neutrophilic inflammation can incite marked dysplastic changes in neighboring epithelial cells, and thus a cytologic diagnosis of squamous cell carcinoma in the presence of inflammation is challenging and must be made with caution.

Sebaceous Gland Hyperplasia and Neoplasms

In decreasing order of prevalence, sebaceous mass lesions include nodular sebaceous hyperplasia, sebaceous adenoma, sebaceous epitheliomas, and sebaceous carcinomas.[1] Cytologic differentiation of sebaceous hyperplasia and sebaceous adenomas is not possible as aspirates of both hyperplastic and adenomatous lesions reveal a uniform population of clustered or individualized sebocytes with abundant cytoplasm containing numerous, punctate, clear vacuoles, small round nuclei, clumped chromatin, and indistinct nucleoli[18,23–25] (Figure 12.7a). Sebaceous

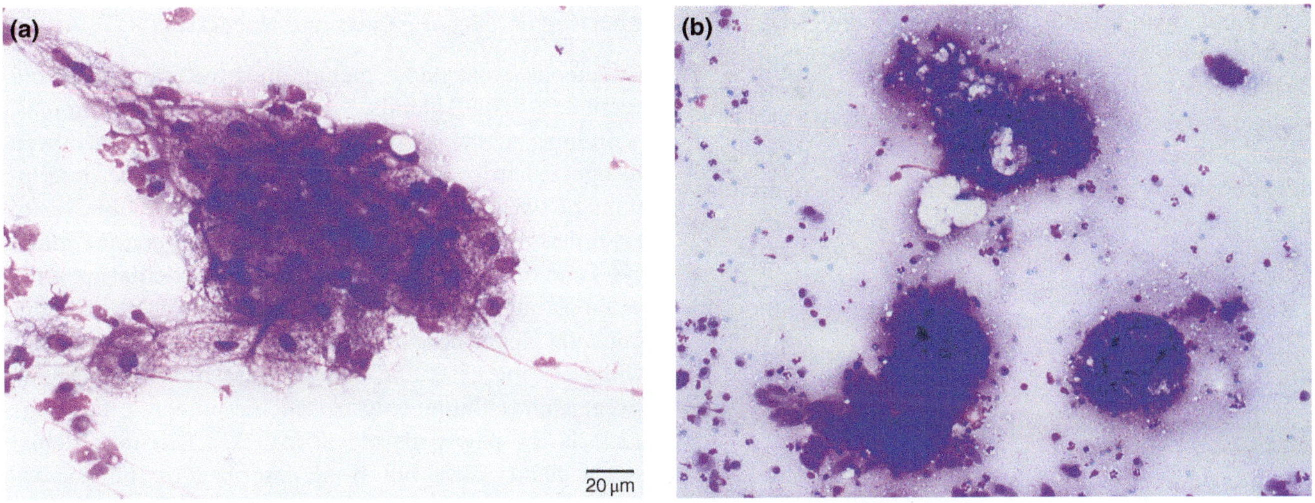

Figure 12.7 (a) FNA of a canine sebaceous adenoma. The cells are polygonal and contain numerous clear, punctate, cytoplasmic vacuoles (Wright–Giemsa, 500×). (b) Cytology image from an inflamed, canine, sebaceous epithelioma. Note that the majority of cells are a uniform population of basilar epithelial cells that have exfoliated in small clusters with only scattered vacuolated, terminally differentiated sebocytes within the top cluster of cells. Numerous neutrophils, small lymphocytes, and scattered macrophages are found in the proteinaceous background (Wright–Giemsa, 200×).

epitheliomas are sebaceous tumors containing a preponderance of cuboidal basilar epithelial reserve cells with few foci of sebaceous differentiation.[8,15] If only the basilar epithelial reserve cells exfoliate, the tumor can only be classified as a "basilar epithelial neoplasm," but frequently, the clusters of basilar cells that exfoliate do contain scattered differentiated sebocytes that would suggest a diagnosis of sebaceous epithelioma (Figure 12.7b). However, owing to sample bias, differentiating sebaceous adenomas from sebaceous epitheliomas by cytology alone usually is not possible.

Sebaceous carcinomas are infrequently encountered but have been described cytologically as exfoliating large numbers of pleomorphic, individualized, or very rarely acinar clusters of round to polygonal cells with variable N:C ratios, marked anisocytosis and anisokaryosis, and multinucleation.[46] Cells have basophilic, finely granular cytoplasm that variably contain clear vacuoles, intracytoplasmic secretory vacuoles, and cannibalized tumor cells.[46] Nuclei are round with fine chromatin and multiple prominent variably shaped and sized nucleoli. The cytologic appearance was considered more compatible with a tumor of mesenchymal origin although an anaplastic carcinoma was a differential diagnosis.[46] Immunohistochemically, increased nuclear survivin expression and the loss of estrogen and progesterone receptors in malignant sebaceous tumors are associated with increasing malignancy and may be useful as new diagnostic markers.[47,48]

Similarly, a single case of canine clear cell adnexal carcinoma has been reported.[49] A clear cell adnexal carcinoma is defined as a primary cutaneous adnexal neoplasm without definitive apocrine, sebaceous, or follicular differentiation.[8] The aspirate in the report was highly cellular and depicted a pleomorphic population of loosely arranged, oval to polygonal to occasionally spindled cells with indistinct margins.[49] Occasionally, cytoplasmic eosinophilic stippling, cytoplasmic globular deposits, or pink needle-shaped cytoplasmic inclusions were noted.[49] The described cells were not clearly of epithelial origin as they did not display obvious cohesion, cellular junctions, or defined cytoplasmic margins.[49] Therefore, it is important to include anaplastic or undifferentiated carcinomas in the cytologic differential diagnoses for cutaneous masses even if typical epithelial features are not observed.

Circumanal (Perianal) Gland Hyperplasia and Neoplasms

Circumanal (perianal) glands are modified sebaceous glands that occur on the tail, perineum, prepuce, thigh, and dorsal lumbosacral area of the dog.[15] Aspirates from circumanal gland proliferations reveal clusters of uniform round to polygonal epithelial cells containing a moderate amount of grainy, basophilic to amphophilic cytoplasm; round nuclei; intermediately coarse chromatin; and typically a single, small round nucleolus. There is similarity in appearance to hepatocytes, thus their alternative moniker of “hepatoid gland tumor.”[6,18,25] Occasionally, circumanal gland tumors may be composed of predominantly basilar reserve cells (circumanal gland epitheliomas) and may exfoliate primarily basilar reserve cells[24] (Figure 12.8a). If lysed or streaming, these basilar cells and their free nuclei could potentially be mistaken for epithelial cells of anal sac apocrine gland origin, particularly if no characteristic hepatoid circumanal gland cells concurrently exfoliate.[24] Similar to other sebaceous masses, cytologic differentiation between hyperplastic and adenomatous lesions is not possible. Additionally, owing to the cytologic overlap between adenoma and well-differentiated carcinomas, lesions are best diagnosed cytologically as “circumanal (perianal) gland tumor.” The best indicator of malignancy is invasion into surrounding tissues that can only be assessed histologically. Therefore, regardless of their cytologic appearance, surgical excision and histopathology of all circumanal (perianal) gland mass lesions should be recommended. That being said, the majority of circumanal gland tumors are benign with benign circumanal gland tumors reported to represent 8–18% of all canine skin tumors,[15,50] while their malignant counterparts are reported to represent 0.25–2.6% of all skin tumors,[15] and thus surgical excision may not be urgent and may be postponed in poor surgical candidates.

Apocrine and Eccrine Cysts and Neoplasms

Cutaneous sweat glands include apocrine (epitrichial) and eccrine (atrichial) glands. Sweat gland cysts, hamartomas, adenomas, adenocarcinomas, and carcinomas have been recognized in cats, dogs, and horses. Cytologic descriptions of sweat gland lesions are limited,[16,18,24] but histologic descriptions are numerous.[8,15,51–55] Apocrine gland cysts and tumors arise from either the epitrichial apocrine sweat glands associated with the hair follicle or those nonfollicular apocrine glands associated with the anal sac, while eccrine cysts and tumors arise from the atrichial sweat glands found only in specific anatomic locations such as the paw pads of carnivores.[55] Eccrine/atrichial sweat glands have not been described in the horse.[56] Eccrine cysts and neoplasms are very rare and will not be discussed further.

Aspiration of apocrine cysts is often unrewarding, yielding only acellular proteinaceous fluid that can be macroscopically clear or brown.[18] Cutaneous epitrichial apocrine tumors arise from either the glandular or ductular portion of the gland, and this will influence their cytologic appearance. Apocrine ductular adenomas and adenocarcinomas exfoliate clusters of pigmented or nonpigmented basilar epithelial cells. Epitrichial apocrine tumors arising from

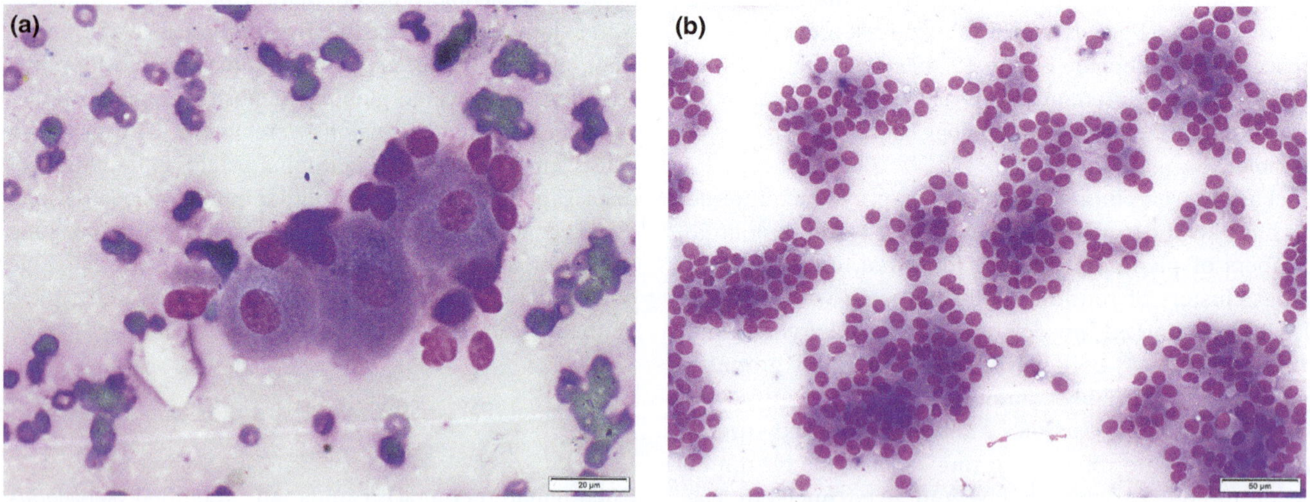

Figure 12.8 (a) FNA of a canine circumanal gland adenoma. Note the three central hepatoid cells containing a moderate amount of grainy, basophilic to amphophilic cytoplasm; round nuclei; intermediately coarse chromatin; and a single, small round nucleolus. There are several basilar reserve cells surrounding the hepatoid cells that display high N:C ratios and contain a scant amount of lightly basophilic cytoplasm and round nuclei with less distinct nucleoli. If present in greater numbers and with few to no hepatoid cells, it may be difficult to differentiate the basilar reserve cells from cells aspirated from an apocrine gland (anal sac) adenocarcinoma. Compare the basilar reserve cells with the cells in (b) (Wright–Giemsa, 1000×). (b) FNA of an apocrine gland (anal sac) adenocarcinoma. Cytology reveals numerous bare nuclei in the background with a population of somewhat basilar appearing epithelial cells that have exfoliated singly and in loosely cohesive clusters. Cells contain a small amount of lightly basophilic cytoplasm with indistinct cellular margins; small round or ovoid nuclei; intermediately coarse chromatin; and indistinct to a single prominent, small, round, basophilic, nucleolus (Wright–Giemsa, 400×).

the glandular portion of the gland exfoliate clusters of cuboidal to columnar secretory epithelial cells that contain a moderate amount of basophilic to amphophilic, grainy cytoplasm; round nuclei; clumped chromatin; and indistinct nucleoli.[24,25] Most canine and feline apocrine sweat gland tumors are benign;[15] however, malignant versions do occur and would be expected to exhibit cytologic criteria of malignancy.

Apocrine gland (anal sac) adenocarcinomas arise from the anal sac apocrine glands and are not associated with hair follicles. While common in dogs, they also infrequently occur in cats.[57–60] Production of parathyroid hormone-related protein (PTHrp) and paraneoplastic hypercalcemia is reported in 26–53% of dogs[61–63] with apocrine gland adenocarcinomas but only one of five cats in one report.[60] These neoplasms are almost all malignant yet exhibit minimal cytologic atypia. Cytology reveals numerous bare nuclei in the background with a population of somewhat basilar appearing epithelial cells that have exfoliated singly and in loosely cohesive clusters. Acinar forms may be seen. Cells contain a small amount of lightly basophilic cytoplasm with indistinct cellular margins; small round or ovoid nuclei; intermediately coarse chromatin; and a single indistinct to prominent, small, round, basophilic nucleolus (Figure 12.8b). The cytologic appearance of apocrine gland (anal sac) adenocarcinomas is often described as a "neuroendocrine-like pattern" (many free nuclei on a background of free cytoplasm) even though the anal sac apocrine glands are not of neuroendocrine origin. An atypical spindle cell morphologic subtype has been described where approximately 75% of aspirated cells were polygonal to oval and had an elliptical or elongate nucleus, while the remaining 25% of cells had a more classic appearance of round to oval nuclei.[64] On cytology both the atypical cells with oval nuclei and the cells with more typical round nuclei appeared to form acinar structures; however, on histology, the two populations were distinct with more cuboidal cells forming glandular structure, while spindled cells formed fascicles.[64]

Carcinomas Metastatic to the Skin

When considering differential diagnoses for epithelial neoplasms in the skin, it is important to remember that the skin can be a metastatic site for carcinomas originating in other tissues. Metastases of bronchogenic adenocarcinomas,[65] mammary adenocarcinoma,[66] intraepidermal adenocarcinoma resembling human extramammary Paget's disease,[67] and vesicular adenocarcinoma[66] have been reported in the literature. Cytologic features of metastatic bronchogenic adenocarcinoma included exfoliation of small clusters, including some acinar forms, of atypical epithelial cells exhibiting marked anisocytosis, high N:C ratios, multinucleated cells, and mitotic activity.[65]

Mesenchymal Cell-Derived Masses Diagnosed by Cytology

Aspiration of a spindle cell population from cutaneous lesions provides a diagnostic challenge to cytologists. Fibroblasts and endothelial cells in areas of fibroplasia and granulation tissue have cytologic features that overlap with those of neoplastic spindle cells in sarcomas. Therefore, aspirates from areas of fibroplasia and granulation tissue cannot be reliably distinguished from aspirates from sarcomas. Histology is required for definitive differentiation.

Reactive and Hyperplastic Lesions

Cytologically, both reactive fibroplasia and granulation tissue are composed of fibroblasts, eosinophilic extracellular matrix or collagen, varying types of inflammatory cells, and/or capillary fragments.

Reactive fibroplasia is a fibroblastic proliferative response occurring secondary to numerous stimuli including chronic inflammation, neoplasia, trauma, and radiation resulting in the formation of fibrous connective tissue and deposition of collagen.[68,69] Lesions are firm and can form at any site of chronic inflammation.

Granulation tissue specifically refers to a form of fibroblastic proliferative response that forms a pink, fleshy, and granular tissue over a wound and is composed of an expansion of fibroblasts, small blood vessels, and an accumulation of connective tissue. Histologically, it is composed of organizing fibroblasts, capillaries that run perpendicular to the organizing fibroblasts and the surface of the wound, edema, inflammatory cells, and extracellular matrix.[70] Granulation tissue forms in response to injury, aiding in wound healing. In some instances, especially in distal limb injury of horses, exuberant granulation tissue can form resulting in "proud flesh."[40]

It is important to note that fibroblasts can range from well-differentiated spindle cells with minimal criteria of malignancy to markedly atypical, plump, and fusiform cells with marked nuclear and cytoplasmic criteria of malignancy (anisocytosis, anisokaryosis, multinucleation, prominent and multiple nucleoli, mitotic figures). Clinical history, such as recent trauma to the area of interest, can be helpful in prioritizing a benign or malignant process.

Benign Tumors of Fibrous Tissue

Benign tumors of fibrous tissue often do not exfoliate well with FNA and are typically not diagnosed via cytology. Examples include fibroma, neurofibroma, collagenous hamartoma, nodular dermatofibrosis, myxoma, and equine sarcoid. Expected cytologic findings include low numbers of relatively well-differentiated spindle cells and variable amounts of eosinophilic extracellular matrix (granular in appearance in the case of myxoma) or collagen.[71] Histology is required for differentiation and definitive diagnosis.

Tumors of Adipose Tissue

Tumors of adipose tissue include benign lipomas, infiltrative lipomas, fibrolipomas, and liposarcomas. Lipomas are benign tumors composed of mature adipocytes that occur in dogs, cats, and rarely horses. In a study from the United Kingdom, lipomas were the second most commonly occurring tumor type in a group of 130 684 dogs. Standardized incidence rate was 318/100 000 dogs/year.[72] In contrast, in a study of 340 feline cutaneous neoplasms diagnosed by histology, less than 1% were lipomas.[11] Lipomas are variably sized, subcutaneous, generally soft, and mobile relative to deeper tissue. They have been reported to commonly occur on the proximal legs, trunk, and gluteal region but can occur in other regions as well.[73] In horses, lipomas occur most commonly on the trunk or neck.[74] As these tumors are benign, depending on location and/or size, continued monitoring or surgical removal are common treatments. Recently, intralesional steroid injections have been shown to decrease the size or resolve lipomas in dogs.[75] Primary literature specifically describing the cytologic appearance of lipomas is lacking; however, expected findings are similar to histologic findings. Adipocytes appear as individualized or aggregated round cells with clear cytoplasm and a peripherally compressed nucleus with dense chromatin. Intermixed capillaries may be seen in large aggregates, and ruptured adipocytes can sometimes appear fusiform. Eosinophilic collagen also can be seen, especially with aspiration of a fibrolipoma. In some instances, adipocytes are lacking, and only lipid droplets are seen. Lipomas also can become mineralized. New methylene blue can be used to stain adipocytes as alcohol-based stains dissolve lipid or lipid is removed during rinsing steps.

Infiltrative lipomas will appear cytologically identical to lipomas but have a more aggressive clinical course. These tumors infiltrate through muscle and other tissues, are difficult to completely excise, and commonly recur.[76] Histology can differentiate an infiltrative lipoma from a non-infiltrative lipoma; however, this can only be achieved if the tissue sample is obtained from a site where the lipoma is invading adjacent tissue. Both computed tomography and magnetic resonance imaging can be used to assess for tissue infiltration and aid in the diagnosis of infiltrative lipoma.[77,78] As the distinction between a lipoma and an infiltrative lipoma impacts prognosis and treatment option, it is important to distinguish between these two clinical entities.[78]

Lipomas may become traumatized resulting in concurrent inflammation and/or fibroplasia that will exfoliate upon aspiration. Aspiration of non-neoplastic causes of panniculitis will also exfoliate variable amounts of inflammation, lipid, and/or fibroplasia.[79] When inflamed, the cytologic appearance of the lipoma would be difficult to differentiate from a primary, nodular, inflammatory lesions affecting the subcutaneous adipose tissue such as idiopathic sterile nodular panniculitis, pancreatic panniculitis, feline pansteatitis, postinjection panniculitis, traumatic panniculitis, or infectious causes of nodular panniculitis.[15]

The cytologic appearance of liposarcomas have been described[80,81] and are discussed in Chapter 16.

Histiocytic Diseases

Histiocytic diseases with cutaneous manifestations represents a biologically, clinically, and microscopically diverse group of disorders. This chapter will discuss the two benign histiocytic neoplasms that can be diagnosed cytologically (xanthoma and histiocytoma) and only one of the malignant histiocytic neoplasms – feline progressive histiocytosis. All other histiocytic neoplasms are discussed in Chapters 16, 23, and 28.

Feline Progressive Histiocytosis

Feline progressive histiocytosis is a disorder of interstitial dendritic cells that begins as a benign process of the skin but progresses to have more malignant features over time. Disease incidence is low in the feline population. In a study of 30 cats, females (intact or neutered) were affected at a slightly higher rate.[82] Age at initial presentation ranged from 2 to 17 years with a mean of 8 years.[82,83] Initially, lesions appear as multiple or solitary intradermal nodules and papules that might change size over time but do not resolve and can progress to larger lesions. Lesions are initially haired to partially alopecic and non-painful but can progress to become ulcerated and painful. Primary nodules most commonly occur on the head (18/30 cats), legs, and feet (21/30 cats) but can also occur on other areas of the body such as the trunk. Over a period of months to years, this disorder progresses to result in clinical illness and internal organ involvement. Long-term prognosis is considered poor, as lesions are poorly responsive to therapy.[82,83]

Initial cytologic characterization was reported as variable, depending on the state of disease progression. Initially, histiocytes appeared well differentiated but became more atypical as the disease progressed.[82] A recent study characterized the cytomorphology of these lesions in more detail.[84] Samples tended to be highly cellular and composed of round to polygonal to rarely spindyloid cells with indistinct cell margins and absent phagocytic behavior. Rarely, cells formed large and cohesive groups. Cells contained moderate to large amounts of clear to light blue and slightly granular cytoplasm that was rarely vacuolated. Nuclei were often eccentrically located and oval to kidney-shaped. Chromatin was finely clumped with rarely visible single nucleoli. Anisocytosis and anisokaryosis were mild to moderate, and rarely, binucleation or multinucleated giant cells were present. Mitotic activity was variable. Small numbers of lymphocytes, nondegenerate neutrophils, or mast cells were observed.[82,84]

Additional diagnostics such as immunocytochemistry or biopsy with immunohistochemistry (IHC) are required for definitive diagnosis, although it is important to note that late-stage feline progressive histiocytosis and histiocytic sarcoma can be difficult to differentiate via microscopy even with immunostaining as marker positivity for CD1a and CD11/CD18 overlap.[83] Clinical presentation and history are important for differentiation of feline progressive histiocytosis from other inflammatory and neoplastic histiocytic diseases. Feline progressive histiocytosis is described as a slowly progressing disease that begins in the skin before disseminating to internal organs, whereas histiocytic sarcoma would have a more aggressive clinical course.[82] Additionally, cytologic atypia may be minimal in early lesions of feline progressive histiocytosis, whereas more atypia would be expected in histiocytic sarcoma.[83,84] Using IHC, atypical cells in feline progressive histiocytosis are expected to stain positive for CD1a, CD1c, CD18, and MHCII. CD5 expression can be variably positive, and E-cadherin can be positive in small numbers of cells. Using immunocytochemistry, the atypical cells stain positive for CD1a, CD1c, CD18, CD11b, and MHCII.[82,84]

Xanthoma

Xanthomas are benign cutaneous or subcutaneous masses composed of macrophages that occur in dogs, cats, horses, and other veterinary species.[85–88] Disease incidence is considered uncommon.[85,86] Xanthomas can be primary (idiopathic) or secondary to disorders of lipoprotein metabolism. The underlying physiology of xanthoma formation has not been fully elucidated but is thought to be secondary to the accumulation of lipids in tissue followed by macrophage ingestion. These lipid-filled macrophages are often referred to as foam cells on histology.[88] Disease conditions associated with xanthoma development include diabetes mellitus in dogs and cats, hypothyroidism and hyperadrenocorticism in dogs, primary hyperlipidemia in dogs and cats, inherited disorders of lipid metabolism in dogs and cats, and pituitary pars intermedia dysfunction in horses.[85,87,89–92] Glucocorticoid administration is also implicated in dogs and cats.[88,93] Lesions may resolve when causes of lipid accumulation are eliminated.[93] Lesions appear as white or yellow (rarely pink to red) papules, plaques, or pustules with erythematous borders and can become ulcerated.[85,86,93,94] Cutaneous xanthomata often occur on the head, pinnae, and neck but can occur on other areas such as the feet or ventrum.[85,93,95] Non-cutaneous xanthomatous lesions are reported to occur in the oral, esophageal, and gastric mucosa; adrenal gland; and liver.[85,96]

Cytology of xanthomas has been reported to consist of individualized and aggregated round cells with low N:C ratio, vacuolated cytoplasm, and oval nuclei with dense chromatin. Minimal atypia was noted.[97] Large numbers of cholesterol clefts can be seen on histology, but cholesterol crystals were not reported in the single cytologic description in the literature.[88,97]

Histology is required for definitive diagnosis of a xanthoma and to rule out other causes of histiocytic/macrophagic inflammation such as fungal infection, foreign body reaction, or atypical mycobacteriosis. Frozen tissue or cytology slides can be stained with Oil Red O to confirm lipid. IHC for CD18 (high expression), lysozyme, and muscarinic acetylcholine receptor M1 (ACM1) can be used to support a macrophage origin of these cells.[85,97]

Cutaneous Histiocytoma

Cutaneous histiocytomas are generally benign tumors thought to arise from epidermal Langerhans cells.[98] In a study from the United Kingdom, they were the most commonly occurring tumor type in a group of 130 684 dogs with a standardized incidence rate of 337/100 000 dogs/year.[72] Overrepresented dog breeds affected by this tumor include Boxers and Dachshunds, while Poodles are reported to have a lower risk. In general, purebred dogs are more commonly affected than mixed breed dogs.[99] Young dogs are more commonly affected than older dogs, with one study reporting approximately 50% of these tumors occurring in dogs under 2 years of age.[99] Histiocytomas are classically described as hairless, round to domed to button-like, raised, erythematous, and sometimes ulcerated dermal/epidermal nodules with plaque-like variations also reported.[100] Histiocytomas typically present as solitary lesions, although dogs with multiple concurrent nodules have been reported.[98–100] Histiocytomas most commonly occur on the head, with the pinna being the most frequently affected site, although tumors can occur on many other areas of the body including the neck, tail, limbs, and trunk. They are non-painful unless inflamed or infected. If left untreated, these tumors generally regress over a period of months via $CD8^+$ cytotoxic T-cell-mediated involution.[98] Regrowth at removal sites is possible, but not common.[98,99] Rare cases of lymph node involvement of canine cutaneous histiocytomas, deemed migratory histiocytomas, have also been reported.[98]

Aspirated cells are generally round to ovoid with a moderate to high N:C ratio. Their cytoplasm is lightly basophilic and can stain similar or somewhat lighter in color than the proteinaceous background, giving them what is sometimes referred to as a "fried-egg" appearance (Figure 12.9). Small numbers of cells can contain punctate vacuoles or small granules. Nuclei are round to ovoid to indented and frequently eccentrically located with lightly stippled to granular chromatin. Nucleoli are not a prominent feature. Anisocytosis and anisokaryosis are mild to moderate, and binucleation can be seen. Variable numbers of small lymphocytes may be present, depending on the stage of tumor regression.[7,101]

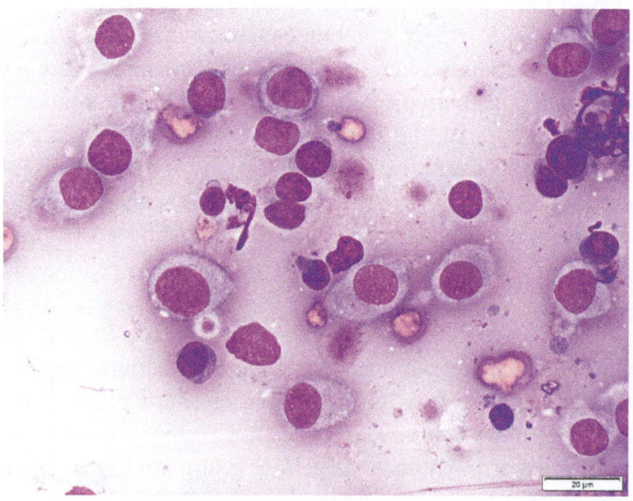

Figure 12.9 Cytology from a canine cutaneous histiocytoma. Aspirated cells are round with a moderate to high N:C ratio. Their cytoplasm is lightly basophilic and is lighter than the proteinaceous background giving them what is sometimes referred to as a "fried-egg" appearance. Nuclei are round to ovoid and frequently eccentrically located with lightly stippled to granular chromatin. Nucleoli are not a prominent feature. Anisocytosis and anisokaryosis are mild. Several small lymphocytes and a plasma cell are present (Wright–Giemsa, 1000×).

In some instances, histiocytomas can be difficult to differentiate from other round cell neoplasms, especially plasmacytomas, and histology with IHC may be required for definitive diagnosis. IHC may be of particular value when histiocytic cells invade the epidermis, mimicking epitheliotropic T-cell lymphoma.[102] Immunohistochemical immunophenotyping of histiocytomas reveals expression of CD1a (dendritic cell differentiation), CD11c/CD18 (β_2-integrins), CD45 (leukocyte common antigen), MHCII, and E-cadherin (cell adhesion molecule expressed in Langerhans cells). E-cadherin expression may not be present in all tumors. CD90 (interstitial dendritic cell) and CD3 (T-lymphocyte marker) expression are expected to be negative.[83,98,99]

Cutaneous histiocytomas have also been reported in cats and in a heifer.[103,104] Cytologic findings are not reported; however, clinical course, histology, and IHC findings in the cats and clinical course and histology in the heifer were similar to those in the dog and consistent with a diagnosis of cutaneous histiocytoma.[103,105]

Canine Transmissible Venereal Tumor

Canine transmissible venereal tumors (TVTs), also known as Sticker's sarcoma, are naturally occurring, contagious tumors characterized as histiocytic, reticuloendothelial, or macrophage in origin.[106–112] Tumor cells have 57–64 chromosomes as opposed to the typical 78 chromosomes of canine cells.[107,113,114] Tumors are described as cauliflower-like and are red, friable, and often associated with hemorrhage or blood-tinged discharge.[109,115] Tumors most commonly occur on the external genitalia but have been reported outside of the genital tract such as in the nasal cavity[115,116] or third eyelid.[117,118] Tumors can metastasize within the reproductive tract and to numerous sites including regional and distant lymph nodes and other organs.[115,116,119–121] There is no sex or breed association, although in one study, intact dogs were more commonly affected and tumor incidence was highest in dogs 2–5 years of age.[122,123] Tumor cells spread via direct transplantation on mucous membranes or damaged skin, either through coitus, licking, biting, or sniffing, and act as an allograft within the canine species, regardless of major histocompatibility complex compatibility.[108,124,125] This may be partially achieved by downregulation of dog leukocyte antigens on tumor cells.[126] Tumor regression can occur spontaneously, often over a six-month period, and this may be mediated via T lymphocytes. Treatment with vincristine, radiation, and/or surgical excision is often recommended, especially if clinical signs such as hemorrhage or secondary infection are present, to prevent transmission, or in cases of metastasis or atypical tumor location.[110,115,123,127,128]

Cytologic preparations of TVTs are often highly cellular. Cells can be individualized to highly aggregated. Cells are reported to be 14–30 μm in diameter with moderate to high N:C ratio. Cytoplasm is lightly basophilic, finely granular and often contains variable numbers of punctate, clear vacuoles. Nuclei are round to oval with coarsely stippled chromatin and often have a large, single nucleolus (Figure 12.10). Multinucleation may be present as well as mitotic figures.[101,106,125,127] *Leishmania* amastigotes have been cytologically identified within the cytoplasm of TVT cells.[106,108,129,130]

Additional diagnostics may be required for definitive tumor identification, as many round cell tumors can appear cytologically similar to TVT, especially when vacuoles are scant or absent. With IHC, TVT cells are expected to be vimentin positive; variably positive for lysozyme, alpha-1-antitrypsin, and neuron-specific enolase (NSE); positive for ACM1; and negative for cytokeratin, alpha smooth muscle actin, S-100, kappa and lambda light chains and IgG (except in perivascular tumor cells), IgM, and CD3.[109,110,112] Polymerase chain reaction (PCR) for a long interspersed nuclear element (LINE) insertion in association with the c-myc gene is considered diagnostic, as this is not present in other tumors.[125,131,132]

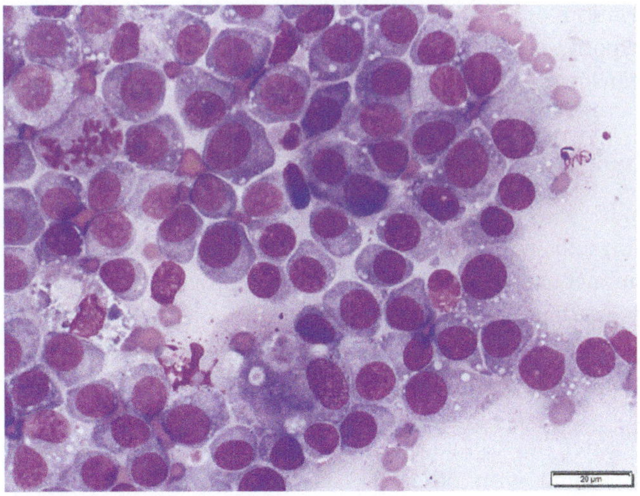

Figure 12.10 FNA of a canine TVT. Neoplastic round cells are individualized and contain a small volume of basophilic, finely granular cytoplasm often with variable numbers of punctate, clear vacuoles. The nuclei are round to oval with coarsely stippled chromatin and often have a large, single nucleolus. Note the aberrant mitotic figure in the upper left corner (Wright–Giemsa, 1000×).

Cutaneous Lymphoma

Cutaneous lymphoma is composed of neoplastic lymphocytes that may infiltrate the epidermis, dermis, and/or adnexal structures[133] and whose etiology is unknown. Cutaneous lymphoma can be divided into two major categories in veterinary species: epitheliotropic and non-epitheliotropic cutaneous lymphoma. The latter includes infiltration of the dermis from primary or disseminated/multicentric lymphoma.[133,134]

Epitheliotropic Lymphoma

As indicated by its name, epitheliotropic cutaneous lymphoma is characterized by neoplastic lymphocytes with tropism for the epidermal layer.[133–135] This form of lymphoma has three major histologic subclassifications: mycosis fungoides, Sezary syndrome, and pagetoid reticulosis, although other classifications based on clinical presentation have been proposed.[134,136,137] Disease manifestation can range from indolent to aggressive.[136] All three subclassifications have been reported in dogs, while mycosis fungoides and Sezary syndrome have been reported in cats.[133] In dogs and cats, older animals tend to be affected, and there is no breed or sex predilection.[136,138,139] Incidence in cats is reported to be extremely low with one study reporting an incidence of 0.08% of all reported feline cutaneous tumors in a 17-year period.[137] Differentiating between the three subclassifications requires histology and in the case of Sezary syndrome hematology. All three variants are primarily composed of $CD8^+$ T lymphocytes, which is in contrast to human variants, which are primarily $CD4^+$.[133] Additionally, the majority of tumors express T-cell receptor gamma/delta.[102] Overall prognosis is generally poor with a median survival time of six months in dogs despite therapy.[134,136] Survival time in cats is variable with a mean of 10.25 months; however, survival times as short as 1–6 months also are reported.[140]

Cytologically, cutaneous epitheliotropic lymphoma can be mistaken for chronic inflammation as a heterogeneous population of lymphocytes may be seen, or alternatively, cells can appear monomorphic or pleomorphic.[135,141–143] Clefted nuclei have been reported.[143] Definitive diagnosis requires histology; however, PCR for antigen receptor rearrangement and flow cytometry of cutaneous lesions and peripheral blood can be utilized as complimentary diagnostics for clonality determination and immunophenotyping, respectively.[143] In cats, cutaneous lymphocytosis, considered a benign condition, can exhibit a monomorphic population indicating the need for careful evaluation of the entire clinical picture.[140,144]

Mycosis Fungoides

Mycosis fungoides is the most common variant of cutaneous lymphoma in dogs.[135,139] The "patch, plaque, and nodule form"[134] is common although nodules can be present from the onset of disease, and other lesions such as crusts or depigmentation can also occur.[133–135,139] Aside from cutaneous manifestation, this form also predominates at mucocutaneous junctions.[133,135] Histologically, small to intermediately sized lymphocytes with notched nuclei will broadly invade the epidermis and dermis or appear in small packets (Pautrier's aggregates) in dogs, while in cats, large lymphocytes also can be seen.[133,135,137] In dogs, there also is a predilection for adnexal structures.[133,135] As discussed previously, the majority of cases are composed of $CD8^+$ T lymphocytes, and many cases lack CD5 expression.[102,133,135] Rare concurrent c-kit expression has also been reported.[145] A link between atopic dermatitis and mycosis fungoides has been proposed;[146] however, another study of 25 dogs did not support this association.[136]

Sezary Syndrome

Sezary syndrome presents with similar cutaneous lesions as mycosis fungoides with the addition of lymphadenopathy and circulating neoplastic lymphocytes.[135,147] This condition is often associated with severe pruritus.[135,143] Sezary cells in peripheral blood are described as small to intermediate to large in size and often have round to cleaved nuclei, with homologous lymphocytes seen in cutaneous lesions on cytology.[143,148]

Pagetoid Reticulosis

Initially, lymphocytes are highly restricted to the epidermis or adnexal epithelium.[102,134] As the disease progresses, dermal invasion occurs and confounds distinction from mycosis fungoides.[102,134]

Non-Epitheliotropic Lymphoma

Non-epitheliotropic lymphoma is uncommon in dogs[133] and tends to present more often as nodules or masses as opposed to crusts and scales.[133,135,138] Affected dogs and cats tend to be older, approximately 8 years of age and 11.5 years of age, respectively.[138] Initially, feline leukemia virus was considered a possible causative agent; however, this is now considered unlikely.[149] In dogs, cytologic samples have been reported to contain small to large lymphocytes with round to clefted to irregular nuclei and variably prominent nucleoli[142] (Figure 12.11). Histologically, in dogs, lymphocytes are large and monomorphic and may contain numerous cytoplasmic vacuoles. Lymphocytes can be present in nodules or sheets and can invade vessels. Eosinophilic infiltrate can be observed.[133,138] Lymphocytes tend to be more variably size in cats.[138] Lymphocytes in both dogs and cats also tend to be $CD3^+$, consistent with a T-lymphocyte phenotype.[133,138] Recently, cutaneous lymphoma at previous vaccine injection sites has been reported in 17 cats.[149] Interestingly, the majority of these lymphomas were non-epitheliotropic, large-cell lymphomas with B-cell phenotype. Chronic inflammation and possible reactivation of feline leukemia virus in select cases were hypothesized as possible inducers of malignant transformation.[149]

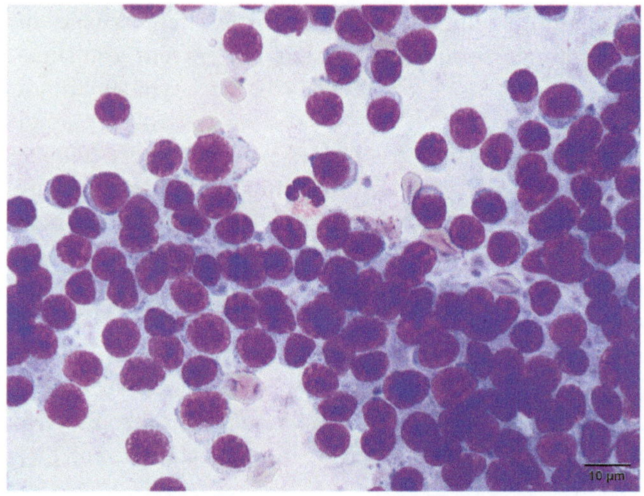

Figure 12.11 FNA from one of multiple raised, alopecic, pink dermal masses in a dog. An expanded population of monomorphic medium to large lymphocytes has exfoliated. Cells contain a small to mildly increased amount of lightly basophilic cytoplasm and occasionally display aberrant cytoplasmic blebbing. Their nuclei are large and round or rarely clefted with intermediately clumped chromatin and variably distinct nucleoli. An eosinophil is present in the center of the image (Wright–Giemsa, 1000×).

Equine Cutaneous Lymphoma

In horses, cutaneous lymphoma is considered a rare condition and may represent primary cutaneous lymphoma or cutaneous involvement of multicentric or alimentary lymphoma.[150–152] The most common form of cutaneous lymphoma is non-epitheliotropic T-cell-rich, large B-cell lymphoma, and affected horses generally present with multiple dermal/subcutaneous nodules.[151,153] In one study, Quarter Horses had an increased incidence of this subtype compared with other breeds.[151] Cutaneous T-cell lymphoma is the second most commonly diagnosed cutaneous lymphoma with thoroughbreds disproportionately represented.[151] It often presents as a solitary lesion and appears histologically similar to mycosis fungoides in dogs with epitheliotropism.[151] Other cutaneous lymphoma subtypes include diffuse large B-cell lymphoma and anaplastic

T-cell lymphoma.[151] On cytology, lymphocytes are primarily large with round, reniform or lobulated nuclei with immature chromatin and prominent, sometimes multiple, nucleoli.[40] Because many small lymphocytes are present in T-cell-rich large B-cell lymphoma, a predominance of small lymphocytes with fewer numbers of pleomorphic large lymphocytes is expected in FNA from these lesions.

Miscellaneous Masses Diagnosed by Cytology

Hygroma

Hygromas are fluid-filled bursas that develop in the subcutaneous space over bony prominences, often after prolonged recumbence. Given their size, giant-breed dogs may be predisposed; however, these masses can form in any size dog. Commonly affected sites include the lateral elbow and other areas prone to pressure.[154] Hygromas appear as fluctuant or semi-firm subcutaneous swellings. Overlying skin may be haired, ulcerated, or alopecic. Aspiration generally yields viscous fluid that varies in color depending on the presence or absence of hemorrhage and chronicity. In uncomplicated hygromas, cytology reveals small numbers of macrophages and small lymphocytes on a thick background.[16,18] Increased neutrophils are seen if inflammation is present. Small numbers of fibroblasts also can be seen as the wall of the bursa is composed of fibroplasia.[154] Treatment may involve decompression via aspiration, pressure wraps, or infrequently surgical intervention.

Seroma

Seromas are subcutaneous fluid-filled pockets that develop at sites of trauma-induced tissue dead space, such as secondary to surgical incisions. They appear cytologically similar to hygromas. Treatment may involve fluid aspiration or compression bandages.

Hematoma

Hematomas are subcutaneous fluid-filled pockets of hemorrhage that develop at sites of previous trauma. Typical cytologic findings will vary depending on the chronicity of the lesion. Aspiration of actively bleeding, peracute lesions typically reveals only peripheral blood including erythrocytes, blood-associated leukocytes, and platelets, and thus, differentiation from a traumatic aspirate containing iatrogenic hemorrhage may not be possible. With increasing chronicity of the hematoma, platelets will disappear, erythrocyte numbers will decrease, and the number of erythrophagocytic macrophages and macrophages containing heme breakdown product (hemosiderin and/or hematoidin) will increase. It must be noted that hematomas and vascular neoplasms such as hemangiomas or hemangiosarcomas appear cytologically similar, and interpretation relies on knowledge of the chronicity of the lesion and any history of trauma to the area.[16,18]

Calcinosis Circumscripta

Calcinosis circumscripta (also known as tumoral calcinosis or calcium gout) lesions are caused by abnormal calcium deposition in soft tissue.[155] The etiology of calcinosis circumscripta has yet to be completely elucidated, but four major types of calcification are thought to occur: (i) dystrophic calcification, characterized by normal serum calcium and phosphorous with site-specific tissue trauma as the cause; (ii) idiopathic calcification; (iii) metastatic calcification, secondary to diseases causing hypercalcemia and/or hyperphosphatemia such as chronic renal disease; and (iv) iatrogenic calcification, related to treatment or surgery (such as fracture repair). Iatrogenic causes can also be classified as dystrophic.[156,157] Large-breed dogs are more commonly affected, and German shepherds are overrepresented, as well as Labrador retrievers and rottweilers.[157,158] There is no sex predilection,[158] and younger dogs (<2 year of age) are more commonly affected.[157,158] Deposits are most often individual and occur on the lateral metatarsus, pelvic phalanges, and elbow.[158] Bilateral and symmetric lesions have been reported.[158] Ear lesions occur in Boxers, especially at sites of ear cropping.[157] Foot lesions have been reported in association with renal disease.[157] In horses, calcium deposits are often periarticular (particularly on the lateral stifle), and incidence may be high in standardbreds.[159,160] A literature review of 18 equine cases revealed the majority of horses were aged 1.5–4 years.[159] There has been some discussion in the literature regarding the interchangeability of the terms tumoral calcinosis and calcinosis circumscripta in horses as tumoral calcinosis may be secondary to metabolic dysfunction while calcinosis circumscripta occurs secondary to dystrophic calcification; however, this remains to be resolved.[160,161] Soft tissue mineralization observed with imaging such as radiographs can aid in diagnosis.[162] Recurrence at sites of surgical removal is not reported.[158]

Grossly, lesions range from cystic and flocculent to firm subcutaneous masses that are generally non-painful. Alopecia has been reported in association with calcinosis circumscripta.[156] Lesions may be ulcerated or discharge a thick, white, and chalky material.[155,158]

Cytologically, calcinosis circumscripta is characterized by white and chalky material when unstained

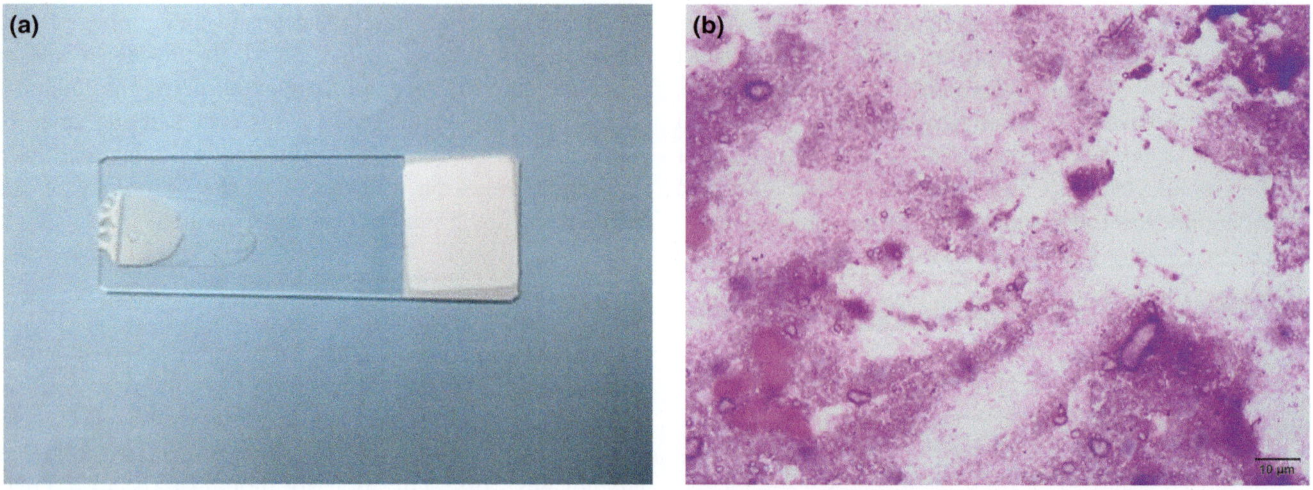

Figure 12.12 (a) Aspirate from a calcinosis circumscripta lesion. Note the chalky appearance of the unstained material on the microscope slide. (b) FNA of cutaneous calcinosis circumscripta from a dog. Characteristic finely granular to amorphous eosinophilic to purple crystalline material occupies the background with scattered larger, clearer crystalline mineral fragments just above the plane of focus. Few erythrocytes are noted in the lower left of the image (Wright–Giemsa, 1000×).

(Figure 12.12a), and amorphous, granular, and nonstaining to basophilic and sometimes refractile material along with granulomatous inflammation (macrophages and giant cells) on stained slides (Figure 12.12b).[163–165] Von Kossa stain and alizarin red S can be used on both cytology and histology samples for the detection of calcium. Alcian blue and periodic acid-Schiff also strongly stain the amorphous mineral material on histology.[163]

References

1 Vail, D.M. and Withrow, S.J. (eds.) (2007). Tumors of the skin and subcutaneous tissues. In: *Withrow & MacEwen's Small Animal Clinical Oncology*, 4e, 375–401. St. Louis, MO: Saunders Elsevier.

2 Eich, C.S., Whitehair, J.G., Moroff, S.D., and Heeb, L.A. (2000). The accuracy of intraoperative cytopathological diagnosis compared with conventional histopathological diagnosis. *J Am Anim Hosp Assoc* 36: 16–18.

3 Ghisleni, G., Roccabianca, P., Ceruti, R. et al. (2006). Correlation between fine-needle aspiration cytology and histopathology in the evaluation of cutaneous and subcutaneous masses from dogs and cats. *Vet Clin Pathol* 35: 24–30.

4 Cohen, M., Bohling, M.W., Wright, J.C. et al. (2003). Evaluation of sensitivity and specificity of cytologic examination: 269 cases (1999–2000). *J Am Vet Med Assoc* 222: 964–967.

5 Yumusak, N. and Kutsal, O. (2016). A comparative study between fine needle aspiration biopsy (FNAB) findings and histopathology in the evaluation of canine skin and skin adnexal tumors. *Ankara Üniv Vet Fak Derg* 63: 393–400.

6 MacNeill, A.L. (2011). Cytology of canine and feline cutaneous and subcutaneous lesions and lymph nodes. *Top Companion Anim Med* 26: 62–76.

7 Sharkey, L.C., Dial, S.M., and Matz, M.E. (2007). Maximizing the diagnostic value of cytology in small animal practice. *Vet Clin North Am Small Anim Pract* 37: 351–372, vii.

8 Goldschmidt, M.H., Dunstan, R.W., Stannard, A.A. et al. (1998). *Histological Classification of Epithelial and Melanocytic Tumors of the Skin of Domestic Animals*. Washington, DC: Armed Forces Institute of Pathology.

9 Masserdotti, C. and Ubbiali, F.A. (2002). Fine needle aspiration cytology of pilomatricoma in three dogs. *Vet Clin Pathol* 31: 22–25.

10 Bostock, D.E. (1986). Neoplasms of the skin and subcutaneous tissues in dogs and cats. *Br Vet J* 142: 1–19.

11 Miller, M.A., Nelson, S.L., Turk, J.R. et al. (1991). Cutaneous neoplasia in 340 cats. *Vet Pathol* 28: 389–395.

12 Schaffer, P.A., Wobeser, B., Martin, L.E. et al. (2013). Cutaneous neoplastic lesions of equids in the central United States and Canada: 3,351 biopsy specimens from 3,272 equids (2000–2010). *J Am Vet Med Assoc* 242: 99–104.

13 Villamil, J.A., Henry, C.J., Bryan, J.N. et al. (2011). Identification of the most common cutaneous neoplasms in dogs and evaluation of breed and age distributions for selected neoplasms. *J Am Vet Med Assoc* 239: 960–965.

14 Abramo, F., Pratesi, F., Cantile, C. et al. (1999). Survey of canine and feline follicular tumours and tumour-like lesions in central Italy. *J Small Anim Pract* 40: 479–481.

15 Gross, T.L., Ihrke, P.J., Walder, E.J., and Affolter, V.K. (2005). *Skin Diseases of the Dog and Cat: Clinical and Histopathologic Diagnosis*, 2e. Ames, IA: Blackwell Publishing.

16 Tyler, R.D., Cowell, R.L., and Meinkoth, J.H. (2008). Cutaneous and subcutaneous lesions. In: *Diagnostic Cytology and Hematology of the Dog and Cat*, 3e (eds. R.L. Cowell, R.D. Tyler, J.H. Meinkoth and D.B. DeNicola), 78–111. St. Louis, MO: Mosby Elsevier.

17 Masserdotti, C. (2006). Architectural patterns in cytology: correlation with histology. *Vet Clin Pathol* 35: 388–396.

18 Raskin, R.E. and Meyer, D.J. (2010). *Canine and Feline Cytology a Color Atlas and Interpretation Guide*. St. Louis, MO: Saunders Elsevier.

19 Alleman, A.R. and Bain, P.J. (2000). Diagnosing neoplasia: the cytologic criteria of malignancy. *Vet Med* 95: 204–223.

20 De Vico, G., Sfacteria, A., Maiolino, P., and Mazzullo, G. (2002). Comparison of nuclear morphometric parameters in cytologic smears and histologic sections of spontaneous canine tumors. *Vet Clin Pathol* 31: 16–18.

21 Kidney, B.A. and Meachem, M.D. (2014). Morphometric studies in veterinary cytology. *Vet Clin Pathol* 43: 305–309.

22 Moriello, K.A. and Rosenthal, R.C. (1990). Clinical approach to tumors of the skin and subcutaneous tissues. *Vet Clin North Am Small Anim Pract* 20: 1163–1190.

23 Bohn, A.A., Wills, T., and Caplazi, P. (2006). Basal cell tumor or cutaneous basilar epithelial neoplasm? Rethinking the cytologic diagnosis of basal cell tumors. *Vet Clin Pathol* 35: 449–453.

24 Johnson, M.C. and Myers, A.N. (2017). Cytology of skin neoplasms. *Vet Clin North Am Small Anim Pract* 47: 85–110.

25 Shelly, S.M. (2003). Cutaneous lesions. *Vet Clin North Am Small Anim Pract* 33: 1–46.

26 Stockhaus, C., Teske, E., Rudolph, R., and Werner, H.G. (2001). Assessment of cytological criteria for diagnosing basal cell tumours in the dog and cat. *J Small Anim Pract* 42: 582–586.

27 Emanuelli, M.P. and Bohn, A.A. (2014). What is your diagnosis? Dermal mass in a dog. *Vet Clin Pathol* 43: 285–286.

28 Adedeji, A.O., Affolter, V.K., and Christopher, M.M. (2017). Cytologic features of cutaneous follicular tumors and cysts in dogs. *Vet Clin Pathol* 46: 143–150.

29 Asakawa, M.G., Lewis, S.M., Buckles, E.L., and Stokol, T. (2015). What is your diagnosis? Cutaneous mass in a dog. *Vet Clin Pathol* 44: 607–608.

30 Diters, R.W. and Walsh, K.M. (1984). Feline basal cell tumors: a review of 124 cases. *Vet Pathol* 21: 51–56.

31 Jackson, K., Boger, L., Goldschmidt, M., and Walton, R.M. (2010). Malignant pilomatricoma in a soft-coated Wheaten Terrier. *Vet Clin Pathol* 39: 236–240.

32 Duclos, D.D., Hargis, A.M., and Hanley, P.W. (2008). Pathogenesis of canine interdigital palmar and plantar comedones and follicular cysts, and their response to laser surgery. *Vet Dermatol* 19: 134–141.

33 Ginel, P.J., Zafra, R., Lucena, R., and Bautista, M.J. (2007). Multiple generalized follicular cysts in a stallion. *Vet Dermatol* 18: 456–459.

34 Park, J.K., Hong, I.H., Ki, M.R. et al. (2010). Multiple perianal infundibular follicular cysts in a dog. *Vet Dermatol* 21: 303–306.

35 Goldschmidt, M., Pena, L., Rasotto, R., and Zappulli, V. (2011). Classification and grading of canine mammary tumors. *Vet Pathol* 48: 117–131.

36 Stewart, J. and Monti, P. (2015). What is your diagnosis? Perianal mass in a dog. *Vet Clin Pathol* 44: 615–616.

37 Munday, J.S. and Kiupel, M. (2010). Papillomavirus-associated cutaneous neoplasia in mammals. *Vet Pathol* 47: 254–264.

38 Nagata, M. and Rosenkrantz, W. (2013). Cutaneous viral dermatoses in dogs and cats. *Compend Contin Educ Vet* 35: E1.

39 Sprague, W. and Thrall, M.A. (2001). Recurrent skin mass from the digit of a dog. *Vet Clin Pathol* 30: 189–192.

40 Tyler, R.D., Meinkoth, J.H., Cowell, R.L. et al. (2002). Cutaneous and subcutaneous lesions, masses, cysts, and fistulous tracts. In: *Diagnostic Cytology and Hematology of the Horse*, 2e (eds. R.L. Cowell and R.D. Tyler), 19–42. St. Louis, MO: Mosby.

41 Munday, J.S., Gibson, I., and French, A.F. (2011). Papillomaviral DNA and increased p16CDKN2A protein are frequently present within feline cutaneous squamous cell carcinomas in ultraviolet-protected skin. *Vet Dermatol* 22: 360–366.

42 Munday, J.S., Kiupel, M., French, A.F., and Howe, L. (2008). Amplification of papillomaviral DNA sequences from a high proportion of feline cutaneous in situ and invasive squamous cell carcinomas using a nested polymerase chain reaction. *Vet Dermatol* 19: 259–263.

43 Boon, G.D., Rebar, A.H., and DeNicola, D.B.A. (1982). Cytologic comparison of Romanowsky stains and Papanicolaou-type stains I. Introduction, methodology and cytology of normal tissues. *Vet Clin Pathol* 11: 22–30.

44 Rebar, A.H., Boon, G.D., and DeNicola, D.B. (1982). A cytologic comparison of Romanowsky stains and Papanicolaou-type stains II. Cytology of inflammatory and neoplastic lesions. *Vet Clin Pathol* 11: 16–25.

45 Grandi, F., Monteiro, L.N., Fernandes, T.R. et al. (2011). What is your diagnosis? Cutaneous mass in the mammary region of a dog. Acantholytic squamous cell carcinoma (ASCC). *Vet Clin Pathol* 40: 101–102.

46 Dickinson, R.M. and Young, K.M. (2005). Cutaneous mass aspirate from a Golden Retriever: "glandular guile". *Vet Clin Pathol* 34: 421–424.

47 Bongiovanni, L., Suter, M.M., Malatesta, D. et al. (2012). Nuclear survivin expression as a potentially useful tool for the diagnosis of canine cutaneous sebaceous lesions. *Vet Dermatol* 23: 394-e73.

48 Ginel, P.J., Lucena, R., Millan, Y. et al. (2010). Expression of oestrogen and progesterone receptors in canine sebaceous gland tumours. *Vet Dermatol* 21: 297–302.

49 Piviani, M., Sanchez, M.D., and Patel, R.T. (2012). Cytologic features of clear cell adnexal carcinoma in 3 dogs. *Vet Clin Pathol* 41: 405–411.

50 Bevier, D.F. and Goldschmidt, M.H. (1981). Skin tumors in the dog. Part I: epithelial tumors and tumor-like lesions. *Compend Contin Educ Dent* 3: 389–398.

51 Cihocki, L.M., Divers, T.J., Johnson, A.L. et al. (2007). A case of multiple epitrichial sweat gland ductal carcinomas in a horse. *Vet Dermatol* 18: 134–137.

52 Heimann, M.H. and Ngendahayo, P. (2007). Sweat gland hamartoma resembling human syringocystadenoma papilliferum in two young cats. *Vet Dermatol* 18: 451–455.

53 Kusters, A.H., Peperkamp, K.H., and Hazewinkel, H.A. (1999). Atrichial sweat gland adenocarcinoma in the dog. *Vet Dermatol* 10: 51–54.

54 Simko, E., Wilcock, B.P., and Yager, J.A. (2003). A retrospective study of 44 canine apocrine sweat gland adenocarcinomas. *Can Vet J* 44: 38–42.

55 Whitley, D.B. and Mansell, J.E. (2012). Multiple eccrine poromas in the paw of a dog. *Vet Dermatol* 23: 167–170, e134.

56 Scott, D.W. and Miller, W.H. (2003). *Equine Dermatology*. St. Louis, MO: W.B. Saunders.

57 Petterino, C. and Woodger, N. (2014). What is your diagnosis? Perianal gland mass in a cat. Anal sac gland carcinoma. *Vet Clin Pathol* 43: 611–612.

58 Chun, R., Jakovljevic, S., Morrison, W.B. et al. (1997). Apocrine gland adenocarcinoma and pheochromocytoma in a cat. *J Am Anim Hosp Assoc* 33: 33–36.

59 Parry, N.M. (2006). Anal sac gland carcinoma in a cat. *Vet Pathol* 43: 1008–1009.

60 Shoieb, A.M. and Hanshaw, D.M. (2009). Anal sac gland carcinoma in 64 cats in the United Kingdom (1995–2007). *Vet Pathol* 46: 677–683.

61 Bennett, P.F., DeNicola, D.B., Bonney, P. et al. (2002). Canine anal sac adenocarcinomas: clinical presentation and response to therapy. *J Vet Intern Med* 16: 100–104.

62 Turek, M.M., Forrest, L.J., Adams, W.M. et al. (2003). Postoperative radiotherapy and mitoxantrone for anal sac adenocarcinoma in the dog: 15 cases (1991–2001). *Vet Comp Oncol* 1: 94–104.

63 Williams, L.E., Gliatto, J.M., Dodge, R.K. et al. (2003). Carcinoma of the apocrine glands of the anal sac in dogs: 113 cases (1985–1995). *J Am Vet Med Assoc* 223: 825–831.

64 Sakai, H., Murakami, M., Mishima, H. et al. (2012). Cytologically atypical anal sac adenocarcinoma in a dog. *Vet Clin Pathol* 41: 291–294.

65 Petterino, C., Guazzi, P., Ferro, S., and Castagnaro, M. (2005). Bronchogenic adenocarcinoma in a cat: an unusual case of metastasis to the skin. *Vet Clin Pathol* 34: 401–404.

66 Hubert, B. and Magnol, J.P. (2002). Four examples of metastatic canine cutaneous nodules. *Vet Dermatol* 13: 211–229.

67 Hargis, A.M., Baldessari, A.E., and Walder, E.J. (2008). Intraepidermal adenocarcinoma in the perianal skin of two cats, a condition resembling human extramammary Paget's disease. *Vet Dermatol* 19: 31–37.

68 Ackermann, M.R. (2012). Inflammation and healing. In: *Pathologic Basis of Veterinary Disease*, 5e (eds. J.F. Zachary and M.D. McGavin), 89–146. St. Louis, MO: Elsevier Mosby.

69 Mauldin, E.A. and Peters-Kennedy, J. (2016). Integumentary system. In: *Jubb, Kennedy, & Palmer's Pathology of Domestic Animals*, 6e (ed. M.G. Maxie), 509–605. St. Louis, MO: Elsevier.

70 Kumar, V., Abbas, A.K., and Aster, J.C. (2015). Inflammation and repair. In: *Robbins and Cotran Pathologic Basis of Disease*, 9e (eds. V. Kumar, A.K. Abbas and J.C. Aster), 69–111. Philadelphia, PA: Saunders Elsevier.

71 Zanatta, M., Bettini, G., Scarpa, F. et al. (2013). Nodular dermatofibrosis in a dog without a renal tumour or a mutation in the folliculin gene. *J Comp Pathol* 148: 248–251.

72 Dobson, J.M., Samuel, S., Milstein, H. et al. (2002). Canine neoplasia in the UK: estimates of incidence rates from a population of insured dogs. *J Small Anim Pract* 43: 240–246.

73 Goldschmidt, M.H. and Hendrick, M.J. (2002). Tumors of the skin and soft tissues. In: *Tumors in Domestic Animals*, 4e (ed. D.J. Meuten). Ames, IA: Iowa State Press.

74 Knottenbelt, D.C., Patterson-Kane, J.C., and Snalune, K.L. (eds.) (2015). Tumors of the skin. In: *Clinical Equine Oncology*, 567–568. New York, NY: Elsevier.

75 Lamagna, B., Greco, A., Guardascione, A. et al. (2012). Canine lipomas treated with steroid injections: clinical findings. *PLoS One* 7: e50234.

76 Bergman, P.J., Withrow, S.J., Straw, R.C., and Powers, B.E. (1994). Infiltrative lipoma in dogs: 16 cases (1981–1992). *J Am Vet Med Assoc* 205: 322–324.

77 Agut, A., Anson, A., Navarro, A. et al. (2013). Imaging diagnosis-infiltrative lipoma causing spinal cord and lumbar nerve root compression in a dog. *Vet Radiol Ultrasound* 54: 381–383.

78 McEntee, M.C. and Thrall, D.E. (2001). Computed tomographic imaging of infiltrative lipoma in 22 dogs. *Vet Radiol Ultrasound* 42: 221–225.

79 O'Kell, A.L., Inteeworn, N., Diaz, S.F. et al. (2010). Canine sterile nodular panniculitis: a retrospective study of 14 cases. *J Vet Intern Med* 24: 278–284.

80 Lanevschi, A., Lapointe, J.M., Belanger, J.F., and Noël, D. (1999). Fine needle aspirate of a subcutaneous mass on the forelimb of a dog. *Vet Clin Pathol* 28: 46.

81 Piseddu, E., De Lorenzi, D., Freeman, K., and Masserdotti, C. (2011). Cytologic, histologic, and immunohistochemical features of lingual liposarcoma in a dog. *Vet Clin Pathol* 40: 393–397.

82 Affolter, V.K. and Moore, P.F. (2006). Feline progressive histiocytosis. *Vet Pathol* 43: 646–655.

83 Moore, P.F. (2014). A review of histiocytic diseases of dogs and cats. *Vet Pathol* 51: 167–184.

84 Pinto da Cunha, N., Ghisleni, G., Scarampella, F. et al. (2014). Cytologic and immunocytochemical characterization of feline progressive histiocytosis. *Vet Clin Pathol* 43: 428–436.

85 Balme, E., Thuilliez, C., Lejeune, T. et al. (2009). Multiple atypical mucosal xanthomas in a dog similar to human verruciform xanthoma. *J Vet Diagn Invest* 21: 124–128.

86 Grieshaber, T.L., McKeever, P.J., and Conroy, J.D. (1991). Spontaneous cutaneous (Eruptive) xanthomatosis in two cats. *J Am Anim Hosp Assoc* 27: 509–512.

87 Miller, W.H. and Scott, D.W. (eds.) (2011). Endocrine, nutritional, and miscellaneous hair coat disorders. In: *Equine Dermatology*, 2e, 364. St. Louis, MO: Saunders Elsevier.

88 Ravens, P.A., Vogelnest, L.J., and Piripi, S.A. (2013). Unique presentation of normolipaemic cutaneous xanthoma in a cat. *Aust Vet J* 91: 460–463.

89 Jones, B.R., Wallace, A., Hancock, W. et al. (1985). Cutaneous xanthomata associated with diabetes mellitus in a cat. *J Small Anim Pract* 26: 33–41.

90 Jones, B.R., Wallace, A., Harding, D.R. et al. (1983). Occurrence of idiopathic, familial hyperchylomicronaemia in a cat. *Vet Rec* 112: 543–547.

91 Kwochka, K.W. and Short, B.G. (1984). Cutaneous xanthomatosis and diabetes mellitus following long-term therapy with megestrol acetate in a cat. *Compend Contin Educ Vet* 6: 185–192.

92 Wisselink, M.A., Koeman, J.P., Wensing, T. et al. (1994). Hyperlipoproteinaemia associated with atherosclerosis and cutaneous xanthomatosis in a cat. *Vet Q* 16: 199–202.

93 Vogelnest, L.J. (2001). Cutaneous xanthomas with concurrent demodicosis and dermatophytosis in a cat. *Aust Vet J* 79: 470–475.

94 Chastain, C.B. and Graham, C.L. (1978). Xanthomatosis secondary to diabetes mellitus in a dog. *J Am Vet Med Assoc* 172: 1209–1211.

95 Vitale, C.B., Ihrke, P.J., and Gross, T.L. (1998). Diet-induced alterations in lipid metabolism and associated cutaneous xanthoma formation in 5 cats. In: *Advances in Veterinary Dermatology* (eds. K.W. Kwochka, T. Willemse and C. von Tscharner), 243–249. Oxford: Butterworth-Heinemann.

96 Gumbrell, R.C. (1972). A case of multiple xanthomatosis and diabetes mellitus in a dog. *N Z Vet J* 20: 240–242.

97 Banajee, K.H., Orandle, M.S., Ratterree, W. et al. (2011). Idiopathic solitary cutaneous xanthoma in a dog. *Vet Clin Pathol* 40: 95–98.

98 Moore, P.F., Schrenzel, M.D., Affolter, V.K. et al. (1996). Canine cutaneous histiocytoma is an epidermotropic Langerhans cell histiocytosis that expresses CD1 and specific beta 2-integrin molecules. *Am J Pathol* 148: 1699–1708.

99 Taylor, D.O., Dorn, C.R., and Luis, O.H. (1969). Morphologic and biologic characteristics of the canine cutaneous histiocytoma. *Cancer Res* 29: 83–92.

100 Bender, W.M. and Muller, G.H. (1989). Multiple, resolving, cutaneous histiocytoma in a dog. *J Am Vet Med Assoc* 194: 535–537.

101 Duncan, J.R. and Prasse, K.W. (1979). Cytology of canine cutaneous round cell tumors. Mast cell tumor, histiocytoma, lymphosarcoma and transmissible venereal tumor. *Vet Pathol* 16: 673–679.

102 Moore, P.F., Affolter, V.K., Graham, P.S., and Hirt, B. (2009). Canine epitheliotropic cutaneous T-cell lymphoma: an investigation of T-cell receptor immunophenotype, lesion topography and molecular clonality. *Vet Dermatol* 20: 569–576.

103 Day, M.J., Lopatkin, I., Lucke, V.M., and Whitbread, T.J. (2000). Multiple cutaneous histiocytomas in a cat. *Vet Dermatol* 11: 305–310.

104 Sutton, R.H. and McLennan, M.W. (1987). Cutaneous histiocytoma in a heifer. *J Comp Pathol* 97: 463–468.

105 Sharkey, L.C. and Wellman, M.L. (2011). Diagnostic cytology in veterinary medicine: a comparative and evidence-based approach. *Clin Lab Med* 31: 1–19.

106 Albanese, F., Poli, A., Millanta, F., and Abramo, F. (2002). Primary cutaneous extragenital canine transmissible venereal tumour with *Leishmania*-laden

neoplastic cells: a further suggestion of histiocytic origin? *Vet Dermatol* 13: 243–246.

107 Ganguly, B., Das, U., and Das, A.K. (2016). Canine transmissible venereal tumour: a review. *Vet Comp Oncol* 14: 1–12.

108 Kegler, K., Habierski, A., Hahn, K. et al. (2013). Vaginal canine transmissible venereal tumour associated with intra-tumoural *Leishmania* spp. amastigotes in an asymptomatic female dog. *J Comp Pathol* 149: 156–161.

109 Marchal, T., Chabanne, L., Kaplanski, C. et al. (1997). Immunophenotype of the canine transmissible venereal tumour. *Vet Immunol Immunopathol* 57: 1–11.

110 Mozos, E., Mendez, A., Gomez-Villamandos, J.C. et al. (1996). Immunohistochemical characterization of canine transmissible venereal tumor. *Vet Pathol* 33: 257–263.

111 Ostrander, E.A., Davis, B.W., and Ostrander, G.K. (2016). Transmissible tumors: breaking the cancer paradigm. *Trends Genet* 32: 1–15.

112 Sandusky, G.E., Carlton, W.W., and Wightman, K.A. (1987). Diagnostic immunohistochemistry of canine round cell tumors. *Vet Pathol* 24: 495–499.

113 Murray, M., James, Z.H., and Martin, W.B. (1969). A study of the cytology and karyotype of the canine transmissible venereal tumour. *Res Vet Sci* 10: 565–568.

114 Prier, J.E. (1966). Chromosome pattern of canine transmissible sarcoma cells in culture. *Nature* 212: 724–726.

115 Rogers, K.S., Walker, M.A., and Dillon, H.B. (1998). Transmissible venereal tumor: a retrospective study of 29 cases. *J Am Anim Hosp Assoc* 34: 463–470.

116 Gurel, A., Kuscu, B., Gulanber, E.G., and Arun, S.S. (2002). Transmissible venereal tumors detected in the extra-genital organs of dogs. *Isr J Vet Med* 57: 1–8.

117 Komnenou, A.T., Thomas, A.L., Kyriazis, A.P. et al. (2015). Ocular manifestations of canine transmissible venereal tumour: a retrospective study of 25 cases in Greece. *Vet Rec* 176: 523.

118 Milo, J. and Snead, E. (2014). A case of ocular canine transmissible venereal tumor. *Can Vet J* 55: 1245–1249.

119 Bastan, A., Baki Acar, D., and Cengiz, M. (2008). Uterine and ovarian metastasis of transmissible venereal tumor in a bitch. *Turk J Vet Anim Sci* 32: 65–66.

120 Caniatti, M., da Cunha, N.P., Avallone, G. et al. (2012). Diagnostic accuracy of brush cytology in canine chronic intranasal disease. *Vet Clin Pathol* 41: 133–140.

121 Chikweto, A., Kumthekar, S., Larkin, H. et al. (2013). Genital and extragenital canine transmissible venereal tumor in dogs in Grenada, West Indies. *Open J Vet Med* 3: 111–114.

122 Das, U. and Das, A.K. (2000). Review of canine transmissible venereal sarcoma. *Vet Res Commun* 24: 545–556.

123 Higgins, D.A. (1966). Observations on the canine transmissible venereal tumor as seen in the Bahamas. *Vet Rec* 79: 67–71.

124 Cohen, D. (1985). The canine transmissible venereal tumor: a unique result of tumor progression. *Adv Cancer Res* 43: 75–112.

125 Park, M.S., Kim, Y., Kang, M.S. et al. (2006). Disseminated transmissible venereal tumor in a dog. *J Vet Diagn Invest* 18: 130–133.

126 Murgia, C., Pritchard, J.K., Kim, S.Y. et al. (2006). Clonal origin and evolution of a transmissible cancer. *Cell* 126: 477–487.

127 Gonzalez, C.M., Griffey, S.M., Naydan, D.K. et al. (2000). Canine transmissible venereal tumour: a morphological and immunohistochemical study of 11 tumours in growth phase and during regression after chemotherapy. *J Comp Pathol* 122: 241–248.

128 Wood, J.P. (2013). Canine transmissible venereal tumor. In: *Withrow and MacEwen's Small Animal Clinical Oncology*, 5e (eds. S.J. Withrow, D.M. Vail and R.L. Page), 692–696. St. Louis, MO: Saunders Elsevier.

129 Catone, G., Marino, G., Poglayen, G. et al. (2003). Canine transmissible venereal tumour parasitized by *Leishmania infantum*. *Vet Res Commun* 27: 549–553.

130 Carreira, V.S., Ferrari, H.F., Langohr, I.M. et al. (2014). *Leishmania* sp. amastigotes identification in canine transmissible venereal tumor. *Case Rep Vet Med*; 4 pages. http://dx.doi.org/10.1155/2014/603852.

131 Liao, K.W., Lin, Z.Y., Pao, H.N. et al. (2003). Identification of canine transmissible venereal tumor cells using in situ polymerase chain reaction and the stable sequence of the long interspersed nuclear element. *J Vet Diagn Invest* 15: 399–406.

132 VonHoldt, B.M. and Ostrander, E.A. (2006). The singular history of a canine transmissible tumor. *Cell* 126: 445–447.

133 Moore, P.F. and Olivry, T. (1994). Cutaneous lymphomas in companion animals. *Clin Dermatol* 12: 499–505.

134 Fontaine, J., Bovens, C., Bettenay, S., and Mueller, R.S. (2009). Canine cutaneous epitheliotropic T-cell lymphoma: a review. *Vet Comp Oncol* 7: 1–14.

135 Moore, P.F., Olivry, T., and Naydan, D. (1994). Canine cutaneous epitheliotropic lymphoma (mycosis fungoides) is a proliferative disorder of $CD8^+$ T cells. *Am J Pathol* 144: 421–429.

136 Fontaine, J., Heimann, M., and Day, M.J. (2010). Canine cutaneous epitheliotropic T-cell lymphoma: a review of 30 cases. *Vet Dermatol* 21: 267–275.

137 Fontaine, J., Heimann, M., and Day, M.J. (2011). Cutaneous epitheliotropic T-cell lymphoma in the cat: a review of the literature and five new cases. *Vet Dermatol* 22: 454–461.

138 Day, M.J. (1995). Immunophenotypic characterization of cutaneous lymphoid neoplasia in the dog and cat. *J Comp Pathol* 112: 79–96.

139 Wilcock, B.P. and Yager, J.A. (1989). The behavior of epidermotropic lymphoma in twenty-five dogs. *Can Vet J* 30: 754–756.

140 Pariser, M.S. and Gram, D.W. (2014). Feline cutaneous lymphocytosis: case report and summary of the literature. *J Feline Med Surg* 16: 758–763.

141 Tobey, J.C., Houston, D.M., Breur, G.J. et al. (1994). Cutaneous T-cell lymphoma in a cat. *J Am Vet Med Assoc* 204: 606–609.

142 Choi, U.S., Jeong, S.M., Kang, M.S. et al. (2004). Cutaneous lymphoma in a juvenile dog. *Vet Clin Pathol* 33: 47–49.

143 Rutgen, B.C., Flickinger, I., Wolfesberger, B. et al. (2016). Cutaneous T-cell lymphoma: Sezary syndrome in a Boxer. *Vet Clin Pathol* 45: 172–178.

144 Gilbert, S., Affolter, V.K., Gross, T.L. et al. (2004). Clinical, morphological and immunohistochemical characterization of cutaneous lymphocytosis in 23 cats. *Vet Dermatol* 15: 3–12.

145 Shiomitsu, K., Bauer, R.W., Grasperge, B.J. et al. (2012). Cutaneous epitheliotropic lymphoma with dual CD3 and c-kit expression in a dog. *Vet Clin Pathol* 41: 594–598.

146 Santoro, D., Marsella, R., and Hernandez, J. (2007). Investigation on the association between atopic dermatitis and the development of mycosis fungoides in dogs: a retrospective case-control study. *Vet Dermatol* 18: 101–106.

147 Foster, A.P., Evans, E., Kerlin, R.L., and Vail, D.M. (1997). Cutaneous T-cell lymphoma with Sezary syndrome in a dog. *Vet Clin Pathol* 26: 188–192.

148 Thrall, M.A., Macy, D.W., Snyder, S.P., and Hall, R.L. (1984). Cutaneous lymphosarcoma and leukemia in a dog resembling Sezary syndrome in man. *Vet Pathol* 21: 182–186.

149 Roccabianca, P., Avallone, G., Rodriguez, A. et al. (2016). Cutaneous lymphoma at injection sites: pathological, immunophenotypical, and molecular characterization in 17 cats. *Vet Pathol* 53: 823–832.

150 Littlewood, J.D., Whitwell, K.E., and Day, M.J. (1995). Equine cutaneous lymphoma: a case report. *Vet Dermatol* 6: 105–111.

151 Miller, C.A., Durham, A.C., Schaffer, P.A. et al. (2015). Classification and clinical features in 88 cases of equine cutaneous lymphoma. *J Vet Diagn Invest* 27: 86–91.

152 Wilson, R.G., Sutton, R.H., Groenendyk, S., and Seawright, A.A. (1985). Alimentary lymphosarcoma in a horse with cutaneous manifestations. *Equine Vet J* 17: 148–150.

153 de Bruijn, C.M., Veenman, J.N., Rutten, V.P. et al. (2007). Clinical, histopathological and immunophenotypical findings in five horses with cutaneous malignant lymphoma. *Res Vet Sci* 83: 63–72.

154 Ginn, P.E., Mansell, J.E., and Rakich, P.M. (2007). Skin and appendages. In: *Pathology of Domestic Animals*, 5e (ed. M.G. Maxie), 605. St. Louis, MO: Saunders Elsevier.

155 Roudebush, P., Maslin, W.R., and Cooper, R.C. (1988). Canine tumoral calcinosis. *Compend Contin Educ Vet Pract* 10: 1162–1164.

156 O'Brien, C.R. and Wilkie, J.S. (2001). Calcinosis circumscripta following an injection of proligestone in a Burmese cat. *Aust Vet J* 79: 187–189.

157 Tafti, A.K., Hanna, P., and Bourque, A.C. (2005). Calcinosis circumscripta in the dog: a retrospective pathological study. *J Vet Med A Physiol Pathol Clin Med* 52: 13–17.

158 Scott, D.W. and Buerger, R.G. (1988). Idiopathic calcinosis circumscripta in the dog: a retrospective analysis of 130 cases. *J Am Vet Med Assoc* 24: 651–658.

159 Goulden, B.E. and O'Callaghan, M.W. (1980). Tumoral calcinosis in the horse. *N Z Vet J* 28: 217–219.

160 Toth, F., Schumacher, J., and Newman, S. (2009). Calcinosis circumscripta in the antebrachiocarpal joint of a horse. *Equine Vet Educ* 21: 584–588.

161 Stone, W.C., Wilson, D.G., Dubielzig, R.R. et al. (1990). The pathologic mineralization of soft tissue, calcinosis circumscripta in horses. *Compend Contin Educ Vet Pract* 12: 1643–1648.

162 Lewis, D.G. and Kelly, D.F. (1990). Calcinosis circumscripta in dogs as a cause of spinal ataxia. *J Small Anim Pract* 31: 36–38.

163 Bettini, G., Morini, M., Campagna, F., and Preziosi, R. (2005). True grit: the tale of a subcutaneous mass in a dog. *Vet Clin Pathol* 34: 73–75.

164 Marcos, R., Santos, M., Oliveira, J. et al. (2006). Cytochemical detection of calcium in a case of calcinosis circumscripta in a dog. *Vet Clin Pathol* 35: 239–242.

165 Sharkey, L.C., Gliatto, J.M., and Gallagher, J.G. (1999). Deep tissue mass aspirate from a young German shepherd dog. *Vet Clin Pathol* 28: 147–149.

13

Cutaneous Mast Cell Tumors

Maxey L. Wellman and Cheryl London

Introduction

Mast cells are generated from hematopoietic precursors in the bone marrow and migrate to various tissues, including multiple epithelial surfaces such as skin and the gastrointestinal tract.[1] Mast cell differentiation and proliferation is dependent on the growth factor, stem cell factor (SCF), that binds to the receptor tyrosine kinase KIT.[2–4] Mast cells are involved in wound healing, anti-parasite and innate immune responses, and attenuation of several insect and spider venoms, mediated in part by the contents of mast cell granules.[1] These granules contain multiple bioactive substances including heparin, histamine, tumor necrosis factor-α, and several proteases, although the composition of mast cell granules is variable, dependent on species and tissue distribution.[1,5,6] For example, in dogs, mast cells found in the skin contain chymase and tryptase, whereas mast cells in the gastrointestinal tract contain primarily chymase.[5,7] Neoplasia of mast cells occurs in multiple species, although it is most common in dogs and cats. Given the widespread distribution of normal mast cells, tumors can develop in a variety of tissues, although the skin is the most common location. The clinical findings, cytology, histologic type, biologic behavior, treatment, and prognosis of cutaneous mast cell tumors differ among species and thus will be discussed in separate species-specific sections.

Mast Cell Tumors in Dogs

Incidence

Mast cell tumors (MCTs) are considered the most common skin tumor in dogs, comprising about 20% of all cutaneous neoplasms.[6,8] The mean age of occurrence is 8–9 years, but there is a wide age distribution, and MCTs have been reported in dogs as young as 3 weeks of age.[9] There is no apparent gender predilection.[5,10,11] Numerous breeds are at increased risk: Boxers, Boston Terriers, English Bulldogs, Pugs, Labrador Retrievers, Golden Retrievers, Cocker Spaniels, Schnauzers, Staffordshire Terriers, Beagles, Rhodesian Ridgebacks, Weimaraners, and Shar-Peis. However, MCTs also occur commonly in several other breeds and in mixed breed dogs.[5,6,12,13] Although the reason for the high incidence of MCT in dogs is not currently known, recent data implicate specific gene loci involving hyaluronidase genes in Golden Retrievers.[14]

Clinical Findings

Cutaneous MCTs usually occur as single masses in the skin or subcutaneous tissue, although some dogs present with multiple MCTs.[11,15–17] Cutaneous MCTs are typically found on the trunk, on the limbs, and in the perineal region; the head and neck are less frequently involved.[6,18] The clinical appearance of these tumors is quite variable, and any cutaneous mass has the potential to be a MCT. Well-differentiated tumors can be small, slow-growing, non-encapsulated, non-ulcerated masses with minimal alopecia, whereas less differentiated tumors can be large, rapidly growing, ulcerated masses with inflammation and edema of adjacent tissue (Figure 13.1). Subcutaneous MCT may be large and soft and as such initially may be misdiagnosed as a lipoma.[5,6] Degranulation and release of histamine and heparin from manipulation during examination may result in tumor swelling and/or erythema and wheal formation of surrounding tissue (Darier's sign) (Figure 13.1b). Owners sometimes describe increasing and decreasing tumor size, likely from similar spontaneous or trauma-induced degranulation. Degranulation also can cause hemorrhage, vascular necrosis, edema, and collagenolysis. Localized hemorrhage during surgery has been reported in dogs with MCT undergoing resection, likely related to release of histamine, heparin, and other vasoactive granule contents.[5,16,19–23]

Veterinary Cytology, First Edition. Edited by Leslie C. Sharkey, M. Judith Radin, and Davis Seelig.

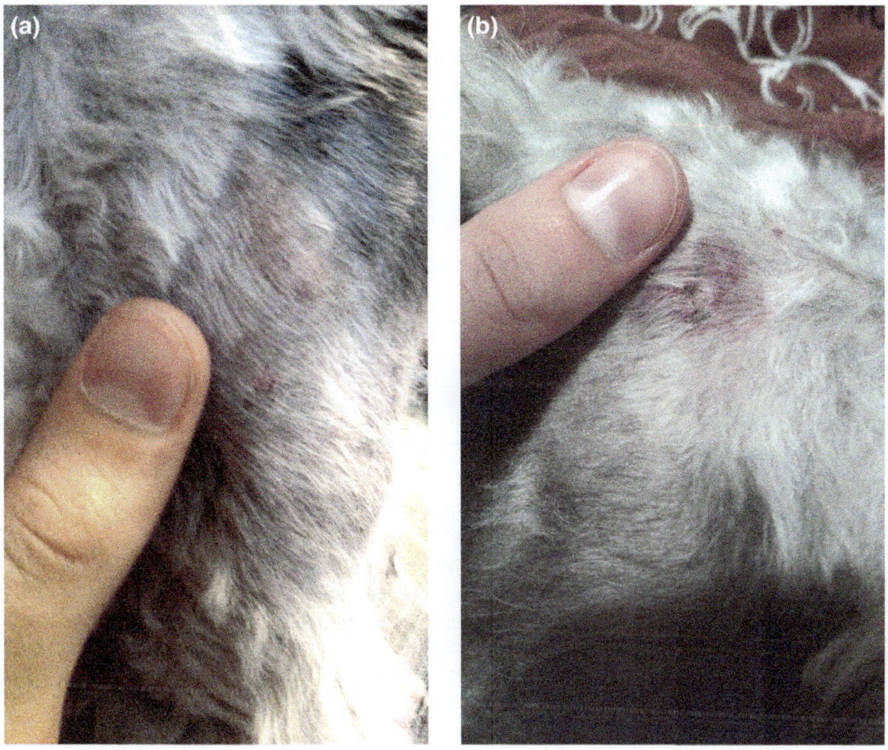

Figure 13.1 Mast cell tumor from a dog. (a) Before aspiration the mass appears raised and pink. (b) After aspiration, there is noticeable erythema around the mass (*Source:* Images courtesy of Camille McAloney).

Sample Collection

Cytology often is helpful in the diagnosis of cutaneous and subcutaneous MCT. Samples are collected using routine fine-needle aspiration (FNA), which provides an accurate diagnosis in most cases of cutaneous MCT in dogs.[24] Slides are stained routinely with Wright's stain, Wright–Giemsa stain or commercially available quick stains such as Diff-Quik®.[23] Incisional biopsy/needle biopsy of these tumors is typically not recommended due to their propensity for bleeding; therefore this should only be performed if FNA cannot provide a definitive diagnosis of a MCT, because knowing this information would be critical to develop a treatment plan.

Cytology

MCTs are classified as round cell tumors because of cell shape. Like most round cell tumors, MCTs typically exfoliate readily, and samples often are very cellular.[25,26] The cytologic diagnosis of MCT usually is straightforward and has been shown to have a 96–100% agreement with the histologic diagnosis of MCT.[27–29] Most are 10–35 μm, individual round cells with round, centrally located nuclei that have condensed chromatin and inconspicuous nucleoli. Nuclei may stain poorly, especially if the mast cells are heavily granulated.[23] The most characteristic feature is abundant basophilic cytoplasm containing numerous granules that typically stain purple (metachromatic) with Wright–Giemsa (Figure 13.2) and, in many cases,

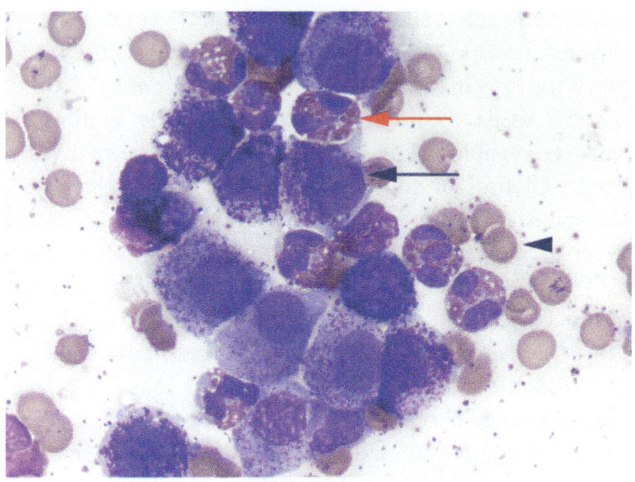

Figure 13.2 Mast cell tumor from a dog. There are numerous mast cells (black arrow), most of which are well granulated. There also are numerous eosinophils (red arrow). The blood in the background (black arrowhead indicates an RBC for size comparison) is typical of aspirates of mast cell tumors (Wright's stain, 1000×).

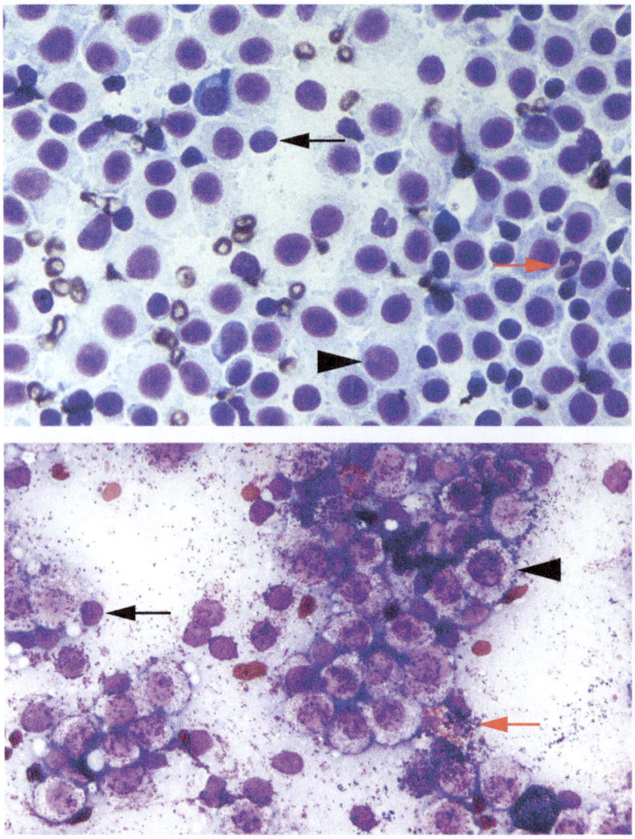

Figure 13.3 Mast cell tumor from a dog stained with Diff-Quik® (top panel) and Wright's stain (bottom panel). The mast cells (black arrowhead) are well granulated, but the granules are more difficult to see with Diff-Quik® than with Wright's stain. There are rare eosinophils (red arrows) and rare small lymphocytes (black arrow) (1000×).

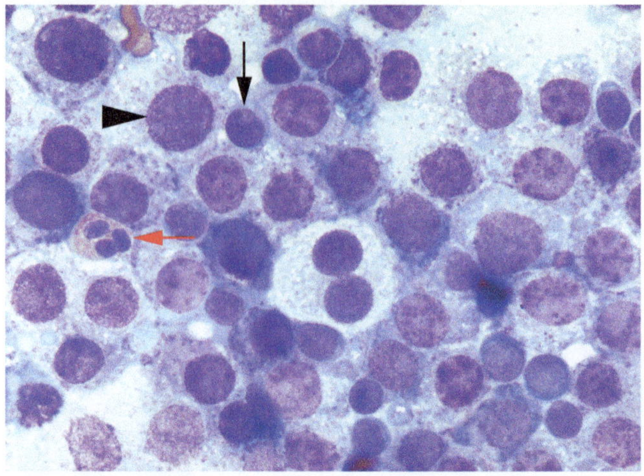

Figure 13.4 Mast cell tumor from a dog. There is moderate to marked variation in cell size, nuclear size, and nuclear to cytoplasmic ratio and moderate variation in granularity among the neoplastic mast cells. Nucleoli are sometimes visible (black arrowhead), and there is one binucleated mast cell in the center. There are several small lymphocytes (black arrow indicating one of these) and one eosinophil (red arrow) (Wright's stain, 1000×).

commercial quick stains like Diff-Quik®.[23] However, the granules in some MCT do not stain well with Diff-Quik®, even if the time in the fixative is increased (Figure 13.3).[26,30] In some cases, granules that stained poorly with Diff-Quik® are visible if slides are subsequently stained with Wright–Giemsa or toluidine blue.[1,5,23,31] Toluidine blue stains mast cell granules blue on cytology smears and may detect more mast cells than Wright–Giemsa stain, especially when scanning aspirates from the spleen or liver for metastasis.[31,32]

In poorly differentiated tumors, the mast cells may be more difficult to definitively identify as the cells often have fewer granules. There may be uneven distribution of granules in the cytoplasm, and the size of the granules may be more variable. There may be variation in nuclear contour, visible nucleoli, and binucleated and multinucleated cells. There may be moderate to marked variation in cell size, nuclear size, and nuclear to cytoplasmic ratio (N:C) (Figure 13.4).[33] Rarely, there is phagocytosis of RBCs or WBCs by neoplastic mast cells.[34,35] Mast cells typically have a "fried egg" appearance, but poorly differentiated mast cells may be challenging to differentiate from other anaplastic round cell tumors based on cytology and routine staining.

In dogs, MCT can be accompanied by variable numbers of eosinophils and large, spindle-shaped cells interpreted as reactive fibroblasts. These spindle cells are characterized by abundant basophilic cytoplasm and round to oval nuclei with fine chromatin and single or multiple nucleoli.[23] They can exhibit moderate variation in cell size, nuclear size, and nuclear to cytoplasmic ratio. There also may be minimal to abundant extracellular eosinophilic material consistent with collagen (Figure 13.5).[23]

Several classification schemes based on cytology have been described, most of which are based on the 2-tier (low-grade and high-grade MCTs) and 3-tier (grade I or low grade, grade II or intermediate grade, and grade III or high grade) histologic grading schemes described below.[23,36–39] Several recent studies have assessed the applicability of some of the criteria used in the histologic grading schemes to FNA of MCT, including granularity, anisokaryosis, binucleated and multinucleated cells, bizarre nuclei, and mitotic figures.[25,33,37] Although cytology had a high sensitivity (85–88%) and specificity (94–97%) in comparison with histologic grading in all of these studies, findings were inconsistent about which criteria are most closely associated with histologic grading. In addition, several high-grade MCTs based on histologic grading were incorrectly classified by cytology as low-grade tumors, and several low-grade MCTs based on histologic grading were

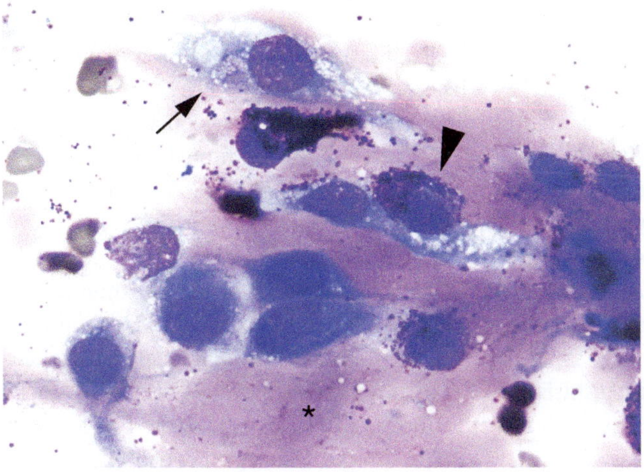

Figure 13.5 Mast cell tumor from a dog. There are several well-granulated mast cells (black arrowhead) and several spindle-shaped fibroblasts (black arrow). Note the variation in cell size and nuclear size and the prominent nucleoli in the fibroblasts. There is abundant eosinophilic extracellular material that is interpreted as collagen (*) (Wright's stain, 1000×).

incorrectly classified as high grade on cytology.[25,33,37] Given that misclassification can be extremely problematic for treatment and prognosis, MCT grade should always be based on histopathologic classification, in addition to other molecular and immunohistochemical markers known to provide prognostic value.

Histopathology

The biologic behavior of cutaneous MCTs in dogs varies from benign to markedly invasive and metastatic.[8,40–42] In general, histologic grading correlates with prognosis, and the 3-tier and 2-tier schemes are the most widely used with both typically reported by anatomic pathologists following surgical removal of the tumor.[21,43–47]

The Patnaik system classifies cutaneous mast cell tumors into three grades based on cellularity, cellular morphology, invasiveness, mitotic activity, and stromal reaction.[24,40,46] This 3-tier system evaluated survival time as a prognostic indicator, and subsequent studies have shown an inconsistent prognosis, especially for dogs with grade II and grade III tumors.[8,48–52] In addition, subsequent studies have shown only 62–74% agreement in assignment of histologic grade among pathologists using this system.[33,46,53,54] The more recently proposed 2-tier grading system assigns a low or high grade using primarily nuclear criteria (Table 13.1).[44] This 2-tier system more consistently predicted clinical behavior, and there is increased concordance among pathologists compared with the Patnaik system (77–97% agreement with the 2-tier system).[33,40,44,46,55,56] Most dogs (90%) with cutaneous MCT have low-grade tumors according to the 2-tier classification system, and the median survival time for these dogs is greater than two years compared with a median survival time of less than four months for dogs with high-grade tumors.[24,44]

Table 13.1 Comparison of the 3-tier and 2-tier histologic grading systems for cutaneous MCT in dogs.

Patnaik 3-tier grading system[46]			Kiupel 2-tier grading system[44]	
Grade I (low grade)	**Grade II (intermediate grade)**	**Grade III (high grade)**	**Low grade**	**High grade**
Least cellular		Most cellular		
Superficial dermis	Superficial and deep dermis, subcutis, adjacent muscle			
Minimal edema or necrosis	Edema and necrosis			
Round cells, round nuclei	Pleomorphic cells with indented nuclei, visible nucleoli	Irregularly shaped nuclei, multiple nucleoli, multinucleated cells	None of the criteria described for high-grade MCT	Any of these criteria: Karyomegaly in ≥10% of tumor cells
<2 mitoses/10 HPF	0–2 mitoses/HPF	3–6 mitoses/HPF		≥3 multinucleated cells/10 HPF 3 bizarre nuclei/10 HPF ≥7 mitoses/HPF
Unlikely to metastasize or recur following surgical excision	Variable behavior	Invasive, metastasize, recur following surgical excision	Median survival greater than two years	Median survival less than four months

HPF, high power field; MCT, mast cell tumor.

Several studies have compared these two grading systems, but no consensus has been reached about which one provides the most consistent grading and prognostic information.[40,45,55,56] This is important because neither predicts the behavior of all MCTs.[24,44,57]

Most MCTs originate in the dermis and extend into the subcutis.[40] However, some MCTs are restricted to subcutaneous tissue. These subcutaneous MCTs are considered as a subset of cutaneous MCTs by many pathologists.[40,58,59] Although there is no specific classification scheme for subcutaneous MCTs, most dogs with subcutaneous MCTs have long survival times with low rates of recurrence and metastasis, similar to low-grade MCTs, even in the face of incomplete excision.[58,59]

Cytochemistry and Immunohistochemistry

MCTs typically are positive for chloroacetate esterase, omega-exonuclease, vimentin, tryptase, chymase, monocyte chemoattractant protein (MCP-1), interleukin-8 (IL-8), and CD117 (KIT).[5,23,44,60–64] The interleukin-2 receptor subunit CD25 is expressed most strongly by cells in grade I MCT compared with decreased levels in grade III MCT. CD25 is not expressed on nonneoplastic resting cutaneous mast cells and is weakly expressed on only small numbers of presumably activated mast cells in dogs with allergic dermatitis. This is similar to the absence of CD25 expression on nonneoplastic mast cells and expression on neoplastic mast cells in people.[65]

Proliferation Markers

Increases in several cellular proliferation markers are associated with shorter survival times in dogs with cutaneous MCT. The number of mitotic figures, which indicate cells in the M phase of the cell cycle, can be assessed on routinely stained cytology smears or histologic sections. The presence of mitotic figures on cytology smears and high numbers of mitotic figures (≥5–7 mitoses/10 high power field [HPF]) on histologic sections have been associated with poor prognosis.[24,33,44,66,67] Ki67, determined by immunohistochemistry, is used to assess cells in all phases of the active cell cycle (growth fraction), and argyrophilic nucleolar organizer regions (AgNOR), measured by silver staining, is used to assess proliferation rate. Although each can be assessed separately, MCT with a Ki67 × AgNOR score ≥54 is associated with increased risk of metastasis and MCT-related mortality.[24,68] Proliferating cell nuclear antigen (PCNA), determined by immunohistochemistry, indicates cells in the S phase of the cell cycle, but probably is not as reliable as the proliferation markers described above.[5,44,47,58,59,66–73]

Molecular Abnormalities

Neoplastic mast cells from all dogs with cutaneous MCT express the KIT receptor tyrosine kinase. Although the pattern of staining for the KIT protein has been shown to have some prognostic implication, it may be more helpful for prognosis and treatment to determine whether there is a mutation in the *KIT* gene.[5,24,74] Neoplastic mast cells from 20 to 40% of dogs with cutaneous MCT have activating mutations in the *KIT* gene, in particular exon 11 of the juxtamembrane domain or exon 8 of the extracellular domain. Mutations in exon 11 are linked to increased risk of local recurrence, metastasis, and a worse prognosis, perhaps because of SCF-independent activation of KIT and unregulated KIT signal transduction.[74–78] The prognostic significance of exon 8 mutations is currently unknown, but as with exon 11 mutations, these induce ligand independent activation of KIT.[24,55,75,79] Polymerase chain reaction (PCR) tests are available for determining the presence of these mutations. This is important because MCTs with activating mutations in *KIT* are more likely to respond to therapy with tyrosine kinase inhibitors than MCT without these mutations.[24,78]

Prognostic Factors

Numerous prognostic factors have been described for cutaneous MCT in dogs, the most consistent of which is histologic grading. Other factors include age, breed, tumor location, duration and size of the tumor, and the presence of clinical signs associated with mast cell disease. Older dogs and male dogs may have a worse prognosis compared with younger dogs and female dogs, depending on treatment. Boxers, Pugs, and dogs of Bulldog descent tend to have low- or intermediate-grade tumors and thus a better prognosis.[5,71,79] Dogs with MCT confined to the skin have a better prognosis than if there is local lymph node involvement or metastasis to other tissues, although prognosis associated with lymph node involvement is controversial.[5,41,80,81] Cutaneous MCT occurring in the preputial or perineal region, in the scrotum or on digits, or in the perioral region or on the muzzle have been reported to have a worse prognosis.[82–84] However, recent data suggest that perineal tumors may not be as aggressive as previously described.[82,84] Additionally, although MCTs of the muzzle do have a high rate of metastasis to the local lymph nodes, survival times with aggressive therapy exceed one year. Subcutaneous MCTs often exhibit a more benign biologic behavior, with surgical excision typically curative.[23,58,82–84] MCTs that have been present for greater than six months have a better prognosis than more rapidly growing tumors, and large tumors and tumors that have recurred locally have a worse prognosis following surgical removal.[5,15] Ulceration, erythema, and pruritus of the tumor may be associated with a worse prognosis.[5,15,41] There is controversy about whether dogs with multiple MCTs have a worse prognosis than dogs with a single MCT.[5,15,41,42,45]

Additional prognostic factors include vascularity, nuclear morphology, ploidy, and proliferation indices. Increased microvessel density, irregular nuclear shape, and increased nuclear area, mean diameter, and perimeter are associated with a higher grade, invasiveness, and a worse prognosis.[38,39,85,86] Aneuploid tumors are associated with higher-grade tumors and shorter survival times, and increased indicators of cell proliferation are predictive of shorter postsurgical survival.[44,47,58,59,66,69–73,86,87] As mentioned above, specific mutations in the *KIT* gene are associated with a poor prognosis.[5,88,89]

Clinical Staging

Any MCT is capable of metastasis, so clinical staging is recommended. Clinical staging includes assessment of the primary tumor (size, number of tumors, location, etc.) and evaluation for local and systemic metastasis (Table 13.2).[5,24,90] Evaluation of metastasis can be challenging because sentinel lymph nodes may not be the closest lymph node to the tumor, and it is often difficult to distinguish neoplastic mast cells from nonneoplastic mast cells simply based on FNA cytology.[24,91,92] Small numbers of mast cells (1–16 mast cells/slide) occur in normal lymph nodes, and mast cells can be increased with inflammation.[5,93,94] Toluidine blue may facilitate recognition of mast cells in cytology smears and histologic sections.[32,95] Proposed recommendations for metastasis based on cytology and histology of lymph nodes are shown in Table 13.3.[94,95] The discrepancy between detection of metastasis using cytology or histology may be as high as 20%, with more cases of metastasis detected by histologic evaluation.[94] Importantly, a new grading system to assess local lymph nodes based on histopathologic evaluation following removal has been shown to be prognostic for outcome.[95]

As with lymph nodes, the cytologic diagnosis of metastasis to the spleen and liver can be challenging. Mast cells are present in splenic aspirates from normal dogs. Although the number of mast cells per aggregate of splenic cells and the number of isolated mast cells per slide are higher in dogs with cutaneous MCT, there is overlap between dogs with MCT and normal dogs, and a cutoff value for what is consistent with metastasis cannot be easily determined.[96] Small numbers of mast cells (<1 mast cell/100 hepatocytes) are normal in aspirates of hepatic tissue, and increased numbers of mast cells occur with nonneoplastic diseases like hepatic fibrosis and reactive hepatitis.[96–98] Importantly, the granules in splenic and hepatic mast cells may be difficult to see with routine staining.[32,96–98] Immersing the slides in 0.1% toluidine blue for 30 seconds at room temperature, rinsing in tap water, and air-drying the slides can

Table 13.2 Criteria for staging cutaneous MCT in dogs.[5,24,90]

Stage 1	Stage 2	Stage 3	Stage 4
Single tumors confined to the dermis with no evidence of metastasis	Multiple dermal masses or a large infiltrating mass with or without metastasis to regional lymph nodes	Single tumors confined to the dermis with involvement of regional lymph nodes	Metastasis to distant lymph nodes or other tissues

Table 13.3 Recommendations for determining metastasis of MCT to lymph nodes.

Criteria for fine-needle aspirates (Krick[94])		Criteria for histologic sections (Weishaar[95])	
		Non-metastatic (HN)	<3 scattered, individual mast cells/HPF in sinuses and/or parenchyma
Possible metastasis	2–3 aggregates of 2–3 mast cells	Pre-metastatic (HN1)	>3 individual mast cells in a minimum of 4 HPF in sinuses and/or parenchyma
Probable metastasis	>3 aggregates of 2–3 mast cells and/or 2–5 aggregates of >3 mast cells	Early metastasis (HN2)	Aggregates of >3 mast cells in sinuses and/or parenchyma
Certain metastasis	Large numbers of mast cells and/or aggregates of poorly differentiated mast cells and/or >5 aggregates of >3 mast cells	Overt metastasis (HN3)	Discrete foci, nodules, sheets, or masses of mast cells that disrupt or efface normal lymph node architecture

HN, histopathologic lymph node; HPF, high power field.

be done to more easily detect mast cells in and may be helpful in detecting metastasis. Mast cell granules stain brightly eosinophilic with toluidine blue.[32]

Although complete staging includes a complete blood count (CBC), serum biochemical profile, cytology of regional lymph nodes, abdominal ultrasound with cytology of the spleen and liver, and thoracic radiographs (if indicated), a less extensive work-up may be applicable to tumors amenable to wide surgical excision in dogs without negative prognostic indicators.[5] In these cases, a CBC, serum biochemical profile, and cytology of the regional lymph node (regardless of size) may be adequate. Buffy coat smears are no longer recommended, and bone marrow aspirates are typically not performed as increased numbers of mast cells in blood and bone marrow occur more often in dogs with diseases other than MCT.[99–101] Although bone marrow metastasis is associated with a worse prognosis, involvement of bone marrow in the absence of metastasis to lymph nodes, spleen, or liver is unlikely in dogs with cutaneous MCT.[5,100–103]

Treatment

Most dogs with low-grade and intermediate-grade cutaneous MCT have long-term survival after complete surgical excision of the tumor.[5,15,45,49,51,52] Recommendations for surgical margins vary, and tumor grade often is undetermined at the time of surgery. However, low-grade MCTs with low proliferation indices are unlikely to recur, and survival times may not differ even if the tumor is incompletely excised.[24,45,51,70,104] If histologic evaluation of a cutaneous MCT indicates that surgical margins are complete, the tumor is low or intermediate grade, and there are no negative prognostic indicators (i.e. recent rapid growth, tumor ulceration, lymph node metastasis, *KIT* mutation positive, etc.), then no further therapy may be indicated.[5] For those low-grade MCTs with no negative prognostic indicators that cannot be completely removed, adjuvant local radiation therapy is often quite effective at preventing disease recurrence. However, for those MCTs with negative prognostic indicators or for those that are high grade, treatment recommendations may include a combination of surgery, radiation therapy, chemotherapy, and/or tyrosine kinase inhibitors.[5,105,106]

Mast Cell Tumors in Cats

Incidence

MCTs are the second most common tumor of the skin in cats, comprising 20% of skin tumors, although incidence may vary worldwide.[5,107–109]

Clinical Findings

Cats with the more common mastocytic form of MCT typically present with a single, raised, firm, white or erythematous, hairless dermal nodule, 0.5–3 cm in diameter, with intermittent pruritus, erythema, and Darier's sign.[110] MCT can be ulcerated, or be a flat, pruritic plaque-like lesion, or a discrete subcutaneous nodule. Some cats present with multiple cutaneous MCTs. The mean age is 8–9 years, and there is no sex predilection.[108,109,111,112] The less common atypical or histiocytic form of MCT occurs in cats <4 years of age as multiple, nonpruritic, firm, hairless, pink subcutaneous nodules that may be ulcerated. Atypical or histiocytic MCT can spontaneously regress.[111–113] Siamese cats may be predisposed to both forms of cutaneous MCT.[113] Cutaneous MCTs in cats occur most commonly on the head and neck, especially on the pinnae or at the base of the ear. They also can occur on the trunk, limbs, and other various sites.[108,110,111]

Cytology

The cytologic diagnosis of cutaneous MCT in most cats is straightforward because the granules stain readily with Wright–Giemsa. Eosinophils, reactive fibroblasts, and collagen fibrils are less commonly present than in MCT in dogs. Erythrophagocytosis has been reported.[114] The cytologic diagnosis of histiocytic MCT can be challenging because the majority of the cells may be histiocytes, with only 20% mast cells and occasional aggregates of lymphocytes and eosinophils. These can be misinterpreted as an inflammatory reaction because of the mixed population of cells.[112,113]

Histopathology

There is no consensus regarding the histologic classification of cutaneous MCT in cats. They are typically described as mastocytic or histiocytic (atypical), and the mastocytic tumors can be compact (confined to the dermis and superficial subcutis) or diffuse (less discrete and can infiltrate the deeper subcutis).[108,115] However, most cutaneous MCTs in cats are compact aggregates of well-differentiated mast cells. Some MCTs in cats are described as pleomorphic, with marked cytomegaly, karyomegaly, and nuclear pleomorphism, and they can be compact or diffuse, although most are compact.[108,112,115,116] There currently is not a histologic grading system for MCT in cats as the majority of these tumors tend to exhibit a more benign course. Indeed, most studies indicate that pleomorphism is not associated with a more aggressive clinical behavior.[108,111,115,116] The only potential prognostic indicator is increased mitotic index, although this remains somewhat controversial.[117]

Immunohistochemistry

The neoplastic mast cells are positive for vimentin, α-1 antitrypsin, and KIT.[118]

Molecular Abnormalities

Similar to dogs, MCTs in cats are associated with activating mutations in *KIT*, although these are almost exclusively due to mutations in exons 8 and 9 of the gene. As with the canine mutations, these have been shown to induce ligand-independent KIT activation.[119–122]

Prognostic Factors

The histologic grading system used in dogs does not provide prognostic information in cats. However, well-differentiated, compact tumors tend to be benign, whereas multiple tumors (>5 tumors), a high mitotic index (>5/10 HPF), high KIT immunoreactivity, and a high Ki67 index have been correlated with a poorer prognosis.[111,117,123–125]

Clinical Staging

A CBC and serum biochemical profile are recommended, as are a careful evaluation for additional tumors, lymphadenopathy, and involvement of other tissues, in particular the spleen, liver, and gastrointestinal tract.

Treatment

Most cats with cutaneous MCTs are cured by surgical excision. Anaplastic tumors or those with a high mitotic index may be more likely to recur or metastasize, and adjuvant treatment following surgical excision may be warranted.[116,126,127] Radiation therapy, particularly in the form of strontium 90, can be particularly effective for those tumors on the head and neck that cannot be completely removed.[128] There is limited information on chemotherapy for cutaneous MCT in cats, although KIT inhibitors have demonstrated benefit in cats whose tumors are known to possess an activating *KIT* mutation.[119,120,127]

Mast Cell Tumors in Horses

Incidence

MCTs are uncommon skin tumors in horses, comprising 2–10% of skin tumors. They occur more commonly in males with no apparent breed predilection. The mean age is 7 years, but there is a wide distribution of age.[123]

Clinical Findings

MCTs in horses most commonly occur as focal masses, but multiple masses have been reported.[123,129] They occur most commonly on the head, neck, and legs. They typically are immovable, non-painful, non-puritic masses involving the dermis or subcutis. Subcutaneous edema and draining tracts have been described.[129] MCT in horses can be quite variable in size (0.5–20 cm), with variable alopecia, hyperpigmentation, and ulceration. Most are slowly progressive, but sudden rapid growth has been described. Dystrophic mineralization can be present, and granuloma formation and fibrosis can occur.[123,129,130] Rare malignant forms of MCT can be associated with eosinophilia, hyperfibrinogenemia, pruritus, metastasis to lymph nodes, and joint involvement.[131,132]

Cytology

The cytology of cutaneous MCT in most horses reveals primarily mast cells, but a predominance of eosinophils has been described.[129] In most cases, the mast cells appear well differentiated. However, in rare cases of mast cell neoplasia, the cells exhibit moderate to marked anisokaryosis, prominent nucleoli, increased or variable nuclear to cytoplasmic ratios, and a high mitotic index.[123]

Histopathology

There are multifocal to coalescing aggregates of well-differentiated mast cells admixed with variable numbers of eosinophils that often invade into adjacent tissues. There may be extensive reactive fibroplasia, abundant collagen, dystrophic mineralization, and areas of necrosis. Neoplastic mast cells typically are round to polygonal, but spindeloid forms have been described.[123,129,130]

Immunohistochemistry

The neoplastic mast cells are positive for tryptase, chymase, and KIT.[123,129]

Prognostic Factors and Treatment

No reliable prognostic factors for MCT in horses have been described. Most are benign and are treated with surgical excision, and recurrence is uncommon.[123,129]

References

1. Kumar, V. and Sharma, A. (2010). Mast cells: emerging sentinel innate immune cells with diverse role in immunity. *Mol Immunol* 48: 14–25.
2. Galli, S.J., Zsebo, K.M., and Geissler, E.N. (1994). The KIT ligand, stem cell factor. *Adv Immunol* 55: 1–95.
3. Roskoski, R. Jr. (2005). Structure and regulation of KIT protein-tyrosine kinase: the stem cell factor receptor. *Biochem Biophys Res Commun* 338: 1307–1315.
4. Roskoski, R. Jr. (2005). Signaling by KIT protein-tyrosine kinase: the stem cell factor receptor. *Biochem Biophys Res Commun* 337: 1–13.
5. London, C.A. and Séguin, B. (2003). Mast cell tumors in the dog. *Vet Clin North Am Small Anim Pract* 33: 473–489.
6. Thamm, D.H. and Vail, D.M. (2007). Mast cell tumors. In: *Withrow and MacEwen's Small Animal Clinical Oncology* (eds. S.J. Withrow and D.M. Vail), 402–424. St Louis, MO: Saunders-Elsevier.
7. Noviana, D., Mamba, K., Makimura, S., and Horii, Y. (2004). Distribution, histochemical and enzyme histochemical characterization of mast cells in dogs. *J Mol Histol* 35: 123–132.
8. Blackwood, L., Murphy, S., Buracco, P. et al. (2012). European consensus document on mast cell tumours in dogs and cats. *Vet Comp Oncol* 10: e1–e29.
9. Davis, B.J., Page, R., Sannes, P.L., and Meuten, D.J. (1992). Cutaneous mastocytosis in a dog. *Vet Pathol* 29: 363–365.
10. Finnie, J.W. and Bostock, D.E. (1979). Skin neoplasia in dogs. *Aust Vet J* 55: 602–604.
11. Rothwell, T.L., Howlett, C.R., Middleton, D.J. et al. (1987). Skin neoplasms of dogs in Sydney. *Aust Vet J* 64: 161–164.
12. Peters, J.A. (1969). Canine mastocytoma: excess risk as related to ancestry. *J Natl Cancer Inst* 42: 435–443.
13. White, C.R., Hohenhaus, A.E., Kelsey, J., and Procter-Gray, E. (2011). Cutaneous MCTs: associations with spay/neuter status, breed, body size, and phylogenetic cluster. *J Am Anim Hosp Assoc* 47: 201–216.
14. Arendt, M.L., Melin, M., Tonomura, N. et al. (2015). Genome-wide association study of Golden Retrievers identifies germ-line factors predisposing to mast cell tumors. *PLoS Genet* 11: 1–21.
15. Mullins, M.N., Dernell, W.S., Withrow, S.J. et al. (2006). Evaluation of prognostic factors associated with outcome in dogs with multiple cutaneous mast cell tumors treated with surgery with and without adjuvant treatment: 54 cases (1998–2004). *J Am Vet Med Assoc* 228: 91–95.
16. Tams, T.R. and Macy, D.W. (1981). Canine mast cell tumors. *Compend Contin Educ Pract Vet* 27: 259–263.
17. Van Pelt, D.R., Fowler, J.D., and Leighton, F.A. (1986). Multiple cutaneous mast cell tumors in a dog: a case report and brief review. *Can Vet J* 27: 259–263.
18. Cohen, D., Reif, S.S., Brodey, R.S., and Keiser, H. (1974). Epidemiological analysis of the most prevalent sites and types of canine neoplasia observed in a veterinary hospital. *Cancer Res* 34: 2859–2868.
19. Fox, L.E., Rosenthal, R.C., Twedt, D.C. et al. (1990). Plasma histamine and gastrin concentration in 17 dogs with mast cell tumors. *J Vet Intern Med* 4: 242–246.
20. Howard, E.B., Sawa, T.R., Nielsen, S.W., and Kenyon, A.J. (1969). Mastocytoma and gastroduodenal ulceration. Gastric and duodenal ulcers in dogs with mastocytoma. *Pathol Vet* 6: 146–158.
21. Hotendorf, G.H., Nielsen, S.W., and Kenyon, A.J. (1965). Canine mastocytoma: I. Blood coagulation time in dogs with mastocytoma. *Pathol Vet* 2: 129–141.
22. O'Keefe, D.A., Couto, C.G., Burke-Schwartz, C., and Jacobs, R.M. (1987). Systemic mastocytosis in 16 dogs. *J Vet Intern Med* 1: 75–80.
23. Raskin, R.E. (2016). Round or discrete cells. In: *Canine and Feline Cytology: A Color Atlas and Interpretation Guide*, 3e (eds. R.E. Raskin and D.J. Meyer), 78–82. St. Louis, MO: Saunders Elsevier.
24. Sledge, D.G., Webster, J., and Kiupel, M. (2016). Canine cutaneous mast cell tumors: a combined clinical and pathologic approach to diagnosis, prognosis, and treatment selection. *Vet J* 215: 43–54.
25. Hergt, F., von Bomhard, W., Kent, M.S., and Hirschberger, J. (2016). Use of a 2-tier histologic grading system for canine cutaneous mast cell tumors on cytology specimens. *Vet Clin Pathol* 45: 1–7.
26. Jackson, D.E., Selting, K.A., Spoor, M.S. et al. (2012). Evaluation of fixation time using Diff-Quik for staining of canine mast cell tumor aspirates. *Vet Clin Pathol* 42: 99–102.
27. Baker-Gabb, M., Hunt, G.B., and France, M.P. (2003). Soft tissue sarcomas and mast cell tumours in dogs; clinical behaviour and response to surgery. *Aust Vet J* 81: 732–738.
28. Duncan, J.R. and Prasse, K.W. (1979). Cytology of canine cutaneous round cell tumors. Mast cell tumor, histiocytoma, lymphosarcoma and transmissible venereal tumor. *Vet Pathol* 16: 673–679.
29. Griffiths, G.L., Lumsden, J.H., and Valli, V.E.O. (1984). Fine needle aspiration cytology and histologic correlation in canine tumors. *Vet Clin Pathol* 13: 13–17.
30. Allison, R.W. and Velguth, K.E. (2010). Appearance of granulated cells in blood films stained by automated aqueous versus methanolic Romanowsky methods. *Vet Clin Pathol* 39: 99–104.
31. Cannas Simoes, J.P. and Schoning, P. (1994). Canine mast cell tumors: a comparison of stain techniques. *J Vet Diagn Invest* 6: 458–465.

32 Masserdotti, C. (2013). Proportions of mast cells in normal canine hepatic cytologic specimens: comparison of 2 staining methods. *Vet Clin Pathol* 42: 522–525.

33 Camus, M.S., Priest, H.L., Koehler, J.W. et al. (2016). Cytologic criteria for mast cell tumor grading in dogs with evaluation of clinical outcome. *Vet Pathol* 53: 1117–1123.

34 Barger, A.M., Skowronski, M.C., and MacNeill, A.L. (2012). Cytologic identification of erythrophagocytic neoplasms in dogs. *Vet Clin Pathol* 41: 587–589.

35 Meléndez-Laso, A., Cazzini, P., Camus, M. et al. (2015). Cell cannibalism by malignant neoplastic cells: three cases in dogs and a literature review. *Vet Clin Pathol* 44: 287–294.

36 Barbosa, D.F.L., Paraveti, M.D., and Strefezzi, R.F. (2014). Reproducibility of nuclear morphometry parameters from cytologic smears of canine cutaneous mast cell tumors-intra-and interobserver variability. *Vet Clin Pathol* 43: 469–472.

37 Scarpa, F., Sabattini, S., and Bettini, G. (2016). Cytological grading of canine cutaneous mast cell tumours. *Vet Comp Oncol* 14: 245–251.

38 Strefezzi Rde, F., Xavier, J.G., and Catao-Dias, J.L. (2003). Morphometry of canine cutaneous mast cell tumors. *Vet Pathol* 40: 268–275.

39 Strefezzi Rde, F., Xavier, J.G., Kleeb, S.R., and Catão-Dias, J.L. (2009). Nuclear morphometry in cytopathology: a prognostic indicator for canine cutaneous mast cell tumors. *J Vet Diagn Invest* 21: 821–825.

40 Sabattini, S., Scarpa, F., Berlato, D., and Bettini, G. (2015). Histologic grading of canine mast cell tumor: is 2 better than 3? *Vet Pathol* 52: 70–73.

41 Thamm, D.H., Mauldin, E.A., and Vail, D.M. (1999). Prednisone and vinblastine chemotherapy for canine mast cell tumor: 41 cases (1992–1997). *J Vet Intern Med* 13: 491–497.

42 Thamm, D.H., Turek, M.M., and Vail, D.M. (2006). Outcome and prognostic factors following adjuvant prednisone/vinblastine chemotherapy for high-risk canine mast cell tumour: 61 cases. *J Vet Med Sci* 68: 581–587.

43 Bostock, D.E. (1973). The prognosis following surgical removal of mastocytomas in dogs. *J Small Anim Pract* 14: 27–41.

44 Kiupel, M., Webster, J.D., Bailey, K.L. et al. (2011). Proposal of a 2-tier histologic grading system for canine cutaneous mast cell tumors to more accurately predict biological behavior. *Vet Pathol* 48: 147–155.

45 Murphy, S., Sparkes, A.H., Smith, K.C. et al. (2004). Relationships between the histological grade of cutaneous mast cell tumours in dogs, their survival and the efficacy of surgical resection. *Vet Rec* 154: 743–746.

46 Patnaik, A.K., Ehler, W.J., and MacEwen, E.G. (1984). Canine cutaneous mast cell tumor: morphologic grading and survival time in 83 dogs. *Vet Pathol* 21: 469–474.

47 Simoes, J.P.C. and Schoning, P. (1994). Canine mast cell tumors: a comparison of staining techniques. *J Vet Diagn Invest* 6: 458–465.

48 Hume, C.T., Kiupel, M., Rigatti, L. et al. (2011). Outcomes of dogs with grade 3 mast cell tumors: 43 cases (1997–2007). *J Am Anim Hosp Assoc* 47: 37–44.

49 Michels, G.M., Knapp, D.W., DiNicola, D.B. et al. (2002). Prognosis following surgical excision of canine cutaneous mast cell tumors with histopathologically tumor-free versus nontumor-free margins: a retrospective study of 31 cases. *J Am Anim Hosp Assoc* 38: 458–466.

50 Schultheiss, P.C., Gardiner, D.W., Rao, S. et al. (2011). Association of histologic tumor characteristics and size of surgical margins with clinical outcome after surgical removal of cutaneous mast cell tumors in dogs. *J Am Vet Med Assoc* 238: 1464–1469.

51 Séguin, B., Leibman, N.F., Bregazzi, V.S. et al. (2001). Clinical outcome of dogs with grade-II mast cell tumors treated with surgery alone: 55 cases (1996–1999). *J Am Vet Med Assoc* 218: 1120–1123.

52 Weisse, C., Shofer, F.S., and Sorenmo, K. (2002). Recurrence rates and sites for grade II canine cutaneous mast cell tumors following complete surgical excision. *J Am Anim Hosp Assoc* 38: 71–73.

53 Northrup, N.C., Harmon, B.G., Gieger, T.L. et al. (2005). Variation among pathologists in the histologic grading of canine cutaneous mast cell tumors. *J Vet Diagn Invest* 17: 245–248.

54 Northrup, N.C., Howerth, E.W., Harmon, B.G. et al. (2005). Variation among pathologists in the histologic grading of canine cutaneous mast cell tumors with uniform use of a single grading reference. *J Vet Diagn Invest* 17: 561–564.

55 Takeuchi, Y., Fujino, Y., Watanabe, M. et al. (2013). Validation of the prognostic value of histopathological grading or c-KIT mutation in canine cutaneous mast cell tumours: a retrospective cohort study. *Vet J* 196: 492–498.

56 Vascellari, M., Giantin, M., Capello, K. et al. (2013). Expression of Ki67, BCL-2, and COX-2 in canine cutaneous mast cell tumors: association with grading and prognosis. *Vet Pathol* 50: 110–121.

57 Stefanello, D., Buracco, P., Sabattini, S. et al. (2015). Comparison of 2- and 3-category histologic grading systems for predicting the presence of metastasis at the time of initial evaluation in dogs with cutaneous mast cell tumors: 386 cases (2009–2014). *J Am Vet Med Assoc* 246: 765–769.

58 Thompson, J.J., Pearl, D.L., Yager, J.A. et al. (2011). Canine subcutaneous mast cell tumor: characterization and prognostic indices. *Vet Pathol* 48: 156–168.

59 Thompson, J.J., Yager, J.A., Best, S.J. et al. (2011). Canine subcutaneous mast cell tumors: cellular proliferation and KIT expression as prognostic indices. *Vet Pathol* 48: 169–181.

60 Fernandez, N.J., West, K.H., Jackson, M.L., and Kidney, B.A. (2005). Immunohistochemical and histochemical stains for differentiating canine cutaneous round cell tumors. *Vet Pathol* 42: 437–445.

61 Mederle, O., Mederle, N., Bocan, E.V. et al. (2010). VEGF expression in dog mastocytoma. *Rev Med Chir Soc Med Nat Iasi* 114: 185–188.

62 Preziosi, R., Morini, M., and Sarli, G. (2005). Expression of the KIT protein (CD117) I primary cutaneous mast cell tumors of the dog. *J Vet Diagn Invest* 16: 554–561.

63 Rabanal, R.H., Fondevila, D.M., Montane, V. et al. (1989). Immunocytochemical diagnosis of skin tumours of the dog with special reference to undifferentiated types. *Res Vet Sci* 47: 129–133.

64 Sandusky, G.E., Carlton, W.W., and Wightman, K.A. (1987). Diagnostic immunohistochemistry of canine round cell tumors. *Vet Pathol* 24: 495–499.

65 Meyer, A., Gruber, A.D., and Klopfleisch, R. (2012). CD25 is expressed by canine cutaneous mast cell tumors but not by cutaneous connective tissue mast cells. *Vet Pathol* 49: 988–997.

66 Elston, L.B., Sueiro, F.A., Cavalcanti, J.N., and Metze, K. (2009). The importance of the mitotic index as a prognostic factor for survival of canine cutaneous mast cell tumors: a validation study. *Vet Pathol* 46: 362–364.

67 Romansik, E.M., Reilly, C.M., Kass, P.H. et al. (2007). Mitotic index is predictive for survival for canine cutaneous mast cell tumors. *Vet Pathol* 44: 335–341.

68 Webster, J.D., Yuzbasiyan-Gurkan, V., Miller, R.A. et al. (2007). Cellular proliferation in canine cutaneous mast cell tumors: associations with c-KIT and its role in prognostication. *Vet Pathol* 44: 298–308.

69 Berlato, D., Murphy, S., Monti, P. et al. (2013). Comparison of mitotic index and Ki67 index in the prognostication of canine cutaneous mast cell tumours. *Vet Comp Oncol* 2: 143–150.

70 Abadie, J.J., Amardeilh, M.A., and Delverdier, M.E. (1999). Immunohistochemical detection of proliferating cell nuclear antigen and Ki-67 in mast cell tumors from dogs. *J Am Vet Med Assoc* 15: 1629–1634.

71 Bostock, D.E., Crocker, J., Harris, K., and Smith, P. (1989). Nucleolar organizer regions as indicators of post-surgical prognosis in canine spontaneous mast cell tumours. *Br J Cancer* 59: 915–918.

72 Kravis, L.D., Vail, D.M., Kisseberth, W.C. et al. (1996). Frequency of argyrophilic nucleolar organizer regions in fine-needle aspirates and biopsy specimens from mast cell tumors in dogs. *J Am Vet Med Assoc* 209: 1418–1420.

73 Scase, T.J., Edwards, D., Miller, J. et al. (2006). Canine mast cell tumors: correlation of apoptosis and proliferation markers with prognosis. *J Vet Intern Med* 20: 151–158.

74 Webster, J.D., Yuzbasiyan-Gurkan, V., Kaneene, J.B. et al. (2006). The role of c-KIT in tumorigenesis: evaluation in canine cutaneous mast cell tumors. *Neoplasia* 8: 104–111.

75 Downing, S., Chien, B.M., Kass, P.H. et al. (2002). Prevalence and importance of internal tandem duplications in exons 11 and 12 of c-KIT in mast cell tumors of dogs. *Am J Vet Res* 12: 1718–1723.

76 Jones, C.L., Grahn, R.A., Chien, M.B. et al. (2004). Detection of c-KIT mutations in canine mast cell tumors using fluorescent polyacrylamide gel electrophoresis. *J Vet Diagn Invest* 16: 95–100.

77 Letard, S., Yang, Y., Hanssens, K. et al. (2008). Gain-of-function mutations in the extracellular domain of KIT are common in canine mast cell tumors. *Mol Cancer Res* 6: 1137–1145.

78 London, C.A., Galli, S.J., Yuuki, T. et al. (1999). Spontaneous canine mast cell tumors express tandem duplications in the proto-oncogene c-KIT. *Exp Hematol* 27: 689–697.

79 McNiel, E.A., Prink, A.L., and O'Brien, D. (2004). Evaluation of risk and clinical outcome of mast cell tumours in pug dogs. *Vet Comp Oncol* 4: 2–8.

80 Chaffin, K. and Thrall, D.E. (2002). Results of radiation therapy in 19 dogs with cutaneous mast cell tumor and regional lymph node metastasis. *Vet Radiol Ultrasound* 43: 392–395.

81 LaDue, T., Price, G.S., Dodge, R. et al. (1998). Radiation therapy for incompletely resected canine mast cell tumors. *Vet Radiol Ultrasound* 39: 57–62.

82 Cahalane, A.K., Payne, S., Barber, L.G. et al. (2004). Prognostic factors for survival of dogs with inguinal and perineal mast cell tumors treated surgically with or without adjunctive treatment: 68 cases (1994–2002). *J Am Vet Med Assoc* 225: 401–408.

83 Hillman, L.A., Garrett, L.D., de Lorimier, L.P. et al. (2010). Biological behavior of oral and perioral mast cell tumors in dogs: 44 cases (1996–2006). *J Am Vet Med Assoc* 237: 936–942.

84 Sfiligoi, G., Rassnick, K.M., Scarlett, J.M. et al. (2005). Outcome of dogs with mast cell tumors in the inguinal or perineal region versus other cutaneous locations: 124 cases (1990–2001). *J Am Vet Med Assoc* 226: 1468–1374.

85 Patruno, R., Marech, I., Zizzo, N. et al. (2014). c-KIT expression, angiogenesis, and grading in canine mast cell tumour: a unique model to study c-KIT driven human malignancies. *Biomed Res Int* 2014 (730246).

86 Preziosi, R., Sarli, G., and Paltrinieri, M. (2004). Prognostic value of intratumoral vessel density in cutaneous mast cell tumors of the dog. *J Comp Pathol* 130: 143–151.

87 Ayl, R.D., Couto, C.G., Hammer, A.S. et al. (1992). Correlation of DNA ploidy to tumor histologic grade, clinical variables, and survival in dogs with mast cell tumors. *Vet Pathol* 29: 386–390.

88 Amagai, Y., Matsuda, A., Jung, K. et al. (2015). A point mutation in the extracellular domain of KIT promotes tumorigenesis of mast cell via ligand-independent auto-dimerization. *Sci Rep* 12: 9975–9982.

89 Casagrande, T.A.C., Barros, L.M., Fukumasu, H. et al. (2013). The value of molecular expression of KIT and KIT ligand analysed using real-time polymerase chain reaction and immunohistochemistry as a prognostic indicator for canine cutaneous mast cell tumours. *Vet Comp Oncol* 13: 1–10.

90 Blackwood, L., Murphy, S., and Pator, J. (2013). Response to letter by Dr. Schulman regarding "European consensus document on mast cell tumors in dogs and cats". *Vet Comp Oncol* 11: 164–165.

91 Worley, D.R. (2014). Incorporation of sentinel lymph node mapping in dogs with mast cell tumours: 20 consecutive procedures. *Vet Comp Oncol* 12: 215–226.

92 Baginski, H., Davis, G., and Bastian, R.P. (2014). The prognostic value of lymph node metastasis with grade 2 MCTs in dogs: 55 cases (2001–2010). *J Am Anim Hosp Assoc* 50: 89–95.

93 Bookbinder, P.F., Butt, M.T., and Harvey, H.J. (1992). Determination of the number of mast cells in lymph node, bone marrow, and buffy coat cytologic specimens from dogs. *J Am Vet Med Assoc* 200: 1648–1650.

94 Krick, E.L., Billings, A.P., Shofer, F.S. et al. (2009). Cytological lymph node evaluation in dogs with mast cell tumours: association with grade and survival. *Vet Comp Oncol* 7: 130–138.

95 Weishaar, K.M., Thamm, D.H., Worley, D.R., and Kamstock, D.A. (2014). Correlation of nodal mast cells with clinical outcome in dogs with mast cell tumour and a proposed classification system for evaluation of node metastasis. *J Comp Pathol* 151: 329–338.

96 Finora, K., Leibman, N.F., Fettman, M.J. et al. (2006). Cytological comparison of fine-needle aspirates of liver and spleen of normal dogs and of dogs with cutaneous mast cell tumours and an ultrasonographically normal appearing liver and spleen. *Vet Comp Oncol* 4: 178–183.

97 Masserdotti, C. and Bertazzolo, W. (2008). Cytologic features of hepatic fibrosis in dogs: description of 11 cases. *Vet Dermatol* 22: 9–14.

98 Meyer, D.J. (2001). The Liver. In: *Atlas of Canine and Feline Cytology* (eds. R.E. Raskin and D.J. Meyer), 227–228. St. Louis, MO: Saunders Elsevier.

99 Aubry, O.A., Spangler, E.A., Schleis, S.E., and Smith, A.N. (2012). Evaluation of bone marrow aspirates from multiple sites for staging of canine lymphoma and mast cell tumours. *Vet Comp Oncol* 12: 58–66.

100 Cayatte, S.M., McManus, P.M., Miller, W.H., and Scott, D.W. (1995). Identification of mast cell in buffy coat preparations from dogs with inflammatory skin diseases. *J Am Vet Med Assoc* 206: 325–326.

101 McManus, P.M. (1999). Frequency and severity of mastocytemia in dogs with and without mast cell tumors: 120 cases (1995–1997). *J Am Vet Med Assoc* 215: 355–357.

102 Endicott, M.M., Charney, S.C., McKnight, J.A. et al. (2007). Clinicopathological findings and results of bone marrow aspiration in dogs with cutaneous mast cell tumors: 157 cases (1999–2002). *Vet Comp Oncol* 5: 31–37.

103 Stockham, S.L., Basel, D.L., and Schmidt, D.A. (1986). Mastocytemia in dogs with acute inflammatory disease. *Vet Clin Pathol* 15: 16–21.

104 Smith, J., Kiupel, M., Farrelly, J. et al. (2017). Recurrence rates and clinical outcome for dogs with grade II mast cell tumours with a low AgNOR count and Ki67 index treated with surgery alone. *Vet Comp Oncol* 15: 36–45.

105 Burton, J.H., Venable, R.O., Vail, D.M. et al. (2015). Pulse-administered toceranib phosphate plus lomustine for treatment of unresectable mast cell tumors in dogs. *J Vet Intern Med* 29: 1098–1104.

106 Giantin, M., Vascellari, M., Morello, E.M. et al. (2012). c-KIT messenger RNA and protein expression and mutations in canine cutaneous mast cell tumors: correlations with post-surgical prognosis. *J Vet Diagn Invest* 24: 116–126.

107 Brodey, R.S. (1970). Canine and feline neoplasia. *Adv Vet Sci Comp Med* 14: 309–354.

108 Carpenter, J.L., Andrews, L.K., and Holzworth, J. (1987). Tumors and tumor-like lesions. In: *Diseases of the Cat: Medicine and Surgery* (ed. J. Holzworth). Philadelphia, PA: W.B. Saunders.

109 Miller, M.A., Nelson, S.L., Turk, J.R. et al. (1991). Cutaneous neoplasia in 340 cats. *Vet Pathol* 28: 389–395.

110 Macy, D.W. (1986). Canine and feline mast cell tumors: biologic behavior, diagnosis, and therapy. *Semin Vet Med Surg* 1: 72–83.

111 Buerger, R.G. and Scott, D.W. (1987). Cutaneous mast cell neoplasia in cats: 14 cases (1975–1985). *J Am Vet Med Assoc* 190: 1440–1444.

112 Wilcock, B.P., Yager, J.A., and Zink, M.C. (1986). The morphology and behavior of feline cutaneous mastocytomas. *Vet Pathol* 23: 320–324.

113 Chastain, C.B., Turk, M.A., and O'Brien, D. (1988). Benign cutaneous mastocytomas in two litters of Siamese kittens. *J Am Vet Med Assoc* 193: 959–960.

114 Madewell, B.R., Gunn, C., and Gribble, D.H. (1983). Mast cell phagocytosis of red blood cells in a cat. *Vet Pathol* 20: 638–640.

115 Holzinger, E.A. (1973). Feline cutaneous mastocytomas. *Cornell Vet* 63: 87–93.

116 Johnson, T.O., Schulman, F.Y., Lipscomb, T.P., and Yantis, L.D. (2002). Histopathology and biologic behavior of pleomorphic cutaneous mast cell tumors in fifteen cats. *Vet Pathol* 39: 452–457.

117 Sabattini, S. and Bettini, G. (2010). Prognostic value of histologic and immunohistochemical features in feline cutaneous mast cell tumors. *Vet Pathol* 47: 643–653.

118 Rodriquez-Cariño, C., Fondevila, D., Segalés, J., and Rabanal, R.M. (2009). Expression of KIT receptor in feline cutaneous mast cell tumors. *Vet Pathol* 46: 878–883.

119 Isotani, M., Tamura, K., Yagihara, H. et al. (2006). Identification of a c-KIT exon 8 internal tandem duplication in a feline mast cell tumor case and its favorable response to the tyrosine kinase inhibitor imatinib mesylate. *Vet Immunol Immunopathol* 114: 168–172.

120 Isotani, M., Yamada, O., Lachowicz, J.L. et al. (2009). Mutations in the fifth immunoglobulin-like domain of KIT are common and potentially sensitive to imatinib mesylate in feline mast cell tumours. *Br J Haematol* 148: 144–153.

121 Hadzijusufovic, E., Peter, B., Rebuzzi, L. et al. (2009). Growth-inhibitory effects of four tyrosine kinase inhibitors on neoplastic feline mast cells exhibiting a KIT exon 8 ITD mutation. *Vet Immunol Immunopathol* 132: 243–250.

122 Dank, G., Chien, M.B., and London, C.A. (2002). Activating mutations in the catalytic or juxtamembrane domain of c-KIT in splenic mast cell tumors of cats. *Am J Vet Res* 63: 1129–1133.

123 Kiupel, M. (2017). Mast cell tumors. In: *Tumors in Domestic Animals*, 5e (ed. D.J. Meuten), 176–202. Ames, IA: Wiley-Blackwell.

124 Litster, A.L. and Sorenmo, K.U. (2006). Characterisation of the signalment, clinical and survival characteristics of 41 cats with mast cell neoplasia. *J Feline Med Surg* 8: 177–183.

125 Molander-McCrary, H., Henry, C.J., Potter, K. et al. (1998). Cutaneous mast cell tumors in cats: 32 cases (1991–1994). *J Am Anim Hosp Assoc* 34: 281–284.

126 Lepri, E., Ricci, G., Leonardi, L. et al. (2003). Diagnostic and prognostic feature of feline cutaneous mast cell tumours: a retrospective analysis of 40 cases. *Vet Res Commun* 27 (Suppl 1): 707–709.

127 London, C.A. and Thamm, D.H. (2013). Mast cell tumors. In: *Withrow and MacEwen's Small Animal Clinical Oncology* (eds. S.J. Withrow, D.M. Vail and R.L. Page), 335–355. St Louis, MO: Saunders-Elsevier.

128 Turel, J.M., Farrelly, J., Page, R.L., and MC, M.E. (2006). Evaluation of strontium 90 irradiation in treatment of cutaneous mast cell tumors in cats: 35 cases (1992–2002). *J Am Vet Med Assoc* 228: 898–901.

129 Millward, L.M., Hamberg, A., Mathews, J. et al. (2010). Multicentric mast cell tumors in a horse. *Vet Clin Pathol* 39: 365–370.

130 Brown, H.M., Cuttino, E., and LeRoy, B.E. (2007). A subcutaneous mass on the neck of a horse. *Vet Clin Pathol* 36: 109–113.

131 Reppas, G.P. and Canfield, P.J. (1996). Malignant mast cell neoplasia with local metastasis in a horse. *N Z Vet J* 44: 22–25.

132 Riley, C.B., Yovich, J.V., and Howell, J.M. (1991). Malignant mast cell tumours in horses. *Aust Vet J* 68: 346–347.

14

Plasma Cell Tumors

Maxey L. Wellman and William C. Kisseberth

Introduction

Incidence

Plasma cell neoplasms can be categorized as multiple myeloma, plasma cell leukemia, solitary plasma cell tumors of bone, and extramedullary plasmacytomas.[1] Extramedullary plasmacytomas can occur in the skin or other soft tissues. In dogs, cutaneous plasmacytomas comprise the majority (73–86%) of extramedullary plasma cell tumors.[2,3] Other sites include mucocutaneous junctions, the oral cavity and gastrointestinal tract, and other soft tissues.[2–5] Cutaneous plasmacytomas are relatively uncommon in dogs, accounting for 1.5% of all cutaneous neoplasms.[2,6–9] Cutaneous and mucocutaneous plasmacytomas associated with aggressive forms of multiple myeloma, and progression of cutaneous plasmacytoma to multiple myeloma or plasma cell leukemia, are rare in dogs.[1,9–13]

In cats, extramedullary plasmacytomas might be more commonly associated with multiple myeloma or plasma cell neoplasia involving visceral organs than in dogs. However, the terminology used for cats with plasma cell neoplasia sometimes is confusing, and not all cases have been critically evaluated as to whether there was bone marrow involvement. Cutaneous plasma cell neoplasms in cats often are classified as myeloma-related tumors and have been included in case series of plasma cell tumors involving other tissues. In a retrospective study of cats with multiple myeloma, one cat had a single cutaneous plasma cell tumor, and one cat had multiple cutaneous plasma cell tumors.[14] Another study included cats with multiple myeloma, plasma cell neoplasia involving abdominal organs, and cutaneous plasmacytomas. None of the cats with bone marrow infiltration or plasma cell neoplasia involving abdominal organs had cutaneous masses.[15] There are isolated case reports of cats with cutaneous plasmacytomas.[8,16,17] Progression to multiple myeloma has been reported but not clearly documented.[17]

Extramedullary plasmacytomas also are rare in horses and can involve the skin but more typically involve the liver, spleen, or lymph nodes. One unusual case involving cranial nerves has been reported.[7,18,19]

In people, cutaneous plasmacytomas not associated with multiple myeloma are called primary cutaneous plasmacytomas, and these are much less common than secondary cutaneous plasmacytomas, which are associated with multiple myeloma.[20] The diagnosis of primary cutaneous extramedullary plasmacytomas in people is based on criteria established by the International Myeloma Working Group, which include demonstrating a monoclonal proliferation of plasma cells, the absence of M protein in serum and/or urine, normal magnetic resonance imaging of the spine and pelvis, and no related end organ damage such as hypercalcemia, renal insufficiency, or anemia.[21–24] There is a much higher incidence of visceral metastasis and progression to multiple myeloma in people with primary cutaneous plasmacytomas than in dogs and cats with cutaneous plasmacytomas.[2,25,26]

The etiology of cutaneous and mucocutaneous plasmacytomas is unknown. Cutaneous plasmacytomas at sites of local trauma have been reported in people, but not in domestic animals.[24] However, cutaneous and mucocutaneous plasmacytomas have been reported in areas of chronic inflammation in dogs.[27,28] Multiple cutaneous plasmacytomas also have been described in dogs on immunosuppressive therapy; the tumors resolved with discontinuation or diminishing the dose of the immunosuppressive drug.[8]

Clinical Findings

Cutaneous plasmacytomas typically are small (1–2 cm), smooth, firm, raised pink to red, sparsely haired or alopecic, dermal or rarely subcutaneous nodules (Figure 14.1).[2,3,7,8,29,30] In dogs, these typically are single tumors, most commonly involving the skin or subcutaneous

Veterinary Cytology, First Edition. Edited by Leslie C. Sharkey, M. Judith Radin, and Davis Seelig.

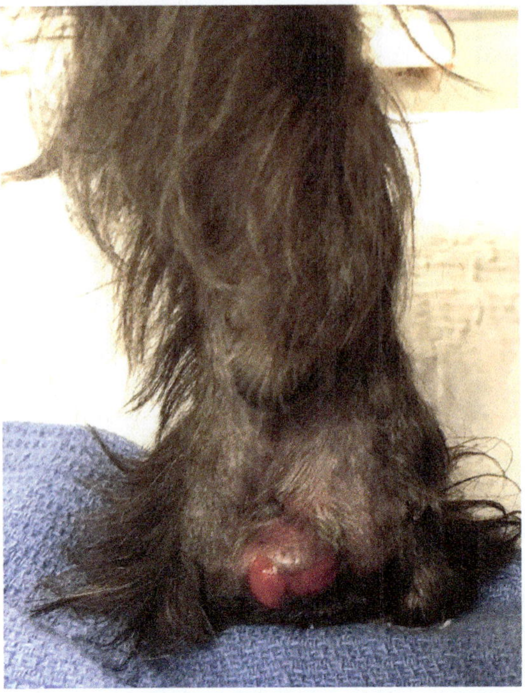

Figure 14.1 Plasmacytoma on the plantar surface near the foot pad from a mixed breed dog. The firm, smooth dermal mass is raised, red, and alopecic.

tissues on the head, ear pinnae, ear canal, lips, trunk, digits, limbs, and perineum.[2–4,8,9,30–34] The gross appearance and site predilection can be similar to histiocytomas.[5] Location does not appear to affect prognosis for cutaneous and mucocutaneous plasmacytomas, but the presence of multiple masses may be associated with more aggressive clinical behavior.[1,4,10,12] Cutaneous and mucocutaneous plasmacytomas occur in a wide variety of breeds. However, Cocker Spaniels, Airedale Terriers, Kerry Blue Terriers, Standard Poodles, Yorkshire Terriers, and Scottish Terriers may have an increased incidence.[4,7,8,29,34] The mean age of occurrence is 8–10 years, but tumors have been reported in dogs as young as 1 year of age.[2,4,6,8,35] There is no sex predilection.[8] In seven cats with cutaneous or subcutaneous plasmacytomas, head and neck were the most common location. Almost half of these cats had multiple masses.[15]

Typically no other clinical signs or laboratory abnormalities are present in dogs with cutaneous or mucocutaneous plasmacytomas.[9] However, the true incidence of monoclonal gammopathies in dogs with cutaneous and mucocutaneous plasmacytomas is unknown. Most dogs with cutaneous and mucocutaneous plasmacytomas do not have hyperproteinemia or hyperglobulinemia, and more sensitive and specific diagnostic tests such as capillary zone protein electrophoresis, immunofixation electrophoresis, and immunoelectrophoresis are not commonly performed. Cats with cutaneous masses involving plasma cells are more likely to have paraproteinemia, rapid tumor progression, and plasma cell infiltration of multiple organs.[15–17,36,37] An IgG-secreting monoclonal gammopathy has been reported in a horse with an extramedullary plasmacytoma.[19]

Sample Collection

Cytology often is helpful in the diagnosis of extramedullary plasmacytomas. Samples are collected using either routine fine-needle aspiration or a non-aspiration technique. Slides are stained routinely with Wright's stain, Wright–Giemsa stain, or commercially available quick stains such as Diff-Quik®.[38]

Cytology

Aspirates typically are markedly cellular with a relatively uniform population of individualized cells. Morphologic features are similarly variable in dogs, cats, and horses with plasmacytomas. In some tumors, the cells resemble normal plasma cells, which typically are 10–25 μm in diameter round cells with distinct borders (Figure 14.2).[1] Nuclei are round, central, or eccentric and have moderately condensed chromatin and inconspicuous nucleoli. There is abundant basophilic cytoplasm that sometimes contains a perinuclear clear area that represents the Golgi. Binucleated cells often are a characteristic feature.[1,29,30] It may be difficult to distinguish well-differentiated

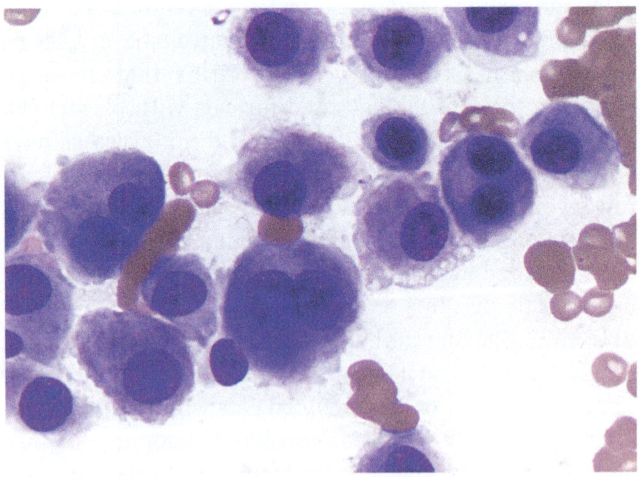

Figure 14.2 Plasmacytoma from a dog. The plasma cells have abundant basophilic cytoplasm that sometimes contains a perinuclear clear area, most clearly visible in the binucleated plasma cells. Nuclei are round and have moderately condensed chromatin. Nucleoli are visible in several nuclei. The binucleated plasma cells are a characteristic feature of plasmacytomas (Wright's stain, 1000×).

plasmacytomas from inflammatory lesions with a predominance of plasma cells.[27] Although most plasmacytomas are characterized by a relative paucity of inflammatory cells, nonneoplastic lymphoid cells and macrophages also may be present.[27,28]

Plasma cell lineage may be less apparent in some cutaneous and mucocutaneous plasmacytomas. Cells may appear more pleomorphic, cell shape may vary more, and cytoplasmic borders may be less distinct (Figure 14.3). Nuclei may be indented or lobulated with less condensed chromatin and visible nucleoli. There may be other features of malignancy, such as moderate or marked anisocytosis and anisokaryosis, binucleated and multinucleated cells, and cells with giant nuclei.[29] Erythrophagocytosis and leukophagocytosis have been reported uncommonly in extramedullary plasmacytomas.[39] Variable amounts of amyloid, which appears as extracellular, amorphous, eosinophilic material with routine staining, have been reported in about 10% of cases.[2,7]

In some aspirates, there may be a mixed population of well-differentiated and poorly differentiated plasma cells.[29] Recognition that the cytologic features can be suggestive of a malignant neoplasm is important because almost all cutaneous plasmacytomas are benign and are cured by surgical excision. Differential diagnoses include lymphoma, histiocytoma, histiocytic sarcoma, amelanotic melanoma, neuroendocrine tumor, and peripheral nerve sheath tumor.[40,41] Histologic evaluation with immunohistochemical staining may be helpful to confirm the cytologic diagnosis, especially for tumors that appear less differentiated.

Histopathology

In general, plasmacytomas are non-encapsulated, well-demarcated, expansile masses beneath the epidermis and infiltrating the dermal and subcutaneous tissues (Figure 14.4).[1,4,5,42] Occasionally, there is infiltration into the epidermis.[28] Cells are arranged diffusely or in nests, packets, and cords supported by a fine fibrovascular stroma.[1,28,30] There may be infiltration with lymphocytes (T cells) and macrophages.[28]

Plasmacytomas in dogs have been classified into several cell types based on histology and routine staining. The histologic features are described below, although these morphologic differences may not have clinical or prognostic significance.[5] The cleaved and asynchronous types are the most common.[2,43] Although one population typically predominates, there may be a transition from one type to another in various regions of the tumor. The histologic classification does not correlate with clinical behavior in dogs, except for the polymorphous blastic type, which may act more aggressively.[4,43] In cats, well-differentiated tumors are associated with increased survival duration compared with poorly differentiated tumors.[15,44,45]

In the mature type, tumor cells resemble mature plasma cells. Round to oval cells have eccentric nuclei with clumped chromatin and eosinophilic cytoplasm that may contain a perinuclear clear area. Multinucleated cells are rare, and the mitotic index is very low (Figure 14.4).[4,43] In the hyaline type, tumor cells have eccentric crescent shaped nuclei with visible nucleoli and abundant lightly

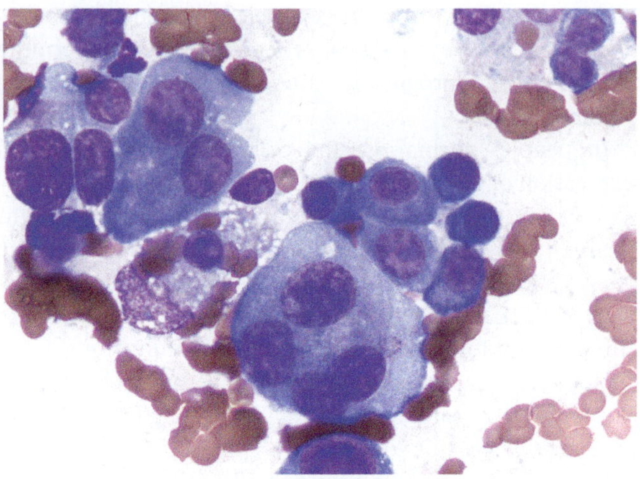

Figure 14.3 Plasmacytoma from a dog. These cells appear more pleomorphic than the cells in Figure 14.2. Notice the marked variation in cell size, nuclear size, and nuclear to cytoplasmic ratio. Nuclei have irregularly condensed chromatin and single or multiple nucleoli. There is a binucleated cell and a multinucleated cell (Wright's stain, 1000×).

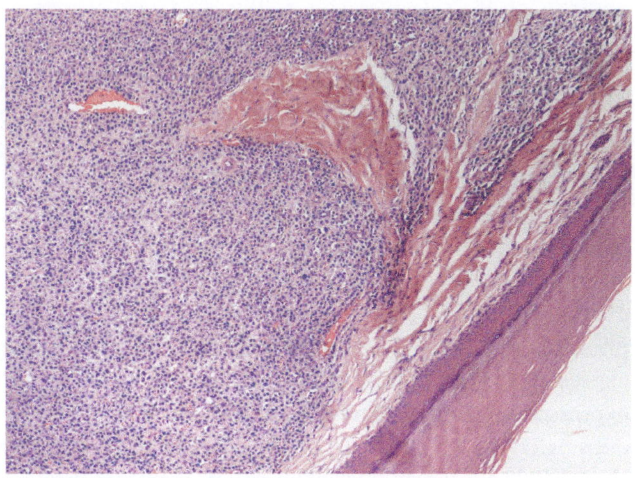

Figure 14.4 Plasmacytoma from a dog. Notice the non-encapsulated, well-demarcated, expansile mass beneath the epidermis and infiltrating the dermal and subcutaneous tissues. The tumor cells resemble mature plasma cells, multinucleated cells are rare, and the mitotic index is very low, most consistent with the mature form (hematoxylin and eosin, 100×).

eosinophilic cytoplasm that may contain a perinuclear clear area. Multinucleated cells are rare and there is a low mitotic index.[4,43] In the cleaved type, nuclei are cleaved or convoluted with finely granulated chromatin and inconspicuous nucleoli. There is abundant pale cytoplasm with indistinct borders. Multinucleated giant cells and mitotic figures are few to numerous.[4,43]

In the asynchronous type, large, eccentric nuclei have prominent nucleoli. There is abundant basophilic cytoplasm with a prominent perinuclear clear area. Nuclear to cytoplasmic asynchrony is prominent. Multinucleated cells can be numerous and there are low numbers of mitotic figures.[4,43] In the monomorphous blastic type, there is a monomorphic population of round to oval cells with large nuclei that have lightly staining chromatin and small, central, prominent nucleoli. There are low numbers of multinucleated cells and mitotic figures.[4,43] In the polymorphous blastic type, there is a pleomorphic population of large, round to oval cells and mature or cleaved type of cells. The cytoplasm is eosinophilic, and there is no perinuclear clear area. Prominent, centrally located nucleoli are present in some cells. There are high numbers of multinucleated cells and numerous mitotic figures.[4,43]

The small cell type reported in people with plasmacytomas has not been reported in dogs.[4,43] A different classification has been proposed for extramedullary plasma cell tumors in cats, which includes cutaneous plasmacytomas. This classification is based on the percentage of plasmablasts, which has prognostic implications.[46]

Immunohistochemistry

Immunohistochemical detection of various surface molecules may be helpful in differentiation of plasmacytomas from other round cell tumors, especially for anaplastic plasmacytomas, but antigen expression is variable. CD18, the common β chain of the β_2 integrin family, is expressed in high levels by monocytes, macrophages, and dendritic cells, but not on plasma cells in plasmacytomas.[28] CD45A is present on B cells and most plasma cells, but also is expressed on mast cells and some cutaneous T-cell lymphocytes.[28] CD20, a transmembrane phosphoprotein expressed on several stages of B lymphocytes, is not expressed on normal or neoplastic plasma cells, at least in dogs.[2] CD79a, which is part of the B-cell antigen receptor complex, is expressed by early B-cell progenitors through plasma cells, including some neoplastic plasma cells.[2,46,47] CD138, a transmembrane proteoglycan, is relatively specific for plasma cells in people.[48] Expression of this marker has been evaluated in two dogs with plasmacytomas. In one dog, neoplastic cells were CD138 positive, but in the other dog, neoplastic cells were negative.[1,27] CD138 expression has not been evaluated in cats with plasmacytomas.

Multiple myeloma oncogene 1/interferon regulatory factor 4 (MUM1/IRF4) is required for immunoglobulin light chain rearrangement during B lymphocyte maturation and is expressed by a subset of germinal center B cells and by plasma cells, activated T cells, and some macrophages and dendritic cells.[2] In people, the majority of cutaneous plasmacytomas express MUM1/IRF4.[2] In one large case series of dogs, MUM1/IRF4 was a very sensitive and specific immunohistochemical stain for plasmacytomas. In this study, 93.5% of plasmacytomas were positive for MUM1/IRF4, compared with 56.2% positive for CD79a and 19.4% positive for CD20. Another study reported a higher percentage (81.3%) of plasmacytomas expressing CD79a, but fewer cases were evaluated.[28] MUM/1RF4 also may be positive in some B-cell lymphomas and anaplastic lymphomas.[2] Although a high percentage of melanomas in people express MUM1/IRF4, none of the melanocytic tumors from dogs were positive.[2] Histiocytic sarcoma, mast cell tumors, and T-cell epitheliotropic lymphoma are negative for MUM1/RF4,[2] but cutaneous canine histiocytomas may be positive.[49]

Plasma cells typically are characterized by light chain restriction.[45,50] In dogs with cutaneous plasmacytomas, lambda light chain restriction is much more common than kappa light chain restriction, which also is the case for normal plasma cells.[51–53] Too few cases have been evaluated to determine if kappa or lambda light chain restriction is more common in cats with plasmacytomas.[44,47,50,52] Expression of cyclin D1 is rare in cutaneous plasmacytomas compared with multiple myeloma in dogs.[4] Too few cases expressing cyclin D1 have been reported to determine whether it has prognostic value in dogs with cutaneous plasmacytomas.

In people, normal plasma cells show heterogeneous expression of CD19, CD45, CD56, and CD79a, high expression of CD38 and CD138, and either kappa or lambda light chain expression and are negative for CD3 and CD20.[48,54,55] Neoplastic plasma cells can have multiple aberrant expression patterns.[54,55] Several additional markers used to detect minimal residual disease in people with multiple myeloma include CD27, CD56, CD81, and CD117, but most of these have not been evaluated in animals.[48] Strong CD56 expression may be specific for neoplastic proliferation of plasma cells in people with multiple myeloma, compared with negative CD56 expression in reactive proliferations of plasma cells.[56] Similar markers to distinguish between reactive plasma cells and neoplastic plasma cells have not yet been identified in domestic animals. Although polymerase chain reaction can determine if there is clonal rearrangement of the immunoglobulin heavy chain variable region gene, which may be useful in supporting a diagnosis of plasmacytoma in difficult cases, clonality alone does not establish a diagnosis of neoplasia.[3,42]

There may be infiltration of plasmacytomas with CD3-positive T cells and CD18-positive macrophages or dendritic cells.[28] Focal or diffuse immunoglobulin-type amyloid deposition has been associated with cutaneous and mucocutaneous plasmacytomas in dogs, cats, and horses, and in these areas, there may be macrophages and multinucleated giant cells.[4,16,17,53,57–60] The presence of amyloid did not have prognostic value in dogs.[4]

Treatment and Prognosis

Most cutaneous plasmacytomas in dogs are benign tumors and are cured by surgical excision.[3,4,9,29,31,33,61] For non-resectable or incompletely excised tumors, radiation therapy or chemotherapy may be considered. Local recurrence and nodal or distant metastasis are uncommon, and progression to multiple myeloma is rare.[3,4,11,29,62] Surgical excision may be curative in cats with only cutaneous masses, but involvement of the bone marrow and internal organs likely is more common in cats with cutaneous plasmacytomas.[15] If there are clinical findings or laboratory abnormalities indicating that a patient may have systemic plasma cell neoplasia, a bone marrow aspirate, serum electrophoresis, abdominal ultrasound, and skeletal survey radiographs or magnetic resonance imaging may be helpful for further evaluation. Cutaneous plasma cell tumors associated with bone marrow or organ involvement likely have a more aggressive clinical course.[1,15]

In dogs, prognosis for solitary plasmacytomas is not correlated with tumor location, histologic classification, or the presence of amyloid.[3,4] In cats, prognosis is less well defined. Surgical excision and chemotherapy can result in long-term control, but metastasis and progression to multiple myeloma have been reported.[3,17] The prognosis in people is worse if there are multiple skin lesions, large lesions (>5 cm), or immunoglobulin-A-secreting tumors or the patient is immunocompromised. More than half of human patients relapse or progress to multiple myeloma.[63]

References

1 Mayer, M.N., Kerr, J.E., Grier, C.K., and VS, M.D. (2008). Immunoglobulin A multiple myeloma with cutaneous involvement in a dog. *Can Vet J* 49: 694–702.

2 Ramos-Vera, J.A., Miller, M.A., and Valli, V.E.O. (2007). Immunohistochemical detection of multiple myeloma 1/interferon regulatory factor 4 (MUM1/RF-4) in canine plasmacytoma: comparison with CD79a and CD20. *Vet Pathol* 44: 875–844.

3 Vail, D.M. (2007). Plasma cell neoplasms. In: *Withrow and MacEwen's Small Animal Clinical Oncology* (eds. S.J. Withrow and D.M. Vail), 769–784. St. Louis, MO: Saunders Elsevier.

4 Cangul, I.T., Wijnen, M., van Garderen, E., and van den Ingh, T.S. (2002). Clinico-pathological aspects of canine cutaneous and mucocutaneous plasmacytomas. *J Vet Med* 49: 307–312.

5 Hendrick, M.J. (2017). Mesenchymal tumors of the skin and soft tissues. In: *Tumors in Domestic Animals* (ed. D.J. Meuten), 171–172. Ames, IA: Wiley-Blackwell.

6 Goldschmidt, M.H. and Shofer, F.S. (eds.) (1992). Cutaneous plasmacytomas. In: *Skin Tumors of the Dog and Cat*, 265–270. Oxford: Pergamon Press.

7 Gross, T.E., Ihrke, P.J., and Walder, E.J. (eds.) (2005). Lymphocytic tumors: cutaneous plasmacytoma. In: *Skin Diseases of the Dog and Cat*, 2e, 866–872. Ames, IA: Blackwell Science.

8 Miller, W.H. Jr., Griffin, C.E., and Campbell, K.L. (eds.) (2013). Neoplastic and non-neoplastic tumors. In: *Muller and Kirk's Small Animal Dermatology*, 143. St. Louis, MO: Elsevier.

9 Rakich, P.H., Latimer, K.S., Weiss, R., and Steffens, W.L. (1989). Mucocutaneous plasmacytomas in dogs: 75 cases (1980–1987). *J Am Vet Med Assoc* 194: 803–810.

10 Fukumoto, S., Hanazono, K., Kawasaki, N. et al. (2012). Anaplastic atypical myeloma with extensive cutaneous involvement in a dog. *J Vet Med Sci* 74: 111–115.

11 Lester, S.J. and Mesfin, G.M. (1980). A solitary plasmacytoma in a dog with progression to a disseminated myeloma. *Can Vet J* 21: 284–286.

12 Rout, E., Shank, A.M. et al. (2017). Progression of cutaneous plasmacytoma to plasma cell leukemia in a dog. *Vet Clin Pathol* 46: 77–84.

13 Walton, G.S. and Gopinath, C. (1972). Multiple myeloma in a dog with some unusual features. *J Small Anim Pract* 13: 703–708.

14 Patel, R.T., Caceras, A., French, A.F., and PM, M.M. (2005). Multiple myeloma in 16 cats: a retrospective study. *Vet Clin Pathol* 34: 341–352.

15 Mellor, P.J., Haugland, S., Murphy, S. et al. (2006). Myeloma-related disorders in cats commonly present as extramedullary neoplasms in contrast to myeloma in human patients: 24 cases with clinical follow-up. *J Vet Intern Med* 20: 1376–1383.

16 Carothers, M.A., Johnson, G.C., DiBartola, S.P. et al. (1989). Extramedullary plasmacytoma and immunoglobulin-associated amyloidosis in a cat. *J Am Vet Med Assoc* 195: 1593–1597.

17 Radhakrishnan, A., Risbon, R.E., Patel, R.T. et al. (2004). Progression of a solitary, malignant cutaneous plasma-cell tumour to multiple myeloma in a cat. *Vet Comp Oncol* 2: 36–42.

18 Linke, R.O., Geisel, O., and Mann, K. (1991). Equine cutaneous amyloidosis derived from an immunoglobulin lambda-light chain. Immunohistochemical, immunochemical and chemical results. *Biol Chem Hoppe Seyler* 372: 835–843.

19 McConkey, S., López, A., and Pringle, J. (2000). Extramedullary plasmacytoma in a horse with ptyalism and dysphagia. *J Vet Diagn Invest* 12: 282–284.

20 Kazakov, D.V., Belousova, I.E., Müller, B. et al. (2002). Primary cutaneous plasmacytoma: a clinicopathological study of two cases with a long-term follow-up and review of the literature. *J Cutan Pathol* 29: 244–248.

21 De Larrea, C.F., Kyle, R.A., Durie, B.G.M. et al. (2012). Plasma cell leukemia: consensus statement on diagnostic requirements, response criteria, and treatment recommendations by the international myeloma working group. *Leukemia* 27: 780–791.

22 Ertuk, K.T., Tastekin, D., Gundogdu, G. et al. (2016). Is it solitary plasmacytoma or nonsecretory myeloma? A must-be-solved dilemma. *Biomed Pharmacother* 77: 27–29.

23 Finsinger, P., Grammatico, S., Chisni, M. et al. (2015). Clinical features and prognostic factors in solitary plasmacytoma. *Br J Haematol* 172: 554–560.

24 Mosea, A. and Millwaters, M. (2016). Cutaneous plasmacytoma adjacent to Bowenoid actinic keratosis on the scalp: is there a link? *Int J Surg Case Rep* 21: 52–54.

25 Weedon, D. (ed.) (2002). Plasmacytomas and multiple myeloma. In: *Skin Pathology*, 1062–1063. Edinburgh: Churchill Livingstone.

26 Wong, K.F., Chan, J.K.C., Li, L.P.K. et al. (1994). Primary cutaneous plasmacytoma: report of two cases and review of the literature. *Am J Dermatopathol* 16: 392–397.

27 Perlmann, E., Dagli, M.L.Z., Martins, M.C. et al. (2009). Extramedullary plasmacytoma of the third eyelid gland in a dog. *Vet Ophthalmol* 12: 102–105.

28 Schrenzel, M.D., Naydan, D.K., and Moore, P.F. (1998). Leucocyte differentiation in canine cutaneous and oral plasmacytomas. *Vet Dermatol* 9: 33–41.

29 Caruso, K., Meinkoth, J.H., Cowell, R.L. et al. (2003). A distal colonic mass in a dog. *Vet Clin Pathol* 32: 27–30.

30 Gupta, A., Fry, J.L., Meindel, M., and Gumber, S. (2014). Cutaneous extramedullary solitary digital plasmacytoma in a dog. *J Am Vet Med Assoc* 244: 163–166.

31 Baer, K.E., Patnaik, A.K., Gilbertson, S.R., and Hurvitz, A.I. (1989). Cutaneous plasmacytomas in dogs: a morphologic and immunohistochemical study. *Vet Pathol* 26: 216–221.

32 Breuer, W., Colbatzky, F., Platz, S., and Hermanns, W. (1993). Immunoglobulin-producing tumours in dogs and cats. *J Comp Pathol* 109: 203–216.

33 Brunnert, S.R. and Altman, N.H. (1991). Identification of immunoglobulin light chains in canine extramedullary plasmacytomas by thioflavin T and immunohistochemistry. *J Vet Diagn Invest* 3: 245–251.

34 Clark, G.N., Berg, J., Engler, S.J., and Bronson, R.T. (1992). Extramedullary plasmacytomas in dogs: results of surgical excision in 131 cases. *J Am Anim Hosp Assoc* 28: 105–111.

35 Kyriazidou, A., Brown, P.J., and Lucke, V.M. (1989). An immunohistochemical study of canine extramedullary plasma cell tumours. *J Comp Pathol* 100: 259–266.

36 Dust, A., Norris, A.M., and Valli, V.E.O. (1982). Cutaneous lymphosarcoma with IgG immunoglobulin monoclonal gammopathy, serum hyperviscosity and hypercalceaemia in a cat. *Can Vet J* 23: 235–239.

37 Harbison, M.L. (1987). Plasma cell myeloma and plasmacytoma. In: *Diseases of the Cat: Medicine and Surgery* (ed. J. Holzworth), 442–444. Philadelphia, PA: W.B. Saunders.

38 Wellman, M.L. and Radin, M.J. (2018). Hematology and cytology. In: *McCurnin's Clinical Textbook for Veterinary Technicians*, 9e (eds. J.M. Bassert, O.M. Samples and A.D. Beal), 367–390. St. Louis, MO: Elsevier.

39 Yearley, J.H., Stanton, C., Olivery, T., and Dean, G.A. (2007). Phagocytic plasmacytoma in a dog. *Vet Clin Pathol* 36: 293–296.

40 Raskin, R. (2016). Skin and subcutaneous tissues. In: *Canine and Feline Cytology. A Color Atlas and Interpretation Guide*, vol. 82 (eds. R.E. Raskin and D.J. Meyer). St. Louis, MO: Elsevier.

41 Tremblay, N., Lanevschi, A., Doré, M. et al. (2005). Of all the nerve! A subcutaneous forelimb mass in a cat. *Vet Clin Pathol* 34: 417–420.

42 Van Wettere, A.J., Linder, K.E., Suter, S.E., and Olby, N.J. (2009). Solitary intracerebral plasmacytoma in a dog: microscopic, immunohistochemical, and molecular features. *Vet Pathol* 46: 949–951.

43 Platz, S.J., Breuer, W., Pfleghaar, S. et al. (1999). Prognostic value of histopathological grading in canine extramedullary plasmacytomas. *Vet Pathol* 36: 23–27.

44 Igase, M., Shimokawa Miyama, T., Kambayashi, S. et al. (2016). Bimodal immunoglobulin A gammopathy in a cat with feline myeloma-related disorders. *J Vet Med Sci* 78: 691–695.

45 Majzoub, M., Breuer, W., Platz, S.J. et al. (2003). Histopathologic and immunophenotypic characterization of extramedullary plasmacytomas in nine cats. *Vet Pathol* 40: 249–253.
46 Mellor, P.J., Haugland, S., Smith, K.C. et al. (2008). Histopathologic, immunohistochemical, and cytologic analysis of feline myeloma related disorders: further evidence for primary extramedullary development in the cat. *Vet Pathol* 45: 159–173.
47 Fernandez, N.J., West, K.H., Jackson, M.L., and Kidney, B.A. (2005). Immunohistochemical and histochemical stains for differentiating canine cutaneous round cell tumors. *Vet Pathol* 42: 437–445.
48 Flores-Montero, J., de Tute, R., Paiva, B. et al. (2016). Immunophenotype of normal vs. myeloma plasma cells: toward antibody panel specifications for MRD detection in multiple myeloma. *Cytometry B Clin Cytom* 90: 61–72.
49 Stilwell, J.M. and Rissi, D.R. (2018). Immunohistochemical labeling of multiple myeloma oncogene 1/interferon regulatory factor 4 (MUM1/IRF-4) in canine cutaneous histiocytoma. *Vet Pathol* 55: 517–520.
50 Greenberg, M.J., Schatzberg, S.J., deLahunta, A. et al. (2004). Intracerebral plasma cell tumor in a cat: a case report and literature review. *J Vet Intern Med* 18: 581–585.
51 Arun, S.S., Breuer, W., and Hermanns, W. (1996). Immunohistochemical examination of light-chain expression (λ/κ ratio) in canine, feline, equine, bovine and porcine plasma cells. *J Vet Med A* 43: 573–576.
52 Kryriazidou, A., Brown, P.J., and Lucke, V.M. (1989). Immunohistochemical staining of neoplastic and inflammatory plasma cell lesions in feline tissues. *J Comp Pathol* 100: 337–341.
53 Platz, S.J., Breuer, W., Geisel, O. et al. (1997). Identification of lambda light chain amyloid in eight canine and two feline extramedullary plasmacytomas. *J Comp Pathol* 116: 45–54.
54 Conway, E.J., Wen, J., Feng, Y. et al. (2009). Phenotyping studies of clonotypic B lymphocytes from patients with multiple myeloma by flow cytometry. *Arch Pathol Lab Med* 133: 1594–1599.
55 Muccio, V.E., Saraci, E., Saraci, E. et al. (2016). Multiple myeloma: new surface antigens for the characterization of plasma cell in the era of novel agents. *Cytometry B Clin Cytom* 90: 81–90.
56 Ioannou, M.G., Stathakis, E., Lazaris, A.C. et al. (2009). Immunohistochemical evaluation of 95 bone marrow reactive plasmacytoses. *Pathol Oncol Res* 15: 25–29.
57 Geisel, O., Stiglmair-Herb, M., and Linke, R.P. (1990). Myeloma associated with immunoglobulin lamda-light chain derived amyloid in a dog. *Vet Pathol* 27: 374–376.
58 Rowland, P.H. and Linke, R.P. (1994). Immunohistochemical characterization of lamda light-chain-derived amyloid in one feline and five canine plasma cell tumors. *Vet Pathol* 31: 390–393.
59 Rowland, P.H., Valentine, B.A., Stebbins, K.E., and Smith, C.A. (1991). Cutaneous plasmacytomas with amyloid in six dogs. *Vet Pathol* 28: 125–130.
60 Schwartzman, R.M. (1984). Cutaneous amyloidosis associated with a monoclonal gammopathy in a dog. *J Am Vet Med Assoc* 185: 102–104.
61 Lucke, V.M. (1987). Primary cutaneous plasmacytomas in the dog and cat. *J Small Anim Pract* 28: 49–55.
62 Trigo, F.J. and Hargia, A.M. (1983). Canine cutaneous plasmacytoma with regional lymph node metastasis. *Vet Med Small Anim Clin* 78: 1749–1751.
63 Walby, M.L., Ahluwalia, J., and Mehregan, D.R. (2016). Primary cutaneous plasmacytoma in an HIV-positive patient. *Int J Dermatol* 55: 464–467.

15

Melanoma

Helen Michael

Introduction

Melanocytes are neural crest-derived cells arising from a common precursor with Schwann cells. The majority of melanocytes are associated with skin and hair follicles, although they are also found in diverse tissues including eye, inner ear, meninges, heart, and mucosal surfaces. Melanocytes can give rise to both benign and malignant lesions. The terminology for melanocytic lesions in different species is not consistent. Confusingly, the term "melanoma" is often used in veterinary medicine to refer to both benign and malignant melanocytic lesions, while that term is reserved for malignant lesions in humans. Benign melanocytic lesions in dogs are sometimes called melanocytomas, but these lesions do not correlate clinically or histologically with the subset of human melanocytic lesions called "pigmented epithelioid melanocytomas."[1]

Melanomas and melanocytomas can arise in a variety of different anatomic locations that can affect diagnosis and prognosis for the patients. In veterinary species, melanocytic lesions are most common in dogs and horses and uncommon in cats. The prognosis and common sites vary by species. Generally, melanocytic lesions can be cutaneous, intraocular (arising from the iris, ciliary body, or choroid), mucosal or from the nail bed. Occasional primary melanomas are reported from unusual sites, including the tibia of a dog.[2]

Local invasion is common in melanomas at all sites in all species. Melanomas that involve the epidermal/dermal junction and epidermis often spread within the epithelial layers, leading to melanoma nests in the epidermis in mucosal or cutaneous melanomas. At epithelial sites, melanomas can also cause epidermal hyperplasia and dysplasia. Osseous and cartilaginous metaplasia, including matrix production by the tumor, has been rarely reported histologically and cytologically in canine and human melanoma.[3–6]

Melanomas can metastasize to diverse sites in all species. Lymph node, lung, and liver are the most common sites.[7] Brain and bone metastasis are less common,[8–10] and other abdominal organs, prostate, and myocardium have rarely been reported.[7,11]

Melanoma is a common malignancy in dogs.[8,12] Mucosal melanoma (primarily in the oral cavity) is the most common site in dogs, followed by lip, haired skin, digit, and rarely uveal.[8] Anatomic location has long been considered a major prognostic determinant in dogs. Mucosal melanomas (primarily in the oral cavity) are the most common site for canine melanoma and have historically been considered universally malignant,[13,14] but additional data suggest that a small subset of oral and lip tumors that are histologically well differentiated can behave in a clinically benign fashion.[15] Digital melanoma arising from the nail bed also has a poor prognosis and is metastatic in approximately 60% of cases and frequently invades into the bone.[16,17] Melanomas also can arise in the anal sac and appear to be associated with a poor clinical outcome.[18] Canine uveal melanomas (primarily from the iris and ciliary body) are usually benign or localized and only 4–5% metastasize.[19] Ninety-five percent of cutaneous melanocytic lesions are benign.[8] Breed predilections vary with the location of the melanoma. Oral melanomas are most common in German Shepherd dogs and Boxers, while lip melanomas are most common in Golden Retrievers, Irish Setters, and Cocker Spaniels.[3,17] Cutaneous melanomas are most common in heavily pigmented breeds, including Rottweilers, Schnauzers, and Scottish Terriers.[8]

Equine melanocytic lesions are common and are most frequently reported in the skin, eye, and mucosal or visceral locations.[8,20,21] Cutaneous melanomas are most common and account for up to 15% of equine skin tumors.[8] Age and gray coat color is a predisposing factor, and cutaneous melanomas are reported in 80% of older gray horses.[8] There are four classifications of equine

Veterinary Cytology, First Edition. Edited by Leslie C. Sharkey, M. Judith Radin, and Davis Seelig.
 Published 2021 by John Wiley & Sons, Inc.

cutaneous melanocytic tumors: dermal melanoma, dermal melanomatosis, anaplastic melanoma, and melanocytic nevi.[22] Benign melanocytic nevi occur in young horses of all colors, while dermal melanoma and melanomatosis affect older gray horses, and anaplastic melanoma occurs in older non-gray horses.[22,23] Most melanomas in gray horses are clinically benign and have a relatively benign cytologic and histologic appearance with high melanin production.[22] Differentiation between dermal melanoma and melanomatosis is based on clinical rather than pathologic features.[22] In gray horses, nevi can undergo malignant transformation, and malignant transformation is seen in up to 14% of dermal melanomas.[24,25] Anaplastic melanomas have been described in non-gray horses and have a poor prognosis.[8,22,23] Cutaneous equine melanocytic lesions can arise from a variety of locations and are most common on the ventral surface of the tail in all colors[8,23] and genitals.[8,26,27] Mucosal and ocular melanomas occur in horses of all colors and have been described throughout the respiratory, gastrointestinal, and genitourinary tracts.[8,21]

In cats, melanomas are uncommon, are usually uveal or cutaneous with rare oral melanomas, and are usually malignant.[8,28] Cutaneous melanomas account for 0.5% of skin tumors and are most common on the head, tail, distal extremities, and lumbar region.[8] Approximately 50% of feline cutaneous melanomas are metastatic.[8] Feline uveal melanomas are most commonly diffuse iridial melanomas, followed by ciliary body and rarely choroid melanomas.[29] Feline uveal melanomas metastasize in 30–50% of cases, and patients with extension of anterior lesions into the choroid or adjacent ocular tissue have a worse prognosis.[30] Bone metastases have been reported from bone cytology in a case of uveal melanoma,[31] and bone marrow aspiration in a case of limbal melanoma.[32]

Melanocytic or pigment cell lesions have been reported in a variety of other species, as well. Sinclair miniature pigs and Duroc pigs are predisposed to melanoma and can have congenital melanocytic lesions.[8] In cattle, melanocytic lesions appear to be benign, but metastasis has been reported, while melanomas are frequently metastatic in sheep and goats.[8] Melanomas are rarely noted in other species, including ferrets,[33,34] rabbits,[35,36] and birds.[37–39]

Sample Collection

Melanoma samples are often collected as fine-needle aspirates and generally exfoliate well. Intranasal melanoma can be detected using nasal flushes, rhinoscopy,[40] or brush cytology.[41] Generally, sampling of melanomas is considered safe, with few contraindications in the literature. There is a potential for a risk of seeding or enhanced metastatic capability reported in human oral melanoma following biopsy.[42]

Diagnosis of Melanoma and Melanocytoma

Cutaneous Melanoma

Normal cutaneous melanocytes are dendritic cells located individually between epithelial cells, in the superficial dermis, or in the hair follicle. Melanin is packaged within melanosomes by melanocytes and transferred to keratinocytes. Melanin granules vary from rod shape to granular[43] and stain greenish to brown or black with standard cytologic stains[44] and appear small and relatively fine in normal melanocytes.

Any melanocytic proliferation should be carefully evaluated to determine if it is a benign or malignant melanocytic lesion. Malignant melanomas usually have more pronounced criteria of malignancy. Benign melanocytic lesions are generally well organized with low mitotic counts of <2/10 high power fields (HPF) and minimal criteria of malignancy.[15,17] Melanoma cells in any species can assume a variety of appearances and tissue architectures. Histologically and cytologically, melanoma cells can be found in epithelioid clusters (Figure 15.1), as individual

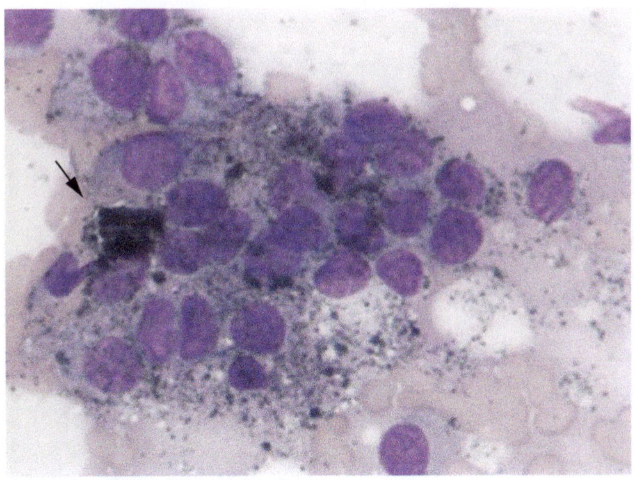

Figure 15.1 Epithelioid melanoma with a cluster of moderately pigmented melanocytes. Melanoma cells are plump to polygonal with variably distinct cell margins and moderate amounts of fine to chunky melanin granules. Clear vacuoles are seen in some of the melanocytes. Anisocytosis and anisokaryosis are moderate, and some nuclei have prominent nucleoli. A melanophage (arrow) containing dense, chunky melanin obscuring nuclear detail is seen on the edge of the cluster (modified Wright–Giemsa, 500×).

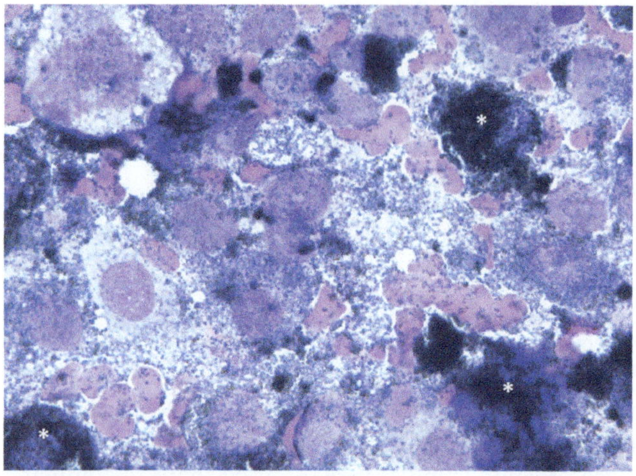

Figure 15.2 Pleomorphic pigmented melanoma with marked anisocytosis and anisokaryosis. Numerous melanin granules are seen in the cells and free in the background. Within melanoma cells, melanin granules are primarily located around the nuclei. Melanin-laden macrophages (asterisks) are also seen containing dense melanin granules obscuring the nuclei and cellular detail (modified Wright–Giemsa, 500×).

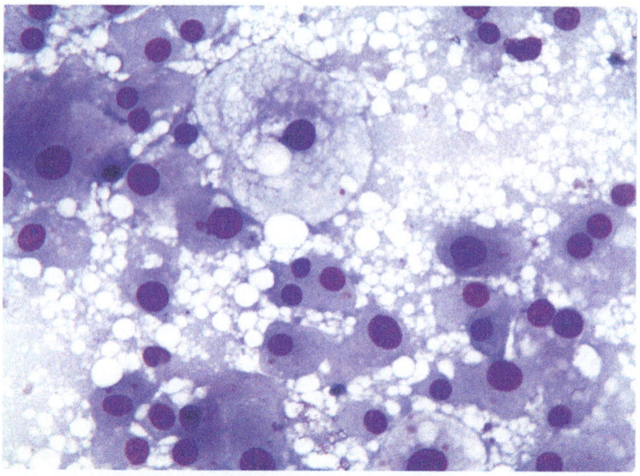

Figure 15.4 Balloon cell melanoma from a dog. The melanoma cells exhibit moderate anisokaryosis, and binucleated and multinucleated cells are seen. Chromatin is coarsely stippled to coarse with one to several prominent nucleoli. Cytoplasm is often abundant in amount, can appear vacuolated, and can contain magenta granules (Wright's stain, 500×. *Source:* Image courtesy of M. Judith Radin).

spindloid cell (Figure 15.2), round cells (Figure 15.3), or a mixture of these cell types.[28,44–46] Melanoma should be considered for any tumor that cannot be easily classified. Melanoma cells often have large nuclei and can have variable nuclear to cytoplasmic ratios and large prominent nucleoli. Anisocytosis and anisokaryosis are often marked, and melanomas may appear anaplastic.[47] Multinucleation,

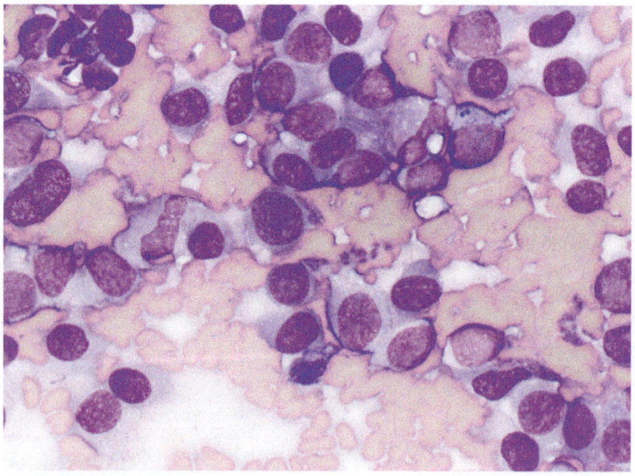

Figure 15.3 Poorly pigmented metastatic melanoma in a lymph node. The melanoma cells have a small to moderate amount of basophilic to amphophilic cytoplasm, sometimes with clear vacuolization. A single cell contains low numbers of fine to chunky melanin granules. There is moderate anisocytosis and anisokaryosis, and many cells have large, prominent nucleoli. Low numbers of lymphocytes and plasma cells are present (modified Wright-Giemsa, 500×).

vacuolization of nuclei and giant cells can also be seen in melanomas.[40,48,49] Melanin content of both tumors and individual cells can vary from highly pigmented to amelanotic.[28,49] While degree of pigmentation was associated with mitotic index, it was not found to be correlated with prognosis.[14] Amelanotic cells may appear vacuolated, and clear cell or balloon cell variants can have large amounts of clear cytoplasm (Figure 15.4) and have been reported in dogs and cats.[8,50]

Immune cells can be seen in melanomas. Melanin-containing macrophages (melanophages) are commonly seen in melanin-containing lesions and are generally large macrophages containing phagosomes packed with melanin (Figure 15.1).[43,44] Low numbers of lymphocytes are also common in melanomas.[51,52] Inflammation, particularly neutrophilic, can be seen, especially with ulceration or necrosis in mucosal or cutaneous tumors.[53]

Uveal Melanoma

The proposed canine uveal melanocytic lesion classification divides tumors into benign melanocytomas and melanomas at risk for metastasis.[19] Canine uveal melanocytomas generally contain primarily polyhedral, highly pigmented melanocytes with minimal criteria of malignancy.[19,54] Uveal melanomas consist of a combination of spindle cells and polyhedral cells with varying levels of pigmentation and/or a mitotic rate of ≥4/10 HPF.[19,54] An additional classification of "melanocytoma-like melanoma" is characterized by smaller, more highly pigmented cells and 0–1 mitoses/10 HPF but has some criteria of malignancy.[55]

Metastatic uveal melanomas can have a fairly benign appearance even at metastatic sites, so patients should be monitored for metastasis following surgical excision or enucleation.[29] Anterior uveal melanomas can be associated with glaucoma, hyphema, and uveitis.[8,19] Exfoliated melanoma or melanocytoma cells can be seen in the anterior uveal chamber.[19]

Lymph Node Evaluation

Evaluation of draining lymph nodes is appropriate in most cases of malignant melanoma, and the size of lymph nodes is not predictive of the presence or absence of metastatic disease in dogs and cats.[56–58] Normal lymph nodes can contain melanocytes, melanophages, or pigment granules, which can complicate cytologic and histologic diagnosis of metastatic melanoma.[8,58–60] Melanophages can be seen in lymph nodes draining an area with hyperpigmentation or lesions associated with free melanin (pigmentary incontinence).[8] Skin hyperpigmentation and pigmentary incontinence do not necessarily indicate a melanocytic disorder and can occur with skin infections, chronic inflammation, endocrine disorders, and sun exposure.[61] Additionally, reactive fibroblasts can be mistaken for spindloid amelanotic melanoma, leading to false-positive diagnoses.[45,62] Lymph node metastases may be amelanotic, and a large human study found that only 27% of lymph node melanoma metastases contained pigment.[45] Melanocytes can be part of the normal resident population in lymph nodes or lymph node nevi.[63–65] The causes of these melanocytic proliferations are not clearly understood.[65] This potential for benign melanocytic populations within the lymph node complicates the diagnosis of metastatic melanoma, and the significance of these cells and the best ways to definitively differentiate them from metastatic melanocytic cells remain controversial.[66] The diagnosis of metastatic melanoma should rely on finding melanocytic cells with clear criteria of malignancy, such as anisocytosis, anisokaryosis, and large nucleoli.[45] Diagnosis of melanoma within a lymph node should only be made when malignant melanoma cells are clearly noted within the lymph node, and histology, immunocytochemistry (ICC), or immunohistochemistry (IHC) should be considered to confirm the identity of amelanotic cells.

Melanoma Effusions

Melanoma cells and melanophages can sometimes be found in peritoneal and pleural fluid.[8,20,67] Fluid analysis usually is consistent with a modified transudate or exudate.[8] Melanoma cells in fluid can be variably pigmented and can be as cytologically variable as tissue melanoma cells.

Differential Diagnoses

Pigmented basal cell tumors and schwannomas or peripheral nerve sheath tumors are potential differential diagnoses for pigmented lesions. Melanotic schwannomas are rare but can appear similar to spindloid melanomas.[68] Clear cell adnexal carcinomas containing melanin have been reported in dogs.[69] Amelanotic melanomas can appear similar to round cell tumors, soft tissue sarcomas, or carcinomas. Melanoma should be considered for any tumor that is difficult to classify or anaplastic.[47]

Histologic Correlation

The histologic appearance of melanomas is as varied as the cytologic appearance. They can arise from the dermis, epidermal/dermal junction, or mucosa. For tumors with epithelial involvement (cutaneous or mucosal), nests of neoplastic cells often can be seen within the epidermis and may extend beyond the edges of the nodular tumor component (Figure 15.5).[8,70] Epidermal hyperplasia and ulceration also are commonly seen.[8,70] Histologically, melanomas also can have epithelial, sarcomatous, round cell or mixed appearances.[8,14]

Diagnostic Accuracy of Cytology for Diagnosis of Melanoma

Cytology is a useful tool for diagnosis of melanoma. Studies of the value of cytology in diagnosing canine melanoma have found 100% sensitivity and specificity for pigmented melanoma and variable sensitivity (67–100%) and specificity (85–100%) for amelanotic melanoma.[71–73]

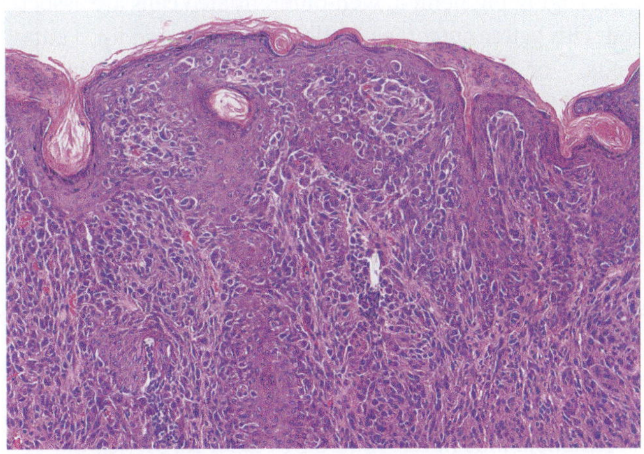

Figure 15.5 Histology of a cutaneous amelanotic melanoma from a mouse showing epithelial melanoma nests, epithelial hyperplasia, and disruption of the hair follicle morphology. Melanoma cells exhibit moderate anisocytosis and anisokaryosis, prominent nucleoli, and occasional mitotic figures. Lymphocytic infiltration is seen (hematoxylin and eosin, 20×).

Combination of routine cytology and ICC increases sensitivity.[73]

The sensitivity and specificity of cytologic diagnosis of melanoma metastasis in lymph nodes is unclear. The correlation between cytologic and histologic diagnosis for lymph node evaluation has not been thoroughly studied, but appears fair to poor.[57,58,73] Przezdziecki et al.[73] found that cytology gave the correct diagnosis in 4/6 cases of metastatic amelanotic melanoma. On the other hand, Grimes et al.[58] found poor to fair correlation for diagnosis of lymph node melanoma metastasis between cytology and histopathology (weighted kappa scores of 0.007–0.24) and between the original and reviewed cytologic (weighted kappa = 0.24) and histologic (weighted kappa = 0.18) diagnoses. Similarly, studies of fine needle aspiration in lymph node evaluation of human patients have varying results but generally conclude that aspiration of sentinel nodes is valuable.[45,62,74,75]

Predictive Prognostic Features

Anatomic location and proliferation within the tumor are prognostically important in species-specific ways (see Introduction). Canine melanoma has been most thoroughly evaluated for prognostic information. For canine oral, cutaneous, and digital melanomas, histologic evidence of increased mitotic index (≥3/10 HPF and ≥4/10 HPF for cutaneous and oral, respectively), greater nuclear atypia (in epithelioid melanomas), deep invasion, and higher Ki67 labeling are correlated with decreased survival for canine[76,77] and feline melanomas.[78] No consistent association between predominant cell type and survival has been found for dogs.[77] The role of pigmentation in survival is not entirely clear. Highly pigmented, well-differentiated cells are associated with better outcomes for dogs with oral and lip,[15] cutaneous,[79] or ocular tumors.[55] However, lower amount of pigment is not sufficient for prognostication.[77] In dogs, well-differentiated, highly pigmented oral and lip, cutaneous, and ocular tumors have a higher survival rate, but amelanotic tumors do not universally have a poor prognosis.[77]

The Role of Special Stains in Melanoma Diagnosis

In some cases, melanin can be differentiated from other pigments. Melanin can be positively identified with Schmorl's, Fontana-Masson, or Warthin-Starry stains.[80–82] Melanin pigment can interfere with the interpretation of IHC for Ki67 or other markers, and melanin granules can be bleached with potassium permanganate and oxalic acid[83] or hydrogen peroxide[84] or stained with azure B.[85]

IHC diagnosis of amelanotic melanomas may require a panel of antibodies, since expression of individual melanoma markers can be lost in poorly differentiated melanomas. In addition to vimentin, there are a variety of melanocyte markers including Melan-A, tyrosinase, tyrosinase-related protein (TRP)-1, TRP-2, HMB-45, PNL2, S100, and MiTF.[47] Melan-A is both sensitive and specific for melanocytic origin,[47] but labeling can be seen in steroid-producing cells, salivary and alveolar epithelium, and testicular cells. Tyrosinase, TRP-1, and TRP-2 are sensitive and relatively specific labels.[47] PNL2 in combination with Melan-A and either tyrosinase[86] or TRP-1 and TRP-2[47] shows around 100% sensitivity for melanoma diagnosis. S100 is commonly used in human melanoma diagnosis but is nonspecific in diagnosis of canine and feline melanoma since it also labels normal tissues and other tumors.[47,85] S100 labeling may be useful in equine melanomas.[87] Rarely, labeling of melanoma cells with cytokeratins has been reported in human and equine melanomas.[25] Alkaline phosphatase positivity has been reported in some melanomas with IHC and ICC.[88–90]

Cytology can be complemented with ICC for Melan-A and S100 to aid in the diagnosis of amelanotic canine melanoma.[73,91,92] Cytologic preparations can be destained and subsequently stained with Fontana-Masson to identify melanin granules.[93]

References

1 Zembowicz, A., Carney, J.A., and Mihm, M.C. (2004). Pigmented epithelioid melanocytoma: a low-grade melanocytic tumor with metastatic potential indistinguishable from animal-type melanoma and epithelioid blue nevus. *Am J Surg Pathol* 28: 31–40.

2 Stefanello, D., Romussi, S., Signorelli, P. et al. (2008). Primary osseous melanoma in the tibia of a dog. *J Am Anim Hosp Assoc* 44: 139–143.

3 Chenier, S. and Dore, M. (1999). Oral malignant melanoma with osteoid formation in a dog. *Vet Pathol* 36: 74–76.

4 Oyamada, T., Tanaka, H., Park, C.H. et al. (2007). Pathology of canine oral malignant melanoma with cartilage and/or osteoid formation. *J Vet Med Sci* 69: 1155–1161.

5 Kerr, M.E. and Burgess, H.J. (2013). What is your diagnosis? Gingival mass in a dog. *Vet Clin Pathol* 42: 115–116.

6 Ellis, A.E., Harmon, B.G., Miller, D.L. et al. (2010). Gingival osteogenic melanoma in two dogs. *J Vet Diagn Invest* 22: 147–151.

7 Day, M.J. and Lucke, V.M. (1995). Melanocytic neoplasia in the cat. *J Small Anim Pract* 36: 207–213.

8 Smith, S.H., Goldschmidt, M.H., and McManus, P.M. (2002). A comparative review of melanocytic neoplasms. *Vet Pathol* 39: 651–678.

9 Proulx, D.R., Ruslander, D.M., Dodge, R.K. et al. (2003). A retrospective analysis of 140 dogs with oral melanoma treated with external beam radiation. *Vet Radiol Ultrasound* 44: 352–359.

10 Rovesti, G.L., Guandalini, A., and Peiffer, R. (2001). Suspected latent vertebral metastasis of uveal melanoma in a dog: a case report. *Vet Ophthalmol* 4: 75–77.

11 Delgado, E., Silva, J.X., Pissarra, H. et al. (2016). Late prostatic metastasis of an uveal melanoma in a miniature Schnauzer dog. *Clin Case Rep* 4: 647–652.

12 Boerkamp, K.M., Teske, E., Boon, L.R. et al. (2014). Estimated incidence rate and distribution of tumours in 4,653 cases of archival submissions derived from the Dutch golden retriever population. *BMC Vet Res* 10: 34.

13 Bolon, B., Calderwood Mays, M.B., and Hall, B.J. (1990). Characteristics of canine melanomas and comparison of histology and DNA ploidy to their biologic behavior. *Vet Pathol* 27: 96–102.

14 Bostock, D.E. (1979). Prognosis after surgical excision of canine melanomas. *Vet Pathol* 16: 32–40.

15 Esplin, D.G. (2008). Survival of dogs following surgical excision of histologically well-differentiated melanocytic neoplasms of the mucous membranes of the lips and oral cavity. *Vet Pathol* 45: 889–896.

16 Marino, D.J., Matthiesen, D.T., Stefanacci, J.D., and Moroff, S.D. (1995). Evaluation of dogs with digit masses: 117 cases (1981–1991). *J Am Vet Med Assoc* 207: 726–728.

17 Schultheiss, P.C. (2006). Histologic features and clinical outcomes of melanomas of lip, haired skin, and nail bed locations of dogs. *J Vet Diagn Invest* 18: 422–425.

18 Vinayak, A., Frank, C.B., Gardiner, D.W. et al. (2017). Malignant anal sac melanoma in dogs: eleven cases (2000 to 2015). *J Small Anim Pract* 58: 231–237.

19 Wilcock, B.P. and Peiffer, R.L. Jr. (1986). Morphology and behavior of primary ocular melanomas in 91 dogs. *Vet Pathol* 23: 418–424.

20 Tarrant, J., Stokol, T., Bartol, J. et al. (2001). Diagnosis of malignant melanoma in a horse from cytology of body cavity fluid and blood. *Equine Vet J* 33: 531–534.

21 Caston, S.S. and Fales-Williams, A. (2010). Primary malignant melanoma in the oesophagus of a foal. *Equine Vet Educ* 22: 387–390.

22 Valentine, B.A. (1995). Equine melanocytic tumors: a retrospective study of 53 horses (1988 to 1991). *J Vet Intern Med* 9: 291–297.

23 Valentine, B.A., Calderwood Mays, M.B., and Cheramie, H.S. (2014). Anaplastic malignant melanoma of the tail in non-grey horses. *Equine Vet Educ* 26.

24 MacGillivray, K.C., Sweeney, R.W., and Del Piero, F. (2002). Metastatic melanoma in horses. *J Vet Intern Med* 16: 452–456.

25 Patterson-Kane, J.C. and Ginn, P.E. (2003). Dermal malignant melanoma in a horse with multifocal pancytokeratin expression. *J Vet Diagn Invest* 15: 54–56.

26 Seltenhammer, M.H., Simhofer, H., Scherzer, S. et al. (2003). Equine melanoma in a population of 296 grey Lipizzaner horses. *Equine Vet J* 35: 153–157.

27 Fluery, C., Berard, F., LeBlond, A. et al. (2000). The study of cutaneous melanomas in Camargue-type gray-skinned horses: epidemiological survey. *Pigm Cell Melanoma Res* 13: 47–51.

28 Patnaik, A.K. and Mooney, S. (1988). Feline melanoma: a comparative study of ocular, oral, and dermal neoplasms. *Vet Pathol* 25: 105–112.

29 Semin, M.O., Serra, F., Mahe, V. et al. (2011). Choroidal melanocytoma in a cat. *Vet Ophthalmol* 14: 205–208.

30 Kalishman, J.B., Chappell, R., Flood, L.A., and Dubielzig, R.R. (1998). A matched observational study of survival in cats with enucleation due to diffuse iris melanoma. *Vet Opthalmol* 1: 25–29.

31 Planellas, M., Pastor, J., Torres, M.D. et al. (2010). Unusual presentation of a metastatic uveal melanoma in a cat. *Vet Ophthalmol* 13: 391–394.

32 Betton, A., Healy, L.N., English, R.V., and Bunch, S.E. (1999). Atypical limbal melanoma in a cat. *J Vet Intern Med* 13: 379–381.

33 Tunev, S.S. and Wells, M.G. (2002). Cutaneous melanoma in a ferret (*Mustela putorius furo*). *Vet Pathol* 39: 141–143.

34 d'Ovidio, D., Rossi, G., and Meomartino, L. (2016). Oral malignant melanoma in a ferret (*Mustela putorius furo*). *J Vet Dent* 33: 108–111.

35 von Bomhard, W., Goldschmidt, M.H., Shofer, F.S. et al. (2007). Cutaneous neoplasms in pet rabbits: a retrospective study. *Vet Pathol* 44: 579–588.

36 Brandao, J., Blair, R., Kelly, A. et al. (2015). Amelanotic melanoma in the rabbit: a case report with an overview of immunohistochemical characterization. *J Exot Pet Med* 24: 193–200.

37 Guthrie, A.L., Gonzalez-Angulo, C., Wigle, W.L., and TW, D.M. (2010). Radiation therapy of a malignant melanoma in a thick-billed parrot (*Rhynchopsitta pachyrhyncha*). *J Avian Med Surg* 24: 299–307.

38 Kusewitt, D.F., Reece, R.L., and Miska, K.B. (1997). S-100 immunoreactivity in melanomas of two marsupials, a bird, and a reptile. *Vet Pathol* 34: 615–618.

39 Irizarry-Rovira, A.R., Lennox, A.M., and Ramos-Vara, J.A. (2007). Malignant melanoma in a zebra finch (*Taeniopygia*

guttata): cytologic, histologic, and ultrastructural characteristics. *Vet Clin Pathol* 36: 297–302.

40 Balint, E.M., Dumitrescu, F., Mihai, I., and Manolescu, N. (2016). Methods for diagnosing some malignant neoplasms of the canine nasal mucosa. *Bull Univ Agri Sci Vet Med* 73: 356–359.

41 Caniatti, M., da Cunha, N.P., Avallone, G. et al. (2012). Diagnostic accuracy of brush cytology in canine chronic intranasal disease. *Vet Clin Pathol* 41: 133–140.

42 Umeda, M., Komatsubara, H., Shigeta, T. et al. (2008). Treatment and prognosis of malignant melanoma of the oral cavity: preoperative surgical procedure increases risk of distant metastasis. *Oral Surg Oral Med Oral Pathol Oral Radiol Endod* 106: 51–57.

43 Wellings, S.R. and Siegel, B.V. (1963). Electron microscopic studies on the subcellular origin and ultrastructure of melanin granules in mammalian melanomas. *Ann N Y Acad Sci* 100: 548–568.

44 Barton, C.L. (1987). Cytologic diagnosis of cutaneous neoplasia: an algorithmic approach. *Compend Small Anim* 9: 20–33.

45 Murali, R., Doubrovsky, A., Watson, G.F. et al. (2007). Diagnosis of metastatic melanoma by fine-needle biopsy: analysis of 2,204 cases. *Am J Clin Pathol* 127: 385–397.

46 Luna, L.D., Higginbotham, M.L., Henry, C.J. et al. (2000). Feline non-ocular melanoma: a retrospective study of 23 cases (1991–1999). *J Feline Med Surg* 2: 173–181.

47 Smedley, R.C., Lamoureux, J., Sledge, D.G., and Kiupel, M. (2011). Immunohistochemical diagnosis of canine oral amelanotic melanocytic neoplasms. *Vet Pathol* 48: 32–40.

48 Woyke, S., Domagala, W., Czerniak, B., and Strokowska, M. (1980). Fine needle aspiration cytology of malignant melanoma of the skin. *Acta Cytol* 24: 529–538.

49 Schobert, C.S., Labelle, P., and Dubielzig, R.R. (2010). Feline conjunctival melanoma: histopathological characteristics and clinical outcomes. *Vet Ophthalmol* 13: 43–46.

50 Wilkerson, M.J., Dolce, K., DeBey, B.M. et al. (2003). Metastatic balloon cell melanoma in a dog. *Vet Clin Pathol* 32: 31–36.

51 Tominaga, M., Horiuchi, Y., Ichikawa, M. et al. (2010). Flow cytometric analysis of peripheral blood and tumor-infiltrating regulatory T cells in dogs with oral malignant melanoma. *J Vet Diagn Invest* 22: 438–441.

52 Dow, S.W., Elmslie, R.E., Willson, A.P. et al. (1998). In vivo tumor transfection with superantigen plus cytokine genes induces tumor regression and prolongs survival in dogs with malignant melanoma. *J Clin Invest* 101: 2406–2414.

53 Millanta, F., Fratini, F., Corazza, M. et al. (2002). Proliferation activity in oral and cutaneous canine melanocytic tumours: correlation with histological parameters, location, and clinical behaviour. *Res Vet Sci* 73: 45–51.

54 Labelle, A.L. and Labelle, P. (2013). Canine ocular neoplasia: a review. *Vet Ophthalmol* 16 (Suppl 1): 3–14.

55 Zoroquiain, P., Mayo-Goldberg, E., Alghamdi, S. et al. (2016). Melanocytoma-like melanoma may be the missing link between benign and malignant uveal melanocytic lesions in humans and dogs: a comparative study. *Melanoma Res* 26: 565–571.

56 Williams, L.E. and Packer, R.A. (2003). Association between lymph node size and metastasis in dogs with oral malignant melanoma: 100 cases (1987–2001). *J Am Vet Med Assoc* 222: 1234–1236.

57 Langenbach, A., McManus, P.M., Hendrick, M.J. et al. (2001). Sensitivity and specificity of methods of assessing the regional lymph nodes for evidence of metastasis in dogs and cats with solid tumors. *J Am Vet Med Assoc* 218: 1424–1428.

58 Grimes, J.A., Matz, B.M., Christopherson, P.W. et al. (2017). Agreement between cytology and histopathology for regional lymph node metastasis in dogs with melanocytic neoplasms. *Vet Pathol* 54: 579–587.

59 Hutt, J.H., Dunn, K.A., Scase, T.J., and Shipstone, M.A. (2015). A preliminary survey of the histopathological features of skin from the planum nasale and adjacent skin of dogs unaffected by dermatological or respiratory disease. *Vet Dermatol* 26: 359–362, e378–e379.

60 Grindem, C.B. (1994). What is your diagnosis? Lymph node aspirate from a dog with carcinoma. *Vet Clin Pathol* 23: 72.

61 Desai, S.R. (2014). Hyperpigmentation therapy: a review. *J Clin Aesthet Dermatol* 7: 13–17.

62 Hall, B.J., Schmidt, R.L., Sharma, R.R., and Layfield, L.J. (2013). Fine-needle aspiration cytology for the diagnosis of metastatic melanoma: systematic review and meta-analysis. *Am J Clin Pathol* 140: 635–642.

63 Bautista, N.C., Cohen, S., and Anders, K.H. (1994). Benign melanocytic nevus cells in axillary lymph nodes. A prospective incidence and immunohistochemical study with literature review. *Am J Clin Pathol* 102: 102–108.

64 Holt, J.B., Sangueza, O.P., Levine, E.A. et al. (2004). Nodal melanocytic nevi in sentinel lymph nodes. Correlation with melanoma-associated cutaneous nevi. *Am J Clin Pathol* 121: 58–63.

65 Piana, S., Tagliavini, E., Ragazzi, M. et al. (2015). Lymph node melanocytic nevi: pathogenesis and differential diagnoses, with special reference to p16 reactivity. *Pathol Res Pract* 211: 381–388.

66 Reed, D., Kudchadkar, R., Zager, J.S. et al. (2013). Controversies in the evaluation and management of atypical melanocytic proliferations in children, adolescents, and young adults. *J Natl Compr Cancer Netw* 11: 679–686.

67 Metcalfe, L.V., O'Brien, P.J., Papakonstantinou, S. et al. (2013). Malignant melanoma in a grey horse: case presentation and review of equine melanoma treatment options. *Ir Vet J* 66: 22.

68 Patnaik, A.K., Erlandson, R.A., and Lieberman, P.H. (1984). Canine malignant melanotic schwannomas: a light and electron microscopic study of two cases. *Vet Pathol* 21: 483–488.

69 Schulman, F.Y., Lipscomb, T.P., and Atkin, T.J. (2005). Canine cutaneous clear cell adnexal carcinoma: histopathology, immunohistochemistry, and biologic behavior of 26 cases. *J Vet Diagn Invest* 17: 403–411.

70 Simpson, R.M., Bastian, B.C., Michael, H.T. et al. (2014). Sporadic naturally occurring melanoma in dogs as a preclinical model for human melanoma. *Pigment Cell Melanoma Res* 27: 37–47.

71 Ghisleni, G., Roccabianca, P., Ceruti, R. et al. (2006). Correlation between fine-needle aspiration cytology and histopathology in the evaluation of cutaneous and subcutaneous masses from dogs and cats. *Vet Clin Pathol* 35: 24–30.

72 Griffiths, G.L., Lumsden, J.H., and Valli, V.E. (1984). Fine needle aspiration cytology and histologic correlation in canine tumors. *Vet Clin Pathol* 13: 13–17.

73 Przezdziecki, R., Czopowicz, M., and Sapierzynski, R. (2015). Accuracy of routine cytology and immunocytochemistry in preoperative diagnosis of oral amelanotic melanomas in dogs. *Vet Clin Pathol* 44: 597–604.

74 Voit, C., Kron, M., Schafer, G. et al. (2006). Ultrasound-guided fine needle aspiration cytology prior to sentinel lymph node biopsy in melanoma patients. *Ann Surg Oncol* 13: 1682–1689.

75 van Rijk, M.C., Teertstra, H.J., Peterse, J.L. et al. (2006). Ultrasonography and fine-needle aspiration cytology in the preoperative evaluation of melanoma patients eligible for sentinel node biopsy. *Ann Surg Oncol* 13: 1511–1516.

76 Bergin, I.L., Smedley, R.C., Esplin, D.G. et al. (2011). Prognostic evaluation of Ki67 threshold value in canine oral melanoma. *Vet Pathol* 48: 41–53.

77 Smedley, R.C., Spangler, W.L., Esplin, D.G. et al. (2011). Prognostic markers for canine melanocytic neoplasms: a comparative review of the literature and goals for future investigation. *Vet Pathol* 48: 54–72.

78 Roels, S., Tilmant, K., and Ducatelle, R. (1999). PCNA and Ki67 proliferation markers as criteria for prediction of clinical behaviour of melanocytic tumours in cats and dogs. *J Comp Pathol* 121: 13–24.

79 Laprie, C., Abadie, J., Amardeilh, M.F. et al. (2001). MIB-1 immunoreactivity correlates with biologic behaviour in canine cutaneous melanoma. *Vet Dermatol* 12: 139–147.

80 Warkel, R.L., Luna, L.G., and Helwig, E.B. (1980). A modified Warthin-Starry procedure at low pH for melanin. *Am J Clin Pathol* 73: 812–815.

81 Levene, A. (1980). On the histological diagnosis and prognosis of malignant melanoma. *J Clin Pathol* 33: 101–124.

82 Gibson, L.E. and Goellner, J.R. (1988). Amelanotic melanoma: cases studied by Fontana stain, S-100 immunostain, and ultrastructural examination. *Mayo Clin Proc* 63: 777–782.

83 Cattoretti, G., Becker, M.H., Key, G. et al. (1992). Monoclonal antibodies against recombinant parts of the Ki-67 antigen (MIB 1 and MIB 3) detect proliferating cells in microwave-processed formalin-fixed paraffin sections. *J Pathol* 168: 357–363.

84 Liu, C.H., Lin, C.H., Tsai, M.J. et al. (2013). Melanin bleaching with dilute hydrogen peroxide: a simple and rapid method. *Appl Immunohistochem Mol Morphol* 21: 275–279.

85 Ramos-Vara, J.A., Miller, M.A., Johnson, G.C. et al. (2002). Melan A and S100 protein immunohistochemistry in feline melanomas: 48 cases. *Vet Pathol* 39: 127–132.

86 Ramos-Vara, J.A. and Miller, M.A. (2011). Immunohistochemical identification of canine melanocytic neoplasms with antibodies to melanocytic antigen PNL2 and tyrosinase: comparison with Melan A. *Vet Pathol* 48: 443–450.

87 LeRoy, B.E., Knight, M.C., Eggleston, R. et al. (2005). Tail-base mass from a "horse of a different color". *Vet Clin Pathol* 34: 69–71.

88 Ryseff, J.K. and Bohn, A.A. (2012). Detection of alkaline phosphatase in canine cells previously stained with Wright–Giemsa and its utility in differentiating osteosarcoma from other mesenchymal tumors. *Vet Clin Pathol* 41: 391–395.

89 Frieling, G.W., Al-Zaid, T., and Prieto, V.G. (2014). Placental alkaline phosphatase positivity in metastatic melanoma. *Am J Dermatopathol* 36: 189–190.

90 Williams, M.V. and Hook, R.R. (1984). Properties of an alkaline phosphatase from Sinclair swine melanoma. *J Invest Dermatol* 82: 526–531.

91 Hoinghaus, R., Hewicker-Trautwein, M., and Mischke, R. (2008). Immunocytochemical differentiation of canine mesenchymal tumors in cytologic imprint preparations. *Vet Clin Pathol* 37: 104–111.

92 Hoinghaus, R., Mischke, R., and Hewicker-Trautwein, M. (2002). Use of immunocytochemical techniques in canine melanoma. *J Vet Med A Physiol Pathol Clin Med* 49: 198–202.

93 Marcos, R., Santos, M., Santos, N. et al. (2009). Use of destained cytology slides for the application of routine special stains. *Vet Clin Pathol* 38: 94–102.

16

Soft Tissue Sarcomas

Jennifer D. Steinberg and John Keating

Sample Collection

Soft tissue sarcomas encompass a broad class of tumors derived from extraskeletal mesenchymal tissues, with fibrosarcoma, angiosarcoma, perivascular wall tumors, liposarcoma, and peripheral nerve sheath tumors being notable examples. Sample collection with a 20–22 G needle using the needle only, or needle and syringe with continuous negative pressure, typically yields aspirates of sufficient cellularity for cytologic interpretation. Tumor type may have an inherent influence on diagnostic yield, depending on the cellularity, amount and type of stroma, and the tendency of cells to exfoliate. Certain soft tissue sarcomas, particularly perivascular wall tumors and vaccine-associated fibrosarcomas, possess cystic compartments; however, neoplastic cells often do not exfoliate into the fluid. In the experience of the author, removal of all or as much fluid as possible, followed by aspiration of a remnant "tissue" component, can improve diagnostic yield by increasing the likelihood of cellular exfoliation from the sampled tissue. Aspiration of lesions that contain multiple or large foci of necrosis can lead to equivocal results. Necrosis more commonly occurs in high-grade tumors but also can be seen in lesions that have undergone diagnostic or therapeutic intervention and in lesions located in areas vulnerable to trauma or self-trauma.[1,2] In such situations, multiple, separate aspirations at different sites within the lesion may enhance viable tissue recovery. Typically, fine-needle aspiration of soft tissue sarcomas should yield samples of moderate to high cellularity with the possible exception of highly vascular/hemorrhagic and sclerotic/collagenized lesions.[3]

Histopathologic diagnosis can be made on examination of core, wedge, or excisional samples. Excisional samples in particular can provide information regarding peripheral infiltration, excision margins, and the presence of vascular invasion. Grading schemes of individual soft tissue sarcoma subtypes vary but generally involve evaluation for mitotic rate, pleomorphism, and the presence of necrosis to classify neoplasms as low, intermediate, or high grade. Classification of tumors most commonly can be accomplished with routine histochemical stain (e.g., hematoxylin and eosin), but other methods such as immunohistochemical staining and evaluation of proliferation indices may aid in diagnostic accuracy.

Perivascular Wall Tumors

Canine perivascular wall tumors (PWTs) comprise a heterogeneous group of neoplasms arising from nonendothelial components of the vascular wall.[4] Until recently, such lesions had been uniformly classified as canine hemangiopericytomas (HEPs) despite discrepancies in biologic behavior and immunohistochemical staining profiles when compared with the analogous human tumor.[5–7] Using immunohistochemistry and electron microscopy, Avallone et al. demonstrated that canine PWTs include vascular myomas, myosarcomas, myopericytomas, and, less commonly, HEPs.[8]

Cytologically, PWTs consist of spindle-shaped to stellate cells that are present individually and in aggregates.[6,8] The cells typically contain variable amounts of basophilic, often vacuolated cytoplasm with indistinct cytoplasmic membranes, and round to ovoid nuclei.[6,8] The chromatin is finely to coarsely granular. Nucleoli, when visible, are basophilic, round to ovoid, and occasionally multiple. Anisocytosis and anisokaryosis vary from mild to moderate, attributable in part to the presence of multinucleate "crown" cells (Figure 16.1a). When present, binucleated and multinucleated cells and capillary structures are additional features, supporting an interpretation of PWT.[8]

Veterinary Cytology, First Edition. Edited by Leslie C. Sharkey, M. Judith Radin, and Davis Seelig.

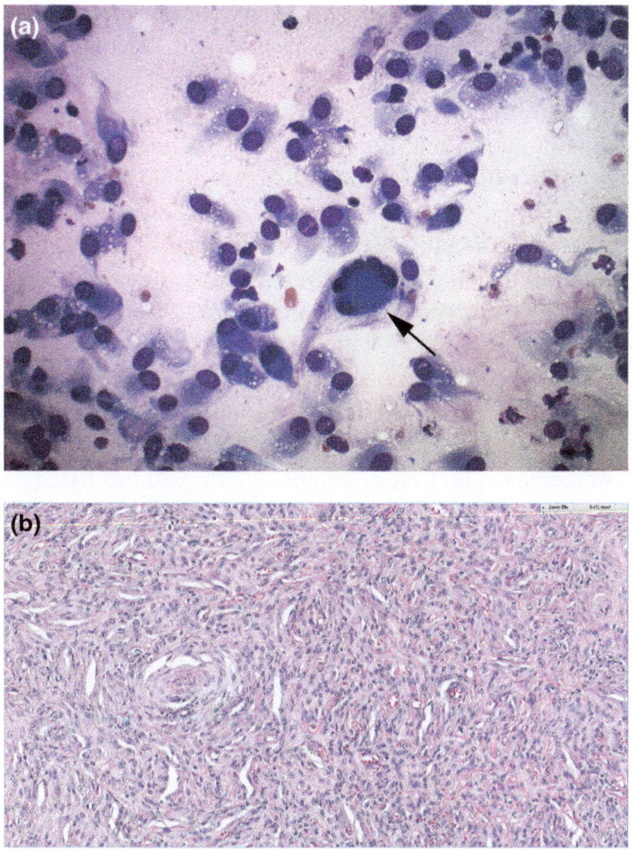

Figure 16.1 Perivascular wall tumor from a dog. (a) Cytology. Loose aggregates of spindle-shaped cells. Note the multinucleate crown cell (arrow) (modified Wright stain 500×). (b) Myopericytoma. Histopathology demonstrates prominent perivascular and storiform growth patterns (hematoxylin and eosin, 200×. *Source:* Histopathology image courtesy of Dave Getzy).

While PWTs may have a characteristic microscopic appearance, cytologic evaluation does not allow distinction among the different tumor types.[8] Definitive characterization requires histopathology and immunohistochemistry. Histopathology allows for evaluation of tumor architecture including the appearance of vascular (placentoid, staghorn, capillary, and whorling) and nonvascular (storiform, bundles, solid, myxoid, and Verocay-like) components. The hallmark of the myopericytoma is the multilayered concentric growth of tumor cells around vessels (perivascular whorling: Figure 16.1b), whereas this feature is conspicuously absent in HEPs.[4,8] Hemangiopericytomas contain numerous capillaries with staghorn and/or myxoid growth pattern.[8] Vascular myomas exhibit perivascular whorling to a lesser extent; however, most cells are present in interlacing bundles originating from the tunica media of medium-sized to large-sized vessels.[8]

All PWTs stain positively for vimentin; however, the contractile protein expression profile may permit further differentiation.[8] The concurrent evaluation of cytology, histology, and immunophenotype allowed for the diagnosis of a specific type of PWT in 85% of canine patients.[8] For example, vascular myomas tend to stain positively for desmin, calponin, CD34, and heavy caldesmon with less intense and less consistent smoothelin reactivity. Myopericytomas usually express pan-actin, calponin, and desmin but lack smoothelin and heavy caldesmon staining. Canine HEPs reliably stain positively for pan-actin, and α-smooth muscle actin (α-SMA), and inconsistently with CD34, calponin, and cell membrane ganglioside (CMG-3G5).[5,8] HEPs are negative for desmin, smoothelin, and heavy caldesmon.[8]

Angiosarcoma

Angiosarcomas arise from vascular endothelial cells of the hemic and less frequently the lymphatic systems and occur commonly in dogs, less frequently in cats, and rarely in large animal species.[9–11] In canine patients, dermal angiosarcomas commonly appear on the ventral abdominal and preputial regions, whereas hypodermal and muscular variants show no site predilections.[12] In cats cutaneous tumors occur most frequently on the head and subcutaneous tumors on the flank, abdominal, and inguinal regions.[10] A juvenile form of hemangiosarcoma occurs in young horses, manifesting as cutaneous masses or swellings on the distal limbs.[9]

Cytologic samples typically contain moderate to large amounts of peripheral blood, while nucleated cellularity varies. The spindle-shaped to polygonal to epithelioid neoplastic cells are present individually and in aggregates and clusters (Figure 16.2a). The cells contain moderate to large amounts of basophilic, often vacuolated cytoplasm and round to ovoid to indented nuclei.[13–16] The chromatin is finely granular, and nucleoli are variable in size, shape, and number. There is moderate to marked anisocytosis and anisokaryosis in this population.[13–16] Cytologic features suggestive, though not pathognomonic, for angiosarcoma, include the presence of extramedullary hematopoiesis, erythrophagocytosis by tumor cells, and the presence of apoptotic leukocytes.[13] Some tumors may exhibit vasoformative features, defined as intracytoplasmic lumens and microacinar lumen formation, though blood-filled vascular channels can only be definitively visualized on histopathologic sections.[15,17]

Cytologic differentiation between benign lesions (hemangiomas and lymphangiomas) and some malignant variants, such as sarcomas with high vascularity and low cellularity, can pose significant challenges. While there are myriad

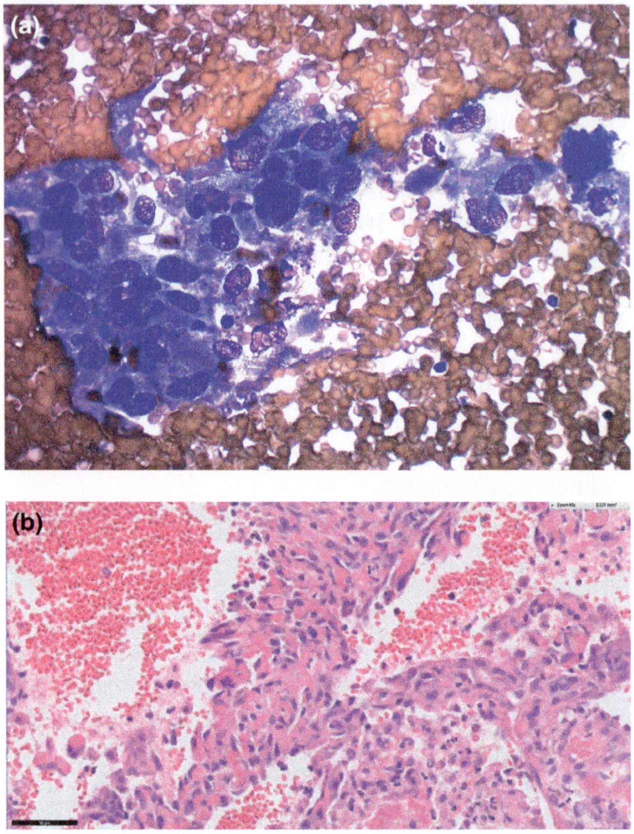

Figure 16.2 Subcuticular hemangiosarcoma from a dog. (a) Cytology. Aggregates of pleomorphic, vacuolated spindle-shaped cells within abundant blood (modified Wright stain, 500×). (b) Same tumor, histopathology. Neoplastic cells form blood-filled vascular spaces (hematoxylin and eosin, 400×. *Source:* Histopathology image courtesy of Tammy Johnson).

publications in the veterinary literature devoted to making this distinction on a histologic basis, the same cannot be said for cytologic analysis.[18] In human patients, cytologic samples from hemangiomas consist of variable numbers of spindle-shaped cells arranged in aggregates and compact three-dimensional coiled tissue arcades, present in a background of abundant blood.[19,20] The cells contain small to moderate amounts of basophilic cytoplasm with long wispy tails and ovoid to angulated nuclei. The chromatin is coarsely granular, and nucleoli are rarely visible. The spindle-shaped endothelial cells exhibit minimal anisocytosis and anisokaryosis.[19,20] Interestingly, though aspirates contain significant amounts of peripheral blood, human hemangiomas inconsistently show evidence of intralesional pathologic hemorrhage, e.g., hemosiderin laden macrophages and erythrophagia.[20] Aspiration of lymphangiomas yield variable numbers of lymphocytes and activated macrophages.[18]

Histologically, angiosarcomas vary from predominantly solid to microvascular to pseudocystic, with vascular spaces or channels lined by variably pleomorphic, atypical endothelium, and supported by sparse, smudgy, bright eosinophilic stroma (Figure 16.2b).[21,22] Tumors may contain subpopulations of cells indistinguishable from normal endothelium, with flattened profiles and small, flattened nuclei. Additional indicators of malignancy include the presence of bulging, tombstone-like profile along the endothelial linings, cellular and nuclear pleomorphism, the presence of enlarged nuclei/nucleoli, and/or increased mitotic index that includes atypical mitoses.[22]

In human medicine, tumors of endothelial origin are no longer subdivided into hemangiosarcomas and lymphangiosarcomas as they often cannot be differentiated based on morphologic features alone as well as the mixed phenotype of some tumors.[21] Both lymphangiosarcomas and hemangiosarcomas stain positively with CD31 and exhibit variable factor VIII reactivity.[13,23] Prospero-related homeobox gene-1 (Prox-1) is a marker specific to lymphatic endothelium that can be used to determine the histogenesis of vascular lesions.[23,24] Determining the origin of endothelial tumors may have some utility as cutaneous lymphangiosarcomas seem to follow a more aggressive clinical course in veterinary patients relative to the human counterparts.[23–27]

Liposarcoma

Liposarcomas originate from lipoblasts, the precursor cells to mature adipocytes, and do not arise from malignant transformation within preexisting lipomas or infiltrative lipomas.[28,29] Though considered the most common sarcoma in adult human patients, liposarcomas occur relatively infrequently in dogs and sporadically in other species.[30–32] In human patients identification of subtype has prognostic significance as biologic behavior differs among the well-differentiated, myxoid, and pleomorphic histologic variants.[28] In contrast to the benign lipoma, liposarcomas tend to involve the subcutis and/or deeper musculature. Tumors in dogs occur in the axial and appendicular regions with similar frequency.[33]

Cytologically, pleomorphic liposarcomas consist of moderate to large numbers of spindle-shaped to polygonal to ovoid cells that are present individually and in variably sized aggregates, often within a lipid-rich background. The aggregates may surround fine fibrovascular stroma. The cells contain moderate to large amounts of basophilic to eosinophilic granular cytoplasm with variable numbers of discrete, cytoplasmic vacuoles, and round to ovoid nuclei.[34,35] The vacuoles may take up much of the cell

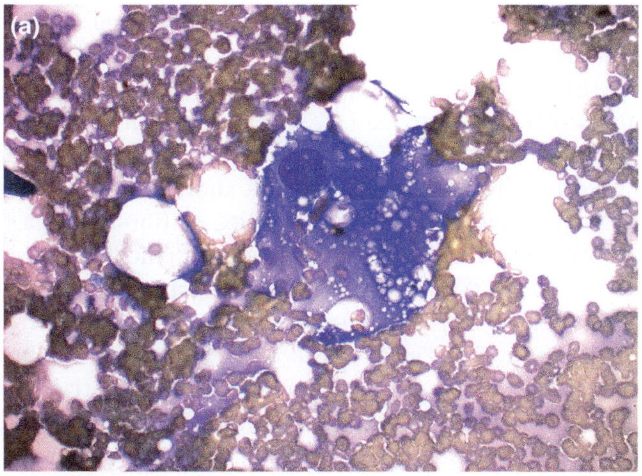

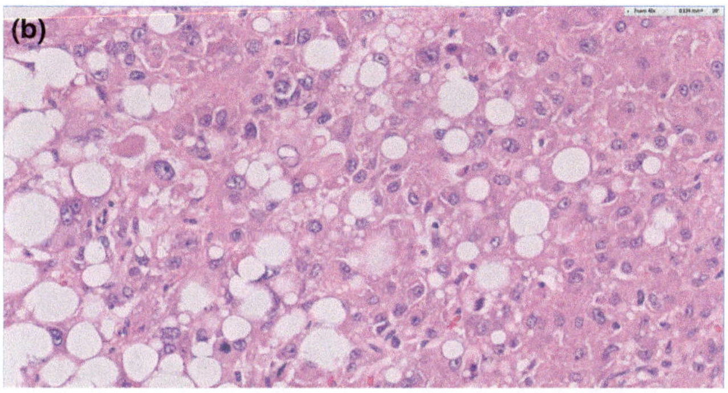

Figure 16.3 Pleomorphic liposarcoma from a dog. (a) Cytology. Atypical, multinucleate adipocytes contain variably sized, discrete lipid vacuoles (modified Wright stain, 500×). (b) Same tumor, histopathology. Sheets of pleomorphic adipocytes similar to those seen in the cytologic sample (hematoxylin and eosin, 400×. *Source:* Histopathology image courtesy of Alison Righton).

volume (Figure 16.3a). The chromatin is finely to coarsely granular, and nucleoli, when visible, are basophilic and variable in size, shape, and number. Well-differentiated tumors exhibit mild anisocytosis and anisokaryosis, whereas pleomorphic variants display atypia in the form of multinucleation with nuclear asymmetry and karyomegaly.[35,36] In myxoid liposarcomas, the neoplastic cells are present in densely cellular aggregates supported by a branching capillary network within a myxomatous background (Figure 16.4).[29,37] The cells are ovoid to spindle-shaped with small amounts of basophilic cytoplasm. Lipoblasts, when present, are univacuolar with a signet ring appearance.[29,37] The cytologic diagnosis of well-differentiated liposarcomas (WDL) can present an insurmountable challenge, as atypical cells (lipoblasts) may be so rare in some tumors they escape detection despite extensive tissue sampling.[37] In human patients, WDLs that occur in the subcutis are nonmetastasizing lesions and are not

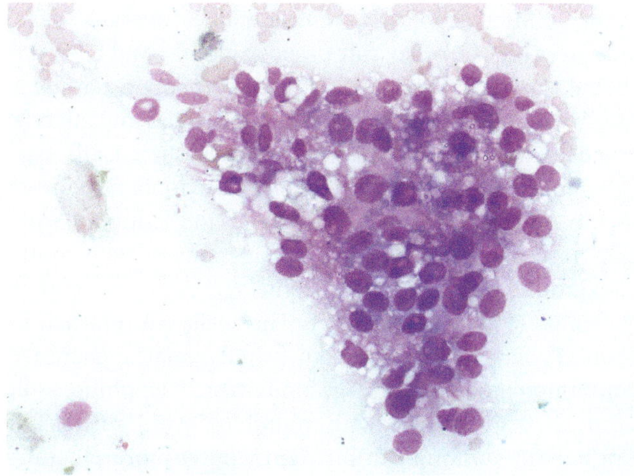

Figure 16.4 Liposarcoma from a dog. Recurrent mass on left forelimb. The cells in this lesion are less pleomorphic than those in Figure 16.3a. Note the thickness of the background, which is consistent with a myxoid liposarcoma (Diff-Quik, 500×).

associated with tumor-related death.[37] Use of Oil Red O stain for lipid may aid in differentiation of pleomorphic and myxoid liposarcomas from sebaceous carcinomas or other tumors that contain vacuolated cells.[38]

Histologically, liposarcomas are composed of variable numbers of plump, spindle-shaped to stellate cells with pale basophilic cytoplasm and single or multiple sharply demarcated cytoplasmic vacuoles that may distort cellular architecture and, as with nonneoplastic adipocytes, marginalize and compress the cell nucleus (Figure 16.3b).[37] Mitotic activity is low, but most mitotic figures are abnormal in appearance.[39] Stroma is generally negligible, while intralesional inflammation (especially macrophages and foam cells) in response to adipocyte necrosis may be significant.[39]

Malignant Peripheral Nerve Sheath Tumors

Malignant peripheral nerve sheath tumors (MPNSTs) arise from peripheral nerves or replicate the various elements of the nerve sheath including Schwann cell, perineural myofibroblasts, and fibroblasts.[40] These neoplasms occur with the greatest frequency in dogs, but have been reported in cats, in a myriad of large and small mammals, and in nonmammals.[41–45] In canine patients, MPNSTs have a predilection for the brachial plexus, whereas those in feline patients have an affinity for the limbs and head.[42,46]

A diagnosis of MPNST via fine-needle aspirate poses no shortage of investigative challenges. For example, patients may present with only neurologic deficits and no palpable mass.[42] Microscopically, considerable overlap exists among MPNSTs, other soft tissue sarcomas and even epithelial tumors.[47] Cytologic features that support a neural origin include a spindled cellular profile and slender ovoid to wavy to comma-shaped nuclei.[48–50] Cells typically have scant amounts of basophilic cytoplasm, appearing in tridimensional fascicles and individually. Some tumors contain fibrillary to collagenous stroma in the background and admixed with the aggregates of neoplastic cells (Figure 16.5a).[48,50] The cells in epithelioid MPNSTs have a plasmacytoid to polygonal appearance, containing moderate to large amounts of basophilic, often vacuolated cytoplasm with round to ovoid nuclei.[49–51] Epithelioid variants exhibit significantly more pleomorphism in the form of multinucleation, moderate anisocytosis and anisokaryosis, prominent nucleoli, and variable mitotic activity.[46,48–51]

Histologically, some MPNSTs share the primary features of fibrosarcomas, i.e., spindle cells and collagenous stroma, but are differentiated by the organization of the cells into stacks, whorls, and short bundles rather than the more typical long bundles of fibrosarcoma.[40] Other MPNSTs contain more abundant pale basophilic, mucinous to myxoid stroma with a microcystic appearance. Features of classic schwannomas may be present, with distinct Antoni A areas or loose Antoni B areas (Figure 16.5b).[41] Antoni A areas are characterized by densely cellular, fibrillar stacks, sometimes with the extremely characteristic, orderly palisading of Verocay bodies.[41]

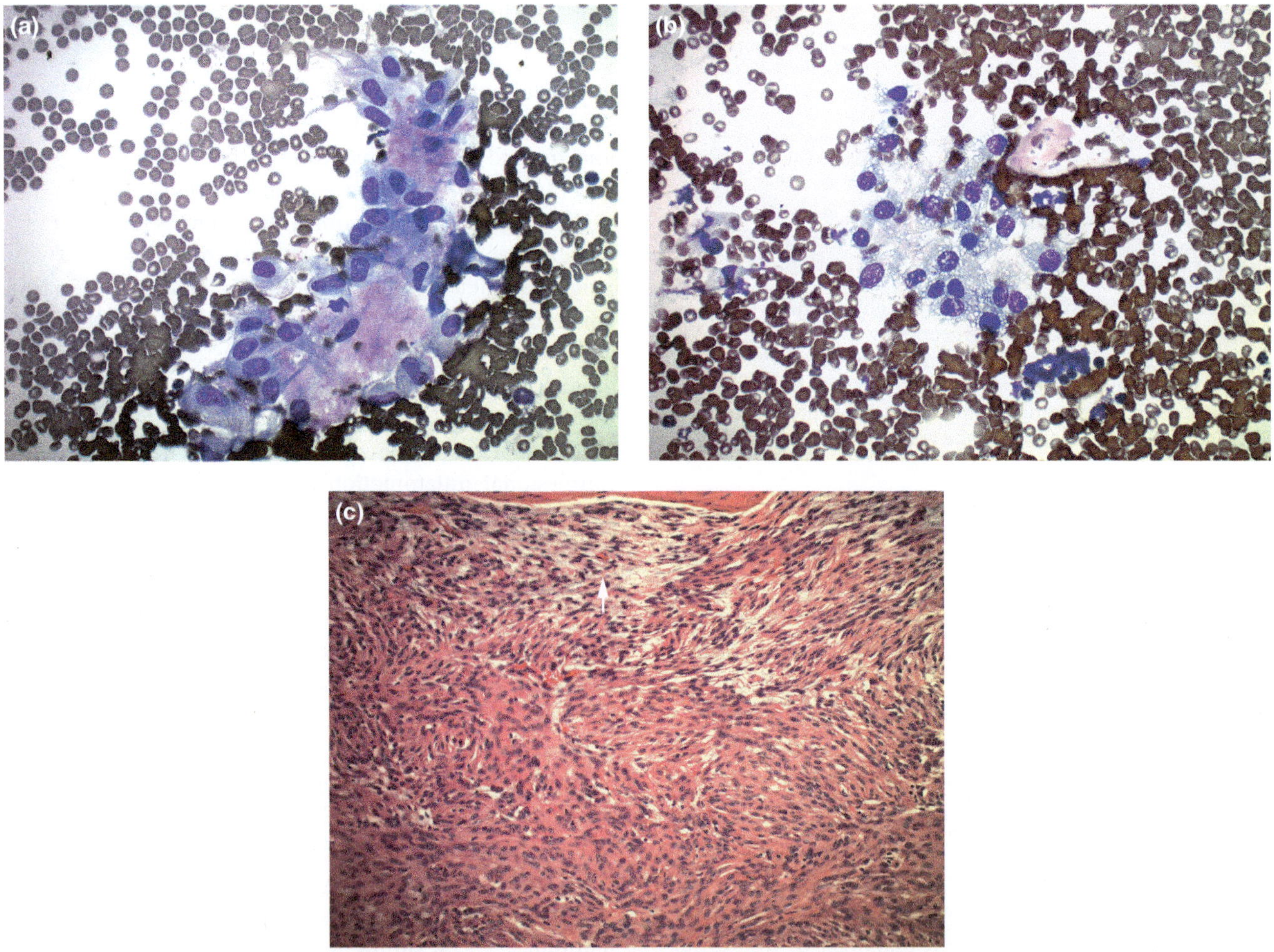

Figure 16.5 Malignant peripheral nerve sheath tumor, grade II from a dog. (a) Cytology. Aggregate of spindle-shaped cells and fibrillar eosinophilic matrix material. Nuclei are ovoid to indented (comma shaped) (modified Wright stain, 500×). (b) Cytology of the same tumor. In this image, the cells have more abundant basophilic, vacuolated cytoplasm, and round to ovoid nuclei (modified Wright stain, 500×). (c) Histopathology of the same tumor. Note the interlacing bundles/fascicles of spindle-shaped cells in Antoni A (majority of image) and Antoni B (arrow) formations (hematoxylin and eosin, 200×).

Further complicating the diagnostic process is the inconsistency of immunohistochemical analyses. Feline tumors are uniformly positive for vimentin and S-100, while 75% stain positively for glial fibrillary acidic protein (GFAP).[46] Canine MPNSTs also stain positively for vimentin; however, S-100 immunoreactivity varies from 45 to 76%.[43,52] GFAP staining is usually absent in canine MPNSTs, whereas 64% of lesions exhibit variable nerve growth factor receptor (NGFR) positivity.[43,52] Fibrillary and/or collagenous stroma in some tumors coincides with laminin and collagen IV staining,[53] though the actual tumor cells in canine MPNSTs stain neither for laminin nor α-SMA,which may help distinguish MPNSTs from PWTs.[51] The majority of canine tumors express PGP 9.5, a member of the ubiquitin hydrolase family of proteins.[43] PGP 9.5 is also present in a variety of neuroectodermal and epithelial tissues, thus limiting the marker's specificity.[43] Bovine MPNSTs exhibit variable reactivity for S-100 and weak 2′,3′-cyclic nucleotide-3′-phosphohydrolase, the latter being a specific Schwann cell marker.[54,55] Bovine MPNSTs possibly have an underlying viral etiology.[54,55]

Fibrosarcoma

Fibrosarcoma (FSA) originates from a neoplastic proliferation of fibroblasts and occurs in cats, dogs, and horses with sporadic reports in new world camelids and other exotic species.[56–59] Most lesions arise in the subcutis, with a predilection for the trunk and legs in cats and dogs.[60] Intradermal FSAs, an uncommon variant, occur most frequently on the pinnae of feline patients.[60] Though FSAs tend to invade locally, metastasis is rare, and therefore, wide and complete surgical excision generally carries a favorable prognosis.[60–62]

The veterinary literature on the cytologic appearance of fibrosarcomas consists of a handful of case reports describing tumors in individual patients. The tumor cells have a spindle-shaped to fusiform appearance and contain moderate amounts of basophilic cytoplasm with ovoid to elongate nuclei.[59,63–65] The cells are present individually and in aggregates (Figures 16.6a and 16.7). The chromatin is finely to coarsely granular, and nucleoli, when visible, are basophilic, round to ovoid, and occasionally multiple. The cells exhibit mild to moderate anisocytosis and anisokaryosis. Variable amounts of hypereosinophilic fibrillar matrix material (collagen) are present in the background and admixed with the cellular aggregates. In keloidal variants, the collagen has a hyalinized, refractile appearance.[63] Some tumors may contain scant mastocytic infiltrates. Similar appearing cells occur

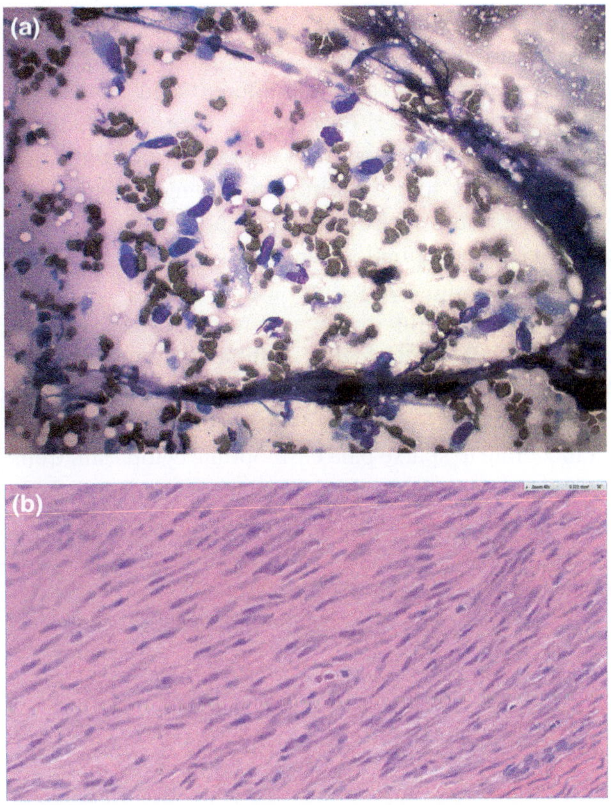

Figure 16.6 Fibrosarcoma from a cat. (a) Cytology. Individualized spindle-shaped cells and scant amounts of collagen. Nuclei are ovoid to slightly indented. Note the similarity of these cells to those in Figure 16.5a (modified Wright stain, 500×). (b) Same tumor, histopathology. Bundles and sheets of elongated spindle-shaped cells supported by fibrous stroma (hematoxylin and eosin, 200×. *Source:* Histopathology image courtesy of Vincent Carroll).

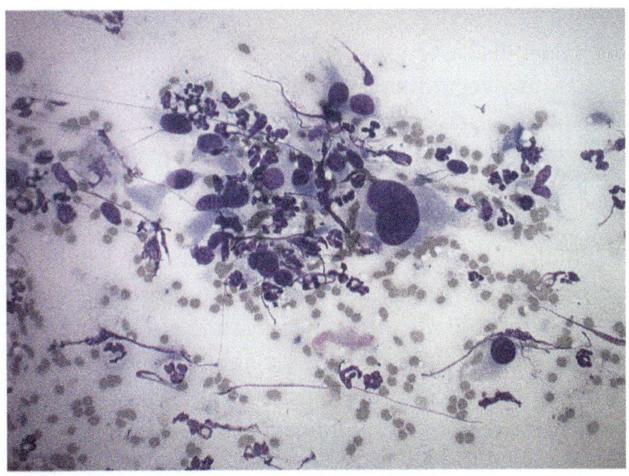

Figure 16.7 Dermal fibrosarcoma from a cat. Sample was obtained from a mass encompassing the dorsal and ventral aspect of the left pinna. Despite the inflammation, the degree of atypia exhibited by the spindle-shaped cells is beyond what would be expected from reactive change and more consistent with malignant transformation (modified Wright stain, 500×).

in scirrhous or desmoplastic portions of mast cell tumors and foci of nodular fasciitis.[3,57,66]

Differentiating between well-differentiated fibrosarcomas and fibromas based on cytologic appearance can be problematic, and the veterinary literature regarding this topic is tragically sparse. In human patients the cytologic features associated with fibromas include low cellularity, bland fibroblastic spindle-shaped cells, hyalinized collagenous matrix, and rarely myxoid material.[67] The mesenchymal cells contain variable amounts of cytoplasm and elongated, ovoid nuclei that exhibit minimal nuclear pleomorphism.[67]

Histologically, FSAs consist of large spindle-shaped cells with moderate to sparse pale eosinophilic cytoplasm. Cells are arranged in variably sized interlacing bundles to form irregular, often multinodular masses within the subcutis.[60] Variable amounts of collagenous stroma support these neoplastic cells (Figure 16.6b). Ulceration, necrosis, and hemorrhage are common secondary features.[60]

Vaccine Associated Sarcomas

As one might expect, post vaccinal sarcomas arise at sites of previous vaccine administration, most frequently in cats but also in ferrets and putatively in dogs.[68–70] The lesions occur most commonly in the subcutis and often contain cavitations within central areas of the tumors. Larger masses can contain extensive fluid-filled spaces. Similar lesions have occurred at sites of microchip implantation and retained surgical sponges in both cats and dogs.[71–74]

There is a distressing lack of information in the veterinary literature regarding the cytologic appearance of vaccine-associated sarcomas. Postvaccinal sarcomas possess microscopic features typical of fibrosarcomas (spindle-shaped cells with variable pleomorphism in fascicular or storiform arrangements) (Figure 16.8); however, they can have unique histologic characteristics that, especially in aggregate, may help distinguish them from non-vaccine-related lesions.[68] For example, approximately 50% of primary tumors contain neoplastic multinucleate giant cells.[69,75] Primary and recurrent tumors typically contain prominent perivascular lymphocytic inflammatory infiltrates located at the periphery of the lesions. More notably but less consistently, macrophages may contain blue–gray material (presumptive adjuvant).[69,75] Cytologically, vaccine-derived material appears basophilic and crystalline (IMRAB 3 TF®, Merial, Duluth, GA) or eosinophilic and

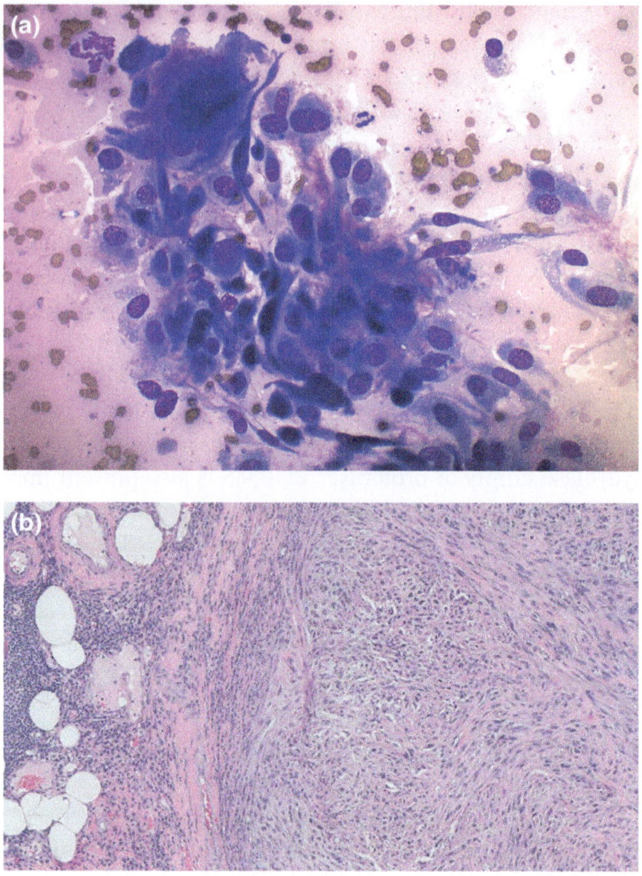

Figure 16.8 Vaccine associated sarcoma from a cat. (a) Cytology from a mass located on the hip at the site of FeLV vaccine administration. Note the aggregates of atypical spindle-shaped cells and the multinucleate giant cells (modified Wright stain, 500×). (b) Histopathology. Intersecting bundles of spindle-shaped cells with adjacent area of peritumoral lymphocytic inflammatory infiltrate (hematoxylin and eosin, 100×. *Source:* Histopathology image courtesy of David Pinson).

globular (Rabvac® 1, and Fel-O-Vax® Lv-K, Boehringer Ingelheim Vetmedica, Inc., St. Joseph, MN).[76]

Most vaccine-associated sarcomas are classified as fibrosarcomas based on histologic appearance and vimentin staining; however, at least 43% of the tumors demonstrate variable α-SMA positivity, implying a myofibroblastic origin.[67,73] The positive cells typically contain abundant pink cytoplasm with large, often lobular nuclei, though multinucleate giant cells can stain positive for α-SMA.[73] Additionally, the multinucleate giant cells exhibit immunoreactivity for Ki-67 and lack reactivity for CD18.[73] The lymphoid infiltrates consist of primarily T cells with fewer B cells and plasma cells.[73]

Sarcoid

Sarcoids represent a unique, virally induced epithelial and mesenchymal cell proliferation, occurring most often in horses, but occasionally in cats. In equine patients, cutaneous lesions occur commonly on the abdominal, cervical, paragenital, and pectoral regions.[77] Feline lesions occur as solitary or multiple nodules located on the face, digits, tip of the tail, and ears.[60] Very few descriptions of the cytological appearance of sarcoids exist in the veterinary literature. They purportedly consist of spindle-shaped cells with variably coarse chromatin and small nucleoli (Figure 21.2).[78] While the majority of sarcoids exhibit positivity for bovine papilloma virus (BPV), PCR for BPV cannot be used to differentiate equine sarcoids from other soft tissue sarcomas, as viral DNA also has been detected in a variety of soft tissue tumors including fibrosarcomas, PNSTs, fibromas, and myxosarcomas.[77,79] Please refer to Chapter 21 for more detailed information regarding the cytology of sarcoids.

References

1 Kandel, L.H.R., Davis, A., Bell, R. et al. (1994). Histological necrosis in soft tissue sarcoma following preoperative irradiation. *J Surg Oncol* 57: 111–114.

2 MacDermed, D.M., Miller, L.L., Peabody, T.D. et al. (2010). Primary tumor necrosis predicts distant control in locally advanced soft tissue sarcomas following preoperative concurrent chemoradiotherapy. *Int J Radiat Oncol Biol Phys* 76: 1147–1153.

3 Geisinger, K.R. and Abdul-Karim, F.W. (2014). Fine-needle aspiration biopsy of soft tissue tumors. In: *Enzinger and Weiss's Soft Tissue tumors*, 6e (eds. J.R. Goldblum, A.L. Folpe and S.W. Weiss), 110–126. Philadelphia, PA: Saunders.

4 Goldblum, J., Folpe, A., and Weiss, S. (2014). Perivascular tumors. In: *Enzinger and Weiss's Soft Tissue Tumors*, 6e (eds. J.R. Goldblum, A.L. Folpe and S.W. Weiss), 749–765. Philadelphia, PA: Saunders.

5 Mazzei, M., Millanta, F., Citi, S. et al. (2002). Hemangiopericytoma: histological spectrum, immunohistochemical characterization and prognosis. *Vet Dermatol* 13: 15–21.

6 Caniatti, M., Ghisleni, G., Ceruti, R. et al. (2001). Cytological features of canine hemangiopericytoma in fine needle aspiration biopsy. *Vet Rec* 149: 242–244.

7 Pérez, J., Bautista, M., Rollón, E. et al. (1996). Immunohistochemical characterization of hemangiopericytomas and other spindle cell tumors in the dog. *Vet Pathol* 33: 391–397.

8 Avallone, G., Helmbold, P., Caniatti, M. et al. (2007). The spectrum of canine cutaneous perivascular wall tumors: morphologic, phenotypic and clinical characterization. *Vet Pathol* 44: 607–620.

9 Cian, F., Stewart, J., Minshall, G.J., and Wright, I.M. (2015). What is your diagnosis? Swelling of the left antebrachium and carpus in a horse. *Vet Clin Pathol* 44: 609–610.

10 Johannes, C., Henry, C., Turnquist, S.E. et al. (2007). Hemangiosarcoma in cats: 53 cases (1992–2002). *J Am Vet Med Assoc* 231: 1851–1856.

11 Johns, I., Stephen, J.O., Del Piero, F. et al. (2005). Hemangiosarcoma in 11 young horses. *J Vet Intern Med* 19: 564–570.

12 Ward, H., Fox, L.E., Calderwood-Mays, M.B. et al. (1994). Cutaneous hemangiosarcoma in 25 dogs: a retrospective study. *J Vet Intern Med* 8: 345–348.

13 Bertazzolo, W., Dell'Orco, M., Bonfanti, U. et al. (2005). Canine angiosarcoma: cytologic, histologic, and immunohistochemical correlations. *Vet Clin Pathol* 34: 28–34.

14 Didier, M. and Bertazzolo, W. (2015). Corner diagnostico, citologia. *Veterinaria (Cremona)* 29: 51–52.

15 Boucher, L.D., Swanson, P.E., Stanley, M.W. et al. (2000). Cytology of angiosarcoma. Findings in fourteen fine-needle aspiration biopsy specimens and one pleural fluid specimen. *Am J Clin Pathol* 114: 210–219.

16 Bird, K.E., Farrar, W.P., and Whitney, M.S. (1996). What is your diagnosis? *Vet Clin Pathol* 25: 90–92.

17 Minimo, C., Zakowski, M., and Lin, O. (2002). Cytologic findings of malignant vascular neoplasms: a study of twenty-four cases. *Diagn Cytopathol* 26: 349–355.

18 Post, K., Clark, E.G., and Gent, I.B. (1991). Cutaneous lymphangioma in a young dog. *Can Vet J* 32: 747–748.

19 Khurana, K.K. and Mortelliti, A.J. (2001). The role of fine-needle aspiration biopsy in the diagnosis and management of juvenile hemangioma of the parotid gland and cheek. *Arch Pathol Lab Med* 125: 1340–1343.

20 Layfield, L.J. and Mooney, E.E. (1998). Not by blood alone: diagnosis of hemangiomas by fine-needle aspiration. *Diagn Cytopathol* 19: 250–254.

21 Goldblum, J., Folpe, A., and Weiss, S. (2014). Malignant vascular tumors. In: *Enzinger and Weiss's Soft Tissue Tumors*, 6e (eds. J.R. Goldblum, A.L. Folpe and S.W. Weiss), 703–732. Philadelphia, PA: Saunders.

22 Ihrke, P.J., Walder, E.J., and Affolter, V.K. (2005). Vascular tumors. In: *Skin Diseases of the Dog and Cat*, 2e (eds. T.L. Gross, P.J. Ihrke and E.J. Walder), 735–758. Ames, IA: Blackwell.

23 Gerding, J.C., Gilger, B.C., Montgomery, S.A., and Clode, A.B. (2015). Presumed primary ocular lymphangiosarcoma with metastasis in a miniature horse. *Vet Ophthalmol* 18: 502–509.

24 Jackson, D.E., Berent, L.M., Cohn, L.A., and Senter, D.A. (2011). Locally invasive lymphangiosarcoma in a young domestic shorthair. *J Feline Med Surg* 13: 796–799.

25 Puff, C., Herder, V., Philipp, A., and Baumgärtner, W. (2008). Lymphangiosarcoma in the nictitating membrane of a horse. *J Vet Diagn Invest* 20: 108–110.

26 Webb, J.A., Boston, S.E., Armstrong, J., and Moens, N.M. (2004). Lymphangiosarcoma associated with primary lymphedema in a Bouvier des Flandres. *J Vet Intern Med* 18: 122–124.

27 Hinrichs, U., Puhl, S., Rutteman, G.R. et al. (1999). Lymphangiosarcomas in cats: a retrospective study of 12 cases. *Vet Pathol* 36: 164–167.

28 Goldblum, J., Folpe, A., and Weiss, S. (2014). Liposarcoma. In: *Enzinger and Weiss's Soft Tissue Tumors*, 6e (eds. J.R. Goldblum, A.L. Folpe and S.W. Weiss), 484–523. Philadelphia, PA: Saunders.

29 Messick, J.B. and Radin, M.J. (1989). Cytologic, histologic, and ultrastructural characteristics of a canine myxoid liposarcoma. *Vet Pathol* 26: 520–522.

30 Doria-Torra, G., Martínez, J., Domingo, M. et al. (2015). Liposarcoma in animals: literature review and case report in a domestic pig (*Sus scrofa*). *J Vet Diagn Invest* 27: 196–202.

31 Kondo, H., Wickins, S.C., Conway, J.A. et al. (2012). Cranial mediastinal liposarcoma in a horse. *Vet Pathol* 49: 1040–1042.

32 Cramer, S.D., Porter, K.L., Rochat, M.C., and Lamm, C.G. (2011). Pathology in practice. Liposarcoma. *J Am Vet Med Assoc* 239: 757–759.

33 Baez, J.L., Hendrick, M.J., Shofer, F.S. et al. (2004). Liposarcomas in dogs: 56 cases (1989–2000). *J Am Vet Med Assoc* 224: 887–891.

34 Piseddu, E., De Lorenzi, D., Freeman, K., and Masserdotti, C. (2011). Cytologic, histologic, and immunohistochemical features of lingual liposarcoma in a dog. *Vet Clin Pathol* 40: 393–397.

35 Romsland, T.D., Wills, T.B., Haldorson, G.J. et al. (2011). What is your diagnosis? Lingual mass in a dog. *Vet Clin Pathol* 40: 561–562.

36 Lanevschi, A., Lapointe, J.M., Bélanger, J.F., and Noël, D. (1999). Fine needle aspirate of a subcutaneous mass on the forelimb of a dog. *Vet Clin Pathol* 28: 46–48.

37 Wakely, P.E. (1999). Myxoid soft tissue tumors: correlation of cytopathology and histopathology. *Ann Diagn Pathol* 3: 227–242.

38 Masserdotti, C., Bonfanti, U., De Lorenzi, D., and Ottolini, N. (2006). Use of Oil Red O stain in the cytologic diagnosis of canine liposarcoma. *Vet Clin Pathol* 35: 37–41.

39 Ihrke, P.J., Walder, E.J., and Affolter, V.K. (2005). Lipocytic tumors. In: *Skin Diseases of the Dog and Cat*, 2e (eds. T.L. Gross, P.J. Ihrke and E.J. Walder), 760–777. Ames, IA: Blackwell.

40 Goldblum, J., Folpe, A., and Weiss, S. (2014). Malignant peripheral nerve sheath tumors. In: *Enzinger and Weiss's Soft Tissue Tumors*, 6e (eds. J.R. Goldblum, A.L. Folpe and S.W. Weiss), 855–879. Philadelphia, PA: Saunders.

41 Buza, E.L., Menzies, R.A., Goldschmidt, M.H., and Durham, A.C. (2012). Malignant peripheral nerve sheath tumor in a cat with nodal and pulmonary metastases. *J Vet Diagn Invest* 24: 781–784.

42 Da Costa, R.C., Parent, J.M., Dobson, H. et al. (2008). Ultrasound-guided fine needle aspiration in the diagnosis of peripheral nerve sheath tumors in 4 dogs. *Can Vet J* 49: 77–81.

43 Gaitero, L., Añor, S., Fondevila, D., and Pumarola, M. (2008). Canine cutaneous spindle cell tumors with features of peripheral nerve sheath tumors: a histopathological and immunohistochemical study. *J Comp Pathol* 139: 16–23.

44 Snyder, L.A., Linder, K.E., and Neel, J.A. (2007). Malignant peripheral nerve sheath tumor in a hamster. *J Am Assoc Lab Anim Sci* 46: 55–57.

45 Tremblay, N., Lanevschi, A., Doré, M. et al. (2005). Of all the nerve! A subcutaneous forelimb mass on a cat. *Vet Clin Pathol* 34: 417–420.

46 Schulman, F.Y., Johnson, T.O., Facemire, P.R., and Fanburg-Smith, J.C. (2009). Feline peripheral nerve sheath tumors: histologic, immunohistochemical, and clinicopathologic correlation (59 tumors in 53 cats). *Vet Pathol* 46: 1166–1180.

47 Ciau, N., Eisele, D.W., and van Zante, A. (2014). Epithelioid schwannoma of the facial nerve masquerading as pleomorphic adenoma: a case report. *Diagn Cytopathol* 42: 58–62.

48 Wakely, P.E., Syed, A.Z., and Bishop, J.A. (2012). The cytopathology of malignant peripheral nerve sheath tumor: a report of 55 fine-needle aspiration cases. *Cancer Cytopathol* 120: 334–341.

49 Klijanienko, J., Caillaud, J.M., Legace, R., and Vielh, P. (2002). Cytohistologic correlations of 24 malignant peripheral nerve sheath tumor (MPNST) in 17 patients: the Institut Curie experience. *Diagn Cytopathol* 27: 103–108.

50 Jimenez-Hefferman, J.A., Lopez-Ferrer, P., Vicandi, B. et al. (1999). Cytologic features of malignant peripheral nerve sheath tumors. *Acta Cytol* 43: 175–183.

51 Reis-Filho, J., Pope, L., Balderrama, M. et al. (2002). Epithelioid malignant peripheral nerve sheath tumour: case report and review of the previously published cases. *Cytopathology* 13: 54–63.

52 Chijiwa, K., Uchida, K., and Tateyama, S. (2004). Immunohistochemical evaluation of canine peripheral nerve sheath tumours and other soft tissue sarcomas. *Vet Pathol* 41: 307–318.

53 Suzuki, S., Uchida, K., and Nakayama, H. (2014). The effects of tumor location on diagnostic criteria for canine malignant peripheral nerve sheath tumors (MPNSTs) and the markers for distinction between canine MPNSTs and canine perivascular wall tumors. *Vet Pathol* 51: 722–736.

54 Nielsen, A.B., Jensen, H.E., and Leifsson, P.S. (2011). Immunohistochemistry for 2′,3′-cyclic nucleotide-3′-phosphohydrolase in 63 bovine peripheral nerve sheath tumors. *Vet Pathol* 48: 796–802.

55 Murcia, P.R., Delhon, G., González, M.J. et al. (2008). Cluster of cases of malignant schwannoma in cattle. *Vet Rec* 163: 331–335.

56 Higginbotham, M.L., McCaw, D.L., Anderson, D.E. et al. (2015). Treatment of a maxillary fibrosarcoma in an adult alpaca. *J Am Vet Med Assoc* 246: 674–680.

57 Goldblum, J., Folpe, A., and Weiss, S. (eds.) (2014). Borderline and malignant fibroblastic/myofibroblastic tumors. In: *Enzinger and Weiss's Soft Tissue Tumors*, 6e, 288–340. Philadelphia, PA: Saunders.

58 Findlay, J.A., Singer, E.R., Milner, P.I., and Leeming, G.H. (2014). Use of immunohistochemical staining and electron microscopy to aid in diagnosis of soft tissue sarcomas associated with the fetlock joint in two horses. *J Vet Diagn Invest* 26: 465–469.

59 Steele, H. (2001). Subcutaneous fibrosarcoma in an aged guinea pig. *Can Vet J* 42: 300–302.

60 Ihrke, P.J., Walder, E.J., and Affolter, V.K. (2005). Fibrous tumors. In: *Skin Diseases of the Dog and Cat*, 2e (eds. T.L. Gross, P.J. Ihrke and E.J. Walder), 710–734. Ames, IA: Blackwell.

61 Bacon, N.J., Dernell, W.S., Ehrhart, N. et al. (2007). Evaluation of primary re-excision after recent inadequate resection of soft tissue sarcomas in dogs: 41 cases (1999–2004). *J Am Vet Med Assoc* 230: 548–554.

62 Dillon, C.J., Mauldin, G.N., and Baer, K.E. (2005). Outcome following surgical removal of nonvisceral soft tissue sarcomas in cats: 42 cases (1992–2000). *J Am Vet Med Assoc* 227: 1955–1957.

63 Little, L.K. and Goldschmidt, M. (2007). Cytologic appearance of a keloidal fibrosarcoma in a dog. *Vet Clin Pathol* 36: 364–367.

64 Story, M.R., Gaughan, E.M., Andrews, G.A., and Balch, S. (2005). Fibrosarcoma over the tarsal groove of a 14-month-old Quarter horse. *Vet Comp Orthop Traumatol* 18: 115–118.

65 Johnson, J.G. 3rd, Blair, R., Brandão, J. et al. (2014). Atypical fibrosarcoma in the skin of a Roborovski hamster (*Phodopus roborovskii*). *Vet Clin Pathol* 43: 281–284.

66 McEntee, M.F. (1991). Equine cutaneous mastocytoma: morphology, biological behaviour and evolution of the lesion. *J Comp Pathol* 104: 71–78.

67 Nasit, J.G. and Dhruva, G. (2015). Fibroma of the tendon sheath: a diagnostic dilemma on fine-needle aspiration cytology. *J Cytol* 32: 207–209.

68 Hendrick, M.J. and Brooks, J.J. (1994). Postvaccinal sarcomas in the cat: histology and immunohistochemistry. *Vet Pathol* 31: 126–129.

69 Munday, J.S., Stedman, N.L., and Richey, L.J. (2003). Histology and immunohistochemistry of seven ferret vaccination-site fibrosarcomas. *Vet Pathol* 40: 288–293.

70 Vascellari, M., Melchiotti, E., Bozza, M., and Mutinelli, F. (2003). Fibrosarcomas at presumed sites of injection in dogs: characteristics and comparison with non-vaccination site fibrosarcomas and feline post-vaccinal fibrosarcomas. *J Vet Med, A* 50: 286–291.

71 Haddad, J.L., Goldschmidt, M.H., and Patel, R.T. (2010). Fibrosarcoma arising at the site of a retained surgical sponge in a cat. *Vet Clin Pathol* 39: 241–246.

72 Rayner, E.L., Scudamore, C.L., Francis, I., and Schöniger, S. (2010). Abdominal fibrosarcoma associated with a retained surgical swab in a dog. *J Comp Pathol* 143: 81–85.

73 Daly, M.K., Saba, C.F., Crochik, S.S. et al. (2008). Fibrosarcoma adjacent to the site of microchip implantation in a cat. *J Feline Med Surg* 10: 202–205.

74 Vascellari, M., Melchiotti, E., and Mutinelli, F. (2006). Fibrosarcoma with typical features of postinjection sarcoma at site of microchip implant in a dog: histologic and immunohistochemical study. *Vet Pathol* 43: 545–548.

75 Couto, S.S., Griffey, S.M., Duarte, P.C., and Madewell, B.R. (2002). Feline vaccine-associated fibrosarcoma: morphologic distinctions. *Vet Pathol* 39: 33–41.

76 Scruggs, J.L. and LeBlanc, C.J. (2015). Identification of blue staining vaccine-derived material in inflammatory lesions using cultured canine macrophages. *Vet Clin Pathol* 44: 152–156.

77 Martens, A., De Moor, A., Demeulemeester, J., and Ducatelle, R. (2000). Histopathological characteristics of five clinical types of equine sarcoid. *Res Vet Sci* 69: 295–300.

78 Tyler, R.D., Meinkoth, J.H., Cowell, R.L. et al. (2002). Cutaneous and subcutaneous lesions. In: *Diagnostic Cytology and Hematology of the Horse*, 2e (eds. R.L. Cowell and R.D. Tyler), 19–42. St. Louis, MO: Mosby.

79 Epperson, E.D. and Castleman, W.L. (2017). Bovine papillomavirus DNA and S100 profiles in sarcoids and other cutaneous spindle cell tumors in horses. *Vet Pathol* 54: 44–52.

Part IV

Ear and Eye

17

Ear Cytology

Susan Lowum, Sandra Nogueira Koch, and Leslie C. Sharkey

Introduction

This chapter focuses on external ear canal cytology of otitis with a brief review of other conditions amenable to cytologic evaluation. Diseases of the pinnae have been reviewed.[1] Otitis externa is common in dogs and cats.[2] Clinical signs of otitis include odor, scratching or rubbing of ears and head, head shaking, pain or sensitivity, behavior changes, and hearing loss. Animals present with erythema, inflammation, otic discharge, ulcerated ear canals, pinnal alopecia, excoriation, and crusts. Chronic cases exhibit pinnal hyperkeratosis, hyperpigmentation, lichenification, ear canal hyperplasia, and stenosis.

Predisposing causes include allergy and other immune-mediated disease, parasites, keratinization disorders, hypothyroidism, inflammatory polyps, neoplasia, and foreign objects.[3] Ear conformation, excessive moisture, and iatrogenic irritation can contribute.[3,4] Otic cytology is an effective diagnostic tool routinely used in patients with ear disease.

Sample Collection and Slide Preparation

Samples are collected after otoscopic examination but prior to cleaning or treatment. Even with unilateral signs, separate samples should be collected from each ear to allow comparison and for early recognition of subclinical pathology.[5] Most cases of otitis externa are bilateral with clinically relevant differences in cytological findings between ears.[3,6,7] Cotton-tipped swabs target the junction of the vertical and horizontal ear canals.[6–8] For larger dogs, the otoscope enables visualization of the horizontal canal, and the sampling swab can be passed through the cone. Sampling complications are uncommon; however proper head position and restraint is important to avoid trauma. Sampling from masses is similar to other sites (Chapter 1).

Heat fixation of slides is common, but does not impact yeast recovery.[9,10] Modified Wright's stain such as Diff-Quik (Baxter Scientific Products, McGaw Park, Illinois) is commonly used and has good agreement with rapid Gram stains for organism detection.[11] If parasites are suspected, a separate slide is prepared by collecting a large quantity of otic exudate and mixing with mineral oil on an unfixed and unstained slide for examination at low magnification.[7]

If repeat collection is required, there is good agreement for identification and quantitation of bacteria for two serially collected smears, but the second smear may fail to contain yeast.[4] Samples can be obtained deeper in the horizontal canal from patients anesthetized for flushes or video otoscopy. If otitis media is suspected with an intact tympanum, samples should be collected via myringotomy since microbial populations differ between compartments.[5,6] Highly cellular samples can be prepared from external ear canal masses of anesthetized cats via gentle aspiration with a soft rubber catheter after washing of the canal with warm saline.[12]

Normal Histologic Architecture

The pinnae consist of a cartilaginous core covered by haired skin and numerous small muscles for mobility.[13] The external ear canal is similar; however hair is variably sparse depending on breed, becoming scant deeper in the canal. Sebaceous and ceruminous glands are present in the external canal. The middle and inner ear sections are anatomically complex, containing epithelial and mesenchymal structures and closely associated with major nerves such as the facial and vestibulocochlear cranial nerves.[13]

Veterinary Cytology, First Edition. Edited by Leslie C. Sharkey, M. Judith Radin, and Davis Seelig.

Diagnostic Approach and Normal Cytology of the External Canal

After low power scanning, 5–10 high power fields are examined, and the average yeast, bacteria, and leukocyte counts and morphology are recorded.[5,7] Normal cytology includes cornified squamous epithelial cells (Figure 17.1), which may contain melanin granules that can be confused with bacteria.[7] Small numbers of commensal cocci (*Staphylococcus* and *Streptococcus* spp.) can be present, while rods are rarely present in healthy ears, except for *Corynebacterium* sp.[7,14] Leukocytes are always abnormal, so bacteria in the presence of leukocytes signal infection. A few *Malassezia* spp. can be normal; however, overgrowth signals opportunistic pathology.

Conditions of the External Canal Diagnosed by Cytology

Malassezia

With predisposing factors, *Malassezia pachydermatis* is the most common cause of mycotic otitis externa.[7,15,16] *Malassezia* is more commonly seen in ears with otitis than in normal ears.[5,15,17,18] *Malassezia* is a basophilic staining yeast from 2.0×4.0 up to 6.0×7.0 µm.[19] Unipolar broad-based budding creates a "footprint," "snowman," "peanut," or "bowling pin" morphology (Figure 17.2a); however, ellipsoid or globose shapes are described. Concurrent suppurative inflammation is uncommon.[5–7]

Cytologic semiquantitative assessment of organism burden is recommended with thresholds of 2 or fewer yeast organisms per 400× field considered normal.[20] Mean counts of >5 yeast/field in dogs and >12 in cats are abnormal.[20] Using these values, cytology had a specificity of 95% in dogs and 100% for mycotic otitis in cats compared with culture results. The sensitivity was only 50% for dogs and 63% in cats due to some cases of otitis externa being exclusively bacterial. Another study suggested a threshold of 10 total yeast in the sum of five 400× fields for a diagnosis of yeast otitis.[15] *Malassezia* culture is not recommended due to low organism recovery.[15] Ultimately, cytologic findings must be integrated with history and clinical signs for diagnosis.

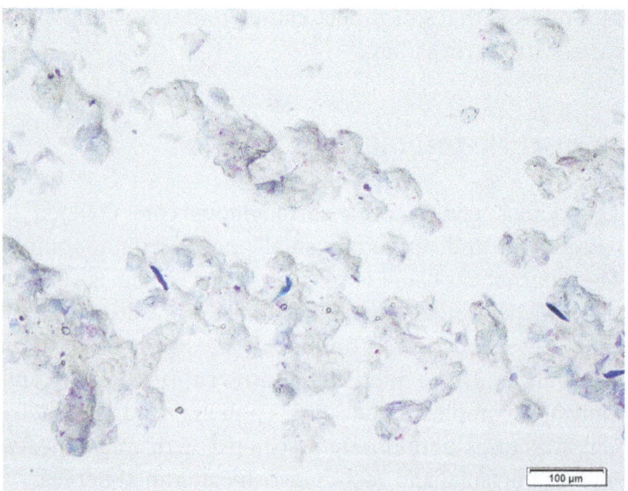

Figure 17.1 Cytology from normal canine ear canal swab showing cornified squamous epithelial cells (Wright's, 500×).

Other Less Common Mycotic Infections

Candida spp. and *Aspergillus* spp. are uncommon causes of otitis externa with risk factors such as immunosuppression and otic foreign bodies. *Candida albicans* is a normal resident of the gastrointestinal tract and skin of dogs and cats.[5] *Candida* spp. are thin-walled, round to oval, with a halo around the yeast body and can form short, tubular, and septate pseudohyphae. *Aspergillus* spp. are saprophytic environmental fungi and septate hyphae can be seen on cytology. A recent study showed that *Aspergillus* spp. otitis is more typically seen as unilateral otitis externa in cats and larger breed dogs.[21] *Aspergillus fumigatus* was the most common isolate overall and was the dominant isolate in cats. *Aspergillus niger* and *Aspergillus terreus* were the most commonly isolated species from dogs.

Bacteria

Bacteria are also common commensals, many of which are potentially pathogenic. The most common pathogens are coagulase-positive *Staphylococcus* spp., B-hemolytic *Streptococcus* spp., *Pseudomonas* spp., *Proteus* spp., and *Escherichia coli*.[7] Mixed infections are common, including yeast. Cytology generally reveals large numbers of extracellular bacteria (Figure 17.2b). Proposed semiquantitative cytologic criteria use a normal threshold of <5/400× field in dogs and <4 in cats, whereas >25 in dogs and >15 in cats suggest overgrowth or infection.[5,20] For 1000×, <2 bacteria/field is normal, and >10 is abnormal.[5] Using these mean count criteria to differentiate normal from bacterial otitis externa ears yielded 95% specificity and 50% sensitivity in dogs and 100% specificity and 63% sensitivity in cats when compared with culture.[20]

Leukocytes are only present in cytological samples from abnormal ears and are rarely associated with bacterial overgrowth; intracellular bacteria tend to be the most pathogenic.[5] Leukocytes in the external canal increase the suspicion for concurrent otitis media, warranting cytology and

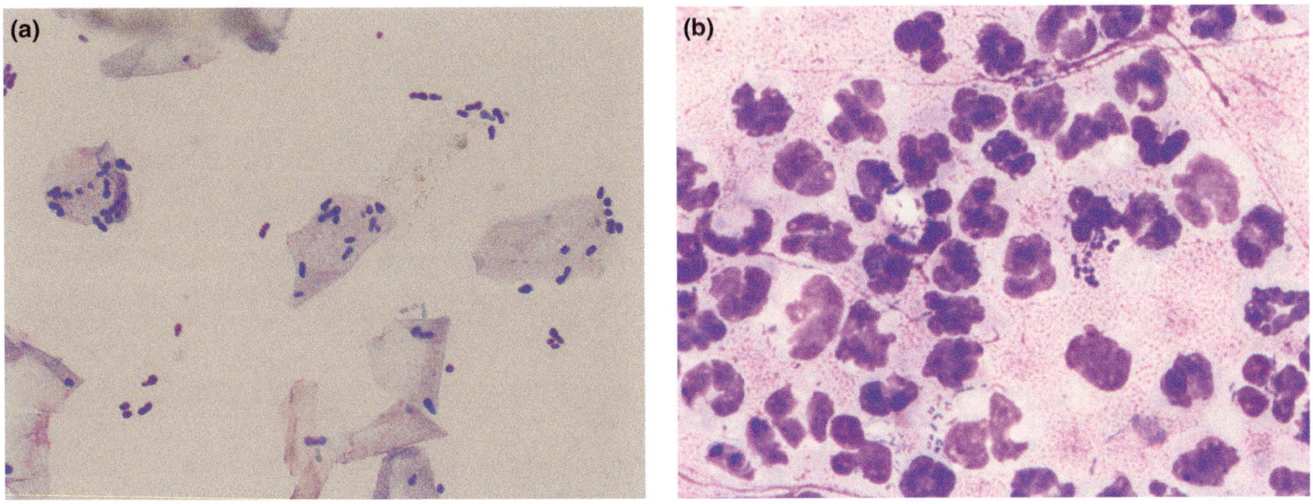

Figure 17.2 (a) Squamous epithelial cells with many *Malassezia* sp. organisms characterized by broad-based, budding yeast organisms (Wright's, 500×). (b) Bacterial infection showing degenerate neutrophils with cocci and rods (Wright's, 1000×).

culture and susceptibility samples from the external canal and the middle ear because of the likelihood of concurrent infection, which is four times more common in chronic than acute disease.[5,7]

When routine therapy is ineffective or whenever rods are present, culture and sensitivity are indicated.[22] Culture should never be used as the sole diagnostic test in diagnosing or monitoring response to treatment due to commensal bacteria and because of variability in culture results between paired samples.[23] Cytology has been reported to both over- and underdiagnose bacterial infection compared with culture. In normal ears Gram-positive cocci bacteria were identified by cytology in 42% of the dogs, but only 25% by culture, while a study of otitis externa in dogs revealed 68% agreement with culture, culture revealing more organisms in 80% of cases and fewer in 20% of cases, concluding that cytology may be a more realistic reflection of major pathogens.[5,23]

Parasites

Otodectes cynotis (ear mite) accounts for up to 50% of otitis externa in cats and 10% in dogs, typically associated with dry reddish-brown to black granular discharge.[3,7,24] It is not species specific and is highly contagious. Secondary bacterial and/or yeast infections often occur.

O. cynotis is a large-bodied mite easily observed on unstained smears on low power (Figure 17.3). It has a psoroptiform body type similar to *Sarcoptes* spp., but is larger with short unjointed pedicles extending from the legs.[7] Adult females are approximately 280 μm wide and 450 μm long. Males are slightly smaller. Other life stages observed include protonymph, larva, and eggs. Identification of a single egg or mite of any life stage provides a definitive diagnosis. Absence of mites does not exclude infection and a miticidal treatment trial should be implemented in suspected cases.[5] Other mites occasionally found on cytologic preparations include *Demodex* spp., *Sarcoptes scabiei, Notoedres cati, Eutrombicula alfreddugesi*, and *Neotrombicula autumnalis.*[5,7]

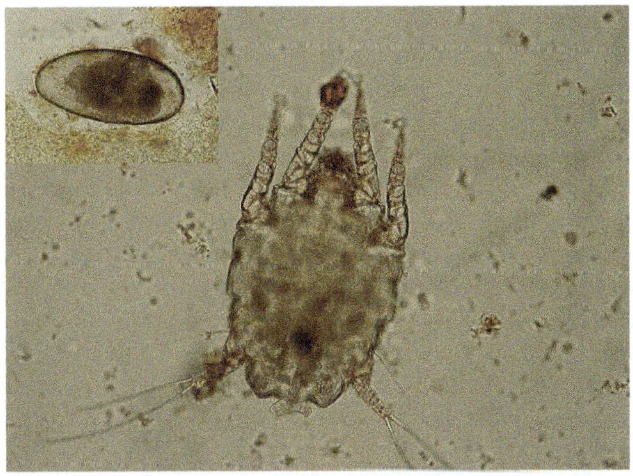

Figure 17.3 Ear mite (*O. cynotis*) on an unstained smear of ear canal secretions. (100×) Inset demonstrates an egg.

Noninfectious Inflammatory Diseases

The most common noninfectious diseases are atopic dermatitis and allergic/irritant contact otitis from topical medications. Uncommon noninfectious inflammatory diseases of the ear canal include juvenile cellulitis, an immune-mediated disease causing exudative otitis externa in puppies three weeks to six months old, and pemphigus foliaceus, an autoimmune dermatitis characterized by sterile epidermal pustules, often affecting the pinnae but occasionally the external canal. Cytologic findings from pemphigus cases include non-degenerate neutrophils, eosinophils, and acantholytic keratinocytes. Diagnoses are confirmed histologically.[7]

Neoplasia of the Ear

The ear is susceptible to many neoplasms due to the complexity of the anatomy. Unilateral disease is more common, but bilateral is documented.[24] Common tumors include polyps, papillomas, basal cell tumors, histiocytomas, mast cell tumors, ceruminous gland neoplasms, squamous cell carcinomas, and carcinoma of undetermined origin; sporadic rare tumors are described.[25–31]

Polyps are inflammatory lesions with a characteristic gross appearance and are histologically characterized by fibrovascular stroma with associated mixed inflammation covered by stratified squamous or ciliated epithelium.[32,33] Characteristic cytologic features include mixed inflammation, multinucleated giant cells, and polygonal to oval epithelial cells occurring as individualized cells or in small sheets of monolayered cells. Limited data suggests accurate cytologic diagnosis in cats.[12] Cholesteatomas (aural epidermoid cysts) are nonneoplastic but expansile and destructive cystic lesions of the canine middle ear associated with inflammation or trauma.[34] Histologically, cholesteatomas consist of hyperplastic hyperkeratotic epithelial cells without adnexa surrounded by a fibrous layer accompanied by inflammation.[35] Cytologic findings are reported to include numerous anucleate keratinized squamous epithelial cells, few mature spindle cells, scattered non-degenerate neutrophils, and fewer macrophages; bacteria may be present.[34]

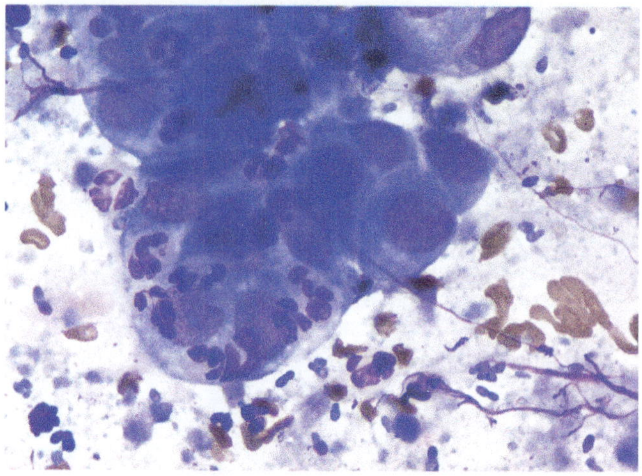

Figure 17.4 Cytology from a small pink mass of the external ear canal of a 12-year-old domestic short-haired cat with a ceruminous gland carcinoma. Atypical epithelial cells are accompanied by neutrophils with scattered *Malassezia* sp. in the background (Wright's, 1000×. *Source:* Image courtesy of Maxey Wellman).

Hyperplastic, benign neoplastic, and malignant neoplastic lesions of ceruminous and sebaceous glands occur in the external ear canal of dogs and cats.[36] An association with chronic inflammation has been postulated, particularly for ceruminous gland lesions.[37] Ceruminous gland adenocarcinoma cytology in cats consists of numerous highly anaplastic epithelial cells often forming papillary, tubular, or acinar arrangements with associated suppurative inflammation (Figure 17.4). Nuclear molding and normal mitotic figures are common; black intracytoplasmic granular material is ubiquitous.[12] Ceruminous cystomatosis in cats has a variable cytologic appearance, sometimes overlapping in atypia with adenocarcinoma; thus histopathology is recommended for diagnosis to avoid false-positive diagnosis of malignancy.[12] Malignant lesions appear to predominate in both dogs and cats.[38]

References

1 Matousek, J.L. (2004). Diseases of the ear pinna. *Vet Clin North Am Small Anim Pract* 34: 511–540.

2 Banfield Pet Hospital (2011). State of Pet Health Report 2011. https://www.banfield.com/Banfield/media/PDF/Downloads/soph/Banfield-State-of-Pet-Health-Report_2011.pdf (accessed 3 December 2019).

3 Saridomichelakis, M.N., Farmaki, R., Leontides, L.S., and Koutinas, A.F. (2007). Aetiology of canine otitis externa: a retrospective study of 100 cases. *Vet Dermatol* 18: 341–347.

4 Lehner, G., Louis, C.S., and Mueller, R.S. (2010). Reproducibility of ear cytology in dogs with otitis externa. *Vet Rec* 167: 23–26.

5 Gotthelf, L.N. (2005). Cytology and histopathology of the ear in health and disease. In: *Small Animal Ear Diseases: An Illustrated Guide*, 2e, 42–75. St. Louis, MO: Elsevier/Saunders.

6 Cole, L.K., Kwochka, K.W., Kowalski, J.J., and Hillier, A. (1998). Microbial flora and antimicrobial susceptibility patterns of isolated pathogens from the horizontal ear canal and middle ear in dogs with otitis media. *J Am Vet Med Assoc* 212: 534–538.

7 Angus, J.C. (2004). Otic cytology in health and disease. *Vet Clin North Am Small Anim Pract* 34: 411–424.

8 Dickson, D.B. and Love, D.N. (1983). Bacteriology of the horizontal ear canal of dogs. *J Small Anim Pract* 24: 413–421.

9 Toma, S., Cornegliana, L., Persico, P., and Noli, C. (2006). Comparison of 4 fixation and staining methods for the cytologic evaluation of ear canals with clinical evidence of ceruminous otitis externa. *Vet Clin Pathol* 35: 194–198.

10 Griffin, J.S., Scott, D.W., and Herb, H.N. (2007). Malassezia otitis externa in the dog: the effect of heat-fixing otic exudate for cytological analysis. *J Am Vet Med Assoc* 54: 424–427.

11 Bouassiba, C., Osthold, W., and Mueller, R.S. (2013). Comparison of four different staining methods for ear cytology of dogs with otitis externa. *Tierarztl Prax Ausg K Klientiere Heimtiere* 41: 7–15.

12 De Lorenzi, D., Bonfanti, U., Masserdotti, C., and Tranquillo, M. (2005). Fine-needle biopsy of external ear canal masses in the cat: cytologic results and histologic correlations in 27 cases. *Vet Clin Pathol* 34: 100–105.

13 Njaa, B.L., Cole, L.K., and Tabacca, N. (2012). Practical otic anatomy and physiology of the dog and cat. *Vet Clin North Am Small Anim Pract* 42: 1109–1126.

14 Kowalski, J.J. (1988). The microbial environment of the ear canal in health and disease. *Vet Clin North Am Small Anim Pract* 18: 743–754.

15 Cafarchia, C., Gallo, S., Capelli, G., and Otranto, D. (2005). Occurrence and population size of *Malassezia* spp. in the external ear canal of dogs and cats both healthy and with otitis. *Mycopathologia* 160: 143–149.

16 Miller, W.H., Griffin, C.E., and Campbell, K. (eds.) (2012). Fungal and algal skin diseases. In: *Muller and Kirk's Small Animal Dermatology*, 7e, 223–283. St. Louis, MO: Elsevier.

17 Bond, R., Saijonmaa-Koulumies, L.E., and Lloyd, D.H. (1995). Population sizes and frequency of *Malassezia pachydermatis* at skin and mucosal sites on healthy dogs. *J Small Anim Pract* 36: 147–150.

18 Crespo, M.J., Abarca, M.L., and Cabanes, F.J. (2002). Occurrence of *Malassezia* spp. in the external ear canals of dogs and cats with and without otitis externa. *Med Mycol* 40: 115–121.

19 Guillot, J. and Bond, R. (1999). *Malassezia pachydermatis*: a review. *Med Mycol* 37: 295–306.

20 Ginel, P.J., Lucena, R., Rodriquez, J.C., and Ortega, J. (2002). A semiquantitative cytological evaluation of normal and pathological samples from the external ear canal of dogs and cats. *Vet Dermatol* 13: 151–156.

21 Goodale, E.C., Outerbridge, C.A., and White, S.D. (2016). Aspergillus otitis in small animals: a retrospective study of 17 cases. *Vet Dermatol* 27: 3–e2.

22 Blue, J.L. and Wooley, R.E. (1977). Antibacterial sensitivity patterns of bacteria isolated from dogs with otitis externa. *J Am Vet Med Assoc* 171: 362–363.

23 Graham-Mize, C.A. and Rosser, E.J. (2004). Comparison of microbial isolates and susceptibility patterns from the external ear canal of dogs with otitis externa. *J Am Anim Hosp Assoc* 40: 102–108.

24 Glaze, M.B. (2012). Diseases of eyelids, claws, anal sacs, and ears. In: *Muller and Kirk's Small Animal Dermatology*, 7e (eds. W.H. Miller, C.E. Griffin and K. Campbell), 741–757. St. Louis, MO: Elsevier.

25 Zur, G. (2005). Bilateral ear canal neoplasia in three dogs. *Vet Dermatol* 16: 276–280.

26 London, C.A., Dubielzeig, R.R., Vail, D.M. et al. (1996). Evaluation of dogs and cats with tumors of the ear canal: 145 cases (1978–1992). *J Am Vet Med Assoc* 208: 1413–1418.

27 Park, J.K., Lee, S.K., Park, S.J. et al. (2010). Fibroma with osseous metaplasia of external auditory canal in a dog. *J Vet Diagn Invest* 22: 635–638.

28 Van Goethem, B., Bosmans, T., and Chiers, K. (2010). Surgical resection of a mature teratoma on the head of a young cat. *J Am Anim Hosp Assoc* 46: 121–126.

29 Romanucci, M., Alatesta, D., Marinelli, A. et al. (2011). Aural carcinoma with chondroid metaplasia at metastatic sites in a dog. *Vet Dermatol* 22: 373–377.

30 Mineshige, T., Sugahara, G., Ohmuro, T. et al. (2015). Lymphangiosarcoma with bone formation of the auricle in a dog. *J Vet Med Sci* 77: 739–742.

31 Mineshige, T., Kawarai, S., Yauchi, T. et al. (2016). Cutaneous epitheliotropic T-cell lymphoma with systemic dissemination in a dog. *J Vet Diagn Invest* 28: 327–331.

32 Pratschke, K.M. (2003). Inflammatory polyps of the middle ear in 5 dogs. *Vet Surg* 32: 292–296.

33 Fan, T.M. and de Lorimier, L.P. (2004). Inflammatory polyps and aural neoplasia. *Vet Clin North Am Small Anim Pract* 34: 489–509.

34 Newman, A.W., Estey, C.M., McDonough, S. et al. (2014). Cholesteatoma and meningoencephalitis in a dog with chronic otitis externa. *Vet Clin Pathol* 44: 157–163.

35 Banco, B., Grieco, V., Di Giancamillo, M. et al. (2014). Canine aural cholesteatoma: a histological and immunohistological study. *Vet J* 200: 440–445.

36 Sula, M.J.M. (2012). Tumors and tumorlike lesions of dog and cat ears. *Vet Clin North Am Small Anim Pract* 42: 1161–1178.

37 Vickers, T.W., Clifford, D.L., Garcelon, D.K. et al. (2015). Pathology and epidemiology of ceruminous gland tumors among endangered Santa Catalina Island foxes (Urocyon littoralis catalinae) in the Channel Islands, USA. *PLoS One* 10 (11): e0143211.

38 Moisan, P.G. and Watson, G.L. (1996). Ceruminous gland tumors in dogs and cats: a review of 124 cases. *J Am Anim Hosp Assoc* 32: 449–453.

18

Collection of Ophthalmic Cytology Specimens

Michala de Linde Henriksen and Christine C. Lim

Introduction

Cytology is an important diagnostic technique in ophthalmic disease. However, collection from ocular and periocular tissues can be technically challenging due to the delicate nature of the tissues and the potential for iatrogenic injury. This chapter will describe guidelines for safe collection as well as indications and contraindications for collection.

Sample Collection

In most cases, samples can be collected from dogs and cats using only local anesthetic without sedation. Topical anesthesia such as proparacaine 0.5% ophthalmic solution is strongly recommended, especially when using spatulas or scalpels for collection. In horses, sedation and auriculopalpebral blocks are recommended as well. For all species, the head should be positioned by an experienced assistant to allow quick collection of diagnostic samples; movement must be minimized (Figure 18.1). For horses, the assistant should stand on the opposite side of sample to avoid interfering with sample collection (Figure 18.2).[1,2]

Scraping

In advance of sample collection, implements and slides should be arranged so that they are readily available to minimize time between collection and slide preparation. We recommend three slides for Wright–Giemsa and one for Gram staining. Instruments used to collect cytology from ocular tissue include the cytobrush, Kimura spatula, the blunt end of a sterile scalpel blade, and a cotton swab, each producing samples of different characteristics (Figure 18.3).[1–3]

Cytobrush

The cytobrush is the tool of choice for most clinicians. Samples are highly cellular with good cellular preservation and there is minimal tissue damage. Many types of cytobrush are available; the authors' preference is the "Microbrush International regular-green size 2.0 mm" disposable micro-applicators (Microbrush International, Grafton, WI). This cytobrush has a short, round head with softer brush hairs than other products. The cytobrush should be rotated several times over the area of interest before rolling the brush over the slides (Figure 18.4). In our experience, one cytobrush-collected cell sample can provide enough samples to distribute over two microscope glass slides.[1,2]

Kimura Spatula

Although not stocked in most general practices, the Kimura spatula is excellent for sampling periocular tissue, conjunctiva, and cornea. A sterile spatula is used to scrape the tissue in one direction; the spatula is then gently smeared across the surface of the slides (Figure 18.5). Samples are generally very cellular but can be unevenly distributed and cells can be damaged.[1,2,4]

Scalpel Blade

The blunt end of a sterile scalpel blade such as a no. 15. Bard-Parker blade can be used for cytology sampling (Figure 18.6). The blunt end of the blade is used in the same manner as the Kimura spatula.

Cotton Swab

The swab is rolled across the surface of the tissue to be sampled and then across the slide. Although relatively atraumatic, the number of cells obtained using cotton

Veterinary Cytology, First Edition. Edited by Leslie C. Sharkey, M. Judith Radin, and Davis Seelig.

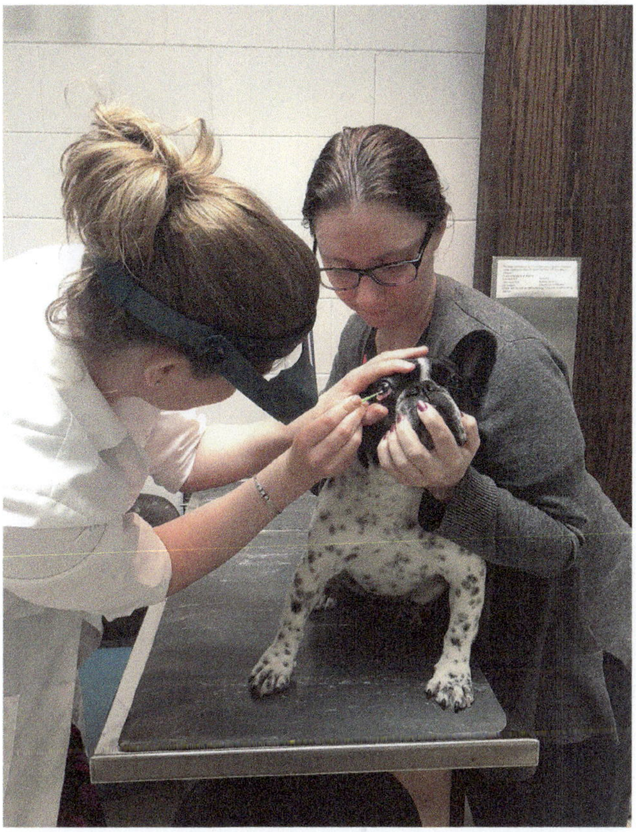

Figure 18.1 The head of the animal should be positioned by an experienced assistant to allow quick collection of diagnostic samples. Movement of the animal must be minimized by the handler, and the person collecting the sample must have a good view of the eye to minimize risk of causing excessive trauma. Magnification and a good light source also are important.

swabs is low, so other techniques are generally recommended (Figure 18.6).[4]

Fine-Needle Aspiration

Fine-needle aspiration can be used to collect cytology samples from periocular masses according to the usual protocol with some special considerations. Any instrument near the globe could potentially cause blunt or penetrating damage, emphasizing the need for appropriate analgesia and restraint. Typically, aseptic preparation with a 5% Betadine solution is followed by a local block if needed, using lidocaine 2%, via a small-bore needle (e.g. 25 or 27 G). Because injection of local anesthetic will alter cell morphology, the anesthetic should be injected around but not directly into the site of interest.[5,6]

Aqueous/Vitreous Paracentesis

Cytologic analysis of aqueous or vitreous humor is a beneficial diagnostic test for some ophthalmic diseases. These procedures are not without risk; ocular paracentesis induces uveitis.[7,8] In dogs, 27 and 30 G needles are recommended over 25 G needles as the larger needle induces significantly more uveitis than the smaller needles.[9] Both procedures can also cause more severe complications such as endophthalmitis, trauma to the iris or lens, or retinal detachment and therefore should only be performed by a

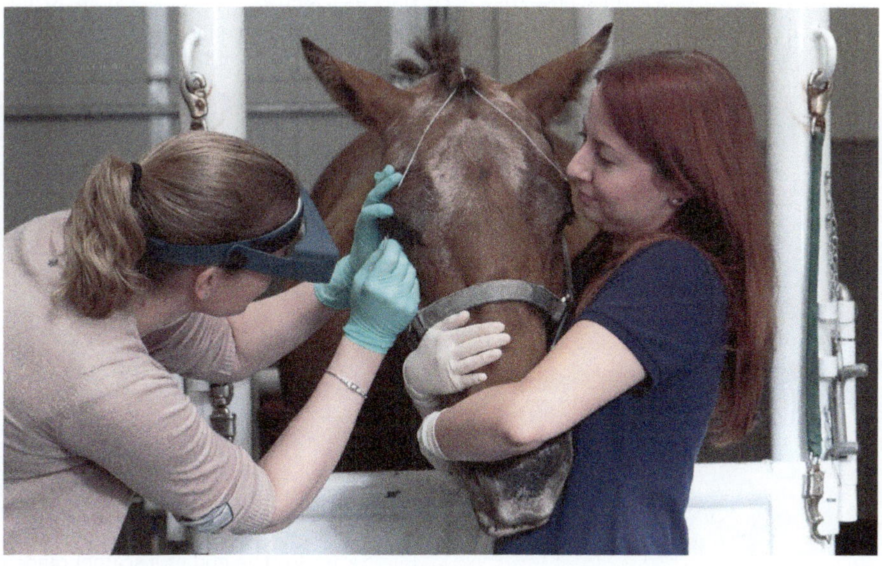

Figure 18.2 Cytology collection from the conjunctiva and cornea from horses should be performed with the assistant holding the sedated horse on the opposite side of the horse head.

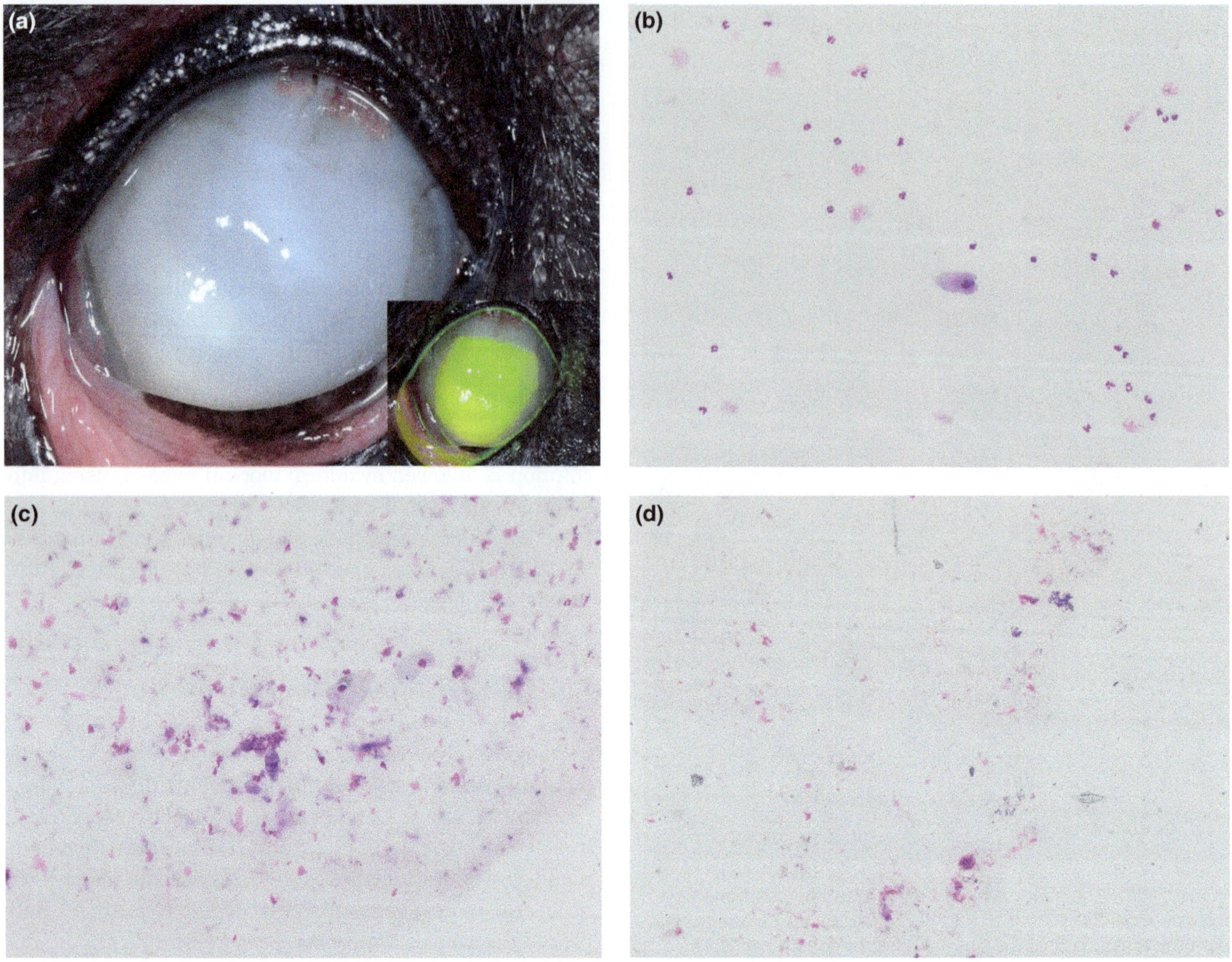

Figure 18.3 (a) A large melting corneal ulceration in a dog with corneal edema, cellular infiltration, and corneal vascularization. Inserted picture shows same melting corneal ulceration after fluorescein stain of the eye. (b) Cytology collected with a cytobrush collected from the melting corneal ulceration shown in (a). Note the intact neutrophils and corneal epithelial cells. (c) Cytology collected with the blunt end of a scalpel blade from the melting corneal ulceration shown in (a). Note the more numerous corneal epithelial cells with this type of cytology collection compared with the cytobrush. However, no intact neutrophils are present, and abundant debris is seen. (d) Cytology collected with a cotton swap from the melting corneal ulceration in (a). Note how only debris is present with no intact neutrophils or epithelial cells. This cotton swab slide illustrates why this collection method is not recommended (b–d: Wright's, 100×).

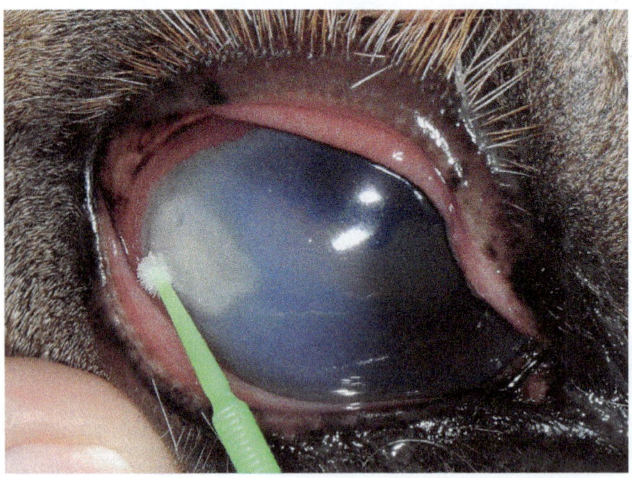

Figure 18.4 The cytobrush is an easy way of collecting conjunctival and corneal cytology with minimal tissue trauma and high quality samples.

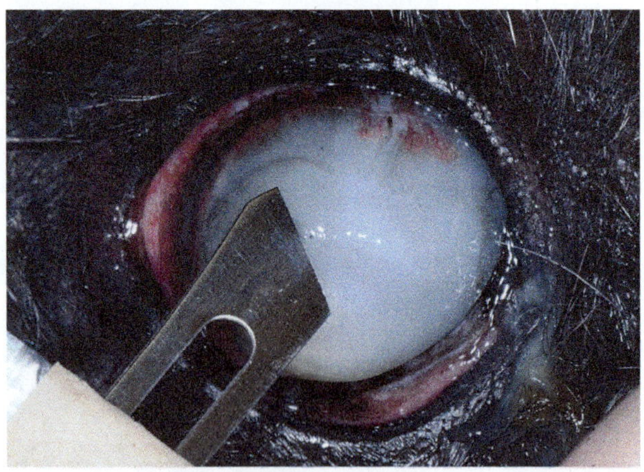

Figure 18.5 The end of a scalpel blade can be used to collect cytology from the conjunctiva and cornea but has a higher risk of traumatizing the tissue than the cytobrush and Kimura spatula. The scalpel blade also collects a large amount of normal conjunctival or corneal epithelial cells and often disrupts inflammatory cells (Figure 18.3c).

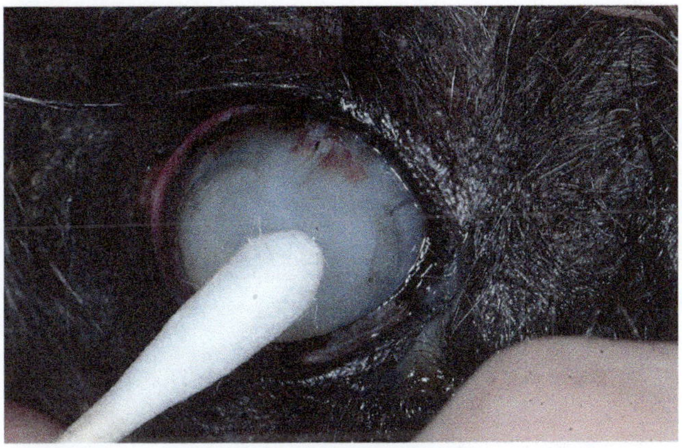

Figure 18.6 The cotton swab is a safe cytology collection method, but is not recommended due to poor sample quality (Figure 18.3d).

veterinary ophthalmologist. The complication rate following aqueous paracentesis performed by board-certified physician ophthalmologists was found to be less than 1%.[10] Veterinary studies have shown minimal risks associated with aqueous paracentesis in dogs and cats.[11] Although cytologic analysis of aqueous samples is often nondiagnostic, when interpreted in context with other diagnostic testing, it appears to be most useful for diagnosing lymphoma compared with other neoplastic and infectious/inflammatory diseases.[11,12] In an equine study, where aqueous humor was collected via aqueous paracentesis before and after intravitreous triamcinolone injection, four out of 12 eyes developed bacterial endophthalmitis.[13] The authors of this study recommend using correct ocular aseptic surgery preparation, sterile technique, and topical and systemic antibiotic before and after ocular paracentesis in horses. Consultation with specific veterinary ophthalmology textbooks is recommended for detailed descriptions of the technique for aqueous or vitreous paracentesis.[1,2]

Aqueous and vitreous humor samples submitted for cytology and/or culture and sensitivity should be placed into an ethylenediaminetetraacetic acid (EDTA) tube for cytology and a sterile plain red top tube for culture and sensitivity. Both aqueous humor and vitreous can be useful for detecting systemic and ocular diseases and, in addition to cytology and culture and sensitivity, can also be used for protein measurement, polymerase chain reaction and antibody titers (e.g. *Leptospira* spp. in horses with equine recurrent uveitis).[1,2,6]

References

1. Gilger, B.C. and Stoppini, R. (2011). Equine ocular examination: routine and advanced diagnostic techniques. In: *Equine Ophthalmology* (ed. B.C. Gilger), 1–51. Maryland Heights, MO: Elsevier.
2. Featherstone, H.J. and Heinrich, C.L. (2013). Ophthalmic examination and diagnostics. Part 1: The eye examination and diagnostic procedures. In: *Veterinary Ophthalmology*, 2e (eds. K.N. Gelatt, B.C. Gilger and T.J. Kern), 533–613. Ames, IA: Wiley-Blackwell.
3. Hodges, J. (2013). Using cytology to increase small animal practice revenue. *Vet Clin North Am Small Anim Pract* 43: 1385–1408.
4. Bauer, G.A., Spiess, B.M., and Lutz, H. (1996). Exfoliative cytology of conjunctiva and cornea in domestic animals: a comparison of four collecting techniques. *Vet Comp Ophthalmol* 6: 181–186.
5. Stone, E.A. (1995). Biopsy: principles, technical considerations, and pitfalls. *Vet Clin North Am Small Anim Pract* 25: 33–45.
6. Meinkoth, J.H. and Cowell, R.L. (2002). Sample collection and preparation in cytology: increasing diagnostic yield. *Vet Clin North Am Small Anim Pract* 32: 1187–1207.
7. Pinard, C.L., Gauvin, D., Moreau, M. et al. (2011). Measurements of canine aqueous humor inflammatory mediators and the effect of carprofen following anterior chamber paracentesis. *Vet Ophthalmol* 14: 296–303.
8. Rankin, A.J., Krohn, S.G., Glickman, N.W. et al. (2002). Laser flaremetric evaluation of experimentally induced blood-aqueous barrier disruption in cats. *Am J Vet Res* 63: 750–756.
9. Allbaugh, R.A., Roush, J.K., Rankin, A.J., and Davidson, H.J. (2011). Fluorophotometric and tonometric evaluation of ocular effects following aqueocentesis performed with needles of various sizes in dogs. *Am J Vet Res* 72: 556–561.
10. Trivedi, D., Denniston, A.K., and Murray, P.I. (2011). Safety profile of anterior chamber paracentesis performed at the slit lamp. *Clin Exp Ophthalmol* 39: 725–728.
11. Linn-Pearl, R.N., Powell, R.M., Newman, H.A., and Gould, D.J. (2015). Validity of aqueocentesis as a component of anterior uveitis investigation in dogs and cats. *Vet Ophthalmol* 18: 326–334.
12. Wiggans, K.T., Vernau, W., Lappin, M.R. et al. (2014). Diagnostic utility of aqueocentesis and aqueous humor analysis in dogs and cats with anterior uveitis. *Vet Ophthalmol* 17: 212–220.
13. Yi, N.Y., Davis, J.L., Salmon, J.H., and Gilger, B.C. (2008). Ocular distribution and toxicity of intravitreal injection of triamcinolone acetonide in normal equine eyes. *Vet Ophthalmol* 11 (S1): 15–19.

19

Ocular Cytology of the Dog

Cathy Trumel, Jean-Yves Douet, and Fanny Granat

Introduction

Cytologic evaluation of specimens collected from canine eyes can be helpful in both the diagnosis and management of ocular diseases. Cytologic analysis is a quick and simple method that can provide a specific diagnosis. It is often used in conjunction with other tests, such as bacterial culture, to optimize diagnosis and management. Conjunctival and corneal cytology in cases of suspected inflammatory lesions or fine-needle aspiration (FNA) in cases of suspected infectious uveitis or neoplasia of the globe and surrounding structures has been described in dogs. But no primary information is available for the sclera and the lens, so these topics will not be developed in this chapter. Gross identification of lesions is common, so the chapter will be enriched with images that might augment cytologic interpretation, particularly as more clinicians are including photos of lesions with cytology submission forms.

Eyelid and Adnexa

Normal Structure

The outer surface of the eyelid is covered by haired, keratinized squamous stratified epithelium. The dorsal and ventral eyelids meet at the lateral and medial canthus. Several rows of lashes are observed at the free margin of the upper eyelid of the dog. Sebaceous glands such as Meibomian gland are found along the eyelid margin. All epidermal and dermal lesions occurring elsewhere on the body can occur on the haired skin of the eyelid. See Chapters 11 and 12 for more detail on general cutaneous and subcutaneous lesions.

Inflammation

Inflammation of the eyelids (blepharitis) can involve the skin, glands, and one or both eyelids and sometimes can extend to generalized dermatological disease or can present as a localized lesion such as a granuloma or pseudotumor. If blepharitis is accompanied by conjunctivitis, it is likely to be considered an ophthalmic disease; however, if it is associated primarily with other dermatologic signs, it may be considered a skin disease and may be best addressed by a dermatologist.[1] Many noninfectious causes of blepharitis in the dog are immune mediated, occur with concurrent conjunctivitis, and include clinical signs of pruritus, redness, and ocular discharge. Histopathology is required for definitive diagnosis and the role of cytology is currently quite limited. Based on histologic characteristics, cytology should be characterized by variable, primarily non-suppurative inflammation.

Autoimmune conditions include medial canthal ulcerative blepharitis and pemphigus complex. Vogt–Koyanagi–Harada-like (or uveodermatologic) syndrome is an autoimmune disease targeting melanocytes in which intraocular signs can be accompanied by blepharitis and other mucocutaneous lesions. Canine juvenile cellulitis can involve the eyelids, periocular tissues, and face. Cellulitis is bilateral and manifests as acute onset swelling, pustules, and mandibular lymphadenopathy in puppies less than 8 months old. Cytology of the eyelid lesions reflects suppurative to pyogranulomatous inflammation but lacks microorganisms.[1,2,3] Differential diagnoses are demodicosis, dermatophytosis, distemper, drug reaction, and pyoderma. Blepharitis and conjunctivitis can be allergic and are sometimes related to atopy, and pruritus-related trauma can result in secondary bacterial infections.[1]

Veterinary Cytology, First Edition. Edited by Leslie C. Sharkey, M. Judith Radin, and Davis Seelig.

Chalazia present as yellow subconjunctival cystic masses under the eyelids that can be associated with blepharitis. They represent accumulating lipid secretions of the tarsal gland that eventually rupture, resulting in granulomatous inflammation and sometimes secondary bacterial infection. Cytology is rarely performed due to the characteristic gross appearance.

Infectious blepharitis can be caused by bacterial (*Staphylococcus* and *Streptococcus* spp.), mycotic (*Microsporum* and *Trichophyton* spp.), parasitic (*Cuterebra*), and protozoal (*Leishmania* spp.) infections that share features with the generalized cutaneous disease (Chapters 3, 11, and 12). *Malassezia* spp. are lipophilic yeast organisms that have been detected on the eyelid skin of approximately 5% of healthy dogs but might contribute to blepharitis (see Figure 17.2a). They were found in increased frequency cytologically using tape preparations in dogs with blepharitis, dogs with mucoid or mucopurulent ocular discharge, or dogs being treated with aqueous-based ophthalmic medications. The potential pathogenic role of the yeast is currently unclear. In leishmaniasis, eyelid lesions are considered to be *Leishmania* dermatitis; this will be addressed further in the section on conjunctiva.[3] Canine herpesvirus-1 (CHV-1) can cause blepharitis but is most often associated with conjunctivitis and will be discussed further in the section "Viral Conjunctivis."[4]

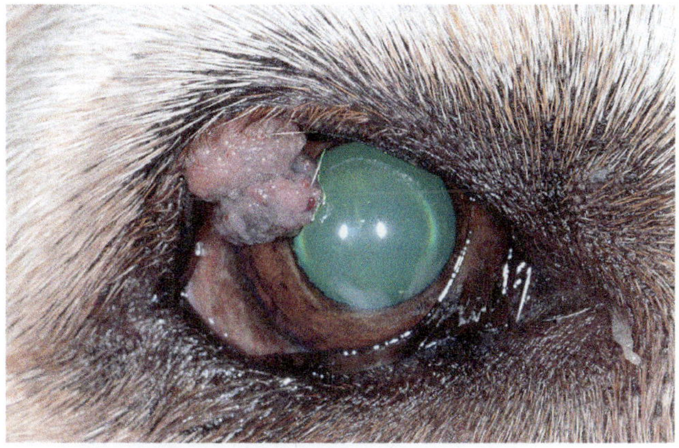

Figure 19.1 Upper eyelid Meibomian adenoma in a dog. The mass is pink in color with pigmentation and has a lobular appearance involving the eyelid margin. The mass is causing discomfort and potential risk of corneal ulcerations due to rubbing on the cornea (*Source:* Image courtesy of Michala de Linde Henriksen).

Neoplasia

Many neoplasms occur on canine eyelids, most of which are benign and of epithelial origin. Gross identification is common. Meibomian gland adenomas are the most common eyelid tumors in older dogs, although they are rare in other species.[5] These tumors arise from the inner aspect of the eyelid, characteristically forming exophytic masses emerging from the eyelid margin (Figure 19.1). They are infrequently aspirated cytologically but are histologically composed of well-differentiated sebaceous tissue and are expected to appear similar to sebaceous adenomas on cytologic examination. Meibomian carcinomas are rare.[6] A related but rare neoplasm, lobular orbital adenoma, was reported as an upper eyelid swelling in a dog. Cytology consisted of well-differentiated foamy epithelial cells exhibiting "windrowing," similar to salivary origin secretory tissue.[7] Papillomas (Figure 19.2) and squamous cell carcinomas of the eyelid can also occur in dogs and are described elsewhere (Chapters 12 and 21).

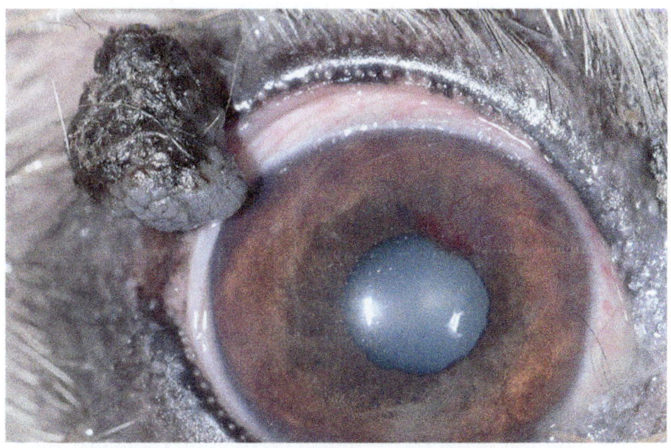

Figure 19.2 Gross photo of an upper eyelid pigmented and lobular papilloma. The papilloma is located at the eyelid margin; cytology or histopathology is required to confirm the diagnosis. The mass is rubbing on the cornea causing corneal vascularization and corneal hemorrhage and could potentially cause a corneal ulceration (*Source:* Image courtesy of Michala de Linde Henriksen.)

Benign melanocytomas are common in the eyelids of dogs, usually presenting as brown to black round masses. Interestingly, melanocytic tumors are rare in the eyelids of cats. Cytologic findings of melanocytic neoplasms are described in detail in Chapter 15, although it should be noted that even histology can have limitations in predicting the biological behavior of melanocytic neoplasia in some cases.[8] Generally, the typical cytologic criteria of malignancy are applied to melanocytic tumors. Histiocytomas and mast cell tumors are identified in the canine eyelid and are described in more detail in Chapters 12 and 13. Unilateral granular cell tumors of the eyelid have been described in a report of eight dogs. Histology was reported to be identical to similar tumors in the oral cavity; however, cytology was not reported.[9]

Conjunctivae and Nictitating Membrane

Normal Architecture and Cytology

The palpebral conjunctiva is composed of pseudostratified columnar mucous epithelium that then reverses direction at the fornix and transforms into the stratified squamous non-keratinized epithelium of the bulbar conjunctiva heading toward the cornea. Lymphoid aggregates are observed in the subepithelial connective tissue particularly on the nictitating membrane.[10]

Cytology of normal conjunctiva in dogs has not been well described and has not been correlated with histology as has been done in the horse.[11] Impression cytology of the conjunctiva has been described as containing sheets of epithelial cells. Cells from the basal, intermediate, and superficial layer were observed, occasionally containing perinuclear or dispersed brown cytoplasmic melanin granules in the superficial and intermediate cells, which were the most numerous.[12] A few goblet cells and keratinized cells were identified in 60 and 33% of specimens, respectively. Small numbers of neutrophils (33% of samples), lymphocytes, and monocytes (20% of samples) were observed. A small amount of mucus represented by dark-pink-staining strands was also observed in half of the specimens.[12]

These findings were quite similar to the results obtained from conjunctival scraping of the central palpebral conjunctiva from the lower eyelid using a Kimura spatula.[13] There was some discrepancy for goblet cells, which were only observed on the scraping performed from the fornix, likely due to the heterogeneous distribution of canine conjunctival goblet cells. Lower nasal fornix and adjacent sites, lower middle fornix, and lower nasal tarsal conjunctiva had the most goblet cells.[14] Moreover, bacteria were sometimes observed but were epicellular.[3] One study also described columnar cells, probably from the pseudostratified columnar mucous epithelium.[15]

Inflammation

Cytology is rarely performed in canine conjunctivitis and literature is scant.[13] Texts suggest that conjunctivitis without any other ocular signs in dogs is most often non-infectious and a manifestation of allergy, desiccation, or mechanical irritation. Clinically, the conjunctiva responds to insult with a limited number of mechanisms. Chemosis, hyperemia, blepharospasm, and cellular exudation characterize acute conjunctivitis. The presence of a mucopurulent discharge would be more suggestive of an infection.

Infectious

Infectious conjunctivitis with or without keratoconjunctivitis sicca (KCS) or keratitis is rare except as a manifestation of systemic diseases such as distemper, CHV-1 infection, ehrlichiosis, leishmaniosis, toxoplasmosis, Rocky Mountain spotted fever, and fungal diseases.[16] Cytology is rarely reported for diagnosis, probably because infectious agents are inconsistently observed.[17]

Bacterial Conjunctivitis

Primary bacterial conjunctivitis is uncommon in dogs. It generally occurs secondary to eyelid abnormalities, KCS, or trauma. Bacterial conjunctivitis is usually caused by *Staphylococcus* spp. and other Gram-positive organisms. Cytology is helpful to confirm the bacterial component. It is characterized by a large number of neutrophils, few mononuclear cells, and numerous bacteria (Figure 19.3).[13,18] In bacterial conjunctivitis, neutrophils remain the predominant cells even in chronic disease, but an increased number of mononuclear cells with degenerating cellular debris are observed.[13,18]

Viral Conjunctivitis

Canine distemper is a cause of viral conjunctivitis and KCS in dogs and other species. Mononuclear cells predominate early in infection, consisting of small and large lymphocytes as well as macrophages. After the primary antiviral mononuclear cell response, a neutrophilic predominance is observed, probably due to secondary bacterial conjunctivitis with increased neutrophils, goblet cells, plasma cells, and debris. Giant cells are also observed during all the stages of the disease.[13] Distemper inclusions are

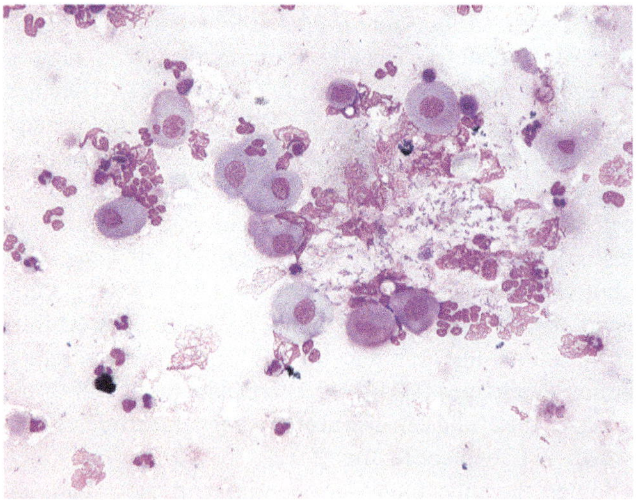

Figure 19.3 Conjunctival brushing from a dog with neutrophilic bacterial conjunctivitis. Degenerative neutrophils, numerous bacterial rods, and few epithelial cells are seen (May-Grünwald–Giemsa, 400×).

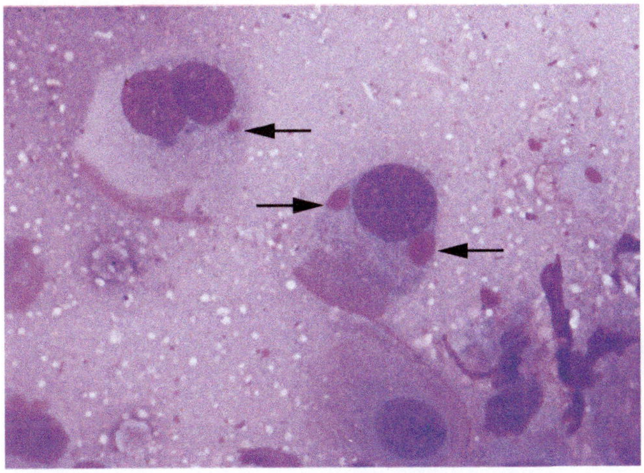

Figure 19.4 Conjunctival brushing from a dog with keratoconjunctivitis sicca secondary to distemper. Well-defined, homogeneous, azurophilic intracytoplasmic inclusions of different size are found in epithelial cells (arrows). There is a granular background rich in debris (May-Grünwald–Giemsa, 1000×).

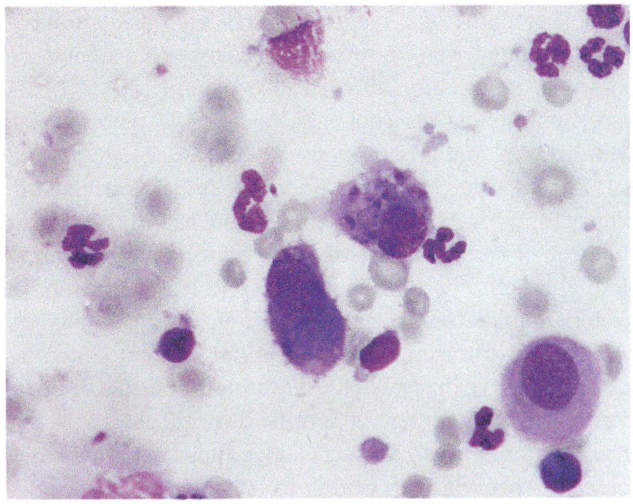

Figure 19.5 Conjunctival brushing from a dog with conjunctivitis secondary to leishmaniasis. Few red blood cells, neutrophils, lymphocytes, and three epithelial cells are observed. Multiple *Leishmania* amastigotes are observed in the cytoplasm of a cell and one is free on the background (May-Grünwald–Giemsa, 1000×).

infrequently found in the cytoplasm of conjunctival cells (Figure 19.4).[19,20] Because of the low sensitivity of cytology, direct immunofluorescence or polymerase chain reaction (PCR) testing of conjunctival samples is preferred for definitive diagnosis.[21] A virologic survey performed on 30 dogs with idiopathic conjunctivitis showed that CHV-1 and canine adenovirus-2 (CAV-2) could be common agents of conjunctivitis in dogs, including adults; cytology was not reported in this study.[20] CHV-1 presents similarly to other types of primary canine conjunctivitis, with the exception that many dogs will also exhibit petechial hemorrhages and ulceration of the conjunctiva.[4] Since detection of intranuclear inclusion bodies is unreliable, cytology is more often performed to exclude other etiologies. Recommended confirmatory testing for CHV-1 includes PCR, virus isolation, electron microscopy, or immunofluorescent antibody assay.[4]

Protozoal Conjunctivitis

Protozoal conjunctivitis has been reported in dogs as a sign of systemic disease. Primary ocular presentation can be associated with preexisting ocular surface disease (KCS, pigmentary keratitis, Meibomian adenitis) or immunosuppression (treatment with tacrolimus or cyclosporine).[22] In a survey of the prevalence of ocular lesions due to leishmaniasis in Italy, ocular manifestations were observed in two-third of the affected dogs. Anterior uveitis was the most frequent manifestation, but blepharitis and granulomatous nodular lesions in the cornea, the conjunctiva, and the eyelid were also observed. Cytology of nodular lesions of the cornea, conjunctiva, and eyelids was performed in a subset of eight dogs from a larger study of owned and shelter dogs with leishmania in Italy, and organisms were present in all samples (Figure 19.5, Chapter 3).[3] In a retrospective study of protozoal infections localized to the conjunctiva and the cornea of dogs treated with local immunosuppression, cytology results for a case of suspected *Toxoplasma gondii* infection included a granulomatous conjunctivitis and protozoal tachyzoites with rare pseudocysts (Chapter 3).[22]

Nematode Conjunctivitis

Ocular onchocercosis is a currently rare but emerging disease of predominantly adult dogs most often presenting as unilateral or asymmetrical conjunctival and/or episcleral nodules, although other ocular, retrobulbar, and periocular tissues can be involved.[23] Aberrant presentation around the larynx of a dog was reported, and cervical spinal lesions have been reported in people.[24] This disease is caused by *Onchocerca lupi* and has been rarely been reported in cats. It is zoonotic and is related to human river blindness.[25] Although sporadic, the disease range in dogs is expanding and is currently reported in the United States, Canada, Iran, Turkey, Spain, Romania, and Greece.[26–30] In the United States, southwestern states such a Colorado, Utah, California, and Nevada have been the focus of investigations. Diagnosis is often by identification of thread-like white nematodes on the surface of or just underneath the conjunctiva during examination or biopsy procedures. The nematodes have unique structural and genetic features that aid in diagnosis, including characteristic cuticular ridges on the external layer with striae on the internal layer. Histopathologic examination reveals granulation tissue and coiled well-preserved or degenerating nematode parasites; granulation tissue can be composed of fibroblasts, epithelioid macrophages, eosinophils, plasma cells, lymphocytes, and granulocytes.[26,27] Since cytology has not yet been reported, potential findings can be inferred from biopsy samples. Microfilaria can be detected in the skin of the head or ears, so skin snips are performed for examination, although microfilaria do not appear to be present in peripheral blood samples.[25] Anecdotally, medical imaging, particularly ultrasound, has potential value to identify lesions that are inaccessible to routine physical examination.[31] The development of specific serologic tests is under investigation; however, affected dogs appear to be negative for heartworm antigen testing for *Dirofilaria immitis*.[23,32] As with *D. immitis*, *Wolbachia* bacterial endosymbionts might offer a therapeutic target. These lesions may have some similarity to those described associated with *Dracunculus insignis* lesions in dogs that are characterized by the presence of larvae and inflammatory cells; however, these lesions typically occur on the limbs and trunk of dogs.[33,34]

Thelazia callipaeda is another nematode parasite of the eye that infects dogs, cats, and people and is increasingly common in Europe, although as of this writing has yet to be reported in North America to the best of our knowledge.[35–37] Organisms reside in the conjunctiva, nictitating membrane, sclera, and cornea, and dogs can be subclinical or present with conjunctivitis to corneal ulceration. Often dogs have follicular conjunctivitis, mucoid to purulent ocular discharge, and lymphoid hyperplasia. Identification of nematodes is by gross and molecular characterization using PCR.[38]

Noninfectious

Among the noninfectious causes of conjunctivitis in the dog, allergic conjunctivitis is often observed as a component of atopic dermatitis, although it can occur as an isolated manifestation.[1] Eosinophils and lymphocytes are observed in smears, which appears to be a unique cytologic finding.[17] The presence of a single eosinophil is considered diagnostic.[13] Furiani et al. have shown statistically significant higher numbers of epithelial cells, especially keratinized epithelial cells, in cytology, probably secondary to squamous metaplasia in atopic dogs.[39] Follicular conjunctivitis occurs secondary to chronic antigenic stimulation with no evidence of infectious disease. Clinically, dogs present with prominent conjunctival follicles. Follicular conjunctivitis is cytologically characterized by lymphocytes, which should be predominantly mature (Figure 19.6).[1,40] Conjunctivitis can also be observed after an irritation due to toxic chemicals, smoke, and massive amounts of particulate matter; cytologic findings are not well described. Foreign materials including cactus glochids, tarantula hairs, and setae of the pine processionary caterpillar can embed in the conjunctiva, leading to conjunctivitis and keratoconjunctivitis.[41,42] Pine processionary caterpillar setae also contain thaumetopoein, an urticating protein.

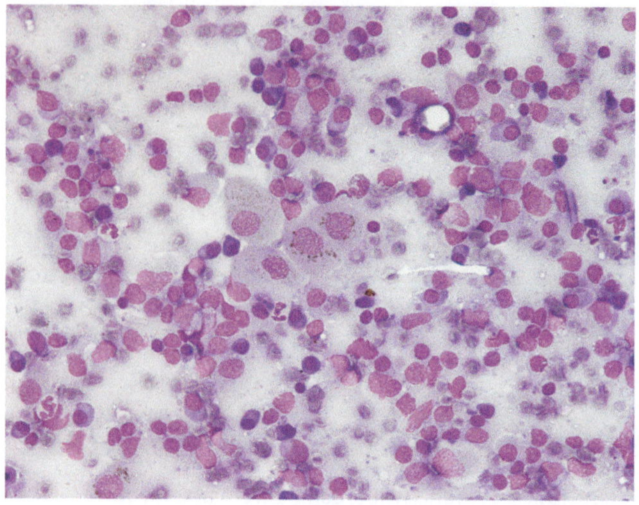

Figure 19.6 Conjunctival brushing from a dog with follicular conjunctivitis. Numerous lymphocytes, blasts, plasma cells, and few neutrophils are observed. Several epithelial cells contain melanin granules (center) (May-Grünwald–Giemsa, 400×).

Conjunctivitis can also be associated with deficient tear production, and there is variation in the literature describing the cytologic characteristics of KCS. Scrapings from dogs with chronic untreated KCS were characterized by increased amounts of mucus, goblet cells, and keratinization, while samples from dogs with acute KCS revealed bacteria, neutrophils, mucus, and debris.[13] Impression cytology of the bulbar or palpebral conjunctiva of dogs with immune-mediated KCS confirmed squamous metaplasia with keratinization and possible inflammatory cell infiltrate consisting primarily of neutrophils, but goblet cells were not observed. This observation was confirmed by a periodic acid-Schiff staining method.[43,44] Corneal and conjunctival cell metaplasia in KCS patients increased proportional to the decrease in Schirmer tear test values.[44]

Ligneous membranitis (or conjunctivitis) is an uncommon chronic membranous/pseudomembranous to proliferative and ulcerative conjunctivitis (Figure 19.7). Dogs typically present at a young age, and it is most frequently associated with congenital plasminogen deficiency, although Doberman pinschers may be an exception.[45] Ocular, oral, and genital lesions are most commonly observed. Histologically, lesions consist of hyperplastic epithelium covering expansion of the substantia propria by amorphous eosinophilic hyaline material consistent with fibrin that stains blue with Mallory PTAH stain and negatively for Congo red, excluding amyloid.[46] Cytology can consist of amorphous eosinophilic material consistent with fibrin, with or without mixed inflammatory cells.[46,47]

Neoplasia

Conjunctival neoplasia is relatively uncommon in dogs. Discrete cell neoplasms are probably the most frequent neoplasms diagnosed by FNA. Mast cell tumors of the conjunctiva are uncommon and are usually low or intermediate grade, but their diagnosis and staging are easily accomplished by FNA. Histology is recommended for confirmation and grading (see Chapter 13).[48] A study of ocular manifestations of transmissible venereal tumor (TVT) in dogs found unilateral multilobular irregular masses predominantly on the nictitating conjunctiva, but also on the upper and lower eyelids.[49] In 22/25 dogs, there was no genital manifestation. Cytologic features of ocular TVT cells include individualized large round cells with foamy cytoplasm, a high nuclear to cytoplasmic ratio (N:C), clumped chromatin, one or two prominent nucleoli, and mitotic figures.[49,50] Retrievers, Rottweilers, and Cocker Spaniels are more commonly affected by conjunctival melanoma than other breeds, and the most common site of origin is the bulbar surface of the nictitating membrane. Malignant forms are more often observed and are characterized histologically by lightly pigmented polygonal to spindle-shaped cells with a high mitotic index (Chapter 15).[7] Conjunctival lymphoma can be a component of more generalized disease. Monocentric extranodal conjunctival lymphoma is rare in dogs; a single case report indicated that cytology failed to diagnose the lymphoma, but details were lacking (Figure 19.8).[51]

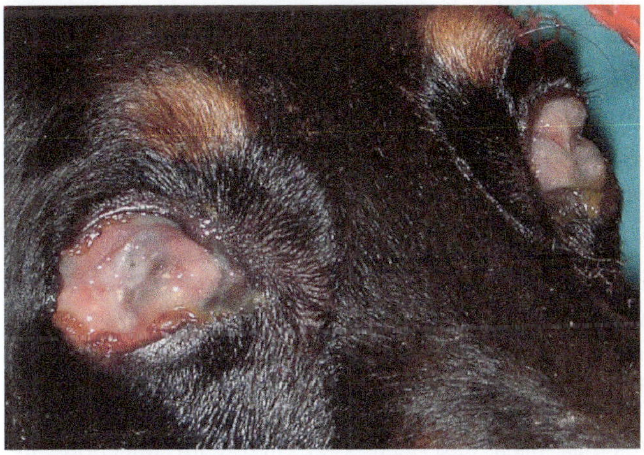

Figure 19.7 Gross photo of bilateral ligneous conjunctivitis in a dog. Severe proliferation of the conjunctiva can be appreciated in both eyes, causing the hyperemic and chemotic conjunctiva to cover the corneas. Mucopurulent discharge is present as well (*Source:* Image courtesy of Michala de Linde Henriksen).

Meibomian adenoma, conjunctival papilloma, squamous cell carcinoma (Chapter 12), preneoplastic telangiectasia, hemangioma, hemangiosarcoma (Chapter 28), and hibernoma can affect the conjunctiva; most are cytologically similar to the lesions in other anatomic locations.[52] A recent large retrospective study of canine and feline third eyelid gland neoplasms demonstrated that the most

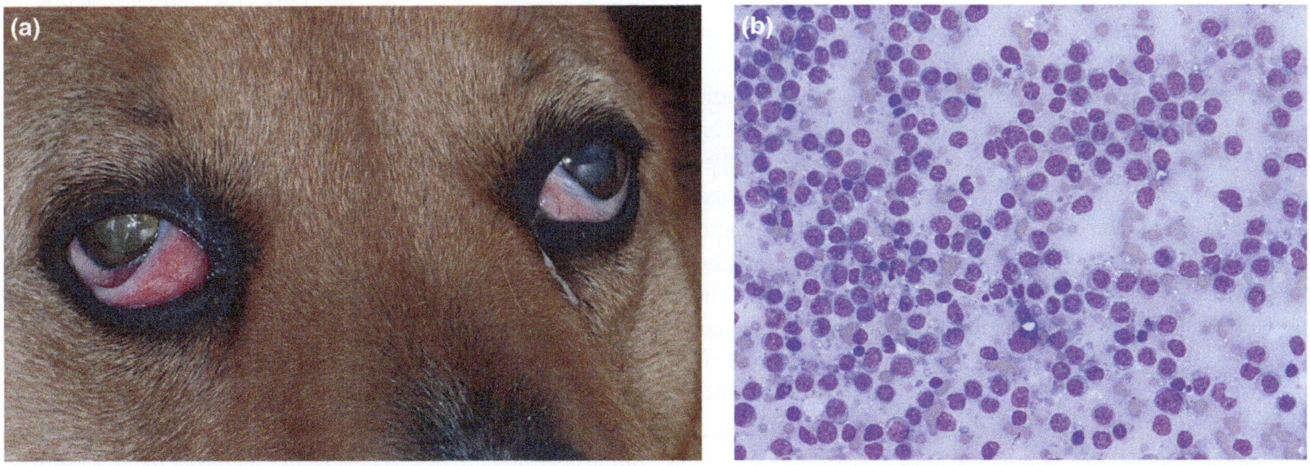

Figure 19.8 (a) Gross photo of bilateral lymphoma causing thickening of the conjunctiva of the third eyelids. The conjunctiva is severely hyperemic and chemotic. Lymphatic tissue on the posterior aspect of the third eyelid has developed an almost mass effect due to the severe thickening of the conjunctival tissue (*Source:* Image courtesy of Michala de Linde Henriksen). (b) Conjunctival brushing from a dog with ocular lymphoma. A monomorphic population of medium to large lymphocytes is characterized by clumped chromatin, eccentric nuclei, and medium blue cytoplasm with occasional clear and round small vacuoles. Few cells have prominent nucleoli (May-Grünwald–Giemsa, 400×).

common tumors in dogs were adenocarcinoma (85%), adenoma (14%), and squamous cell carcinoma (1%).[53] Although cytologic features were not described, histology of the adenocarcinomas revealed secretory features such as acinar or duct formation and secretory product accompanied by poor cellular differentiation and desmoplastic mesenchymal tissue, whereas adenomas were well differentiated. Individual reports of other tumors include myoepithelioma, melanocytoma, and plasmacytoma.[54–56]

Cornea

Normal Architecture and Cytology

The cornea is composed of three layers. The most superficial layer is a stratified squamous non-keratinized epithelium, the middle layer is the corneal stroma, and the innermost layer is a single layer of flattened cuboidal epithelial cells (the corneal endothelium) overlying the basement membrane (Descemet's membrane).[57] Non-keratinized squamous cells with no pigment are observed on scraping from normal cornea.

Inflammation

Inflammation of the cornea is classified as ulcerative or non-ulcerative keratitis. Corneal ulcer or ulcerative keratitis is the most frequent ocular disease in dogs. Many infectious causes are similar to those described for the conjunctiva. Corneal ulcers can result from eyelid abnormalities, foreign bodies, trauma, and KCS; however, bacterial, or less frequently fungal, infections can occur. Diagnosis of bacterial or mycotic infection of corneal ulcers is made via cytologic examination and microbiologic culture. Use of both microbial culture and cytologic evaluation of corneal specimens maximizes identification of infectious keratitis; however, cytologic diagnosis frequently correlates with microbial culture.[58] The most prevalent bacterial isolates were *Streptococcus* spp. and *Staphylococcus* spp. A syndrome of infectious crystalline keratopathy is defined grossly by the presence of branching fine white crystalline anterior stromal opacities accompanied by cytologic identification of bacteria, primarily Gram-positive cocci in corneal samples. The most frequently cultured bacteria are *Streptococcus* spp. and *Staphylococcus* spp.[59]

Canine keratomycosis usually occurs in dogs predisposed because of endocrinopathy, preexisting corneal disease, intraocular surgery, or prolonged use of topical antibiotics or corticosteroids. Cytology is characterized by neutrophilic and macrophagic infiltrate with fungal hyphae and normal to hyperplastic corneal epithelial cells sometimes associated with bacteria and yeast.[60–62] Common fungal isolates include *Aspergillus* spp., *Candida* spp., and *Scedosporium* spp. (Chapter 3).[50] Although infrequent and not often diagnosed cytologically, parasitic keratitis has been described associated with infections by *Leishmania* spp., *T. gondii*, *O. lupi*, *T. callipaeda*, and unidentified microfilarial organisms.[63]

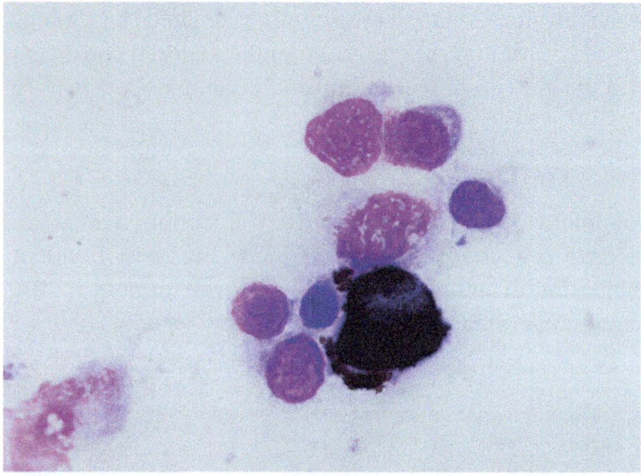

Figure 19.9 Corneal brushing from a dog with pigmentary superficial keratitis. An epithelial cell containing a very large amount of melanin granules is associated with a few lymphocytes and a plasma cell (May-Grünwald–Giemsa, 1000×).

Noninfectious keratitis includes pigmentary keratitis syndrome in brachycephalic dogs and pigmentary superficial keratitis secondary to chronic corneal irritation (Figure 19.9). Chronic superficial keratitis (pannus) has a breed predisposition in German Shepherds, Shepherd crosses, and Greyhounds and is suspected to be an autoimmune keratopathy with a genetic basis.[64] Neurogenic keratitis can occur secondary to trigeminal or facial nerve defects.[65] Cytology in such cases is rarely performed and has not been described in case reports or experimental studies.

Neoplasia

Among the corneal tumors, squamous cell carcinoma has been described in dogs with chronic corneal irritation.[66] Papilloma, corneal lymphoma, hemangioma, hemangiosarcoma, and limbal melanoma also have been reported, but no cytological descriptions are available in case reports or experimental studies.[67] Limbal melanocytic tumors are usually benign and are a frequent form of ocular melanoma. German shepherd dogs, Labrador retrievers, and Golden retrievers are predisposed. They have histologically benign features and are heavily pigmented.[7]

Miscellaneous Diseases

Corneal epithelial inclusion cysts occur as raised, yellow fluid-filled, white to pink corneal masses. They are typically chronic and non-painful and are of posttraumatic origin. Even though cytology for this condition has not been specifically described, it could be used to exclude other differential diagnoses such as abscesses or neoplasia. Noninfectious and nonneoplastic keratopathies such as corneal dystrophy, corneal degeneration, or lipid keratopathy have not been cytologically described in case reports or experimental studies, probably because clinical aspects are sufficient to suspect the disease.[65]

Iris and Ciliary Body

Uveal mass aspiration is uncommonly performed because of possible complications; therefore, the cytology literature is extremely limited. More details on collection procedures and complications are in Chapter 18.

Normal Architecture and Cytology

The anterior uvea is composed of the iris, a muscle diaphragm controlling the quantity of light reaching the posterior segment, and the ciliary body, which produces aqueous humor. The iris separates the anterior and posterior chambers and can be divided into an anterior face, mainly composed of endothelial cells, fibroblasts, and melanocytes, and a posterior face, composed of two highly pigmented epithelial layers and muscle.[57,67,68] No inflammatory cells are present in the normal iris. The ciliary body consists of muscle, stroma, and pigmented epithelium.[57,68] In dogs, the melanin granules of melanocytes are lanceolate.[68] Cytology of the normal iris and ciliary body has not been well described, although some texts extrapolate probable findings based on the histologic structure.[69]

Inflammation

Anterior uveitis is defined as an inflammation of iris and ciliary body, but to our knowledge, there is no relevant cytology literature in this area because sampling of the solid tissues is not usually performed. In such conditions, aqueous and/or vitreous should be cytologically evaluated.

Neoplasia

Anterior uveal tumors are quite uncommon and can be primary or secondary to metastasis. Many different tumors can arise from the uvea, but aspiration of intraocular masses is not frequently performed (Chapter 18).[70]

Melanocytic Tumors (Benign or Malignant)

These tumors are the most common canine primary intraocular tumors and arise from the iris or ciliary body. They are often locally invasive with loss of vision but are infrequently metastatic.[7,69–72] The cytologic diagnosis tumors is challenging because of the normal presence of melanocytes in uvea, and anecdotal evidence suggests poor exfoliation.[72] Histologically, heavily pigmented round cells with distinct borders, a round nucleus, small to medium nucleoli, and a low mitotic index are observed along with a few spindle cells.[7,73] A high mitotic index can occur with malignant melanoma.[72] See Chapter 15 for a more comprehensive discussion of melanoma.

Iridociliary Epithelial Tumors

These represent the second most frequent canine primary intraocular tumor, with approximately equal incidence of adenoma and adenocarcinoma. These tumors arise from the iris or ciliary body, are of neuroectodermal origin, and can be pigmented or non-pigmented.[70] Oncocytic change can occur.[74] Cytology has been reported to be helpful in the diagnosis of iridociliary tumors in people, but there is little in the veterinary literature (Figure 19.10).[75] One case report described cytological features of an iridociliary adenoma, including an abundant epithelial cell population characterized by cuboidal to columnar shape and the formation of papillary clusters or palisades.[76] These structures were often arranged around an eosinophilic fibrillar material corresponding to a basement membrane protein produced by

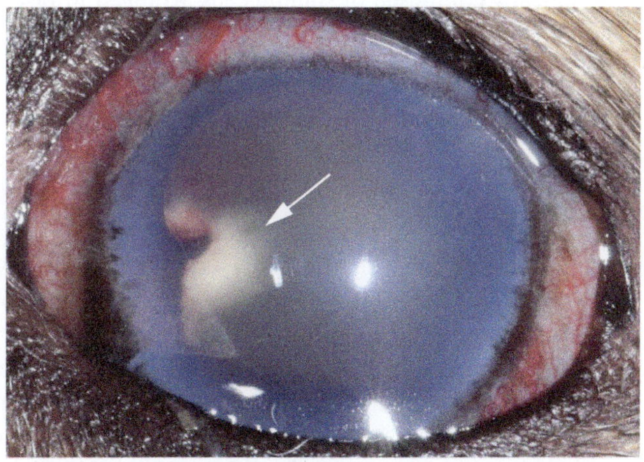

Figure 19.10 Gross photo of a ciliary body adenoma extending into the pupil in a dog (white arrow). The yellow vascularized mass can be appreciated behind the medial aspect of the iris from 8 to 10 o'clock causing a dyscoria pupil with posterior synechiae. Other ophthalmic findings are moderate to severe episcleral injection, diffuse moderate corneal edema, and a mydriatic pupil due to secondary glaucoma. The final diagnosis of ciliary body adenoma was verified with histopathology (*Source:* Image courtesy of Michala de Linde Henriksen).

non-pigmented iridociliary epithelial tumor cells. Neoplastic cells had a moderate N:C with scantly vacuolated basophilic cytoplasm and a round to ovoid nucleus with finely granular chromatin and rarely a nucleolus. Anisocytosis and anisokaryosis were mild to moderate. Histological examination was necessary to achieve the final diagnosis of iridociliary adenoma, since cytologic differential diagnoses included iridociliary adenoma, well-differentiated iridociliary adenocarcinoma, and medulloepithelioma.[76] Caution is indicated based on observations that even biopsy cannot reliably distinguish adenomas from adenocarcinomas in dogs without evidence of scleral invasion, which may be sample dependent.[75]

Lymphoma

Solitary intraocular lymphoma is uncommon.[77] Ocular signs are quite frequent in canine lymphoma that is diagnosed by examination of other infiltrated organs that are easier to sample.[77] The cytological examination of these primary intraocular or metastatic lymphomas is equivalent to lymphoma elsewhere (Chapter 27).[68]

Other Primary Tumors

Spindle cell tumors, primitive neuroectodermal tumors, and medulloepithelioma have been described.[78–82] Intraocular spindle cell tumors of dogs are rare and include peripheral nerve sheath tumors and metastatic sarcoma with hemangiosarcoma, osteosarcoma, and anaplastic mesenchymal tumors. Schwannomas were characterized in a study of 13 blue-eyed dogs with uveal tumors and were histologically composed of spindle cells arranged in fascicles and whorls.[81]

Aqueous Humor

Normal Cytology

Aqueocentesis has the potential for complications (Chapter 18) and is often nonspecific in canine anterior uveitis.[83] However, aqueous humor evaluation can be valuable for the diagnosis of some neoplastic conditions in dogs, especially lymphoma.[84,85] Normal aqueous humor fluid is clear, colorless, and characterized by low protein concentration, which can only be measured by microtechniques such as pyrogallol red technique similar to those used for cerebrospinal fluid.[86] The mean protein concentration is 36.4 mg/dL (range: 21–65 mg/dL), and the mean direct cell count is 8.2 cells/μL (range: 0–37 cells/μL) in unmodified aqueous humor.[87] Consequently, aqueous paracentesis should be processed immediately after collection to avoid cell degradation, and the fluid requires sedimentation or cytocentrifugation similar to cerebrospinal fluid to obtain adequately cellular smears for evaluation. Occasional degenerate or smudged cells, mononuclear cells, and/or melanocytes are identified.[69,84,87]

Hemorrhage

Hyphema is usually associated with underlying conditions such as trauma, neoplasia, inflammatory uveitis, hypertension, and coagulopathies due to thrombocytopenia or clotting disorders.[88,89] Classical signs of acute or chronic hemorrhage are present (Figure 19.11), so aqueous humor resembles blood and can contain some macrophages with erythrophagocytosis and/or presence of hemosiderin pigments.[69,84] If there is no sign of trauma, a complete minimum laboratory database (complete blood count, serum biochemistry, and urinalysis) should be performed, and screening for coagulopathy and infectious diseases may ultimately be required.[88]

Ocular Melanosis

This condition is best characterized in Cairn Terriers and manifests as bilateral expansion of pigmented cells in the anterior uveal structures, potentially leading to glaucoma.[90] There is progressive thickening of the iris root, development of pigment plaques in the sclera, iridal changes with the presence of pigmented particles in the aqueous sometimes associated with uveitis, and ultimately glaucoma. Anecdotally, rafts of pigmented cells can be identified cytologically in the aqueous humor (Figure 19.12).

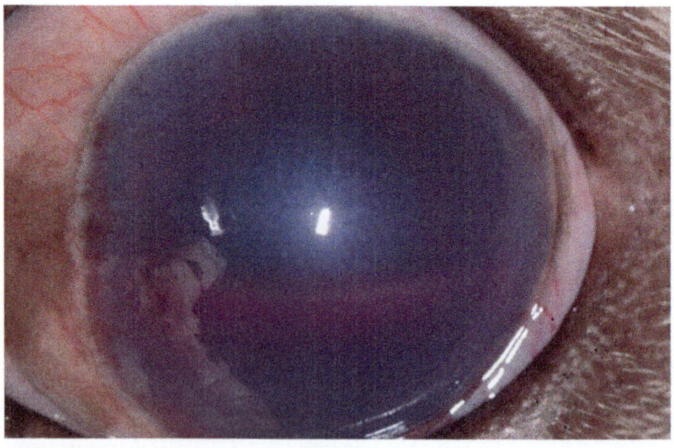

Figure 19.11 Gross photo of anterior uveitis with hyphemia taking up approximately 40% of the anterior chamber. The pupil is miotic due to ciliary body spasm. Other ophthalmic findings are hyperemia of the conjunctiva, diffuse mild to moderate corneal edema, and perilimbal corneal vascularization. The dog was diagnosed with immune-mediated thrombocytopenia (*Source:* Image courtesy of Michala de Linde Henriksen).

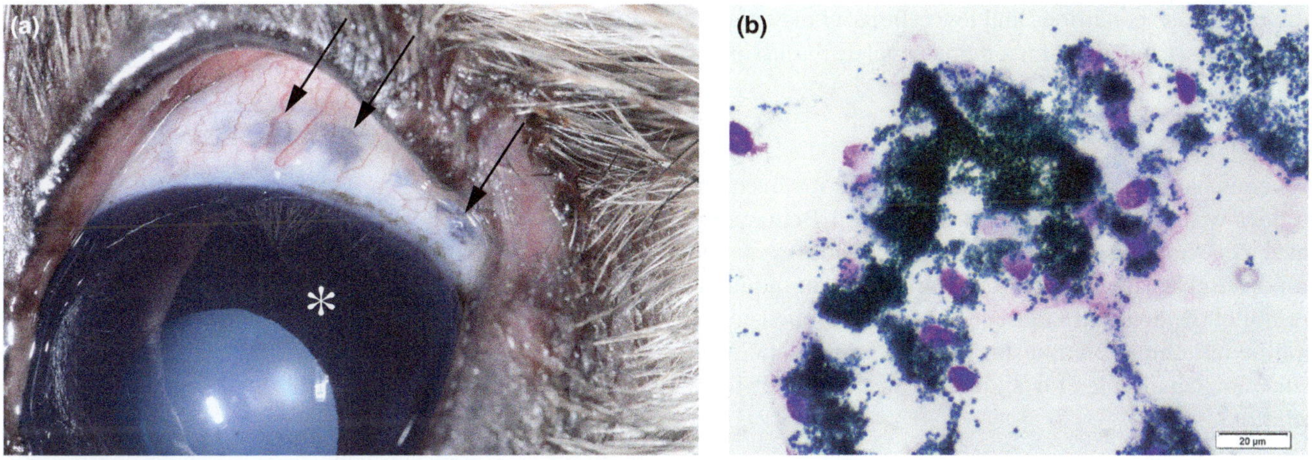

Figure 19.12 (a) Ocular melanosis in a Cairn Terrier. Ophthalmic findings for this ocular genetic disease is hyperpigmentation of the uvea causing pigmented plaques on the sclera (black arrows), hyperpigmentation of the iris (white asterisk), and anterior uveitis with pigmented cells floating in the aqueous humor. The end-stage result of this disease is secondary glaucoma (*Source:* Image courtesy of Michala de Linde Henriksen). (b) Rafts of well-differentiated, heavily pigmented cells in the aqueous humor of a dog with ocular melanosis (Wright–Giemsa, 500×. *Source:* Image courtesy of Leslie Sharkey).

Inflammation

Causes of anterior uveitis in the dog are numerous and include trauma, lens induced, infectious (bacterial, algal, fungal, protozoal, rickettsial, parasitic, viral), immune mediated, metabolic, neoplastic, paraneoplastic, or idiopathic.[91,92] With anterior uveitis, there is a disruption of the blood–aqueous barrier, allowing inflammatory proteins and cells to access the aqueous humor, increasing cellularity and protein concentration.[84,92] The protein concentration appears to be higher in acute (less than four weeks) than chronic (greater than four weeks) uveitis, with a mean of 3.5 g/dL ($n = 12$, range: 0.3–6.6) and 1.8 g/dL ($n = 5$, range: 0.1–4.5), respectively.[84] Cytological examination of aqueous humor is frequently nonspecific for primary inflammatory and/or infectious uveitis in small animals.[92,93] Nevertheless, aqueous humor aspiration is occasionally diagnostic for infectious etiologies such as bacterial and fungal infections and can provide samples for ancillary testing (e.g. bacterial and fungal culture and PCR).[84,91] Mycotic agents include *Blastomyces dermatitidis*, *Coccidioides immitis*, *Histoplasma capsulatum*, and *Cryptococcus neoformans* and less frequently *Aspergillus* and *Candida* spp. (Chapter 3). Parasitic agents include nematodes (larva migrans and filariasis) as described for conjunctiva and aberrant migration of cuterebra. Protozoal agents include *Leishmania infantum*, *T. gondii*, *Neospora caninum*, and *Trypanosoma evansi*. Rickettsial agents include *Ehrlichia canis* and *Rickettsia rickettsiae*. Viral agents include CAV-1. Specific bacteria include *Brucella canis*, *Bartonella vinsonii*, and *Leptospira* organisms. Algal agents include *Prototheca* spp.[92]

Inflammation can be primarily neutrophilic, mononuclear, mixed, or eosinophilic. In one study, acute uveitis (less than four weeks) was often associated with a higher neutrophil to mononuclear cell ratio than chronic uveitis.[84] There is a possible correlation between the duration of disease and the number of plasma cells, but not with other types of inflammatory cells.[93] Neutrophilic inflammation is seen with infectious uveitis due to bacterial, protozoal (*Leishmania* spp.), viral, algal (*Prototheca* spp.), fungal (*Blastomyces* spp.), and noninfectious uveitis (e.g. lens-induced, intraocular foreign body and suspected idiopathic).[69,92,94] Bacterial endophthalmitis induces neutrophilic and mixed inflammation, while suspected idiopathic uveitis had been associated mainly with mononuclear or mixed and occasionally neutrophilic or no evident inflammation.[85,93] Dogs with idiopathic and dysimmune uveitis are less likely to have signs of systemic illness.[91]

Neoplasia

Lymphoma

Aqueous humor aspiration can be useful for the diagnosis of neoplastic uveitis, primarily round cell tumors such as lymphoma.[83,84,92] In high-grade lymphoma with ocular involvement, variable numbers of monomorphic lymphoid blast cells are commonly observed, but not in every case.[84,85,93] Aqueous protein concentration is high in some cases, with a mean of 3.0 g/dL.[84] PCR for antigen receptor rearrangement (PARR) has been performed in rare cases.[95] Clonality could be assessed in few cases, but unfortunately not in other archived cytocentrifuged slides of aqueous humor. Storage conditions and low cellularity may impact results.[85] See Chapter 27 for a more complete discussion of lymphoma.

Mast Cell Tumor

Aqueous paracentesis demonstrated ocular involvement in dogs with a multifocal recurrent grade III cutaneous mast cell tumor, a recurrent subcutaneous mast cell tumor, and a large cell carcinoma.[85,93,96] The aqueous humor of the dogs with mast cell disease exhibited eosinophilic inflammation and some atypical neoplastic mast cells. See Chapter 13 for additional discussion of mast cell tumors.

Miscellaneous Tumors

Some primary ocular neoplasms are unlikely to be diagnosed by aqueous cytology (e.g. anterior uveal adenoma, iridociliary adenocarcinoma, and anterior uveal melanoma), since only an inflammatory component could be identified.[85] Uveitis can occur with systemic neoplasia such as lymphoma even when there is no evidence of direct involvement of the tumor in the eye. Thus, a search for underlying neoplasia in dogs with uveitis is recommended.[97]

Vitreous Body

Vitreous aspiration is rarely performed and not commonly recommended because of the higher risk of complications than for aqueous humor aspiration, such as local hemorrhage, inflammation, and retinal- or lens-induced lesions (Chapter 18).[98]

Normal Structure and Cytology

Vitreous humor is a gelatinous structure filling the posterior cavity of the ocular globe. It is composed mainly of water (about 99%) and to a lesser extent of collagen and hyaluronic acid.[68,99] Vitreous is inhomogeneous in dogs and cats, being fluid at the periphery and denser at the center of the posterior cavity. Like aqueous, it is low in protein and cellularity with only few hyalocytes producing hyaluronic acid.[98] Therefore, vitreous paracentesis should be processed similarly to aqueous fluid. To our knowledge, no study has thoroughly described the cytological characteristics of unmodified vitreous humor. According to some textbooks, fluid can be acellular or contain only rare erythrocytes, have scarce melanin pigment free or in cells, and has a granular eosinophilic background.[69,94,100] Lens fibers and retinal cells can also be aspirated inadvertently or occur secondary to lens or retinal diseases.[69,94,100]

Inflammation

Causes of vitreal inflammation in the dog are numerous and often secondary to inflammation or infection of adjacent structures (e.g. uvea, choroid, retina, and optic nerve), perforation, trauma, retinal detachment, and intraocular hemorrhage or neoplasia.[99] Vitreous aspiration for cytology and culture is more likely to yield a diagnosis than aqueous humor evaluation in endophthalmitis, especially if due to an infectious agent.[99,101] However, sampling is only recommended as a last resort after other options are exhausted. Texts indicate that neutrophilic inflammation is commonly observed with bacterial, mycotic, parasitic, and algal endophthalmitis, as well as with lens- or trauma-induced endophthalmitis.[94] Infectious agents were occasionally observed without signs of inflammation in few case reports of infectious endophthalmitis (e.g. blastomycosis and cryptococcosis).[102,103]

Several cases of mycotic or algal infections inducing endophthalmitis are described in the literature, including blastomycosis, cryptococcosis, aspergillosis, histoplasmosis, coccidioidomycosis, and protothecosis (see Chapter 3 for more detail on the cytology of specific organisms).[91,99,102,104–108] Ocular protothecosis is a component of systemic disease in about two thirds of cases. Case reports of protothecosis with ocular involvement in dogs describe a proteinaceous background with variable numbers of degenerate neutrophils and extracellular and/or intracellular microorganisms consistent with *Prototheca* spp., although concurrent inflammation can be absent.[102,104,106] Reactive macrophages, few lymphocytes, melanocytes, free melanin pigment, retinal cells, and/or lens fibers were sometimes observed in vitreous smears.[102,104,106] Culture of vitreous fluid was positive for *Prototheca zopfii* in one case.[104] In one case of ocular and systemic cryptococcosis in a dog, vitreous paracentesis showed mononuclear inflammation mainly composed of lymphocytes and few macrophages and plasma cells associated with the presence of organisms suggestive of *Cryptococcus* spp.[103,109]

Neoplasia

Diagnosis of neoplasia by cytologic examination of vitreous in dogs has not been described in the veterinary literature to the best of our knowledge. Vitreous tumors are rare and often the result of extension of uveal neoplasms.

Retina

The retina is very rarely aspirated, and retinal cells are more often observed after inadvertent sampling during examination of vitreous or associated with retinal detachment due to various causes (e.g. inflammation, neoplasia, and hemorrhage).

Normal Structure and Cytology

The retina is located between the vitreous and choroid, and its main function is to transmit light stimuli to the brain. Histologically, the retina is divided into ten distinct layers, from outermost to innermost layers: (i) retinal pigmented epithelium, (ii) rod and cone layer, (iii) outer limiting membrane, (iv) outer nuclear layer, (v) outer plexiform layer, (vi) inner nuclear layer, (vii) inner plexiform layer, (viii) ganglion cell layer, (ix) nerve fiber layer, and (x) inner limiting membrane.[62] One study described normal retinal cytological findings after inadvertent puncture of the retina during investigation of a meningioma around the optic nerve.[110] Cytologically, some specific cells of the retina can be recognized including retinal pigmented cells, photoreceptors of the outer and inner nuclear layer, ganglion cells, and nerve fibers. Retinal pigmented cells are polygonal epithelial cells containing numerous melanin granules that are ovoid to lanceolate shaped.[69,110] Photoreceptors of the outer nuclear layer are easily recognized on cytological smear because of their unique bilobed and cleaved nuclei. The chromatin of these nuclei is clumped and very dense and clearly divided by a linear white cleavage. The outer segments of these photoreceptors are moreover characterized by medium gray rod-shaped structure.[110]

Abnormal Findings

Cytology is not commonly performed to explore diseases of retina, but signs of inflammation, infection, hemorrhage, and neoplasia could be logically expected on cytological samples. One study reported a diagnosis of protothecosis through a subretinal aspirate, and another case series indicated diagnosis via cytology of retinal exudate.[102,111] Many organisms and retinal cells were observed on a smear of subretinal fluid.

Orbital Cavity

The orbit is a complex cavity delineated by bone and soft tissue boundaries. In the dog, conditions involving this region result from infectious, inflammatory, and neoplastic diseases. Cytology is valuable for the diagnosis of inflammatory lesions and to a lesser extent for neoplasms.[112]

Inflammation

Orbital infection occurs secondary to foreign bodies, extension from tooth root abscesses, sinusitis, and osteomyelitis or from hematogenous spread. Bacterial or fungal agents can be involved. Inflammation can be noninfectious and associated with optic nerve involvement in granulomatous meningoencephalitis. In dogs, FNA from bacterial infections has been described with observation of neutrophils and bacteria.[112] *Staphylococcus* spp., *Escherichia coli*, *Pasteurella multocida*, *Bacteroides*, *Clostridium*, and *Pasteurella* spp. have been isolated.[113]

Neoplasia

Orbital neoplasia can be primary or secondary. Primary tumors can originate from any anatomic structure of the orbit and the surrounding bone. Secondary neoplasia is caused either by metastasis or by extension from tumors involving nearby structures.[114] Among primary orbital tumors, meningioma and lobular orbital adenoma have been cytologically described. Among secondary orbital tumors, lymphoma, mast cell tumors, squamous cell carcinoma, and adenocarcinoma of the nictitating membrane have been cytologically described.[5,112,114,115]

Meningioma

Of the primary orbital tumors, retrobulbar meningioma is a common nervous system tumor that arises from the meninges covering the optic nerve within the orbit.[114] Meningiomas have variable microscopic appearance and are classified according to their histomorphological characteristics (Chapter 48). According to Montoliu et al., due to their distinctive morphological features, optic nerve meningiomas should be considered a distinct entity.[116] They consist of lobules and sheets of epithelioid cells with abundant eosinophilic cytoplasm, showing a meningothelial/transitional pattern; rare cases have a granular cell component with frequent multiple areas of myxoid, cartilaginous, and osseous metaplasia (Figure 19.13).[116] Cytology of a slow-growing meningioma involving the optic nerve consisted of cells with irregular and indistinct shape and size with moderate to abundant amounts of cytoplasm and round nuclei displaying mild anisokaryosis and small to indistinct nucleoli. There was an unusually distinct and extensive whorl formation.[110,117] A case of meningoepitheliomatous meningioma manifesting as a retrobulbar mass consisted of a neoplastic cell population of round to polygonal to occasionally elongated cells with a moderate amount of lightly basophilic to gray cytoplasm.[114] Nuclei were round to ovoid with one or more small distinct nucleoli and a coarse granular chromatin pattern. Moderate anisocytosis and mild to moderate anisokaryosis were present.

Lobular Orbital Adenoma

A case of lobular orbital adenoma consisted of clusters of epithelial cells associated with a finely granular streaming

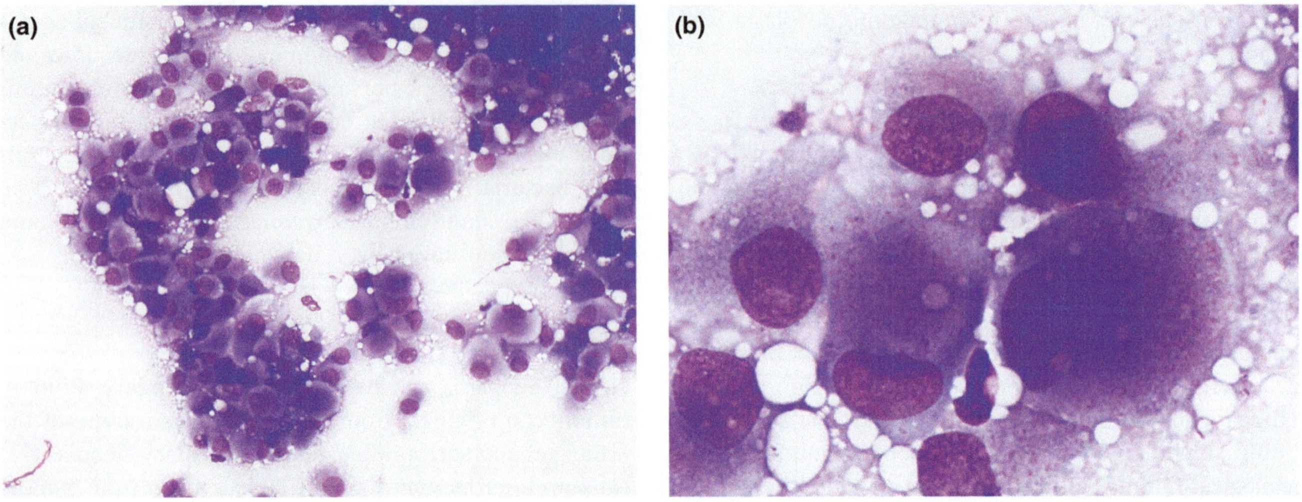

Figure 19.13 (a) Rafts of round to oval somewhat cohesive cells from an histologically confirmed orbital meningioma exhibiting moderate to marked anisocytosis and mild to moderate anisokaryosis (Wright–Giemsa, 200×). (b) Higher magnification demonstrates abundant finely granular amphophilic cytoplasm (Wright–Giemsa, 1000×. *Source:* Images courtesy of Leslie Sharkey)

eosinophilic matrix with red blood cells in a windrowing pattern.[5] Cells were round to polygonal with relatively indistinct cell margins, contained a moderate to abundant amount of foamy, basophilic to amphophilic cytoplasm, and had a round to oval central nucleus. No atypia was observed. Morphology was similar to well-differentiated lacrimal or salivary gland tissue.

Conclusion

Canine ocular cytology can be useful in screening lesions and sometimes in making definitive diagnoses. Given the relatively noninvasiveness of most sampling techniques and rapid turnaround times, we advocate for routine use in the diagnosis of eye disease in the dog.

References

1 Pena, M.T. and Leiva, M. (2008). Canine conjunctivitis and blepharitis. *Vet Clin North Am Small Anim Pract* 38: 233–249.

2 Martens, S.M. (2016). Juvenile cellulitis in a 7-week-old golden retriever dog. *Can Vet J* 57: 202–203.

3 Pietro, S.D., Bosco, V.R., Crino, C. et al. (2016). Prevalence, type, and prognosis of ocular lesions in shelter and owned-client dogs naturally infected by *Leishmania infantum*. *Vet World* 9: 633–637.

4 Ledbetter, E.C. (2013). Canine herpesvirus-1 ocular diseases of mature dogs. *N Z Vet J* 61: 193–201.

5 Bussieres, M., Krohne, S.G., Stiles, J., and Townsend, W.M. (2005). The use of carbon dioxide laser for the ablation of meibomian gland adenomas in dogs. *J Am Anim Hosp Assoc* 41: 227–234.

6 Goldschmidt, M.H. and Goldschmidt, K.H. (2017). Epithelial and melanocytic tumors of the skin. In: *Tumors in Domestic Animals*, 5e (ed. D.J. Meuten). Ames, IA: Wiley Blackwell.

7 Schappa, J.T., Peterson, A., Dubielzig, R.R. et al. (2014). What is your diagnosis? Upper eyelid swelling in a dog. *Vet Clin Pathol* 43: 111–112.

8 Wang, A.L. and Kern, T. (2015). Melanocytic ophthalmic neoplasms of the domestic veterinary species: a review. *Top Companion Anim Med* 30: 148–157.

9 Bolzan, A.A., Brunelli, A.T.J., Castro, M.B. et al. (2005). Conjunctival impression cytology in dogs. *Vet Ophthalmol* 8: 401–405.

10 Lu, J.E. and Dubielzig, R. (2012). Canine eyelid granular cell tumor: a report of eight cases. *Vet Ophthalmol* 15: 406–412.

11 Wilcock, B.P and Njaa, B.L. (2016). Special senses. In: Pathology of Domestic Animals, 6e (eds. K.V. Jubb, P.C. Kennedy and N. Palmer). St-Louis, MO: Elsevier.

12 Bourges-Abella, N., Raymond-Letron, I., Diquelou, A. et al. (2007). Comparison of cytologic and histologic evaluations of the conjunctiva in the normal equine eye. *Vet Ophthalmol* 10: 12–18.

13 Lavach, J.D., Thrall, M.A., Benjamin, M.M., and Severin, G.A. (1977). Cytology of normal and inflamed conjunctivas in dogs and cats. *J Am Vet Med Assoc* 170: 722–727.

14 Moore, C.P., Wilsman, N.J., Nordheim, E.V. et al. (1987). Density and distribution of canine conjunctival goblet cells. *Invest Ophthalmol Vis Sci* 28: 1925–1932.

15 Cullen, C.L., Ihle, S.L., Webb, A.A., and McCarville, C. (2005). Keratoconjunctival effects of diabetes mellitus in dogs. *Vet Ophthalmol* 8: 215–224.

16 Hendrix, D.V.H. (2013). Diseases and surgery of the canine conjunctiva and nictitating membrane. In: *Veterinary Ophthalmology*, 5e (eds. K.N. Gelatt, B.C. Gilger and T.J. Kern), 945–975. Ames, IA: Wiley-Blackwell.

17 Pena, M.T., Roura, X., and Davidson, M.G. (2000). Ocular and periocular manifestations of leishmaniasis in dogs: 105 cases (1993–1998). *Vet Ophthalmol* 3: 35–41.

18 Murphy, J.M. (1988). Exfoliative cytologic examination as an aid in diagnosing ocular diseases in the dog and cat. *Semin Vet Med Surg* 3: 10–14.

19 Erno, H. (1964). On the diagnosis of distemper, with special reference to the intravital demonstration of cytoplasmic inclusion bodies in the third eyelid. *Nord Vet Med* 16: 522.

20 Ledbetter, E.C., Hornbuckle, W.E., and Dubovi, E.J. (2009). Virologic survey of dogs with naturally acquired idiopathic conjunctivitis. *J Am Vet Med Assoc* 235: 954–959.

21 Athanasiou, L.V., Kantere, M.C., Kyriakis, C.S. et al. (2018). Evaluation of a direct immunofluorescent assay and/or conjunctival cytology for detection of canine distemper virus antigen. *Viral Immunol* 31: 272–275.

22 Beckwith-Cohen, B., Gasper, D.J., Bentley, E. et al. (2016). Protozoal infections of the cornea and conjunctiva in dogs associated with chronic ocular surface disease and topical immunosuppression. *Vet Ophthalmol* 19: 206–213.

23 Otranto, D., Giannelli, A., Trumble, N.S. et al. (2015). Clinical case presentation and a review of the literature of canine onchocercosis by *Onchocerca lupi* in the United States. *Parasit Vectors* 8: 89–97.

24 Alho, A.M., Cruz, L., Coehlo, A. et al. (2016). Aberrant laryngeal location of *Onchocerca lupi* in a dog. *Parasitol Int* 65: 218–220.

25 Gracio, A.J.S., Richter, J., Komnenou, A.T., and Grácio, M.A. (2015). Onchocerciasis caused by *Onchocerca lupi*: an emerging zoonotic infection. Systematic review. *Parasitol Res* 4: 2401–2413.

26 Szell, Z., Erdelyi, I., Sreter, T. et al. (2001). Canine occular onchocersosis in Hungary. *Vet Parasitol* 97: 243–249.

27 Komnenou, A., Eberhard, M.L., Kaldrymidou, E. et al. (2002). Subconjunctival filariasis due to *Onchocerca* sp. in dogs: report of 23 cases in Greece. *Vet Ophthalmol* 5: 119–126.

28 Miro, G., Montoya, A., Checa, R. et al. (2016). First detection of *Onchocerca lupi* infection in dogs in southern Spain. *Parasit Vectors* 9: 290–293.

29 Tudor, P., Turcitu, M., Mateescu, M. et al. (2016). Zoonotic ocular onchocerciasis cause by *Onchocerca lupi* in dogs in Romania. *Parasitol Res* 115: 859–862.

30 Verocai, G.G., Conboy, G., Lejeune, M. et al. (2016). *Onchocerca lupi* nematodes in dogs exported from the United States to Canada. *Emerg Infect Dis* 22: 1477–1479.

31 Franchini, D., Giannelli, A., Di Paola, G. et al. (2014). Image diagnosis of zoonotic onchocercosis by *Onchocerca lupi*. *Vet Parasitol* 203: 91–95.

32 Giannelli, A., Cantacessi, C., Graves, P. et al. (2014). A preliminary investigation of serological tools for the detection of *Onchocerca lupi* infection in dogs. *Parasitol Res* 113: 1989–1991.

33 Langlais, L. (2003). Dracunculosis in a German Shepherd dog. *Can Vet J* 44: 681–682.

34 Stowe, D.M., Bidwell, A., and Patel, R. (2016). What is your diagnosis? Subcutaneous mass from a dog. *Vet Clin Pathol* 45: 507–508.

35 Pimenta, P., Cardoso, L., Pereira, M.J. et al. (2013). Canine ocular thelaziosis caused by *Thelazia callipaeda* in Portugal. *Vet Ophthalmol* 16: 312–315.

36 Graham-Brown, J., Gilmore, P., Colella, V. et al. (2017). Three cases of imported eyeworm infection in dogs: a new threat for the United Kingdom. *Vet Rec* 181: 346–351.

37 Papadopoulos, E., Komnenou, A., Thomas, A. et al. (2018). Spreading of *Thelazia callipaeda* in Greece. *Transbound Emerg Dis* 65: 248–252.

38 Caron, Y., Premont, J., Losson, B., and Grauwels, M. (2013). *Thelazia callipaeda* ocular infection in two dogs in Belgium. *J Small Anim Pract* 54: 205–208.

39 Furiani, N., Scarampella, F., Martino, P.A. et al. (2011). Evaluation of the bacterial microflora of the conjunctival sac of healthy dogs and dogs with atopic dermatitis. *Vet Dermatol* 22: 490–496.

40 Glaze, M.B. (1991). Ocular allergy. *Semin Vet Med Surg* 6: 296–302.

41 Costa, D., Esteban, J., Sanz, F. et al. (2016). Ocular lesions produced by pine processionary caterpillar setae (*Thaumetopoea pityocampa*) in dogs: a descriptive study. *Vet Ophthalmol* 19: 493–497.

42 Reed, Z., Doering, C., and Barrett, P.M. (2016). Tarantula hair keratoconjunctivitis with concurrent fungal infection in a rat terrier. *J Am Anim Hosp Assoc* 52: 392–397.

43 Bounous, D., Krenzer, K., Kaswan, R. et al. (1998). Conjunctival impression cytology from dogs with keratoconjunctivitis sicca. In: *Lacrimal Gland, Tear Film, and Dry Eye Syndromes*, 2e (eds. D.A. Sullivan, D.A. Dartt and M.A. Meneray). New York, NY: Springer.

44 Balicki, I., Radziejewski, K., and Bielecki, W. (2011). Evaluation of corneal and conjunctival epithelium with the use of impression cytology in mixed-breed dogs diagnosed with keratoconjunctivitis sicca. *Bull Vet Inst Pulawy* 55: 493–499.

45 Moyer, M.A., Scott, K., and Cianciolo, R.E. (2016). Features and outcome of a glomerulonephropathy associated with ligneous conjunctivitis in a Doberman pinscher dog. *Can Vet J* 57: 501–506.

46 Torres, M.D., Leiva, M., Tabar, M.D. et al. (2009). Ligneous conjunctivitis in a plasminogen-deficient dog: clinical management and 2-year follow-up. *Vet Ophthalmol* 12: 248–253.

47 Mason, S.L., Fisher, C., Ressel, L. et al. (2016). Presentation, clinical pathological and post-mortem findings in three related Scottish terriers with ligneous membranitis. *J Small Anim Pract* 57: 271–276.

48 Fife, M., Blocker, T., Fife, T. et al. (2011). Canine conjunctival mast cell tumors: a retrospective study. *Vet Ophthalmol* 14: 153–160.

49 Komnenou, A.T., Thomas, A.L.N., Kyriazis, A.P. et al. (2015). Ocular manifestations of canine transmissible venereal tumor: a retrospective study of 25 cases in Greece. *Vet Rec* 176: 523.

50 Boscos, C.M., Ververidis, H.N., Tondis, D.K. et al. (1998). Ocular involvement of transmissible venereal tumor in a dog. *Vet Ophthalmol* 1: 167–170.

51 Vascellari, M., Multari, D., and Mutinelli, F. (2005). Unicentric extranodal lymphoma of the upper eyelid conjunctiva in a dog. *Vet Ophthalmol* 8: 67–70.

52 Stuckey, J.A., Rankin, A.J., Romkes, G. et al. (2015). Subconjunctival hibernoma in a dog. *Vet Ophthalmol* 18: 78–82.

53 Dees, D.D., Schobert, C.S., Dubielzig, R.R., and Stein, T.J. (2016). Third eyelid gland neoplasms of dogs and cats: a retrospective histopathologic study of 145 cases. *Vet Ophthalmol* 19: 138–143.

54 Bondoc, A., Izawa, T., Hirata, S. et al. (2014). Myoepithelioma of the gland of the third eyelid in a dog. *J Comp Pathol* 151: 186–189.

55 Dees, D.D., Maclaren, N.E., Teixeira, L. et al. (2013). An unusual case of ocular melanosis and limbal melanocytoma with benign intraorbital extension in a dog. *Vet Ophthalmol* 16: 117–122.

56 Perlmann, E., Dagli, M.L., Martins, M.C. et al. (2009). Extramedullary plasmacytoma of the third eyelid gland in a dog. *Vet Ophthalmol* 12: 102–105.

57 Wilcock, B.P. and Njaa, B.L. (2016). Special senses. In: *Jubb, Kennedy, and Palmer's Pathology of Domestic Animals*, 6e (ed. M.G. Maxie). St. Louis, MO: Elsevier.

58 Massa, K.L., Murphy, C.J., Hartmann, F.A. et al. (1999). Usefulness of aerobic microbial culture and cytologic evaluation of corneal specimens in the diagnosis of infectious ulcerative keratitis in animals. *J Am Vet Med Assoc* 215: 1671–1674.

59 Ledbetter, E.C., McDonough, P.L., and Kim, K. (2017). Infectious crystalline keratopathy in dogs and cats: clinical, in vivo, confocal microscopic, histopathologic, and microbiological features of eight cases. *Vet Ophthalmol* 20: 250–258.

60 Scott, E.M. and Carter, R.T. (2014). Canine keratomycosis in 11 dogs: a case series (2000–2011). *J Am Anim Hosp Assoc* 50: 112–118.

61 Rampazzo, A., Kuhnert, P., Howard, J., and Bornand, V. (2009). *Hormographiella aspergillata* keratomycosis in a dog. *Vet Ophthalmol* 12: 43–47.

62 Ben-Shlomo, G., Plummer, C., Barrie, K., and Brooks, D. (2010). Curvularia keratomycosis in a dog. *Vet Ophthalmol* 13: 126–130.

63 Morales, A., Perlmann, E., Abelha, A.N.V. et al. (2018). Keratitis due to microfilariae in dogs: a newly recognized disease. *Vet Ophthalmol* 21: 305–311.

64 Jokinen, P., Rusanen, E.M., Kennedy, L.J., and Lohi, H. (2011). MHC class II risk haplotype associated with canine chronic superficial keratitis in German Shepherd dogs. *Vet Immunol Immunopathol* 140: 37–41.

65 Ledbetter, E.C. and Gilger, B.C. (2013). Diseases and surgery of the canine cornea and sclera. In: *Veterinary Ophthalmology*, 5e (eds. K.N. Gelatt, B.C. Gilger and T.J. Kern). Ames, IA: Wiley-Blackwell.

66 Dreyfus, J., Schobert, C.S., and Dubielzig, R.R. (2011). Superficial corneal squamous cell carcinoma occurring in dogs with chronic keratitis. *Vet Ophthalmol* 14: 161–168.

67 Aly, K.H., Abd-Elhafez, E., Ali, M., and Abd-Elmaksoud, A. (2009). Histomorphometric analysis of the irides of dogs, camels, buffalos and donkeys. *Res Vet Sci* 86: 1–6.

68 Samuelson, D.A. (2013). Ophthalmic anatomy. In: *Veterinary Ophthalmology*, 5e (eds. K.N. Gelatt, B.C. Gilger and T.J. Kern). Ames, IA: Wiley-Blackwell.

69 Raskin, R.E. (2016). Eyes and adnexa. In: *Canine and Feline Cytology*, 3e (eds. R.E. Raskin and D.J. Meyer). St. Louis, MO: W.B. Saunders.

70 Dubielzig, R.R. (1990). Ocular neoplasia in small animals. *Vet Clin North Am Small Anim Pract* 20: 837–848.

71 Cook, C.S. and Wilkie, D.A. (1999). Treatment of presumed iris melanoma in dogs by diode laser photocoagulation: 23 cases. *Vet Ophthalmol* 2: 217–225.

72 Rovesti, G.L., Guandalini, A., and Peiffer, R. (2001). Suspected latent vertebral metastasis of uveal melanoma in a dog: a case report. *Vet Ophthalmol* 4: 75–77.

73 Wilcock, B.P. and Peiffer, R.L. (1986). Morphology and behavior of primary ocular melanomas in 91 dogs. *Vet Pathol* 23: 418–424.

74 Okawauchi, M., Tsuboi, M., Nibe, K. et al. (2016). Iridociliary adenocarcinoma with oncocytic change in a dog. *J Vet Med Sci* 78: 883–887.

75 Beckwith-Cohen, B., Bentley, E., and Dubielzig, R.R. (2015). Outcome of iridociliary epithelial tumour biopsies in dogs: a retrospective study. *Vet Rec* 176: 147–152.

76 Petterino, C., Bjornson, S., and Hayes, S. (2014). What is your diagnosis? An intraocular mass in a dog. *Vet Clin Pathol* 43: 289–290.

77 Wiggans, K.T., Skorupski, K.A., Reilly, C.M. et al. (2014). Presumed solitary intraocular or conjunctival lymphoma in dogs and cats: 9 cases (1985–2013). *J Am Vet Med Assoc* 244: 460–470.

78 Regan, D.P., Dubielzig, R.R., Zeiss, C.J. et al. (2013). Primary primitive neuroectodermal tumors of the retina and ciliary body in dogs. *Vet Ophthalmol* 16 (Suppl 1): 87–93.

79 Duke, F.D., Teixeira, L.B.C., Galle, L.E. et al. (2015). Malignant uveal schwannoma with peripheral nerve extension in a 12-week-old color-dilute Labrador retriever. *Vet Pathol* 52: 181–185.

80 Duke, F.D., Brudenall, D.K., Scott, E.M. et al. (2013). Metastatic uveal schwannoma of blue-eyed dogs. *Vet Ophthalmol* 16: 141–144.

81 Zarfoss, M.K., Klauss, G., Newkirk, K. et al. (2007). Uveal spindle cell tumor of blue-eyed dogs: an immunohistochemical study. *Vet Pathol* 44: 276–284.

82 Alekseandersen, M., Bjerkas, E., Heiene, R., and Heegaard, S. (2004). Malignant teratoid medulloepithelioma with brain and kidney involvement in a dog. *Vet Ophthalmol* 7: 407–411.

83 Featherstone, H. and Scurrell, E. (2015). Ocular sampling in the dog and cat. *In Pract* 37: 510–539.

84 Olin, D.D. (1977). Examination of the aqueous humor as a diagnostic aid in anterior uveitis. *J Am Vet Med Assoc* 171: 557–559.

85 Linn-Pearl, R.N., Powell, R.M., Newman, H.A., and Gould, D.J. (2015). Validity of aqueocentesis as a component of anterior uveitis investigation in dogs and cats. *Vet Ophthalmol* 18: 326–334.

86 Behr, S., Trumel, C., Palanche, F., and Braun, J.P. (2003). Assessment of a pyrogallol red technique for total protein measurement in the cerebrospinal fluid of dogs. *J Small Anim Pract* 44: 530–533.

87 Hazel, S.J., Thrall, M.A., Severin, G.A. et al. (1985). Laboratory evaluation of aqueous humor in the healthy dog, cat, horseand cow. *Am J Vet Res* 46: 657–659.

88 Telle, M.R. and Betbeze, C. (2015). Hyphema: considerations in the small animal patient. *Top Companion Anim Med* 30: 97–106.

89 Graham, K.L., Korckenberger, M.B., and Billson, F.M. (2018). Intraocular sarcoma associated with lens capsule rupture and persistent hyperplastic primary vitreous in a dog. *Vet Ophthalmol* 21: 188–193.

90 Peterson-Jones, S.M., Forcier, J., and Mentzer, A.L. (2007). Ocular melanosis in the Cairn Terrier: clinical description and investigation of mode of inheritance. *Vet Ophthalmol* 10 (Suppl 1): 63–69.

91 Massa, K.L., Gilger, B.C., Miller, T., and Davidson, M.G. (2002). Causes of uveitis in dogs: 102 cases (1989–2000). *Vet Ophthalmol* 5: 93–98.

92 Hendrix, D.V.H. (2007). Diseases and surgery of the canine anterior uvea. In: *Veterinary Ophthalmology*, 4e (ed. K.N. Gelatt). Ames, IA: Blackwell.

93 Wiggans, K.T., Vernau, W., Lappin, M.R. et al. (2014). Diagnostic utility of aqueocentesis and aqueous humor analysis in dogs and cats with anterior uveitis. *Vet Ophthalmol* 17: 212–220.

94 Young, K.M. (2013). Eyes and associated structures. In: *Cowell and Tyler's Diagnostic Cytology and Hematology of the Dog and Cat*, 4e (eds. A. Valenciano and R. Cowell). St. Louis, MO: Elsevier Health Sciences.

95 Pate, D.O., Gilger, B.C., Suter, S.E., and Clode, A.B. (2011). Diagnosis of intraocular lymphosarcoma in a dog by use of a polymerase chain reaction assay for antigen receptor rearrangement. *J Am Vet Med Assoc* 238: 625–630.

96 Boostrom, B.O., Good, K.L., Maggs, D.J. et al. (2014). Unilateral intraocular mastocytosis and anterior uveitis in a dog with subcutaneous mast cell tumors. *Vet Ophthalmol* 17: 131–138.

97 Schwartz, B., Rom, M.E., Bealka, N., and Qi, Y. (2002). Dose response of dexamethasone for the enhanced ocular hypotensive response to epinephrine in rabbits with prior dexamethasone treatment. *J Ocul Pharmacol Ther* 18: 133–139.

98 Featherstone, H.J. and Heinrich, C.L. (2013). Ophthalmic examination and diagnostics. Part 1: The eye examination and diagnostic procedures. In: *Veterinary Ophthalmology*, 5e (eds. K.N. Gelatt, B.C. Gilger and T.J. Kern). Ames, IA: Wiley-Blackwell.

99 Bocve, M.H. and Stades, F.C. (2013). Diseases and surgery of the canine vitreous. In: *Veterinary Ophthalmology*, 5e (eds. K.N. Gelatt, B.C. Gilger and T.J. Kern). Ames, IA: Wiley-Blackwell.

100 Barger, A.M. and Schlicher, K. (2016). Ocular Cytology. In: *Small Animal Cytologic Diagnosis* (eds. A.M. Barger and A.L. MacNeill). Boca Raton, FL: CRC press, Taylor & Francis Group.

101 Brightman, A., Brown, M., Johnson, B. et al. (1986). Vitreous centesis as a diagnostic procedure. *Proceedings of the Annual Meeting of the American College of Veterinary Ophthalmologists*, New Orleans, LA (11–14 October 1986).

102 Rizzi, T.E., Cowell, R.L., Meinkoth, J.H., and Gilmour, M.A. (2006). More than meets the eye: subretinal aspirate from an acutely blind dog. *Vet Clin Pathol* 35: 111–113.

103 Gelatt, K.N., McGill, L.D., and Perman, V. (1973). Ocular and systemic cryptococcosis in a dog. *J Am Vet Med Assoc* 162: 370–375.

104 Schultze, A.E., Ring, R.D., Morgan, R.V., and Patton, C.S. (1998). Clinical, cytologic and histopathologic manifestations of protothecosis in two dogs. *Vet Ophthalmol* 1: 239–243.

105 Arceneaux, K.A., Taboada, J., and Hosgood, G. (1998). Blastomycosis in dogs: 115 cases (1980–1995). *J Am Vet Med Assoc* 213: 658–664.

106 Beribe, F., Miglio, A., Cassarani, M.P. et al. (2014). What is your diagnosis? Systemic lymphadenopathy and blindness in a dog from Italy. *Vet Clin Pathol* 43: 605–606.

107 Stenner, V.J., Mackay, B., King, T. et al. (2007). Protothecosis in 17 Australian dogs and a review of the canine literature. *Med Mycol* 45: 249–266.

108 Narfstrom, K. and Petersen-Jones, S.M. (2013). Diseases and surgery of the canine fundus. In: *Veterinary Ophthalmology*, 5e (eds. K.N. Gelatt, B.C. Gilger and T.J. Kern). Ames, IA: Wiley-Blackwell.

109 Gelatt, K.N., Chrisman, C.L., Samuelson, D.A. et al. (1991). Ocular and systemic aspergillosis in a dog. *J Am Anim Hosp Assoc* 27: 427–431.

110 Tvedten, H. and Hillström, A. (2013). Cytologic appearance of retinal cells included in a fine-needle aspirate of a meningioma around the optic nerve of a dog. *Vet Clin Pathol* 42: 234–237.

111 Shank, A.M., Dubielzig, R.D., and Teixeira, L.B. (2015). Canine ocular protothecosis: a review of 14 cases. *Vet Ophthalmol* 18: 437–442.

112 Boydell, P. (1991). Fine needle aspiration biopsy in the diagnosis of exophthalmos. *J Small Anim Pract* 32: 542–546.

113 Spiess, B.M. and Pot, S.A. (2013). Diseases and surgery of the canine orbit. In: *Veterinary Ophthalmology*, 5e (eds. K.N. Gelatt, B.C. Gilger and T.J. Kern), 793–832. Ames, IA: Wiley-Blackwell.

114 Regan, D.P., Kent, M., Mathes, R. et al. (2011). Clinicopathologic findings in a dog with a retrobulbar meningioma. *J Vet Diagn Invest* 23: 857–862.

115 Attali-Soussa, K., Jegou, J.P., and Clerc, B. (2001). Retrobulbar tumors in dogs and cats: 25 cases. *Vet Ophthalmol* 4: 19–27.

116 Montoliu, P., Anor, S., Vidal, E., and Pumarola, M. (2006). Histological and immunohistochemical study of 30 cases of canine meningioma. *J Comp Pathol* 135: 200–207.

117 Tvedten, H. and Falkeno, U. (2015). Cytologic appearance of a meningioma recurring over 4 years after initial diagnosis. *Vet Clin Pathol* 44: 474.

20

Ocular Cytology of the Cat

Christine C. Lim and Jennifer L. Brazzell

Introduction

Ocular cytology is relatively easy to perform, and the most common uses and indications for ocular cytology in the cat include (i) conjunctival and corneal scrapings, impressions, or brushings to determine the type and etiology of conjunctivitis and keratitis; (ii) aspirates of aqueous or vitreous humor in cases of suspected septic uveitis or endophthalmitis; and (iii) aspiration of solid tissue or cystic masses of the globe and surrounding structure.[1–4] Using sharp or pointy collection tools to obtain cytology specimens near the sensitive and relatively unforgiving ocular anatomy must be done carefully to avoid iatrogenic trauma. Details and recommendations for collection of samples are described in Chapter 18. This chapter is a broad description of feline-specific ocular and periocular diseases, their clinical presentations, and cytological and histological characteristics.

Eyelid and Adnexa

Normal Structure, Cytology, and Collection

The outer surface of the eyelid is covered by a haired, keratinized squamous epithelium (Figure 20.1). At the lid margin, the haired skin reflects back on itself to become the palpebral conjunctiva. The lid margin itself is hairless; ducts of sebaceous glands (Meibomian or tarsal glands) exit along the eyelid margin. Specialized sebaceous glands (glands of Zeis) and apocrine glands (glands of Moll) are associated with the eyelashes. All epidermal and dermal lesions occurring elsewhere on the body can occur on the haired skin of the eyelid. Chapters 11 and 12 discuss cutaneous inflammatory, infectious, and neoplastic lesions that also can affect the haired skin of the eyelid (Table 20.1). Collection techniques are described in Chapter 18.

Inflammation

Blepharitis and conjunctivitis usually occur concurrently. Refer to the section "Conjunctiva, Nictitating Membrane, and Cornea" for discussion of conjunctivitis, with the knowledge that conjunctivitis and blepharitis share similar differential diagnoses.

Neoplasia

Aspiration or incisional biopsy of all feline eyelid mass lesions is encouraged prior to attempting complete excision. Benign lesions requiring less aggressive surgical resection (e.g. mast cell tumors or apocrine hidrocystomas) can be distinguished from other tumors that can appear clinically similar but that may require more aggressive medical and/or surgical therapy (e.g. lymphoma, adenocarcinomas, and peripheral nerve sheath tumors).

Apocrine Hidrocystoma (Apocrine Cystadenoma)

Apocrine hidrocystoma is an eyelid lesion unique to the cat. Long-haired breeds such as Persians and Himalayans are overrepresented,[5–8] but short-haired breeds also can be affected.[9] One study identified apocrine hidrocystomas as an infrequent neoplasm (3/43 samples evaluated).[10] Macroscopically, apocrine hidrocystomas are fairly unique in appearance, presenting as single or multiple fluid-filled, non-painful masses (Figure 20.2). Aspiration of the cyst yields dark brown to black turbid fluid. Microscopic examination of the fluid reveals numerous large, vacuolated macrophages in a proteinaceous background that occasionally contains cholesterol crystals. Macrophages from the lesions are reported to contain phagocytosed brown to black amorphous material that is assumed to represent apocrine secretory product similar to that described in association with ceruminous cysts and tumors.[8,11] This material must be distinguished from melanin or hemosiderin. Melanin tends to

Veterinary Cytology, First Edition. Edited by Leslie C. Sharkey, M. Judith Radin, and Davis Seelig.

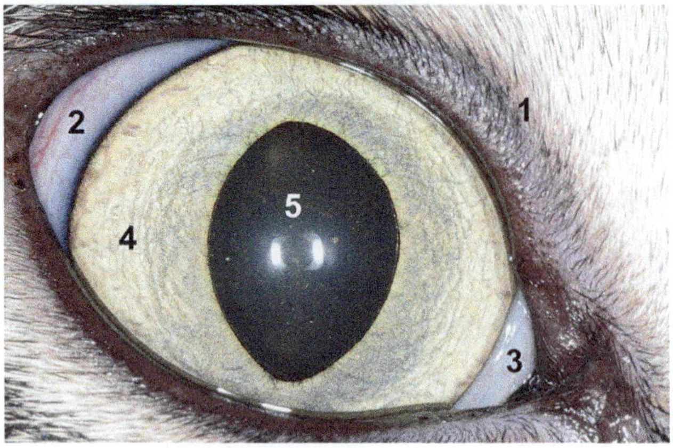

Figure 20.1 Structures of the feline eye. 1. Eyelid/adnexa. 2. Sclera and cornea. 3. Conjunctiva and nictitating membrane. 4. Iris and ciliary body. 5. Intraocular contents: aqueous and vitreous humors, lens.

be black brown and more discretely globular or rod shape (Figure 20.3), while hemosiderin appears blue black and somewhat more amorphous. The unique appearance of the cystic lesions combined with the presence of macrophages containing the amorphous brown to black material supports a clinical diagnosis of apocrine hidrocystoma.

Mast Cell Tumor

Eyelids are a frequent site for the development of feline cutaneous mast cell tumors. Feline cutaneous mast cell tumors tend to behave in a more benign fashion than those of their canine counterparts. Strontium 90 irradiation or surgical excision of eyelid and periocular mast cell tumors in cats is often curative, even following incomplete surgical excision.[12,13] Additional information on mast cell tumors is available in Chapter 13.

Other Neoplasms

Other neoplasms described in the feline eyelid, in order of decreasing frequency, include squamous cell carcinoma (SCC) (Chapter 12), hemangiosarcoma (Chapter 28), adenocarcinoma, peripheral nerve sheath tumor (Chapter 16), lymphoma (Chapter 27), and hemangioma.[10,14] Vascular tumors and SCC are reported to occur more frequently in white-haired cats or non-pigmented skin, with neoplastic transformation postulated to occur secondary to damage caused by solar irradiation.[10,14,15] Melanocytic tumors of the feline eyelid appear to be very rare.[16]

Conjunctiva, Nictitating Membrane, and Cornea

Normal Structure, Cytology, and Collection

In health, the conjunctival surface is composed of nonkeratinized stratified squamous epithelium interspersed with goblet cells. The deeper substantia propria contains lymphoid tissue, nerves, blood vessels, lymphatics, and collagen. Conjunctival samples from healthy cats consist of a mixture of nonkeratinized epithelial cells, goblet cells (especially if scraping in ventral conjunctival fornix, where these cells are most plentiful), and occasional neutrophils, lymphocytes, and monocytes (Figure 20.4).[1,17] Occasional bacteria, melanin granules, and mucus also can be present in samples from normal tissues.[1,17] Mast cells and eosinophils should not be seen in samples collected from healthy feline conjunctivae.

The corneal epithelium is also composed of nonkeratinized stratified squamous cells but lacks goblet cells. Stroma makes up the majority of the corneal thickness. It is composed of collagen lamella arranged in a highly ordered fashion. The stroma contains nerve fibers but lacks blood vessels and lymphatics. The deepest layer of the cornea consists of Descemet's membrane, which is the basement membrane of the corneal endothelium, and the overlying single layer of flattened endothelial cells. Cytologic samples from healthy corneas can contain epithelial cells, lymphocytes, polymorphonuclear cells, nuclei, keratin, mucous, and bacteria.[18] Topical anesthetic may be needed for conjunctival sampling but is definitely required for corneal sampling. Details are addressed in Chapter 18.

Inflammation

Compared with dogs, feline conjunctival smears are more cellular, and inflamed conjunctivae yield more cells than normal conjunctivae.[1] The most common indication for ocular surface cytology in cats is conjunctivitis, with or without concurrent keratitis; keratoconjunctivitis is also the most common ophthalmic presenting complaint in feline practice. Various etiologies for conjunctivitis often present similarly with unilateral or bilateral ocular discharge, conjunctival hyperemia, chemosis, and lymphoid follicle development such that a specific diagnosis cannot be established based on clinical signs alone. Concurrent upper respiratory disease can also be present. When keratitis is also present, underlying feline herpesvirus (FHV-1) can be presumed,[19] but secondary involvement of other infectious agents cannot be excluded. Therefore, the main goals of cytology are to determine the underlying cause of the conjunctivitis and if secondary infections are present.

Infectious

Infectious agents are responsible for the majority of cases of feline conjunctivitis/keratoconjunctivitis; FHV-1 and *Chlamydia felis* are considered the most common etiologic agents for feline ocular surface inflammation, with mixed infections possible.[20–22] When keratitis is concurrently

Table 20.1 Common pathologies of the feline eye.

Lesion	Affected ocular structures	Typical clinical appearance	Amenable to cytologic diagnosis?
Neoplastic conditions			
Adenocarcinoma	1, 2, 3, 4, 6	Extraocular: raised, infiltrative, irregular, may be ulcerated. Intraocular: smooth pink mass arising from the ciliary body	Yes, for extraocular masses
Apocrine cystadenoma	1	Single to multiple blue-black cysts on eyelid margins	Yes, if lesion is large enough to aspirate. Cyst wall does not exfoliate but may see characteristic apocrine secretions within macrophages
Feline restrictive myofibroblastic sarcoma	6	Enophthalmos or exophthalmos, decreased retropulsion, restricted movement of globe and periocular tissues, thickened eyelids	No, poorly exfoliative
Fibrosarcoma	2, 6	Corneal: Raised fibrovascular mass Orbit: poorly defined, infiltrative, effacing connective tissue of orbit often produces exophthalmos	No, often poorly exfoliative and cytologic differentiation of neoplastic spindle cells from reactive ones difficult
Hemangioma/ hemangiosarcoma	1, 2, 6	Small, raised mass arising from the ocular surface, most often the leading edge of the nictitans or lateral bulbar conjunctiva	No, may see hemorrhage but neoplastic cells poorly exfoliative
Lymphoma	1, 2, 3, 4, 5, 6	Conjunctival: hyperemia, "meaty" thickening of conjunctiva rather than chemosis Intraocular: similar to anterior uveitis, iris bombe	Yes for extraocular lesions, intraocular lesions often do not exfoliate into the humors
Mast cell tumor	1, 3, 6	Dermal: domed, hairless, may be ulcerated. Conjunctival: white to pink mass accompanying conjunctivitis	Yes
Melanoma	1, 2, 3, 4, 6	Conjunctival: black thickening of conjunctiva, with or without overt conjunctival hyperemia Iridal: Brown to black iridal discoloration of variable distribution across the iris, with or without overt mass formation; hyperpigmented areas may have altered texture when compared with unaffected areas	Yes
Peripheral nerve sheath tumor	1, 6	Nodular to diffuse and poorly defined, subcutaneous, firm, infiltrates and effaces connective tissue of eyelid	No, often poorly exfoliative and cytologic differentiation of neoplastic spindle cells from reactive ones difficult
Squamous cell carcinoma	1, 2, 3, 6	Corneal: similar to keratitis (neovascularization, edema, fibrosis) but may also be raised, pink, fleshy	Yes
Inflammatory and infectious			
Acute bullous keratopathy	2	Blepharospasm, epiphora, conjunctival hyperemia, chemosis, keratomalacia, keratoconus, sometimes corneal vascularization	No, clinical appearance is characteristic; cytology performed to rule out concurrent bacterial infection
Aspergillosis	5, 6	Exophthalmos, dorsolateral deviation of the globe, decreased globe retropulsion, and raised third eyelid, with or without hyperemia and keratitis may also be present. Signs of upper respiratory disease are usually present	Yes

(*Continued*)

Table 20.1 (Continued)

Lesion	Affected ocular structures	Typical clinical appearance	Amenable to cytologic diagnosis?
Corneal sequestrum	2	Brown to black plaque on corneal surface, corneal ulceration with or without corneal vascularization and conjunctivitis (chemosis, conjunctival hyperemia), with or without epiphora/discharge and blepharospasm	No, clinical appearance is characteristic; cytology performed to rule out concurrent bacterial infection
Eosinophilic	1, 2, 3	Blepharospasm, epiphora, conjunctival hyperemia, chemosis, white to tan plaques on corneal and conjunctival surface, corneal vascularization, corneal white cell infiltrate, corneal edema	Yes
Lipogranulomatous	1, 3	Blepharospasm, epiphora, conjunctival hyperemia, chemosis, round white to tan conjunctival masses of varying sizes, affecting eyelid margin/palpebral conjunctiva of white/light-colored cats	Yes
Local irritation/medication reaction	1, 2, 3	Blepharospasm, conjunctival hyperemia, chemosis, epiphora/ocular discharge, eyelid swelling and erythema, sometimes alopecia	No
Mastocytic	3	Proliferative or nodular conjunctivitis, with or without concurrent keratitis or nictitans lesions. White to tan conjunctival plaques and conjunctival ulceration may also be seen	Yes
Neutrophilic	1, 2, 3, 4, 5, 6	Conjunctivitis: Blepharospasm, epiphora/ocular discharge, conjunctival hyperemia (they say this is more pronounced with FHV-1 vs *C. felis*), chemosis (they say this is more pronounced with *C. felis* vs FHV-1), sometimes conjunctival follicles (*C. felis*), with or without keratitis Anterior uveitis: Blepharospasm, epiphora, corneal edema, aqueous flare, miosis, rubeosis iridis, iridal congestion; cats may not develop overt redness to eye like the dog; may additionally see iridal nodules, hypopyon, anterior chamber fibrin, hyphema, keratic precipitates	Yes, indicates presence/absence of inflammation but often not etiologic cause (bacterial cocci/rods/fungal elements may be noted; may rarely see *Mycoplasma*/*C. mydia*, herpesvirus inclusions)

1, eyelid/adnexa; 2, cornea; 3, conjunctiva/nictitating membrane; 4, iris/ciliary body; 5, aqueous/vitreous humor; 6, orbit.

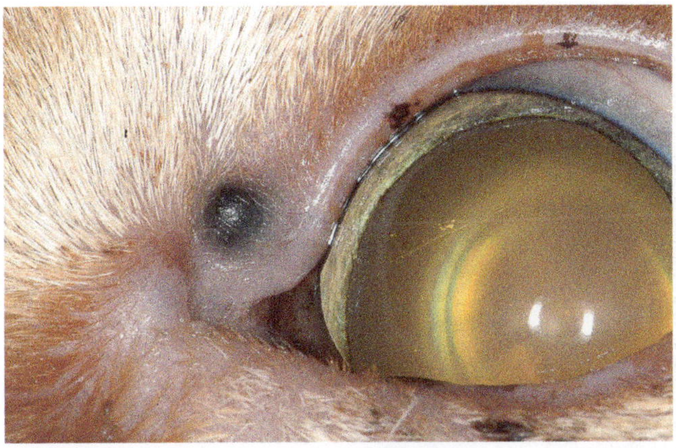

Figure 20.2 Apocrine hidrocystoma affecting the upper left eyelid in a 15-year-old, spayed female domestic short-haired cat. A discrete, smooth, round black mass located adjacent to the eyelid margin is the typical appearance for this eyelid neoplasm.

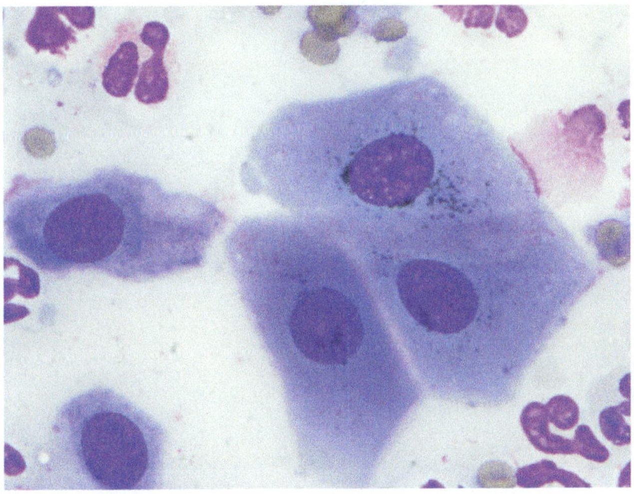

Figure 20.3 Corneal scraping. Superficial squamous cells contain uniform, brown-black, rod-shaped melanin granules. Few neutrophils, eosinophils, and erythrocytes are present in the background. This sample was taken from a patient with a clinical diagnosis of eosinophilic keratoconjunctivitis (Wright–Giemsa, 1000×).

present, FHV-1 is presumed to be the cause, as *C. felis* is a conjunctival, not corneal, pathogen.[19,23] *Mycoplasma* spp. and feline calicivirus are considered infrequent causes of feline conjunctivitis. Various chlamydial agents isolated from cats with conjunctivitis have an unclear role in disease.[24–26] Non-mycoplasmal or chlamydial primary bacterial conjunctivitis is considered to be a rare cause of feline conjunctivitis,[20,27–31] as are fungal[32–34] and parasitic[35–37] etiologies. However, bacterial and fungal organisms have been associated with feline corneal ulceration.[28,38–40]

Diagnosis is based more often on clinical suspicion than laboratory testing due to the low sensitivity of cytology for

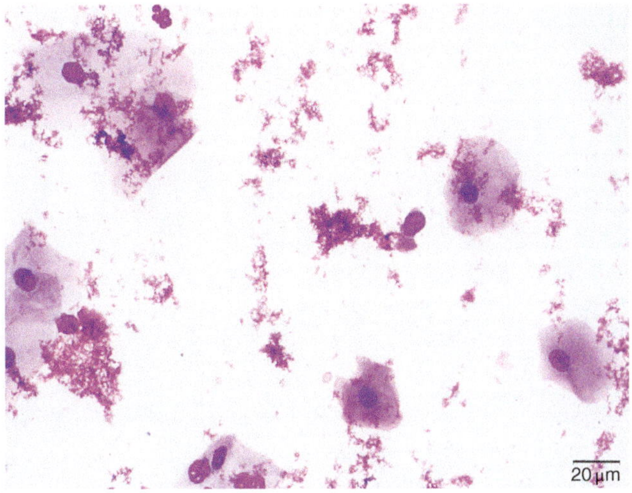

Figure 20.4 Conjunctival swab taken from a normal conjunctiva. Superficial squamous cells predominate. A single columnar epithelial cell and a single disrupted neutrophil are also present on the stippled proteinaceous/mucinous background (Wright–Giemsa, 1000×).

organism detection and the challenges associated with interpreting results of virus isolation, cell culture, immunofluorescent antibody testing, and polymerase chain reaction testing. This is partly because the various etiologies produce similar patterns of inflammation, especially in chronic cases.[41] FHV-1, *C. felis*, and *Mycoplasma* spp. all produce a predominantly neutrophilic inflammatory response with lesser numbers of mononuclear cells.[17,23,42] Eosinophil predominant inflammation has been associated with some FHV-1 keratoconjunctivitis. Giant cells are sometimes seen with herpetic and chlamydial conjunctivitis, and plasma cells are sometimes seen with chlamydial conjunctivitis, but the inflammatory patterns are not specific enough to determine which infectious agent is causal.

Etiology specific cellular inclusions are found in a minority of samples; however, cytology has the potential to identify specific agents such as FHV-1, *C. felis*, and *Mycoplasma felis*. Care must be taken not to mistake infectious inclusions for melanin granules (Figure 20.3), drug inclusions, or other artifacts with similar appearance. Inability to identify the inclusions of infectious agents does not exclude these etiologies.[29,41] The likelihood of observing herpetic intranuclear viral inclusions is low, but these can be seen in the first week after infection[29,41,42] with routine staining[43] or more frequently with Papanicolaou's or Pappenheim's stains.[29,44]

Chlamydial inclusions (Figure 20.5a) are most likely to be detected cytologically between days 7 and 14 following infection.[23] Inclusions are basophilic and appear adjacent to the nucleus in the cytoplasm of epithelial cells and neutrophils.[23,29,44] They can appear in clusters of small, round

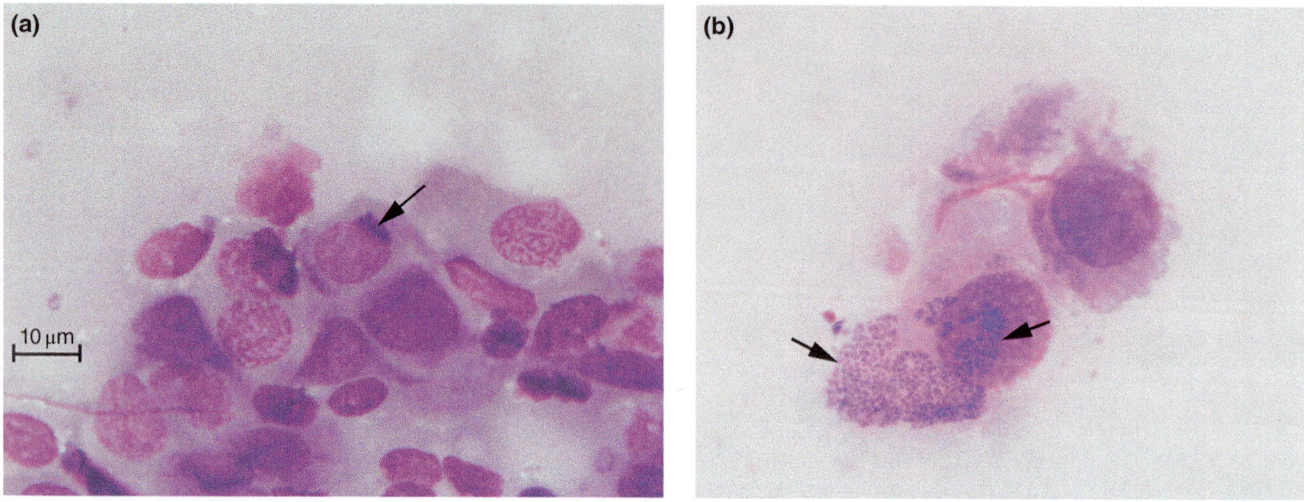

Figure 20.5 (a) Feline conjunctival scrape. An epithelial cell contains *C. felis* organisms. (b) Feline conjunctival scrape. A colony of *M. felis* organisms (arrows) are on the surface of an epithelial cell (Wright–Giemsa, 1000×. *Source:* Images courtesy of Karen Young).

inclusions ranging in diameter from 0.5 to 1 µm, or as larger, crescent-shaped or circular single inclusions 3–5 µm diameter.[23,24,29] Chlamydial inclusions are easily detected with routine Wright–Giemsa stain,[17,23,44] but immunoperoxidase or immunofluorescence staining can increase sensitivity.[45] Identification of numerous chlamydial inclusions in samples taken from cats with acute disease is specific for infection with *C. felis.*[29] However, observation of "suspected" chlamydial inclusions may lead to false positives if nonspecific material is overinterpreted.[29]

Mycoplasmal inclusions (Figure 20.5b) are also visible on routine Wright–Giemsa stain.[46] They are basophilic, 0.2–0.8 µm in diameter, and located in clusters within epithelial cytoplasm or between cells.[46] In contrast to chlamydial inclusions, mycoplasmal inclusions occur near epithelial cell membranes rather than adjacent to nuclei.[29]

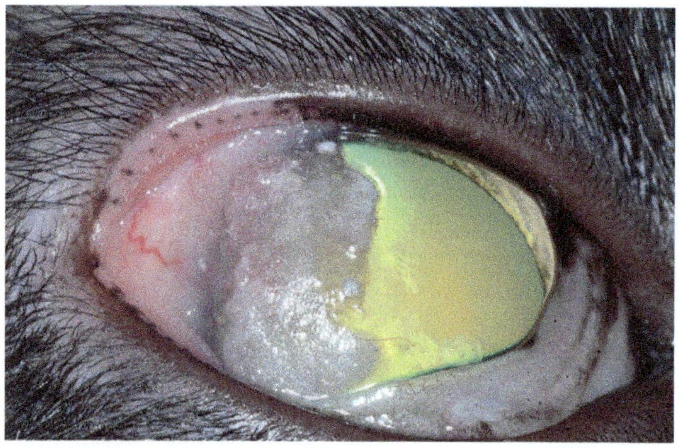

Figure 20.6 Clinical features of conjunctival disease. There is moderate chemosis and conjunctival hyperemia. In addition to the conjunctival abnormalities, there is depigmentation of the upper lateral eyelid margin, white cell plaques on the lateral 1/3 of the cornea, and superficial corneal vascularization.

Noninfectious

While it may be difficult to cytologically differentiate between the more common causes of feline conjunctivitis and keratoconjunctivitis, less common causes of feline conjunctivitis and keratoconjunctivitis have more specific cytologic patterns that facilitate diagnosis.

Eosinophilic Keratoconjunctivitis

Eosinophilic keratoconjunctivitis is characterized clinically by ocular discharge, conjunctival hyperemia, corneal vascularization, corneal edema, corneal white cell infiltrate, and tan to white plaques that are raised from the surfaces of the conjunctiva and cornea.[47–50] Other abnormalities that can also be present include corneal ulceration and depigmentation of the eyelids (Figure 20.6).[49–51] One or both eyes are affected.[47,49–51] The disease is suspected to be immune-mediated.[48,51] Some affected cats will test positive for FHV-1, especially those with concurrent corneal ulceration, but the pathogenic role of this organism is unclear.[49,51–53] The characteristic appearance of conjunctiva and corneal plaques allows a presumptive diagnosis to be made, but definitive diagnosis requires corneal cytology, preferably via direct sampling of the corneal plaques to maximize diagnostic yield. Typical cytological findings include a mixture of eosinophils, mast cells, neutrophils, and epithelial cells that can be hyperplastic (Figure 20.7a) or dysplastic (Figure 20.7b).[47,49,51,53] Lymphocytes, goblet cells, and mucous can also be present.[49–51,53] Inflammatory conditions often elicit

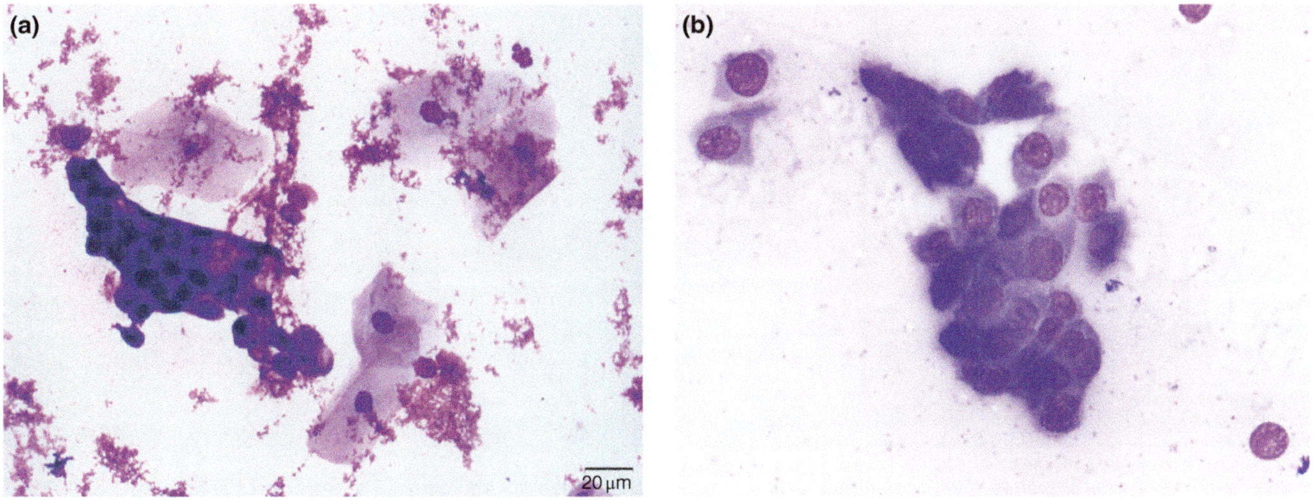

Figure 20.7 (a) Conjunctival scraping. Angular superficial squamous cells predominate, but a single cluster of deeply basophilic, cuboidal basilar epithelial cells is also noted, suggesting a hyperplastic response. Note the magenta colored amorphous artifact likely related to topical treatment of the eye with a petrolatum product (Wright–Giemsa, 1000×). (b) Conjunctival scraping. This dysplastic cluster of cuboidal to polygonal, cohesive conjunctival epithelial cells that has exfoliated displays mild pleomorphism in the form of anisocytosis and anisokaryosis. Small nucleoli, ropy chromatin, cellular encroachment, and slight nuclear molding are noted. Numerous eosinophil granules are noted in the background. Sample was collected from a patient with a clinical diagnosis of eosinophilic keratitis (Wright–Giemsa, 500×).

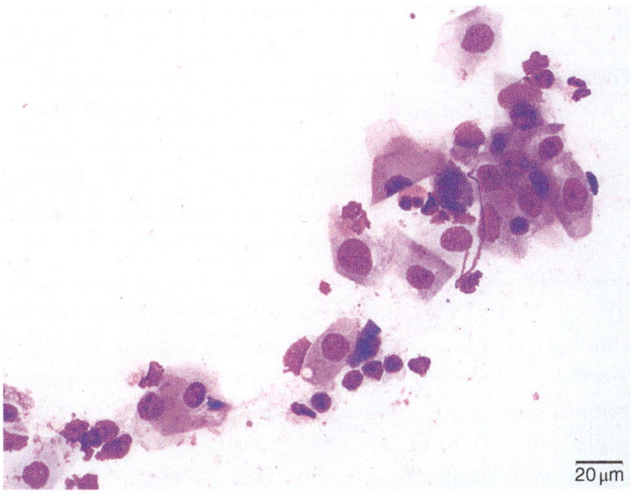

Figure 20.8 Corneal scraping of a cat with eosinophilic and lymphocytic keratitis. Numerous angular superficial squamous cells with small round nuclei and oval intermediate squamous cells with larger round nuclei predominate. Low numbers of eosinophils and small lymphocytes are present. The presence of eosinophils supports a diagnosis of eosinophilic keratoconjunctivitis. The presence of lymphocytes suggests some chronicity to the lesion (Wright–Giemsa, 500×).

hyperplastic and dysplastic responses in corneal and conjunctival epithelium, and morphology should be interpreted cautiously to avoid overinterpretation as evidence of epithelial neoplasia. The diagnosis is confirmed when eosinophils or their granules are observed (Figure 20.8).[47,48] The observation of mast cells can lead to a misdiagnosis of mast cell tumor.[47,48] Eosinophilic keratoconjunctivitis does not appear to be related to the dermatologic eosinophilic granuloma complex.

Epitheliotropic Mastocytic Conjunctivitis

This is a benign conjunctivitis occurring rarely in cats.[54] An underlying allergy has been postulated.[54] Clinically, it is characterized by proliferative or nodular conjunctivitis, with or without concurrent keratitis or nictitans lesions.[54] White to tan conjunctival plaques and conjunctival ulceration also can be seen.[54] Cytology is not helpful in obtaining a definitive diagnosis due to the similar findings for other causes of feline conjunctivitis such as eosinophilic keratoconjunctivitis, *C. felis*, and conjunctival mast cell tumors.[54] Rather, histopathologic visualization of intraepithelial mast cells is required for diagnosis.[54] Mast cells tend to be well-differentiated with basophilic to amphophilic granular cytoplasm, with metachromatic granules stained by toluidine blue, Giemsa, or both.[54] Common concurrent histologic changes include papillary epithelial proliferation, marked conjunctival edema, and infiltration of the substantia propria with lymphocytes, plasma cells, eosinophils, and neutrophils.[54] Testing for FHV-1 is usually negative.[54]

Lipogranulomatous Conjunctivitis

This is a very uncommon cause of feline conjunctivitis, presenting as white, opaque, nodular swellings that are 1–5 mm in diameter within the palpebral conjunctiva (Figure 20.9a). The average age of onset is approximately

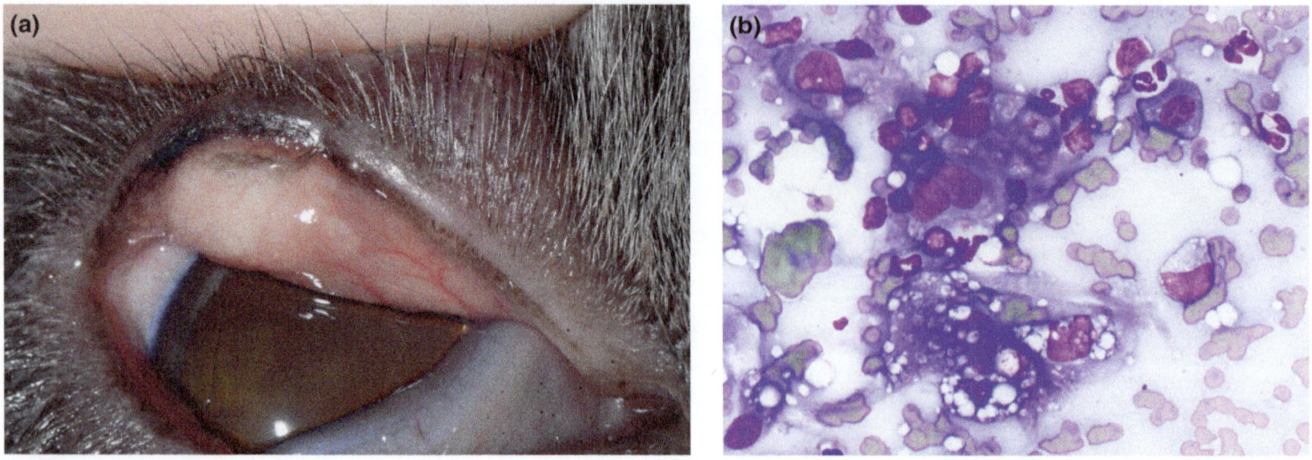

Figure 20.9 (a) A white, opaque, nodular swelling is present within the palpebral conjunctiva. The lesion was confirmed histologically as lipogranulomatous conjunctivitis (*Source:* Image courtesy of Michala de Linde Henriksen). (b) Cytology of this same case contained a mixed population of inflammatory cells including neutrophils, small and medium lymphocytes, and macrophages, some of which contained clear, punctate lipid vacuoles (Wright–Giemsa, 1000×. *Source:* Image courtesy of Leslie Sharkey).

11 years.[55,56] Cats with white skin are disproportionately affected.[56] Histologically, variably sized clear spaces are seen within the conjunctival lamina propria; special stains confirm these contain lipid.[55] Surrounding the spaces are flattened macrophages, multinucleated giant cells, and some accumulations of lymphocytes, plasma cells, and rare neutrophils.[55] Goblet cell hyperplasia is also sometimes seen.[55,56] Lesions tend to occur near the Meibomian glands.[55,56] Cytologic findings have not been reported in the primary literature, but based on histopathology are expected to consist of macrophage predominant inflammation with lesser numbers of lymphocytes, plasma cells, and few neutrophils characteristic of a foreign body response. Representative cytology from a histologically confirmed lesion is demonstrated in Figure 20.9b.

Medication Effects

Local irritation in response to topically applied medications has also been reported,[57,58] although the frequency of this has not been defined. In one study assessing the effects of an ointment vehicle, cytology from cats that developed conjunctivitis following application of the ointment was described only as inflammation without evidence of epithelial metaplasia or intra- or extracellular bacteria.[57]

Acute Bullous Keratopathy

Acute bullous keratopathy (ABK) causes rapidly progressive corneal edema and bulla formation.[59] The cause is unknown; corneal dystrophy and administration of anti-inflammatory medications have been implicated.[59,60] As ABK progresses, keratoconus develops; the cornea thins and without treatment eventually ruptures.[61] The clinical appearance of ABK is very similar to the collagenolysis that is characteristic of melting corneal ulcers in dogs. However, with ABK, there is minimal, neutrophilic corneal inflammation and no evidence of infectious organisms.[61,62]

Corneal Sequestrum

This disease consists of necrosis of the corneal stroma occurring in response to chronic corneal trauma.[61] FHV-1 may play a role in development of sequestra,[52,63,64] as may *Toxoplasma gondii*.[63] Clinically, sequestra are characterized by light brown to black corneal discoloration, most often affecting the central cornea.[61,65] Concurrent corneal ulceration and keratitis of variable severity are present. Cytology is usually only performed to confirm or negate secondary bacterial infection. Samples obtained from a mineralized sequestrum yielded nondegenerate neutrophils, normal epithelial cells, and small numbers of secondarily invading and infecting bacterial cocci.[66]

Neoplasia

Neoplasms affecting the feline ocular surface are uncommon. Reported tumors of the cornea and limbus include SCC, hemangioma, mast cell tumor, melanoma, and fibrosarcoma.[67–74] Reported conjunctival neoplasms include SCC, lymphoma, melanoma, and hemangioma.[71,75–78] Reported neoplasms of the nictitans include adenocarcinoma ($n = 15$; 83.3%) followed by SCC ($n = 3$; 16.7%).[79] Of note is that feline nictitating membrane malignancies are reported to behave more aggressively than their canine counterparts, with shorter survival times and higher metastasis and recurrence rates.[79] Cytology images of ocular SCC can be found in Chapter 21; mast cell tumors are addressed in Chapter 13, melanoma in Chapter 15, and fibrosarcoma in Chapter 16.

Squamous Cell Carcinoma

This tumor affects the conjunctiva, nictitating membrane, and cornea.[71,73] It is aggressive with the potential for intraocular and/or orbital invasion[73,79] and often presents as a chronic keratitis unresponsive to therapy, with or without a mass effect.[71,73] The cytologic appearance of ocular SCC is similar to its counterpart occurring elsewhere (Table 20.1). Briefly, squamous cells are variably mature and exfoliate singly or in sheets. They vary from round to angular depending on the degree of differentiation. Less mature, rounder, more basilar cells contain a small amount of basophilic cytoplasm, while larger, angular, more mature cells are characterized by light blue, keratinized cytoplasm. Angular keratinized cells can contain large, round nuclei indicative of asynchronous maturation of nuclei relative to cytoplasm – a criterion of malignancy characteristic of SCCs. Other features often identified in SCCs include emperipolesis, "tear-drop-" or "tadpole-"shaped squamous cells, and perinuclear punctate vacuoles assumed to represent colorless and atypical keratohyalin granules (Figure 20.10). SCCs are frequently inflamed, and variable numbers of neutrophils typically appear with neoplastic cells. In addition, lymphocytic inflammation has been described associated with this neoplasm.[71,73]

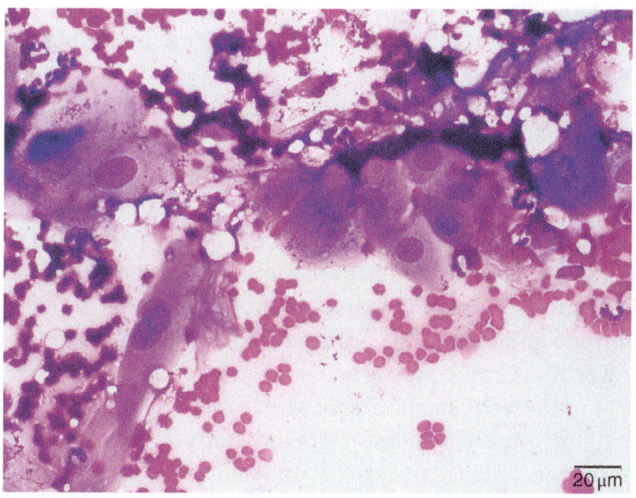

Figure 20.10 Aspirate of squamous cell carcinoma in the nictitating membrane in a cat. A population of keratinized squamous cells of various morphology (angular, polygonal, "tadpole" shaped) has exfoliated singly and in poorly cohesive sheets. Cells show atypia including anisocytosis, nuclear pleomorphism, multinucleation, nuclear-to-cytoplasmic asynchronous maturation, and prominent nucleoli. Erythrocytes and scattered neutrophils are present in the background. Neutrophil emperipolesis is observed in the angular cell on the far right of the image (Wright–Giemsa, 500×).

Conjunctival Lymphoma

This malignancy most often presents as a swelling of the upper palpebral conjunctiva.[75,80–82] The cytologic appearance of lymphoma is similar to its counterpart in other parts of the body and is described in detail elsewhere (Chapter 27) (Table 20.1). Briefly, an immature population of large round cells (1.5–2.5 times the diameter of a neutrophil) is present. Immunohistochemistry shows that most are B cell in origin.[75,80–82]

Conjunctival Melanoma

This is an uncommon neoplasm in the cat. It originates from the palpebral conjunctiva, the conjunctiva overlying the third eyelid, or the bulbar conjunctiva.[16,67,77,78,83] Although benign lesions have been documented,[69,77] all conjunctival melanocytic neoplasms should be considered malignant with a high likelihood of distant metastasis until proven otherwise.[78,83,84] Cytologic findings are similar to melanoma aspirates in other tissues and are described thoroughly in other chapters (Table 20.1). The cytologic appearance of melanotic neoplasms from any body site, including the eye, is highly variable and depends on the differentiation and pigmentation of the cells (Chapter 15). Cells can be round, spindled, or epithelioid with a small to moderate amount of lightly basophilic cytoplasm with variably distinct cytoplasmic margins. Pigmentation can be absent, consist of a light cytoplasmic dusting of fine brown-black melanin pigment, or reflect dense pigmentation that obscures the nucleus. Nuclei are large and round to oval with open chromatin and large, angular, prominent nucleoli. When present in pairs, the nucleoli give the nucleus the appearance of a "pig nose." One cytologic description of a conjunctival mass, ultimately diagnosed as benign conjunctival melanoma, described neutrophilic inflammation with some lymphocytes and plasma cells, as well as melanophages.[77] Difficulty differentiating between melanophages and neoplastic cells is reported;[77] however, anecdotally, melanophages tend to contain larger, chunkier, irregular melanin pigment, while melanocytes tend to contain finer, more uniform, round- or rod-shaped melanin granules. Because of significant overlap in the appearance of benign and well-differentiated malignant melanotic neoplasms, cytology is limited to a diagnosis of "melanotic neoplasm." Histologic examination of the lesion is required for definitive determination of biological behavior. Histologically, conjunctival melanomas are composed of predominantly round cells or a mixture of round and spindle cells; exclusively spindle cell tumors are not described.[78] Most tumors are abundantly pigmented, but they can be poorly pigmented as well.[78] Necrosis and inflammatory cells have been reported.[77] Risk of recurrence or metastasis cannot be determined by histologic tumor morphology; however,[78] criteria of malignancy (such as prominent nucleoli, anisocytosis, anisokaryosis, and mitotic figures) have been suggested as the best indicators of prognosis in feline melanotic tumors.[77]

Hemangioma and Hemangiosarcoma

Both of these tumors can affect the conjunctiva and the cornea in cats. Affected cats tend to be lightly pigmented; exposure to ultraviolet light is thought to play a role in tumor development.[71,72,76,85] Conjunctival hemangioma and hemangiosarcoma are red to brown, smooth to multilobulated, exophytic nodules most often arising from the leading edge of the third eyelid.[71,76,85] Corneal tumors present as raised, vascular, hemorrhagic corneal masses with associated keratitis.[71,72] A gross image of ocular hemangiosarcoma in a horse is presented in Chapter 21. Due to the small size of these masses, aspiration for cytology is not possible in the cat, further complicated by the fact that sampling of these vascular tumors often yields only blood. Histologically, tumors are characterized by spindle-shaped to polygonal neoplastic endothelial cells forming vascular spaces in which erythrocytes can be seen.[71,72,85] Neoplastic cells contain minimal cytoplasm, demonstrate nuclear pleomorphism, have variably prominent nucleoli, and can have an increased mitotic index.[72,85] Differentiation between hemangioma and hemangiosarcoma is based on histologic degree of differentiation and local tissue invasion.[76]

Iris and Ciliary Body

Normal Structure, Cytology, and Collection

The uveal tract is composed of the iris and ciliary body anteriorly and the choroid posteriorly. The iris is the most anterior part of the uveal tract; the base is attached to the anterior ciliary body. It is composed of a loose connective tissue stroma containing fibroblasts, melanocytes, blood vessels, and circumferentially arranged bundles of smooth muscles. The anterior iris has no epithelial surface but rather is covered by a discontinuous layer of fibroblasts and melanocytes that allows fluid exchange with the anterior chamber. The posterior surface is covered by a bilayer of epithelial cells consisting of a basal layer of pigmented myoepithelial cells and a superficial layer of pigmented columnar cells.[86,87] The ciliary body joins the choroid to the base of the iris. It is composed of loose connective tissue, elastic fibers, smooth muscle (ciliary muscle), and blood vessels and is lined by a bilayer of epithelial cells consisting of a pigmented basal layer and a non-pigmented surface layer of columnar cells.[86,87] Cytology of intraocular disease is performed much less often than for extraocular disease. When done, it is usually combined with other diagnostics to determine an underlying cause of anterior uveitis. Aspiration of vitreous inflammation or intraocular masses appears to be extremely uncommon; enucleation with histopathology is the most common diagnostic test when intraocular masses are present.

Inflammation

Causes of uveitis are numerous and include endogenous causes such as corneal ulceration, ocular trauma, cataract, and lens luxation and exogenous causes such as metastatic malignancy and infectious disease.[88,89] Idiopathic uveitis, the most common cause of uveitis, accounts for between 40 and 70% of cases and is a diagnosis of exclusion.[88–90] The most commonly implicated infectious diseases include feline leukemia virus, feline immunodeficiency virus, feline infectious peritonitis, *Bartonella* spp., *T. gondii*, cryptococcosis, histoplasmosis, blastomycosis, and coccidioidomycosis.[89–94] Other, rare, reported etiologies include intraocular parasites,[95–97] *Burkholderia pseudomallei*,[98] and septic peritonitis.[99] In the case of uveitis secondary to septic peritonitis, the authors hypothesize that uveitis may have been either secondary to hematogenous spread of bacterial organisms from the abdomen to the eye or the effect of circulating bacterial toxins and inflammatory mediators on the uvea.

Examination of the aqueous humor usually does not identify a specific etiology for the anterior uveitis in cats, but can identify the type and chronicity of inflammatory infiltrate.[100,101] Acute and chronic inflammation can be differentiated cytologically based on the higher proportion of polymorphonuclear cells to mononuclear cells with acute inflammation and the mainly mononuclear cells found in chronic inflammation.[100] In addition, protein levels are lower for chronic versus acute inflammation[100]; however, due to the very small sample size, protein concentrations are not routinely measured. One study of the aqueous humor in 37 dogs and cats found that cytology was only helpful in the diagnosis in three cases, none of them feline.[100] A more recent study also only revealed general trends, such as aqueous humor plasma cell numbers correlating with clinically visible keratic precipitates and disease duration, aqueous humor erythrocyte number correlating with clinical hyphema, and higher numbers of larger, reactive lymphocytes and plasma cells in the aqueous humor of cats with idiopathic uveitis.[101] As with the previous study, aqueous humor cytology did not lead to the diagnosis of the underlying cause of uveitis for any feline patient.[101]

To the authors' knowledge, specific cytologic findings from intraocular aspirates have not been reported, with the exception of *B. pseudomallei*.[98] Vitreous samples taken from one feline patient revealed high cellularity fluid dominated by degenerate neutrophils, with few lymphocytes and macrophages.[98] Gram-negative bacilli were visible both extra- and intracellularly.[98]

Neoplasia

The most common feline intraocular tumors are diffuse iris melanoma and lymphoma. Aqueocentesis is rarely performed to diagnose ocular melanoma due to the highly suggestive clinical appearance of brown iridal hyperpigmentation, with or without overt mass formation. By contrast, lymphoma often presents as a persistent uveitis,[102,103] for which aqueocentesis is more likely to be employed as part of a diagnostic workup. It is possible to visualize neoplastic lymphocytes in smears prepared from aqueocenteses based on the experience of the author (JB). Other intraocular neoplasms are rare. Reported intraocular tumors, which present as ocular masses or as uveitis, include iridociliary epithelial tumors, bronchogenic carcinoma, histiocytic sarcoma, melanocytoma, extramedullary plasmacytoma, osteosarcoma, fibrosarcoma, uveal spindle cell tumor similar to the spindle cell tumor of blue-eyed dogs (schwannoma), and posttraumatic ocular sarcoma.[104–115] Posttraumatic ocular sarcoma occurs in eyes with a history of trauma (including intraocular gentamicin injection for treatment of glaucoma), especially if the lens is disrupted, and is often found in phthisical eyes.[106,108,116–118] Cytologic descriptions of intraocular neoplasms other than lymphoma have not been reported in cat. Primary and metastatic intraocular neoplasms tend to be poorly exfoliative, and aspirates of aqueous and vitreous humor for the diagnosis of neoplastic disease may be of limited diagnostic value due to low cellularity. Direct aspiration of intraocular masses is infrequently attempted, and cytologic evaluation of feline intraocular masses has not been reported.

Aqueous and Vitreous Humor

Normal Structure, Cytology, and Collection

Vitreous humor and aqueous humor are transparent, gel-like, and colorless fluids that fill the space between the retina and the lens and the lens and cornea, respectively. In healthy eyes, aqueous humor is expected to be acellular with low protein content.[100,119] Collection techniques are described in Chapter 18.

Hyphema

Hyphema is a pooling or collection of blood inside the anterior chamber. Diagnosis of hyphema is typically made clinically as the presence of blood in the anterior chamber can readily be identified during an ophthalmic examination. Cytologic evaluation of hyphema is not specifically described in the literature but would be expected to be similar to cytologic evaluation of hemorrhagic effusions with abundant erythrocytes and variable numbers of macrophages, some of which may be erythrophagocytic or contain hemosiderin.

Inflammation

Although uncommon, aspiration of aqueous and vitreous humors is occasionally performed as part of a diagnostic workup for uveitis or in an attempt to identify an intraocular mass. Both cellularity and protein content tend to increase In the presence of disease.[100,119] These changes are described in the previous section "Iris and Ciliary Body." Regarding overall diagnostic utility however, aqueous humor cytology tends to be unhelpful in determining an etiologic diagnosis for anterior uveitis in cats.[120]

Neoplasia

Vitreocentesis or aqueocentesis can be attempted in order to diagnose intraocular neoplasia but has been found to be of limited utility for this purpose in cats.[120]

Retina

Normal Structure, Cytology, and Collection

The retina extends from the optic nerve and runs anteriorly to merge with the ciliary epithelial layers. It is composed of 10 histologically identifiable layers of specialized cells: the inner limiting membrane, the nerve fiber layer, the ganglion cell layer, the inner plexiform layer, the inner nuclear layer, the outer plexiform layer, the outer nuclear layer, the outer limiting membrane, the photoreceptor layer, and the retinal pigmented epithelium.[87] While the retina is very well described histologically, normal cytology of the feline retina has not been described.

Inflammation

Retinitis is rarely clinically diagnosed in cats. Cytology of feline retinitis has not been described.

Neoplasia

Primary retinal neoplasia is exceedingly rare and to the authors' knowledge has not been reported in cats. Cytology of feline retinal neoplasms has not been described.

Orbit

Generic signs of orbital disease include exophthalmos, raised third eyelid, chemosis, conjunctival hyperemia, periocular tissue swelling, decreased globe retropulsion, and sometimes enophthalmos. Most are associated with an orbital mass effect and do not point to a specific etiology. The most common causes of orbital disease in cat include inflammation of infectious origin and orbital neoplasia.

Inflammation

Sino-orbital aspergillosis (SOA) appears to be diagnosed with increasing frequency recently. It can be a progression of sinonasal aspergillosis,[121] and brachycephalic cats are disproportionately affected.[122] Clinical signs include exophthalmos, dorsolateral deviation of the globe, decreased globe retropulsion, and raised third eyelid.[122–127] Conjunctival hyperemia and keratitis also can be present.[121,124,125] Signs of upper respiratory disease are usually present.[121,126] Treatment with systemic steroids can be associated with improvement or worsening of clinical signs.[124,126] Cytology taken from diseased orbital tissues sometimes yields fungal hyphae and mixed inflammatory infiltrate (Chapter 3).[124] However, etiologic agents are frequently absent, and failure to identify fungal hyphae on cytology should not rule out SOA.[22,123,125,126] Fungal culture and histopathology from affected areas are recommended to increase the sensitivity for detecting organisms.[121,126] Histologic changes include visualization of fungal hyphae up to 5 μm in width and granulomatous, pyogranulomatous, eosinophilic, or lymphoplasmacytic inflammation.[122,124–127] Scattered neutrophils, eosinophils, and mast cells can also be present.[126] Staining with Gomori methenamine silver or periodic acid–Schiff is recommended to visualize fungal hyphae.

Orbital bacterial cellulitis resulting from external trauma/puncture wounds, extension from the oral and nasal cavities, or penetration of the orbit during dental extractions is not uncommon.[128] Aspiration of the lesion is expected to produce purulent material composed of degenerate neutrophils and often a mixed population of bacterial organisms (Figure 20.11).

Neoplasia

The most common orbital tumor in cats is SCC.[129] Aspirates are typically high yield and diagnostic and are cytologically similar to SCC of the ocular surfaces as described above. Other orbital tumors described include but are not limited to lymphoma, melanoma, mast cell tumors, hemangiosarcoma, chondroma, fibrosarcoma, meningioma, peripheral nerve sheath tumor, and adenocarcinoma of the lacrimal and salivary glands. Although they can present clinically as orbital disease (Figure 20.12), many of these tumors are a result of extension from other structures within or

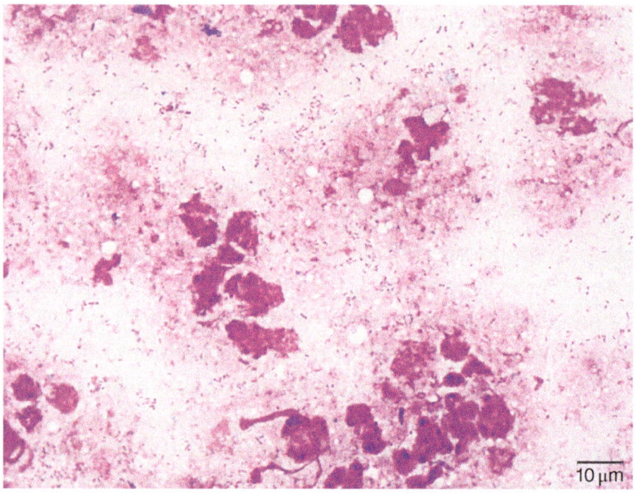

Figure 20.11 Orbital aspirate. A myriad of extracellular rod-shaped bacteria are found in the stippled proteinaceous background. Numerous markedly degenerated neutrophils (so degenerate that they are barely recognizable as such) have exfoliated (Wright–Giemsa, 1000×).

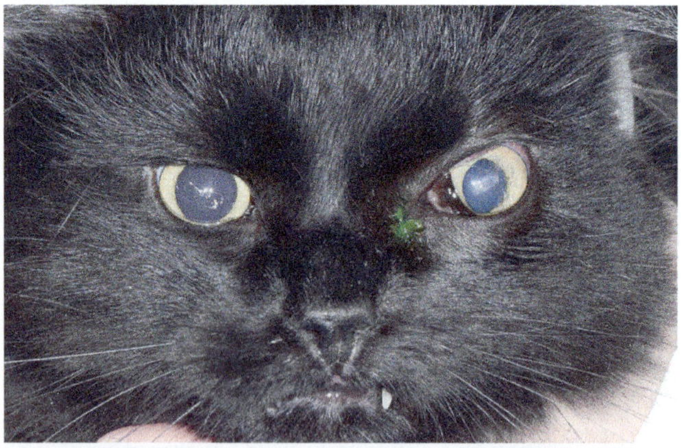

Figure 20.12 Clinical features of orbital disease. There is left-sided ocular discharge, third eyelid elevation, and episcleral hyperemia. The left globe is exophthalmic and displaced dorsally and laterally. The direction of globe displacement suggests a mass-like lesion ventral and medial to the globe. This patient was ultimately diagnosed with sino-orbital aspergillosis.

surrounding the eye, oral cavity, or nasal sinus. In one study of 21 histopathologically confirmed orbital neoplasms, 14% of orbital neoplasms were primary, 71% were invading the orbit from adjacent tissues, and 14% were a manifestation of multicentric disease.[129]

Feline restrictive myofibroblastic sarcoma (FROMS) is another proliferative process previously referred to as feline orbital pseudotumor. It is characterized clinically by a slowly progressive restriction of the eyelids and globe, leading to lagophthalmos and secondary keratoconjunctivitis and corneal ulceration.[130–132] Entropion can also result.[131,132] The condition can present unilaterally or bilaterally. However, unilateral cases almost inevitably become bilateral with time due to infiltration of neoplastic cells along fascial planes.[130,131,133] The invasive nature of this neoplasm often leads to involvement of the lips and oral cavity as well.[131–133] In one case, neoplastic spindle cells invaded into the bones of the maxilla, hard palate, gingiva, and nasal cavity.[132] Cytology has not been reported. Diagnosis is made histologically, usually of enucleation, exenteration, or necropsy specimens. Microscopy reveals bland spindle cell infiltration and invasion along fascial planes with entrapment and atrophy of normal orbital tissues.[131,133] The densest infiltration occurs at the limbus or the palpebral conjunctiva near the fornix.[133] Mitotic index is low.[133] Lymphoplasmacytic inflammation is observed at the margins between neoplastic and normal tissues.[131,133] Immunohistochemistry reveals strong labeling for smooth muscle actin, S-100 protein, and vimentin in most samples.[132,133] These findings may lead to a misdiagnosis of reactive fibrosis; however, compared with reactive fibrosis, the inflammation associated with FROMS is minimal.[133] Submission of samples taken from the anterior and superior episclera, conjunctival substantia propria near the fornix, thickened skin, or grossly abnormal orbital tissue, along with adequate clinical history, will decrease the potential for misdiagnosis.[133] If enucleation or exenteration is performed, the globe should be submitted with all surrounding soft tissues in place.[133]

Conclusion

Feline ocular cytology is most commonly employed to determine the type and etiology of conjunctivitis, keratitis, uveitis, and endophthalmitis and to diagnose solid tissue or cystic masses of the globe and surrounding structures.

References

1. Willis, M., Bounous, D.I., Hirsh, S. et al. (1997). Conjunctival brush cytology: evaluation of a new cytological collection technique in dogs and cats with a comparison to conjunctival scraping. *Vet Comp Ophthalmol* 7: 74–81.
2. Venancio, S.A.S., Vieira, A.B., Alencar, N.X., and AMB, S. (2012). Avaliação da técnica de esfoliação com escova citológica para coleta de células conjuntivais em gatos sadios: comparação entre a face palpebral da membrana nictitante e a conjuntiva palpebral. *Pesqui Vet Bras* 32: 1199–1204.
3. Eordogh, R., Schwendenwein, I., Tichy, A., and Nell, B. (2015). Impression cytology: a novel sampling technique for conjunctival cytology of the feline eye. *Vet Ophthalmol* 18: 276–284.
4. Perazzi, A., Bonsembiante, F., Gelain, M.E. et al. (2017). Cytology of the healthy canine and feline ocular surface: comparison between cytobrush and impression technique. *Vet Clin Pathol* 46: 164–171.
5. Chaitman, J., van der Woerdt, A., and Bartick, T.E. (1999). Multiple eyelid cysts resembling apocrine hidrocystomas in three Persian cats and one Himalayan cat. *Vet Pathol* 36: 474–476.
6. Giudice, C., Muscolo, M.C., Rondena, M. et al. (2009). Eyelid multiple cysts of the apocrine gland of Moll in Persian cats. *J Feline Med Surg* 11: 487–491.
7. Cantaloube, B., Raymond-Letron, I., and Regnier, A. (2004). Multiple eyelid apocrine hidrocystomas in two Persian cats. *Vet Ophthalmol* 7: 121–125.
8. Kahane, N., Ofri, R., Prager, O. et al. (2014). Aprocrine hidrocystoma in four Persian cats. *Isr J Vet Med* 69: 29–34.
9. Sivagurunathan, A., Goodhead, A.D., and Du Plessis, E.C. (2010). Multiple eyelid apocrine hidrocystoma in a domestic short-haired cat. *J S Afr Vet Assoc* 81: 65–68.
10. Newkirk, K.M. and Rohrbach, B.W. (2009). A retrospective study of eyelid tumors from 43 cats. *Vet Pathol* 46: 916–927.
11. Raskin, R.E. (2010). Skin and subcutaneous tissues. In: *Canine and Feline Cytology A color Atlas and Interpretation Guide*, 2e (eds. R.E. Raskin and D.J. Meyer), 55. St. Louis, MO: Elsevier.
12. Turrel, J.M., Farrelly, J., Page, R.L., and MC, M.E. (2006). Evaluation of strontium 90 irradiation in treatment of cutaneous mast cell tumors in cats: 35 cases (1992–2002). *J Am Vet Med Assoc* 228: 898–901.

13 Montgomery, K.W., van der Woerdt, A., Aquino, S.M. et al. (2010). Periocular cutaneous mast cell tumors in cats: evaluation of surgical excision (33 cases). *Vet Ophthalmol* 13: 26–30.

14 Hartley, C., Ladlow, J., and Smith, K.C. (2007). Cutaneous haemangiosarcoma of the lower eyelid in an elderly white cat. *J Feline Med Surg* 9: 78–81.

15 Dorn, C.R., Taylor, D.O., and Schneider, R. (1971). Sunlight exposure and risk of developing cutaneous and oral squamous cell carcinomas in white cats. *J Natl Cancer Inst* 46: 1073–1078.

16 Wang, A.L. and Kern, T. (2015). Melanocytic ophthalmic neoplasms of the domestic veterinary species: a review. *Top Companion Anim Med* 30: 148–157.

17 Lavach, J.D., Thrall, M.A., Benjamin, M.M., and Severin, G.A. (1977). Cytology of normal and inflamed conjunctivas in dogs and cats. *J Am Vet Med Assoc* 170: 722–727.

18 Featherstone, H.J. and Heinrich, C.L. (2013). Ophthalmic examination and diagnostics. In: *Veterinary Ophthalmology*, 5e (eds. K.N. Gelatt, B.C. Gilger and T.J. Kern). Ames, IA: Wiley-Blackwell.

19 Sykes, J.E. (2005). Feline chlamydiosis. *Clin Tech Small Anim Pract* 20: 129–134.

20 Nasisse, M.P., Guy, J.S., Stevens, J.B. et al. (1993). Clinical and laboratory findings in chronic conjunctivitis in cats: 91 cases (1983–1991). *J Am Vet Med Assoc* 203: 834–837.

21 Low, H.C., Powell, C.C., Veir, J.K. et al. (2007). Prevalence of feline herpesvirus 1, *Chlamydophila felis*, and *Mycoplasma* spp DNA in conjunctival cells collected from cats with and without conjunctivitis. *Am J Vet Res* 68: 643–648.

22 Hartmann, A.D., Hawley, J., Werckenthin, C. et al. (2010). Detection of bacterial and viral organisms from the conjunctiva of cats with conjunctivitis and upper respiratory tract disease. *J Feline Med Surg* 12: 775–782.

23 Hoover, E.A., Kahn, D.E., and Langloss, J.M. (1978). Experimentally induced feline chlamydial infection (feline pneumonitis). *Am J Vet Res* 39: 541–547.

24 von Bomhard, W., Polkinghorne, A., Lu, Z.H. et al. (2003). Detection of novel chlamydiae in cats with ocular disease. *Am J Vet Res* 64: 1421–1428.

25 Richter, M., Matheis, F., Gonczi, E. et al. (2010). *Parachlamydia acanthamoebae* in domestic cats with and without corneal disease. *Vet Ophthalmol* 13: 235–237.

26 Sibitz, C., Rudnay, E.C., Wabnegger, L. et al. (2011). Detection of *Chlamydophila pneumoniae* in cats with conjunctivitis. *Vet Ophthalmol* 14 (Suppl 1): 67–74.

27 Fox, J.G. and Galus, C.B. (1977). Salmonella-associated conjunctivitis in a cat. *J Am Vet Med Assoc* 171: 845–847.

28 Lamagna, B., Paciello, O., Ragozzino, M. et al. (2009). Isolated lepromatous conjunctivo-corneal granuloma in a cat from Italy. *Vet Ophthalmol* 12: 97–101.

29 Hillstrom, A., Tvedten, H., Kallberg, M. et al. (2012). Evaluation of cytologic findings in feline conjunctivitis. *Vet Clin Pathol* 41: 283–290.

30 Walther, B., Wieler, L.H., Vincze, S. et al. (2012). MRSA variant in companion animals. *Emerg Infect Dis* 18: 2017–2020.

31 Fyfe, J.A., McCowan, C., O'Brien, C.R. et al. (2008). Molecular characterization of a novel fastidious mycobacterium causing lepromatous lesions of the skin, subcutis, cornea, and conjunctiva of cats living in Victoria, Australia. *J Clin Microbiol* 46: 618–626.

32 Schubach, T.M., Schubach, A., Okamoto, T. et al. (2004). Evaluation of an epidemic of sporotrichosis in cats: 347 cases (1998–2001). *J Am Vet Med Assoc* 224: 1623–1629.

33 Tofflemire, K. and Betbeze, C. (2010). Three cases of feline ocular coccidioidomycosis: presentation, clinical features, diagnosis, and treatment. *Vet Ophthalmol* 13: 166–172.

34 Labelle, A.L., Hamor, R.E., Barger, A.M. et al. (2009). *Aspergillus flavus* keratomycosis in a cat treated with topical 1% voriconazole solution. *Vet Ophthalmol* 12: 48–52.

35 Dorchies, P., Chaudieu, G., Simeon, L.A. et al. (2007). First reports of autochthonous eyeworm infection by *Thelazia callipaeda* (Spirurida, Thelaziidae) in dogs and cat from France. *Vet Parasitol* 149: 294–297.

36 Soares, C., Ramalho Sousa, S., Anastacio, S. et al. (2013). Feline thelaziosis caused by *Thelazia callipaeda* in Portugal. *Vet Parasitol* 196: 528–531.

37 Chatzis, M.K., Andreadou, M., Leontides, L. et al. (2014). Cytological and molecular detection of *Leishmania infantum* in different tissues of clinically normal and sick cats. *Vet Parasitol* 202: 217–225.

38 Gray, L.D., Ketring, K.L., and Tang, Y.W. (2005). Clinical use of 16S rRNA gene sequencing to identify *Mycoplasma felis* and M. gateae associated with feline ulcerative keratitis. *J Clin Microbiol* 43: 3431–3434.

39 Lin, C.T. and Petersen-Jones, S.M. (2008). Antibiotic susceptibility of bacteria isolated from cats with ulcerative keratitis in Taiwan. *J Small Anim Pract* 49: 80–83.

40 Binder, D.R., Sugrue, J.E., and Herring, I.P. (2011). Acremonium keratomycosis in a cat. *Vet Ophthalmol* 14 (Suppl 1): 111–116.

41 Nasisse, M.P., Guy, J.S., Davidson, M.G. et al. (1989). Experimental ocular herpesvirus infection in the cat. Sites of virus replication, clinical features and effects of corticosteroid administration. *Invest Ophthalmol Vis Sci* 30: 1758–1768.

42 Nasisse, M.P. and Weigler, B.J. (1997). The diagnosis of ocular feline herpesvirus infection. *Vet Comp Ophthalmol* 7: 44–51.

43 Volopich, S., Benetka, V., Schwendenwein, I. et al. (2005). Cytologic findings, and feline herpesvirus DNA and *Chlamydophila felis* antigen detection rates in normal cats and cats with conjunctival and corneal lesions. *Vet Ophthalmol* 8: 25–32.

44 Murphy, J.M. (1988). Exfoliative cytologic examination as an aid in diagnosing ocular diseases in the dog and cat. *Semin Vet Med Surg* 3: 10–14.

45 Woodland, R.M., El-Sheikh, H., Darougar, S., and Squires, S. (1978). Sensitivity of immunoperoxidase and immunofluorescence staining for detecting chlamydia in conjunctival scrapings and in cell culture. *J Clin Pathol* 31: 1073–1077.

46 Campbell, L.H., Snyder, S.B., Reed, C., and Fox, J.G. (1973). *Mycoplasma felis*-associated conjunctivitis in cats. *J Am Vet Med Assoc* 163: 991–995.

47 Paulsen, M.E., Lavach, J.D., Severin, G.A., and Eichenbaum, J.D. (1987). Feline eosinophlic keratitis: a review of 15 clinical cases. *J Am Anim Hosp Assoc* 23: 63–69.

48 Pentlarge, V.W. (1991). Eosinophilic conjunctivitis in five cats. *J Am Anim Hosp Assoc* 27: 21–28.

49 Morgan, R.V., Abrams, K.L., and Kern, T.J. (1996). Feline eosinophilic keratitis: a retrospective study of 54 cases: (1989–1994). *Vet Comp Ophthalmol* 6: 131–134.

50 Spiess, A.K., Sapienza, J.S., and Mayordomo, A. (2009). Treatment of proliferative feline eosinophilic keratitis with topical 1.5% cyclosporine: 35 cases. *Vet Ophthalmol* 12: 132–137.

51 Allgoewer, I., Schaffer, E.H., Stockhaus, C., and Vögtlin, A. (2001). Feline eosinophilic conjunctivitis. *Vet Ophthalmol* 4: 69–74.

52 Nasisse, M.P., Glover, T.L., Moore, C.P., and Weigler, B.J. (1998). Detection of feline herpesvirus 1 DNA in corneas of cats with eosinophilic keratitis or corneal sequestration. *Am J Vet Res* 59: 856–858.

53 Dean, E. and Meunier, V. (2013). Feline eosinophilic keratoconjunctivitis: a retrospective study of 45 cases (56 eyes). *J Feline Med Surg* 15: 661–666.

54 Beckwith-Cohen, B., Dubielzig, R.R., Maggs, D.J., and Teixeira, L.B. (2017). Feline epitheliotropic mastocytic conjunctivitis in 15 cats. *Vet Pathol* 54: 141–146.

55 Kerlin, R.L. and Dubielzig, R.R. (1997). Lipogranulomatous conjunctivitis in cats. *Vet Comp Ophthalmol* 7: 177–179.

56 Read, R.A. and Lucas, J. (2001). Lipogranulomatous conjunctivitis: clinical findings from 21 eyes in 13 cats. *Vet Ophthalmol* 4: 93–98.

57 Eordogh, R., Schwendenwein, I., Tichy, A. et al. (2016). Clinical effect of four different ointment bases on healthy cat eyes. *Vet Ophthalmol* 19 (Suppl 1): 4–12.

58 Hume-Smith, K.M., Groth, A.D., Rishniw, M. et al. (2011). Anaphylactic events observed within 4 h of ocular application of an antibiotic-containing ophthalmic preparation: 61 cats (1993–2010). *J Feline Med Surg* 13: 744–751.

59 Glover, T.L., Nasisse, M.P., and Davidson, M.G. (1994). Acute bullous keratopathy in the cat. *Vet Comp Ophthalmol* 4: 66–70.

60 Pierce, K.E., Bartoe, J.T., Wilkie, D.A. et al. (2010). Abstract No.: 046 An association between acute bullous keratopathy and administration of systemic anti-inflammatory/immunosuppressive therapy in cats. Proceedings of the ACVO. *Vet Ophthalmol* 13: 407–423.

61 Lim, C.C. and Maggs, D.J. (2012). Ophthalmology. In: *The Cat* (ed. S.E. Little), 807–845. St. Louis, MO: Saunders/Elsevier.

62 Pattullo, K. (2008). Acute bullous keratopathy in a domestic shorthair. *Can Vet J* 49: 187–189.

63 Cullen, C.L., Wadowska, D.W., Singh, A., and Melekhovets, Y. (2005). Ultrastructural findings in feline corneal sequestra. *Vet Ophthalmol* 8: 295–303.

64 Grahn, B.H., Sisler, S., and Storey, E. (2005). Qualitative tear film and conjunctival goblet cell assessment of cats with corneal sequestra. *Vet Ophthalmol* 8: 167–170.

65 Featherstone, H.J., Franklin, V.J., and Sansom, J. (2004). Feline corneal sequestrum: laboratory analysis of ocular samples from 12 cats. *Vet Ophthalmol* 7: 229–238.

66 Gemensky, A.J. and Wilkie, D.A. (2001). Mineralized corneal sequestrum in a cat. *J Am Vet Med Assoc* 219: 1568–1572. 1550.

67 Betton, A., Healy, L.N., English, R.V., and Bunch, S.E. (1999). Atypical limbal melanoma in a cat. *J Vet Intern Med* 13: 379–381.

68 Larocca, R.D. (2000). Eosinophilic conjunctivitis, herpes virus and mast cell tumor of the third eyelid in a cat. *Vet Ophthalmol* 3: 221–225.

69 Kanai, K., Kanemaki, N., Matsuo, S. et al. (2006). Excision of a feline limbal melanoma and use of nictitans cartilage to repair the resulting corneoscleral defect. *Vet Ophthalmol* 9: 255–258.

70 Plummer, C.E., Kallberg, M.E., Ollivier, F.J. et al. (2008). Use of a biosynthetic material to repair the surgical defect following excision of an epibulbar melanoma in a cat. *Vet Ophthalmol* 11: 250–254.

71 Perlmann, E., da Silva, E.G., Guedes, P.M., and Barros, P.S. (2010). Co-existing squamous cell carcinoma and hemangioma on the ocular surface of a cat. *Vet Ophthalmol* 13: 63–66.

72 Cazalot, G., Regnier, A., Deviers, A. et al. (2011). Corneal hemangiosarcoma in a cat. *Vet Ophthalmol* 14 (Suppl 1): 117–121.

73 Scurrell, E.J., Lewin, G., Solomons, M. et al. (2013). Corneolimbal squamous cell carcinoma with intraocular invasion in two cats. *Vet Ophthalmol* 16 (Suppl 1): 151–154.

74 Strong, T.D., Tangeman, S., Ben-Shlomo, G. et al. (2016). Corneal fibrosarcoma in a cat. *Vet Ophthalmol* 19 (Suppl 1): 131–135.

75 Radi, Z.A., Miller, D.L., and Hines, M.E. 2nd (2004). B-cell conjunctival lymphoma in a cat. *Vet Ophthalmol* 7: 413–415.

76 Pirie, C.G. and Dubielzig, R.R. (2006). Feline conjunctival hemangioma and hemangiosarcoma: a retrospective evaluation of eight cases (1993–2004). *Vet Ophthalmol* 9: 227–231.

77 Payen, G., Estrada, M., Clerc, B., and Chahory, S. (2008). A case of conjunctival melanoma in a cat. *Vet Ophthalmol* 11: 401–405.

78 Schobert, C.S., Labelle, P., and Dubielzig, R.R. (2010). Feline conjunctival melanoma: histopathological characteristics and clinical outcomes. *Vet Ophthalmol* 13: 43–46.

79 Dees, D.D., Schobert, C.S., Dubielzig, R.R., and Stein, T.J. (2016). Third eyelid gland neoplasms of dogs and cats: a retrospective histopathologic study of 145 cases. *Vet Ophthalmol* 19: 138–143.

80 Holt, E., Goldschmidt, M.H., and Skorupski, K. (2006). Extranodal conjunctival Hodgkin's-like lymphoma in a cat. *Vet Ophthalmol* 9: 141–144.

81 McCowan, C., Malcolm, J., Hurn, S. et al. (2014). Conjunctival lymphoma: immunophenotype and outcome in five dogs and three cats. *Vet Ophthalmol* 17: 351–357.

82 Ota-Kuroki, J., Ragsdale, J.M., Bawa, B. et al. (2014). Intraocular and periocular lymphoma in dogs and cats: a retrospective review of 21 cases (2001–2012). *Vet Ophthalmol* 17: 389–396.

83 Roels, S. and Ducatelle, R. (1998). Malignant melanoma of the nictitating membrane in a cat (*Felis vulgaris*). *J Comp Pathol* 119: 189–193.

84 Cook, C.S., Rosenkrantz, W., Peiffer, R.L., and MacMillan, A. (1985). Malignant melanoma of the conjunctiva in a cat. *J Am Vet Med Assoc* 186: 505–506.

85 Multari, D., Vascellari, M., and Mutinelli, F. (2002). Hemangiosarcoma of the third eyelid in a cat. *Vet Ophthalmol* 5: 273–276.

86 Bacha, W.J. and Bacha, L.M. The eye. In: *Color Atlas of Veterinary Histology*, 3e, 2012. Ames, IA: Wiley-Blackwell.

87 Dubielzig, R.R., Ketring, K.L., McLellan, G.J., and Albert, D. (eds.). The uvea. In: *Veterinary Ocular Pathology: A Comparative Review*, 2010. St. Louis, MO: Saunders Elsevier.

88 Davidson, M.G., Nasisse, M.P., English, R.V. et al. (1991). Feline anterior uveitis: a study of 53 cases. *J Am Anim Hosp Assoc* 27: 77–83.

89 Jinks, M.R., English, R.V., and Gilger, B.C. (2016). Causes of endogenous uveitis in cats presented to referral clinics in North Carolina. *Vet Ophthalmol* 19 (Suppl 1): 30–37.

90 Maggs, D.J. (2009). Feline uveitis. An 'intraocular lymphadenopathy'. *J Feline Med Surg* 11: 167–182.

91 Blouin, P. and Cello, R.M. (1980). Experimental ocular cryptococcosis. Preliminary studies in cats and mice. *Invest Ophthalmol Vis Sci* 19: 21–30.

92 Davidson, M.G., Lappin, M.R., English, R.V., and Tompkins, M.B. (1993). A feline model of ocular toxoplasmosis. *Invest Ophthalmol Vis Sci* 34: 3653–3660.

93 Powell, C.C. and Lappin, M.R. (2001). Clinical ocular toxoplasmosis in neonatal kittens. *Vet Ophthalmol* 4: 87–92.

94 Stiles, J. (2014). Ocular manifestations of feline viral diseases. *Vet J* 201: 166–173.

95 Harris, B.P., Miller, P.E., Bloss, J.R., and Pellitteri, P.J. (2000). Ophthalmomyiasis interna anterior associated with *Cuterebra* spp in a cat. *J Am Vet Med Assoc* 216: 352–355. 345.

96 Wyman, M., Starkey, R., Weisbrode, S. et al. (2005). Ophthalmomyiasis (interna posterior) of the posterior segment and central nervous system myiasis: *Cuterebra* spp. in a cat. *Vet Ophthalmol* 8: 77–80.

97 Stiles, J. and Rankin, A. (2006). Ophthalmomyiasis interna anterior in a cat: surgical resolution. *Vet Ophthalmol* 9: 165–168.

98 Parkes, H.M., Shilton, C.M., Jerrett, I.V. et al. (2009). Primary ocular melioidosis due to a single genotype of *Burkholderia pseudomallei* in two cats from Arnhem Land in the Northern Territory of Australia. *J Feline Med Surg* 11: 856–863.

99 Pumphrey, S.A., Pirie, C.G., and Rozanski, E.A. (2011). Uveitis associated with septic peritonitis in a cat. *J Vet Emerg Crit Care (San Antonio)* 21: 279–284.

100 Olin, D.D. (1977). Examination of the aqueous humor as a diagnostic aid in anterior uveitis. *J Am Vet Med Assoc* 171: 557–559.

101 Wiggans, K.T., Skorupski, K.A., Reilly, C.M. et al. (2014). Presumed solitary intraocular or conjunctival lymphoma in dogs and cats: 9 cases (1985–2013). *J Am Vet Med Assoc* 244: 460–470.

102 Giordano, C., Giudice, C., Bellino, C. et al. (2013). A case of oculo-cerebral B-cell lymphoma in a cat. *Vet Ophthalmol* 16: 77–81.

103 Nerschbach, V., Eule, J.C., Eberle, N. et al. (2016). Ocular manifestation of lymphoma in newly diagnosed cats. *Vet Comp Oncol* 14: 58–66.

104 Peiffer, R.L. Jr., Seymour, W.G., and Williams, L.W. (1977). Malignant melanoma of the iris and ciliary body in a cat. *Mod Vet Pract* 58: 854–856.

105 Woog, J., Albert, D.M., Gonder, J.R., and Carpenter, J.J. (1983). Osteosarcoma in a phthisical feline eye. *Vet Pathol* 20: 209–214.

106 Dubielzig, R.R., Everitt, J., Shadduck, J.A., and Albert, D.M. (1990). Clinical and morphologic features of post-traumatic ocular sarcomas in cats. *Vet Pathol* 27: 62–65.

107 Dubielzig, R.R., Steinberg, H., Garvin, H. et al. (1998). Iridociliary epithelial tumors in 100 dogs and 17 cats: a morphological study. *Vet Ophthalmol* 1: 223–231.

108 Dubielzig, R.R. (1984). Ocular sarcoma following trauma in three cats. *J Am Vet Med Assoc* 184: 578–581.

109 Cassotis, N.J., Dubielzig, R.R., Gilger, B.C., and Davidson, M.G. (1999). Angioinvasive pulmonary carcinoma with posterior segment metastasis in four cats. *Vet Ophthalmol* 2: 125–131.

110 Michau, T.M., Proulx, D.R., Rushton, S.D. et al. (2003). Intraocular extramedullary plasmacytoma in a cat. *Vet Ophthalmol* 6: 177–181.

111 Kershaw, O., Linek, J., Linke, R.P., and Gruber, A.D. (2011). Intraocular ALλ amyloidoma with plasma cell neoplasia in a cat. *Vet Ophthalmol* 14 (Suppl 1): 88–92.

112 Semin, M.O., Serra, F., Mahe, V. et al. (2011). Choroidal melanocytoma in a cat. *Vet Ophthalmol* 14: 205–208.

113 Mowat, F.M., Langohr, I.M., Bilyk, O. et al. (2012). Bilateral uveal metastasis of a subcutaneous fibrosarcoma in a cat. *Vet Ophthalmol* 15: 391–397.

114 Scurrell, E., Trott, A., Rozmanec, M., and Belford, C.J. (2013). Ocular histiocytic sarcoma in a cat. *Vet Ophthalmol* 16 (Suppl 1): 173–176.

115 Evans, P.M., Lynch, G.L., and Dubielzig, R.R. (2010). Anterior uveal spindle cell tumor in a cat. *Vet Ophthalmol* 13: 387–390.

116 Stoltz, J.H., Carpenter, J.L., Albert, D.M. et al. (1994). Histologic, immunohistochemical, and ultrastructural features of an intraocular sarcoma of a cat. *J Vet Diagn Invest* 6: 114–116.

117 Zeiss, C.J., Johnson, E.M., and Dubielzig, R.R. (2003). Feline intraocular tumors may arise from transformation of lens epithelium. *Vet Pathol* 40: 355–362.

118 Duke, F.D., Strong, T.D., Bentley, E., and Dubielzig, R.R. (2013). Feline ocular tumors following ciliary body ablation with intravitreal gentamicin. *Vet Ophthalmol* 16 (Suppl 1): 188–190.

119 Hazel, S.J., Thrall, M.A., Severin, G.A. et al. (1985). Laboratory evaluation of aqueous humor in the healthy dog, cat, horse, and cow. *Am J Vet Res* 46: 657–659.

120 Wiggans, K.T., Vernau, W., Lappin, M.R. et al. (2014). Diagnostic utility of aqueocentesis and aqueous humor analysis in dogs and cats with anterior uveitis. *Vet Ophthalmol* 17: 212–220.

121 Hartmann, K., Lloret, A., Pennisi, M.G. et al. (2013). Aspergillosis in cats: ABCD guidelines on prevention and management. *J Feline Med Surg* 15: 605–610.

122 Hamilton, H.L., Whitley, R.D., and McLaughlin, S.A. (2000). Exophthalmos secondary to aspergillosis in a cat. *J Am Anim Hosp Assoc* 36: 343–347.

123 McLellan, G.J., Aquino, S.M., Mason, D.R. et al. (2006). Use of posaconazole in the management of invasive orbital aspergillosis in a cat. *J Am Anim Hosp Assoc* 42: 302–307.

124 Barachetti, L., Mortellaro, C.M., Di Giancamillo, M. et al. (2009). Bilateral orbital and nasal aspergillosis in a cat. *Vet Ophthalmol* 12: 176–182.

125 Giordano, C., Gianella, P., Bo, S. et al. (2010). Invasive mould infections of the naso-orbital region of cats: a case involving *Aspergillus fumigatus* and an aetiological review. *J Feline Med Surg* 12: 714–723.

126 Smith, L.N. and Hoffman, S.B. (2010). A case series of unilateral orbital aspergillosis in three cats and treatment with voriconazole. *Vet Ophthalmol* 13: 190–203.

127 Barrs, V.R., Halliday, C., Martin, P. et al. (2012). Sinonasal and sino-orbital aspergillosis in 23 cats: aetiology, clinicopathological features and treatment outcomes. *Vet J* 191: 58–64.

128 Ramsey, D.T., Marretta, S.M., Hamor, R.E. et al. (1996). Ophthalmic manifestations and complications of dental disease in dogs and cats. *J Am Anim Hosp Assoc* 32: 215–224.

129 Gilger, B.C., McLaughlin, S.A., Whitley, R.D., and Wright, J.C. (1992). Orbital neoplasms in cats: 21 cases (1974–1990). *J Am Vet Med Assoc* 201: 1083–1086.

130 Miller, S.A., van der Woerdt, A., and Bartick, T.E. (2000). Retrobulbar pseudotumor of the orbit in a cat. *J Am Vet Med Assoc* 216: 356–358. 345.

131 Billson, F.M., Miller-Michau, T., Mould, J.R., and Davidson, M.G. (2006). Idiopathic sclerosing orbital pseudotumor in seven cats. *Vet Ophthalmol* 9: 45–51.

132 Thomasy, S.M., Cissell, D.D., Arzi, B. et al. (2013). Restrictive orbital myofibroblastic sarcoma in a cat-cross-sectional imaging (MRI & CT) appearance, treatment, and outcome. *Vet Ophthalmol* 16 (Suppl 1): 123–129.

133 Bell, C.M., Schwarz, T., and Dubielzig, R.R. (2011). Diagnostic features of feline restrictive orbital myofibroblastic sarcoma. *Vet Pathol* 48: 742–750.

21

Ocular Cytology of the Horse

Michala de Linde Henriksen and Leslie C. Sharkey

Introduction

Ocular disease is common in the equine, with estimates that 5–10% of horses have problems that affect vision or function.[1,2] The challenges and expenses associated with managing these diseases in horses are significant and unique to the horse compared with small animal species. Cytology, especially of the more superficial structures of the eye, is a key diagnostic tool in both ambulatory and specialty equine practice that can facilitate early treatment, improve prognosis, and reduce treatment costs.[1,2] We have focused on the most common ophthalmic diseases in horses in which cytology would be recommended as an important diagnostic component.

Eyelid and Adnexa

Normal Structure and Cytology

For normal anatomy of the mammalian eyelid and adnexa, please see Chapter 20. Chapter 12 also covers general lesions of the skin and subcutis in common domestic species.

Inflammation

Eyelid Abscessation (Dacryoadenitis)

Acute eyelid abscessation, or dacryoadenitis,[3,4] manifests as a periocular swelling in the lateral–dorsal aspect of the eyelid with or without a history or evidence of trauma.[4] Culture and cytology from the swollen area are recommended for initial diagnostics. Two case reports describe cytologic findings consisting of neutrophils without eosinophils.[3,4] Ultrasound or computed tomography can help determine the extent of the involvement.[3,4]

Lacrimal Cyst (Dacryops)

Lacrimal cysts, or dacryops, are swellings of the nasolacrimal duct in the medial–ventral area of the eyelid. Cytology is recommended for preliminary diagnosis and to rule out neoplasia. Although suppurative inflammation was reported by the referring veterinarian in a published case, the histologic description of the lesion would predict a more typical appearance of a low cellularity high protein cystic fluid with macrophages, variable mixed inflammatory cells, cholesterol crystals, and potential mild resolving hemorrhage in uncomplicated lesions.[5] Diagnosis can be confirmed using computed tomography dacryocystorhinogram with contrast.[5,6]

Blepharitis

Inflammation of the eyelids (blepharitis) in horses can occur concurrently with evidence of trauma and/or conjunctivitis.[2] Infectious and noninfectious causes such as pemphigus foliaceous and allergic and actinic causes should be ruled out.[7] Collection of samples for cytology and microbial culture are recommended; however, histology may be necessary in some cases for definitive diagnosis.[7]

Neoplasia

Squamous cell carcinoma (SCC) and sarcoids are the two most common equine eyelid tumors, although many tumors can potentially occur in this region.[2,8] Adnexal neoplasia must be distinguished from nodular or ulcerated inflammatory lesions, including foreign body reactions and parasitic lesions.[8] Mast cell tumors are rare in horses compared with other domestic species, but they have been reported in the periorbital skin.[9] For extensive lesions, imaging studies may be warranted. Likewise, cytologic evaluation of regional lymphoid tissue for evidence of metastatic disease can be beneficial. Interestingly, ocular and

Veterinary Cytology, First Edition. Edited by Leslie C. Sharkey, M. Judith Radin, and Davis Seelig.

adnexal tumors other than sarcoid appear to be uncommon in donkeys.[10]

Squamous Cell Carcinoma

SCC is the most common eyelid mass in horses and is also common in the conjunctiva, third eyelid, and cornea.[8] Overall, SCC was the second most diagnosed tumor in horses in the United Kingdom.[11] Horses lacking periocular pigmentation, especially in areas of high UV light exposure are at risk, although chronic irritation of any etiology can promote SCC formation.[2,8] Periocular SCC should be considered with any erosive, erythematous, cobblestone-like, or cauliflower-like raised periocular mass (Figure 21.1).[8] Progressive local invasion can have fatal consequences, with larger size or occurrence on the eyelids, cornea, and limbus having poorer prognosis.[8,12] Local recurrence after treatment varies from 25 to 67%. SCC has been subdivided into four histologic types (plaque, papillomatous, noninvasive, and invasive SCC).[2,13] Cytologically, SCC has been categorized as well-differentiated, moderately differentiated, and poorly differentiated phenotypes.[14] Well-differentiated tumors are often inflamed, with large polyhedral or spindloid squamous cells with a "flaked" morphology that sometimes

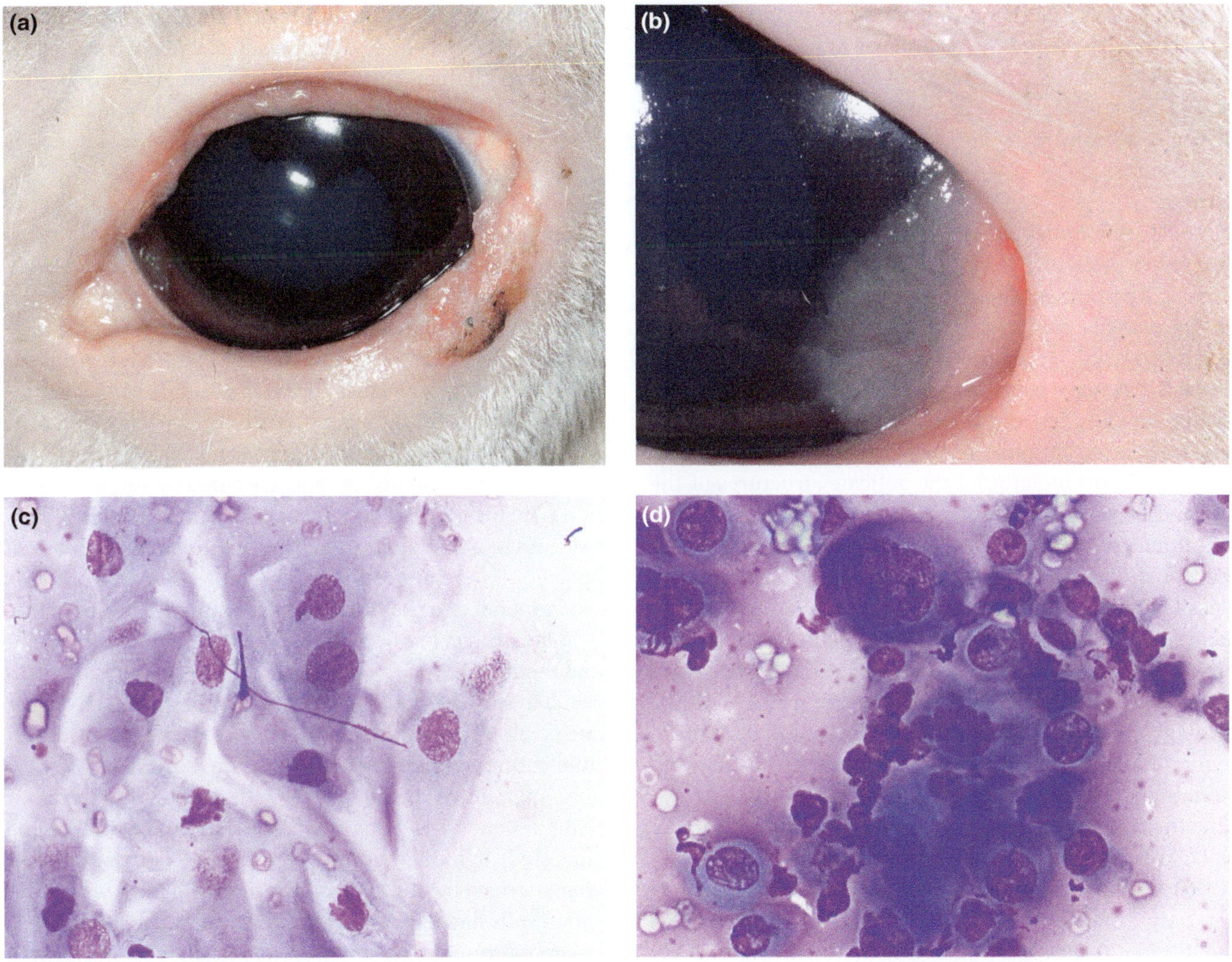

Figure 21.1 Squamous cell carcinoma (SCC) in the lower eyelid of a horse. (a) Gross photo of a paint horse that is non-pigmented in the periocular region and has developed a SCC lesion encompassing a third of the eyelid from the lateral aspect. (b) SCC also occurs in the cornea, often in the lateral aspect as an irregular pink vascular plaque. (c) Superficial impression smears or scrapings sometimes consist of more mature squamous cells that are either normal, hyperplastic, or better differentiated than the bulk of the lesion and thus poorly reflective of the deeper underlying neoplastic cells. These cells are slightly atypical in that they have retained relatively immature nuclei for the cytoplasmic characteristics. (d) Anaplastic cells characterized by less abundant, basophilic cytoplasm and one or more immature nuclei with up to several prominent nucleoli were observed with deeper sampling. Anisocytosis and anisokaryosis can be dramatic. Some degree of neutrophilic inflammation can be observed (c and d: Wright–Giemsa, 500×).

contain keratohyalin granules and variable keratinization. Up to 30% of cells can be round, and caudate or tadpole cells are seen. Moderately differentiated tumors contain >50% round or oval cells, often in sheets, and are characterized by less abundant cytoplasm than well-differentiated tumors and moderate nuclear atypia. Poorly differentiated tumors are often ulcerated and inflamed with a predominance of round to oval cells that often exhibit marked anisocytosis, anisokaryosis, and prominent nucleoli (Figure 21.1). Emperipolesis of neutrophils is observed in many cases of well-differentiated and moderately differentiated SCC. In all subtypes, there is dyssynchrony of nuclear and cytoplasmic maturation. Differential diagnoses include papillomas, other epithelial neoplasms with squamous differentiation, and reactive non-neoplastic lesions with secondary hyperplasia and dysplasia.[14] For this reason, cytologic diagnoses of SCC in the equine eye should be considered preliminary and should be confirmed histologically.

Sarcoids

Sarcoids are cutaneous tumors of fibroblastic origin that often have proliferative epithelial components.[15] Quarter Horses, Appaloosas, and Arabians are postulated to have an increased risk, whereas standardbreds have a decreased risk.[8] Metastasis is very uncommon, but recurrence is frequent, especially with more invasive lesions. Eyelid sarcoids can cause corneal friction and damage, and treatment options can be limited due to the constraints of working around the delicate structures of the eye and because the eyelids are very important for normal function of the eye.[7,8,15,16] Early diagnosis and treatment can decrease recurrence. Grossly, sarcoids are classified as occult, verrucose, nodular (A, non-ulcerated, or B, ulcerated), fibroblastic (A, pedunculated, or B, broad based), or mixed,[15,17] and diagnosis is sometimes made based on clinical criteria alone (Figure 21.2). While cytology has been used to diagnose equine sarcoids, reports indicate problems with poor sample quality, presumably due to minimal exfoliation.[18] According to text references, cytology samples contain scattered spindle cells, which is considered nonspecific (Figure 21.2).[19] Histopathologic diagnosis is recommended, but cytology can help differentiate sarcoids from other more exfoliative tumors like melanoma and lymphoma. Even biopsy diagnosis can be challenging in some cases, with variable histopathologic features that do not always correlate well with the five clinical subtypes. In particular, histologic diagnosis of the occult and nodular types can be challenging.[20] The immunohistochemical detection of bovine papilloma virus DNA (BPV-DNA) and increased density of dermal fibroblasts are diagnostic criteria.[20] Reports of immunocytochemical detection of BPV-DNA could not be found.

Lymphoma

Lymphoma is the most common systemic hemolymphatic neoplasm in horses.[21,22] Periocular eyelid lymphoma in horses is usually the cutaneous type and is often the first sign of the disease,[21,23] although it may be the only location. Lymphoma of the third eyelid, cornea, sclera, and/or conjunctiva has a fair to good prognosis in the horse provided the affected tissue is completely excised. Lymphoma of the eyelids and cutaneous tissue carries a poor prognosis for the horse.[21] The clinical presentation includes eyelid swelling or variably sized masses.[24–28] There is minimal specific information about the cytologic diagnosis of periocular lymphoma, since diagnosis is usually accomplished by histopathology or cytology of other affected tissues (Figure 21.3). See Chapter 27 for a more detailed discussion of lymphoma and Chapter 12 for cutaneous manifestations.

Melanoma

A retrospective study of melanoma in gray-skinned horses showed that only 24% had melanoma of the eyelids; however, the periocular skin is the most common site for melanocytic neoplasia involving the eye and adnexa in the horse.[29–31] Adnexal melanomas are often described as slowly progressive, cutaneous, partially alopecic pigmented masses of the adnexal tissue in gray horses (Figure 21.4).[8] Most equine eyelid melanomas are cured by surgical resection. The histology of equine melanocytic neoplasia is variable and of questionable relevance in predicting biological behavior.[29,31] Prior to surgery, a careful systemic workup is recommended to exclude metastatic disease since conjunctival melanoma has been described as potentially recurrent and metastatic.[29,32] Cytologic descriptions of equine melanoma in the literature are rare and do not specifically reference ocular lesions. Melanoma detected in equine pleural fluid contained melanophages and small numbers of variably pigmented melanocytes with multiple criteria of malignancy.[33,34] Cytology of a tail base mass melanoma consisted of individualized or clustered polyhedral cells characterized by multiple criteria of malignancy with occasional cells having scant melanin granules.[35] In all of these cases, the tumors were more biologically aggressive than the typical adnexal melanocytic tumors in the horse. Chapter 15 contains additional information on melanoma.

Papilloma

Viral papillomatosis, also known as grass warts, warts, or verrucae, is caused by *Equus caballus* papilloma virus

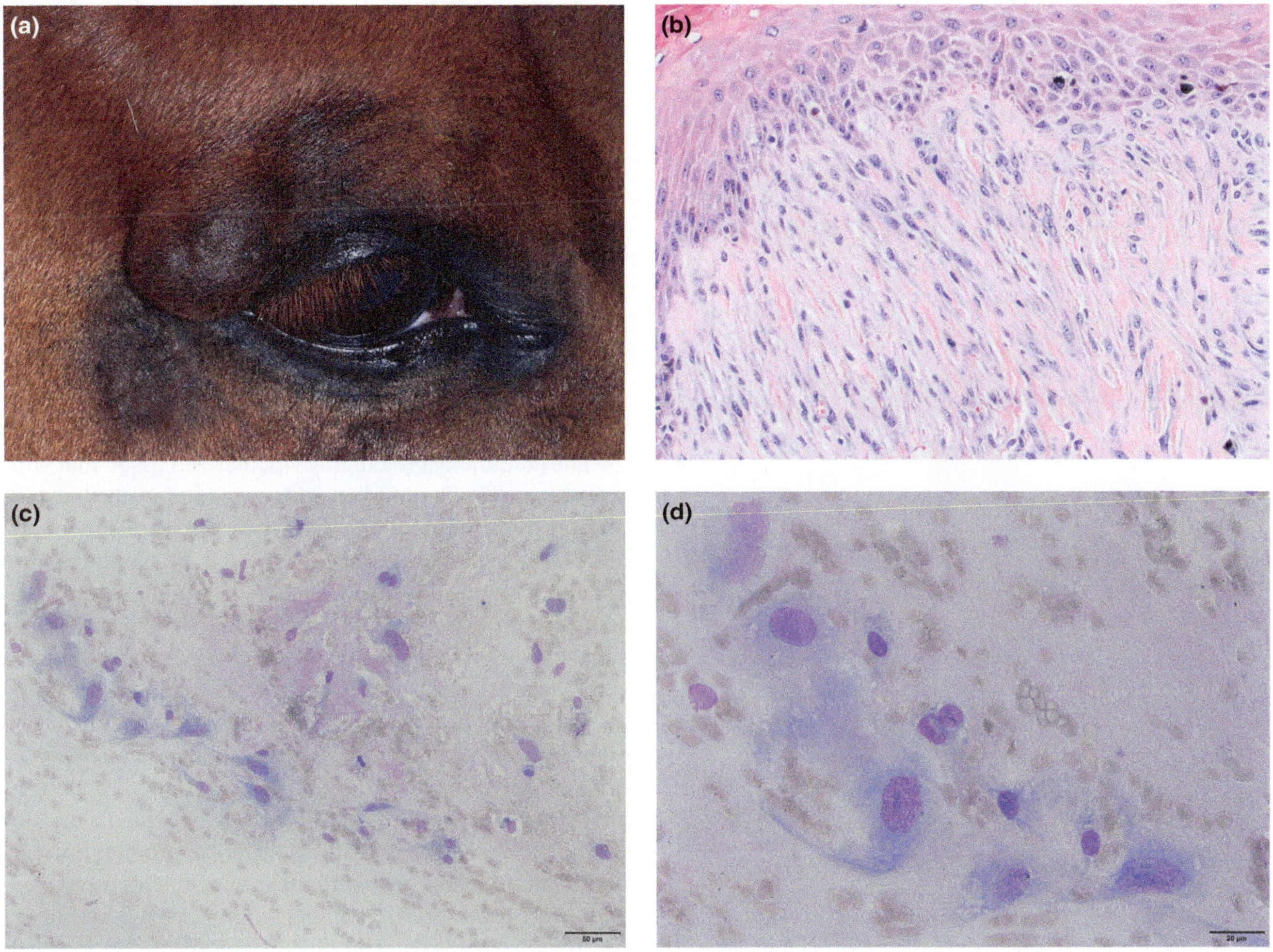

Figure 21.2 (a) Gross photo of a periocular nodular type A sarcoid in the dorsal–lateral canthus. (a) Histologically, sarcoids consist of a thick epidermal layer covering proliferating dermal spindle cells that form interlacing bunches or a herringbone pattern. Nuclear pleomorphism is variable, and stromal is typically scant (hematoxylin & eosin, 100×. *Source:* Image courtesy of Nick Robinson). (c and d) This cytology sample was collected from a preputial sarcoid and reveals a population of plump to elongated spindle cells reflecting the proliferating spindloid cells. An ocular sarcoid is anticipated to appear similar (Wright–Giemsa, 200× and 500×, respectively. *Source:* Images courtesy of Dr. Francisco Conrado).

type and typically affects horses less than 3 years of age.[36] Transmission occurs via direct contact with other infected horses or indirectly through fomites.[37] Papillomas initially appear as one millimeter gray to white papules with a smooth, shiny surface.[37] With progression, lesions increase in size and develop a hyperkeratotic surface. The disease is self-limiting after several months with the development of complete immunity.[37] While most commonly seen on the muzzle and lips, the eyelids, paragenital regions, and distal legs can also be involved.[37] Differential diagnoses include sarcoids and SCC. Cytology can suggest papilloma when there is minimal nuclear atypia,[14] whereas the distinction between papilloma and superficial samples of the epidermal component of sarcoid can be more difficult and a surgical biopsy or even polymerase chain reaction (PCR) analysis can be necessary.[37,38] Non-virus-associated congenital papillomas have been reported in foals, but not associated with the ocular structures.[39]

Adnexal Adenoma

Meibomian adenoma is a benign neoplasm that is common in dogs but rarely described in horses.[40–42] The tumor presents as a white to pinkish mass with a lobular or multinodular appearance located at the eyelid margin in the area of the Meibomian gland openings.[40] Cytology in horses has not been reported, but based on histologic descriptions, lesions are composed of mildly pleomorphic basal cells bounded by thin fibrous connective tissue with relatively frequent mitotic figures.[41]

Conjunctiva and Nictitating Membrane

Normal Structure and Cytology

The equine conjunctiva is similar to the dog and cat in structure. Briefly, depending on the region (proximal to the eyelid margin versus the bulbar surface), the surface consists of stratified squamous keratinized, stratified squamous, or stratified columnar to cuboidal cells, all of which can be observed in normal conjunctival cytology.[43] The presence of superficial lymphoid aggregates can be reflected in cytology samples, and more rarely, deeper sampling can contain goblet cells. Impression cytology sampling is likely to increase the representation of goblet cells in normal horses.[44]

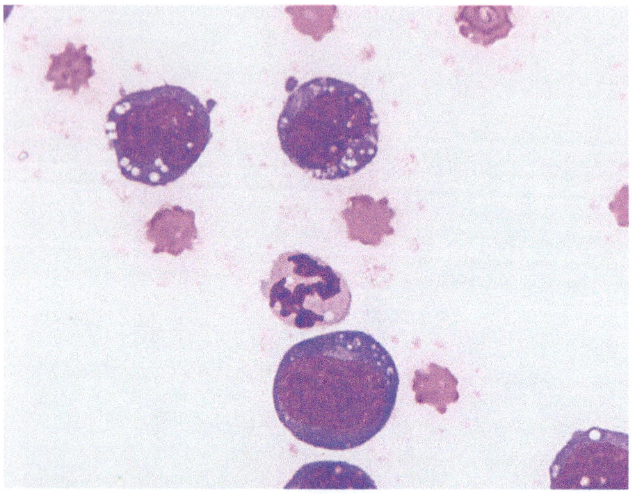

Figure 21.3 Abdominal fluid from a 9-year-old Quarter Horse gelding presenting for swelling of the right eye for 3 weeks. The total nucleated cell count of 130 000/µL. The majority of the cells were large atypical lymphocytes characterized by scant to moderate amounts of deeply basophilic and variably vacuolated cytoplasm and pleomorphic nuclei, resulting in a diagnosis of lymphoma. Necropsy revealed extensive systemic involvement of the skeletal muscles, abdominal organs, heart, and the dorsal rectus muscle (Wright–Giemsa, 1000×).

Inflammation

Conjunctivitis

Conjunctivitis is common in horses but often as an extension of pathology in other structures rather than as a primary condition.[2] Thus, a thorough ophthalmic and general physical exam is indicated for all horses with conjunctivitis. The conjunctiva is a highly vascularized tissue that will show signs of inflammation with swelling (chemosis) and redness (hyperemia) along with serous to purulent ocular discharge.[7,45] Reported causes of primary conjunctivitis include trauma, solar, hypersensitivity, immune-mediated, allergic, and infectious, although other structures associated with the eye can also be affected. Cytology reveals variable populations of inflammatory and normal to hyperplastic epithelial cells, although there is little primary literature on this topic. Primary bacterial conjunctivitis can be caused by many different organisms; therefore culture and sensitivity are important in cases for which this is a diagnostic consideration.[7,46–48] The most common normal flora in the equine conjunctiva are Gram-positive *Staphylococcus* spp.[49,50] Fungal conjunctivitis has been described, but is not common in horses.[2,7,51] Cytologic examination can be beneficial in identification of causative agents, keeping in mind that there is a robust normal microbial flora that in some cases can become opportunistically pathogenic.[2,49–52] Environmental contamination of

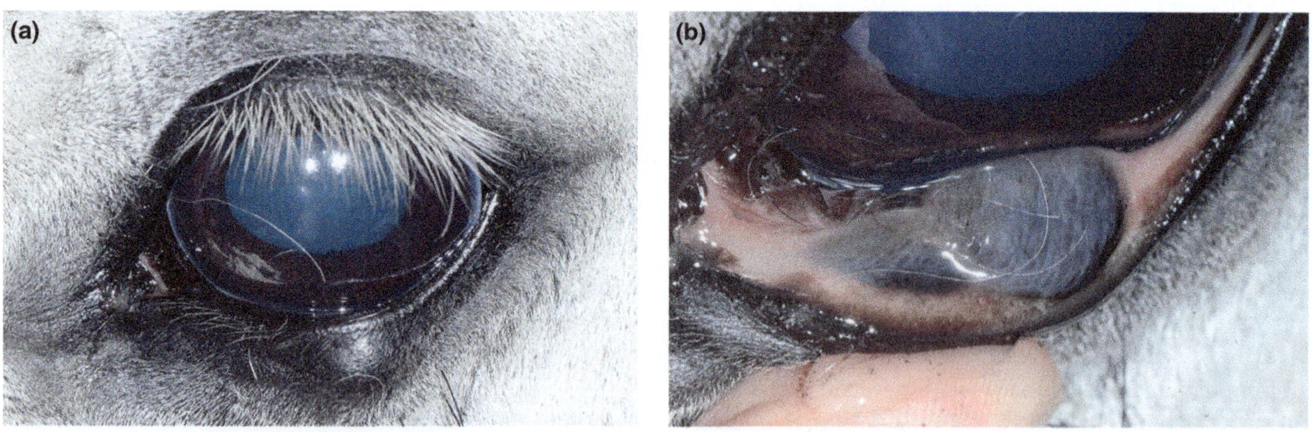

Figure 21.4 Gross photos of an eyelid melanoma in the (a), lower eyelid, and (b), conjunctiva. Cytology samples (not shown) consisted only of dense mats of melanin granules and erythrocytes. This was consistent with but not diagnostic for melanoma due to insufficient numbers of intact nucleated cells.

both cytology and microbial culture samples can occur as well. Common normal fungal flora include *Alternaria* spp., *Aspergillus* spp., *Cladosporium* spp., *Fusarium* spp., *Penicillium* spp., and *Scopulariopsis* spp., while pathogenic fungi include *Aspergillus* spp., *Histoplasma* spp., *Blastomyces* spp., and *Rhinosporidium seeberi* (Figure 21.5). See Chapter 3 for microscopic descriptions and images of the common fungal pathogens. Biopsy may be required to assess the presence of microbes in the context of tissue structure.

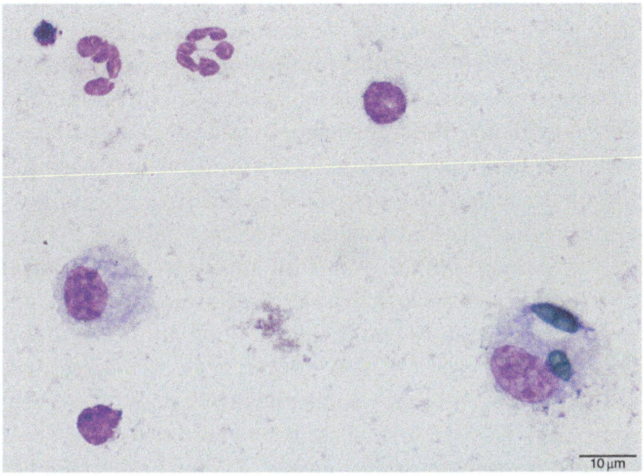

Figure 21.5 *Alternaria* spp. found in equine ocular cytology samples are most often environmental contaminants rather than pathogens. Spores most often appear as green intra- or extracellular structures in eye and airway samples. This sample was an equine bronchoalveolar lavage collected from a horse with equine asthma, but the organism would appear identical as a contaminant in equine ocular samples (Wright–Giemsa, 1000×. *Source:* Image courtesy of Francisco Conrado).

Conjunctival habronemiosis is a common finding in horses and should be considered when multifocal microabscesses are found in the medial canthus conjunctiva (Figure 21.6).[53–55] Conjunctival habronemiosis is caused by infection and immune response to the migration of the larvae of *Habronema* or *Draschia* spp.[55] Diagnosis is sometimes made based on history and the location and gross appearance of lesions, including yellowish granules representing necrotic to mineralized debris surrounding the larvae.[56] Histopathology can be performed to confirm the diagnosis by identification of nodular to diffuse eosinophilic inflammation and the presence of organisms; however one study found that nematode larvae were identified in less than half of biopsy samples.[56] Conjunctival cytology is reported to consist of eosinophils that are often mixed with other inflammatory cells.[56–59] Differential diagnoses include granulation tissue, equine sarcoid, SCC, and other infectious granulomas and neoplasms. Although not definitive, cytology can be used to narrow down possible diagnoses. Equine herpesvirus and influenza virus can also cause conjunctivitis.[55] To our knowledge no cytological studies have been performed to look for viral inclusions in equine conjunctival tissue.

Pseudotumor

Conjunctival pseudotumor or nodular lymphocytic conjunctivitis has been described in horses as a unilateral or bilateral, nodular or smooth, pink, non-ulcerated conjunctival mass that can involve the conjunctiva, third eyelid, and cornea.[60,61] Differential diagnoses include neoplastic lesions and habronema infection. The underlying cause for equine pseudotumors is thought to be an immune-mediated

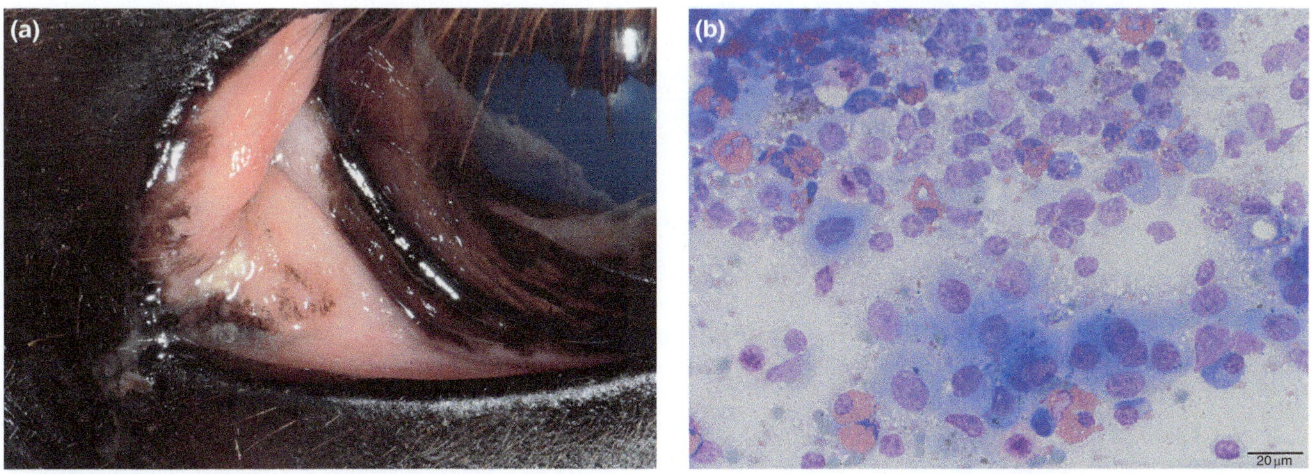

Figure 21.6 (a) A characteristic microabscess is found in the medial/dorsal canthus of the eye of a horse with conjunctival habronemiosis. (b) Cytology from the conjunctiva of a different horse with clinically suspected habronemiosis consists of a mix of macrophages, eosinophils, plasma cells, and epithelial cells (Wright–Giemsa, 500×. *Source:* Image courtesy of Francisco Conrado).

reaction; histologically, the lesions are composed of lymphoid follicles with lymphocytes, plasma cells, and histiocytes.[60,61] Histopathology is definitive; however, cytology can be used for initial screening. Cytologic findings from an impression smear of a biopsy in a horse from a case series of five with conjunctival pseudotumors were reported to consist of a predominance of small lymphocytes with scattered large lymphocytes and occasional lymphoblasts consistent with reactive lymphoid tissue.[62]

Amyloidosis

Amyloidosis of the conjunctiva and cornea is described in horses, most recently in a horse euthanized for a two-year history of nasal amyloidosis.[63] Papillary conjunctival masses were characterized histologically by amyloid and moderate infiltrates of a mixed B- and T-lymphocyte population. Cytology was not performed; however, a cytologic description of equine nasal amyloidosis indicated the presence of fibrillar to granular eosinophilic to gray material within macrophages and multinucleated giant cells (Figure 21.7).[64]

Neoplasia

Many of the equine eyelid neoplasms also occur in the conjunctiva and nictitating membrane, including SCC, melanoma, lymphoma, mast cell tumor, and papilloma.[2] These lesions can involve the cornea by extension. One study of excision of 50 equine nictitating membrane tumors identified 37 SCC, 5 lymphoma, 1 hemangiosarcoma, 1 sarcoma, 1 adenocarcinoma, and 5 non-neoplastic lesions.[28] Recurrence and mortality were high in this study. A pigmented conjunctival SCC was reported in a Thoroughbred that was initially misinterpreted as a melanoma based on coloration, demonstrating the value of microscopy.[65]

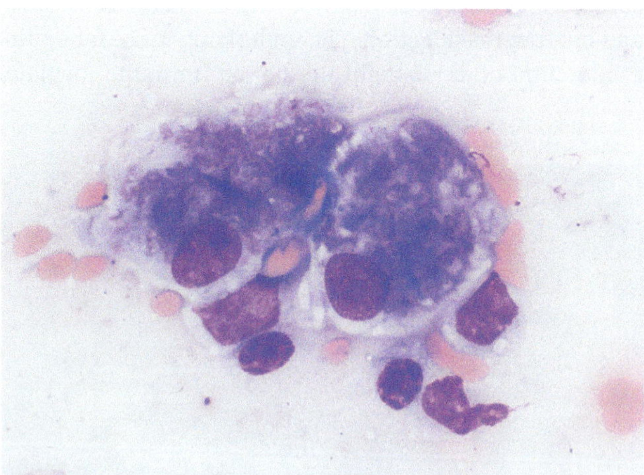

Figure 21.7 Eosinophilic fibrillar material within macrophages was confirmed as amyloid by staining red-orange using Congo red stain and by exhibiting green birefringence with polarized light. Also present are lymphocytes and plasma cells, reflecting concurrent lymphoplasmacytic inflammation. These samples were collected from a 6-year-old Quarter Horse gelding with nasal amyloidosis; however, the cytologic appearance is presumed to be similar in nasal and conjunctival lesions (Wright–Giemsa, 1000×. *Source:* Image courtesy of Mary Leissinger).

Hemangiosarcoma and Angiosarcoma

Horses with hemangiosarcoma typically present with a vascular mass on the third eyelid or conjunctiva (Figure 21.8). Hemangiosarcoma can be a locally aggressive and metastatic tumor that can have a variable prognosis depending on the case.[66,67] Cytology of hemangiosarcoma often consists of variable numbers of plump anaplastic mesenchymal cells sometimes associated with inflammation or evidence of hemorrhage. Cytology of an epithelioid variant of hemangiosarcoma of the third eyelid in a gelding was characterized by clustered to individualized spindloid to oval cells with indistinct cytoplasmic margins.[68] Large nuclei were round to oval with multiple variably sized nuclei; anisocytosis and anisokaryosis were moderate, and a concurrent mature lymphoid cell population was identified.[68] Another gelding presented with a single fused mass of the third eyelid that was histologically defined as being composed of a hemangiosarcoma and a SCC.[66,67,69] In another horse, incisional biopsy of a superior palpebral conjunctival mass rendered a diagnosis of hemangiosarcoma; however eventual enucleation yielded additional diagnostic material and a revised diagnosis of lymphangiosarcoma based on the lack of erythrocytes within neoplastic vascular channels and the presence of normal blood vessels within the neoplasm, features that might not be appreciable cytologically.[70] Hemangiomas occur in the

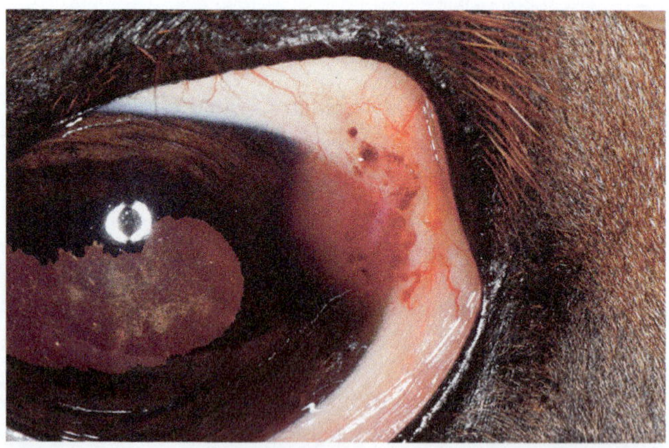

Figure 21.8 Gross appearance of a vascular hemangiosarcoma in the lateral aspect of the conjunctiva and cornea. Cytology (not shown) was unrewarding and consisted only of squamous epithelial cells, reflecting the poorly exfoliative nature of some sarcomas unless more aggressive sampling techniques are used. Cytology of hemangiosarcoma can be seen in Chapter 28.

ocular structures of the horse as well. Angiosarcoma has also been reported in a horse with a lateral limbus mass.[71] Intravascular papillary endothelial hyperplasia is a benign intraluminal proliferation of endothelial cells that has been reported in the conjunctiva of a horse and could be confused with angiosarcoma.[72] Thus, a variety of related spindle cell lesions occur in the conjunctiva and nictitating membrane of the horse that likely cannot be distinguished cytologically and require biopsy for definitive diagnosis.

Other Neoplasms

Mast cell tumors of the nictitating membrane can occur, sometimes extending to involve other structures (see Chapter 13 for more detail).[73] Neurofibrosarcoma is another adnexal neoplasm diagnosed in a horse; however, cytologic findings were not reported.[74] Basal cell tumor of the nictitating membrane has been reported in a horse.[75] Malignant adenocarcinoma is rare with only one equine case of a primary lacrimal adenocarcinoma.[76]

Cornea

Normal Structure and Cytology

The normal equine cornea is 0.8–1 mm thick and composed of 4 layers superficial to deep: epithelial (anterior portion), stroma, Descemet's membrane, and a single layer of endothelial cells.[77,78] Approximately 90% of the thickness of the equine cornea is stroma, composed of collagen fibrils and keratocytes. Descemet's membrane is also composed of collagen fibrils.[78] A single layer of endothelial cells covers Descemet's membrane on the posterior surface of the anterior chamber.[78] The endothelial cells are important in keeping the cornea dehydrated and transparent using ATPase pumps to extract fluid (aqueous humor) that enters the cornea from the anterior chamber.[78] The healthy cornea is avascular and is devoid of inflammatory cells and erythrocytes.[78] Therefore, normal cytology of the equine cornea consists mostly of epithelial cells and occasional collagen fibrils depending on the depth of sampling. Foreign plant and organic material as well as bacteria from the surrounding environment can contaminate slides; however, the presence of rare (or single) hyphal structures or bacteria should be interpreted as strong evidence of infection if there are suggestive corneal lesions.

Inflammation

Inflammatory and infectious corneal diseases are common in horses. Inflammation of the cornea (keratitis) has many etiologies. Clinical subtypes include ulcerative keratitis, divided into simple (acute, superficial, noninfected, healed within three to five days), complicated (infected corneal ulceration, chronic underlying irritation, indolent corneal ulceration), and non-ulcerative keratitis (corneal stromal abscess or immune-mediated keratitis [IMMK]).[78–81]

Simple (Noninfected) Ulcerative Keratitis

Cytology of simple noninfected ulcerative keratitis is usually not performed since these ulcerations heal within three to five days with appropriate treatment.[79,82] When cytology is performed, samples consist of normal corneal epithelial cells indicative of a simple corneal ulceration. A few neutrophils may be present but should raise concern for possible infection. Culture and sensitivity should be performed in any case with the potential for infection, and the eye should be treated as a complicated ulceration until proven not to be.

Complicated Ulcerative Keratitis

Infected Ulcerative Keratitis

Infected ulcerative keratitis is associated with a variety of clinical manifestations, including superficial or deep ulceration with stromal loss or keratomalacia (melting corneal ulceration). Cellular infiltration with leukocytes can be appreciated as a yellow to cream-colored discoloration of the ulcerated corneal tissue and surroundings (Figure 21.9).[79,82]

Bacterial Bacterial infections with Gram-negative organisms such as *Pseudomonas aeruginosa, Klebsiella* spp., and *Enterobacter* spp. and Gram-positive organisms such as *Staphylococcus* and *Streptococcus* spp. (e.g. *Streptococcus equi* subspecies *zooepidemicus*) are regularly identified, and methicillin resistance has been identified (Figure 21.9).[83–87] Bacterial infections of the cornea can cause vision-threatening complications, including keratomalacia (melting corneal ulceration), deep corneal ulcerations, and iris prolapse.[84,88,89] Cytology, Gram stain, and culture/sensitivity are important diagnostic tools. Cytology sometimes identifies bacteria not demonstrated using culture, particularly when there is a history of antimicrobial therapy with fastidious organisms.[86,90,91] Although commonly seen, inflammatory cells are not always present or prominent despite an infectious cause. For example, in a series of four horses with *Listeria monocytogenes* associated keratoconjunctivitis, characteristic rod-shaped bacteria formed short chains in association with corneal epithelial cells, but neutrophils were not seen.[92]

Fungal Fungal ulcerative keratitis is common in horses and is always a consideration with non-healing corneal ulceration; however there is regional variation in the prevalence and organisms most frequently identified.[79,82,93] Predisposing factors include exposure to environmental fungal flora, prominent eyes with large protruding corneas at risk for trauma, slow corneal vascularization and healing

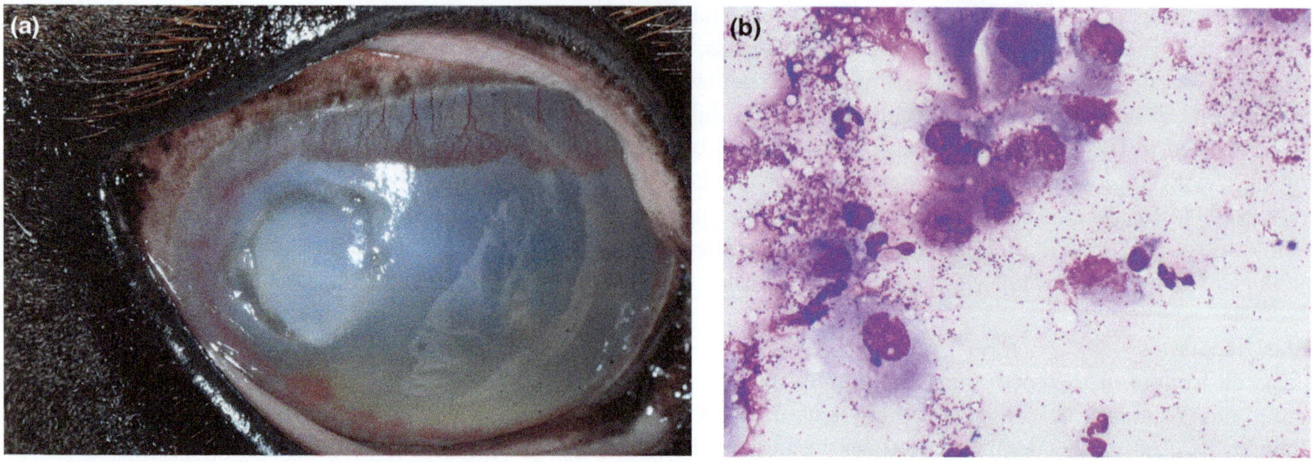

Figure 21.9 Infectious ulcerative keratitis is a common finding in horses. (a) Gross image of a corneal ulceration. The ulcerated area has inflammatory cell infiltration that imparts a yellow/creamy color and indicates high possibility of an infection. Other clinical signs are corneal vascularization and diffuse moderate to severe corneal edema. These signs indicate a severe corneal lesion causing secondary uveitis. (b) Cytology samples consisted of large numbers of extracellular and intracellular small cocci, moderate numbers of poorly preserved neutrophils, and scattered hyperplastic epithelial cells. Bacterial culture grew *Streptococcus zooepidemicus* (Wright–Giemsa, 1000×).

compare with other species, and the use of topical steroids.[79,82,94] Because it can be difficult to distinguish bacterial from fungal keratitis grossly, corneal cytology is an important rapid screening test. However, microscopy does not identify fungal elements in all cases, so fungal culture is also recommended along with histopathology if possible (Figure 21.10).[84,95] Unfortunately, fungal culture requires up to two to three weeks for a final result. Other techniques, such as PCR, are being investigated, but are not yet considered substitutes for standard diagnostic techniques.[96,97] A retrospective study of keratomycosis in 35 horses (36 eyes) from Switzerland identified fungal elements in the vast majority of involved eyes (34/36), while 14 samples had abundant predominantly neutrophilic inflammation, and bacteria were seen in 5 out of 36 eyes.[98] *Aspergillus* spp., *Fusarium* spp., and *Candida* spp. are the most common fungi causing ulcerative fungal keratitis in horses;[99,100] however many types of fungi have been implicated. *Histoplasma* spp. keratitis was reported to be cytologically characterized by neutrophilic and histiocytic inflammation with classic intra- and extracellular globular fungal bodies (see Chapter 3 for images and additional description).[101] *Mortierella wolfii*, typically a cause of systemic disease in cattle, was described as a cause of keratomycosis in a horse and was characterized by the presence of nonseptate fungal hyphae with corneal epithelial cells.[102] This fungus has also been reported as a cause of keratomycosis in Japan.[103] More common hyphae such as *Aspergillus* spp., *Fusarium* spp., and *Penicillium* spp. are septate. In an unusual microscopic presentation, a corneal scraping from a Quarter Horse with fungal culture and PCR confirmed *Fusarium* infection was cytologically characterized by a predominance of microconidia with smaller numbers of septate hyphae.[95] This can be observed more frequently in devascularized or necrotic tissue and is important because microconidia can be misidentified as yeast or protozoa, leading to delayed treatment. Keratomycosis resulting from *Cladorrhinum bulbillosum* was described in a Percheron cross gelding; preliminary diagnosis was by cytology; however, the details were not reported.[104]

In general, common cytologic findings include fungal hyphae that take up stain, or can appear as nonstaining filaments in thicker areas of cytologic preparations; in some cases, numerous elements are present, while in other cases they may be very rare. More common hyphae such as *Aspergillus* spp., *Fusarium* spp., and *Penicillium* spp. are septate (Figure 21.10). Variable numbers of inflammatory cells can be present. Fungal spores are likely more indicative of contamination than infection.[105] A non-ulcerated form of equine subepithelial keratomycosis has been described in 21 horses, with cytologic identification of fungi in 10 cases.[106] Differential diagnoses include IMMK and subepithelial herpes keratitis.

Viral Keratoconjunctivitis/Keratitis Viral keratoconjunctivitis/keratitis presents clinically as chemosis and hyperemia of the conjunctiva, with a multifocal superficial punctate or dendritic pattern of corneal ulcerations that varies in staining positively with rose bengal and fluorescein staining depending on the depth of the lesions.[78,79]

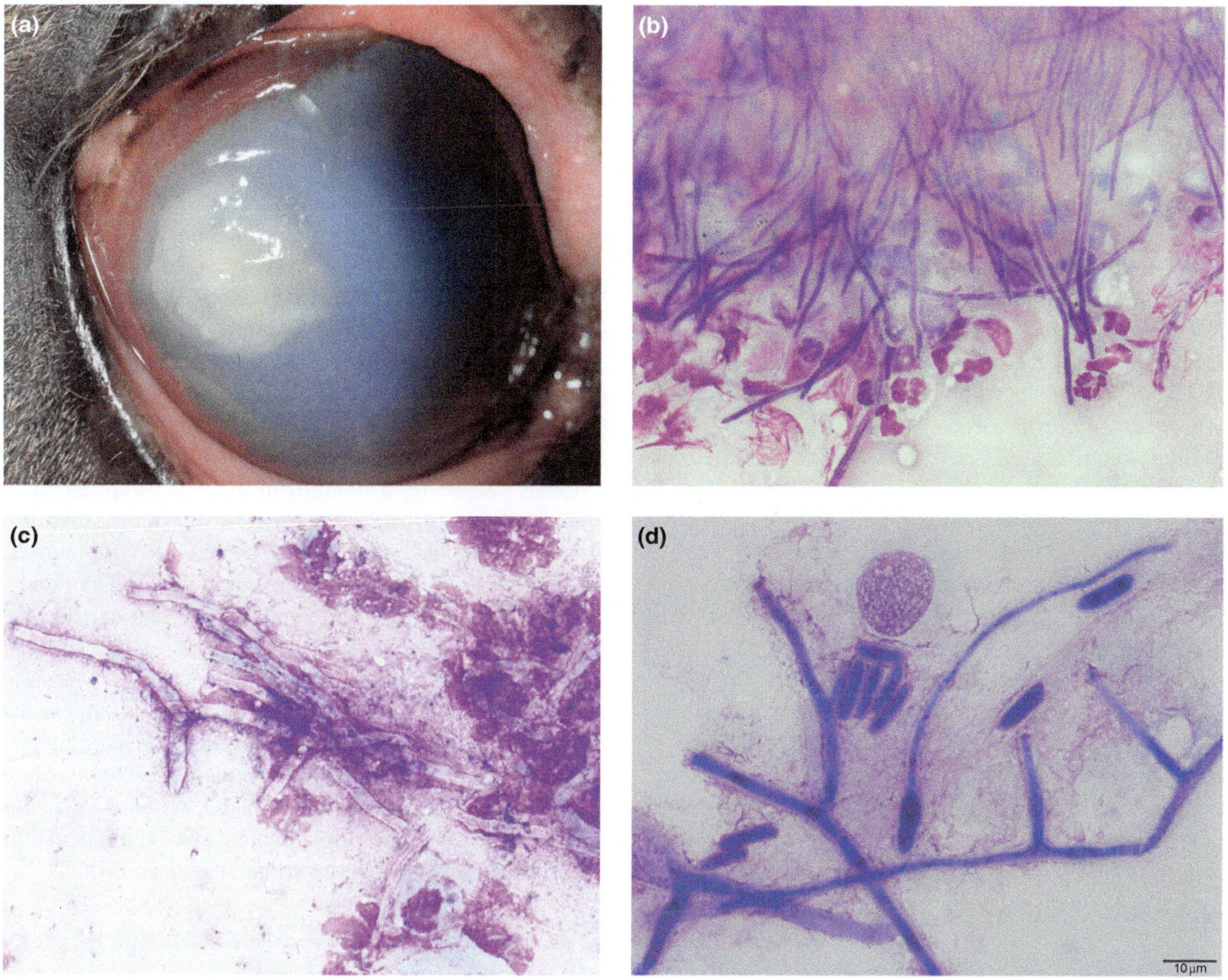

Figure 21.10 (a) A yellow fungal plaque in the lateral aspect of the cornea of a horse. Other ophthalmic findings are corneal vascularization as well as diffuse moderate to severe corneal edema in the lateral aspect of the cornea. (b) Cytology from this lesion reveals large mats of well-stained septate fungal hyphae mixed with a neutrophilic infiltrate (Wright–Giemsa, 500×). Fungal culture grew *Penicillium* sp. (c) Cytology from a different horse illustrates that some fungal hyphae do not take up stain well and may be visualized as nonstaining linear structures (Wright–Giemsa, 500×). (d) Cytology from a fungal corneal ulcer in a Quarter Horse gelding demonstrates well-stained septate branching fungal hyphae. The elongated structures are consistent with macroconidia. Fungal culture grew *Fusarium* spp. (Wright–Giemsa, 1000×. *Source:* Image courtesy of Francisco Conrado).

Equine herpesvirus-2 has been implicated as an infectious agent for equine keratoconjunctivitis; other viruses are rare.[105,107,108] Superficial fungal keratitis and epithelial/superficial IMMK can have identical clinical presentations; cytology and culture/sensitivity are therefore important to help rule out fungal etiology, but otherwise cytology is not rewarding for the diagnosis of viral infection.[105,107] A conjunctival swab is recommended over a conjunctival biopsy for viral DNA testing.[108]

Chronic Underlying Irritation

Chronic underlying irritation causing complicated ulcerative keratitis is well characterized in dogs and cats where entropion, distichiae, ectopic cilia, or conjunctival/corneal foreign body cause ulceration.[17] Congenital/hereditary entropion is less common in horses and is mainly seen in premature or dehydrated foals and due to trauma.[17,109] Other underlying causes for complicated ulcerative keratitis in horses have been described. A unilateral choristoma of the nictitating membrane in a horse resulted in a deep corneal stromal ulcer associated with trauma from hairs contacting the cornea.[110] Cytology of the corneal lesion revealed severe neutrophilic inflammation and corneal epithelial cells. No fungal elements were identified cytologically despite low growth of *Candida* sp. that was ultimately determined to be nonpathogenic. Similar cytology was recorded from a corneal ulcer occurring secondary to a third eyelid dermoid.[111]

Indolent Corneal Ulceration

The term indolent corneal ulceration (also known in dogs as spontaneous chronic corneal epithelial defect) is applied when a lesion does not heal within the expected time frame, generally a minimum of 7–10 days depending on the size of the ulceration.[79,105,112] Indolent corneal ulcerations are defined by epithelial loss with intact stroma, non-adherent epithelial edges, and lack of cellular infiltration and infectious agents; the etiology in horses is often unclear.[105,112,113] Cytology and culture/sensitivity are used to help exclude infectious etiologies since indolent corneal ulcerations require a different treatment approach than infected lesions.[79,113,114]

Non-Ulcerative Keratitis: Corneal Stromal Abscess

Corneal stromal abscesses in horses present clinically as a white to yellow corneal opacity, frequently associated with uveitis, corneal vascularization, and edema.[2,115] These lesions are painful and can cause blindness.[115,116] The pathogenesis is postulated to be entrapment of bacteria or fungi in the corneal stroma associated with trauma or a healed ulcer.[115] Because the lesion is covered with intact corneal epithelial, superficial sampling of the cornea for cytology and culture/sensitivity can be unrewarding, although fungal organisms can be detected in some cases.[115,117] Histopathology is often performed as part of surgical treatment.[2,115]

Non-ulcerative Keratitis: Immune-Mediated Keratitis

IMMK refers to a group of primary non-ulcerative, noninfectious conditions clinically characterized by progressive or chronic corneal vascularization, cellular infiltration, and corneal edema.[79–81,118] IMMK is subdivided into five types, four of which are based on anatomic localization (epithelial, superficial stromal, mid-stromal, and endothelial) and are typically unilateral. The last type is called eosinophilic keratitis and is often bilateral.[118,119] Because the corneal surface is intact in IMMK, collection of samples for cytology and culture/sensitivity is not always recommended. Cytology can be used to confirm a clinical impression of eosinophilic keratitis via the identification of eosinophils, along with variable numbers of mast cells, lymphocytes, plasma cells, and neutrophils from the plaque-like lesions most often under the third eyelid, or to help exclude the presence of infectious etiologies (Figure 21.11).[78,79,119,120] Corneal ulceration can occur concurrently with eosinophilic keratitis. Corneal scraping cytology for superficial IMMK has been reported (12 eyes) to include lymphocytes as the predominant cell type, although neutrophils were seen in a very small number of cases.[80] Microorganisms were not identified.[80] Corneal biopsy may be indicated for diagnosis of superficial, midstromal, and deep IMMK.[121]

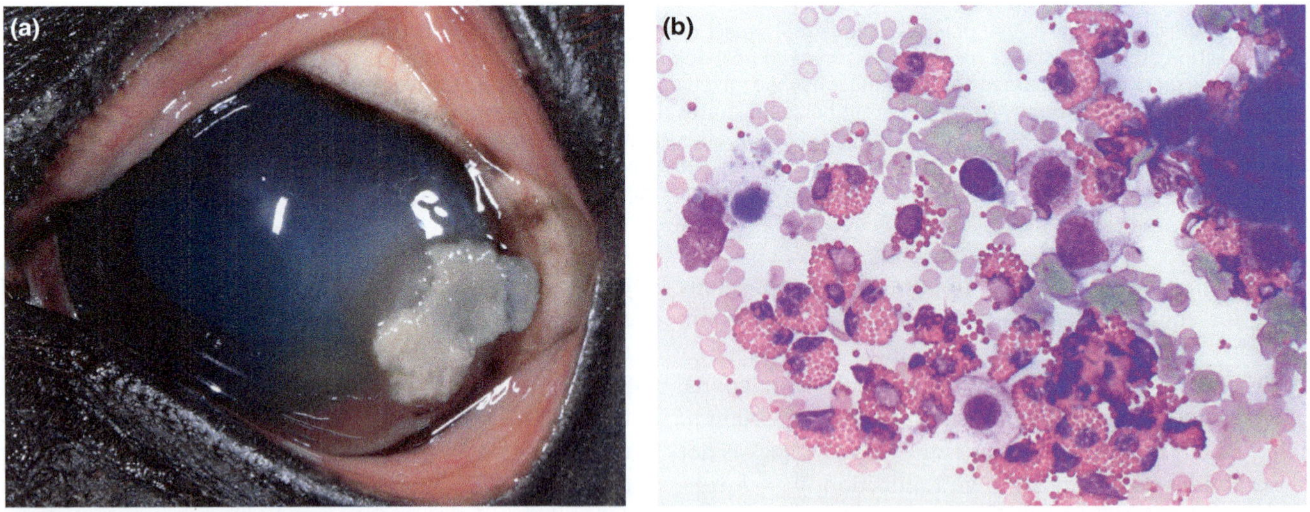

Figure 21.11 (a) Corneal ulceration associated with eosinophilic keratitis is characterized by a "cake-frosting" appearance. Eosinophilic keratitis lesions not only are often found under the third-eyelid but also can occur at other locations in the cornea as can be seen in this example of a lesion in the lateral–ventral aspect of the cornea. Grossly, eosinophilic keratitis can easily be mistaken for fungal keratitis, and cytology is an important diagnostic tool to verify or exclude diagnosis (*Source:* Image courtesy of Mary Lassaline). (b) Cytology reveals numerous eosinophils and free granules mixed with occasional lymphocytes and epithelial cells (Wright–Giemsa, 500×).

Neoplasia

Squamous Cell Carcinoma

SCC is the most common corneal neoplasm in horses, and the lateral limbus is the most frequent location.[79,122] Corneal SCC is typically a raised, white-pink, proliferative mass that is amenable to cytologic examination (Figure 21.1).[79,122,123] The intrastromal form occurs as an infiltrate and requires biopsy, particularly to distinguish it from chronic active stromal keratitis such as mid-stromal IMMK.[78,79,123] There is the potential for deeper infiltration of the uveoscleral meshwork and iridocorneal angle.[124] There may be a genetic component to the disease in some horses, including limbal SCC in Haflingers.[125] The cytologic appearance should be similar to SCC in other locations.

Mast Cell Tumor

Mast cell tumors occur in the equine cornea, sometimes by extension from other tissues. They are relatively uncommon, and differential diagnoses include SCC, stromal abscess, eosinophilic keratitis, parasitic granuloma, orbital fat prolapse, inclusion cyst, or granulation tissue.[73,79,126,127] Specific cytologic criteria for diagnosis in this tissue could not be identified in the literature. The prognosis for corneal mast cell tumors is good for the globe and life, and no recurrence has been reported in the few cases that have been published.[73,126,127]

Other Neoplasms

Hemangiosarcoma, hemangioma, and lymphangiosarcoma do not commonly involve the cornea (Figure 21.8); however, they are reported, and cytology is anticipated to be similar to other anatomic locations.[70,79] Long-term survival after surgical removal was reported in one case.[128] Primary corneal B-cell lymphoma has been reported in the horse, putatively arising from IMMK; cytology was not reported.[129] Isolated corneoscleral lymphoma appears to be rare, while this tissue may be involved more often if the lymphoma is present in other tissues.[22] Melanoma of the sclera and cornea (also known as limbal or epibulbar melanoma) is another rare finding in horses that is not associated with breed or coat color.[79,130,131] Clinically, melanomas most often present as raised pigmented and firm masses located at the limbus and potentially infiltrating the cornea.[79] UV radiation, chemical exposure, trauma, or chronic irritation could be the underlying factors for scleral and corneal melanomas.[79] Cytology from epibulbar melanoma can be performed by either scraping the surface or fine-needle aspiration (FNA) from the raised mass; epibulbar melanoma has been reported in a foal.[130] It is important to exclude staphyloma and iris prolapses before an FNA is collected due to risk of globe perforation and contamination of the anterior segment.

Uvea, Aqueous Humor, and Vitreous

Normal Structure and Cytology

Cytology sampling of intraocular tissue (e.g. uvea) and fluid (aqueous and vitreous) is rare in horses due to potential complications from the collection procedure. The anterior uvea (iris and ciliary body) and posterior uvea (choroid) are very vascular tissues; thus aspiration can result in hyphema, vitreal hemorrhage, and possible glaucoma and retinal detachment. The eye is an immunologically privileged organ lacking lymphatics and characterized by a blood–ocular barrier that excludes leukocytes and blood-borne pathogens from the normal eye, resulting in essentially acellular aqueous humor and vitreous.[28]

Inflammation

Aqueous Humor and Vitreous

Inflammation of the uvea (uveitis) is subdivided into anterior, posterior, and panuveitis. As described in the canine and feline ophthalmology chapters, uveitis will cause a breakdown of the blood–ocular barrier with subsequent presence of protein (flare), leukocytes, fibrin, and/or erythrocytes in the aqueous humor and/or vitreous.[28,132] Uveitis in animals can result from multiple underlying causes, for example, trauma and lens induced uveitis as well as infectious, neoplastic or immune-mediated causes.[28,133] Equine recurrent uveitis (ERU) is a specific equine immune-mediated disease that can sometimes be an indication for sampling aqueous humor or vitreous (see section on ERU below). Intraocular infection (endophthalmitis) will also cause severe uveitis and cytology from aqueous humor or vitreous can be beneficial for identification of a possible infectious etiology.[134]

Equine Recurrent Uveitis

ERU is a common ophthalmic disease affecting 2–25% of horses, potentially causing blindness in 1–10% of all horses in the United States.[135,136] ERU causes of the anterior and/or posterior uvea resulting in complications such as glaucoma, chronic inflammation cataracts, retinal detachment, and phthisis bulbi.[136,137] The pathogenesis of ERU is attributed to an immune-mediated response most likely due to infectious agents such as *Leptospira* spp.[136,138–141] Also, genetic predisposition has been verified and breeds as Appaloosa and warmbloods are predisposed.[136,142,143] Cytology and culture/sensitivity is recommended on any aqueous humor and vitreous collected from equine eyes with ERU, primarily to exclude other processes.

Endophthalmitis

Endophthalmitis is the inflammation of the intraocular contents exclusive of the cornea and sclera with effusion of the inflammatory cells into aqueous humor and vitreous.[144] Endophthalmitis is usually caused by a bacterial or fungal infection.[22,144,145] Trauma to the globe with penetration of a foreign body through the cornea and a ruptured corneal ulceration with retrograde bacterial migration are the most common causes for endophthalmitis in adult horses (Figure 21.12),[22,89] whereas sepsis in foals can cause endophthalmitis.[145–147] Intraocular surgery is the most common reason for endophthalmitis in humans, especially after cataract surgery, which also occurs in horses.[148–151] Aqueous paracentesis carries a significant risk for septic endophthalmitis in horses, and this procedure should therefore be used sparingly and only be performed by veterinary ophthalmologists or clinicians experienced in the technique.[152,153] The clinical appearance of septic endophthalmitis is a severe painful eye with severe intraocular flare, hypopyon, and fibrin. Many cases will have a miotic pupil due to severe uveitis, as well as elevated intraocular pressure due to obstruction of the iridocorneal angle with inflammatory cells and debris.[18,144] Prognosis for septic endophthalmitis is poor for the globe, and most cases culminate in enucleation. Culture/sensitivity and cytology can sometimes provide a definitive diagnosis and facilitate planning.[18]

Intraocular Neoplasia

Primary intraocular neoplastic lesions as well as secondary uveitis complicating systemic neoplasia are reported in horses.[154–156] Anterior uveal melanocytic tumors are the most common intraocular neoplastic lesion in horses, and they are most frequently found in young gray horses.[156–158] Other reported intraocular neoplastic lesions in horses are retinoblastoma, medulloepithelioma, and primary lymphoma lesions as well as secondary uveitis to systemic lymphoma.[154,155,159,160] Metastatic intraocular adenocarcinoma of suspected pulmonary origin has also been reported in a horse.[76]

FNA of intraocular masses is not recommended in affected horses due to high risk of complications such as intraocular hemorrhage (hyphema), secondary glaucoma, lens capsule rupture, endophthalmitis, and potential systemic spread of neoplastic cells through the iridocorneal angle.[6,159,161] Aqueous and vitreous paracentesis is an alternative method to collect cells from the anterior chamber.[6] As indicated previously, this method should only be performed by veterinary ophthalmologists or by experienced clinicians since blinding complications can occur with aqueous and vitreous paracentesis.[6,152] Reports from horses with multicentric lymphoma and primary uveal lymphoma indicate that aqueous paracentesis and cytological examination provides a useful antemortem diagnostic tool for these two types of lymphoma in horses.[154,155]

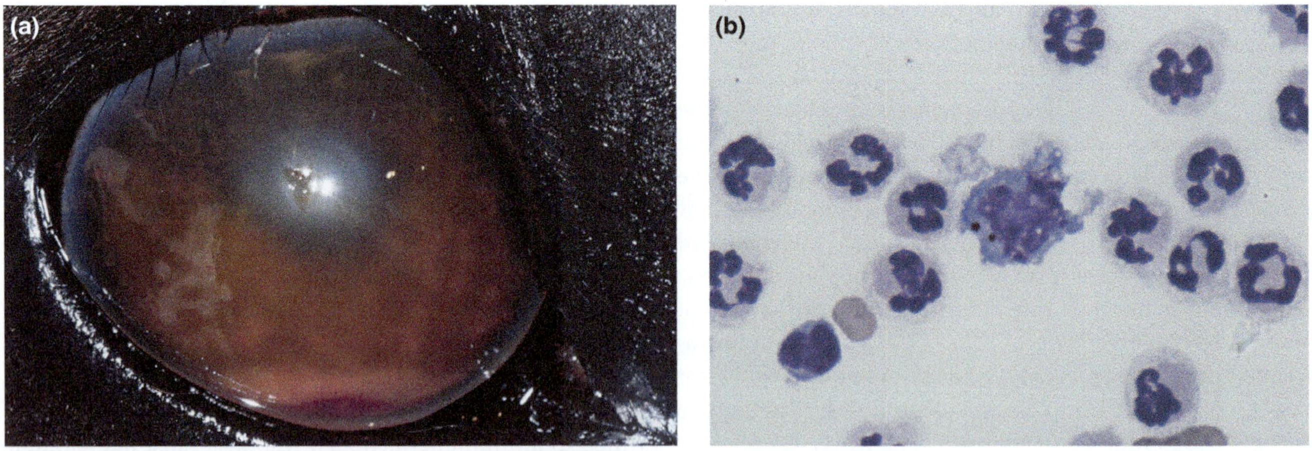

Figure 21.12 (a) The endophthalmitis in this horse was due to a full thickness penetration by a foreign body of plant origin. The foreign body can be seen in the center of the cornea. Other ophthalmic findings are diffuse mild corneal edema and limbal corneal vascularization, miotic pupil, mixed hypopyon and hyphema in the ventral aspect of the anterior chamber, and a yellow/orange discoloration to the aqueous humor due to fibrin and proteins (flare). (b) Cytoprep concentrated samples from the aqueous humor (collected post enucleation) were very cellular, consisting of numerous nondegenerate neutrophils with fewer macrophages and lymphocytes. Scattered melanin granules were present intracellularly in macrophages; care should be taken not to confuse these with cocci. Bacteria were not identified cytologically, and no culture was submitted from this case (Wright–Giemsa, 500×).

Orbit

Diseases of the equine orbit are uncommon but, like all ocular disease, can have serious consequences. Orbital disease can present as changes in the size, shape, or position of the globe; epiphora; third eyelid elevation; and changes in airflow through the nostrils.[162] Trauma, inflammation, and neoplasia can affect the equine orbit. Imaging including radiographs and ultrasound can be helpful, but often, computed tomography and magnetic resonance studies are valuable in characterizing lesions and potentially guiding cytologic sampling.[163]

Normal Structure and Cytology

A recent review of orbital disease in the horse describes the normal equine orbit as being composed of a bony rim formed by the frontal, lacrimal, zygomatic, and temporal bones with a medial wall consisting of the sphenoid and palatine bones.[162] The globe is positioned anteriorly with the rest of the space occupied by extraocular muscles, connective tissue, and adipose tissue. The orbit is adjacent to the oral cavity, guttural pouches, and sinus cavities diseases of these structures can extend to the orbit.[162] The normal cytology of the equine orbit has not been formally described, but can be inferred based on the anatomy.

Inflammation

Inflammatory conditions of the orbit can be due to wounds, extension of inflammation or infection from adjacent structures such as the sinuses, or via septic emboli.[162] Parasitic causes are reported but rare. Hydatid cyst disease of the equine orbit is reported in Europe, so caution is recommended in aspirating lesions because of the potential to cause marked inflammation in regional tissues.

Neoplasia

Neuroendocrine tumors are reported to be the most common primary orbital tumor, with sarcomas and adenocarcinomas also reported.[162] Extra-adrenal paraganglioma has been described in six horses, with exophthalmia and nonpainful eyes.[164] Unfortunately, cytologic evaluation of these lesions is not reported.

Conclusion

Cytology from ocular abnormalities in the horse is a very useful tool for the equine veterinarian as well as for the veterinary ophthalmologist to diagnose specific diseases and constitute correct treatment. Knowledge about normal and abnormal findings for the different ophthalmic structures is important. It is also very important to acknowledge comfort level for the different collection procedures (especially aqueous and vitreous paracentesis) due to the delicate ocular tissue and severe complications that can follow a wrongly performed cytology collection.

References

1 Dwyer, A.E. (2012). Ophthalmology in equine ambulatory practice. *Vet Clin Equine* 28: 155–174.
2 Bauer, B.S. (2015). Ocular pathology. *Vet Clin North Am Equine Pract* 31: 425–448.
3 Greenberg, S.M., Plummer, C.E., Brooks, D.E. et al. (2011). Unilateral orbital lacrimal gland abscess in a horse. *Vet Ophthalmol* 14 (1): 55–60.
4 Reimer, J.M. and Latimer, C.S. (2011). Ultrasound findings in horses with severe eyelid swelling, and recognition of acute dacryoadenitis: 10 cases (2004–2010). *Vet Ophthalmol* 14 (2): 86–92.
5 Dawson, C., Dixon, J., Lam, R. et al. (2016). Differential diagnosis, investigation, and management of a periocular swelling close to the nasolacrimal duct in a horse: a case report of Dacryops. *Vet Ophthalmol* 19 (5): 427–431.
6 Gilger, B.C. and Stoppini, R. (2011). Equine ocular examination: routine and advanced diagnostic techniques. In: *Equine Ophthalmology*, (ed. Gilber, B.C.), 2e, 1–51. Maryland Heights, MO: Saunders.
7 Giuliano, E.A. (2011). Equine ocular adnexal and nasolacrimal disease. In: *Equine Ophthalmology*, (ed. Gilber, B.C.), 2e, 133–180. Maryland Heights, MO: Saunders.
8 Giuliano, E.A. (2010). Equine periocular neoplasia: current concepts in aetiopathogenesis and emerging treatment modalities. *Equine Vet J* 42 (37): 9–18.
9 Mair, T.S. and Krudewig, C. (2008). Mast cell tumours (mastocytosis) in the horse: a review of the literature and report of 11 cases. *Equine Vet Educ* 20: 177–182.
10 Davis, C.R., Valentine, B.A., Gordon, E. et al. (2016). Neoplasia in 125 donkeys (*Equus asinus*): literature review and a survey of five veterinary schools in the United States and Canada. *J Vet Diagn Invest* 28: 662–670.

11 Knowles, E.J., Tremaine, W.H., Pearson, G.R., and Mair, T.S. (2016). A database survey of equine tumours in the United Kingdom. *Equine Vet J* 48: 280–284.

12 Dugan, S.J., Roberts, S.M., Curtis, C.R., and Severin, G.A. (1991). Prognostic factors and survival of horses with ocular/adnexal squamous cell carcinoma: 147 cases (1978–1988). *J Am Vet Med Assoc* 15 (2): 298–303.

13 Gilger, B.C. (2013). Equine ophthalmology. In: *Veterinary Ophthalmology*, (eds. Gelatt, K.N., Gilger, B.C., Kern, T.J.), 5e, 1560–1609. Ames, IA: Wiley-Blackwell.

14 Garma-Avina, A. (1994). The cytology of squamous cell carcinomas in domestic animals. *J Vet Diagn Invest* 6: 238–246.

15 Knottenbelt, D.C. and Kelly, D.F. (2000). The diagnosis and treatment of periorbital sarcoid in the horse; 445 cases from 1974–1999. *Vet Ophthalmol* 3: 169–191.

16 Komaromy, A.M., Andrew, S.E., Brooks, D.E. et al. (2004). Periocular sarcoid in a horse. *Vet Ophthalmol* 7 (3): 141–146.

17 Giuliano, E.A. (2017). Diseases of the adnexa and nasolacrimal system. In: *Equine Ophthalmology*, (ed. Gilber, B.C.), 3e, 197–251. Ames, IA: Wiley Blackwell.

18 Zachar, E.K., Burgess, H.J., and Wobeser, B.K. (2016). Fine-needle aspiration in the diagnosis of equine skin disease and the epidemiology of equine skin cytology submissions in a western Canadian diagnostic laboratory. *Can Vet J* 57: 629–634.

19 Giuliano, E.A. and Moore, C.P. (2001). Eyes and ocular adnexa. In: *Diagnostic Cytology and Hematology of the Horse*, (ed. Cowell, R., and Tyler, R.), 2e, 43–64. St. Louis, MO: Elsevier.

20 Martens, A., De Moor, A., Demeulemeester, J., and Ducatelle, R. (2000). Histopathological characteristics of five clinical types of equine sarcoid. *Res Vet Sci* 69: 295–300.

21 Schnoke, A.T., Brooks, D.E., Wilkie, D.A. et al. (2013). Extraocular lymphoma in horses. *Vet Ophthalmol* 16 (1): 35–42.

22 Taintor, J. and Schleis, S. (2011). Equine lymphoma. *Equine Vet J* 23 (4): 205–213.

23 Johnson, P.J. (1998). Dermatologic tumors (excluding sarcoids). *Vet Clin North Am Equine Pract* 14 (3): 625–658.

24 Murphy, C.J., Lavoie, J.P., Groff, J. et al. (1989). Bilateral eyelid swelling attributable to lymphosarcoma in a horse. *J Am Vet Med Assoc* 194 (7): 939–942.

25 Rebhun, W.C. and Del Piero, F. (1998). Ocular lesions in horses with lymphosarcoma: 21 cases (1977–1997). *J Am Vet Med Assoc* 212 (6): 852–854.

26 Lawn, K. (2005). Sudden death due to thoracic lymphoma in a standardbred racing horse. *Can Vet J* 46: 528–529.

27 Rendle, D.I., Hughes, K.J., Farish, C., and Kessell, A. (2012). Multicentric T-cell lymphoma presenting as inferior palpebral swelling in a standarbred mare. *Aust Vet J* 90 (12): 485–489.

28 Scherrer, N.M., Lassaline-Utter, M., and McKenna, B.C. (2014). Characterization and outcome following excision of masses in the nictitating membranes of horses: 50 cases (1998–2912). *J Am Vet Med Assoc* 245 (7): 812–815.

29 Phillips, J.C. and Lembcke, L.M. (2013). Equine melanocytic tumors. *Vet Clin North Am Equine Pract* 29: 673–687.

30 Fleury, C., Berard, F., Balme, B., and Thomas, L. (2000). The study of cutaneous melanomas in Camargue-type gray-skinned horses (1): clinical-pathological characterization. *Pigment Cell Res* 13: 39–46.

31 Wang, A.L. and Kern, T. (2015). Melanocytic ophthalmic neoplasms of the domestic veterinary species. *Top Companion Anim Med* 30: 148–157.

32 Moore, C.P., Collins, B.K., Linton, L.L., and Collier, L.L. (2000). Conjunctival malignant melanoma in horses. *Vet Ophthalmol* 3: 201–206.

33 Tarrant, J., Stokol, T., Bartol, J. et al. (2001). Diagnosis of malignant melanoma in a horse from cytology of body cavity fluid and blood. *Equine Vet J* 33: 531–535.

34 Metcalfe, L.V.A., O'Brien, P.J., Papakonstantinou, S. et al. (2013). Malignant melanoma in a grey horse: case presentation and review of equine melanoma treatment options. *Ir Vet J* 66: 22–27.

35 LeRoy, B.E., Knight, M.C., Eggleston, R. et al. (2005). Tail-base mass from a "horse of a different color". *Vet Clin Pathol* 34: 69–71.

36 O'Banion, M.K., Reichmann, M.E., and Sundberg, J.P. (1986). Coning and characterization of an equine cutaneous papillomavirus. *Virology* 152 (1): 100–109.

37 Torres, S.M. and Koch, S.N. (2013). Papillomavirus-associated diseases. *Vet Clin North Am Equine Pract* 29: 643–655.

38 Postey, R.C., Appleyard, G.D., and Kidney, B.A. (2007). Evaluation of equine papillomas, aural plaques, and sarcoids for the presence of equine papillomavirus DNA and papillomavirus antigen. *Can J Vet Res* 71: 28–33.

39 White, K.S., Fuji, R.N., Valentine, B.A., and Bildfell, R.J. (2004). Equine congenital papilloma: pathological findings and results of papillomavirus immunohistochemistry in five cases. *Vet Dermatol* 15: 240–244.

40 Maggs, D.J. (2008). Eyelids. In: *Slatter's Fundamentals of Veterinary Ophthalmology*, (eds. Maggs, D.J., Miller, P.E., and Ofri, R.), 4e, 107–134. St. Louis, MO: Saunders.

41 Choi, S.K., Park, J.K., Jeon, W.B. et al. (2013). Meibomian epithelioma of the lower eyelid in a thoroughbred horse. *Pak Vet J* 33 (2): 244–247.

42 Kerr, K.M. and Alden, C.L. (1974). Equine neoplasia: a ten year survey. *Proc Annu Meet Am Assoc Vet Lab Diagn* 17: 183–187.

43 Bourges-Abella, N., Raymond-Letron, I., Diquelou, A. et al. (2007). Comparison of cytologic and histologic evaluations of the conjunctiva in the normal equine eye. *Vet Ophthalmol* 10 (1): 12–18.

44 Braus, B.K., Lehenauer, B., Tichy, A. et al. (2017). Impression cytology as diagnostic tool in horses with and without ocular surface disease. *Equine Vet J* 49: 438–444.

45 Brooks, D.E. (2010). Equine conjunctival diseases: a commentary. *Equine Vet Educ* 22: 382–386.

46 Huntington, P.J., Coloe, P.J., Bryden, J.D., and Macdonald, F. (1987). Isolation of a *Moraxella* sp. from horses with conjunctivitis. *Aust Vet J* 6 (4): 118–119.

47 Evans, K., Smith, M., McDonough, P., and Wiedmann, M. (2004). Eye infections due to *Listeria monocytogenes* in three cows and one horse. *J Vet Diagn Invest* 16: 464–469.

48 Gaede, W., Reckling, K., Schliephake, A. et al. (2010). Detection of *Chlamydophilia caviae* and *Streptococcus equi* subsp. zooepidemicus in horses with signs of rhinitis and conjunctivitis. *Vet Microbiol* 142: 440–444.

49 Johns, I.C., Baxter, K., Booler, H. et al. (2011). Conjunctival bacterial and fungal flora in healthy horses in the UK. *Vet Ophthalmol* 14 (3): 195–199.

50 Andrew, S.E., Nguyen, A., Jones, G.L., and Brooks, D.E. (2003). Seasonal effects on the aerobic bacterial and fungal conjunctival flora of normal thoroughbred brood mares in Florida. *Vet Ophthalmol* 6 (1): 45–50.

51 Berzina, I., Trumble, N.S., Novicki, T., and Sharkey, L.C. (2011). Subconjunctival mycetoma caused by *Scedosporium apiospermum* infection in a horse. *Vet Clin Pathol* 40: 84–88.

52 Voelter-Ratson, K., Monod, M., Unger, M. et al. (2014). Evaluation of the conjunctival fungal flora and its susceptibility to antifungal agents in healthy horse in Switzerland. *Vet Ophthalmol* 17 (1): 31–36.

53 Rebhun, W.C., Mirro, E.J., Georgi, M.E., and Kern, T.J. (1981). Habronemic blepharoconjunctivitis in horses. *J Am Vet Med Assoc* 179 (5): 469–472.

54 Gasthuys, F.M., van Heerden, M., and Vercruysse, J. (2004). Conjunctival habronemiosis in a horse in Belgium. *Vet Rec* 154 (24): 757–758.

55 Davis JL. Ocular manifestations of systemic diseases. *Equine Ophthalmol*, 2. Maryland Heights, MO: Elsevier 2011;443-469.

56 Pusterla, N., Watson, J.L., Wilson, W.D. et al. (2003). Cutaneous and ocular habronemiasis in horses: 63 cases (1988–2002). *J Am Vet Med Assoc* 222: 978–982.

57 Prasad, A., Kumar, V., and Patel, J.S. (2017). Bilateral conjunctival habronemiasis with blepharoconjunctivitis in a Marwari horse. *Intas Polivet* 18: 216–218.

58 Pugh, D.G., Hu, X.P., and Blagburn, B. (2014). Habronemiasis: biology, signs, and diagnosis, and treatment and prevention of the nematodes and vector flies. *J Equine Vet Sci* 34: 241–248.

59 Yarmut, Y., Brommer, H., Weisler, S. et al. (2008). Ophthalmic and cutaneous habronemiasis in a horse: case report and review of the literature. *Is J Vet Med* 63: 87–90.

60 Stoppini, R., Gilger, B.C., Malarkey, D.E. et al. (2005). Bilateral nodular lymphocytic conjunctivitis in a horse. *Vet Ophthalmol* 8 (2): 129–134.

61 Saroglu, M., Aktas, M., Olgun, D., and Arun, S.S. (2005). Limbal pseudotumor in a cob pony. *Vet Ophthalmol* 8 (2): 135–138.

62 Moore, C.P., Grevan, V.L., Champagne, E.S. et al. (2000). Equine conjunctival pseduotumors. *Vet Ophthalmol* 3: 57–63.

63 Ostevik, L., Gunnes, G., de Souza, G. et al. (2014). Nasal and ocular amyloidosis in a 15 year old horse. *Acta Vet Scand* 56: 50–59.

64 Leissinger, M.K., McCauley, C., Fowlkes, N., and Grasperge, B.J. (2017). What is your diagnosis? Nasal lesion in a horse. *Vet Clin Pathol* 46: 361–362.

65 McCowan, C. and Stanley, R.G. (2004). Pigmented squamous cell carcinoma of the conjunctiva of a horse. *Vet Ophthalmol* 7: 421–423.

66 Gearhart, P.M., Steficek, B.A., and Petersen-Jones, S.M. (2007). Hemangiosarcoma and squamous cell carcinoma in the third eyelid of a horse. *Vet Ophthalmol* 10 (2): 121–126.

67 Arenas-Gamboa, A.M. and Mansell, J. (2011). Epithelioid haemangiosarcoma in the ocular tissue of horses. *J Comp Pathol* 144: 328–333.

68 Gupta, A., Bhaskaran, M., Storey, E. et al. (2012). What is your diagnosis? Fine-needle aspiration of a third eyelid mass in a paint horse. *Vet Clin Pathol* 41 (2): 299–300.

69 Sansom, J., Donaldson, D., Smith, K. et al. (2006). Haemangiosarcoma involving the third eyelid in the horse: a case series. *Equine Vet J* 38: 277–282.

70 Gerding, J.C., Gilger, B.C., Montgomery, S.A., and Clode, A.B. (2015). Presumed primary ocular lymphangiosarcoma with metastasis in a miniature horse. *Vet Ophthalmol* 18 (6): 505–509.

71 Schultze, A.E., Morgan, R.V., and Patton, C.S. (1996). What is your diagnosis? A 9-year old American paint horse. *Vet Clin Pathol* 25: 91–92.

72 Herrera, H.D., Duchene, A.G., Croxatto, J.O. et al. (2003). Intravascular papillary endothelial hyperplasia of the conjunctiva in a horse. *Vet Ophthalmol* 6: 269–272.

73 Halse, S., Pizzirani, S., Parry, N.M.A., and Burgess, K.E. (2014). Mast cell tumor invading the cornea in a horse. *Vet Ophthalmol* 17 (3): 221–227.

74 Strubbe, D.T. (2001). Periocular neurofibrosarcoma in a horse. *Vet Ophthalmol* 4 (4): 237–241.

75 Baril, C. (1973). Basal cell tumour of third eyelid in a horse. *Can Vet J* 14: 66–67.

76 Matheis, F.L., Birkmann, K., Ruetten, M. et al. (2013). Ocular manifestations of a metastatic adenocarcinoma in a horse. *Vet Ophthalmol* 16 (3): 214–218.

77 Williams, L.B. and Pinard, C.L. (2013). Corneal ulcers in horses. *Compend Cont Educ* 35: E4.

78 Brooks, D.E., Matthews, A., and Clode, A.B. (2017). Diseases of the cornea. In: *Equine Ophthalmology*, (ed. Gilber, B.C.), 3e, 252–368. Ames, IA: Wiley Blackwell.

79 Clode, A.B. (2011). Disease and surgery of the cornea. In: *Equine Ophthalmology*, (ed. Gilber, B.C.), 2e, 181–266. Maryland Heights, MO: Elsevier.

80 Gilger, B.C., Michau, T.M., and Salmon, J.H. (2005). Immune-mediated keratitis in horses: 19 cases (1998–2004). *Vet Ophthalmol* 8 (4): 233–239.

81 Gilger, B.C., Stoppini, R., Wilkie, D.A. et al. (2014). Treatment of immune-mediated keratitis in horses with episcleal silicone matrix cyclosporine deliver devices. *Vet Ophthalmol* 17 (1): 23–30.

82 Brooks, D.E. (2004). Inflammatory stromal keratopathies: medical management of stromal keratomalacia, stromal abscesses, eosinophilic keratitis, and band keratopathy in the horse. *Vet Clin North Am Equine Pract* 20: 345–360.

83 Keller, R.L. and Hendrix, D.V.H. (2005). Bacterial isolates and antimicrobial susceptibilities in equine bacterial ulcerative keratitis (1993–2004). *Equine Vet J* 37 (3): 207–211.

84 Clode, A.B. (2010). Therapy of equine infectious keratitis: a review. *Equine Vet J* 42 (37): 19–23.

85 Sanchez, S., Studer, M., Currin, P. et al. (2001). Listeria keratitis in a horse. *Vet Ophthalmol* 4: 217–219.

86 Sauer, P., Andrew, S.E., and Lassaline, M. (2003). Changes in antibiotic resistance in equine bacterial ulcerative keratitis (1991–2000): 65 horses. *Vet Ophthalmol* 6: 309–313.

87 Suter, A., Voleter, K., Hartnack, S. et al. (2018). Septic keratitis in dogs, cats, and horses in Switzerland; associated bacteria and antibiotic susceptibility. *Vet Ophthalmol* 21 (1): 66–75.

88 Mancuso, L.A., Lassaline, M., and Scherrer, N.M. (2016). Porcine urinary bladder extracellular matrix grafts (ACell Vet® Corneal Discs) for keratomalacia in 17 equids (2012–2013). *Vet Ophthalmol* 19 (1): 3–10.

89 Henriksen, MdL., Plummer, C.E., Mangan, B. et al. (2012). Visual outcome after corneal transplantation for corneal perforation and iris prolapse in 37 horses: 1998–2010. *Equine Vet J* 44 (43): 115–119.

90 Henriksen, MdL., Sharkey, L., Esser, M., and Costello, J. (2019). A clinical management of superficial complicated corneal ulcerations infected with newly identified fastidious bacteria with unknown antibiotic sensitivity in three horses. *Equine Vet Educ* 31 (6): 303–309.

91 Messa, K.L., Murphy, C.J., Hartmann, F.A. et al. (1999). Usefulness of aerobic microbial culture and cytologic evaluation of corneal specimens in the diagnosis of infectious ulcerative keratitis in animals. *J Am Vet Med Assoc* 215 (11): 1671–1674.

92 Revold, T., Abayneh, T., Brun-Hansen, H. et al. (2015). Listeria monocytogenes associated kerato-conjunctivitis in four horses in Norway. *Acta Vet Scand* 57: 76–87.

93 Reed, Z., Thomasy, S.M., Good, K.L. et al. (2013). Equine keratomycoses in California from 1987–2010 (47 cases). *Equine Vet J* 45: 361–366.

94 Pearce, J.W., Giuliano, E.A., and Moore, C.P. (2009). In vitro susceptibility patterns of *Aspergillus* and *Fusarium* species isolated from equine ulcerative keratomycosis cases in the Midwestern and southern United States with inclusion of the new antifungal agent voriconazole. *Vet Ophthalmol* 12 (5): 318–324.

95 Bradford, K.A., Allison, R.W., and Love, B.C. (2012). What is your diagnosis? Corneal scraping from an ulcerative lesion in a quarter horse. *Vet Clin Pathol* 41 (4): 601–602.

96 Zeiss, C., Neaderland, M., Yang, F. et al. (2013). Fungal polymerase chain reaction testing in equine ulcerative keratitis. *Vet Ophthalmol* 16 (5): 341–351.

97 Ledbetter, E.C., Irby, N.L., and Kim, S.G. (2011). In vivo confocal microscopy of equine fungal keratitis. *Vet Ophthalmol* 14 (1): 1–9.

98 Voelter-Ratson, K., Pot, S.A., Florin, M., and Spiess, B.M. (2013). Equine keratomycosis in Switzerland: a retrospective evaluation of 35 horses (January 2000–August 2011). *Equine Vet J* 45: 608–612.

99 Brooks, D.E., Andrew, S.E., Dillavou, C.L. et al. (1998). Antimicrobial susceptibility patterns of fungi isolated from horses with ulcerative keratomycosis. *Am J Vet Res* 59 (2): 138–142.

100 Richter, M., Hauser, B., Kaps, S., and Spiess, B.M. (2003). Keratitis due to *Histoplasma* spp. in a horse. *Vet Ophthalmol* 6 (2): 99–103.

101 Wada, S., Ode, H., Hobo, S. et al. (2011). Mortirella wolfi keratomycosis in a horse. *Vet Ophthalmol* 14: 267–270.

102 Wada, S., Hobo, S., Ode, H. et al. (2013). Equine keratomycosis in Japan. *Vet Ophthalmol* 16: 1–9.

103 Chopin, J.B., Sigler, L., Connole, M.D. et al. (1997). Keratomycosis in a Percheron cross horse caused by *Cladorrhinum bulbillosum*. *J Med Vet Mycol* 35: 53–55.

104 Cutler, T.J. (2004). Corneal epithelial disease. *Vet Clin North Am Equine Pract* 20 (2): 319–343.

105 Brooks, D.E., Plummer, C.E., Mangan, B.G., and Ben-Shlomo, G. (2013). Equine subepithelial keratomycosis. *Vet Ophthalmol* 16: 93–96.

106 Kershaw, O., von Oppen, T., Glitz, F. et al. (2001). Detection of equine herpesvirus type 2 (EHV-2) in horses with keratoconjunctivitis. *Virus Res* 80: 93–99.

107 Hollingsworth, S.R., Pusterla, N., Kass, P.H. et al. (2015). Detection of equine herpesvirus in horses with idiopathic keratoconjunctivitis and comparison of three sampling techniques. *Vet Ophthalmol* 18 (5): 416–421.

108 Brooks, D.E., Andrew, S.E., Denis, H.M. et al. (2000). Rose Bengal positive epithelial microerosions as a manifestation of equine keratomycosis. *Vet Ophthalmol* 3: 83–86.

109 Gornik, K.R., Pirie, C.G., and Bearner, G.L. (2015). Unilateral choristoma of the nictitating membrane in a horse. *J Am Vet Med Assoc* 246 (2): 231–235.

110 Greenberg, S.H., Plummer, C.E., Brooks, D.E. et al. (2012). Third eyelid dermoid in a horse. *Vet Ophthalmol* 15 (2): 351–354.

111 Hempstead, J.E., Clode, A.B., Borst, L.B., and Gilger, B.C. (2014). Histopathological features of equine superficial, nonhealing, corneal ulcers. *Vet Ophthalmol* 17 (1): 46–52.

112 Lassaline-Utter, M., Cutler, T.J., Michau, T.M., and Nunnery, C.M. (2014). Treatment of nonhealing corneal ulcers in 60 horses with diamond burr debridement (2010–2013). *Vet Ophthalmol* 17 (1): 76–81.

113 Brunott, A., Boeve, M.H., and Velden, M.A. (2007). Grid keratotomy as a treatment for superficial nonhealing corneal ulcers in 10 horses. *Vet Ophthalmol* 10 (3): 162–167.

114 Henriksen, MdL., Andersen, P.H., Plummer, C.E. et al. (2013). Equine corneal stromal abscesses: an evaluation in the understanding of pathogenesis and treatment during the past 30 years. *Equine Vet J* 25 (6): 315–323.

115 Henriksen, MdL., Andersen, P.H., Mietelka, K. et al. (2014). Equine deep stromal abscesses (51 cases – 2004–2009). Part 2: The histopathology and immunohistochemical aspect with attention to the histopathologic diagnosis, vascular response, and infectious agents. *Vet Ophthalmol* 17 (1): 14–22.

116 Hamilton, H.L., McLaughllin, S.A., Whitley, E.M. et al. (1994). Histological findings in corneal stromal abscesses of 11 horses: correlation with cultures and cytology. *Equine Vet J* 26: 448–453.

117 Matthews, A. and Gilger, B.C. (2009). Equine immune-mediated keratopathies. *Vet Ophthalmol* 12 (1): 10–16.

118 Lassaline-Utter, M., Miller, C., and Wotman, K.L. (2014). Eosinophilic keratitis in 46 eyes of 27 horses in the Mid-Atlantic United States (2008–2012). *Vet Ophthalmol* 17 (5): 311–320.

119 Edwards, S., Clode, A.B., and Gilber, B.C. (2015). Equine eosinophilic keratitis in horses: 28 cases (2003–2013). *Clin Case Rep* 3: 1000–1006.

120 Pate, D.O., Clode, A.B., Olivry, T. et al. (2012). Immunohistochemical and immunopathologic characterization of superficial stromal immune-mediated keratitis in horses. *Am J Vet Res* 73 (7): 1067–1073.

121 Clode, A.B., Miller, C., McMullen, R.J., and Gilger, B.C. (2012). A retrospective comparison of surgical removal of subsequent CO_2 laser ablation versus topical administration of mitomycin C as therapy for equine corneolimbal squamous cell carcinoma. *Vet Ophthalmol* 15 (4): 254–262.

122 Kafarnik, C., Rawlings, M., and Dubielzig, R.R. (2009). Corneal stromal invasive squamous cell carcinoma: a retrospective morphological description in 10 horses. *Vet Ophthalmol* 12 (1): 6–12.

123 Kaps, S., Richter, M., Philipp, M. et al. (2005). Primary invasive ocular squamous cell carcinoma in a horse. *Vet Ophthalmol* 8: 193–197.

124 Lassaline, M., Cranford, T.L., Latimer, C.A., and Bellone, R.R. (2015). Limbal squamous cell carcinoma in Haflinger horses. *Vet Ophthalmol* 18: 404–408.

125 Ward, D.A., Lakritz, J., and Bauer, R.W. (1993). Scleral mastocytosis in a horse. *Equine Vet J* 25 (1): 79–80.

126 Bosch, G. and Klein, W.R. (2005). Superficial keratectomy and cryosurgery as therapy for limbal neoplasm in 13 horses. *Vet Ophthalmol* 8 (4): 241–246.

127 Pinn, T.L., Cushing, T., Valentino, L.M., and Koch, S.A. (2011). Corneal invasion by hemangiosarcoma in a horse. *Vet Ophthalmol* 14 (3): 200–204.

128 Vallone, L.V., Neaderland, M.H., Ledbetter, E.C., and Dubielzig, R.R. (2016). Suspected malignant transformation of B lymphocytes in the equine cornea from immune-mediated keratitis. *Vet Ophthalmol* 2: 172–179.

129 McMullen, R.J., Clode, A.B., Kumar, A. et al. (2008). Epibulbar melanoma in a foal. *Vet Ophthalmol* 11 (1): 44–50.

130 Ramadan, R.O. (1975). Primary ocular melanoma in a young horse. *Equine Vet J* 7 (1): 49–50.

131 English, R. and Gilger, B.C. (2017). Ocular immunology. In: *Veterinary Ophthalmology*, (eds. Gelatt, K.N., Gilger, B.C., Kern, T.J.), 5e, 273–299. Ames, IA: Wiley Blackwell.

132 Powell, C.C. and Lappin, M.R. (2001). Cause of feline uveitis. *Compend Contin Educ Pract Vet* 23: 128–141.

133 McMullen, R.J. and Gilger, B. (2017). Disease and surgery of the lens. In: *Equine Ophthalmology*, (ed. Gilber, B.C.), 3e, 416–452. Ames, IA: Wiley Blackwell.

134 Gerding, J.C. and Gilger, B.C. (2016). Prognosis and impact of equine recurrent uveitis. *Equine Vet J* 48 (3): 290–298.

135 Gilger, B.C. and Deeg, C. (2011). Equine recurrent uveitis. In: *Equine Ophthalmology*, (ed. Gilber, B.C.), 2e, 317–349. Maryland Heights, MO: Elsevier Saunders.

136 Allbaugh, R.A. (2017). Equine recurrent uveitis: a review of clinical assessment and management. *Equine Vet Educ* 29 (5): 279–288.

137 Polle, F., Storey, E., Eades, S. et al. (2014). Role of intraocular *Leptospira* infections in the pathogenesis of equine recurrent uveitis in the southern United States. *J Equine Vet Sci* 34: 1300–1306.

138 Faber, N.A., Crawford, M., LeFebvre, R.B. et al. (2000). Detection of *Leptospira* spp. in aqueous humor of horses with naturally acquired recurrent uveitis. *J Clin Microbiol* 38: 2731–2733.

139 Pearce, J.W., Galle, L.E., Kleiboeker, S.B. et al. (2007). Detection of *Leptospira* interrogans DNA and antigen in fixed equine eyes affected with end-stage equine recurrent uveitis. *J Vet Diagn Invest* 19: 686–690.

140 Gilger, B.C., Salmon, J.H., Yi, N.Y. et al. (2008). Role of bacteria in the pathogenesis of recurrent uveitis in horses from the southeastern United States. *Am J Vet Res* 69: 1329–1335.

141 Kulbrock, M., Lehner, S., Metzger, J. et al. (2013). A genome-wide association study indentifies risk loci to equine recurrent uveitis in German warmblood horses. *PLoS One* 8 (8): e71619.

142 Fritz, K.L., Kaese, H.J., Valberg, S.J. et al. (2014). Genetic risk factors for insidious equine recurrent uveitis in Appaloosa horses. *Anim Genet* 45: 392–399.

143 Wilcock, B.P. (2008). General pathology of the eye. In: *Slatter's Fundamentals of Veterinary Ophthalmology*, (ed. Maggs, D.J., Miller, P.E., Ofri, R.), 4e, 62–80. St. Louis, MO: Elsevier Saunders.

144 Reilly, L.K. and Palmer, J.E. (1994). Systemic candidiasis in four foals. *J Am Vet Med Assoc* 205: 464–466.

145 Blogg, J.R., Barton, M.D., Graydon, R., and Cust, R.E. (1983). Blindness caused by *Rhodococcus equi* infection in a foal. *Equine Vet J* 15 (2): 25–26.

146 Labelle, A.L., Hamor, R.E., Townsend, W.M. et al. (2011). Ophthalmic lesions in neonatal foals evaluated for nonophthalmic disease at referral hospital. *J Am Vet Med Assoc* 239: 486–492.

147 Millichamp, N.J. and Dziezyc, J. (2000). Cataract phacofragmentation in horses. *Vet Opthalmol* 3: 157–164.

148 Cao, X., Liu, A., Zhang, J. et al. (2007). Clinical analysis of endophthalmitis after phacoemulsification. *Can J Ophthalmol* 42: 844–848.

149 Colitz, C.M.H. and McMullen, R.J. (2011). Disease and surgery of the lens. In: *Equine Ophthalmology*, (ed. Gilber, B.C.), 2e, 282–316. Maryland Heights, MO: Elsevier Saunders.

150 Brooks, D.E., Plummer, C.E., Carastro, S.M., and Utter, M.E. (2014). Visual outcomes of phacoemulsification cataract surgery in horses: 1990–2013. *Vet Ophthalmol* 17 (1): 117–128.

151 Yi, N.Y., Davis, J.L., Salmon, J.H., and Gilger, B.C. (2008). Ocular distribution and toxicity of intravitreal injection of triamcinolone acetonide in normal equine eyes. *Vet Ophthalmol* 11 (1): 15–19.

152 Stoppini, R. and Gilger, B.C. (2017). Equine ocular examination basic techniques. In: *Equine Ophthalmology*, (ed. Gilber, B.C.), 3e, 1–39. Ames, IA: Wiley-Blackwell.

153 Germann, S.E., Richter, M., Schwarzwald, C.C. et al. (2008). Ocular and multicentric lymphoma in a young race horse. *Vet Ophthalmol* 11 (1): 51–56.

154 Trope, G.D., McCowan, C.T., Tyrrell, D. et al. (2014). Solitary (primary) uveal T-cell lymphoma in a horse. *Vet Ophthalmol* 17: 139–145.

155 Scotty, N.C., Barrie, K.B., Brooks, D.E., and Taylor, D. (2008). Surgical management of a progressive iris melanocytoma in a mustang. *Vet Ophthalmol* 11: 75–80.

156 Murphy, J. and Young, S. (1979). Intraocular melanoma in a horse. *Vet Pathol* 16: 539–542.

157 Latimer, C.A. and Wyman, M. (1983). Sector iridectomy in the management of iris melanoma in a horse. *Equine Vet J* 15 (2): 101–104.

158 Knottenbelt, D.C., Hetzel, U., and Roberts, V. (2007). Primary intraocular primitive neuroectodermal tumor (retinoblastoma) causing unilateral blindness in a gelding. *Vet Ophthalmol* 10: 348–356.

159 Leiva, M., Felici, F., Carcalho, A. et al. (2013). Benign intraocular teroid medulloepithelioma causing glaucoma in an 11-year-old Arabian mare. *Vet Ophthalmol* 16: 297–302.

160 Singh, A.D. and Biscotti, C.V. (2012). Fine needle aspiration biopsy of ophthalmic tumors. *Saudi J Ophthalmol* 26: 117–123.

161 Pucket, J.D. (2017). Equine orbital disease: a review. *Equine Vet Educ* 29: 452–458.

162 D'Aout, C., Nisolle, J.F., Navez, M. et al. (2015). Computed tomography and magnetic resonance anatomy of the normal orbit and eye of the horse. *Anat Histol Embryol* 44: 370–377.

163 Miesner, T., Wilkie, D., Gemensky-Metzler, A. et al. (2009). Extra-adrenal paraganglioma of the equine orbit: six cases. *Vet Ophthalmol* 12: 263–268.

164 Henriksen, MdL., Plummer, C.E., and Brooks, D.E. (2013). Modified Kuhnt-Szwmanowski surgical procedure for secondary cicatricial ectropion in a horse. *Vet Ophthalmol* 16 (4): 276–281.

Part V

Musculoskeletal System

22

Muscle

Catherine J. Benson

Introduction

Various processes, including degenerative, nutritional, toxic, immune-mediated, infectious, and neoplastic conditions involving muscle have been described in-depth histologically.[1] However, cytology of skeletal, smooth, and cardiac muscle is most often performed when a mass is suspected in these tissues. Determining the extent of invasion by neoplastic or inflammatory cells into skeletal muscle deep to tissue such as the dermis or into smooth muscle beneath the mucosa is often difficult to determine unless histopathology is performed.

Normal

Cytologically, skeletal muscle cells form aggregates with deeply basophilic cytoplasm containing cross striations and peripheralized nuclei. Nuclei are oval and relatively uniform in shape and size; they have stippled chromatin and a single variably distinct nucleolus (Figure 22.1). Normal skeletal muscle can be inadvertently aspirated.[2] Histologically, smooth muscle cells are classically described as being elongated with a central elongated oval blunt-ended nucleus with stippled chromatin and multiple nucleoli.[3,4] Cytologically, these cells are similar appearing to other mesenchymal cells, although the central cigar-shaped nucleus is a characteristic.[5,6] Cardiac myocytes are histologically similar to skeletal muscle myocytes with cross striations, but the nucleus is centrally located.[3] Cytology of cardiac muscle is usually limited to impression smears performed at necropsy. This can be done in cases of suspected neoplasia or in cases when infectious organisms such as fungi are suspected.

Support for muscle fibers is by a connective tissue network composed of the endomysium (containing capillaries), perimysium (containing larger blood vessels and nerves), and epimysium.[1]

Inflammation

Characterization of myositis is limited in fine-needle aspirates due to the lack of tissue architecture as compared with histopathology, although organisms, inflammatory cells, and degenerating muscle tissue can be appreciated cytologically in some cases (Figure 22.2). Using a combination of cytology, histopathology, and immunohistochemistry, cutaneous neosporosis with secondary suppurative inflammation (dermatitis, panniculitis, and myositis) has been described in a dog with ulcerative skin lesions.[7]

Degeneration

Degenerative processes have not been well characterized cytologically, and these changes are often best seen on histopathology. However, the mineral in calcinosis circumscripta has been described cytologically as clear to purple extracellular refractile material. This was found histologically to extend into adjacent skeletal muscle[8]. See Chapter 12 for additional discussion and a cytologic image.

Neoplasia

The determinants of primary neoplastic processes in muscle are dictated by the histologic components. Neoplasms originating in adjacent tissue such as subcutaneous soft tissue sarcomas, subcutaneous mast cell tumors (Figure 22.3), infiltrative lipomas (Figure 22.4), and carcinomas can on occasion invade into the muscle.[1] While uncommon compared with other organs, metastases to skeletal muscle from carcinomas can occur.[1]

Veterinary Cytology, First Edition. Edited by Leslie C. Sharkey, M. Judith Radin, and Davis Seelig.

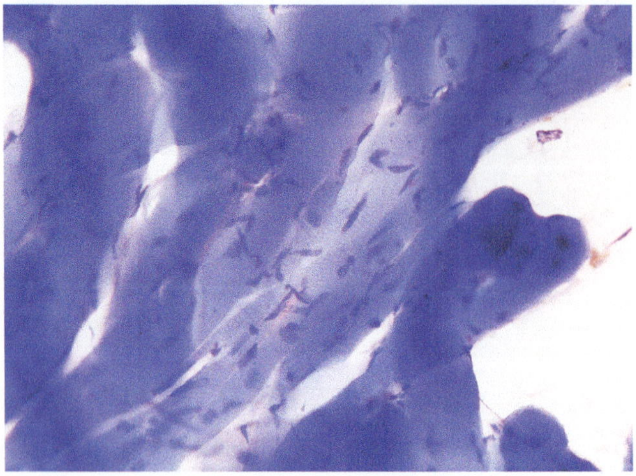

Figure 22.1 Cytology of normal skeletal muscle in a dog. Note the deeply basophilic cytoplasm and prominent cross striations (Wright–Giemsa, 500×. *Source:* Image courtesy of William Gow).

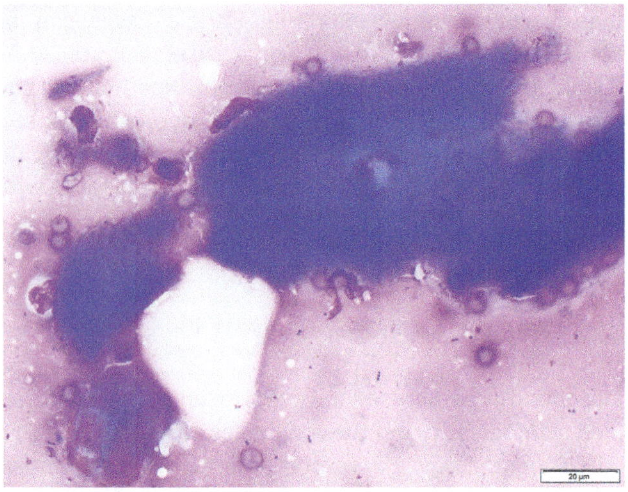

Figure 22.2 Cytology of degenerating muscle tissue with small numbers of chaining cocci from an adult female dog presenting with a painful swelling and edema of her right rear leg. Computed tomography showed diffuse infiltrate around the muscles. The dog responded to antimicrobial therapy (Wright–Giemsa, 500×. *Source:* Image courtesy of Leslie Sharkey).

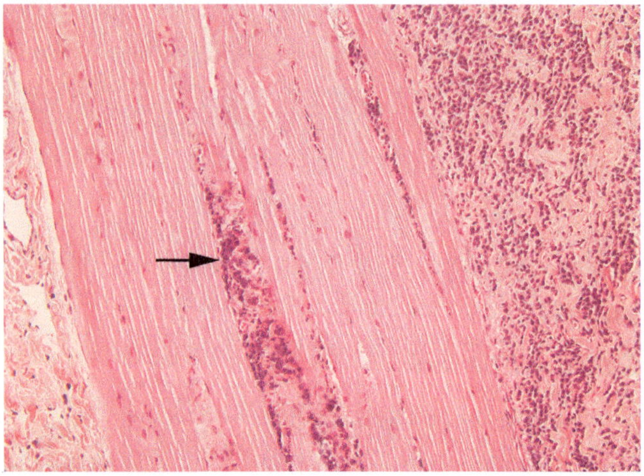

Figure 22.3 Histologic section showing a longitudinal section of skeletal muscle that is invaded by neoplastic round mast cells (arrow). Note the more eosinophilic elongated skeletal myocytes that often have indistinct cell margins and oval nuclei (hematoxylin & eosin, 200×. *Source:* Image courtesy of William Gow).

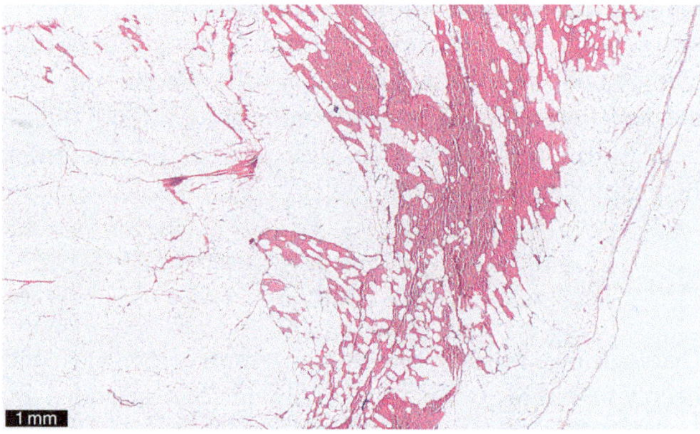

Figure 22.4 Histologic section of an infiltrative lipoma. Note the bulk of the mass (left side of photomicrograph) is composed of sheets of mature adipocytes. These mature-appearing adipocytes with large clear lipid vacuoles are also present multifocally as aggregates within the residual skeletal muscle (hematoxylin & eosin, scale bar = 1 mm).

Skeletal Muscle

Primary Tumors

Given the limited cell types within this tissue, there are few primary tumors of skeletal muscle. Primary neoplasms of skeletal and cardiac muscle are rare in domestic animals.[1]

Rhabdomyoma

Two reports of the cytologic features of rhabdomyomas have been reported in dogs, both in the larynx, where they occur most commonly in this species. In pigs, they can occur in the heart.[1,9,10] The cytologic description of the neoplastic cells in the two case reports of canine rhabdomyomas is somewhat different. One case described the neoplastic population as having two different morphologies.[9] One population consisted of smaller rounded to polygonal cells with pale cytoplasm that were individualized or that were in aggregates. They had a single round to oval nucleus. The population of larger cells had fine granular basophilic cytoplasm. Nuclei had coarsely clumped chromatin like the smaller cells, but the cells also had prominent nucleoli, which was not a prominent feature of the smaller cells. In the other case, only one cell morphology was described, which was that of large, round cells with similar features to those described in the other case report.[10] Anisocytosis was marked, anisokaryosis was mild, and multinucleated cells were reported in both cases.

Differential diagnoses for rhabdomyomas include rhabdomyosarcomas, oncocytomas, and granular cell tumors.[9–11] These are often differentiated with histopathology, histochemical staining, and immunohistochemistry.

Rhabdomyosarcoma

There are three main types of rhabdomyosarcomas: embryonal, alveolar, and pleomorphic in descending order of frequency.[1,12] While histopathology is needed to subtype rhabdomyosarcomas, familiarity with the various morphologies is important when considering differential diagnoses for cytological preparations. Limited case reports in the veterinary literature have described the cytologic features of rhabdomyosarcomas corresponding to the various histologic types.

Embryonal rhabdomyosarcomas are subdivided into a round cell variant composed of varying proportions of smaller and larger (myoblast-like) round cells and the botryoid variant that has more elongated myotube-like cells.[1,12] A subcutaneous round cell variant of a canine embryonal rhabdomyosarcoma was described as having two populations of round individualized cells.[12] The large 30–50 μm diameter cells had ample basophilic cytoplasm and large paracentric nuclei. Multinucleation, marked pleocytosis, and occasional mitotic figures were noted. Chromatin was finely granular. The smaller 10–15 μm diameter cells resembled lymphoid cells with scant cytoplasm and round nuclei with condensed chromatin. Cross striations were not seen in either population. Differential diagnoses included round cell neoplasms of histiocytic or plasma cell origin.

A botryoid embryonal rhabdomyosarcoma in the bladder of a young dog was described cytologically to have elongated ribbon-shaped myotubular-like cells with basophilic cytoplasm and cross striations typical of muscle origin.[13] The cells had oval nuclei with prominent nucleoli and clumped chromatin, while strap cells had multiple linear nuclei. Although cross striations help identify tumors as skeletal muscle in origin, the lack of cross striations does not preclude this diagnosis.[13]

Two cytological descriptions of alveolar rhabdomyosarcomas have been reported, both oral masses in young dogs.[14,15] Neoplastic cells were described as 5–25 μm diameter round cells with moderate pale blue cytoplasm resembling lymphoid cells. Nuclei were round with stippled or clumped chromatin and one to two indistinct nucleoli. Mitotic figures were sometimes frequent. Various differential diagnoses were considered, which included round cell neoplasms, primitive neuroectodermal tumors, and other anaplastic neoplasms.

Pleomorphic rhabdomyosarcomas have more irregularly arranged plump spindle cells. Given the varying morphologies of cells, tumors of the pleomorphic type can be difficult to differentiate from embryonal rhabdomyosarcomas.[1,12] Cytology of pleomorphic rhabdomyosarcomas has been described based on lesions of a bovine stifle and in the tongue of a dog.[11,16] Both cases had two cell populations of equal distribution. One population consisted of larger pleomorphic 50–80 or 12–30 μm mesenchymal cells with variable nuclear to cytoplasmic ratios.[11,16] Morphologically the cells varied between being oval, spindle shaped, and plump. These larger cells had a moderate to large amount of intracytoplasmic granular pink to magenta material within abundant basophilic cytoplasm. This granular material was stained in the bovine case with periodic acid–Schiff (PAS), and it was positive indicative of polysaccharides. Most cells had a single round to oval nucleus with coarse to granular chromatin, and nucleoli were prominent but varied from being multiple to singular.[11,16] Both cases had marked anisocytosis and anisokaryosis, occasional strap cells with linear nuclei and elongated multinucleated and binucleated cells, and a second population of round cells that resembled small lymphocytes. These lymphoid-appearing cells were similar to the smaller cells in the round cell variant of the embryonal rhabdomyosarcoma. Cross striations were not seen in the neoplastic cells in either case. Differential diagnoses for the tongue mass were similar to those listed above for rhabdomyomas.[9–11] An anaplastic invasive and metastatic pleomorphic rhabdomyosarcoma in a young dog with multiple subcutaneous and soft tissue masses has also been described, but the cytologic features were not noted.[17]

A subcutaneous rhabdomyosarcoma with markedly pleomorphic fusiform to stellate mesenchymal cells arranged in groups and individually has been reported in a dog in association with a pacemaker generator implant.[18] Marked anisocytosis and anisokaryosis were evident. Occasional multinucleated cells and rare strap cells with linear nuclei were seen. The mitotic index on histologic evaluation was high at 28/10 high power fields.

A primary ureteral giant cell tumor in a dog had strap-like cells on impression smear.[19] While a pleomorphic rhabdomyosarcoma could not be fully excluded, immunohistochemistry for various muscle markers was negative.[19]

Secondary Tumors

Multiple secondary tumors invading skeletal muscle have been described cytologically, which were confirmed using histopathology. In dogs these include a myxosarcoma,[20] angiosarcomas,[21] a malignant pilomatricoma,[22] a lingual liposarcoma that cytologically resembled a granular cell tumor,[23] and an atypical anal sac adenocarcinoma with cytologically more elongated and oval nuclei.[24] Neoplastic cells from lingual granular cell tumors, which stain positively with PAS, have been described cytologically.[25]

In other species, these include an equine angiosarcoma of the extraocular skeletal muscle,[26] a thyroid follicular adenocarcinoma in a ferret,[27] and a schwannoma in a goldfish.[28]

While most lipomas are benign, some lipomas infiltrate into and between skeletal muscle fibers, segregating, entrapping, and in some cases replacing muscle fibers on histopathology (Figure 22.4).[29] Cytologically, infiltrative lipomas and intermuscular lipomas (which are neither subcutaneous nor infiltrative lipomas but which have been reported to occur in the thigh region in dogs) appear as normal mature adipocytes with minimal pleomorphism and are otherwise similar to simple lipomas.[30]

Smooth Muscle

Smooth muscle tumors can occur in the spleen, gastrointestinal and urogenital tracts, skin (arrector pilae muscles), and liver.[6,31] Leiomyosarcomas can have variable cellularity with cells that are individualized or are arranged in aggregates. Cells often have indistinct cell margins, and nuclei are often cigar shaped with one to two nucleoli. Pleomorphism is moderate. Cigar-shaped central nuclei in mesenchymal cells with moderate pleomorphism and increased cellularity are characteristics of leiomyosarcomas.[5,6] Leiomyomas are often difficult to distinguish cytologically from leiomyosarcomas, but the neoplastic cells tend to have less pleomorphism compared with those of leiomyosarcomas; histologic distinction is based on assessment of invasion, necrosis, and mitotic index.[5,6]

Various histologic descriptions of myofibroblastic tumors, some of which are sarcomas (myofibrosarcomas) and some of which have been termed either inflammatory myofibroblastic tumors or inflammatory pseudotumors have been reported to occur in both humans and in animals. They are considered to be of modified fibroblastic origin with cells that stain positively with vimentin with a subpopulation that stain positively for smooth muscle actin. These mesenchymal cells are negative or have minority subpopulation that are positive for desmin.[6,32–35]

Cardiac Muscle

Various tumors have been described to occur in cardiac muscle including rhabdomyomas, rhabdomyosarcomas, lymphoma, hemangiosarcomas, and other sarcomas.[36] Cytologically, these are similar to tumors that occur in other tissues.

Additional Diagnostics

Histology

Histology is recommended, when clinically indicated, to further characterize or confirm cytologic findings. Rhabdomyosarcomas are similar to other mesenchymal origin tumors with sometimes haphazardly arranged spindle-shaped, plump, and polygonal cells, but the presence of multinucleated "strap" cells and cross striations is often considered specific for skeletal muscle origin.[6,11,16–18] Necrosis can be present in some rhabdomyosarcomas.[17] Occasionally, a second smaller population of cells is described.[16] In the case reports with concurrent cytologic descriptions, the mitotic index on histology varied between 0–5/40× field[16] and 28 in 10/high power fields.[18] In addition to rhabdomyosarcomas, rhabdomyomas and smooth muscle tumors have also been previous described histologically.[6]

Ancillary Testing

In some cases, special stains and other ancillary tests on biopsy samples are needed to further characterize some tumors.

Immunocytochemistry

Vimentin, cytokeratin, lymphoid markers, histiocytic markers, endothelial markers, and muscle markers may be needed to further characterize a mass, given the varying morphologies of cells that can be present in some muscle neoplasms. Smooth muscle actin and desmin can, although not frequently, be performed at some laboratories to aid in further diagnosis. These markers can be used in conjunction with other markers such as CD18 for histiocytic sarcoma or Factor VIII/von Willebrand factor for hemangiosarcomas prior to surgery. Additional detail on cytochemical staining is presented in Chapter 7.

Histochemical Staining

Mallory's phosphotungstic acid hematoxylin stain (PTAH) can be used to show cross striations in skeletal muscle cells,[10,11,13,17] although in the bovine pleomorphic rhabdomyosarcoma, PTAH staining was negative.[16] Most neoplastic cells in rhabdomyomas are negative for PAS, although a few positively staining cells can be seen in some tumors.[6,10]

Immunohistochemistry

Skeletal muscle cells classically stain positive for vimentin[12,14,16–18] and desmin[12,14,17] and are negative for smooth muscle actin.[9,11,12,14,16,18] Desmin was negative in the bovine pleomorphic rhabdomyosarcoma.[16] Skeletal muscle cells often stain positive with myoglobin,[10,12] although not always,[14] and they have been reported to stain positive with myogenin and MyoD1.[14,16] The large cells in the canine laryngeal rhabdomyosarcoma were positive for myoglobin and desmin, but the small cells were negative.[9] Smaller cells in the canine glossal pleomorphic rhabdomyosarcoma were positive for vimentin and were weakly stained with MyoD1, while the larger cells were positive for desmin and had variable positivity for myoglobin.[11] Smooth muscle cells can stain with vimentin, desmin, and smooth muscle actin.[6]

Electron Microscopy

Mitochondria and cytoplasmic myofilaments denoting rhabdomyoblasts were seen with electron microscopy in the round cell variant of the embryonal rhabdomyosarcoma.[12] In the bovine pleomorphic rhabdomyosarcoma, neoplastic cells had abundant glycogen depicted as electron dense beta granules.[16]

Conclusion

Although muscle is infrequently sampled for cytologic evaluation, a number of inflammatory and neoplastic disorders can be evaluated. Histopathologic confirmation, sometimes requiring special staining, is often beneficial.

References

1 Cooper, B.J. and Valentine, B.A. (2016). Muscle and tendon. In: *Jubb, Kennedy, and Palmer's Pathology of Domestic Animals. Vol. 1*,(ed. Maxie, M.G.), 6e, 164–249. St. Louis, MO: Elsevier.

2 Barger, A.M. (2010). Musculoskeletal system. In: *Canine and Feline Cytology: A Color Atlas and Interpretation Guide*, (eds. Raskin, R.E., Meyer D.J.), 2e, 318. St. Louis, MO: Saunders Elsevier.

3 Eurell, J.A. (1998). Muscle. In: *Textbook of Veterinary Histology*, (eds. Dellmann, R.E., Eurell, J.), 5e, 80–88. Philadelphia, PA: Lippincott Williams & Wilkins.

4 Aughey, E. and Frye, F. (2001). Muscle. In: *Comparative Veterinary Histology with Clinical Correlates*, (eds. Aughey, E., Frye, F.L.), 1e, 65–70. London: Manson Publishing Ltd.

5 Messick, J.B., Haddad, T., Kitchell, B. et al. (2001). Abdominal mass in a dog. *Vet Clin Pathol* 30: 25–27.

6 Cooper, B.J. and Valentine, B.A. (2002). Tumors of muscle. In: *Tumors in Domestic Animals*, (ed. Meuten, D.J.), 4e, 319–363. Ames, IA: Blackwell Publishing.

7 Gupta, A., Stroup, S., Dedeaux, A. et al. (2011). What is your diagnosis? Fine-needle aspirate of ulcerative skin lesions in a dog. *Vet Clin Pathol* 40: 401–402.

8 Sharkey, L.C., Gliatto, J.M., and Gallagher, J.G. (1999). Deep tissue mass aspirate from a young German Shepherd dog. *Vet Clin Pathol* 28: 147–149.

9 Barnhart, K. and Lewis, B. (2000). Laryngopharyngeal mass in a dog with upper airway obstruction. *Vet Clin Pathol* 29: 47–50.

10 Dunbar, M.D., Ginn, P., Winter, M. et al. (2012). Laryngeal rhabdomyoma in a dog. *Vet Clin Pathol* 41: 590–593.

11 Chapman, S., Nabity, M., and Calise, D. (2008). What is your diagnosis? Lingual mass in a dog. *Vet Clin Pathol* 37: 133–139.

12 Avallone, G., Pinto da Cunha, N., Palmieri, C. et al. (2010). Subcutaneous embryonal rhabdomyosarcoma in a dog: cytologic, immunocytochemical, histologic, and ultrastructural features. *Vet Clin Pathol* 39: 499–504.

13 Alleman, A.R., Raskin, R.E., Uhl, E.W. et al. (1991). What is your diagnosis? *Vet Clin Pathol* 20: 49–50.

14 Murakami, M., Sakai, H., Iwatani, N. et al. (2010). Cytologic, histologic, and immunohistochemical features of maxillofacial alveolar rhabdomyosarcoma in a juvenile dog. *Vet Clin Pathol* 39: 113–118.

15 Snyder, L.A. and Michael, H. (2011). Alveolar rhabdomyosarcoma in a juvenile Labrador Retriever: case report and literature review. *J Am Anim Hosp Assoc* 47: 443–446.

16 Bisby, T.M., Pratt, S.M., Fenton, K. et al. (2009). What is your diagnosis? Perifemoral mass in a cow. *Vet Clin Pathol* 38: 343–347.

17 Fallin, C.W., Fox, L.E., Papendick, R.E. et al. (1995). What is your diagnosis? *Vet Clin Pathol* 24: 100–101.

18 Thieman-Mankin, K.M., Dunbar, M.D., Toplon, D. et al. (2014). Rhabdomyosarcoma associated with the lead wire of a pacemaker generator implant. *Vet Clin Pathol* 43: 276–280.

19 Rigas, J.D., Smith, T.J., Gorman, E. et al. (2012). Primary ureteral giant cell sarcoma in a Pomeranian. *Vet Clin Pathol* 41: 141–146.

20 Grindem, C.B., Riley, J., Sellon, R., and Davis, B. (1990). Myxosarcoma in a dog. *Vet Clin Pathol* 19: 119–121.

21 Bertazzolo, W., Dell'Orco, M., Bonfanti, U. et al. (2005). Canine angiosarcoma: cytologic, histologic, and immunohistochemical correlations. *Vet Clin Pathol* 34: 28–34.

22 Jackson, K., Boger, L., Goldschmidt, M., and Walton, R.M. (2010). Malignant pilomatricoma in a soft-coated Wheaten Terrier. *Vet Clin Pathol* 39: 236–240.

23 Piseddu, E., De Lorenzi, D., Freeman, K., and Masserdotti, C. (2011). Cytologic, histologic, and immunohistochemical features of lingual liposarcoma in a dog. *Vet Clin Pathol* 40: 393–397.

24 Sakai, H., Murakami, M., Mishima, H. et al. (2012). Cytologically atypical anal sac adenocarcinoma in a dog. *Vet Clin Pathol* 41: 291–294.

25 Jergens, A.E., Jones Hostetter, S., and Andreasen, C.B. (2016). Oral cavity, gastrointestinal tract, and associated structures. In: *Canine and Feline Cytology: A Color Atlas and Interpretation Guide*, (eds. Raskin, R.E., Meyer, D.J.), 3e, St. Louis, MO: Elsevier; 222, 226.

26 Schultze, A.E., Morgan, R.V., and Patton, C.S. (1996). What is your diagnosis? *Vet Clin Pathol* 25 (79): 91–92.

27 Wills, T.B., Bohn, A.A., Finch, N.P. et al. (2005). Thyroid follicular adenocarcinoma in a ferret. *Vet Clin Pathol* 34: 405–408.

28 Sirri, R., Diana, A., Scarpa, F. et al. (2015). Ultrasonographic and pathologic study of schwannoma in a Goldfish (*Carassius auratus*). *Vet Clin Pathol* 44: 586–591.

29 Gleiser, C.A., Jardine, J.H., Raulston, G.L., and Gray, K.N. (1979). Infiltrating lipomas in the dog. *Vet Pathol* 16: 623–624.

30 Thomas, M.J., Withrow, S.J., Dernell, W.S., and Powers, B.E. (1999). Intermuscular lipomas of the thigh region in dogs: 11 cases. *J Am Anim Hosp Assoc* 35: 165–167.

31 Kapatkin, A.S., Mullen, H.S., Matthiesen, D.T., and Patnaik, A.K. (1992). Leiomyosarcoma in dogs: 44 cases (1983–1988). *J Am Vet Med Assoc* 7: 1077–1079.

32 Dubielzig, R.R., Hawkins, K.L., and Miller, P. (1993). Myofibroblastic sarcoma originating at the site of rabies vaccination in a cat. *J Vet Diagn Invest* 5: 637–638.

33 Knight, C., Fan, E., Riis, R., and McDonough, S. (2009). Inflammatory myofibroblastic tumors in two dogs. *Vet Pathol* 46: 273–276.

34 Silva, J.F., Palhares, M.S., Maranhãno, R.P.A. et al. (2012). Myofibroblastic sarcoma in the limb of a horse. *J Equine Vet Sci* 32: 197–200.

35 Goldblum, J., Folpe, A., and Weiss, S. (2014). Borderline and malignant fibroblastic/myofibroblastic tumors. In: *Enzinger and Weiss's Soft Tissue Tumors*, (eds. Goldbum, J.R., Folpe, A.L., and Weiss, S.W.), 6e, 288–340. Philadelphia, PA: Saunders/Elsevier.

36 Robinson, W. and Robinson, N.A. (2016). Cardiovascular system. In: *Jubb, Kennedy, and Palmer's Pathology of Domestic Animals. Vol. 3*, (ed. Maxie, M.G.), 6e, 52–53. St. Louis, MO: Elsevier.

23

Bone and Periarticular Structures

Jessica Lawrence and Elspeth Milne

Introduction

Cytologic approaches have become increasingly utilized more routinely in the evaluation of musculoskeletal diseases. While histopathology is often required for definitive diagnosis, cytology can provide clinically valuable information. Healthy bone is difficult to aspirate, but inflammatory and neoplastic lesions of the bone and periarticular structures can often be successfully aspirated. It is important to correlate physical examination and radiographic findings with cytologic findings.

Sample Collection

Lesions with soft tissue components, lytic or proliferative bone changes, and/or mineralization can be aspirated using similar techniques to those employed for any soft tissue mass. Non-aspiration (stab or woodpecker) collection works well for most masses; however, needle aspiration may be useful for lesions that are initially unrewarding following non-aspiration attempts.[1–4] A large gauge needle (16–20 G) can allow more successful aspiration in lesions that exfoliate poorly. Thorough palpation is often sufficient to guide aspiration, while regional radiographs, ultrasound, or advanced imaging (fluoroscopy, computed tomography [CT]) can be helpful in directing aspiration in challenging regions[5–8] (Figure 23.1a). If aspirate attempts are unsuccessful, impression smears following biopsy are often highly cellular and may yield a diagnosis. Prior to making an impression smear, it is important to adequately blot any blood from the surface to improve cellular imprints. Cells also can be gently scraped from the surface using a spatula or blade. Operator comfort and experience with bone aspirates also play a role in the likelihood of obtaining an adequate sample for analysis; similarly, it may be beneficial to have samples analyzed by cytopathologists accustomed to evaluating osseous samples.

Normal Cytology

Normal bone is composed of osteocytes within lacunae with surrounding osteoblasts and osteoclasts in low numbers within the extracellular matrix (ECM). Osteoid, which appears cytologically and histologically as amorphous, pink material, is produced by osteoblasts, while the periosteal tissue consists of thick fibrous tissue. Cytologically, normal bone consists of samples with low or no cellularity. Cells are most often identified as either periosteal mesenchymal cells or osteoblasts, characterized as round cells with an eccentrically located nucleus and occasionally prominent nucleolus. Care should be taken to avoid bone marrow aspiration during aspiration of bone lesions, as samples can become contaminated if the medullary space is inadvertently penetrated.[9,10] Similar to bone, normal cartilage consists of elliptical chondrocytes within lacunae surrounded by ECM (chondroid) with peripherally located round chondroblasts responsible for the production of homogeneous, pink chondroid. The normal anatomy of periarticular structures is complex and consists of muscle, dense collagenous connective tissue (ligaments, tendons, fascia, and joint capsules), cartilage, osteochondral junction, and a subchondral bone plate.

Bone and Cartilage

Hyperplasia and Cystic Changes

Hyperplastic lesions affecting bone or cartilage are rare in dogs and cats and often require histopathologic evaluation for definitive diagnosis. Hyperplastic or cystic conditions include multiple cartilaginous exostosis (MCE), bone cyst, intraosseous epidermoid cyst, and fibrous dysplasia.

MCE occurs in growing dogs and can be diagnosed as an incidental finding. It occurs following new bone formation by endochondral ossification, but lesions typically

Veterinary Cytology, First Edition. Edited by Leslie C. Sharkey, M. Judith Radin, and Davis Seelig.

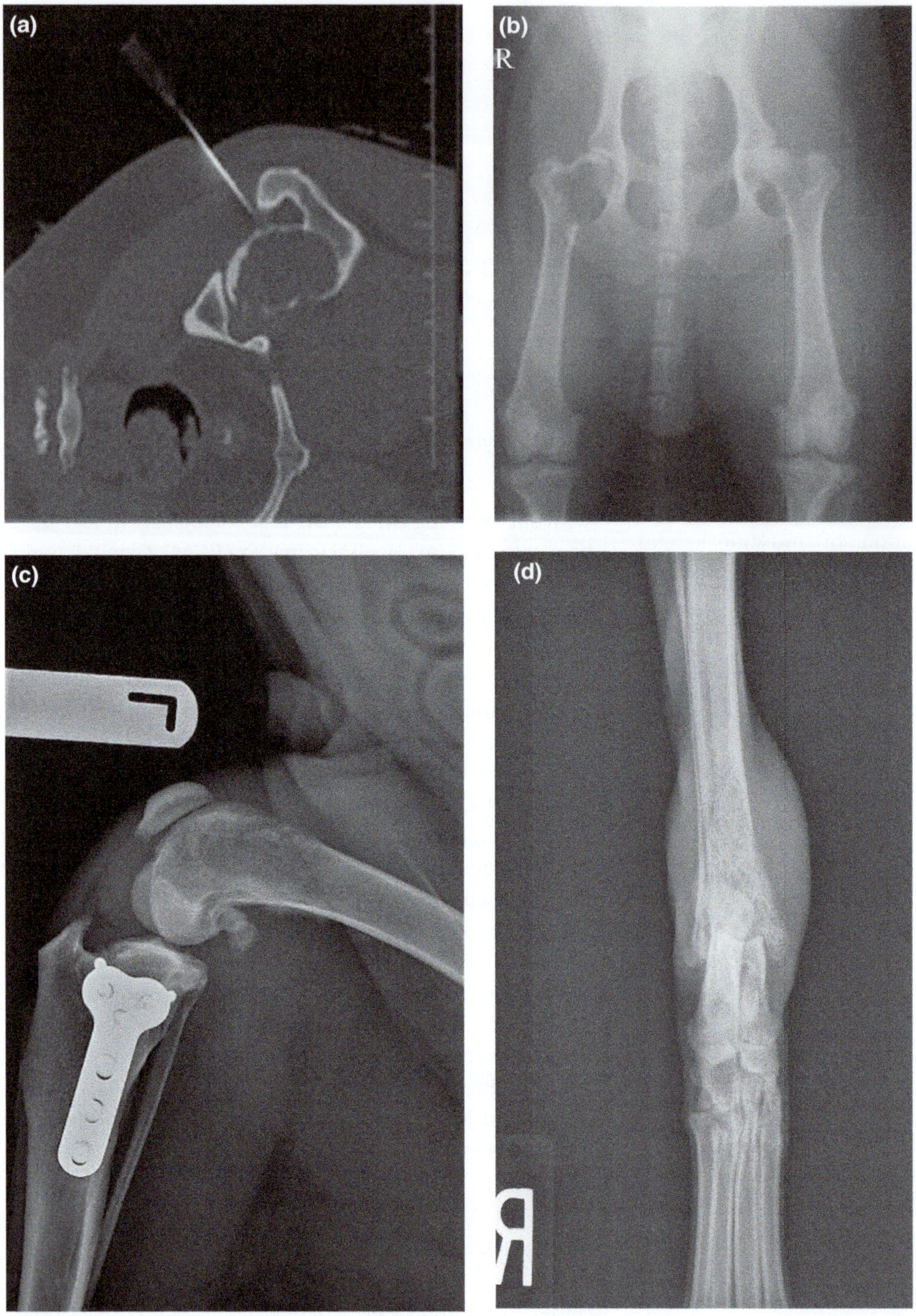

Figure 23.1 (a) Axial image of a CT scan from a 10-year-old Beagle with right pelvic pain, demonstrating a CT-guided fine-needle aspirate of a lytic lesion that was subsequently diagnosed as an osteosarcoma. (b) The corresponding dorsoventral radiograph from a 10-year-old Beagle with right pelvic pain. The radiograph demonstrates an expansile lytic mass affecting the right femoral head that was diagnosed as an osteosarcoma. (c) Dorsoplantar tarsal radiograph from a Boxer dog with coccidioidomycosis, demonstrating a mixed lytic and proliferative bone lesion of the distal tibia with associated soft tissue swelling (*Source:* Image courtesy of Tobias Schwarz). (d) Lateral radiograph of the left stifle from an 8-year-old Flat-Coated Retriever with histiocytic sarcoma, demonstrating a large area of moth-eaten bone lysis centered around the femoral epicondylar region. There is surrounding irregular periosteal reaction along the cranial margins of the trochlear ridge. Primary differentials initially included a primary bone tumor (osteosarcoma and chondrosarcoma) and osteomyelitis.

stabilize at skeletal maturity.[11] Aspirates are poorly cellular and reflective of normal bone; however, malignant transformation may occur.[12] Radiographs demonstrate a nonaggressive proliferative osseous mass on a bone surface. A presumptive diagnosis can be made when radiographs are correlated with the history and clinical examination, but definitive diagnosis requires biopsy. A hereditary form of multiple exostoses has been studied in horses and is similar to hereditary multiple exostoses in humans, predominantly affecting the long bones, ribs, and pelvis.[13,14]

Bone cysts are rare, benign, usually solitary lesions that include simple bone cysts (true cysts in which epithelium lines a fluid-filled sac), subchondral bone cysts, juxtacortical bone cysts, or aneurysmal bone cysts.[15] Horses with osteochondrosis may develop pseudocysts and cysts within the subchondral bone, which are important causes of lameness in this species.[16,17] Dogs with simple bone cysts often present with lameness at a young age, as lesions typically occur in the metaphysis of long bones.[15,18] Because the cortical bone remains intact over the cyst, aspiration can be low yield, thus few cysts have been cytologically analyzed. Successful aspiration will be consistent with a cyst. Aneurysmal bone cysts consist of blood, but reactive osteoblasts and osteoclasts can also be present with associated bone remodeling and lysis. Aneurysmal cysts can mimic primary bone tumors radiographically; therefore if features of malignancy are present on radiographs, aspirates can help guide further diagnostics.

Inflammation

Inflammatory lesions affecting bone are typically similar to those in other tissues. Neutrophils tend to be the predominant cell type with intermediate numbers of activated macrophages and multinucleated giant cells, but relative numbers depend on the underlying process. Because inflammatory lesions are associated with bone proliferation and remodeling, it is common for small numbers of reactive osteoblasts and osteoclasts to be present in cytologic samples. Reactive osteoblasts tend to be smaller and more uniform with fewer features of malignancy compared with neoplastic osteoblasts. However, osteomyelitis can rarely occur concurrently with osteosarcoma, and the possibility of underlying neoplasia in aspirates with evidence of inflammation should not be summarily dismissed, particularly if organisms are not identified.[19] Furthermore, the rate of correlation between cytologic and histologic diagnosis of non-neoplastic bone lesions in dogs is low.[20] Bacterial or fungal osteomyelitis can be presumptively diagnosed prior to culture results when organisms are identified.[21]

Bacterial Osteomyelitis

Bacterial osteomyelitis is usually of exogenous origin in dogs and cats, including bite wounds, postsurgical infections and foreign bodies; hematogenous infections are rare.[22] Common species are *Actinomyces* spp., *Nocardia* spp., *Staphylococcus* spp., *Escherichia coli*, and *Streptococcus* spp. and less commonly enteric bacteria, *Corynebacterium* spp. and anaerobes.[23] In cats, osteomyelitis can occasionally be caused by *Bartonella* spp. and *Mycobacterium* spp.[24,25] Single-species infections are more common than mixed. Inflammation in bacterial osteomyelitis is usually neutrophilic to pyogranulomatous, and the presence of intracellular bacteria confirms the diagnosis. Sterile osteomyelitis causing non-weight-bearing lameness as the presenting complaint has also been described secondary to pancreatic neoplasia in two dogs, with inflammation and necrosis of adipose tissue in the medullary cavity of long bones in conjunction with multifocal panniculitis.[26] In young horses and ruminants, hematogenous infections predominate as part of a systemic septic process.[27,28]

Fungal Osteomyelitis

Fungal causes of osteomyelitis include *Blastomyces dermatitidis*, *Coccidioides immitis*, *Cryptococcus neoformans*, *Histoplasma capsulatum*, and less often *Sporothrix* spp., *Aspergillus* spp., *Penicillium* spp., and *Geomyces* spp. (Figure 23.1c and Figure 23.2). The microscopic characteristics of fungi are described in Chapter 3. Osteomyelitis, especially in the appendicular skeleton, is the commonest form of disseminated *Coccidioides* infection in dogs.[29] Fungal infections generally cause pyogranulomatous but sometimes neutrophilic inflammation. Variable numbers of organisms

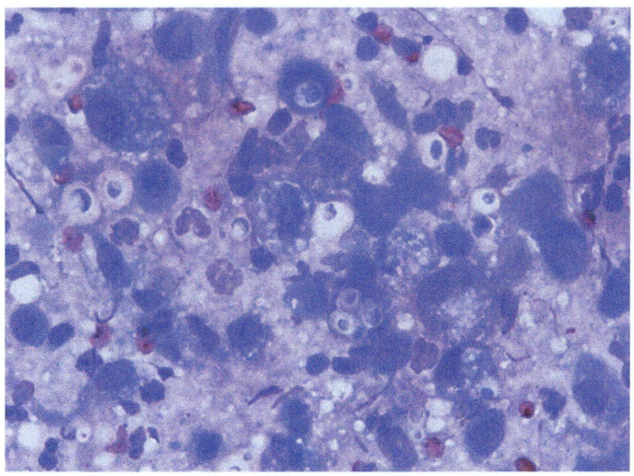

Figure 23.2 FNA of a lytic bone lesion on the distal humerus of a 4-year-old mixed breed dog. Numerous round *C. neoformans* yeasts are present, with degenerate neutrophils and vacuolated macrophages (May-Grünwald–Giemsa, 600×. *Source:* Image courtesy of Paola Cazzini).

may be present in fungal infections, and their absence does not exclude infection. However, cytology is considered sensitive for the diagnosis of cryptococcosis.[30] Fungal stains applicable to cytologic preparations include Grocott's methenamine silver and periodic acid–Schiff, and culture and polymerase chain reaction analysis can aid speciation.

Protozoal Osteomyelitis

Protozoal osteomyelitis is relatively uncommon. In *Leishmania infantum* infection, the appendicular skeleton is mainly affected. Lesions are often destructive with bone remodeling and pyogranulomatous to granulomatous inflammation with infiltration of macrophages, histiocytes, lymphocytes, plasma cells, and neutrophils.[31] Similar lesions with the presence of typical amastigotes intracellularly within macrophages also occur in *Leishmania donovani* infection.[32] *Hepatozoon americanum* frequently causes proliferative lesions of the periosteum of the proximal long bones, but inflammation is not a significant feature.[33] Conversely, *Hepatozoon canis* rarely involves the skeleton, but neutrophilic inflammation and intracellular meronts have been described in aspirates of proliferative bone lesions when they occur.[34]

Neoplasia

Osseous neoplasia is relatively common in small animals but rare in horses and farm animals, and cytology can be useful when distinguishing neoplastic from non-neoplastic conditions.[7,8,20,35–38] Immunocytochemical (ICC) and cytochemical stains may help further differentiate tumor type in some cases although definitive diagnosis rests on histopathologic evaluation.[15,39–41] Comparatively, despite concerns that nondiagnostic specimens are possible, studies in humans have suggested there is utility in performing fine-needle aspirate (FNA) initially or in conjunction with biopsy for tumors or tumor-like lesions affecting bone.[42–45]

Benign Bone and Cartilage Neoplasia

Osteomas and chondromas are rare in animals, usually appearing as well circumscribed, dense bone lesions that are rarely painful on palpation. Histologically, lesions are consistent with reactive bone or cartilage. Aspiration of benign lesions is often unrewarding due to low cellularity and difficulty distinguishing reactive osteoblasts or chondroblasts from neoplastic cells. Biopsy is typically needed for definitive diagnosis although cytology can guide further diagnostics.

Malignant Bone and Cartilage Neoplasia

Osteosarcoma

Osteosarcoma is the most common primary bone tumor in dogs and cats, although primary bone tumors in cats are rare overall. Up to 85% of primary bone tumors in dogs are osteosarcomas, with the remaining tumor types including chondrosarcoma, fibrosarcoma, hemangiosarcoma, multilobular osteochondrosarcoma, and solitary osseous plasma cell tumors.[15] Cytology of neoplastic bone lesions in dogs yields a presumptive diagnosis in greater than 80% of cases, although only small studies have been published.[6–8] Definitive diagnosis relies on histopathology. While canine osteosarcoma occurs more commonly in the proximal humerus and distal radius, any bone can be affected (Figure 23.1a and b). Aspirates from a suspected tumor should be collected from the center of the lesion and are often moderately to highly cellular (Figure 23.3a and b).[6,37] Malignant osteoblasts occur individually or in aggregates. Cells can vary from round/oval, to polygonal, to fusiform, and they can resemble reactive osteoblasts. Some tumors display abundant criteria of malignancy including anisocytosis, anisokaryosis, and multiple and/or large nucleoli.[4,39] The nucleus is often eccentrically located, while the cytoplasm of osteoblasts is typically basophilic and contains clear vacuoles and/or small pink granules. Erythrophagia by neoplastic cells has been reported.[46] Pink, proteinaceous, homogeneous material (osteoid) is variably present. Lytic bone lesions (or mixed lytic–proliferative lesions) often have abundant giant multinucleated cells that are typically consistent with osteoclasts; however, some malignant osteoblasts can appear as giant multinucleated cells (Figure 23.3b). The histologic subtype likely influences the cytologic appearance. Samples that lack inflammation and contain a uniform population of osteoblasts or a population with minimal pleomorphism should be interpreted cautiously and in light of the clinical picture.

Osteosarcoma can sometimes be difficult to distinguish from other tumors affecting bone, such as chondrosarcoma and fibrosarcoma, due to the similarity of clinical and radiographic features and the ability of malignant osteoblasts to appear as round, oval, or fusiform cells. There are a variety of histologic subtypes in canine osteosarcoma, each with diverse and heterogeneous features including osteoblastic, chondroblastic, fibroblastic, telangiectatic, and giant cell and poorly differentiated.[47] Cytochemical staining of neoplastic cells for alkaline phosphatase (ALP) activity with nitroblue tetrazolium chloride/5-bromo-4-chloro-3-indolyl phosphate toluidine salt (NBT/BCIP) may increase the sensitivity of differentiating osteosarcoma from other tumors.[39,41] Both stained and unstained slides can be submitted for ALP staining, increasing its utility as additional FNA attempts are not required.[41] However, it is important to note that reactive osteoblasts will stain positive for ALP, as can some other tumor types (see Chapter 7 for additional details); thus staining may be best on carefully selected samples. The exact role for ALP staining is not yet determined.[48]

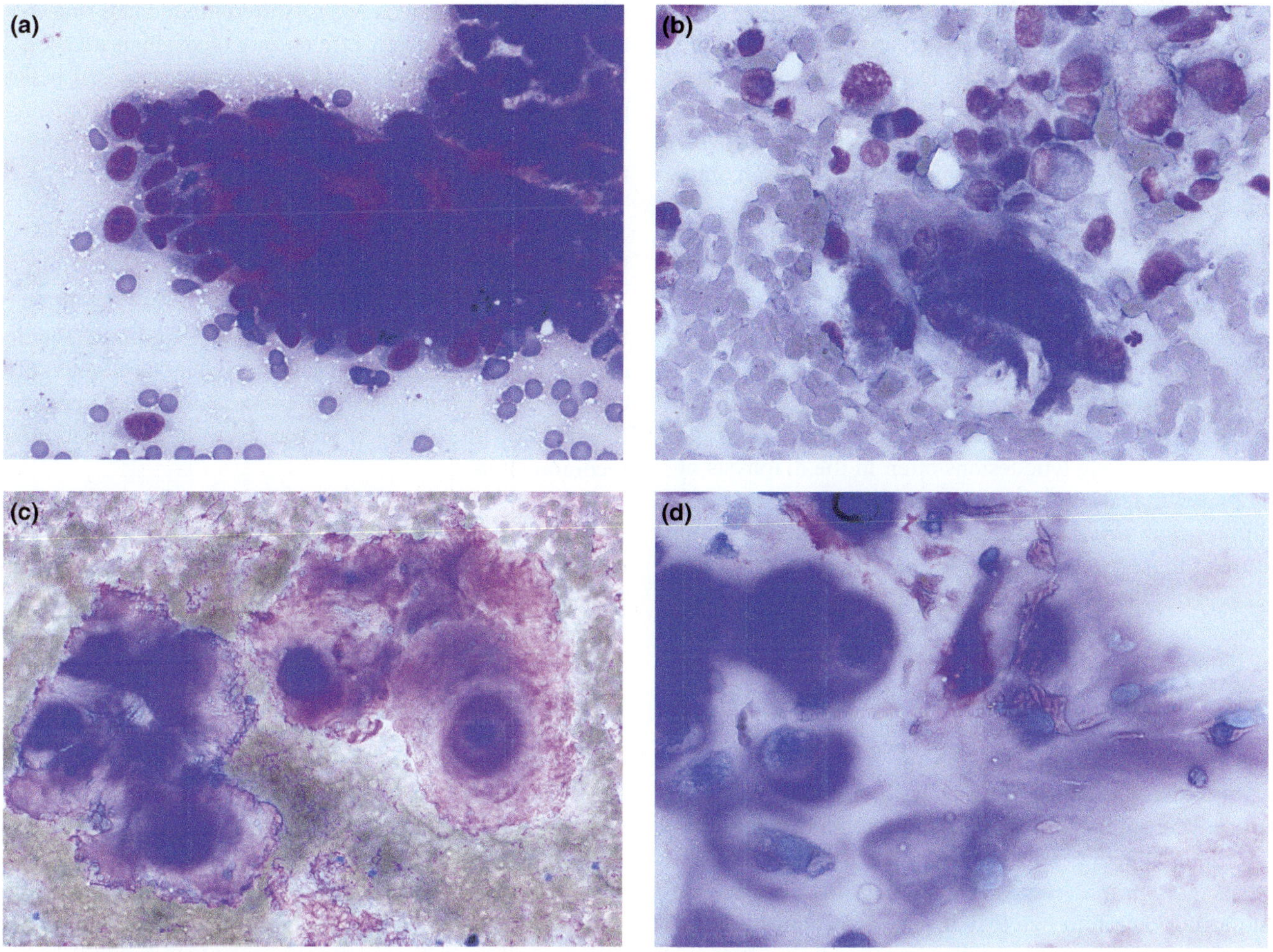

Figure 23.3 (a) FNA of a lytic bone lesion from the distal radius of a 6-year-old Irish wolfhound. A dense aggregate of atypical osteoblasts with multiple prominent nucleoli and associated pink osteoid is present. Histology confirmed an osteosarcoma. (b) FNA of a lytic bone lesion on the distal tibia of a 6-year-old greyhound. Atypical osteoblasts including a large multinucleated tumor cell are present consistent with the giant cell form of osteosarcoma. (c) FNA of a large mass in the lumbar vertebra of an 11-year-old Lhasa Apso dog with a chondrosarcoma. Large, round atypical chondroblasts are surrounded by pink chondroid. (d) FNA of the same vertebral chondrosarcoma as in (c). Large, round atypical chondroblasts are present. The smooth pink/blue extracellular material is chondroid (May-Grünwald–Giemsa, 400×).

Chondrosarcoma

Chondrosarcoma is the second most common tumor of bone, often affecting the nasal cavity, long bones, ribs, pelvis, and various extraskeletal tissues.[15] Cytologically, chondrosarcomas tend to have abundant eosinophilic amorphous matrix (interpreted as chondroid), occasionally leading to understaining of chondroblasts (Figure 23.3c and d). Differentiating true osteoid from chondroid matrix is difficult to impossible on cytology, and chondroblastic osteosarcoma can mimic features of chondrosarcoma, making it difficult to definitively confirm the cell of origin of the tumor without histology.[43] Likewise, while there are some radiographic features that may help narrow the list of differentials for a bone tumor (e.g. an intramedullary metaphyseal lesion is more likely osteosarcoma than chondrosarcoma), many radiographic signs overlap and can be mimicked by malignant and benign processes.[49] Chondroblasts vary from round, to ovoid, to fusiform with basophilic cytoplasm and large nuclei that are often eccentrically located. Similar to osteosarcoma, fine, pink cytoplasmic granules can be present in some cells. Features of malignancy can be prominent, although well-differentiated tumors appear more uniform. In humans, low-grade chondrosarcoma can be difficult to differentiate from chondroma, and a combination of clinical presentation, radiologic appearance, and cytologic interpretation is needed to guide further diagnostic approaches.[43,50]

Other Primary Bone Sarcomas

Fibrosarcomas and hemangiosarcomas occur with some regularity in bone, and cytologic features of these tumors types are similar to their appearance in more common sites of occurrence.[15] Both tend to consist of fusiform cells with varying degrees of pleomorphism. As with osteosarcoma, hemangiosarcoma can exhibit erythrophagia.[46] In lytic lesions, osteoclasts can be present and help confirm bone origin or involvement.

Other Bone Tumors

Some tumors arising in bone marrow, such as multiple myeloma and lymphoma, also can cause bone lysis. Radiographically, hematopoietic tumors affecting bone create round, purely lytic lesions often in the diaphysis of long bones, dorsal spinous processes of vertebrae, and ribs but may occur anywhere.[51] Because lysis is a predominant feature of these tumors, highly cellular samples consisting of sheets of plasma cells or malignant lymphocytes often are obtained. Cellular morphology of plasma cell tumors and lymphoma is described elsewhere (Chapters 14 and 27). It is unusual for cases with systemic hematopoietic neoplasia to present as primary bone tumors, although lameness may be a primary clinical complaint in some dogs and cats.[52,53] Although plasma cell tumors are usually multicentric, solitary osseous plasmacytoma is a rare primary tumor affecting bone in humans, dogs, and cats.[51,54,55] Lesions can mimic osteosarcoma clinically and radiographically; therefore cytology can be informative. Some malignant osteoblasts resemble plasma cells, so careful consideration of differential diagnoses is warranted, and additional ICC staining can be indicated.

Some tumors are more likely to invade bone by extension and therefore are not true primary bone tumors. Tumors affecting the soft tissue of the oral cavity, such as malignant melanoma, squamous cell carcinoma, or fibrosarcoma, often locally invade bone and present with lytic–proliferative lesions affecting the bones of the head. Definitive diagnosis usually requires biopsy due to the degree of oral inflammation; however, cytology can be suggestive of tumor type. Periarticular histiocytic sarcoma also locally invades bone, causing destructive lesions that can be mistaken for primary bone neoplasia (Figures 23.1d and 23.4a, b).[56]

Metastatic Tumors

Virtually any tumor can metastasize to bone hematogenously, although it is well recognized that urogenital tumors in dogs and cats, such as prostate carcinoma and mammary carcinoma, are more likely to metastasize to bone.[15,57,58] Epithelial tumors are typically easily identifiable and often resemble neoplastic cells from the site of origin; however, metastatic cells can also be less differentiated and thus difficult to differentiate from other tumor types (Figure 23.4c).[59] ICC stains can provide more information, and cell pellet blocks created from bone marrow FNAs appear promising for immunohistochemical methods to diagnose micrometastasis to bone.[60]

Periarticular Tissue

Cytologic findings in inflammatory and neoplastic conditions affecting periarticular tissues are generally consistent with the underlying process or tumor type, and if a mass or thickening is present, cytologic evaluation is recommended.

Neoplasia

Tumors commonly identified near joints include histiocytic sarcomas, synovial myxoma, synovial sarcoma, and other sarcomas.[61] Cytologically, histiocytic sarcomas display marked pleomorphism including anisocytosis, anisokaryosis, multinucleation, coarse chromatin patterns, and bizarre mitotic figures. Cells not only are most often round to ovoid but also can be spindle shaped; cytological samples often show marked variations in tumor cell shape. The cytoplasm is basophilic and sometimes vacuolated, and nuclei are round to indented with one or more nucleoli and often a coarse chromatin. Inflammatory cells including lymphocytes (commonly T lymphocytes), neutrophils, and normal histiocytes are commonly identified concurrently.[62]

Synovial cell tumors are more frequent in dogs than cats and are more commonly spindle shaped or consist of a mixed population of spindle-shaped and epithelioid cells (Figure 23.4d).[63] The nature of the epithelioid cells is controversial; they may either be truly epithelial or represent aberrant expression of cytokeratin by neoplastic mesenchymal cells.[63] ICC can be helpful, particularly if biopsy for histopathological and immunohistochemical interpretation is not performed. Immunostaining is recommended to aid in the diagnosis of periarticular tumors as staining patterns can support a definitive diagnosis. Synovial cell sarcoma typically stains vimentin$^+$ with variable cytokeratin staining; histiocytic sarcomas are typically vimentin$^+$, CD18+, CD3−, and CD79a (or another B-lymphocyte antibody) negative, while pleomorphic or poorly differentiated sarcomas (anaplastic sarcoma with giant cells, previously malignant fibrous histiocytoma) are actin$^+$, desmin$^-$, and S100$^-$.[62,64–67] It can be difficult, even with ICC, to differentiate periarticular tumors, and full staging is vital to exclude disseminated histiocytic sarcoma or metastatic sarcoma.

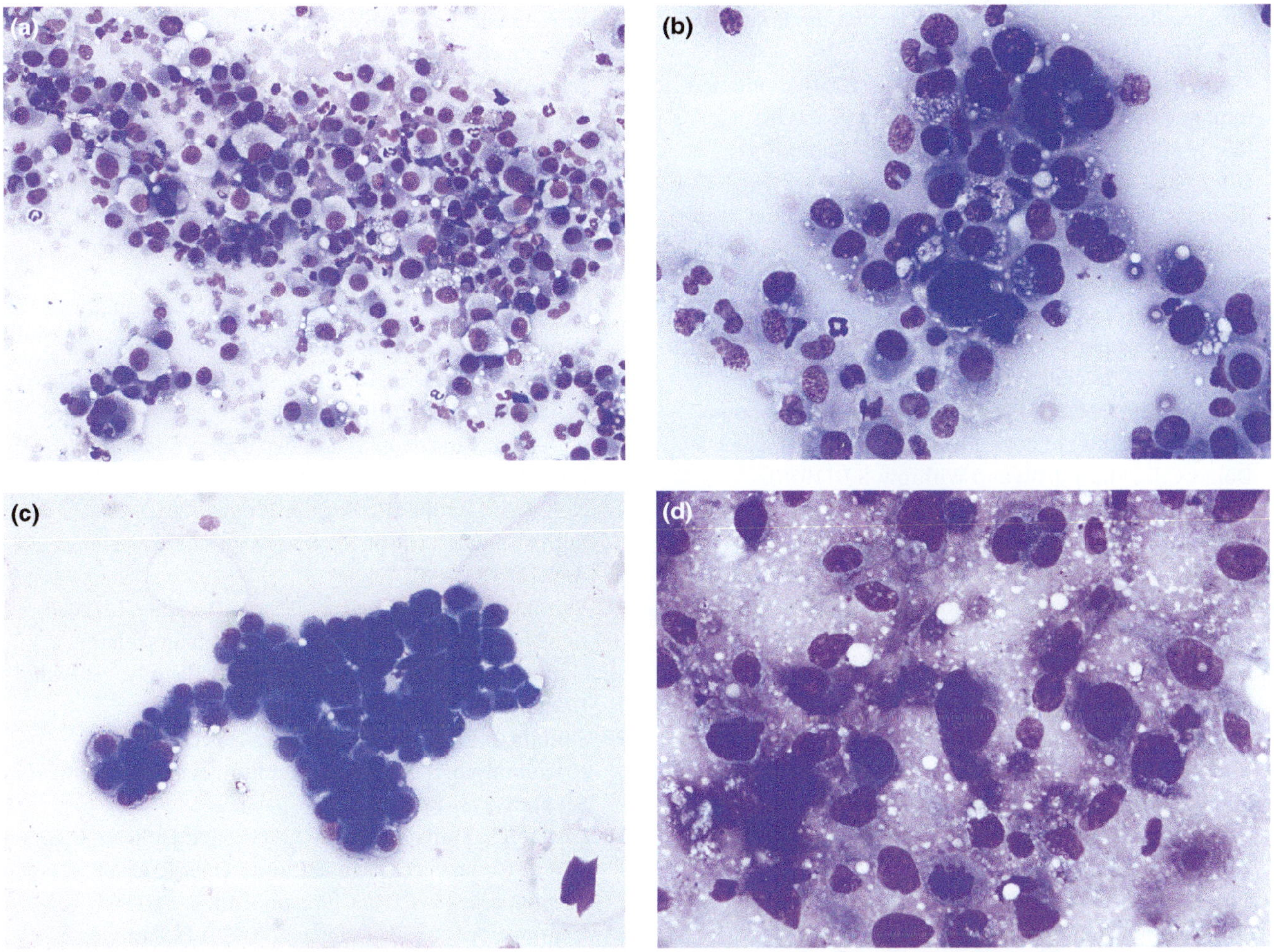

Figure 23.4 (a) FNA of a periarticular histiocytic sarcoma from the elbow of a 9-year-old Labrador retriever dog. There are numerous atypical, discreet, round to polyhedral histiocytes with abundant, pale blue, often vacuolated cytoplasm. Some histiocytes are multinucleated (May-Grünwald–Giemsa, 200×). (b) FNA of a periarticular histiocytic sarcoma from the same case as (a). Multinucleated tumor cells are present (May-Grünwald–Giemsa, 400×). (c) FNA from the vertebral body of L6 from an 8-year-old Scottish terrier with metastasis of a urethral transitional cell carcinoma to bone. There is a cluster of large, cohesive epithelial cells (May-Grünwald–Giemsa, 200×. *Source:* Image courtesy of Chiara Piccinelli). (d) FNA from a 2-year-old domestic short-haired cat with a lytic bone lesion involving the tarsocrural joint. There are round, stellate, and fusiform cells with prominent nucleoli, and one mitotic figure is shown. Histopathology and immunohistochemistry confirmed a synovial cell sarcoma (Wright–Giemsa, 400×. *Source:* Image courtesy of Paola Cazzini).

References

1 Meinkoth, J.H. and Cowell, R.L. (2002). Sample collection and preparation in cytology: increasing diagnostic yield. *Vet Clin North Am Small Anim Pract* 32: 1187–1207.

2 Menard, M. and Papageorges, M. (1997). Fine needle biopsies: how to increase diagnostic yield. *Compend Contin Educ Pract Vet* 19: 738–740.

3 Meyer, D.J. (2016). The acquisition and management of cytology specimens. In: *Canine and Feline Cytology*, (ed. Raskin R.E. and Meyer D.J.), 3e, 1–15. St. Louis, MO: Elsevier.

4 Fielder, S.E. (2014). The musculoskeletal system. In: *Diagnostic Cytology and Hematology of the Dog and Cat*, (eds. Cowell R.L., Tyler R.D., Meinkoth J.H., DeNicola D.B.), 4e, 216–221. St. Louis, MO: Elsevier.

5 Menard, M. and Papageorges, M. (1995). Technique for ultrasound-guided fine needle biopsies. *Vet Rad Ultrasound* 36: 137–138.

6 Sammi, V.F., Nyland, T.G., Werner, L.L., and Baker, T.W. (1999). Ultrasound-guided fine-needle aspiration biopsy of bone lesions: a preliminary report. *Vet Rad Ultrasound* 40: 82–86.

7 Britt, T., Clifford, C., Barger, A. et al. (2007). Diagnosing appendicular osteosarcoma with ultrasound-guided

fine-needle aspiration: 36 cases. *J Small Anim Pract* 48: 145–150.

8 Vignoli, M., Ohlerth, S., Rossi, F. et al. (2004). Computed tomography-guided fine-needle aspiration and tissue-core biopsy of bone lesions in small animals. *Vet Rad Ultrasound* 45: 125–130.

9 Bommer, K.K., Ramzy, I., and Mody, D. (1997). Fine-needle aspiration biopsy in the diagnosis and management of bone lesions: a study of 450 cases. *Cancer* 81: 148–156.

10 Akerman, M. and Domanski, H. (2011). Bone. In: *Fine Needle Aspiration Cytology*, (eds. Orell S.R., Sterret G.F.), 5e, 412–427. Philadelphia, PA: Elsevier.

11 Gee, B.R. and Doige, C.E. (1970). Multiple cartilaginous exostoses in a litter of dogs. *J Am Vet Med Assoc* 156: 53–59.

12 Doige, C.E., Pharr, J.W., and Withrow, S.J. (1978). Chondrosarcoma arising in multiple cartilaginous exostosis in a dog. *J Am Anim Hosp Assoc* 15: 605–611.

13 Shupe, J.L., Leone, N.C., Gardner, E.J., and Olson, A.E. (1981). Hereditary multiple exostoses. Hereditary multiple exostoses in horses. *Am J Pathol* 104: 285–288.

14 Li, J.K., Moloney, B.K., Shupe, J.L. et al. (1989). DNA polymorphism analysis of hereditary multiple exostoses in horses. *Am J Vet Res* 50: 978–983.

15 Ehrhart, N.P., Ryan, S.D., and Fan, T.M. (2013). Tumors of the skeletal system. In: *Small Animal Clinical Oncology*, (eds. Withrow S.J., Vail D.M., Page R.L.), 5e, 463–503. St. Louis, MO: Elsevier.

16 Olstad, K., Ostevik, L., Carlson, C.S., and Ekman, S. (2015). Osteochondrosis can lead to formation of pseudocysts and true cysts in the subchondral bone of horses. *Vet Pathol* 52: 862–872.

17 Trotter, G.W. and McIlwraith, C.W. (1981). Osteochondritis dissecans and subchondral cystic lesions and their relationship to osteochondrosis in the horse. *Equine Vet Sci* 1: 157–162.

18 Schrader, S.C., Burk, R.L., and Liu, S.K. (1983). Bone cysts in two dogs and a review of similar cystic bone lesions in the dog. *J Am Vet Med Assoc* 182: 490–495.

19 Boston, S., Singh, A., Murphy, K., and Nykamp, S. (2010). Osteosarcoma masked by osteomyelitis and cellulitis in a dog. *Vet Comp Orthop Traumatol* 23: 336–371.

20 Berzina, I., Sharkey, L.C., Matise, I., and Kramek, B. (2008). Correlation between cytologic and histopathologic diagnoses of bone lesions in dogs: a study of the diagnostic accuracy of bone cytology. *Vet Clin Pathol* 37: 332–338.

21 Bubenik, L.J. (2005). Infections of the skeletal system. *Vet Clin North Am Small Anim Pract* 35: 1093–1109.

22 Rabillard, M., Souchu, L., Niebauer, G.W., and Gauthier, O. (2011). Haematogenous osteomyelitis: clinical presentation and outcome in three dogs. *Vet Comp Orthop Traumatol* 24: 146–150.

23 Sequiera, E.G.M., Rahal, S.C., Ribeiro, M.G. et al. (2014). Exogenous bacterial osteomyelitis in 52 dogs: a retrospective study of etiology and *in vitro* antimicrobial susceptibility. *Vet Q* 34: 201–204.

24 Varanat, M., Travis, A., Lee, W. et al. (2009). Recurrent osteomyelitis in a cat due to infection with *Bartonella vinsonii* subsp. *berkhoffii* genotype II. *J Vet Intern Med* 23: 1273–1277.

25 Lo, A.J., Goldschmidt, M.H., Aronson, L.R. (2012). Osteomyelitis of the coxofemoral joint due to Mycobacterium species in a feline renal transplant patient. *J Fel Med Surg* 14: 919–923.

26 Gear, R.N.A., Bacon, N.J., Langley-Hobbs, S. et al. (2006). Panniculitis, polyarthritis and osteomyelitis associated with pancreatic neoplasia in two dogs. *J Small Anim Pract* 47: 400–404.

27 Neil, K.M., Axon, J.E., Begg, A.P. et al. (2010). Retrospective study of 108 foals with septic osteomyelitis. *Aust Vet J* 88: 4–12.

28 Verschooten, F., Vermeiren, D., and Devriese, L. (2000). Bone infection in the bovine appendicular skeleton: a clinical, radiographic, and experimental study. *Vet Radiol Ultrasound* 41: 250–260.

29 Shubitz, L.F. (2007). Comparative aspects of coccidiomycosis in animals and humans. *Ann N Y Acad Sci* 1111: 395–403.

30 Lester, S.J., Malik, R., Bartlett, K.H., and Duncan, C.G. (2011). Cryptococcosis: update and emergence of *Cryptococcus gattii*. *Vet Clin Pathol* 40: 4–17.

31 Koutinas, A.F. and Koutinas, C.K. (2014). Pathologic mechanisms underlying the clinical findings in canine leishmaniosis due to *Leishmania infantum/chagasi*. *Vet Pathol* 51: 527–538.

32 de Souza, A.I., Juliano, R.S., Gomes, T.S. et al. (2005). Osteolytic osteomyelitis associated with visceral leishmaniasis in a dog. *Vet Parasitol* 129: 51–54.

33 Panciera, R.J., Mathew, J.S., Ewing, S.A. et al. (2000). Skeletal lesions of canine hepatozoonosis caused by *Hepatozoon americanum*. *Vet Pathol* 37: 225–230.

34 Marchetti, V., Lubas, G., Baneth, G. et al. (2009). Hepatozoonosis in a dog with skeletal involvement and meningoencephalomyelitis. *Vet Clin Pathol* 38: 121–125.

35 Cohen, M., Bohling, M., Wright, J.C. et al. (2003). Evaluation of sensitivity and specificity of cytologic examination: 269 cases (1999–2000). *J Am Vet Med Assoc* 222: 964–967.

36 Loukopoulos, P., Rozmanec, M., and Sutton, R.H. (2005). Cytological versus histopathological diagnosis in canine osteosarcoma. *Vet Rec* 157: 784.

37 Reinhardt, S., Stockhaus, C., Teske, E. et al. (2005). Assessment of cytological criteria for diagnosing osteosarcoma in dogs. *J Small Anim Pract* 46: 65–70.

38 Bush, J.M., Fredrickson, R.L., and Ehrhart, E.J. (2007). Equine osteosarcoma: a series of 8 cases. *Vet Pathol* 44: 247–249.

39 Barger, A., Graca, R., Bailey, K. et al. (2005). Use of alkaline phosphatase staining to differentiate canine osteosarcoma from other vimentin-positive tumors. *Vet Pathol* 42: 161–165.
40 Neihaus, S.A., Locke, J.E., Barger, A.M. et al. (2011). A novel method of core aspirate cytology compared to fine-needle aspiration for diagnosing canine osteosarcoma. *J Am Anim Hosp Assoc* 47: 317–323.
41 Ryseff, J.K. and Bohn, A.A. (2012). Detection of alkaline phosphatase in canine cells previously stained with Wright–Giemsa and its utility in differentiating osteosarcoma from other mesenchymal tumors. *Vet Clin Pathol* 41: 391–395.
42 Jorda, M., Rey, L., Hanly, A., and Ganjei-Azar, P. (2000). Fine-needle aspiration cytology of bone: accuracy and pitfalls of cytodiagnosis. *Cancer* 90: 47–54.
43 Layfield, L.J. (2009). Cytologic diagnosis of osseous lesions: a review with emphasis on the diagnosis of primary neoplasms of bone. *Diagn Cytopathol* 37: 299–310.
44 Layfield, L.J., Dodd, L.G., Hirschowitz, S., and Crabtree, S.N. (2010). Fine-needle aspiration of primary osseous lesions: a cost effectiveness study. *Diagn Cytopathol* 38: 239–243.
45 Koscick, R.L., Petersigle, C.A., Makley, J.T., and Abdul-Karim, F.W. (1998). CT-guided fine needle aspiration and needle core biopsy of skeletal lesions. Complementary diagnostic techniques. *Acta Cytol* 42: 697–702.
46 Barger, A.M., Skowronski, M.C., and MacNeill, A.L. (2012). Cytologic identification of erythrophagocytic neoplasms in the dog. *Vet Clin Pathol* 41: 587–589.
47 Nagamine, E., Hirayama, K., Matsuda, K. et al. (2015). Diversity of histologic patterns and expression of cytoskeletal proteins in canine skeletal osteosarcoma. *Vet Pathol* 52: 977–984.
48 Stokol, T., Schaefer, D.M., Shuman, M. et al. (2015). Alkaline phosphatase is a useful cytochemical marker for the diagnosis of acute myelomonocytic and monocytic leukemia in the dog. *Vet Clin Pathol* 44: 79–93.
49 Yarmish, G., Klein, M.J., Landa, J. et al. (2010). Imaging characteristics of primary osteosarcoma: nonconventional subtypes. *Radiographics* 30: 1653–1672.
50 Layfield, L.J., Armstrong, K., Zaleski, S., and Eckardt, J. (1993). Diagnostic accuracy and clinical utility of fine-needle aspiration cytology in the diagnosis of clinically primary bone lesions. *Diagn Cytopathol* 9: 168–173.
51 Vail, D.M., Pinkerton, M.E., and Young, K.M. (2013). Hematopoietic tumors. In: *Small Animal Clinical Oncology*, (eds. Withrow S.J., Vail D.M., Page R.L.), 5e, 608–678. St. Louis, MO: Elsevier.
52 Matus, R.E., Leifer, C.E., MacEwan, E.G., and Hurvitz, A.I. (1986). Prognostic factors for multiple myeloma in the dog. *J Am Vet Med Assoc* 188: 1288–1291.
53 Patel, R.T., Caceres, A., French, A.F., and PM, M.M. (2005). Multiple myeloma in 16 cats: a retrospective study. *Vet Clin Pathol* 34: 341–352.
54 Dimopoulos, M.A. and Hamilos, G. (2002). Solitary bone plasmacytoma and extramedullary plasmacytoma. *Curr Treat Options in Oncol* 3: 255–259.
55 Dagan, R., Morris, C.G., Kirwan, J., and Mendenhall, W.M. (2009). Solitary plasmacytoma. *Am J Clin Oncol* 32: 612–617.
56 Schultz, R.M., Puchalski, S.M., Kent, M., and Moore, P.F. (2007). Skeletal lesions of histiocytic sarcoma in nineteen dogs. *Vet Radiol Ultrasound* 48: 539–543.
57 Cooley, D.M. and Waters, D.J. (1998). Skeletal metastasis as the initial clinical manifestation of metastatic carcinoma in 19 dogs. *J Vet Intern Med* 12: 288–293.
58 Cornell, K.K., Bostwick, D.G., Cooley, D.M. et al. (2000). Clinical and pathologic aspects of spontaneous canine prostate carcinoma: a retrospective analysis of 76 cases. *Prostate* 45: 173.
59 Barger, A.M. (2016). Musculoskeletal system. In: *Atlas of Canine and Feline Cytology*, (ed. Raskin R.E., Meyer D.J.), 3e, 353–368. St. Louis, MO: Elsevier.
60 Taylor, B.E., Leibman, N.F., Luong, R. et al. (2013). Detection of carcinoma micrometastasis in bone marrow of dogs and cats using conventional and cell block cytology. *Vet Clin Pathol* 42: 85–91.
61 Craig, L.E., Julian, M.E., and Ferracone, J.D. (2002). The diagnosis and prognosis of synovial tumors in dogs: 35 cases. *Vet Pathol* 39: 66–73.
62 Moore, P.F. (2014). A review of histiocytic diseases in dogs and cats. *Vet Pathol* 51: 167–184.
63 Cazzini, P., Frontera-Acevedo, K., Garner, B. et al. (2015). Morphologic, molecular, and ultrastructural characterization of a feline synovial cell sarcoma and derived cell line. *J Vet Diagn Invest* 27: 369–376.
64 Affolter, V.K. and Moore, P.F. (2002). Localized and disseminated histiocytic sarcoma of dendritic cell origin in dogs. *Vet Pathol* 39: 74–83.
65 Morris, J.S., McInnes, E.F., Bostock, D.E. et al. (2002). Immunohistochemical and histopathologic features of 14 malignant fibrous histiocytomas from Flat-Coated Retrievers. *Vet Pathol* 39: 473–479.
66 Fox, D.B., Cook, J.L., Kreeger, J.M. et al. (2002). Canine synovial cell sarcoma: a retrospective assessment of described prognostic criteria in 16 cases (1994–1999). *J Am Anim Hosp Assoc* 38: 347–355.
67 Dei Tos, A.P. (2006). Classification of pleomorphic sarcomas: where are we now? *Histopathology* 48: 51–62.

Part VI

Respiratory System

24

Upper Respiratory Tract of the Dog and Cat

Janet Beeler-Marfisi, Alice Defarges Bichot, and Dorothee Bienzle

Introduction

The nose and associated mucosae are primarily responsible for olfaction, humidification and warming of inhaled air, filtration of particulates, processing of antigens, and biotransformation of xenobiotics. These functions protect the more distal lower airways, leaving the URT relatively more exposed to potential injury. In this chapter, structure and function of the URT in health is briefly reviewed, approaches to cytologic diagnosis of disease are outlined, and specific conditions are summarized.

Upper Airway Anatomy

The upper airways extend from the external nares to the nasopharyngeal ostium immediately cranial to the larynx and include the nasal cavity, paranasal sinuses, auditory tubes, and nasopharynx.[1] There are several types of URT epithelium: stratified squamous epithelium in the nasal vestibule, non-ciliated cuboidal to columnar epithelium in a narrow transitional zone between the vestibule and the nasal cavity, and pseudostratified ciliated epithelium in the majority of the main nasal cavity.[2] Mucus-producing goblet cells are interspersed among epithelial cells. Olfactory neuroepithelium lines the ethmoid conchae of the caudal and caudodorsal nasal cavity and includes highly specialized olfactory sensory neurons.[2] The sinuses are lined by ciliated epithelium.[3] Dogs and cats have individual lymphocytes and antigen-presenting cells within the epithelial cell layer and in the lamina propria of the nasal cavity, but in health they lack organized nasal-associated lymphoid tissue (NALT).[4,5] However, NALT can be induced by inhaled antigenic challenge in dogs[6] and by fungal infection in cats.[7] When present, NALT is composed of aggregates of lymphocytes covered by ciliated cuboidal epithelium, goblet cells, and non-ciliated cuboidal cells with luminal microvilli (M cells) that mediate uptake, processing, and presentation of luminal antigen to underlying lymphocytes.[2]

The dog has a small lingual tonsil at the base of the tongue, paired palatine tonsils at the lateral aspect of the oropharynx, and pharyngeal tonsils in the nasopharynx.[8] Tonsils are composed of either diffuse lymphoid aggregates or lymphocytes organized into primary and secondary follicles and covered by keratinized stratified squamous epithelium (lingual tonsil), non-keratinized stratified squamous epithelium (palatine tonsils) or pseudostratified columnar epithelium (pharyngeal tonsil). The epithelium overlying most tonsils includes numerous lymphocytes, and such epithelium is also termed "lymphoepithelium."[2] The cat not only has tonsils in the same locations as the dog but also has paraepiglottic tonsils that either consist of a few loose aggregates of lymphocytes only apparent microscopically or are fully developed macroscopically visible tonsils.[8] All oropharyngeal and nasopharyngeal tonsils are components of the mucosa-associated lymphoid tissue (MALT).[8]

Nasal Microorganisms

The bacterial microbiome of the nasal cavity and URT of dogs and cats in health and disease as determined by quantitative amplification of a segment of bacterial ribosomal RNA (rRNA) was recently described.[9–12] Assessment of bacterial sequences in specific body locations with RNA sequencing is a very different approach than former culture-based identification and has yielded different insights on the microbiome in animals (and humans), some of which are relevant to interpretation of cytologic samples. For instance, bacterial sequences are present in sites such as the lower respiratory tract that were previously considered devoid of bacteria in health. However, detection of bacterial sequences is not synonymous with the presence

Veterinary Cytology, First Edition. Edited by Leslie C. Sharkey, M. Judith Radin, and Davis Seelig.

of replication-competent organisms that produce toxins and other pathogenic factors. The frequency and diversity of bacterial sequences is greater at sites proximal rather than distal to external surfaces. For example, oropharyngeal swabs yielded a greater number of distinct sequences than bronchoalveolar lavage. Variation in the microbiome associated with factors such as host genetics, age, diet, sex, and environment has not been established, and repeatability of molecular microbial analysis is incompletely defined.

Therefore, attributing pathogenic roles to bacteria observed in cytologic preparations from the URT should continue to consider the presence of concurrent inflammation and/or tissue necrosis, bacteria within phagocytes, variation in bacterial morphology, and interference with the physical or functional epithelial barrier.

The predominant organisms isolated by bacterial culture from the nose of healthy dogs were *Streptococcus* spp.,[13] *Staphylococcus* spp.,[13,14] *Pasteurella multocida, Bordetella bronchiseptica, Pseudomonas* spp., and coliform species.[14] Less common organisms were *Neisseria canis*,[13] *Capnocytophagia* spp.,[15] *Alternaria* spp., and *Cladosporium* spp.[16] Molecular studies largely agree with culture-based findings and suggest that bacterial sequences representing the families of *Moraxellaceae, Porphyromonas, Bacteroides,* and *Pseudomonadaceae* are also prevalent in oropharyngeal and nasal samples.[10] However, culture-based identification of bacteria also evolved from a limited range of stains and biochemical tests to analysis of colonies by mass spectrometric and molecular methods.[17] Furthermore, culture conditions, especially of more fastidious organisms such as *Mycoplasma* spp., are not standardized. Hence, in animals with respiratory tract disease, clinical, cytologic, and microbial results must be integrated to gauge the potential role of an organism in causing disease.

Descriptions of URT bacterial culture results are sparse for healthy cats. In 214 nasal swabs from clinically healthy cats where bacteria lacking a cell wall (*Mollicutes*) were specifically targeted, predominantly *Mycoplasma gatae* and less frequent *Mycoplasma felis* and *Acholeplasma laidlawii* were recovered.[18] In that study, *Mycoplasma* spp. were much more highly concentrated in the throat but were absent in the lower airway and other organs.[18] Oropharyngeal examination of 71 shelter cats considered free of URT infection frequently isolated *B. bronchiseptica* and *Mycoplasma* spp.; however *Chlamydia felis* was rare.[19] Bacterial rRNA sequence analysis of feline nasal samples yielded 375 unique operational taxonomic units with high similarity to bacteria previously identified in diseased cats,[10] but that conflicted with culture results of healthy cats.[18,19] In healthy cats and those with feline upper respiratory tract disease (FURTD), *Moraxella* spp. had the highest relative abundance, followed by *Bradyrhizobiaceae* and *Neisseriaceae* (both identified to the level of family only), *Alloiococcus, Sediminibacterium, Staphylococcus,* and *Pseudomonas* species.[10] Cats with neoplasia had a predominance of *Bradyrhizobiaceae, Moraxella, Prevotella, Phyllobacterium, Bibersteinia* (family *Pasteurellaceae*), and *Pasteurella* species, and these were of similar abundance in cats with FURTD. Mycoplasmal DNA was only found in cats with neoplasia and FURTD, and chlamydial DNA was only retrieved from cats with FURTD.[10] Cats with FURTD also had the highest abundance of *Moraxella* spp. of any group, and the next most common sequences belonged to *Bradyrhizobiaceae, Staphylococcus, Pasteurella,* and *Sediminibacterium* spp.

While genomic analysis suggests a very wide range of bacterial organisms in the nose of healthy and diseased dogs and cats, there was marked individual variation, and most organisms identified frequently by culture were also present at high frequency in genomic analysis.[9,10] Association of specific bacterial species with particular diseases remains limited, since organisms were generally identified in swabs collected from the surface of the nasal epithelium, and may not be capable of causing disruption of the physical or functional epithelial barrier without cofactors.

Clinical Findings in Upper Respiratory Tract Disease

There is considerable overlap in the presenting signs and advanced imaging results of different types of URT in dogs and cats (Tables 24.1 and 24.2). Therefore, diagnosis of the specific underlying process is often challenging and more likely successful if results from physical examination, anterograde rhinoscopy, retroflex nasopharyngoscopy,[22,35] advanced imaging, cytology, and histopathologic samples are assessed in combination.[22,35–37] Bacterial and in particular fungal culture can be useful.[22] When fungal rhinitis is suspected, brush or squash preparations of endoscopic biopsies are more likely to be diagnostic than nasal secretions or swabs obtained without lesion visualization.[38] Nasal flush fluid has been suggested to be more rewarding than biopsy specimens for bacterial culture in cats.[39]

Marked inflammation associated with rhinitis can cause endoscopic changes suggestive of neoplasia.[35,40] Radio graphically, soft tissue opacity and bony lysis are features of some types of neoplasia and rhinitis in dogs (Table 24.1),[22,41] but in cats, radiographic changes tend to be more severe with neoplasia than rhinitis (Table 24.2).[29,42] In cases of fungal rhinitis, fungal plaques or proliferative

Table 24.1 Frequency of clinical and imaging changes in dogs with upper respiratory tract disease.

	Percent abnormal; number assessed		
	Neoplasia	**Chronic rhinitis**	**Fungal rhinitis**
Nasal discharge	54; 54[20]	100; 33[21]	100; 8[22]
Epistaxis or hemorrhagic	78; 228[3,20,22]	3; 33[21]	38; 8[22]
Mucopurulent or purulent	26; 35[22]	12; 33[21]	87; 23[22,23]
Facial deformity	35; 193[3,20]	±[a]	NS[b]
Rhinoscopic mass	94; 35[22]	±	NS
Rhinoscopic fungal plaque	NS	NS	84; 69[22–24]
Advanced imaging			
Unilateral disease	32; 113[3,25]	9; 33[21]	74; 69[22–24]
Bilateral disease	42; 113[3,25]	18; 33[21]	28; 69[22–24]
Bone lysis	52; 247[3,20,22,25,26]	18; 33[21]	99; 69[22–24]
Septal changes	61; 104[20,26]	NS	NS
Soft tissue opacity	88; 85[22,26]	100; 33[21]	94; 69[22–24]
Median duration of clinical signs (days)	82199[3,20,27]	NS	141; 46[24]

[a] Possible occurrence.
[b] Not specified.

Table 24.2 Frequency of clinical and imaging changes in cats with upper respiratory tract disease.

	Percent abnormal; number assessed		
	Neoplasia	**Chronic rhinitis**	**Fungal rhinitis**
Sneezing	36; 177[28–30]	52; 27[29]	67; 6[31]
Respiratory noise	45; 177[28–30]	44; 27[29]	Common[a]
Nasal discharge	60; 315[28–30,32,33]	90; 31[29,32]	78; 9[31,32]
Unilateral	51; 95[29,30,32]	32; 31[29,32]	Common
Bilateral	44; 95[29,30,32]	61; 31[29,32]	Common
Epistaxis or hemorrhagic	24; 315[28–30,32,33]	29; 31[29,32]	30; 6[31]
Mucopurulent or purulent	52; 92[28–30,32]	48; 31[29,32]	Common
Facial deformity	22; 300[28–30,33]	4; 27[29]	±[b]
Rhinoscopic mass	58; 80[29,30,34]	0; 27[29]	NS[c]
Bone lysis on advanced imaging	58; 117[28–30]	59; 27[29]	NS
Median duration of clinical signs (days)	60; 144[28–30]	210; 27[29]	NS

[a] Not further specified.
[b] Possible occurrence.
[c] Not specified.

lesions can be observed on rhinoscopy, offering obvious targets for sampling (Figure 24.1).[43] Rhinosporidiosis can present with a polypoid[44] or protruding lesion,[45] and sporangia can be visible as small white nodules beneath the surface of the lesion.[46]

Age

Neoplasms can occur in the URT of juvenile to geriatric dogs[47] and cats;[28,29] however, the average age of affected dogs and cats was 9.8[3,22,25,35,37,41,47,48] and 9.5 years,[28–30,32,33,49]

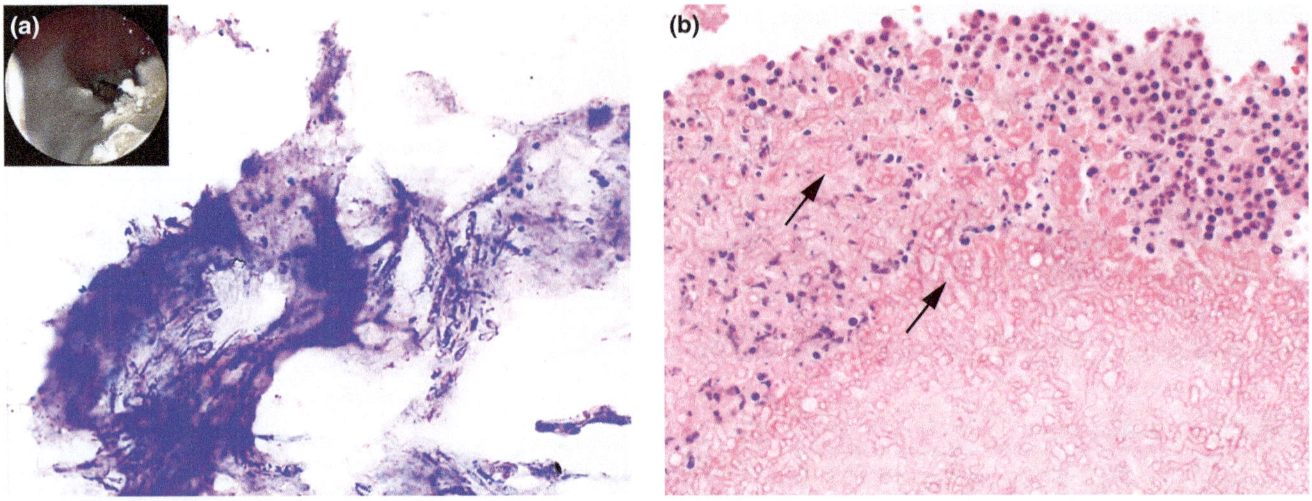

Figure 24.1 (a) Squash preparation of nasopharyngeal material retrieved endoscopically from a dog with chronic sneezing. Embedded in cell debris and mucus are numerous fungal hyphae with parallel walls and basophilic granular internal structure (Wright stain, 630×). Inset: Endoscopic view of fungal plaque. (b) Endoscopic biopsy of nasopharyngeal lesion. There is cell debris with leukocytes and innumerable, parallel sided, septate, approximately 5 μm diameter, non-pigmented, branching fungal hyphae (arrows). The surface epithelial barrier is absent (hematoxylin & eosin stain, 200×).

respectively. The age of animals with nasal cancer overlaps extensively with that of animals with chronic rhinitis.

Sampling

Cytologic evaluation can be rewarding for specific nasal lesions. Transmissible venereal tumor affecting the nose in dogs[20,50,51] (Figure 24.2) and nasal lymphoma in cats are readily diagnosed (Figure 24.3).[30,49] However, samples of nasal discharge sometimes reflect superficial septic suppurative inflammation but fail to capture the underlying lesion. Imprint[20] and squash preparations of biopsies[34] are often suitable to identify etiologic agents and neoplasms, but samples are challenging to obtain and need to be allocated carefully to cytology and histology. Swabs, aspirates, flush, and brush cytologic samples[50] can all yield diagnostic

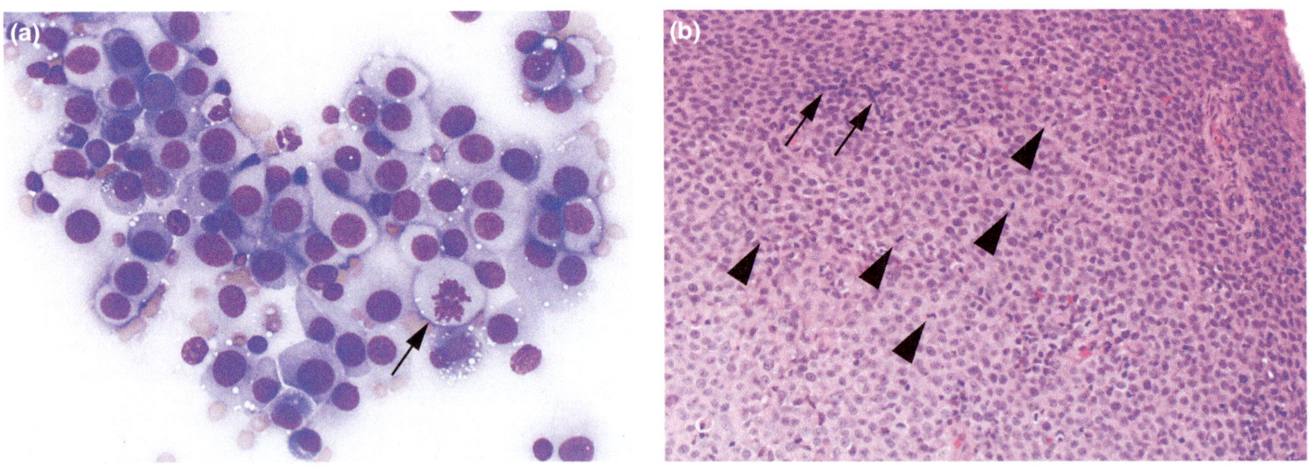

Figure 24.2 (a) Impression smear of a nasal transmissible venereal tumor. Cells are round and of medium size with distinct cytoplasmic borders and pale gray to blue cytoplasm. Occasional cells have punctate vacuoles. Nuclei are round to oval with finely granular chromatin and often have a distinct, medium-sized nucleolus. There is moderate anisocytosis, anisokaryosis, and mitotic activity (arrow) (Wright stain, 630×). (b) Histologically the tumor consists of sheets of medium to large round cells with abundant eosinophilic and frequently vacuolated cytoplasm. Nuclei are round to oval with a single prominent central nucleolus. There are twofold anisokaryosis, numerous mitotic cells (arrowheads), and scattered foci of small lymphocytes (arrows). Mucosal epithelium is attenuated (hematoxylin & eosin, 200×).

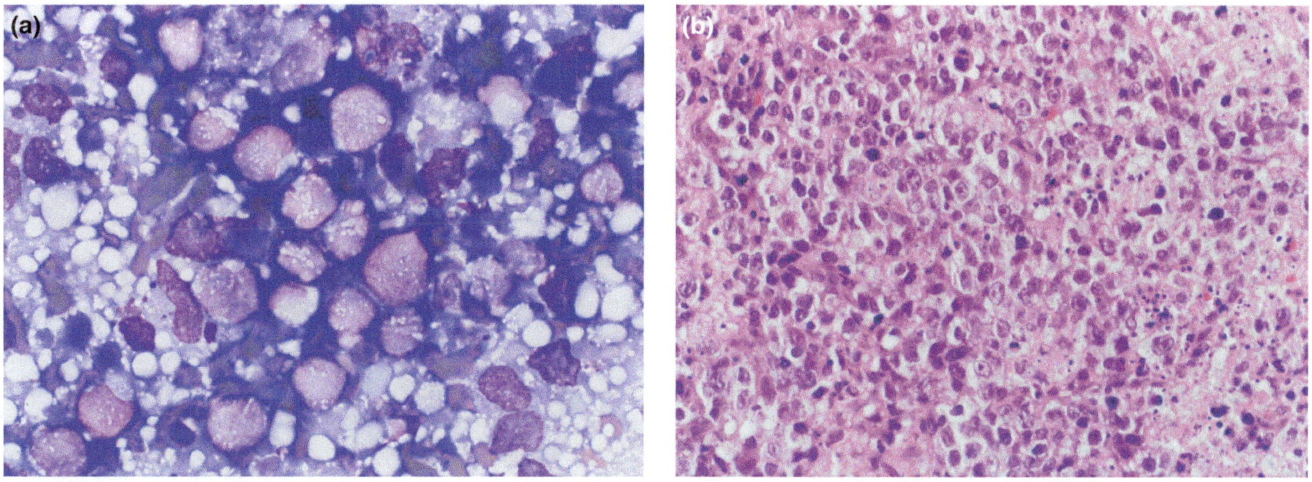

Figure 24.3 Nasal mass in a 12-year-old cat. The cat had mucopurulent nasal discharge for 1.5 years. Two biopsies obtained during that time showed only suppurative rhinitis. (a) An imprint of a third biopsy consists of extensive necrotic cell debris and a few intact large lymphocytes with cytoplasmic and nuclear vacuolar change (Wright stain, 630×). (b) Histologically, this is an immunoblastic B-cell lymphoma that was positive for CD79a. Extensive necrosis and apoptosis are also apparent (hematoxylin & eosin, 400×).

material but usually require repeated and aggressive sampling to maximize diagnostic yield. It is important to stress that even with histologic assessment, an etiologic diagnosis can remain elusive. Obtaining biopsies from multiple sites can increase diagnostic success.[32,37,41]

Conditions of the Upper Respiratory Tract

Epistaxis

Epistaxis is diagnosed grossly, but cytology samples can reflect hemorrhage when present. Unilateral epistaxis usually arises from focal neoplasia, severe rhinitis, or trauma to a single nasal cavity. Bilateral epistaxis is more often associated with hemorrhage arising caudal to the nasal cavity (e.g. nasopharynx or lungs) due to a bleeding diathesis, pulmonary contusion, neoplasm, granuloma, hypertension, and vasculitis or due to progressive, severe unilateral nasal cavity disease.

Parasites

Parasites found in the nasal cavity and sinuses include the nasal mite *Pneumonyssoides caninum* (synonym: *Pneumonyssus caninum*),[52–55] the capillarid nematode *Eucoleus boehmi*,[56–61] larvae of the sheep botfly *Oestrus* ovis,[62] larvae of the lagomorph and rodent botfly *Cuterebra* sp.,[63] the pentastome tongue worm *Linguatula serrata*,[64,65] and the gapeworm *Mammomonogamus* spp.[66–68]

P. caninum affects canids worldwide but is most often reported to affect dogs in Scandinavian countries.[53] The mite typically resides in the caudal nasal cavity and paranasal sinuses and is therefore not easily visualized. Clinical signs reflect irritation of the mucosa in these locations and consist of sneezing, reverse sneezing, and epistaxis.[53]

E. boehmi is a slender serpentine worm grossly visible beneath the mucosa of the nasal cavity and paranasal sinuses and causes eosinophilic and lymphoplasmacytic rhinitis with goblet cell hyperplasia in the conchae.[69,70] Both adults and eggs may be noted in the URT, the eggs having similar morphology (bipolar plugged eggs) to the canid lungworm *Eucoleus aerophilus*.[70]

There are a few reports of infection with larvae of the sheep botfly *O. ovis* causing clinical signs of URT disease in dogs[71] and one report in a cat.[72] Infection appears to be rare, associated with extensive exposure to sheep, and is curable.[71,72] Diagnosis is based on identifying in situ nasopharyngeal or expelled larvae.[71,72] On the other hand, myiasis due to infection with *Cuterebra* larvae is relatively common in many parts of the world, including North America, and can result in serious systemic illness.[63] *Cuterebra* larvae infect aberrant canine or feline hosts via the mucosa or injured skin and then migrate to a subcutaneous site where a warble hosting further larval development forms.[63] Aberrant migration with warble formation in trachea, nasal cavity, or surrounding subcutaneous tissues can result in respiratory signs including epistaxis, sneezing, gagging, and coughing (and involvement of the central nervous system).[63] Diagnosis is by observing the larvae.[63]

As the name implies, *L. serrata* are tongue-shaped, large (adults are ~6 cm in length) arthropod parasites noted in many parts of the world.[65,73,74] Canids are definitive hosts, and adult worms reside in the nasal cavity following migration from the gastrointestinal tract. Infected dogs have sinusitis and coughing, but clinical features of infection are not described in detail. Canine infection has not been reported in North America. While the nymphs of this parasite have been observed in the lungs of cats,[75] it does not appear to be found in the URT of this species. *L. serrata* has zoonotic potential, causing visceral linguatuliasis in humans.[75]

Mammomonogamus sp. are gapeworms of the *Syngamus* family reported from the Caribbean islands[66] and a North Pacific island.[68] Permanently conjoined large female and small male adult worms live in the nares, nasopharynx, or middle ear of cats. Infection is associated with sneezing, coughing,[66] and headshaking,[68] and eggs are observed in feces.[67,68] Most parasitic infections of the URT in dogs and cats are of undetermined pathogenicity. Diagnosis typically depends on observing the organisms grossly in the URT, or eggs or parasite components in cytologic or histologic samples.

Noninfectious Rhinitis

The diagnosis of noninfectious rhinitis in dogs and cats is based largely on excluding other causes of URT disease. Lymphoplasmacytic rhinitis is most common in dogs, and immune-mediated, allergic, and infectious etiologies are suspected.[21] One study found a partial Th1 immune response in dogs with lymphoplasmacytic rhinitis and a Th1 response in dogs with aspergillosis.[76] Mixed lymphoplasmacytic and neutrophilic inflammation appears most common in cats with acute or chronic rhinitis.[77]

Bacterial Rhinitis

Primary bacterial rhinitis is unusual in dogs and cats. *C. felis* infection in cats can cause URT signs similar to those of viral infections,[78] but conjunctivitis is the major clinical sign. There are a few reports of rhinosinusitis due to primary *Streptococcus equi* subspecies *zooepidemicus*[79–81] and single case reports of primary *Nocardia* sp.[82] and *Capnocytophagia* sp.[15] infections. In a population of rescue cats infected with a highly pathogenic beta-hemolytic *Streptococcus*, systemic disease and purulent rhinitis were noted.[83] Thus, while bacterial rhinosinusitis associated with neutrophilic inflammation and phagocytosed bacteria occurs, it appears infrequent and should not preclude vigorous efforts to rule out underlying disease.

Fungal Rhinitis

Fungal rhinitis is more common in dogs than cats.[84] Infection can occur associated with foreign body penetration, other concurrent nasal disease (including neoplasia), defective mucosal immunity, and inhalation of large numbers of fungal spores.[24,85] Dolichocephalic and mesocephalic canine breeds are predisposed to sinonasal aspergillosis,[23] whereas brachycephalic breeds are predisposed in cats.[85] While evidence of immunocompromise is rare in cats with URT fungal infection, immunosuppression might be permissive of systemic spread.[85]

Aspergillus fumigatus is the most frequently isolated agent of noninvasive fungal rhinitis in both dogs and cats.[23,85,86] While invasive sino-orbital fungal infections are generally caused by cryptic forms of *Aspergillus* spp. such as *Aspergillus felis* in cats,[31] sino-cutaneous *Fusarium* sp. infection has been reported.[87] Cryptic *Aspergillus* species are morphologically indistinguishable from *A. fumigatus* but are molecularly distinct. Differentiation of cryptic from non-cryptic *Aspergillus* spp. is important because higher dosages of antifungal drugs are required for the treatment of cryptic forms.[85]

Advanced imaging, rhinoscopy, cytology, histology, fungal culture, real-time polymerase chain reaction (PCR), panfungal or specific PCR on formalin-fixed paraffin-embedded tissues,[88] fungal serology, and serum agar immunodiffusion can contribute to the diagnosis of fungal infections. Fungal plaques are often observed by rhinoscopy in dogs[22–24] (Figure 24.1) and cats[85] with nasal aspergillosis. Sinuscopy is specifically recommended when computed tomographic images indicate sinus disease but when fungal plaques are not identified on rhinoscopy.[24,85] Positive findings on two, or preferably three, of these tests is sufficient for diagnosis of nasal aspergillosis.[23]

Cytologic samples of nasal aspergillosis generally yield a mixture of necrotic cell debris and fungal hyphae, with or without inflammatory cells (Figure 24.1). *Aspergillus* spp. are recognized by having 2–5 μm diameter, parallel-walled, dichotomously branching and septate hyphae.[85,89] Histologically, aspergillosis in dogs induces either a severe chronic lymphoplasmacytic[4] or pyogranulomatous inflammatory response in the lamina propria.[22] Inflammation causes turbinate destruction and lysis of other bony structures[90] noted radiographically and histologically. Histologic descriptions of feline noninvasive sinonasal aspergillosis are varied, including lymphoplasmacytic,[85] granulomatous,[91] and mixed cell[92] inflammation with histiocytic, eosinophilic, or neutrophilic infiltrates.[31,85] Invasive forms cause either granuloma formation[31] or pyogranulomatous inflammation with lymphoplasmacytic rhinitis in areas of uninfected nasal mucosa.[93] Regardless of invasiveness, histologic sampling must access several sites and obtain tissues deep to fungi. The frequency of identification of hyphae in cytologic versus histologic samples of nasal aspergillosis is undetermined.

Blastomycosis

Infection with *Blastomyces dermatitidis* is acquired by inhalation of spores but usually manifests as systemic rather than URT disease.[94,95] However, the nasal cavity is often affected in blastomycosis of the central nervous system.[96] Cytologically, *B. dermatitidis* yeast are recognized as basophilic round structures 8–25 µm in diameter, with a double-contoured wall, and broad-based budding. Histologic findings include pyogranulomatous rhinitis and nasopharyngitis[94] with intralesional round to slightly oval structures that have a refractile wall. The structures can be empty or contain basophilic nuclear material (Chapter 3). Blastomycosis is readily diagnosed cytologically, but availability of sensitive and specific immunoassays to detect antibodies and fungal antigens is increasing. Critical assessment of diagnostic methods in high and low prevalence settings would be helpful.[97]

Cryptococcosis

Cryptococcus gattii and Cryptococcus neoformans are primary pathogens of dogs, cats, and other species with a worldwide distribution.[43] While *Cryptococcus* spp. infection is generally considered sporadic, outbreaks involving *C. gattii* have been reported.[98] *C. gattii* is more virulent than *C. neoformans*, and cats appear two to four times more susceptible to infection than dogs.[43] This could reflect actual higher susceptibility but could be attributed to that fact that dogs most commonly present with systemic disease, including neurological involvement, resulting in euthanasia prior to definitive diagnosis.[43] In cats, infection is more often restricted to the URT. Concurrent infection with feline leukemia virus or feline immunodeficiency virus does not appear to increase risk of developing cryptococcosis, but might hamper the ability to clear infection.[43,99] While humans also develop cryptococcosis, infection is from environmental exposure and not zoonotic transmission.[100] Exposure and colonization without clinical signs are considered to be relatively common for *C. neoformans*. Pathogenicity might be related to inhalation of high numbers of basidiospores or strain-specific virulence factors.[43] Treatment does not prevent carriage or reinfection, and disease recrudescence, even a decade later, is possible.[43,101] Cryptococcal capsular antigen can be measured in serum, cerebrospinal fluid, and urine. Positive titers imply tissue invasion but not necessarily presence of viable organisms,[43] nor does the titer correlate with disease severity.[43]

Cytologic evaluation of lesion imprints, aspirates, or fluid is generally rewarding since organisms are frequently present and readily recognized as round to oval, homogeneous yeast with narrow-based budding and a thick nonstaining capsule (Figure 24.4).[43] Culture and a latex agglutination assay for cryptococcal antigen in serum can be useful diagnostic adjuncts when infection is suspected, but organisms are not observed.[102,103] The degree and type of inflammation associated with *Cryptococcus* spp. is highly variable and might relate to capsule thickness.[100] Host inflammatory response is variable, being absent or characterized by abundant neutrophils and macrophages, or a predominance of eosinophils.[104] The capsule of *Cryptococcus* spp. is

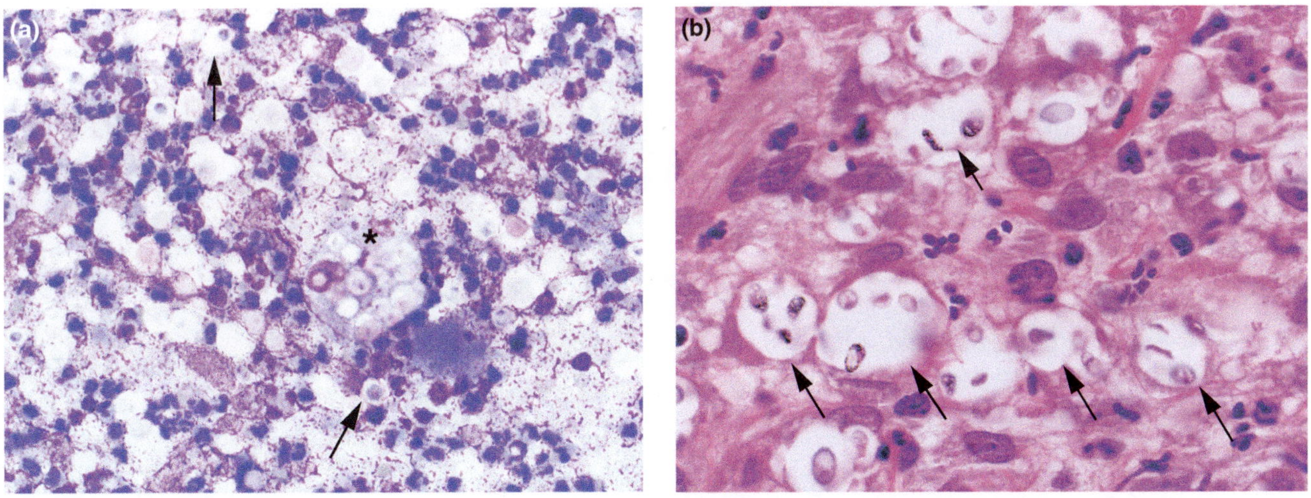

Figure 24.4 (a) Nasal exudate from a cat contains abundant cellular debris, lytic neutrophils, occasional macrophages, and *Cryptococcus* sp. organisms with variably thick capsules (arrows). One macrophage contains phagocytosed organisms (asterisk) (Wright stain, 630×). (b) Histologic section with numerous *Cryptococcus* organisms (arrows) surrounded by epithelioid macrophages, neutrophils, and occasional lymphocytes (granulomatous inflammation with intralesional *Cryptococcus* sp.) (hematoxylin & eosin, 200×).

composed of polysaccharide, and the variable outer glycans can escape innate immune recognition, while the inner more conserved structural glycans are more likely to elicit immune responses.[105,106] The capsule can be highlighted by India ink negative staining[107] or positive staining with Alcian Blue and mucicarmine.[108] Periodic acid–Schiff and Gomori methenamine silver both stain the yeast body but not the capsule.[108] Within macrophages, *Cryptococcus* spp. can appear as small stippled basophilic yeast forms that resemble *Histoplasma* sp., *Trichosporon* sp., and other yeasts.[43] However, the thickness of the capsule and narrow-based budding are distinctive. In histologic sections, *Cryptococcus* spp. can present as "pseudocysts" containing round to oval yeast structures surrounded by variably thick, negative staining areas and marked granulomatous inflammation (Figure 24.4b).[109]

Rhinosporidiosis

Rhinosporidium seeberi is a widely distributed pathogen of dogs, cats, and other species. This non-culturable organism has been tentatively placed phylogenetically among the lower aquatic fungi.[110] Endemic in India, Sri Lanka, and Argentina, rhinosporidiosis is only sporadic in people and animals elsewhere. Exposure to water appears common in affected dogs,[46,111–114] and feline cases originate from outdoor cats with access to water in the eastern United States.[44,115] Most animals present with sneezing or nasal discharge and polypoid masses in the nasal cavity.[46] Masses can be several centimeters in diameter, composed of sporangia and associated inflammatory cells. Cytologically, aspirates and impression smears usually yield sufficient diagnostic material.[112] Immature endospores are round, pale structures of 2–4 μm diameter that can have a central pink-purple area and one to two small, round, dark basophilic elements. Mature endospores are thicker-walled, round structures, 5–15 μm in diameter that appear eosinophilic with globular internal structures, or darkly basophilic with no apparent internal detail (Figure 24.5). Organisms are associated with a pyogranulomatous reaction or lymphoplasmacytic and suppurative inflammation.[111,112]

Histologically, juvenile sporangia are the most numerous form and are nucleated, single-walled structures, 15–75 μm in diameter. Intermediate sporangia are the least numerous, double walled, 100–150 μm in diameter, and contain immature endospores.[46] Mature sporangia are single walled, measure up to 1000 μm in diameter[116] and contain both immature and mature endospores[46]. While *Rhinosporidium* is morphologically distinct, when sporangia are infrequent, there is some resemblance to *Coccidioides immitis*.[112] However, the endospores of *R. seeberi* are larger and more numerous than those of *C. immitis*.[116] Additionally, the thick-walled sporangia and endospores of *R. seeberi* stain positively with mucicarmine, whereas the sporangia and spores of *C. immitis* do not.[116]

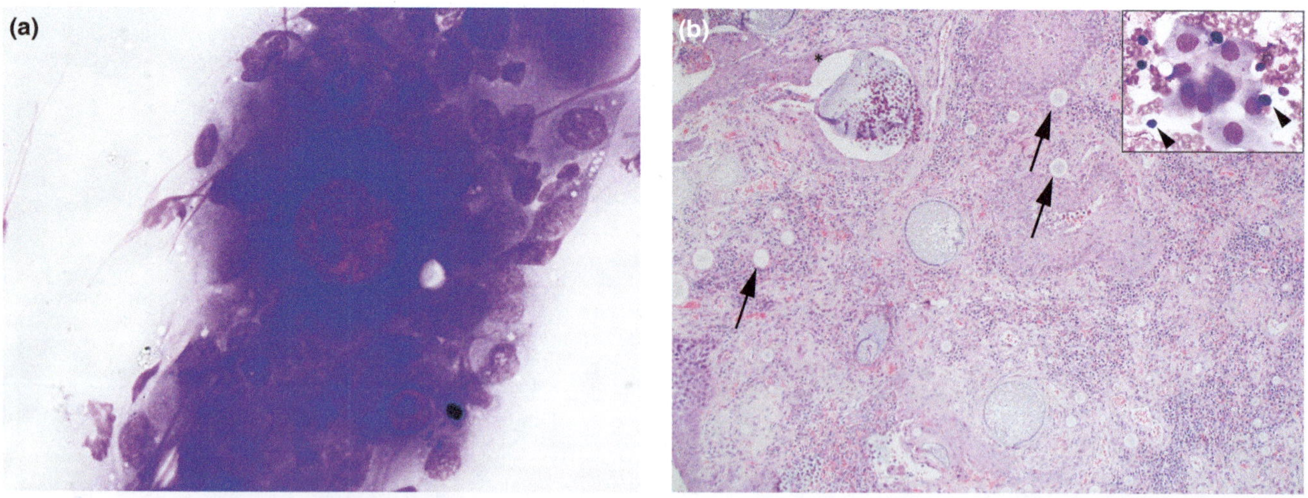

Figure 24.5 (a) Aspirate of a nasal mass from a dog. Among neutrophils, macrophages and fibroblasts are two juvenile sporangia of *R. seeberi* with granular basophilic cytoplasm and nucleus (Wright stain, 630×). (b) Histologic section shows thickened mucosal epithelium, granulomatous inflammation, and *R. seeberi* elements in various stages of development. There is a ruptured mature sporangium releasing endoconidia (asterisk) and multiple juvenile sporangia (10–70 μm diameter, arrows). Juvenile sporangia have a thick cell wall and granular cytoplasm with one to several eosinophilic nuclei (hematoxylin & eosin, 100×). Inset: Free endoconidia (arrowheads) with thick capsule among squamous epithelial cells.

Additional Fungal, Algal, and Oomycetal organisms

There are rare reports of *Sporothrix schenckii*[117] and *Scedosporium apiospermum*[118] causing mycotic rhinitis in dogs. Rarely, other fungi have been reported in feline URT mycosis including *Alternaria* spp.,[119] *Candida parapsilosis*,[120] *Metarhizium anisopliae*,[121] and *S. apiospermum*.[7] Algal (*Prototheca wickerhamii*[122]) and oomycetal (*Pythium insidiosum*[123]) URT infections have also been reported rarely. The general diagnostic approaches outlined above apply, but limitations in definitive identification of fungi based solely on morphology should be considered.[124]

Viral Rhinitis and Sinusitis

Viral rhinitis in the absence of tonsillitis and pharyngitis is uncommon in dogs. Canine influenza, canine parainfluenza, canine respiratory coronavirus, and herpes virus in young and adult dogs can manifest with rhinitis as part of the canine infectious respiratory disease complex.[125] Pneumonia is rare in canine herpesvirus 1 infection.[126] Canine influenza A subtype H3N8 caused kennel-associated outbreaks of respiratory disease in 2004.[127] Subtype H3N2 has circulated in North American dogs since 2015 and in Asian dogs prior to that. Infection causes URT disease and only rarely pneumonia.[127] A single report of avian origin-influenza infection in cats described avian influenza subtype H5N1 affecting cats in a Thai zoo.[128]

Cats are commonly affected by feline herpesvirus-1, the agent of feline rhinotracheitis, and feline calicivirus. Both viruses are considered primary causes of URT disease in cats and infect epithelial cells.[129,130] Infection disrupts epithelial barrier function in the URT, increasing susceptibility to secondary invasive infection with oropharyngeal bacteria such as *P. multocida*, *B. bronchiseptica*, and others. Limited host immune response and viral persistence lead to chronic necrosuppurative inflammation, nasal discharge, and possible osteolysis. *C. felis* is a primary bacterial cause of rhinitis in cats, but conjunctivitis is a more pronounced clinical feature of infection (Chapter 20).[131] *Mycoplasma* spp.[19,32,132–134] and *B. bronchiseptica*[132,133,135,136] are inconsistently primary causes of URT disease in cats. Overall, while rhinitis and sinusitis are relatively common in cats, cytology is of limited value for diagnosis of viral and bacterial causes of URT disease. Cats with experimentally induced asthma can develop eosinophilic rhinitis;[26] however, this has not been demonstrated in cats with naturally occurring asthma (Table 24.3).

Table 24.3 Frequency of detection of viruses in cats with upper respiratory disease.

	Percent positive; number assessed		
	Neoplasia	Chronic rhinitis	Fungal rhinitis
FeLV antigen serology	8; 106[28–30,49]	0; 27[29]	0; 11[31]
FeLV IHC p27	44; 39[49]	—	—
FeLV IHC gp70	31; 39[49]	—	—
FeLV IHC p27 and gp70	20; 39[49]	—	—
FIV antibody serology	10; 106[28–30,49]	7; 27[29]	0; 14[31]
Feline calicivirus virus, isolation	0; 6[29]	18; 11[29]	—
Feline herpesvirus-1 virus, isolation	0; 6[29]	18; 11[29]	—

FeLV, feline leukemia virus; FIV, feline immunodeficiency virus.

Neoplasia

Primary neoplasms of the URT are relatively uncommon in small animals (Tables 24.4 and 24.5). In dogs, URT neoplasms account for approximately 2%[33] and in cats for up to 8%[145] of all tumors. Tumors are commonly locally invasive.[33,174] At the time of diagnosis, spread to local lymph nodes and lung metastases are present in up to 24 and 2% of cases, respectively.[3] Metastasis is uncommon in cats with nasal carcinomas,[33] but nasal lymphoma can be associated with multicentric disease.[30,145] In dogs, epithelial tumors account for approximately 73% of all URT neoplasms, and the majority of these are adenocarcinomas followed by other carcinomas (Table 24.4). Various sarcomas can also affect the nose in dogs but are less common than epithelial tumors. In cats, lymphoma accounts for nearly 75% of all URT neoplasms, and epithelial tumors and sarcomas are much less common (Table 24.5).

Sex does not have an appreciable effect on nasal tumors in dogs,[22,25,37,47] but medium to large breed dogs are more commonly affected.[3,20,37,47,174,184] The proportional representation of specific breeds appears to reflect popular trends rather than specific breed predisposition.[3,20,37,47,174,184] On the other hand, cats with nasal tumors are slightly more often male (56%[29,49] to 64%[28]) and of domestic or European short-haired type.[28,29,33,49,158,185] The efficacy of cytologic samples for diagnosis of nasal neoplasia in dogs is uncertain[37,47] but likely more rewarding if samples from multiple and varied sites (>9 has been suggested[22]) are obtained. Cytology is robust for the diagnosis of lymphoma in cats with cytologic samples sufficient for diagnosis in approximately 50%[49] to 71%[30] of cases.

Table 24.4 Frequency of upper respiratory tract neoplasms in dogs (n = 802).

	No. of cases	Percent	References
Adenocarcinoma	274	34	3,20,22,25,26,35,37,47,137–148
Carcinoma	172	21	3,20,22,26,37,47,137–145,148
Chondrosarcoma	69	9	20,22,26,35,37,47,139,140,143,145,149
Transitional carcinoma	51	6	3,20,22,37,137,138,144,147,148,150
Squamous cell carcinoma	50	6	3,20,22,26,37,47,139–142,144,145,147,148,151–153
Other, sarcoma[a]	38	5	20,22,26,37,47,139,145,154–157
Osteosarcoma	34	4	20,47,143–145,149
Lymphoma	29	4	20,26,48,158
Other, benign[b]	23	3	20,22,35,37,159–162
Neuroendocrine carcinoma	18	2	20,22,35,148,163–165
Olfactory neuroblastoma	15	2	26,166,167
Transmissible venereal tumor	15	2	51,146,168–170
Other, malignant[c]	14	2	35,145,171,172

[a] Angioleiomyosarcoma, fibrosarcoma, hemangiosarcoma, myxosarcoma, unspecified sarcoma.
[b] Adenoma, angiofibroma, inflammatory myofibroblastic tumor, neuroepithelioma, oncocytoma, papilloma, respiratory epithelial adenomatoid hamartoma.
[c] Liposarcoma, mast cell tumor, paranasal meningioma.

Table 24.5 Frequency of upper respiratory tract neoplasms in cats (n = 600).

	No. of cases	Percent	References
Lymphoma	440	73	28–30,33,34,42,49,136,173–175
Carcinoma	37	6	29,33,34,42,136,148,176
Adenocarcinoma	36	6	29,33,136,148
Squamous cell carcinoma	19	3	29,33,148
Other, benign[a]	18	3	33,177–179
Other sarcoma[b]	17	3	29,33,34,42,180,181
Olfactory neuroblastoma	12	2	33,166,182
Fibrosarcoma	11	2	29,33
Chondrosarcoma	6	1	33,183
Other, malignant[c]	4	1	33,148

[a] Adenoma, basal cell tumor, fibroma, neurofibroma, oncocytoma, plasmacytoma.
[b] Hemangiosarcoma, histiocytic sarcoma, melanoma, osteosarcoma.
[c] Mast cell tumor, neuroendocrine carcinoma.

Carcinoma

Adenocarcinoma and carcinoma are the most common nasal neoplasms reported in dogs (Table 24.4), but both are uncommon in cats (Table 24.5). Cytologically, these tumors range from very well differentiated with clear features of respiratory epithelium, such as columnar shape and apical cilia, to being composed of anaplastic cells not amenable to more specific classification. Adenocarcinomas can distort facial features and are characterized by the appearance of acinar and tubular structures and carcinomas by a lack of glandular differentiation (Figure 24.6). Both types of neoplasm usually exfoliate in clusters and include a few poorly intact individual cells. Nuclei are basally located in columnar cells, more central in others, and usually round to oval in shape.

In dogs, squamous and transitional cell carcinoma account for approximately 6% each (Table 24.4), and in cats

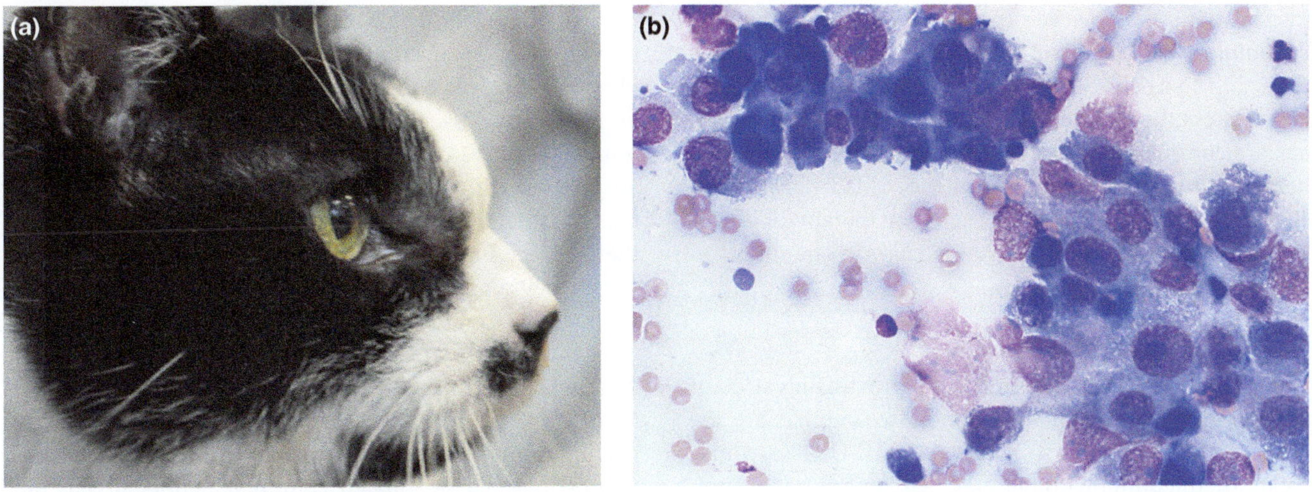

Figure 24.6 (a) Cat with facial protrusion due to a nasal carcinoma (*Source:* Image courtesy of Steve Patten). (b) Aspirate of the nasal mass shows cohesive cuboidal to squamous cells with basophilic cytoplasm, high nuclear to cytoplasmic ratio, moderate anisokaryosis and prominent nucleoli (Wright stain, 630×).

squamous cell carcinoma comprises approximately 3% of nasal cancers (Table 24.5). Cytologically, these tumors appear similar to those from other locations. Olfactory neuroblastoma is an uncommon tumor in both species, and cytologic descriptions are lacking.[194] Histologically, this tumor is defined by small cells that have scant cytoplasm; because cells may form structures that mimic tubules and acini, it is sometimes misdiagnosed as adenocarcinoma.[33] The median survival time (MST) of dogs with untreated nasal carcinoma is short (approximately 90 days).[3] Dogs that had concurrent epistaxis[3] and metastatic disease[25] or were diagnosed with nasal osteosarcoma[47] also had a poor prognosis (88,[3] 117,[25] and 93[47] days, respectively).

Lymphoma

Lymphoma is an uncommon URT neoplasm in dogs accounting for approximately 4% of all URT cancers (Table 24.4).[48] Among the few reports of canine URT lymphoma,[20,48,174,186] intermediate to high-grade B-cell lymphomas were most common.[48] Lymphoma is the most common URT neoplasm in cats and more often affects the nasal cavity than the nasopharynx (Figure 24.3). Nasal lymphoma is readily diagnosed cytologically, and large cell phenotype appears to predominate.[30,49,158] There are discrepant reports on the frequency of B-cell compared with T-cell type. Across several studies with a total of 105 cases using antibodies to CD3 and CD79a, 86 were classified as B cell (82%) and 20 as T cell (19%) (Table 24.6).[28,30,49,158] However, other authors reported 45 B-cell and 54 T-cell lymphomas out of 119 cases (38 and 45%, respectively, Table 24.6).[145] A third group also identified a predominance of B-cell tumors[33] using an antibody to BLA.36, which is not considered definitive marker because it is also expressed by a subset of T-cell lymphomas.[187,188] These differences might reflect regional variation, different immunohistochemical protocols, or divergent interpretations.

As with other feline lymphomas, virtually all URT lymphomas have diffuse architecture.[30,33,49,158] The mucosae are not always sufficiently intact in biopsy specimens to permit

Table 24.6 Immunohistochemical results in 259 cases of feline upper respiratory tract lymphoma.

	n	CD3$^+$/79a$^-$	CD3$^-$/79a$^+$	CD3$^-$/79a$^+$/MHCII$^+$	CD3$^-$/79a$^-$	CD3$^-$/79a$^-$/MHCII$^+$	CD3$^+$/79a$^+$	BLA.36$^+$/CD3$^-$	BLA.36$^-$/CD3$^+$
Day[174]	18	0	—	17	—	1	—	—	—
Haney[28]	3	0	3	—	—	—	—	—	—
Little[30]	45	7	32	—	—	—	6	—	—
Mukaratirwa[33]	35	—	—	—	—	—	—	25	10
Nagata[136]	119	54	45	—	4	—	15	1	—
Santagostino[49]	39	3	34	—	2	—	—	—	—

classification;[30,158] however, epitheliotropism can be noted in a minority of cases and could be either B-cell or T-cell type.[30,33,49] Epitheliotropism of B-cell lymphoma is uncommon at sites other than the nasal cavity. Feline URT lymphomas are considered aggressive,[28,29,49] and in the absence of therapy[49] or with glucocorticoids alone,[29] MST ranged from 28[29] to 53[49] days. Chemotherapy, radiation therapy, or a combination of both improved MST to 172 days in one study.[28]

Sarcoma

As a group, sarcomas account for approximately 18% of nasal tumors in dogs, of which chondrosarcomas are the most frequent (Table 24.4, Figure 24.7).[195] URT sarcomas in cats are uncommon (Table 24.5). Sarcoma cytomorphology is similar to that in tumors at other anatomic sites (Chapter 16). Of note is that anaplastic sarcomas and anaplastic carcinomas can be impossible to differentiate using either cytology or histology; thus specific diagnosis often depends on immunochemical assays.[33]

Otic and Nasopharyngeal Polyps and Nasal Hamartomas

Polypoid growths are rare in dogs and can originate from the middle ear, nasopharynx, and nose.[189] In cats, nasopharyngeal polyps arise from the nasopharynx, auditory tube, or tympanic cavity where they are often noted associated with chronic inflammatory or infectious processes.[177] However, as DNA or RNA from suspected inciting agents can be isolated from both healthy cats and those with polyps,[190] the role of infectious agents is unclear. In younger cats, nasopharyngeal polyps can be congenital, arising from remnant branchial arch tissue, or in older cats from inflammation or trauma (Figure 24.8).[177] Histologically, inflammatory polyps are covered with ciliated pseudostratified columnar epithelial cells surrounding a fibrovascular core. Within the polyp, there can be increased vascularity and inflammatory infiltrates, including lymphoid aggregates.[177] These are distinct from feline nasal hamartomas affecting young cats.[189,191,192] Cats with nasal hamartoma often present with stertorous breathing, sneezing, and intermittent epistaxis[189,191] and, in more severe cases, can have facial deformity and a mass protruding from the nose.[189] Histologically, nasal hamartomas may be covered by ciliated columnar epithelial cells and contain woven bone and irregularly shaped, blood-filled spaces lined by endothelial cells.[192] These are surrounded by a variable amount of connective tissue stroma with a scant lymphocytic infiltrate.[191] Cytologic evaluation of polyp samples is useful to rule out fungal infection and neoplasia, but classification requires architectural assessment.

Other Conditions Mimicking Neoplasia

Other conditions mimicking neoplasia can affect the URT of dogs and cats. These are more common in dogs and include cysts that arise in the orbit or sinuses and that can extend into the nasal cavity.[193] There are rare instances of idiopathic turbinate osseous hyperplasia noted in a dog[27] and osteopetrosis-like hypertrophy of the nasal turbinates in a cat.[137]

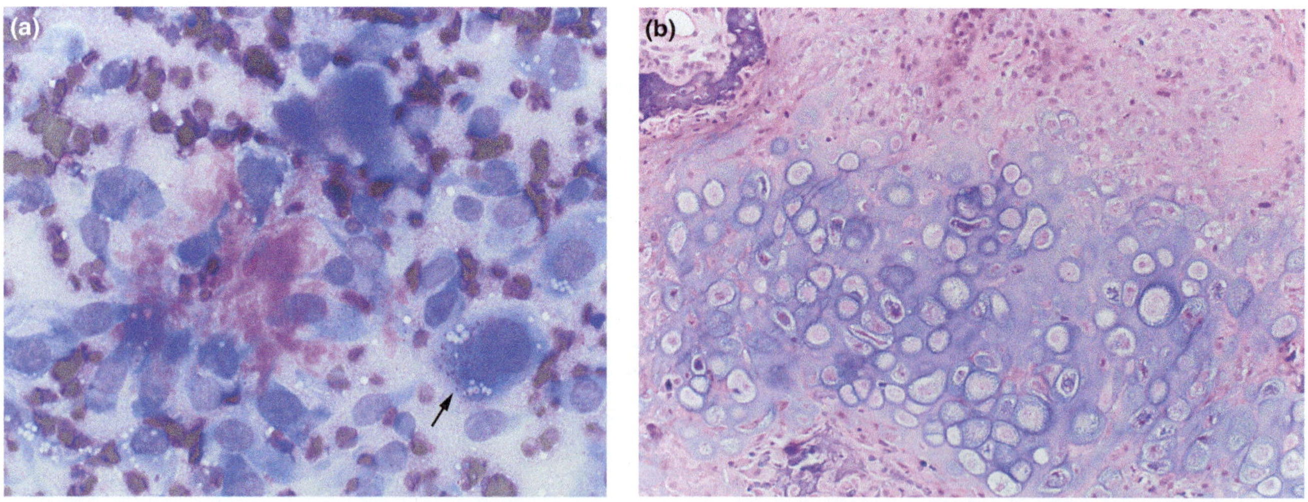

Figure 24.7 (a) Fine-needle aspirate of a nasal chondrosarcoma in a dog. Individual and aggregated basophilic spindle cells are associated with pink extracellular material. Some cells have pink to azurophilic granules (lysosomes, arrow). There is marked anisocytosis, anisokaryosis, and anisonucleoliosis (Wright stain, 630×). (b) Histologic section with spindle cells that surround and transition into irregular islands of variably basophilic, chondromatous matrix. Neoplastic cells have a chondroblastic to fibroblastic phenotype and are associated with eosinophilic extracellular matrix (hematoxylin & eosin, 200×).

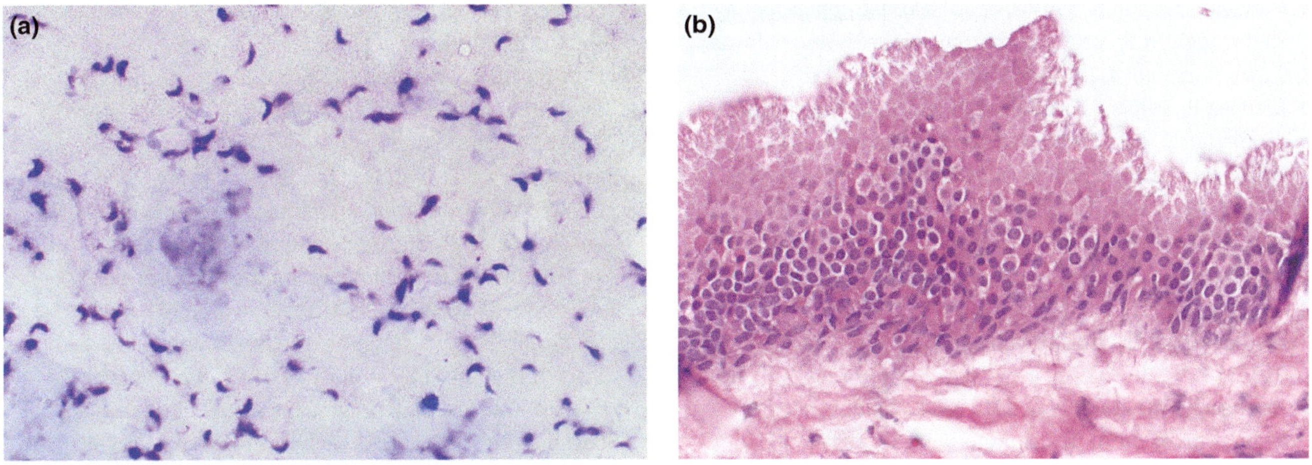

Figure 24.8 Samples from a soft mass on the palate of a 14-year-old cat with a history of chronic sneezing. (a) An aspirate consists of proteinaceous fluid with numerous curved structures interpreted to be dislodged cilia. There were no intact cells (Wright stain, 630×). (b) Histologically, the cystic mass is lined by ciliated stratified squamous epithelium. The cyst was considered acquired and of branchial origin (hematoxylin & eosin, 200×. *Source:* Images courtesy of Karlee Craig).

Conclusion

Establishing a diagnosis in cases of URT disease in dogs and cats is often challenging, and multiple attempts and application of different investigative modalities are usually necessary. Cytology is a very useful component of such investigation but may not be sufficient as the only approach.

References

1 Weeden, A.M. and Degner, D.A. (2016). Surgical approaches to the nasal cavity and sinuses. *Vet Clin North Am Small Anim Pract* 46: 719–733.

2 Harkema, J.R., Carey, S.A., and Wagner, J.G. (2006). The nose revisited: a brief review of the comparative structure, function, and toxicologic pathology of the nasal epithelium. *Toxicol Pathol* 34: 252–269.

3 Rassnick, K.M., Goldkamp, C.E., Erb, H.N. et al. (2006). Evaluation of factors associated with survival in dogs with untreated nasal carcinomas: 139 cases (1993–2003). *J Am Vet Med Assoc* 229: 401–406.

4 Peeters, D., Day, M.J., and Clercx, C. (2005). An immunohistochemical study of canine nasal aspergillosis. *J Comp Pathol* 132: 283–288.

5 Cesta, M.F. (2006). Normal structure, function, and histology of mucosa-associated lymphoid tissue. *Toxicol Pathol* 34: 599–608.

6 Haley, P.J. (2003). Species differences in the structure and function of the immune system. *Toxicology* 188: 49–71.

7 Leperlier, D., Vallefuoco, R., Laloy, E. et al. (2010). Fungal rhinosinusitis caused by *Scedosporium apiospermum* in a cat. *J Feline Med Surg* 12: 967–971.

8 Casteleyn, C., Breugelmans, S., Simoens, P., and Van den Broeck, W. (2011). The tonsils revisited: review of the anatomical localization and histological characteristics of the tonsils of domestic and laboratory animals. *Clin Dev Immunol* 2011: 472460.

9 Dorn, E.S., Tress, B., Suchodolski, J.S. et al. (2017). Bacterial microbiome in the nose of healthy cats and in cats with nasal disease. *PLoS One* 12: e0180299.

10 Tress, B., Dorn, E.S., Suchodolski, J.S. et al. (2017). Bacterial microbiome of the nose of healthy dogs and dogs with nasal disease. *PLoS One* 12: e0176736.

11 Ericsson, A.C., Personett, A.R., Grobman, M.E. et al. (2016). Composition and predicted metabolic capacity of upper and lower airway microbiota of healthy dogs in relation to the fecal microbiota. *PLoS One* 11: e0154646.

12 Vientos-Plotts, A.I., Ericsson, A.C., Rindt, H. et al. (2017). Dynamic changes of the respiratory microbiota and its relationship to fecal and blood microbiota in healthy young cats. *PLoS One* 12: e0173818.

13 Clapper, W.E. and Meade, G.H. (1963). Normal flora of the nose, throat, and lower intestine of dogs. *J Bacteriol* 85: 643–648.

14 Kuehn, N.F. (2017). Overview of respiratory diseases of small animals. Merck Veterinary Manual. https://www.merckvetmanual.com/respiratory-system/respiratory-diseases-of-small-animals/overview-of-respiratory-diseases-of-small-animals. Accessed: 01-January-2020

15 Frey, E., Pressler, B., Guy, J. et al. (2003). *Capnocytophaga* sp. Isolated from a cat with chronic sinusitis and rhinitis. *J Clin Microbiol* 41: 5321–5324.

16 Mercier, E., Peters, I.R., Billen, F. et al. (2013). Potential role of *Alternaria* and *Cladosporium* species in canine lymphoplasmacytic rhinitis. *J Small Anim Pract* 54: 179–183.

17 Sauget, M., Valot, B., Bertrand, X., and Hocquet, D. (2017). Can MALDI-TOF mass spectrometry reasonably type bacteria? *Trends Microbiol* 25: 447–455.

18 Tan, R., Lim, E., and Ishak, B. (1977). Ecology of mycoplasmas in clinically healthy cats. *Aust Vet J* 53: 515–518.

19 Bannasch, M.J. and Foley, J.E. (2004). Epidemiologic evaluation of multiple respiratory pathogens in cats in animal shelters. *J Feline Med Surg* 7: 109–119.

20 Clercx, C., Wallon, J., Gilbert, S. et al. (1996). Imprint and brush cytology in the diagnosis of canine intranasal tumours. *J Small Anim Pract* 37: 423–427.

21 Lobetti, R. (2014). Idiopathic lymphoplasmacytic rhinitis in 33 dogs. *J S Afr Vet Assoc* 85: 1151.

22 Lobetti, R.G. (2009). A retrospective study of chronic nasal disease in 75 dogs. *J S Afr Vet Assoc* 80: 224–228.

23 Saunders, J.H., Clercx, C., Snaps, F.R.R. et al. (2004). Radiographic, magnetic resonance imaging, computed tomographic, and rhinoscopic features of nasal aspergillosis in dogs. *J Am Vet Med Assoc* 225: 1703–1712.

24 Johnson, L.R., Drazenovich, T.L., Herrera, M.A., and Wisner, E.R. (2006). Results of rhinoscopy alone or in conjunction with sinuscopy in dogs with aspergillosis: 46 cases (2001–2004). *J Am Vet Med Assoc* 228: 738–742.

25 Henry, C.J., Brewer, W.G., Tyler, J.W. et al. (1998). Survival in dogs with nasal adenocarcinoma: 64 cases (1981–1995). *J Vet Intern Med* 12: 436–439.

26 Venema, C.M., Williams, K.J., Gershwin, L.J. et al. (2012). Histopathologic and morphometric evaluation of the nasal and pulmonary airways of cats with experimentally induced asthma. *Int Arch Allergy Immunol* 160: 365–376.

27 Rutherford, S., Whitbread, T., and Ness, M. (2011). Idiopathic osseous hyperplasia of the nasal turbinates in a Welsh terrier. *J Small Anim Pract* 52: 492–496.

28 Haney, S.M., Beaver, L., Turrel, J. et al. (2009). Survival analysis of 97 cats with nasal lymphoma: a multi-institutional retrospective study (1986–2006). *J Vet Intern Med* 23: 287–294.

29 Henderson SM, Bradley K, Day MJ, et al. Investigation of nasal disease in the cat: a retrospective study of 77 cases. *J Feline Med Surg*. 2004;6:245–257.

30 Little, L., Patel, R., and Goldschmidt, M. (2007). Nasal and nasopharyngeal lymphoma in cats: 50 cases (1989–2005). *Vet Pathol* 44: 885–892.

31 Barrs, V.R., Halliday, C., Martin, P. et al. (2012). Sinonasal and sino-orbital aspergillosis in 23 cats: aetiology, clinicopathological features and treatment outcomes. *Vet J* 191: 58–64.

32 Demko, J.L. and Cohn, L.A. (2007). Chronic nasal discharge in cats: 75 cases (1993–2004). *J Am Vet Med Assoc* 230: 1032–1037.

33 Mukaratirwa, S., Van Der Linde-Sipman, J.S., and Gruys, E. (2001). Feline nasal and paranasal sinus tumours: clinicopathological study, histomorphological description and diagnostic immunohistochemistry of 123 cases. *J Feline Med Surg* 3: 235–245.

34 De Lorenzi, D., Bertoncello, D., and Bottero, E. (2008). Squash-preparation cytology from nasopharyngeal masses in the cat: cytological results and histological correlations in 30 cases. *J Feline Med Surg* 10: 55–60.

35 Pietra, M., Spinella, G., Pasquali, F. et al. (2010). Clinical findings, rhinoscopy and histological evaluation of 54 dogs with chronic nasal disease. *J Vet Med Sci* 11: 249–255.

36 Harris, B.J., Lourenço, B.N., Dobson, J.M., and Herrtage, M.E. (2014). Diagnostic accuracy of three biopsy techniques in 117 dogs with intra-nasal neoplasia. *J Small Anim Pract* 55: 219–224.

37 Mason, S.L., Maddox, T.W., Lillis, S.M., and Blackwood, L. (2013). Late presentation of canine nasal tumours in a UK referral hospital and treatment outcomes. *J Small Anim Pract* 54: 347–353.

38 Lorenzi, D.D., Bonfanti, U., Masserdotti, C. et al. (2006). Diagnosis of canine nasal aspergillosis by cytological examination: a comparison of four different collection techniques. *J Small Anim Pract* 47: 316–319.

39 Johnson, L.R. and Kass, P.H. (2009). Effect of sample collection methodology on nasal culture results in cats. *J Feline Med Surg* 11: 645–649.

40 Johnson, L.R., Clarke, H.E., Bannasch, M.J., and De Cock, H.E. (2004). Correlation of rhinoscopic signs of inflammation with histologic findings in nasal biopsy specimens of cats with or without upper respiratory tract disease. *J Am Vet Med Assoc* 225: 395–400.

41 Meler, E., Dunn, M., and Lecuyer, M. (2008). A retrospective study of canine persistent nasal disease: 80 cases (1998–2003). *Can Vet J* 49: 71–76.

42 Nemanic, S., Hollars, K., Nelson, N.C., and Bobe, G. (2015). Combination of computed tomographic imaging characteristics of medial retropharyngeal lymph nodes and nasal passages aids discrimination between rhinitis and neoplasia in cats. *Vet Radiol Ultrasound* 56: 617–627.

43 Lester, S.J., Malik, R., Bartlett, K.H., and Duncan, C.G. (2011). Cryptococcosis: update and emergence of *Cryptococcus gattii*. *Vet Clin Pathol* 40: 4–17.

44 Brenseke, B.M. and Saunders, G.K. (2010). Concurrent nasal adenocarcinoma and rhinosporidiosis in a cat. *J Vet Diagn Invest* 22: 155–157.

45 Wallin, L.L., Coleman, G.D., Froeling, J., and Parker, G.A. (2001). Rhinosporidiosis in a domestic cat. *Med Mycol* 39: 139–141.

46 Easley, J.R., Meuten, D.J., Levy, M.G. et al. (1986). Nasal rhinosporidiosis in the dog. *Vet Pathol* 23: 50–56.

47 Kubicek, L., Milner, R., An, Q. et al. (2016). Outcomes and prognostic factors associated with canine sinonasal tumors treated with curative intent cone-based stereotactic radiosurgery (1999–2013). *Vet Radiol Ultrasound* 57: 331–340.

48 George, R., Smith, A., Schleis, S. et al. (2016). Outcome of dogs with intranasal lymphoma treated with various radiation and chemotherapy protocols: 24 cases. *Vet Radiol Ultrasound* 57: 306–312.

49 Santagostino, S.F., Mortellaro, C.M., Boracchi, P. et al. (2015). Feline upper respiratory tract lymphoma. *Vet Pathol* 52: 250–259.

50 Caniatti, M., Da Cunha, N., Avallone, G. et al. (2012). Diagnostic accuracy of brush cytology in canine chronic intranasal disease. *Vet Clin Pathol* 41: 133–140.

51 Papazoglou, L.G., Koutinas, A.F., Plevraki, A.G., and Tontis, D. (2001). Primary intranasal transmissible venereal tumour in the dog: a retrospective study of six spontaneous cases. *J Vet Med A* 48: 391–400.

52 Bredal, W.P. (1998). The prevalence of nasal mite (*Pneumonyssoides caninum*) infection in Norwegian dogs. *Vet Parasitol* 76: 233–237.

53 Gunnarsson, L.K., Zakrisson, G., Egenvall, A. et al. (2001). Prevalence of *Pneumonyssoides caninum* infection in dogs in Sweden. *J Am Anim Hosp Assoc* 37: 331–337.

54 Movassaghi, A.R. and Mohri, M. (1998). Nasal mite of dogs *Pneumonyssus* (*Pneumonyssoides*) *caninum* in Iran. *Vet Rec* 142: 551–552.

55 Traldi, G., Principato, M., and Faravelli, G. (1989). *Pneumonyssoides caninum*: a mite from the nasal cavities and frontal sinuses of the dog. A case report. *Parassitologia* 31: 173–176.

56 Alho, A., Mouro, S., Pissarra, H. et al. (2016). First report of *Eucoleus boehmi* infection in a dog from Portugal. *Parasitol Res* 115: 1721–1725.

57 Baan, M., Kidder, A.C., Johnson, S.E., and Sherding, R.G. (2010). Rhinoscopic diagnosis of *Eucoleus boehmi* infection in a dog. *J Am Anim Hosp Assoc* 47: 60–63.

58 Campbell, B.G. and Little, M.D. (1991). Identification of the eggs of a nematode (*Eucoleus boehmi*) from the nasal mucosa of North American dogs. *J Am Vet Med Assoc* 198: 1520–1523.

59 Cesare, A., Veronesi, F., Di Regalbono, A. et al. (2015). PCR-based assay for the mitochondrial cox1 specific amplification of *Eucoleus böhmi*. *Vet Parasitol* 211: 67–70.

60 Magi, M., Guardone, L., Prati, M.C. et al. (2012). First report of *Eucoleus boehmi* (syn. *Capillaria boehmi*) in dogs in north-western Italy, with scanning electron microscopy of the eggs. *Parasite* 19: 433–435.

61 Schoning, P., Dryden, M.W., and Gabbert, N.H. (1993). Identification of a nasal nematode (*Eucoleus boehmi*) in greyhounds. *Vet Res Commun* 17: 277–281.

62 Luján, L., Vázquez, J., Lucientes, J. et al. (1998). Nasal myiasis due to *Oestrus ovis* infestation in a dog. *Vet Rec* 142: 282–283.

63 Rutland, B.E., Byl, K.M., Hydeskov, H.B. et al. (2017). Systemic manifestations of *Cuterebra* infection in dogs and cats: 42 cases (2000–2014). *J Am Vet Med Assoc* 251: 1432–1438.

64 Meshgi, B. and Asgarian, O. (2003). Prevalence of *Linguatula serrata* infestation in stray dogs of Shahrekord, Iran. *J Vet Med B Infect Dis Vet Public Health* 50: 466–467.

65 Mitchell, S., Bell, S., Wright, I. et al. (2016). Tongue worm (*Linguatula* species) in stray dogs imported into the UK. *Vet Rec* 179: 259–260.

66 Gattenuo, T., Ketzis, J., and Shell, L. (2014). Fenbendazole treatment for *Mammomonogamus* species infection of a domestic cat on St. Kitts, West Indies. *J Feline Med Surg* 16: 864–866.

67 Ketzis, J., Shell, L., Chinault, S. et al. (2015). The prevalence of *Trichuris* spp. infection in indoor and outdoor cats on St. Kitts. *J Infect Dev Ctries* 9: 111–113.

68 Tudor, E.G., Lee, A.C., Armato, D.G., and Bowman, D.D. (2008). *Mammomonogamus auris* infection in the middle ear of a domestic cat in Saipan, Northern Mariana Islands, USA. *J Feline Med Surg* 10: 501–504.

69 Lopez, A., Aburto, E., Jones, K. et al. (2016). *Eucoleus boehmi* Infection in the nasal conchae and paranasal sinuses of red fox (*Vulpes vulpes*) on Prince Edward Island, Canada. *J Wildl Dis* 52: 279–285.

70 Manzocchi, S., Spiranelli, E., and Bertazzolo, W. (2016). What is your diagnosis? Nasal cavity imprint from a dog. *Vet Clin Pathol* 45: 719–720.

71 Mcgarry, J., Penrose, F., and Collins, C. (2012). *Oestrus ovis* infestation of a dog in the UK. *J Small Anim Pract* 53: 192–193.

72 Webb, S.M. and Grillo, V.L. (2010). Nasal myiasis in a cat caused by larvae of the nasal bot fly, *Oestrus ovis*. *Aust Vet J* 88: 455–457.

73 Villedieu, E., Sanchez, R.F., Jepson, R.E., and Ter Haar, G. (2017). Nasal infestation by *Linguatula serrata* in a dog in the UK: a case report. *J Small Anim Pract* 58: 183–186.

74 Shamsi, S., McSpadden, K., Baker, S., and Jenkins, D.J. (2017). Occurrence of tongue worm, *Linguatula cf. serrata* (*Pentastomida: Linguatulidae*) in wild canids and livestock in south-eastern Australia. *Int J Parasitol Parasites Wildl* 6: 271–277.

75 Esmaeilzadeh, S. and Mohammadian, B. (2008). *Linguatula serrata* nymph in a cat. *Iran J Vet Med* 9: 387–389.

76 Peeters, D. and Clercx, C. (2007). Update on canine sinonasal aspergillosis. *Vet Clin North Am Small Anim Pract* 37: 901–916.

77 Michiels, L., Day, M.J., Snaps, F. et al. (2003). A retrospective study of non-specific rhinitis in 22 cats and the value of nasal cytology and histopathology. *J Feline Med Surg* 5: 279–285.

78 Schulz, C., Hartmann, K., Mueller, R.S. et al. (2015). Sampling sites for detection of feline herpesvirus-1, feline calicivirus and *Chlamydia felis* in cats with feline upper respiratory tract disease. *J Feline Med Surg* 17: 1012–1019.

79 Piva, S., Zanoni, R.G., Specchi, S. et al. (2010). Chronic rhinitis due to *Streptococcus equi* subspecies *zooepidemicus* in a dog. *Vet Rec* 167: 177–178.

80 Blum, S., Elad, D., Zukin, N. et al. (2010). Outbreak of *Streptococcus equi* subsp. *zooepidemicus* infections in cats. *Vet Microbiol* 144: 236–239.

81 Britton, A.P. and Davies, J.L. (2010). Rhinitis and meningitis in two shelter cats caused by *Streptococcus equi* subspecies *zooepidemicus*. *J Comp Pathol* 143: 70–74.

82 Nakanishi, A., Hita, T., Akiyama, K. et al. (2015). Suppurative granulomatous sinorhinitis associated with *Nocardia* spp. infection in a cat. *J Vet Med Sci* 77: 597–599.

83 Morrow, B.L., McNatt, R., Joyce, L. et al. (2016). Highly pathogenic beta-hemolytic streptococcal infections in cats from an institutionalized hoarding facility and a multi-species comparison. *J Feline Med Surg* 18: 318–327.

84 Barrs, V.R., Ujvari, B., Dhand, N.K. et al. (2015). Detection of *Aspergillus*-specific antibodies by agar gel double immunodiffusion and IgG ELISA in feline upper respiratory tract aspergillosis. *Vet J* 203: 285–289.

85 Barrs, V.R. and Talbot, J.J. (2014). Feline aspergillosis. *Vet Clin North Am Small Anim Pract* 44: 51–73.

86 Talbot, J.J., Johnson, L.R., Martin, P. et al. (2014). What causes canine sino-nasal aspergillosis? A molecular approach to species identification. *Vet J* 200: 17–21.

87 Vascellari, M., Carminato, A., Danesi, P. et al. (2011). Pathology in practice. Severe, chronic, pyogranulomatous rhinosinusitis with necrosis and fungal septate hyphae consistent with *Fusarium* spp infection. *J Am Vet Med Assoc* 238: 449–451.

88 Meason-Smith, C., Edwards, E.E., Older, C.E. et al. (2017). Panfungal polymerase chain reaction for identification of fungal pathogens in formalin-fixed animal tissues. *Vet Pathol* 54: 640–648.

89 Hartmann, K., Lloret, A., Pennisi, M. et al. (2013). Aspergillosis in cats. *J Feline Med Surg* 15: 605–610.

90 Day, M.J. (2009). Canine sino-nasal aspergillosis: parallels with human disease. *Med Mycol* 47: S315–S323.

91 Kano, R., Takahashi, T., Hayakawa, T. et al. (2015). The first case of feline sinonasal aspergillosis due to *Aspergillus fischeri* in Japan. *J Vet Med Sci* 77: 1183–1185.

92 Tomsa, K., Glaus, T.M., Zimmer, C., and Greene, C.E. (2003). Fungal rhinitis and sinusitis in three cats. *J Am Vet Med Assoc* 222: 1380–1384.

93 Barachetti, L., Mortellaro, C.M., Giancamillo, M. et al. (2009). Bilateral orbital and nasal aspergillosis in a cat. *Vet Ophthalmol* 12: 176–182.

94 Wehner, A., Crochik, S., Howerth, E.W., and Koenig, A. (2008). Diagnosis and treatment of blastomycosis affecting the nose and nasopharynx of a dog. *J Am Vet Med Assoc* 233: 1112–1116.

95 Hecht, S., Adams, W.H., Thomas, W.B., and Smith, J.R. (2011). Clinical and imaging findings in five dogs with intracranial blastomycosis (*Blastomyces dermatiditis*). *J Am Anim Hosp Assoc* 47: 241–249.

96 Bentley, T.R., Reese, M.J., Heng, H. et al. (2013). Ependymal and periventricular magnetic resonance imaging changes in four dogs with central nervous system blastomycosis. *Vet Radiol Ultrasound* 54: 489–496.

97 Mourning, A.C., Patterson, E.E., Kirsch, E.J. et al. (2015). Evaluation of an enzyme immunoassay for antibodies to a recombinant *Blastomyces* adhesin-1 repeat antigen as an aid in the diagnosis of blastomycosis in dogs. *J Am Vet Med Assoc* 247: 1133–1138.

98 Hagen, F., Ceresini, P.C., Polacheck, I. et al. (2013). Ancient dispersal of the human fungal pathogen *Cryptococcus gattii* from the Amazon rainforest. *PLoS One* 8: e71148.

99 Vorathavorn, V.I., Sykes, J.E., and Feldman, D.G. (2013). Cryptococcosis as an emerging systemic mycosis in dogs. *J Vet Emerg Crit Care* 23: 489–497.

100 Bojarczuk, A., Miller, K.A., Hotham, R. et al. (2016). *Cryptococcus neoformans* intracellular proliferation and capsule size determines early macrophage control of infection. *Sci Rep* 6: 21489.

101 Kluger, E.K., Karaoglu, H.K., Krockenberger, M.B. et al. (2006). Recrudescent cryptococcosis, caused by *Cryptococcus gattii* (molecular type VGII), over a 13-year period in a Birman cat. *Med Mycol* 44: 561–566.

102 Trivedi, S.R., Malik, R., Meyer, W., and Sykes, J.E. (2011). Feline cryptococcosis impact of current research on clinical management. *J Feline Med Surg* 13: 163–172.

103 Trivedi, S.R., Sykes, J.E., Cannon, M.S. et al. (2011). Clinical features and epidemiology of cryptococcosis in cats and dogs in California: 93 cases (1988–2010). *J Am Vet Med Assoc* 239: 357–369.

104 Windsor, R.C., Sturges, B.K., Vernau, K.M., and Vernau, W. (2009). Cerebrospinal fluid eosinophilia in dogs. *J Vet Intern Med* 23: 275–281.

105 Zaragoza, O., Rodrigues, M.L., Jesus, M. et al. (2009). The capsule of the fungal pathogen *Cryptococcus neoformans*. *Adv Appl Microbiol* 68: 133–216.

106 Snarr BD, Qureshi ST, Sheppard DC. Immune recognition of fungal polysaccharides. *J Fungi (Basel)*. 2017;3:E47.

107 Philip, K.J., Kaur, R., Sangeetha, M. et al. (2012). Disseminated cryptococcosis presenting with generalized lymphadenopathy. *J Cytol* 29: 200–202.

108 Marcos, R., Malhão, F., Santos, J. et al. (2016). The cryptic *Cryptococcus*. *Vet Clin Pathol* 45: 532–533.

109 Headley, S., Santis, G., De Alcântara, B. et al. (2015). *Cryptococcus gattii*-induced infections in dogs from southern Brazil. *Mycopathologia* 180: 265–275.

110 Vilela, R. and Mendoza, L. (2012). The taxonomy and phylogenetics of the human and animal pathogen *Rhinosporidium seeberi*: a critical review. *Rev Iberoam Micol* 29: 185–199.

111 Caniatti, M., Roccabianca, P., Scanziani, E., and Finazzi, M. (1998). Nasal rhinosporidiosis in dogs: four cases from Europe and a review of the literature. *Vet Rec* 142: 334–338.

112 Hill, S.A., Sharkey, L.C., Hardy, R.M. et al. (2010). Nasal rhinosporidiosis in two dogs native to the upper Mississippi river valley region. *J Am Anim Hosp Assoc* 46: 127–131.

113 Miller, R.I. and Baylis, R. (2009). Rhinosporidiosis in a dog native to the UK. *Vet Rec* 164: 210–210.

114 Mosier, D.A. and Creed, J.E. (1984). Rhinosporidiosis in a dog. *J Am Vet Med Assoc* 185: 1009–1010.

115 Moisan, P.G. and Baker, S.V. (2001). Rhinosporidiosis in a cat. *J Vet Diagn Invest* 13: 352–354.

116 Sinha, A., Phukan, J.P., Bandyopadhyay, G. et al. (2012). Clinicopathological study of rhinosporidiosis with special reference to cytodiagnosis. *J Cytol* 29: 246–249.

117 Schubach, T.M.P., Schubach, A., Okamoto, T. et al. (2006). Canine sporotrichosis in Rio de Janeiro, Brazil: clinical presentation, laboratory diagnosis and therapeutic response in 44 cases (1998–2003). *Med Mycol* 44: 87–92.

118 Coleman, M.G. and Robson, M.C. (2005). Nasal infection with *Scedosporium apiospermum* in a dog. *N Z Vet J* 53: 81–83.

119 Tennant, K., Patterson-Kane, J., Boag, A.K., and Rycroft, A.N. (2004). Nasal mycosis in two cats caused by *Alternaria species*. *Vet Rec* 155: 368–370.

120 Lamm, C.G., Grune, S.C., Estrada, M.M. et al. (2013). Granulomatous rhinitis due to *Candida parapsilosis* in a cat. *J Vet Diagn Invest* 25: 596–598.

121 Muir, D., Martin, P., Kendall, K., and Malik, R. (1998). Invasive hyphomycotic rhinitis in a cat due to *Metarhizium anisopliae*. *Med Mycol* 36: 51–54.

122 Endo, S., Sekiguchi, M., Kishimoto, Y. et al. (2010). The first case of feline *Prototheca wickerhamii* infection in Japan. *J Vet Med Sci* 72: 1351–1353.

123 Bissonnette, K.W., Sharp, N.J., Dykstra, M.H. et al. (1991). Nasal and retrobulbar mass in a cat caused by *Pythium insidiosum*. *J Med Vet Mycol* 29: 39–44.

124 Hibbett, D., Abarenkov, K., Koljalg, U. et al. (2016). Sequence-based classification and identification of fungi. *Mycologia* 108: 1049–1068.

125 Joffe, D.J., Lelewski, R., Weese, J.S. et al. (2016). Factors associated with development of canine infectious respiratory disease complex (CIRDC) in dogs in 5 Canadian small animal clinics. *Can Vet J* 57: 46–51.

126 Kumar, S., Driskell, E.A., Cooley, A.J. et al. (2015). Fatal canid herpesvirus 1 respiratory infections in 4 clinically healthy adult dogs. *Vet Pathol* 52: 681–687.

127 Voorhees, I., Glaser, A.L., Toohey-Kurth, K. et al. (2017). Spread of canine influenza A(H3N2) virus, United States. *Emerg Infect Dis* 23: 1950–1957.

128 Beeler, E. (2009). Influenza in dogs and cats. *Vet Clin North Am Small Anim Pract* 39: 251–264.

129 Monne Rodriguez, J.M., Leeming, G., Kohler, K., and Kipar, A. (2017). Feline herpesvirus pneumonia: investigations into the pathogenesis. *Vet Pathol* 54: 922–932.

130 Spiri, A.M., Theze, J., Meli, M.L. et al. (2016). Genetic diversity and phenotypic associations of feline caliciviruses from cats in Switzerland. *J Gen Virol* 97: 3253–3266.

131 Masubuchi, K., Nosaka, H., Iwamoto, K. et al. (2002). Experimental infection of cats with *Chlamydophila felis*. *J Vet Med Sci* 64: 1165–1168.

132 Burns, R.E., Wagner, D.C., Leutenegger, C.M., and Pesavento, P.A. (2011). Histologic and molecular correlation in shelter cats with acute upper respiratory infection. *J Clin Microbiol* 49: 2454–2460.

133 Johnson, L.R., Foley, J.E., De Cock, H.E. et al. (2005). Assessment of infectious organisms associated with chronic rhinosinusitis in cats. *J Am Vet Med Assoc* 227: 579–585.

134 Veir, J.K., Ruch-Gallie, R., Spindel, M.E., and Lappin, M.R. (2008). Prevalence of selected infectious organisms and comparison of two anatomic sampling sites in shelter cats with upper respiratory tract disease. *J Feline Med Surg* 10: 551–557.

135 Helps, C.R., Lait, P., Damhuis, A. et al. (2005). Factors associated with upper respiratory tract disease caused by feline herpesvirus, feline calicivirus, *Chlamydophila felis* and *Bordetella bronchiseptica* in cats: experience from 218 European catteries. *Vet Rec* 156: 669–673.

136 Egberink, H., Addie, D., Belak, S. et al. (2009). *Bordetella bronchiseptica* infection in cats. ABCD guidelines on prevention and management. *J Feline Med Surg* 11: 610–614.

137 Fujita, M., Takaishi, Y., Nagae, H. et al. (2007). Osteopetrosis-like disease in a cat with respiratory distress. *J Vet Med Sci* 69: 687–690.

138 Lux, C.N., Culp, W.T.N., Johnson, L.R. et al. (2017). Prospective comparison of tumor staging using computed tomography versus magnetic resonance imaging findings in dogs with nasal neoplasia: a pilot study. *Vet Radiol Ultrasound* 58: 315–325.

139 Belshaw, Z., Constantio-Casas, F., Brearley, M.J. et al. (2011). COX-2 expression and outcome in canine nasal carcinomas treated with hypofractionated radiotherapy. *Vet Comp Oncol* 9: 141–148.

140 Borzacchiello, G., Paciello, O., and Papparella, S. (2004). Expression of cyclooxygenase-1 and -2 in canine nasal carcinomas. *J Comp Pathol* 131: 70–76.

141 Confer, A.W. and Depaoli, A. (1978). Primary neoplasms of the nasal cavity, paranasal sinuses and nasopharynx in the dog: a report of 16 cases from the files of the AFIP. *Vet Pathol* 15: 18–30.

142 Drees, R., Forrest, L.J., and Chappell, R. (2009). Comparison of computed tomography and magnetic resonance imaging for the evaluation of canine intranasal neoplasia. *J Small Anim Pract* 50: 334–340.

143 Impellizeri, J.A. and Esplin, G.D. (2008). Expression of cyclooxygenase-2 in canine nasal carcinomas. *Vet J* 176: 408–410.

144 Kleiter, M., Malarkey, D.E., Ruslander, D.E., and Thrall, D.E. (2004). Expression of cyclooxygenase-2 in canine epithelial nasal tumors. *Vet Radiol Ultrasound* 45: 255–260.

145 Nagata, K., Lamb, M., Goldschmidt, M.H. et al. (2014). The usefulness of immunohistochemistry to differentiate between nasal carcinoma and lymphoma in cats: 140 cases (1986–2000). *Vet Comp Oncol* 12: 52–57.

146 Lana, S.E., Dernell, W.S., Larue, S.M. et al. (1997). Slow release cisplatin combined with radiation for the treatment of canine nasal tumors. *Vet Radiol Ultrasound* 38: 474–478.

147 Langova, V., Mutsaers, A.J., Illips, B., and Straw, R. (2004). Treatment of eight dogs with nasal tumours with alternating doses of doxorubicin and carboplatin in conjunction with oral piroxicam. *Aust Vet J* 82: 676–680.

148 Mylonakis, M.E., Saridomichelakis, M.N., Lazaridis, V. et al. (2008). A retrospective study of 61 cases of spontaneous canine epistaxis (1998 to 2001). *J Small Anim Pract* 49: 191–196.

149 Ninomiya, F., Suzuki, S., Tanaka, H. et al. (2008). Nasal and paranasal adenocarcinomas with neuroendocrine differentiation in dogs. *Vet Pathol* 45: 181–187.

150 Vanherberghen, M., Day, M.J., Delvaux, F. et al. (2009). An immunohistochemical study of the inflammatory infiltrate associated with nasal carcinoma in dogs and cats. *J Comp Pathol* 141: 17–26.

151 Patnaik, A.K., Lieberman, P.H., Erlandson, R.A., and Liu, S.K. (1984). Canine sinonasal skeletal neoplasms: chondrosarcomas and osteosarcomas. *Vet Pathol* 21: 475–482.

152 Paiva, S.C.C.S., Werner, J., Montiani-Ferreira, F. et al. (2013). Transitional carcinoma with extensive invasion of the bony orbit in a dog. *Arq Bras Med Vet Zoo* 65: 1017–1023.

153 Bosward, K.L., Kessell, A.E., and Lucy, R.J. (2004). Squamous cell carcinoma with sarcomatous stroma in the nasal cavity of a dog. *Aust Vet J* 82: 553–555.

154 De Vos, J., Vega, R.S., Noorman, E., and de Vos, P. (2012). Primary frontal sinus squamous cell carcinoma in three dogs treated with piroxicam combined with carboplatin or toceranib. *Vet Comp Oncol* 10: 206–213.

155 Rogers, K.S., Walker, M.A., and Helman, R.G. (1996). Squamous cell carcinoma of the canine nasal cavity and frontal sinus: eight cases. *J Am Anim Hosp Assoc* 32: 103–110.

156 Fujita, M., Takaishi, Y., Yasuda, D. et al. (2008). Intranasal hemangiosarcoma in a dog. *J Vet Med Sci* 70: 525–528.

157 Fukuda, S., Kobayashi, T., Robertson, I.D. et al. (2014). Computed tomographic features of canine nonparenchymal hemangiosarcoma. *Vet Radiol Ultrasound* 55: 374–379.

158 Day, M.J., Henderson, S.M., Belshaw, Z., and Bacon, N.J. (2004). An immunohistochemical investigation of 18 cases of feline nasal lymphoma. *J Comp Pathol* 130: 152–161.

159 Hicks, D.G. and Fidel, J.L. (2006). Intranasal malignant melanoma in a dog. *J Am Anim Hosp Assoc* 42: 472–476.

160 Mcghie, J.A., Fitzgerald, L., and Hosgood, G. (2015). Angioleiomyosarcoma in the nasal vestibule of a dog: surgical excision via a modified lateral approach. *J Am Anim Hosp Assoc* 51: 130–135.

161 Burgess, K.E., Green, E.M., Wood, R.D., and Dubielzig, R.R. (2011). Angiofibroma of the nasal cavity in 13 dogs. *Vet Comp Oncol* 9: 304–309.

162 Hara, K., Shimada, A., Morita, T. et al. (2002). Olfactory neuroepithelioma in a dog: an immunohistochemical and electron microscopic study. *J Vet Med Sci* 64: 391–393.

163 Leroith, T., Binder, E.M., Graham, H.A., and Duncan, R.B. (2009). Respiratory epithelial adenomatoid hamartoma in a dog. *J Vet Diagn Invest* 21: 918–920.

164 Swinbourne, F., Kulendra, E., Smith, K. et al. (2014). Inflammatory myofibroblastic tumour in the nasal cavity of a dog. *J Small Anim Pract* 55: 121–124.

165 Koehler, J.W., Weiss, R.C., Aubry, O.A. et al. (2012). Nasal tumor with widespread cutaneous metastases in a golden retriever. *Vet Pathol* 49: 870–875.

166 Patnaik, A.K., Ludwig, L.L., and Erlandson, R.A. (2002). Neuroendocrine carcinoma of the nasopharynx in a dog. *Vet Pathol* 39: 496–500.

167 Sako, T., Shimoyama, Y., Akihara, Y. et al. (2005). Neuroendocrine carcinoma in the nasal cavity of ten dogs. *J Comp Pathol* 133: 155–163.

168 Brosinski, K., Janik, D., Polkinghorne, A. et al. (2012). Olfactory neuroblastoma in dogs and cats: a histological and immunohistochemical analysis. *J Comp Pathol* 146: 152–159.

169 Ueno, H., Kobayashi, Y., and Yamada, K. (2007). Olfactory esthesioneuroblastoma treated with orthovoltage radiotherapy in a dog. *Aust Vet J* 85: 271–275.

170 Ginel, P., Molleda, J.M., Novales, M. et al. (1995). Primary transmissible venereal tumour in the nasal cavity of a dog. *Vet Rec* 136: 222–223.

171 Parent, R., Teuscher, E., Morin, M. et al. (1983). Presence of the canine transmissible venereal tumor in the nasal cavity of dogs in the area of Dakar (Senegal). *Can Vet J* 24: 287–288.

172 Rogers, K.S., Walker, M.A., and Dillon, H.B. (1998). Transmissible venereal tumor: a retrospective study of 29 cases. *J Am Anim Hosp Assoc* 34: 463–470.

173 Naganobu, K., Ogawa, H., Uchida, K. et al. (2000). Mast cell tumor in the nasal cavity of a dog. *J Vet Med Sci* 62: 1009–1011.

174 Avner, A., Dobson, J.M., Sales, J.I., and Herrtage, M.E. (2008). Retrospective review of 50 canine nasal tumours evaluated by low-field magnetic resonance imaging. *J Small Anim Pract* 49: 233–239.

175 Patnaik, A.K., Lieberman, P.H., Erlandson, R.A. et al. (1986). Paranasal meningioma in the dog: a clinicopathologic study of ten cases. *Vet Pathol* 23: 362–368.

176 Beam, S.L., Rassnick, K.M., Moore, A.S., and McDonough, S.P. (2003). An immunohistochemical study of cyclooxygenase-2 expression in various feline neoplasms. *Vet Pathol* 40: 496–500.

177 Lamb, C.R., Sibbing, K., and Priestnall, S.L. (2016). Pathologic basis for rim enhancement observed in computed tomographic images of feline nasopharyngeal polyps. *Vet Radiol Ultrasound* 57: 130–136.

178 Louwerens, M., London, C.A., Pedersen, N.C., and Lyons, L.A. (2005). Feline lymphoma in the post-feline leukemia virus era. *J Vet Intern Med* 19: 329–335.

179 Psalla, D., Geigy, C., Konar, M. et al. (2008). Nasal acinic cell carcinoma in a cat. *Vet Pathol* 45: 365–368.

180 Doughty, R.W., Brockman, D., Neiger, R., and McKinney, L. (2006). Nasal oncocytoma in a domestic shorthair cat. *Vet Pathol* 43: 751–754.

181 You, M.-H., Kim, Y.-B., Woo, G.-H. et al. (2011). Nasopharyngeal oncocytoma in a cat. *J Vet Diagn Invest* 23: 391–394.

182 Scavelli, T.D., Patnaik, A.K., Mehlhaff, C.J., and Hayes, A.A. (1985). Hemangiosarcoma in the cat: retrospective evaluation of 31 surgical cases. *J Am Vet Med Assoc* 187: 817–819.

183 Wong, V.M., Snyman, H.N., Ackerley, C., and Bienzle, D. (2012). Primary nasal histiocytic sarcoma of macrophage–myeloid cell type in a cat. *J Comp Pathol* 147: 209–213.

184 Mellanby, R.J., Stevenson, R.K., Herrtage, M.E. et al. (2002). Long-term outcome of 56 dogs with nasal tumours treated with four doses of radiation at intervals of seven days. *Vet Rec* 151: 253–257.

185 Lamb, C.R., Richbell, S., and Mantis, P. (2003). Radiographic signs in cats with nasal disease. *J Feline Med Surg* 5: 227–235.

186 Kaldrymidou, E., Papaioannou, N., Poutahidis, T.H. et al. (2000). Malignant lymphoma in nasal cavity and paranasal sinuses of a dog. *J Vet Med A* 47: 457–462.

187 Felisberto, R., Matos, J., Alves, M. et al. (2017). Evaluation of *Pax*5 expression and comparison with BLA.36 and CD79αcy in feline non-Hodgkin lymphoma. *Vet Comp Oncol* 15: 1257–1268.

188 Pohlman, L.M., Higginbotham, M.L., Welles, E.G., and Johnson, C.M. (2009). Immunophenotypic and histologic classification of 50 cases of feline gastrointestinal lymphoma. *Vet Pathol* 46: 259–268.

189 Greci, V. and Mortellaro, C. (2016). Management of otic and nasopharyngeal, and nasal polyps in cats and dogs. *Vet Clin North Am Small Anim Pract* 46: 643–661.

190 Klose, T.C., Macphail, C.M., Schultheiss, P.C. et al. (2010). Prevalence of select infectious agents in inflammatory aural and nasopharyngeal polyps from client-owned cats. *J Feline Med Surg* 12: 769–774.

191 Chambers, B.A., Laksito, M.A., Fliegner, R.A. et al. (2010). Nasal vascular hamartoma in a Domestic Shorthair cat. *Aust Vet J* 88: 107–111.

192 Greci, V., Mortellaro, C.M., Olivero, D. et al. (2011). Inflammatory polyps of the nasal turbinates of cats: an argument for designation as feline mesenchymal nasal hamartoma. *J Feline Med Surg* 13: 213–219.

193 Zemljič, T., Matheis, F.L., Venzin, C. et al. (2011). Orbito-nasal cyst in a young European short-haired cat. *Vet Ophthalmol* 14: 122–129.

194 Parker, V.J., Morrison, J., and Yaeger, M.J. (2010). Olfactory neuroblastoma in a cat. *J Feline Med Surg* 12: 867–871.

195 Durham, A.C., Popovitch, C.A., and Goldschmidt, M.H. (2008). Feline chondrosarcoma: a retrospective study of 67 cats (1987–2005). *J Am Anim Hosp Assoc* 44: 124–130.

25

Lower Respiratory Tract of the Dog and Cat

Alice Defarges Bichot and Dorothee Bienzle

Introduction

The lower respiratory tracts (LRT) of the dog and cat are susceptible to a range of infectious, degenerative, and neoplastic conditions, some of which induce intraluminal or parenchymal inflammation. Cells and other constituents within the lumen of lower airways are readily collected for cytological analysis with different lavage techniques and are useful for classifying inflammation; identifying infectious agents or accumulated lipid, protein, or crystals; and diagnosing neoplasia. Correspondingly, parenchymal lung lesions localized by imaging can be sampled by direct aspiration, depending on the size of the animal, often yielding diagnostic specimens. Special considerations for cytological analysis of lesions in the LRT pertain to standardization of techniques for lavages and aspiration; integration of cytological findings with imaging; microbiological, molecular, and other assays; and appreciation of the limits of cytology to distinguish hyperplastic from neoplastic cells. This chapter briefly reviews the anatomy of the LRT followed by different sampling techniques. Associated cytology findings in health and disease are reviewed, organisms and degenerative conditions most frequently associated with LRT disease are described and illustrated, and evidence for cytological approaches in the diagnosis of specific neoplasms is considered.

Anatomy and Immunology

The LRT consists of the trachea, bronchi, bronchioles, and alveoli. The trachea extends from the larynx to the carina and, in dogs and cats, is composed of incomplete cartilaginous rings supported by connective tissue and smooth muscle.[1,2] The tracheal epithelium is ciliated and pseudostratified with interspersed goblet cells. Bronchial cartilaginous rings are complete, and after the third to fourth bronchial branching, the airways no longer have cartilaginous support and are termed bronchioles. Bronchioles are surrounded by smooth muscle, supported by attachment to lung parenchyma and lined by ciliated and non-ciliated cuboidal to columnar epithelium. The bronchial epithelium includes serous and mucus-secreting cells. Terminal bronchioles branch into respiratory bronchioles lacking ciliated cells, and those further divide into alveolar ducts, alveolar sacs, and alveoli.[3] Flat (squamous) epithelial cells (type I pneumocytes) with fewer interspersed cuboidal epithelial cells (type II pneumocytes) line the alveoli, and capillaries intimately surround the alveoli. In lung from healthy dogs, mast cells, macrophages, dendritic cells, and lymphocytes are present primarily in the subepithelial lamina propria of trachea and bronchi with occasional intraepithelial lymphocytes and mast cells.[4] In the lower airway, T lymphocytes outnumber B lymphocytes, and IgA-expressing lymphocytes outnumber IgG- and IgM-expressing lymphocytes.[4] Bronchus-associated lymphoid tissue, common in other species, is absent in dog and cat lung.[4] Cells of bronchial, bronchiolar, or alveolar epithelium may be present in lavage samples if the tissue is injured or if excessive negative pressure is applied during lavage.[5] Luminal leukocytes are largely absent in the conducting airways, but macrophages are prominent in alveoli.[6] Parenchymal lung disease often also affects the airways and luminal leukocytes.[7,8]

Diagnostic Approach

Clinical Signs and Physical Examination

The most commonly recognized clinical signs of tracheobronchial disease are coughing, stertorous noisy inspiratory sounds, stridulous or wheezing expiratory sounds, and occasionally cyanosis. Patients with pulmonary parenchymal disorders can have a variety of clinical

Veterinary Cytology, First Edition. Edited by Leslie C. Sharkey, M. Judith Radin, and Davis Seelig.

signs related either to respiratory dysfunction or systemic disease. Common manifestations are cough, exercise intolerance, tachypnea, excessive panting, and respiratory distress; less common manifestations are hemoptysis, collapse or syncope, and cyanosis. Lameness may be a presenting sign in cats with bronchial carcinoma that has metastasized to digits.[9] The most common clinical signs in dogs with hypertrophic osteoarthropathy associated with either metastatic or primary pulmonary neoplasia or with pulmonary infection were leg swelling and lameness.[10,11] Physical examination is important to detect tracheal sensitivity, abnormal lung sounds, heart murmurs, stertor, stridor, dyspnea, and increased body temperature. Some respiratory infections also affect other organs; therefore, a full physical examination should be performed in all animals with pulmonary disease.

Diagnostic Evaluation of Respiratory Disease

Localizing pulmonary disease requires integration of physical and imaging findings, visualization of large airways, and evaluation of specific airway or tissue samples. The distribution of lung disease can reflect the inciting cause: disease affecting primarily the airways suggests exposure by inhalation, while interstitial lung disease usually arises from non-airway tissues such as alveolar and interlobular septae or vasculature. Results of a complete blood cell count are often normal, but eosinophilia can characterize parasitic infestations, eosinophilic bronchopneumopathy (dogs), and asthma (cats), and neutrophilia with a left shift can reflect bacterial or fungal bronchopneumonia and necrotic pulmonary neoplasms.[12–14]

Molecular and serologic tests are available to detect many infectious agents and allergens. Tests are selected based on history, clinical, or microscopic findings. Bacterial and fungal agents are often recognized microscopically in cytology samples and can be further identified by microbial culture, antibody assays, or antigen detection in blood or urine.[14,15] Alternatively, viral respiratory infections rarely generate pathognomonic cytologic findings and require identification by viral culture, polymerase chain reaction (PCR), or serology. Many laboratories offer PCR panels for respiratory infectious agents, which is helpful because multiple organisms are often present. However, for microbial culture and PCR, it is essential to submit samples (lavage, aspirate, or biopsy) that are likely to contain organisms.

Imaging is crucial to localize lung lesions and to suggest an etiology. Thoracic radiography can suggest an etiology based on patterns such as alveolar (bronchopneumonia), bronchial (bronchitis, asthma), or nodular (blastomycosis, parasitic infection, neoplasm) patterns.[16–19] Consolidated lung lobes or enlarged lymph nodes are also readily detected by radiography. Radiography was moderately sensitive for identifying lung tumors in cats (67%, $n = 79$) and dogs (77%, $n = 210$),[20,21] and for diagnosing bronchiectasis, thromboembolism, hyperinflation, and atelectasis.[22,23] Computed tomography (CT) provides greater detail for identifying lung tumors and conditions such as bronchiectasis and can be used to guide fine-needle aspiration (FNA) and biopsy.[24–28] Methods for transbronchial biopsy of parenchymal nodules during real-time CT have been described in dogs, but are not yet widely used in animals.[29] Ultrasound-guided FNA of focal parenchymal lung lesions is a valuable technique that yielded cytologic findings highly correlated with histopathology and autopsy diagnosis.[30] Contrast-enhanced ultrasonography provides greater detail on lesion edges and poorly perfused regions than regular ultrasonography and yielded diagnostic samples in all 40 cases with noncardiac thoracic disorders.[31] Although imaging is essential to investigate lung disease, it is usually insufficient to confirm a specific disease and initiate therapy. Microscopy evaluation of the respiratory tract is required for definitive diagnoses.

Types of Lower Airway Samples

Techniques commonly employed to obtain samples for cytology and/or culture include tracheal wash, either by transtracheal wash (TTW) or transoral tracheal wash (TOTW), bronchoalveolar lavage (BAL), with or without bronchial brushing, and transthoracic lung aspiration (Table 25.1). TTW and lung aspiration are performed awake with or without sedation, while TOTW and BAL require general anesthesia.

Tracheal Wash

Tracheal wash collects material from the tracheal lumen in a sterile manner to obtain cytologic confirmation of suspected inflammation, infection, allergy, parasitic infestation, or neoplasia. Tracheal washes are performed via either a transoral (also called endotracheal) or transtracheal approach, depending on clinician preference and patient characteristics. The transoral approach can be more suitable for small dogs and cats where placement of a needle in the intertracheal ring space is difficult, or if the animal is fractious and general anesthesia is necessary.[32] For this procedure, brief general anesthesia is induced with injectable agents, an endotracheal tube is placed, a rubber catheter (8 Fr) is fed through the endotracheal tube, and saline is infused and re-aspirated, while coupage and tracheal palpation are applied to encourage coughing.[33] Alternatively, the caudal aspect of the animal can be elevated, and the draining fluid collected as it exits from the

Table 25.1 Techniques for sampling the lower respiratory tract.

	Advantages	Limitations
Tracheal wash	Readily performed with minimal specialized equipment Identification of bacterial and/or mycotic infection, aspirated material	Restricted to trachea and large bronchi; possible pharyngeal contamination with transoral approach May need sedation or general anesthesia
Tracheobronchial brush cytology	Sampling of directly visualized tracheobronchial lesions	Need for special equipment and expertise General anesthesia required
Bronchoalveolar lavage	Identification of alveolar cells, infectious agents, and other constituents Samples suitable for culture to characterize infection Can sample multiple lung regions	Need for special equipment (bronchoscopic BAL) and expertise May need to lavage multiple lung regions General anesthesia required
Ultrasound- or CT-guided transthoracic aspiration of masses or parenchyma	Direct identification of neoplastic cells, fungal and bacterial agents	Expertise and imaging equipment required Risk of pneumothorax if lesion distant from pleura

BAL, bronchoalveolar lavage; CT, computed tomography.

endotracheal tube.[34] This procedure is practical and easy to perform with equipment available in general practice but is more prone to oropharyngeal contamination and can yield less sample volume than TTW since the cough reflex is suppressed by anesthesia.[34]

For TTW, a local anesthetic and light sedation, if needed, are administered before percutaneous puncture either between mid-tracheal rings or through the cricothyroid ligament with a through-the-needle catheter. Insertion of the needle between tracheal rings is easier in more anterior locations since muscle coverage increases toward the thoracic inlet. One milliliter of sterile warmed saline per kilogram of body weight (maximum 10 mL) is injected through the catheter and immediately re-aspirated. Washes reflecting luminal content of trachea and large bronchi in health contain few leukocytes, a small amount of mucus, and no surfactant.[12,35,36] Complications of TTW are uncommon, but consist of subcutaneous emphysema, pneumomediastinum, pneumothorax, airway bleeding, and cellulitis.[7] Transient bronchoconstriction and a mild neutrophil influx into the airways can occur.[35]

Bronchoalveolar Lavage (BAL)

Indications for BAL include chronic cough, bronchial or interstitial changes on thoracic radiographs, and lung masses. Protocols for BAL in cats and dogs with and without bronchoscopic guidance have been described.[5,37–40] In non-bronchoscopic BAL, a soft sterile rubber catheter is introduced through an endotracheal tube and wedged in a bronchus for infusion and re-aspiration of saline without visualization of the airway. This technique can be readily performed in small dogs and cats with minimal equipment to lavage the dependent caudal lung lobe (e.g. the left caudal lung lobe when the patient is in left lateral recumbency, and vice versa); therefore animals should be positioned appropriately.[37,41]

In bronchoscopic BAL, a flexible fiber-optic bronchoscope is guided into a chosen bronchus and gently wedged into position. Then, aliquots of sterile saline are injected through the biopsy channel and immediately re-aspirated with a syringe or pump.[5] Multiple samples can be obtained in this manner from one or more sites. The recommended volume of saline for infusion is 1–3 mL/kg of body weight or 5–20 mL per site in dogs and 3–10 mL aliquots per site in cats.[12,32,39,42,43] A "foamy" appearance of the aspirated fluid indicates presence of surfactant and therefore lavage of distal airways. Ideally, >50% of infused volume is recovered by BAL, and the proportion of fluid retrieved as well as any complications during the procedure should be indicated on cytology submission forms.[5,32] The advantages of bronchoscopy for BAL are that abnormalities of the airways can be visualized for direct brushing and/or biopsy and that the bronchoscope can be wedged in specific regions of the lung for lavage of defined segments.[7] However, even use of very narrow diameter pediatric endoscopes in small patients requires removal of the endotracheal tube, which increases the risk of oxygen desaturation and prolonged recovery.[44]

Both non-bronchoscopic and bronchoscopic BAL are considered safe in healthy cats and those with respiratory disease, although transient hypoxemia, bronchoconstriction, and exacerbation of respiratory insufficiency can occur.[7,39,45] Despite widespread veterinary use of BAL, neither lavage technique nor lavage fluid volume is standardized for dogs or cats, and decisions are made based on clinician preferences. In healthy dogs, BAL repeated at five- to seven-week intervals did not significantly change cell concentration or composition, but cynomolgus monkeys had airway neutrophilia 24 hours after lavage.[43,46]

Tracheobronchial Brushing

Tracheobronchial brushing allows cytological evaluation of visible endobronchial lesions.[47–49] Specimens are obtained with an endoscopic brush passed through the biopsy channel of the endoscope, moved forth and back along the bronchial wall, withdrawn, and rolled on glass slides. Alternatively, a protected sterile culture swab or cytology brush can also be introduced directly through the oral cavity and larynx into the trachea for specimen retrieval. Agreement of tracheobronchial brush cytology with BAL cytology was good for detecting the presence of inflammation, but the type of inflammation identified frequently differed between techniques.[49] In dogs with chronic cough, bronchial brushing cytology was more likely to reveal inflammation than BAL cytology.[48] Bronchial brushing also has utility in detecting *Bordetella* organisms adherent to epithelial cells.[50] Possible reasons for discrepant cytology findings of bronchial brushing and BAL are restricted mural origin by the former versus representation of intraluminal constituents of multiple bronchioles and alveoli by the latter technique. Brush cytology should be considered a useful adjunct but not a replacement for BAL. Brush cytology can be particularly useful when a hypocellular BAL sample is anticipated because of retrieval of low volume or surfactant-poor fluid or when a bronchoscope of appropriate size for lower airways is unavailable.

Transthoracic Lung Aspiration

This technique is useful when lymphadenopathy, lung lobe consolidation, or discrete lung masses are identified by radiography or ultrasonography. Non-sedated patients should be placed in sternal recumbency. If the patient is struggling or fractious, sedation can minimize procedural risks. Proper restraint is critical, but general anesthesia is typically not required. Local anesthetic can be injected at the anterior aspect of the intercostal space since intercostal vessels and nerves are located at the posterior aspect of ribs. Aspiration is usually performed with ultrasound or CT guidance; however, blind aspirates have also been reported.[20,27,31,51] An area of skin approximately 4 × 6 cm over the site to be aspirated is clipped and prepared aseptically. Several aspiration techniques are described. Once the chest cavity has been entered with the needle, slight negative pressure is applied to the syringe, and the needle tip is advanced to the appropriate depth as estimated by imaging, withdrawn slightly, and readvanced through the lesion while maintaining negative pressure.[30] Alternatively, the needle is placed in the lesion and advanced and retracted several times without negative pressure before removal.[52] Retracting and advancing the needle at slightly different angles ("fanning") might enhance the likelihood of obtaining a representative sample but was also more likely to induce bleeding.[52] Speed is critical to minimize clotting, which distorts cells and can render cellular samples nondiagnostic. Therefore, rapid preparation of slides, even before appearance of cellular material in the needle hub, should be attempted.[52] If non-hemorrhagic fluid is aspirated, it should be transferred to a tube without additive. If blood-tinged fluid is aspirated, the sample should be quickly placed in a small (3 mL) EDTA tube to minimize clotting. If overtly hemorrhagic fluid is aspirated, the procedure should be halted and reattempted at another site.

The reported proportion of lung aspirates yielding sufficient cellular material for cytopathologic interpretation varies from 65 to 85%.[27,51,53] Compared with histopathology, cytopathology had >80% sensitivity and specificity for diagnosis of 18 and 28 lung neoplasms from dogs and cats, respectively.[27,51,53] Aspiration of solid lung masses was also highly sensitive and specific for neoplasms and blastomycosis in dogs and cats,[30] and cytopathology agreed with histopathology in 82% of 45 cat lung carcinomas.[20] Obtaining adequate samples was the main limitation for cytologic diagnosis of lung tumors in another study of dogs, but direct aspiration was nevertheless considered a successful diagnostic method.[21]

Clinically important adverse effects from image-guided aspiration or tissue biopsy of lung parenchyma are rare,[30] although subclinical pneumothorax or hemorrhage detected by CT was noted in 43% of 30 cases.[27] In one study, non-guided pulmonary needle aspiration was associated with severe pneumothorax, intrapulmonary hemorrhage, hemoptysis, or death in 2, 1, 2, and 5 cases, respectively, of 32 cases.[51] However, several dogs that died had also extrapulmonary diseases such as lymphoma, disseminated intravascular coagulation, and myocarditis; therefore, such findings may not be representative of all patients selected for FNA.[51] Adequate platelet mass and coagulation times, lesion location proximal to the thoracic wall, and image guidance for aspiration are likely to minimize adverse effects. Post-procedure monitoring of respiratory and cardiac function is important.

Deep Oral Swab

In humans, throat swabs are considered suitable to identify lower airway infection. In dogs, culture and sensitivity results from deep oral swabs are poorly correlated with those from TTOW, likely due to oral contamination or failure to obtain a representative sample. This sample type is therefore not recommended.[33]

Sample Handling and Analysis

Standardized processing of fluids is important for repeatable results and for comparison between studies and institutions (Table 25.2). Cell and protein concentrations are typically not determined for tracheal washes and for BAL fluid (BALF) only in some laboratories. The volume of saline infused and retrieved is highly variable, and therefore the degree of dilution is inconsistent.[40] At our institution, cell concentration in BALF is measured with an electrical

Table 25.2 Handling, processing, and assessing bronchoalveolar lavage fluid.

Variable	Recommendation
Sample handling	Cytology: Assess fluid from each BAL site individually Pool sequential lavage fluids from the same site Microbiology: Pool samples from all lavage sites
Time to process	Ideally within one hour. If this is not possible, place sample on ice or store at 4 °C and process within four hours
Filtration	Do not filter fluid
Total nucleated cell count	Manual hemocytometer count on whole fluid or single cell particle counting on whole fluid
Cytologic evaluation	Cytocentrifuge 100–200 µL (depending on estimated cell concentration) of sample for 5 minutes Prepare 1–2 featheredge smears from centrifuged cell pellet Stain slides with Romanowsky-type stain Differentially count at least 200 and ideally 400–500 cells on cytocentrifuge preparation Enumerate each type of leukocyte, epithelial cells, and erythrocytes as separate categories Evaluate cell pellet smear for similarity in cell distribution to cytocentrifuge slide Identify infectious agents Recommend additional stains, culture, molecular, or other assays, as appropriate
Additives	Adding fixatives and/or preservatives to BALF is not recommended Effect of adding serum to BALF is unknown

BAL, bronchoalveolar lavage; BALF, bronchoalveolar lavage fluid.

impedance particle counter. Subjectively, microscopic correlation with the number of cells on cytospin preparations is generally reasonable in samples from medium to large dogs, but less consistent in small dog or cat samples. A possible reason is that aspiration of lavage fluid is more likely to result in high negative pressure in small diameter airways, thereby inducing collapse of non-cartilaginous bronchioles, which in turn reduces fluid retrieval.[54] Protein concentration in BALF is very low and not routinely measured. Therefore, qualitative assessment of cells is the mainstay of TTW and BAL interpretation. The laboratory should prepare at least one cytocentrifuged slide and one featheredge film of centrifuged cell pellets. The turbidity of the BALF can be used as an approximate guide to adjust the volume to yield cytocentrifuge preparations with a single cell layer. Two hundred microliter is suitable for clear BAL and TTW fluid, while 100 µL can yield better quality thin preparations from turbid (abnormal) samples.[5] For cell pellet slides, the fluid should be centrifuged for 10 minutes at 500–600 g, the supernatant discarded, and the cell pellet resuspended in the small amount of fluid remaining in the tube for preparation of featheredge smears. The cytocentrifuge preparation generally yields superior cell preservation and is more suitable for differential counting compared to cell pellet smears, but the cell differential count may differ slightly between preparations.[42] Hence, both types of slides should be prepared and reviewed.

Appropriately collected BALF should reflect luminal cells of the respiratory bronchioles and alveoli. Cell concentration in lavage fluid is determined in many institutions although different volumes and different methods of infusing and retrieving fluid render it challenging to establish firm reference intervals associated with health. Most studies assessing BALF in healthy animals report <500 cells/µL (0.5×10^9/L), >70% alveolar macrophages, and <10% lymphocytes, neutrophils, eosinophils, or mast cells (Figure 25.1).[12,43,47] In healthy dogs and cats, epithelial cells comprise <1% of cells in BALF, and a higher proportion can be associated with excessive negative pressure during the procedure, an incompletely immobilized patient, or injured epithelium such as in viral infections.[5,12,43,48,55–57] Ciliated epithelial cells indicate exfoliation from trachea, bronchi, or proximal bronchioles. Cuboidal epithelial cells are likely non-ciliated epithelial (club) cells from the distant bronchioles, and flat epithelial cells are likely type I pneumocytes from the alveoli. Presence of *Simonsiella* bacteria or keratinized squamous epithelial cells indicates oropharyngeal contamination and/or aspiration of gastric content. A paucity of alveolar macrophages raises concern that alveoli were not lavaged. Low BAL cell concentration can indicate lavage of large rather than small airways. Hence, cytological evaluation of

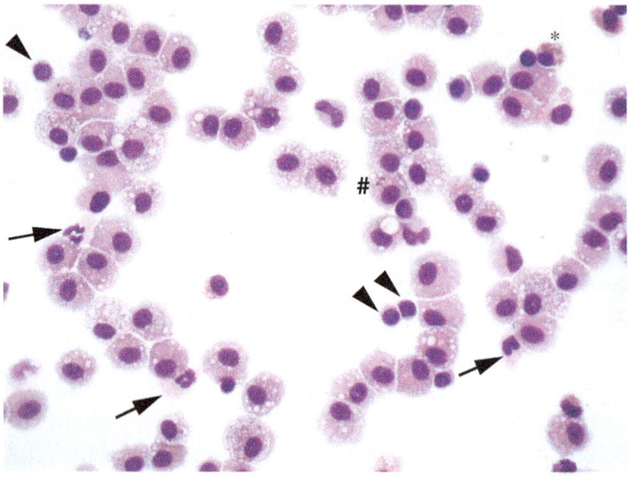

Figure 25.1 Cytocentrifuge preparation of BAL from a clinically healthy dog. The predominant cells (92%) are alveolar macrophages with light pink cytoplasm and variable degree of vacuolation. There are also a few small lymphocytes (arrowheads), neutrophils (arrows), and eosinophils (*). One macrophage contains small aggregates of pigment (#) that may represent environmental particulate carbon inhalation. Note absence of erythrocytes and epithelial cells (Wright stain, 400×).

any BAL slides is indicative of whether the sample is representative of the lower airways.

Defining parameters for analysis is important for cytologic interpretation of BAL. The American Thoracic Society recommends that at least 400 cells should be differentially counted, and for reproducible assessment of the proportion of all cells in BALF from dogs with bronchopneumonia, differential counting of 500 cells was recommended.[58,59] There is variability in the "normal values" reported from different institutions, which is particularly marked for the proportion of eosinophils in cat BALF. Such differences likely reflect variability in the definition and origin of "clinically normal animals," in the BAL procedure, in the manner of processing of fluid, and in microscopic assessment. In studies from Europe, control cats consistently had <8% eosinophils in BAL,[42,60] while in studies from North America eosinophil proportions of 10[61], 18[62], and 26%[12] are reported for clinically normal cats. Therefore, caution is required when considering the "normal" proportion of eosinophils in cat BAL.

At our institution, we prepare one cytocentrifuge slide with cells in monolayer and two slides of a centrifuged fluid pellet with a featheredge. At least 200 consecutive leukocytes on the cytocentrifuged slide are differentially counted for samples with concentration of <300 cells/μL, and epithelial cells and erythrocytes are enumerated in separate categories. If the cell concentration is >300 cells/μL, at least 400 consecutive leukocytes are counted. The cell pellet smears are reviewed for similarity to the cytocentrifuge preparation in cell composition.

Cytologic Features of Lower Respiratory Tract Samples

Tracheal Wash and Brushing

In healthy animals, cells dislodged during tracheobronchial washing are few and consist almost exclusively of a few ciliated columnar and non-ciliated cuboidal epithelial cells, a few goblet cells, and rare macrophages or other leukocytes.[32,35] Tracheal washes are suitable for diagnosing mycotic infections,[12,14] aspiration pneumonia,[63] suppurative inflammation, and bacterial infection associated with bronchiectasis[17,64] and for obtaining samples for viral PCR testing.[65] Tracheal or bronchial brushings in healthy dogs consist almost entirely of epithelial cells, while >7% leukocytes were noted in dogs with cough.[48] Bronchial brushing was suitable for diagnosis of *Bordetella* and *Aspergillus* infection.[50,66] Tracheobronchial brushing yielded results discordant with BAL regarding the type or presence of inflammation in 54% of 34 dogs and 4 of 5 cats with chronic cough.[49] Hence, it has to be considered that brushings are likely to detect focal mural lesions, that BAL reflects more widespread luminal inflammation, and that results from these techniques will yield distinct though complementary information about the respiratory tract.

Bronchoalveolar Lavage

BAL samples are generally considered hypocellular if the concentration is <500 and <400 cells/μL in dogs and cats, respectively,[12] although in other studies of normal dogs counts were <300 cells/μL (Table 25.3).[5,43,47] Alveolar macrophages are the predominant cell type in BAL from healthy animals. Alveolar macrophages are large cells with abundant pale pink cytoplasm that frequently is vacuolated and may contain phagocytized material (Figure 25.1). The nucleus of alveolar macrophages is round to oval and located central or slightly eccentric. Alveolar macrophages phagocytose particulate matter and microorganisms that reach the alveoli, regulate activation of innate and adaptive immune responses, and absorb and catabolize surfactant (Figure 25.2).[67] Occasional binucleate alveolar macrophages may be an incidental finding, while multinucleate forms are associated with cell activation and increased phagocytosis in conditions such as endogenous lipid pneumonia, mycobacterial infection, and lycoperdonosis (pyogranulomatous bronchointerstitial pneumonia from inhalation of mushroom spores).[8,68–70] Other cell types present in BAL in low numbers are lymphocytes,

Table 25.3 Expected nucleated cell concentration and proportion of cell types in bronchoalveolar lavage fluid.

	Cells/μL	Macrophage (%)	Lymphocyte (%)	Eosinophil (%)	Neutrophil (%)	Mast cell (%)
Dog	<400–600	70–100	<7	<6	<5	<1
Cat	<400	70–100	<5	<10	<7	<2

Approximate ranges as identified in studies of healthy animals using a variety of techniques.

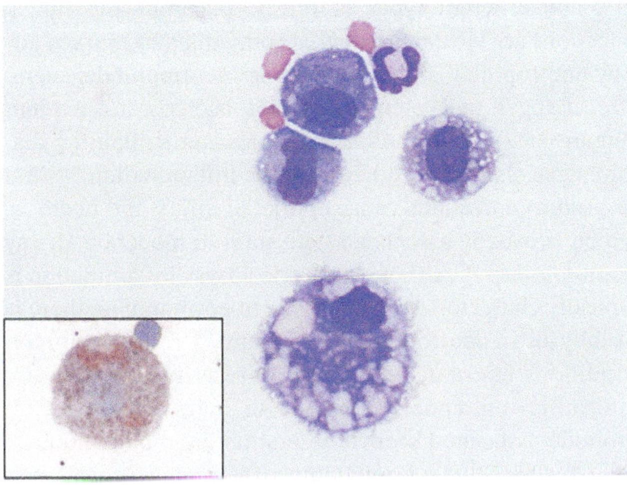

Figure 25.2 Cytocentrifuge preparation of BAL from a clinically normal dog. There are macrophages with variable cytoplasmic vacuolation, occasional erythrocytes, and one neutrophil (Wright stain, 1000×). Inset: Material in large macrophage vacuoles stains positive with Oil Red O and likely consists of pinocytosed surfactant phospholipid.

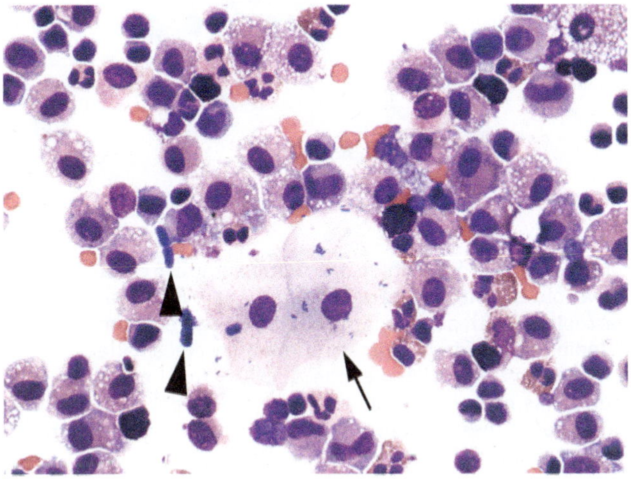

Figure 25.3 Cytocentrifuge preparation of BAL from a dog with cough. The sample consists predominantly of macrophages, but there are also squamous epithelial cells with rod-shaped bacteria (arrow), erythrocytes, eosinophils, and neutrophils. Similar bacteria are free in the background. The arrangement of multiple "stacked up" bacterial cells (arrowheads) is typical of *Simonsiella* bacteria that are commensal organisms of the oropharynx. Their presence indicates that the lavage included the oropharynx. Absence of degenerate neutrophils, phagocytosed bacteria, and food material makes aspiration pneumonia unlikely (Wright stain, 630×).

neutrophils, eosinophils, and mast cells.[40,42] Squamous epithelial cells and bacteria such as *Simonsiella* spp. are not a normal finding in BAL (Figure 25.3) and indicate either inadvertent sampling of the oropharynx, aspiration pneumonia, or tracheoesophageal fistula.[6,71,72]

Erythrocytes are also not normally present in BAL and indicate iatrogenic trauma or acute hemorrhage. If free erythrocytes are accompanied by erythrophagocytosis and hemosiderin pigment in macrophages, *in vivo* pulmonary hemorrhage due to a primary lung lesion, cardiac disease, or chronic injury is likely (Figure 25.4 and 25.5). Tracheal wash hemosiderosis was very common in cats with a variety of inflammatory and neoplastic airway diseases, including rhinitis, and with cardiac disease.[16,73] In dogs, infection with *Angiostrongylus* sp., certain strains of *Streptococcus zooepidemicus*, H3N2 influenza, and herpesvirus 1 resulted pulmonary hemorrhage that was occasionally fatal.[74–77]

Inflammation of the Lower Respiratory Tract

Inflammation of the LRT is identified by increased concentration or altered proportions of inflammatory cells in BALF. Inflammatory cells consist of lymphocytes, plasma

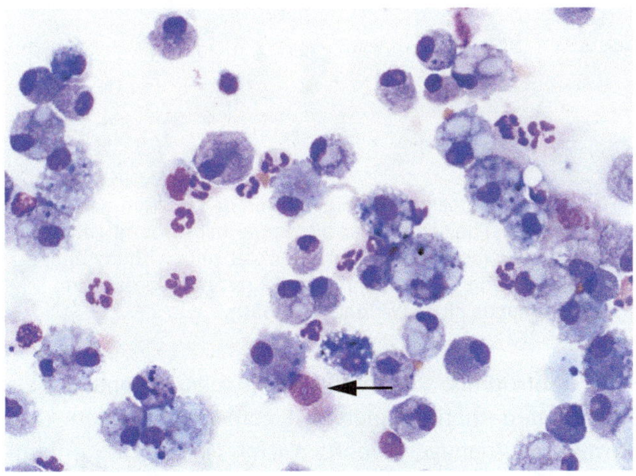

Figure 25.4 Cytocentrifuge preparation of BAL from a 6-year-old cat with myocardial disease. There are numerous macrophages with globular bluish cytoplasmic material and pigment (hemosiderin), non-lytic neutrophils, a few erythrocytes, and one ciliated epithelial cell (arrow) (Wright stain, 630×).

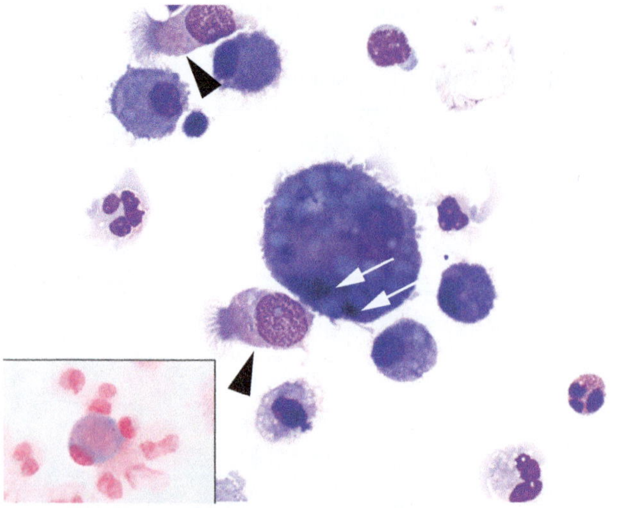

Figure 25.5 Cytocentrifuge preparation of BAL from a 6-year-old cat with myocardial disease. There is one giant macrophage with abundant phagocytosed aggregate material including hemosiderin pigment (arrows), several smaller macrophages, two ciliated epithelial cells (arrowheads), two neutrophils, one eosinophil, and two small lymphocytes (Wright stain, 1000×). Inset: Prussian blue staining confirms the pigment as hemosiderin.

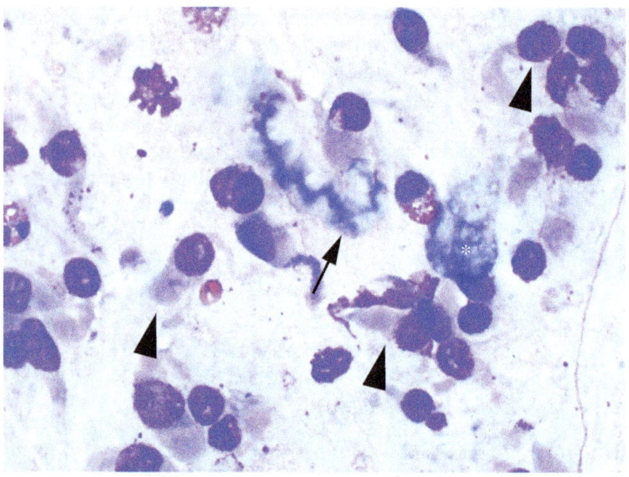

Figure 25.6 Cytocentrifuge preparation of BAL from a dog with chronic cough. The sample has a granular background, columnar epithelial cells (arrowheads), intact goblet cells with distended cytoplasm (*), and Curschmann's spirals (arrow) representing dislodged mucus plugs (Wright stain, 630×).

cells, neutrophils, eosinophils, mast cells, basophils, or a combination thereof. Increased cell concentration with normal macrophage proportion can also indicate inflammation. Other indicators of LRT disease are Curschmann's spirals composed of dislodged mucus plugs from subepithelial mucous gland ducts or bronchioles (Figure 25.6) and goblet cell hyperplasia that occurs in bronchiectasis, bronchopneumonia, and microlithiasis.[7,17,24,78] Goblet cell hyperplasia can manifest with increased mucus apparent on bronchoscopy and numerous goblet cells and excessive mucus on BAL or brush slides. Inflammation identified in BAL samples should be classified according to the predominant cell type or as mixed.

Neutrophilic Inflammation

Airway neutrophilic inflammation is a common response to many different types of injury. Bacterial and fungal infections are virtually always accompanied by marked airway neutrophilia, and in many cases neutrophil degenerative changes and phagocytosis of bacteria are evident (Figure 25.7).[38,50,65,66] Aspiration of water containing diatom algae also induced neutrophilic inflammation.[63] Viral respiratory infections cause epithelial injury and necrosis, which is usually associated with mild to moderate airway neutrophilia.[57,65] Although allergic airway inflammation is typically characterized by prominent eosinophilia, there is usually also a neutrophilic component.[45,60,79] Less common conditions associated with mild airway neutrophilia are idiopathic pulmonary fibrosis in dogs and cats,[80,81] bromide-associated bronchointerstitial lipid pneumonia,[82] bronchiectasis,[16,23] bronchomalacia and tracheal collapse,[64] microlithiasis,[78] and neoplasia.[16] A purulent exudate is sometimes seen during endoscopy (Figure 25.7) and corresponds to neutrophilic inflammation in BAL.[32,39,83]

In the presence of bacteria and their toxins, neutrophils undergo degenerative changes that sometimes result in dispersed nuclear material. The dispersed nuclear material

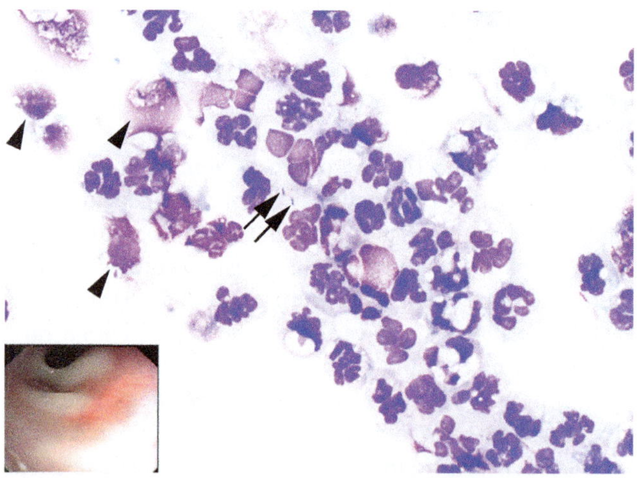

Figure 25.7 Cell pellet smear of a TTW from a 1-year-old cat with intermittent cough. Cells consist of variably lytic neutrophils. Occasional neutrophils contain phagocytosed rod-shaped bacteria (arrows). Lysed nuclear material assumes a fibrillar matrix suggestive of neutrophil extracellular traps (NETs, arrowheads). Bacterial culture yielded *Escherichia coli* (Wright stain, 630×). Inset: Purulent material identified during endoscopy of trachea.

often appears fibrillar and consists primarily of chromatin bound to cytoplasmic proteins. The physical and biochemical properties of such nuclear material serve to trap bacteria, and hence such structures have been termed "neutrophil extracellular traps" (NETs).[84] Disintegrated neutrophils frequently observed in bacterial lung infections have morphology akin to NETs and likely result from a similar pathogenic mechanism (Figure 25.7).[85] The presence of degenerating neutrophils in BAL should prompt bacterial and/or fungal culture, even if bacteria are not microscopically identified. Fungal infections can manifest with plaque during endoscopy, and the inflammatory response is typically a mixture of neutrophils and macrophages, sometimes including multinucleate giant cells (Figure 25.8).[12]

Lymphocytic Inflammation

Causes of increased lymphocytes in BAL are incompletely defined. Lymphocytes and/or plasma cells may reflect immune stimulation, which could be associated with infectious and noninfectious causes. Presence of morphologically abnormal lymphocytes on BAL slides was more sensitive for pulmonary involvement in multicentric lymphoma than radiography.[86]

Eosinophilic Inflammation

Eosinophilic inflammation is usually associated with clinical disease and most often implies allergic or parasitic tracheobronchitis.[13,45,87] The proportion of eosinophils in BAL reported for clinically healthy cats is highly variable, rendering interpretation sometimes difficult.[37,42,60,62] We have observed up to 20% eosinophils in group-housed clinically normal laboratory cats but rarely >10% in individually owned and housed cats. Hence, it is possible that group housing is associated with subclinical allergic airway disease in cats, and we consider >10% eosinophils in BAL from companion cats to be abnormal. The proportion of BAL eosinophils in healthy dogs has been reported as <11%[43,48] but is most often <5%.[79,87] Eosinophilic and neutrophilic inflammation frequently occur together (Figure 25.9), and in dogs with allergic pneumopathy, eosinophils with round nuclei may be observed.[13]

Granulomatous Inflammation

Granulomatous inflammation usually originates in and affects predominantly the lung interstitium, but luminal leukocytes collected during airway lavages can reflect interstitial disease.[58] Multinucleate giant cells and increased number or proportion of macrophages and neutrophils characterize granulomatous inflammation (Figure 25.8). Epithelioid macrophages, named for their granular eosinophilic cytoplasm and tendency to cluster akin to epithelial cells at sites of granuloma formation, can be observed (Figure 25.10). Neutrophils, plasma cells, lymphocytes, and eosinophils are frequently also increased. Typical causes of granulomatous inflammation are infection with fungi such as *Blastomyces*, *Histoplasma*,

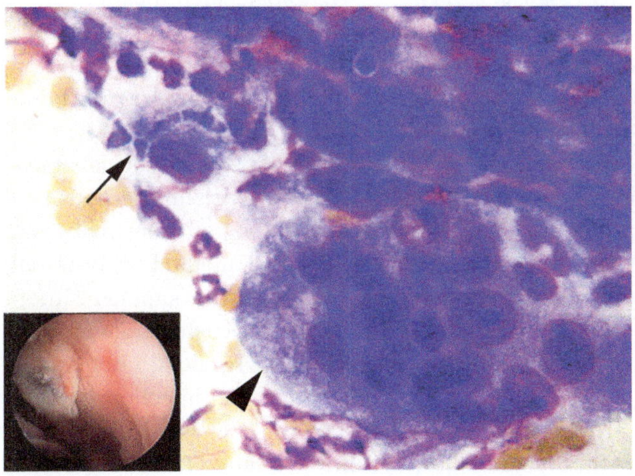

Figure 25.8 Aspirate of a nodular lung lesion from a 3-year-old dog with fever and cough. There is a large multinucleate cell (arrowhead), smaller macrophages, degenerate neutrophils, erythrocytes, and fungal hyphae consistent with *Aspergillus* (arrow) (Wright stain, 630×). Inset: A fungal plaque was apparent during endoscopy.

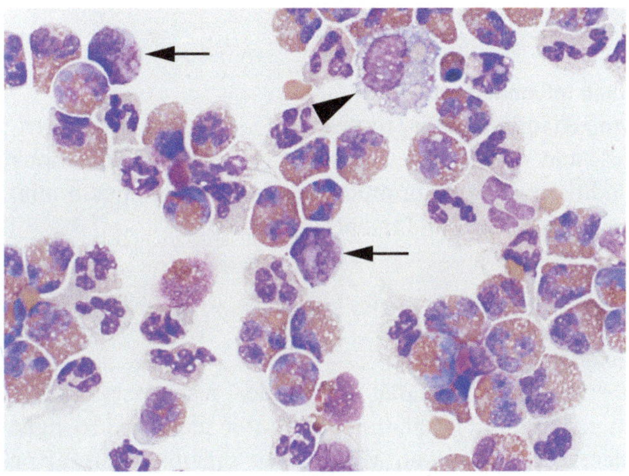

Figure 25.9 Cytocentrifuge preparation of BAL from a 10-year-old dog with a one-month history of pancreatitis and cough. The dog had marked blood eosinophilia and basophilia and a diffuse bronchial pattern with bronchiectasis on radiographs. On bronchoscopy an irregular mucosa, purulent exudate, and possible nodules were noted. The BAL consists predominantly of eosinophils and neutrophils, although basophils (arrows) and macrophages with phagocytosed eosinophil granules (arrowhead) are also apparent. Parasites were not identified in the BAL or by fecal examination, and the dog clinically responded to immunosuppressive therapy (Wright stain, 630×).

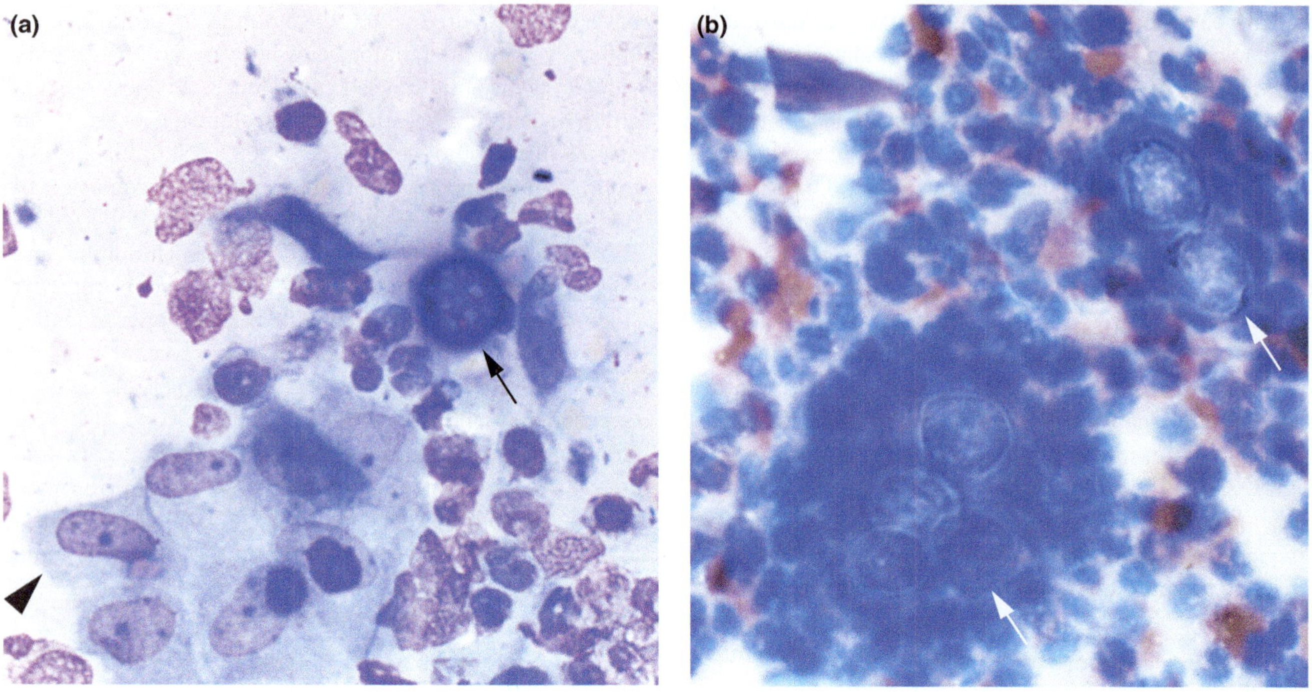

Figure 25.10 Direct aspirate of nodular lung lesions in dogs. (a) A single *Blastomyces* organism (arrow) is surrounded by lytic neutrophils and a cluster of epithelioid macrophages (arrowhead). (b) Budding *Blastomyces* organisms (arrows) have an apparent halo with microscopic focus above cells (Wright stain, 400×).

Coccidioides, and *Aspergillus* spp.; inhalation of puffball mushroom spores; and infection with *Mycobacteria* spp. (Figure 25.10).[8,70,88,89]

Mixed Inflammation

A mixed inflammatory response of non-degenerate neutrophils and macrophages characterizes some noninfectious conditions such as bromide-associated lipid pneumonia, lung lobe torsion, and tracheal collapse.[64,73,90]

Specific Conditions of the Lower Respiratory Tract

Bacterial Pneumonia

Most bacteria associated with clinical respiratory disease are acquired by inhalation and can be identified by light microscopy. However, *Mycoplasma* organisms are at or near the level of light microscopic resolution, are difficult to visualize, and are usually identified by culture or PCR.[91] Dogs are most often infected with *Mycoplasma cynos*, but since healthy and diseased dogs have similar rates of detection of organisms, *M. cynos* is generally not considered a primary pathogen.[50] The role of *Mycoplasma* spp. in respiratory disease of cats is not clear. Organisms have been identified by culture and PCR of upper and lower respiratory tract samples from diseased cats, but most often in conjunction with other bacterial or viral pathogens.[38,92] Nevertheless, in some cases, mycoplasmal infection has been considered the sole cause of pneumonia.[93,94]

Bordetella bronchiseptica organisms are relatively small but recognizable on light microscopy. They typically adhere to cilia and are only sometimes phagocytosed by neutrophils (Figure 25.11).[50,57,95] Cytologic identification of *B. bronchiseptica* in samples that contained epithelial cells was more sensitive than culture, and a low concentration of *B. bronchiseptica* was present in BAL samples from clinically healthy dogs.[50]

Successful culture of bacteria varies between laboratories depending on incorporation of enrichment steps and specific media, which will affect apparent sensitivity and specificity in relation to cytological methods.[96] Bacterial culture results from tracheal wash samples should be interpreted in light of cytologic findings since the larger airways are not sterile and positive culture results do not distinguish between airway colonization and infection. In general, cytologic identification of bacteria has 70–90% sensitivity and >95% specificity relative to culture detection of bacteria, and inclusion of Gram-stained slides may yield greater sensitivity.[6,91]

Many other bacteria such as *Pasteurella* sp., *Streptococcus* sp., and *Enterobacteriaceae* can be identified in cases of LRT disease.[18,24,38,77,91,97] Aspiration pneumonia typically

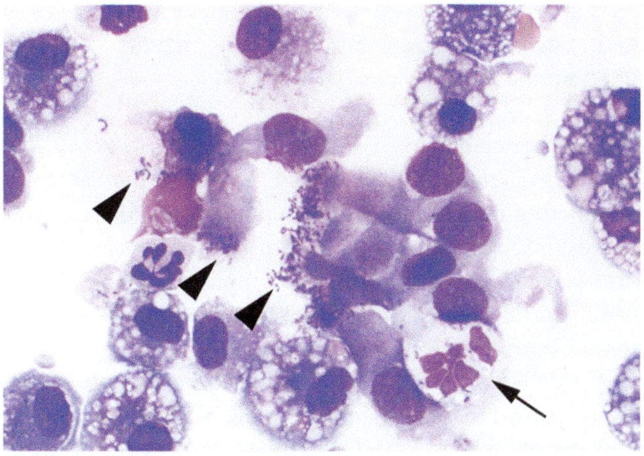

Figure 25.11 Cytocentrifuge preparation of BAL from a 10-month-old Yorkshire terrier. The cell concentration was 1.2×10^9/L. *B. bronchiseptica* are attached to cilia on the epithelial cells (arrowheads) and are phagocytosed by neutrophils (arrow) (Wright stain, 1000×).

manifests with a mixed bacterial infection, marked suppurative inflammatory response, squamous epithelial cells from the oropharynx or upper gastrointestinal tract, and sometimes food materials (Figure 25.12).[63]

Fungal Pneumonia

Mycotic agents that spread to or primarily infect the lung such as *Blastomyces dermatitidis, Histoplasma capsulatum, Coccidioides immitis, Cryptococcus neoformans,* and *Pneumocystis carinii* are more likely to be found in the pulmonary interstitium than in the airways or alveoli (also see Chapter 3). Depending on the extent of infection and inflammation, airway lavage can fail to retrieve fungal components, and direct parenchymal aspiration of nodular lesions can be more rewarding.[14,30] *Blastomyces* and *Histoplasma* are dimorphic fungi that are usually present as yeast rather than hyphae in airway samples. *Blastomyces* are readily recognized cytologically as dark blue, thick-walled, round, broad-based budding yeast that are 10–20 µm in diameter and often imbedded in aggregates of mucus and necrotic debris (Figure 25.10). *Histoplasma* are 1–4 µm round to oval yeast with lightly basophilic protoplasm surrounded by an apparent halo. Organisms usually occur in multiples in macrophages and neutrophils or extracellularly.

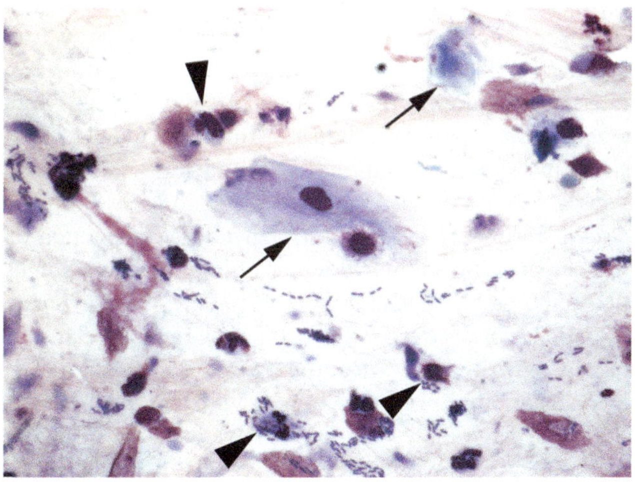

Figure 25.12 Cytocentrifuge preparation of BAL from an 8-year-old bulldog with fever. The sample contains abundant cell debris, mucus, nucleate and anucleate keratinized squamous cells (arrows), degenerated neutrophils with phagocytosed bacteria (arrowhead), and numerous extracellular bacteria. The dog had aspiration pneumonia due to poor laryngeal function (Wright stain, 630×).

Coccidioides spherules (sporangia) vary in size from 20 to 100 µm in diameter, have an irregular thick wall, and contain numerous small endospores. Infection is regionally endemic in arid regions of the Southwestern United States and Central and South America and manifests with cough, skin lesions, or systemic illness.[89] Organisms are cytologically readily identified at low magnification but are inconsistently present in airway lavages.[12] Direct aspiration of radiographically identified lung masses, skin lesions, or enlarged lymph nodes can be more diagnostically rewarding.

Cryptococcosis occurs secondary exposure by inhalation of desiccated yeast and more often affects the upper than lower respiratory tract. Cats are more frequently infected than dogs.[98] *Cryptococcus* spp. are round, 8–30 µm in diameter, and have a thick, nonstaining mucinous capsule. Both *C. neoformans* and *C. gattii* cause disease, but in California the former is more common in dogs and the latter more common in cats.[98] Different species of *Cryptococcus* are cytologically indistinguishable. Among cats with cryptococcal upper respiratory tract infection, approximately 30% also had pulmonary lesions.[38]

Pneumocystis spp. are unicellular fungal organisms that cause pneumonia in a wide variety of species.[99] The organism appears to colonize the lung of clinically healthy animals, and in animals with immune defects, it proliferates to cause interstitial pneumonia.[99] Clinical respiratory disease in dogs is most often reported in certain breeds such as Cavalier King Charles spaniels, miniature Dachshunds, and Pomeranians, and in some cases an underlying immune defect has been characterized.[100–102] The organism infecting dogs has been termed *Pasteurella canis*.[103] Immunosuppression from glucocorticoid treatment or feline leukemia virus infection can result in clinical disease in cats.[104,105] *Pneumocystis* spp. cannot be cultured; therefore, diagnosis depends on cytological identification, typical imaging findings, and/or PCR.[103] Infection results in macrophage activation, which

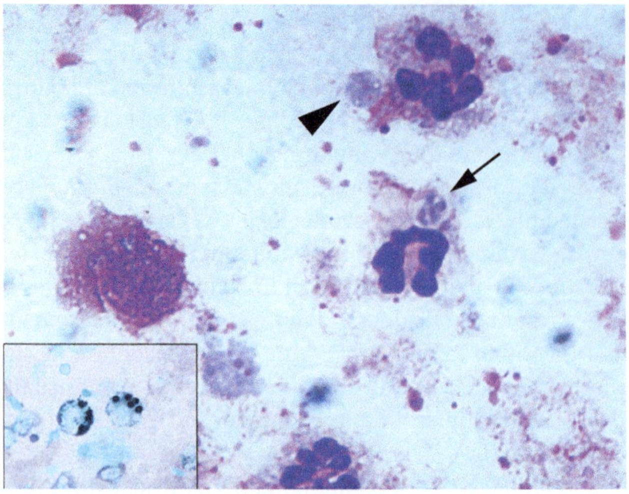

Figure 25.13 Cytocentrifuge preparation of BAL from a 4-year-old mixed breed dog with intermittent cough and exercise intolerance. The preparation has a granular background. Small round structures with internal structures (arrow) are consistent with *Pneumocystis* spp. cyst forms. Spore cases are also apparent (arrowhead). Inset: The organism was confirmed by methenamine silver staining (Wright stain, 1000×).

manifests with increased macrophage BAL cell concentration, increased cell size, and extensive cytoplasmic vacuolation. In some cases neutrophilic inflammation predominates. *Pneumocystis* organisms stain poorly with Romanowsky stains, and their presence is typically suspected by finding granular gray-bluish extracellular material in BAL cytospin preparations (Figure 25.13). Various morphotypes such as cysts, trophozoites, and disintegrating components may be observed. Cysts are 5–10 µm in diameter, contain four to eight basophilic bodies, and stain with methenamine silver.

Viral Pneumonia

Infectious respiratory disease is usually caused by multiple organisms and often includes multiple viruses and bacteria.[55,65,97] Hence, airway changes from infection with a single type of virus are poorly characterized. Luminal cell debris and neutrophilic inflammation were present in canine respiratory coronavirus and in feline cowpox virus infection in the absence of bacterial infection, and histologic changes in airway epithelium were pronounced.[55,106] In dogs, the main viral causes of pneumonia are distemper, adenovirus, and herpesvirus, but parainfluenza and coronavirus are also frequently detected in conjunction with bacterial pneumonia.[75,97,107] Adenovirus, poxvirus, and herpesvirus may cause nuclear inclusions, while distemper inclusions can be nuclear or cytoplasmic.[75,106,107] Virally injured epithelial cells may be more readily dislodged during lavage, but viral inclusions in respiratory epithelial cells are rarely observed. In cats, coronavirus, herpesvirus, and cowpox virus may be sole agents of viral pneumonia.[18,56,106]

Protozoal Pneumonia

Toxoplasma gondii is a protozoal organism that can cause necrotizing interstitial pneumonia in cats. Clinical disease is most often associated with immunosuppression but has also been reported in immune competent cats.[38,108,109] In dogs, *Toxoplasma* can be a component of infectious pneumonia but is rarely the sole agent.[110] Cytologic examination of BAL can show increased neutrophils and tachyzoites, but organisms are more frequent in pulmonary parenchyma.[108,109] Tachyzoites are 1–4 µm crescent-shaped structures with basophilic cytoplasm and a central metachromatic nucleus.

Neospora caninum affects mostly young dogs and causes systemic illness including pneumonia and neurologic disease.[111,112] Tachyzoites in lung aspirates or lavages are morphologically indistinguishable from those of *T. gondii*, and infection causes pyogranulomatous inflammation.[111] Protozoal speciation requires immunochemical or molecular assays.[113]

Pulmonary Parasites

Airway lavages can be helpful to identify parasite larvae or eggs. Many metazoan infestations are associated with eosinophilic inflammatory responses, but some cases of concurrent verminous and bacterial infection in cats had neutrophil- rather than eosinophil-predominant inflammation in BAL samples.[38] The larval stages of *Aelurostrongylus abstrusus* are readily identifiable in samples from cats but are released only intermittently from parenchymal location into airways.[38,87] Direct lung aspirates of sonographically identified lesions can also yield diagnostic samples in *A. abstrusus* infection.[114] Other parasites that can be identified in feline lung samples are *Toxocara cati, Paragonimus kellicotti, Eucoleus aerophilus, Oslerus rostratus*, and *Troglostrongylus brevior*, though the frequency of infestation varies according to region, domesticity, and type of housing.[115–119] *Dirofilaria immitis* causes pulmonary disease secondary to cardiac infestation in cats, but in experimental infection BAL eosinophilia was an inconsistent finding.[120] Pneumonia with a bronchointerstitial pattern and BAL eosinophilia developed in cats experimentally infected with *T. cati*.[121]

Parasites that can be identified cytologically in lung samples from dogs include *Angiostrongylus vasorum, P. kellicotti, Crenosoma vulpis, Toxocara canis, and E. aerophilus*.[74,122] Similar to *A. abstrusus*, larvae of *A. vasorum* have a distinct appearance.[87,123] *P. kellicotti* can induce formation of inflammatory cysts that are most commonly

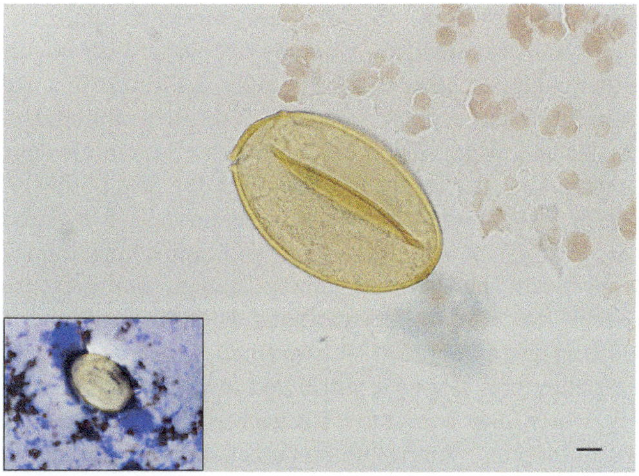

Figure 25.14 Aspirate of a lung mass from an 11-year-old Labrador retriever with a six-month history of gagging, occasional hemoptysis, weight loss, and blood eosinophilia. In the unstained direct smear, a large egg with an operculum consistent with *P. kellicotti* is apparent (bar = 10 µm). Inset: Egg morphology is less readily appreciated in this stained preparation (Wright stain, 200×). Clinical signs resolved after appropriate anthelminthic therapy.

located in the caudal lung lobe. If eggs are present in lung washes, they have a typical operculated appearance (Figure 25.14). *D. immitis* infestation of pulmonary arteries results in pulmonary hypertension, and adulticide treatment may be associated with pulmonary thromboembolism, but organisms are not present in airways.[124]

Lack of direct parasite detection by microscopy can be due to intermittent presence of organisms in airways or nonrepresentative sampling; therefore, appropriate fecal examination and serologic testing should be performed if animals have lung lavage eosinophilia and respiratory signs suggestive of parasitism.

Neoplasms of the Lung

Primary Epithelial Lung Tumors

Primary lung tumors in dogs and cats most commonly originate from epithelium of the airways or alveoli.[20,21,28] In general, location of the primary (largest) mass in the periphery of the lung corresponds to alveolar or distal bronchiolar origin and location in the hilar region to bronchial origin.[26,28] On histopathology, tumors are classified according to architectural patterns such as papillary, acinar, solid, or mixed glandular and composition of squamous (with or without keratinization), cuboidal, and glandular cells.[20,125]

In cats, epithelial pulmonary tumors are most often located in the caudal lung lobes and classified as bronchiolar or bronchial adenocarcinoma.[20,125] The majority of feline pulmonary carcinomas metastasize, most commonly within the lung, but involvement of pleural cavity, lymph nodes, and distal organs is also frequent.[20,125] Cytologic assessment of aspirates, thoracocentesis, and endoscopic bronchiolar brushing samples was highly sensitive and specific for diagnosis of pulmonary neoplasia,[20,27,30] though in one study BAL cytology was not considered to reliably distinguish between epithelial hyperplasia due to bronchitis and epithelial neoplasia.[7] Pulmonary carcinomas metastatic to digits often affect multiple digits, include goblet and ciliated cells, and usually lack keratinization.[9,126,127] Approximately one third of pulmonary carcinomas in cats involve the pleural space and are associated with pleural effusion and a worse prognosis.[20,125,128] Tracheal wash hemosiderosis is common not only in pulmonary neoplasms of cats but also in other conditions.[73] Occasional lung carcinomas in cats are associated with endogenous lipid pneumonia characterized by lipid-filled macrophages, type II pneumocyte hyperplasia, and cholesterol crystal formation.[129] The pathogenesis is thought to involve epithelial injury with subsequent type II pneumocyte proliferation, excessive cholesterol-rich surfactant production, and small airway obstruction.[129] Thyroid transcription factor (TTF)-1 is a sensitive and specific immunohistochemical marker of feline neoplastic and benign lung and thyroidal epithelial cells, but expression is weak or absent in poorly differentiated tumors.[125,130] Surfactant protein A (SPA) immunohistochemistry, in combination with TTF-1, identified >80% of primary feline lung tumors.[125]

Pulmonary epithelial tumors in dogs are less common than in cats, affect cranial and caudal lung lobes more equally than in cats, most often present as a single mass, and are most often histologically classified as bronchioalveolar carcinoma, adenocarcinoma, or anaplastic carcinoma.[19,26,131] Metastasis of pulmonary carcinomas is less common in dogs than cats, and evidence of cell differentiation and absence of clinical signs are associated with better prognosis.[132] Similar as in cats, TTF-1 detection is highly specific for pulmonary and thyroidal epithelium but only for those lung carcinomas that include glandular cells.[133] Thyroid carcinoma metastatic to lung is difficult to distinguish from primary lung carcinoma by histomorphology and TTF-1 immunohistochemistry, but SPA and napsin are more sensitive and specific markers for pulmonary origin.[134] Direct aspiration was considered a successful diagnostic method for tumors that could be reached with a transthoracic approach,[21,27,30] and BAL cytology yielded a definitive or supportive diagnosis in 10 of 14 lung carcinomas.[37] However, in a study of dogs with primary lung tumors, tracheal washing generated a definitive diagnoses in only one of six cases.[132] Comparing the cytopathologic and histopathologic interpretation, there was very good agreement for diagnosis of pulmonary carcinoma in samples from dogs and cats.[30,53]

Cytological criteria of malignancy in epithelial lung tumors are similar to those in other epithelial tissues. Neoplastic cells typically are larger than benign cells, have higher nuclear to cytoplasmic ratio (N:C), prominent and often multiple nucleoli, and more intense cytoplasmic staining (hyperchromasia; Figure 25.15).[30,135] Distinction of primary from metastatic lung carcinomas is difficult on cytopathology and also often challenging on histopathology. Presence of cilia or secretory products such as thyroidal colloid allows identification of bronchial or thyroidal epithelium, respectively, but lack of histopathologic assessment often precludes confident assignment of tumor origin.[136] Cell cannibalism, whereby neoplastic cells engulf either benign or other neoplastic cells, is a feature of some pulmonary carcinomas.[135,137] Cilia, indicative of bronchial or tracheal origin, are infrequently observed in cytology preparations, which is consistent with the distal bronchiolar or alveolar origin of most lung carcinomas in dogs and cats. With CT, 56 and 16% of feline and canine lung tumors, respectively, had foci of mineralization, but presence thereof in cytology preparations is undetermined.[26,28] Heterogeneous contrast enhancement in large primary lung tumors in dogs was attributed to variable blood supply, which may correlate with necrosis and neutrophilic inflammation.[26] Rarely, pulmonary carcinomas ectopically

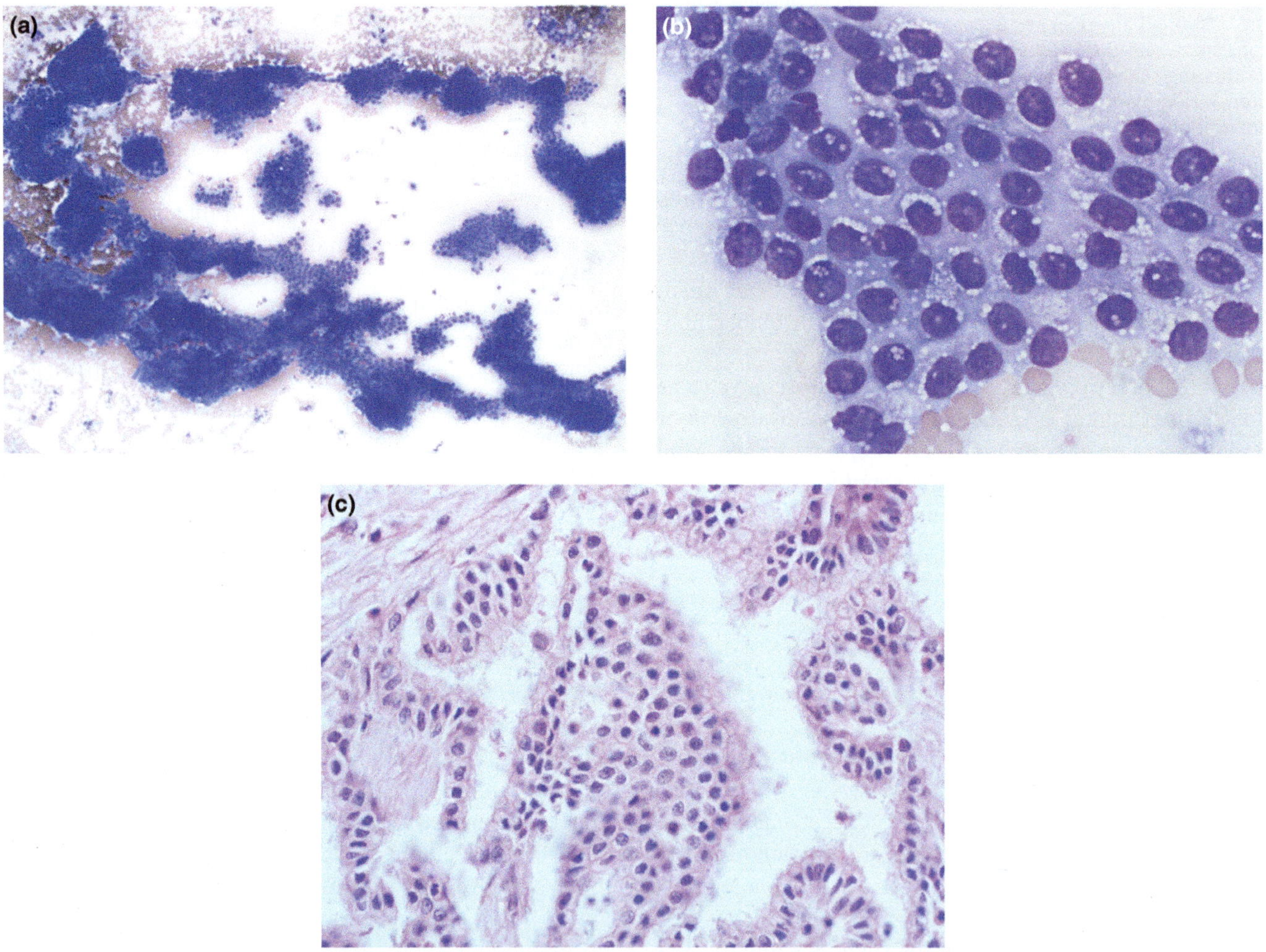

Figure 25.15 Large right caudal lung lobe mass from a 7-year-old dog. (a) On aspiration the mass readily exfoliated, and cells were tightly adherent to each other and arranged in long papillary structures (Wright stain, 100×). (b) At higher magnification there was minimal anisocytosis and anisokaryosis, and cells had mild hyperchromasia and moderately high N:C (Wright stain, 630×). (c) Histologically, the mass was expansile but encapsulated and arranged in trabeculae with collagenous cores. There were approximately twofold anisocytosis and anisokaryosis and rare mitotic figures (hematoxylin & eosin, 400×). Cytologic interpretation was likely carcinoma; histologic interpretation was adenocarcinoma, papillary type with minimal dysplasia.

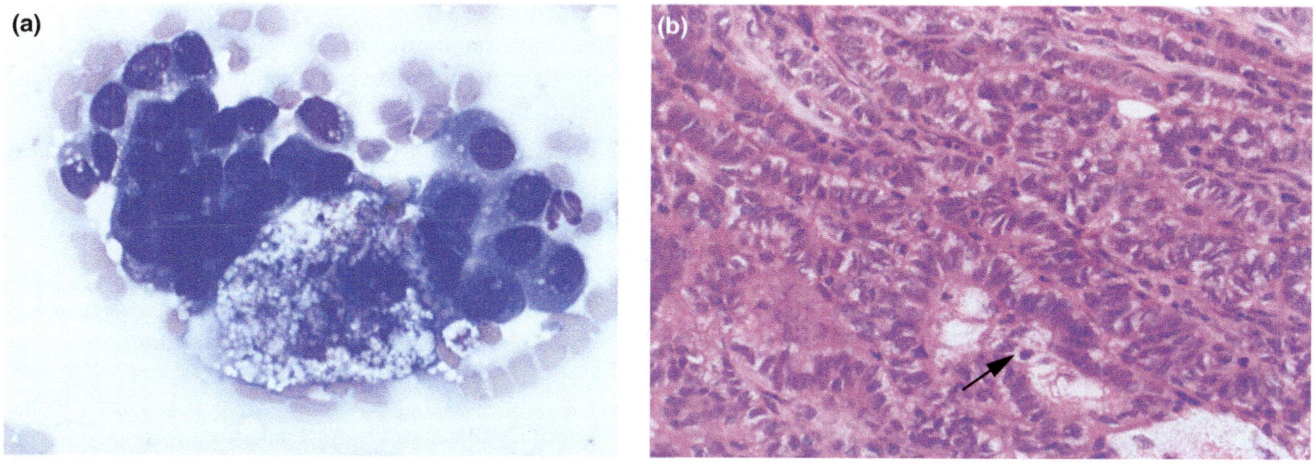

Figure 25.16 Large right caudal lung lobe mass from a 10-year-old dog. (a) On cytology there were clusters of angular, hyperchromatic epithelial cells with high N:C. Individual, highly vacuolated large macrophages are seen (Wright stain, 1000×). (b) Histologically, the mass was expansile and partially encapsulated, contained large areas of necrosis and intravascular tumor cell aggregates. The mass was composed of fronds of columnar to cuboidal hyperchromatic epithelial cells supported by a fibrovascular stalk. There were individual highly vacuolated macrophages (arrow) (hematoxylin & eosin, 400×). Cytologic interpretation was carcinoma, and histologic interpretation was adenocarcinoma, papillary subtype with multiple satellite masses, and metastases.

produce growth factors, such as granulocyte colony-stimulating factor or granulocyte–macrophage colony-stimulating factor, resulting in marked leukocytosis.[138,139] Thus, cytologic assessment of lung mass lesions is overall a very useful and noninvasive diagnostic test. However, large lung tumors can be very heterogeneous and consist of different architectural arrangements, necrosis, mineralization, and intra-lung metastases. Therefore, aspirates will be poorly representative of such heterogeneity and may have to be supplemented by tissue biopsy (Figure 25.16).

Primary Non-epithelial Lung Tumors

Histiocytic sarcoma is the most common non-epithelial primary lung tumor in dogs.[19] Radiographically, histiocytic sarcomas are often larger than pulmonary carcinomas and are characterized by internal air bronchograms.[19] Predilection of large breed dogs to histiocytic sarcoma is well known, but small dogs are also affected.[140,141] In most cases, histiocytic sarcoma cells are readily diagnosed by cytology due to a distinct appearance consisting of plump, irregular to spindle-shaped cells with gray-blue cytoplasm, and occasional phagocytosed cell debris or whole cells.[142] Multinucleation, anisonucleosis, atypical mitoses, and concurrent mixed inflammation are common additional features.

Pulmonary Langerhans cell histiocytosis is an uncommon but fatal lung neoplasm of cats where infiltration of the lung with histiocytes leads to progressive respiratory failure.[140,143] Cells have features of atypia, and the condition usually also involves non-pulmonary organs.[143]

Only one type of lymphoma of primary pulmonary origin has been described though the lung is frequently affected in multicentric lymphoma.[144] Angiocentric lymphoma, also called lymphomatoid granulomatosis, is an uncommon neoplasm of typically young dogs and rarely reported in cats.[145,146] At diagnosis, the tumor is usually widespread within the lung, and most dogs are clinically ill and have neutrophilia and/or eosinophilia. Cytologically, tumors are made up of large atypical lymphocytes admixed with small lymphocytes, eosinophils, neutrophils, and plasma cells. The large lymphocytes are considered to be the neoplastic cells and express antigens of B lymphocytes. The constellation of young age, advanced pulmonary disease, mass lesions, and a cytologically mixed lung sample allow a high suspicion of this type of lymphoma, but for definitive diagnoses an angiocentric distribution should be demonstrated by histopathology.[145]

Carcinoids are rare tumors that may arise from neuroendocrine cells in the airway epithelium. Similar to other neuroendocrine tumors, cells aspirated from a canine lung carcinoid are fragile and exhibit mostly bare nuclei.[147] The histological appearance is characteristic, and immunohistochemical detection of chromogranin A or neuron-specific enolase confirms neuroendocrine origin.

Conclusion

Cytological assessment is a very rewarding diagnostic step in the investigation of LRT disease. A definitive diagnosis of infection or neoplasia can be derived in many instances, and samples for microbiological and other assays are readily obtained. However, although there is an abundance of publications on different aspects of LRT disease, there is nevertheless a shortage of adequately powered and properly controlled prospective studies of diagnostic approaches. The diagnostic value of cytology samples may be enhanced by the use of standardized techniques and implementation of ancillary methods such as immunocytochemistry and cell block cytology.[148]

References

1 Amis, T.C. and McKiernan, B.C. (1986). Systematic identification of endobronchial anatomy during bronchoscopy in the dog. *Am J Vet Res* 47: 2649–2657.

2 Caccamo, R., Twedt, D.C., Buracco, P., and BC, M.K. (2007). Endoscopic bronchial anatomy in the cat. *J Feline Med Surg* 9: 140–149.

3 Patra, A.L. (1986). Comparative anatomy of mammalian respiratory tracts: the nasopharyngeal region and the tracheobronchial region. *J Toxicol Environ Health* 17: 163–174.

4 Peeters, D., Day, M.J., and Clercx, C. (2005). Distribution of leucocyte subsets in bronchial mucosa from dogs with eosinophilic bronchopneumopathy. *J Comp Pathol* 133: 128–135.

5 Woods, K.S., Defarges, A.M., Abrams-Ogg, A.C. et al. (2014). Comparison of bronchoalveolar lavage fluid obtained by manual aspiration with a handheld syringe with that obtained by automated suction pump aspiration from healthy dogs. *Am J Vet Res* 75: 85–90.

6 Peeters, D.E., McKiernan, B.C., Weisiger, R.M. et al. (2000). Quantitative bacterial cultures and cytological examination of bronchoalveolar lavage specimens in dogs. *J Vet Intern Med* 14: 534–541.

7 Johnson, L.R. and Vernau, W. (2011). Bronchoscopic findings in 48 cats with spontaneous lower respiratory tract disease (2002–2009). *J Vet Intern Med* 25: 236–243.

8 Alenghat, T., Pillitteri, C.A., Bemis, D.A. et al. (2010). Lycoperdonosis in two dogs. *J Vet Diagn Invest* 22: 1002–1005.

9 Wobeser, B.K., Kidney, B.A., Powers, B.E. et al. (2007). Diagnoses and clinical outcomes associated with surgically amputated feline digits submitted to multiple veterinary diagnostic laboratories. *Vet Pathol* 44: 362–365.

10 Withers, S.S., Johnson, E.G., Culp, W.T. et al. (2015). Paraneoplastic hypertrophic osteopathy in 30 dogs. *Vet Comp Oncol* 13: 157–165.

11 Caywood, D.D., Kramek, B.A., Feeney, D.A., and Johnston, G.R. (1985). Hypertrophic osteopathy associated with a bronchial foreign body and lobar pneumonia in a dog. *J Am Vet Med Assoc* 186: 698–700.

12 Hawkins, E.C., DeNicola, D.B., and Kuehn, N.F. (1990). Bronchoalveolar lavage in the evaluation of pulmonary disease in the dog and cat. State of the art. *J Vet Intern Med* 4: 267–274.

13 Baldwin, F. and Becker, A.B. (1993). Bronchoalveolar eosinophilic cells in a canine model of asthma: two distinctive populations. *Vet Pathol* 30: 97–103.

14 Crews, L.J., Feeney, D.A., Jessen, C.R. et al. (2008). Utility of diagnostic tests for and medical treatment of pulmonary blastomycosis in dogs: 125 cases (1989–2006). *J Am Vet Med Assoc* 232: 222–227.

15 Garcia, R.S., Wheat, L.J., Cook, A.K. et al. (2012). Sensitivity and specificity of a blood and urine galactomannan antigen assay for diagnosis of systemic aspergillosis in dogs. *J Vet Intern Med* 26: 911–919.

16 Norris, C.R., Griffey, S.M., Samii, V.F. et al. (2002). Thoracic radiography, bronchoalveolar lavage cytopathology, and pulmonary parenchymal histopathology: a comparison of diagnostic results in 11 cats. *J Am Anim Hosp Assoc* 38: 337–345.

17 Hawkins, E.C., Basseches, J., Berry, C.R. et al. (2003). Demographic, clinical, and radiographic features of bronchiectasis in dogs: 316 cases (1988–2000). *J Am Vet Med Assoc* 223: 1628–1635.

18 Macdonald, E.S., Norris, C.R., Berghaus, R.B., and Griffey, S.M. (2003). Clinicopathologic and radiographic features and etiologic agents in cats with histologically confirmed infectious pneumonia: 39 cases (1991–2000). *J Am Vet Med Assoc* 223: 1142–1150.

19 Barrett, L.E., Pollard, R.E., Zwingenberger, A. et al. (2014). Radiographic characterization of primary lung tumors in 74 dogs. *Vet Radiol Ultrasound* 55: 480–487.

20 Hahn, K.A. and McEntee, M.F. (1997). Primary lung tumors in cats: 86 cases (1979–1994). *J Am Vet Med Assoc* 211: 1257–1260.

21 Ogilvie, G.K., Haschek, W.M., Withrow, S.J. et al. (1989). Classification of primary lung tumors in dogs: 210 cases (1975–1985). *J Am Vet Med Assoc* 195: 106–108.

22 Norris, C.R., Griffey, S.M., and Samii, V.F. (1999). Pulmonary thromboembolism in cats: 29 cases (1987–1997). *J Am Vet Med Assoc* 215: 1650–1654.

23 Norris, C.R. and Samii, V.F. (2000). Clinical, radiographic, and pathologic features of bronchiectasis in cats: 12 cases (1987–1999). *J Am Vet Med Assoc* 216: 530–534.

24 Johnson, L.R. (2016). Laryngeal structure and function in dogs with cough. *J Am Vet Med Assoc* 249: 195–201.

25 Cannon, M.S., Johnson, L.R., Pesavento, P.A. et al. (2013). Quantitative and qualitative computed tomographic characteristics of bronchiectasis in 12 dogs. *Vet Radiol Ultrasound* 54: 351–357.

26 Marolf, A.J., Gibbons, D.S., Park, R.D., and Podell, B.K. (2011). Computed tomographic appearance of primary lung tumors in dogs. *Vet Radiol Ultrasound* 52: 168–172.

27 Zekas, L.J., Crawford, J.T., and O'Brien, R.T. (2005). Computed tomography-guided fine-needle aspirate and tissue-core biopsy of intrathoracic lesions in thirty dogs and cats. *Vet Radiol Ultrasound* 46: 200–204.

28 Aarsvold, S., Reetz, J.A., Reichle, J.K. et al. (2015). Computed tomographic findings in 57 cats with primary pulmonary neoplasia. *Vet Radiol Ultrasound* 56: 272–277.

29 Silvestri, G.A., Herth, F.J., Keast, T. et al. (2014). Feasibility and safety of bronchoscopic transparenchymal nodule access in canines: a new real-time image-guided approach to lung lesions. *Chest* 145: 833–838.

30 Wood, E.F., O'Brien, R.T., and Young, K.M. (1998). Ultrasound-guided fine-needle aspiration of focal parenchymal lesions of the lung in dogs and cats. *J Vet Intern Med* 12: 338–342.

31 Linta, N., Baron Toaldo, M., Bettini, G. et al. (2017). The feasibility of contrast enhanced ultrasonography (CEUS) in the diagnosis of non-cardiac thoracic disorders of dogs and cats. *BMC Vet Res* 13: 141.

32 Finke, M.D. (2013). Transtracheal wash and bronchoalveolar lavage. *Top Companion Anim Med* 28: 97–102.

33 Sumner, C.M., Rozanski, E.A., Sharp, C.R., and Shaw, S.P. (2011). The use of deep oral swabs as a surrogate for transoral tracheal wash to obtain bacterial cultures in dogs with pneumonia. *J Vet Emerg Crit Care* 21: 515–520.

34 Creevy, K.E. (2009). Airway evaluation and flexible endoscopic procedures in dogs and cats: laryngoscopy, transtracheal wash, tracheobronchoscopy, and bronchoalveolar lavage. *Vet Clin North Am Small Anim Pract* 39: 869–880.

35 Kaneko, T., Massion, P.R., Hara, M., and Nadel, J.A. (1996). Ragweed antigen causes interleukin-8 production in sensitized dog trachea. *Am J Respir Crit Care Med* 153: 136–140.

36 Hawkins, E.C., DeNicola, D.B., and Plier, M.L. (1995). Cytological analysis of bronchoalveolar lavage fluid in the diagnosis of spontaneous respiratory tract disease in dogs: a retrospective study. *J Vet Intern Med* 9: 386–392.

37 Hawkins, E.C., Kennedy-Stoskopf, S., Levy, J. et al. (1994). Cytologic characterization of bronchoalveolar lavage fluid collected through an endotracheal tube in cats. *Am J Vet Res* 55: 795–802.

38 Foster, S.F., Martin, P., Allan, G.S. et al. (2004). Lower respiratory tract infections in cats: 21 cases (1995–2000). *J Feline Med Surg* 6: 167–180.

39 Johnson, L.R. and Drazenovich, T.L. (2007). Flexible bronchoscopy and bronchoalveolar lavage in 68 cats (2001–2006). *J Vet Intern Med* 21: 219–225.

40 Woods, K.S., Defarges, A.M., Abrams-Ogg, A.C. et al. (2013). Comparison between manual aspiration via polyethylene tubing and aspiration via a suction pump with a suction trap connection for performing bronchoalveolar lavage in healthy dogs. *Am J Vet Res* 74: 523–529.

41 McCarthy, G. and Quinn, P.J. (1986). The development of lavage procedures for the upper and lower respiratory tract of the cat. *Irish Vet J* 17: 6–9.

42 Dehard, S., Bernaerts, F., Peeters, D. et al. (2008). Comparison of bronchoalveolar lavage cytospins and smears in dogs and cats. *J Am Anim Hosp Assoc* 44: 285–294.

43 Rajamäki, M.M., Järvinen, A.K., Saari, S.A., and Maisi, P.S. (2001). Effect of repetitive bronchoalveolar lavage on cytologic findings in healthy dogs. *Am J Vet Res* 62: 13–16.

44 Hawkins, E.C. and DeNicola, D.B. (1989). Collection of bronchoalveolar lavage fluid in cats, using an endotracheal tube. *Am J Vet Res* 50: 855–859.

45 Allerton, F.J., Leemans, J., Tual, C. et al. (2013). Correlation of bronchoalveolar eosinophilic percentage with airway responsiveness in cats with chronic bronchial disease. *J Small Anim Pract* 54: 258–264.

46 Haley, P.J., Muggenburg, B.A., Rebar, A.H. et al. (1989). Bronchoalveolar lavage cytology in cynomolgus monkeys and identification of cytologic alterations following sequential saline lavage. *Vet Pathol* 26: 265–273.

47 Rebar, A.H., DeNicola, D.B., and Muggenburg, B.A. (1980). Bronchopulmonary lavage cytology in the dog: normal findings. *Vet Pathol* 17: 294–304.

48 Hawkins, E.C., Rogala, A.R., Large, E.E. et al. (2006). Cellular composition of bronchial brushings obtained from healthy dogs and dogs with chronic cough and cytologic composition of bronchoalveolar lavage fluid obtained from dogs with chronic cough. *Am J Vet Res* 67: 160–167.

49 Zhu, B.Y., Johnson, L.R., and Vernau, W. (2015). Tracheobronchial brush cytology and bronchoalveolar lavage in dogs and cats with chronic cough: 45 cases (2012–2014). *J Vet Intern Med* 29: 526–532.

50 Canonne, A.M., Billen, F., Tual, C. et al. (2016). Quantitative PCR and cytology of bronchoalveolar lavage fluid in dogs with *Bordetella bronchiseptica* infection. *J Vet Intern Med* 30: 1204–1209.

51 Teske, E., Stokhof, A.A., Ingh, T.V.D. et al. (1991). Transthoracic needle aspiration biopsy of the lung in dogs with pulmonary diseases. *J Am Anim Hosp Assoc* 27: 289–294.

52 Menard, M. and Papageorges, M. (1995). Ultrasound corner technique for ultrasound-guided fine needle biopsies. *Vet Radiol Ultrasound* 36: 137–138.

53 DeBerry, J.D., Norris, C.R., Samii, V.F. et al. (2002). Correlation between fine-needle aspiration cytopathology and histopathology of the lung in dogs and cats. *J Am Anim Hosp Assoc* 38: 327–336.

54 Verbanck, S. (2012). Physiological measurement of the small airways. *Respiration* 84: 177–188.

55 Mitchell, J.A., Cardwell, J.M., Renshaw, R.W. et al. (2013). Detection of canine pneumovirus in dogs with canine infectious respiratory disease. *J Clin Microbiol* 51: 4112–4119.

56 McGregor, G.F., Sheehan, K., and Simko, E. (2016). Pneumonia and gastritis in a cat caused by feline herpesvirus-1. *Can Vet J* 57: 147–150.

57 Dambro, N.N., Grad, R., Witten, M.L. et al. (1992). Bronchoalveolar lavage fluid cytology reflects airway inflammation in beagle puppies with acute bronchiolitis. *Pediatr Pulmonol* 12: 213–220.

58 Meyer, K.C., Raghu, G., Baughman, R.P. et al. (2012). An official American Thoracic Society clinical practice guideline: the clinical utility of bronchoalveolar lavage cellular analysis in interstitial lung disease. *Am J Respir Crit Care Med* 185: 1004–1014.

59 De Lorenzi, D., Masserdotti, C., Bertoncello, D., and Tranquillo, V. (2009). Differential cell counts in canine cytocentrifuged bronchoalveolar lavage fluid: a study on reliable enumeration of each cell type. *Vet Clin Pathol* 38: 532–536.

60 Kirschvink, N., Kersnak, E., Leemans, J. et al. (2007). Effects of age and allergen-induced airway inflammation in cats: radiographic and cytologic correlation. *Vet J* 174: 644–651.

61 Norris, C.R., Decile, K.C., Berghaus, L.J. et al. (2003). Concentrations of cysteinyl leukotrienes in urine and bronchoalveolar lavage fluid of cats with experimentally induced asthma. *Am J Vet Res* 64: 1449–1453.

62 Padrid, P.A., Feldman, B.F., Funk, K. et al. (1991). Cytologic, microbiologic, and biochemical analysis of bronchoalveolar lavage fluid obtained from 24 healthy cats. *Am J Vet Res* 52: 1300–1307.

63 Benson, C.J., Edlund, M.B., Gray, S. et al. (2013). The presence of diatom algae in a tracheal wash from a German Wirehaired Pointer with aspiration pneumonia. *Vet Clin Pathol* 42: 221–226.

64 Johnson, L.R. and Pollard, R.E. (2010). Tracheal collapse and bronchomalacia in dogs: 58 cases (7/2001–1/2008). *J Vet Intern Med* 24: 298–305.

65 Viitanen, S.J., Lappalainen, A., and Rajamäki, M.M. (2015). Co-infections with respiratory viruses in dogs with bacterial pneumonia. *J Vet Intern Med* 29: 544–551.

66 De Lorenzi, D., Bonfanti, U., Masserdotti, C. et al. (2006). Diagnosis of canine nasal aspergillosis by cytological examination: a comparison of four different collection techniques. *J Small Anim Pract* 47: 316–319.

67 Hussell, T. and Bell, T.J. (2014). Alveolar macrophages: plasticity in a tissue-specific context. *Nat Rev Immunol* 14: 81–93.

68 Jones, D.J., Norris, C.R., Samii, V.F., and Griffey, S.M. (2000). Endogenous lipid pneumonia in cats: 24 cases (1985–1998). *J Am Vet Med Assoc* 216: 1437–1440.

69 Foster, S.F., Martin, P., Davis, W. et al. (1999). Chronic pneumonia caused by Mycobacterium thermoresistibile in a cat. *J Small Anim Pract* 40: 433–438.

70 Leissinger, M.K., Garber, J.B., Fowlkes, N. et al. (2015). Mycobacterium fortuitum lipoid pneumonia in a dog. *Vet Pathol* 52: 356–359.

71 Kaminen, P.S., Viitanen, S.J., Lappalainen, A.K. et al. (2014). Management of a congenital tracheoesophageal fistula in a young Spanish water dog. *BMC Vet Res* 10: 16.

72 Kogan, D.A., Johnson, L.R., Jandrey, K.E., and Pollard, R.E. (2008). Clinical, clinicopathologic, and radiographic findings in dogs with aspiration pneumonia: 88 cases (2004–2006). *J Am Vet Med Assoc* 233: 1742–1747.

73 DeHeer, H.L. and McManus, P. (2005). Frequency and severity of tracheal wash hemosiderosis and association with underlying disease in 96 cats: 2002–2003. *Vet Clin Pathol* 34: 17–22.

74 Di Cesare, A., Traversa, D., Manzocchi, S. et al. (2015). Elusive *Angiostrongylus vasorum* infections. *Parasit Vectors* 8: 438.

75 Kumar, S., Driskell, E.A., Cooley, A.J. et al. (2015). Fatal canid herpesvirus 1 respiratory infections in 4 clinically healthy adult dogs. *Vet Pathol* 52: 681–687.

76 Watson, C.E., Bell, C., and Toohey-Kurth, K. (2017). H3N2 canine influenza virus infection in a dog. *Vet Pathol* 54: 527–530.

77 Velineni, S., Timoney, J.F., Russell, K. et al. (2014). Clones of *Streptococcus zooepidemicus* from outbreaks of hemorrhagic canine pneumonia and associated immune responses. *Clin Vaccine Immunol* 21: 1246–1252.

78 Brummer, D.G., French, T.W., and Cline, J.M. (1989). Microlithiasis associated with chronic bronchopneumonia in a cat. *J Am Vet Med Assoc* 194: 1061–1064.

79 Clercx, C. and Peeters, D. (2007). Canine eosinophilic bronchopneumopathy. *Vet Clin North Am Small Anim Pract* 37: 917–935.

80 Krafft, E., Heikkilä, H.P., Jespers, P. et al. (2011). Serum and bronchoalveolar lavage fluid endothelin-1 concentrations as diagnostic biomarkers of canine idiopathic pulmonary fibrosis. *J Vet Intern Med* 25: 990–996.

81 Cohn, L.A., Norris, C.R., Hawkins, E.C. et al. (2004). Identification and characterization of an idiopathic pulmonary fibrosis-like condition in cats. *J Vet Intern Med* 18: 632–641.

82 Bertolani, C., Hernandez, J., Gomes, E. et al. (2012). Bromide-associated lower airway disease: a retrospective study of seven cats. *J Feline Med Surg* 14: 591–597.

83 Nutt, L.K., Webb, J.A., Prosser, K.J., and Defarges, A. (2014). Management of dogs and cats with endotracheal tube tracheal foreign bodies. *Can Vet J* 55: 565–568.

84 Brinkmann, V. and Zychlinsky, A. (2012). Neutrophil extracellular traps: is immunity the second function of chromatin? *J Cell Biol* 198: 773–783.

85 Jeffery, U. and LeVine, D.N. (2018). Canine neutrophil extracellular traps enhance clot formation and delay lysis. *Vet Pathol* 55: 116–123.

86 Hawkins, E.C., Morrison, W.B., DeNicola, D.B., and Blevins, W.E. (1993). Cytologic analysis of bronchoalveolar lavage fluid from 47 dogs with multicentric malignant lymphoma. *J Am Vet Med Assoc* 203: 1418–1425.

87 Barçante, J.M., Barçante, T.A., Ribeiro, V.M. et al. (2008). Cytological and parasitological analysis of bronchoalveolar lavage fluid for the diagnosis of *Angiostrongylus vasorum* infection in dogs. *Vet Parasitol* 158: 93–102.

88 Couto, S.S. and Artacho, C.A. (2007). Mycobacterium fortuitum pneumonia in a cat and the role of lipid in the pathogenesis of atypical mycobacterial infections. *Vet Pathol* 44: 543–546.

89 Shubitz, L.F. (2007). Comparative aspects of coccidioidomycosis in animals and humans. *Ann N Y Acad Sci* 1111: 395–403.

90 Bailiff, N.L. and Norris, C.R. (2002). Clinical signs, clinicopathological findings, etiology, and outcome associated with hemoptysis in dogs: 36 cases (1990–1999). *J Am Anim Hosp Assoc* 38: 125–133.

91 Johnson, L.R., Queen, E.V., Vernau, W. et al. (2013). Microbiologic and cytologic assessment of bronchoalveolar lavage fluid from dogs with lower respiratory tract infection: 105 cases (2001–2011). *J Vet Intern Med* 27: 259–267.

92 Burns, R.E., Wagner, D.C., Leutenegger, C.M., and Pesavento, P.A. (2011). Histologic and molecular correlation in shelter cats with acute upper respiratory infection. *J Clin Microbiol* 49: 2454–2460.

93 Foster, S.F., Barrs, V.R., Martin, P., and Malik, R. (1998). Pneumonia associated with *Mycoplasma* spp in three cats. *Aust Vet J* 76: 460–464.

94 Trow, A.V., Rozanski, E.A., and Tidwell, A.S. (2008). Primary mycoplasma pneumonia associated with reversible respiratory failure in a cat. *J Feline Med Surg* 10: 398–402.

95 Taha-Abdelaziz, K., Bassel, L.L., Harness, M.L. et al. (2016). Cilia-associated bacteria in fatal *Bordetella bronchiseptica* pneumonia of dogs and cats. *J Vet Diagn Invest* 28: 369–376.

96 Johnson, L.R., Drazenovich, N.L., and Foley, J.E. (2004). A comparison of routine culture with polymerase chain reaction technology for the detection of *Mycoplasma* species in feline nasal samples. *J Vet Diagn Invest* 16: 347–351.

97 Priestnall, S.L., Mitchell, J.A., Walker, C.A. et al. (2014). New and emerging pathogens in canine infectious respiratory disease. *Vet Pathol* 51: 492–504.

98 Trivedi, S.R., Sykes, J.E., Cannon, M.S. et al. (2011). Clinical features and epidemiology of cryptococcosis in cats and dogs in California: 93 cases (1988–2010). *J Am Vet Med Assoc* 239: 357–369.

99 Sokulska, M., Kicia, M., Wesołowska, M., and Hendrich, A.B. (2015). Pneumocystis jirovecii—from a commensal to pathogen: clinical and diagnostic review. *Parasitol Res* 114: 3577–3585.

100 Kanemoto, H., Morikawa, R., Chambers, J.K. et al. (2015). Common variable immune deficiency in a Pomeranian with *Pneumocystis carinii* pneumonia. *J Vet Med Sci* 77: 715–719.

101 Watson, P.J., Wotton, P., Eastwood, J. et al. (2006). Immunoglobulin deficiency in Cavalier King Charles Spaniels with Pneumocystis pneumonia. *J Vet Intern Med* 20: 523–527.

102 Lobetti, R. (2000). Common variable immunodeficiency in miniature dachshunds affected with *Pneumonocystis carinii* pneumonia. *J Vet Diagn Invest* 12: 39–45.

103 Danesi, P., Ravagnan, S., Johnson, L.R. et al. (2017). Molecular diagnosis of Pneumocystis pneumonia in dogs. *Med Mycol* 55: 828–842.

104 Shiota, T., Shimada, Y., Kurimoto, H., and Oikawa, H. (1990). *Pneumocystis carinii* infection in corticosteroid-treated cats. *J Parasitol* 76: 441–445.

105 Hagler, D.N., Kim, C.K., and Walzer, P.D. (1987). Feline leukemia virus and *Pneumocystis carinii* infection. *J Parasitol* 73: 1284–1286.

106 McInerney, J., Papasouliotis, K., Simpson, K. et al. (2016). Pulmonary cowpox in cats: five cases. *J Feline Med Surg* 18: 518–525.

107 Damián, M., Morales, E., Salas, G., and Trigo, F.J. (2005). Immunohistochemical detection of antigens of distemper, adenovirus and parainfluenza viruses in domestic dogs with pneumonia. *J Comp Pathol* 133: 289–293.

108 Brownlee, L. and Sellon, R.K. (2001). Diagnosis of naturally occurring toxoplasmosis by bronchoalveolar lavage in a cat. *J Am Anim Hosp Assoc* 37: 251–255.

109 Davidson, M.G., Rottman, J.B., English, R.V. et al. (1993). Feline immunodeficiency virus predisposes cats to acute generalized toxoplasmosis. *Am J Pathol* 143: 1486–1497.

110 Headley, S.A., Alfieri, A.A., Fritzen, J.T. et al. (2013). Concomitant canine distemper, infectious canine

hepatitis, canine parvoviral enteritis, canine infectious tracheobronchitis, and toxoplasmosis in a puppy. *J Vet Diagn Invest* 25: 129–135.

111 Greig, B., Rossow, K.D., Collins, J.E., and Dubey, J.P. (1995). *Neospora caninum* pneumonia in an adult dog. *J Am Vet Med Assoc* 206: 1000–1001.

112 Prandini da Costa Reis, R., Crisman, R., Roser, M. et al. (2016). Neonatal neosporosis in a 2-week-old Bernese mountain dog infected with multiple *Neospora caninum* strains based on MS10 microsatellite analysis. *Vet Parasitol* 221: 134–138.

113 Dubey, J.P. and Schares, G. (2011). Neosporosis in animals: the last five years. *Vet Parasitol* 180: 90–108.

114 Gambino, J., Hiebert, E., Johnson, M., and Williams, M. (2016). Diagnosis of *Aelurostrongylus abstrusus* verminous pneumonia via sonography-guided fine-needle pulmonary parenchymal aspiration in a cat. *JFMS Open Rep* 2: 2055116916646584.

115 Broman, M.M. and Miller, M.A. (2016). Pathology in practice. *J Am Vet Med Assoc* 248: 1253–1255.

116 Traversa, D. and Di Cesare, A. (2014). Cardio-pulmonary parasitic nematodes affecting cats in Europe: unraveling the past, depicting the present, and predicting the future. *Front Vet Sci* 1: 11.

117 Varcasia, A., Brianti, E., Tamponi, C. et al. (2015). Simultaneous infection by four feline lungworm species and implications for the diagnosis. *Parasitol Res* 114: 317–321.

118 Pennisi, M.G., Hartmann, K., Addie, D.D. et al. (2015). Lungworm disease in cats: ABCD guidelines on prevention and management. *J Feline Med Surg* 17: 626–636.

119 Riggio, F., Mannella, R., Ariti, G., and Perrucci, S. (2013). Intestinal and lung parasites in owned dogs and cats from central Italy. *Vet Parasitol* 193: 78–84.

120 Ray Dillon, A., Tillson, D.M., Wooldridge, A. et al. (2014). Effect of pre-cardiac and adult stages of *Dirofilaria immitis* in pulmonary disease of cats: CBC, bronchial lavage cytology, serology, radiographs, CT images, bronchial reactivity, and histopathology. *Vet Parasitol* 206: 24–37.

121 Dillon, A.R., Tillson, D.M., Hathcock, J. et al. (2013). Lung histopathology, radiography, high-resolution computed tomography, and bronchio-alveolar lavage cytology are altered by *Toxocara cati* infection in cats and is independent of development of adult intestinal parasites. *Vet Parasitol* 193: 413–426.

122 Barutzki, D. (2013). Nematode infections of the respiratory tract in dogs in Germany. *Tierarztl Prax Ausg K Kleintiere Heimtiere* 41: 326–336; quiz 337.

123 Houpin, E., McCarthy, G., Ferrand, M. et al. (2016). Comparison of three methods for the detection of *Angiostrongylus vasorum* in the final host. *Vet Parasitol* 220: 54–58.

124 Kramer, L., Grandi, G., Passeri, B. et al. (2011). Evaluation of lung pathology in *Dirofilaria immitis*-experimentally infected dogs treated with doxycycline or a combination of doxycycline and ivermectin before administration of melarsomine dihydrochloride. *Vet Parasitol* 176: 357–360.

125 D'Costa, S., Yoon, B.I., Kim, D.Y. et al. (2012). Morphologic and molecular analysis of 39 spontaneous feline pulmonary carcinomas. *Vet Pathol* 49: 971–978.

126 van der Linde-Sipman, J.S. and van den Ingh, T.S. (2000). Primary and metastatic carcinomas in the digits of cats. *Vet Q* 22: 141–145.

127 Goldfinch, N. and Argyle, D.J. (2012). Feline lung-digit syndrome: unusual metastatic patterns of primary lung tumours in cats. *J Feline Med Surg* 14: 202–208.

128 Maritato, K.C., Schertel, E.R., Kennedy, S.C. et al. (2014). Outcome and prognostic indicators in 20 cats with surgically treated primary lung tumors. *J Feline Med Surg* 16: 979–984.

129 Jerram, R.M., Guyer, C.L., Braniecki, A. et al. (1998). Endogenous lipid (cholesterol) pneumonia associated with bronchogenic carcinoma in a cat. *J Am Anim Hosp Assoc* 34: 275–280.

130 Kujawa, A., Olias, P., Böttcher, A., and Klopfleisch, R. (2014). Thyroid transcription factor-1 is a specific marker of benign but not malignant feline lung tumours. *J Comp Pathol* 151: 19–24.

131 Burgess, H.J. and Kerr, M.E. (2009). Cytokeratin and vimentin co-expression in 21 canine primary pulmonary epithelial neoplasms. *J Vet Diagn Invest* 21: 815–820.

132 McNiel, E.A., Ogilvie, G.K., Powers, B.E. et al. (1997). Evaluation of prognostic factors for dogs with primary lung tumors: 67 cases (1985–1992). *J Am Vet Med Assoc* 211: 1422–1427.

133 Ramos-Vara, J.A., Miller, M.A., and Johnson, G.C. (2005). Usefulness of thyroid transcription factor-1 immunohistochemical staining in the differential diagnosis of primary pulmonary tumors of dogs. *Vet Pathol* 42: 315–320.

134 Beck, J., Miller, M.A., Frank, C. et al. (2017). Surfactant protein A and napsin A in the immunohistochemical characterization of canine pulmonary carcinomas: comparison with thyroid transcription factor-1. *Vet Pathol* 54: 767–774.

135 Ferreira, F.C., Soares, M.J., Carvalho, S. et al. (2015). Four cases of cell cannibalism in highly malignant feline and canine tumors. *Diagn Pathol* 10: 199.

136 Verrilli, A.M., Hohenhaus, A.E., Le Roux, A.B., and Donovan, T.A. (2016). What is your diagnosis? Primary pulmonary neoplasia. *J Am Vet Med Assoc* 248: 493–496.

137 Meléndez-Lazo, A., Cazzini, P., Camus, M. et al. (2015). Cell cannibalism by malignant neoplastic cells: three cases in dogs and a literature review. *Vet Clin Pathol* 44: 287–294.

138 Dole, R.S., MacPhail, C.M., and Lappin, M.R. (2004). Paraneoplastic leukocytosis with mature neutrophilia in a cat with pulmonary squamous cell carcinoma. *J Feline Med Surg* 6: 391–395.

139 Sharkey, L.C., Rosol, T.J., Gröne, A. et al. (1996). Production of granulocyte colony-stimulating factor and granulocyte-macrophage colony-stimulating factor by carcinomas in a dog and a cat with paraneoplastic leukocytosis. *J Vet Intern Med* 10: 405–408.

140 Moore, P.F. (2014). A review of histiocytic diseases of dogs and cats. *Vet Pathol* 51: 167–184.

141 Clarke, L.L., Kelly, L.S., Garner, B., and Brown, C.A. (2017). Atypical cytologic presentation of a histiocytic sarcoma in a Cavalier King Charles Spaniel dog. *J Vet Diagn Invest* 29: 541–543.

142 Mastrorilli, C., Spangler, E.A., Christopherson, P.W. et al. (2012). Multifocal cutaneous histiocytic sarcoma in a young dog and review of histiocytic cell immunophenotyping. *Vet Clin Pathol* 41: 412–418.

143 Busch, M.D., Reilly, C.M., Luff, J.A., and Moore, P.F. (2008). Feline pulmonary Langerhans cell histiocytosis with multiorgan involvement. *Vet Pathol* 45: 816–824.

144 Geyer, N.E., Reichle, J.K., Valdés-Martínez, A. et al. (2010). Radiographic appearance of confirmed pulmonary lymphoma in cats and dogs. *Vet Radiol Ultrasound* 51: 386–390.

145 Needle, D.B., Hollinger, C., Singer, L.M. et al. (2015). Pathology in practice. Lymphomatoid granulomatosis of lung tissue and mediastinal lymph node in a dog. *J Am Vet Med Assoc* 247: 1113–1116.

146 Valentine, B.A., Blue, J.T., Zimmer, J.F. et al. (2000). Pulmonary lymphomatoid granulomatosis in a cat. *J Vet Diagn Invest* 12: 465–467.

147 Choi, U.S., Alleman, A.R., Choi, J.H. et al. (2008). Cytologic and immunohistochemical characterization of a lung carcinoid in a dog. *Vet Clin Pathol* 37: 249–252.

148 Saqi, A. (2016). The state of cell blocks and ancillary testing: past, present, and future. *Arch Pathol Lab Med* 140: 1318–1322.

26

Respiratory Cytology of the Horse

Melissa Dawn Meachem and Julia Bettina Montgomery

Introduction

Cytological analysis of upper airway samples (nasal passages, nasopharynx, guttural pouches) is only infrequently performed in horses. Both swabs and washes can be obtained using either a blind technique or endoscopic guidance. Use of videoendoscopy enables visual assessment at the time of sampling and allows for easier access to the guttural pouches. Routine sampling sites of the equine lower airways include the trachea via transtracheal wash ((T)TW) or aspirate and the bronchial tree via bronchoalveolar lavage (BAL).

Clinical Indications for Sampling

Upper Airway

Relevant historical and clinical examination findings that warrant sampling include inappetence, fever, nasal discharge (serous to mucopurulent), and/or coughing. Horses with strangles can show signs of respiratory distress if the retropharyngeal lymph nodes are so enlarged that they occlude the airway. Often more than one horse will be affected and sampling of in-contact horses is recommended. Sampling of the upper airway is often performed to collect specimens for viral polymerase chain reaction (PCR) analysis or bacterial PCR and/or culture for upper respiratory pathogens such as equine influenza, equine herpes viruses (EHV) 1 and 4, or strangles (*Streptococcus equi* ssp. *equi*).[1] Many diagnostic laboratories will offer an "upper airway panel" that also includes equine rhinovirus (rhinitis virus). Analysis of guttural pouch washes is often required for the identification of strangles carriers that can shed the organism without obvious clinical signs.[2]

Lower Airway

The sampling site of choice should be determined by the clinical question. (T)TW cytology and culture should be performed to assess for bacterial or fungal pneumonia. BAL cytology is recommended over (T)TW cytology to aid in the diagnosis of equine asthma.[3–5] Due to sample collection method, culture of BAL fluid is not recommended because upper airway contamination cannot be avoided with the commonly used blind sampling techniques. Relevant historical and clinical examination findings that warrant sampling include respiratory symptoms such as coughing and nasal discharge. Horses with bacterial or fungal pneumonia are frequently febrile with a mucoid to mucopurulent nasal discharge and have an increased respiratory rate and/or effort at rest. Other common clinical findings indicative of pneumonia include increased tracheal mucus (tracheal rattle), as well as crackles and/or wheezes over the lung fields. The complete absence of sounds can be indicative of pleural effusion (pleuritis or pleuropneumonia).

The most common clinical signs associated with non-septic lower airway inflammation in mild to moderate equine asthma, formerly described as inflammatory airway disease (IAD), are exercise intolerance and coughing without other obvious clinical signs at rest.[6] Horses with severe equine asthma, formerly known as recurrent airway obstruction (RAO), can present similarly but usually also have some degree of increased respiratory effort at rest ("heaves") as well as a history of recurrence. Auscultation of the lung is usually unremarkable in horses with mild to moderate equine asthma. Horses with severe equine asthma frequently have increased tracheal mucus and auscultable wheezes. Rebreathing examination is recommended as part of the respiratory workup, unless the horse is in obvious

Veterinary Cytology, First Edition. Edited by Leslie C. Sharkey, M. Judith Radin, and Davis Seelig.

respiratory distress at rest. BAL can further aid in the diagnosis of exercise-induced pulmonary hemorrhage (EIPH) in the absence of overt clinical signs such as epistaxis.

Sample Collection Techniques

Nasal and Nasopharyngeal Swabs

Nasal swabs are obtained from the mucosa just inside the nasal passages using longer guarded swabs. These samples are not routinely used for cytological analysis in horses. For EHV-1 PCR, nasal swabs are recommended over nasopharyngeal samples.[1]

Guttural Pouch Lavage and Swab

Similar to the nasal cavity, guttural pouches of horses are rarely sampled for cytological analysis. Samples are frequently collected to aid in a diagnosis of strangles and identify inapparent strangles carriers. Guttural pouch lavage is considered to be more sensitive than guttural pouch swab.[2,7] Commercial guttural pouch lavage catheters are available. Another option is to use uterine insemination pipettes, which have been bent at a 45° angle on one end, to access the guttural pouch. Successful access to the guttural pouch should be confirmed by concurrent upper airway endoscopy, with the catheter inserted through the nostril on the same side as the guttural pouch of interest, and the endoscope inserted through the other nostril. It is difficult to enter the guttural pouch with an endoscope/catheter inserted through the opposite nostril, i.e. accessing the right guttural pouch from the left side. It is easiest to reach the guttural pouch by passing the catheter along the nasal septum.

Transtracheal and Tracheal Wash (Aspirate)

Collection of tracheal secretions can either be performed transtracheal (TTW) or through the biopsy channel of a videoendoscope (tracheal wash [TW]). For the latter, a two-stage sampling catheter should be used to avoid upper airway contamination of the sample, especially if the sample is also intended for bacterial culture. To obtain a TTW or TW sample, 10–20 mL of sterile saline is instilled into the trachea through the sampling catheter and aspirated. The sample will pool at the most dependent part of the trachea (thoracic inlet).

Bronchoalveolar Lavage

BAL can be performed using a cuffed BAL tube (blind technique) or a 3-m videoendoscope. Only the latter technique will allow for confirmation of the site within the lung from where the sample has been obtained. Regardless of technique, a standardized (250–500 mL) amount of saline is instilled and retrieved. Different sampling methodologies have been published.[3] The current consensus is that the most important factor for interpretation of the results is consistency in collection methodology and analysis.[6] Bronchial collapse in horses with severe equine asthma can affect the amount of fluid that can be retrieved.[8] Timing of BAL should be consider when also testing lung function as the BAL procedure has a temporary effect on lung function.[9]

Sample and Slide Preparation

Sample Processing

Immediately after collection, (T)TW and BAL fluid should be placed into an ethylenediaminetetraacetic acid (EDTA) tube to preserve cellular morphology and prevent clotting. Multiple aliquots can be combined without significantly altering the diagnostic outcome, although the proportion of mast cells is higher in initial aliquots.[10] If indicated by history, clinical signs, or gross appearance of the fluid, a portion of the sample should also be placed into a plain tube (lacking anticoagulant) to facilitate bacterial culture and sensitivity.

Washes and lavage samples should be processed as soon as possible to reduce sample storage changes such as neutrophil aging mimicking degenerative changes and *in vitro* phagocytosis of erythrocytes, extracellular bacteria, and debris. Samples to be processed within 8–24 hours of collection should be refrigerated or placed on ice to prevent bacterial overgrowth and to ensure adequate cell preservation.[11] For longer processing delays, a fixative (equal volume of 10% buffered formalin or 40% ethanol) can be added to the sample immediately following collection, although resulting cellular morphology is often less than ideal.[11]

The gross appearance of the fluid should be noted as it can be helpful in indicating the clinical process(es) occurring, as well as adequacy of the sample collection technique. Normal BAL fluid is clear or mildly turbid and can appear foamy when alveolar spaces containing surfactant are sampled. A clear sample lacking foam suggests sampling of the large airways or trachea.[3] Floccular material reflects mucus and cellular debris, whereas a pink or brown tinge indicates recent or chronic hemorrhage, respectively.[3]

A total nucleated cell count (TNCC) can be performed on wash and lavage samples using an automated analyzer or manually with a hemocytometer, although diagnostic usefulness is questionable owing to the variable recovery of fluid, unknown dilution factor, and cell entrapment in mucus. Reported TNCCs of BAL fluid from normal horses range from <0.3 to 1.32×10^6 cells/mL.[10,12] Use of a standard volume and sampling procedure can help improve accuracy of the TNCC.[10] Frequently, a qualitative estimate on stained direct smears is performed to identify samples with low, normal, or increased cellularity.

Slide Preparation

Direct, line, squash, and concentrated preparations are typically examined. Clinicians are strongly encouraged to prepare direct smears shortly after sample collection to help differentiate *in vivo* from *in vitro* changes, especially if the sample is to be sent to an external laboratory. If flocculent or mucoid material is present grossly, a squash prep of the material should be made as cells and organisms are frequently embedded in the mucus (Figure 26.1). Given the dilute nature of TTW and BAL samples, concentration of the cellular elements helps improve diagnostic yield; a cytocentrifuge (cytospin) is preferred. If not available, a sediment smear can be prepared as follows: centrifuge at 300g for 10 minutes, pour off the supernatant, and prepare a direct smear from the resuspended pellet.[3] Compared with cytospin preparations, visualization of cellular detail can be more problematic with direct and sediment smears owing to cellular condensation, and the relative proportions of mast cells, eosinophils, and macrophages can also be lower.[3,13]

Slide Staining

Air-dried smears are typically stained by Romanowsky-type stains. Fast or aqueous-based Romanowsky stains (for example, Diff-Quik®) are easy to use and provide rapid results; however, they often stain mast cell granules poorly, leading to underestimation of mast cell numbers.[4] A second smear should be stained with toluidine blue to allow for mast cell differential counts.[14] Alternatively, metachromatic or methanol-based Romanowsky stains, such as Wright's or Wright–Giemsa, will reliably identify equine mast cells and are frequently used in automated stainers in clinical pathology laboratories.[4] Other stains that can be used include Gram stain to identify bacteria, periodic acid–Schiff stain to highlight fungal organisms, and Perl's Prussian blue stain to highlight iron.

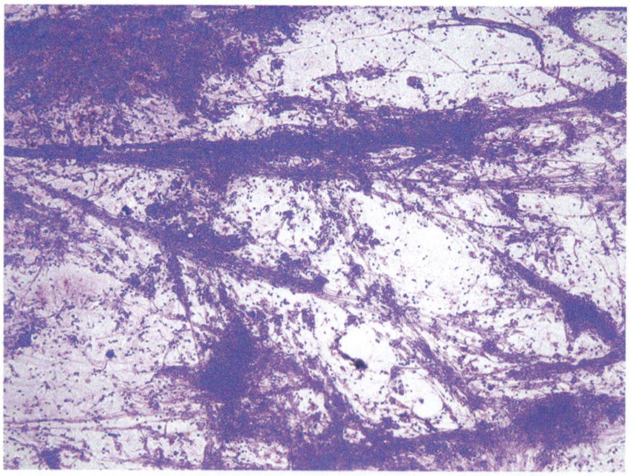

Figure 26.1 Squash preparation of mucoid material in a transtracheal wash from a horse with severe equine asthma. The background contains streaming eosinophilic mucus enmeshing abundant inflammatory cells (Wright–Giemsa, 200×).

Normal Cytological Findings of the Upper Respiratory Tract

Cellular Elements

Swabs and flushes from the upper respiratory system contain low numbers of exfoliated epithelial cells characteristic of the region sampled. The rostral nasal cavity is lined by stratified squamous epithelium. Cytologically, squamous cells appear as large platelike cells with abundant pale basophilic cytoplasm, angular borders, and small condensed nuclei. Caudal to the vestibule, the majority of the nasal cavity is lined by pseudostratified respiratory epithelium composed of ciliated and nonciliated columnar epithelial cells admixed with abundant goblet cells. Columnar cells are elongate with a basally located round nucleus and, if present, fine cilia on their apical surface forming an eosinophilic brush border. Mucus-producing goblet cells are also columnar shaped but lack cilia and contain many large magenta mucin granules in their apical portion (Figure 26.2a). The nasopharynx is lined by ciliated pseudostratified columnar epithelium with areas of stratified squamous epithelium. The mucosa of the guttural pouches and paranasal sinuses is composed of pseudostratified ciliated columnar and cuboidal epithelium with sparse goblet cells. Cuboidal cells have a high nuclear to cytoplasmic ratio (N:C), moderate amounts of basophilic granular cytoplasm, and round centrally located nuclei.

Lymphoid nodules are present throughout the submucosa of the upper respiratory tract and are particularly abundant in the nasopharynx. These small localized collections of lymphocytes respond to antigenic stimulation, and hyperplasia can occur. Other underlying structures that inadvertently might be sampled include glands within the lamina propria (e.g. nasal and Bowman's glands in the nasal cavity), adipose tissue, bone, and cartilage.

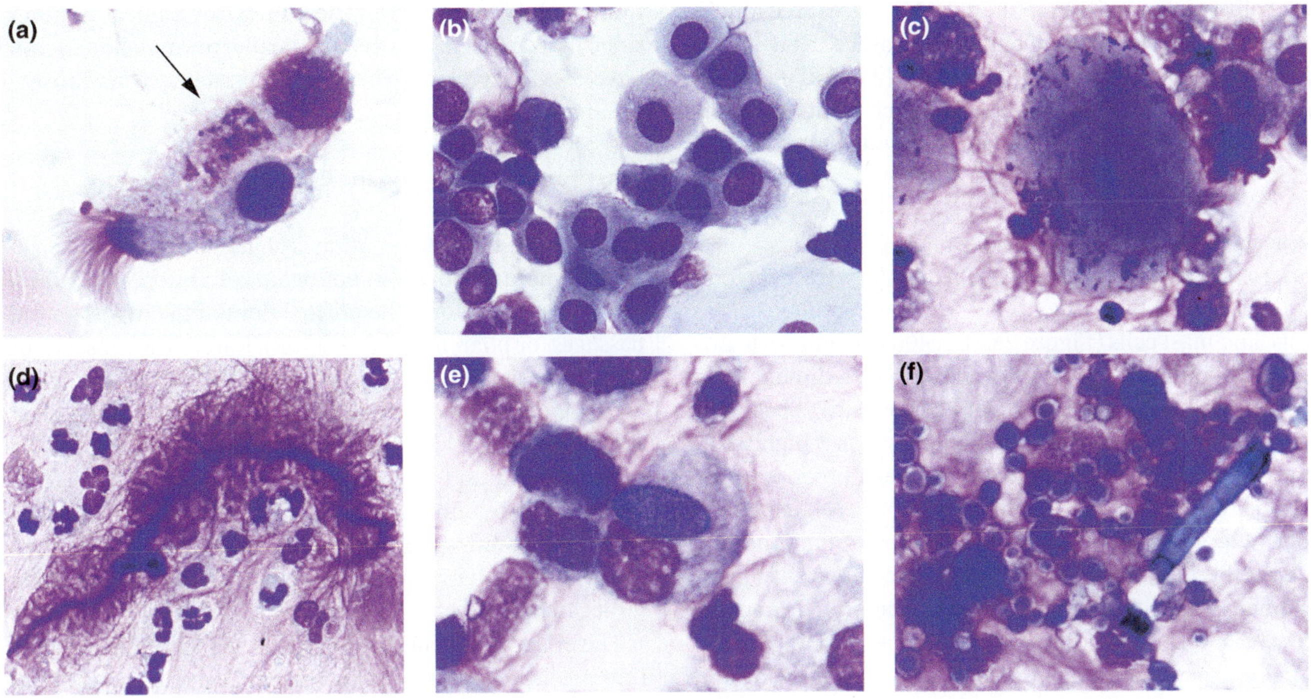

Figure 26.2 (a) Goblet cell (arrow) and ciliated columnar respiratory epithelial cell. The apical portion of goblet cells contains mucin granules. (b) Cuboidal epithelial cells line the smaller bronchioles and may be seen in BAL samples. (c) Squamous epithelial cell with adherent mixed bacteria reflecting oropharyngeal contamination of the sample. (d) Curschmann's spiral in a transtracheal wash from a horse with severe equine asthma. (e) Phagocytosed pollen grain within a macrophage. (f) Inhaled environmental contaminants include fungal spores and fragments of hyphae (Wright–Giemsa, 1000×).

Noncellular Elements

Low numbers of a mixed population of extracellular bacteria can be seen in samples collected from the upper respiratory tract of normal horses. These bacteria are considered normal microflora and do not induce an inflammatory response. Small amounts of amorphous to streaming magenta mucous material can also be seen.

Normal Cytological Findings of the Lower Respiratory Tract

Cellular Elements

Respiratory Epithelial Cells

The trachea, bronchi, and larger bronchioles are lined by ciliated columnar epithelial cells that frequently exfoliate into (T)TW and occasionally into BAL samples. Goblet cells are not commonly observed, but can increase in number with chronic pulmonary irritation. The large size of the mucin granules helps to differentiate these cells from mast cells, which have finer granules. Cuboidal epithelial cells line the smaller bronchioles and can be seen in both (T)TW and BAL samples (Figure 26.2b). Both columnar and cuboidal respiratory epithelial cells can exfoliate individually and in small sheets (Figure 26.3). Predominance of epithelial cells accompanied by low numbers of leukocytes suggests poor technique with principal sampling of the

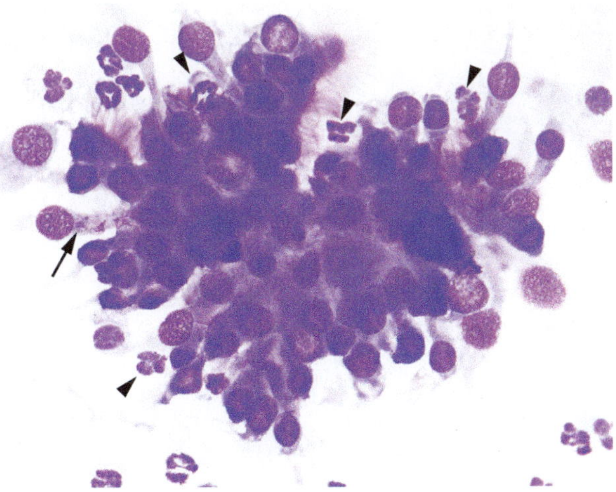

Figure 26.3 Ciliated columnar respiratory epithelial cells with admixed goblet cells (arrow) and neutrophils (arrowheads) in a transtracheal wash from a horse (Wright–Giemsa, 1000×).

larger airways as opposed to the alveolar space. Free mucin granules from ruptured goblet cells may be seen in the background of the smear and must be differentiated from bacterial cocci. Similarly, cilia can detach from columnar cells during sample storage and free cilia must not be confused with bacterial rods.

Leukocytes and Differential Cell Count

Other cells present in the lower respiratory tract include alveolar macrophages, lymphocytes, neutrophils, eosinophils, and mast cells (Figure 26.4). A 400-cell leukocyte differential count performed on a cytospin or sediment slide is advocated for equine BAL fluid to ensure repeatability.[3,15] An alternative 5-field method in which 5 highly cellular fields are evaluated at 500× has been proposed; this method resulted in greater reliability of mast cell enumeration.[15] Flocculent material should also be examined as part of the differential cell count as cell populations entrapped in mucus can differ from those in concentrated preparations. Caution must be exercised when performing differential leukocyte counts performed on BAL fluid with low cellularity or gross oropharyngeal contamination as these samples may not reflect the true disease process. The cytology of normal equine TW samples typically consists of <32% neutrophils, 24% macrophages, 8% lymphocytes, <1% eosinophils, and 34% epithelial cells.[16]

Based on the current consensus statement on IAD, normal BAL cytology is defined as ≤5% neutrophils, ≤2% mast cells, and ≤1% eosinophils.[6] Since publication of the first IAD consensus statement in 2007, several studies have identified >5% neutrophils in clinically normal horses, and it has been suggested that 10% is a better cutoff.[16] Table 26.1 contains differential cell counts from equine BAL samples from various studies. It is absolutely vital that cytology findings be interpreted in the context of clinical findings since it is recognized that clinically normal horses can have BAL cytology findings consistent with airway inflammation.

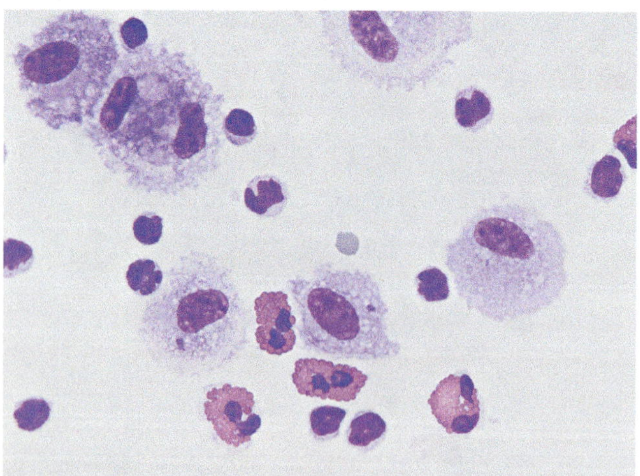

Figure 26.4 Macrophages, lymphocytes, and eosinophils in a bronchoalveolar sample from a horse (Wright–Giemsa, 600×).

Other Factors Influencing the Cytology of the Lower Respiratory Tract

Oropharyngeal contamination is characterized by the presence of mature squamous epithelial cells often with adherent bacteria that form the normal flora of the mouth, nasal passages, or pharynx (Figure 26.2c). Rarely, the presence of such material reflects a true biological process, such as aspiration of oropharyngeal material into the airway or bronchoesophageal fistula. The presence of neutrophilic inflammation and a supportive clinical history could be helpful to differentiate these processes. Care must be taken when interpreting aged samples with evidence of oropharyngeal contamination, as *in vitro* phagocytosis of bacteria can occur.

The effect of repeated sampling on TW and BAL cytology findings has been studied in horses. One study performed in healthy Standardbred horses found that repeated sampling at 24 hour intervals did not affect TW or BAL cytology findings.[23] In another study, BAL neutrophil percentage increased in horses sampled twice 48 hours apart; however, they remained within the reference range.[24] Another study, performed in both exercising and rested Thoroughbreds, showed a decreasing number of neutrophils in BAL fluid collected once a week for 10 weeks.[25]

Normal BAL cytology does not appear to differ in healthy animals based on age. Season can have an indirect effect on airway cytology due to changes in air quality (dust, mold, smoke), temperature (cold air-induced bronchoconstriction), and housing (outdoors vs. indoors).[26–29] Stabling has been associated with an increase of BAL neutrophil percentage and increased expression of pro-inflammatory cytokines in normal racehorses.[30] The effect of season and environment on airway cytology has been most extensively studied in horses with non-septic lower airway inflammation (equine asthma syndrome). Especially for severe equine asthma, environmental factors such as dust or moldy hay are known to result in disease exacerbations of predisposed horses.[6] As a result of the association with stabling, severe equine asthma is generally more frequently observed in the winter months; however, one disease phenotype has been associated with hot and humid weather (formerly known as summer pasture associated RAO).[6] For this reason, as previously mentioned, results must be interpreted within the clinical context, and an abnormal airway cytology in a clinically healthy horse without a history of poor performance is likely clinically insignificant and does not warrant treatment.

Table 26.1 Differential cell count (%) bronchoalveolar lavage findings in normal horses from the published literature.

		Neutrophils	Lymphocytes	Macrophages	Eosinophils	Mast cells	Epithelial cells
Couëtil et al.[16]	$n = 9$, mean (SD)	6.8 (2.7)	31.4 (13.0)	57.1 (10.3)	0.3 (0.5)	1.5 (0.8)	NS
Derksen et al.[17]	$n = 10$, mean (SE)	8.9 (1.2)	43 (2.7)	45 (2.8)	<1	1.2 (0.3)	3.5 (0.7)
Miskovic et al.[18]	$n = 9$, median (range)	8 (3–28)	36 (18–50)	50 (38–65)	NS	NS	NS
Christmann et al.[19]	$n = 15$, mean (SD)	4.6 (3.18)	42.87 (12.32)	52.53 (12.13)	NS	NS	NS
Costa et al.[20]	Summer: $n = 6$, mean (SD)	8 (3)	52 (4)	34 (2)	NS	2.2 (0.6)	NS
Costa et al.[20]	Winter: $n = 6$, mean (SD)	4 (2)	39 (6)	50 (2)	NS	1.8 (0.6)	NS
Koblinger et al.[8]	$n = 33$, mean (SD)	4.3 (2.6)	46.3 (11.6)	47.9 (12.0)	0.1 (0.2)	1.4 (0.4)	NS
Hare and Viel[21]	$n = 6$, median (range)	0.4 (0.2–1.4)	31.5 (19–35)	67.7 (61–78.8)	0.3 (0–1)	1 (0–2.8)	0 (0–0.6)
Naylor et al.[22]	$n = 9$, mean (SD)	4.4 (3.3)	38.8 (12.6)	48.2 (10.8)	1.3 (4.0)	7.3 (4.7)	NS
Hoffman[3]	Literature summary	<5	30–50	50–70	<0.1	<2	Rare

SD, standard deviation; SE, standard error; NS, not specified.

When interpreting airway cytology findings, it is important to consider how much sampling of one site (within one lung; left versus right lung) reflects the overall clinical picture. Although statistically significant differences in neutrophil and mast cell percentages between the right and left lung have been shown, their clinical impact is questionable.[31,32] As mentioned previously, sampling of a specific site within the lung can only be accomplished with videoendoscopy. For reasons of practicality, obtaining several samples from one horse could be more relevant in a research setting than in clinical cases, especially since the observed differences were often small. Lung atelectasis following general anesthesia has also been shown to result in a transient increase in BAL neutrophils.[33]

Noncellular Elements

Mucus

A small amount of mucus is a normal finding in (T)TW and BAL samples. Mucus can appear as finely stippled amorphous to streaming eosinophilic material, often entrapping cells. Curschmann's spirals are tight spirals of inspissated mucus that form in the small bronchioles secondary to excessive production or decreased clearance of mucus (Figure 26.2d). Increased mucus can be seen in chronic inflammatory conditions such as severe equine asthma.

Other Foreign Material

Various other contaminants can be observed in TTW and BAL samples, including starch granules from surgical gloves, keratin bars from the skin of the horse or sample collector, and environmental inhalants such as pollen (Figure 26.2e), mold spores, and fragments of saprophytic fungi such as *Alternaria* spp. (Figure 26.2f). The latter can be phagocytosed by macrophages with numbers paralleling degree of exposure to particulates in forage, stable dust, and other environmental sources. Black carbonaceous material can be seen in horses with smoke inhalation and those that live in heavily polluted environments.[34] Silicosis results in a chronic granulomatous pneumonia and can be diagnosed by the presence of intracytoplasmic birefringent crystalline material within pulmonary macrophages.[35]

Abnormal Cytological Findings of the Respiratory Tract

Neutrophilic, Macrophagic, and Mixed Inflammation

General Principles of Interpretation

Neutrophilic inflammation is typically associated with acute processes but can also be observed in more chronic conditions that have an active focus. Increased neutrophils warrant close examination for infectious organisms, especially if the cells are degenerate. However, since similar karyolytic changes will occur with sample aging, the preparation of direct preparations at the time of collection is always helpful. Septic neutrophilic inflammation can be due to bacterial, fungal, or less commonly, viral infection. Well-preserved neutrophils can occasionally be seen in septic conditions if numbers of infectious organisms are low and slides are prepared soon after collection. Thus, culture of fluid samples is often performed if there is evidence of neutrophilic inflammation even in the absence of cytologically apparent infectious agents.

Low numbers of alveolar macrophages are often seen with suppurative inflammation and can begin to predominate in chronic disease and with certain etiological agents. Binucleated and occasional multinucleated forms can be noted, and cells can contain phagocytosed debris and other contaminants.

Infectious Etiologies

Bacteria

In adult horses, bacterial pneumonia and pleuropneumonia are typically associated with immunosuppression.[36,37] Most organisms reflect opportunistic bacteria that are normal residents of the upper respiratory tract, with β-hemolytic streptococci, such as *S. equi* subspecies *zooepidemicus* (*Streptococcus zooepidemicus*), being most common.[38] *S. zooepidemicus* is a common cause of bacterial pneumonia in both adult horses and foals. Cytologically, it can appear as individual, pairs, or short chains (usually less than four) of Gram-positive coccoid bacteria. Definitive diagnosis requires bacterial culture of TW samples. Culture results should always be interpreted in the context of clinical signs and cytologic findings, as positive cultures can reflect infection, transient lower airway colonization, or oropharyngeal contamination. Fluid samples should be submitted for both aerobic and anaerobic culture as anaerobic bacteria can be isolated from approximately one third of cases and mixed aerobic and anaerobic infections are common.[38] If pneumonia is suspected, a (T)TW is the preferred sample over BAL for both cytological examination and culture, as BAL fluid can be normal in some horses with confirmed pneumonia and pleuropneumonia.[39] *Actinobacillus equuli,* a Gram-negative oval to rod-shaped bacterium, is another frequent cause of bacterial pneumonia in horses. Definitive etiological diagnosis requires bacterial culture of TW samples. Strangles (*S. equi* subspecies *equi*) usually does not affect the lower respiratory tract (with the exception of bastard strangles). Strangles is usually diagnosed by nasopharyngeal swab PCR or culture/PCR of guttural pouch washes. Cytologically, *S. equi* is morphologically indistinguishable from *S. zooepidemicus*, although it can occur in longer chains.

Bacterial infection is associated with an increased relative proportion of neutrophils, often approaching 100%. Neutrophils frequently appear degenerate with large swollen nuclei and can display cytoplasmic vacuolation. The presence of intracellular bacteria is helpful to confirm sepsis, provided that the sample was processed promptly to minimize *in vitro* phagocytosis. Bacterial morphology and Gram stain can aid in the selection of initial antimicrobial therapy but are not a substitute for culture and sensitivity.[36] Aspiration pneumonia is characterized by severe neutrophilic inflammation together with oropharyngeal material and typically a mixed bacterial population. The diagnosis should be supported by history and clinical signs with the possibility of sample contamination excluded. Common causes of aspiration pneumonia in horses include choke and dysphagia.

Bacterial pneumonia is relatively common in foals and can be part of a systemic septic process in neonates with Gram-negative aerobes frequently isolated.[29] *Rhodococcus equi* is a Gram-positive obligate intracellular bacterium that causes bacterial pneumonia and pulmonary abscesses in foals between 3 weeks and 6 months of age. A definitive diagnosis of *R. equi* is made based on bacteriological culture of TW obtained from affected foals. Cytologically, *R. equi* is a small, pleomorphic, intracellular bacteria that can appear coccoid to rod shaped and is often described as a watermelon seed with a thin peripheral clear halo. It is a Gram-positive facultative intracellular pathogen that can be found within both neutrophils and macrophages. Confirmation of the diagnosis requires either culture or positive identification of the VapA gene by PCR of (T)TW samples.[29,30] Due to the ubiquity of *R. equi* in the environment, the organism can be isolated from normal foals; however, false-positive diagnosis can be avoided by ensuring the presence of concurrent supportive cytological and thoracic imaging findings. A mixed infection with other anaerobes does not affect prognosis but warrants culture and sensitivity testing in all cases.[36,37,40]

Fungi

Fungal respiratory infections can occur in the paranasal sinuses, guttural pouches, and lungs. Primary pathogenic fungi include dimorphic yeast, such as *Blastomyces dermatitidis*, *Histoplasma capsulatum*, *Coccidioides immitis*, *Cryptococcus neoformans*, and *Conidiobolus coronatus*, and tend to result in upper respiratory tract infections in normal horses.[41–43] Fungal pneumonia is typically associated with opportunistic fungal species, such as *Aspergillus* spp., *Penicillium* spp., *Mucor* spp., *Acremonium* spp., and *Fusarium* spp. It is reported mostly in immunocompromised animals with leukopenia, neutropenia, and/or devitalized tissue.[41,42] Guttural pouch mycosis should be considered as a differential diagnosis in horses with epistaxis. Clinical diagnosis is made by endoscopy of the guttural pouches. Sampling of fungal plaques is generally avoided due to their close association with the internal carotid artery.

Respiratory fluid samples from horses with mycotic pneumonia typically contain abundant neutrophils and macrophages, with multinucleated giant cells sometimes observed.[41,44] Fungal hyphae and spores in large numbers accompanied by numerous intracellular forms help to support the diagnosis. Repeated positive culture or histological evidence of hyphal tissue invasion is needed to confirm invasive fungal disease.[44] Fungal elements, including spores and hyphae, are commonly observed in (T)TW and rarely in BAL samples of many normal horses and reflect inhalation of saprophytic fungi, such as *Alternaria* spp., from the barn environment.[41] Inhaled fungal contaminants are phagocytosed by mononuclear cells; however, they rarely incite an inflammatory response. Environmental contaminants and other opportunistic fungi can be cultured in a low number of normal horses; thus culture results should not be interpreted in isolation.[44]

Aspergillus spp. is the most common fungal pathogen of the equine lower respiratory tract. In cytologic samples it appears as fragments and mats of broad, septate hyphae with parallel walls, and acute right-angled branching.[44] As the morphological appearance of *Aspergillus* is not unique, culture or PCR is required for confirmation. A PCR system has recently been developed that is able to identify three major pathogenic species of *Aspergillus* (*Aspergillus fumigatus, Aspergillus niger*, and *Aspergillus flavus*) and differentiate them from common contaminant species.[45] Serological titers are of limited use due to the prevalence of exposure to *Aspergillus* in the environment. The use of fungal urine antigen tests in the equine does not appear to have been evaluated at this time.

Pneumocystis jirovecii (formerly *Pneumocystis carinii*) is an opportunistic fungal pathogen resulting in interstitial pneumonia in immunocompromised foals and rarely adult horses.[46] The organism resides primarily in the alveolar spaces and can be recovered in BAL fluid and by percutaneous aspiration or lung biopsy. Several forms are typically visible: the trophic form is small (1–4 µm), light staining, and pyriform to elongate; intermediate cysts are round and contain 2–8 nuclei (early, intermediate, and late precysts, respectively), and mature cysts are round, 8–10 µm in diameter with 8 intracystic nuclei.[47] *P. jirovecii* invokes a neutrophilic to macrophagic to mixed inflammatory response, and aggregates of cysts and trophozoites are described as having a granular, foamy, or honeycomb-like appearance.[46] *P. jirovecii* cannot be cultured, and diagnosis is typically based on cytologic or histologic identification of characteristic organisms.[34,39] Special staining, such as Gomori methenamine silver, can help to highlight the cyst form. Immunohistochemistry, fluorescent *in situ* hybridization and PCR are currently being explored to aid in diagnosis.[46–48]

Viruses

Viral infections that have been implicated as a cause of interstitial pneumonia in horses include equine viral arteritis, adenovirus in Arabian severe combined immunodeficiency (SCID) foals, influenza A virus, and equine herpes viruses (EHV-1, EHV-4, and EHV-5). Typical findings on (T)TW and BAL samples include increased numbers of neutrophils and macrophages.[42] Fungal and bacterial cultures are negative for significant organisms in uncomplicated cases, although horses can develop secondary bacterial pneumonia.[42,49] Definitive diagnosis is made by PCR evaluation of nasal or nasopharyngeal samples.[42]

Equine multinodular pulmonary fibrosis is a recently described condition in horses that has been associated with EHV-5.[50,51] Cytology of BAL and (T)TW samples from affected horses reveal neutrophilic inflammation; neutrophils are typically greater than 50–70% and can be either degenerate or non-degenerate. Visible infectious organisms are not observed, and fungal/bacterial culture results are negative or consistent with sample contamination.[52–54] Eosinophilic intranuclear viral inclusion bodies within macrophages in BAL samples have rarely been reported.[55] A tentative diagnosis can be made in horses with radiographic evidence of nodular interstitial pneumonia and PCR identification of EHV-5 from BAL fluid. However, EHV-5 can often be identified in BAL and (T)TW samples in a low number of unaffected horses; thus histopathological evaluation of lung tissue is needed for a definitive diagnosis.[56] Characteristic histopathologic changes include marked pulmonary interstitial fibrosis with preservation of alveolar-like architecture, infiltration of mixed inflammatory cells, and the presence of intranuclear viral inclusion bodies within macrophages.[51]

Non-Septic Etiologies (Equine Asthma Syndrome)

A diagnosis of mild to moderate or severe equine asthma should be made based on BAL cytology in conjunction with history and clinical signs.[6] BAL neutrophilia is the cytological hallmark of equine asthma, which can occur in horses of all ages. In younger horses, it is more frequently characterized by increased percentages of eosinophils and/or mast cells on BAL cytology, while BAL neutrophilia is more commonly seen in older horses.

The correlation between (T)TW and BAL cytology is often poor in horses with mild to moderate or severe equine asthma, and (T)TW differentials are highly variable compared with BAL; thus, BAL is the superior method to assess small airway inflammation. Mild to moderate equine asthma is generally diagnosed on the basis of a BAL sample with mild neutrophilia (>5% but <20%), eosinophilia (>1%), mastocytosis (>2%), or a combination of these. Horses with neutrophilic BAL cytology tend to be older, with a cough and greater levels of hypoxemia when exercising, whereas horses with mastocytosis are more likely to have airway hypersensitivity to histamine bronchoprovocation and increased amounts of mucus on BAL cytology. BAL cytology in horses with severe equine asthma is primarily neutrophilic (>20%, often approaching 100%) with mast cells rarely identified, abundant mucus, occasional

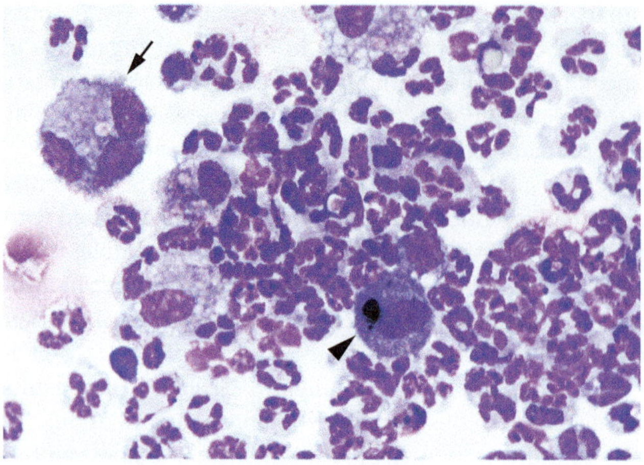

Figure 26.5 Bronchoalveolar lavage from a horse with severe equine asthma. The sample contains predominantly non-degenerate neutrophils and low numbers of macrophages and small lymphocytes. Note the multinucleated macrophage (arrow) and hemosiderophage (arrowhead) (Wright–Giemsa, 600×).

Curschmann's spirals, and frequent mold spores or pollen grains engulfed by alveolar macrophages (Figure 26.5).

Mild to moderate and severe equine asthma has overlapping clinical and cytological features that arise from pulmonary response to organic dust and noxious gases encountered in the barn environment.[57] Contributors to mild to moderate equine asthma are thought to include high levels of environmental particulates, viral disease (EHV-2, equine rhinitis A virus), air pollution, genetic predisposition, and bacterial infection (either primary or secondary as a result of poor airway clearance). Severe equine asthma likely arises from a complex interaction between innate and acquired immunity, environment, and genetic susceptibility. Histopathologic changes include mucosal inflammatory cell infiltrates, luminal exudate, bronchiolar hyperplasia, and goblet cell metaplasia. Up to 80% of clinically normal horses can have evidence of mild peribronchiolitis.[58]

S. zooepidemicus and *Streptococcus pneumoniae* could play an important etiological role in the pathogenesis of mild to moderate equine asthma in young horses.[59] Prevalence in horses with no bacterial growth (tracheal samples) was 4% compared with 80% in horses with $\geq 10^5$ colony forming units of bacteria/mL. Mixed infections were common. *S. pneumoniae* was detected in 23% of 2-year-old or younger horses with mild to moderate equine asthma but was not detected in older animals. *S. zooepidemicus* was isolated in 66% of horses with mild to moderate equine asthma (30% of samples having $\geq 10^3$ colony forming units/mL) and was not affected by the age of the horse.[59]

Another characteristic of equine asthma is airway hypersensitivity (AHS), which does not always appear to correlate with BAL cytology in affected horses. Some horses had abnormal pulmonary function in the absence of cytological evidence of inflammation and vice versa. This finding led some researchers to postulate that AHS and airway inflammation are not always related and/or that these discordant horses reflect early manifestation of disease.[60]

Severe equine asthma has a better understood environmental link (exposure to moldy hay, endotoxin, exotoxin, fungal spores, etc.). Exposure to organic particulates causes transient airway neutrophilia in most horses, but only those with severe equine asthma will develop clinical signs. Severe equine asthma also has a potential genetic basis with differences in interleukin-4 receptor gene and Th2 response observed in affected horses.[61]

Tilley et al. proposed a system for staging severe equine asthma (stage 1–4) based on endoscopic mucous score (accumulation, localization, viscosity, color), BAL neutrophil percentage (<20, 21–40, 41–60, >41), clinical signs score (cough, nostril flare, and abdominal lift), and thoracic radiographic changes.[62,63]

Based on one study, radiographic scoring is not useful in diagnosis of mild to moderate equine asthma and does not correlate with BAL cytology or lung function testing.[63] Histopathologic examination of lungs from horses with severe equine asthma reveals inflammatory infiltrate around the airways, profound airway remodeling with goblet cell and epithelial hyperplasia, variable airway smooth muscle hypertrophy or hyperplasia, and alveolar fibrosis.

Eosinophilic and Mast Cell Inflammation

Unlike mast cells, which are primarily restricted to the distal small airways and alveoli, eosinophils tend to be equally distributed throughout the equine respiratory tract.[4] However, high numbers of eosinophils are occasionally only present in (T)TW samples and can be focally distributed or entrapped in mucus. Thus, it is best to examine both (T)TW and BAL samples, including squash preps of mucoid material, when evaluating numbers of mast cells and eosinophils. Eosinophilic inflammation in (T)TW and BAL samples can be seen with parasitic, allergic, or hyperreactive inflammatory lower airway disease and rarely with hypereosinophilic syndromes such as paraneoplastic hypereosinophilia, idiopathic chronic eosinophilic pneumonia, and multisystemic eosinophilic epitheliotrophic disease (MEED).[64]

Parasitic pneumonia in adult horses is most often caused by migrating larvae of *Dictyocaulus arnfieldi* and has rarely been associated with *Echinococcus granulosus* (hydatidosis), *Habronema* (aberrant migration), and *Dirofilaria immitis*.[58] First stage larvae of *D. arnfieldi* can occasionally be identified in T(TW) and BAL samples from horses;

larvae are approximately 450 μm in length with dark granular food material in intestinal cells and a small spiked tail. In foals, *Parascaris equorum* is the most common etiologic agent, with a few reports of *Strongyloides westeri* and *Strongylus vulgaris*.[65] (T)TW and BAL cytology can reveal an increased proportion of eosinophils, potentially greater than 80%. Parasitic larvae and eggs are sometimes seen. Eggs of *P. equorum* are approximately 100 μm, thick shelled with a rough proteinaceous coat, and contain a single cell. Larvae of *S. vulgaris* are large with a very long filamentous extension of the sheath, short esophagus, and 28–32 well-defined, rectangular intestinal cells; eggs are typical of nematode species with a thin shell surrounding a central group of cells. In comparison, strongyloides larvae lack a sheath and have an esophagus almost half the length of the body; eggs of *S. westeri* are small, 40–52 × 32–40 μm, and larvated.

Secondary suppurative bacterial pneumonia can be a potential sequela and occasionally mask eosinophilic inflammation.[66] Examination of the feces for parasite eggs or larvae should be performed via centrifugal flotation or the modified Baermann technique. Horses with *D. arnfieldi* infection typically have a history of close association with donkeys or mules, the natural host for the lungworm.

Mild pulmonary eosinophilia and mastocytosis have been reported in a subset of horses with mild to moderate equine asthma. Affected horses tend to be younger (average age 3 years) racehorses evaluated for poor performance rather than cough, with Thoroughbreds overrepresented.[4,67] Median BAL eosinophils were reported as 3.5% (range 0–12%) and mast cells at 3% (range 0–10%). Mild increase in BAL eosinophils can also be seen in horses with severe equine asthma (mean 2.6%, range 0–10%); however, the significance of mild eosinophilia and mastocytosis is not easily interpreted.[62] Clinically normal racehorses can have increased BAL eosinophilia in the summer compared with winter (mean of 2.25% versus 0.13%, respectively).[30] Transient pulmonary eosinophilia has also been reported in a small group of Standardbred horses in training.[68] BAL cytology revealed significantly elevated eosinophils (5–37%) that were not associated with clinical signs and that resolved within two months without specific treatment. These studies highlight the importance of interpretation of cytological findings within the context of history and clinical signs.

A predominance of eosinophils in BAL fluid samples also can be seen with equine idiopathic chronic eosinophilic pneumonia. This uncommon condition is characterized by peripheral eosinophilia, diffuse miliary or granular interstitial pattern on radiography, and pulmonary infiltration by eosinophils observed histologically with limited extrapulmonary involvement. The reported mean percentage of eosinophils in BAL fluid is 28% (range 4–40%).[64] Severe eosinophilic pulmonary disease has also been described in horses with MEED, but these horses will likely also have eosinophilic lesions in other organ systems, such as the skin and gastrointestinal tract.[69–71]

Hemosiderosis

The presence of erythrophagia and hemosiderin-laden macrophages (hemosiderophages) reflects acute or more chronic hemorrhage. Common causes include EIPH, inhalation of blood from bleeding neoplasms or other lesions in the upper respiratory cavity, and epistaxis. Iatrogenic bleeding during the sampling procedure warrants prompt processing of the sample to avoid *in vitro* erythrophagia, which can confound interpretation. Many normal horses will have a low number of erythrocytes and hemosiderophages in BAL samples even at rest.[72,73]

EIPH is an important performance limiting disease in racehorses.[74,75] The currently accepted pathogenic mechanism is stress-induced damage of the pulmonary capillaries created by an imbalance between high intra-capillary pressure and low intra-alveolar pressure during exercise.[76] Recent research has also demonstrated venous remodeling.[77] All horses undergoing strenuous activity can demonstrate a degree of pulmonary hemorrhage, with up to 20% hemosiderophages reported in BAL fluid from normal horses after a single bout of strenuous exercise.[73] Increased hemosiderophages were seen one week after exercise and remained elevated for three weeks; thus time delays between bleeding and sample collection must also be taken into consideration. The exact proportion of hemosiderophages needed to diagnose EIPH is not clear; however, finding greater than 50% hemosiderophages in BAL fluid samples is generally considered to be significant.[72,76] In addition, the individual cellular hemosiderin content tends to be higher in alveolar macrophages in EIPH compared with normal horses.[72] EIPH can be a progressive disease with histological evidence of bronchiolitis, proliferation of bronchial arterial vessels, and fibrosis in moderate to severe cases.[76] Eosinophilic infiltrates can be observed in advanced cases. Due to the difference in clinical severity, EIPH does not always present with epistaxis. In many cases, endoscopy and/or BAL cytology is required for a definitive diagnosis.[74]

Atypical Cells

BAL and (T)TW samples are generally of limited utility for the diagnosis of pulmonary neoplasia in the horse because tumor cells are rarely present in the airways.[78,79] Percutaneous aspiration, cytological assessment of pleural fluid, and lung biopsy are typically better suited for ante mortem diagnosis.[79] Concurrent septic and non-septic neutrophilic inflammation can be present. Respiratory epithelial cells can undergo dysplastic or metaplastic changes secondary to chronic inflammation, and this can be difficult to differentiate cytologically from neoplasia. Common dysplastic features include a more cuboidal to round appearance, increased N:C, visible nucleoli, and increased cytoplasmic basophilia. Neoplastic epithelial cells tend to display greater criteria of malignancy, such as multiple nucleoli and marked anisokaryosis; however, there can be significant morphological overlap. Primary epithelial lung tumors, including pulmonary and bronchial carcinomas and adenocarcinomas, are exceedingly rare in horses, often with single case reports in the literature.[79] Other primary tumors include bronchial myxoma, leiomyosarcoma, blastoma, pleural mesothelioma, chondrosarcoma, bronchogenic squamous cell carcinoma, and granular cell tumor.[79–81] Of these, granular cell tumors are the most common, typically occurring as single or multiple creamy white firm nodules adjacent to bronchi or bronchioles with extension into and occlusion of the lumen. Tumor cells are round to polyhedral with abundant eosinophilic cytoplasm filled with coarse eosinophilic granules.[81] Immunohistochemical studies support a Schwann cell origin, and staining for glial fibrillary acidic protein, myelin basic protein, and luxol fast blue with periodic acid-Schiff counterstain for myelin can be helpful to confirm the diagnosis on histological specimens.[82] Hypertrophic osteopathy has been reported as a paraneoplastic complication of granular cell tumor in some horses.[79]

Metastatic pulmonary neoplasia is relatively more common than primary disease, with lymphoma and disseminated hemangiosarcoma being most frequently reported.[79] Other tumor types that metastasize to the thoracic cavity include adenocarcinoma, squamous cell carcinoma, fibrosarcoma, malignant melanoma, mastocytoma, and undifferentiated sarcoma.

Conclusion

In conclusion, cytological evaluation of the equine respiratory tract is an invaluable tool for the diagnosis of infectious and non-septic processes, as well as EIPH. Choice of sampling site (TTW versus BAL) should be guided by the suspect diagnosis, and results should be interpreted in conjunction with history and clinical findings. Microbiologic assessment of samples for infectious disease often complements the cytologic evaluation.

References

1 Lunn, D.P., Davis-Poynter, N., Flaminio, M.J.B.F. et al. (2009). Equine herpesvirus-1 consensus statement. *J Vet Intern Med* 23: 450–461.

2 Boyle, A.G., Timoney, J.F., Newton, J.R. et al. (2018). *Streptococcus equi* infections in horses: guidelines for treatment, control, and prevention of strangles – revised consensus statement. *J Vet Intern Med* 32: 633–647.

3 Hoffman, A.M. (2008). Bronchoalveolar lavage: sampling technique and guidelines for cytologic preparation and interpretation. *Vet Clin North Am Equine Pract* 24: 423–435.

4 Hughes, K.J., Malikides, N., Hodgson, D.R., and Hodgson, J.L. (2003). Comparison of tracheal aspirates and bronchoalveolar lavage in racehorses 1. Evaluation of cytological stains and the percentage of mast cells and eosinophils. *Aust Vet J* 81: 681–684.

5 Malikides, N., Hughes, K.J., Hodgson, D.R., and Hodgson, J.L. (2003). Comparison of tracheal aspirates and bronchoalveolar lavage in racehorses 2. Evaluation of the diagnostic significance of neutrophil percentage. *Aust Vet J* 81: 685–687.

6 Couëtil, L.L., Cardwell, J.M., Gerber, V. et al. (2016). Inflammatory airway disease in horses - revised consensus statement. *J Vet Intern Med* 30: 503–515.

7 Mallicote, M.M. (2015). Update on *Streptococcus equi* subsp equi infections. *Vet Clin North Am Equine Pract* 31: 27–41.

8 Koblinger, K., Nicol, J., McDonald, K. et al. (2011). Endoscopic assessment of airway inflammation in horses. *J Vet Intern Med* 25: 1118–1126.

9 Léguillette, R. and Lavoie, J.P. (2006). Effects of the bronchoalveolar lavage procedure on lung function in horses with clinical exacerbation of recurrent airway obstruction. *Am J Vet Res* 67: 1929–1933.

10 Pickles, K., Pirie, R.S., Rhind, S. et al. (2002). Cytological analysis of equine bronchoalveolar lavage fluid. Part 1: Comparison of sequential and pooled aliquots. *Equine Vet J* 34: 288–291.

11 Pickles, K., Pirie, R.S., Rhind, S. et al. (2002). Cytological analysis of equine bronchoalveolar lavage fluid. Part 3: The effect of time, temperature and fixatives. *Equine Vet J* 34: 297–301.

12 Mair, T.S., Stokes, C.R., and Bourne, F.J. (1987). Cellular content of secretions obtained by lavage from different levels of the equine respiratory tract. *Equine Vet J* 19: 458–462.

13 Pickles, K., Pirie, R.S., Rhind, S. et al. (2002). Cytological analysis of equine bronchoalveolar lavage fluid. Part 2: Comparison of smear and cytocentrifuged preparations. *Equine Vet J Suppl* 34: 402–407.

14 Leclere, M., Desnoyers, M., Beauchamp, G., and Lavoie, J.P. (2006). Comparison of four staining methods for

detection of mast cells in equine bronchoalveolar lavage fluid. *J Vet Intern Med* 20: 377–381.

15 Fernandez, N.J., Hecker, K.G., Gilroy, C.V. et al. (2013). Reliability of 400-cell and 5-field leukocyte differential counts for equine bronchoalveolar lavage fluid. *Vet Clin Pathol* 42: 92–98.

16 Couëtil, L.L., Rosenthal, F.S., DeNicola, D.B., and Chilcoat, C.D. (2001). Clinical signs, evaluation of bronchoalveolar lavage fluid, and assessment of pulmonary function in horses with inflammatory respiratory disease. *Am J Vet Res* 62: 538–546.

17 Derksen, F.J., Brown, C.M., Sonea, I. et al. (1989). Comparison of transtracheal aspirate and bronchoalveolar lavage cytology in 50 horses with chronic lung disease. *Equine Vet J* 21: 23–26.

18 Miskovic, M., Couëtil, L.L., and Thompson, C.A. (2007). Lung function and airway cytologic profiles in horses with recurrent airway obstruction maintained in low-dust environments. *J Vet Intern Med* 21: 1060–1066.

19 Christmann, U., Hite, R.D., Witonsky, S.G. et al. (2009). Influence of age on surfactant isolated from healthy horses maintained on pasture. *J Vet Intern Med* 23: 612–618.

20 Costa, L.R., Eades, S.C., Venuqopal, C.S., and Moore, R.M. (2009). Plasma and pulmonary fluid endothelin in horses with seasonal recurrent airway obstruction. *J Vet Intern Med* 23: 1239–1246.

21 Hare, J.E. and Viel, L. (1998). Pulmonary eosinophilia associated with increased airway responsiveness in young racing horses. *J Vet Intern Med* 12: 163–170.

22 Naylor, J.M., Clark, E.G., and Clayton, H.M. (1992). Chronic obstructive pulmonary disease: usefulness of clinical signs, bronchoalveolar lavage, and lung biopsy as diagnostic and prognostic aid. *Can Vet J* 33: 591–598.

23 Koblinger, K., Hecker, K., Nicol, J. et al. (2013). Bronchial collapse during bronchoalveolar lavage in horses is an indicator of lung inflammation. *Equine Vet J* 46: 50–55.

24 Tee, S.Y., Dart, A.J., MacDonald, M.H. et al. (2012). Effects of collecting serial tracheal aspirate and bronchoalveolar lavage samples on the cytological findings of subsequent fluid samples in healthy Standardbred horses. *Aust Vet J* 90: 247–251.

25 Sweeney, C.R., Rossier, Y., Ziemer, E.L., and Lindborg, S.R. (1994). Effect of prior lavage on bronchoalveolar lavage fluid cell populations of lavaged and unlavaged lung segments in horses. *Am J Vet Res* 55: 1501–1504.

26 Clark, C.K., Lester, G.D., Vetro, T., and Rice, B. (1995). Bronchoalveolar lavage in horses: effect of exercise and repeated sampling on cytology. *Aust Vet J* 72: 249–252.

27 Millerick-May, M.L., Karmaus, W., Derksen, F.J. et al. (2012). Local airborne particulate concentration is associated with visible tracheal mucus in Thoroughbred racehorses. *Equine Vet J* 45: 85–90.

28 Davis, M.S. (2005). Cold weather exercise and airway cytokine expression. *J Appl Physiol* 98: 2132–2136.

29 Davis, M.S., Royer, C.M., McKenzie, E.C. et al. (2006). Cold air-induced late-phase bronchoconstriction in horses. *Equine Vet J* 38 (S36): 535–539.

30 Holcombe, S.J., Jackson, C., Gerber, V. et al. (2001). Stabling is associated with airway inflammation in young Arabian horses. *Equine Vet J* 33: 244–249.

31 Riihimäki, M., Raine, A., Elfman, L., and Pringle, J. (2008). Markers of respiratory inflammation in horses in relation to seasonal changes in air quality in a conventional racing stable. *Can J Vet Res* 72: 432–439.

32 Sweeney, C.R., Rossier, Y., Ziemer, E.L., and Lindborg, S. (1992). Effects of lung site and fluid volume on results of bronchoalveolar lavage fluid analysis in horses. *Am J Vet Res* 53: 1376–1379.

33 Depecker, M., Richard, E.A., Pitel, P.H. et al. (2014). Bronchoalveolar lavage fluid in Standardbred racehorses: influence of unilateral/bilateral profiles and cut-off values on lower airway disease diagnosis. *Vet J* 199: 150–156.

34 Ito, S., Hobo, S., and Kasashima, Y. (2003). Bronchoalveolar lavage fluid findings in the atelectatic regions of anesthetized horses. *J Vet Med Sci* 65: 1011–1013.

35 Kirkland, K.D., Goetz, T.E., Foreman, J.H. et al. (1993). Smoke inhalation injury in a pony. *J Vet Emerg Crit Care* 3: 83–89.

36 Berry, C.R., O'Brien, T.R., Madigan, J.E., and Hager, D.A. (1991). Thoracic radiographic features of silicosis in 19 horses. *J Vet Intern Med* 5: 248–256.

37 Reus, S.M. and Cohen, N.D. (2015). Update on bacterial pneumonia and pleuropneumonia in the adult horse. *Vet Clin North Am Equine Pract* 31: 105–120.

38 Reus, S.M. and Cohen, N.D. (2015). Update on bacterial pneumonia in the foal and weanling. *Vet Clin North Am Equine Pract* 31: 121–135.

39 Sweeney, C.R., Holcome, S.J., Barningham, S.C., and Beech, J. (1991). Aerobic and anaerobic bacterial isolates from horses with pneumonia or pleuropneumonia and antimicrobial sensitivity patterns of the aerobes. *J Am Vet Med Assoc* 198: 839–842.

40 Rossier, Y., Sweeney, C.R., and Ziemer, E.L. (1991). Bronchoalveolar lavage fluid cytologic findings in horses with pneumonia or pleuropneumonia. *J Am Vet Med Assoc* 198: 1001–1004.

41 Cohen, N.D. (2014). *Rhodococcus equi* foal pneumonia. *Vet Clin North Am Equine Pract* 30: 609–622.

42 Stewart, A.J. and Cuming, R.S. (2015). Update on fungal respiratory disease in horses. *Vet Clin North Am Equine Pract* 31: 43–62.

43 Wilkins, P.A.W. (2015). Update on interstitial pneumonia. *Vet Clin North Am Equine Pract* 31: 137–157.

44 Riley, C.B., Bolton, J.R., Mills, J.N., and Thomas, J.B. (1992). Cryptococcosis in seven horses. *Aust Vet J* 69: 135–139.

45 Higgins, J.C. and Pusterla, N. (2006). Fungal pneumonia in horses. *Clin Tech Equine Pract* 5: 218–224.

46 Sugita, C., Makimura, K., Uchida, K. et al. (2004). PCR identification system for the genus *Aspergillus* and three major pathogenic species: *Aspergillus fumigatus*, *Aspergillus flavus* and *Aspergillus niger*. *Med Mycol* 42: 433–437.

47 Franklin, R.P., Long, M.T., MacNeill, A. et al. (2002). Proliferative interstitial pneumonia, *Pneumocystis carinii* infection, and immunodeficiency in an adult Paso Fino horse. *J Vet Intern Med* 16: 607–611.

48 Thomas, C.F. and Limper, A.H. (2007). Current insights into the biology and pathogenesis of Pneumocystis pneumonia. *Nat Rev Microbiol* 5: 298–308.

49 Peters, S.E., Wakefield, A.E., Whitwell, K.E., and Hopkin, J.M. (1994). *Pneumocystis carinii* pneumonia in thoroughbred foals: identification of a genetically distinct organism by DNA amplification. *J Clin Microbiol* 32: 213–216.

50 Begg, A.P., Reece, R.L., Hum, S. et al. (2011). Pathological changes in horses dying with equine influenza in Australia, 2007. *Aust Vet J* 89: 19–22.

51 Williams, K.J., Maes, R., Del Piero, F. et al. (2007). Equine multinodular pulmonary fibrosis: a newly recognized herpesvirus-associated fibrotic lung disease. *Vet Pathol* 44: 849–862.

52 Williams, K.J., Robinson, N.E., Lim, A. et al. (2013). Experimental induction of pulmonary fibrosis in horses with the gammaherpesvirus equine herpesvirus 5. *PLoS One* 8: e77754.

53 Niedermaier, G., Poth, T., and Gehlen, H. (2010). Clinical aspects of multinodular pulmonary fibrosis in two warmblood horses. *Vet Rec* 166: 426–430.

54 Soare, T., Leeming, G., Morgan, R. et al. (2011). Equine multinodular pulmonary fibrosis in horses in the UK. *Vet Rec* 169: 313–313.

55 Spelta, C.W., Axon, J.E., Begg, A. et al. (2013). Equine multinodular pulmonary fibrosis in three horses in Australia. *Aust Vet J* 91: 274–280.

56 Schwarz, B., Schwendenwein, I., and van den Hoven, R. (2013). Successful outcome in a case of equine multinodular pulmonary fibrosis (EMPF) treated with valacyclovir. *Equine Vet Educ* 25: 389–392.

57 Fortier, G., Pronost, S., Miszczak, F. et al. (2009). Identification of equid herpesvirus-5 in respiratory liquids: a retrospective study of 785 samples taken in 2006–2007. *Vet J* 182: 346–348.

58 Ivester, K.M., Couëtil, L.L., and Zimmerman, N.J. (2014). Investigating the link between particulate exposure and airway inflammation in the horse. *J Vet Intern Med* 28: 1653–1665.

59 Mazan, M.R. (2015). Update on noninfectious inflammatory diseases of the lower airway. *Vet Clin North Am: Equine Pract* 31: 159–185.

60 Wood, J.L.N., Newton, J.R., Chanter, N., and Mumford, J.A. (2005). Association between respiratory disease and bacterial and viral infections in British racehorses. *J Clin Microbiol* 43: 120–126.

61 Wichtel, M., Gomez, D., Burton, S. et al. (2016). Relationships between equine airway reactivity measured by flowmetric plethysmography and specific indicators of airway inflammation in horses with suspected inflammatory airway disease. *Equine Vet J* 48: 466–471.

62 Robinson, N.E., Karmaus, W., Holcombe, S.J. et al. (2006). Airway inflammation in Michigan pleasure horses: prevalence and risk factors. *Equine Vet J* 38: 293–299.

63 Tilley, P., Luis, J.P.S., and Ferreira, M.B. (2012). Correlation and discriminant analysis between clinical, endoscopic, thoracic X-ray and bronchoalveolar lavage fluid cytology scores, for staging horses with recurrent airway obstruction (RAO). *Res Vet Sci* 93: 1006–1014.

64 Mazan, M.R., Vin, R., and Hoffman, A.M. (2005). Radiographic scoring lacks predictive value in inflammatory airway disease. *Equine Vet J* 37: 541–545.

65 Bell, S.A., Drew, C.P., Wilson, W.D., and Pusterla, N. (2008). Idiopathic chronic eosinophilic pneumonia in 7 horses. *J Vet Intern Med* 22: 648–653.

66 Boyle, A.G. and Houston, R. (2006). Parasitic pneumonitis and treatment in horses. *Clin Tech Equine Pract* 5: 225–232.

67 Henton, J.E. and Geiser, D.R. (1982). *Dictyocaulus arnfieldi* in foal pneumonia: a case report. *J Equine Vet Sci* 5: 170–171.

68 Nolen-Walston, R.D., Harris, M., and Agnew, M.E. (2013). Clinical and diagnostic features of inflammatory airway disease subtypes in horses examined because of poor performance: 98 cases (2004–2010). *J Am Vet Med Assoc* 242: 1138–1145.

69 Riihimäki, M., Lilliehöök, I., Raine, A. et al. (2008). Clinical alterations and mRNA levels of IL-4 and IL-5 in bronchoalveolar cells of horses with transient pulmonary eosinophilia. *Res Vet Sci* 85: 52–55.

70 La Perle, K., Piercy, R.J., Long, J.F., and Blomme, E.A.G. (1998). Multisystemic, eosinophilic, epitheliotropic disease with intestinal lymphosarcoma in a horse. *Vet Pathol* 35: 144–146.

71 Pucheu-Haston, C.M. and Del Piero, F. (2013). Equine multi-systemic eosinophilic epitheliotropic disease. *Equine Vet Educ* 25: 614–617.

72 Singh, K., Holbrook, T.C., Gilliam, L.L. et al. (2006). Severe pulmonary disease due to multisystemic eosinophilic epitheliotropic disease in a horse. *Vet Pathol* 43: 189–193.

73 Doucet, M.Y. and Viel, L. (2002). Alveolar macrophage graded hemosiderin score from bronchoalveolar lavage in horses with exercise-induced pulmonary hemorrhage and controls. *J Vet Intern Med* 16: 281–286.

74 Meyer, T.S., Fedde, M.R., Gaughan, E.M. et al. (1998). Quantification of exercise-induced pulmonary haemorrhage with bronchoalveolar lavage. *Equine Vet J* 30: 284–288.

75 Hinchcliff, K.W., Couëtil, L.L., Knight, P.K. et al. (2015). Exercise induced pulmonary hemorrhage in horses: American College of Veterinary Internal Medicine consensus statement. *J Vet Intern Med* 29: 743–758.

76 Hinchcliff, K.W., Jackson, M.A., Morley, P.S. et al. (2005). Association between exercise-induced pulmonary hemorrhage and performance in Thoroughbred racehorses. *J Am Vet Med Assoc* 227: 768–774.

77 Sullivan, S. and Hinchcliff, K.W. (2015). Update on exercise-induced pulmonary hemorrhage. *Vet Clin North Am Equine Pract* 31: 187–198.

78 Williams, K.J., Robinson, N.E., DeFeijter-Rupp, H. et al. (2013). Distribution of venous remodeling in exercise-induced pulmonary hemorrhage of horses follows reported blood flow distribution in the equine lung. *J Appl Physiol* 114: 869–878.

79 Davis, E.G. and Rush, B.R. (2011). Diagnostic challenges: equine thoracic neoplasia. *Equine Vet Educ* 25: 96–107.

80 Binanti, D., Stancari, G., Fantinato, E. et al. (2013). A case of bronchoalveolar carcinoma in a mare. *J Equine Vet Sci* 33: 751–755.

81 Mair, T.S., Rush, B.R., and Tucker, R.L. (2004). Clinical and diagnostic features of thoracic neoplasia in the horse. *Equine Vet Educ* 16: 30–36.

82 Kagawa, Y., Hirayama, K., Tagami, M. et al. (2001). Immunohistochemical analysis of equine pulmonary granular cell tumours. *J Comp Pathol* 124: 122–127.

Part VII

Hemolymphatic System

27

Lymph Nodes

Stefano Comazzi, Luca Aresu, Jenna H. Burton, and Paul R. Avery

Introduction

Lymph node cytology is indicated and commonly performed when lymphadenopathy, whether a single node, regional, or generalized enlargement, is identified. Collection of peripheral lymph node samples is quick, simple, relatively inexpensive, and minimally invasive to the patient. The most commonly performed techniques are either fine-needle aspiration biopsy (FNAB) or fine-needle capillary biopsy (FNCB). Sampling of lymph nodes within the thoracic or abdominal cavity generally requires ultrasound guidance to ensure adequate sample collection. Causes of lymphadenopathy diagnosed cytologically include neoplasia (lymphoproliferative diseases and metastatic neoplasia), reactive lymphoid hyperplasia, lymphadenitis, and primary infectious processes. Even when lymph nodes are of normal shape and size on palpation, FNAB or FNCB should be performed as a staging test for lymph nodes that drain neoplastic masses.

Sample Collection

To perform a non-aspiration FNCB of peripheral lymph nodes, the lymph node is manually stabilized, and a small-gauge hypodermic needle (generally 21–23 G) is inserted through the skin and into the lymph node. The needle is redirected several times in the lymph node without withdrawing it from the skin. Cells move into the needle by capillary pressure. Once the needle has been redirected several times or when blood appears in the hub of the needle, the needle is withdrawn, attached to an air-filled syringe, and the contents are expelled on a glass slide, preferably near the frosted end. The sample smears can be prepared by gently placing a second glass slide onto the aspirate sample and quickly pulling the two slides apart parallel to each other (Figure 50.1). This technique takes some practice, as too much downward pressure will cause the cells to rupture and too little pressure can result in a thick preparation, potentially limiting the diagnostic quality of the sample in both situations. The second slide used in making the FNCB slide preparation should be examined prior to discarding it, as some cellular material may remain on this slide that can be useful for diagnostic evaluation.

Alternatively, FNAB can be performed with the needle attached to a syringe to apply suction to withdraw cells from the lymph node. The lymph node is stabilized, the needle inserted into the lymph node, the plunger of the syringe withdrawn to create a vacuum, and the needle redirected several times within the lymph node. The pressure on the plunger must be released gently before the removal of the needle from the lymph node; otherwise the sample will be aspirated into the syringe making retrieval of the sample material difficult. Once withdrawn from the lymph node, the syringe should be removed from the needle, filled with air, reattached to the needle, and the sample gently expelled on to a glass slide. The material can then be dispersed on the slide using the methods described above.

Either procedure can be repeated several times to ensure adequate quantity of sample for submission. If more than one lymph node is enlarged, multiple lymph nodes should be sampled and submitted for analysis. Cells generally exfoliate easily from lymph nodes, and FNCB may result in higher quality cytologic peripheral lymph node samples as compared with FNAB.[1,2]

Systematic evaluation of the optimal needle gauge and syringe size to use for either FNCB or FNAB of lymph nodes has not been performed, yet likely impacts sample quality and diagnostic yield. In general, larger gauge needles (18–20 G) yield a larger sample but are more likely to contribute to blood contamination and hemodilution of the sample. Use of larger syringes (≥10 mL) for FNAB not

Veterinary Cytology, First Edition. Edited by Leslie C. Sharkey, M. Judith Radin, and Davis Seelig.

only can result in increased sample yield but also generates greater pressure during the aspiration process resulting in rupture of fragile neoplastic cells.

Complications from FNAB or FNCB are not well reported, yet clinical experience suggests that the risk of adverse effects is low. Mild bleeding, bruising, or momentary discomfort may occur; FNCB may be associated with less discomfort than FNAB as the application of suction can be uncomfortable.[2]

Specificity of lymph node cytology for a variety of lesions in people has been reported to be >94% when using histopathology as a gold standard.[3] The sensitivity rates were more variable, depending on the underlying lesion, and ranged from 30 to 97%.[3] While no formal evaluation of the diagnostic yield, accuracy, or specificity of lymph node cytology for lymphoma has been conducted in veterinary medicine, several studies have examined the detection of metastatic disease (see section "Metastatic Neoplasia"). Lymph node cytology has been reported to be nondiagnostic in up to 30% of cases in veterinary medicine.[4] It should be noted that >50% of the clinicians submitting samples in this study did not evaluate the cytologic samples in-house to assess the diagnostic quality prior to sending them to an external laboratory. Staining and in-house evaluation of one of the cytology slides prior to submission to a clinical pathologist would likely increase diagnostic yield and decrease clinician and client frustration with nondiagnostic results. If in-house assessment of the cytologic sample is performed, a minimum number of slides should be stained (ideally only one) and the stained slide should be submitted with the unstained slides to the diagnostic laboratory.

Sampling Considerations for Ancillary Testing

Ancillary tests such as immunocytochemistry (ICC), polymerase chain reaction for antigen receptor rearrangement (PARR), and flow cytometry can be helpful in diagnosing and characterizing lymphoid malignancies. The potential need for these tests should be kept in mind when sample collection is performed. Unstained slides may be required to perform some ICC tests. If it is anticipated that ICC is needed for immunophenotyping, sufficient lymph node cytology slides, ideally seven to eight slides, should be submitted for both cytology and ICC. DNA for PARR can be obtained directly from the glass slide even if the sample has previously been stained, so in general, additional slides do not need to be submitted for this test. Sufficient DNA for PARR can typically be isolated from two or more moderately to highly cellular slides.

Flow cytometry is performed on live cells in suspension so samples for this test need special consideration. Prior to lymph node aspiration, 1 mL of 0.9% NaCl, lactated Ringer's solution, Normosol-R, or other isotonic solution is combined with 0.1 mL of serum from the same animal or same species in a sterile tube without additives (red top tube). To ensure a cellular sample, it is recommended that the lymph node sample be collected by FNAB, and the contents in the hub of the aspiration needle gently expelled into the prepared solution in the red top tube and the needle rinsed with the saline/serum solution. Several FNAB should be collected and combined in the tube to ensure adequate cellularity of the sample. To maximize cell viability and minimize the risk of a nondiagnostic result, samples should be kept at 4 °C until shipped and then shipped overnight to the laboratory with cold packs on the same day as collection.

Normal Lymph Node

A discussion of the normal organization and architecture of a lymph node is instructive in understanding the changes seen with lymph node hyperplasia. Secondary lymphoid organs including peripheral lymph nodes are colonized by B cells, which have matured in the bone marrow, and T cells, which have matured in the thymus. Lymph nodes can be divided into three general regions: cortex, paracortex, and medulla (Figure 27.1).

Naïve B cells reside in the cortex and, upon activation by antigen-specific T cells, are transformed into blasts that enter the follicles to initiate the formation of a germinal center. Activated B cells that enter the primary follicle form centroblasts, which eventually migrate to the more peripheral zone of the germinal center to become centrocytes. Centrocytes can become memory cells and reside in the mantle zone around the germinal center or leave the germinal center to form the marginal zone around the periphery of the mantle zone. Some centrocytes differentiate into immunoglobulin-secreting plasma cells within the germinal centers.[5] In mice, short-lived plasma cells are produced approximately three days after immunization, whereas long-lived plasma cells are produced within coalescing germinal centers by day 6 and can continue to generate plasma cells for weeks.[6] Macrophages are part of the germinal center and phagocytize the many B cells that undergo apoptosis during proliferation and differentiation and are then described as "tingible body macrophages."[7] T lymphocytes enter the lymph nodes through the endothelial venule and, if activated, populate the paracortical areas as T immunoblasts.[8] The medulla is composed of the lymph draining sinuses where macrophages and mast cells are commonly found and the medullary cords where immunoblasts and plasma cells localize after formation in the germinal centers.[7,9]

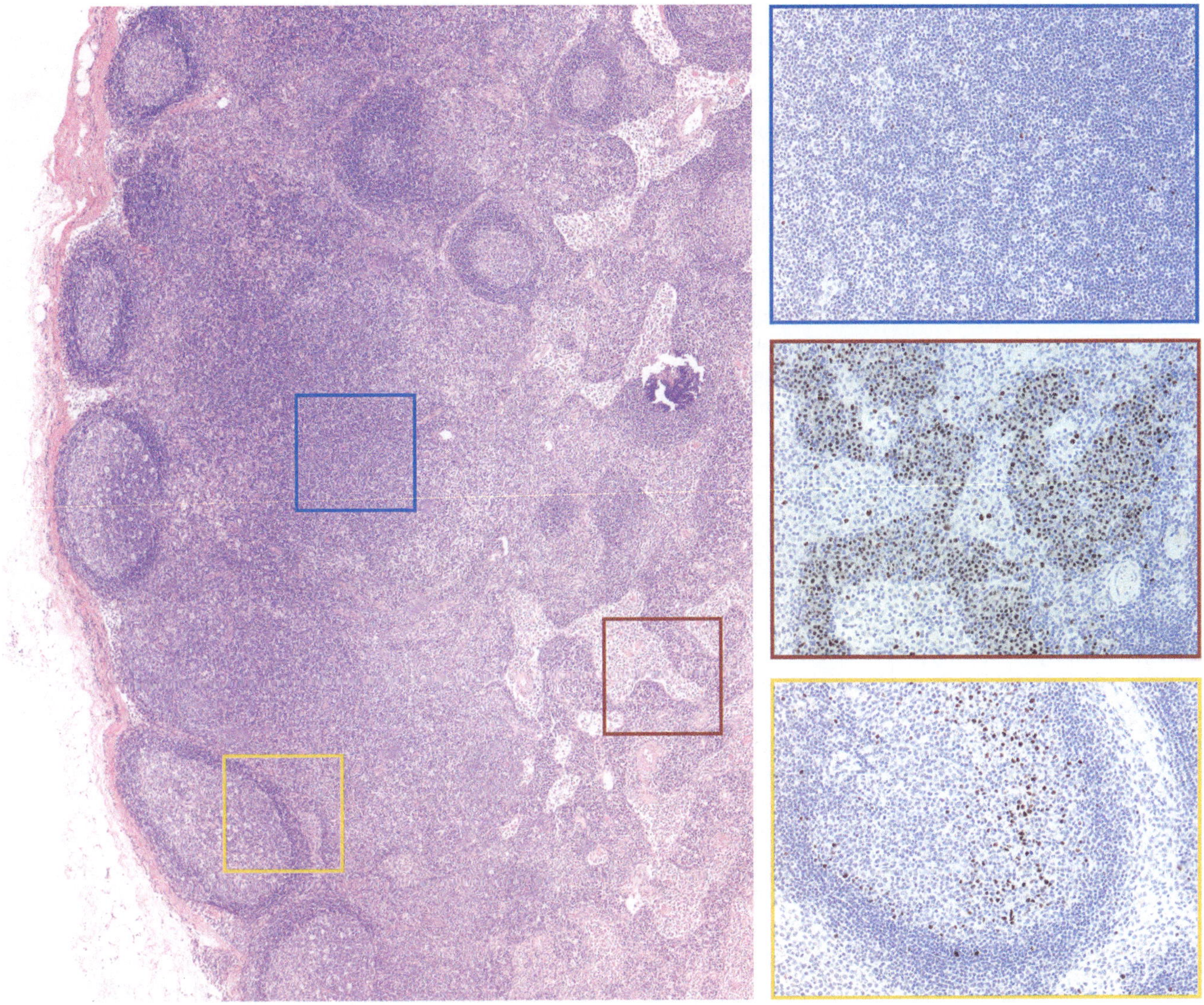

Figure 27.1 Histology of reactive lymphoid hyperplasia highlighting the distribution of plasma cells. The yellow box includes a germinal center within the cortex, the blue box is located in the paracortical region, and the red box includes medullary cords within the medulla. Immunohistochemical staining with Mum1 labels plasma cells brown. Plasma cells are seen in variable numbers within germinal centers and in large numbers within the medullary cords. Relatively few plasma cells are found in the paracortical region. GC = germinal center (Large image: hematoxylin & eosin, 40×. Small boxes: Mum1 stain, 200×).

Normal Lymph Node Cytology

Because aspiration cytology removes any architectural context, cytologists describe normal cytology based on the relative proportions of visibly distinct lymphocyte subsets. Some lymphocyte subsets are visually unique, whereas many are cytologically indistinguishable and grouped together based on size and presence or absence of nucleoli. Small lymphocytes (both B and T cell) predominate in any normal lymph node. A recent study examining cytospin and imprint preparations from 11 canine lymph nodes harvested from dogs without any evidence of inflammatory or neoplastic diseases documented a median of 85.5% cytologically small lymphocytes.[10] This is expected because small B cells are found in primary follicles, the mantle zone of secondary follicles, and the medullary cords, while small T cells comprise many of the cells throughout the paracortex. Small lymphocytes are generally described as cells that are approximately 7–10 μm, are smaller than a neutrophil, and contain a round nucleus approximately 1× to 1.5× the size of an erythrocyte with dense/clumped chromatin and a scant rim of cytoplasm.[11,12] There are smaller numbers of intermediate-sized lymphocytes, which are composed of the follicular centrocytes and marginal zone B cells. These cells are described as approximately 9–15 μm in diameter or as being similar in size to a neutrophil, and containing a nucleus approximately 2× to 2.5× the size of a red blood cell.[11,13] Rutgen et al. documented a median value of 3.7% medium-sized lymphocytes in normal canine lymph nodes.[10] Larger lymphoid blasts are normally seen in small numbers and are derived from follicular centroblasts and T and B immunoblasts found in the paracortex and scattered in the medullary cords. Blastic cells are often defined by the presence of one or more prominent nucleoli. Plasma cells are found in small numbers in the medullary cords in resting lymph nodes and have been shown in one study to have a median value of 4.7% in normal canine lymph nodes.[10] Another study of clinically normal dogs only documented 1 of 32 dogs as having greater than 4–6% plasma cells based on cytology.[14] Macrophages are seen in small numbers in lymph nodes from clinically normal dogs with 1.4% documented by cytology.[10] Using flow cytometry, a mean of 2.4% (95% confidence interval (CI) = 1.7–3.0%)[14] or 5.5% (±6.8%)[10] macrophages was documented. Macrophages generally reside in the medullary region and subcapsular sinus.

Reactive Lymphoid Hyperplasia

In human medicine, the term reactive lymphoid hyperplasia is commonly used to encompass nonneoplastic, reversible enlargement of the lymph node secondary to antigenic stimulation. Histologically, this term is used to describe changes that include follicular hyperplasia, interfollicular/paracortical hyperplasia, sinus histiocytosis, and medullary plasma cell hyperplasia in various combinations and proportions.[15] In people, follicular hyperplasia is described as the most common form of hyperplasia although it is unclear if this is true in animals.[16,17] It is also common for some degree of paracortical and/or sinus hyperplasia to accompany follicular hyperplasia.[18] The full details of antigen-dependent antibody production are beyond the scope of this chapter, but reactive lymphoid hyperplasia is a dynamic process that, depending on the timing relative to antigen exposure, can influence the cytologic findings. T cells that enter the lymph node and are activated by antigen will become T lymphoblasts in the paracortex. Primary follicles in unstimulated lymph nodes consist primarily of small B cells, which are transformed into IgM positive lymphoblasts in the paracortex as they interact with antigen-specific T lymphoblasts within one to two days of antigen exposure (reviewed in[19]). Approximately three to four days after antigen exposure, these activated B cells can either move into extrafollicular regions and differentiate into short-lived plasma cells or initiate the formation of a germinal center.[20–22] At this early stage in a hyperplastic process, germinal centers may consist entirely of centroblasts, whereas the number of smaller centrocytes expands with time.[23,24] Plasma cells begin to form in the germinal centers approximately six days after antigenic stimulation in mice and then migrate to the medullary cords where they become long-lived plasma cells.[9] In experimental rodent models, germinal center formation peaks during the second week after antigen exposure and declines back to a resting status by three to five weeks post challenge.[22]

Cytology of Reactive Lymphoid Hyperplasia

Because lymph node hyperplasia can manifest with temporal and regional expansions of lymphocyte populations and because the specific region sampled can vary with aspiration, the cytologic features can be somewhat variable (Figure 27.2). In a large study of human cases of reactive lymphadenopathy, the cytologic criteria included "the usual predominant component of small lymphocytes accompanied by a variable number of typical follicle center cells (centrocytic, centroblastic, or immunoblastic cells) and of cells belonging to the plasma cell series (plasmablasts, plasmacytoid cells, or mature plasma cells)."[25] This would correspond to follicular expansion and generally appear cytologically as primarily small lymphocytes with a condensed, dark chromatin; a variable expansion of plasma cells; and an expanded population of intermediate-sized lymphocytes with inconspicuous nucleoli (centrocytes) and of larger cells with one to three peripheral nucleoli and scant cytoplasm (centroblasts) or one centrally located nucleolus and moderate amounts of cytoplasm (immunoblasts).[8,16] Interfollicular or paracortical expansions consist primarily of the small lymphocytes found in the paracortex, possibly with variably increased numbers of large immunoblasts, plasma cells, histiocytes, and eosinophils.[18,24] An aspirate from within the medullary cords and sinuses would likely contain small lymphocytes, large numbers of plasma cells, and increased numbers of macrophages and mast cells.[24]

Veterinary Terminology

In veterinary medicine, some have advocated distinguishing lymph node hyperplasia from lymph node reactivity based on cytology, whereas other authors have grouped the two processes together.[11–13,26] The distinction between a hyperplastic lymph node and a reactive lymph node is based on the presumption that a hyperplastic lymph node will yield a relatively normal distribution of lymphocytes possibly with a mild expansion of intermediate or large lymphocytes, whereas a reactive lymph node has an increased proportion of plasma cells as a signature feature.[12,13] Given the temporal and regional expansion of lymphocyte subsets in a lymph node responding to antigen

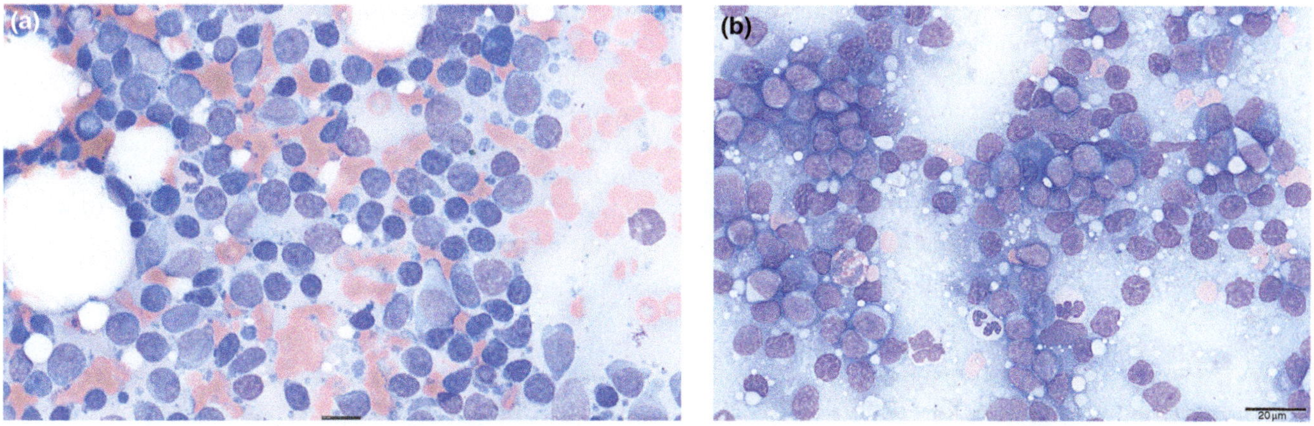

Figure 27.2 Variation in the cellular distribution in reactive lymphoid hyperplasia is illustrated in these aspirates from the enlarged regional lymph nodes of two dogs with primary sarcomas. There was no cytologic evidence of metastasis. (a) There is an expansion of intermediate-sized lymphocytes with and without prominent nucleoli (possibly a mix of centrocytes and centroblasts from an emerging germinal center) and rare plasma cells. (b) There is a pronounced expansion of plasma cells (arrows) in addition to an expanded population of intermediate-sized lymphocytes without nucleoli (centrocytes), which suggests sampling from a more developed germinal center or possibly from the medullary cords (Wright–Geimsa, 500×).

and the lack of control over which region is sampled during aspiration, it seems reasonable to expect variation in the cytologic picture across lymph nodes within the full spectrum of reactive lymphoid hyperplasia. Sampling the paracortical region early in reactive lymphoid hyperplasia might yield an aspirate with relatively few plasma cells, whereas an aspirate from a follicle/medullary cord or an aspirate taken a few days later from the same lymph node would likely yield notable numbers of plasma cells (Figure 27.2).

Potential Regional Variability

The distribution of lymphocyte subtypes varies with anatomic location in people. Lymph nodes draining areas of consistent antigenic exposure might be expected to have larger numbers of germinal centers than other lymph nodes. Larger germinal center volumes are documented in normal human cervical and mesenteric lymph nodes when compared with axillary, cubital, and popliteal lymph nodes.[27] Others reviewing human cytology have stated that "cervical lymph nodes have numerous secondary lymphoid follicles, and the smears show germinal center cells."[8] This is consistent with the Authors' experience that mandibular lymph nodes of dogs often appear to have an expanded population of intermediate-sized lymphocytes with variably prominent nucleoli, which may correspond to follicular centrocytes and centroblasts. Mandibular lymph nodes in mice have also been reported to have considerable numbers of plasma cells within the medullary cords.[28] Sinus histiocytosis has been described as a normal finding in murine mesenteric lymph nodes with increased numbers of pigment-laden macrophages noted.[28]

Lymphadenitis

The term "lymphadenitis" is used to describe increased inflammatory cells within a lymph node. There are commonly mentioned cytologic criteria for defining lymphadenitis in veterinary medicine and these generally consist of >5% neutrophils for suppurative lymphadenitis, >3% eosinophils for eosinophilic lymphadenitis, and >3% macrophages for histiocytic lymphadenitis although the exact origin of these numbers is unclear.[11,26,29] A recent study examining cytology from the popliteal lymph nodes of 11 dogs that had been euthanized for reasons other than hematopoietic malignancies or severe inflammatory disease revealed that median values for neutrophils, eosinophils, and macrophages were 1.4, 2, and 1.4%, respectively.[10] By flow cytometry, CD14 expression revealed a mean of 2.4% monocytes/macrophages (95% CI = 1.7–3.0%) in the lymph nodes of 29 clinically healthy dogs.[14] This same study also identified 7/29 dogs with what was described as moderate to severe eosinophilic inflammation (>4–6% eosinophils by cytology). This finding highlights the potential difficulty in correlating physical health with cytologic normality. Subjective assessment of the relative contribution of any significant peripheral blood contamination, particularly in reference to neutrophils, needs to be considered when examining clinical samples.

Cytologic evidence of increased inflammatory cells can be seen in lymph node draining areas of primary inflammation and can be associated with a concurrent reactive lymphoid hyperplasia. Dermatopathic lymphadenitis consisting of increased numbers of pigment-laden macrophages and/or eosinophils is described in people with primary skin lesions.[15] Foreign body responses also are associated with increased number of macrophages that are likely aspirated from the medullary sinuses of the draining lymph nodes.[15] When inflammation becomes more prominent or begins to dominate the cytologic picture, infection within the lymph node becomes a differential. A complete discussion of all forms of infectious lymphadenitis is not possible, but diseases where cytologic detection of inflammatory patterns can be useful in establishing clinically important differentials will be highlighted.

Infectious Lymphadenitis

Blastomyces and *Coccidioides*

The finding of significant pyogranulomatous inflammation within a lymph node often elicits a search for an underlying fungal infection. Blastomycosis and coccidioidomycosis are reported to induce pyogranulomatous lymphadenitis. Dogs are more commonly affected than cats.[30,31] *Blastomyces dermatitidis* typically enters the body through inhalation of spores where it can then spread systemically to multiple organs including lymph nodes.[32] Peripheral lymphadenopathy is reported in approximately 50–60% of canine cases.[32,33] The pattern of inflammation seen within lymph nodes has most commonly been described as pyogranulomatous with smaller numbers of cases having suppurative responses (>95% neutrophils) or lymphoid hyperplasia.[34] Multinucleated giant cells are commonly described.[34] The frequency of detecting organisms in lymph node aspirates appears relatively high; in three studies, 14/17, 19/24, and 36/54 cases had demonstrable organisms.[32,34,35] *B. dermatitidis* are round to oval yeast ranging from 10 to 20 μm^2 in size with thick, double walls and can demonstrate broad-based budding (Figure 3.1).[34] *Coccidioides immitis* can produce a similar pattern of pyogranulomatous lymphadenitis, and it too enters the body primarily through inhaled spores.[36] Systemic spread can occur to lymph nodes, but peripheral lymphadenopathy has been described as uncommon. In one retrospective study, only 3 of 20 dogs had detectable peripheral lymphadenopathy (1 generalized, 1 mandibular, and 1 prescapular), and 3 of 14 dogs with abdominal ultrasound findings had mesenteric or sublumbar lymphadenopathy.[37] Histologic confirmation of fungal lymphadenitis was confirmed in the dog with popliteal lymphadenopathy. Cats will commonly have non-healing skin lesions with respiratory disease as a slightly less frequent manifestation, and again, peripheral lymphadenopathy appears relatively uncommon.[38,39] Only 8 of 48 cats in a retrospective study were described as having localized lymphadenopathy.[39] Hilar or sternal lymphadenopathy is much more common as a sequela to the respiratory component of the infection.[37,40] *C. immitis* organisms are identified as large (10–70 m^2 or larger), round, double-walled spherules, which contain numerous small endospores (Figure 3.2).[36,41] The spherules often collapse during fixation, and distinct folds in the capsule can then be appreciated.[41] The large size and endospores are distinctive features from *Blastomyces*, yet some authors caution that immature spherules that lack obvious endospores can be mistaken for other fungal organisms.[36,42] The frequency with which organisms can be identified from lymph node aspirates is unclear, but spherules were demonstrated in the lymph nodes of 4/8 dogs in one study (2 peripheral, 1 hilar, and 1 sternal).[42] Draining skin lesions and pleural fluids have been described as consistently yielding visible organisms.[36–38]

Leishmania

Leishmania spp. infect both dogs and cats, and the regional incidence of disease is quite high in certain parts of the world. Cutaneous and lymph node involvement are common, and aspiration cytology of lymph nodes to identify amastigotes is commonly employed to diagnose the disease (Figures 19.5 and 34.10). The sensitivity for detecting organisms in lymph node aspirates approaches 93% in clinically ill animals with sufficient cellular material, while detection rates drop below 30% in asymptomatically infected dogs.[43,44] The pattern of lymph node changes has been described as both lymphoid hyperplasia and granulomatous lymphadenitis.[44,45] In a study of 32 dogs with clinical Leishmaniasis, cytologic evidence of lymphoid hyperplasia was the most prevalent finding (78.1% of cases) followed by smaller numbers of cases that had a histiocytic component (18.8%) defined as >3% macrophages and suppurative inflammation (3.1%) defined as >5% neutrophils.[44] Lymphoid hyperplasia was defined as >50% small lymphocytes and >5% plasma cells or no detectable cytologic changes in the context of an enlarged lymph node. Subclinically infected dogs had lymph node cytology results that were reported as normal in 95.8% of cases with only a single animal demonstrating lymphoid hyperplasia.

Tularemia

Tularemia caused by *Francisella tularensis* is an uncommon cause of lymphadenopathy in veterinary patients, but the zoonotic potential merits discussion of expected findings. Dogs appear to be relatively resistant to infection although transient fever and lymphadenopathy have been reported.[46,47] Because cats are more likely to be exposed through hunting infected rodents and rabbits, they are more prone to clinical disease. Regional or generalized lymphadenopathy is reported in cats with tularemia. In cats, histologic descriptions of peripheral lymph nodes predominate and describe caseous to liquefying necrosis with neutrophils and macrophages and variation in the degree of necrosis in lesser affected nodes.[48–51] Human case series of aspiration cytology reveals prominent cytolysis and necrotic background material with suppurative inflammation.[52,53] Fewer cases have evidence of multinucleated giant cells suggesting some degree of granulomatous inflammation. In studies in people, there tends to be an early suppurative "abscess" phase followed by more emerging granulomatous inflammation in the ensuing weeks.[54] From a total of 89 human cases across two studies, FNAB in eight cases revealed only reactive lymphoid hyperplasia highlighting the possible early detection of disease in these cases.[52,53] This may be relevant to the small number of descriptions of lymph node cytology in dogs and cats. One report described a cytologic picture of lymphoid hyperplasia in a cat who had been exposed to a rabbit seven days earlier.[55] A case report of canine tularemia revealed mild mandibular lymphadenopathy that was cytologically described as reactive hyperplasia with moderate numbers of neutrophils. Rare, partially degraded bacterial rods were seen within neutrophils.[46]

Yersinia pestis

Similar to tularemia, *Yersinia pestis* infection or plague is a relatively uncommon disease seen primarily in cats but important to recognize as a potentially zoonotic clinical differential. Most cases in the United States have been reported in western states, primarily California, Colorado, and New Mexico.[56] Despite being potential reservoirs for transmission, dogs have been reported to be less susceptible to disease than cats, but case series of clinical plague in dogs have been reported.[57,58] Cats commonly have lymphadenopathy, and in two studies, 71–75% of the enlarged peripheral lymph nodes were submandibular lymph nodes.[59,60] This is likely due to oral exposure to infected rodent or rabbit hosts, and lymphadenopathy is often bilateral.[59] Histologically, the inflammation in the lymph nodes from infected cats is typically described as marked, acute, necrotizing inflammation.[56] Bacteria are gram-negative coccobacilli and have been described as numerous in histologic sections of infected lymph nodes.[56] There are limited descriptions of lymph node cytology but most clinical descriptions of cases involve abscessation of lymph nodes that would be consistent with severe, suppurative lymphadenitis.[59,61–63] There is a lack of information about how prevalent the bacteria are in cytologic preparations, but given the abundance described in histologic sections, detectable coccobacilli might be anticipated. In a case series of 62 dogs that were clinically ill with plague, only 23% had lymphadenopathy, but similar to cats, mandibular lymph nodes were most commonly involved, although cytologic findings were not specifically discussed.[58]

Bartonella spp.

Bartonella spp. are zoonotic gram-negative bacilli bacteria. While cats are considered the primary reservoir for *Bartonella henselae*, *Bartonella* spp. have been detected with increasing frequency in dogs based on both DNA amplification and serology.[64] Cats are typically asymptomatic when infected with *Bartonella* spp. The frequency with which *Bartonella* results in lymphadenopathy in dogs is unclear, but there are reports of three dogs with antibiotic-responsive, suppurative, pyogranulomatous, or granulomatous lymphadenitis with concurrent amplification of *Bartonella* DNA by polymerase chain reaction.[65,66,67] Visceral and peripheral lymph nodes were involved, and aspiration cytology in one case revealed degenerate neutrophils, macrophages, and multinucleated giant cells,[65] while another revealed primarily degenerate neutrophils[67] and a third described large mononuclear cells as the predominant inflammatory cell type.[66] The pattern of lymphadenitis reported in people with cat scratch disease or *Bartonella* infection is similar in that early lesions may have small foci of neutrophils and necrosis followed by progressive necrotizing granulomas.[16]

Lymphoid Neoplasia

Lymphoma Classification

The current and historical veterinary literature reveals varied approaches toward lymphoma subtyping and an understanding of the origins and evolution of these lymphoma classification schemes is instructive. The classification, or subtyping, of lymphoma denotes the process by which the generic diagnosis of "lymphoma" is refined to a more specific and uniquely defined entity (e.g., diffuse large B-cell lymphoma) through the application of light microscopy, immunophenotyping, genetic analysis, and the incorporation of clinical features.[68,69] The aim of classification is to better delineate specific tumor biological behavior, response to therapy, and prognosis. Moreover, classification provides clinicians and scientists with a uniform language that is independent of country and institution. The development of lymphoma classification schemes is, in part, driven by the availability of diagnostic technologies, which, in the case of veterinary medicine, includes species cross-reactive reagents (e.g., cell phenotyping antibodies). In veterinary medicine, the approach toward lymphoma classification has largely emphasized the adaptation of human-derived schemes. Owing to the microscopic similarities with humans, their high prevalence of lymphoma, and the availability of reagents, the major efforts have been oriented on canine lymphoma.

The first human classification scheme was developed in the 1960s and divided tumors based on their histopathologic growth pattern (i.e., diffuse vs nodular). Although insufficient in terms of scope (lymphoblastic lymphomas and Hodgkin lymphoma were ignored), the Rappaport scheme incorporated clinical behavior and demonstrated that diffuse lymphomas were generally characterized by a poor prognosis, whereas nodular lymphomas often had an indolent behavior.[70] Approximately a decade later, coincident with the emergence of immunophenotyping techniques, two parallel classification systems were developed in the United States and in Europe, namely, the Lukes and Collins Classification and Kiel Classification schemes, respectively. The Lukes and Collins classification, in contrast to the Rappaport scheme, emphasized immunophenotype and cytomorphology in lieu of growth pattern.[71] Similarly, the Kiel classification, which has been updated several times since its inception, is based on cytomorphology, immunological criteria, and comparison of neoplastic cells to their normal counterpart with limited emphasis on growth pattern.[72]

Initial attempts to introduce lymphoma classification to veterinary medicine emerged in the late 1990s when the updated Kiel classification was applied to canine lymphoma.[73] The early adoption of a canine-adapted Kiel scheme, which places limited emphasis on growth pattern, was favored owing to the recognition that the majority of canine lymphomas demonstrate a diffuse architecture at the time of diagnosis. Early results showed good interobserver reproducibility and agreement with histopathology,[74] allowed identification of unique lymphoma subtypes such as medium-sized macronucleolated cell lymphoma and small clear cell lymphoma, and demonstrated prognostic relevance.[75–77] However, the complexity of the Kiel scheme, the limited clinical significance of many of its entities, and the minimal emphasis given to nodular subtypes makes its application unsuitable for many lymphoma subtypes, including follicular lymphoma and mantle cell lymphoma.

In order to produce a reproducible, prognostically relevant scheme in human medicine, the National Cancer Institute developed the Working Formulation (WF) in 1982, which was intended to serve as a translational tool between preexisting classifications.[78] In the WF, lymphoma subtypes are grouped by clinical aggressiveness into low, intermediate, and high-grade malignancies. While popular for its clinical usefulness, the interobserver reproducibility was somewhat low and some entities, including marginal and mantle cell lymphoma, did not find adequate inclusion in the classification. Attempts to apply the WF to canine lymphoma were carried out, but poor reproducibility strengthened the need for a new classification scheme.[79]

Most recently, the International Lymphoma Study Group developed the Revised European American classification of Lymphoid neoplasms (REAL), which aimed to integrate all available patient (clinical features and outcome) and tumor (tumor topography/architecture, cell morphology, immunophenotype, and tumor genetic/molecular) characteristics to subtype lymphoma. In collaboration with the World Health Organization (WHO), the REAL classification scheme eventually expanded to include all hematopoietic tumors.[80] Notable characteristics of the REAL/WHO classification are (i) a high inter- and intraobserver reproducibility (>85%), (ii) the flexibility to incorporate new discoveries or techniques through regular update, and (iii) the combining of some entities (acute lymphoblastic leukemia/lymphoblastic lymphoma and chronic lymphocytic leukemia/small lymphocytic lymphoma) into unique subtypes. The WHO classification scheme was first applied to canine samples in 2002 and was demonstrated to have an 83% agreement for 300 canine lymphoma cases and 87% agreement for the 5 most common types of canine lymphoma (T-zone lymphoma, lymphoblastic T-cell lymphoma, peripheral T-cell lymphoma not otherwise specified, marginal zone lymphoma, and diffuse large B-cell lymphoma).[81,82] There are currently 20 recognized subtypes of canine and feline lymphoma according to WHO scheme.[81] While there have been a number of publications comparing veterinary-adapted versions of the Kiel, WF, and WHO, there is increasing global adoption of the latter owing to its incorporation of histopathology and immunophenotyping.[73,79,83,84]

Role of Cytology in the Diagnosis and Classification of Lymphoma

In most clinical veterinary settings, owing to low cost, limited degree of invasiveness, safety, and generally high diagnostic yield, FNAB or FNCB is often the first-line approach in dogs with lymphadenomegaly.[85] No studies comparing the diagnostic performance of cytology (with or without immunophenotyping) with histology are available in veterinary medicine, but accuracy of cytology for the general diagnosis of canine lymphoma is reported as high, likely due to the diffuse nature of most forms of veterinary lymphoma (>80% of cases).[73,86] Generally, histology is reserved as a second step (e.g., for confirmation, for subtyping, or to obtain tissue for further therapy). A similar approach has been adopted in humans, in which FNAB is considered the first-line lymphoma diagnostic followed by immunophenotyping with histopathology recognized as the gold standard technique.[87–89]

Except for the Kiel classification, all the aforementioned classification schemes emphasize histopathology and immunophenotyping. With the identification of subtype-specific immunophenotypes, there is an increasing recognition of the utility of FNAB plus flow cytometry for the diagnosis and subtyping of some forms of canine lymphoma (e.g., T-zone lymphoma),[90,91] although histology remains the gold standard for classification for many canine lymphomas.[92] For feline lymphoma, owing to the lack of extensive study on their classification, the role of cytology is even more unknown, but given the higher incidence of nodular, low grade, and mixed cell cases, histopathology may be even more important.[93] However, some specific feline subtypes, such as large granular lymphocyte lymphoma and Hodgkin-like lymphoma, have been recognized and well described (see sections "Large Granular Lymphocyte Lymphoma" and "Hodgkin-Like Lymphoma").

Common Subtypes of Lymphoma

Lymphoblastic Lymphoma

Lymphoblastic lymphoma (LBL) is a rare subtype of lymphoma arising from precursor cells. According to the current WHO guidelines, the term of "lymphoblast" should only be used to define precursor cells with well-defined morphological features. The cytology of LBL is characterized by a monotonous population of small to medium cells (nuclei not larger than two erythrocytes) with scarce unipolar, sometimes vacuolated and weakly basophilic cytoplasm. The nucleus is round to often indented with irregular nuclear margins, fine chromatin, and poorly visible or inconspicuous nucleoli. Mitotic index is high, thus confirming the high grade of malignancy. Histologically, LBL is characterized by medium-sized blast cells that may be very uniform or show varying degrees of anisocytosis. The cytoplasm is scarcely visible or indistinct by hematoxylin and eosin-stained sections. Nuclei are rounded or convoluted with smooth or finely granular chromatin. Nucleoli are usually small and inconspicuous, and the mitotic index is often high (>10/high-powered field [HPF]). The use of immunohistochemistry is needed for immunophenotyping, and neoplastic cells may express lineage-specific cluster of differentiation (CD) markers (CD79a and CD20 for B cell; CD3 and/or CD5 for T-cell lineage), may be double negative ($CD4^-$ and $CD8^-$), or may be double positive ($CD4^+$ and $CD8^+$) T cells.[76] Neoplastic cells can express the precursor marker CD34, thus confirming bone marrow origin. LBL is often characterized by a very aggressive behavior, especially with the B subtype.[11] In a study of lymphoma in the Boxer dog breed, T-cell LBL is associated with a longer survival than other subtypes of lymphoma.[94] Mediastinal localization is frequent, often associated with hypercalcemia and T-cell phenotype. Notably, according to the current WHO classification, the distinction between stage V lymphoblastic lymphoma and lymphoblastic leukemia originating in the bone marrow with secondary lymph node invasion has been reconsidered in favor of two different presentations of the same disease.

Diffuse Large B-Cell Lymphoma

Diffuse large B-cell lymphoma (DLBCL) is the most common canine lymphoma subtype.[81] According to morphology and the Kiel classification, canine DLBCL can be separated into two distinct subtypes, the centroblastic and immunoblastic subtypes, both of which are recognizable on both cytologic and histologic preparations.[83,92] On cytology, centroblastic lymphoma is characterized by the proliferation of medium to large lymphoid cells (centroblasts) containing moderately abundant blue cytoplasm and, characteristically, a round nucleus with several prominent, peripherally located nucleoli.[81] Additional cell types include small numbers of large immunoblasts (described below), medium-sized lymphocytes, and a variable population of residual small lymphocytes. Mitoses are moderate to frequent, ranging from 2 to >5/HPF. Based on cytology alone, it may be challenging to differentiate primary centroblastic lymphoma from forms of nodular lymphoma, including marginal lymphoma in transformation and follicular lymphoma.[83] The second cytologic variant of DLBCL is immunoblastic lymphoma. This neoplasm is characterized by the proliferation of large cells (immunoblasts) containing a small amount of deeply basophilic cytoplasm and a round nucleus with a single, central, prominent nucleolus. This subtype is less common in the dog while it is more frequent in the cat.[83,93] Aspiration cytology of DLBCL typically reveals intermediate-sized to large deeply basophilic lymphoid blasts that contain one to multiple large, prominent nucleoli (Figure 27.3). Neoplastic cells in both subtypes stain positive for B-cell markers (CD21, CD79a, CD20, and surface immunoglobulins). Flow cytometry may be useful to stage the infiltration of large B cells in peripheral blood and bone marrow, and this may be of prognostic interest.[95]

Histologically, DLBCL is characterized by a diffuse proliferation of medium to large neoplastic lymphoid cells with nuclear size more than twice the size of red blood cells. The centroblast variant is most frequent and is characterized by large, non-cleaved cells resembling the

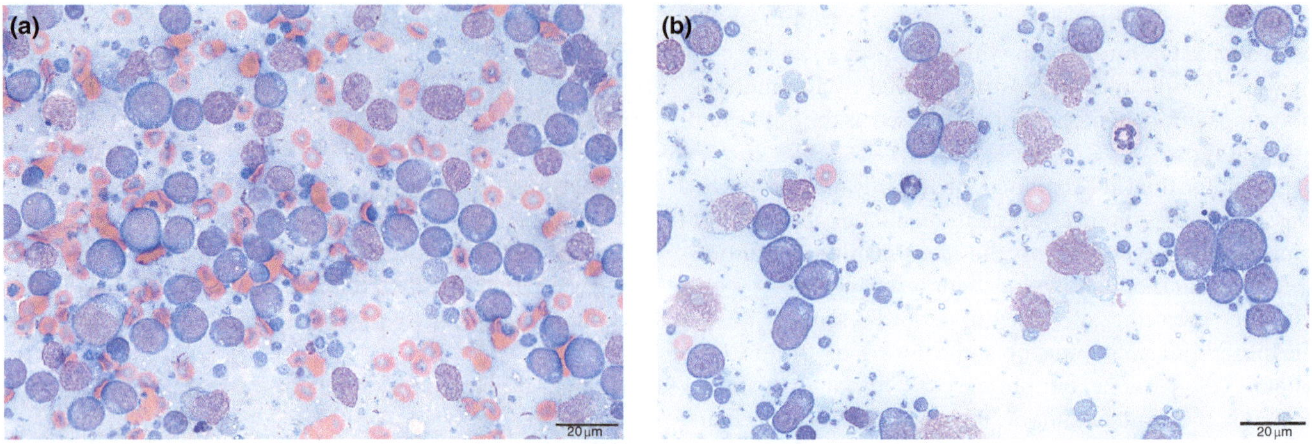

Figure 27.3 Aspirates of lymph nodes from two cases of histologically confirmed canine diffuse large B-cell lymphoma. There is a marked expansion of deeply basophilic lymphoid blasts that range from 8 to 20 μm^2 in size. These cells contain round nuclei with dispersed chromatin and one to multiple, large, prominent nucleoli (Wright–Geimsa, 500×).

proliferating cells of the germinal center with oval to round vesicular nuclei, fine chromatin, multiple nucleoli, and scanty amphophilic to basophilic cytoplasm.[83,92] The immunoblast variant in dogs is less frequent with cells containing predominantly a single and centrally located nucleolus. By immunohistochemistry, DLBCLs express CD79, CD20, and the nuclear transcription factor PAX5.

Beyond morphology, human DLBCL is commonly subdivided according to gene expression data into germinal center (GC) and non-GC types (this latter category comprised mostly from activated B cells). These subtypes, which can be segregated according to several immunohistochemistry-based algorithms, are linked to distinct prognoses and therapies.[96,97] These subtypes are described in the dog using gene expression profiling and NF-kB expression patterns, and the authors suggest that the non-GC subtype is the most frequent in dog.[98,99] However, the clinical utility and reproducibility of this classification scheme is uncertain as cases cannot currently be reliably differentiated using morphology or immunohistochemistry.[99]

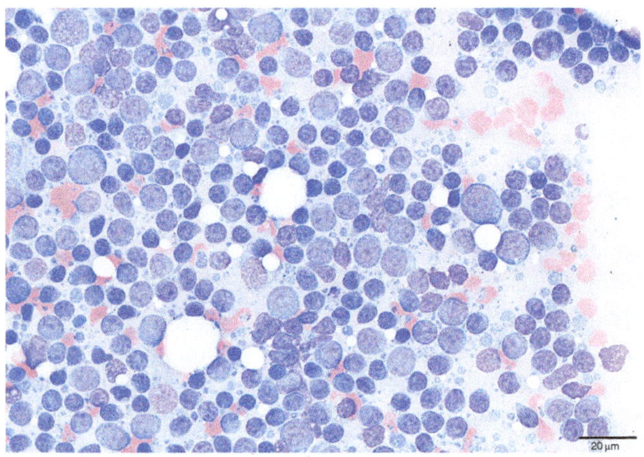

Figure 27.4 Aspirate of a lymph node from a histologically confirmed canine marginal zone lymphoma. There is an expansion of intermediate to large, deeply basophilic lymphoid blasts that range from 8 to 12 μm^2 in size (arrows). These cells contain a round nucleus with a central, large, single nucleolus. The ability to use cytology to reliably differentiate MZL from DLBCL has not been rigorously explored (Wright–Geimsa, 500×).

Marginal Zone Lymphoma

Marginal zone lymphoma (MZL) is a mature B-cell neoplasm that is stratified into clinically unique nodal, splenic, or extranodal forms. Based on limited clinical reports, there may be behavioral differences between the various subtypes of MZL and other forms of B-cell lymphoma. Splenic MZL is a nodular form of lymphoma showing a less aggressive behavior and a good prognosis after splenectomy.[100,101] Despite the generally reported "indolent" designation, the outcome of nodal MZL has recently been shown to be more guarded, and systemic involvement appears frequent.[102] Nodal MZL is characterized by a node that has focally retained the normal architecture but is infiltrated by a neoplastic population composed of lymphocytes resembling cells of the marginal zone. Cytology of MZL is similar irrespective of the tissue of origin and is characterized by a homogeneous population of medium-sized lymphoid cells (nuclei about the size of two erythrocytes) with round nuclei and a single prominent, central, large nucleolus (Figure 27.4).[102] Centroblasts and immunoblasts are rarely found but tend to increase in number during progression. Mitotic index is low to intermediate with few or no mitoses,[75] and Ki67 positivity is low.[103,104] The sensitivity and specificity of cytologic morphology to distinguish canine MZL from DLBCL has not been investigated. Histologically, the neoplastic cells in MZL are medium in size and show a distinctive appearance characterized by intermediate-sized nucleus, a prominent single central nucleolus and abundant lightly stained cytoplasm. Mitoses are rare or absent. By immunohistochemistry, MZLs express CD79a, CD20, PAX5, and CD21. As nodal MZL progresses, the residual remnant follicles are effaced, leading to a more diffuse appearance, and accordingly, the term "marginal zone lymphoma late stage" has been proposed.[81] In the most advanced cases, an increased percentage of lymphoid blasts can be seen, which may suggest transformation to DLBCL.[105]

Peripheral T-Cell Lymphoma Not Otherwise Specified

Peripheral T-cell lymphoma not otherwise specified (PTCL-NOS) describes high-grade, aggressive variants of nodal T-cell lymphoma. Although different cytological presentations may be found and the updated Kiel classification describes different morphological entities, the current WHO scheme annotates them in a single entity due to the lack of clinical differences among them. The most common cytologic picture of PTCL-NOS is the pleomorphic mixed small and large subtype, which is characterized by a dominant population of pleomorphic cells, often with moderate amounts of lightly basophilic cytoplasm. Nuclei in these cells are pleomorphic, ranging from indented to multilobated to cerebriform or with a "flowerlike" appearance, and contain smooth chromatin with variably prominent nucleoli (Figure 27.5). Mitotic index is generally medium to high. The residual population of nonneoplastic lymphoid cells is often scarce but some reactive plasma cells can be recognized. Other cytological subtypes are rare, including high-grade T-cell lymphoma with plasmacytoid appearance and T-cell immunoblastic lymphoma,[83] both of which can be difficult to diagnose based only on morphology. The former can be difficult to differentiate from a plasma cell tumor, whereas the latter can resemble the analogous B form. In both of these cases, mitotic index is high, and the clinical behavior is very aggressive.

T-Zone Lymphoma

T-zone lymphoma (TZL) is a unique variant of canine T-cell lymphoma characterized by an indolent behavior, low grade, frequent blood involvement, and a characteristic cytologic, histologic, and flow cytometric pattern.[90,106] Cytologically, TZL is characterized by a proliferation of small to medium cells with moderately abundant clear cytoplasm, an often unipolar extension of the cytoplasm ("hand mirror" shape), and a round nucleus with condensed chromatin and a generally inapparent nucleolus (Figure 27.6). Mitotic index is low, and reactive plasma cells are frequent.[73] This peculiar cytological pattern has been previously named as "small clear cell lymphoma" and, while the cytomorphology is very suggestive, a diagnosis of TZL must be confirmed through either histology or flow cytometry. Histologically, TZL is characterized by a nodular to diffuse pattern of infiltration of the paracortex and separation and compression of the residual primary and secondary follicles. In nodular disease, mild expansion of the residual follicles may be observed. The neoplastic cells are small to intermediate in size, lack internal nuclear detail, and have shallow nuclear indentations. Few

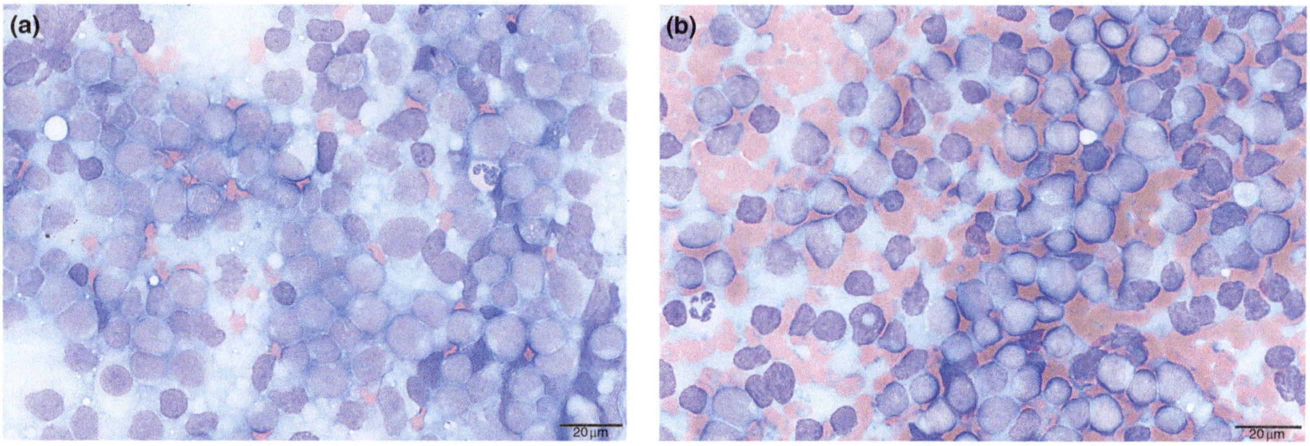

Figure 27.5 Aspirates of lymph nodes from two cases of histologically confirmed canine peripheral T-cell lymphoma not otherwise specified. There is a marked expansion of intermediate to large lymphocytes that range from 10 to 20 μm^2 in size. These cells contain round to oval to indented nuclei with occasional faint nucleoli. The nuclear chromatin pattern is smooth, and the cytoplasm is lightly basophilic and variably abundant (Wright–Geimsa, 500×).

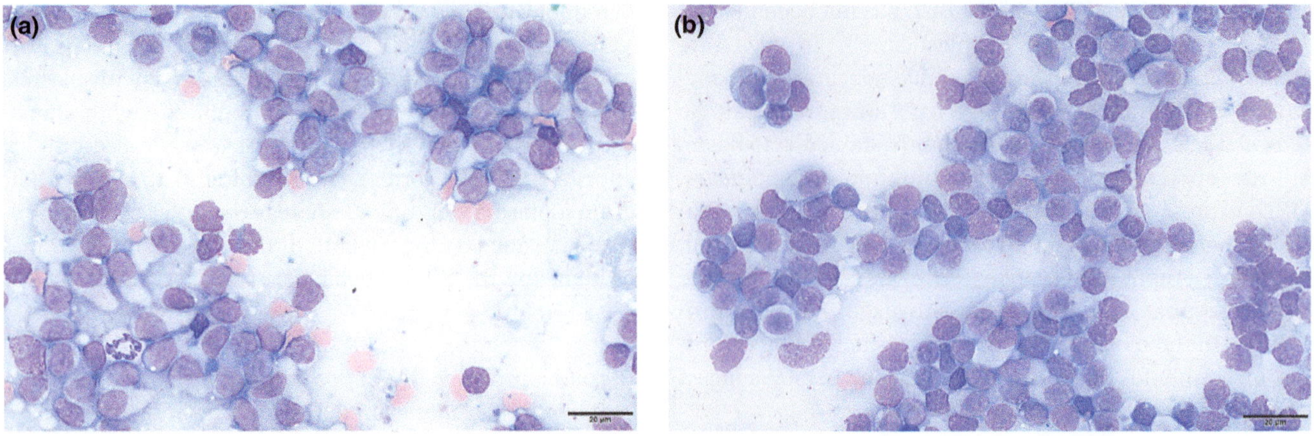

Figure 27.6 Aspirates from two cases of histologically confirmed canine T-zone lymphoma. There is an expansion of intermediate-sized lymphocytes that range from 12 to 20 μm^2 in size. These cells contain uniform, small, round nuclei without nucleoli. The moderate to abundant light cytoplasm, which can form unipolar cytoplasmic extensions, is one of the characteristic features. Flow cytometry can be used to confirm the cytologic suspicion (Wright–Geimsa, 500×).

macrophages and tingible bodies are usually observed. The number of mitoses is low (0–3/HPF). Notably, canine TZL is associated with a unique flow cytometric immunophenotype. Specifically, the neoplastic cells demonstrate a recurrent aberrant pattern with diminished to absent expression of the common leukocyte antigen CD45, co-expression of T lineage markers (CD5 and CD3) with CD21, and variable CD4 and CD8 expression.[90,91]

Follicular Lymphoma

Follicular lymphoma (FL) is a rare form of canine lymphoma, accounting for less than 1% of cases.[81,83] While no studies have examined its utility in the diagnosis of canine FL, it is likely that cytology alone is insufficient as a stand-alone tool, particularly in differentiating FL from follicular hyperplasia or from other forms of lymphoma. Although histopathology and immunohistochemistry remain mandatory for final diagnosis, FL may be suspected based on the presence of a prevalent mixed population of centrocytes (small cells with angular nuclei and scant amounts of pale cytoplasm), centroblasts, and follicular dendritic cells without an increased number of plasma cells and in the absence of a progressive differentiation among the cells.[83] Histologically, FL recapitulates normal lymph node architecture through a nodular pattern of tumor growth. Neoplastic follicles are differentiated from normal follicles by the former's lack of a well-defined mantle zone, polarization, or tingible body macrophages. Within the follicles, FL is characterized by a nodular proliferation of centrocytes and centroblasts.[81] Based upon the proportion of centroblasts, FL can be assigned a grade of 1–3, but the significance of this in veterinary medicine is unknown. As with other B-cell neoplasms, PARR may be useful to confirm clonality, and the neoplastic cells are positive for CD79 and CD20. Similarly to humans, canine FL may evolve to DLBCL.[105] Notably, although human FL is characterized by a stereotypic t(14;18) chromosomal translocation resulting in constitutive expression of the anti-apoptotic bcl2 protein, such a translocation has not been identified in dogs with FL.[107]

Large Granular Lymphocyte Lymphoma

Large granular lymphocyte (LGL) lymphoma, although lacking a specific human counterpart, is described in both the dog (largely involving the spleen and liver) and the cat (largely involving the alimentary tract).[108–111] The cytology of LGL lymphoma is characterized by neoplastic medium-sized lymphoid cells with moderately abundant gray to light blue cytoplasm containing azurophilic granules. The characteristic granules are seen in Wright's stained samples, are often located in a perinuclear area in the dog, can vary in size from fine to large globular granules, and may be surrounded by a clear halo. Neoplastic cell nuclei are round to indented with variably mature (smooth to clumped) chromatin and variably prominent nucleoli. On histologic samples, the neoplastic cells are medium-sized and pleomorphic, have variably sized and shaped nuclei, and contain the characteristic cytoplasmic eosinophilic granules. Immunophenotypically, canine LGL lymphoma is most commonly composed of $CD8^+$ T cells, although $CD4^-$, $CD8^-$, $TCR\delta\Delta^+$, or $CD3^-$ variants are described.[112] In the cat, a $CD8^+$ immunophenotype is frequently reported.[109] In the dog, prognosis varies from quite good in the differentiated forms (mainly as chronic lymphocytic leukemia), to very poor in less differentiated high-grade lymphomas. In cats with LGL lymphoma, survival and response to therapy are reported to be poor.[108,113]

Hodgkin-Like Lymphoma

Hodgkin-like lymphoma (HLL) is a rare subtype of "T-cell-rich B-cell" lymphoma that is sporadically reported in the cat.[93,114,115] Clinically, HLL typically presents with involvement of a single or a few lymph nodes of the neck or head. There is limited published information on the cytology of HLL, but the recognition of occasional Reed–Sternberg cells may be suggestive of HLL.[115] Reed–Sternberg cells are large cells with clear cytoplasm that are often binucleated with ovoid nuclei and prominent large nucleoli (Figure 27.7). Morphologically, the remainder of the lymphoid population is heterogeneous and composed of small lymphocytes, plasma cells, and large macrophages containing cellular debris. Histologically, HLL is characterized by regional to diffuse nodal infiltration by a mixed population of small lymphocytes, lymphoblasts, eosinophils, large histiocytoid cells, and small numbers of Reed–Sternberg cells. Immunophenotype shows a prevalent population of small reactive T cells, although the neoplastic population is assumed to be B cell in origin. The presumed neoplastic Reed–Sternberg cells in cats demonstrate variable staining for CD79a and BLA.36 but are negative for CD3 and macrophage markers.[115]

Equine Lymphoma

Lymphoma is one of the more common malignancies in horses, but overall frequency and nodal presentation is less prevalent than in dogs and cats.[116–118] Equine lymphoma shows a highly variable presentation, and clinical course and relatively few case reports have been described over the years. From several case reports, LGL cytologic appearance of neoplastic cells in equids emerges, but larger case series focused on cytological features of neoplastic cells in equine lymphoma are still lacking.[119–121] A retrospective histologic study of 31 cases of equine lymphoma demonstrated a mix of B- and T-cell tumors with frequent cutaneous, splenic, and mediastinal involvement.[122] Lymph nodes were described as involved in 10 of the 31 cases. More recently, a larger number of horses affected by lymphoma and tumors were classified according to the WHO histologic guidelines.[117] T-cell-rich large B-cell lymphoma was the most frequent histotype, accounting for 43% of the 203 cases, whereas PTCL and DLBCL comprised 22 and 12.5% of cases, respectively. Similar to earlier reports, mediastinal, alimentary and cutaneous forms were frequently described with only a small number of cases ($n = 9$) having primary nodal involvement.[117] Specific cytologic features were not described. The roles of cytology in the diagnosis of equine lymphoma and the utility of ancillary techniques such as flow cytometry remain to be elucidated.

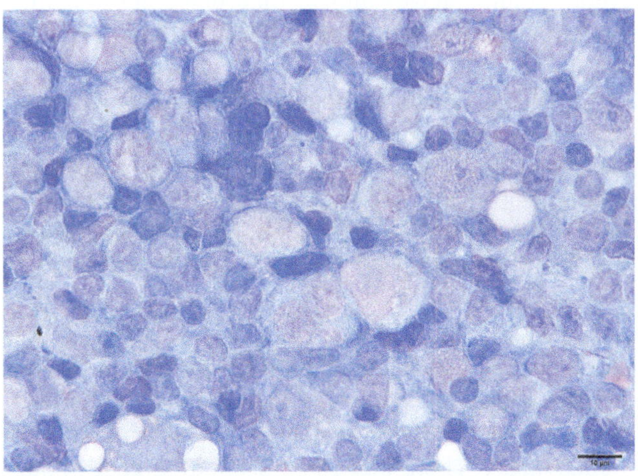

Figure 27.7 Aspirates from a histologically confirmed feline Hodgkin-like lymphoma. There is an expanded population of very large cells that range from 15 to 30 μm^2 in size. These cells contain pleomorphic nuclei with variably prominent nucleoli. Occasional cells are binucleate (arrow), resembling Reed–Sternberg cells described in people with Hodgkin lymphoma. A background population of normal small lymphocytes is present (Wright–Geimsa, 500×).

Metastatic Neoplasia

Aspiration of regional lymph nodes is often performed in the initial staging of primary tumors. Studies have demonstrated the utility of assessing regional lymph nodes with aspiration cytology in dogs and cats even when the lymph nodes palpate normally.[123–127] The ease with which metastatic disease can be diagnosed depends on the degree of lymph node involvement. This ranges from straightforward when the lymph node has been largely effaced with an overtly neoplastic population (Figure 27.8) to much more problematic when small numbers of individual cells such as mast cells or melanocytes are noted in a lymph node draining a mast cell tumor or melanoma. In a study examining a variety of primary tumors in both dogs and cats, cytologic assessment of the regional lymph node was 100% sensitive and 96% specific when compared with excisional lymph node histology.[123] When specifically examining oral tumors in both dogs and cats, cytologic results of lymph node aspiration concurred with the histology in 90.5% of cases.[126] In both of these studies, the vast majority of tumors were epithelial or mesenchymal in origin, which aids in identifying neoplastic cells among the background lymphocytes.

Sentinel Versus Draining Lymph Node

Determining which lymph node is the actual sentinel lymph node is critical for evaluating metastasis and presents some challenges.[128] To date, most staging procedures

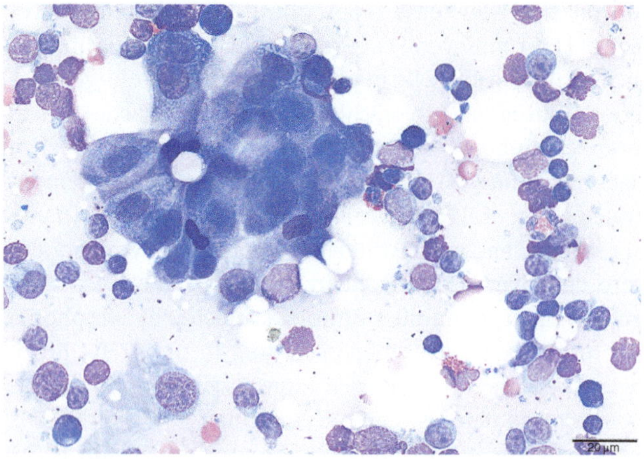

Figure 27.8 Cytologic evidence of metastasis in the medial iliac lymph node from a dog with transitional cell carcinoma of the bladder. There is a population of pleomorphic, cohesive epithelial cells intermixed with a heterogeneous population of lymphocytes. There were numerous such clusters in this aspirate (Wright–Geimsa, 500×).

in veterinary medicine involve sampling the regional lymph node(s) based on accessibility and an assumption of tumor drainage. True sentinel lymph nodes are defined as the first lymph nodes to drain a specific region of the body and, as such, are the most important lymph node in the assessment of early tumor dissemination.[129] Lymphatic drainage patterns in the head and neck, mammary glands, limbs, and prostate are described as variable in both normal dogs and dogs with tumors.[130–135] Lymphatic pathways in the head of dogs have been shown to be complex with multiple lymph nodes receiving drainage from both ipsilateral and contralateral regions of the head.[135] Sentinel lymph node mapping using vital dyes, and lymphoscintigraphy is a technique commonly used in human medicine and has been described in specific situations in preclinical and veterinary studies (reviewed in Refs.[128,130]). In a small subset of dogs with mast cell tumors, it was determined that the true sentinel lymph node was distinct from the closest regional lymph node in 8 of 19 dogs.[136] In dogs with metastatic oral and maxillofacial tumors, the mandibular lymph nodes are involved in only 55% of cases, yet these are the most commonly assessed lymph nodes when tumors occur in the head.[126] Techniques to routinely detect sentinel lymph nodes in a veterinary clinical setting would likely contribute to an enhanced sensitivity in detecting metastatic disease.

Histologic Scoring of Metastasis

Sentinel lymph node assessment in human medicine has led to the histologic description of isolated tumor cells (ITCs), micrometastasis, and macrometastasis. Macrometastasis is typically defined as a metastasis of >2 mm in diameter and micrometastasis as 0.2–2.0 mm, while ITCs consist of a metastasis of <0.2 mm or <200 tumor cells.[137] Immunohistochemistry to detect epithelial or mesenchymal antigens improves the detection rate for micrometastasis and ITCs.[138] The significance of ITCs, micrometastasis, and macrometastasis in human medicine is still emerging for various forms of neoplasia. Contradictory data exist about the prognostic significance of micrometastasis in several human tumors including squamous cell carcinoma and mammary tumors.[139–142] A recent meta-analysis has shown that the presence of micrometastasis is associated with a worse outcome in colorectal cancer, whereas ITCs have no apparent impact on outcome.[143] There are similar studies involving invasive human breast cancer where ITCs alone did not influence outcome.[144,145] Very few veterinary studies examining these subcategories have been published, but two studies relevant to canine mammary tumors are summarized below. Determining the potential significance of ITCs and micrometastasis for various veterinary malignancies could impact how the finding of rare metastatic cells on cytology is incorporated into treatment planning. A complete review of all tumor types is beyond the scope of this chapter, and in this section, we will discuss some of the more common veterinary oncology situations where draining lymph nodes are sampled.[146]

Mast Cell Tumors

Several studies have shown that detecting regional lymph node metastasis of canine mast cell tumors (clinically Stage II) is a negative prognostic indicator.[147–151] One study comparing 55 dogs with metastatic Grade 2 mast cell tumors (MCT) to 35 dogs without evidence of metastasis failed to identify a statistically significant impact on survival.[124] However, this study did identify a survival benefit to surgical removal of the metastatic lymph node providing another possible impetus for aspiration cytology.

The histologic definition of canine MCT metastasis has not been universally adopted but Weishaar et al. proposed a four-tier grading system based on the number and aggregation of mast cells in lymph node sinuses and parenchyma.[152] There was a significant difference in outcome when the two lower histologic grades were compared with the two higher grades.[152] Conclusive cytologic evidence of mast cell metastasis would therefore provide an early, noninvasive measure of biologic behavior that could aid both clinician and client in subsequent decision-making. It is known that normal canine lymph nodes can contain few to several mast cells, often in the medullary regions, so their simple presence is not evidence of neoplastic dissemination.[153] Previous studies using various cytologic criteria to define metastasis (the increased mast cell numbers in >2 HPFs, the degree of cytologic differentiation, and the presence of clusters or sheets of mast cells) have yielded conflicting results on the clinical impact of cytologically classifying animals as having Stage II disease.[148,150,154] Although not a primary goal of the paper, one study documented complete histologic concordance using a cytologic classification system based on clustering, "large" numbers of mast cells or atypical morphology in 50 dogs diagnosed with cytologic evidence of metastasis that had subsequent lymph node biopsy.[155] While instructive in cases where cytology was highly suggestive of metastasis, the true sensitivity of lymph node cytology was not addressed. A small study with both cytology and histology that did not report specific cytologic criteria indicates that metastatic status of four out of five cases was correctly assigned.[136]

In an attempt to further codify the cytologic indicators of mast cell tumor metastasis, Krick et al. developed specific criteria and applied them to a retrospective cohort of 152 dogs with regional lymph node aspirates.[149] The system that they used divided lymph node cytology results into five categories: (i) normal, (ii) reactive lymphoid hyperplasia, (iii) possible metastasis, (iv) probable metastasis, and (v) certain metastasis. Normal lymph nodes lacked mast cells, whereas nodes with reactive lymphoid hyperplasia contained rare, individual mast cells admixed with other cellular evidence of reactivity. "Possible metastasis" was utilized to categorize samples where there were two to three incidences of mast cells in aggregates of two to three cells, whereas "probable metastasis" included samples with >3 foci of two to three cell aggregates and/or two to five aggregates of more than three mast cells. "Certain metastasis" was reserved for samples that displayed effacement of the lymphoid tissue by mast cells, and/or aggregated, pleomorphic mast cells (criteria included anisocytosis, anisokaryosis, variable, or decreased granulation) and/or >5 aggregates of more than three mast cells (Figure 27.9). When only the "certain metastasis" category was used to define Stage II tumors, there was a significant difference in survival times between dogs with Stage I and Stage II tumors. There was no difference in the survival times between those dogs categorized as "possible metastasis" and those categorized as normal or reactive, whereas those categorized as "probable metastasis" had a significantly shorter survival than the normal and reactive categories. The lack of a gold standard technique such as lymph node biopsy precluded the authors from confirming metastasis and from calculating positive and negative predictive values in this study.

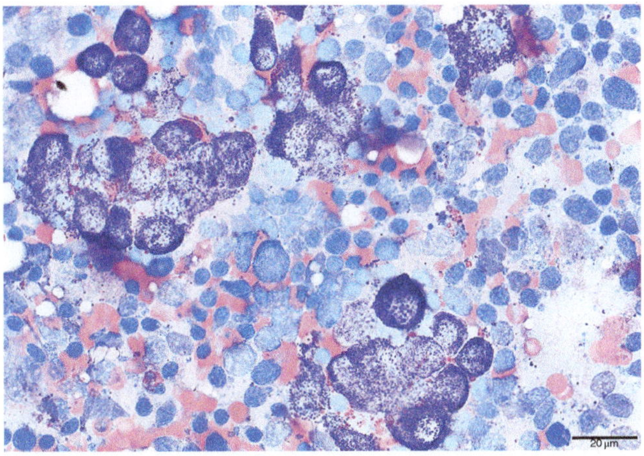

Figure 27.9 Cytologic evidence of metastatic mast cell tumor in a canine lymph node aspirate. There are several clusters of variably granular, pleomorphic mast cells intermixed with a heterogeneous population of lymphocytes. This dog had a grade II mast cell tumor that was incompletely excised (Wright–Geimsa, 500×).

Melanoma

One of the difficulties in determining the metastatic status of melanomas is distinguishing macrophages with phagocytized melanin pigment (melanophages) from true melanocytes in the aspirated sample (Figure 27.10). Melanophages are typically found in the lymph node sinuses and can be seen when there is inflammation associated with any pigmented region of the body. In human medicine, dermatopathic lymphadenitis is a term used to describe the accumulation of melanin-laden macrophages in association with cytologic evidence of paracortical hyperplasia in lymph nodes that are draining regions of exfoliative dermatitis.[15] Typically, the identification of melanophages is based on the irregular and globular nature of the pigment and the typical cytologic features of macrophages such as abundant cytoplasm with cytoplasmic vacuolization. Additional difficulties determining the cell of origin of the neoplastic cells can occur in amelanotic or poorly pigmented melanomas. ICC with the antibodies Melan-A and S-100 is shown to be helpful in determining melanocytic origin in some of these poorly pigmented metastatic tumors.[156,157]

Using the WHO staging system for canine oral melanoma, dogs with lymph node metastasis are classified as having Stage III melanoma. Most studies have demonstrated that dogs with Stage III disease, which also includes tumor size >4 cm, have a worse outcome than those with Stage I or II melanoma.[158–160] Conflicting evidence exists as to whether lymph node metastasis influences patient outcome independent of tumor size.[159,161,162]

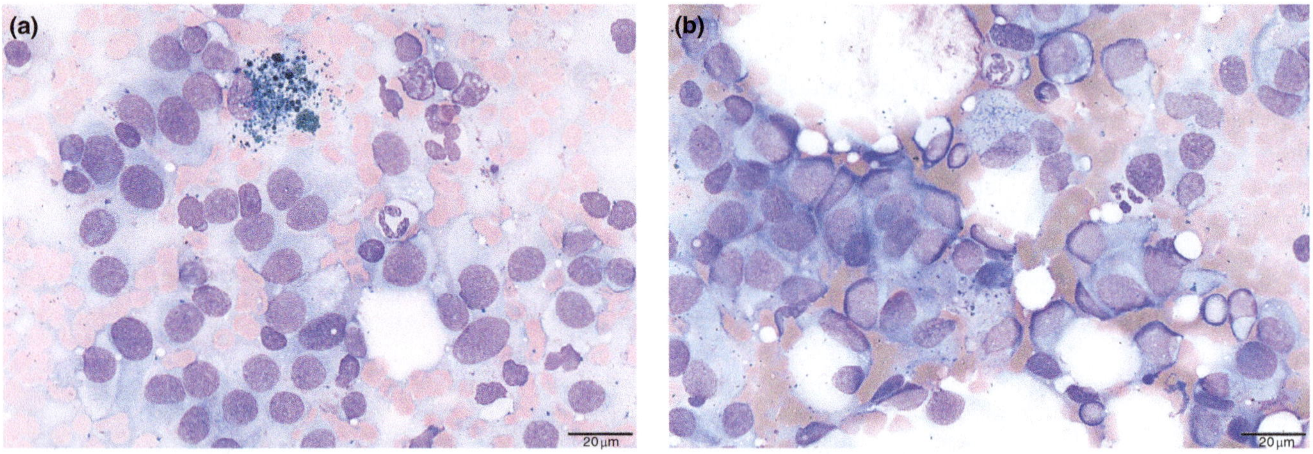

Figure 27.10 Aspirate of the mandibular lymph node from a dog with an oral mass that illustrates the potential difficulty in distinguishing melanocytes from melanophages. There is an atypical, loosely aggregated, spindle cell population with rare small lymphocytes in the background. (a) The pigmented cell (arrow) potentially represents a macrophage with phagocytized melanin. (b) This pigmented cell (arrow) is more convincingly part of the same cell population as the more numerous unpigmented atypical cells. The oral mass was confirmed as a poorly pigmented melanoma by histology and positive staining for Melan-A (Wright–Geimsa, 500×).

Cytologic criteria for diagnosing metastatic melanomas in veterinary species have not been comprehensively described. In a small subset of cases selected from primary oral masses with poor cytologic differentiation, four out of six dogs were correctly identified as having poorly pigmented melanoma metastasis while the remaining two cases required ICC with Melan-A, cytokeratin, and vimentin to confirm melanocytic origin.[157] In a recent study comparing the correlation between cytology and histopathology in diagnosing canine metastatic melanoma in 27 dogs, cytologic evidence of metastasis was defined as >5 melanin-containing cells that were spindle shaped, exhibited cohesiveness, and/or had distinct features of malignancy.[127] Malignant features included anisocytosis, anisokaryosis, variation and/or increase in nuclear to cytoplasmic ratio, multinucleation, and increased mitotic activity. Samples were deemed equivocal if there were >5 melanin-containing cells, but these cells were individualized and round without the aforementioned criteria of malignancy. Correlation between cytologic and histologic diagnosis of metastasis was found to be poor in this study. Of the nine dogs without cytologic evidence of metastasis, three were found to have histologic evidence of metastasis. Of the four dogs reaching the cytologic threshold for metastasis, only two dogs had this finding confirmed histologically. Interestingly, 15/16 dogs with equivocal findings with increased numbers of non-pleomorphic melanin-containing cells were free of histologic evidence of metastatic disease. There are some limitations of this study due largely to the retrospective nature, but it highlights some of the difficulty in accurately predicting melanoma metastases using cytology alone.

Mammary Tumors

In dogs, the existing classification system places all animals with histologic or cytologic evidence of mammary tumor metastasis as Stage IV.[163] The classification system does not currently take into account the location of the lymph node(s) relative to the mammary chain or the size of the metastatic foci. There is some conflicting evidence as to the impact on survival of mammary tumor lymph node metastasis in dogs.[164–168] A recent study examining histology of both the inguinal and axillary lymph nodes from 90 dogs with mammary tumors found that detection of metastasis has a significant impact on survival.[167] Additional factors associated with survival time include the number of lymph nodes involved and whether the metastasis is determined to be a micrometastasis or a macrometastasis (defined as metastatic foci >2 mm in diameter). Dogs with micrometastasis had a similar outcome to those without evidence of metastasis, whereas the presence of macrometastasis was associated with an inferior outcome. Interestingly, the presence of ITCs was associated with a worse prognosis than either no metastasis or micrometastasis. However, there were small numbers of animals in the ITC group, and a third of these dogs had aggressive histologic variants such as carcinosarcomas and solid carcinomas. Szczubial et al. similarly found that dogs with mammary micrometastasis did not have significantly altered outcome, whereas macrometastasis was associated with shortened disease-free interval and overall survival.[168] The presence of individual tumor cells was not evaluated in this study. Matos et al. demonstrated that micrometastases could be more readily detected using pan cytokeratin antibodies in canine tissue sections, but their presence was not assessed for impact on outcome.[138]

The fact that small numbers of metastatic mammary tumor cells may not have a significant impact on outcome in dogs influences the interpretation of cytologic findings. While small numbers of atypical mammary epithelial cells may suggest true metastasis, the disruption of cells and the loss of tissue architecture during cytologic preparation make it difficult to determine the actual tumor burden. There are currently no studies of cytology examining relative mammary tumor cell numbers or organizational pattern as has been done for the cytology of mast cell tumor metastasis.

Conclusion

Lymph node cytology is a noninvasive technique that often provides valuable clinical information. Reactive lymphoid hyperplasia is commonly seen and can have a variable cytologic appearance depending on the underlying stimulus and time course. Lymphadenitis can be due to both noninfectious and infectious causes, and the cytologic pattern of inflammation with or without identifiable organisms can be useful in creating important clinical differentials. Lymphoma is often confirmed with cytology and the cellular morphology can suggest the subtype. Subtyping is important as prognosis can vary dramatically, and additional techniques such as histology or immunophenotyping are needed for final classification. There is sometimes contradictory information about the clinical relevance of metastatic disease in some common veterinary tumors, and standardization of cytologic detection has only been explored in few tumor types. Cytology remains an important staging tool and will likely have even higher utility as we employ sentinel lymph node mapping and further standardize the cytologic criteria for determining metastatic status.

References

1. Akhtar, S.S., Imran-Ul-Huq, S.S., Faiz-U-Din, M., and Reyes, L.M. (1997). Efficacy of fine-needle capillary biopsy in the assessment of patients with superficial lymphadenopathy. *Cancer* 81: 277–280.
2. Sajeev, S. and Siddaraju, N. (2009). A comparative analysis of fine-needle capillary cytology vs. fine-needle aspiration cytology in superficial lymph node lesions. *Diagn Cytopathol* 37: 787–791.
3. Prasad, R.R.A., Narasimhan, R., Sankaran, V., and Veliath, A.J. (1996). Fine-needle aspiration cytology in the diagnosis of superficial lymphadenopathy: an analysis of 2,418 cases. *Diagn Cytopathol* 15: 382–386.
4. Skeldon, N. and Dewhurst, E. (2009). The perceived and actual diagnostic utility of veterinary cytological samples. *J Small Anim Pract* 50: 180–185.
5. Falini, B., Fizzotti, M., Pucciarini, A. et al. (2000). A monoclonal antibody (MUM1p) detects expression of the MUM 1/IRF4 protein in a subset of germinal center B cells, plasma cells, and activated T cells. *Blood* 95: 2084–2092.
6. Ho, F., Lortan, J.E., Maclnnan, I.C.M., and Khan, M. (1986). Distinct short-lived and long-lived antibody producing cell populations. *Eur J Immunol* 16: 1297–1301.
7. Willard-Mack, C.L. (2006). Normal structure, function, and histology of lymph nodes. *Toxicol Pathol* 34: 409–424.
8. Pambuccian, S.E. and Bardales, R.H. (2011). *Lymph Node Cytopathology*, Essentials in Cytopathology, 1–287.
9. Fooksman, D.R., Schwickert, T.A., Victora, G.D. et al. (2010). Development and migration of plasma cells in the mouse lymph node. *Immunity* 33: 118–127.
10. Rutgen, B.C., Konig, R., Hammer, S.E. et al. (2015). Composition of lymphocyte subpopulations in normal canine lymph nodes. *Vet Clin Pathol* 44: 58–69.
11. Raskin, R. and Meyer, D.J. (2010). *Canine and Feline Cytology: A Color Atlas and Interpretation Guide*, 2e. St. Louis, MO: Saunders Elsevier.
12. MacNeill, A.L. (2011). Cytology of canine and feline cutaneous and subcutaneous lesions and lymph nodes. *Top Companion Anim Med* 26: 62–76.
13. Cowell, R.L., Dorsey, K.E., and Meinkoth, J.H. (2003). Lymph node cytology. *Vet Clin North Am Small Anim Pract* 33: 47 67.
14. Gibson, D., Aubert, I., Woods, J.P. et al. (2004). Flow cytometric immunophenotype of canine lymph node aspirates. *J Vet Intern Med* 18: 710–717.
15. Monaco, S.E., Khalbuss, W.E., and Pantanowitz, L. (2012). Benign non-infectious causes of lymphadenopathy: a review of cytomorphology and differential diagnosis. *Diagn Cytopathol* 40: 925–938.
16. Cibas, E.S. and Ducatman, B.S. (2009). *Cytology: Diagnostic Principles and Clinical Correlates*, 3e. Philadelphia, PA: Saunders Elsevier.
17. Hicks, J. and Flaitz, C. (2002). Progressive transformation of germinal centers: review of histopathologic and clinical features. *Int J Pediatr Otorhinolaryngol* 65: 195–202.
18. Weiss, L.M. and O'Malley, D. (2013). Benign lymphadenopathies. *Mod Pathol* 26: S88–S96.

19 Goodnow, C.C., Vinuesa, C.G., Randall, K.L. et al. (2010). Control systems and decision making for antibody production. *Nat Immunol* 11: 681–688.
20 Jacob, J., Kassir, R., and Kelsoe, G. (1991). Insitu studies of the primary immune response to (4-hydroxy-3-nitrophenyl)acetyl. I. The architecture and dynamics of responding cell populations. *J Exp Med* 173: 1165–1175.
21 Chan, T.D., Gatto, D., Wood, K. et al. (2009). Antigen affinity controls rapid T-dependent antibody production by driving the expansion rather than the differentiation or extrafollicular migration of early plasmablasts. *J Immunol* 183: 3139–3149.
22 Wolniak, K.L., Shinall, S.M., and Waldschmidt, T.J. (2004). The germinal center response. *Crit Rev Immunol* 24: 39–65.
23 Liu, Y.J., Zhang, J., Lane, P.J. et al. (1991). Sites of specific B cell activation in primary and secondary responses to T cell-dependent and T cell-independent antigens. *Eur J Immunol* 21: 2951–2962.
24 Vandervalk, P. and Meijer, C.J.L.M. (1987). The histology of reactive lymph nodes. *Am J Surg Pathol* 11: 866–882.
25 Stani, J. (1987). Cytologic diagnosis of reactive lymphadenopathy in fine needle aspiration biopsy specimens. *Acta Cytol* 31: 8–13.
26 Cowell, R.L. and Valenciano, A.C. (2014). *Cowell and Tyler's Diagnostic Cytology and Hematology of the Dog and Cat*, 4e. St. Louis, MO: Elsevier.
27 Luscieti, P., Hubschmid, T., Cottier, H. et al. (1980). Human lymph node morphology as a function of age and site. *J Clin Pathol* 33: 454–461.
28 Elmore, S.A. (2006). Histopathology of the lymph nodes. *Toxicol Pathol* 34: 425–454.
29 Mills, J.N. (1989). Lymph node cytology. *Vet Clin North Am Small Anim Pract* 19: 697–717.
30 Bromel, C. and Sykes, J.E. (2005). Epidemiology, diagnosis, and treatment of blastomycosis in dogs and cats. *Clin Tech Small Anim Pract* 20: 233–239.
31 Shubitz, L.E. (2007). Comparative aspects of coccidioidomycosis in animals and humans. *Ann N Y Acad Sci* 1111: 395–403.
32 Arceneaux, K.A., Taboada, J., and Hosgood, G. (1998). Blastomycosis in dogs: 115 cases (1980–1995). *J Am Vet Med Assoc* 213: 658–664.
33 Legendre, A.M., Walker, M., Buyukmihci, N., and Stevens, R. (1981). Canine blastomycosis: a review of 47 clinical cases. *J Am Vet Med Assoc* 178: 1163–1168.
34 Garma-Avina, A. (1995). Cytologic findings in 43 cases of blastomycosis diagnosed ante-mortem in naturally infected dogs. *Mycopathologia* 131: 87–91.
35 Crews, L.J., Feeney, D.A., Jessen, C.R. et al. (2008). Utility of diagnostic tests for and medical treatment of pulmonary blastomycosis in dogs: 125 cases (1989–2006). *J Am Vet Med Assoc* 232: 222–227.
36 Graupmann-Kuzma, A., Valentine, B.A., Shubitz, L.F. et al. (2008). Coccidioidomycosis in dogs and cats: a review. *J Am Anim Hosp Assoc* 44: 226–235.
37 Johnson, L.R., Herrgesell, E.J., Davidson, A.P., and Pappagianis, D. (2003). Clinical, clinicopathologic, and radiographic findings in dogs with coccidioidomycosis: 24 cases (1995–2000). *J Am Vet Med Assoc* 222: 461–466.
38 Simoes, D.M., Dial, S.M., Coyner, K.S. et al. (2016). Retrospective analysis of cutaneous lesions in 23 canine and 17 feline cases of coccidiodomycosis seen in Arizona, USA (2009–2015). *Vet Dermatol* 27: 346–352.
39 Greene, R.T. and Troy, G.C. (1995). Coccidioidomycosis in 48 cats: a retrospective study (1984–1993). *J Vet Intern Med* 9: 86–91.
40 Crabtree, A.C., Keith, D.G., and Diamond, H.L. (2008). Relationship between radiographic hilar lymphadenopathy and serologic titers for *Coccidioides* sp. in dogs in an endemic region. *Vet Radiol Ultrasound* 49: 501–503.
41 Shubitz, L.F. and Dial, S.M. (2005). Coccidioidomycosis: a diagnostic challenge. *Clin Tech Small Anim Pract* 20: 220–226.
42 Armstrong, P.J. and Dibartola, S.P. (1983). Canine coccidioidomycosis: a literature review and report of 8 cases. *J Am Anim Hosp Assoc* 19: 937–946.
43 Saridomichelakis, M.N., Mylonakis, M.E., Leontides, L.S. et al. (2005). Evaluation of lymph node and bone marrow cytology in the diagnosis of canine leishmaniasis (*Leishmania infantum*) in symptomatic and asymptomatic dogs. *Am J Trop Med Hyg* 73: 82–86.
44 Mylonakis, M.E., Papaioannou, N., Saridomichelakis, M.N. et al. (2005). Cytologic patterns of lymphadenopathy in dogs infected with *Leishmania infantum*. *Vet Clin Pathol* 34: 243–247.
45 Moreira, P.R., Vieira, L.M., de Andrade, M.M. et al. (2010). Immune response pattern of the popliteal lymph nodes of dogs with visceral leishmaniasis. *Parasitol Res* 107: 605–613.
46 Meinkoth, K.R., Morton, R.J., and Meinkoth, J.H. (2004). Naturally occurring tularemia in a dog. *J Am Vet Med Assoc* 225: 545–547.
47 Gustafson, B.W. and DeBowes, L.J. (1996). Tularemia in a dog. *J Am Anim Hosp Assoc* 32: 339–341.
48 Baldwin, C.J., Panciera, R.J., Morton, R.J. et al. (1991). Acute tularemia in three domestic cats. *J Am Vet Med Assoc* 199: 1602–1605.
49 Rhyan, J.C., Gahagan, T., and Fales, W.H. (1990). Tularemia in a cat. *J Vet Diagn Invest* 2: 239–241.
50 Spagnoli, S.T., Kuroki, K., Schommer, S.K. et al. (2011). Pathology in practice. *Francisella tularensis*. *J Am Vet Med Assoc* 238: 1271–1273.

51 Berman-Booty, L.D., Cui, J., Horvath, S.J., and Premanandan, C. (2010). Pathology in practice. Tularemia. *J Am Vet Med Assoc* 237: 163–165.

52 Tuncer, E., Onal, B., Simsek, G. et al. (2014). Tularemia: potential role of cytopathology in differential diagnosis of cervical lymphadenitis: multicenter experience in 53 cases and literature review. *APMIS* 122: 236–242.

53 Markoc, F., Koseoglu, R.D., Koc, S., and Gurbuzler, L. (2014). Tularemia in differential diagnosis of cervical lymphadenopathy: cytologic features of tularemia lymphadenitis. *Acta Cytol* 58: 23–28.

54 Asano, S. (2012). Granulomatous lymphadenitis. *J Clin Exp Hematopathol* 52: 1–16.

55 Woods, J.P., Crystal, M.A., Morton, R.J., and Panciera, R.J. (1998). Tularemia in two cats. *J Am Vet Med Assoc* 212: 81–83.

56 Watson, R.P., Blanchard, T.W., Mense, M.G., and Gasper, P.W. (2001). Histopathology of experimental plague in cats. *Vet Pathol* 38: 165–172.

57 Orloski, K.A. and Lathrop, S.L. (2003). Plague: a veterinary perspective. *J Am Vet Med Assoc* 222: 444–448.

58 Nichols, M.C., Ettestad, P.J., Vinhatton, E.S. et al. (2014). Yersinia pestis infection in dogs: 62 cases (2003–2011). *J Am Vet Med Assoc* 244: 1176–1180.

59 Eidson, M., Thilsted, J.P., and Rollag, O.J. (1991). Clinical, clinicopathologic, and pathologic features of plague in cats: 119 cases (1977–1988). *J Am Vet Med Assoc* 199: 1191–1197.

60 Eidson, M., Tierney, L.A., Rollag, O.J. et al. (1988). Feline plague in New Mexico: risk factors and transmission to humans. *Am J Public Health* 78: 1333–1335.

61 Orloski, K.A. and Eidson, M. (1995). Yersinia pestis infection in three dogs. *J Am Vet Med Assoc* 207: 316–318.

62 Rollag, O.J., Skeels, M.R., Nims, L.J. et al. (1981). Feline plague in New Mexico. Report of five cases. *J Am Vet Med Assoc* 179: 1381–1383.

63 Rosser, W.W. (1987). Bubonic plague. *J Am Vet Med Assoc* 191: 406–409.

64 Guptill, L. (2010). Bartonellosis. *Vet Microbiol* 140: 347–359.

65 Drut, A., Bublot, I., Breitschwerdt, E.B. et al. (2014). Comparative microbiological features of *Bartonella henselae* infection in a dog with fever of unknown origin and granulomatous lymphadenitis. *Med Microbiol Immunol* 203: 85–91.

66 Pappalardo, B.L., Brown, T., Gookin, J.L. et al. (2000). Granulomatous disease associated with Bartonella infection in 2 dogs. *J Vet Intern Med* 14: 37–42.

67 Tucker, M.D., Sellon, R.K., Tucker, R.L. et al. (2014). Bilateral mandibular pyogranulomatous lymphadenitis and pulmonary nodules in a dog with *Bartonella henselae* bacteremia. *Can Vet J* 55: 970–974.

68 Jin, M. and Wakely, P.E. Jr. (2018). Lymph node cytopathology: essential ancillary studies as applied to lymphoproliferative neoplasms. *Cancer Cytopathol* 126 (Suppl 8): 615–626.

69 Li, S., Young, K.H., and Medeiros, L.J. (2018). Diffuse large B-cell lymphoma. *Pathology* 50: 74–87.

70 Rappaport, H. (1966). *Atlas of Tumor Pathology. Sect. 3, Fasc. 8, Tumors of the hematopoietic system*. Washington, DC: Armed Forces Institute of Pathology.

71 Lukes, R.J. and Collins, R.D. (1974). Immunologic characterization of human malignant lymphomas. *Cancer* 34 (4 Suppl): 1488–1503.

72 Lennert, K. and Feller, A.C. (1992). *Histopathology of Non-Hodgkin Lymphomas: (Based on the Updated Kiel Classification)*, 2e. Berlin: Springer-Verlag.

73 Fournel-Fleury, C., Magnol, J.P., Bricaire, P. et al. (1997). Cytohistological and immunological classification of canine malignant lymphomas: comparison with human non-Hodgkin's lymphomas. *J Comp Pathol* 117: 35–59.

74 Teske, E. and van Heerde, P. (1996). Diagnostic value and reproducibility of fine-needle aspiration cytology in canine malignant lymphoma. *Vet Q* 18: 112–115.

75 Magnol, J.P., Fournel, C., Marchal, T. et al. (1995). Malignant lymphoma with medium-sized macronucleolated cells in the dog: involvement of an original cell from the marginal zone of the reactive lymph node. *Bull Acad Natl Med* 179: 51–65.

76 Fournel-Fleury, C., Ponce, F., Felman, P. et al. (2002). Canine T-cell lymphomas: a morphological, immunological, and clinical study of 46 new cases. *Vet Pathol* 39: 92–109.

77 Ponce, F., Magnol, J.P., Ledieu, D. et al. (2004). Prognostic significance of morphological subtypes in canine malignant lymphomas during chemotherapy. *Vet J* 167: 158–166.

78 (1982). National Cancer Institute sponsored study of classifications of non-Hodgkin's lymphomas: summary and description of a working formulation for clinical usage. The Non-Hodgkin's Lymphoma Pathologic Classification Project. *Cancer* 49: 2112–2135.

79 Teske, E., Wisman, P., Moore, P.F., and van Heerde, P. (1994). Histologic classification and immunophenotyping of canine non-Hodgkin's lymphomas: unexpected high frequency of T cell lymphomas with B cell morphology. *Exp Hematol* 22: 1179–1187.

80 Harris, N.L., Jaffe, E.S., Diebold, J. et al. (1999). World Health Organization classification of neoplastic diseases of the hematopoietic and lymphoid tissues: report of the Clinical Advisory Committee meeting-Airlie House, Virginia, November 1997. *J Clin Oncol* 17: 3835–3849.

81 Valli, V.E., San Myint, M., Barthel, A. et al. (2011). Classification of canine malignant lymphomas according

to the World Health Organization criteria. *Vet Pathol* 48: 198–211.
82 Valli, V.E. and Armed Forces Institute of Pathology, American Registry of Pathology, Oncology WHO CCfWRoC (2002). *Histological Classification of Hematopoietic Tumors of Domestic Animals*. Washington, DC: Armed Forces Institute of Pathology, in cooperation with the American Registry of Pathology and the World Health Organization Collaborating Center for Worldwide Reference on Comparative Oncology.
83 Ponce, F., Marchal, T., Magnol, J.P. et al. (2010). A morphological study of 608 cases of canine malignant lymphoma in France with a focus on comparative similarities between canine and human lymphoma morphology. *Vet Pathol* 47: 414–433.
84 Vezzali, E., Parodi, A.L., Marcato, P.S., and Bettini, G. (2010). Histopathologic classification of 171 cases of canine and feline non-Hodgkin lymphoma according to the WHO. *Vet Comp Oncol* 8: 38–49.
85 Marconato, L., Gelain, M.E., and Comazzi, S. (2013). The dog as a possible animal model for human non-Hodgkin lymphoma: a review. *Hematol Oncol* 31: 1–9.
86 Comazzi, S. and Gelain, M.E. (2011). Use of flow cytometric immunophenotyping to refine the cytological diagnosis of canine lymphoma. *Vet J* 188: 149–155.
87 Dey, P., Amir, T., Al Jassar, A. et al. (2006). Combined applications of fine needle aspiration cytology and flow cytometric immunophenotyping for diagnosis and classification of non-Hodgkin lymphoma. *CytoJournal* 3: 24.
88 Hehn, S.T., Grogan, T.M., and Miller, T.P. (2004). Utility of fine-needle aspiration as a diagnostic technique in lymphoma. *J Clin Oncol* 22: 3046–3052.
89 Bangerter, M., Brudler, O., Heinrich, B. et al. (2007). Fine needle aspiration cytology and flow cytometry in the diagnosis and subclassification of non-Hodgkin's lymphoma based on the World Health Organization classification. *Acta Cytol* 51: 390–398.
90 Seelig, D.M., Avery, P., Webb, T. et al. (2014). Canine T-zone lymphoma: unique immunophenotypic features, outcome, and population characteristics. *J Vet Intern Med* 28: 878–886.
91 Martini, V., Poggi, A., Riondato, F. et al. (2015). Flow-cytometric detection of phenotypic aberrancies in canine small clear cell lymphoma. *Vet Comp Oncol* 13: 281–287.
92 Valli, V.E., Kass, P.H., San Myint, M., and Scott, F. (2013). Canine lymphomas: association of classification type, disease stage, tumor subtype, mitotic rate, and treatment with survival. *Vet Pathol* 50: 738–748.
93 Valli, V.E., Jacobs, R.M., Norris, A. et al. (2000). The histologic classification of 602 cases of feline lymphoproliferative disease using the National Cancer Institute working formulation. *J Vet Diagn Invest* 12: 295–306.
94 Lurie, D.M., Milner, R.J., Suter, S.E., and Vernau, W. (2008). Immunophenotypic and cytomorphologic subclassification of T-cell lymphoma in the boxer breed. *Vet Immunol Immunopathol* 125: 102–110.
95 Marconato, L., Martini, V., Aresu, L. et al. (2013). Assessment of bone marrow infiltration diagnosed by flow cytometry in canine large B cell lymphoma: prognostic significance and proposal of a cut-off value. *Vet J* 197: 776–781.
96 Hans, C.P., Weisenburger, D.D., Greiner, T.C. et al. (2004). Confirmation of the molecular classification of diffuse large B-cell lymphoma by immunohistochemistry using a tissue microarray. *Blood* 103: 275–282.
97 Chang, C.C., McClintock, S., Cleveland, R.P. et al. (2004). Immunohistochemical expression patterns of germinal center and activation B-cell markers correlate with prognosis in diffuse large B-cell lymphoma. *Am J Surg Pathol* 28: 464–470.
98 Gaurnier-Hausser, A., Patel, R., Baldwin, A.S. et al. (2011). NEMO-binding domain peptide inhibits constitutive NF-kappaB activity and reduces tumor burden in a canine model of relapsed, refractory diffuse large B-cell lymphoma. *Clin Cancer Res* 17: 4661–4671.
99 Richards, K.L., Motsinger-Reif, A.A., Chen, H.W. et al. (2013). Gene profiling of canine B-cell lymphoma reveals germinal center and postgerminal center subtypes with different survival times, modeling human DLBCL. *Cancer Res* 73: 5029–5039.
100 Stefanello, D., Valenti, P., Zini, E. et al. (2011). Splenic marginal zone lymphoma in 5 dogs (2001–2008). *J Vet Intern Med* 25: 90–93.
101 O'Brien, D., Moore, P.F., Vernau, W. et al. (2013). Clinical characteristics and outcome in dogs with splenic marginal zone lymphoma. *J Vet Intern Med* 27: 949–954.
102 Cozzi, M., Marconato, L., Martini, V. et al. (2018). Canine nodal marginal zone lymphoma: descriptive insight into the biological behaviour. *Vet Comp Oncol* 16: 246–252.
103 Fournel-Fleury, C., Magnol, J.P., Chabanne, L. et al. (1997). Growth fractions in canine non-Hodgkin's lymphomas as determined in situ by the expression of the Ki-67 antigen. *J Comp Pathol* 117: 61–72.
104 Poggi, A., Miniscalco, B., Morello, E. et al. (2015). Flow cytometric evaluation of ki67 for the determination of malignancy grade in canine lymphoma. *Vet Comp Oncol* 13: 475–480.
105 Comazzi, S., Aresu, L., and Marconato, L. (2015). Transformation of canine lymphoma/leukemia to more aggressive diseases: anecdotes or reality? *Front Vet Sci* 2: 42.

106 Martini, V., Marconato, L., Poggi, A. et al. (2016). Canine small clear cell/T-zone lymphoma: clinical presentation and outcome in a retrospective case series. *Vet Comp Oncol* 14 (suppl 1): 117–126.

107 Thomas, R., Demeter, Z., Kennedy, K.A. et al. (2017). Integrated immunohistochemical and DNA copy number profiling analysis provides insight into the molecular pathogenesis of canine follicular lymphoma. *Vet Comp Oncol* 15: 852–867.

108 Finotello, R., Vasconi, M.E., Sabattini, S. et al. (2018). Feline large granular lymphocyte lymphoma: an Italian Society of Veterinary Oncology (SIONCOV) retrospective study. *Vet Comp Oncol* 16: 159–166.

109 Roccabianca, P., Vernau, W., Caniatti, M., and Moore, P.F. (2006). Feline large granular lymphocyte (LGL) lymphoma with secondary leukemia: primary intestinal origin with predominance of a CD3/CD8(alpha)(alpha) phenotype. *Vet Pathol* 43: 15–28.

110 Suwa, A. and Shimoda, T. (2018). Lymphoma-associated hemophagocytic syndrome in six dogs. *J Vet Med Sci* 80: 1271–1276.

111 Keller, S.M., Vernau, W., Hodges, J. et al. (2013). Hepatosplenic and hepatocytotropic T-cell lymphoma: two distinct types of T-cell lymphoma in dogs. *Vet Pathol* 50: 281–290.

112 McDonough, S.P. and Moore, P.F. (2000). Clinical, hematologic, and immunophenotypic characterization of canine large granular lymphocytosis. *Vet Pathol* 37: 637–646.

113 Krick, E.L., Little, L., Patel, R. et al. (2008). Description of clinical and pathological findings, treatment and outcome of feline large granular lymphocyte lymphoma (1996–2004). *Vet Comp Oncol* 6: 102–110.

114 Steinberg, J.D. and Keating, J.H. (2008). What is your diagnosis? Cervical mass in a cat. *Vet Clin Pathol* 37: 323–327.

115 Walton, R.M. and Hendrick, M.J. (2001). Feline Hodgkin's-like lymphoma: 20 cases (1992–1999). *Vet Pathol* 38: 504–511.

116 Miller, M.A., Moore, G.E., Bertin, F.R., and Kritchevsky, J.E. (2016). What's new in old horses? Postmortem diagnoses in mature and aged equids. *Vet Pathol* 53: 390–398.

117 Durham, A.C., Pillitteri, C.A., San Myint, M., and Valli, V.E. (2013). Two hundred three cases of equine lymphoma classified according to the World Health Organization (WHO) classification criteria. *Vet Pathol* 50: 86–93.

118 Knowles, E.J., Tremaine, W.H., Pearson, G.R., and Mair, T.S. (2016). A database survey of equine tumours in the United Kingdom. *Equine Vet J* 48: 280–284.

119 Mastrorilli, C., Cesar, F., Joiner, K. et al. (2015). Disseminated lymphoma with large granular lymphocyte morphology diagnosed in a horse via abdominal fluid and transtracheal wash cytology. *Vet Clin Pathol* 44: 437–441.

120 Zimmerman, B., Jones, S., and Rotstein, D.S. (2004). Large granular lymphoma in a mule. *Vet Rec* 155: 462–463.

121 Quist, C.F., Harmon, B.G., Mahaffey, E.A., and Collatos, C. (1994). Large granular lymphocyte neoplasia in an aged mare. *J Vet Diagn Invest* 6: 111–113.

122 Kelley, L.C. and Mahaffey, E.A. (1998). Equine malignant lymphomas: morphologic and immunohistochemical classification. *Vet Pathol* 35: 241–252.

123 Langenbach, A., McManus, P.M., Hendrick, M.J. et al. (2001). Sensitivity and specificity of methods of assessing the regional lymph nodes for evidence of metastasis in dogs and cats with solid tumors. *J Am Vet Med Assoc* 218: 1424–1428.

124 Baginski, H., Davis, G., and Bastian, R.P. (2014). The prognostic value of lymph node metastasis with grade 2 MCTs in dogs: 55 Cases (2001–2010). *J Am Anim Hosp Assoc* 50: 89–95.

125 Williams, L.E. and Packer, R.A. (2003). Association between lymph node size and metastasis in dogs with oral malignant melanoma: 100 cases (1987–2001). *J Am Vet Med Assoc* 222: 1234–1236.

126 Herring, E.S., Smith, M.M., and Robertson, J.L. (2002). Lymph node staging of oral and maxillofacial neoplasms in 31 dogs and cats. *J Vet Dent* 19: 122–126.

127 Grimes, J.A., Matz, B.M., Christopherson, P.W. et al. (2017). Agreement between cytology and histopathology for regional lymph node metastasis in dogs with melanocytic neoplasms. *Vet Pathol* 54: 579–587.

128 Uren, R.F., Howman-Giles, R., Chung, D., and Thompson, J.F. (2015). Imaging sentinel lymph nodes. *Cancer J* 21: 25–32.

129 Balch, C.M. and Lange, J.R. (2001). Lymphatic mapping and sentinel node lymphadenectomy for cancer: an overview. *Ann Surg Oncol* 8 (9 Suppl): 1S–4S.

130 Tuohy, J.L., Milgram, J., Worley, D.R., and Dernell, W.S. (2009). A review of sentinel lymph node evaluation and the need for its incorporation into veterinary oncology. *Vet Comp Oncol* 7: 81–91.

131 Wells, S., Bennett, A., Walsh, P. et al. (2006). Clinical usefulness of intradermal fluorescein and patent blue violet dyes for sentinel lymph node identification in dogs. *Vet Comp Oncol* 4: 114–122.

132 Smith, M.M. (1995). Surgical approach for lymph node staging of oral and maxillofacial neoplasms in dogs. *J Am Anim Hosp Assoc* 31: 514–518.

133 Pereira, C.T., Rahal, S.C., de Carvalho Balieiro, J.C. et al. (2003). Lymphatic drainage on healthy and neoplastic mammary glands in female dogs: can it really be altered? *Anat Histol Embryol* 32: 282–290.

134 Stroup, S.P., Kane, C.J., Farchshchi-Heydari, S. et al. (2012). Preoperative sentinel lymph node mapping of the prostate using PET/CT fusion imaging and Ga-68-labeled tilmanocept in an animal model. *Clin Exp Metastasis* 29: 673–680.

135 Belz, G.T. and Heath, T.J. (1995). Lymph pathways of the medial retropharyngeal lymph node in dogs. *J Anat* 186: 517–526.

136 Worley, D.R. (2014). Incorporation of sentinel lymph node mapping in dogs with mast cell tumours: 20 consecutive procedures. *Vet Comp Oncol* 12: 215–226.

137 Tsuda, H. (2015). Histological examination of sentinel lymph nodes: significance of macrometastasis, micrometastasis, and isolated tumor cells. *Breast Cancer* 22: 221–229.

138 Matos, A.J., Faustino, A.M., Lopes, C. et al. (2006). Detection of lymph node micrometastases in malignant mammary tumours in dogs by cytokeratin immunostaining. *Vet Rec* 158: 626–630.

139 Sato, F., Shimada, Y., Li, Z. et al. (2001). Lymph node micrometastasis and prognosis in patients with oesophageal squamous cell carcinoma. *Br J Surg* 88: 426–432.

140 Zingg, U., Montani, M., Busch, M. et al. (2009). Prognostic influence of immunohistochemically detected lymph node micrometastasis and histological subtype in pN0 oesophageal cancer. *Eur J Surg Oncol* 35: 593–599.

141 Kahn, H.J., Hanna, W.M., Chapman, J.A. et al. (2006). Biological significance of occult micrometastases in histologically negative axillary lymph nodes in breast cancer patients using the recent American Joint Committee on Cancer breast cancer staging system. *Breast J* 12: 294–301.

142 Tan, L.K., Giri, D., Hummer, A.J. et al. (2008). Occult axillary node metastases in breast cancer are prognostically significant: results in 368 node-negative patients with 20-year follow-up. *J Clin Oncol* 26: 1803–1809.

143 Slothaak, D.A., Sahami, S., van der Zaag-Loonen, H.J. et al. (2014). The prognostic value of micrometastases and isolated tumour cells in histologically negative lymph nodes of patients with colorectal cancer: a systematic review and meta-analysis. *Eur J Surg Oncol* 40: 263–269.

144 Reed, J., Rosman, M., Verbanac, K.M. et al. (2009). Prognostic implications of isolated tumor cells and micrometastases in sentinel nodes of patients with invasive breast cancer: 10-year analysis of patients enrolled in the prospective East Carolina University/ Anne Arundel Medical Center Sentinel Node Multicenter Study. *J Am Coll Surg* 208: 333–340.

145 Grube, B.J., Hansen, N.M., Ye, X., and Giuliano, A.E. (2002). Tumor characteristics predictive of sentinel node metastases in 105 consecutive patients with invasive lobular carcinoma. *Ame J Surg* 184: 372–376.

146 Sapierzynski, R., Czopowicz, M., and Jagielski, D. (2017). Metastatic lymphadenomegaly in dogs – cytological study. *Pol J Vet Sci* 20: 731–736.

147 Cahalane, A.K., Payne, S., Barber, L.G. et al. (2004). Prognostic factors for survival of dogs with inguinal and perineal mast cell tumors treated surgically with or without adjunctive treatment: 68 cases (1994–2002). *J Am Vet Med Assoc* 225: 401–408.

148 Thamm, D.H., Turek, M.M., and Vail, D.M. (2006). Outcome and prognostic factors following adjuvant prednisone/vinblastine chemotherapy for high-risk canine mast cell tumour: 61 cases. *J Vet Med Sci* 68: 581–587.

149 Krick, E.L., Billings, A.P., Shofer, F.S. et al. (2009). Cytological lymph node evaluation in dogs with mast cell tumours: association with grade and survival. *Vet Comp Oncol* 7: 130–138.

150 Sfiligoi, G., Rassnick, K.M., Scarlett, J.M. et al. (2005). Outcome of dogs with mast cell tumors in the inguinal or perineal region versus other cutaneous locations: 124 cases (1990–2001). *J Am Vet Med Assoc* 226: 1368–1374.

151 Hume, C.T., Kiupel, M., Rigatti, L. et al. (2011). Outcomes of dogs with grade 3 mast cell tumors: 43 cases (1997–2007). *J Am Anim Hosp Assoc* 47: 37–44.

152 Weishaar, K.M., Thamm, D.H., Worley, D.R., and Kamstock, D.A. (2014). Correlation of nodal mast cells with clinical outcome in dogs with mast cell tumour and a proposed classification system for the evaluation of node metastasis. *J Comp Pathol* 151: 329–338.

153 Bookbinder, P.F., Butt, M.T., and Harvey, H.J. (1992). Determination of the number of mast cells in lymph node, bone marrow, and buffy coat cytologic specimens from dogs. *J Am Vet Med Assoc* 200: 1648–1650.

154 Gieger, T.L., Theon, A.P., Werner, J.A. et al. (2003). Biologic behavior and prognostic factors for mast cell tumors of the canine muzzle: 24 cases (1990–2001). *J Vet Intern Med* 17: 687–692.

155 Stefanello, D., Buracco, P., Sabattini, S. et al. (2015). Comparison of 2- and 3-category histologic grading systems for predicting the presence of metastasis at the time of initial evaluation in dogs with cutaneous mast cell tumors: 386 cases (2009–2014). *J Am Vet Med Assoc* 246: 765–769.

156 Hoinghaus, R., Mischke, R., and Hewicker-Trautwein, M. (2002). Use of immunocytochemical techniques in canine melanoma. *J Vet Med A Physiol Pathol Clin Med* 49: 198–202.

157 Przezdziecki, R., Czopowicz, M., and Sapierzynski, R. (2015). Accuracy of routine cytology and immunocytochemistry in preoperative diagnosis of oral amelanotic melanomas in dogs. *Vet Clin Pathol* 44: 597–604.

158 Kawabe, M., Mori, T., Ito, Y. et al. (2015). Outcomes of dogs undergoing radiotherapy for treatment of oral malignant melanoma: 111 cases (2006–2012). *J Am Vet Med Assoc* 247: 1146–1153.

159 Tuohy, J.L., Selmic, L.E., Worley, D.R. et al. (2014). Outcome following curative-intent surgery for oral melanoma in dogs: 70 cases (1998–2011). *J Am Vet Med Assoc* 245: 1266–1273.

160 Theon, A.P., Rodriguez, C., Griffey, S., and Madewell, B.R. (1997). Analysis of prognostic factors and patterns of failure in dogs with periodontal tumors treated with megavoltage irradiation. *J Am Vet Med Assoc* 210: 785–788.

161 Proulx, D.R., Ruslander, D.M., Dodge, R.K. et al. (2003). A retrospective analysis of 140 dogs with oral melanoma treated with external beam radiation. *Vet Radiol Ultrasound* 44: 352–359.

162 Boston, S.E., Lu, X., Culp, W.T. et al. (2014). Efficacy of systemic adjuvant therapies administered to dogs after excision of oral malignant melanomas: 151 cases (2001–2012). *J Am Vet Med Assoc* 245: 401–407.

163 Lana, S.E., Rutteman, G.R., and Withrow, S.J. (2007). Tumors of the mammary gland. In: *Withrow & MacEwen's Small Animal Clinical Oncology* (eds. S.J. Withrow, D.M. Vail and R.L. Page), 619–636. St. Louis, MO: Saunders Elsevier.

164 Hellmen, E., Bergstrom, R., Holmberg, L. et al. (1993). Prognostic factors in canine mammary tumors: a multivariate study of 202 consecutive cases. *Vet Pathol* 30: 20–27.

165 Yamagami, T., Kobayashi, T., Takahashi, K., and Sugiyama, M. (1996). Prognosis for canine malignant mammary tumors based on TNM and histologic classification. *J Vet Med Sci* 58: 1079–1083.

166 Perez Alenza, M.D., Pena, L., del Castillo, N., and Nieto, A.I. (2000). Factors influencing the incidence and prognosis of canine mammary tumours. *J Small Anim Pract* 41: 287–291.

167 de Araujo, M.R., Campos, L.C., Ferreira, E., and Cassali, G.D. (2015). Quantitation of the regional lymph node metastatic burden and prognosis in malignant mammary tumors of dogs. *J Vet Intern Med* 29: 1360–1367.

168 Szczubial, M. and Lopuszynski, W. (2011). Prognostic value of regional lymph node status in canine mammary carcinomas. *Vet Comp Oncol* 9: 296–303.

28

Spleen

Davis Seelig

Normal Structure

The spleen is a highly vascularized lymphoid organ with a parenchyma that is divided into red and white pulp. This anatomic and functional division is architecturally determined by a network of dense, collagenous trabeculae composed of elastic fibers and smooth muscle that is contiguous with the surrounding serous capsule. The white pulp is composed of lymphatic tissue organized about, and intimately associated with, branches of the splenic artery. The lymphatic tissue is subdivided into lymph nodules (i.e. splenic corpuscles), which are interspersed among the splenic arterioles, and the periarterial lymphatic sheaths (PALs) that surround the splenic arterioles. Structurally, splenic corpuscles are similar to lymph node nodules. The red pulp, which is the region between the white pulp and collagenous trabeculae, is composed of splenic sinuses, phagocytic cells (macrophages and dendritic cells), and hematopoietic precursors.[1,2]

Indications for Cytology

Indications for cytology include diffuse splenic enlargement (i.e. splenomegaly), architectural abnormalities as detected by advanced imaging (e.g. single or multifocal masses or abnormal splenic texture), or staging of multicentric neoplasia (e.g. mast cell neoplasia and lymphoma).[3] From a clinical perspective, the chief differential diagnoses for splenic masses include benign (nodular hyperplasia, hematoma, hemangioma, and inflammation) and malignant (hemangiosarcoma, lymphoma, non-angiomatous sarcomas, and metastatic neoplasia) processes. For splenomegaly, clinical considerations include infectious disease (e.g. ehrlichiosis or bacterial endocarditis), splenic congestion (e.g. congestive heart failure, hepatic cirrhosis, and splenic vein thrombosis), splenic hyperplasia (e.g. associated with immune-mediated hemolytic anemia or thrombocytopenia), and infiltrative disease (e.g. leukemia, lymphoma, and mast cell neoplasia).

Prevalence of Splenic Pathology

There are a number of retrospective studies documenting the frequency of splenic pathology in veterinary medicine. Owing to its confirmatory nature, these publications are based upon samples compared with histopathology. While histopathology is considered to have higher diagnostic accuracy than cytology, this approach may introduce sampling bias into the prevalence data, resulting in an underrepresentation of diseases that might be sufficiently diagnosed by fine-needle aspiration (FNA) (e.g. benign processes and round cell neoplasms, including lymphoma) and an overrepresentation of conditions that require surgical intervention (e.g. hemangiosarcoma, hematoma, and vascular disturbances).

There is significant variation in the reported prevalence of splenic pathologies across veterinary medicine, which likely represents the unique inclusion/exclusion criteria of each publication. In a series of 1480 canine biopsy specimens, splenic hyperplasia was the most common finding (25% of submissions), followed by hemangiosarcoma (10%) and hematoma (9%).[4] A similar feline study of 455 cases identified mast cell neoplasia as the most frequent finding (15%), followed by lymphoma (9%) and myeloid neoplasia (6%), with hemangiosarcoma representing only 3% of cases.[5] In a review of 87 canine splenic biopsies, the most common diagnosis was hemangiosarcoma (20%), followed by hematoma (18%); nonspecific benign changes, including congestion, hemorrhage, and extramedullary hematopoiesis (EMH) (16%); and non-angiomatous sarcoma (15%).[6] In a study of 51

Veterinary Cytology, First Edition. Edited by Leslie C. Sharkey, M. Judith Radin, and Davis Seelig.

histopathologically confirmed canine cases from Australia, hemangiosarcoma was the most frequent diagnosis (33%) followed by benign hyperplasia (29%).[7] In a study of 32 samples (29 dogs and 3 cats), benign hyperplasia (lymphoid and hematopoietic) was the most common finding (16%), followed by lymphoma (13%) and mast cell neoplasia (9%). In this series, only two cases of hemangiosarcoma were identified (6%).[8] In a series of 100 dogs with splenomegaly, the most common diagnosis was hemangiosarcoma (43%), followed by lymphoid hyperplasia (12%) and hematoma (11%).[9] In a review of 57 canine splenectomy samples, angiomatous neoplasia (combining hemangiosarcoma with hemangioma) was the most common diagnosis, representing 75% of the cases.[10] In 105 dogs undergoing splenectomy for incidentally detected masses, the most common diagnoses were nodular lymphoid hyperplasia (35%), hemangiosarcoma (17%), and hematoma (15%).[11] Lastly, in a study of splenic FNA in dogs and cats, based upon 15 cases with confirmatory histopathology, benign processes (e.g. hyperplasia, hematoma, and congestion) were the most common finding (27%) followed by hemangiosarcoma (13%) and mast cell neoplasia (13%).[12]

When small breed dogs are specifically examined, a similar pattern emerges. In a study of 45 small breed dogs (defined as <16 kg or 35.2 lb) undergoing splenectomy, the most common diagnoses were lymphoid hyperplasia, hematoma, and/or EMH (38%) followed by hemangiosarcoma (31%).[13] In a second study of 105 small dogs (defined as ≤27.8 kg or 61.3 lb), the most frequent diagnosis was hemangiosarcoma (42%) followed by hematoma (33%) and nodular hyperplasia (26%).[14] Similar large-scale prevalence studies are not available for other veterinary species.

Sampling Collection

The approach toward sampling the spleen is similar to the sampling of other visceral organs (Chapter 1). Several studies have demonstrated that splenic aspiration is safe, with no complications reported across three canine and feline studies.[8,12,15] Moreover, splenic cytology samples are generally useful, with diagnostic quality rates from 87 to 100% reported.[8,12,16] While similar data are not reported in veterinary medicine, the influence of sampling proficiency has been documented in human medicine. Operators who performed more than 100 ultrasound-guided splenic FNAs had significantly higher diagnostic accuracy as compared with those with less than 100 FNAs.[17] Notably, a study comparing collection techniques in the ultrasound-guided sampling of dog and cat spleens revealed that samples collected via a non-aspiration technique yielded samples that were more cellular, had less blood contamination, and had similar cell morphology compared with those collected via an aspiration technique.[18]

Normal Cytology

Correlated with its vascularity and functions as a erythrocyte reservoir and a secondary lymphoid organ, normal splenic cytology samples contain large numbers of erythrocytes (the hematocrit of the spleen is reported to be 80–90%) with variable numbers of stromal elements, lymphocytes, and hematopoietic precursors (Figure 28.1).[19] One study describes 1000 nucleated cell differential counts from 12 splenic samples and reports the most frequent cell type to be small lymphocytes (64%) with fewer mature neutrophils (18%), large lymphocytes (9%), and ≤2% each of neutrophil precursors, eosinophils, and their precursors, erythroid precursors, macrophages, monocytes, plasma cells, and stromal cells.[20] Additionally, cytology samples can have significant numbers of well-differentiated mast cells. A study of splenic FNAs from 32 clinically normal dogs reported up to 91 mast cells per slide or up to 904 mast cells across 4 slides.[21] In light of these findings, it can be challenging to diagnosis metastatic mast cell neoplasia using FNA (Chapter 13). The stromal component of the spleen consists of clumps of uniform mesenchymal cells that often contain macrophages and variable amounts of hemosiderin.

Diagnostic Accuracy of Splenic Cytology

There are a number of cytohistologic correlation studies describing the diagnostic accuracy of splenic cytology. However, it is important to note that many of the processes

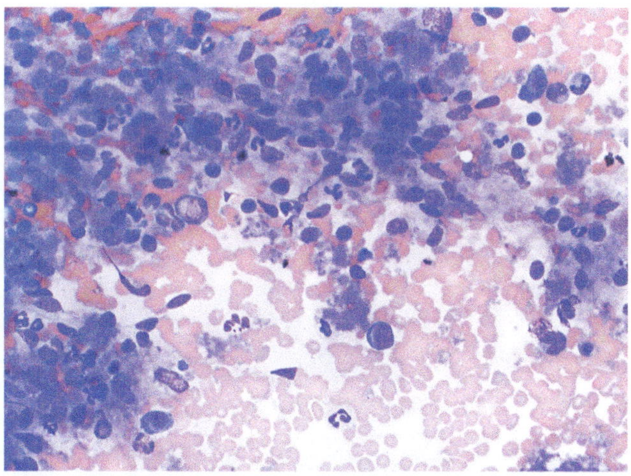

Figure 28.1 Dog, normal spleen. Normal splenic constituents consist of clumps of splenic stroma, small numbers of lymphocytes, and scattered hematopoietic precursors. Owing to its function as a red blood cell reserve organ, splenic cytology samples contain large numbers of erythrocytes (Wright–Giemsa, 400×).

that result in clinically detectable splenic pathology are not amenable to a cytologic diagnosis. This includes alteration in blood flow (congestion, hemorrhage, infarction, and thrombosis), fibrosis, splenic rupture, splenic torsion, and any lesion that may be composed of blood-filled spaces (e.g. hematoma, hemangioma, and hemangiosarcoma). Across 4 studies representing 76 canine and feline samples, the diagnostic accuracy rate of splenic cytology ranges from 38 to 100%.[7,8,12,22] In the study with the lowest rate of agreement, the authors propose that the sampling of discreet masses may have resulted in overrepresentation of cytologically inconclusive/nondiagnostic angiomatous neoplasia.[22]

Benign Conditions

Benign lesions can present as either generalized splenomegaly or as nodular conditions. Benign splenic pathologies include nodular hyperplasia of the red and white pulp, extramedullary hematopoiesis, hematoma, infarction, necrosis, hemorrhage, thrombosis, amyloidosis, and congestion. Across 8 studies, benign processes range from 24 to 71% in canine and feline splenic samples.[4,6–9, 11–13]

Splenic Hyperplasia

Benign splenic hyperplasia represents 16–38% of splenic disease in small animal patients.[4,6–9, 11–13] Splenic hyperplasia represents the proliferation of normal splenic constituents (lymphoid, hematopoietic, or inflammatory cells) in response to a broad spectrum of inflammatory conditions.[3] Cytologically, splenic lymphoid hyperplasia (often referred to as reactive lymphoid hyperplasia or nodular lymphoid hyperplasia) is often similar to lymphoid hyperplasia seen within lymph nodes and is characterized by increased numbers of small, medium, and large lymphoid cells and plasma cells (including "flame" cells or Mott cells), macrophages, mast cells, and plump stromal cells.[3] Notably, robust hyperplasia can contain a predominant population of large lymphocytes, making the distinction between hyperplasia and lymphoid neoplasia challenging.[23,24] In such cases, additional testing, including flow cytometry, polymerase chain reaction for antigen receptor rearrangement (PARR), and/or histopathology, may be needed. Extramedullary hematopoiesis is reported in up to 24% of FNA samples from dogs and cats with splenomegaly or splenic masses and is cytologically characterized by variable proportions of erythrocyte, granulocyte, and platelet precursors (Figure 28.2).[12] Lastly, histiocytic hyperplasia, represented by increased numbers of macrophages (which may be cytophagic) is reported in patients with immune- and non-immune-mediated hemolytic anemia, immune-mediated thrombocytopenia, and erythroparasitic diseases.[3]

Siderotic Nodules

Siderotic nodules or siderotic plaques are regions of chronic, organizing hemorrhage that are often found along the splenic margins and result from trauma, neoplasia, or age-related change.[25,26] Siderotic nodules are considered to be incidental lesions but can be sampled during imaging studies or during surgery. Grossly, they appear as yellow-to-brown plaques along the margins of the spleen.

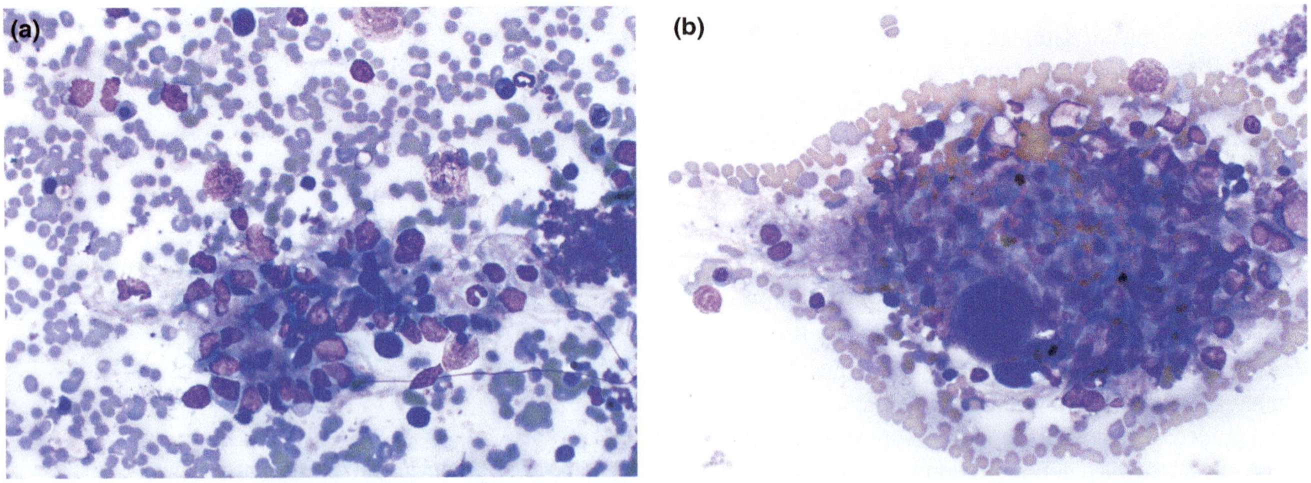

Figure 28.2 Dog, spleen. Extramedullary hematopoiesis (EMH). (a) EMH is characterized by mixed hematopoietic precursors, including immature cells of the myeloid and erythroid lineage. These cells are often found individualized or organized about splenic stroma. (b) In addition to myeloid and erythroid precursors, megakaryocytes are commonly seen with splenic EMH (Wright–Giemsa, 400×).

Microscopically, siderotic nodules are heterogeneous and composed of a variably proportioned mixture of macrophages (which can exhibit leukophagia and erythrophagia), multinucleated giant cells, mixed lymphocytes, hematopoietic precursors, and splenic stromal cells. Reflective of their hemorrhagic origin, they also contain variable amounts of hemosiderin and/or hematoidin. Siderotic nodules also can contain structures known as Gamna–Gandy bodies. In a series of seven canine cases, these are described as being "generally 2–5 μm diameter, 10–35 μm long, refractile, clear, pale-tan or pale yellow, wavy or straight, and tubular structures."[26] Gamna–Gandy bodies can be found within the cytoplasm of macrophages and multinucleated giant cells. Similar structures have been cytologically described in the aspirate of a feline splenic mass.[27] In light of their potential morphologic similarities, Gamna–Gandy bodies may need to be distinguished from fungal hyphae through cytochemical staining. In contrast to fungal organisms, Gamna–Gandy bodies stain positive for calcium (using alizarin red S stains), iron (using Perl's Prussian blue), and are negative for Gomori methenamine silver, acid-fast, and calcofluor white stains.[26,27]

Neoplasms

The involvement of the spleen in both primary and metastatic neoplasia is common. In the two largest studies, malignant processes constitute 21 and 37% of canine and feline cases, respectively.[4,5] As the cytology of non-splenic origin neoplasms is covered elsewhere, this section will focus on the most common primary splenic malignancies.

Splenic Lymphoma

Splenic lymphoma can be classified as either primary or secondary, according to the extent and, if known, origin and progression of the disease. Primary splenic lymphoma is defined as lymphoma confined to the spleen, whereas secondary splenic lymphoma denotes splenic involvement as part of multicentric disease (Figure 28.3). According to the current veterinary-adapted version of the WHO lymphoma classification scheme, three subtypes of lymphoma are most likely to represent primary splenic disease, namely, hepatosplenic, marginal zone, and mantle cell lymphoma.[28] Other subtypes of lymphoma are described in Chapter 27. Other variants of lymphoid neoplasia reported using canine splenic cytology include Mott cell lymphoma, plasma cell neoplasia, and acute leukemia.[29,30]

Definitive criteria for the diagnosis of splenic lymphoma have not been published. There are two reports that define splenic involvement of lymphoma as >5% lymphoblasts in canine patients previously diagnosed with multicentric lymphoma; however, this cutoff has not been vigorously evaluated nor examined for its utility in the new diagnosis of splenic lymphoma.[31,32] A retrospective study comparing cytology with PARR clonality testing demonstrated a blast percentage of greater than 40% in 8 of 10 PARR-positive splenic aspirates.[24] Notably, while four PARR-negative

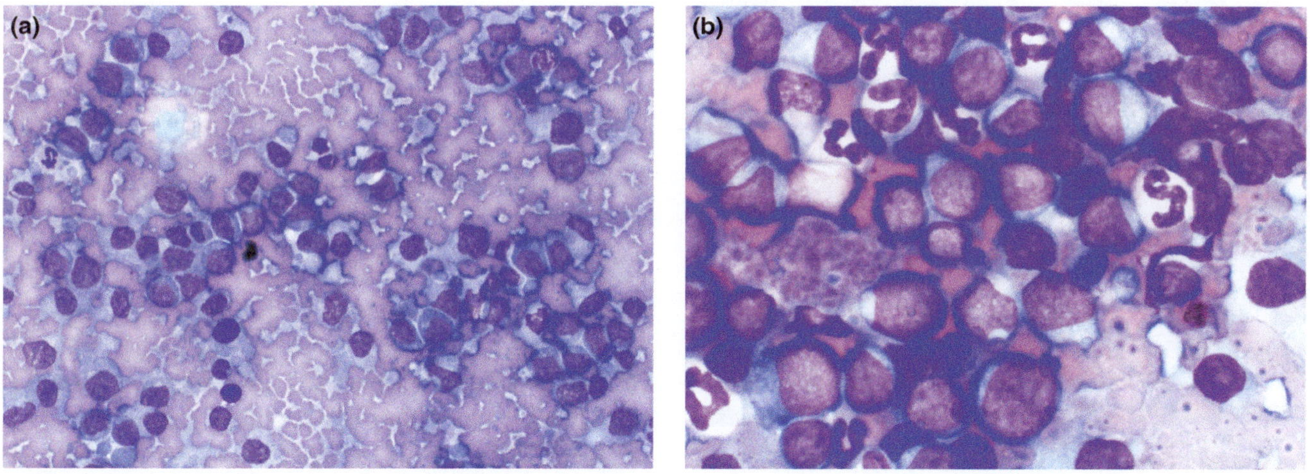

Figure 28.3 Dog, spleen. Lymphoma. (a) Aspirate is from a dog with a history of splenomegaly. The samples contained >90% large, atypical lymphoid cells. The atypical lymphoid cells contain round to reniform, eccentrically positioned nuclei with coarse chromatin, moderate anisokaryosis, and a prominent perinuclear clear zone (Wright–Giemsa, 400×). (b) Aspirate is from a dog with a history of splenomegaly and peripheral and visceral lymphadenopathy. There are >80% large, atypical lymphoid cells among a background of residual small and intermediate-sized lymphocytes and scattered erythroid precursors. The atypical lymphoid cells contain round to reniform, eccentrically positioned nuclei with smooth chromatin and moderate anisokaryosis (Wright–Giemsa, 1000×).

samples in this study also had a blast count greater than 40%, these patients already had a clinical diagnosis of lymphoma. When samples were grouped as either PARR-positive and/or clinically positive for lymphoma, a blast percentage of 40% had 100% specificity for the presence of lymphoma. All samples interpreted as cytologically benign (e.g. hyperplasia and/or EMH) were PARR negative.[24]

Hepatosplenic Lymphoma

Hepatosplenic lymphoma (HSL) is a rare variant of lymphoma that is reported in the dog, cat, and horse (Chapter 34).[33–38] Canine patients with HSL commonly present with generalized splenomegaly, regenerative anemia, thrombocytopenia, hypoalbuminemia, and mild increases in alkaline phosphatase, gamma-glutamyl transferase, and total bilirubin.[33] Cytologically, the neoplastic cells are described as intermediate to large in size with a moderate amount of pale to medium blue cytoplasm, fine pink to magenta cytoplasmic granules, round to oval to irregular nuclei, stippled chromatin, and variably prominent nucleoli (Figure 28.4).[33] One case report describes more atypical nuclear morphology, including bizarre nucleoli, binucleated and multinucleated cells, moderate to marked anisokaryosis, and atypical mitoses.[36] Neoplastic cell engulfment of erythrocytes is frequently reported. Similar to the liver, the neoplastic cells in the spleen are centered on sinusoids, specifically of the red pulp.[33] In a canine report, neoplastic cells were γδT cells ($CD3^+$, $CD8\alpha^+$, $CD18^+$, $CD45^+$, $CD45ra^+$, $TCR\gamma\delta^+$, and $CD79a^-$).[37]

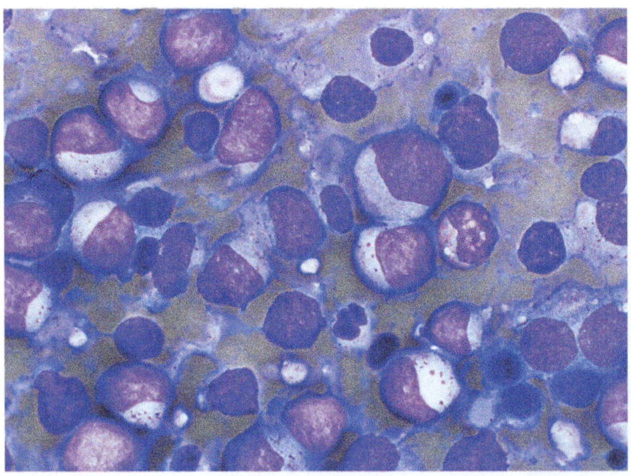

Figure 28.4 Dog, spleen. Lymphoma. Aspirate is from a dog with a history of hepatosplenomegaly. The neoplastic lymphocytes are large in contrast to the few normal neutrophils and erythroid precursors and contain a moderate amount of pale blue cytoplasm with modest numbers of variably sized, red granules. The PARR assay identified a clonal T-cell receptor rearrangement, and the clinical diagnosis was hepatosplenic lymphoma (Wright–Giemsa, 1000×).

In the single feline report, a definitive diagnosis of HSL was not obtained, but was suspected based upon histologic pattern of tissue involvement and the T-cell immunophenotype.[34] Similar to the dog, neoplastic cell engulfment of erythrocytes was described. In an equine report, a presumptive diagnosis of HSL in a case of T-cell lymphoma was made based upon clinicopathologic, gross, and histologic findings.[38]

Marginal Zone Lymphoma

Splenic marginal zone lymphoma (MZL) is an uncommon form of lymphoma (0.2–1.0% of canine lymphomas) that has been reported only in the dog.[39,40] It is one of the three subtypes of MZL (in addition to nodal MZL and mucosal-associated lymphoid tissue lymphoma) and represents a neoplasm derived from memory lymphocytes of the marginal zone. Clinically, canine splenic MZL presents as either a solitary mass or multiple splenic nodules, and affected dogs may have a hemoabdomen.[41,42] While the cytologic features of splenic MZL have not been published, histologically, it is composed of medium-sized lymphocytes with vesicular nuclei, peripheralized chromatin, and a single nucleolus. Immunophenotypically, cells are $CD79a^+$, $CD20^+$, and $CD3^-$.[41,42]

Mantle Cell Lymphoma

Among veterinary species, splenic mantle cell lymphoma (MCL) has only been reported in the dog. In contrast to human MCL, which is a multicentric disease characterized by generalized peripheral lymphadenopathy and frequent extranodal involvement, 80% of the published canine cases appear to be of splenic origin.[39–41,43]

There are no published cytologic reports of canine splenic MCL, but histologically, the neoplastic cells are small-to-intermediate in size, contain a small amount of cytoplasm, and have a round to clefted nucleus with coarse chromatin that lack nucleoli. Like other canine B-cell lymphomas, MCL is characterized by CD79a and CD20 expression.[43]

Angiomatous Sarcomas

The angiomatous neoplasms (i.e. angiomas and angiosarcomas) represent endothelium-origin neoplasms, including those of vascular (hemangioma and hemangiosarcoma) or lymphatic origin (lymphangioma and lymphangiosarcoma). Across veterinary species, the former are much more common. In the dog, the prevalence of hemangiosarcoma and hemangioma based on splenic histopathology ranges from 6 to 43% and 9 to 18% of case submissions, respectively.[4,6–14] In the cat, vascular neoplasms are uncommon with hemangiosarcoma reported to be 3% of splenic histology case submissions.[5] Similar to other tissues (Chapter 16), the cytologic

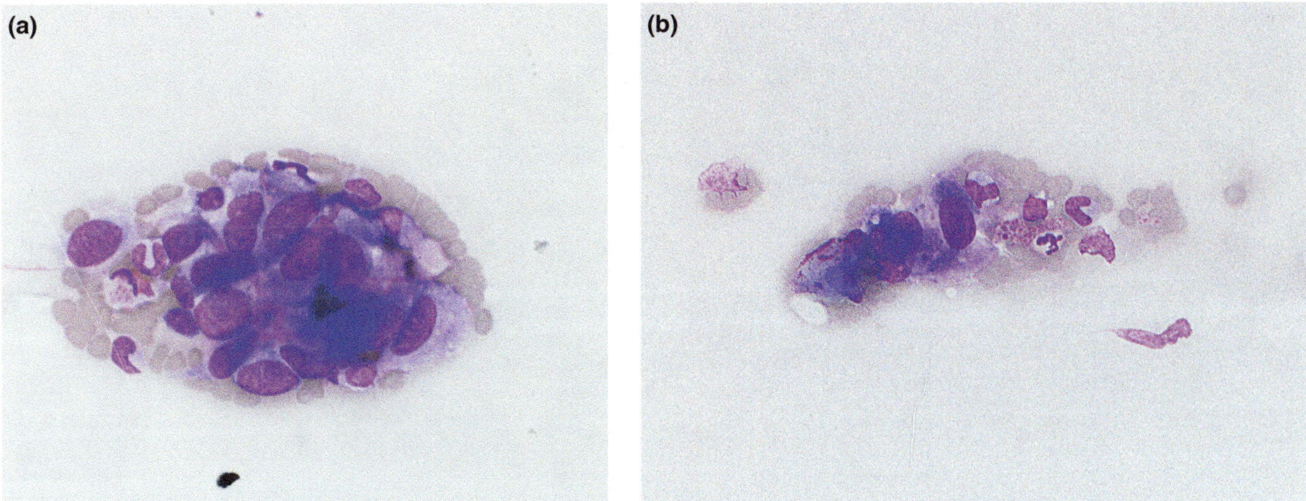

Figure 28.5 Dog, spleen. Aspirate is from a cavitated splenic mass that was histologically confirmed as a hemangiosarcoma. (a) Typical of most hemangiosarcoma aspirates, the samples were of low cellularity and consisted predominantly of peripheral blood and associated elements. On the feathered edge, small numbers of plump, atypical mesenchymal cells were identified (both individually and in clusters). (b) Rarely, the atypical mesenchymal cells contain intracytoplasmic pigment consistent with hemosiderin (Wright–Giemsa, 1000×).

findings in hemangiosarcoma include spindle cells that exhibit a varying degree of atypia. The presence of intracytoplasmic pigment consistent with hemosiderin is a common finding (Figure 28.5).[23,44] However, as large areas of hemangiosarcoma may be composed of acellular, blood-filled spaces, the genesis of a definitive diagnosis by cytology and differentiation between hemangioma and hematoma is often very difficult. Lymphangioma and lymphangiosarcoma of the spleen are very uncommon.[45,46]

Non-angiomatous Neoplasia

The non-angiomatous, nonlymphoid sarcomas are uncommon splenic neoplasms in veterinary species. Across all species, reported neoplasms include leiomyoma, lipoma–myelolipoma (Chapter 35), undifferentiated sarcoma, liposarcoma (Chapter 16), neurofibrosarcoma, malignant fibrous histiocytoma, mast cell neoplasia (Chapter 13), extraskeletal osteosarcoma (Chapter 23), leiomyosarcoma (Chapter 32), and myxosarcoma.[13,47–49]

Histiocytic Proliferative Diseases

The histiocytic proliferative disorders are a group of diseases that have historically been linked owing to their shared cytomorphologic features but in actuality represent a biologically and phenotypically diverse spectrum of neoplastic and nonneoplastic conditions that originate from macrophages, dendritic cells, or Langerhans cells. This chapter will focus on those histiocytic proliferative diseases with notable splenic involvement. Additional relevant material is presented in Chapter 12 and review articles.[50]

Histiocytic Sarcoma

Histiocytic sarcoma (HS) is a neoplasm believed to originate from interstitial dendritic cells and appears capable of arising in any tissue.[51] When found at only a single site (e.g. the spleen), the neoplasm is referred to as localized HS or simply as HS; however, when extension beyond one site occurs (i.e. multicentric disease), the currently accepted term is disseminated histiocytic sarcoma (previously known as malignant histiocytosis).[50] HS is primarily reported in the dog, although it has also been described in the cat, horse, cow, and ferret.[52–58] In the dog, although HS has been identified in many breeds, there is overrepresentation of Bernese mountain dogs, flat-coated retrievers, and Rottweilers.[51,59–61]

The splenic version of HS typically presents as an ill-defined mass lesion that may be white to tan in color.[50] Cytologically, HS usually exfoliates large numbers of large pleomorphic cells that often demonstrate dramatic cytologic and nuclear atypia with frequent multinucleated cells and cells with bizarre mitotic figures (Figure 28.6).[62] The neoplastic cells occasionally demonstrate erythrophagia and leukophagia. Owing to the morphologic overlap between the bizarre tumor cells in HS and other malignant neoplasms, including carcinoma, lymphoma, and sarcoma, additional staining may be needed for lineage assignment.

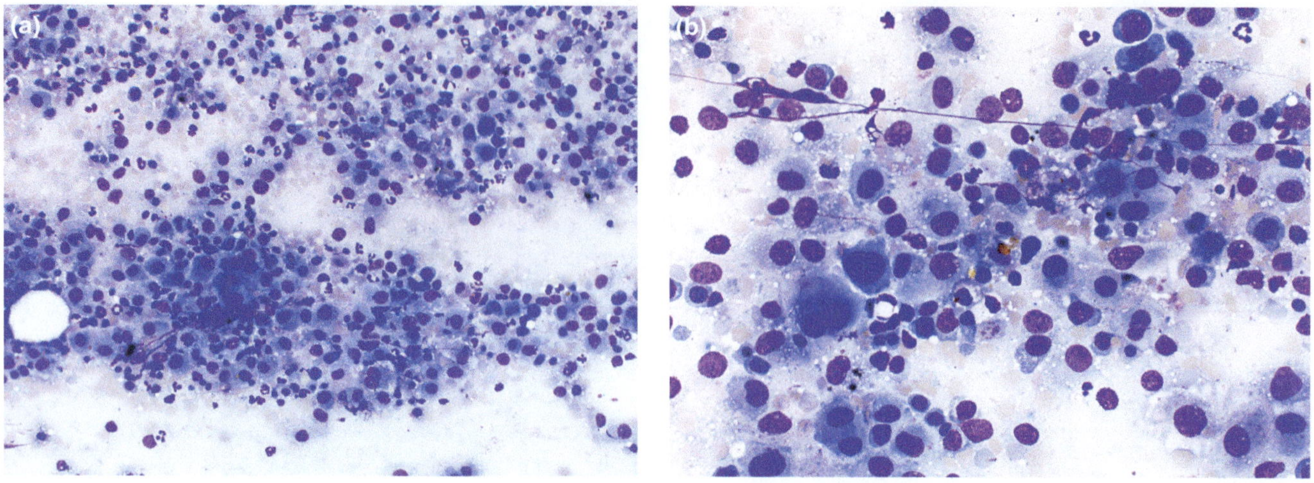

Figure 28.6 Dog, spleen. Histiocytic sarcoma. (a) Samples are of high cellularity and consist of large, atypical round cells dispersed throughout a background of mixed normal splenic elements (Wright-Giemsa, 200×). (b) Neoplastic cells exhibit marked anisocytosis and anisokaryosis with multinucleation and evidence of erythrophagia (i.e. intracellular hematoidin pigment) (Wright–Giemsa, 1000×).

On unfixed, fresh samples, interstitial dendritic cells express CD1a, MHC Class II, and CD11c/CD18.[51]

Hemophagocytic Histiocytic Sarcoma

Hemophagocytic histiocytic sarcoma (HHS) is a neoplasm of macrophage origin that has been reported in a dog, cat, and cow.[55,57,63] In contrast to non-hemophagocytic HS, HHS tends to result in generalized splenic enlargement rather than defined mass lesions and may not demonstrate the marked atypia and pleomorphism that is characteristic of HS. In a case series of 17 patients, affected dogs frequently presented with a Coombs negative regenerative anemia (94%), thrombocytopenia (88%), hypoalbuminemia (94%), and hypocholesterolemia (69%).[63] Grossly, the spleen of all dogs was characterized by generalized enlargement with few to many, variably sized masses. Similarly, in both cat and dog case reports, animals were anemic and demonstrated significant splenomegaly.[55,57] Histologically, the neoplastic cells in all affected species vary in the magnitude of their atypia but include multinucleated giant cells and erythrophagocytosis.[54,57,63] Cytologic appearance has been described only in one case of feline HHS. In that report, the cells were described as large, round, and moderately pleomorphic cells with variably sized magenta granules and occasionally phagocytosed erythrocytes, lymphocytes, and platelets.[55] In alignment with their proposed cell of origin (a splenic red pulp macrophage), the neoplastic cells demonstrate a unique immunophenotype, namely, $CD45^+$, MHC-II^+, $CD18^+$, and $CD11d^+$.[63] In the single feline case report, the neoplastic cells were MHC-II^+, $CD18^+$, $CD11b^+$, and $CD11d^-$.[55] The single bovine case report describes erythrophagocytic histiocytes expressing CD18, MHC-II, lysozyme, and CD68.[57]

Fibrohistiocytic Nodule

The diagnosis fibrohistiocytic nodule (FHN) was originally reported in series of 98 canine splenic lesions.[64] This report describes a series of nodular lesions composed of mixed proportions of histiocytic cells, spindle cells, hematopoietic precursors, plasma cells, and/or lymphocytes that were subsequently graded according to the percentage of lymphocytes within the lesions as Grade 1 (70–99% lymphoid cells), Grade 2 (40–69% lymphoid cells), and Grade 3 (0–39% lymphoid cells). Notably, tumor grade had prognostic significance with the one year survival rates for the Grade 3 lesions (32%) being significantly worse than the Grades 1 and 2 nodules (87%). The cytologic findings of FHN were not described. A subsequent study reevaluated the diagnosis of FHN through the application of additional immunohistochemical staining and reclassified 31 cases of canine splenic FHN as 13 cases of benign nodular hyperplasia, 5 cases of lymphoma, 8 cases of stromal sarcoma, and 6 cases of HS. In light of this latter report, which reveals its lack of specificity, the term FHN should no longer be used in diagnostic pathology.

Inflammatory Disease

Inflammatory splenic disease (splenitis) is an uncommon condition in veterinary species. Based upon published histopathology studies, the prevalence of splenitis is 2–8% in the dog and 9% in the cat.[5,6,65] Infectious causes of splenitis include *Aspergillus terreus, Cryptococcus neoformans, Candida albicans, Aspergillus caninus, Penicillium purpurogenum, Neospora caninum, Hepatozoon canis, Trypanosoma cruzi, Leishmania chagasi, Bacillus anthracis, Listeria monocytogenes, Mycobacterium avium, Mycobacterium tuberculosis*, and *Staphylococcus* spp.[65–79]

References

1 Banks, W.J. (ed.) (1993). Lymphatic system and immunit. In: *Applied Veterinary Histology*, 3e. St. Louis, MO: Mosby-Year Book.

2 Ferri, F., Zini, E., Auriemma, E. et al. (2017). Splenitis in 33 dogs. *Vet Pathol* 54: 147–154.

3 Christopher, M.M. (2003). Cytology of the spleen. *Vet Clin North Am Small Anim Pract* 33: 135–152.

4 Spangler, W.L. and Culbertson, M.R. (1992). Prevalence, type, and importance of splenic diseases in dogs: 1,480 cases (1985–1989). *J Am Vet Med Assoc* 200: 829–834.

5 Spangler, W.L. and Culbertson, M.R. (1992). Prevalence and type of splenic diseases in cats: 455 cases (1985–1991). *J Am Vet Med Assoc* 201: 773–776.

6 Day, M.J., Lucke, V.M., and Pearson, H. (1995). A review of pathological diagnoses made from 87 canine splenic biopsies. *J Small Anim Pract* 36: 426–433.

7 Christensen, N., Canfield, P., Martin, P. et al. (2009). Cytopathological and histopathological diagnosis of canine splenic disorders. *Aust Vet J* 87: 175–181.

8 Ballegeer, E.A., Forrest, L.J., Dickinson, R.M. et al. (2007). Correlation of ultrasonographic appearance of lesions and cytologic and histologic diagnoses in splenic aspirates from dogs and cats: 32 cases (2002–2005). *J Am Vet Med Assoc* 230: 690–696.

9 Johnson, K.A., Powers, B.E., Withrow, S.J. et al. (1989). Splenomegaly in dogs. Predictors of neoplasia and survival after splenectomy. *J Vet Intern Med* 3: 160–166.

10 Frey, A.J. and Betts, C.W. (1977). Retrospective survey of splenectomy in dog. *J Am Anim Hosp Assoc* 13: 730–734.

11 Cleveland, M.J. and Casale, S. (2016). Incidence of malignancy and outcomes for dogs undergoing splenectomy for incidentally detected nonruptured splenic nodules or masses: 105 cases (2009–2013). *J Am Vet Med Assoc* 248: 1267–1273.

12 O'Keefe, D.A. and Couto, C.G. (1987). Fine-needle aspiration of the spleen as an aid in the diagnosis of splenomegaly. *J Vet Intern Med* 1: 102–109.

13 Corbin, E.E., Cavanaugh, R.P., Schwartz, P. et al. (2017). Splenomegaly in small-breed dogs: 45 cases (2005–2011). *J Am Vet Med Assoc* 250: 1148–1154.

14 Sherwood, J.M., Haynes, A.M., Klocke, E. et al. (2016). Occurrence and clinicopathologic features of splenic neoplasia based on body weight: 325 dogs (2003–2013). *J Am Anim Hosp Assoc* 52: 220–226.

15 Osborne, C.A., Perman, V., and Stevens, J.B. (1974). Needle biopsy of the spleen. *Vet Clin North Am* 4: 311–316.

16 Christiansen, S.M., Hungerbuhler, S.O., and Mischke, R. (2016). Relevance of cytology of the canine spleen: a retrospective study. *Prakt Tierarzt* 97: 668–679.

17 Civardi, G., Vallisa, D., Berte, R. et al. (2001). Ultrasound-guided fine needle biopsy of the spleen: high clinical efficacy and low risk in a multicenter Italian study. *Am J Hematol* 67: 93–99.

18 Leblanc, C.J., Head, L.L., and Fry, M.M. (2009). Comparison of aspiration and nonaspiration techniques for obtaining cytologic samples from the canine and feline spleen. *Vet Clin Pathol* 38: 242–246.

19 MacDonald, I.C., Schmidt, E.E., and Groom, A.C. (1991). The high splenic hematocrit: a rheological consequence of red cell flow through the reticular meshwork. *Microvasc Res* 42: 60–76.

20 Swisher, S.N. and Dale, W.A. (1955). Splenic aspiration biopsy in the dog. *Blood* 10: 812–819.

21 Finora, K., Leibman, N.F., Fettman, M.J. et al. (2006). Cytological comparison of fine-needle aspirates of liver and spleen of normal dogs and of dogs with cutaneous mast cell tumours and an ultrasonographically normal appearing liver and spleen. *Vet Comp Oncol* 4: 178–183.

22 Eich, C.S., Whitehair, J.G., Moroff, S.D., and Heeb, L.A. (2000). The accuracy of intraoperative cytopathological diagnosis compared with conventional histopathological diagnosis. *J Am Anim Hosp Assoc* 36: 16–18.

23 Raskin, R.E. (2010). Lymphoid system. In: *Canine and Feline Cytology: A Color Atlas and Interpretation Guide*, 2e (eds. R.E. Raskin and D.J. Meyer). St. Louis, MO: W.B. Saunders.

24 Williams, M., Avery, A., and Olver, C.S. (2006). Diagnosing lymphoid hyperplasia vs lymphoma in canine splenic aspirates. *Vet Pathol* 43: 809.

25 Cole, P.A. (2012). Association of canine splenic hemangiosarcomas and hematomas with nodular lymphoid hyperplasia or siderotic nodules. *J Vet Diagn Invest* 24: 759–762.

26 Moore, A.R., Leavell, S.E., Conrado, F.O. et al. (2017). Cytologic features and staining characteristics of Gamna–Gandy bodies from seven canine fine-needle aspirate preparations. *J Vet Diagn Invest* 29: 920–925.

27 Ryseff, J.K., Duncan, C., Sfiligoi, G., and Avery, P.R. (2014). Gamna–Gandy bodies: a case of mistaken identity in the spleen of a cat. *Vet Clin Pathol* 43: 94–100.

28 Seelig, D.M., Avery, A.C., Ehrhart, E.J., and Linden, M.A. (2016). The comparative diagnostic features of canine and human lymphoma. *Vet Sci* 3: 11.

29 De Zan, G., Zappulli, V., Cavicchioli, L. et al. (2009). Gastric B-cell lymphoma with Mott cell differentiation in a dog. *J Vet Diagn Invest* 21: 715–719.

30 Yearley, J.H., Stanton, C., Olivry, T., and Dean, G.A. (2007). Phagocytic plasmacytoma in a dog. *Vet Clin Pathol* 36: 293–296.

31 Joetzke, A.E., Eberle, N., Nolte, I. et al. (2012). Flow cytometric evaluation of peripheral blood and bone marrow and fine-needle aspirate samples from multiple sites in dogs with multicentric lymphoma. *Am J Vet Res* 73: 884–893.

32 Nerschbach, V., Eberle, N., Joetzke, A.E. et al. (2016). Splenic and hepatic ultrasound and cytology in canine lymphoma: effects of findings on stage migration and assessment of prognosis. *Vet Comp Oncol* 14 (1): 82–94.

33 Keller, S.M., Vernau, W., Hodges, J. et al. (2013). Hepatosplenic and hepatocytotropic T-cell lymphoma: two distinct types of T-cell lymphoma in dogs. *Vet Pathol* 50: 281–290.

34 Carter, J.E., Tarigo, J.L., Vernau, W. et al. (2008). Erythrophagocytic low-grade extranodal T-cell lymphoma in a cat. *Vet Clin Pathol* 37: 416–421.

35 Jaffe, E.S. (2006). Pathobiology of peripheral T-cell lymphomas. *Hematology Am Soc Hematol Educ Program*: 317–322.

36 Cienava, E.A., Barnhart, K.F., Brown, R. et al. (2004). Morphologic, immunohistochemical, and molecular characterization of hepatosplenic T-cell lymphoma in a dog. *Vet Clin Pathol* 33: 105–110.

37 Fry, M.M., Vernau, W., Pesavento, P.A. et al. (2003). Hepatosplenic lymphoma in a dog. *Vet Pathol* 40: 556–562.

38 Roccabianca, P., Paltrinieri, S., Gallo, E., and Giuliani, A. (2002). Hepatosplenic T-cell lymphoma in a mare. *Vet Pathol* 39: 508–511.

39 Ponce, F., Marchal, T., Magnol, J.P. et al. (2010). A morphological study of 608 cases of canine malignant lymphoma in France with a focus on comparative similarities between canine and human lymphoma morphology. *Vet Pathol* 47: 414–433.

40 Valli, V.E., Kass, P.H., San Myint, M., and Scott, F. (2013). Canine lymphomas: association of classification type, disease stage, tumor subtype, mitotic rate, and treatment with survival. *Vet Pathol* 50: 738–748.

41 van Stee, L.L., Boston, S.E., Singh, A. et al. (2015). Outcome and prognostic factors for canine splenic lymphoma treated by splenectomy (1995–2011). *Vet Surg* 44: 976–982.

42 Stefanello, D., Valenti, P., Zini, E. et al. (2011). Splenic marginal zone lymphoma in 5 dogs (2001–2008). *J Vet Intern Med* 25: 90–93.

43 Flood-Knapik, K.E., Durham, A.C., Gregor, T.P. et al. (2013). Clinical, histopathological and immunohistochemical characterization of canine indolent lymphoma. *Vet Comp Oncol* 11: 272–286.

44 Bertazzolo, W., Dell'Orco, M., Bonfanti, U. et al. (2005). Canine angiosarcoma: cytologic, histologic, and immunohistochemical correlations. *Vet Clin Pathol* 34: 28–34.

45 Sanchez, B., Nieto, A., de Ruiz Leon, M.A. et al. (2002). Metastatic lymphangiosarcoma in a horse. *Vet Pathol* 39: 266–268.

46 Barnes, J.C., Taylor, S.M., Clark, E.G. et al. (1997). Disseminated lymphangiosarcoma in a dog. *Can Vet J* 38: 42–44.

47 Langenbach, A., Anderson, M.A., Dambach, D.M. et al. (1998). Extraskeletal osteosarcomas in dogs: a retrospective study of 169 cases (1986–1996). *J Am Anim Hosp Assoc* 34: 113–120.

48 Spangler, W.L., Culbertson, M.R., and Kass, P.H. (1994). Primary mesenchymal (nonangiomatous/nonlymphomatous) neoplasms occurring in the canine spleen: anatomic classification, immunohistochemistry, and mitotic activity correlated with patient survival. *Vet Pathol* 31: 37–47.

49 Gower, K.L., Liptak, J.M., Culp, W.T. et al. (2015). Splenic liposarcoma in dogs: 13 cases (2002–2012). *J Am Vet Med Assoc* 247: 1404–1407.

50 Moore, P.F. (2014). A review of histiocytic diseases of dogs and cats. *Vet Pathol* 51: 167–184.

51 Affolter, V.K. and Moore, P.F. (2002). Localized and disseminated histiocytic sarcoma of dendritic cell origin in dogs. *Vet Pathol* 39: 74–83.

52 Scurrell, E., Trott, A., Rozmanec, M., and Belford, C.J. (2013). Ocular histiocytic sarcoma in a cat. *Vet Ophthalmol* 16 (1): 173–176.

53 Pinard, J., Wagg, C.R., Girard, C. et al. (2006). Histiocytic sarcoma in the tarsus of a cat. *Vet Pathol* 43: 1014–1017.

54 Ide, K., Setoguchi-Mukai, A., Nakagawa, T. et al. (2009). Disseminated histiocytic sarcoma with excessive hemophagocytosis in a cat. *J Vet Med Sci* 71: 817–820.

55 Friedrichs, K.R. and Young, K.M. (2008). Histiocytic sarcoma of macrophage origin in a cat: case report with a literature review of feline histiocytic malignancies and comparison with canine hemophagocytic histiocytic sarcoma. *Vet Clin Pathol* 37: 121–128.

56 Paciello, O., Passantino, G., Costagliola, A. et al. (2013). Histiocytic sarcoma of the nasal cavity in a horse. *Res Vet Sci* 94: 648–650.

57 Matsuda, K., Nomoto, H., Kawamura, Y. et al. (2010). Hemophagocytic histiocytic sarcoma in a Japanese black cow. *Vet Pathol* 47: 339–342.

58 Warschau, M., Hoffmann, M., Dziallas, P. et al. (2017). Invasive histiocytic sarcoma of the lumbar spine in a ferret (*Mustela putorius furo*). *J Small Anim Pract* 58: 115–118.

59 Kennedy, K., Thomas, R., and Breen, M. (2016). Canine histiocytic malignancies: challenges and opportunities. *Vet Sci* 3: 2.

60 Dobson, J., Hoather, T., McKinley, T.J., and Wood, J.L. (2009). Mortality in a cohort of flat-coated retrievers in the UK. *Vet Comp Oncol* 7: 115–121.

61 Dobson, J., Villiers, E., Roulois, A. et al. (2006). Histiocytic sarcoma of the spleen in flat-coated retrievers with regenerative anaemia and hypoproteinaemia. *Vet Rec* 158: 825–829.

62 Rossi, S., Gelain, M.E., and Comazzi, S. (2009). Disseminated histiocytic sarcoma with peripheral blood involvement in a Bernese Mountain dog. *Vet Clin Pathol* 38: 126–130.

63 Moore, P.F., Affolter, V.K., and Vernau, W. (2006). Canine hemophagocytic histiocytic sarcoma: a proliferative disorder of CD11d$^+$ macrophages. *Vet Pathol* 43: 632–645.

64 Spangler, W.L. and Kass, P.H. (1998). Pathologic and prognostic characteristics of splenomegaly in dogs due to fibrohistiocytic nodules: 98 cases. *Vet Pathol* 35: 488–498.

65 Collett, M.G., Doyle, A.S., Reyers, F. et al. (1987). Fatal disseminated cryptococcosis and concurrent ehrlichiosis in a dog. *J S Afr Vet Assoc* 58: 197–202.

66 Schroeder, H. and van Rensburg, I.B. (1993). Generalised *Listeria monocytogenes* infection in a dog. *J S Afr Vet Assoc* 64: 133–136.

67 Richardson, E.F. and Brown, N.O. (1996). Hematological and biochemical changes and results of aerobic bacteriological culturing in dogs undergoing splenectomy. *J Am Anim Hosp Assoc* 32: 199–210.

68 Reis, A.B., Teixeira-Carvalho, A., Giunchetti, R.C. et al. (2014). Cellular immunophenotypic profile in the splenic compartment during canine visceral leishmaniasis. *Vet Immunol Immunopathol* 157: 190–196.

69 Pastor, J., Pumarola, M., Cuenca, R., and Lavin, S. (1993). Systemic aspergillosis in a dog. *Vet Rec* 132: 412–413.

70 Nabity, M.B., Barnhart, K., Logan, K.S. et al. (2006). An atypical case of *Trypanosoma cruzi* infection in a young English Mastiff. *Vet Parasitol* 140: 356–361.

71 Hoskins, J.D., Bunge, M.M., Dubey, J.P., and Duncan, D.E. (1991). Disseminated infection with *Neospora caninum* in a ten-year-old dog. *Cornell Vet* 81: 329–334.

72 Campora, L., Corazza, M., Zullino, C. et al. (2011). *Mycobacterium avium* subspecies hominissuis disseminated infection in a Basset Hound dog. *J Vet Diagn Invest* 23: 1083–1087.

73 Brown, M.R., Thompson, C.A., and Mohamed, F.M. (2005). Systemic candidiasis in an apparently immunocompetent dog. *J Vet Diagn Invest* 17: 272–276.

74 Baneth, G. (2011). Perspectives on canine and feline hepatozoonosis. *Vet Parasitol* 181: 3–11.

75 Abdellatif, A., Gunther, C., Peppler, C., and Kramer, M. (2014). A rare case of splenic abscess with septic peritonitis in a German Shepherd dog. *BMC Vet Res* 10: 201.

76 Allen, J., Hartley, A.N., and Neel, J.A. (2018). What is your diagnosis? Splenic aspirate from a dog. *Vet Clin Pathol* 47 (4): 674–675.

77 Kim, M.C., Kim, J., Kang, W. et al. (2016). Systemic infection of *Mycobacterium avium* subspecies hominissuis and fungus in a pet dog. *J Vet Med Sci* 78: 157–160.

78 Zanatta, R., Miniscalco, B., Guarro, J. et al. (2006). A case of disseminated mycosis in a German Shepherd dog due to *Penicillium purpurogenum*. *Med Mycol* 44: 93–97.

79 O'Toole, D., Tharp, S., Thomsen, B.V. et al. (2005). Fatal mycobacteriosis with hepatosplenomegaly in a young dog due to *Mycobacterium avium*. *J Vet Diagn Invest* 17: 200–204.

29

Thymus

Cleverson D. Souza and Meredeth Crandall McEntire

Normal Structure and Function

The thymus, located in the cranial mediastinum, is a primary lymphoid organ critical for T-lymphocyte development.[1,2] The thymus is primarily composed of two cell types. The thymic epithelial cells arise from the third and sometimes the fourth pharyngeal pouches during embryonic development. Lymphoid thymocytes migrate as hematopoietic precursors from the bone marrow during late-stage thymic epithelial development.[3] The thymus is prominent in young animals but decreases in size during pubertal involution.[2]

Histologically, the thymus is similar across species and is divided into many lobules with lymphocyte-rich cortices and less cellular medullae (Figure 29.1). Early T-lymphocyte develop in the cortex, expressing neither cluster of differentiation (CD)4 nor CD8, so are characterized as double-negative ($CD4^-CD8^-$) cells. As these $CD4^-CD8^-$ T lymphocytes develop, they migrate toward the medulla, become double positive ($CD4^+CD8^+$), and finally mature as single-positive ($CD4^+CD8^-$ or $CD4^-CD8^+$) lymphocytes.[4] The uniquely double-positive ($CD4^+CD8^+$) T lymphocyte predominates in the normal thymus.[5] In addition to terminally maturing T lymphocytes, the thymic medulla also contains low numbers of thymic epithelial cells that form a diffuse reticular network as well as Hassall's corpuscles (Figure 29.2). The organ-specific Hassall's corpuscles are composed of concentric layers of flattened, keratinized reticular epithelial cells.[1] Presentation of self-antigen by thymic epithelial cells permits negative selection of autoreactive T lymphocytes and the maintenance of central tolerance.[1]

Sampling for Cytology

In veterinary medicine, thymic enlargements or masses are typically sampled via ultrasound or computed tomography guided percutaneous fine-needle aspirate (FNA).[6] Depending on the size of the animal and the mass, a 1.5–2.5 in., 22–25 G needle can be used to collect quality samples for cytologic review by employing either an aspiration or non-aspiration technique (Chapter 1). This type of percutaneous FNA is considered feasible and accepted as a diagnostic for thymic disease in human medicine but is being replaced to some extent by ultrasound-guided core needle biopsy or endoscopic ultrasound-guided FNA.[7]

Diseases of the Thymus

The most common thymic diseases in domestic animals are thymomas and thymic lymphoma. Uncommon thymic lesions, which are the subject of scattered case reports, include cysts,[8–19] thymolipomas,[20,21] and thymofibrolipomas,[22] squamous cell carcinomas,[23,24] lymphangiosarcomas,[25] carcinoids,[26] hemorrhage,[16,27,28] and antigen- or developmental arrest-induced hyperplasia.[16,28]

Thymoma

Thymomas are tumors arising from thymic epithelial cells.[29,30] They are reported most often in older dogs, dairy goats, cattle, and rabbits, with fewer cases reported in cats and horses.[23,31–44] Located most often in the cranial mediastinum, they can occur in any area through which thymic progenitor cells pass during embryonic development, such as the cervical region or pericardial sac.[31,45]

There are three basic histological classifications based on the ratio of lymphocytic and epithelial components (L : E) including epithelial (L : E < 30%), mixed lymphoepithelial (L : E 30–70%), and lymphocyte-rich (L : E > 70%) thymomas.[6,30,46] Evidence for the effect of histologic subtype on patient survival is mixed, with some reports concluding that lymphocyte-rich thymomas are associated with longer survival times[47,48] and others suggesting that the subtype

Veterinary Cytology, First Edition. Edited by Leslie C. Sharkey, M. Judith Radin, and Davis Seelig.

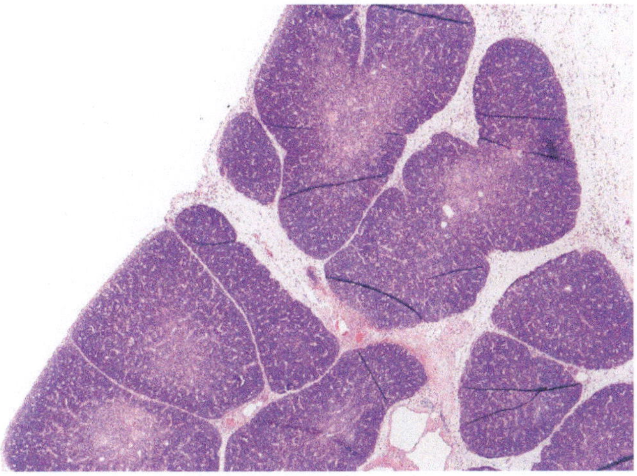

Figure 29.1 Normal thymus of a one-week-old dog. The thymus has a thin capsule of connective tissue that projects inward as septa, partially dividing the organ into lobules. The parenchyma of each lobule is organized into a cortex and a medulla. The dense cortical area is composed mostly of small undifferentiated lymphocytes, while the medulla exhibits paler staining and is less densely populated by lymphoid and stromal cells (hematoxylin & eosin, 40×).

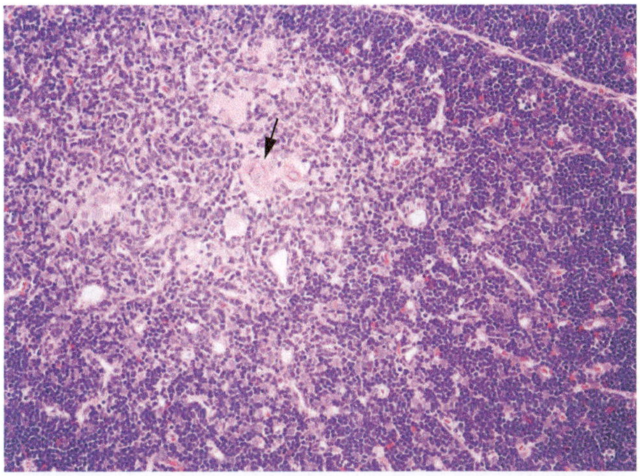

Figure 29.2 Same dog as Figure 29.1. The medulla contains two defined Hassall's corpuscles, characterized by perivascular cuffs of epithelial cells that become calcified and/or keratinized. Numerous small lymphocytes and lesser numbers of stromal cells are present (hematoxylin & eosin, 50×).

has no association with survival.[37] Irrespective of its microscopic appearance, accurate prognostication depends on an assessment of a tumor's clinical behavior and invasiveness into surrounding tissues and thus its benignancy or malignancy.[8,37,49]

Thymomas are associated with an increased incidence of immune-mediated paraneoplastic conditions and other tumor types.[16,50] The exact mechanism is uncertain, but abnormal thymic epithelial cells or damage induced by tumor growth is suspected to diminish the ability of the thymus to maintain self-tolerance and tumor surveillance, thus creating increased opportunity for immune-mediated diseases and other tumors to develop, respectively.[50] Immune-mediated and paraneoplastic conditions reported to occur with thymoma include myasthenia gravis,[16,41,51–53] myositis,[16,54,55] pemphigus foliaceous,[16] superficial necrolytic dermatitis,[16] exfoliative dermatitis,[56] erythema multiforme,[57] and hypercalcemia.[16] Up to 50% of patients with thymomas have symptoms of myasthenia gravis or megaesophagus with lower incidences of the other reported conditions.[37,50]

Cytology of the Thymoma

Cytologically, thymomas are composed of (i) a mixed, predominantly small lymphocyte population, (ii) low numbers of loosely aggregated epithelial cells, and (iii) well-differentiated mast cells.[47] The individual thymic epithelial cells vary in size and shape (round, oval, polyhedral, or spindle) with round to oval nuclei, indistinct nucleoli, moderate amounts of basophilic cytoplasm, and often indistinct cell margins (Figure 29.3). In addition to these epithelial cells and a mixed lymphoid population, mast cells are observed in 53% of FNA thymoma samples based on one retrospective study.[48] Increased numbers of perivascular, medullary mast cells are present in human thymomas compared with normal adult or fetal thymuses and may play a role in endothelial cell and tumor proliferation.[58] Less common cytologic findings include areas of mixed inflammation,

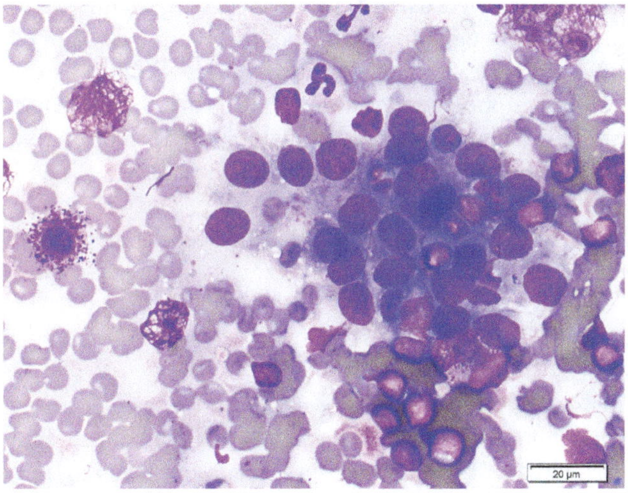

Figure 29.3 Thymoma, mixed epithelial/lymphocytic type, from a 12-year-old Labrador retriever presenting for difficulty breathing. Epithelial thymic cells (center) have indistinct cell borders with round to elongated nuclei, finely stippled chromatin patterns, and high nuclear to cytoplasmic ratios (N:C). Small lymphocytes, a single well-differentiated mast cell, and smudged nuclei also are seen (Wright's, 100×. *Source:* Image courtesy of Daniel Heinrich).

cystic fluid, necrosis, rare melanocytes, mesenchymal cells, malignant squamous epithelial cells resulting from abnormal differentiation, and aggregations of homogeneous eosinophilic stromal-like material.[37,42,43,59,60] Sampling a malignant thymoma may yield overtly malignant epithelial cells with increased N:C, cytoplasmic basophilia, anisocytosis, and anisokaryosis, but biologically malignant forms can also present without major cytological abnormalities.[6]

Additional Diagnostics for the Diagnosis of Thymoma

Cytology is often diagnostic for thymomas. Diagnostic success in canine case series has ranged from 7 of 17 cases[48] to 7 of 9 cases[59] with 100% positive predictive values reported for rabbits.[44] The correlation between cytology and histopathologic subtype is low ($r = 0.55$), likely due to the comparatively low exfoliation and low numbers of thymic epithelial cells as compared with lymphocytes.[6,44,48,59] Based on cytology alone, mistaken diagnoses of lymphoma, metastatic mast cell disease, and branchial cysts have occurred.[5,9,61] Flow cytometry has been shown to be a useful tool in the diagnosis of canine mediastinal masses, including both thymoma and lymphoma. In a case series of 13 canine mediastinal masses, 6/6 thymomas could be identified by flow cytometry through the detection of greater than 10% double-positive ($CD4^+$, $CD8^+$) small T lymphocytes. Moreover, 7/7 cases of lymphoma could be identified through a combination of flow cytometry and polymerase chain reaction for antigen receptor rearrangement (PARR) testing.[5] A similar population of $CD4^+CD8^+$ cells was detected using flow cytometry in a feline thyomoma.[45] Although rare, thymomas in dogs and cats can be associated with a paraneoplastic polyclonal, mature T-lymphocyte lymphocytosis upward of 20 000/μL in published reports.[62,63] Flow cytometric evaluation of two such canine lymphocytoses revealed a predominantly (53%) $CD4^-CD8^-$ double-negative population in one[62] and a mixed $CD4^+CD8^-$, $CD4^-CD8^+$, and $CD4^-CD8^-$ population in the other.[63]

Thymic Lymphoma

Thymic lymphoma is most commonly reported in dogs, young feline leukemia virus positive cats, and bovine leukosis virus (BLV) negative beef cattle between 6 and 18 months of age, with rare reports in horses.[46,64] Most canine and feline case reports do not discriminate between primary thymic and mediastinal lymphoid lymphoma, but more than 85% of mediastinal cases arise from T lymphocytes.[46,65,66] Most cases of thymic lymphomas are due to a clonal expansion of large lymphocytes that can be readily identified cytologically, but small cell and mixed cell lymphomas have been described and may necessitate ancillary diagnostics such as flow cytometry and PARR testing for confirmation.[5,16,48,61] In dogs, mediastinal lymphoma is predominantly a $CD4^+$ disease, although $CD4^+CD8^+$ and $CD21^+CD3^+$ variants are reported.[5] Discriminating the benign population of $CD4^+CD8^+$ cells found in thymoma from the malignant variant in lymphoma can be accomplished by flow cytometry, where the latter population is characterized by higher forward scatter (i.e. large size) as compared with the small lymphocytes in the former.[5] Both thymic lymphoma and thymoma can be associated with a paraneoplastic hypercalcemia, but it is a relatively common finding for thymic lymphoma[24] and rare for thymomas (2 of 23 dogs).[37]

Uncommon Thymic Conditions

Thymic branchial cysts are developmental abnormalities arising from persistent vestigial remnants of a branchial cleft or pouch.[10,11,67] Cervical and mediastinal branchial cysts are rare, often incidental findings in dogs and cats,[8,9,12–18] with an increased frequency of asymptomatic cysts in aged Beagles (nearly 50% of Beagles affected by microscopically detectable cysts by 2.5 years).[19] Ultrasound or computed tomography detection of a single or multilocular mediastinal cystic lesion with relatively little associated solid tissue is suggestive of, but not diagnostic for, a thymic cyst. Cytologic findings supporting the presence of a branchial cyst include low numbers of mature squamous epithelial cells, neutrophils, macrophages, small lymphocytes, and cholesterol crystals,[17] although increased cellularity due to inflammation induced by cyst rupture can also be seen.[11,13]

Thymolipomas and thymofibrolipomas are benign, typically large, mesenchymal neoplasms in the cranial mediastinum composed of mature adipose tissue and thymic tissue and, with the latter, abundant fibrous connective tissue.[20–22] These tumors are rare in dogs and cats, and while the cytology has not been explicitly described, the collection of a mixed, predominantly mature lymphoid population and adipocytes should prompt their consideration.

Squamous cell carcinomas, whose cytologic features have been described elsewhere (Chapter 12), and thymoma-associated squamous cell carcinoma have been described in horses, cows, dogs, and rats.[23,24] A thymic carcinoid was identified incidentally during a necropsy of a captive Bengal tiger euthanized due to a distal aortic thromboembolism.[26] Cytology was not described, but the features of carcinoids have been described elsewhere in detail (Chapter 32). Cranial mediastinal lymphangiosarcoma has been reported within a single case series of twelve cats.[25] Lymphangiosarcoma and hemangiosarcoma cannot be discriminated cytologically, but their features have been described elsewhere herein (Chapter 28). Immunohistochemical detection of prospero-related homeobox gene-1 (PROX-1) and lymphatic vessel endothelial receptor-1 (LYVE-1) has been useful to exclude hemangiosarcoma in the diagnosis of lymphatic endothelial neoplasms in horses and dogs.[68,69]

While rare, hemorrhage and hematoma formation within the thymus occurs primarily in young dogs. Causes include anticoagulant rodenticide toxicity, collar- and car-related trauma, and idiopathia. The propensity for intra-thymic hemorrhage in young dogs is unclear, but a sudden rise in blood pressure is suspected to rupture thin-walled vessels in a regressing thymus. The vessels in an involuted thymus are sclerotic and do not appear to rupture as easily.[16,27,28] Cytologic evidence of previous hemorrhage, such as macrophagic inflammation with erythrophagia, hemosiderin, and/or hematoidin, in a young dog should prompt consideration of intra-thymic hemorrhage. Thymic hyperplasia has been reported in cattle, cats, dogs, birds, rabbits, and tortoises.[16] Repeated vaccinations in cattle, rabbits, and birds can result in thymic hyperplasia,[64] while other causes in cattle include BLV infection and congenital impaired T-lymphocyte differentiation.[70]

References

1 Press, C. and Landsverk, T. (2006). Immune system. In: *Dellmann's Textbook of Veterinary Histology*, 6e (eds. J.A. Eurell and B.L. Frappier), 134–152. Ames, IA: Wiley-Blackwell.

2 Faisca, P., Henriques, J., Dias, T.M. et al. (2011). Ectopic cervical thymic carcinoma in a dog. *J Small Anim Pract* 52: 266–270.

3 Larsen, W. (2001). *Human Embryology*, 3e, 366–367. St. Louis, MO: Elsevier.

4 Fry, M.M. and MD, M.G. (2012). Bone marrow, blood cells, and the lymphatic system. In: *Pathologic Basis of Veterinary Disease*, 5e (eds. J.F. Zachary and M.G. MD), 698–770. St. Louis, MO: Elsevier Mosby.

5 Lana, S., Plaza, S., Hampe, K. et al. (2006). Diagnosis of mediastinal masses in dogs by flow cytometry. *J Vet Intern Med* 20: 1161–1165.

6 Dell'Orco, M., Bertazzolo, W., Caniatti, M. et al. (2008). Cytologic features of 11 cases of canine and feline thymoma and correlation with a human histologic classification. *Veterinaria* 22: 23–37.

7 Tomaszek, S., Wigle, D.A., Keshavjee, S., and Fischer, S. (2009). Thymomas: review of current clinical practice. *Ann Thorac Surg* 87: 1973–1980.

8 Robinson, W.C., Cantwell, H.D., Crawley, R.R. et al. (1977). Invasive thymoma in a dog: a case report. *J Am Anim Hosp Assoc* 13: 95–97.

9 Malik, R., Gabor, L., Hunt, G.B. et al. (1997). Benign cranial mediastinal lesions in three cats. *Aust Vet J* 75: 183–187.

10 Fahmy, S. (1974). Cervical thymic cysts: their pathogenesis and relationship to branchial cysts. *J Laryngol Otol* 88: 47–60.

11 Kadhim, A.L., Sheahan, P., Colreavy, M.P., and Timon, C.V. (2004). Pearls and pitfalls in the management of branchial cyst. *J Laryngol Otol* 118: 946–950.

12 Karbe, E. and Nielsen, S.W. (1965). Branchial cyst in a dog. *J Am Vet Med Assoc* 147: 637–640.

13 Liu, S., Patnaik, A.K., and Burk, R.L. (1983). Thymic branchial cysts in the dog and cat. *J Am Vet Med Assoc* 182: 1095–1098.

14 Clark, D.M., Kostolich, M., and Mosier, D. (1989). Branchial cyst in a dog. *J Am Vet Med Assoc* 194: 67–68.

15 Parnell, P.G. and Andreasen, C.B. (1992). What is your diagnosis? *Vet Clin Pathol* 21: 9–10.

16 Day, M.J. (1997). Review of thymic pathology in 30 cats and 36 dogs. *J Small Anim Pract* 38: 393–403.

17 Zekas, L.J. and Adams, W.M. (2002). Cranial mediastinal cysts in nine cats. *Vet Radiol Ultrasound* 43: 413–418.

18 Levien, A.S., Summers, B.A., Szladovits, B. et al. (2010). Transformation of a thymic branchial cyst to a carcinoma with pulmonary metastasis in a dog. *J Small Anim Pract* 51: 604–608.

19 Newman, A.J. (1971). Cysts of branchial arch origin in the thymus of the Beagle. *J Small Anim Pract* 12: 681–685.

20 Vilafranca, M. and Font, A. (2005). Thymolipoma in a cat. *J Feline Med Surg* 7: 125–127.

21 Ramírez, G.A., Spattini, G., Altimira, J. et al. (2008). Clinical and histopathological features of a thymolipoma in a dog. *J Vet Diagn Invest* 20: 360–364.

22 Morini, M., Bettini, G., Diana, A. et al. (2009). Thymofibrolipoma in two dogs. *J Comp Pathol* 141: 74–77.

23 Carpenter, J.L. and Valentine, B.A. (1992). Squamous cell carcinoma arising in two feline thymomas. *Vet Pathol* 29: 541–543.

24 Anilkumar, T.V., Voigt, R.P., Quigley, P.J. et al. (1994). Squamous cell carcinoma of the feline thymus with widespread apoptosis. *Res Vet Sci* 56: 208–215.

25 Hinrichs, U., Puhl, S., Rutteman, G.R. et al. (1999). Lymphangiosarcomas in cats: a retrospective study of 12 cases. *Vet Pathol* 36: 164–167.

26 Powe, J., Castleman, W., and Fiorello, C. (2005). A thymic carcinoid in a Bengal tiger (*Panthera tigris*). *J Zoo Wildl Med* 36: 531–533.

27 Van der Linde-Sipman, J.S. and van Dijk, J.E. (1987). Hematomas in the thymus in dogs. *Vet Pathol* 24: 59–61.

28 Liggett, A.D., Thompson, L.J., Frazier, K.S. et al. (2002). Thymic hematoma in juvenile dogs associated with anticoagulant rodenticide toxicosis. *J Vet Diagn Invest* 14: 416–419.

29 Parker, G.A. and Casey, H.W. (1976). Thymomas in domestic animals. *Vet Pathol* 13: 353–364.

30 Ströbel, P., Marx, A., Zettl, A., and Müller-Hermelink, H.K. (2005). Thymoma and thymic carcinoma: an update of the WHO classification 2004. *Surg Today* 35: 805–811.

31 Patnaik, A.K., Lieberman, P.H., Erlandson, R.A., and Antonescu, C. (2003). Feline cystic thymoma: a clinicopathologic, immunohistologic, and electron microscopic study of 14 cases. *J Feline Med Surg* 5: 27–35.

32 Altman, N.H. and Streett, C.S. (1968). Bovine thymoma: case report. *Am J Vet Res* 29: 2411–2414.

33 Watson, A.D. and Farrow, B.R. (1971). True thymoma in the dog: a case report. *Vet Rec* 89: 460–463.

34 Hadlow, W.J. (1978). High prevalence of thymoma in the dairy goat: report of 17 cases. *Vet Pathol* 15: 153–169.

35 Momotani, E., Nakamura, N., and Shoya, S. (1981). Morphologic evidence of the histogenesis of epithelial thymoma in a cow. *Am J Vet Res* 42: 114–121.

36 Bellah, J.R., Stiff, M.E., and Russell, R.G. (1983). Thymoma in the dog: two case reports and review of 20 additional cases. *J Am Vet Med Assoc* 183: 306–311.

37 Aronsohn, M.G., Schunk, K.L., Carpenter, J.L., and King, N.W. (1984). Clinical and pathologic features of thymoma in 15 dogs. *J Am Vet Med Assoc* 184: 1355–1362.

38 Middleton, D.J., Ratcliffe, R.C., and Xu, F.N. (1985). Thymoma with distant metastases in a cat. *Vet Pathol* 22: 512–514.

39 Whiteley, L.O., Leininger, J.R., Wolf, C.B., and Ames, T.R. (1986). Malignant squamous cell thymoma in a horse. *Vet Pathol* 23: 627–629.

40 Furuoka, H., Taniyama, H., Matsui, T. et al. (1987). Malignant thymoma with multiple metastases in a mare. *Jpn J Vet Sci* 49: 577–579.

41 Scott-Moncrieff, J.C., Cook, J.R. Jr., and Lantz, G.C. (1990). Acquired myasthenia gravis in a cat with thymoma. *J Am Vet Med Assoc* 196: 1291–1293.

42 Andreasen, C.B., Mahaffey, E.A., and Latimer, K.S. (1991). What is your diagnosis? *Vet Clin Pathol* 20: 15–16.

43 Ecco, R., Langohr, I.M., Túry, E. et al. (2006). Mixed thymoma in a cow. *J Vet Diagn Invest* 18: 503–507.

44 Künzel, F., Hittmair, K.M., Hassan, J. et al. (2012). Thymomas in rabbits: clinical evaluation, diagnosis, and treatment. *J Am Anim Hosp Assoc* 48: 97–104.

45 Lara-Garcia, A., Wellman, M., Burkhard, M.J. et al. (2008). Cervical thymoma originating in ectopic thymic tissue in a cat. *Vet Clin Pathol* 37: 397–402.

46 Jacobs, R., Messick, J., and Valli, V.E. (2002). Tumors of the hemolymphatic system. In: *Tumors in Domestic Animals*, 4e, 119–198. Ames, IA: Wiley-Blackwell.

47 Zitz, J.C., Birchard, S.J., Couto, G.C. et al. (2008). Results of excision of thymoma in cats and dogs: 20 cases (1984–2005). *J Am Vet Med Assoc* 232: 1186–1192.

48 Atwater, S.W., Powers, B.E., Park, R.D. et al. (1994). Thymoma in dogs: 23 cases (1980–1991). *J Am Vet Med Assoc* 205: 1007–1013.

49 Robinson, M. (1974). Malignant thymoma with metastases in a dog. *Vet Pathol* 11: 172–180.

50 Cameron, R.B., Loehrer, P.J., and Thomas, C.R. (2005). Neoplasms of the mediastinum. In: *Cancer: Principles and Practice*, 1e. Philadelphia, PA: JB Lippincott.

51 Shelly, S., Agmon-Levin, N., Altman, A., and Shoenfeld, Y. (2001). Thymoma and autoimmunity. *Cell Mol Immunol* 8: 199–202.

52 Okumura, M., Fujii, Y., Shiono, H. et al. (2008). Immunological function of thymoma and pathogenesis of paraneoplastic myasthenia gravis. *Gen Thorac Cardiovasc Surg* 56: 143–150.

53 Uchida, K., Awamura, Y., Nakamura, T. et al. (2002). Thymoma and multiple thymic cysts in a dog with acquired myasthenia gravis. *J Vet Med Sci* 64: 637–640.

54 Stewart, H.L. and Snell, K.C. (1968). Thymomas and thymic hyperplasia in *Praomys* (*Mastomys*) natalensis. Concomitant myositis, myocarditis, and sialodacryoadenitis. *J Natl Cancer Inst* 40: 1135–1159.

55 McNeil, P.H. (1980). A thymoma as a cause of oesophageal obstruction in a dog. *N Z Vet J* 28: 143–145.

56 Rottenberg, S., Von Tscharner, C., and Roosje, P.J. (2004). Thymoma-associated exfoliative dermatitis in cats. *Vet Pathol* 41: 429–433.

57 Tepper, L.C., Spiegel, I.B., and Davis, G.J. (2011). Diagnosis of erythema multiforme associated with thymoma in a dog and treated with thymectomy. *J Am Anim Hosp Assoc* 47: e19–e25.

58 Raica, M., Cimpean, A.M., Nico, B. et al. (2010). A comparative study of the spatial distribution of mast cells and microvessels in the foetal, adult human thymus and thymoma. *Int J Exp Pathol* 91: 17–23.

59 Rae, C.A., Jacobs, R.M., and Couto, C.G. (1989). A comparison between the cytological and histological

characteristics in thirteen canine and feline thymomas. *Can Vet J* 30: 497.

60 Choi, Y.W., McAdams, H.P., Jeon, S.C. et al. (2001). Idiopathic multilocular thymic cyst: CT features with clinical and histopathologic correlation. *Am J Roentgenol* 177: 881–885.

61 Carter, R.F., Valli, V.E., and Lumsden, J.H. (1986). The cytology, histology, and prevalence of cell types in canine lymphoma classified according to the National Cancer Institute Working Formulation. *Can J Vet Res* 50: 154–164.

62 Burton, A.G., Borjesson, D.L., and Vernau, W. (2014). Thymoma-associated lymphocytosis in a dog. *Vet Clin Pathol* 43: 584–588.

63 Batlivala, T.P., Bacon, N.J., Avery, A.C. et al. (2010). Paraneoplastic T-cell lymphocytosis associated with thymoma in a dog. *J Small Anim Pract* 37: 267–282.

64 Valli, V.E. (2007). Hematopoietic system. In: *Jubb, Kennedy, and Palmer's Pathology of Domestic Animals*, 5e, 107–324. Philadelphia, PA: Saunders Elsevier.

65 Ruslander, D.A., Gebhard, D.H., Tompkins, M.G. et al. (1997). Immunophenotypic characterization of canine lymphoproliferative disorders. *In Vivo* 11: 169–172.

66 Vail, D.M., Moore, A.S., Ogilvie, G.K., and Volk, L.M. (1998). Feline lymphoma (145 cases): proliferation indices, CD3 immunoreactivity and their association with prognosis in 90 cats receiving therapy. *J Vet Intern Med* 12: 349–354.

67 McGeady, T.A., Quinn, P.J., FitzPatrick, E.S. et al. (2006). Endocrine system. In: *Veterinary Embryology*, 1e, 286–294. Ames, IA: Wiley-Blackwell.

68 Junginger, J., Rotting, A., Staszyk, C. et al. (2010). Identification of equine cutaneous lymphangioma by application of a lymphatic endothelial cell marker. *J Comp Pathol* 143: 57–60.

69 Halsey, C.H., Worley, D.R., Curran, K. et al. (2016). The use of novel lymphatic endothelial cell-specific immunohistochemical markers to differentiate cutaneous angiosarcomas in dogs. *Vet Comp Oncol* 14: 236–244.

70 Fantinato, E., Pravettoni, D., Forlani, A. et al. (2013). Severe thymic hyperplasia in a newborn calf associated with impaired T-cell differentiation. *J Vet Diagn Invest* 25: 603–607.

Part VIII

Gastrointestinal Tract

30

Oral Cavity

Jill Schappa Faustich, Kevin S. Stepaniuk, Nicholas A. Robinson, and Cesar Piedra-Mora

Introduction

The veterinary literature describing the cytology of frequently encountered oral lesions is limited to scant case reports of common malignant tumors or small case series of rare diagnoses.[1] Cytology can guide selection of further diagnostics and suggest treatment and referral options even though histology is typically required for diagnostic confirmation. This chapter focuses on the characteristics of common oral lesions, and integration of clinical history, gross appearance, and imaging findings to support clinical decision-making.

Normal Tissue Architecture and Cytology

Anatomy and Histology

The oral cavity is composed of the vestibule and the oral cavity proper. The lips form the rostral and most of the lateral external boundaries of the vestibule, while the cheeks form the caudal portion of the lateral walls. The oral cavity proper is bounded dorsally by the hard palate and a small part of the rostral soft palate. The rostral and lateral boundaries are the dental arches and teeth, while the tongue and the mucosa ventral and lateral to it form the floor of the cavity. The palate separates the oral cavity from the nasal cavity and nasopharynx.

The lips form the junction between the skin and the digestive system. In general, the mucosa of the oral cavity in dogs and cats is covered by nonkeratinized stratified squamous epithelium, while the underlying lamina propria and submucosa blend together. The oropharyngeal palatine glands are covered by stratified squamous epithelium. The gingiva surrounds the teeth and is composed of dense fibrous tissue covered by smooth, highly vascularized mucosa. The periodontium includes the periodontal ligament, the cementum of the root, and the alveolar bone, which give structural support to the teeth. The tongue consists of skeletal muscle lined by stratified squamous epithelium, keratinized and thick dorsally, and nonkeratinized and thin ventrally. Salivary glands originate from the oral ectoderm and grow into the underlying mesoderm as large aggregates of compound glands. Major salivary glands include parotid, mandibular, and sublingual glands. Minor are labial, lingual, buccal, palatine, molar (in cats), and zygomatic glands.

The palatine tonsils are pharyngeal lymphoid structures covered by stratified squamous epithelium. In dogs and cats, they are found in crypts or recesses at the dorsolateral aspect of the caudal oropharynx. The epithelium is variably infiltrated with lymphocytes, neutrophils, and macrophages. Lymphoid nodules beneath the epithelium frequently have a germinal center and a mantle of small lymphocytes. The teeth are not amenable to cytologic examination and are evaluated by gross inspection and dental imaging, which thus will not be discussed further.

Oral cytology samples include the mucosa, gingiva, and bone. Gingiva refers to the tissue immediately surrounding the tooth. Mucosal lesions are located on the buccal surfaces, tongue, palate, soft palate, tonsil, and pharynx. Because many lesions involve both the mucosa and gingiva, these tissues are discussed together followed by separate sections describing entities specific to the mucosa, gingiva, tongue, tonsil, and bone.

Normal Cytology

Common cytologic observations include a granular eosinophilic proteinaceous background, keratinized and nonkeratinized squamous epithelial cells, mixed extracellular bacteria, mixed inflammatory cells, melanin, and scattered mature mesenchymal cells (Figure 30.1).

Veterinary Cytology, First Edition. Edited by Leslie C. Sharkey, M. Judith Radin, and Davis Seelig.

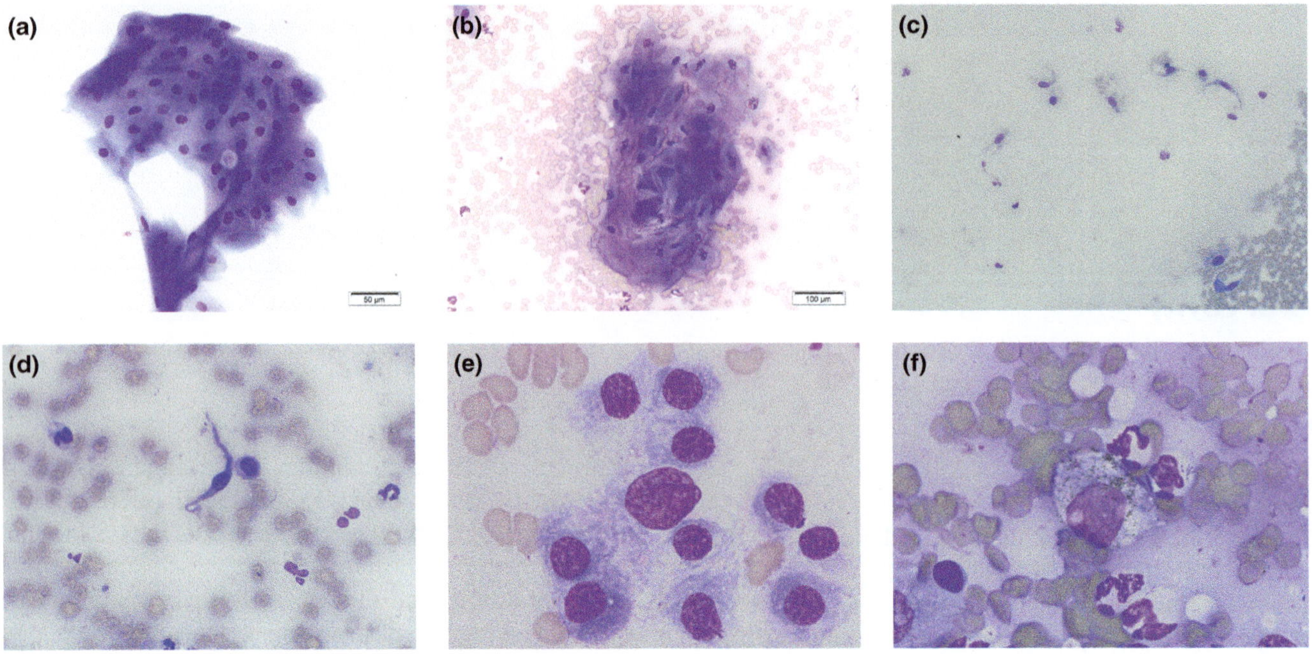

Figure 30.1 Common background findings in oral mass aspirates. (a and b) Hyperplastic and reactive squamous epithelial cells. (c) Small numbers of mesenchymal cells. (d) Well-differentiated mesenchymal cell. (e) Plasmacytic inflammation. (f) Septic neutrophilic inflammation and a squamous epithelial cell with melanin granules (Wright–Giemsa, (a–c) 200×, (d) 600×, (e and f) 1000×).

In the author's experience, commensal bacteria vary from scattered individual organisms to large thick mats of variably sized cocci, rods, coccobacilli, and occasionally large chaining rods. *Simonsiella* spp. (*Conchiformibius* spp.) often adheres to squamous epithelial cells (Figure 30.2). Squamous epithelial hyperplasia and mesenchymal hyperplasia are common secondary processes. Squamous epithelial hyperplasia is characterized by cytoplasmic basophilia, cytoplasmic vacuolization, and increased anisocytosis and anisokaryosis (Figure 30.1a and b). Oral mesenchymal cells vary from individualized to small aggregates of thin elongated spindloid cells with a single oval to cigar-shaped nucleus to plumper cells with increased basophilic cytoplasm and 1–2 nuclei sometimes containing a few prominent nucleoli (Figure 30.1c and d).[2]

Sample Collection

Gross examination is the critical first step in the evaluation of the oral cavity. Although much of the oral cavity is technically visible, patient compliance impacts the feasibility and quality of the examination. Sedation or anesthesia is likely to be required for even a cursory examination in some patients.

Indications

For better outcomes, recognition of oral masses in dogs and cats requires a thorough oral examination to identify growths when small, before they become a presenting complaint to the veterinarian. All oral masses in cats and most oral masses in dogs have underlying neoplastic, infectious, and/or inflammatory pathology requiring a diagnosis for appropriate treatment. Oral ulcers and swellings (e.g. salivary pathology) also require cytological and/or histopathological sampling.

Methods

For safe collection of representative samples, general anesthesia or heavy sedation with intubation might be needed. Oral lesions are sampled by fine-needle aspiration (FNA) and incisional or excisional biopsy. Impression smears for cytologic examination can be prepared from biopsy samples for preliminary diagnosis; however, in the authors'

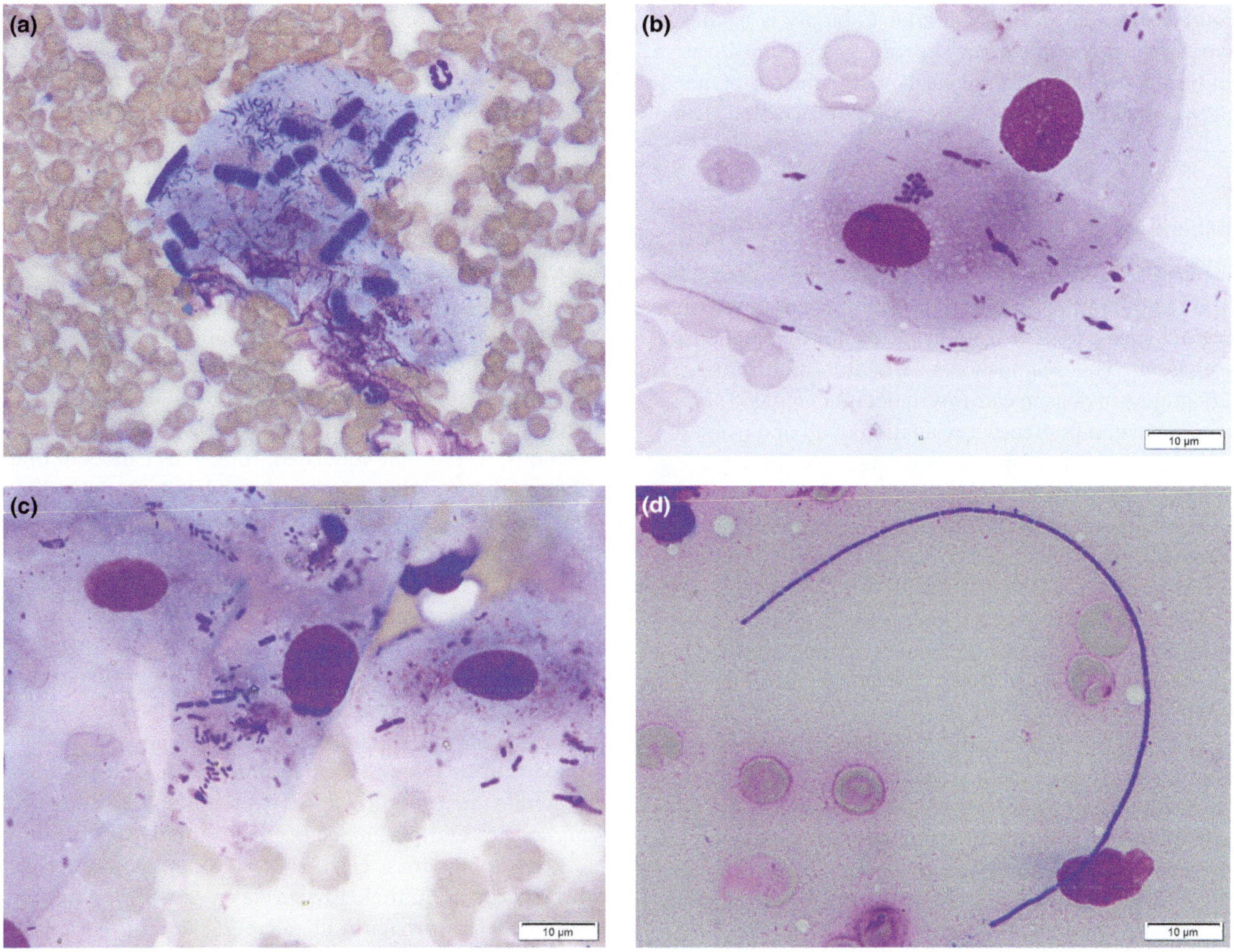

Figure 30.2 The background of oral cytology samples often contains a mixed population of bacteria. (a) *Simonsiella* adhered to the surface of a squamous epithelial cell (Wright–Giemsa, 200×). (b and c) Mixed bacterial population attached to squamous epithelial cells. (d) Commonly noted chaining bacteria (Wright–Giemsa, 1000×).

experience, superficial impression smears are rarely diagnostic. Incisional biopsies should be obtained within the visual clinical margins of the mass, avoiding disruption of normal tissue during sample collection.[3] Excisional biopsies are planned in the marginal zone of the tumor (zone of inflammation) or in normal tissue for wide excision. Incisional biopsies are collected using a scalpel blade or punch biopsy device. Firmer mineralized tissue can require a bone curette via the soft tissue biopsy site or access through a mucoperiosteal flap. Rarely, a Michele Trephine is needed. The oral mucosa should be sutured closed with an appropriate oral absorbable suture, such as poliglecaprone 25. A common pitfall is a collection of a superficial sample reflecting only overlying hyperplastic and/or chronically inflamed oral mucosa and gingiva rather than deeper inciting pathology. FNA can be nondiagnostic for poorly exfoliative lesions. Evaluation of regional lymph nodes, thoracic radiographs or computed tomography (CT), and abdominal ultrasound contribute to complete staging for many malignant oral tumors.

Safety

Complications from oral biopsy are uncommon when best practices are applied. Sample collection should avoid obvious regions of necrosis. Significant hemorrhage is rare if regional anatomical neurovascular bundles such as the inferior alveolar, infraorbital, and maxillary neurovascular bundles are avoided. Imaging prior to biopsy is helpful to plan if bone and teeth require removal. Many invasive tumors involve and replace bone; however, the risk of maxillofacial fracture is very low with proper collection techniques.

Imaging

Lesions involving the mandibles and maxilla or associated with teeth require intraoral radiographs or alternative imaging such as CT or cone-beam CT for comprehensive assessment. The diagnostic value of full-mouth intraoral radiographs in dogs in cats is well documented and should be part of a comprehensive evaluation of all oral masses.[4,5] With the exception of masses restricted to soft tissues (e.g. tongue, cheek), all oral masses adjacent to the maxilla, mandible, hard palate, and dentition require imaging. Interpretation of skull radiographs is challenging due to superimposition of maxillofacial structures; therefore, dental radiography and/or CT is preferred. Magnetic resonance imaging is beneficial in oral cavity and maxillofacial soft tissue tumors involving the tongue and salivary system.

CT is valuable in assessment of oral masses and cone-beam CT may prove more valuable in the future, particularly with odontogenic masses. Cone-beam CT provides excellent detail of the teeth and maxillofacial skeleton but currently is rare in clinical practice. Likewise, conventional CT is mostly limited to academic institutions and large private specialty practices. However, digital dental radiography is available and affordable in most small animal practices and should be part of the diagnostic evaluation for oral masses.

Lesions Involving the Mucosa and Gingiva

Inflammation

Inflammation is described according to the structures involved, for example, gingivitis, periodontitis, glossitis, and pharyngitis. Historically, terminology has been inconsistent, and oral inflammation was generically termed stomatitis. Stomatitis refers to the inflammation of the entire mouth, extending beyond the gingiva and mucogingival junction to include the caudal pharynx, palatoglossal folds, palatal mucosa, and buccal mucosa. This term is reserved for a feline-specific immune dysregulation defined by a clinical pattern of caudal oral mucosal inflammation (caudal mucositis).[6] Gingivitis refers to the first stage of periodontitis; the free gingiva is edematous and red and bleeds with periodontal probing, mild trauma, or spontaneously. Gingivitis is ubiquitous in dogs and cats, caused by dental plaque biofilm. Some breeds (e.g. Boxer, Bulldog) develop fibrous gingivitis.[7,8] The degree of visible gingivitis does not necessarily correlate to the extent of subgingival periodontitis and hidden periodontium attachment loss; radiographs are required to assess the extent of gingivitis and stage of periodontal disease.[9] Inflammation and loss of tissue attachment to the periodontium (i.e. gingiva, periodontal ligament, cementum, and alveolar bone) is periodontitis.[10] Glossitis is lingual inflammation, often secondary to contact with infected mandibular dentition such as in chronic ulcerative paradental stomatitis.[11] Pharyngeal inflammation (pharyngitis) can be traumatic, infectious, or immune-mediated. Infectious causes of oral inflammation are uncommon. Fungal lesions, including *Blastomyces, Cryptococcus, Sporothrix schenckii*, and *Candida albicans*, can present as oral masses or necrotic lesions (Chapter 3).[6,12–14] Periodontal and endodontic abscesses with surrounding inflammation in the mucosa or gingiva occur with chronic periodontal and endodontic infection. A case of transmissible venereal tumor with concurrent Leishmaniasis was reported in the oral cavity of a dog.[15]

Many intraoral inflammatory lesions appear similar cytologically as low cellularity samples consisting of non-degenerate neutrophils and/or predominantly mature lymphocytes and plasma cells. Small numbers of eosinophils, basophils, mast cells, and large mononuclear cells can be present. Epithelial hyperplasia and fibroplasia are common. Hemorrhage and necrotic debris are present uncommonly with commensal bacteria.[2]

Oral inflammation can precipitate reactive mass lesions that can be mistaken for neoplasia. As neoplasia can cause ulcerations and inflammation, discrimination of non-neoplastic and neoplastic lesions can be challenging both grossly and cytologically.[2] For example, sublingual foreign body-induced inflammation in cats appears clinically and sometimes cytologically similar to squamous cell carcinoma (SCC).[16] Concurrent epithelial and mesenchymal hyperplasia and inflammation are frequent cytologic observations in oral lesions, so definitive differentiation of hyperplasia and neoplasia can be impossible.[2] Results require interpretation in the context of clinical findings and histopathology is often required for definitive diagnosis.

Ulcers

Viruses, chemicals, uremia, immune-mediated disease, electricity, contact mucositis (adjacent to teeth) and some toxins (e.g. *Dieffenbachia* plants) cause ulcerative oral lesions. Most are acute, but chronic ulcers occur with neoplasia or traumatic occlusion, when a malocclusion causes sublingual or buccal granulomas. Acute ulcers often have a red zone of inflammation, whereas chronic ulcers typically do not. Location can sometimes be helpful in assessing the underlying cause. For example, contact mucositis will be adjacent to teeth, and uremic ulcers often occur in areas of high epithelial cell turnover like the tongue. In the author's experience, cytology samples from ulcers are characterized by moderate to high cellularity, containing non-degenerate neutrophils and fewer small lymphocytes, plasma cells, large mononuclear cells, mast cells, and eosinophils. Ulcers are often associated with concurrent epithelial and mesenchymal reactivity.[2] Consideration should also be given to possible concurrent neoplasia such as SCC, canine acanthomatous ameloblastoma (CAA), sarcoma, or a plasma cell tumor with secondary ulceration.[16,17]

Feline-Specific Conditions

Eosinophilic Granuloma Complex Eosinophilic granuloma complex can occur on the lips as an indolent ulcer or ulcerated mass.[18] Microscopic confirmation of a diagnosis is required because malignant tumors (e.g. SCC), amyloid-producing odontogenic tumors (APOTs), feline inductive odontogenic tumors (FIOT), and proliferative inflammatory lesions can have a similar clinical presentation.[16] Cytology should consist of eosinophils with fewer macrophages, neutrophils, mast cells, lymphocytes, plasma cells, and fibroblasts.[6,18–22]

Feline Caudal Mucositis Feline caudal mucositis is a frustrating oral condition with a possible immune-mediated pathogenesis. This "stomatitis" must be differentiated from periodontitis, epitheliotropic lymphoma, autoimmune conditions, and eosinophilic granulomas. Aggressive periodontitis and adult onset periodontitis can be mistaken for "stomatitis." Caudal mucositis is a defining clinical pattern of inflammation for diagnosis of "stomatitis." Severe periodontitis, juvenile gingivitis, juvenile onset periodontitis, and aggressive periodontitis often only involve the gingiva (gingivitis) with or without extension past the mucogingival junction into the mucosa (buccal mucositis). Stomatitis is commonly associated with widely distributed periodontitis and external inflammatory root resorption.[9] Cytology would be inflammatory based on the reported histologic features.[6]

Hyperplasia and Neoplasia

Epithelial

Important intraoral proliferative epithelial lesions include hyperplasia (Figure 30.1a and b), mucosal polyps/tags, odontogenic tumors, squamous papilloma, and SCC. Squamous epithelial and gingival epithelial hyperplasias are often secondary to oral inflammation, feline tooth resorption, and neoplasia.

Sublingual mucosal hyperplasia or sublingual and buccal granulomas comprise a specific oral lesion in dogs. These "gum-chewer" lesions occur secondary to chronic self-trauma from chewing the buccal or lingual mucosa. The gross appearance can mimic other more serious masses. Cytologically, these should appear similar to other hyperplastic mucosal lesions. Mucosal polyps and tags are similar and relatively uncommon lesions of the oral cavity. The difference between the two lesions is primarily histologic. Tags consist of a simple epithelium-covered projection of propria submucosa, whereas polyps contain a fibrovascular core with a hyperplastic epithelial covering. Cytologically, these are low cellularity, and are most commonly diagnosed as either inflammation or mesenchymal hyperplasia. Biopsy is recommended for definitive diagnosis.[2]

Oral papillomatosis (viral and non-viral) often occurs in juvenile or immunosuppressed dogs. Papillomavirus is persistent on environmental fomites and contagious to susceptible hosts. Lesions are pedunculated and cauliflower-like (Figure 30.3a and b). Most oral papilloma lesions undergo complete spontaneous regression. However, large aggregations may require surgical removal. Oral papillomatosis is not a significant cause of oral SCCs in dogs but may be in cats.[23–25] Cytologic features include moderate numbers of keratinized and nonkeratinized, well-differentiated to mildly reactive appearing squamous cells. Moderate inflammation, predominantly non-degenerate neutrophils and large mononuclear cells, evidence of hemorrhage, and pigmentary incontinence are also possible, similar to inflammatory or other hyperplastic lesions (Figure 30.3c–f).[2]

SCC is the most common oral tumor in the cat and second in the dog.[26–30] One study found SCC was more common in spayed females, dogs between 10 and 15 years of age, English Springer Spaniels, and Shetland Sheepdogs.[31] SCC occurs in the tonsillar and non-tonsillar regions, commonly the mandibular and maxillary oral mucosa and bone, and is the most common lingual tumor in the cat.[32,33] Lesions are grossly variable and include ulcerative, proliferative, expansile, infiltrative, proliferative, and firm presentations.[15,31] Imaging can reveal lysis or invasion of bone with or without osteoproliferation.[16,33] Cytology samples are cellular with classic features, including variable cohesiveness of epithelial cells, cytoplasmic to nuclear dyssynchrony of maturation, perinuclear vacuolization, and increased nucleus to cytoplasm ratio. Concurrent septic or aseptic neutrophilic inflammation, fibroplasia, hemorrhage, and bone remodeling can occur.[2,26] Markedly hyperplastic squamous epithelial cells can be difficult to differentiate from neoplastic cells, especially with concurrent

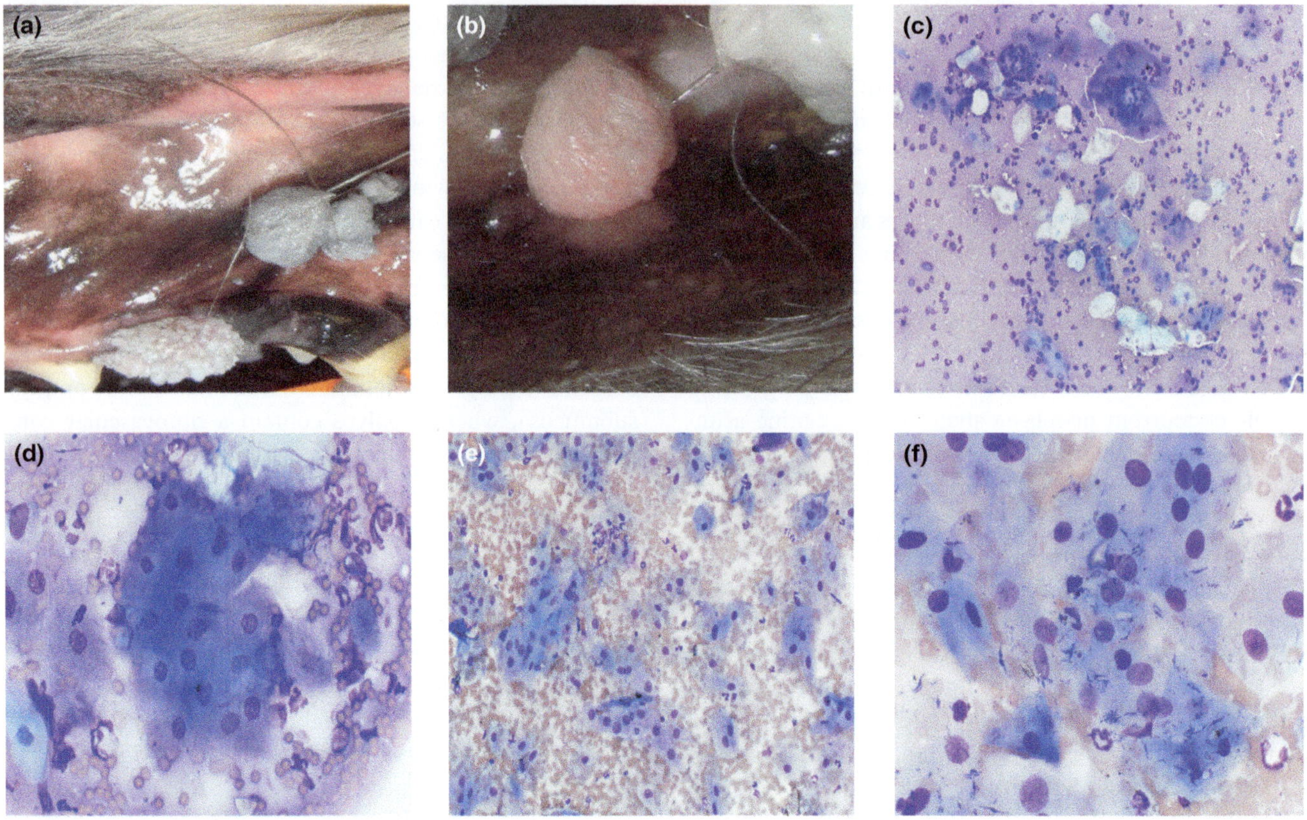

Figure 30.3 Squamous papilloma. (a and b) Gross photos of squamous papilloma in two dogs. (c and d) Cytology of a viral papilloma characterized by blood, neutrophils, keratinocytes, and uniform nucleated squamous epithelial cells (Wright–Giemsa, (c) 200×, (d) 600×). (e and f) Cytology of a non-viral papilloma containing blood with mature squamous cells and epicellular bacteria (Wright–Giemsa, (e) 200×, (f) 600×).

septic inflammation (Figure 30.7e and f).[2] Deep sampling can facilitate accurate diagnosis, but interpretation requires careful integration of cytology with the clinical picture, and biopsy confirmation is often recommended.

Mesenchymal

Sarcomas present as ulcerated or non-ulcerated firm swellings of the maxillary or mandibular mucosa invading the underlying bone.[16] They can be expansile soft tissue lesions or remain hidden in the maxillofacial bones.[9] Associated bone lysis can leave teeth floating in masses with regular or irregular margins. When sufficiently cellular, sarcoma FNAs are characteristic of similar lesions elsewhere (Chapter 16), consisting of elongate to plump individualized and aggregated mesenchymal cells that can be associated with variable amount of wispy pink extracellular material. Cells contain moderate amounts of basophilic cytoplasm, a single round to oval or elongated nucleus, and occasionally prominent nucleoli. Anisocytosis and anisokaryosis are often mild to moderate. Mild mixed inflammation (septic or non-septic) and evidence of bone remodeling (the presence of well-differentiated osteoblasts and osteoclasts with or without eosinophilic extracellular material) are common. Interpretation as inflammation with fibroplasia can occur if the mesenchymal population is poorly represented or if cells are very well differentiated. Cytologically, it can be difficult to distinguish a sarcoma from focal fibroplasia and peripheral odontogenic fibroma (POF).[2]

Oral fibrosarcoma is reported to be the third most common tumor in the dog and second in the cat.[29,34] Tumors are firm and raised, often with a "benign" clinical appearance resembling POF, fibroma, or ameloblastic fibroma. One variant is histologically low-grade but biologically aggressive, particularly on the maxilla. Local invasion is common and advanced imaging is recommended for treatment planning.[35] Radiographs show minimal bone changes or a geographic to moth-eaten pattern of bone loss.[36] FNAs of fibrosarcomas are variably cellular, typically at least moderately diagnostic.[2] The background is often granular and eosinophilic with small numbers of mixed inflammatory cells. A uniform population of elongated thin to plump individualized and aggregated mesenchymal cells is present. Cells contain scant, lightly basophilic cytoplasm; single to occasionally multiple oval to cigar-shaped nuclei; stippled chromatin; and occasionally 1–2 small nucleoli.

Cytologic atypia is often minimal. Differentiating these tumors from other predominantly mesenchymal samples, such as a sarcoma, POF, and focal fibrous hyperplasia (FFH) can be challenging.[2] High cellularity and robust criteria of malignancy favor a diagnosis of fibrosarcoma, but extreme caution is required in interpreting samples composed of mature cells.[2]

Round Cell

Melanoma is the most common oral "round cell" tumor and is the most commonly reported canine oral neoplasm.[26,37–42] Lesions are grossly variable, pigmented or amelanotic, flat, raised, firm, friable lesions that can invade bone.[29,43] Tumors are locally aggressive and often highly metastatic.[44] The maxilla and mandible are common locations, but melanoma occurs in all mucosal tissues.[43] Cytologically, oral melanoma appears similar to other locations and consists of round to spindle-shaped cells with fine, dark green to black cytoplasmic granules that vary depending on tumor differentiation (Chapter 15). Concurrent squamous epithelial and mesenchymal cell hyperplasia occur.[2,26] Rarely, oral melanomas are osteogenic or have osteocartilagenous differentiation, which cytologically appears as eosinophilic extracellular matrix and/or intracellular eosinophilic granules.[45–47] Poorly pigmented melanomas displaying marked criteria of malignancy are likely malignant; however, histopathology is recommended in cases of cytologically well-differentiated appearing melanomas to evaluate the potential for aggressive biologic behavior. Differentiating poorly pigmented or granular round cell tumors from each other can be challenging. Immunocytochemistry using cytokeratin, vimentin, and melan-A has a sensitivity and specificity of 100% when combined with cytology.[48]

Other oral round cell tumors include plasma cell tumors, mast cell tumors, transmissible venereal tumor, and epitheliotropic lymphoma.[26] Similar to many oral masses, the gross appearance of plasmacytomas is variable (ulcerated and non-ulcerated, flat or raised). They are cytologically similar to plasma cell tumors in other locations (Chapter 14).[49,50] Intraoral mast cell tumors are very uncommon; however, they can appear along the mucocutaneous junctions of the oral cavity (Chapter 13).[51–53] Oral lymphoma is rare but can present clinically as gingivitis, mucositis, glossitis, erosions, ulcerations, or masses.[31,54–56] Most are epitheliotropic T-cell lymphomas localized to the oral cavity, multifocal (skin, adnexal structures, mucocutaneous junctions), or systemically disseminated.[54,56,57] Cytology is similar to other locations (Chapter 27), and concurrent eosinophilia can be present.[58] No oral lymphoma cases were reported in a recent review of feline epitheliotropic lymphoma.[59]

Proliferative Lesions Specific to the Gingiva

The terminology of proliferative gingival lesions in veterinary medicine has undergone multiple revisions and can be confusing.[60–62] The most common and misleading of these terms is epulis, a generic term meaning "growth on the gingiva," often used to describe reactive and neoplastic oral masses including FFH, CAA, and POF. The term also encompasses malignant tumors of non-odontogenic origin; thus, the authors do not recommend it.[63,64] Proliferative gingival lesions should be classified as either reactive lesions or odontogenic tumors.

Reactive Lesions

Tumor-like reactive gingival lesions include FFH, pyogenic granuloma, and peripheral giant cell granuloma. FFH in dogs is common, while the others are rare.[63,64] A proliferative gingival lesion due to *Cryptococcus neoformans* was described surrounding a feline canine tooth.[65]

FFH is often referred to as fibrous epulis, fibromatous epulis, and gingival hypertrophy. FFH is composed of reactive tissue and should not be confused with "fibromatous epulis" (i.e. POF).[61,63] FFH occurs secondary to underlying periodontal disease, breed (e.g. Boxer, Bulldog), or medication (e.g. cyclosporine, amlodipine, phenytoin). FFH appears as a localized proliferation of gingival tissue similar to gingival hyperplasia, most commonly in the rostral aspect of the maxilla.[61] Intraoral radiography is relatively normal in the absence of significant periodontal disease. Cytology is often poorly cellular, consisting of few well-differentiated uniform thin elongated predominantly individualized mesenchymal cells and few to moderate inflammatory cells. Less commonly, plump mesenchymal cells predominate. Mesenchymal cells contain small amounts of lightly basophilic cytoplasm, a single oval to cigar-shaped nucleus, stippled chromatin, and occasionally 1–2 small nucleoli. Anisocytosis and anisokaryosis are mild; criteria of malignancy are minimal.[2] Associated inflammation is neutrophilic to mixed, with or without bacteria. Mild squamous hyperplasia and rarely evidence of tissue degeneration (cholesterol crystals, mineralization, lipid vacuolization) are present.[2] Low cellularity and frequent concurrent inflammation and epithelial hyperplasia confound definitive diagnosis, particularly in distinguishing FFH from inflammation, squamous or gingival hyperplasia, or well-differentiated mesenchymal neoplasia.[2]

Pyogenic granulomas represent exuberant vascular granulation tissue in response to injury, local irritation, and/or infection.[63,64,66–68] They are sessile or pedunculated, ulcerated or bleeding, and bright red or blue gingival masses found in the region of the caudal mandible and mandibular first molars.[66,68,69] Peripheral giant-cell granulomas (formerly giant-cell epulis) are similar to pyogenic granulomas with characteristic giant cells with multiple nuclei and eosinophilic cytoplasm.[60,70,71]

Odontogenic Tumors Odontogenic tumors are oral neoplasms arising from tooth-forming embryologic tissues and include epithelial, mesenchymal, and mixed origin tumors.[62,63] They are considered benign but are often locally invasive or expansile. Although several subtypes of each category exist, the most common are CAA and POF.[61,62]

CAA (formerly acanthomatous epulis) is an epithelial tumor arising from the enamel organ. Because CAAs aggressively invade bone, accurate diagnosis and wide surgical excision are essential.[72] CAA can occur throughout the dental arcades, but there is a predilection for the mandibular incisor and premolar regions.[61,73] Predisposed breeds include Shetland Sheepdogs, Golden Retrievers, Akitas, and Cocker Spaniels.[61,73] Lesions can grow rapidly, can ulcerate, are firm and/or friable, and often displace surrounding teeth (Figure 30.4a and b). Transformation or association with malignant SCC is rarely reported. In our experience, cytology samples from biopsy confirmed CAA have low to moderate cellularity, with variably sized clusters of organized, uniform, and basaloid epithelial cells that sometimes form rows. Nuclei are single, round, and basally located and have hyperchromatic chromatin. Anisocytosis and anisokaryosis are minimal (Figure 30.5).[2,62] A proteinaceous background sometimes contains small amounts of eosinophilic extracellular material and mild mixed inflammation with or without bacterial infection. Few to moderate, stellate to plump, uniform mesenchymal cells are present. It can be difficult to distinguish CAA from POF cytologically, especially if the epithelial component is prominent due to sample bias (Figure 30.7a and b). Additionally, POFs can have nests of basaloid epithelial cells that appear cytologically similar to CAA.[2,64,73,74] CAA must be differentiated from SCC, given that CAA samples often contain large numbers of hyperplastic squamous epithelial cells.[2,27] Differentiation of CAA from SCC can be challenging even histologically; however, positive calretinin staining supports a diagnosis of SCC.[27]

Rarely encountered epithelial odontogenic tumors include ameloblastoma and APOT.[61,75] Ameloblastomas originate from odontogenic epithelium, whereas CAAs develop from the epithelial rests of gingiva.[71] Cytologically, ameloblastoma and CAA appear similar, and histopathology is required for diagnosis; however, CAA is much more common.[62,63] APOTs are rare in dogs and cats and, given overlapping histologic features, might be classified as calcifying epithelial odontogenic tumor and keratinizing ameloblastoma.[61,71] These present as unencapsulated gingival masses similar to other odontogenic tumors in the dog, while in cats, it can mimic SCC or fibrosarcoma.[71,75] Based on histopathological description, these tumors would be expected to appear cytologically similar to a CAA with the presence of amyloid.[62,75]

POFs (sometimes incorrectly referred to as fibromatous epulis or ossifying epulis) are tumors arising from the tooth-forming mesenchyme or periodontal ligament. These are slow-growing firm masses that can displace teeth, but, in contrast to CAAs, do not destroy bone. They are often epithelialized and located in the gingival tissues, more commonly in the rostral maxilla (Figure 30.4c–f).[61,73] Radiographically, they have a non-aggressive appearance with minimal bone loss. Multiple POFs can occur in cats as generalized, firm, multilobulated, non-ulcerated masses of the mandibular and maxillary gingiva.[76] Cytology is characterized by low to moderate cellularity, consisting of few well-differentiated elongated mesenchymal cells (Figure 30.6). Scattered plump spindloid cells can also be present and rarely predominate. Common concurrent processes are mild mixed inflammation and squamous epithelial hyperplasia. Mineral, cholesterol crystals, and scant eosinophilic extracellular material are seen in the background.[2] It is challenging to use cytology to distinguish POF from other similar mesenchymal lesions (FFH, fibroma, fibrosarcoma) and from CAA because POF can also contain odontogenic epithelium (Figure 30.7c and d).[2,73,74] In general, the appearance of eosinophilic extracellular material is more supportive of a mesenchymal origin lesion; however, CAAs also can contain similar material that further complicates cytologic differentiation.[2,73] Misdiagnosis of inflammation or epithelial hyperplasia is possible if the mesenchymal component is underrepresented.[2] Clinical history, gross appearance, and radiographic findings can support a probable diagnosis in these cases. On intraoral radiographs, non-odontogenic tumors are more commonly associated with external inflammatory tooth resorption compared with odontogenic tumors.[77] However, histopathology is required for definitive diagnosis.

Odontogenic tumors of mixed (both mesenchymal and epithelial components) origin include odontoma and feline inductive odontogenic tumor (FIOT). Given that these lesions occur most commonly in the jaw, they will be discussed below.

Lingual Lesions

Lingual lesions occur infrequently. Neoplasia is most common, followed by glossitis, then calcinosis circumscripta.[78–80] Most neoplasms are malignant and include melanoma, SCC, hemangiosarcoma, and

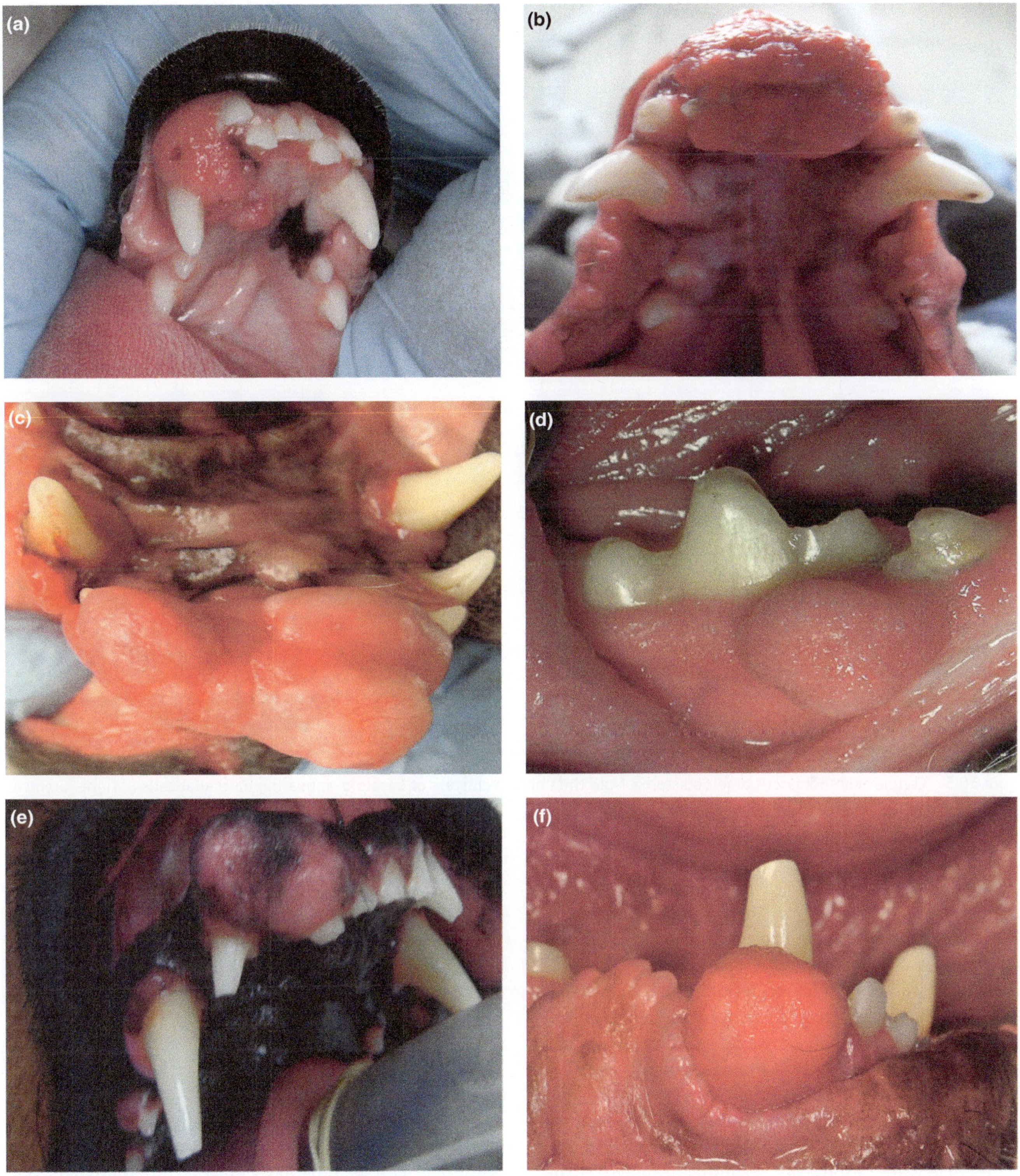

Figure 30.4 Gross photos of common odontogenic tumors. (a and b) Canine acanthomatous ameloblastoma (CAA). These masses have a predilection for the mandibular incisor and premolar regions, often displace the surrounding teeth, and are locally invasive. (c–f) Canine peripheral odontogenic fibroma (POF). Masses are firm, are located in the gingival tissues primarily in the rostral maxilla, and do not invade bone.

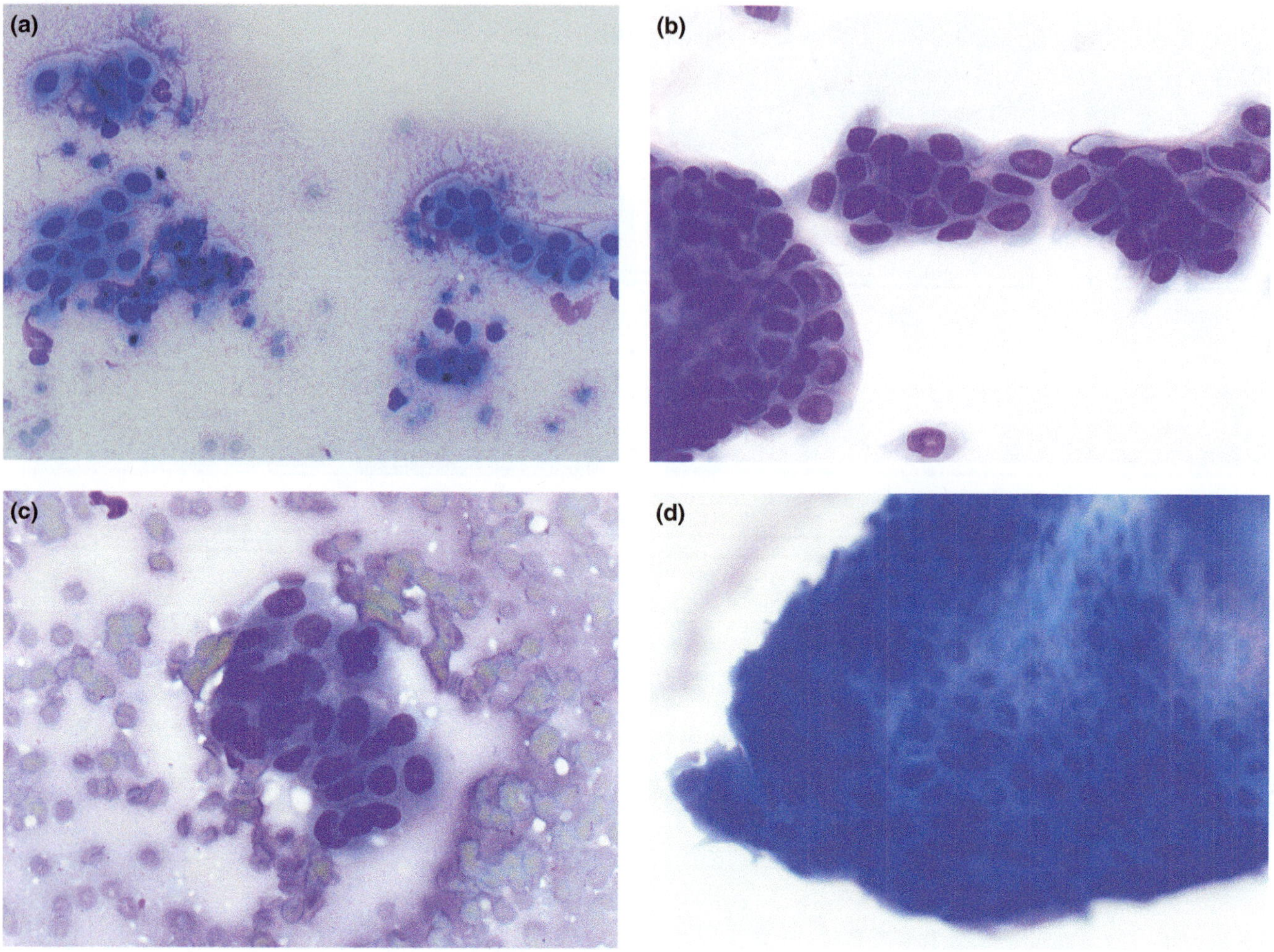

Figure 30.5 Canine acanthomatous ameloblastoma. Note the uniform clusters of basaloid-appearing epithelial cells (Wright–Giemsa, (a) 400×, (b) 500×, (c) 500×, (d) 600×).

fibrosarcoma.[30,71,80–83] Benign tumors include squamous papilloma, granular cell tumor, and plasmacytoma.[80,83] Rarely reported tumors include dermoid cyst, adenocarcinoma, fibroma, liposarcoma, peripheral nerve sheath tumor, hemangioma, rhabdomyoma, rhabdomyosarcoma, osteoma, and lymphoma.[83–98] Cytologic findings are similar to those noted in other locations.

Granular cell tumors are most common at the base of the tongue in older dogs but can occur on the gingiva, lips, and palate.[99] They are rare in cats.[99] Tumors are raised, firm, red, granular, or smooth masses that are white on cut section.[100] Cytology consists of large epithelioid cells with acidophilic granular cytoplasm, a central to eccentric nucleus, and 1–2 nucleoli.[71,100–106] Positive staining with periodic acid–Schiff, cytokeratin, S-100, vimentin, and neuron-specific enolase is reported.[99,100,107]

The cause of glossitis is often not identified, but trauma, infectious agents, foreign bodies, ulcers, eosinophilic granulomas, reactive histiocytosis, and trauma (bite wounds, electrical burns, and caustic agents) have been implicated.[78–80,108] Infectious causes include bacteria (*Pasteurella multocida*), viruses (feline calicivirus, feline herpesvirus-1, canine calicivirus, canine distemper), mycoses (*Candida* spp.), and *Leishmania,* resulting in nodular, papular, or ulcerative lesions.[78,80,108–114] Granulomatous inflammation associated with leishmaniasis must be differentiated from neoplasia and eosinophilic granuloma.[113,115] Lingual ulcers can be associated with uremia, an exaggerated response to tooth plaque (contact mucosal ulceration), and the viruses mentioned above. Uremic ulcers also appear as necrosis or generalized sloughing.[78] Though often nondiagnostic, cytology can demonstrate a proteinaceous background,

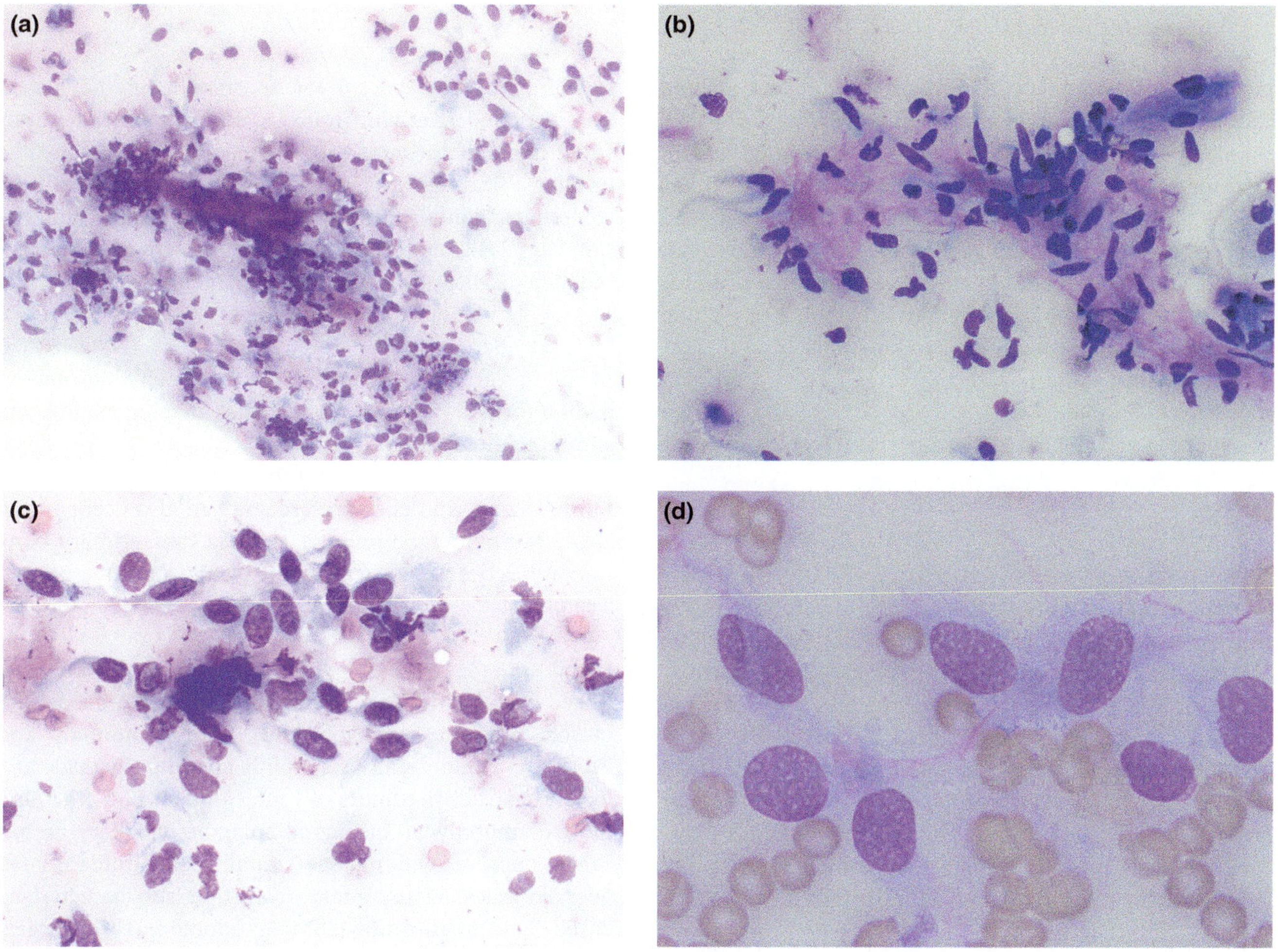

Figure 30.6 Canine peripheral odontogenic fibroma (POF). Note aggregates of well-differentiated mesenchymal cells often associated with extracellular eosinophilic material (Wright–Giemsa, (a) 100×, (b) 400×, (c) 500×, (d) 1000×).

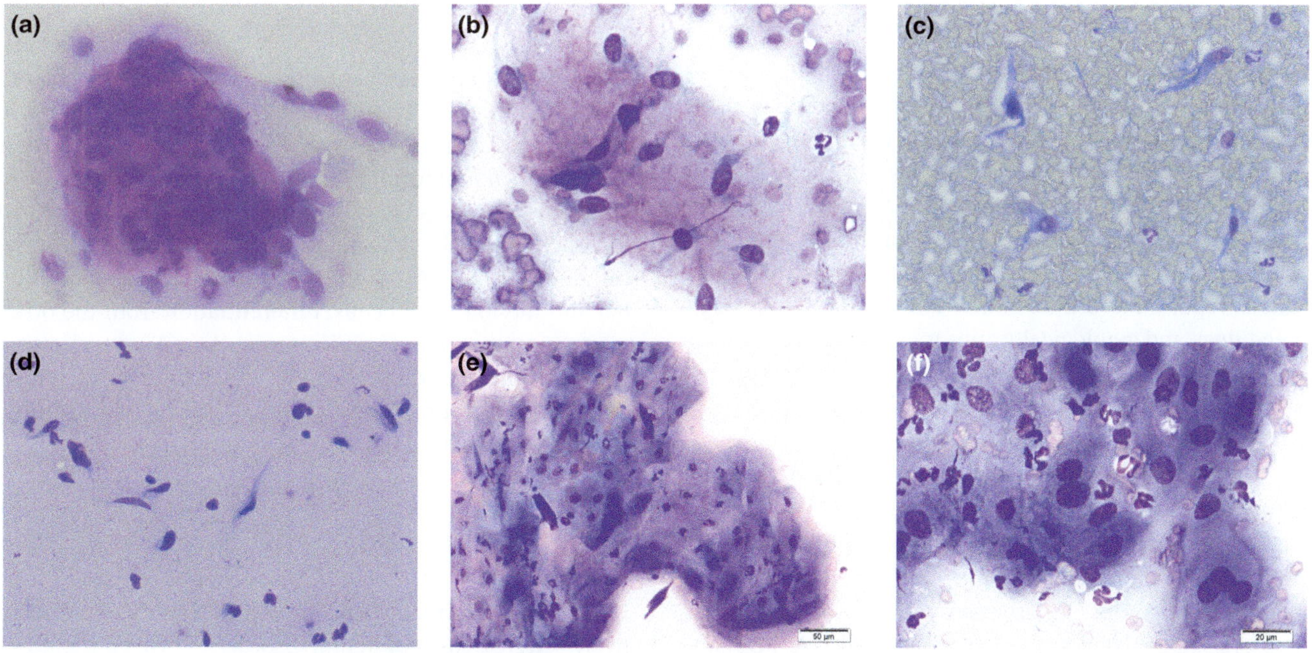

Figure 30.7 Common oral cytology diagnostic dilemmas. Because of cytologic similarities, care must be taken when differentiating between (a) canine peripheral odontogenic fibroma (POF) and (b) canine acanthomatous ameloblastoma with aspiration of an area of periodontal ligament, between (c) resident mesenchymal cells and (d) low-grade fibrosarcoma, and between (e) gingival hyperplasia and (f) well-differentiated squamous cell carcinoma (Wright–Giemsa, (a, b, and f) 500×, (c–e) 200×).

mixed inflammation including lymphocytes and plasma cells, and squamous and mesenchymal hyperplasia.[2]

Calcinosis circumscripta (CC) is a syndrome of ectopic calcium salt deposition manifesting as solitary nodular lesions and is reportedly more common in young, male, large-breed dogs.[80] CC can be dystrophic (trauma, foreign body reaction, neoplasia), metastatic, idiopathic, or iatrogenic.[116–120] Cytologic characteristics include a basophilic background with mineral, foamy macrophages, and giant cells.[118] Positive staining with alizarin red S and von Kossa stain are supportive.[118]

Tonsil

Tonsillar lesions are relatively uncommon and are similar to other lymphoid tissues (Chapter 27).[71] Lymphoid hyperplasia is common.[71] Tonsillitis can occur as part of a general oral condition, in response to a foreign body in the tonsillar crypts, or from infection with agents such as *Listeria monocytogenes*.[121] SCC and lymphoma are common.[15,71,82,122–124] The tonsillar region of cats should be routinely examined for SCC since tumors can be difficult to visualize and can be an incidental finding on oral examination with early disease.[124] Rarely reported benign lesions include cysts and lymphangiomatous or inflammatory polyps.[71,125,126]

Mandibular and Maxillary Bone Lesions

Inflammation

Osteomyelitis is associated with severe periodontal disease, un-sutured extraction sites, foreign material that penetrated the mucosa and bone, and rarely with *Cryptococcus* spp. infections.[12,127] Cytology samples are moderately to highly cellular, consisting of mixed inflammatory cells, few mesenchymal cells with variable morphology, and rare osteoblasts and osteoclasts.[2] Mandibular periostitis ossificans is reported as a mandibular swelling in young large-breed dogs and cytologically appears as serosanguinous or cyst-like fluid.[128]

Hyperplasia and Neoplasia

Epithelial

Odontogenic cysts include any cyst arising from the tooth tissue and are not well described in the veterinary literature.[129] Dentigerous, inflammatory, and neoplasia-associated cysts, associated with tumors such as CAA, POF, and FIOT, are possible.[130–133] Clinically, they often appear as a swelling in the oral cavity with smooth, epithelialized, non-ulcerated overlying mucosa. Radiographically, cysts show regional lucency within the mandible or maxilla. Cytologic findings are generic, except that epithelial cells sometimes contain fine magenta cytoplasmic granulation.[134,135] Histology and advanced imaging are recommended for diagnosis and treatment planning.[136]

Mesenchymal

Maxillofacial osteosarcoma is less common than appendicular forms.[9,29,137–139] Cytologic and imaging features are similar to those reported elsewhere (Chapter 23). However, bone lysis is also seen with other tumors such as CAA.[2] Fibrosarcoma and chondrosarcoma can also occur in the jaw.[29] Multilobular tumor of bone, a rare primary bone tumor, has been reported to cytologically appear similar to a sarcoma.[140]

Mixed

Mixed tumors affecting the jaw include odontoma, ameloblastic fibroma, ameloblastic fibro-odontoma, and FIOT.[141–145] Odontomas are rapidly growing expansile and locally destructive tumors of young animals and are found most commonly in the mandibular or maxillary arch.[71] These encapsulated masses contain fully differentiated dental tissues. Odontomas are further subcharacterized based on disorganization (complex odontoma) or organization into toothlike structures called denticles (compound odontoma).[62,64,71,146–148] Both ameloblastic fibro-odontoma and odontoma have some degree of tooth formation, whereas ameloblastic fibroma does not.[62,149] FIOT are rare locally invasive tumors generally located in the rostral maxilla of young cats.[60,62,71,142,150] In the author's experience, clinical appearance can be mistaken for an eosinophilic granuloma, decreasing the chances of curative surgical treatment and survival. A single cytology report identified monomorphic, tightly packed, columnar to cuboidal epithelial-like cells and individual spindle-shaped mesenchymal cells associated with an eosinophilic extracellular matrix.[151] As all of these tumors consist of epithelial and mesenchymal cells, differentiation from the other more common odontogenic tumors based on aspiration alone would be difficult.[2,71,142,150] Definitive diagnosis requires integration with clinical history, radiographic findings, and histopathology.

Equine Oral Lesions

Equine oral tumors are uncommon in a study of consecutively referred cases of dental disorders.[152] Given the infrequency of these lesions, the literature is minimal, and use of cytology in the diagnosis of equine oral lesions is almost nonexistent. Overall, similar lesions as in small animals occur with similar histopathological and cytological appearances. Inflammatory lesions include mandibular bone abscesses, trauma with granulation tissue, oral ulceration, and FFH.[153–157] The most commonly reported equine odontogenic tumors are ameloblastoma, cementoma, and odontoma.[158–166] Cementomas are of mesenchymal origin and are characterized by proliferation of cementoblasts and deposition of cementum-like matrix with collagen fibers around the tooth root.[167,168] All three present as firm to bony swellings in the upper or lower jaw, with ameloblastoma favoring the mandibular region, while cementoma and odontoma favor the maxillary cheek teeth or premaxilla.[167–169] Odontomas are more frequent in young horses, whereas ameloblastoma and cementoma tend to occur in older animals.[160,167,168] Rarely reported odontogenic tumors include mandibular odontoameloblastoma, ameloblastic fibro-odontoma, and odontogenic myxoma.[161,164,170] Non-odontogenic neoplasms reported in the equine oral cavity include SCC, sarcoid, melanoma, fibroma, fibrosarcoma, and hemangiosarcoma.[153,167,168,171–175] Peripheral nerve sheath tumors, mast cell tumors, lymphoma, choristomas, and malignant glomus tumor are rarely reported.[176–180] SCC is the most commonly documented and tends to behave aggressively in the equine oral cavity. Sarcoids appear as ulcerated subcutaneous nodules on the cheek or within the lips. Solitary oral sarcoids are rare, usually presenting with masses in other locations. Melanomas frequently occur on the lip but can be anywhere in the oral cavity.[12,68–168] Melanoma must be differentiated from granulomas (parasitic, foreign body, trauma, etc.) that appear grossly similar.[167,168] Oral fibroma and fibrosarcoma are most often noted along the maxillary cheek teeth and must be differentiated from other mesenchymal lesions such as granulation tissue, sarcoids, fibromatous epulis of periodontal ligament origin, and gingival fibrous hyperplasia.[71,181,182] Oral hemangiosarcoma in horses is malignant and often ulcerated, thus requiring differentiation from foreign body reactions, SCC, and *Gastrophilus* spp. ulcers.[71,171] Jaw lesions consist of bone cysts, hamartomas, ossifying fibromas, metastatic carcinoma, osteosarcoma, undifferentiated sarcoma, leiomyosarcoma, and lymphoma.[153,182–194] Tongue lesions include SCC, adenocarcinoma, rhabdomyosarcoma, mast cell tumor, lymphoma, and chondrosarcoma.[71,190,195–198]

Conclusions

Cytology of oral lesions can facilitate clinical management, especially in the case of malignant oral tumors such as melanoma and SCC. Cytology can aid in the diagnosis of odontogenic tumors; however, low cellularity and differentiation between subtypes can be difficult. Sampling bias and the frequent occurrence of secondary processes complicate interpretation. Given these cytologic challenges, there is often the need to incorporate a thorough clinical history, gross appearance, and imaging findings to arrive at a probable diagnosis. Biopsy is ultimately recommended in most cases for definitive diagnosis.

References

1. Niemiec, B.A. (2008). Oral pathology. *Top Companion Anim Med* 23: 59–71.
2. Schappa, J., Sharkey, L., Seelig, D. et al. (2014). Validation and optimization of cytology for the screening of oral lesions in dogs and cats. Proceedings of the 16th ESVCP Annual Congress, Milan, Italy (October 1–4, 2014).
3. Arzi, B. and Verstraete, F.J.M. (2012). Clinical staging and biopsy of maxillofacial tumors. In: *Oral and Maxillofacial Surgery in Dogs and Cats*, (eds. Verstraete, F.J.M., Lommer, M.J.), 373–380. Edinburgh: Saunders Elsevier.
4. Verstraete, F.J., Kass, P.H., and Terpak, C.H. (1998). Diagnostic value of full-mouth radiography in cats. *Am J Vet Res* 59: 692–695.
5. Verstraete, F.J., Kass, P.H., and Terpak, C.H. (1998). Diagnostic value of full-mouth radiography in dogs. *Am J Vet Res* 59: 686–691.
6. Lommer, M.J. (2013). Oral inflammation in small animals. *Vet Clin North Am Small Anim Pract* 43: 555–571.
7. Lewis, J.R. and Reiter, A.M. (2005). Management of generalized gingival enlargement in a dog case report and literature review. *J Vet Dent* 22: 160–169.
8. Sitzman, C. (2000). Simultaneous hyperplasia, metaplasia, and neoplasia in an 8 year-old boxer dog: a case report. *J Vet Dent* 17: 27–30.
9. Farcas, N., Lommer, M.J., Kass, P.H., and Verstraete, F.J. (2014). Dental radiographic findings in cats with chronic gingivostomatitis (2002–2012). *J Am Vet Med Assoc* 244: 339–345.
10. Tsugawa, A.J., Verstraete, F.J., Kass, P.H., and Görrel, C. (2003). Diagnostic value of the use of lateral and occlusal radiographic views in comparison with periodontal probing for the assessment of periodontal attachment of the canine teeth in dogs. *Am J Vet Res* 64: 255–261.
11. Anderson, J.G., Peralta, S., Kol, A. et al. (2017). Clinical and histopathologic characterization of canine chronic ulcerative stomatitis. *Vet Pathol* 54: 511–519.

12 Block, K. and Battig, J. (2017). Cryptococcal maxillary osteomyelitis and osteonecrosis in a 18-month-old dog. *J Vet Dent* 34: 76–85.

13 Jadhav, V.J. and Pal, M. (2006). Canine mycotic stomatitis due to *Candida albicans*. *Rev Iberoam Micol* 23: 233–234.

14 Madrid, I.M., Mattei, A.S., Fernandes, C.G. et al. (2012). Epidemiological findings and laboratory evaluation of sporotrichosis: a description of 103 cases in cats and dogs in southern Brazil. *Mycopathologia* 173: 265–273.

15 Levy, E., Mylonakis, M.E., Saridomichelakis, M.N. et al. (2006). Nasal and oral masses in a dog. *Vet Clin Pathol* 35: 115–118.

16 Bilgic, O., Duda, L., Sánchez, M.D., and Lewis, J.R. (2015). Feline oral squamous cell carcinoma: clinical manifestations and literature review. *J Vet Dent* 32: 30–40.

17 Stepaniuk, K., Legendre, L., and Watson, S. (2011). Acquired myasthenia gravis associated with oral sarcoma in a dog. *J Vet Dent* 28: 242–249.

18 Bredal, W.P., Gunnes, G., Vollset, I., and Ulstein, T.L. (1996). Oral eosinophilic granuloma in three cavalier King Charles spaniels. *J Small Anim Pract* 37: 499–504.

19 Buckley, L. and Nuttall, T. (2012). Feline eosinophilic granuloma complex(ities): some clinical clarification. *J Feline Med Surg* 14: 471–481.

20 Bloom, P.B. (2006). Canine and feline eosinophilic skin diseases. *Vet Clin North Am Small Anim Pract* 36: 141–160.

21 Pedersen, N.C. (1992). Inflammatory oral cavity diseases of the cat. *Vet Clin North Am Small Anim Pract* 22: 1323–1345.

22 Sykes, J.M., Garner, M.M., Greer, L.L. et al. (2007). Oral eosinophilic granulomas in tigers (*Panthera tigris*): a collection of 16 cases. *J Zoo Wildl Med* 38: 300–308.

23 Munday, J.S. (2014). Papillomaviruses in felids. *Vet J* 199: 340–347.

24 Munday, J.S., Thomson, N.A., and Luff, J.A. (2017). Papillomaviruses in dogs and cats. *Vet J* 225: 23–31.

25 Sundberg, J.P., Van Ranst, M., Montali, R. et al. (2000). Feline papillomas and papillomaviruses. *Vet Pathol* 37: 1–10.

26 Bonfanti, U., Bertazzolo, W., Gracis, M. et al. (2015). Diagnostic value of cytological analysis of tumours and tumour-like lesions of the oral cavity in dogs and cats: a prospective study on 114 cases. *Vet J* 205: 322–327.

27 Fulton, A., Arzi, B., Murphy, B. et al. (2014). The expression of calretinin and cytokeratins in canine acanthomatous ameloblastoma and oral squamous cell carcinoma. *Vet Comp Oncol* 12: 258–265.

28 Mestrinho, L.A., Pissarra, H., Carvalho, S. et al. (2017). Comparison of histological and proliferation features of canine oral squamous cell carcinoma based on intraoral location: 36 cases. *J Vet Dent* 34: 92–99.

29 Rejec, A., Butinar, J., Gawor, J., and Petelin, M. (2017). Evaluation of complete blood count indices (NLR, PLR, MPV/PLT, and PLCRi) in healthy dogs, dogs with periodontitis, and dogs with oropharyngeal tumors as potential biomarkers of systemic inflammatory response. *J Vet Dent* 34: 231–240.

30 Sabhlok, A. and Ayl, R. (2014). Palliative radiation therapy outcomes for cats with oral squamous cell carcinoma (1999–2005). *Vet Radiol Ultrasound* 55: 565–570.

31 Nemec, A., Murphy, B., Kass, P.H., and Verstraete, F.J. (2012). Histological subtypes of oral non-tonsillar squamous cell carcinoma in dogs. *J Comp Pathol* 147: 111–120.

32 Fulton, A.J., Nemec, A., Murphy, B.G. et al. (2013). Risk factors associated with survival in dogs with nontonsillar oral squamous cell carcinoma 31 cases (1990–2010). *J Am Vet Med Assoc* 243: 696–702.

33 Soltero-Rivera, M.M., Krick, E.L., Reiter, A.M. et al. (2014). Prevalence of regional and distant metastasis in cats with advanced oral squamous cell carcinoma: 49 cases (2005–2011). *J Feline Med Surg* 16: 164–169.

34 Stebbins, K.E., Morse, C.C., and Goldschmidt, M.H. (1989). Feline oral neoplasia: a ten-year survey. *Vet Pathol* 26: 121–128.

35 Ciekot, P.A., Powers, B.E., Withrow, S.J. et al. (1994). Histologically low-grade, yet biologically high-grade, fibrosarcomas of the mandible and maxilla in dogs: 25 cases (1982–1991). *J Am Vet Med Assoc* 204: 610–615.

36 Ghirelli, C.O., Villamizar, L.A., and Pinto, A.C. (2013). Comparison of standard radiography and computed tomography in 21 dogs with maxillary masses. *J Vet Dent* 30: 72–76.

37 Esplin, D.G. (2008). Survival of dogs following surgical excision of histologically well-differentiated melanocytic neoplasms of the mucous membranes of the lips and oral cavity. *Vet Pathol* 45: 889–896.

38 Liptak, J.M. and Withrow, S.J. (2007). Oral tumors: oral melanoma. In: *Withrow & MacEwen's Small Animal Clinical Oncology*, (eds. Withrow, S.J., Vail, D.M.), 4e, 455–475. St. Louis: Sounders Elsevier.

39 Ramos-Vara, J.A., Beissenherz, M.E., Miller, M.A. et al. (2000). Retrospective study of 338 canine oral melanomas with clinical, histologic, and immunohistochemical review of 129 cases. *Vet Pathol* 37: 597–608.

40 Sapierzynski, R., Malicka, E., Bielecki, W. et al. (2007). Oral tumors in dogs and cats: retrospective review of 143 cases. *Med Weter* 63: 1196–1199.

41 Smedley, R.C., Lamoureux, J., Sledge, D.G., and Kiupel, M. (2011). Immunohistochemical diagnosis of canine oral amelanotic melanocytic neoplasms. *Vet Pathol* 48: 32–40.

42 Smith, S.H., Goldschmidt, M.H., and McManus, P.M. (2002). A comparative review of melanocytic neoplasms. *Vet Pathol* 39: 651–678.
43 Kawabe, M., Mori, T., Ito, Y. et al. (2015). Outcomes of dogs undergoing radiotherapy for treatment of oral malignant melanoma: 111 cases (2006–2012). *J Am Vet Med Assoc* 247: 1146–1153.
44 Bradley, R.L., MacEwen, E.G., and Loar, A.S. (1984). Mandibular resection for removal of oral tumors in 30 dogs and 6 cats. *J Am Vet Med Assoc* 184: 460–463.
45 Ellis, A.E., Harmon, B.G., Miller, D.L. et al. (2010). Gingival osteogenic melanoma in two dogs. *J Vet Diagn Invest* 22: 147–151.
46 Kerr, M.E. and Burgess, H.J. (2013). What is your diagnosis? Gingival mass in a dog. *Vet Clin Pathol* 42: 115–116.
47 Oyamada, T., Tanaka, H., Park, C.H. et al. (2007). Pathology of canine oral malignant melanoma with cartilage and/or osteoid formation. *J Vet Med Sci* 69: 1155–1161.
48 Przeździecki, R., Czopowicz, M., and Sapierzyński, R. (2015). Accuracy of routine cytology and immunocytochemistry in preoperative diagnosis of oral amelanotic melanomas in dogs. *Vet Clin Pathol* 44: 597–604.
49 Wright, Z.M., Rogers, K.S., and Mansell, J. (2008). Survival data for canine oral extramedullary plasmacytomas: a retrospective analysis (1996–2006). *J Am Anim Hosp Assoc* 44: 75–81.
50 Smithson, C.W., Smith, M.M., Tappe, J. et al. (2012). Multicentric oral plasmacytoma in 3 dogs. *J Vet Dent* 29: 96–110.
51 Elliott, J.W., Cripps, P., Blackwood, L. et al. (2016). Canine oral mucosal mast cell tumours. *Vet Comp Oncol* 14: 101–111.
52 Hillman, L.A., Garrett, L.D., de Lorimier, L.P. et al. (2010). Biological behavior of oral and perioral mast cell tumors in dogs: 44 cases (1996–2006). *J Am Vet Med Assoc* 237: 936–942.
53 Pabilonia, K.L., Podell, B.K., and Powers, B.E. (2013). Pathology in practice. Mast cell tumor (MCT) of the oral mucosa with submandibular lymph node metastasis in a dog. *J Am Vet Med Assoc* 243: 795–797.
54 Berlato, D., Schrempp, D., Van Den Steen, N., and Murphy, S. (2012). Radiotherapy in the management of localized mucocutaneous oral lymphoma in dogs: 14 cases. *Vet Comp Oncol* 10: 16–23.
55 Bhang, D.H., Choi, U.S., Kim, M.K. et al. (2006). Epitheliotropic cutaneous lymphoma (mycosis fungoides) in a dog. *J Vet Sci* 7: 97–99.
56 Mineshige, T., Kawarai, S., Yauchi, T. et al. (2016). Cutaneous epitheliotropic T-cell lymphoma with systemic dissemination in a dog. *J Vet Diagn Invest* 28: 327–331.
57 Moore, P.F., Olivry, T., and Naydan, D. (1994). Canine cutaneous epitheliotropic lymphoma (mycosis fungoides) is a proliferative disorder of CD8+ T cells. *Am J Pathol* 144: 421–429.
58 Shiomitsu, K., Bauer, R.W., Grasperge, B.J. et al. (2012). Cutaneous epitheliotropic lymphoma with dual CD3 and c-kit expression in a dog. *Vet Clin Pathol* 41: 594–598.
59 Fontaine, J., Heimann, M., and Day, M.J. (2011). Cutaneous epitheliotropic T-cell lymphoma in the cat: a review of the literature and five new cases. *Vet Dermatol* 22: 454–461.
60 Bell, C.M. and Soukup, J.W. (2014). Nomenclature and classification of odontogenic tumors – Part 2: Clarification of specific nomenclature. *J Vet Dent* 31: 234–243.
61 Fiani, N., Verstraete, F.J., Kass, P.H., and Cox, D.P. (2011). Clinicopathologic characterization of odontogenic tumors and focal fibrous hyperplasia in dogs: 152 cases (1995–2005). *J Am Vet Med Assoc* 238: 495–500.
62 Gardner, D.G. (1992). An orderly approach to the study of odontogenic tumours in animals. *J Comp Pathol* 107: 427–438.
63 Gardner, D.G. (1996). Epulides in the dog: a review. *J Oral Pathol Med* 25: 32–37.
64 Verstraete, F.J., Ligthelm, A.J., and Weber, A. (1992). The histological nature of epulides in dogs. *J Comp Pathol* 106: 169–182.
65 Odom, T. and Anderson, J.G. (2000). Proliferative gingival lesion in a cat with disseminated cryptococcosis. *J Vet Dent* 17: 177–181.
66 Gracis, M., Molinari, E., and Ferro, S. (2015). Caudal mucogingival lesions secondary to traumatic dental occlusion in 27 cats: macroscopic and microscopic description, treatment and follow-up. *J Feline Med Surg* 17: 318–328.
67 Lewis, J.R. and Tsugawa, A.J. (2004). Gingival hyperplasia and granulation tissue associated with a feline dental resorptive lesion. *J Vet Dent* 21: 23–25.
68 Riehl, J., Bell, C.M., Constantaras, M.E. et al. (2014). Clinicopathologic characterization of oral pyogenic granuloma in 8 cats. *J Vet Dent* 31: 80–86.
69 Soukup, J.W. and Bell, C.M. (2014). Nomenclature and classification of odontogenic tumors – Part 1: Historical review. *J Vet Dent* 31: 228–232.
70 Desoutter, A.V., Goldschmidt, M.H., and Sánchez, M.D. (2012). Clinical and histologic features of 26 canine peripheral giant cell granulomas (formerly giant cell epulis). *Vet Pathol* 49: 1018–1023.
71 White, S.D. (1987). Diseases of the lips and oral cavity of domestic animals. *Clin Dermatol* 5: 190–201.
72 Goldschmidt, S.L., Bell, C.M., Hetzel, S., and Soukup, J. (2017). Clinical characterization of canine

acanthomatous ameloblastoma (CAA) in 263 dogs and the influence of postsurgical histopathological margin on local recurrence. *J Vet Dent* 34: 241–247.

73 Yoshida, K., Yanai, T., Iwasaki, T. et al. (1999). Clinicopathological study of canine oral epulides. *J Vet Med Sci* 61: 897–902.

74 Arzi, B., Murphy, B., Nemec, A. et al. (2011). Expression of cytokeratins in the epithelium of canine odontogenic tumours. *J Comp Pathol* 145: 345–351.

75 Bock, P., Hach, V., and Baumgärtner, W. (2011). Oral masses in two cats. *Vet Pathol* 48: 906–910.

76 Colgin, L.M., Schulman, F.Y., and Dubielzig, R.R. (2001). Multiple epulides in 13 cats. *Vet Pathol* 38: 227–229.

77 Nemec, A., Murphy, B.G., Jordan, R.C. et al. (2014). Oral papillary squamous cell carcinoma in twelve dogs. *J Comp Pathol* 150: 155–161.

78 Buelow, M.E., Marretta, S.M., Barger, A., and Lichtensteiger, C. (2011). Lingual lesions in the dog and cat: recognition, diagnosis, and treatment. *J Vet Dent* 28: 151–162.

79 Cornegliani, L., Gracis, M., Ferro, S. et al. (2011). Sublingual reactive histiocytosis in a dog. *J Vet Dent* 28: 164–170.

80 Dennis, M.M., Ehrhart, N., Duncan, C.G. et al. (2006). Frequency of and risk factors associated with lingual lesions in dogs: 1,196 cases (1995–2004). *J Am Vet Med Assoc* 228: 1533–1537.

81 Culp, W.T., Ehrhart, N., Withrow, S.J. et al. (2013). Results of surgical excision and evaluation of factors associated with survival time in dogs with lingual neoplasia: 97 cases (1995–2008). *J Am Vet Med Assoc* 242: 1392–1397.

82 Fidel, J., Lyons, J., Tripp, C. et al. (2011). Treatment of oral squamous cell carcinoma with accelerated radiation therapy and concomitant carboplatin in cats. *J Vet Intern Med* 25: 504–510.

83 Syrcle, J.A., Bonczynski, J.J., Monette, S., and Bergman, P.J. (2008). Retrospective evaluation of lingual tumors in 42 dogs: 1999–2005. *J Am Anim Hosp Assoc* 44: 308–319.

84 Baratt, R.M., Rawlinson, J., Roth-Johnson, L., and Jones, C.J. (2015). Lingual malignant peripheral nerve sheath tumor in a Chinese Pug dog. *J Vet Dent* 32: 165–172.

85 Brockus, C.W. and Myers, R.K. (2004). Multifocal rhabdomyosarcomas within the tongue and oral cavity of a dog. *Vet Pathol* 41: 273–274.

86 Burton, J.H., Powers, B.E., and Biller, B.J. (2014). Clinical outcome in 20 cases of lingual hemangiosarcoma in dogs: 1996–2011. *Vet Comp Oncol* 12: 198–204.

87 Chapman, S., Nabity, M., and Calise, D. (2008). What is your diagnosis? Lingual mass in a dog. *Vet Clin Pathol* 37: 133–139.

88 Fernandez, M., Grau-Roma, L., Roura, X., and Majó, N. (2012). Lingual osteoma in a dog. *J Small Anim Pract* 53: 480–482.

89 Harris, L.J., Rout, E.D., Hughes, K.L. et al. (2018). Clinicopathologic features of lingual canine T-zone lymphoma. *Vet Comp Oncol* 16: 131–139.

90 Lascelles, B.D., McInnes, E., Dobson, J.M., and White, R.A. (1998). Rhabdomyosarcoma of the tongue in a dog. *J Small Anim Pract* 39: 587–591.

91 Liptak, J.M., Canfield, P.J., and Hunt, G.B. (2000). Dermoid cyst in the tongue of a dog. *Aust Vet J* 78: 160–161.

92 Montinaro, V. and Boston, S.E. (2013). Tongue rotation for reconstruction after rostral hemiglossectomy for excision of a liposarcoma of the rostral quadrant of the tongue in a dog. *Can Vet J* 54: 591–594.

93 Piseddu, E., De Lorenzi, D., Freeman, K., and Masserdotti, C. (2011). Cytologic, histologic, and immunohistochemical features of lingual liposarcoma in a dog. *Vet Clin Pathol* 40: 393–397.

94 Rivera, R.Y. and Carlton, W.W. (1992). Lingual rhabdomyoma in a dog. *J Comp Pathol* 106: 83–87.

95 Romsland, T.D., Wills, T.B., Haldorson, G.J. et al. (2011). What is your diagnosis? Lingual mass in a dog. *Vet Clin Pathol* 40: 561–562.

96 Rütgen, B.C., Flickinger, I., Wolfesberger, B. et al. (2016). Cutaneous T-cell lymphoma: Sézary syndrome in a Boxer. *Vet Clin Pathol* 45: 172–178.

97 Schoofs, S.H. (1997). Lingual hemangioma in a puppy: a case report and literature review. *J Am Anim Hosp Assoc* 33: 161–165.

98 Thuilliez, C., Watrelot-Virieux, D., Chanut, F. et al. (2008). Presumed primary muscular lymphoma in a dog. *J Vet Diagn Invest* 20: 824–826.

99 Patnaik, A.K. (1993). Histologic and immunohistochemical studies of granular cell tumors in seven dogs, three cats, one horse, and one bird. *Vet Pathol* 30: 176–185.

100 Rallis, T.S., Tontis, D.K., Soubasis, N.H. et al. (2001). Immunohistochemical study of a granular cell tumor on the tongue of a dog. *Vet Clin Pathol* 30: 62–66.

101 Irizarry-Rovira, A.R., Lennox, A.M., and Ramos-Vara, J.A. (2008). Granular cell tumor in the testis of a rabbit: cytologic, histologic, immunohistochemical, and electron microscopic characterization. *Vet Pathol* 45: 73–77.

102 Liu, C.H., Liu, C.I., Liang, S.L. et al. (2004). Intracranial granular cell tumor in a dog. *J Vet Med Sci* 66: 77–79.

103 Mishra, S., Kent, M., Haley, A. et al. (2012). Atypical meningeal granular cell tumor in a dog. *J Vet Diagn Invest* 24: 192–197.

104 Rossi, G., Tarantino, C., Taccini, E. et al. (2007). Granular cell tumour affecting the left vocal cord in a dog. *J Comp Pathol* 136: 74–78.

105 Sharkey, L.C., McDonnell, J.J., and Alroy, J. (2004). Cytology of a mass on the meningeal surface of the left brain in a dog. *Vet Clin Pathol* 33: 111–114.

106 Spoor, M.S., Kim, D.Y., Kanazono, S. et al. (2013). What is your diagnosis? Impression smears of a cerebral mass from a dog. *Vet Clin Pathol* 42: 240–241.

107 Geyer, C., Hafner, A., Pfleghaar, S., and Hermanns, W. (1992). Immunohistochemical and ultrastructural investigation of granular cell tumours in dog, cat, and horse. *Zentralbl Veterinarmed B* 39: 485–494.

108 Lobprise, H.B. and Wiggs, R.B. (1993). Anatomy, diagnosis and management of disorders of the tongue. *J Vet Dent* 10: 16–23.

109 Blavier, A., Keroack, S., Denerolle, P. et al. (2001). Atypical forms of canine leishmaniosis. *Vet J* 162: 108–120.

110 Foglia Manzillo, V., Paparcone, R., Cappiello, S. et al. (2009). Resolution of tongue lesions caused by *Leishmania infantum* in a dog treated with the association miltefosine-allopurinol. *Parasit Vectors* 2 (1): S6.

111 Font, A., Roura, X., Fondevila, D. et al. (1996). Canine mucosal leishmaniasis. *J Am Anim Hosp Assoc* 32: 131–137.

112 Parpaglia, M.L., Vercelli, A., Cocco, R. et al. (2007). Nodular lesions of the tongue in canine leishmaniosis. *J Vet Med A Physiol Pathol Clin Med* 54: 414–417.

113 Tangalidi, M.K., Oikonomidis, I.L., Psalla, D. et al. (2016). Nodular granulomatous glossitis as the sole clinical sign in canine leishmaniosis. *Vet Clin Pathol* 45: 710–714.

114 Viegas, C., Requicha, J., Albuquerque, C. et al. (2012). Tongue nodules in canine leishmaniosis: a case report. *Parasit Vectors* 5: 120.

115 Saari, S., Rasi, J., and Anttila, M. (2000). Leishmaniosis mimicking oral neoplasm in a dog: an unusual manifestation of an unusual disease in Finland. *Acta Vet Scand* 41: 101–104.

116 Collados, J., Rodríguez-Bertos, A., Peña, L. et al. (2002). Lingual calcinosis circumscripta in a dog. *J Vet Dent* 19: 19–21.

117 Jeong, W., Noh, D., Kwon, O.D. et al. (2004). Calcinosis circumscripta on lingual muscles and dermis in a dog. *J Vet Med Sci* 66: 433–435.

118 Marcos, R., Santos, M., Oliveira, J. et al. (2006). Cytochemical detection of calcium in a case of calcinosis circumscripta in a dog. *Vet Clin Pathol* 35: 239–242.

119 Mouzakitis, E., Papazoglou, L.G., Loukopoulos, P.G. et al. (2015). Carbon dioxide laser excision of lingual calcinosis circumscripta in a dog. *J Vet Dent* 32: 177–179.

120 Tafti, A.K., Hanna, P., and Bourque, A.C. (2005). Calcinosis circumscripta in the dog: a retrospective pathological study. *J Vet Med A Physiol Pathol Clin Med* 52: 13–17.

121 Läikkö, T., Båverud, V., Danielsson-Tham, M.L. et al. (2004). Canine tonsillitis associated with *Listeria monocytogenes*. *Vet Rec* 154: 732.

122 Grant, J. and North, S. (2016). Evaluation of the factors contributing to long-term survival in canine tonsillar squamous cell carcinoma. *Aust Vet J* 94: 197–202.

123 Kanehara, T., Matsui, N., Murakami, M. et al. (2016). B-cell lymphoma with Mott cell differentiation in a cat. *Vet Clin Pathol* 45: 356–360.

124 Mas, A., Blackwood, L., Cripps, P. et al. (2011). Canine tonsillar squamous cell carcinoma: a multi-centre retrospective review of 44 clinical cases. *J Small Anim Pract* 52: 359–364.

125 Degner, D.A., Bauer, M.S., and Ehrhart, E.J. (1994). Palatine tonsil cyst in a dog. *J Am Vet Med Assoc* 204: 1041–1042.

126 Miller, A.D., Alcaraz, A., and McDonough, S.P. (2008). Tonsillar lymphangiomatous polyp in an adult dog. *J Comp Pathol* 138: 215–217.

127 Bell, C.M. and Soukup, J.W. (2015). Histologic, clinical, and radiologic findings of alveolar bone expansion and osteomyelitis of the jaws in cats. *Vet Pathol* 52: 910–918.

128 Blazejewski, S.W., Lewis, J.R., Gracis, M. et al. (2010). Mandibular periostitis ossificans in immature large breed dogs: 5 cases (1999–2006). *J Vet Dent* 27: 148–159.

129 Verstraete, F.J.M., Zin, B.P., Kass, P.H. et al. (2011). Clinical signs and histological findings in dogs odontogenic cysts: 41 cases (1995–2010). *J Am Vet Med Assoc* 239: 1470–1476.

130 Druet, M.S., Husson, J.C., Gaillot, H.A., and Arzi, B. (2017). Diagnostic imaging in veterinary dental practice. *J Am Vet Med Assoc* 251: 1139–1142.

131 Kuyama, K., Hayashi, K., Fufita, S.F. et al. (2009). Immunohistochemical analysis of a dentigerous cyst in a dog. *J Vet Dent* 26: 106–109.

132 LaDeuceur, E.E., Walker, K.S., Mohr, F.C., and Murphy, B. (2014). Odontogenic keratocyst in a cat. *J Comp Pathol* 151: 212–216.

133 Tjepkema, J., Soukup, J.W., and Bell, C. (2017). Suspected lateral periodontal cyst presenting concurrently with canine acanthomatous ameloblastoma in a 2-year-old Standard Poodle. *J Vet Dent* 34: 141–147.

134 McEntire, M.C., Rigas, J.D., Farnsworth, R.K. et al. (2015). What is your diagnosis? Oral soft tissue and cystic lesion in a dog. *Vet Clin Pathol* 44: 327–328.

135 Singh, S., Garg, N., Gupta, S. et al. (2011). Fine needle aspiration cytology in lesions of oral and maxillofacial region: diagnostic pitfalls. *J Cytol* 28: 93–97.

136 Vicari, E.D., Stepaniuk, K., and Goldstein, G. (2014). Diagnostic imaging in veterinary dental practice. *J Am Vet Med Assoc* 245: 889–891.

137 Coyle, V.J., Rassnick, K.M., Borst, L.B. et al. (2015). Biological behaviour of canine mandibular osteosarcoma. A retrospective study of 50 cases (1999–2007). *Vet Comp Oncol* 13: 89–97.

138 Farcas, N., Arzi, B., and Verstraete, F.J. (2014). Oral and maxillofacial osteosarcoma in dogs: a review. *Vet Comp Oncol* 12: 169–180.

139 Selmic, L.E., Ryan, S.D., Ehrhart, N.P., and Withrow, S.J. (2013). Bilateral appendicular bone tumors in four dogs. *J Am Anim Hosp Assoc* 49: 135–141.

140 McCartney, J. (1997). What is your diagnosis? Mass on the hard palate of a dog. *Vet Clin Pathol* 26: 70.

141 Boyd, R.C. (2002). Ameloblastic fibro-odontoma in a German shepherd dog. *J Vet Dent* 19: 148–150.

142 Gardner, D.G. and Dubielzig, R.R. (1995). Feline inductive odontogenic tumor (inductive fibroameloblastoma)-a tumor unique to cats. *J Oral Pathol Med* 24: 185–190.

143 Gardner, D.G. (1998). Ameloblastomas in cats: a critical evaluation of the literature and the addition of one example. *J Oral Pathol Med* 27: 39–42.

144 Miles, C.R., Bell, C.M., Pinkerton, M.E., and Soukup, J.W. (2010). Maxillary ameloblastic fibroma in a dog. *Vet Pathol* 48: 823–826.

145 Nyska, A. and Dayan, D. (1995). Ameloblastic fibroma in a young cat. *J Oral Pathol Med* 24: 233–236.

146 Head, K.W., Else, R.W., and Dubielzig, R.R. (2002). Tumors of the alimentary tract. In: *Tumors in Domestic Animals*, (ed. Meuten, D.J.), 4e, 402–407. Ames, IA: Iowa State Press.

147 Poulet, F.M., Valentine, B.A., and Summers, B.A. (1992). A survey of epithelial odontogenic tumors and cysts in dogs and cats. *Vet Pathol* 29: 369–380.

148 Sowers, J.M. and Gengler, W.R. (2005). Diagnosis and treatment of maxillary compound odontoma. *J Vet Dent* 22: 26–34.

149 Gardner, D.G. (1996). Ameloblastic fibromas and related tumors in cattle. *J Oral Pathol Med* 25: 119–124.

150 Beatty, J.A., Charles, J.A., Malik, R. et al. (2000). Feline inductive odontogenic tumour in a Burmese cat. *Aust Vet J* 78: 452–455.

151 Leite-Filho, R.V., Tagliari, N.J., Grandi, F. et al. (2017). Cytologic features of a feline inductive odontogenic tumor. *Vet Clin Pathol* 46: 516–519.

152 Dixon, P.M., Tremaine, W.H., Pickles, K. et al. (2000). Equine dental disease. Part 3: A long-term study of 400 cases: disorders of wear, traumatic damage and idiopathic fractures, tumours and miscellaneous disorders of the cheek teeth. *Equine Vet J* 32: 9–18.

153 Dixon, P.M. and Dacre, I. (2005). A review of equine dental disorders. *Vet J* 169: 165–187.

154 Handy, L.H., Peyton, L.C., Calderwood-Mays, M.B., and Ackerman, N. (1993). Focal gingival hyperplasia in a horse. *J Am Vet Med Assoc* 202: 1287–1288.

155 Rodrigues, J.B., Requicha, J.F., Bastos, E. et al. (2015). Focal gingival hyperplasia in a donkey (*Equus asinus*). *J Vet Dent* 32: 54–56.

156 Smyth, G.B. (1991). Bone abscess in the mandible of a quarter horse gelding. *Cornell Vet* 81: 239–243.

157 Vengust, M., Baird, J.D., van Dreumel, T. et al. (2008). Equid herpesvirus 2-associated oral and esophageal ulceration in a foal. *J Vet Diagn Invest* 20: 811–815.

158 Brounts, S.H., Hawkins, J.F., Lescun, T.B. et al. (2004). Surgical management of compound odontoma in two horses. *J Am Vet Med Assoc* 225: 1423–1427.

159 De Cock, H.E., Labelle, P., and Magdesian, K.G. (2003). Ameloblastic carcinoma in a horse. *J Comp Pathol* 128: 210–215.

160 Gardner, D.G. (1994). Ameloblastomas in the horse: a critical review and report of an additional example. *J Oral Pathol Med* 23: 41–44.

161 Knowles, S., Blas-Machado, U., Butler, A.M. et al. (2010). Ameloblastic fibro-odontoma associated with a retained molar in an Oldenburg mare. *J Vet Diagn Invest* 22: 987–990.

162 Lingard, D.R. and Crawford, T.B. (1970). Congenital ameloblastic odontoma in a foal. *Am J Vet Res* 31: 801–804.

163 Mendez-Angulo, J.L., Tatarniuk, D.M., Ruiz, I., and Ernst, N. (2014). Extensive rostral mandibulectomy for treatment of ameloblastoma in a horse. *Vet Surg* 43: 222–226.

164 Murphy, B., Bell, C., Koehne, A., and Dubielzig, R.R. (2017). Mandibular odontoameloblastoma in a rat and a horse. *J Vet Diagn Invest* 29: 536–540.

165 Roberts, M.C., Groenendyk, S., and Kelly, W.R. (1978). Ameloblastic ondontoma in a foal. *Equine Vet J* 10: 91–93.

166 Rosol, T.J., Nagode, L.A., Robertson, J.T. et al. (1994). Humoral hypercalcemia of malignancy associated with ameloblastoma in a horse. *J Am Vet Med Assoc* 204: 1930–1933.

167 Knottenbelt, D.C., Patterson-Kane, J.C., and Snalune, K.L. (2015). Bone and dental region neoplasms. In: *Clinical Equine Oncology*, (eds. Knottenbelt, D.C., Patterson-Kane, J.C., and Snalune, K.L.), 323–329. Edinburgh: Elsevier.

168 Knottenbelt, D.C., Patterson-Kane, J.C., and Snalune, K.L. (2015). Tumours of the alimentary tract and abdominal cavity. In: *Clinical Equine Oncology*, (eds. Knottenbelt, D.C., Patterson-Kane, J.C., and Snalune, K.L.), 430–436. Edinburgh: Elsevier.

169 Kreutzer, R., Wohlsein, P., Staszyk, C. et al. (2007). Dental benign cementomas in three horses. *Vet Pathol* 44: 533–536.

170 Chandra, A.M., Buergelt, C.D., and Ethell, M.T. (1999). Odontogenic myxoma of the mandible in a filly. *J Vet Diagn Invest* 11: 274–277.

171 Dunkel, B.M., Del Piero, E., Kraus, B.M. et al. (2004). Congenital cutaneous, oral, and periarticular hemangiosarcoma in a 9-day-old Rocky Mountain horse. *J Vet Intern Med* 18: 252–255.

172 Faragalla, F. (2002). Oral squamous cell carcinoma in a pregnant mare. *J Vet Dent* 19: 86–87.

173 Orsini, J.A., Nunamaker, D.M., Jones, C.J., and Acland, H.M. (1991). Excision of oral squamous cell carcinoma in a horse. *Vet Surg* 20: 264–266.

174 Pérez, J., Mozos, E., Martín, M.P., and Day, M.J. (1999). Immunohistochemical study of the inflammatory infiltrate associated with equine squamous cell carcinoma. *J Comp Pathol* 121: 385–397.

175 Schuh, J.C. (1986). Squamous cell carcinoma of the oral, pharyngeal and nasal mucosa in the horse. *Vet Pathol* 23: 205–207.

176 Oikawa, M., Ohishi, H., Katayama, Y. et al. (2003). Extranodal lymphoblastic lymphoma of suspected B-cell lineage in the gingiva of a racehorse, accompanied by mandibular osteolysis. *J Vet Med A Physiol Pathol Clin Med* 50: 151–155.

177 Peters, M., Grafen, J., Kuhnen, C., and Wohlsein, P. (2016). Malignant glomus tumour (glomangiosarcoma) with additional neuroendocrine differentiation in a horse. *J Comp Pathol* 154: 309–313.

178 Seeliger, F., Hess, O., Pröpsting, M.J. et al. (2007). Confocal laser scanning analysis of an equine oral mast cell tumor with atypical expression of tyrosine kinase receptor C-KIT. *Vet Pathol* 44: 225–228. Erratum in: *Vet Pathol* 2007; 44: 427.

179 Snook, E.R. and Wakamatsu, N. (2011). Diagnostic exercise: oral tumor in an aged mare. *Vet Pathol* 48: 785–787.

180 Steinbach, T.J., Reischauer, A., Kunkemöller, I., and Mense, M.G. (2004). An oral choristoma in a foal resembling hairy polyp in humans. *Vet Pathol* 41: 698–700.

181 Horbal, A. and Dixon, P.M. (2016). Gingival fibrosarcoma in a horse. *J Vet Dent* 33: 243–248.

182 Pirie, R.S. and Dixon, P.M. (1993). Mandibular tumours in the horse: a review of the literature and 7 case reports. *Equine Vet Educ* 5: 287–294.

183 Bush, J.M., Fredrickson, R.L., and Ehrhart, E.J. (2007). Equine osteosarcoma: a series of 8 cases. *Vet Pathol* 44: 247–249.

184 Camus, A.C., Burba, D.J., Valdes, M.A., and Taylor, H.W. (1996). Intraosseous epidermoid cyst in a horse. *J Am Vet Med Assoc* 209: 632–633.

185 Carmalt, J.L. and Linn, K.A. (2013). Large segmental mandibulectomy for treatment of an undifferentiated sarcoma in a horse. *Vet Surg* 42: 433–439.

186 David, F., Levingstone, T.J., Schneeweiss, W. et al. (2015). Enhanced bone healing using collagen-hydroxyapatite scaffold implantation in the treatment of a large multiloculated mandibular aneurysmal bone cyst in a thoroughbred filly. *J Tissue Eng Regen Med* 9: 1193–1199.

187 Greet, T.R., Boys Smith, S.J., and Steven, W.N. (2011). Mandibular lymphoma in a three-year-old thoroughbred filly. *Vet Rec* 168: 80.

188 MacGillivray, K.C., Graham, T.D., and Parente, E.J. (2003). Multicentric leiomyosarcoma in a young male horse. *J Am Vet Med Assoc* 223: 1017–1021, 986.

189 Morse, C.C., Saik, J.E., Richardson, D.W., and Fetter, A.W. (1988). Equine juvenile mandibular ossifying fibroma. *Vet Pathol* 25: 415–421.

190 Rhind, S.M. and Dixon, P.M. (1999). T cell-rich B cell lymphosarcoma in the tongue of a horse. *Vet Rec* 145: 554–555.

191 Richardson, D.W., Evans, L.H., and Tulleners, E.P. (1991). Rostral mandibulectomy in five horses. *J Am Vet Med Assoc* 199: 1179–1182.

192 Robbins, S.C., Arighi, M., and Ottewell, G. (1996). The use of megavoltage radiation to treat juvenile mandibular ossifying fibroma in a horse. *Can Vet J* 37: 683–684.

193 Stenberg, T., Dowling, B.A., and Dart, A.J. (2004). Mandibular bone cysts in two horses. *Aust Vet J* 82: 417–418.

194 Weber, A., Ligthelm, A.J., and Verstraete, F.J. (1991). Primary intra-osseous carcinoma of the maxilla in a horse. *J Comp Pathol* 104: 443–448.

195 Castleman, W.L., Toplon, D.E., Clark, C.K. et al. (2011). Rhabdomyosarcoma in 8 horses. *Vet Pathol* 48: 1144–1150.

196 Hanson, P.D., Frisbie, D.D., Dubielzig, R.R., and Markel, M.D. (1993). Rhabdomyosarcoma of the tongue in a horse. *J Am Vet Med Assoc* 202: 1281–1284.

197 Laus, F., Rossi, G., Paggi, E. et al. (2014). Adenocarcinoma involving the tongue and the epiglottis in a horse. *J Vet Med Sci* 76: 467–470.

198 Wilson, G.J. and Anthony, N.D. (2007). Chondrosarcoma of the tongue of a horse. *Aust Vet J* 85: 163–165.

31

Esophagus and Stomach

Marian Taulescu, Irina Amorim, and Robert Washabau

Introduction

The esophagus and stomach undergo cytologic examination relatively infrequently. Cytologic examination of endoscopic specimens is a reliable adjunct to mucosal biopsy for the diagnosis of esophageal and gastric diseases because results correlate highly with histologic observations.[1] Several techniques for gastric and esophageal sampling are utilized.[2] Gastric brush cytology is more sensitive in identifying superficial changes and infections (e.g. *Helicobacter* spp.) in dogs and cats, while endoscopic ultrasound-guided fine-needle aspirate (FNA) cytology is extensively used for diagnosis of deep gastric lesions.[3,4] Erosive reflux esophagitis, nonspecific gastritis, gastric malignant epithelial neoplasia, and gastric lymphoma are often diagnosed by cytological examination in dogs and cats.[5–7] In horses, granulomatous and ulcerative parasitic gastritis and gastric squamous carcinoma are more common than other gastroesophageal conditions.[8,9]

The primary purpose of this chapter is to describe the cytological features of normal tissues and pathological conditions of the esophagus and stomach in dogs, cats, and horses. The advantages and disadvantages of sampling techniques, morphological features of numerous specific esophageal and gastric infectious organisms, and additional diagnostic tests are also discussed.

Sample Collection

Endoscopic Exfoliative Cytology

Cytological specimens should be collected after mucosal biopsy, using both brush and touch techniques.[10] Brushing is a safe, inexpensive, rapid, and accurate way to detect bacteria.[10] Gastric brush cytology is more sensitive than urease testing or histopathology in identifying *Helicobacter* spp. in dogs and cats.[3] Endoscopic brushings are limited by only sampling the epithelial surface. Multiple cytologic imprints can be performed by placing the tissue sample between a second glass slide and applying light pressure.

Ultrasound-Guided FNA

Recent advances in equipment and technical ability have made ultrasound a viable method for evaluation of gastrointestinal diseases.[11] In both inflammatory and neoplastic conditions, gastric wall thickening is the most common finding.[12] Endoscopic ultrasound-guided FNA cytology combined with a histologic evaluation of cell blocks provides accurate and efficient tissue diagnosis of a wide variety of deeply seated gastric lesions.[4] However, nondiagnostic samples can occur due to low cellularity (18% in one study of dogs and cats) or necrosis.[13] Agreement between histologic and cytologic diagnoses is lower for FNA (72%) than for impression smears of samples collected during surgery or necropsy (94%).[13]

Laparoscopy and Abdominal Exploration

Surgical collection has the advantage of full-thickness sampling, allowing examination of deep tissue layers. Cytologies are prepared by rolling or touching tissue on a slide before it is preserved in formalin, being sure to avoid disruption of the histopathology sample or contamination of the cytology sample by formalin fumes. The disadvantages are those inherent to the surgical procedure and to the invasive sampling technique.[2]

Gastric Reflux Cytology

This is a method used in horses to evaluate fluid obtained via nasogastric tube. A direct smear is air-dried, stained routinely, and examined microscopically.[14]

Veterinary Cytology, First Edition. Edited by Leslie C. Sharkey, M. Judith Radin, and Davis Seelig.

Normal Histology and Cytology

Esophagus

The esophagus is a tubular organ consisting of mucosa, submucosa, muscularis externa, and serosa. The mucosa is lined by nonkeratinizing stratified squamous epithelium in carnivores and is keratinized in large animals. In horses, this epithelium extends throughout the nonglandular portion of the gastric mucosa. The submucosa contains branched tubuloalveolar seromucous glands. In dogs, the glands occur the entire length of the esophagus, while in other species they are restricted to the cranial third.[15]

Cytologically, squamous cells vary from large, flat, irregular to angular with abundant, lightly basophilic or eosinophilic cytoplasm and small, pyknotic or absent nuclei (superficial layers) to small, rounded cells with moderate deeply basophilic cytoplasm and medium-sized central nucleus (deep layers). Intermediate and superficial squamous cells and rare basal cells can be seen. Deeper specimens contain numerous small, round, and intensely basophilic parabasal cells and scattered submucosal glandular cells.[16] Oropharyngeal contamination is common in esophageal samples, consisting of mixed oral flora, particularly *Simonsiella* spp. (Chapter 30), and respiratory epithelial cells.[2]

Stomach

The stomach wall is composed of mucosa, muscularis mucosa, submucosa, muscularis externa, and serosa. The stomach is lined with glandular and absorptive mucosa. The glandular region is composed of cardia, fundus, corpus, antrum, and pylorus. In horses, a nonglandular component is covered with keratinized stratified squamous epithelium extending from the esophagus to the *margo plicatus*. The glandular mucosa is lined by a simple columnar epithelium of surface mucous cells.[17]

The cardia contains tubular glands composed of mucus-secreting cells with rare neuroendocrine cells. The glands of the fundic region contain surface mucous, neck mucous, parietal, chief, and neuroendocrine cells.[18] Rare stem cells are represented by a few low columnar cells with high nuclear to cytoplasmic ratios (N:C) and lack of granules. The gastric antrum has few parietal or chief cells but contains a separate population of alkaline, mucus-producing cells near the base of gland units. G cells are more numerous in the middle portion of the gastric glands of the antrum; their round nuclei are centrally located in the cell.[19] The fundic glandular epithelium contains chief and parietal cells. The former are smaller and polygonal and contain granular light basophilic cytoplasm. The latter are larger and have a pyramidal shape and granular lightly eosinophilic or vacuolated cytoplasm. Both occur in cytology samples of deeper mucosal tissue.

Normal gastric cytology specimens contain superficial, mucus-secreting epithelial cells in monomorphic honeycomb sheets with clearly defined cell borders. These columnar cells have round to oval basal nuclei and abundant lightly basophilic to eosinophilic finely granular cytoplasm. A luminal mucin vacuole can be present. Variable amounts of mucus manifest as large extracellular coarse globules with variable staining characteristics.

Parietal and chief cells may be present in gastric cytology samples collected from brushing techniques. Fragments of ingesta, oropharyngeal flora, and squamous epithelial cells can be observed.[20]

Conditions Diagnosed by Cytology

Focal masses or increased wall thickness identified by ultrasonography or endoscopy are the most common indications to perform cytological examination of aspirates, impression smears, and brushings.

Esophagus

Hyperplasia

Reactive/Reparative Changes of the Mucosa

In chronic esophageal injuries, squamous cells occur in cohesive sheets with uniform karyomegaly, vesicular chromatin, and prominent nucleoli. Mitotic figures can occur with scattered inflammatory cells.[21]

Esophageal Columnar Cell Metaplasia

Columnar-lined distal esophagus (intestinal metaplasia) represents a progressive replacement of the squamous epithelium with patches of columnar to goblet cells. Experimentally induced and spontaneous lesions have been described in dogs and cats associated with chronic reflux esophagitis.[22] With gastroduodenal esophageal reflux of acid and bile, regenerating epithelium is columnar.[23] Cytologic specimens contain clusters of benign columnar cells and goblet cells with squamous cells.[21] Histologically, metaplastic goblet cells stained intensely with periodic acid-Schiff (PAS) and Alcian blue (pH 2.5).[22] Immunohistochemistry reveals increased homeobox gene CDX2 expression during transformation of distal esophageal squamous mucosa to columnar cells.[24] In humans, this condition is known as Barrett's esophagus and can progress to distal esophageal adenocarcinoma.[25]

Leukoplakia

Leukoplakia (epidermoid metaplasia) is an uncommon condition characterized by solitary or multiple elevated white plaques. Esophageal and gastric leukoplakia has been described in a foal with a history of intensive antibiotic and phenylbutazone therapy. The esophageal mucosa contained many raised white plaques up to 6.0 cm diameter.[26] Plaques were characterized by hyperorthokeratosis with a granular cell layer very similar to normal epidermis. In humans, lesions are often associated with gastric reflux, tobacco smoking, and alcohol consumption and are considered a predisposing factor for squamous cell carcinoma (SCC).[27]

Neoplasia

Esophageal cancer is rare and accounts for less than 0.5% of all cancers in the dog and cat.[28]

Benign

Adenomatous Polyps Progression of esophageal intestinal metaplasia to adenomatous polyp has been reported in a dog with painful swallowing.[22] Histologically, the normal epithelium overlying the mass was replaced by papillary projections covered by columnar epithelium with goblet cells. The columnar epithelial cells had moderately eosinophilic cytoplasm and oval, hyperchromatic, tightly packed basal nuclei.[22] No cytologic findings were described.

Esophageal Papillomas Esophageal tumors associated with papillomavirus infection are rare in dogs, cats, and horses. Canine oral papillomavirus, usually type 1, typically causes transient oral papillomas, which can also develop in the pharynx and esophagus as soft, flat, whitish nodules, several millimeters in diameter, becoming pedunculated or cauliflower-like formations.[29] Cytologically, there is a mild to moderate cellularity resembling normal squamous epithelial cells, possibly containing koilocytes (Chapter 30).

Leiomyomas Leiomyomas most commonly occur in dogs, involve the distal esophagus or gastric cardia, and are associated with chronic regurgitation and megaesophagus. These solitary or multiple tumors occur in the submucosa, usually are covered by intact mucosa, and are diagnosed by FNA (Chapter 22).[30]

Extramedullary Plasmacytomas These caudal esophageal lesions have a good prognosis in dogs and cats. The cytology of esophageal plasma cell neoplasms is similar to plasma cell neoplasia in other sites (Chapter 14).

Malignant

Primary malignant esophageal tumors are rare and include SCC, mesenchymal and lymphoid tumors, and adenocarcinoma of esophageal glands.

Squamous Cell Carcinoma As the most aggressive tumor of the esophageal epithelium in dogs, cats, and horses, SCC most often affects the middle and distal esophagus. Local invasiveness and regional lymphoid metastasis are typical of esophageal SCC. Cellular morphology varies from well differentiated to anaplastic, similar to other sites (Chapter 12). Well-differentiated SCC can be misinterpreted as squamous hyperplasia, but increased cellular atypia and asynchrony of nuclear and cytoplasmic differentiation support a diagnosis of malignancy (Figure 31.1). Poorly differentiated SCC contains smaller, less differentiated cells than other subtypes.[31] Ulcerated tumors have an extensive inflammatory reaction with neutrophils. Neoplastic cells can be binucleated or multinucleated with emperipolesis.[8]

Other Carcinomas Adenosquamous carcinoma has been described in a Japanese cat with regurgitation.[32] Histologic features of both adenocarcinoma and SCC were present. Tubular and glandular neoplastic cells stained positively with anti-cytokeratin antibody.[32] Esophageal adenocarcinoma arising from esophageal glands or from sites of Barrett's esophagus and neuroendocrine carcinoma is uncommon in animals with similar features as those found in other organs. Scirrhous adenocarcinoma of the

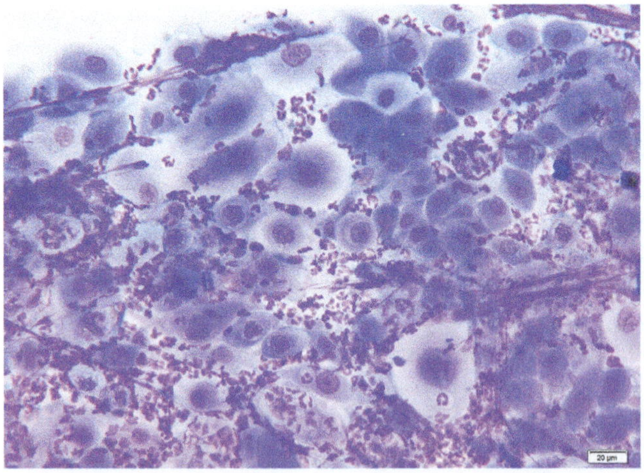

Figure 31.1 Cytology from an esophageal mass in a 10-year-old mixed breed dog with a squamous cell carcinoma. Clusters of neoplastic epithelial cells with asynchronous differentiation are accompanied by large numbers of neutrophils and emperipolesis (Diff-Quik, bar = 20 μm).

esophageal glands associated with hypertrophic osteopathy has been reported in an 8-year-old Irish setter.[33] The cytological features of these lesions were not reported.

Sarcomas Esophageal leiomyosarcomas are more common in dogs and are circumscribed, uniform masses that can infiltrate the wall. Imprint cytology reveals low to moderate numbers of spindle-shaped cells with variably distinct cell borders, occasionally eosinophilic granules, variably N:C, and elongated, blunted, or cigar-shaped nuclei (Chapter 16). Cellular pleomorphism is more prominent than in benign tumors. Submucosal biopsies are required to determine tumor grade.[34]

Esophageal angioleiomyosarcoma was reported in a cat with regurgitation and weight loss.[35] Examination of the smears of the mass lesion revealed a low number of dense clusters of cells with basophilic cytoplasm, spindle-shaped nuclei, minimal anisokaryosis, and finely stippled chromatin. Histologically, the mass was compatible with a spindle cell tumor with a prominent vasoformative component. Immunohistochemistry was positive for α-smooth muscle actin and von Willebrand factor protein and negative for CD117/c-kit protein.[35]

Canine esophageal fibrosarcomas (FSA), osteosarcomas (OSA), and undifferentiated sarcomas arising from granulomatous esophagitis (see "esophageal inflammation") are commonly induced by *Spirocerca lupi*.[36] The tumors are large, protrude into the lumen, and are pedunculated, nodular, or infiltrative with a fibrous or bony consistency. Proper surgical treatment prolongs quality and quantity of life.[36] It is very difficult to cytologically differentiate malignant from benign nodules from *S. lupi*-related esophageal lesions, which resemble FSA and OSA elsewhere in the body.

Other Neoplasms The esophagus can be compressed and infiltrated by extraluminal masses, particularly mediastinal lymphoma or thymoma (Chapter 29). Metastatic lesions are rare in dogs and cats and include thyroid, pulmonary, and gastric carcinomas.[37]

Inflammatory

Noninfectious

The most common causes of ulcerative esophagitis are chemicals, thermal and traumatic injuries (Figure 31.2a), medication retention within the esophageal lumen, and gastroesophageal reflux, usually occurring during anesthesia.[6]

Gastroesophageal reflux secondary to chronic and intermittent vomiting is common in dogs and cats, sometimes causing reflux esophagitis due to the effects of gastric acid, pepsin, bile salts, and pancreatic enzymes.[38] Reflux esophagitis associated with gastrinomas has been described in dogs.[39] Reflux can occur with diminished gastroesophageal sphincter function, preanesthetic agents, or abnormalities of the hiatus. Horses with gastrointestinal motility disorders and ulcerative gastritis commonly develop reflux esophagitis. Endoscopy reveals hyperemia, increased vascularity, ulcers, and erosion, particularly in the distal portion.[40] Transmural changes and esophageal stricture

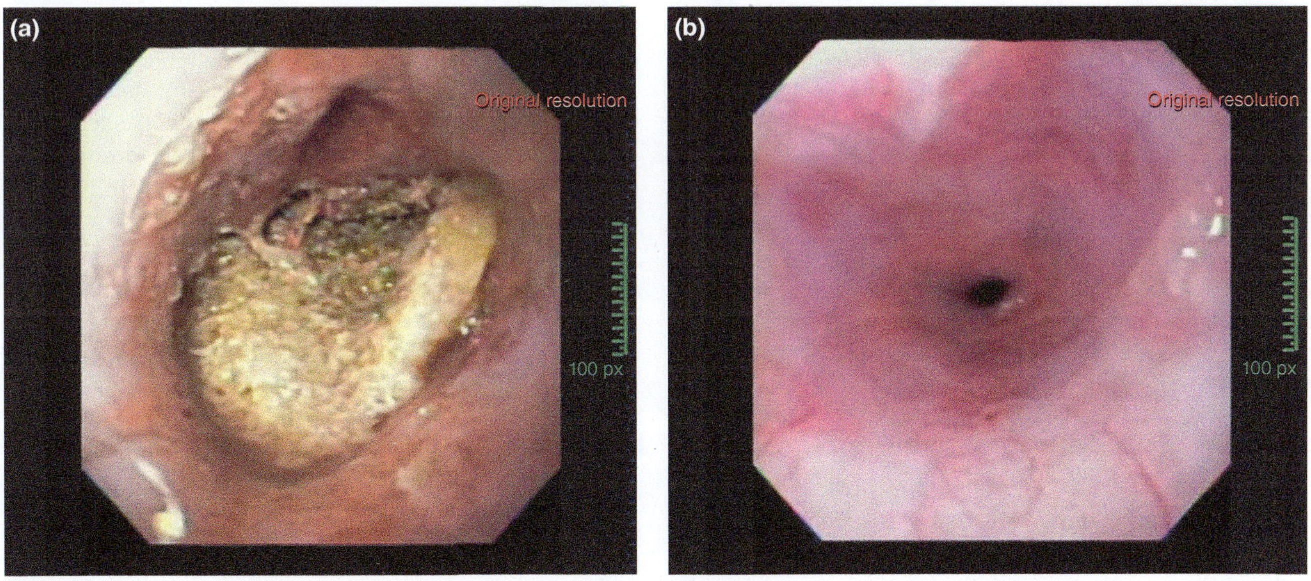

Figure 31.2 (a) Esophageal endoscopy examination in a dog showing an esophageal foreign body with extensive mucosal necrosis and ulceration. (b) Esophageal endoscopy examination in a dog showing a severe circumferential esophageal stricture.

(Figure 31.2b) can occur. Cytology brushing reveals inflammatory cells and squamous epithelial cells, often with columnar or goblet-like morphology (mucous metaplasia) with regenerative changes including enlarged nuclei and prominent nucleoli. Histology is characterized by squamous hyperplasia and dysplasia, erosions, ulcers, lymphocytes, plasma cells, and neutrophils.[40] Gastroesophageal reflux causes Barrett's esophagus with replacement of the distal esophageal squamous epithelium with metaplastic columnar epithelium.[23]

Primary eosinophilic esophagitis has been reported only in a single dog with a history of atopy.[41] Ulcerative lesions were characterized cytologically by many neutrophils and eosinophils and fewer lymphocytes and macrophages in mucus. Histology revealed severe diffuse eosinophilic and neutrophilic ulcerative esophagitis.[41] Eosinophilic esophagitis can accompany eosinophilic gastroenteritis, hypereosinophilic syndrome, mycotic infection, chronic reflux esophagitis, and neoplasia.[42]

Infectious

Herpetic esophagitis in a foal with ulcerative lesions was attributed to equine herpesvirus type 2 based on nuclear inclusions and immunohistochemistry.[43] Calicivirus is another suggested cause of necroulcerative viral esophagitis.

Candida albicans is normal flora of the genital, alimentary, and upper respiratory tract.[44] Immunodeficiency states, prolonged antimicrobial therapy, inanition, proton pump inhibitors, gastric reflux, and diabetes predispose to esophageal candidiasis (thrush).[45,46] A fragile pseudomembrane is characteristic, and brushing cytology is more sensitive than biopsy for diagnosis. Cytology reveals numerous budding yeast and pseudohyphae with cell debris, neutrophils, and regenerative squamous cells (Chapter 3). Gomori's methenamine silver staining is necessary for a definitive diagnosis.[47]

Dysphagia associated with transmural pyogranulomatous and ulcerative esophagitis due to *Pythium insidiosum* infection has been reported in dogs. Large numbers of inflammatory cells, predominately neutrophils, eosinophils, and few macrophages, were observed cytologically.[48] Numerous poorly stained 4–8 μm wide short branching hyphae with infrequent septae are seen. Culture, enzyme-linked immunosorbent assay, immunohistochemistry, or polymerase chain reaction are required to confirm.[49] Systemic infection with *Lagenidium* spp. involving the distal esophagus was identified in dogs.[50] Histology is similar to pythiosis and zygomycosis and is characterized by severe eosinophilic granulomatous inflammation around broad (7–25 μm), infrequently septate hyphae.

Visceral leishmaniasis with acute esophageal necrosis has been described in a dog.[51] The esophageal mucosa was dark and thickened circumferentially with hemorrhage and multifocal ulceration. Severe esophageal necrosis with mixed inflammation and numerous phagocytized amastigotes consistent with *Leishmania chagasi* were observed.[51]

S. lupi is a tropical and subtropical nematode parasite of dogs. Adult forms usually encyst within the wall of the thoracic esophagus, and multiple worm-containing granulomas occur at this level. Adult nematodes can protrude from ulcerations in the esophageal lumen. The male worm is reddish and approximately 6.1 cm long; females are bright red and 10.2 cm in length.[52] Cytology contains nondegenerate neutrophils and activated macrophages with mucus, debris, and scattered small (30 × 15 mm) oval nematode eggs with thick capsules and smooth or longitudinally folded surfaces.[53] Histopathologically, esophageal pyogranulomas with many plasma cells and lymphocytes are surrounded by abundant fibrous tissue. Mesenchymal tumors including FSA and OSA can result.

In horses, *Gasterophilus* spp. larvae can temporarily attach to the distal esophageal mucosa adjacent to the cardia.[54] Chronic ulcerative lesions and occasional esophageal fistula can develop at attachment sites.

Stomach

Hyperplastic and Metaplastic Conditions

Mucous metaplasia and hyperplasia involve mainly the fundus of the stomach and is often associated with chronic inflammation. Mucous metaplasia was reported in dogs with simple diffuse or atrophic forms of gastritis.[55] Cytologic diagnosis of gastric mucosal hyperplasia is suggested by increased mucosal secretory cells with abundant diffuse secretory granules.[31] For confirmation, histopathological analysis is required. Histologically, parietal and chief cells are replaced by foveolar mucus-like cells with retained nuclear polarity and abundant pale eosinophilic cytoplasm. The lamina propria is infiltrated with lymphocytes and plasma cells.[56]

Gastric polyps (GPs) are single or multiple epithelial lesions, projecting above the mucosal surface into the gastric lumen, and are classified either as nonneoplastic (hyperplastic/regenerative and inflammatory) or neoplastic lesions.[57] The hyperplastic polyps consist of elongated, tortuous, and branching foveolae, while inflammatory polyps are characterized by a normal epithelium covering granulation tissue that is infiltrated by mixed inflammatory cells.[58] Nonneoplastic GPs are rare, usually affecting older animals. Possible hereditary predisposition in French bulldogs and an association with chronic gastritis and *Helicobacter* spp. infection have been reported.[58,59] Hyperplastic and inflammatory polyps are cytologically undistinguishable. Cytological findings of GPs are similar to those from gastric ulcer margins, including reparative glandular epithelium with inflammatory cells and necrotic debris. The epithelial cells are uniform and resemble normal gastric epithelial cells, so endoscopic verification of a polypoid lesion is required. In horses, inflammatory and hyperplastic GPs can reach considerable size (14–20 cm long) and cause colic from pyloric and duodenal obstruction.[60,61]

Neoplastic

Benign

Gastric adenomas (adenomatous polyps) are rare benign neoplastic epithelial lesions mainly found in the canine pylorus and defined as circumscribed polyps composed of tubular and/or villous structures lined by dysplastic epithelium.[56,57] Multiple gastric adenomatous polyps are also reported in a bitch, one of which exhibited focal atypia suggestive of malignant transformation.[62] Gastric pyloric adenomatous polyps are also described in horses.[63] Cytology is of limited utility to discriminate between hyperplastic and benign neoplastic lesions because all are characterized by moderate amounts of normal-appearing gastric epithelial cells or minimal atypia.

Gastric leiomyomas are very common in older dogs, arising as single or multiple indolent submucosal masses usually protruding into the lumen.[56] They are typically incidental and rarely cause clinical signs unless ulcerated or causing mechanical obstruction. Gastric leiomyomas were found in two horses as large solitary masses arising from the tunica muscularis of the squamous portion of the stomach. Neither mass infiltrated the gastric serosa nor metastasized.[64] The neoplastic cells of leiomyomas are oval or spindle-shaped and exhibit a thin, elongated cigar-shaped nuclei (Figure 31.3a).[65]

Malignant

Among domestic animals, the highest incidence of gastric cancer is in the dog, accounting for 1% of all reported neoplasms, and it is less frequent in cats.[57,66] Gastric cancer constitutes about 1.5% of equine neoplasms.[67]

Gastric carcinomas often induce localized or diffuse thickening and/or ulceration of the gastric wall, serosal pallor, and reduced rugal folds. In horses, the risk of developing gastric adenocarcinoma is low.[64] However, a unique presentation of a gastric adenocarcinoma with metastasis in the liver and in portal vein caused hepatic encephalopathy in a mare.[68]

FNA has limited value due to poor exfoliation of these lesions.[69] Neoplastic gastric epithelial cells cluster tightly and are large with a round nucleus, one or two prominent nucleoli, and granular cytoplasm (Figure 31.3b).[70] Typical criteria of malignancy include high N:C, marked anisokaryosis, coarse chromatin, and large nucleoli. Occasionally, neoplastic epithelial cells can appear lymphoid. Desmoplasia can result in scattered fibroblasts. Cytoplasmic microvacuolation and/or signet ring cells are strong indicators of malignancy.[71]

Canine gastric mucinous adenocarcinoma with splenic and cutaneous metastases was diagnosed with ultrasound-guided FNA. The tumor was composed of both small cells

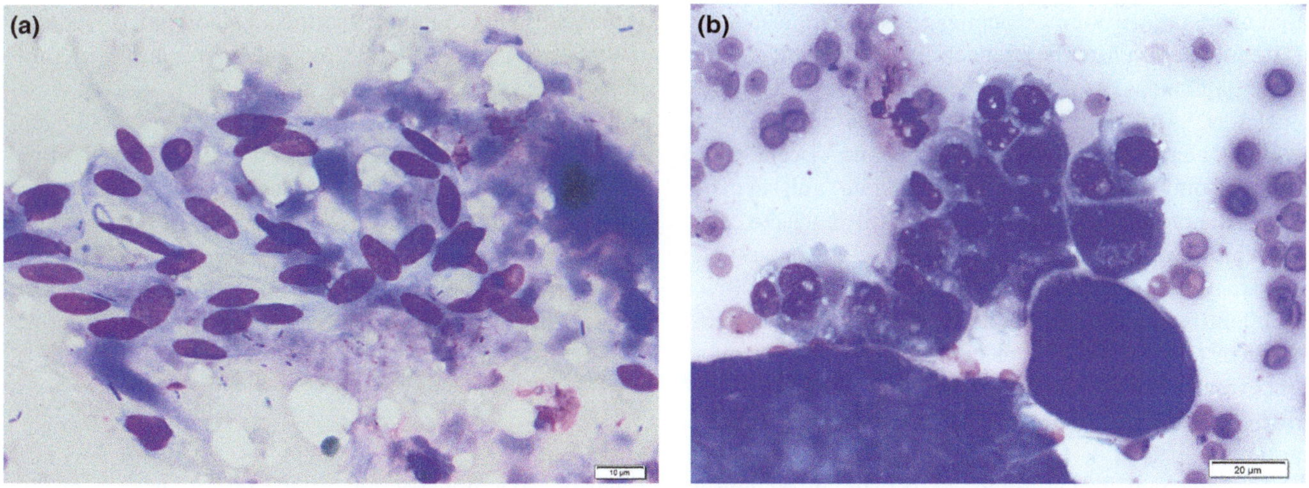

Figure 31.3 (a) Cytology from a gastric (cardia) submucosal leiomyoma in a 16-year-old dog. The neoplastic cells are spindle-shaped with pale blue cytoplasm. The nuclei are elongated and cigar-shaped. There is mild to moderate nuclear atypia (Diff-Quik, bar = 10 µm). (b) Aspirate of a gastric adenocarcinoma from a dog. The large clusters of neoplastic cells exhibiting marked anisocytosis and anisokaryosis, fine cytoplasmic vacuolation, large nuclei, and visible nucleoli suggest a malignant epithelial process. Cells with similar cytological features were found in the gastric lymph nodes (Wright's, bar = 20 µm).

in nests and acinar structures and large histiocytic-like cells with abundant granular to foamy eosinophilic cytoplasm in amorphous eosinophilic extracellular PAS positive material.[72]

SCC is the most common primary gastric neoplasm in horses, accounting for approximately 20% of all equine tumors.[73] It usually occurs as a single ulcerated mass in the nonglandular stomach associated with weight loss and anorexia.[64] Tumors can infiltrate the gastric serosal surface, causing adhesions between the stomach and diaphragm.[73] Metastases can affect the intestine, omentum, liver, and spleen. Gastric brush biopsy or lavage samples shows similar features to esophageal SCC.[8]

Neuroendocrine carcinomas (gastric carcinoids) are rare in dogs and cats, arising from dispersed neuroendocrine cells.[74] In dogs and cats, the gastrointestinal tract is the most common site for development of these tumors.[75] Neuroendocrine cells are loosely cohesive with many free round to oval nuclei with fine chromatin and occasional nucleoli, embedded in a background of pale cytoplasm with indistinct cell margins.[70] Some tumors have basophilic intracytoplasmic granules that can be highlighted with special argyrophilic stains or electron microscopy. Confirmation of histogenesis requires an immunohistochemical panel composed of synaptophysin and chromogranin A.[76]

Mesenchymal tumors originate in the connective tissue of the stomach and generally conform to the cytologic patterns described in Chapter 16. FNA can result in low cellularity; however, impression smears increased the detection of mesenchymal neoplasms from about 44 to 100%.[13]

In contrast to leiomyomas, leiomyosarcomas are more frequent in the intestine, reaching substantial size, with diffuse infiltration into the stomach. Two dogs with gastric leiomyosarcomas developed hepatic and one splenic metastases.[5] An equine gastric leiomyosarcoma extended to the esophagus and involved the hepatic visceral surface.[77] Leiomyosarcomas display moderate anisocytosis and anisokaryosis with mitotic figures. Multinucleate cells and necrosis also suggest malignancy. Leiomyomas and well-differentiated leiomyosarcomas are strongly positive for vimentin, smooth muscle actin, and desmin.[78] A rare variant of a canine gastric pleomorphic leiomyosarcoma was characterized by marked nuclear atypia, high mitotic index, and low immunoreactivity for these common markers.[65]

Gastrointestinal stromal tumors (GIST) are infrequently recognized in the stomach of dogs, and a feline gastric GIST was cytologically diagnosed.[79,80] Smears are highly cellular, containing tight aggregates of spindle-shaped cells with elongated nuclei and sparse delicate and wispy cytoplasm. DOG1 and CD117/KIT immunomarkers are strongly recommended for confirmation of canine GISTs.[81] Only one of 11 equine GISTs was located in the pyloric region of the stomach without metastasis.[82] Equine GISTs share the immunohistochemical profile of canine GISTs, represented by vimentin and CD117/KIT reactivity.[83]

Lymphoma can be present in the stomach of dogs and cats alone or with intestinal involvement (Chapter 32).[69,84] Solitary gastric lymphomas are predominantly large B-cell lymphoblastic tumors and can originate from gastric mucosal-associated lymphoid tissue (MALT).[85] In cats, gastric lymphomas are associated with *Helicobacter* spp. infection.[7] Affected tissue is diffusely thickened, with prominent rugae or a discrete nodular appearance.[86] Small cell gastric lymphoma can be difficult to differentiate from severe lymphocytic inflammation or inflammatory bowel disease based on cytology. A case of equine gastric lymphoma in the submucosa and muscular layers of the stomach with lymph node involvement is described.[64] Further details on the classification and diagnosis of lymphoma can be found in Chapter 27. Gastric plasmacytomas are occasional in dogs and rare in cats and horses. Gastric extramedullary plasmacytoma associated with nonspecific gastrointestinal signs are described in dogs and cats. Cytology is often diagnostic; morphologic details can be found in Chapter 14.[87,88]

Primary gastric mast cell tumors (MCTs) are less frequent in dogs than cats; however, they have been documented, particularly in miniature breeds.[89,90] The gastric mucosa can be tan-colored, thickened, with a nodular or irregular appearance, and ulcerated. Pretreatment with antihistamines is advised prior to aspiration.[91] The cytological features are variable but often characterized by a population of round cells with variable amounts of small purple-staining cytoplasmic granules that exhibit metachromasia with toluidine blue stain. Eosinophils and scattered mesenchymal cells can be present. Mucosal ulceration is often present and usually associated with tumor cell infiltration.[89] Mitotic activity, giant nuclei, or multinucleated giant cells are more frequent in mucosal MCTs. Metastases to the lymph nodes, liver, or spleen at the time of diagnosis is expected. Immunohistochemical staining for c-kit and mast cell tryptase can be used to confirm the nature of the tumor.[89] Differentiation from gastrointestinal eosinophilic sclerosing fibroplasia in cats must be considered.

Inflammatory

Gastritis is a nonspecific inflammatory process of the mucosa resulting from variety of causes. Normal endoscopic appearance of gastric mucosa does not exclude inflammation, but endoscopic visualization of an inflamed area corroborates the cytologic presumption of gastritis.

Infectious

In the stomach of dogs and cats, spiral-shaped organisms are often recognized cytologically with or without inflammation. As mentioned above, brush cytology can gather larger amounts of mucus and superficial epithelial cells, increasing the possibility of identifying *Helicobacter* spp. When present, these bacteria are easily seen entrapped in mucus and between scattered cellular debris, measuring at least as long as the diameter of an erythrocyte. The number of organisms is highly variable, but special stains such as Warthin-Starry or modified Giemsa stain can facilitate identification (Figure 31.4a). Immunohistochemistry using polyclonal antibody against *Helicobacter pylori* may show immunoreactivity with a wide range of organisms belonging to the *Helicobacter* genus (Figure 31.4b). To exclude this infection, at least 10 oil immersion fields in two slides should be analyzed before the specimen is considered negative.[10]

Gastric candidiasis in association with ulceration was diagnosed in five foals with signs of colic, nonresponsive to medical treatment.[92]

P. insidiosum is an aquatic oomycete responsible for gastric pythiosis mainly in dogs, horses and humans, being rare in cats. Cytologically, inflammatory aggregates primarily of neutrophils and eosinophils occur with elongated, thick-walled, sparsely septate, and irregularly branched hyphae (Figure 31.5) in a basophilic proteinaceous background.[93] A singular case of severe multifocal pyogranulomatous gastritis caused by *P. insidiosum* and pulmonary pyogranulomatous pneumonia due to *Blastomyces dermatitidis* was described in 4-year-old Labrador Retriever.[94] Hyphae are 3–5 μm wide and up to 200 μm long. PAS or Gomori methenamine silver and immunohistochemistry using anti-*Pythium* antibodies can be useful.[94]

Histoplasma capsulatum infection is acquired via inhalation or ingestion of infective conidia, which are phagocytosed by macrophages and can be systemically disseminated hematogenously or by lymphatics to many tissues, including the gastrointestinal system in dogs, cats, and horses (Chapter 3).[95,96]

Gastric parasites are uncommon but can be identified endoscopically. Associated inflammation consists of numerous eosinophils and variable numbers of neutrophils. Parasites are seldom observed.[31] Nematodes affecting the proximal gastrointestinal tract of domestic cats include *Cylicospirura* spp., *Ollulanus tricuspis*, *Aonchotheca putorii*, and *Physaloptera preputialis*.[97–100] *Cylicospirura* spp. infection is associated with gastric nodule formation. Cytologically, samples are sparsely cellular with a fine necrotic background and mixed inflammation composed of eosinophils, degenerate neutrophils, and reactive mesenchymal cells. Ovoid, thick-shelled embryonated eggs are approximately 45 μm long and 15 μm wide.[97] *O. tricuspis* feline gastric infection has worldwide distribution and is generally accompanied by chronic inflammation, hypertrophic gastritis, and fibrosis.[101] Endoscopic gastric fluid samples can contain 0.75 mm long microfilariae.

In dogs, gastric infestation by the nematode larvae *S. lupi*, eggs, and adult forms of *Gnathostoma spinigerum* and the trematode *Heterobilharzia americana* have been reported[102–104] The larvae of *S. lupi* penetrate the gastric mucosa, provoking a severe mixed inflammatory and proliferative response. These nodular foci are usually referred

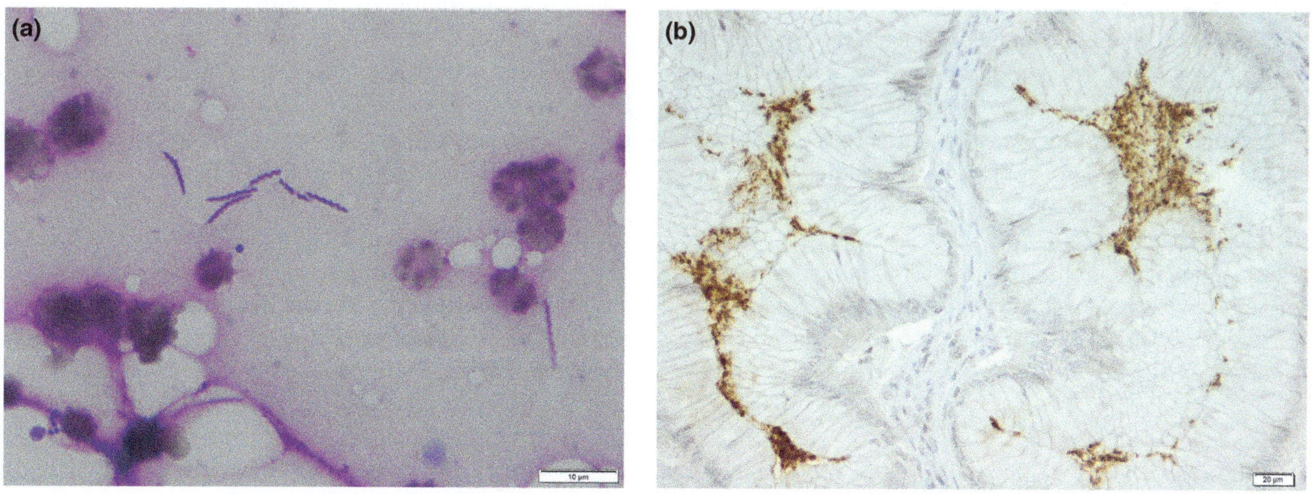

Figure 31.4 (a) Gastric spiral bacteria in a dog. Numerous *Helicobacter*-like spiral-shaped bacteria are embedded in a moderate amount of mucus (Wright's, bar = 10 μm). (b) Large amounts of *Helicobacter* antigen are present in the gastric pits of the pyloric mucosa in a 14-year-old dog (immunoperoxidase–diaminobenzidine stain with Mayer's hematoxylin counterstain, bar = 20 μm).

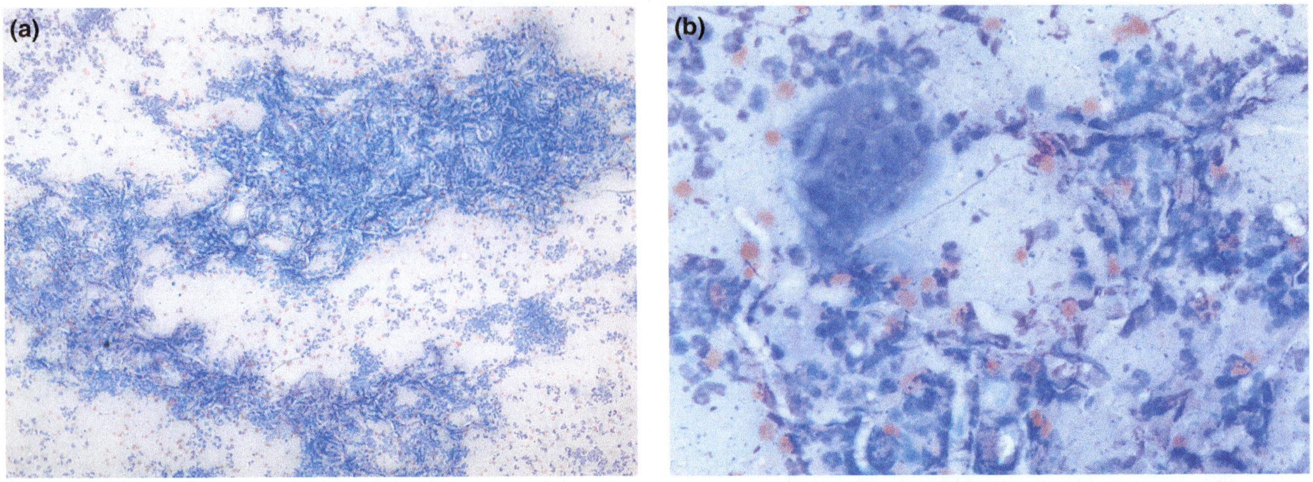

Figure 31.5 (a) Fine-needle aspiration of the gastric wall from a dog with pythiosis. Large aggregates of numerous irregular branched and nonpigmented hyphae consistent with oomycetes are associated with mixed inflammation (Wright's, 100×). (b) Fine-needle aspiration of the gastric wall from a dog with pythiosis. There are large numbers of nonpigmented, nonstaining hyphae with parallel walls and infrequent septation, measuring approximately 6–10 µm in diameter. Multinucleated giant macrophages (foreign body type) are occasionally present (Wright's, 500×).

to as granulomas.[102] In *G. spinigerum* infection, eggs and adults can be lodged in nodules in the submucosa that protrude into the gastric lumen.[103] The trematode parasite *H. americana* was recently associated with granulomatous gastritis circumscribing trapped eggs in one of 32 infected dogs.[104] Gastric infection with *O. tricuspis* has been described in a dog.[105]

Parasites of the equine stomach include *Gasterophilus* spp., *Habronema* spp., *Draschia megastoma*, and *Trichostrongylus axei*.[9] After inhabiting the oral cavity, the larvae of botflies of the genus *Gasterophilus* spp. reach the stomach, where they use chitinous oral hooks to attach and penetrate the squamous mucosa of the cardia. Focal erosions and ulcerations surrounded by a hyperplastic reaction can be detected at the site of attachment. *Habronema muscae* and *Habronema majus* also use various flies as intermediate hosts and have been associated with mild ulceration of gastric mucosa. *D. megastoma* is usually present within inflammatory submucosal nodules in the fundus, especially along the margo plicatus. The fistulated nodules can reach several centimeters, contain necrotic debris and worms, and evoke an eosinophilic granulomatous reaction.[106] *T. axei* may induce chronic gastritis in horses, usually located in the fundus and characterized by small raised plaques of hyperplastic mucosa.[107]

Inflammatory, Noninfectious

Lymphoplasmacytic inflammation is the most common form of chronic gastritis and can be associated with chronic hyperplastic and superficial gastritis, atrophic gastritis, *Helicobacter* spp. infection, parasite infestation, inflammatory bowel disease, or neoplasia.[74] Chronic inflammation is characterized by increased numbers of mature lymphocytes alone or in association with plasma cells and macrophages.

Consistent with the guidelines of the International Gastrointestinal Standardization Group of the World Small Animal Veterinary Association, neutrophils should not be present in normal canine gastric mucosa.[108] They can be present in mechanical or chemical abrasion and more commonly with gastric ulcers or carcinoma.[71] Acute chemical and mechanical gastric injuries are characterized by diffuse congestion, hemorrhage, necrosis, and ulceration. Causes include hyperacidity, ingestion of heavy metals, steroidal and nonsteroidal anti-inflammatory drugs, phosphate fertilizers, foreign bodies, and irritating plants. In horses, blister beetle (*Epicauta* spp.) intoxication induced by cantharidin can cause necrosis and ulceration of the pars esophageal and glandular mucosa of the stomach.[109] Animals with mastocytosis or MCTs can have gastric ulcers.[110] Uremic gastritis is characterized by thickened rugae, edema, and less commonly necrosis, ulceration, and bleeding of the gastric fundus and body with mucosal mineralization.[111] Chronic ulcers are usually larger, with higher edges and signs of adjacent tissue inflammation.[56] Brushings should be obtained from the margin of the ulcer rather than the center. Cytologically, regenerative epithelial cells characterized by enlarged nuclei and prominent nucleoli but with preservation of cohesion and polarity are intimately admixed with neutrophils and granular necrotic debris.

Granulomatous inflammation can be idiopathic or in response to foreign material. Endoscopic appearance ranges from nonspecific minor changes to a nodular and thickened gastric mucosa.[112] *Cryptococcus neoformans* infection resulting in a granulomatous gastritis mimicking carcinoma was reported in a dog.[113]

Eosinophilic gastritis is uncommon in dogs, cats, and horses. In dogs and cats, it is usually a manifestation of a generalized gastrointestinal hypersensitivity reaction (canine eosinophilic gastroenteritis or feline hypereosinophilic syndrome), but it can be isolated to the stomach.[114] Other causes of eosinophilic infiltration of the gastric mucosa can be related to inflammatory bowel disease, infectious agents, and cancer (MCTs or lymphomas).

Feline gastrointestinal eosinophilic sclerosing fibroplasia is a syndrome of unknown etiology, with a possible genetic predisposition in response to bacterial or parasitic antigens.[115,116] This disease usually involves the pyloric region or ileocecal junction and associated lymph nodes, sometimes leading to a mistaken diagnosis of neoplasia.[115,117] Affected cats can present with a focal intramural ulcerated mass often considered surgically non-resectable. Cytology reveals numerous eosinophils and neutrophils, often containing intracytoplasmic rod-shaped or coccoid bacteria with large irregular to spindle-shaped cells and pink extracellular matrix. Small to intermediate-sized lymphocytes, occasional plasma cells, and few degranulated mast cells can be seen.[115]

Scirrhous eosinophilic gastritis of dogs is a rare condition in which the stomach is enlarged with a greatly thickened wall associated with marked infiltration of eosinophils and exuberant granulation tissue formation; marked eosinophilia is usually present.[114,118] In the squamous portion of equine stomach, hyperkeratosis, ulceration, and eosinophilic infiltration may occur in the context of multisystemic eosinophilic epitheliotropic disease.[119]

References

1 Jergens, A.E., Andreasen, C.B., Hagemoser, W.A. et al. (1998). Cytologic examination of exfoliative specimens obtained during endoscopy for diagnosis of gastrointestinal tract disease in dogs and cats. *J Am Vet Med Assoc* 213: 1755–1759.

2 Haddad, J.L., DAM, S., and Neel, J.A. (2013). The gastrointestinal tract. In: *Diagnostic Cytology and Hematology of the Dog and Cat*, 4e, (eds. Valenciano, A.C., Cowell, R.L.), 312–340. St Louis, MO: Elsevier Mosby.

3 Happonen, I., Saari, S., Castren, L. et al. (1996). Comparison of diagnostic methods for detecting gastric *Helicobacter*-like organisms in dogs and cats. *J Comp Pathol* 115: 117–127.

4 Raddaoui, E., Almadi, M.A., Aljebreen, A.M., and Alsaif, F. (2015). Cytologic diagnosis of gastric submucosal lesions by endoscopic ultrasound-guided fine-needle aspiration: a single center experience in Saudi Arabia. *Indian J Pathol Microbiol* 58: 448–452.

5 Swann, H.M. and Holt, D.E. (2002). Canine gastric adenocarcinoma and leiomyosarcoma: a retrospective study of 21 cases (1986–1999) and literature review. *J Am Anim Hosp Assoc* 38: 157–164.

6 Jergens, A. (2005). Diseases of the esophagus. In: *Textbook of Veterinary Internal Medicine*, 6e, (eds. Ettinger, S., Feldman, E.),1298–1309. St Louis, MO: Saunders Elsevier.

7 Bridgeford, E.C., Marini, R.P., Feng, Y. et al. (2008). Gastric *Helicobacter* species as a cause of feline gastric lymphoma: a viable hypothesis. *Vet Immunol Immunopathol* 123: 106–113.

8 Garma-Aviña, A. (1994). The cytology of squamous cell carcinomas in domestic animals. *J Vet Diagn Invest* 6: 238–246.

9 Borgsteede, F.H. and van Beek, G. (1998). Parasites of stomach and small intestine of 70 horses slaughtered in the Netherlands. *Vet Q* 20: 31–34.

10 Leib, M.S. and Duncan, R.B. (2005). Diagnosing gastric *Helicobacter* infections in dogs and cats. *Compend Contin Educ Pract Vet* 27: 221–228.

11 Crystal, M.A., Penninck, D.G., Matz, M.E. et al. (1993). Use of ultrasound-guided fine-needle aspiration biopsy and automated core biopsy for the diagnosis of gastrointestinal diseases in small animals. *Vet Radiol Ultrasound* 34: 438–444.

12 Grooters, A.M., Biller, D.S., Ward, H. et al. (1994). Ultrasonographic appearance of feline alimentary lymphoma. *Vet Radiol Ultrasound* 35: 468–472.

13 Bonfanti, U., Bertazzolo, W., Bottero, E. et al. (2006). Diagnostic value of cytologic examination of gastrointestinal tract tumors in dogs and cats: 83 cases (2001–2004). *J Am Vet Med Assoc* 229: 1130–1133.

14 Patton, K., Wright, A., Kuroki, K., and Beard, L. (2009). Hemorrhagic gastritis associated with renal failure, hemoglobinuria, and isolation of *Clostridium perfringens* in a horse. *J Equine Vet Sci* 29: 633–638.

15 Bacha, W.J. and Bacha, L.M. (2000). *Color Atlas of Veterinary Histology*, 2e. Philadelphia, PA: Lippincott, Williams & Wilkins.

16 Drake, M. (1985). Gastro-esophageal cytology. *Monogr Clin Cytol* 10: 1–9.

17 Dellman, H. and Eurell, J.A. (1998). *Textbook of Veterinary Histology*, 5e. Philadelphia, PA: Lippincott Williams and Wilkins.

18 Wilcock, B. (2013). Histopathology. In: *Canine and Feline Gastroenterology*, (eds. Washabau, R.J., Day, M.J.), 333–385. St. Louis, MO: Saunders Elsevier.

19 Mills, J.C. and Shivdasani, R.A. (2011). Gastric epithelial stem cells. *Gastroenterology* 140: 412–424.

20 Atkinson, B.F. (2004). *Atlas of Diagnostic Cytopathology*, 2e. Philadelphia, PA: W.B. Saunders.

21 Conrad, R., Castelino-Prabhu, S., Cobb, C., and Raza, A. (2012). Role of cytopathology in the diagnosis and management of gastrointestinal tract cancers. *J Gastrointest Oncol* 3: 285–298.

22 Gibson, C.J., Parry, N.M., Jakowski, R.M., and Cooper, J. (2010). Adenomatous polyp with intestinal metaplasia of the esophagus (Barrett esophagus) in a dog. *Vet Pathol* 47: 116–119.

23 Gualtieri, M. and Olivero, D. (2006). Reflux esophagitis in three cats associated with metaplastic columnar esophageal epithelium. *J Am Anim Hosp Assoc* 42: 65–70.

24 Vallböhmer, D., DeMeester, S.R., Peters, J.H. et al. (2006). CDX-2 expression in squamous and metaplastic columnar epithelia of the esophagus. *Dis Esophagus* 19: 260–266.

25 Shaheen, N.J. (2005). Advances in Barrett's esophagus and esophageal adenocarcinoma. *Gastroenterology* 128: 1554–1566.

26 Johnson, J.L., Hultine, J.J., Cook, J.E., and Leipold, H.W. (1980). Leukoplakia of the esophagus and stomach of a foal. *Vet Pathol* 17: 638–640.

27 Singhi, A.D., Arnold, C.A., Crowder, C.D. et al. (2014). Esophageal leukoplakia or epidermoid metaplasia: a clinicopathological study of 18 patients. *Mod Pathol* 27: 38–43.

28 Ridgway, R.L. and Suter, P.F. (1979). Clinical and radiographic signs in primary and metastatic oesophageal neoplasms in the dog. *J Am Vet Med Assoc* 174: 700–704.

29 Wall, M. and Calvert, C.A. (2006). Canine viral papillomatosis. In: *Infectious Disease of the Dog and the Cat*, 3e, (ed. Greene, C.E.), 74–78. St Louis, MO: Elsevier/ Saunders.

30 Kerpsack, S.J. and Birchard, S.J. (1994). Removal of leiomyomas and other noninvasive masses from the cardiac region of the canine stomach. *J Am Anim Hosp Assoc* 30: 500–504.

31 Jergens, A.E., Hostetter, S.J., and Andreasen, C.B. (2016). Oral cavity, gastrointestinal tract, and associated structures. In: *Canine and Feline Cytology: A Color Atlas and Interpretation Guide*, 3e, (eds. Raskin, R.E., Meyer, D.J.), 220–246. St. Louis, MO: Elsevier.

32 Shinozuka, J., Nakayama, H., Suzuki, M. et al. (2001). Esophageal adenosquamous carcinoma in a cat. *J Vet Med Sci* 63: 91–93.

33 Randolph, J.F., Center, S.A., Flanders, J.A., and Diters, R.W. (1984). Hypertrophic osteopathy associated with adenocarcinoma of the esophageal glands in a dog. *J Am Vet Med Assoc* 184: 98–99.

34 Farese, J.P., Bacon, N.J., Ehrhart, N.P. et al. (2008). Oesophageal leiomyosarcoma in dogs: surgical management and clinical outcome of four cases. *Vet Comp Oncol* 6: 31–38.

35 Teo, L.H., Cahalan, S.D., Benigni, L., and Halfacree, Z. (2014). Oesophageal angioleiomyosarcoma in a cat. *J Feline Med Surg* 16: 846–852.

36 Ranen, E., Lavy, E., and Aizenberg, I. (2004). Spirocercosis-associated esophageal sarcomas in dogs. A retrospective study of 17 cases (1997–2003). *Vet Parasitol* 119: 209–221.

37 Slatter, D.H. (2003). *Textbook of Small Animal Surgery*, 3e. Philadelphia, PA: W.B. Saunders.

38 Evander, A., Little, A.G., Riddell, R.H. et al. (1987). Composition of the refluxed material determines the degree of reflux esophagitis in the dog. *Gastroenterology* 93: 280–286.

39 Gal, A., Ridgway, M.D., and Fredrickson, R.L. (2011). An unusual clinical presentation of a dog with gastrinoma. *Can Vet J* 52: 641–644.

40 Han, E., Broussard, J., and Baer, K.E. (2003). Feline esophagitis secondary to gastroesophageal reflux disease: clinical signs and radiographic, endoscopic, and histopathological findings. *J Am Anim Hosp Assoc* 39: 161–167.

41 Mazzei, M.J., Bissett, S.A., Murphy, K.M. et al. (2009). Eosinophilic esophagitis in a dog. *J Am Vet Med Assoc* 235: 61–65.

42 Rothenberg, M.E. (2004). Eosinophilic gastrointestinal disorders (EGID). *J Allergy Clin Immunol* 113: 11–28.

43 Vengust, M., Baird, J.D., van Dreumel, T. et al. (2008). Equid herpesvirus 2-associated oral and esophageal ulceration in a foal. *J Vet Diagn Invest* 20: 811–815.

44 Greene, C.E. and Chandler, F.W. (1998). Candidiasis, torulopsosis, and rhodotorulosis. In: *Infectious Diseases of the Dog and Cat*, 2e, (ed. Greene, C.E.), 414–417. Philadelphia, PA: W.B. Saunders.

45 Kim, Y.H. and Choi, S.Y. (2007). Black esophagus with concomitant candidiasis developed after diabetic ketoacidosis. *World J Gastroenterol* 13: 5662–5663.

46 Choi, J.H., Lee, C.G., Lim, Y.J. et al. (2013). Prevalence and risk factors of esophageal candidiasis in healthy individuals: a single center experience in Korea. *Yonsei Med J* 54: 160–165.

47 Nayar, R. (2014). *Cytopathology in Oncology*. Berlin, Heidelberg: Springer.

48 Patton, C.S., Hake, R., Newton, J., and Toal, R.L. (1996). Esophagitis due to *Pythium insidiosum* infection in two dogs. *J Vet Intern Med* 10: 139–142.

49 Berryessa, N.A., Marks, S.L., Pesavento, P.A. et al. (2008). Gastrointestinal pythiosis in 10 dogs from California. *J Vet Intern Med* 22: 1065–1069.

50 Grooters, A.M., Hodgin, E.C., Bauer, R.W. et al. (2003). Clinicopathologic findings associated with *Lagenidium* sp. infection in 6 dogs: initial description of an emerging oomycosis. *J Vet Intern Med* 17: 637–646.

51 Silva, J.F., Guimarães, L.B., Ribeiro, L.R. et al. (2014). Acute oesophageal necrosis concurrent with *Leishmania chagasi* infection in a dog. *J Comp Pathol* 150: 148–150.

52 Okanishi, H., Matsumoto, J., Aoki, H. et al. (2013). Successful resolution of esophageal granulomas in a dog infected with *Spirocerca lupi*. *J Vet Med Sci* 75: 1629–1632.

53 De Lorenzi, D. and Furlanello, T. (2010). What is your diagnosis? Esophageal nodules in a dog. *Spirocerca lupi* infection. *Vet Clin Pathol* 39: 391–392.

54 Van der Kolk, J.H., Sloet van Oldruitenborgh-Oosterbaan, M.M., and Gruys, E. (1989). Bilateral pleuritis following esophageal fistula in a horse as a complication of a *Gasterophilus* infection. *Tijdschr Diergeneeskd* 114: 769–774.

55 van der Gaag, I. (1988). The histological appearance of peroral gastric biopsies in clinically healthy and vomiting dogs. *Can J Vet Res* 52: 67–74.

56 Amorim, I., Taulescu, M.A., Day, M.J. et al. (2016). Canine gastric pathology: a review. *J Comp Pathol* 154: 9–37.

57 Head, K., Cullen, J.M., Dubielzig, R. et al. (2003). *Histological Classification of Tumors of the Alimentary System of Domestic Animals*. Washington DC: Armed Forces Institute of Pathology in cooperation with the American Registry of Pathology and the World Health Organization Collaborating Center for Worldwide Reference on Comparative Oncology.

58 Taulescu, M.A., Valentine, B.A., Amorim, I. et al. (2014). Histopathological features of canine spontaneous non-neoplastic gastric polyps: a retrospective study of 15 cases. *Histol Histopathol* 29: 65–75.

59 Kuan, S., Hoffmann, K., and Tisdall, P. (2009). Ultrasonographic and surgical findings of a gastric hyperplastic polyp resulting in pyloric obstruction in an 11-week-old French bulldog. *Aust Vet J* 87: 253–255.

60 Morse, C.C. and Richardson, D.W. (1988). Gastric hyperplastic polyp in a horse. *J Comp Pathol* 99: 337–342.

61 Furness, M.C., Snyman, H.N., Abrahams, M. et al. (2013). Severe gastric impaction secondary to a gastric polyp in a horse. *Can Vet J* 54: 979–982.

62 Conroy, J.D. (1969). Multiple gastric adenomatous polyps in a dog. *J Comp Pathol* 79: 465–467.

63 Marley, L.K., Repenning, P., Frank, C.B. et al. (2016). Transendoscopic electrosurgery for partial removal of a gastric adenomatous polyp in a horse. *J Vet Intern Med* 30: 1351–1355.

64 Taylor, S.D., Haldorson, G.J., Vaughan, B., and Pusterla, N. (2009). Gastric neoplasia in horses. *J Vet Intern Med* 23: 1097–1102.

65 Park, C.H., Ishizuka, Y., Tsuchida, Y., and Oyamada, T. (2007). Gastric pleomorphic leiomyosarcoma in a Shetland sheepdog. *J Vet Med Sci* 69: 873–876.

66 Dennis, M.M., Bennett, N., and Ehrhart, E.J. (2006). Gastric adenocarcinoma and chronic gastritis in two related Persian cats. *Vet Pathol* 43: 358–362.

67 Sundberg, J.P., Burnstein, T., Page, E.H. et al. (1977). Neoplasms of equidae. *J Am Vet Med Assoc* 170: 150–152.

68 Patton, K.M., Peek, S.F., and Valentine, B.A. (2006). Gastric adenocarcinoma in a horse with portal vein metastasis and thrombosis: a novel cause of hepatic encephalopathy. *Vet Pathol* 43: 565–569.

69 Willard, M.D. (2012). Alimentary neoplasia in geriatric dogs and cats. *Vet Clin North Am Small Anim Pract* 42: 693–706.

70 Raskin, R.E. and Meyer, D.J. (2001). *Atlas of Canine and Feline Cytology*. Philadelphia, PA: W.B. Saunders.

71 Riondato, F., Miniscalco, B., Berio, E. et al. (2014). Diagnosis of canine gastric adenocarcinoma using squash preparation cytology. *Vet J* 201: 390–394.

72 Dell'Orco, M., Bertazzolo, W., Vergine, M. et al. (2005). Gastric mucinous adenocarcinoma with cutaneous metastases in a dog: diagnosis by fine-needle aspiration cytology. *J Small Anim Pract* 46: 449–453.

73 McKenzie, E.C., Mills, J.N., and Bolton, J.R. (1997). Gastric squamous cell carcinoma in three horses. *Aust Vet J* 75: 480–483.

74 Brown, C., Baker, D., and Barker, I. (2007). Stomach and abomasum. In: *Jubb, Kennedy & Palmer's Pathology of Domestic Animals*, 5e, vol. 2, (ed. Grant Maxie, M.), 52–68. Edinburgh: Elsevier.

75 Sako, T., Uchida, E., Okamoto, M. et al. (2003). Immunohistochemical evaluation of a malignant intestinal carcinoid in a dog. *Vet Pathol* 40: 212–215.

76 Qvigstad, G., Kolbjornsen, O., Skancke, E., and Waldum, H.L. (2008). Gastric neuroendocrine carcinoma associated with atrophic gastritis in the norwegian lundehund. *J Comp Pathol* 139: 194–201.

77 Boy, M.G., Palmer, J.E., Heyer, G., and Hamir, A.N. (1992). Gastric leiomyosarcoma in a horse. *J Am Vet Med Assoc* 200: 1363–1364.

78 LaRock, R.G. and Ginn, P.E. (1997). Immunohistochemical staining characteristics of canine gastrointestinal stromal tumors. *Vet Pathol* 34: 303–311.

79 Russell, K.N., Mehler, S.J., Skorupski, K.A. et al. (2007). Clinical and immunohistochemical differentiation of gastrointestinal stromal tumors from leiomyosarcomas in dogs: 42 cases (1990–2003). *J Am Vet Med Assoc* 230: 1329–1333.

80 Morini, M., Gentilini, F., Pietra, M. et al. (2011). Cytological, immunohistochemical and mutational analysis of a gastric gastrointestinal stromal tumour in a cat. *J Comp Pathol* 145: 152–157.

81 Dailey, D.D., Ehrhart, E.J., Duval, D.L. et al. (2015). DOG1 is a sensitive and specific immunohistochemical marker for diagnosis of canine gastrointestinal stromal tumors. *J Vet Diagn Invest* 27: 268–277.

82 Del Piero, F., Summers, B.A., Cummings, J.F. et al. (2001). Gastrointestinal stromal tumors in equids. *Vet Pathol* 38: 689–697.

83 Muravnick, K.B., Parente, E.J., and Del Fabio, P. (2009). An atypical equine gastrointestinal stromal tumor. *J Vet Diagn Invest* 21: 387–390.

84 Barrs, V. and Beatty, J. (2012). Feline alimentary lymphoma 1. Classification, risk factors, clinical signs and non-invasive diagnostics. *J Feline Med Surg* 14: 182–190.

85 Moore, P.F., Rodriguez-Bertos, A., and Kass, P.H. (2012). Feline gastrointestinal lymphoma: mucosal architecture, immunophenotype, and molecular clonality. *Vet Pathol* 49: 658–668.

86 Penninck, D.G., Moore, A.S., and Gliatto, J. (1998). Ultrasonography of canine gastric epithelial neoplasia. *Vet Radiol Ultrasound* 39: 342–348.

87 Brunnert, S.R., Dee, L.A., Herron, A.J., and Altman, N.H. (1992). Gastric extramedullary plasmacytoma in a dog. *J Am Vet Med Assoc* 200: 1501–1502.

88 Zikes, C.D., Spielman, B., Shapiro, W. et al. (1998). Gastric extramedullary plasmacytoma in a cat. *J Vet Intern Med* 12: 381–383.

89 Ozaki, K., Yamagami, T., Nomura, K., and Narama, I. (2002). Mast cell tumors of the gastrointestinal tract in 39 dogs. *Vet Pathol* 39: 557–564.

90 London, C.A., Malpas, P.B., Wood-Follis, S. et al. (2009). Multi-center, placebo-controlled, double-blind, randomized study of oral toceranib phosphate (SU11654), a receptor tyrosine kinase inhibitor, for the treatment of dogs with recurrent (either local or distant) mast cell tumor following surgical excision. *Clin Cancer Res* 15: 3856–3865.

91 Henry, C. and Herrera, C. (2013). Mast cell tumors in cats: clinical update and possible new treatment avenues. *J Feline Med Surg* 15: 41–47.

92 Gross, T.L. and Mayhew, I.G. (1983). Gastroesophageal ulceration and candidiasis in foals. *J Am Vet Med Assoc* 182: 1370–1373.

93 Fernandes, C.P., Giordani, C., Grecco, F.B. et al. (2012). Gastric pythiosis in a dog. *Rev Iberoam Micol* 29: 235–237.

94 Connolly, S.L., Frank, C., Thompson, C.A. et al. (2012). Dual infection with *Pythium insidiosum* and *Blastomyces dermatitidis* in a dog. *Vet Clin Pathol* 41: 419–423.

95 Bromel, C. and Sykes, J.E. (2005). Histoplasmosis in dogs and cats. *Clin Tech Small Anim Pract* 20: 227–232.

96 Lin Blache, J., Ryan, K., and Arceneaux, K. (2011). Histoplasmosis. *Compend Contin Educ Pract Vet* 33: E1–E10.

97 Ibba, F., Lepri, E., Veronesi, F. et al. (2014). Gastric cylicospirurosis in a domestic cat from Italy. *J Feline Med Surg* 16: 522–526.

98 Cecchi, R., Wills, S.J., Dean, R., and Pearson, G.R. (2006). Demonstration of *Ollulanus tricuspis* in the stomach of domestic cats by biopsy. *J Comp Pathol* 134: 374–377.

99 Curtsinger, D.K., Carpenter, J.L., and Turner, J.L. (1993). Gastritis caused by *Aonchotheca putorii* in a domestic cat. *J Am Vet Med Assoc* 203: 1153–1154.

100 Mohsen, A. and Hossein, H. (2009). Gastrointestinal parasites of stray cats in Kashan, Iran. *Trop Biomed* 26: 16–22.

101 van der Linde-Sipman, J.S., Boersema, J.H., and Berrocal, A. (1992). 3 cases of hypertrophic gastritis associated with a *Ollulanus tricuspis* infection in cats. *Tijdschr Diergeneeskd* 117: 727–729.

102 van der Merwe, L.L., Kirberger, R.M., Clift, S. et al. (2008). *Spirocerca lupi* infection in the dog: a review. *Vet J* 176: 294–309.

103 Maleewong, W., Pariyanonda, S., Sitthithaworn, P. et al. (1992). Seasonal variation in the prevalence and intensity of canine *Gnathostoma spinigerum* infection in northeastern Thailand. *J Helminthol* 66: 72–74.

104 Rodriguez, J., Lewis, B., and Snowden, K. (2014). Distribution and characterization of *Heterobilharzia americana* in dogs in Texas. *Vet Parasitol* 203: 35–42.

105 Daiki, K., Oishi, M., Nakashima, K. et al. (2015). The first report of the ante-mortem diagnosis of *Ollulanus tricuspis* infection in two dogs. *J Vet Med Sci* 77: 1499–1502.

106 Nadalian, M.G., Hosseini, S.H., Tavassoli, A., and Raoufi, A. (1997). Gastritis and gastric perforation due to *Habronema* spp. in the horse. *J Equine Vet Sci* 17: 385–386.

107 Collobert-Laugier, C., Lamidey, C., Brisseau, N. et al. (2000). Prevalence of stomach nematodes (*Habronema* spp, *Draschia megastoma* and *Trichostrongylus axei*) in horses examined post mortem in Normandy. *Rev Med Vet* 151: 151–156.

108 Day, M.J., Bilzer, T., Mansell, J. et al. (2008). Histopathological standards for the diagnosis of gastrointestinal inflammation in endoscopic biopsy samples from the dog and cat: a report from the World Small Animal Veterinary Association Gastrointestinal Standardization Group. *J Comp Pathol* 138 (1): S1–S43.

109 Schmitz, D.G. (1989). Cantharidin toxicosis in horses. *J Vet Intern Med* 3: 208–215.

110 Gelberg, H.B. (2017). Alimentary system and the peritoneum, omentum, mesentery, and peritoneal cavity. In: *Zachary's Pathologic Basis of Veterinary Disease*, 6e, (ed. Zachary, J.F.), 324–411. St. Louis, MO: Elsevier.

111 Peters, R.M., Goldstein, R.E., Erb, H.N., and Njaa, B.L. (2005). Histopathologic features of canine uremic gastropathy: a retrospective study. *J Vet Intern Med* 19: 315–320.

112 Pratt, C.L., Reineke, E.L., and Drobatz, K.J. (2014). Sewing needle foreign body ingestion in dogs and cats: 65 cases (2000–2012). *J Am Vet Med Assoc* 245: 302–308.

113 van der Gaag, I., van Niel, M.H., Belshaw, B.E., and Wolvekamp, W.T. (1991). Gastric granulomatous cryptococcosis mimicking gastric carcinoma in a dog. *Vet Q* 13: 185–190.

114 Hayden, D.W. and Fleischman, R.W. (1977). Scirrhous eosinophilic gastritis in dogs with gastric arteritis. *Vet Pathol* 14: 441–448.

115 Craig, L.E., Hardam, E.E., Hertzke, D.M. et al. (2009). Feline gastrointestinal eosinophilic sclerosing fibroplasia. *Vet Pathol* 46: 63–70.

116 Suzuki, M., Onchi, M., and Ozaki, M. (2013). A case of feline gastrointestinal eosinophilic sclerosing fibroplasia. *J Toxicol Pathol* 26: 51–53.

117 Linton, M., Nimmo, J.S., Norris, J.M. et al. (2015). Feline gastrointestinal eosinophilic sclerosing fibroplasia: 13 cases and review of an emerging clinical entity. *J Feline Med Surg* 17: 392–404.

118 Laisse, C.J., Castro, N.B., Conceição de Oliveira, E. et al. (2016). Scirrhous eosinophilic gastritis in two dogs. *Cienc Rural* 46: 881–884.

119 Bosseler, L., Verryken, K., Bauwens, C. et al. (2013). Equine multisystemic eosinophilic epitheliotropic disease: a case report and review of literature. *N Z Vet J* 61: 177–182.

32

Intestines and Rectum

Ugo Bonfanti

Introduction

Cytological examination of the intestines and rectum is used to screen for many important inflammatory and neoplastic diseases in small animal species; however histology remains the reference standard for diagnosis, particularly for inflammatory conditions. Increasing popularity of ultrasonography and endoscopy allows accurate definition of lesion location and offers less invasive methods to collect cytological specimens than surgery and laparoscopy, although there are limitations. Recent publications review best practices for endoscopic gastrointestinal biopsy and have the potential to impact the accuracy of cytologic preparations.[1] Cytologic examination of these tissues in horses is rarely described in the literature; however lymphoma, adenocarcinoma, and smooth muscle tumors have been reported as common intestinal neoplasms in horses.[2] While technically not of intestinal origin, pedunculated lipomas of the abdomen can cause intestinal pathology in the equine.

Sample Collection

Fine-Needle Aspiration

Fine-needle aspiration (FNA) of intestines and rectum is usually performed with ultrasound or computed tomography guidance.[3] Advanced imaging is particularly useful for lesions of the submucosa and muscularis. In a retrospective study of 83 canine and feline intestinal tumors, complete and complete plus partial agreement between cytology and the definitive histologic diagnosis were 68 and 76%, respectively, with a recovery rate of 82% and higher sensitivity for gastrointestinal tract lymphoma.[4] Studies of FNA for gastrointestinal wall lesions in humans report values for sensitivity, specificity, diagnostic accuracy, predictive positive value, and predictive negative values of approximately 90–91, 100% (no false-positive results), 80–100, 100, and 67%, respectively.[5–7] Very few complications have been described in humans following percutaneous ultrasound-guided FNAs of gastrointestinal tract lesions and include one case of hemoperitoneum, one of sepsis, one of small parietal hematoma, and one of bile peritonitis.[6,8,9] Specific data on complications in veterinary species appear to be lacking.

Endoscopic Brushing and Touch Imprint

Brushings are collected by passing a cytology brush through the accessory channel of the endoscope and rubbing it vigorously on the desired area until slight bleeding occurs and then rolling the brush on a slide. This technique only samples the epithelial surface and is hampered by blood contamination. The touch technique transfers a mucosal specimen from the biopsy forceps to a glass slide using a hypodermic needle to make multiple cytologic imprints. Alternatively, a second slide is placed on the first one, and the application of light pressure creates a squash preparation. A prospective study comparing the diagnostic accuracy of the two techniques (brush and touch) with endoscopic histopathology samples in 85 dogs and 23 cats found the diagnostic accuracy of cytologic examination was high, with ≥70% sensitivity, specificity, and predictive values of positive and negative results for the detection of mucosal lesions. The diagnostic accuracy of the brush technique was equal or superior to that of the touch technique for 84% of specimens. The brush technique was more useful in detecting cellular infiltrates in the lamina propria, whereas the touch technique was more likely to detect mucosal inflammation.[10,11] No severe complications have been reported in the literature.

Veterinary Cytology, First Edition. Edited by Leslie C. Sharkey, M. Judith Radin, and Davis Seelig.

Surgical Biopsies

Imprints from biopsy specimens are one of the most important methods to obtain samples for cytological examination. Touch, roll, or squash preparations can be made, taking care not to disrupt tissue architecture for any samples ultimately being submitted for histology. Endoscopic biopsies are less invasive than surgical biopsy but have the disadvantage of sampling mucosa and submucosa only. In a study of 22 cats, endoscopic biopsy samples were considered useful for diagnosing gastric lymphoma but were considered inadequate for differentiating between inflammatory bowel disease (IBD) and lymphoma of the small intestine.[12,13] A full-thickness histologic biopsy, in particular of the jejunum and ileum, was more useful for IBD diagnosis.[12,13] In contrast, imprints of surgical biopsy allow evaluation of deeper tissues but are more invasive to collect. In a retrospective study of 53 dogs and cats with intestinal tumors, the agreement between the results of cytologic examination of impression smears from surgical biopsies with the histologic diagnosis appeared to be higher.[4] In animals with intestinal neoplasia, complete agreement for imprints from biopsies compared with FNA was 96 and 68%, respectively.[4] While this requires an invasive procedure, cytologic screening of the lesion can provide relatively immediate preliminary results while histology is pending.

Rectal Scraping

Rectal mucosal scraping is an easy, noninvasive method to collect cytological samples when large intestinal diseases are suspected. The objective is to obtain material from the epithelium and the lamina propria to diagnose inflammatory, infectious, or neoplastic diseases. The procedure is performed with a rigid instrument such as an ear curette or a conjunctival scraper. With the aid of a gloved finger, the instrument is inserted cranially to avoid the anus and reach the rectum. Scraping should be firm enough to sample the lamina propria while light enough to avoid perforating a potentially friable rectum. The instrument is removed while protecting the sample with the gloved finger, and the obtained material is used to make a smear or squash preparation.[14,15]

Normal Histological Architecture and Cytology

The small intestine consists of the duodenum, jejunum, and ileum. The mucosal surfaces contain long and thin intestinal microvilli to increase the surface area for absorption. The surface of the small intestine is covered by tall simple columnar epithelial cells and mucus-secreting goblet cells over a core of lamina propria. Deep to the mucosa, the muscularis mucosae consist of two layers of smooth muscle, covered by serosa. The large intestine is composed of columnar epithelium with goblet cells that are abundant in the surface epithelium and in the mucosal glands. Nerves, lymphatic and blood vessels, and lymphoid tissue are concentrated in the submucosal tissues. Muscularis and serosa are present deep to the mucosa, as in the small intestine. The rectum is lined by a simple columnar epithelium with mucosal glands decreasing in number and disappearing entirely approaching the anus.[16]

Normal intestinal cytology consists predominantly of simple columnar epithelium and mucus-producing goblet cells. Columnar cells are rectangular in shape with slightly basophilic cytoplasm with a striated microvillous apical border. The nucleus is round to oval, paracentral to basal, with condensed or reticular chromatin and indistinct nucleoli. Goblet cells, which increase proportionally from the small to the large intestine, are elongated with cytoplasmic mucin granules or vacuoles and a basal nucleus. Extracellular mucus can be diffuse or appear as distinct purple granules. Scattered lymphocytes, plasma cells, elongated mature fibroblasts, rare eosinophils, and few globule leukocytes are also present. Sampling of a Peyer's patch results in a heterogeneous lymphocyte population including small numbers of granular lymphocytes, especially in cats. A mixed population of extracellular bacteria can be present, especially in large intestinal samples.[17–19]

In the small intestine mucosa, villous intraepithelial lymphocytes are less numerous in the dog than the cat, but in the crypts, the number is similar. The number of eosinophils is higher in the crypts than in the villus in dogs. $CD8^+$ T cells are found primarily in the epithelium with fewer in the lamina propria or submucosa. Most intraepithelial lymphocytes are $CD3^+/CD8^+$, while lamina propria T cells are predominantly $CD4^+$. In cats, granular lymphocytes have distinctive eosinophilic granules, express perforin, and have cytotoxic function. Small number of mast cells contributes to immune surveillance, also secreting serotonin and heparin. Certain secretory cells of the mucosal lining of the gastrointestinal tract, either singly or in groups, have the ability to secrete polypeptides and biologically active amines as local hormones. These cells have been termed gastrointestinal endocrine, enteroendocrine argentaffin/argyrophilic, and enterochromaffin cells. At least twelve ultrastructurally distinct gut endocrine cells secrete more than 20 hormones and neurotransmitters from secretory granules, including gastrin, cholecystokinin, secretin, and enteroglucagon. Interstitial cells of Cajal are part of the pacemaker system in the intestinal wall, appearing as c-kit positive cells in the myenteric and deep submucosal plexus of the small intestine and the submucosal plexus of the large intestine.[20–23]

Normal rectal scraping cytology consists of clusters of columnar or polygonal epithelial cells with a mixed population of bacteria, mucin, and debris. Lubricant appears as pink to magenta, granular or fibrillar material that can obscure diagnostic features. Normal anus scrapings contain squamous epithelial cells. When scraping mucosa containing a lymphoid follicle, a mixed population of lymphocytes and plasma cells can be observed.[17–19]

Diseases of the Small and Large Intestines

Hyperplasia

The criteria that differentiate benign and malignant lesions must be carefully evaluated when examining intestinal cytology because of the degree of cellular atypia present with epithelial hyperplasia or metaplasia associated with reparative lesions and regeneration. In reactive change, smears can be quite cellular, with poor cell preservation if there is concurrent degeneration. Frequently, cells increase in size with larger nuclei, but the nuclear to cytoplasmic ratio (N:C) remains within normal limits. Nucleoli can be prominent. Cytoplasm can acquire a squamoid appearance. Evidence of inflammation or necrosis can be observed in the background. Criteria for an interpretation of hyperplasia include preservation of nuclear polarity, uniformity of cell size, and cohesiveness of cells.[19,24]

Neoplasia

Intestinal tumors are relatively rare in dogs and cats, despite the variety of potential neoplasms. Lymphoma is considered the most common intestinal tumor in many reports.[25] Adenocarcinoma is the second most frequent tumor in both species, with mast cell tumors in cats and leiomyosarcomas or gastrointestinal stromal tumors (GISTs) in dogs following.[26–29] Fibrosarcoma, carcinoid, extramedullary plasmacytoma, extraskeletal osteosarcoma, and hemangiosarcoma are rarely reported.[30]

Round Cell Tumors

Lymphoma

Intestinal lymphomas can be either diffuse or nodular. The intestine is the most common anatomic site affected by lymphoma in the cat, representing 39% of all cases in a retrospective study of 477 feline lymphomas.[31] Moreover, lymphoma is the most common intestinal neoplasm in the cat, accounting for 47% of cases in a survey of 1129 feline intestinal neoplasms.[32] In contrast, intestinal lymphoma represents only 7% of all canine lymphomas.[33] It is likely that intestinal T-cell lymphomas originate from diffuse mucosal-associated lymphoid tissue, whereas intestinal B-cell lymphomas principally arise from Peyer's patches and mucosal lymphoid nodules.

As is the case with other anatomic variants, there are a number of different subtypes of intestinal lymphoma, each with unique clinical, microscopic, and immunophenotypic characteristics. In the cat, intestinal lymphoma has traditionally been classified into either (i) small cell (lymphocytic lymphoma/low-grade alimentary lymphoma), (ii) large cell (lymphoblastic lymphoma/high-grade alimentary lymphoma), or (iii) large granular lymphocyte (LGL) forms. More recently, a group used the World Health Organization (WHO) scheme to classify 120 cases of feline intestinal lymphoma according to their most similar human counterpart and identified three variants: (i) enteropathy-associated T-cell lymphoma (EATL) type 1 (transmural, large cell), (ii) EATL type 2 (mucosal, small cell), and (iii) diffuse large B cell.[34]

Irrespective of scheme, there are definitive prognostic implications to histologic classification of feline lymphoma. When classified according to the WHO scheme, cats with mucosal T-cell lymphoma (EATL type 2) had a median survival time of 29 months, whereas cats with transmural T-cell lymphoma (EATL type 1), most of which had an LGL morphology, had a median survival time of 1.5 months.[34] There is conflicting information on the frequency of each of these subtypes, but it appears as though the low-grade/EATL type 2 form of the disease is most common, representing up to 75% of all feline lymphoma, whereas the LGL form of the disease is rare (2–7%). Similar to the cat, three histologic forms of canine intestinal lymphoma have been described: (i) diffuse large B-cell lymphoma, (ii) EATL type 1, and (iii) EATL type 2.[13,35,36] Of these, the T-cell forms of the disease are reported to predominate (75–100%).

Neoplastic cells in intestinal lymphoma exfoliate readily. A monomorphic population of large lymphocytes allows a definitive cytological diagnosis. Large lymphocytes are characterized by oval to irregularly shaped nuclei, with a homogeneous or fine chromatin pattern, one or multiple large nucleoli, and a minimal to moderately abundant, deeply basophilic cytoplasm (Figure 32.1a). Sometimes neoplastic cells are admixed with scattered small, well-differentiated lymphocytes, which can complicate interpretation. Small cell alimentary lymphomas are particularly common in cats. In these cases, the neoplastic lymphocytes lack cytologic atypia and are typically small, with dense chromatin and a small tag of cytoplasm. Diagnosis of small cell alimentary lymphoma requires

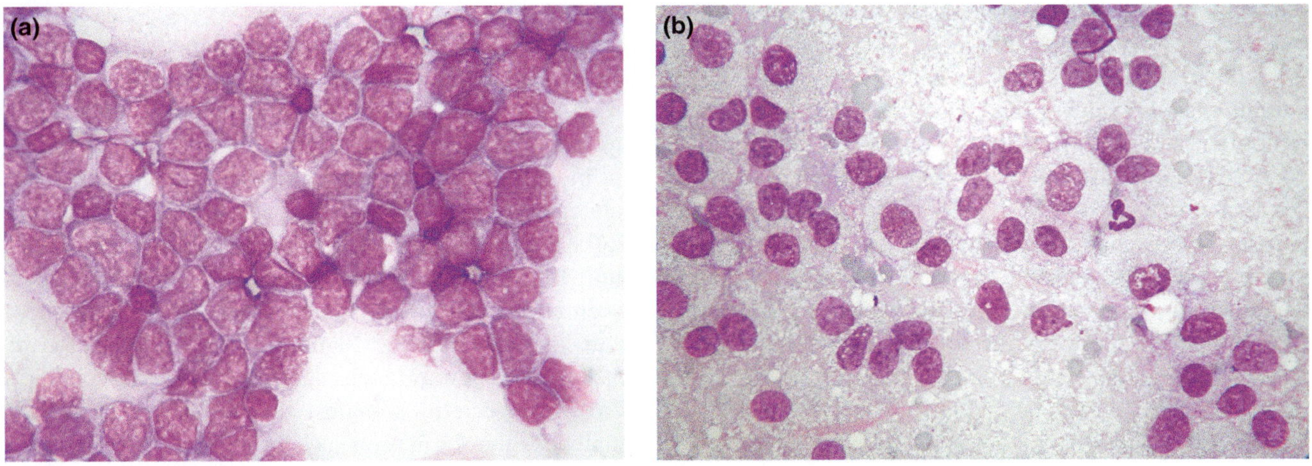

Figure 32.1 (a) Dog, intestinal mass. High-grade lymphoma. Fine-needle biopsy. Cells are round, intermediate to large in size. Nuclei are round to slightly irregular, with smudged chromatin and inconspicuous nucleoli. Cytoplasm is scant and lightly basophilic. Few scattered small lymphocytes are present among the neoplastic cells (May-Grünwald–Giemsa, 1000×). (b) Cat, intestinal mass. Mast cell tumor. Fine-needle biopsy. Cells are round to ovoid in shape, sometimes with indistinct boundaries. Nuclei are single, central to paracentral, round to oval, with finely stippled chromatin. Abundant and finely microvacuolated cytoplasm is evident. A few erythrocytes are in the background (May-Grünwald–Giemsa, 1000×).

concurrent histopathologic evaluation to distinguish this neoplasm from IBD, which has a very similar cytologic appearance.[34,37,38] Moreover, in light of the prognostic significance of histologic subclassification, biopsy with histopathology should be performed in all cases of suspected feline intestinal lymphoma.

More common in cats, neoplastic LGL lymphocytes contain fine to coarse azurophilic or brightly magenta granules ranging from 1 to 20/cell that are located near a nuclear indentation. Phenotypic and molecular studies have assigned feline LGL lymphoma to cytotoxic T-cell lineage based on CD3 and granzyme B expression.[34] LGLs can be mature and small (8–15 μm), characterized by round, frequently indented nuclei with coarsely clumped chromatin, inapparent nucleoli, and an incomplete rim of pale blue cytoplasm with fine granules. In other cases, LGLs are immature large (15–35 μm) cells with pleomorphic nuclei, dispersed chromatin, prominent nucleoli, and a variable volume of cytoplasm containing round, fine to large, irregularly distributed cytoplasmic granules. While usually small, coarse, large (1–2 μm) cytoplasmic granules are occasionally present.[22,39–41] According to the current literature, previously attributed cases of globular leukocyte neoplasms and large granular lymphocytic lymphoma likely represent the same entity.

It can be difficult to distinguish neoplastic lymphocytes if there is significant concurrent inflammation. Differentiation of severe lymphocytic enteritis from lymphoma can be problematic. The distinction between inflammation and neoplasia became less clear following the discovery that the lymphocytic inflammation may predispose to lymphoma development.[42]

Extramedullary Plasmacytoma

Extramedullary plasmacytomas involving the intestinal tract are rare in dogs and cats.[43–47] Primary masses have been reported in the colon, rectum, and ileocecal junction in the dog. Metastasis to the regional lymph nodes, liver, and spleen in association with IgG gammopathy was reported in two dogs.[45,46] Histologically, amyloid can be detected in some cases.[46–48] Caruso et al. described the cytology of a distal colonic mass composed of small to medium-sized round cells with a moderate amount of lavender-pink cytoplasm, exhibiting moderate anisocytosis and anisokaryosis and often with indistinct cytoplasmic borders.[48] Perinuclear clear areas were not a prominent feature. Nuclei were pleomorphic, varied from round to oval to indented or lobulated, and were centrally to eccentrically located. Binucleated and multinucleated cells were noted. Histologically, the neoplasm contained irregular islands of material consistent with amyloid.[48]

Mast Cell Tumors

Feline intestinal mast cell tumors (FIMCT) are considered the third most common tumor following lymphoma and adenocarcinoma, but incidence and behavior are poorly characterized.[29,32,49] They can appear clinically similar to eosinophilic enteritis.[50,51] In a study describing 17 cases of FIMCT, twelve showed Kit protein expression. A significant relationship between Kit pattern and survival was not observed. Mast cells are round to ovoid with single central nucleus. Diagnosis can be confounded when the characteristic cytoplasmic granules fail to stain (Figure 32.1b). In addition, there is evidence that mucosal mast cells (MMC) are not the same as connective mast cells (CTMC). These two subtypes of mast cells have different immunohistochemistry profiles, causing staining difficulties.[52] CTMCs contain tryptase, chymase, and heparin, while MMCs contain tryptase and chondroitin sulfate. In dogs, intestinal mast cell tumors typically are poorly granulated.[29,53] In one report, 5 out of 10 dogs with intestinal mast cell tumors had mast cells detected in circulation.[54]

Epithelial Neoplasia

Adenocarcinoma can present as an annular or constricting lesion or as an intramural mass. Histologic characteristics, which occasionally can be appreciated cytologically, include adeno- (glandular forming), mucinous (>50% mucin), signet ring (>50% of cells have intracellular mucin), and undifferentiated or solid (no evidence of gland formation) forms.[29] Neoplastic cells are often in dense clusters and are characterized by oval to columnar shape, a round nucleus with fine chromatin, 1–2 nucleoli, increased cytoplasmic basophilia, and variable anisocytosis, anisokaryosis, and N:C (Figure 32.2). Prominent desmoplasia can be present, and, if numerous, fibroblasts can complicate the cytologic interpretation. Adenocarcinoma with columnar cells exhibiting a palisading arrangement with necrosis is likely of colonic origin.[17,24,55,56]

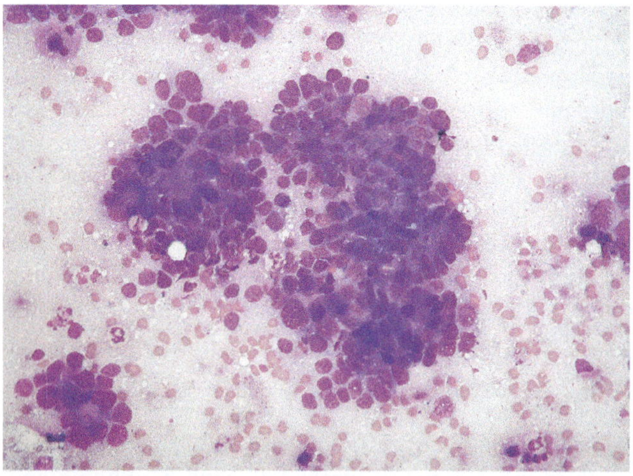

Figure 32.2 Dog, intestinal mass. Adenocarcinoma. Fine-needle biopsy. Aggregates of neoplastic cells are present on a hemorrhagic background. Cells have mild pleomorphism, indistinct borders, moderate anisokaryosis, and lightly basophilic cytoplasm. Microacinar structures are well preserved and evident within the aggregates (May-Grünwald–Giemsa, 400×).

Carcinoid

Carcinoids, also referred to as neuroendocrine tumors, argentaffin tumors, and amine precursor uptake and decarboxylation (APUD) tumors, are rare neoplasms of the large and small intestines. They arise from diffuse enterochromaffin cells rather than the intestinal epithelium, despite histologic similarity to carcinomas. Animals with carcinoid may be affected by a variety of clinical syndromes. Frequent manifestations include hypertension, tachycardia, hyperglycemia, cutaneous flushing, hypotension, bronchospasm, and diarrhea.[57,58] Signs are related to release of substances from tumor cells such as 5-hydroxytryptamine (serotonin), secretin, somatostatin, and gastrin. Cells are usually positive for neuron specific enolase, chromogranin A, and synaptophysin.[59,60] Ultrastructurally, cells are characterized by scattered prominent, round, intracytoplasmic membrane-bound, electron-dense secretory granules with a dense central core, as well as enlarged, irregular mitochondria.[59,61] Carcinoids are often locally invasive with an aggressive and debilitating clinical course, giving a poor prognosis.[20,29,49,62] Smears from carcinoids usually are highly cellular. Cytologic descriptions in the veterinary literature are restricted to a few individual case reports.[17,24,55,60,63] Like other neuroendocrine cells, carcinoids are fragile, and cytologic preparations are characterized by many bare nuclei with fewer intact cells. Intact cells are often uniform, arranged in loosely cohesive clusters with microacinar or cord-like arrangements in a blue to pink background. Necrosis is uncommon. Cells contain finely granular or vacuolated cytoplasm with central round to oval nuclei, dense chromatin, and inconspicuous nuclei.

Mesenchymal Neoplasia

Gastrointestinal Stromal Tumors

GISTs are well documented in humans and are reported in dogs, horses, and a cat.[64,65] Prior to immunohistochemical staining, stromal cell tumors often were misclassified as leiomyosarcomas and leiomyomas originating from smooth muscle or as sarcomas arising in the myenteric plexus. GISTs are thought to arise from multipotential stem cells phenotypically similar to interstitial cells of Cajal and are driven by activating mutations of Kit.[22,66] GISTs are distinguished by high vimentin immunoreactivity, high CD117 (Kit) reactivity, DOG1 positivity, and low smooth muscle actin reactivity.[67–69] In one study, 28/42 leiomyosarcomas in dogs were reclassified as GISTs after histochemical staining; thus the incidence of true leiomyosarcoma is likely lower than previously reported.[70] In the single case in veterinary literature in which cytological features are described, samples were highly cellular and comprised clusters of spindle cells with elongated nuclei, without prominent nuclear atypia, and a sparse, delicate, and wispy cytoplasm with occasional long filamentous extensions.[65] In humans, these tumors can show cytologically both spindled or epithelioid morphology. The cellularity of cytologic preparations ranges from moderate to high. Cells contain blunt-ended nuclei arranged in parallel with a delicate fibrillary cytoplasm. Cells from epithelioid GISTs tend to have eccentric dense cytoplasm with round to oval nuclei. Binucleation and multinucleation can be noted. Nucleoli are inconspicuous.[71–73]

Leiomyomas and Leiomyosarcomas

Cytological characteristics of a canine leiomyosarcoma arising from distal part of the caecum were described.[74] Large tissue fragments were present, and individual cells had indistinct margins. Cells contained oval to elongate or cigar-shaped nuclei with fine chromatin and 1–2 small to medium nucleoli. Moderate anisokaryosis was observed (Figure 32.3). Cytologic differentiation of leiomyomas and leiomyosarcomas is not always possible.[63]

Inflammation

Cytology and histology can be complementary to evaluate inflammation of the intestines and rectum in dogs and cats. IBD occurs in horses but is rarely evaluated cytologically; clinical and histologic characterization is described elsewhere.[75,76] A standardized approach to the collection and evaluation of histopathology samples in small animals has improved the diagnosis of inflammatory gastrointestinal disease.[77] An objective grading system for interpreting endoscopically collected gastrointestinal cytology specimens in dogs and cats has also been proposed.[10]

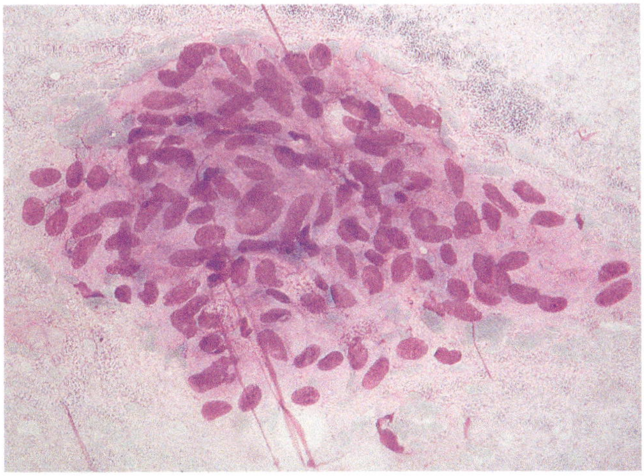

Figure 32.3 Dog, intestinal mass. Leiomyosarcoma. Squash technique. A loose aggregate of neoplastic spindle cells with indistinct borders is seen along with a few red blood cells in the background. Nuclei exhibit mild anisokaryosis, oval to cigar-shaped nuclei, and fine chromatin. The cytoplasm is abundant and lightly eosinophilic (May-Grünwald–Giemsa, 400×).

Criteria for inflammatory cells (neutrophils, lymphocytes, plasma cells, eosinophils, and macrophages), atypical cells, epithelial cells, bacterial flora, hemorrhage, debris, and mucus are included. Inflammatory cells are assigned a score of 0–7 corresponding to numbers of cells/oil immersion field (50× objective) in a minimum of 10 microscopic fields per slide; 2 or higher indicates inflammation. Although bacterial flora is included, overgrowth cannot be confirmed cytologically. Depending on the location (i.e. colonic scrapings), rods and cocci are expected, and the complete absence of bacteria can reflect prolonged antibiotic use or deficient sampling.

Neutrophilic Enterocolitis

Identification of neutrophils, particularly in samples from the distal part of the intestine, indicates active inflammation involving the colon or rectum. Neutrophils entering the more proximal intestinal lumen are destroyed rapidly. Causes of neutrophilic colitis are predominantly bacterial, including *Clostridium perfringens*, *Campylobacter jejuni*, *Salmonella* spp., and *Escherichia coli*. Mild iatrogenic hemorrhage is common in colonic cytology samples, so leukocytes must be interpreted in light of hemodilution, especially when a concurrent peripheral leukocytosis is present.[19]

Lymphocytic–Plasmacytic Enterocolitis

Chronic intestinal disease in the dog is most commonly associated with extensive infiltration of the lamina propria of the small intestine with lymphocytes and plasma cells (Figure 32.4).[77] Causes are not well defined, but some likely represent a local hypersensitivity reaction to dietary components or microbial agents.[78] A monoclonal gammopathy can be associated with this condition.[78] Moderate to severe lymphocytic–plasmacytic infiltrates also can be observed in dogs with intestinal lymphangiectasia and in dogs with bacterial overgrowth in the small intestine.[10,79] A slight increase in the number of granular lymphocytes appears common in nonspecific enteritis, especially in cats.[19,80]

The microscopic distinction, whether cytologic or histologic, between lymphoplasmacytic inflammation and lymphoma can be a diagnostic challenge. While a heterogeneous population of small to medium-sized lymphocytes and plasma cells is the cytologic basis for differentiating feline IBD from lymphoma, it is difficult to distinguish inflammation from early or small cell lymphoma by cytology alone.[80] This distinction is made more challenging because small cell lymphoma can be found coincident with an inflammatory lymphocytic background.[36] In one study, cases were classified as lymphoma by the presence of a monomorphic population of small lymphocytes with few or no plasma cells and large numbers of lymphoglandular bodies.[80] Based on these

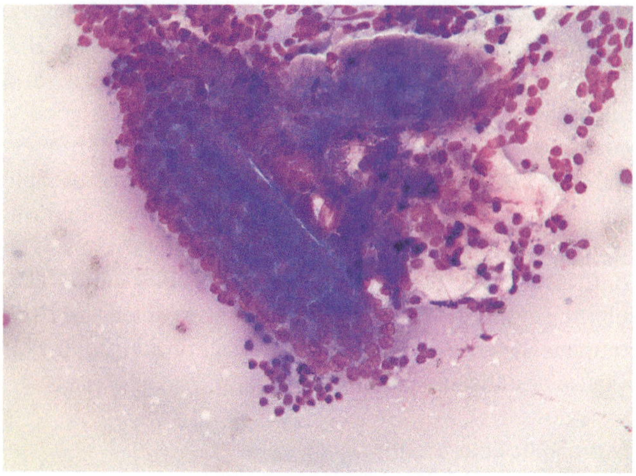

Figure 32.4 Cat, intestinal wall. Inflammatory bowel disease. Squash technique from biopsy specimen. A large cluster of cohesive simple epithelial cells with indistinct boundaries is evident. In addition, a high number of small to medium-sized lymphocytes with high N:C and clumped chromatin are evident in close contact to the epithelial aggregate (May-Grűnwald-Giemsa, 400×).

characteristics sensitivity was low (36%), and specificity was high (87%) with an overall accuracy of 62%.[80]

The published literature on the utility of cytology in the diagnosis of intestinal lymphoma provides mixed results. A review of small intestine endoscopic cytology specimens from 122 dogs and 35 cats reported a sensitivity of 92% and a specificity of 80% in the diagnosis of lymphoma.[11] Similarly, another recent publication found that a "squash and smear" sample preparation technique paired with a novel diagnostic algorithm resulted in a sensitivity of 98.6% and a sensitivity of 73.5% for differentiation between enteritis and lymphoma in dogs.[14] In contrast, a study examining feline endoscopic cytology samples reports a lower sensitivity (60%) and specificity (91%) in the diagnosis of low-grade lymphoma.[81] The addition of ancillary clonality analysis on cytology samples may be informative but has not been robustly studied.

Eosinophilic Enterocolitis

Chronic eosinophilic enterocolitis is characterized by heavy infiltration of the intestinal mucosa with eosinophils along with some lymphocytes and plasma cells. This inflammatory disorder occurs in many breeds of dogs and cats, with a predilection for German shepherds. Circulating eosinophilia and eosinophils in intestinal tissue suggests a hypersensitivity reaction to dietary antigens or parasites or can occur as a paraneoplastic syndrome associated with T-cell lymphoma or mast cell tumors. In cats, eosinophilic inflammation can represent a component of hypereosinophilic syndrome.[82] Cytology of feline gastrointestinal eosinophilic sclerosing fibroplasia is characterized by numerous eosinophils and neutrophils, occasional small to intermediate-sized lymphocytes and plasma cells, few degranulated mast cells, and large irregular- to spindle-shaped cells with pink extracellular matrix.[83]

Infectious Processes

Cryptosporidiosis

Intestinal cryptosporidiosis has been occasionally diagnosed with intestinal imprints (for morphology, see Chapters 3 and 33). *Cryptosporidium* spp. are coccidians that are transmitted among dogs and cats by the ingestion of oocysts in feces. The rupture of those oocysts within the intestines releases sporozoites, which attach to the intestinal epithelium between the cell membrane and the cell cytoplasm. Infiltration of the lamina propria with neutrophils, macrophages, and lymphocytes can result. Thin-walled sporulated oocysts measure approximately 5–7 μm in diameter and can be observed in feces. Modified acid-fast staining of a thin fecal smear can aid in the detection of the organisms.[84]

Coccidiosis

Intestinal coccidiosis is caused by the genus *Isospora*, the most commonly recognized coccidians infecting dogs or cats. Although coccidiosis is frequently diagnosed by demonstrating oocysts in fecal flotation specimens (see Chapter 33), sporozoites, the infective stage, are rarely observed in intestinal imprints taken in acute phases of the disease. Sporozoites have a banana shape with gently pointed ends, a small purple nucleus measuring few microns, and light blue cytoplasm.[85]

Giardiasis

Giardiasis (*Giardia lamblia*) can be diagnosed by finding the trophozoites in imprints from duodenal specimens. They appear as active, binucleated, pear- or teardrop-shaped organisms with four pairs of flagella, measuring approximately 15 × 8 μm (Figure 32.5). Sometimes these organisms are observed in rectal scrapings. Rarely, Giardia can be seen in fecal samples (see Chapter 33), exhibiting the characteristic "falling leaf" motion. Although *Giardia* trophozoites can be confused with tritrichomonas that are similar in size, they can be differentiated from these protozoa based on their motility and morphology (see below).[86]

Diseases of the Rectum

Neoplasia

Lymphoma represents the most common neoplastic disease of the canine rectum that can be diagnosed with rectal scraping.[14,87] The literature suggests that B-cell origin is common, and rectal lymphoma in dogs is associated with a relatively favorable prognosis.[88]

Adenocarcinomas are often pedunculated and polypoid (especially in the distal rectum), cobblestone (middle rectum), or annular (middle rectum) in appearance.[25] These tumors appear cytologically similar to those already described for the small intestine (Figure 32.6).

Extramedullary rectal plasma cell tumors can be associated with monoclonal gammopathy.[45] Plasmacytomas are cytologically characterized by individualized round to oval cells, measuring 15–30 μm in diameter, with moderate to large amount of finely granular and pale basophilic cytoplasm, and a single, round to oval, eccentric nucleus with clumped to reticular chromatin. Binucleated cells can also be observed. Rarely these appear with eosinophilic cytoplasm typical of flame cells, and some neoplastic cells contain a moderate number of golden-brown cytoplasmic hemosiderin granules.[89]

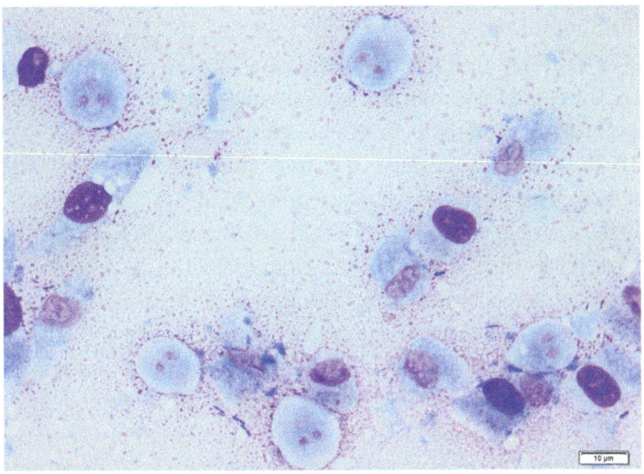

Figure 32.5 Five-month-old dog with chronic vomiting, diarrhea, and weight loss. Endoscopic brush smear from the duodenum reveals numerous trophozoites of *Giardia* spp. Benign epithelial cells and rare bacteria are in the background (Diff-Quik, bar = 10 μm. *Source:* Image courtesy of Marian Taulescu).

Inflammatory and Infectious Diseases

Eosinophilic Colitis and Proctitis

Eosinophilic colitis can involve primarily colon and rectum or be part of a more extensive inflammatory process involving the small intestine as well. Infectious agents, parasites, and food allergies are possible inciting factors. In feline hypereosinophilic and canine eosinophilic gastroenteritis syndromes, there can be large intestinal involvement.[90] Rectal scraping can yield a large number of eosinophils and, if ulcerated, neutrophils, bacteria, and red blood cells.[18] Eosinophilic colitis is a described entity in horses[91,92], and eosinophilic proctitis has been diagnosed cytologically in a pony, with aspirates containing 50% eosinophils as well as neutrophils, epithelial and mesenchymal cells, and few lymphocytes.[93]

Neutrophilic Colitis and Proctitis

Rectal scrapings from ulcerative lesions of different etiologies yield a variable proportion of neutrophils; thus neutrophils are considered a nonspecific finding, especially if blood is present. *Campylobacter* and *Salmonella* spp. can

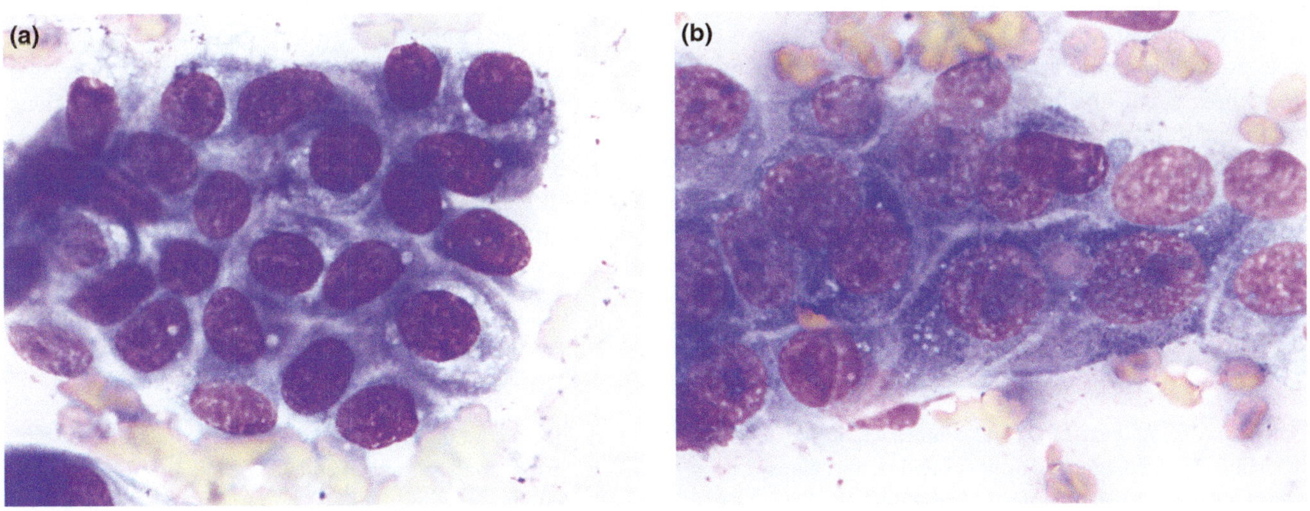

Figure 32.6 Dog, rectal mass. Aspirates from a histologically confirmed anorectal polyp with carcinoma *in situ*. Note the variation of the epithelial populations in this cytology. (a) A cluster of relatively uniform cuboidal epithelial cells characterized by scant to moderate amounts of light basophilic cytoplasm and uniform round to oval to angular nuclei characteristic of well-differentiated epithelial tissue originating from the polyp. (b) A disorganized cluster of anaplastic epithelial cells characterized by a moderate amount of deeply basophilic, lightly vacuolated cytoplasm with round to oval nuclei, and prominent nucleoli presumed to originate from the carcinoma *in situ* (Wright–Giemsa, 1000×. *Source:* Images courtesy of Leslie Sharkey).

be primary bacterial pathogens inducing neutrophilic inflammation. Neutrophilic clostridial colitis can be characterized by a high percentage of large rod-shaped bacteria (*C. perfringens*), which stain blue with a clear center with Romanowsky stains and are Gram-positive. Occasional clostridial organisms can be observed in health, but more than 5/1000× oil field is considered abnormal.[19]

Infectious Agents

Histoplasma capsulatum is a dimorphic, soil-borne fungus that causes large bowel diarrhea. Rectal scraping can detect pyogranulomatous or granulomatous inflammation with intramacrophagic or extracellular yeasts that are 2–5 μm in diameter (Chapter 3).[94,95] *Cryptococcus neoformans* appear as large extracellular round basophilic yeasts measuring 3–7 μm in diameter, with a prominent achromic capsule of variable thickness (see Chapter 3).[96–98] The opportunistic fungal agent, *Cokeromyces recurvatus*, consists of large (30–90 μm) round to oval, deeply basophilic, thick-walled structures, similar in morphology to *Coccidioides immitis*. These yeasts have been seen in some cases of severe mucosal inflammation along with a mixed population of bacteria, and infection may be secondary to immunosuppression.[99] *Cyniclomyces guttulatus* is a yeast frequently present in feces or rectal scrapings in dogs with gastrointestinal symptoms such as chronic diarrhea. It has also been observed in the fecal samples of healthy dogs, presumably after consuming rabbit fecal pellets (Chapter 33). One study concluded that there is no direct evidence that *C. guttulatus* is a primary pathogen and suggested that the yeast might cause chronic diarrhea in a minority of cases, perhaps as an opportunistic infection.[100] Morphologically, these yeasts are elongated, oval to cylindrical in shape, with a thin cell walls and a basophilic internal structure.[100] They are often seen in short, branching chains, appearing in "Y" configurations.

Prototheca zopfii are unicellular colorless algae causing protothecosis, an uncommon cutaneous and systemic disease. With colonization of the large intestines (colon and rectum), acute or chronic large bowel diarrhea occurs, often accompanied by hematochezia and tenesmus. This alga can disseminate to a variety of tissues, apart from colon, including eyes, brain and meninges, kidneys, and bones. Rectal scraping can reveal spheroid, ovoid, bean-shaped, or elliptical organisms ranging in diameter from 1.5 to 30 μm. They have a hyalinized thick nonstaining cell wall (approximately 0.5 μm) with basophilic granular cytoplasm. Organisms are predominantly extracellular, although small forms can be observed within macrophages or neutrophils.[101,102]

Tritrichomonas sp. is the causative agent of feline trichomoniasis, parasitizing the large intestine. A trophozoite measures 10–26 × 3–5 μm, with a single dark nucleus, basophilic cytoplasm with small clear vacuoles, three anterior flagella, and an undulating membrane. On wet mounts, it exhibits rapid forward motion. The sensitivity of a direct fecal smear using specimens from naturally infected cats was only 14% in one study, so false negatives are common with this method. The sensitivity can be improved by analyzing multiple fecal smears.[86,103] *Balantidium coli* is a large ciliated protozoa, measuring 50–150 μm that can infect the canine colon. The diagnosis is based on rectal scraping, coprological identification of motile trophozoites in direct smears, or the detection of cysts with flotation techniques. In rectal scrapings or direct fresh smears, the trophozoites are oval-shaped and show revolving movement by means of cilia, with a macronucleus that may be visible. In stained smears, they are kidney bean shaped, with a prominent macronucleus and a micronucleus that occasionally can be seen.[104] *Entamoeba histolytica* is a commensal ameba of the colonic lumen, which can become pathogenic, invading the intestinal wall and causing inflammation and hemorrhagic large intestine diarrhea. In acute disease, severe diarrhea can develop. Trophozoites, measuring 12–50 μm, are difficult to detect in fecal specimens. Direct smears of fresh feces reveal the sluggish, amoeboid motility of the trophozoites, which constantly change shape when active, moving by means of fingerlike projections of the cytoplasm. In stained smears, the nucleus usually has distributed peripheral chromatin, a nucleolus, and a slightly basophilic cytoplasm that can contain ingested red blood cells. Macrophages in feces are sometimes confused with trophozoites phagocytizing erythrocytes.[104,105]

References

1 Jergens, A.E., Willard, M.D., and Allenspach, K. (2016). Maximizing the diagnostic utility of endoscopic biopsy in dogs and cats with gastrointestinal disease. *Vet J* 214: 50–60.

2 Taylor, S.D., Pusterla, N., Vaughan, B. et al. (2006). Intestinal neoplasia in horses. *J Vet Intern Med* 20: 1429–1436.

3 Crystal, M.A., Penninck, D.G., Matz, M.E. et al. (1993). Use of ultrasound-guided fine-needle aspiration biopsy and automated core biopsy for the diagnosis of gastrointestinal diseases in small animals. *Vet Radiol Ultrasound* 34: 438–444.

4 Bonfanti, U., Bertazzolo, W., Bottero, E. et al. (2006). Diagnostic value of cytologic examination of gastrointestinal tract tumors in dogs and cats: 83 cases (2001–2004). *J Am Vet Med Assoc* 229: 1130–1133.

5 Torp-Pedersen, S., Gronval, S., and Holm, H.H. (1984). Ultrasonically guided fine-needle aspiration biopsy of gastrointestinal mass lesions. *J Ultrasound Med* 3: 65–68.

6 Javid, G., Gulzar, G.M., Khan, B. et al. (1999). Percutaneous sonography-guided fine needle aspiration biopsy of colonscopic biopsy negative colonic lesions. *Indian J Gastroenterol* 18: 146–148.

7 Ballo, M.S. and Guy, C.D. (2001). Percutaneous fine-needle aspiration of gastrointestinal wall lesions with image guidance. *Diagn Cytopathol* 24: 16–20.

8 Tudor, G.R., Rodgers, P.M., and West, K.P. (1999). Bowel lesions: percutaneous US-guided 18-gauge needle biopsy—preliminary experience. *Radiology* 212: 594–597.

9 Marco-Domenech, S.F., Gil-Sanchez, S., Fernandez-Garcia, P. et al. (2001). Sonographically guided percutaneous biopsy of gastrointestinal tract lesions. *Am J Roentgenol* 176: 147–151.

10 Jergens, A.E., Andreasen, C.B., Hagemoser, W.A. et al. (1998). Cytologic examination of exfoliative specimens obtained during endoscopy for diagnosis of gastrointestinal tract disease in dogs and cats. *J Am Vet Med Assoc* 213: 1755–1759.

11 Jergens, A.E., Andreasen, C.B., and Miles, K.G. (2000). Gastrointestinal endoscopic exfoliative cytology: techniques and clinical application. *Compend Contin Educ Pract Vet* 22: 941–952.

12 Evans, S.E., Bonczynski, J.J., Broussars, J.D. et al. (2006). Comparison of endoscopic and full-thickness biopsy specimens for diagnosis of inflammatory bowel disease and alimentary tract lymphoma in cats. *J Am Vet Med Assoc* 229: 1447–1450.

13 Maeda, S., Tsuboi, M., Sakai, K. et al. (2017). Endoscopic cytology for the diagnosis of chronic enteritis and intestinal lymphoma in dogs. *Vet Pathol* 54: 595–604.

14 Webb, J.L., Rakich, P.M., and Latimer, K.S. (2008). The gastrointestinal tract. In: *Diagnostic Cytology and Hematology of the Dog and Cat*, (ed. Cowell R.L., Tyler R.D., Meinkoth J.H., and DeNicola D.B.), 286–297. St. Louis, MO: Elsevier Saunders.

15 Weeden, A.L. and Wamsley, H.L. (2016). Dry-mount fecal cytology. Canine and feline cytology. In: *A Color Atlas and Interpretation Guide*, (ed. Raskin R.E. and Meyer D.J.), 247–258. St. Louis, MO: Elsevier.

16 Aughey, E. and Frye, F.L. (2001). Digestive system. In: *Comparative Veterinary Histology*, (ed. Aughey E. and Frye F.L.), 97–136. London: Manson Publishing.

17 Geisinger, K.R. (1997). Alimentary tract. In: *Comprehensive Cytopathology*, (ed. Bibbo M.), 413–444. Philadelphia, PA: Saunders.

18 Haddad, J.L., Marks, D.A., Stowe, M. et al. (2014). The gastrointestinal tract. In: *Diagnostic Cytology and Hematology of the Dog and Cat*, (ed. Valenciano A.C. and Cowell R.L.), 312–340. St. Louis, MO: Elsevier, Mosby.

19 Jergens, A.E., Jones Hostetter, S., and Andreasen, C.B. (2016). Oral cavity, gastrointestinal tract, and associated structures. In: *Canine and Feline Cytology. A Color Atlas and Interpretation Guide*, (ed. Raskin R.E. and Meyer D.J.), 220–246. St. Louis, MO: Elsevier.

20 Banks, W.J. (1993). Digestive system I: alimentary canal. In: *Applied Veterinary Histology*, (ed. Banks W.J.), 326–359. St. Louis, MO: Mosby.

21 Banks, W.J. (1993). Endocrine system. In: *Applied Veterinary Histology*, (ed. Banks W.J.), 408–428. St. Louis, MO: Mosby.

22 Head, K.W., Cullen, J.M., Dubielzig, R.R. et al. (2003). Tumors of the intestines. In: *Histological Classification of Tumors of the Alimentary System of Domestic Animals*, (ed. Head K.W., Cullen J.M., Dubielzig R.R., Else R.W., Misdorp W., Patnaik A.K., Tateyama S., and van der Gaag I.), 89–110. Washington, DC: AFIP.

23 Washabau, R.J. (2013). Integration of gastrointestinal function. In: *Canine and Feline Gastroenterology*, (ed. Day M.J. and Washabau R.J.), 1–31. St. Louis, MO: Elsevier.

24 DeMay, R.M. (1996). The gastrointestinal tract. In: *The Art and Science of Cytopathology*, (ed. DeMay R.M.), 327–384. Chicago: ASCP Press.

25 Rissetto, K. and Selting, K.A. (2010). Intestinal tumors. In: *Cancer Management in Small Animal Practice*, (ed. Henry C.J. and Higginbotham M.L.), 251–259. St. Louis, MO: Saunders.

26 Dom, C.R., Taylor, D.O.N., Schneider, R. et al. (1968). Survey of animal neoplasms in Alameda and Contra Costa counties, California. II. Cancer morbidity in dogs and cats from Alameda County. *J Natl Cancer Inst* 40: 307–318.

27 Patnaik, A.K., Liu, S.K., and Johnson, G.F. (1976). Feline intestinal adenocarcinoma. *Vet Pathol* 13: 1–10.

28 Crawshaw, J., Berg, J., Sardinas, J.C. et al. (1998). Prognosis for dogs with nonlymphomatous, small intestinal tumors treated by surgical excision. *J Am Anim Hosp Assoc* 34: 451–456.

29 Head, K.W., Else, R.W., and Dubielzig, R.R. (2002). Tumors of the intestines. In: *Tumors in Domestic Animals*, (ed. Meuten D.J.), 461–477. Ames, IA: Iowa State Press.

30 Crow, S.E. (1985). Tumors of the alimentary tract. *Vet Clin North Am Small Anim Pract* 15: 577–587.

31 Louwerens, M., London, C.L., Pedersen, N.C., and Lyons, L.A. (2005). Feline lymphoma in the post-feline leukemia virus era. *J Vet Intern Med* 19: 329–335.

32 Rissetto, K., Villamil, J.A., Selting, K.A. et al. (2011). Recent trends in feline intestinal neoplasia: an epidemiologic study of 1129 cases in the veterinary medical database from 1964 to 2004. *J Am Anim Hosp Assoc* 47: 28–36.

33 Gieger, T. (2011). Alimentary lymphoma in cats and dogs. *Vet Clin North Am Small Anim Pract* 41: 419–432.

34 Moore, P.F., Rodriguez-Bertos, A., and Kass, P.H. (2012). Feline gastrointestinal lymphoma: mucosal architecture, immunophenotype, and molecular clonality. *Vet Pathol* 49: 658–668.

35 Coyle, K.A. and Steinberg, H. (2004). Characterization of lymphocytes in canine gastrointestinal lymphoma. *Vet Pathol* 41: 141–146.

36 Carrasco, V., Rodriguez-Berto, A., and Rodriguez-Franco, F. (2015). Distinguishing intestinal lymphoma from inflammatory bowel disease in canine endoscopic duodenal samples. *Vet Pathol* 52: 668–675.

37 Vail, D.M., Moore, A.S., and Ogilvie, G.K. (1998). Feline lymphoma (145 cases): proliferation indices, cluster of differentiation 3 immunoreactivity, and their association with prognosis in 90 cats. *J Vet Intern Med* 12: 349–354.

38 Russell, K.J., Beatty, J.A., Dhand, N. et al. (2012). Feline low-grade alimentary lymphoma: how common is it? *J Feline Med Surg* 14: 910–912.

39 Franks, P.T., Harvey, J.W., May, M.C. et al. (1986). Feline large granular lymphoma. *Vet Pathol* 23: 200–202.

40 Kariya, K., Konno, A., and Ishida, T. (1997). Perforin-like immunoreactivity in four cases of lymphoma of large granular lymphocytes in the cat. *Vet Pathol* 34: 156–159.

41 Roccabianca, P., Vernau, W., Caniatti, M. et al. (2006). Feline large granular lymphocyte (LGL) lymphoma with secondary leukemia: primary intestinal origin with predominance of a CD3/CD8αα phenotype. *Vet Pathol* 43: 15–28.

42 French, R.A., Seitz, S.E., and Valli, V.E. (1996). Primary epitheliotropic alimentary T-cell lymphoma with hepatic involvement in a dog. *Vet Pathol* 33: 349–352.

43 Loupal, G. and Pfeil, C. (1984). Tumours in the intestines of cats, with particular reference to non-haematopoietic growths. *Berl Munch Tierarztl Wochenschr* 97: 208–213.

44 MacEwen, E.G., Patnaik, A.K., Johnson, G.F. et al. (1984). Extramedullary plasmacytoma of the gastrointestinal tract in two dogs. *J Am Vet Med Assoc* 184: 1396–1398.

45 Trevor, P.B., Saunders, G.K., Waldron, D.R. et al. (1993). Metastatic extramedullary plasmacytoma of the colon and rectum in a dog. *J Am Vet Med Assoc* 203: 406–409.

46 Jackson, M.W., Helfand, S.C., Smedes, S.L. et al. (1994). Primary IgG secreting plasma cell tumor in the gastrointestinal tract of a dog. *J Am Vet Med Assoc* 204: 404–406.

47 Ramos-Vara, J.A., Miller, M.A., Pace, L.W. et al. (1998). Intestinal multinodular A lambda-amyloid deposition associated with extramedullary plasmacytoma in 3 dogs. *J Comp Pathol* 119: 239–249.

48 Caruso, K.J., Meinkoth, J.H., Cowell, R.L. et al. (2003). A distal colonic mass in a dog. *Vet Clin Pathol* 32: 27–30.

49 Selting, K. (2013). Intestinal tumors. In: *Small Animal Clinical Oncology*, (ed. Withrow S.J., Vail D.M., and Page R.L.), 412–423. St. Louis, MO: Elsevier Saunders.

50 Howl, J.H. and Peterson, M.G. (1995). Intestinal mast cell tumor in a cat: presentation as eosinophilic enteritis. *J Am Anim Hosp Assoc* 31: 457–461.

51 Halsey, C.H.C., Powers, B.E., and Kamstock, D.A. (2010). Feline intestinal sclerosing mast cell tumour: 50 cases (1997–2008). *Vet Comp Oncol* 8: 72–79.

52 Munday, J.S., Lohr, C.V., and Dubielzig, R.R. (2017). Tumors of the intestines. In: *Tumors in Domestic Animals*, (ed. Meuten D.J.), 563–587. Ames, IA: Wiley.

53 Ozaki, K., Yamagami, T., Nomura, K., and Narama, I. (2002). Mast cell tumors of the gastrointestinal tract in 39 dogs. *Vet Pathol* 39: 557–564.

54 Takahashi, T., Kadosawa, M., Nagase, S. et al. (2000). Visceral mast cell tumors in dogs: 10 cases (1982–1997). *J Am Vet Med Assoc* 216: 222–226.

55 Leiman, G. (1999). Pancreas, biliary tract and intra-abdominal organs. In: *Manual and Atlas of Fine-Needle Aspiration Cytology*, (ed. Orell S.R., Sterrett G.F., Walters M.N.I., and Whitaker D.), 291–307. London: Churchill Livingstone.

56 Juopperi, T.A., Cesta, M., and Tomlinson, M. (2003). Extensive cutaneous metastases in a dog with duodenal adenocarcinoma. *Vet Clin Pathol* 32: 88–91.

57 Sako, T., Uchida, E., Okamoto, M. et al. (2003). Immunohistochemical evaluation of malignant intestinal carcinoid in a dog. *Vet Pathol* 40: 212–215.

58 Tappin, S., Brown, P., and Ferasin, L. (2008). An intestinal neuroendocrine tumor associated with paroxysmal ventricular tachycardia and melaena in a 10-year-old boxer. *J Small Anim Pract* 49: 33–37.

59 Morrell, C.N., Volk, M.V., and Mankowski, J.L. (2002). A carcinoid tumor in the gallbladder of a dog. *Vet Pathol* 39: 756–758.

60 Choi, U.S., Alleman, A.R., Choi, J.H. et al. (2008). Cytologic and immunohistochemical characterization of a lung carcinoid in a dog. *Vet Clin Pathol* 37: 249–252.

61 Rossmeisl, J.H., Dru Forrester, S., Robertson, J.L., and Cook, W.T. (2002). Chronic vomiting associated with a gastric carcinoid in a cat. *J Am Anim Hosp Assoc* 38: 61–66.

62 Giles, R.C. Jr., Hildebrandt, P.K., and Montgomery, C.A. Jr. (1974). Carcinoid tumor in the small intestine of a dog. *Vet Pathol* 11: 340–349.

63 Baker, R. and Lumsden, J.H. (2000). The gastrointestinal tract. In: *Color Atlas of Cytology of the Dog and Cat*, (ed. Baker R. and Lumsden J.H.), 177–198. St. Louis, MO: Mosby.

64 Del Piero, F., Summers, B.A., Cummings, J.F. et al. (2001). Gastrointestinal stromal cell tumors in Equids. *Vet Pathol* 38: 689–697.

65 Morini, M., Gentilini, F., Pietra, M. et al. (2011). Cytological, immunohistochemical and mutational analysis of a gastric gastrointestinal stromal tumor in a cat. *J Comp Pathol* 145: 152–157.

66 Miettinen, M., Majidi, M., and Lasota, J. (2002). Pathology and diagnostic criteria of gastrointestinal stromal tumors (GISTs): a review. *Eur J Cancer* 38 (5): S39–S51.

67 LaRock, R.G. and Ginn, P.E. (1997). Immunohistochemical staining characteristics of canine gastrointestinal stromal tumors. *Vet Pathol* 34: 303–311.

68 Gillespie, V., Baer, K., Farrelly, J. et al. (2011). Canine gastrointestinal stromal tumors: immunohistochemical expression of CD34 and examination of prognostic indicators including proliferation markers Ki67 and AgNOR. *Vet Pathol* 48: 283–291.

69 Dailey, D.D., Ehrahrt, E.J., Duval, D.L. et al. (2015). DOG1 is a sensitive and specific immunohistochemical marker for diagnosis of canine gastrointestinal stromal cell tumors. *J Vet Diagn Invest* 27: 268–277.

70 Russell, K.N., Mehler, S.J., Skorupski, K.A. et al. (2007). Clinical and immunohistochemical differentiation of gastrointestinal stromal tumors from leiomyosarcomas in dogs: 42 cases (1990–2003). *J Am Vet Med Assoc* 230: 1329–1333.

71 Gu, M., Ghafari, S., Nguyen, P.T., and Lin, F. (2001). Cytologic diagnosis of gastrointestinal stromal tumors of the stomach by endoscopic ultrasound-guided fine-needle aspiration biopsy: cytomorphologic and immunohistochemical study of 12 cases. *Diagn Cytopathol* 25: 343–350.

72 Elliott, D.D., Fanning, C.V., and Caraway, N.P. (2006). The utility of fine-needle aspiration in the diagnosis of gastrointestinal stromal tumors: a cytomorphologic and immunohistochemical analysis with emphasis on malignant tumors. *Cancer* 108: 49–55.

73 Vij, M., Agrawal, V., Kumar, A., and Pandey, R. (2013). Cytomorphology of gastrointestinal stromal tumors and extra-gastrointestinal stromal tumors: a comprehensive morphologic study. *J Cytol* 30: 8–12.

74 Messick, J.B., Haddad, T., Kitchell, B. et al. (2001). Abdominal mass in a dog. *Vet Clin Pathol* 30: 25–27.

75 Schumacher, J., Edwards, J.F., and Cohen, N.D. (2000). Chronic idiopathic inflammatory bowel diseases of the horse. *J Vet Intern Med* 14: 258–265.

76 Kalck, K.A. (2009). Inflammatory bowel disease in horses. *Vet Clin North Am: Large Anim Pract* 25: 303–315.

77 Washabau, R.J., Day, M.J., Willard, M.D. et al. (2010). Endoscopic, biopsy and histopathological guidelines for the evaluation of gastrointestinal inflammation in companion animals. *J Vet Intern Med* 24: 10–26.

78 Tizard, I.R. (2004). Type I hypersensitivity. In: *Veterinary Immunology. An Introduction*, (ed. Tizard I.R.), 308–323. Philadelphia, PA: Saunders.

79 Rutgers, H.C., Batt, R.M., Elwood, C.M., and Lamport, A. (1995). Small intestinal bacterial overgrowth in dogs with chronic intestinal disease. *J Am Vet Med Assoc* 206: 187–193.

80 Sabattini, S., Bottero, E., Turba, M.E. et al. (2016). Differentiating feline inflammatory bowel disease from alimentary lymphoma in duodenal endoscopic biopsies. *J Small Anim Pract* 57: 396–401.

81 Mangelsdorf, S., Teske, E., Bomhard, W., and Stockhaus, C. (2015). Cytology of endoscopically obtained biopsies for the diagnosis of chronic intestinal diseases in cats. *Tierarztl Prax Ausg K Kleintiere Heimtiere* 43: 15–20.

82 Gelberg, H.B. (2007). Alimentary system. In: *Pathologic Basis of Veterinary Disease*, (ed. Zachary J.F. and McGavin M.D.), 301–391. St. Louis, MO: Elsevier, Mosby.

83 Craig, L.E., Hardam, E.E., Hertzke, D.M. et al. (2009). Feline gastrointestinal eosinophilic sclerosing fibroplasia. *Vet Pathol* 46: 63–70.

84 Lappin, M.R. (2014). Cryptosporidiosis. In: *Canine and Feline Infectious Diseases*, (ed. Sykes J.E.), 785–792. St. Louis, MO: Elsevier Saunders.

85 Dubey, J.P. and Greene, C.E. (2012). Enteric coccidiosis. In: *Infectious Diseases of the Dog and Cat*, (ed. Greene C.E.), 828–839. St. Louis, MO: Elsevier Saunders.

86 Lappin, M.R. (2014). Giardiasis. In: *Canine and Feline Infectious Diseases*, (ed. Sykes J.E.), 771–778. St. Louis, MO: Elsevier Saunders.

87 Holt, P.E. and Lucke, V.M. (1985). Rectal neoplasia in the dog: a clinicopathologic review of 31 cases. *Vet Rec* 116: 400–405.

88 Van Den Steen, N., Berlato, D., Polton, G. et al. (2012). Rectal lymphoma in 11 dogs-a retrospective study. *J Small Anim Pract* 53: 586–591.

89 Rannou, B., Hélie, P., and Bédard, C. (2009). Rectal plasmacytoma with intracellular hemosiderin in a dog. *Vet Pathol* 46: 1181–1184.

90 Hendrick, M. (1981). A spectrum of hypereosinophilic syndromes exemplified by six cats with eosinophilic enteritis. *Vet Pathol* 18: 188–200.

91 Edwards, G.B., Kelly, D.F., and Proudman, C.J. (2000). Segmental eosinophilic colitis: a review of 22 cases. *Equine Vet J* 32: 86–93.

92 Archer, D.C., Costain, D.A., and Sherlock, C. (2014). Idiopathic focal eosinophilic enteritis (IFEE), an emerging cause of abdominal pain in horses: the effect of age, time and geographical location on risk. *PLoS One* 9: e112072.

93 Gison, K.T., O'Hara, A.J., and Huxtable, C.R. (2001). Focal eosinophilic proctitis with associated rectal prolapse in a pony. *Aust Vet J* 79: 679–681.

94 Lin Blache, J., Ryan, K., and Arceneaux, K. (2011). Histoplasmosis. *Compend Contin Educ Vet* 3: E1–E11.

95 Sykes, J.E. and Taboada, J. (2014). Histoplasmosis. In: *Canine and Feline Infectious Diseases*, (ed. Sykes J.E.), 587–598. St. Louis, MO: Elsevier Saunders.

96 Honsho, C.S., Mine, S.Y., Orià, A.P. et al. (2003). Generalized systemic cryptococcosis in a dog after immunosuppressive corticotherapy. *Arq Bras Med Vet Zootec* 55: 155–159.

97 Sykes, J.E. and Malik, J. (2012). Cryptococcosis. In: *Infectious Diseases of the Dog and Cat*, (ed. Greene C.E.), 621–634. St. Louis, MO: Elsevier Saunders.

98 Sykes, J.E. and Malik, J. (2014). Cryptococcosis. In: *Canine and Feline Infectious Diseases*, (ed. Sykes J.E.), 599–612. St. Louis, MO: Elsevier Saunders.

99 Parker, V.J., Jergens, A.E., Whitley, E.M., and Frana, T.S. (2011). Isolation of *Cokeromyces recurvatus* from the gastrointestinal tract in a dog with protein-losing enteropathy. *J Vet Diagn Invest* 23: 1014–1016.

100 Mandigers, P.J., Duijvestijn, M.B., Ankringa, N. et al. (2014). The clinical significance of *Cyniclomyces guttulatus* in dogs with chronic diarrhoea, a survey and a prospective treatment study. *Vet Microbiol* 172: 241–247.

101 Stenner, V.J., Mackay, B., King, T. et al. (2007). Protothecosis in 17 Australian dogs and a review of the canine literature. *Med Mycol* 45: 249–266.

102 Sykes, J.E. (2014). Protothecosis. In: *Canine and Feline Infectious Diseases*, (ed. Sykes J.E.), 679–685. St. Louis, MO: Elsevier Saunders.

103 Gookin, J.L., Levy, M.G., Law, J.M. et al. (2001). Experimental infection of cats with *Tritrichomonas foetus*. *Am J Vet Res* 62: 1690–1697.

104 Little, S.E. and Lindsay, D.S. (2012). Laboratory diagnosis of protozoal infections. In: *Infectious Diseases of the Dog and Cat*, (ed. Greene C.E.), 711–717. St. Louis, MO: Elsevier Saunders.

105 Greene, C.E. (2012). Amebiasis. In: *Infectious Diseases of the Dog and Cat*, (ed. Greene C.E.), 792–794. St. Louis, MO: Elsevier Saunders.

33

Fecal Cytology

Cathy Trumel and Olivier Dossin

Introduction

Fecal testing is commonly performed in veterinary gastroenterology. Microscopic assessment is very important, with several techniques available for different diagnostic purposes.[1] Wet-mount fecal cytology is used for identification of motile organisms such as some protozoal trophozoites (e.g. *Giardia* spp., trichomonads), amoebae, nematode larvae (e.g. *Strongyloides* spp.), and selected bacteria (e.g. campylobacter-like organisms, treponeme-like spirochetes) or spores (*Clostridium* spp.). Fecal flotation is routinely used for diagnosis of most intestinal parasites. Fecal sedimentation techniques are used specifically to identify fluke eggs and embryonated nematode eggs (e.g. *Physaloptera* spp., *Spirocerca lupi*). Baermann funnel preparation is used for isolation of nematode larvae such as some lungworm larvae (e.g. *Aelurostrongylus* or *Angiostrongylus* spp.) and small intestinal larvae (e.g. *Strongyloides* spp.). Dry-mount fecal cytology is used for evaluation of cellular infiltrates and assessing flora. This chapter will focus on dry-mount fecal cytology performed using Romanowsky-stained slides. This method is insufficient to distinguish pathogens from nonpathogens. Results should be interpreted cautiously or in the context of clinical presentation and the results of other diagnostic tests including wet-mount fecal cytology, bacterial culture, fecal antigen detection, and other molecular techniques.[2]

Collection

Sampling methods include the collection of fresh fecal material, colonic or rectal saline lavage, and rectal scraping. Fresh fecal material can be obtained during rectal digital examination or using a moistened, cotton-tipped applicator.[1] In this case, the applicator is gently rolled on the slide to prepare a direct thin film, which can be done in parallel with wet-mount cytology. For wet mounts, a drop of room temperature or warm saline is placed on slides; a very small amount of feces is added and mixed with a wooden applicator stick, and then a glass coverslip is applied. Rectal saline lavage is performed with a soft rubber catheter and 6–12 mL of saline in a syringe. After minimal lubrication of the catheter with a water-based lubricant, the catheter is introduced in the rectum, and the saline is injected and aspirated several times. The collected material can be used for wet- and dry-mount evaluation, but contamination with lubricant must be avoided. For all these methods, feces must be fresh, and smears ideally should be prepared under five minutes after collection. Rectal scraping can be done with a swab or a blunt spatula and is more invasive. This method can be used for identification of some infectious agents localized deeper in the mucosa such as fungal agents or the type of cell infiltrate (for more detail, see Chapter 3).[2]

Normal Cytology

Normal fecal cytology is characterized by a polymorphic population of microbial flora predominated by rod-shaped bacteria with rare coccoid bacteria and occasional yeast in a background of mucus and debris. Clusters of columnar epithelial cells or mature squamous cells can be observed on rectal scraping or other invasively collected samples (Figure 33.1). In atraumatic sampling, few to no epithelial cells or blood cells are observed. *Cyniclomyces guttulatus* (formerly *Saccharomycopsis guttulata*) is a normal fungal organism of the gastrointestinal tract in rodents and lagomorphs but can be seen in dogs and less frequently in cats. Cytologically, *C. guttulatus* is a large organism occurring individually or in short, forked, or branching chains. Organisms are approximatively 5–7 × 15–20 µm, oval to cylindrical structures surrounded by a clear wall, with an

Veterinary Cytology, First Edition. Edited by Leslie C. Sharkey, M. Judith Radin, and Davis Seelig.

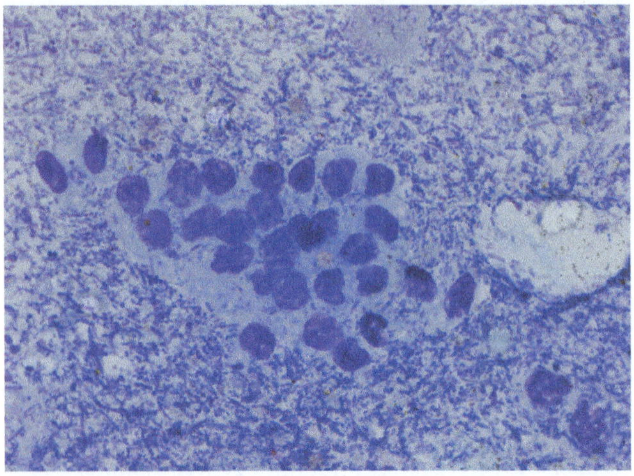

Figure 33.1 Dry-mount fecal cytology from a dog obtained by rectal scraping. Normal fecal cytology. Polymorphic population of microbial flora predominated by rod-shaped bacteria is associated with a cluster of cohesive epithelial cells (May-Grünwald–Giemsa, 1000×).

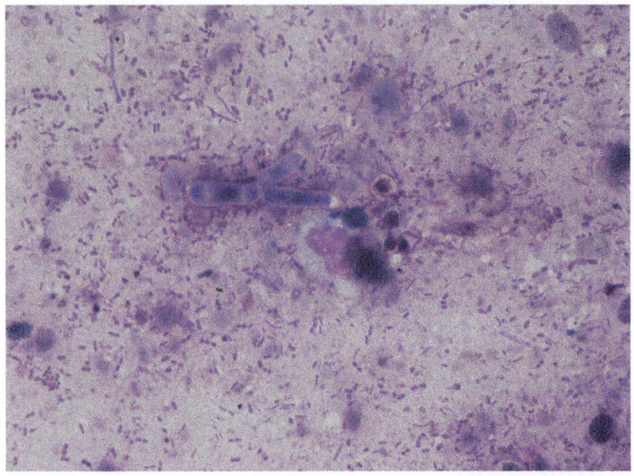

Figure 33.2 Dry-mount fecal cytology from a dog obtained during rectal digital examination. Three fungal spores of *Cyniclomyces guttulatus* are characterized by their large size of approximatively 5–7 × 15–20 μm. They are oval to cylindrical, surrounded by a clear wall, and have an interior that is purple, mottled, or vacuolated, with transverse, clear areas (May-Grünwald–Giemsa, 1000×).

interior that is uniformly purple, mottled, or vacuolated, or has a broad, transverse, poorly staining central region (Figure 33.2). *C. guttulatus* is usually not considered as a pathogen in dogs, but recent studies have suggested that it might be associated with chronic small or large bowel diarrhea in some cases.[3,4]

Conditions Diagnosed by Cytology

Overgrowth

Increased numbers of clostridial spores, yeast, and pathogenic spiral bacteria such as *Campylobacter* spp. can be associated with primary or secondary enteritis. Coccidial merozoites or protozoal trophozoites may be observed in parasitic enteritis. Among the spore-forming bacteria, *Clostridium perfringens* and *Clostridium difficile* are the most frequently reported, but other bacteria such as *Bacillus* spp. could have a similar appearance. *C. perfringens* is a large Gram-positive rod that can have a central spore, giving it a "safety pin" appearance.[5] Sporulation has been associated with enterotoxin production.[5] Typically no more than five spore-forming bacteria per 1000× field should be observed in healthy dogs, and an increased number of spores can be observed in dogs with diarrhea; however, there is no correlation between the spore number and detection of *C. perfringens* enterotoxin.[6] The concurrent presence of excess spore-forming bacteria and neutrophils could be more indicative of infection by *C. perfringens*; however, because evidence is inconclusive,[6–8] an enzyme-linked immunosorbent assay (ELISA) for the enterotoxin and polymerase chain reaction assay for the enterotoxin gene are recommended for a definitive diagnosis of clostridial diarrhea.[9]

Among gull wing-shaped and spiral bacteria, several can be identified, including some spirochetes (treponeme-like bacteria, *Brachyspira* (formerly *Serpulina*) spp., *Helicobacter* spp., *Anaerobiospirillum* spp.) and also *Campylobacter* spp., a Gram-negative rod. They can be identified as campylobacter-like organisms on a Gram-stained fecal smear (Figure 33.3). The campylobacter- and treponeme-like bacteria are thick basophilic spiral organisms, but treponeme-like bacteria show several complete convolutions. *Serpulina* or spiriliform bacteria are thin wing-shaped bacteria.[10] Concurrent observation of neutrophils and an increase in one of these populations of bacteria support a bacterial cause of the diarrhea, typically *Campylobacter* and *Brachyspira* spp.[10] Cytology is not recommended as the sole method of identification of bacteria, so toxin ELISA, culture/sensitivity testing, or molecular techniques are necessary to confirm a suspicion.[9]

Other pathogens have been occasionally diagnosed using dry fecal cytology. Protozoal agents such as *Amoeba* spp. are rarely recognized in dry mounts and are usually diagnosed using fresh wet-mount feces. Non-sporulated endospores of the algae *Prototheca* are morphologically similar to round to oval extracellular fecal yeast but are observed both within macrophages and extracellularly (see Chapter 32).[2] *Histoplasma capsulatum* can be observed within macrophages but sometimes free as an oval or round yeast-like cell of 2–5 μm with a central basophilic

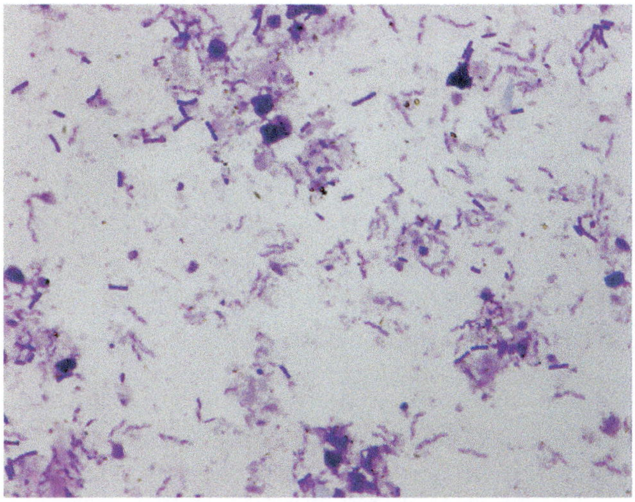

Figure 33.3 Dry-mount fecal cytology from a dog obtained during rectal digital examination. Campylobacter- or treponeme-like organisms appear as numerous thick basophilic spiral bacteria that are sometimes associated with debris (May-Grünwald–Giemsa, 1000×).

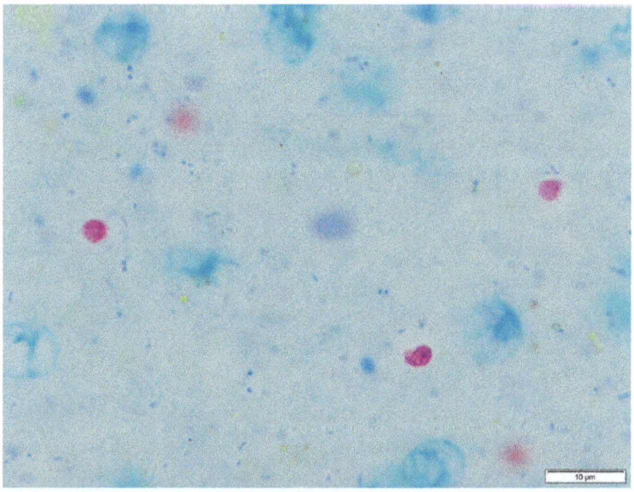

Figure 33.4 Acid-fast staining of a direct fecal smear. There are several 4–6 μm, round oocysts that stain magenta against malachite green counterstained background and are compatible with *Cryptosporidium* spp. (modified Ziehl Neelsen, 1000×. *Source:* Image courtesy of Erin Burton).

body surrounded by a clear halo. Systemic cryptococcosis has been diagnosed in a dog using fecal cytology (see Chapter 3 for more information on these organisms).[11,12]

Cryptosporidium spp. are small coccidian parasites with small oocysts (5 μm) that are passed in feces and are difficult to detect microscopically.[13] A modified Ziehl Neelsen staining technique may help characterize the oocysts as pink to bright red spheres (Figure 33.4; see Chapter 32 for more detail).[13]

Fecal Leukocytes

Dry mounts are used for identification of inflammatory infiltrates. It is generally accepted although not clearly proven that neither inflammatory cells nor blood cells should be found in a dry fecal mount of a healthy dog.[1,2]

Increased numbers of neutrophils can be a sign of bacterial enteritis such as salmonellosis (especially when combined with leukopenia), clostridial colitis, colibacillosis, campylobacteriosis, and other invasive or enterotoxigenic bacteria but also whipworm infestation, chronic primary inflammatory disease (lymphoplasmacytic and eosinophilic enteritis), and neoplasia (Figure 33.5).[1] The absence of fecal neutrophils in a puppy with hemorrhagic diarrhea and peripheral blood neutropenia can be associated with parvoviral enteritis, but the diagnosis requires a specific test.[1]

Eosinophils, sometimes associated with mast cells, can be observed not only in the feces with primary chronic inflammatory bowel disease such as eosinophilic enteritis but also as a component of mixed inflammation in diseases such as fungal, oomycetal, algal, or nematode infections, foreign body, and certain neoplasms such as lymphoma.[2,14] It is reported in textbooks that lymphocytes potentially associated with plasma cells can be observed with any cause of chronic inflammatory primary or secondary bowel disease.[2] Macrophagic inflammation can be observed with various causes of chronic inflammation but may be associated with chronic colitis such as granulomatous colitis or *Leishmania* spp.-associated colitis.[2,15,16]

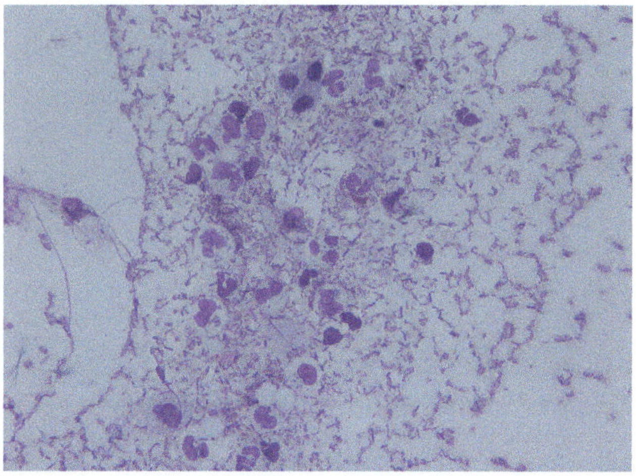

Figure 33.5 Dry-mount fecal cytology from a dog obtained during rectal digital examination. Bacterial enteritis is indicated by increased numbers of neutrophils associated with overgrowth of rod-shaped bacteria. Bacteria are extracellular and phagocytized. Three cohesive epithelial columnar cells are also observed (May-Grünwald–Giemsa, 1000×).

Other Cells

Hyperplastic epithelial cells can be seen with reactive processes, and neoplastic epithelial cells can be observed but must be differentiated from hyperplasia. Other neoplastic conditions such as mast cell tumor, lymphoma, or mesenchymal tumor can be associated with the observation of neoplastic cells. Undigested muscle fibers can be also observed in cases of maldigestion or diarrhea.

References

1 Broussard, J.D. (2003). Optimal fecal assessment. *Clin Tech Small Anim Pract* 18: 218–230.

2 Weeden, A.L. and Wamsley, H.L. (2016). Dry-mount fecal cytology. In: *Canine and Feline Cytology: A Color Atlas and Interpretation Guide*, 3e, (eds. Raskin, R.E., Meyer, D.J.), 247–258. St. Louis, MO: Elsevier.

3 Mandigers, P.J., Duijvestijn, M.B., Ankringa, N. et al. (2014). The clinical significance of *Cyniclomyces guttulatus* in dogs with chronic diarrhoea, a survey and a prospective treatment study. *Vet Microbiol* 172: 241–247.

4 Winston, J.A., Piperisova, I., Neel, J., and Gookin, J.L. (2016). *Cyniclomyces guttulatus* infection in dogs: 19 cases (2006–2013). *J Am Anim Hosp Assoc* 52: 42–51.

5 Marks, S.L. (2012). *Clostridium perfringens*- and *Clostridium difficile*- associated diarrhea. In: *Infectious Diseases of the Dog and Cat*, 4e, (ed. Greene, C.E.), 393–398. St. Louis, MO: Elsevier Saunders.

6 Marks, S.L., Melli, A., Kass, P.H. et al. (1999). Evaluation of methods to diagnose *Clostridium perfringens*-associated diarrhea in dogs. *J Am Vet Med Assoc* 214: 357–360.

7 Marks, S.L., Kather, E.J., Kass, P.H., and Melli, A.C. (2002). Genotypic and phenotypic characterization of *Clostridium perfringens* and *Clostridium difficile* in diarrheic and healthy dogs. *J Vet Intern Med* 16: 533–540.

8 Weese, J.S., Staempfli, H.R., Prescott, J.F. et al. (2001). The roles of *Clostridium difficile* and enterotoxigenic *Clostridium perfringens* in diarrhea in dogs. *J Vet Intern Med* 15: 374–378.

9 Marks, S.L., Rankin, S.C., Byrne, B.A., and Weese, J.S. (2011). Enteropathogenic bacteria in dogs and cats: diagnosis, epidemiology, treatment, and control. *J Vet Intern Med* 25: 1195–1208.

10 Greene, C.E. (2012). *Brachyspira pilosicoli* infection. In: *Infectious Diseases of the Dog and Cat*, 4e, (ed. Greene, C.E.), 391. St. Louis, MO: Elsevier Saunders.

11 Bromel, C. and Sykes, J.E. (2005). Histoplasmosis in dogs and cats. *Clin Tech Small Anim Pract* 20: 227–232.

12 Graves, T.K., Barger, A.M., Adams, B., and Krockenberger, M.B. (2005). Diagnosis of systemic cryptococcosis by fecal cytology in a dog. *Vet Clin Pathol* 34: 409–412.

13 Scorza, V. and Tangtrongsup, S. (2010). Update on the diagnosis and management of *Cryptosporidium* spp. infections in dogs and cats. *Top Companion Anim Med* 25: 163–169.

14 Gorman, E. (2017). Cytology of the gastrointestinal tract. In: *Small Animal Cytologic Diagnosis*, (eds. Barger, A.M., Macneill, A.L.), 317–354. Boca Raton, USA: CRC Press.

15 Adamama-Moraitou, K.K., Rallis, T.S., Koytinas, A.F. et al. (2007). Asymptomatic colitis in naturally infected dogs with Leishmania infantum: a prospective study. *Am J Trop Med Hyg* 76: 53–57.

16 Ferrer, L., Juanola, B., Ramos, J.A. et al. (1991). Chronic colitis due to Leishmania infection in two dogs. *Vet Pathol* 28: 342–343.

Part IX

Liver and Pancreas

34

Nonneoplastic Disorders of the Liver

Carlo Masserdotti

Introduction

Complete characterization of nonneoplastic liver pathology usually requires microanatomical localization of tissue damage and cellular infiltrates, including the orientation relative to portal and centrolobular structures. Cytological examination, largely limited to the cytoplasmic and nuclear changes of individual cells, will often be insufficient for a definitive diagnosis.[1–6] Despite these limitations, the cytologic evaluation of cell morphology, inflammatory cells, pathologic material, and screening for neoplastic features can be valuable in the clinical management of many hepatic diseases.[5–7] The majority of the literature in this area is related to canine and feline liver disease, while there is very little information regarding the use of liver cytology in the horse.

Sample Collection

Clinical signs and hematologic and serum biochemical indicators of liver disease do not always correlate well with microscopic pathology. Likewise, ultrasonographic examination is an important diagnostic modality that can identify abnormalities but cannot reliably differentiate specific causes, with the exception of cholestasis and nodular change.[8–10] In some cases, sample bias can contribute to low sensitivity, which can be partially overcome by sampling from different areas, including multiple liver lobes.[11]

Tru-cut and Menghini needles, fine-needle aspiration (FNA), laparoscopic forceps, and surgical wedge biopsy can all be used to sample hepatic tissue.[12,13] Diagnostic agreement with necropsy is achieved in 66% of needle samples, 60% of laparoscopic cup samples, and 69% of punch samples.[14] A small amount of blood loss is always expected, which can be visualized ultrasonographically or during laparoscopy or surgery. The average amount of blood loss from a liver biopsy is reported to be around 2 mL in normal dogs.[15,16] FNA is widely used to collect cytology samples and is usually performed using a 6 or 12 cc syringe and a 22 G, 1.5–3.5 in. disposable hypodermic or spinal needle. The needle is inserted into the liver via a percutaneous transabdominal approach in small animals or transthoracic in large animals. Large-scale studies of complications associated with liver aspirates in dogs, cats, and horses are lacking, although hemorrhage and accidental perforation of large biliary ducts or cholecystitis are possible.[12] Studies of ultrasound-guided and laparoscopic liver biopsies in dogs, cats, and horses suggest that this procedure is generally safe. Complications following FNA of liver parenchyma include hemorrhage[17] and potential seeding of needle tracts with neoplastic cells.[18] The risk for prolonged or excessive bleeding should be assessed by evaluation of coagulation times prior to performing the procedure.[19–22] Automatic biopsy gun devices tested in cats triggered acute severe shock within 15 minutes of the procedure in approximately 20% of cats.[23]

Normal Structure

Tissue Architecture

The liver is the site of many metabolic processes, based on the function of a single, redundant anatomic subunit: the polygonal hepatic lobule. The angles of the polygon culminate in the portal triads, while the center contains the hepatic vein. The functional unit is the hepatic acinus, which is centered on the line connecting two portal triads and extending outward to the two adjacent central veins. Periportal zone I is composed of hepatocytes nearest to the entering vascular supply and receives the most oxygenated blood, making it least sensitive to ischemic injury but very susceptible to viral or toxic injury. Conversely, the midzonal zone II and the centrilobular zone III are composed of

Veterinary Cytology, First Edition. Edited by Leslie C. Sharkey, M. Judith Radin, and Davis Seelig.

hepatocytes that receive poorly oxygenated blood and are most affected by poor perfusion.

The portal tracts contain a portal vein, hepatic artery, bile duct, and lymph vessels supported by collagenous stroma. Blood flows from the branches of portal vein and hepatic artery into the sinusoids to allow metabolic exchange with the hepatocytes. The sinusoidal lining differs from standard capillaries in being lined by fenestrated endothelial cells supported by a specialized fine basement membrane composed of collagen types III, IV, and XVIII and extracellular matrix that constitute the reticulin meshwork. This structural adaptation allows plasma constituents to pass into a gap between endothelial cells and hepatocytes, called the space of Disse. In this space, metabolites reach the surface of hepatocytes, facilitating uptake and secretion of substances.

The sinusoidal and lateral cytoplasmic membranes cover the basolateral surface of the hepatocyte. The apical membranes of adjacent hepatocytes delineate the bile canaliculi into which the bile is secreted and transported through the terminal ductules (also called canals of Hering), which are lined by ductal cells and hepatocytes. The canal of Hering contains the hepatic progenitor cells, also called oval cells, which are bipotential cells capable of maturation into biliary epithelium or hepatocytes. The terminal ductules enter the limiting plate and, within the portal tract, unite to form the interlobular bile ducts, which are lined with small cuboidal epithelial cells. Interlobular bile ducts anastomose to form the larger intrahepatic bile ducts and are lined with columnar cells. The larger ducts enter the main hepatic ducts that unite in the common bile duct, draining the bile into the duodenum. With the exception of horse and rat, most species have a bile diverticulum, the gallbladder, for storage and concentration of the bile, which communicates with the main hepatic ducts and the common duct via the cystic duct.

In the lumen of sinusoids, there are hepatic macrophages, called Kupffer cells, which remove infectious agents, particulate material, endotoxins, and senescent cells from the portal blood. A small number of resident lymphocytes and plasma cells are recognizable in portal fibrous stroma.[24] In the space of Disse, there are the hepatic stellate cells, also called lipocytes or Ito cells that normally store vitamin A in their characteristic cytoplasmic globules. In canine liver, mast cells occur under the endothelial layer, along the hepatic centrolobular sinusoids, the central veins, and sublobar veins.[25]

Cell Types in Normal Liver

Hepatocytes

The hepatocyte is the predominant cell in FNA samples from normal livers, although anecdotally these cells can also be collected inadvertently while attempting to aspirate other tissues such as the lung. Hepatocytes often exfoliate in large cohesive sheets, sometimes with a trabecular structure. Cells are round to polygonal epithelial cells with bluish to amphophilic cytoplasm crossed by delicate reticular network due to the prominent endoplasmic reticulum (Figure 34.1a). Many cells contain scattered basophilic to blue-green granules, consistent with lipofuscin pigment, the result of cytosolic lipid peroxidation (Figure 34.1b). Nuclei are round, paracentral, or eccentrically located, with granular chromatin and a single prominent nucleolus. In middle-aged or geriatric asymptomatic dogs, binucleated cells occur associated with regenerative changes.[26]

Cholangiocytes

Cholangiocytes, or biliary epithelial cells, are infrequently observed in aspirates of normal livers.[27] These small cuboidal cells have scant lightly basophilic cytoplasm, contain a centrally placed hyperchromatic nucleus, and are arranged in small bidimensional sheets (Figure 34.1c).[18,28] Cholangiocytes that originate from large terminal ducts or gallbladder epithelium are columnar, have round to ovoid hyperchromatic nuclei, and can form a palisading pattern (Figure 34.1d).[29]

Stellate Cells (Ito Cells)

Stellate cells are round and have cytoplasm dilated by nonstaining globules of lipid with a high concentration of vitamin A (Figure 34.2a).[30,31] They are difficult to recognize because they are generally solitary and interspersed among hepatocytes.

Kupffer Cells

Kupffer cells are resident hepatic macrophages.[32,33] In the quiescent form, they cannot be visualized because of the scant amount of pyramidal cytoplasm and hyperchromatic nucleus (Figure 34.2b).[34] As described later, Kupffer cells become easily detectable when activated.

Mast Cells

Mast cells are concentrated in the interlobular connective tissue of the centrolobular region,[25] although they are also described the space of Disse, sometimes in direct contact with stellate cells.[30] They are present in very low numbers and consequently are not usually detectable in normal liver specimens. Mast cells are characterized by cytoplasm filled with small metachromatic or clear granules and a round nucleus (Figure 34.2c), although special stains are necessary to confirm the origin in some cases.[35]

Lymphocytes

T lymphocytes normally occupy the space of Disse and portal triads.[18,24] The presence of a small number of well-differentiated small lymphocytes is considered normal.

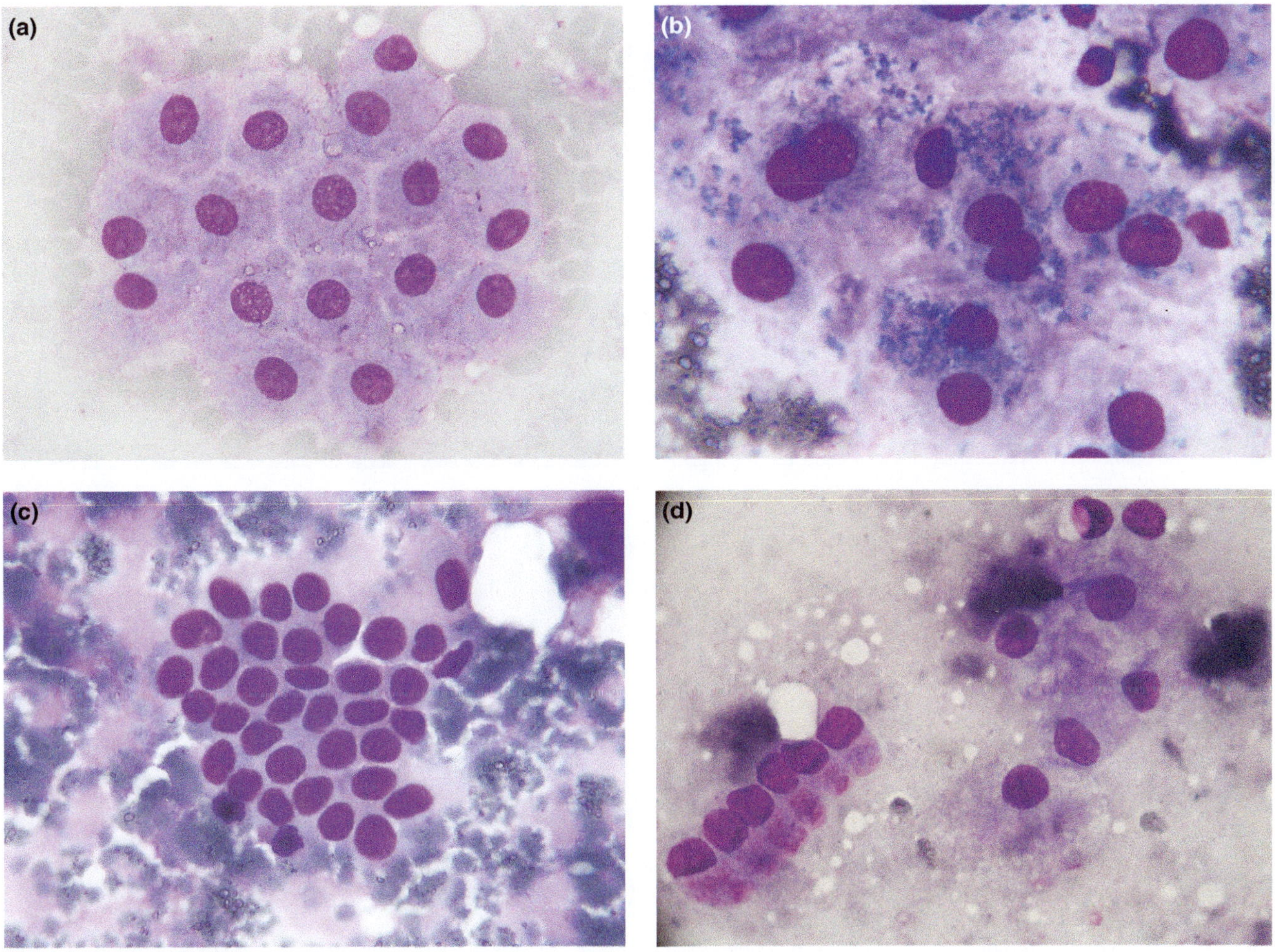

Figure 34.1 (a) Cluster of normal hepatocytes. (b) Lipofuscin pigment accumulation in hepatocytes appears as small blue granules. (c) Normal cholangiocytes from terminal bile ducts have a small amount of cytoplasm, round nuclei, and compact chromatin. (d) Columnar cholangiocytes from large bile ducts (lower left) (May-Grünwald–Giemsa, 1000×).

Mesothelial Cells

Uniform polyhedral mesothelial cells can be obtained as a sampling needle passes through the mesothelial lining of the abdominal cavity.

Hematopoietic Precursors

The liver is a hematopoietic organ during fetal life; hematopoiesis declines after birth but can continue to occur.[36] Increased extramedullary hematopoiesis can be a response to anemia or systemic chronic inflammatory diseases, concurrent with increased bone marrow activity.[37] Hepatic hematopoiesis is generally pathologic in large animal species, while in small animals it can be an incidental finding without specific clinical significance.[37] In cytologic samples, hematopoiesis presents as immature erythroid (often metarubricytes) or myeloid (usually metamyelocytes and band granulocytes) cells (Figure 34.2d), although megakaryocytes can also be present.

Cytoplasmic and Nuclear Changes by Cell Type

Hepatocytes

Anisocytosis

This change describes variation in cell size, predominantly reflecting cytoplasmic volume. Although marked anisocytosis is frequently described in hepatocellular carcinoma (Chapter 35), it can be observed in regenerative processes.[18,38]

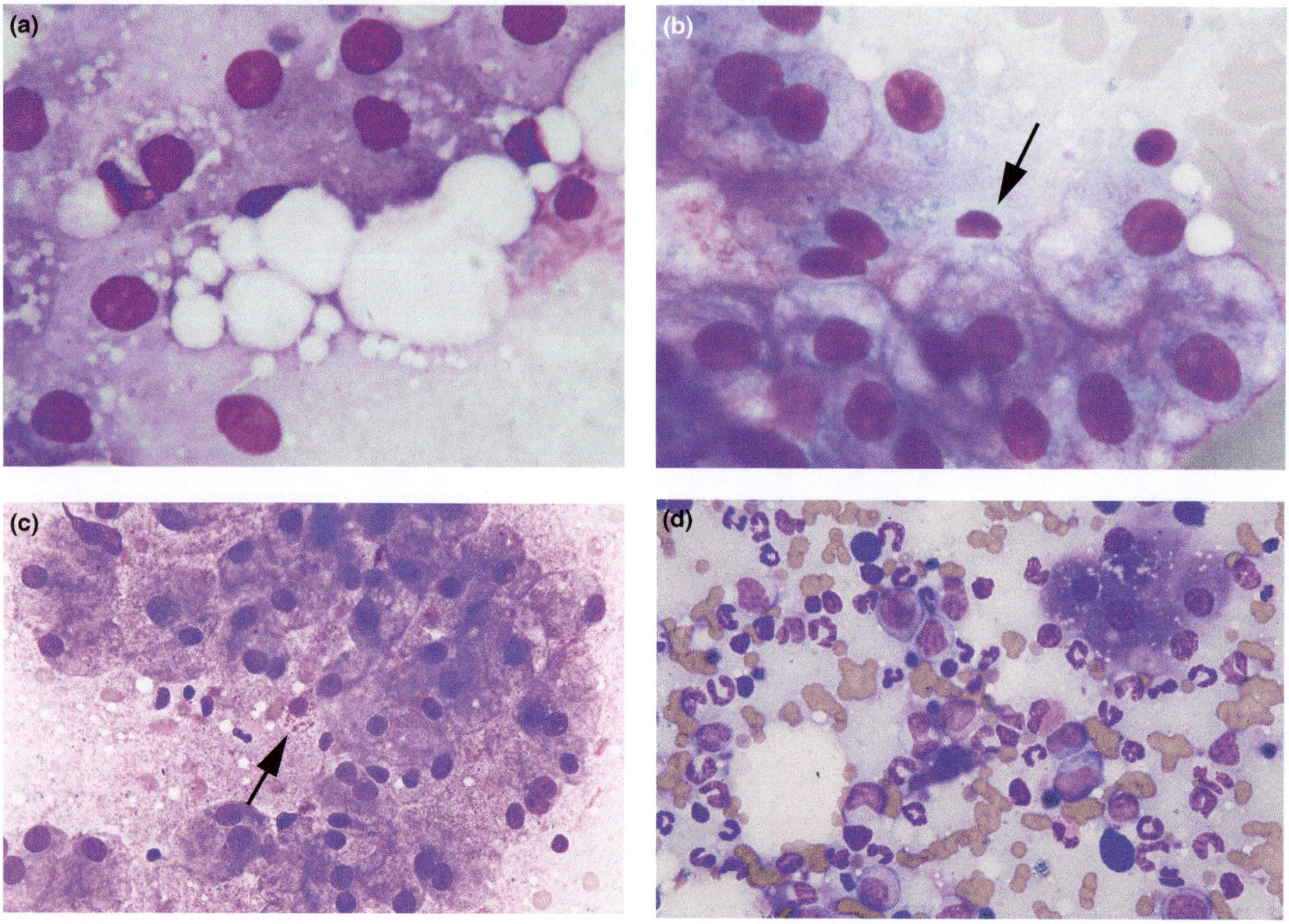

Figure 34.2 (a) Normal stellate cell. The cytoplasm is filled with round achromatic globules that displace the nucleus to the periphery. (b) Normal quiescent Kupffer cell with indistinct, round to ovoid cytoplasm (arrow). (c) Normal mast cell with granulated cytoplasm (arrow) associated with a cluster of hepatocytes. (d) Extramedullary hematopoiesis consisting of myeloid and erythroid precursors (May-Grünwald–Giemsa, (a, b, and d) 1000×, (c) 400×).

Vacuolar Change

The term "vacuolar change" is technically inappropriate since most of the materials that accumulate in the hepatic cytoplasm are not in true membrane-bound vacuoles. Regardless, the terminology is generally accepted, referring to nonstaining material that accumulates in hepatocyte cytoplasm with nonspecific, reversible liver cell damage.[39,40]

Glycogen

Glycogen appears as indistinct nonstaining material dispersed within the cytoplasm (Figure 34.3a). It is virtually indistinguishable from hydropic degeneration and can be confirmed only using special stains such as periodic acid-Schiff (PAS) or periodic acid-Schiff after diastase (PAS-D) (Chapter 7). This change is considered nonspecific and potentially induced by endogenous and exogenous corticosteroid effects,[41,42] other drugs, stress, or chronic disease.[40] Since hepatocyte glycogen content is a function of original glycogen concentration, recent catabolism, and postmortem dissolution, the evaluation in liver tissue is affected by the time of fixation.[37] In cytology smears, the quick air drying of hepatocytes preserves glycogen and reliably reflects cell content. A naturally occurring dog model for glycogen storage disease type Ia was identified in Maltese dogs with a loss-of-function mutation of the gene for glucose-6-phosphatase.[43] Glycogen storage disease type IIIa was described in a Curly-coated Retriever and a German Shepherd dog as an autosomal recessive disease caused by deficiency of glycogen debranching enzyme in liver and muscle.[44]

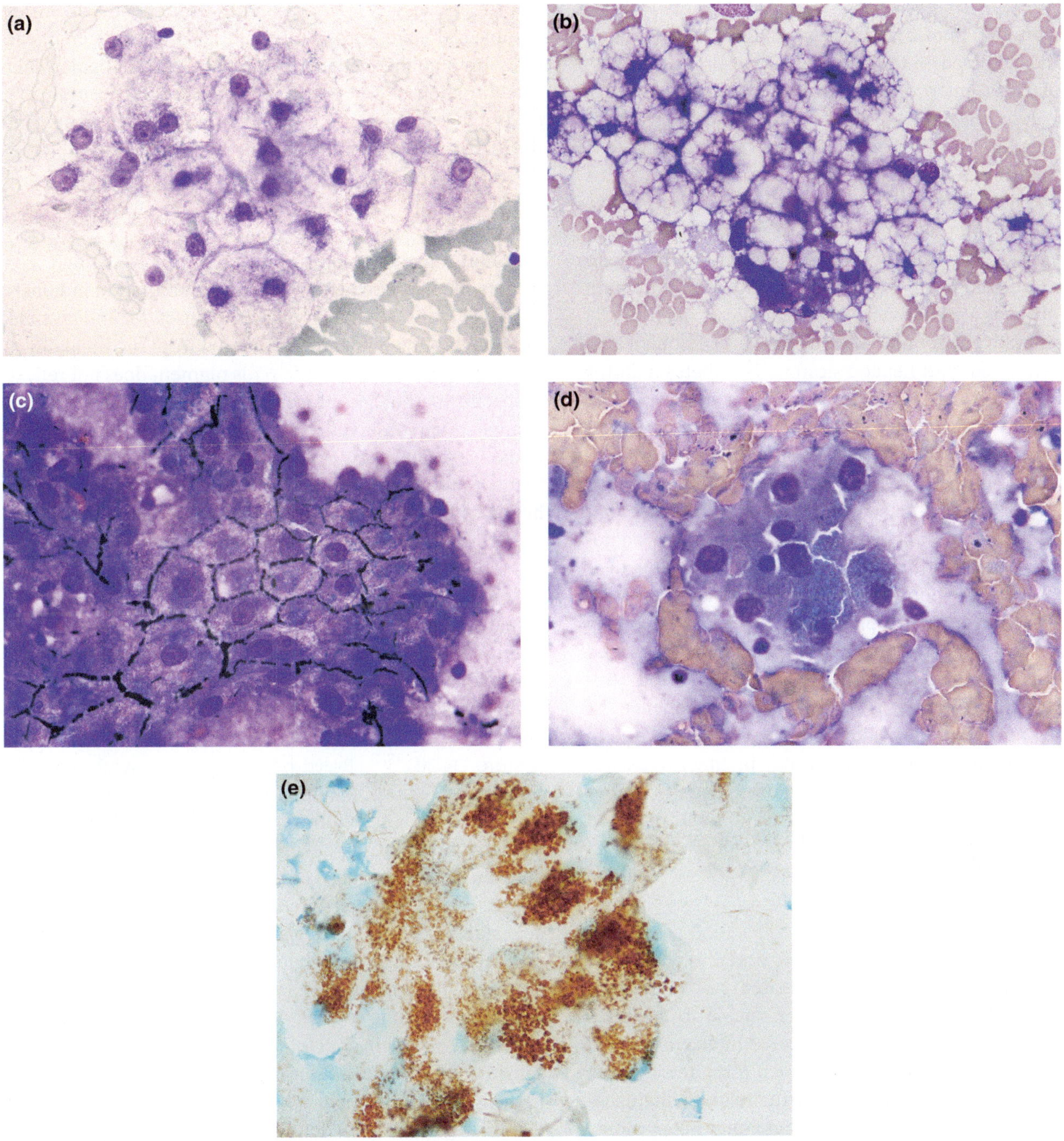

Figure 34.3 (a) Glycogen or water accumulation in hepatocytes is characterized by expansion of the cytoplasm with indistinct clear material. (b) Macrovesicular steatosis. Lipid appears as large achromatic globules with distinct boundaries. (c) Cluster of hepatocytes crossed by linear casts of extracytoplasmic bile. (d) Copper appears as light blue, indistinct granules. (e) Cytoplasmic copper accumulation stains bright orange with rhodanine stain ((a–d) May-Grünwald–Giemsa, 1000×. (e) Rhodanine, 1000×. *Source:* Image (e) courtesy of Russell Moore).

Lipid

The accumulation of triglycerides is called "steatosis" and is subdivided based on the size of the nonstaining cytoplasmic globules as microvesicular steatosis when the globules are smaller than nucleus and as macrovesicular steatosis when they are larger (Figure 34.3b).[39] To differentiate it from other forms of vacuolar change, use of special stains like Oil Red O is required to confirm the lipid nature of the cytoplasmic material, especially with microvesicular steatosis.[45] Lipid accumulation in the cytoplasm can be due to reduced utilization of triglycerides or altered lipoprotein metabolism as a consequence of metabolic, toxic, hypoxic, or degenerative disorders. One of the most frequent diseases associated with hepatic steatosis is diabetes mellitus in the dog and cat. Starvation is another cause of lipid mobilization from adipose tissue and excess accumulation in hepatocytes. In cats, hepatic lipidosis occurs as an idiopathic syndrome associated with reduced caloric intake for unidentified reasons or secondary to other diseases that reduce appetite. In puppies, a condition of juvenile steatosis is associated with severe hypoglycemia.[46] Fatty liver develops when the hepatic uptake of lipids exceeds the oxidation and secretion of lipids by the liver and is usually preceded by high concentrations of plasma non-esterified fatty acids mobilized from adipose tissue. Decreased utilization of triglycerides is typically a consequence of impaired mitochondrial oxidative phosphorylation due to drugs or toxins, usually resulting in microvesicular change.[47] In other cases, microvesicular steatosis can occur secondary to decreased apoprotein synthesis and impaired lipoprotein secretion.[39] Severe hepatic lipidosis in dog can be caused by toxins, such aflatoxicosis.[48]

Water

The accumulation of intracellular water, or hydropic change, is a consequence of decreased cell membrane integrity and occurs when cells are unable to maintain fluid homeostasis. This change is consequence of almost all forms of injury to hepatocytes such toxic and hypoxic damage.[39,49] Hydropic change is virtually undistinguishable from glycogen accumulation by light microscopy alone.

Pigments and Inclusions

Hepatocytes accumulate cytoplasmic material reflective of underlying pathologic conditions. Standard microscopic evaluation can be suggestive, but usually not definitive for identification of the substances and special stains, so advanced techniques may be necessary.[50]

Bile

Bile pigment appears as dark green-blue to blue-black pigment, but special stains, such as Fouchet-Van Gieson stain, are necessary to discriminate it from lipofuscin. More reliable is the presence of bile "plugs," or dark-green linear casts among the hepatocytes reflecting canalicular bile accumulation (Figure 34.3c).[5,18,27,29] Bile casts occur due to obstructive diseases that impair bile flow. Bile casts can reflect extrahepatic biliary lesions or intrahepatic cholestasis resulting from infiltrative disease of the liver.[27]

Lipofuscin

This bluish pigment appears as irregular granules and represents the most frequent pigment accumulation in hepatocytes (Figure 34.1b). Lipofuscin consists of indigestible lipid-containing lysosomes generated from the breakdown of cytoplasmic membranes.[51] This pigment does not reflect a specific pathologic process, but is a mild nonspecific change often observed in hepatocytes of geriatric animals.[52] Special stains are necessary to confirm this pigment,[50] although their presence in the cytoplasm of hepatocytes is quite common and confirmation is generally unnecessary.

Copper

Hepatocellular copper accumulation is very well documented histopathologically. Cytology is used less often to evaluate copper in hepatocytes, which is characterized by relatively subtle light blue-green refractile granules that can be obscured by other concurrent pathology (Figure 34.3d).[18,29] Breed-related genetic syndromes in Bedlington Terriers, Labrador Retrievers, Sky Blue Terriers, and West Highland White Terriers are potential models for human disease.[53] Copper can also accumulate with cholestasis and inflammation.[54] Copper accumulation is very rare in cats[55,56] and has been described in the horse.[57] A rubeanic acid staining procedure for liver cytology samples showed good correlation with histologic assessment in Bedlington Terriers with copper hepatopathy.[58] A protocol for rapid rhodanine staining of both destained Wright–Giemsa and unstained canine liver cytology samples showed increased sensitivity for the detection of copper (Figure 34.3e) compared with Wright–Giemsa stain alone.[59] Grading scores of one through nine were determined using a combination of the proportion of cells containing copper and the degree of copper accumulation in affected cells. Correlation was considered good to excellent between cytologic detection of copper using rhodanine staining and quantitative dry weight hepatic copper concentrations at two clinically relevant concentrations (≥600 and ≥1500 ppm).

Iron and Hemosiderin

Hemosiderin is an insoluble protein with a dark-brown granular appearance that is produced by the macrophagic digestion of hemoglobin. It can accumulate in hepatocytes and macrophages during hemolytic diseases and sometimes in association with portovascular abnormalities. Massive accumulation of iron in hepatocytes and Kupffer cells is termed hemochromatosis, a rare disease described in some birds[60] and Salers cattle.[61] Secondary hemochromatosis can develop as a result of hemolytic anemia associated with pyruvate kinase deficiency,[62] after repeated blood transfusions,[63] or as consequence of massive iron administration.[64]

Other Cytoplasmic Inclusions

These changes are rarely described in the livers of domestic animals. Alpha-1-antitrypsin appears as red globules in cytoplasm and can reflect an hereditary defect in the dog.[65] Protein droplets reflect the accumulation of plasma protein into the cytoplasm of hepatocytes during many diseases, including hepatocellular carcinoma (Figure 34.4).[66]

Degeneration, Necrosis, and Apoptosis

Cellular degeneration and necrosis ranges from scattered individual cell effects to a widespread process. Cytologically, degenerating or necrotic hepatocytes have indistinct cell margins, increased cytoplasmic basophilia, and loss of nuclear detail (Figure 34.5a). Cells are fragile, resulting in dispersal of cytoplasmic debris that can retain recognizable microscopic characteristics or further degradation into indistinct amorphous basophilic debris. Apoptosis, or programmed cell death, causes pyknosis of the nucleus independent of membrane damage. Apoptotic cells are nonspecifically characterized by scanty eosinophilic cytoplasm and shrunken hyperchromatic nuclei undergoing fragmentation (Figure 34.5b). These changes are often accompanied by macrophages with intracytoplasmic material.

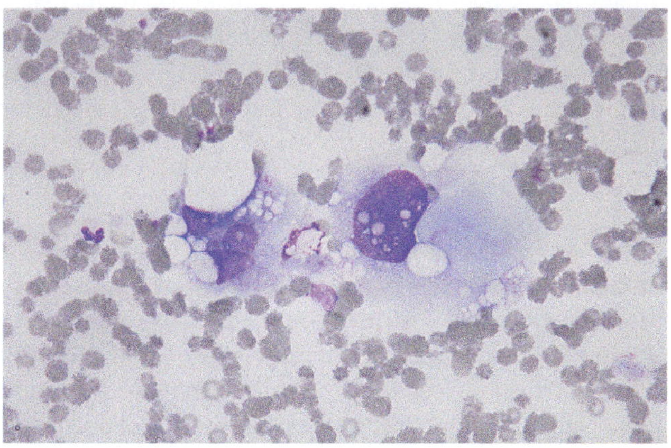

Figure 34.4 Hepatocellular carcinoma. The neoplastic cell on the right contains a large light blue protein droplet (May-Grünwald–Giemsa, 1000×).

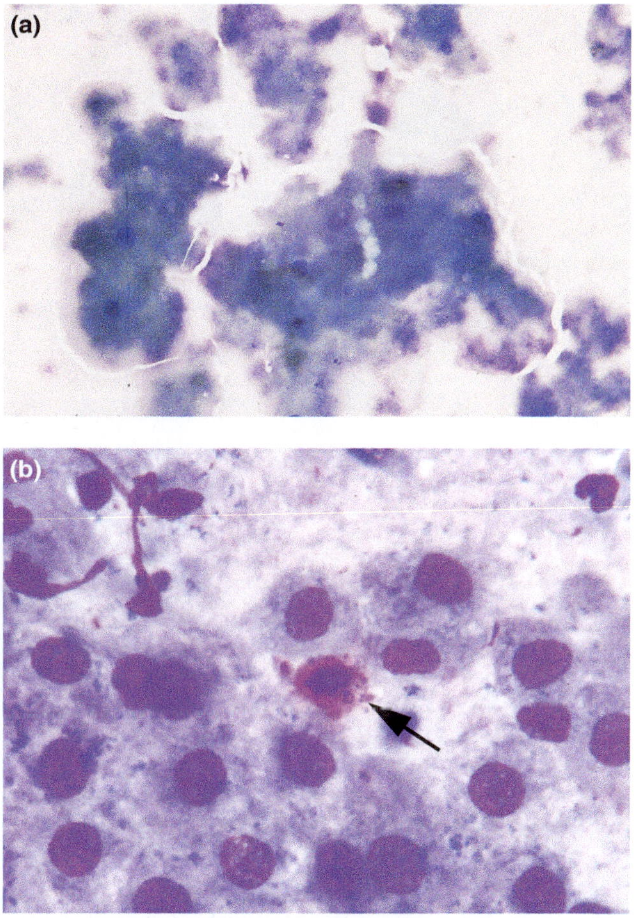

Figure 34.5 (a) Necrotic hepatocytes with indistinct cytoplasmic and nuclear margins. (b) A single apoptotic cell (arrow) contains a small amount of eosinophilic cytoplasm and pyknotic nucleus (May-Grünwald–Giemsa, 1000×).

Nuclear Changes

Anisokaryosis of hepatocytes generally reflects regenerative changes following hepatic injury or nodular regeneration.[38,49] Therefore, it is not reliable for differentiating regenerative changes from well-differentiated hepatocellular carcinoma (Figure 34.6a). Aging does not impact nuclear size.[26,67] Because the volume of cytoplasm increases with age but nuclear size does not, age is associated with a lower nuclear to cytoplasmic ratio. There is also an increase in binucleated cells with aging, which is thought to reflect age-related nodular hyperplasia.[26] Older dogs have normal nucleolar number and morphology, while cholestatic disorders can be associated with increased numbers of hepatocyte nucleoli.[26,27] Intranuclear crystals (brick inclusions) are refractile rectangular crystals that sometimes deform the nuclear outlines and have no known diagnostic significance (Figure 34.6b).[37] Cytoplasmic invaginations of the nucleus appear as clear globular inclusions that contain glycogen and mitochondria by ultrastructural analysis.[37] Glycogen

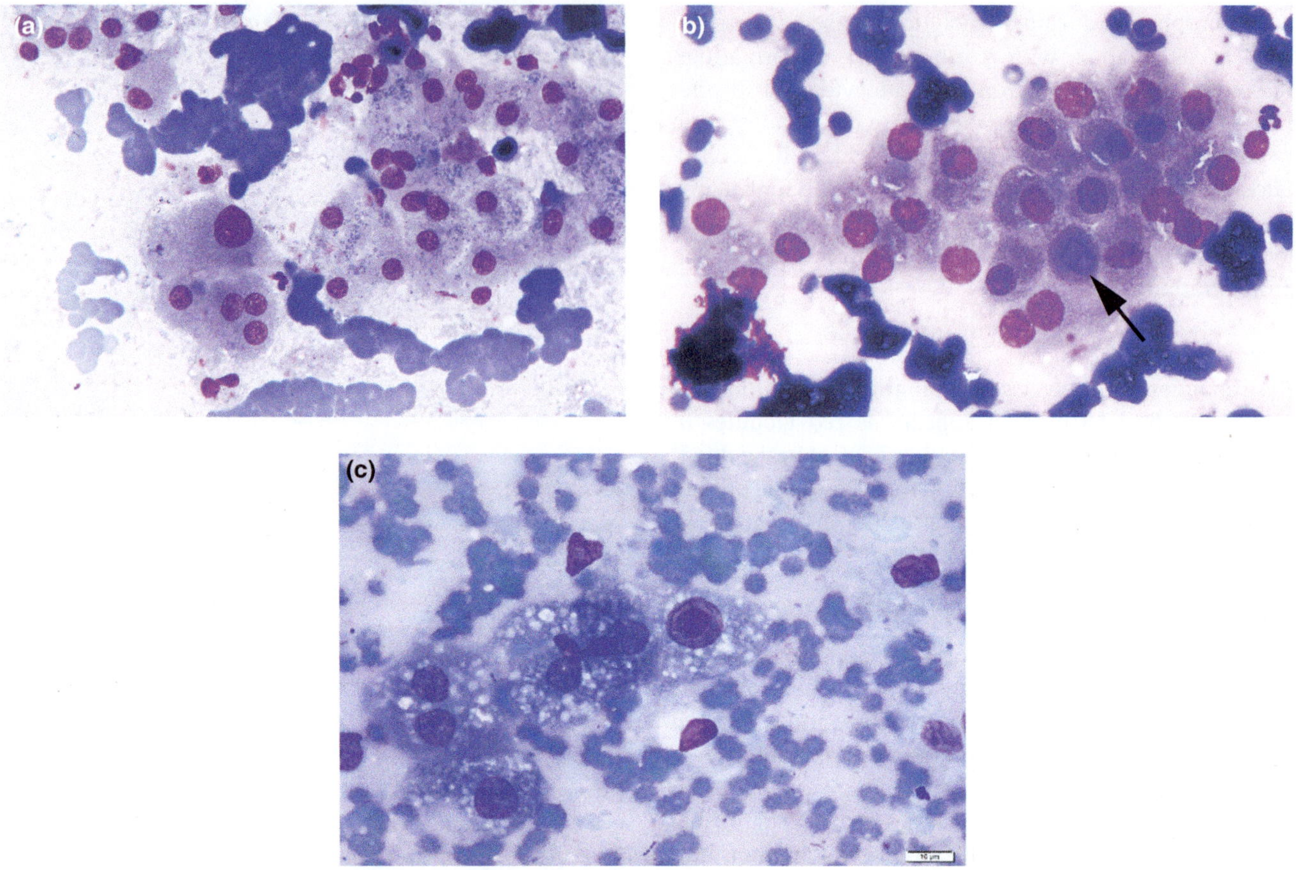

Figure 34.6 (a) Regenerative hepatocytes can display anisokaryosis (May-Grünwald–Giemsa, 1000×). (b) A nuclear brick inclusion appears as a rectangular crystal (arrow) (May-Grünwald–Giemsa, 1000×). (c) Canine adenovirus infection. The nucleus of the cell on the right contains a large, deeply eosinophilic viral inclusion (Wright–Giemsa, 1000×. *Source:* Images courtesy of Marian Taulescu).

pseudoinclusions appear virtually indistinguishable from cytoplasmic invaginations; this change is nonspecific but described in diabetes mellitus and hepatocellular neoplasia.[37] It is important that other nuclear inclusions not to be mistaken for viral inclusions.[29] Viral inclusions are magenta bodies of variable size, generally surrounded by a thin area of marginated chromatin.[18,29] Canine adenovirus 1 and herpesvirus are the most likely viral agents responsible of this change (Figure 34.6c). Lead inclusions are an extremely rare change occasionally described in the dog and appear as intranuclear acid-fast inclusions.[68]

Cholangiocytes

Cholangiocytes can exfoliate in small bidimensional clusters, interspersed among sheets of hepatocytes, especially when there is hyperplasia of ductular epithelium such as in chronic biliary disease (Figure 34.7a).[26,29] They can be a normal feature in small numbers, especially in older dogs. In some instances, the cytoplasm can contain small round clear vacuoles, which can be a feature of reactive hyperplasia, increased secretory activity, or nonspecific accumulation of nonstaining material (Figure 34.7b).[69] Reactive and inflammatory liver diseases are characterized by increased numbers of cholangiocytes, but nuclear atypia was not specifically described in one study of the cytologic features of liver diseases.[27] In contrast, nuclear atypia is considered more typical of neoplastic processes.[27,49]

Stellate Cells

In geriatric cats, an increased number of stellate cells can be observed without any clinical significance (Figure 34.8a).[29] During hepatic injury, stellate cells become activated, lose their vitamin A content, and transform into myofibroblasts that produce collagen and extracellular matrix, leading to hepatic fibrosis and damage to the space of Disse, with consequent impact on

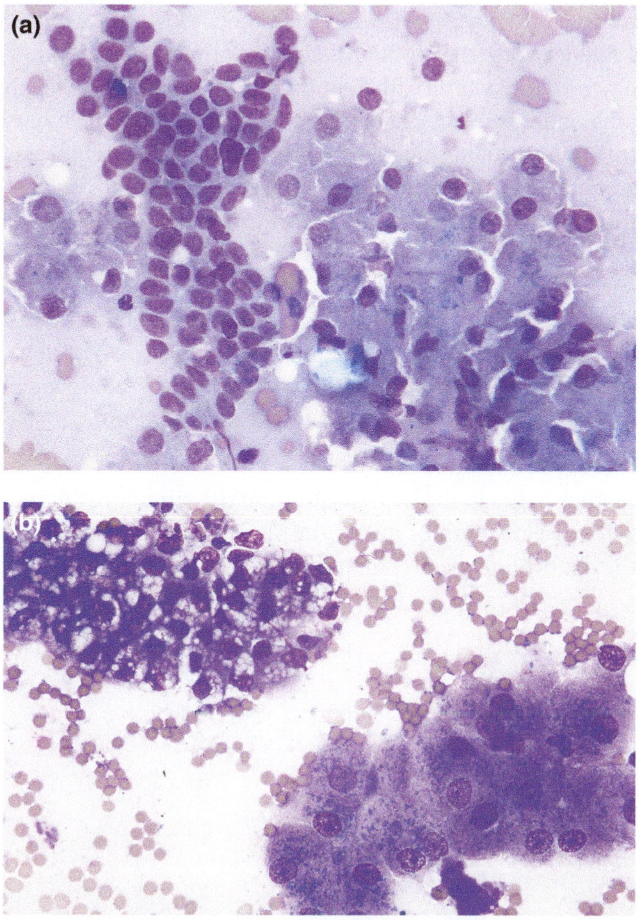

Figure 34.7 (a) Large cluster of hyperplastic cholangiocytes (left) adjacent to normal hepatocytes. (b) A cluster of cholangiocytes has vacuolar cytoplasm (upper left). Nearby normal hepatocytes contain lipofuscin (May-Grünwald–Giemsa, 1000×).

hepatic function. Large numbers of stellate cells with expanded vacuolated cytoplasm can occur during vitamin A toxicity.[70] In such cases, hyperplasia and hypertrophy of stellate cells must be differentiated from hepatic steatosis.

Kupffer Cells

When activated, Kupffer cells are characterized by abundant, frequently vacuolated cytoplasm (Figure 34.8b). The phagocytic activity of these cells removes cellular debris, bacteria from the portal circulation, senescent erythrocytes, bile, toxins, and compounds not visible cytologically. Ceroid, derived from injured hepatocytes, is a golden brown to greenish-yellow pigment rich in oxidized lipids and is one of the most frequent pigments observed in activated Kupffer cells. Kupffer cells exfoliate individually or in small aggregates, representative of the so-called lipogranuloma.[71]

Inflammation and Infectious Agents

Inflammation

Cytology is not a reliable tool for evaluation of inflammatory conditions of the hepatic parenchyma.[1,3,4,10,72,73] The presence of inflammatory cells lacks specificity for the underlying process, particularly in the absence of tissue architecture to inform microanatomic localization.[74] A standardized classification scheme for liver disease in dogs and cats provides guidelines for diagnosis that will facilitate excellent patient care and more translatable research in this important class

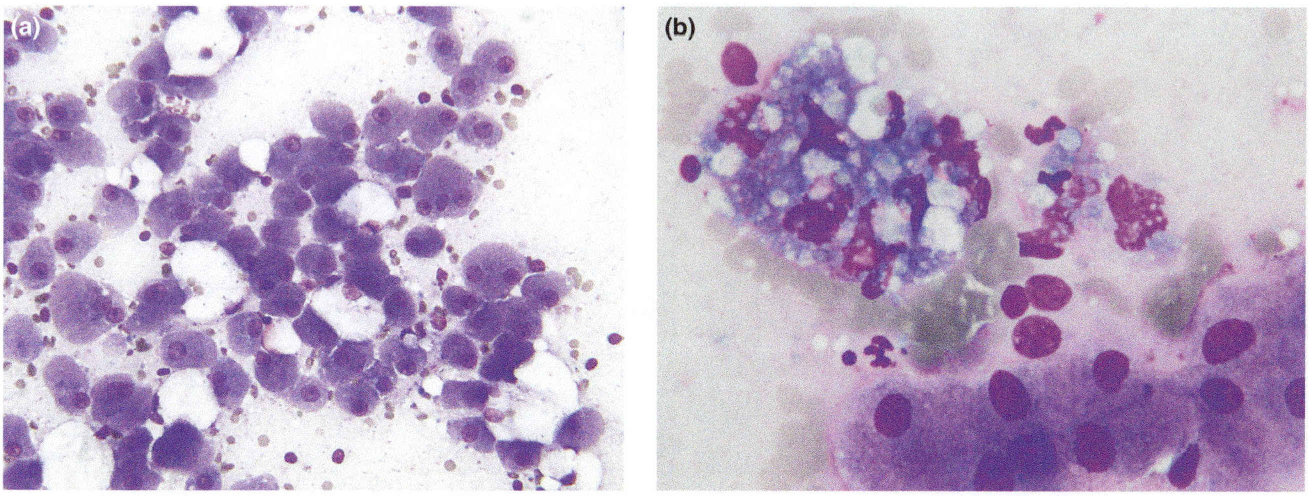

Figure 34.8 (a) Stellate cells with enlarged, achromatic cytoplasm are interspersed among hepatocytes from a cat with stellate cell hyperplasia (May-Grünwald–Giemsa, 400×. *Source:* Image courtesy of Lorenzo Ressel). (b) Activated macrophages in a small cluster have cytoplasm that is filled with achromatic or bluish globules (May-Grünwald–Giemsa, 1000×).

of small animal diseases.[75] Despite acknowledged limitations, cytologic examination can be definitive, for example, in septic suppurative inflammation.[27,73] However, in most instances, the presence of inflammatory cells in hepatic cytology suggests the need for histologic examination, particularly for the diagnosis of chronic inflammatory liver disease. Inflammation can also accompany neoplasia as a secondary process.[27] Moreover, blood contamination can result in variable numbers of leukocytes interspersed among the hepatocytes, leading to uncertainty in interpretation and the need to correlate with peripheral white blood cell concentration.[2]

Neutrophilic Inflammation

Numerous neutrophils indicate potential for a septic process, particularly when degenerate neutrophils are observed (Figure 34.9a). Some cytologists suggest that finding leukocytes within clusters hepatocytes is stronger evidence of true inflammation of the hepatic parenchyma.[27,73] Bacteria can enter the liver parenchyma via portal blood flow or by retrograde contamination of the biliary tree. Unfortunately, cytology cannot discriminate between suppurative hepatitis and cholangitis. Although uncommon, hepatic abscesses can present as hepatic masses with numerous degenerate neutrophils. Ultrasound features are variable, but gas can signal a hepatic abscesses.[76] In dogs, abscesses are typically single lesions, while in cats multifocal abscessation is more common.[77] In both species, cytologic evaluation of peritoneal fluid can aid diagnosis, being indicative of inflammation or revealing a septic process.

Histiocytic Inflammation

Macrophages in the liver derive from the circulating monocytes or activation of quiescent Kupffer cells. They exhibit the morphological changes of typical macrophages

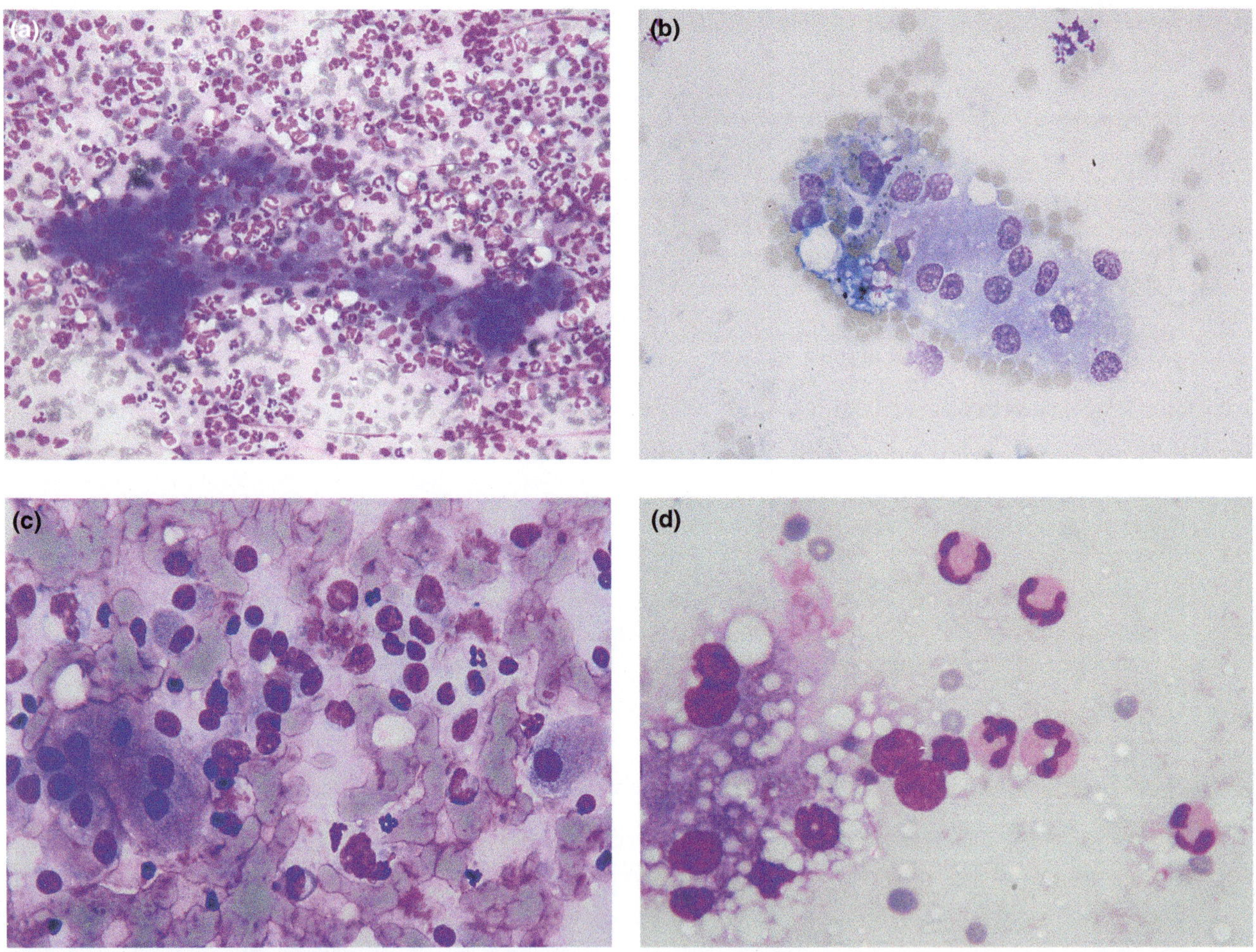

Figure 34.9 (a) Suppurative inflammation. A large number of well-preserved to degenerate neutrophils surround a cluster of hepatocytes (May-Grünwald–Giemsa, 200×). (b) Macrophages exhibiting erythrophagocytosis and hemosiderin (left) are adjacent to normal hepatocytes (May-Grünwald–Giemsa, 1000×). (c) Lymphocytic inflammation. Mature lymphocytes contain a scant amount of blue cytoplasm and nuclei with compact chromatin (May-Grünwald–Giemsa, 1000×). (d) Eosinophilic inflammation (May-Grünwald–Giemsa, 1000×).

described above for Kupffer cells. Increased numbers of activated macrophages, sometimes mixed with neutrophils, lymphocytes, and plasma cells, occur with many infectious diseases, such as *Mycobacterium* spp., *Leishmania* spp., *Cytauxzoon* spp., fungal diseases, and feline infectious peritonitis.[71] Erythrophagocytosis and erythrocyte breakdown products can occur associated with hemorrhage, congestion, or immune-mediated processes (Figure 34.9b).[71]

Lymphocytes and Plasma Cells

Small numbers of well-differentiated lymphocytes can be observed in liver cytology smears from healthy dogs.[26] Lymphocytes and plasma cells, sometimes in association with other inflammatory cells, is a nonspecific finding in chronic liver disease (Figure 34.9c).[27] A predominance of small mature lymphocytes can be present in chronic feline lymphocytic cholangitis, a common disease with slowly progressive course and uncertain etiology, although an immune basis is suspected.[18] Lymphocytes and plasma cells are distributed around clusters of hepatocytes and are sometimes associated with bile plugs and small clusters of normal to hyperplastic cholangiocytes. Lymphocytic inflammation can also be observed in chronic cholangitis, cholangiohepatitis, or chronic mixed hepatitis.[29,73]

Eosinophils

Eosinophilic inflammation is rare in liver disease (Figure 34.9d). Eosinophils can be seen associated with other inflammatory cells, in hypersensitivity and allergic diseases, or with parasitic migration through the liver.[78] Eosinophils can be observed in smears from livers from dogs with eosinophilic syndrome and from cats with eosinophilic enteritis. Eosinophilic inflammation sometimes accompanies drug-induced liver lesions (e.g. trimethoprim/sulfamethoxazole).[78]

Mast Cells

Small numbers of mast cells normally populate the liver parenchyma in a centrolobular distribution. Resident hepatic mast cells have a small hyperchromatic nucleus and shrunken cytoplasm with inconsistently staining granules. With ordinary stains, mast cells can be observed among the hepatocytes. Toluidine blue staining can aid identification, and an expected number of 0.47 mast cells/100 hepatocytes is described.[35] Mast cells predominantly increase in number with nonspecific reactive hepatitis.[27] In inflammatory processes associated with fibrosis, mast cells exfoliate near spindle cells.[79] In contrast, hepatic mast cell tumor is characterized by numerous mast cells that are mostly arranged in small discohesive aggregates.[80]

Infectious Agents

The liver is normally sterile, although some apparently normal dogs have cytological evidence of bacteria in bile smears.[81] Since Kupffer cells are involved in the defense against infections of the liver, compromised anatomy or cell function results in impaired clearance and is alleged to be a predisposing event that facilitates bacterial invasion into hepatic parenchyma.[82] Bacteria most frequently associated with hepatitis are *Escherichia coli*, *Streptococcus* spp., *Staphylococcus* spp., *Enterococcus* spp., and *Clostridium* spp.[83] Other bacteria are recognized as causative agents of hepatic disease, such *Leptospira* spp. and *Helicobacter* spp., although culture is often required to identify organisms.[84,85]

Mycobacterium spp. can cause hepatic disease; organisms appear as small nonstaining rods in the cytoplasm of activated macrophages (Chapter 3).[86,87] *Leishmania* spp. are a causative agent of chronic hepatitis, typically characterized by granulomas in the fibrous support of portal tracts. Cytologically (personal observations) and histologically,[88] well-preserved neutrophils and macrophages containing amastigotes occur in association with hepatocytes (Figure 34.10). Other protozoal agents responsible for hepatic inflammation include *Toxoplasma* spp. and *Sarcocystis canis* in dogs[29,89,90] and *Cytauxzoon felis* in cats.[29] Fungal infections of the hepatic parenchyma are extremely rare; a case of dog with fungal hepatitis and concurrent cobalamin deficiency was described.[91] Recently, an infection with the trematode *Heterobilharzia americana* in a dog was detected by observation of ovoid to round, basophilic, thin-walled eggshell fragments and rare ciliated miracidia.[92] *Mesocestoides* spp. have been identified in FNA of canine liver and mesenteric lymph nodes, without

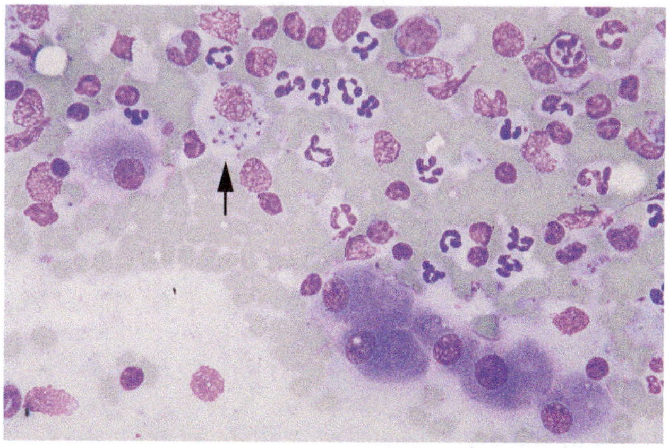

Figure 34.10 A macrophage with expanded cytoplasm contains *Leishmania* amastigotes. (arrow). Moderate numbers of nondegenerate neutrophils and a small cluster of hepatocytes are present (May-Grünwald–Giemsa, 1000×).

evidence of parasites in peritoneal fluid samples.[93] Cytology samples can contain large (200–400 × 500–2000 μm) basophilic vermiform larvae and fragments, tetrathyrdia, and calcareous corpuscles appearing as 15 μm refractile bodies (Figure 52.4). While viruses can infect the liver, cytology has limited potential for diagnosis. Canine infectious hepatitis caused by canine adenovirus-1 is sometimes associated with nuclear inclusions consisting of magenta bodies of various sizes, generally surrounded by a thin area of marginated chromatin (Figure 34.6c).[29] Other viral agents demonstrated or suspected to be causes of hepatic disease are herpesvirus, canine bocavirus, and canine circovirus, but they cannot be detected by cytology.

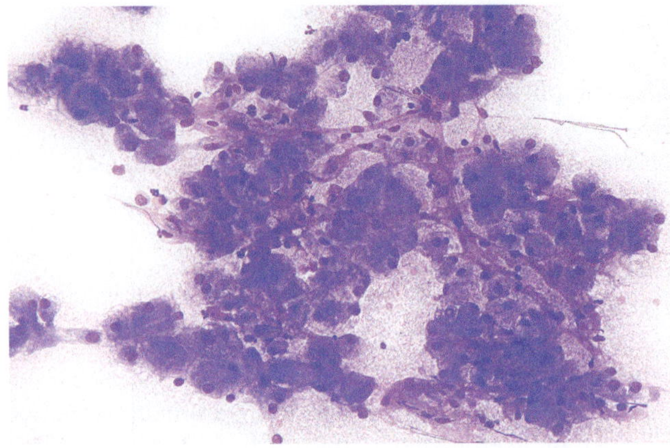

Figure 34.11 Hepatic fibrosis. Spindle cells are interspersed within a large cluster of hepatocytes (May-Grünwald–Giemsa, 400×).

Deposition of Extracellular Material

Fibrosis

Repeated injury of the hepatic parenchyma leads to chronic inflammation, hepatocellular necrosis, and fibrosis, features that are generally evaluated histologically. Hepatic fibrosis creates a diffusion barrier between hepatocytes and sinusoidal structures.[94] Initiation and progression of fibrosis is a consequence of activation of hepatic stellate cells and transdifferentiation of myofibroblasts in response to paracrine stimulation by cytokines released from necrotic or apoptotic hepatocytes, leukocytes, platelets, and Kupffer cells.[95–97] Recently the cytological features of hepatic fibrosis in chronic disease was described.[79] Increased numbers of spindle cells with eosinophilic cytoplasm and elongated nuclei are arranged in thin bundles that cross and interconnect the clusters of hepatocytes (Figure 34.11). Although some spindle cells can be present in smears from normal or non-fibrotic livers, 10.7 spindle cells/100 hepatocytes should be considered a cutoff value indicative of fibrotic changes in cytology samples. The spindle cells sometimes contain brown cytoplasmic granules, which are speculated to represent a precursor of collagen. A variable number of mixed inflammatory cells can be observed, with mast cells frequently located near the spindle cells or scattered among the hepatocytes. Cytological detection of fibrosis is an indication for biopsy to obtain a definitive diagnosis.

Amyloidosis

Amyloid is an acute phase protein produced predominantly by the liver. Functions include transport of cholesterol to the liver for biliary secretion, inflammatory cell recruitment, and induction of enzymes that degrade extracellular matrix.[98] Amyloid production occurs secondary to systemic or localized chronic inflammation, although a familial predisposition is recognized in Abyssinian cats,[99] Siamese cats,[100] and Chinese Shar-Pei dogs.[101,102] The formation of beta-pleated sheets leads to the deposition of amyloid as insoluble protein, mostly in the liver, kidney, pancreas, and spleen. In the liver, amyloid precipitates first in and causes expansion of the space of Disse, with consequent atrophy of hepatocytes and dilation of sinusoids. Histologically, amyloid appears as deposition of dense hyalinized eosinophilic material that stains orange-red with Congo red or Stokes method and is birefringent when examined by a polarizing filter. Cytologically, amyloid appears as pink, fibrillar, or dense, often wispy material interspersed between hepatocytes (Figure 34.12) that sometimes must be differentiated from platelet aggregates.[102]

The Gallbladder

Sampling and Normal Cytology

Gallbladder cytology sampling is often prompted by observing structural abnormalities during imaging studies or exploratory surgery. The procedure usually involves introduction of a 22 G needle with attached extension set, three-way stopcock, and syringe through the ventral aspect of the liver while the patient is in dorsal or lateral recumbency. Fluid is aspirated until the gallbladder is flaccid to minimize potential leakage, and the aspiration

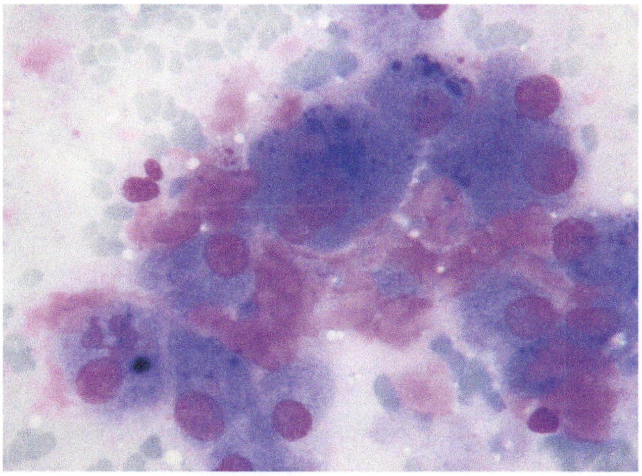

Figure 34.12 Amyloid appears as irregular, wispy, eosinophilic material between hepatocytes (May-Grünwald–Giemsa, 1000×).

site is reevaluated for evidence of free abdominal fluid. Although there is the potential for leakage of bile into the abdominal cavity, this was only documented in two dogs in a large study of dogs and cats and was not observed in another study of 83 cats.[103–105] Rupture is also possible when the wall is under pressure (i.e. mucinous hyperplasia and cholelithiasis) or is altered by ischemia or necrosis in vascular disorders causing infarction.[106] Normal bile fluid is grossly dark green. Microscopically, it is characterized by slightly basophilic granular or amorphous material, sometimes together with aggregates of debris. Needle-shaped, golden to brown bilirubin crystals are sometimes seen.[104] Hepatocytes, mesothelial cells, and individual or short palisades of columnar cholangiocytes from the wall are considered incidental findings.[104]

Hyperplasia and Inflammation

In the author's experience, bile can be too viscous to collect in mucinous hyperplasia, although a very small amount of amorphous basophilic material can be observed on smears. Bile fluid analysis is often performed to evaluate for bactibilia[107,108] and inflammation.[83] In both dogs and cats, bacteria are detected more often than inflammation cytologically.[104,105] While cytology and culture often correlate for the presence of bacteria, results are not concordant in all cases, particularly in dogs.[83,104] There are often differences between the organisms identified cytologically and culture, which has been hypothesized in some cases to relate to the presence of fastidious organisms or overgrowth by a dominant organism.[83,104] For this reason, cytology and bacterial culture are both recommended.[109,110] Inflammation is indicated by the presence of neutrophils with or without degeneration and phagocytic activity, macrophages, and lymphocytes.[104] Spores of the ascomycetes *Cyniclomyces guttulatus* were observed with other bacteria in a dog.[111] Banana-shaped zoites of the protozoa *Isospora* spp. in the dog[104] and ovoid egg fluke of *Platynosomum fastosum* in the cat have been described in bile.[28,112,113]

Advanced Diagnostic Techniques

The evaluation of a liver smears can benefit from the use of stains other than routine Romanowsky-modified stains to highlight some important cytoplasmic and extracytoplasmic features of hepatocytes and Kupffer cells including vacuoles and pigments. Fresh, unstained smears are necessary in obtaining reliable results for clinical interpretation.

Periodic Acid-Schiff

PAS is used to detect polysaccharides such as glycogen and mucosubstances such as glycoproteins, glycolipids, and mucins. In liver samples, it aids in recognition of glycogen accumulation (Figure 34.13a), particularly when used in combination with diastase, an enzyme that breaks down glycogen (PAS-D). Glycogen appears deep purple with PAS and achromatic after the action of diastase (PAS-D). Alpha-1-antitrypsin granules are demonstrated to be PAS positive and diastase resistent.[114]

Oil Red O

Oil Red O is a lysochrome diazo dye used for staining of neutral triglycerides and lipids on frozen sections and some lipoproteins on paraffin sections. In cytology, it is useful in recognition of intracytoplasmic lipids in cases of microvesicular steatosis (Figure 34.13b).[45]

Perl's Prussian Blue

Prussian blue is a common stain used to detect the presence of iron in cytoplasm of hepatocytes and Kupffer cells in cases of iron accumulation (Figure 34.13c).

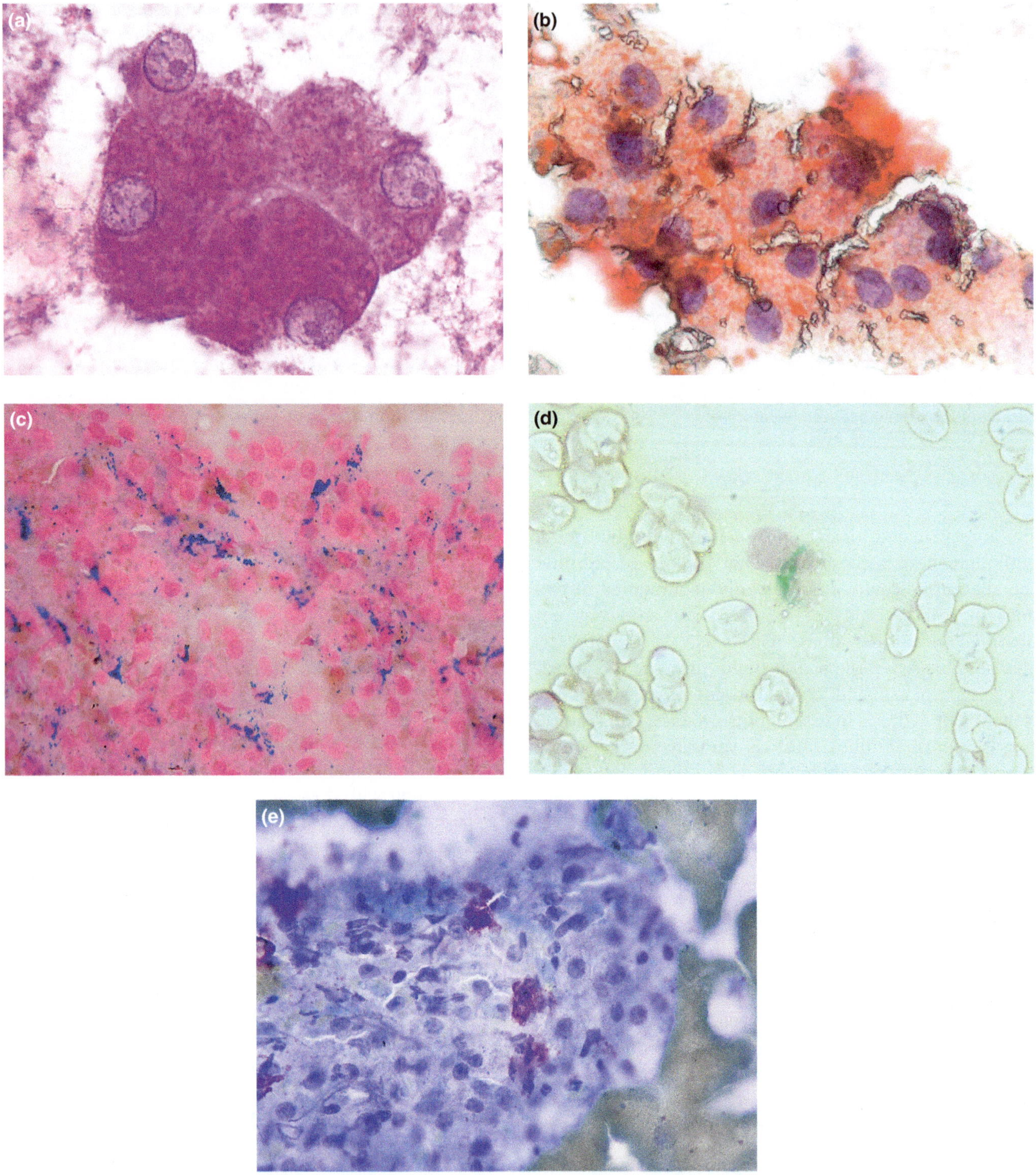

Figure 34.13 Special stains. (a) Glycogen accumulation in the cytoplasm of hepatocytes stains pink with periodic acid-Schiff (PAS) (1000×). (b) Intracytoplasmic lipid stains orange in a case of microvesicular steatosis (Oil Red O, 1000×). (c) Iron pigment is identified as blue staining material (Prussian blue, 1000×). (d) Bile appears bright green in this macrophage (Fouchet-Van Gieson, 1000×). (e) Mast cells within hepatocyte clusters are highlighted by metachromatic staining (Toluidine blue, 1000×).

Congo Red

Congo red stains amyloid as red-orange fibrils that exhibit apple-green birefringence when observed under polarized light.

Fouchet-Van Gieson

This stain is used to differentiate bile from other pigments that have accumulated in the cytoplasm (Figure 34.13d).

Long Ziehl-Neelsen

This stain differentiates lipofuscin from bile or iron pigment. Ceroid is a lipofuscin at an early stage of oxidation and with further oxidation develops into lipofuscin proper. Therefore, to determine if a pigment is ceroid or lipofuscin, Schmorl's method should be performed with the Long Ziehl-Neelsen technique.[115]

Toluidine Blue

This stain helps in recognition of hepatic mast cells (Figure 34.13e).[35]

Rhodanine and Rubeanic Acid

These stains are reliable for detection of copper in hepatocytes, resulting in red-orange stain of the cytoplasmic copper in cytological specimens (Figure 34.3e).[18,59,116]

Conclusion

Although there are significant limitations to the use of cytology for the evaluation of nonneoplastic liver disease, it can be valuable to support diagnosis of some infectious diseases and syndromes of pigment accumulation. Understanding the opportunities and limitations of the technique is important for appropriate utilization.

References

1 Kristensen, A.T., Weiss, D.J., Klausner, J.S., and Hardy, R.M. (1990). Liver cytology in cases of canine and feline hepatic disease. *Compend Contin Educ Pract Vet* 12: 797–808.

2 Burkhard, M.J. and Meyer, D.J. (1996). Invasive cytology of internal organs. *Vet Clin North Am Small Anim Pract* 26: 1203–1222.

3 Menard, M. and Papageorges, M. (1996). Ultrasound-guided liver fine needle biopsies in dogs: results of 600 cases (abstract). *Vet Pathol* 33: 570.

4 Menard, M. and Papageorges, M. (1996). Ultrasound-guided liver fine needle biopsies in cats: results of 307 cases (abstract). *Vet Pathol* 33: 570.

5 Roth, L. (2001). Comparison of liver cytology and biopsy diagnoses in dogs and cats: 56 cases. *Vet Clin Pathol* 30: 35–38.

6 Wang, K.Y., Panciera, D.L., Al-Rukibat, R.K., and Radi, Z.A. (2004). Accuracy of ultrasound-guided fine-needle aspiration of the liver and cytologic findings in dogs and cats: 97 cases (1990–2000). *J Am Vet Med Assoc* 224: 75–78.

7 Cohen, M., Bohling, M.W., Wright, J.C. et al. (2003). Evaluation of sensitivity and specificity of cytologic examination: 269 cases (1999–2000). *J Am Vet Med Assoc* 222: 964–967.

8 Warren-Smith, C.M., Andrew, S., Mantis, P., and Lamb, C.R. (2012). Lack of associations between ultrasonographic appearance of parenchymal lesions of the canine liver and histological diagnosis. *J Small Anim Pract* 53: 168–173.

9 Kemp, S.D., Panciera, D.L., Larson, M.M. et al. (2013). A comparison of hepatic sonographic features and histopathologic diagnosis in canine liver disease: 138 cases. *J Vet Intern Med* 27: 806–813.

10 Bahr, K.L., Sharkey, L.C., Murakami, T., and Feeney, D.A. (2013). Accuracy of US-guided FNA of focal liver lesions in dogs: 140 cases (2005–2008). *J Am Anim Hosp Assoc* 49: 190–196.

11 Kemp, S.D., Zimmerman, K.L., Panciera, D.L. et al. (2015). Histopathologic variation between liver lobes in dogs. *J Vet Intern Med* 29: 58–62.

12 Kerwin, S.C. (1995). Hepatic aspiration and biopsy techniques. *Vet Clin North Am Small Anim Pract* 25: 275–291.

13 Rothuizen, J., Desmet, V.J., Van den Ingh, T.S.G.A.M. et al. (2006). *Sampling and handling of liver tissue. In WSAVA Liver Standardization Group. Standard for Clinical and Histological Diagnosis of Canine and Feline Liver Disease*, 5-14. Saunders Elsevier, Edinburgh, London, New York, Oxford, Philadelphia, St.Louis, Sydney, Toronto.

14 Kemp, S.D., Zimmerman, K.L., Panciera, D.L. et al. (2015). A comparison of liver sampling techniques in dogs. *J Vet Intern Med* 29: 51–57.

15 Rawlings, C.A. and Howerth, E.W. (2004). Obtaining quality biopsies of the liver and kidney. *J Am Anim Hosp Assoc* 40: 352–358.

16 Vasanjee, S.C., Bubenik, L.J., Hosgood, G., and Bauer, R. (2006). Evaluation of hemorrhage, sample size, and

collateral damage for five hepatic biopsy methods in dogs. *Vet Surg* 35: 86–93.
17 Léveillé, R., Partington, B.P., Biller, D.S., and Miyabayashi, T. (1993). Complications after ultrasound-guided biopsy of abdominal structures in dogs and cats: 246 cases (1984–1991). *J Am Vet Med Assoc* 203: 413–415.
18 Arndt, T.P. and Shelly, S.M. (2014). The liver. In: *Diagnostic Cytology of the Dog and Cat*, 4e, (eds. Cowell, R.L., Valenciano, A.C.), 358–359. Elsevier Mosby, St.Louis, MO.
19 Bigge, L.A., Brown, D.J., and Penninck, D.G. (2001). Correlation between coagulation profile findings and bleeding complications after ultrasound-guided biopsies: 434 cases. *J Am Anim Hosp Assoc* 37: 228–233.
20 Johns, I.C. and Sweeney, R.W. (2008). Coagulation abnormalities and complications after percutaneous liver biopsy in horses. *J Vet Intern Med* 22: 185–189.
21 Petre, S.L., McClaran, J.K., Bergman, P.J., and Monette, S. (2012). Safety and efficacy of laparoscopic hepatic biopsy in dogs: 80 cases (2004–2009). *J Am Vet Med Assoc* 240: 181–185.
22 McDevitt, H.L., Mayhew, P.D., Giuffrida, M.A. et al. (2016). Short-term clinical outcome of laparoscopic liver biopsy in dogs: 106 cases (2003–2013). *J Am Vet Med Assoc* 248: 83–90.
23 Proot, S.J.M. and Rothuizen, J. (2006). High complication rate of an automatic tru-cut biopsy gun device for liver biopsy in cats. *J Vet Intern Med* 20: 1327–1333.
24 Weiss, D.J., Gagne, J.M., and Armstrong, P.J. (1995). Characterization of portal lymphocytic infiltrates in feline liver. *Vet Clin Pathol* 24: 91–95.
25 Yamamoto, K. (2000). Electron microscopy of mast cells in the venous wall of canine liver. *J Vet Med Sci* 62: 1183–1188.
26 Stockhaus, C., Teske, E., Van Den Ingh, T., and Rothuizen, J. (2002). The influence of age on the cytology of the liver in healthy dogs. *Vet Pathol* 39: 154–158.
27 Stockhaus, C., Van Den Ingh, T., Rothuizen, J., and Teske, E. (2004). A multistep approach in the cytologic evaluation of liver biopsy samples of dogs with hepatic diseases. *Vet Pathol* 41: 461–470.
28 Flatland, B. (2009). If you have the gall.... *Vet Clin Pathol* 38: 280.
29 Meyer, D.K. (2016). The liver. In: *Canine and Feline Cytology: A Colour Atlas and Interpretation Guide*, 3e, (eds. Raskin, R.E., Meyer, D.J.), 259–283. Elsevier, St. Louis MO.
30 Kobayashi, K., Sakata, K., Miyata, K. et al. (1985). Mast cell-Ito cell pairings found in the Disse's spaces in the liver of the beagle dog. *Arch Histol Jpn* 48: 483–496.
31 Ijzer, J., Roskams, T., Molenbeek, R.F. et al. (2006). Morphological characterization of portal myofibroblasts and hepatic stellate cells in the normal dog liver. *Comp Hepatol* 5: 7.
32 Sakagami, K., Higaki, K., Toda, K. et al. (1989). Role of canine hepatic sinusoidal lining cells in the immune response. *Transplant Proc* 21: 411–415.
33 Boler, R.K. (1969). Fine structure of canine Kupffer cells and their microtubule-containing cytosomes. *Anat Rec* 163: 483–496.
34 Orell, S.R., Sterret, G.F., Walters, M.N.I. et al. (1992). Retroperitoneum, liver and spleen. In: *Manual and Atlas of Fine Needle Aspiration Cytology*, (ed. Orell, S.R.), 247–248. Churchill Livingstone, Edimburgh, London, Madrid, Melbourne, New York and Tokyo.
35 Masserdotti, C. (2013). Proportion of mast cells in normal canine hepatic cytologic specimens: comparison of 2 staining methods. *Vet Clin Pathol* 42: 522–525.
36 Crosbie, O.M., Reynolds, M., McEntee, G. et al. (1999). In vitro evidence for the presence of hematopoietic stem cells in the adult human liver. *Hepatology* 29: 1193–1198.
37 Stalker, M. and Hayes, A. (2007). Liver. In: *Jubb, Kennedy and Palmer's pathology of domestic animals*, 5e, (ed. Maxie, M.G.), 297–388. Philadelphia, PA: Saunders.
38 Shibata, M., Morizane, T., Uchida, T., and Yamagami, T. (1998). Irregular regeneration of hepatocytes and risk of hepatocellular carcinoma in chronic hepatitis and cirrhosis with hepatitis-C-virus infection. *Lancet* 351: 1773–1777.
39 Cullen, J.M., van den Ingh, T.S.G.A.M., van Winkle, T. et al. (2006). Morphological classification of parenchymal disorders of the canine and feline liver: normal histology, reversible hepatocytic injury and hepatic amyloidosis. In: *WSAVA Liver Standardization Group. Standard for Clinical and Histological Diagnosis of Canine and Feline Liver Disease*, (eds. Rothuizen, J., Bunch, S.E., Charles, J.A., Cullen, J.M., Desmet, V.J., Szatmari, V., Twedt, D.C., van den Ing, T.S.G.A.M., van Winkle, T.J., and Washabau, R.J.), 77–83. Saunders Elsevier, Edinburgh, London, New York, Oxford, Philadelphia, St.Louis, Sydney, Toronto.
40 Sepesy, L.M., Center, S.A., Randolph, J.F. et al. (2006). Vacuolar hepatopathy in dogs: 336 cases (1993–2005). *J Am Vet Med Assoc* 229: 246–252.
41 Schaer, M. and Ginn, P.E. (1999). Iatrogenic Cushing's syndrome and steroid hepatopathy in a cat. *J Am Anim Hosp Assoc* 35: 48–51.
42 Kim, Y.H., Lee, Y.B., and Hong, S.S. (1969). Influence of corticosteroids on the hepatic cell and bile secretion. *Yonsei Med J* 10: 10–18.
43 Brix, A.E., Howerth, E.W., McConkie-Rosell, A. et al. (1995). Glycogen storage disease type Ia in two littermate Maltese puppies. *Vet Pathol* 32: 460–465.
44 Yi, H., Thurberg, B.L., Curtis, S. et al. (2012). Characterization of a canine model of glycogen storage disease type IIIa. *Dis Model Mech* 5: 804–811.

45 Masserdotti, C., Bonfanti, U., and De Lorenzi, D. (2004). Oil-red-O stain in cytologic samples of feline hepatic lipidosis. *ESVCP-ESVP Congress Proceedings*, Olsztyn, Poland. (September 15-17, 2004).

46 Van der Linden-Sipman, J.S., Van den Ingh TSGAM, and Van Toor, A.J. (1990). Fatty liver syndrome in puppies. *J Am Anim Hosp Assoc* 26: 9–12.

47 Pessayre, D., Mansouri, A., Berson, A., and Fromenty, B. (2010). Mitochondrial involvement in drug-induced live injury. *Handb Exp Pharmacol*: 311–365.

48 Newman, S.J., Smith, J.R., Stenske, K.A. et al. (2007). Aflatoxicosis in nine dogs after exposure to contaminated commercial dog food. *J Vet Diagn Invest* 19: 168–175.

49 Moore, A.R. and Hoffman, W. (2017). Liver cytology. In: *Small Animal Cytologic Diagnosis*, (eds. Barger, A.M., MacNeill, A.L.), 241–278. Boca Raton, CRC Press, Taylor and Francis Group, London, New York.

50 Scott, M. and Buriko, K. (2003). Characterization of the pigmented cytoplasmic granules common in canine hepatocytes. *Vet Clin Pathol* 34: 281–282.

51 Höhn, A. and Grune, T. (2013). Lipofuscin: formation, effects and role of macroautophagy. *Redox Biol* 1: 140–144.

52 Brunk, U.T. and Terman, A. (2002). Lipofuscin: mechanisms of age-related accumulation and influence on cell function. *Free Radic Biol Med* 33: 611–619.

53 Wu, X., Leegwater, P.A.J., and Fieten, H. (2016). Canine models for copper homeostasis disorders. *Int J Mol Sci* 17: 196.

54 Cedeno, Y., López-Alonso, M., and Miranda, M. (2016). Hepatic concentrations of copper and other metals in dogs with and without chronic hepatitis. *J Small Anim Pract* 57: 703–709.

55 Meertens, N.M., Bokhove, C.A., and Van den Ingh, T.S. (2005). Copper-associated chronic hepatitis and cirrhosis in a European Shorthair cat. *Vet Pathol* 42: 97–100.

56 Whittemore, J.C., Newkirk, K.M., Reel, D.M., and Reed, A. (2012). Hepatic copper and iron accumulation and histologic findings in 104 feline liver biopsies. *J Vet Diagn Invest* 24: 656–661.

57 Ankringe, N., Wijnberg, I.D., Boerma, S., and Ijzer, J. (2012). Copper-associated hepatic cirrhosis in a Friesian horse. *Tijdschr Diergeneeskkd* 137: 310–314.

58 Teske, E., Brinkhuis, B.G.A.M., Bode, P. et al. (1992). Cytological detection of copper for the diagnosis of inherited copper toxicosis in Bedlington Terriers. *Vet Rec* 131: 30–32.

59 Moore, A.R., Coffey, E., and Hamar, D. (2016). Diagnostic accuracy of Wright–Giemsa and rhodanine stain protocols for detection and semi-quantitative grading of copper in canine liver aspirates. *Vet Clin Pathol* 45: 689–697.

60 Mete, A., Hendriks, H.G., Klaren, P.H. et al. (2003). Iron metabolism in mynah birds (*Gracula religiosa*) resembles human hereditary haemochromatosis. *Avian Pathol* 32: 625–632.

61 House, J.K., Smith, B.P., Maas, J., and Lane, V.M. (1994). Hemochromatosis in Salers cattle. *J Vet Intern Med* 8: 105–111.

62 Gultekin, G.I., Raj, K., Foureman, P. et al. (2012). Erythrocytic pyruvate kinase mutations causing hemolytic anemia, osteosclerosis, and secondary hemochromatosis in dogs. *J Vet Intern Med* 26: 935–944.

63 Sprague, W.S., Hackett, T.B., Johnson, J.S., and Swardson-Olver, C.J. (2003). Hemochromatosis secondary to repeated blood transfusions in a dog. *Vet Pathol* 40: 334–337.

64 Lisboa, P.E. (1971). Experimental hepatic cirrhosis in dogs caused by chronic massive iron overload. *Gut* 12: 363–368.

65 Sevelius, E., Andersson, M., and Jönsson, L. (1994). Hepatic accumulation of alpha-1-antitrypsin in chronic liver disease in the dog. *J Comp Pathol* 111: 401–412.

66 Masserdotti, C., Rossetti, E., De Lorenzi, D. et al. (2014). Characterization of cytoplasmic hyaline bodies in a hepatocellular carcinoma of a dog. *Res Vet Sci* 96: 143–146.

67 Masserdotti, C. and Drigo, M. (2012). Retrospective study of cytologic features of well-differentiated hepatocellular carcinoma in dogs. *Vet Clin Pathol* 42: 522–525.

68 Hamir, A.N., Sullivan, N.D., Handson, P.D. (1983). Acid fast inclusions in tissues of dogs dosed with lead. *J Comp Pathol* 93(2): 307–317.

69 Portmann, B.C. and Nakanuma, Y. (2007). Diseases of the bile ducts. In: *MacSween's Pathology of the Liver*, 5e, (eds. Burt, A.D., Portmann, B.C., and Ferrell, L.D.), 517–581. Elsevier, Burt, Portmann and Ferrel. St.Louis, MO.

70 Guerra, J.M., Daniel, A.G., Aloia, T.P. et al. (2014). Hypervitaminosis A-induced hepatic fibrosis in a cat. *J Feline Med Surg* 16: 243–248.

71 van Winkle, T., Cullen, J.M., van den Ingh, T.S.G.A.M. et al. (2006). Morphological classification of parenchymal disorders of the canine and feline liver: hepatic abscesses and granuloma, hepatic metabolic storage disorders and miscellaneous conditions. In: *WSAVA Liver Standardization Group. Standard for Clinical and Histological Diagnosis of Canine and Feline Liver Disease*, (eds. Rothuizen, J., Bunch, S.E., Charles, J.A., Cullen, J.M., Desmet, V.J., Szatmari, V., Twedt, D.C., van den Ing, T.S.G.A.M., van Winkle, T.J., and Washabau, R.J.), 103–116. Saunders Elsevier, Edinburgh, London, New York, Oxford, Philadelphia, St.Louis, Sydney, Toronto.

72 Fondacaro, J.V., Guilpin, V.O., and Powers, B.E. (1999). Diagnostic correlation of liver aspiration cytology with histopathology in dogs and cats with liver disease (abstract). In: *Proceedings of 17th Annual Veterinary Medical Forum*, 719. Chicago: American College of Veterinary Internal Medicine.

73 Weiss, D.J., Blauvelt, M., and Aird, B. (2001). Cytologic evaluation of inflammation in canine liver aspirates. *Vet Clin Pathol* 30: 193–196.

74 Boisclair, J., Doré, M., Beauchamp, G. et al. (2001). Characterization of the inflammatory infiltrate in canine chronic hepatitis. *Vet Pathol* 38: 628–635.

75 Cullen, J.M. (2009). Summary of the world small animal veterinary association standardization committee guide to classification of liver disease in dogs and cats. *Vet Clin North Am Small Anim Pract* 39: 395–418.

76 Schwarz, L.A., Penninck, D.G., and Leveille-Webster, C. (1998). Hepatic abscesses in 13 dogs: a review of the ultrasonographic findings, clinical data, and therapeutic options. *Vet Radiol Ultrasound* 39: 357–365.

77 Sergeeff, J.S., Armstrong, P.J., and Bunch, S.E. (2004). Hepatic abscesses in cats: 14 cases. *J Vet Intern Med* 18: 295–300.

78 van den Ingh, T.S.G.A.M., van Winkle, T., Cullen, J.M. et al. (2006). Morphological classification of parenchymal disorders of the canine and feline liver: hepatocellular death, hepatitis and cirrhosis. In: *WSAVA Liver Standardization Group. Standard for Clinical and Histological Diagnosis of Canine and Feline Liver Disease.* (eds. Rothuizen, J., Bunch, S.E., Charles, J.A., Cullen, J.M., Desmet, V.J., Szatmari, V., Twedt, D.C., van den Ing, T.S.G.A.M., van Winkle, T.J., and Washabau, R.J.), Saunders Elsevier, Edinburgh, London, New York, Oxford, Philadelphia, St.Louis, Sydney, Toronto.

79 Masserdotti, C. and Bertazzolo, W. (2016). Cytologic features of hepatic fibrosis in dogs: a retrospective study on 22 cases. *Vet Clin Pathol* 45: 361–367.

80 Stefanello, D., Valenti, P., Faverzani, S. et al. (2009). Ultrasound guided cytology of spleen and liver: a prognostic tool in cutaneous mast cell tumor. *J Vet Intern Med* 23: 1051–1057.

81 Kook, P.H., Schellenberg, S., Grest, P. et al. (2010). Microbiologic evaluation of gallbladder bile of healthy dogs and dogs with iatrogenic hypercortisolism: a pilot study. *J Vet Intern Med* 24: 224–228.

82 Kolios, G., Valatas, V., and Kouroumalis, E. (2006). Role of Kupffer cells in the pathogenesis of liver disease. *World J Gastroenterol* 12: 7413–7420.

83 Wagner, K.A., Hartmann, F.A., and Trepanier, L.A. (2007). Bacterial culture results from liver, gallbladder, or bile in 248 dogs and cats evaluated for hepatobiliary disease: 1998–2003. *J Vet Intern Med* 21: 417–424.

84 Bishop, L., Strandberg, J.D., Adams, R.J. et al. (1979). Chronic active hepatitis in dogs associated with leptospires. *Am J Vet Res* 40: 839–844.

85 Fox, J.G., Drolet, R., Higgins, R. et al. (1996). *Helicobacter canis* isolated from a dog liver with multifocal necrotizing hepatitis. *J Clin Microbiol* 34: 2479–2482.

86 Turinelli, V., Ledieu, D., Guilbaud, L. et al. (2004). *Mycobacterium tuberculosis* infection in a dog from Africa. *Vet Clin Pathol* 33: 177–181.

87 Oliveira-Filho, J.P., Monteiro, L.N., Delfiol, D.J. et al. (2012). Mycobacterium DNA detection in liver and skin of a horse with generalized sarcoidosis. *J Vet Diagn Invest* 24: 596–600.

88 Rallis, T., Day, M.J., Saridomichelakis, M.N. et al. (2005). Chronic hepatitis associated with canine leishmaniosis (*Leishmania infantum*): a clinicopathological study of 26 cases. *J Comp Pathol* 132: 145–152.

89 Grandi, F., Monteiro, L.N., Salgado, B.S. et al. (2012). What is your diagnosis? Hepatosplenomegaly in a howler monkey (*Alouatta fusca*). *Vet Clin Pathol* 41: 433–434.

90 Allison, R., Williams, P., Lansdowne, J. et al. (2006). Fatal hepatic sarcocystosis in a puppy with eosinophilia and eosinophilic peritoneal effusion. *Vet Clin Pathol* 35: 353–357.

91 Kook, P.H., Drögemüller, M., Leeb, T. et al. (2015). Hepatic fungal infection in a young beagle with unrecognized hereditary cobalamin deficiency (Imerslund-Gräsbeck syndrome). *J Small Anim Pract* 56: 138–141.

92 Le Donne, V., McGovern, D.A., Fletcher, J.M., and Grasperge, B.J. (2016). Cytologic diagnosis of *Heterobilharzia americana* infection in a liver aspirate from a dog. *Vet Pathol* 53: 633–636.

93 Patten, P.K., Rich, L.J., Zaks, K., and Blauvelt, M. (2013). Cestode infection in 2 dogs: cytologic findings in liver and a mesenteric lymph node. *Vet Clin Pathol* 42: 103–108.

94 Gressner, O.A., Weiskirchen, R., and Gressner, A.M. (2007). Evolving concepts of liver fibrogenesis provide new diagnostic and therapeutic options. *Comp Hepatol* 6: 7.

95 Senoo, H. (2004). Structure and function of hepatic stellate cells. *Med Electron Microsc* 37: 3–15.

96 Wynn, T. (2008). Cellular and molecular mechanism of fibrosis. *J Pathol* 214: 199–210.

97 Roth, S., Michel, K., and Gressner, A.M. (1998). Latent transforming growth factor-beta in liver parenchymal cells, its injury-dependent release and paracrine effects on hepatic stellate cells. *Hepatology* 27: 1003–1012.

98 Snyder, P.W. (2007). Amyloidosis. Disease of immunity. In: *Pathological Basis of Veterinary Disease*, 4e, (eds. McGavin, M.D., Zachary, J.F.), 246–250. St. Louis, MO: Mosby, Elsevier.

99 DiBartola, S.P., Tarr, M.J., and Benson, M.D. (1986). Tissue distribution of amyloid deposits in Abyssinian cats with familial amyloidosis. *J Comp Pathol* 96: 387–398.

100 Beatty, J.A., Barrs, V.R., Martin, P.A. et al. (2002). Spontaneous hepatic rupture in six cats with systemic amyloidosis. *J Small Anim Pract* 43: 355–363.

101 Loeven, K.O. (1994). Hepatic amyloidosis in two Chinese Shar Pei dogs. *J Am Vet Med Assoc* 204: 1212–1216.

102 Flatland, B., Moore, R.R., Wolf, C.M. et al. (2007). Liver aspirate from a Shar Pei dog. *Vet Clin Pathol* 36: 105–108.

103 Hogan, M.T., Watne, A., Mossburg, W., and Castaneda, W. (1976). Direct injection into the gallbladder in dogs, using ultrasonic guidance. *Arch Surg* 111: 564–565.

104 Peters, L.M., Glanemann, B., Garden, O.A., and Szladovits, B. (2016). Cytological findings of 140 bile samples from dogs and cats and associated clinical pathological data. *J Vet Intern Med* 30: 123–131.

105 Byfield, V.L., Callahan Clark, J.E., Turek, B.J. et al. (2017). Percutaneous cholecystocentesis in cats with suspected hepatobiliary disease. *J Feline Med Surg* 19: 1254–1260.

106 Holt, D.E., Mehler, S., Mayhew, P.D., and Hendrick, M.J. (2004). Canine gallbladder infarction: 12 cases (1993–2003). *Vet Pathol* 41: 416–418.

107 Lawrence, Y.A., Ruaux, C.G., Nemanic, S., and Milovancev, M. (2015). Characterization, treatment, and outcome of bacterial cholecystitis and bactibilia in dogs. *J Am Vet Med Assoc* 246: 982–989.

108 Tamborini, A., Jahns, H., McAllister, H. et al. (2016). Bacterial cholangitis, cholecystitis, or both in dogs. *J Vet Intern Med* 30: 1046–1055.

109 Boland, L. and Beatty, J. (2017). Feline cholangitis. *Vet Clin North Am Small Anim Pract* 47: 703–724.

110 Otte, C.M.A., Penning, L.C., and Rothuizen, J. (2017). Feline biliary tree and gall bladder disease: aetiology, diagnosis, and treatment. *J Feline Med Surg* 19: 514–528.

111 Neel, J.A., Tarigo, J., and Grindem, C.B. (2006). Gallbladder aspirate from a dog. *Vet Clin Pathol* 35: 467–470.

112 Haney, D.R., Christiansen, J.S., and Toll, J. (2006). Severe cholestatic liver disease secondary to liver fluke (*Platynosomum concinnum*) infection in three cats. *J Am Anim Hosp Assoc* 42: 234–237.

113 Basu, A.K. and Charles, R.A. (2014). A review of the cat liver fluke *Platynosomum fastosum* Kossack, 1910 (Trematoda: Dicrocoeliidae). *Vet Parasitol* 200: 1–7.

114 Talbot, I.C. and Mowat, A.P. (1975). Liver disease in infancy: histological features and relationship to alpha-antitrypsin phenotype. *J Clin Pathol* 28: 559–563.

115 Pearse, A.G.E. (1985). *Histochemistry: Theoretical and Applied*, vol. 2, 211–212. Edinburgh, London: Churchill Livingstone.

116 Thornburg, L.P., Beissenherz, M., Dolan, M., and Raisbeck, M.F. (1985). Histochemical demonstration of copper and copper-associated protein in the canine liver. *Vet Pathol* 22: 327–332.

35

Hepatobiliary Neoplasia and Cancer Staging

Charles E. Wiedmeyer and Jeff Bryan

Introduction

Hepatobiliary neoplasia is an important differential diagnosis for companion animals presenting with liver disease, particularly in older dogs and cats.[1] Liver tumors are quite rare in horses, with the literature mostly restricted to case series and reports.[2,3] Most dogs and cats with hepatobiliary neoplasms have clinical signs at diagnosis, but those signs are often nonspecific, including weight loss, lethargy, ascites, vomiting, diarrhea, polydipsia, or polyuria.[1] Paraneoplastic alopecia has been reported in cats with hepatocellular or bile duct carcinomas.[1,4,5] Hepatomegaly and icterus are clinical findings more specific for hepatic neoplasia, and a majority of dogs and cats have a palpable cranial abdominal mass.[1,6] Signs associated with hepatic encephalopathy such as seizures, weakness, and ataxia also can be observed if there is liver dysfunction.[1]

Dogs and cats with hepatobiliary neoplasms often have nonspecific hematologic and serum biochemical abnormalities. A mild, non-regenerative anemia is present in up to 57% of dogs with hepatic neoplasms; possible etiologies include anemia of chronic disease, sequestration, or iron deficiency.[1] Up to 90% of dogs and 28% of cats with hepatic neoplasms had leukocytosis with neutrophilia, possibly related to necrosis in large tumors.[1,6,7] Other laboratory findings include coagulation profile abnormalities (i.e. prolonged prothrombin time and activated partial thromboplastin time, increased fibrin degradation products, decreases in select coagulation factors), hypoalbuminemia, hyperglobulinemia, increased serum bile acids, and increased liver enzymes.[1,8–11] Hypoglycemia and azotemia also have been reported in selected cases of dogs and cats with hepatic neoplasms; however, the pathophysiology for these laboratory findings is not well characterized in most instances.[6,7]

The prevalence of primary hepatic neoplasms in dogs ranges from 0.6 to 2.6%[1,12,13] and up to 2.9% in cats.[1,13,14] Primary hepatobiliary tumors are usually found in older animals, between 8 and 12 years of age.[13–15] Primary hepatocellular tumors are generally divided into hepatocellular adenomas or carcinomas. Hepatoblastomas have been reported in horses,[3] a dog,[16] and a cat.[17] Histologically, hepatoblastomas are nodules demarcated from adjacent hepatic parenchyma but without an identifiable capsule and arranged in sheets, cords, and nests of neoplastic cells.[17] The neoplastic cells resemble immature hepatocytes and are small, round to ovoid, or spindle shaped with a high nuclear to cytoplasmic ratio (N:C).[16,17] Nuclei have finely granular chromatin with mild anisokaryosis and unremarkable atypia.[16,17] Tumor cells are separated by a fibrovascular stroma and often contain vascular lakes.[16,17] Other neoplasms of the liver can arise from bile duct epithelium (cholangiocellular adenoma or carcinoma), cells of neuroendocrine origin (hepatic carcinoid), stromal cells (sarcomas), and those of the hemolymphatic system (e.g. lymphoma, myeloma-related disorders [MRD]).[12,13,18,19] Tumors originating from hepatic progenitor cells are described as potentially having overlapping morphologic features of multiple cell types, for example, hepatocellular and cholangiocellular.[18,20]

Due to its vascular and lymphatic anatomy, the liver is a common site for metastasis of extrahepatic neoplasms. Between 30.6 and 36.8% of dogs will have metastasis of a non-hepatic neoplasms to the liver.[13] For cats and horses, the prevalence of metastatic neoplasms is not well characterized; however, metastatic neoplasia is more common than primary tumors in equine livers.[21] Metastatic lesions in the liver can occur as a single mass, multiple discrete masses or as a diffuse process.[12,14,15] Metastatic lesions from the mammary glands, spleen, adrenal glands, pancreas, bone, endocrine systems, bladder, and lung are

Veterinary Cytology, First Edition. Edited by Leslie C. Sharkey, M. Judith Radin, and Davis Seelig.

most common in dogs.[12,15] Primary neoplasms of the pancreas and intestinal tract can spread directly to the liver by local extension.[15]

The following chapter will discuss the cytology of primary and metastatic neoplasia of the liver with an emphasis on dogs and cats, although the limited available information for the horse is included.

Collection and Medical Imaging

Liver structure and cytology collection techniques are described in Chapter 34. Imaging studies are used both to characterize lesions and to guide cytologic sampling. The most robust literature is for ultrasound, which has been available longest, is relatively widely accessible, and often does not require anesthesia. While an extensive review is beyond the scope of this chapter, a brief summary of major points is useful for cytologists. In general, ultrasound is not considered definitive for any particular microscopic diagnosis.[22–26] Nodular lesions identifiable by ultrasound can be neoplastic or nonneoplastic. Ultrasonographic characteristics can influence the probability of the categorization but are not definitive. For example, larger lesions (especially >3 cm) and those that occur in association with abdominal effusion are more likely to be malignant.[27,28] Target lesions, while often associated with hepatic malignancy, have also been described associated with nodular hyperplasia, hepatitis, and cirrhosis.[29] It has been suggested that hepatocellular carcinoma (HCC) be considered when a solitary hyperechoic liver lesion is identified.[22] Liver tumors with recognizable cystic components may indicate biliary cystadenomas in cats; however, because other hepatic abnormalities such as hematomas, abscesses, nodular hyperplasia, and other unrelated cystic or metastatic neoplasms can have overlapping ultrasonographic findings, the technique is not definitive.[23]

Ultrasound is even less definitive with diffuse hematologic neoplasms such as lymphoma and mast cell neoplasia.[26,30,31] Neoplastic and inflammatory liver pathology cannot be reliably distinguished, and in some cases, diffuse neoplastic infiltrate can be present in ultrasonographically normal livers in dogs, cats, and horses.[31–34] Therefore, it is recommended that regardless of the ultrasonographic appearance of the liver, fine-needle aspiration be performed if the clinical presentation merits such action.[30,31]

Greater access to magnetic resonance imaging (MRI) and computed tomography in veterinary medicine has demonstrated the potential for improved the differentiation of hepatic masses by imaging.[35–37] Features such as lesion homogeneity, comparative signaling, and patterns of lesion enhancement with contrast can be useful for using advanced imaging to discriminate benign from malignant hepatic lesions based on microscopic diagnosis.[35,36] The current limitations of these techniques are availability, cost, and a requirement for anesthesia. Still, use of advanced imaging techniques combined with fine-needle aspirate can improve diagnostic accuracy.[35–37]

Primary Hepatic Tumors

Hepatocellular Origin

Hepatocellular Adenoma

Hepatocellular adenoma is typically an incidental finding observed more frequently in cats than dogs.[14] Grossly, hepatocellular adenomas are usually singular, sometimes large (up to 20 cm) masses, often with a pedunculated attachment, although nodular, and, rarely, diffuse forms are also reported.[1,15] Histologically and cytologically, these tumors can be difficult to distinguish from nodular hyperplasia and normal hepatocytes. Histologic characteristics include compression of adjacent tissue, encapsulation, and lack of portal tracts or hepatic venules.[15,38] Cytologically, both adenomas and hyperplasia consist of hepatocytes that are well differentiated but can display mild anisocytosis and anisokaryosis, slightly increased N:C, vacuolar degeneration, or greater cytoplasmic basophilia. Additional findings in hyperplastic tissue and adenomas include more frequent binucleation or lipid-laden macrophages.[39] Although a large retrospective study from Japan of over 450 liver biopsies identified hepatocellular adenomas in 8% of canine samples, there is limited material in the primary literature evaluating the cytologic diagnosis, which is considered unreliable due to overlap with normal and hyperplastic hepatocytes.[40]

Hepatocellular Carcinoma

HCC are the most common primary hepatic tumor in dogs and second most common in cats.[14] They have been described in horses; however, cytologic features have not been reported in this species to the best of our knowledge.[3] Like adenomas, HCC are classified as either massive, nodular, or diffuse.[15,41] The massive form is the most common, representing approximately 60% of HCC and typically originating from a single liver lobe with a predilection for the left lobe.[15,41] The nodular type represents approximately 30% of HCC and presents as multiple, discrete, variably sized nodules in all liver lobes. Diffuse tumors make up the remaining 10% of HCC and are non-encapsulated and highly infiltrative. Histologically, HCC have been divided into 11 different groups based on cytologic and architectural characteristics.[41] Further attempts have been made to classify canine and feline tumors according to a human system based on immunohistochemical findings, and results were similar.[18,20,42] Generally, cells have recognizable features of hepatocytes, including granular amphophilic to occasionally vacuolated cytoplasm and round nuclei with granular cytoplasm and prominent nucleoli.[38,39,43–46] When the hepatocytes display prominent criteria of malignancy, a cytologic diagnosis of HCC can be straightforward; however, distinguishing a well-differentiated HCC from nodular hyperplasia can be problematic.[43] One study found HCC to be characterized by a high N:C, cytomegaly, cytoplasmic vacuolization, and increased numbers of nucleoli.[47] Cell crowding, necrosis, and condensed chromatin also can be features.[47] Other features that might distinguish a well-differentiated carcinoma include dissociation of hepatocytes, acinar or palisading cellular arrangements, the presence of bare nuclei, mild anisocytosis and anisokaryosis, multinucleated cells, and increased N:C (Figure 35.1).[43] The morphologic features of the hepatocytes in a pleomorphic HCC include cellular atypia with varying N:C, marked anisocytosis and anisokaryosis, deeply basophilic cytoplasm, variations in nuclear appearance, macronucleoli, and large nucleoli (Figure 35.2).[39] Hyaline bodies, appearing as variably sized homogeneous basophilic cytoplasmic inclusions, have been documented to occur in the dog as they do occasionally in people.[43]

Hepatoblastoma

This tumor has been reported in a small number of fetal, neonatal, and young horses and has been described in mice, pigs, sheep, cattle, camelids, dogs, and cats.[3,17,48–51] Hepatoblastoma is the most common primary hepatic malignancy in children under five years of age, making it

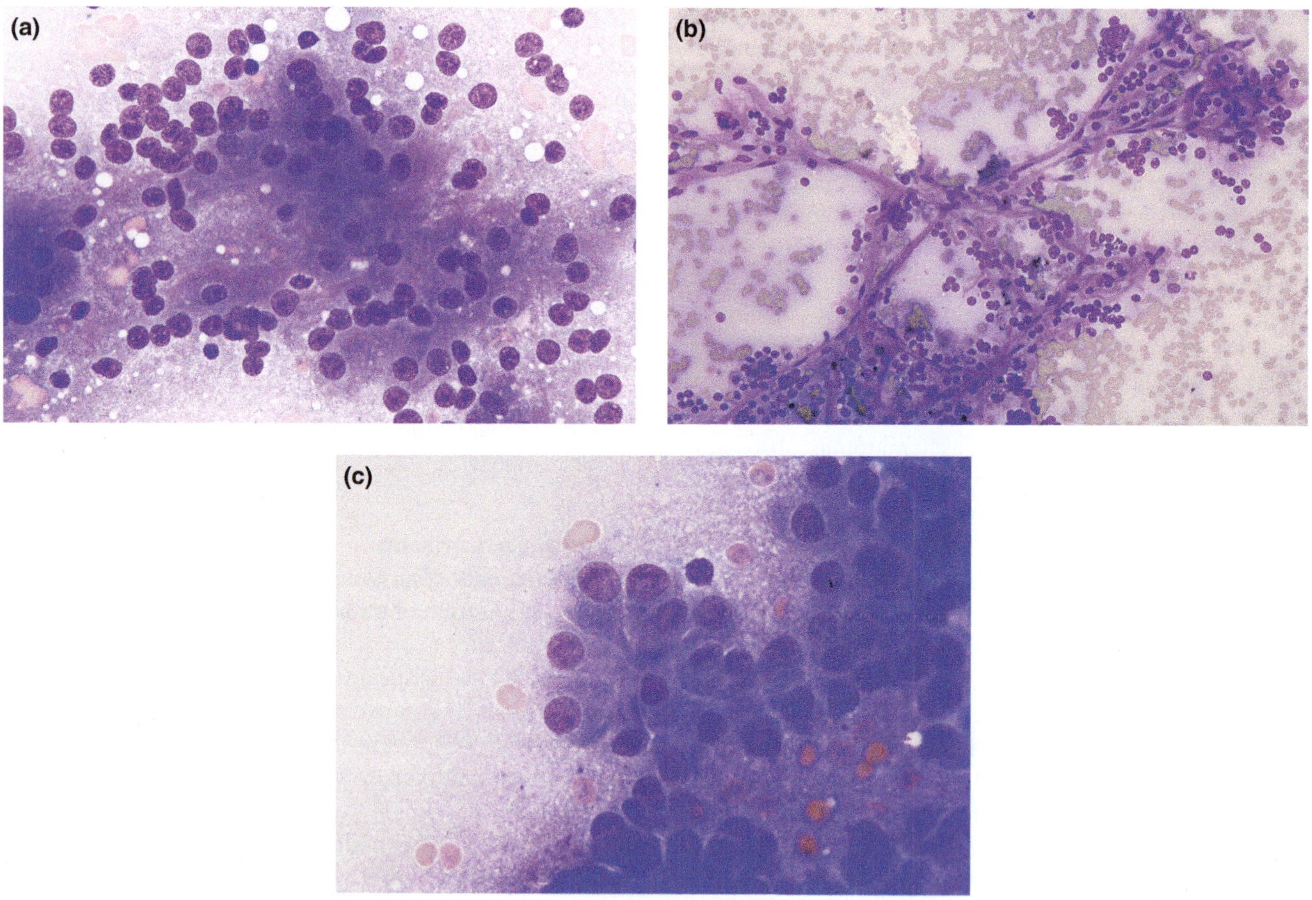

Figure 35.1 Liver aspirates of well-differentiated hepatocellular carcinoma in a dog. (a) A cluster of neoplastic hepatocytes is surrounded by many naked nuclei. Anisokaryosis is minimal in the neoplastic cells. (b) Hepatocytes and naked nuclei are arranged around branched capillaries. Notice the spindle cytoplasm and elongated nuclei of the endotheliocytes. (c) Acinar distribution of neoplastic hepatocytes around a common central area (May-Grünwald Giemsa, (a) and (c) 1000×, (b) 400×. *Source:* Images courtesy of Carlo Masserdotti).

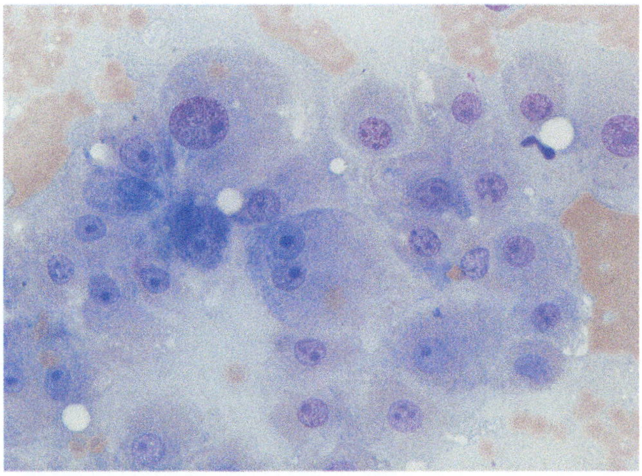

Figure 35.2 Poorly differentiated hepatocellular carcinoma in a mixed breed dog presenting with a hepatic mass. Hepatocytes are characterized by marked anisocytosis and anisokaryosis with prominent, multiple, and variably sized nucleoli (Wright Giemsa, 1000×).

significant from a comparative perspective. These tumors are typically characterized as epithelial or mixed epithelial and mesenchymal, each with several subtypes. Teratoid features have been described in a number of equine cases, as have metastatic lesions, which are uncommon in humans. A single report of cytologic features characterized the smears as consisting of many clusters of well-differentiated hepatocytes with bile plugs and a population of smaller epithelial cells forming dense cords, clusters, and acinar structures.[49] There was an increased N:C (<1 : 2) and single variably sized round nuclei with occasional nucleoli.

Combined Hepatocellular and Cholangiocellular Carcinoma

Combined hepatocellular and cholangiocellular carcinoma is a primary hepatic tumor that is very rare in dogs and horses.[52,53] There have been no reports in cats. Of those described grossly, they presented as multiple varying-sized masses in the liver parenchyma and gallbladder.[6,8,52] Similar to humans, three subgroups based on histology have been identified: (i) glandular or ductal hyperplasia with HCC, (ii) contiguous hepatocellular and ductal carcinoma, and (iii) two tumors arising from different areas.[6,54] Histologically, these tumors have been described as an intermingling of both hepatocellular and cholangiocellular cells that are moderately differentiated with occasionally squamous metaplasia and a high mitotic rate.[52] The hepatocellular component had a trabecular growth pattern, while the cholangiocellular component had tubular and glandular structures.[52] Intraluminal mucin material was observed within tubular structures.[6,52] Immunohistochemical patterns show both cell types as being positive for cytokeratin and antihuman α-smooth muscle actin and variably positive for vimentin. Cholangiocellular cells were positive for antihuman carcinoembryonic antigen, while the hepatocellular component was negative.[52] Using electron microscopy, both types of tumor cells showed several types of filaments including tonofilaments.[52] Cytologic findings have not been published, but likely features can be extrapolated from histopathologic descriptions.

Mesenchymal Neoplasms

Myelolipomas

Myelolipomas are benign primary hepatic tumors in cats.[14] Myelolipomas have been identified in dogs but most often involve the spleen or adrenal gland rather than the liver.[55,56] Reports in the horse were not found. The tumors often present as a solitary mass or a multifocal process affecting several organs.[13] Cytologically, myelolipomas are composed of a mixture of well-differentiated adipocytes and normal hematopoietic elements.[14,56] The hematopoietic cells can consist of erythroid, myeloid, lymphoid, and megakaryocytes in all stages of maturity, resembling extramedullary hematopoiesis.[56] Myelolipomas can be distinguished from extramedullary hematopoiesis by the presence of numerous intermixed mature adipocytes.

Sarcomas

Because primary hepatic neoplasms can arise from any normal cellular constituent in the liver, mesenchymal neoplasms do occur in dogs and cats but are rare, and no reports could be identified in horses.[14,57] Primary hepatic

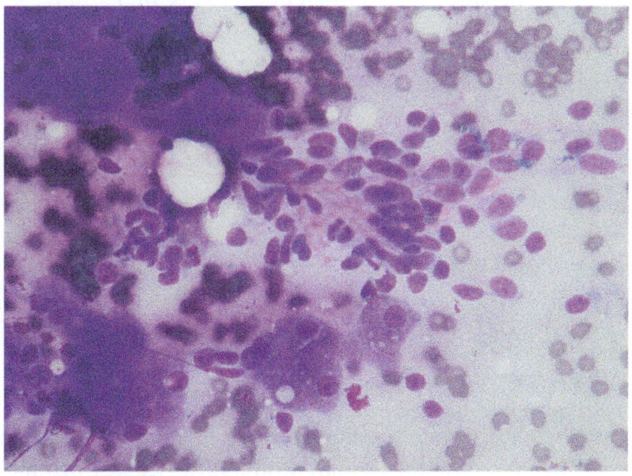

Figure 35.3 Hepatic sarcoma from a dog. A bundle of spindle cells occurs among mature hepatocytes. Spindloid cells are characterized by lightly basophilic cytoplasm and elongated nuclei and are associated with some thin strands of eosinophilic fibrillar matrix material (May-Grűnwald Giemsa, 1000×. *Source:* Image courtesy of Carlo Masserdotti).

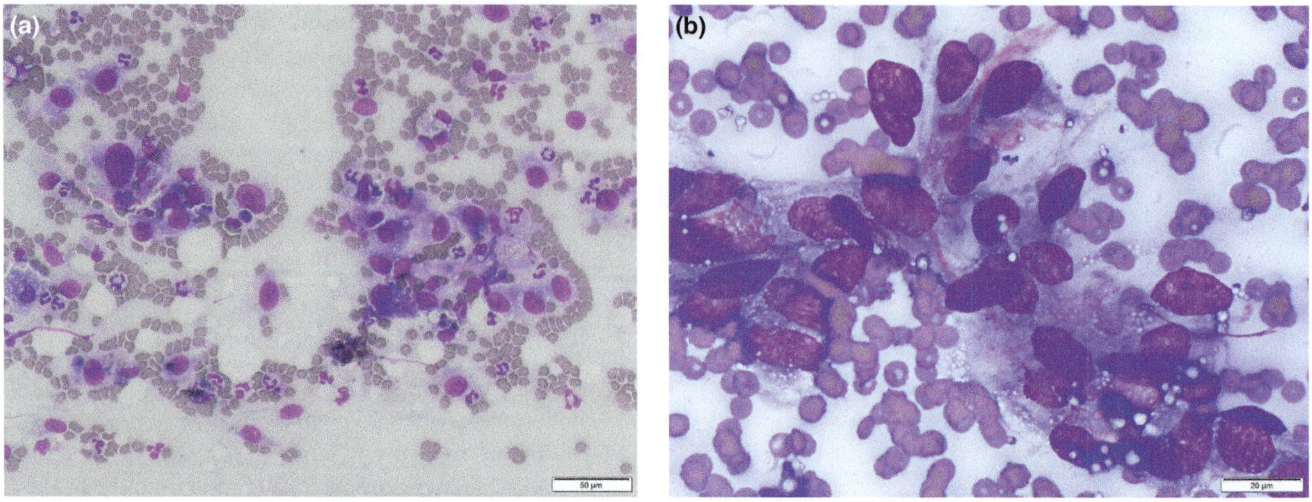

Figure 35.4 Hemangiosarcoma in the liver of a dog. (a) Samples contain many plump to stellate mesenchymal cells on a hemodiluted background along with intermixed blood associated leukocytes. Mesenchymal cells have indistinct cytoplasmic margins and basophilic cytoplasm that often contains numerous punctate cytoplasmic vacuoles. Oval nuclei have prominent multiple nucleoli. Anisocytosis and anisokaryosis are marked in this population. Occasionally, blue-black granular material consistent with iron or hemosiderin is noted within cell cytoplasm. (b) Pink extracellular material consistent with matrix is noted in association with an aggregate of neoplastic mesenchymal cells that exhibit similar features to those described in (a) (Wright Giemsa, (a) 200×, (b) 500×. *Source:* Images courtesy of Daniel Heinrich).

fibrosarcoma, hemangiosarcoma, leiomyosarcoma, liposarcoma, rhabdomyosarcoma, and osteosarcoma have been reported in both dogs and cats (Figures 35.3 and 35.4).[14,58–63] Primary hepatic chondrosarcoma has been reported in a dog, and primary hepatic chondroblastic osteosarcoma in a cat.[64–66] The most common primary hepatic mesenchymal neoplasm is leiomyosarcoma in dogs and hemangiosarcoma in cats.[6,14] Cytologic features of each of these neoplasms are described in Chapters 16, 22, and 23.

Round Cell Neoplasms

Primary Hepatic Lymphoma

Lymphoma is the most common neoplasm overall in dogs and cats.[13,14,67,68] Hepatic involvement is typically a result of multicentric lymphoma, but the liver can be the primary site for the disease.[13,15,67–70] In cats, hepatic lymphoma is most commonly seen as part of abdominal visceral organ disease with few cases affecting solely the liver.[68] Few cases of T-cell (i.e. $CD3^+/CD79a^-$) hepatosplenic lymphoma have been reported in cats, and, in one, the neoplastic cells exhibited marked emperipolesis of erythrocytes.[71] In dogs, small numbers of cases of primary hepatosplenic lymphoma have been described, which are histologically characterized by sinusoidal infiltration.[69,70,72] Hepatosplenic lymphoma has been reported to have a characteristic cytologic appearance, consisting of intermediate to large cells with moderate amounts of basophilic cytoplasm with fine magenta to pink granules having a perinuclear orientation, round to oval to pleomorphic nuclei with stippled chromatin and prominent nucleoli.[70] A case of hepatosplenic T-cell lymphoma has been described in a horse.[73] Hepatocytotropic lymphoma, in which lymphocytes also invade hepatic cords, has been described in two dogs; however, cytologic findings were not reported.[70] Comprehensive cytologic findings of neoplastic lymphocytes are further described in Chapter 27.

Myeloma-Related Disorders in Cats

Extramedullary plasma cell tumors include those neoplasms that originate outside the bone marrow, distinguishing them from multiple myeloma.[74] Extramedullary plasma cell tumors of the skin are addressed in Chapter 14, while non-cutaneous forms will be discussed here. Visceral extramedullary plasma cell tumors are most common in cats but are also recognized in people (Figure 35.5). The term myeloma-related disorder is currently used to describe tumors of extra-marrow plasma cell or immunoglobulin-secreting B-cell lymphocyte origin in both species.[75] Review of the literature can be complicated by inconsistent and sometimes confusing terminology and diagnostic criteria. This discussion will be restricted to the material meeting the criteria outlined above, which is consistent with the hypothesis that primary extramedullary neoplastic transformation occurs in feline MRD.[19] Typically, the spleen and liver are involved.[74] In one retrospective case

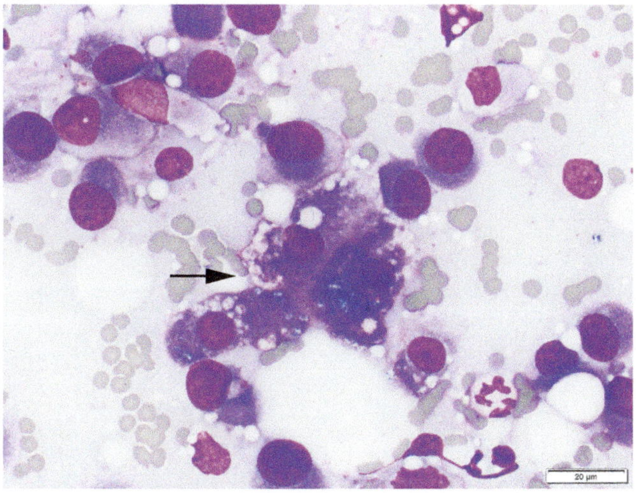

Figure 35.5 Metastatic plasma cell neoplasia in the liver of a cat. A single small cluster of hepatocytes (arrow) is present among numerous atypical plasma cells and a single neutrophil. Plasma cells have distinct margination and basophilic cytoplasm. Nuclei are round and eccentrically located with irregularly clumped chromatin and few faintly visible nucleoli (Wright-Giemsa, 500×. *Source:* Image courtesy of Daniel Heinrich).

series of cats, 5 cats (42%) with abdominal manifestation did not appear to have marrow involvement, 5 cats had both abdominal organ and marrow involvement but the primary site could not be determined, and in 5/10 cats with marrow disease, other organs were not evaluated.[74] In this same case series, all cats with abdominal organ involvement were systemically ill and hyperglobulinemic; 75% had multiorgan involvement and 25% had involvement restricted to a single organ.[74] Another retrospective case series identified hepatic involvement in 8/9 cases in which the liver was examined, corresponding to 31% of the total of 26 cases.

When cytology/histopathology correlation was available, there was almost 100% correlation; this was based on samples from multiple tissues and was not specific to hepatic involvement.[19] Seven cases were cytologically diagnosed with MRD without histologic confirmation; however, all had supportive clinicopathologic evidence. In both people and cats, a better prognosis is associated with well-differentiated tumors. Schemas for morphologic classification of myeloma cells and for categorization of tumors have been published. Criteria for classification of myeloma cells are primarily nuclear since the cytoplasmic characteristics can be quite variable. Briefly, mature cells are classic well-differentiated plasma cells with dense chromatin and no nucleoli. Proplasmacytes are larger with greater anisocytosis and anisokaryosis with indistinct or small nucleoli. Plasmablasts additionally have a high N:C and a large immature nucleus with one or more prominent nucleoli. MRD is considered well differentiated if it contains <15% plasmablasts, intermediate if plasmablasts are 15–49% of cells, and poorly differentiated if plasmablasts are 50% or more of the cells. Other cells include mature plasma cells, proplasmacytes, or lymphoid cells. Confirmatory immunohistochemistry can be performed; cells should be negative for CD3, positive for either light or heavy chain immunoglobulins, and variable for CD79a.[19]

Other Round Cell Neoplasms

Mast cell tumor and histiocytic malignancies occur in the liver with some frequency, but almost always as a component of multiorgan disease. The tissue of origin is often unclear. While primary hepatic genesis cannot be excluded, this chapter will address the other round cell neoplasms in the section on metastatic disease (*see* Metastatic Neoplasia of the Liver).

Neuroendocrine

Hepatic Carcinoid

Carcinoids are uncommon primary tumors in dogs and cats that arise from hepatic neuroendocrine cells found within the biliary epithelium and possibly the hepatic parenchyma (Figure 35.6).[13,14,50,51,76] Most tumors are intrahepatic, but extrahepatic forms have been observed in the gallbladder.[14] Grossly, the tumors are usually diffuse but can have a nodular appearance.[14,76] Primary carcinoids can have an aggressive biological behavior, frequently involve multiple liver lobes, and be metastatic.[14] Three distinct histologic patterns have been described: (i) solid tumors with a fibrovascular stroma, (ii) cells in cords with a fibrovascular stroma, and (iii) an alveolar pattern with

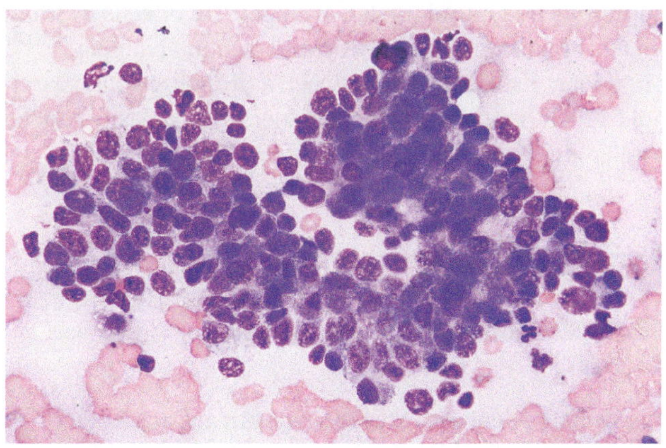

Figure 35.6 Hepatic carcinoid in a dog. A cluster of epithelial cells exhibit scanty, indistinct cytoplasm, round to ovoid nuclei, and clumped chromatin. Some naked nuclei surround the aggregate (May-Grünwald Giemsa, 1000×. *Source:* Image courtesy of Carlo Masserdotti).

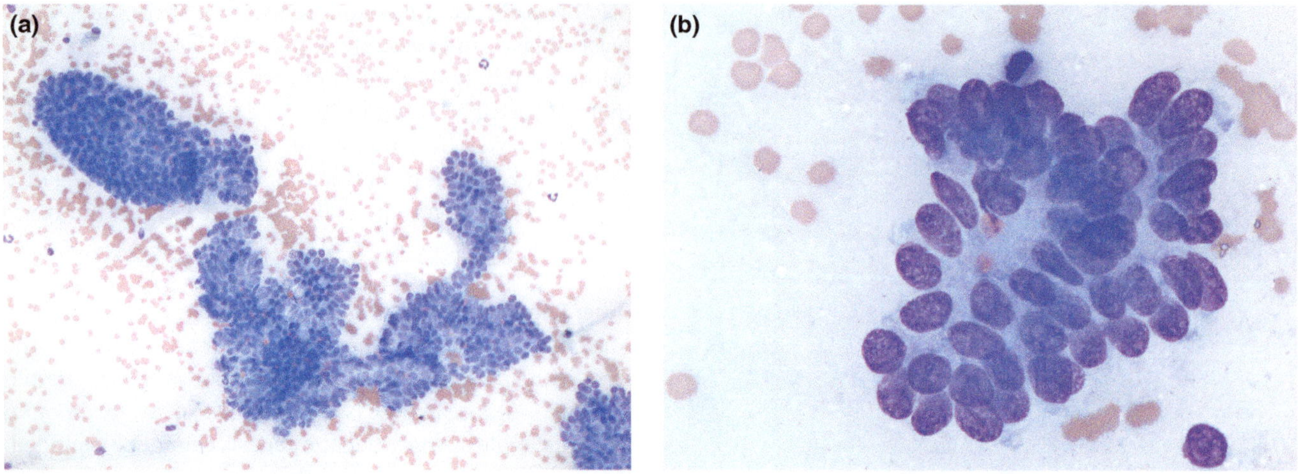

Figure 35.7 Biliary cystadenoma from a dog. (a) Dense sheets of uniform cuboidal epithelial cells are seen in a background of blood (Wright-Giemsa, 100×). (b) Cells are characterized by scant basophilic cytoplasm, uniform oval to angular nuclei, and occasional prominent nucleoli (Wright-Giemsa, 1000×).

rosette-like structures.[76] Tumors were positive for at least one of three immunohistochemical stains: neuron-specific enolase, synaptophysin, and chromogranin A, with most staining positive for neuron-specific enolase.[77] In select cases, intracytoplasmic granules stained diffusely positive for silver stains, and in one cat case, low numbers of neoplastic cells showed immunopositivity to gastrin.[77,78] These immunohistochemical stains are sometimes useful for differentiating these tumors from metastatic carcinomas.[14,77,78] Hepatic carcinoids have been shown to secrete various hormones such as gastrin, insulin, and glucagon.[77–79] Cytologically, the cells have similarities to other neuroendocrine neoplasms (e.g. carotid body tumor, pheochromocytoma, insulinoma) including high cellularity, numerous free round nuclei, arrangement of cells in small sheets or packets, high N:C, and minimal atypia.[38,80,81] Therefore, distinguishing between a primary hepatic carcinoid and a metastatic neuroendocrine neoplasm can be challenging.

Primary Biliary Neoplasms

Biliary Adenomas (Cholangiocellular Adenomas)

True biliary adenomas are rare in dogs, cats, and horses.[50,51] Biliary cystadenomas, also referred to as hepatobiliary cystadenomas, represent greater than 50% of benign hepatic "neoplasms" in cats.[6,7,13–15] There is some ambiguity in the literature regarding terminology because increasingly, biliary cystadenomas in cats are thought to be the result of developmental abnormalities in the ductal plate.[50,51] In cats, they usually affect older animals (greater than 10 years of age) and can occur as focal or multifocal cystic hepatic lesions.[23] Biliary cystadenomas are generally occult unless they reach a large size and compress adjacent organs.[14,23] Histologically, variably sized cystic structures within the mass are lined by mature, uniform simple cuboidal or mildly attenuated epithelium.[57,82] If an aspirate is obtained, the cystic fluid can be acellular, mucinous, hemorrhagic, or clear.[39] Scattered throughout the fluid, inflammatory cells, biliary epithelial cells, or small clusters of uniform hepatocytes can be observed (Figure 35.7).[38,39,83]

Biliary Carcinoma (Cholangiocellular Carcinoma)

Cholangiocellular carcinomas are more common than biliary adenomas and represent the most common and second most common primary hepatic malignancy in cats and dogs, respectively (Figure 35.8).[12,14,15,84,85] Labrador retrievers and female dogs are overrepresented.[6,85] No sex or breed predilection in cats has been noted. *Platynosomum* sp. infection has been associated with the development of cholangiocarcinomas in cats.[86] Several cases of cholangiocellular carcinoma also have been reported in horses.[21,87] The tumors are biologically aggressive and often metastasize to other liver lobes or regional lymph nodes and lungs.[14,84,85] Tumors can be intrahepatic, extrahepatic, or within the gallbladder, with approximately 76% being the intrahepatic form in dogs.[6,12,84,85] In cats, near equal distribution of intrahepatic and extrahepatic forms have been described.[7,85,88] Like HCC, cholangiocellular carcinomas are divided into

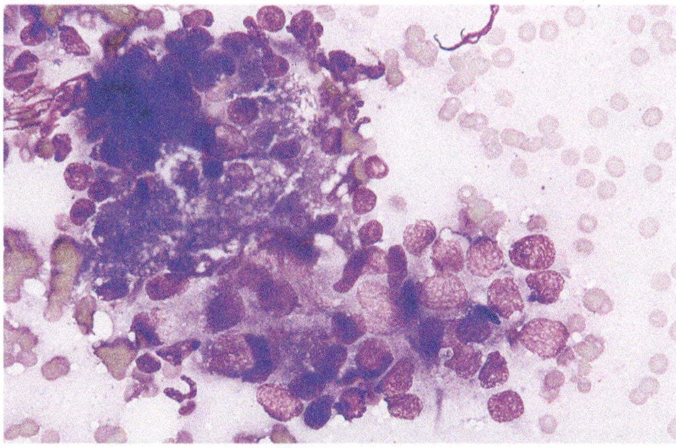

Figure 35.8 Liver aspirate from a dog with cholangiocarcinoma. Well-differentiated vacuolated hepatocytes appear above a cluster of large rounded anaplastic epithelial cells. The neoplastic cells have pale basophilic cytoplasm, round to ovoid nuclei, and clumped chromatin (May-Grünwald Giemsa, 1000×. *Source:* Image courtesy of Carlo Masserdotti).

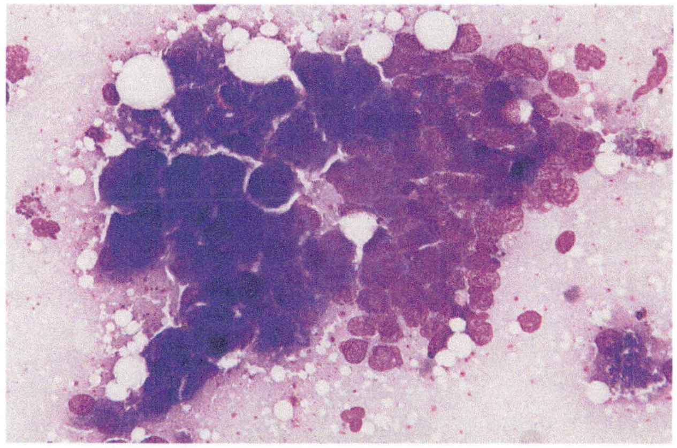

Figure 35.9 Liver aspirate from a cat with metastatic pancreatic carcinoma. A dense sheet of mature hepatocytes with deeply basophilic cytoplasm is present on the left. The large cluster of neoplastic epithelial cells (right) have scanty, sometimes vacuolated cytoplasm, round to angular nuclei, and granular to clumped chromatin (May-Grünwald Giemsa, 1000×. *Source:* Image courtesy of Carlo Masserdotti).

massive, nodular, or diffuse forms, which can be solid or cystic.[84,85] Two histologic subtypes have been described: cholangiocarcinoma and biliary cystadenocarcinoma.[84] Cholangiocarcinomas are characterized by tubular structures lined by cuboidal or columnar epithelial cells, while biliary cystadenocarcinomas display cysts lined by single or multiple layers of epithelial cells admixed with solid sections.[84] In both dogs and cats, neoplastic cells are characterized by relatively scant cytoplasm and moderate to marked nuclear atypia with varying to numerous mitotic figures.[18,20] The neoplasms were nearly 100% positive for K19 immunohistochemical reactivity.[18,20] Although bile cytology has been used to diagnose neoplasia in people with a relatively low sensitivity, reports in the veterinary literature are quite limited.[89]

Other Primary Neoplasms of the Biliary System

Although extremely rare, other primary tumors of the gallbladder may arise. Primary neuroendocrine tumors of the gallbladder and gallbladder lymphoma have been reported in the dog.[90–92]

Metastatic Neoplasia of the Liver

Solid Tissue Tumors

Virtually any cell type can metastasize to the liver via blood vessels or lymphatics or by direct extension or implantation on the capsular surface. Hemangiosarcoma of the spleen and carcinomas of the pancreas and gastrointestinal tract are among the most common metastatic lesions of the liver in dogs and cats (Figures 35.4 and 35.9).[26] Typically, the presence of significant numbers of epithelial cells not consistent with hepatocellular origin can be suggestive of metastatic neoplasia, although tumor subclassification is generally not undertaken based on cytologic features.[47,93] Anecdotally, biliary origin cells can be difficult to distinguish from carcinomas originating outside the hepatobiliary structures. Not all metastatic lesions are characterized by marked cellular atypia, particularly in neuroendocrine tumors. Sensitivity can be affected by sample bias and is generally lower than specificity or positive predictive value for the detection of neoplasia.[93] Sensitivity may be particularly low for sarcomas based on low exfoliative potential and the tendency for the most common sarcoma, hemangiosarcoma, to contain cavities and be hemorrhagic.[93] An additional complication in the cytologic detection of mesenchymal neoplasia in the liver is the potential for hepatic fibrosis to lead to increased numbers of spindle cells in smears, although direct comparisons between fibrotic livers and livers containing sarcoma have not been performed.[94]

Round Cell Neoplasms

Most round cell tumors identified in the liver are presumed to be a component of a multiorgan process, although primary hepatic origin cannot be fully excluded in some cases. Metastatic round cell tumors consist of cells such as lymphocytes, plasma cells, mast cells, and histiocytes (Figure 35.10). These cells also have the potential to increase in association with reactive or inflammatory processes, and strict evidence-based criteria for distinguishing

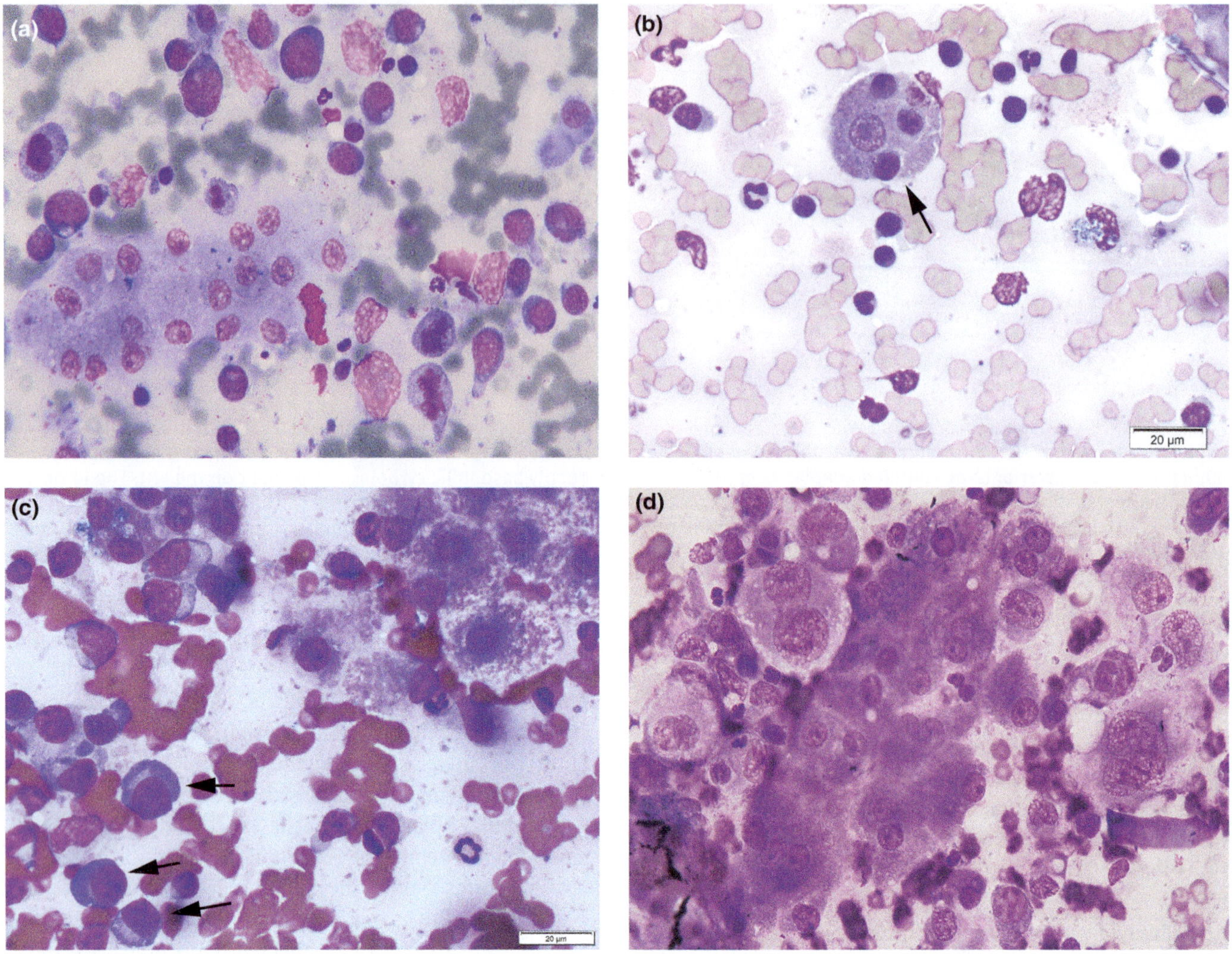

Figure 35.10 (a) Liver aspirate from a dog with hepatic lymphoma. An elongated sheet of mature hepatocytes (left) appears with numerous immature lymphoid cells. These large round cells have deeply basophilic cytoplasm, a single large nucleus, clumped chromatin, and occasional mitotic figures (May-Grünwald Giemsa, 1000×. *Source:* Image courtesy of Carlo Masserdotti). (b) Liver aspirate from a cat with hepatic lymphoma. A single hepatocyte has a slightly eccentrically located oval nucleus with a prominent nucleolus and displays emperipolesis of three neoplastic lymphocytes (arrow). Electron microscopy would be needed to differentiate emperipolesis-like invasion, where the lymphocyte is present within an invagination of cytoplasm, as opposed to true emperipolesis, where lymphocytes are located within hepatocyte cytoplasm. This cat had multicentric lymphoma involving the liver, spleen, and bone marrow (Wright-Giemsa, 500×. *Source:* Image courtesy of Daniel Heinrich). (c) Liver aspirate from a dog with metastatic plasma cell neoplasia. A cluster of hepatocytes (upper right) is characterized by non-lipid vacuolar change. Neoplastic plasma cells exhibit dark basophilic cytoplasm, perinuclear clearing, and faintly visible nucleoli (arrows) (Wright Giemsa, 500×. *Source:* Image courtesy of Daniel Heinrich). (d) Liver aspirate from a dog with histiocytic sarcoma. A cluster of mature but sometimes binucleated hepatocytes (center) is surrounded by large atypical round cells. These cells have vacuolated basophilic cytoplasm and round to lobulated or multiple nuclei characteristic of histiocytic cells. Note the cytophagocytic activity of some of the neoplastic cells (May-Grünwald Giemsa, 1000×. *Source:* Image courtesy of Carlo Masserdotti).

reactive from neoplastic processes are lacking in most cases, particularly when there is minimal cellular atypia (see Chapter 34 for more information on inflammatory liver disease). One study of the cytologic diagnosis of lymphoma in the canine liver determined that the numbers of lymphoblasts should be ≥5% of all nucleated cells in the sample, although the mean value was 50%.[47] Lower numbers of lymphoblasts in some samples were hypothesized to be due to patchy distribution of the neoplastic infiltrate or previous treatment. It was acknowledged that 5% lymphoblasts associated with mature lymphocytes and plasma cells could occur with reactive processes.[47] Lymphoma is addressed in detail in Chapter 27, other than hepatosplenic lymphoma, which is covered in Chapter 28. The cytologic diagnosis of mast cell neoplasia in liver has been proposed to be characterized by sheets or clusters of mast cells, and mast cells with abnormal morphology, including variable granulation; however, mast cells are present in normal livers and increased numbers characterize many hepatic diseases in dogs.[47] Chapter 13 discusses mast cell tumors, including evaluation for metastatic disease. Histiocytic tumors are described in Chapters 12 and 28.

Metastatic Neoplasia of the Gallbladder

Metastatic lesions of the gallbladder appear rare. B-cell lymphoma was identified in a cat with concurrent urinary bladder involvement, and the gallbladder was involved in a case of small cell lymphoma of the gastrointestinal tract in another cat.[95,96]

Conclusion

Hepatic neoplasms can arise from a variety of cell types found in the tissue. Some of these neoplasms have characteristic features and thus can be easily diagnosed via cytology. Challenges arise in distinguishing benign neoplasms of the liver parenchyma and normal or hyperplastic tissue. Also, because the liver is a common site for metastatic lesions, determining a primary hepatic neoplasm from metastatic may be difficult. Uses of imaging, clinical findings, patient history, or histopathology can be helpful for accurate diagnosis of primary hepatic neoplasms.

References

1 Selmic, L.E. (2017). Hepatobiliary neoplasia. *Vet Clin North Am Small Anim Pract* 47: 725–735.

2 Miller, M.A., Moore, G.E., Bertin, F.R., and Kritchevsky, J.E. (2016). What's new in old horses? Postmortem diagnoses in mature and aged equids. *Vet Pathol* 53: 390–398.

3 Beeler-Marfisi, J., Arroyo, L., Caswell, J.L. et al. (2010). Equine primary liver tumors: a case series and review of the literature. *J Vet Diagn Invest* 22: 174–183.

4 Marconato, L., Albanese, F., Viacava, P. et al. (2007). Paraneoplastic alopecia associated with hepatocellular carcinoma in a cat. *Vet Dermatol* 18: 267–271.

5 Pascal-Tenorio, A., Olivry, T., Gross, T. et al. (1997). Paraneoplastic alopecia associated with internal malignancies in the cat. *Vet Dermatol* 8: 47–52.

6 Patnaik, A.K., Hurvitz, A.I., and Lieberman, P.H. (1980). Canine hepatic neoplasms: a clinicopathologic study. *Vet Pathol* 17: 553–564.

7 Post, G. and Patnaik, A.K. (1992). Nonhematopoietic hepatic neoplasms in cats: 21 cases (1983–1988). *J Am Vet Med Assoc* 201: 1080–1082.

8 Trigo, F.J., Thompson, H., Breeze, R.G., and Nash, A.S. (1982). The pathology of liver tumours in the dog. *J Comp Path* 92: 21–39.

9 Bradylak, S., Dodds, W., and Van Vleet, J. (1983). Plasma coagulation factor abnormalities in dogs with naturally occurring hepatic disease. *Am J Vet Res* 44: 2336–2340.

10 Center, S., Baldwin, D., Erb, H., and Tennant, B.C. (1985). Bile acid concentrations in the diagnosis of hepatobiliary disease in the dog. *J Am Vet Med Assoc* 187: 935–940.

11 Liptak, J.M., Dernell, W.S., Monnet, E. et al. (2004). Massive hepatocellular carcinoma in dogs: 48 cases (1992–2002). *J Am Vet Med Assoc* 225: 1225–1230.

12 Hammer, A.S. and Sikkema, D.A. (1995). Hepatic neoplasia in the dog and cat. *Vet Clin North Am Small Anim Pract* 25: 419–435.

13 Balkman, C. (2009). Hepatobiliary neoplasia in dogs and cats. *Vet Clin North Am Small Anim Pract* 39: 617–625.

14 Liptak, J. (2013). Hepatobiliary tumors. In: *Withrow and MacEwen's Small Animal Clinical Oncology*, 5e (eds. Withrow S.J., Vail D.M. and Page R.L.), 405–412. St. Louis, MO: Elsevier.

15 Magne, M.L. and Withrow, S.J. (1985). Hepatic neoplasia. *Vet Clin North Am Small Anim Pract* 15: 243–256.

16 Shiga, A., Shirota, K., Shida, T. et al. (1997). Hepatoblastoma in a dog. *J Vet Med Sci* 59: 1167–1170.

17 Ano, N., Ozaki, K., Nomura, K., and Narama, I. (2011). Hepatoblastoma in a cat. *Vet Pathol* 48: 1020–1023.

18 Van Sprundel, R., van den Ingh, T., Guscetti, F. et al. (2014). Classification of primary hepatic tumours in the cat. *Vet J* 202: 255–266.

19 Mellor, P.J., Haugland, S., Smith, K.C. et al. (2008). Histopathologic, immunohistochemical, and cytologic analysis of feline myeloma-related disorders: further evidence for primary extramedullary development in the cat. *Vet Pathol* 45: 159–173.

20 Van Sprundel, R., van den Ingh, T., Guscetti, F. et al. (2013). Classification of primary hepatic tumors in the dog. *Vet J* 197: 596–606.

21 Conti, M.B., Marchesi, M.C., Zappulla, F. et al. (2008). Clinical findings and diagnosis in a case of cholangiocellular carcinoma in a horse. *Vet Res Commun* 32: S271–S273.

22 Faverzani, S., Chinosi, S., Valenti, P., and Caniatti, M. (2006). Comparison between ultrasonography and cytology of liver focal lesions and parenchyma in the dog and cat. *Vet Res Comm* 30 (Suppl. 1): 293–296.

23 Nyland, T.G., Koblik, P.D., and Tellyer, S.E. (1999). Ultrasonographic evaluation of biliary cystadenomas in cats. *Vet Radiol Ultrasound* 40: 300–306.

24 Kemp, S.D., Panciera, D.L., Larson, M.M. et al. (2013). A comparison of hepatic sonographic features and

histopathologic diagnosis in canine liver disease: 138 cases. *J Vet Intern Med* 27: 806–813.

25 Warren-Smith, G.M.R., Andrew, S., Mantis, P., and Lamb, C.R. (2012). Lack of associations between ultrasonographic appearance of parenchymal lesions of the canine liver and histologic diagnosis. *J Small Anim Pract* 53: 168–173.

26 Larson, M. (2016). Ultrasound imaging of the hepatobiliary system and pancreas. *Vet Clin North Am Small Anim Pract* 46: 453–480.

27 Murakami, T., Feeney, D.A., and Bahr, K.L. (2012). Analysis of clinical and ultrasonographic data by use of logistic regression models for prediction of malignant versus benign causes of ultrasonographically detected focal liver lesions in dogs. *Am J Vet Radiol* 73: 821–829.

28 Guillot, M., D'Anjou, M., Alexander, K. et al. (2009). Can sonographic findings predict the results of liver aspirates in dogs with suspected liver disease? *Vet Radiol Ultrasound* 50: 513–518.

29 Cuccovillo, A. and Lamb, C.R. (2002). Cellular features of sonographic target lesions of the liver and spleen in 21 dogs and a cat. *Vet Radiol Ultrasound* 43: 275–278.

30 Crabtree, A.C., Spangler, E., Beard, D., and Smith, A. (2010). Diagnostic accuracy of gray-scale ultrasonography for the detection of hepatic and splenic lymphoma in dogs. *Vet Radiol Ultrasound* 51: 661–664.

31 Book, A.P., Fidel, J., Wills, T. et al. (2011). Correlation of ultrasound findings, liver and spleen cytology, and prognosis in the clinical staging of high metastatic risk canine mast cell tumors. *Vet Radiol Ultrasound* 52: 548–554.

32 Feeney, D.A., Anderson, K.L., Ziegler, L.E. et al. (2008). Statistical relevance of ultrasonographic criteria in the assessment of diffuse liver disease in dogs and cats. *Am J Vet Radiol* 69: 212–221.

33 Stefanello, D., Valenti, P., Faverzani, S. et al. (2009). Ultrasound-guided cytology of spleen and liver: a prognostic tool in canine cutaneous mast cell tumor. *J Vet Intern Med* 23: 1051–1057.

34 Janvier, V., Evrard, L., Cerri, S. et al. (2016). Ultrasonographic findings in 13 horses with lymphoma. *Vet Radiol Ultrasound* 57: 65–74.

35 Kutara, K., Seki, M., Ishikawa, C. et al. (2014). Triple-phase helical computed tomography in dogs with hepatic masses. *Vet Radiol Ultrasound* 55: 7–15.

36 Clifford, C.A., Pretorius, E.S., Weisse, C. et al. (2004). Magnetic resonance imaging of focal splenic and hepatic lesions in the dog. *J Vet Intern Med* 18: 330–338.

37 Marolf, A.J. (2016). Computed tomography and MRI of the hepatobiliary system and pancreas. *Vet Clin North Am Small Anim Pract* 46: 481–497.

38 Meyer, D.J. (2016). The Liver. In: *Canine and Feline Cytology: A Color Atlas and Interpretation Guide*, (ed. Raskin R.E. and Meyer D.J.), 3e, 259–283. St. Louis, MO: Elsevier.

39 Arndt, T.P. and Shelley, S. (2014). *Cowell and Tyler's Diagnostic Cytology and Hematology of the Dog and Cat*, 4e, 354–371. St. Louis, MO: Elsevier.

40 Hirose, N., Uchida, K., Kanemoto, H. et al. (2014). A retrospective histopathological survey on canine and feline liver diseases at the University of Tokyo between 2006 and 2012. *J Vet Med Sci* 76: 1015–1020.

41 Patnaik, A.K., Hurvitz, A.I., Lieberman, P.H., and Johnson, G.F. (1981). Canine hepatocellular carcinoma. *Vet Pathol* 18: 427–438.

42 Patnaik, A.K. (1992). A morphologic and immunocytochemical study of hepatic neoplasms in cats. *Vet Pathol* 29: 405–415.

43 Masserdotti, C. and Drigo, M. (2012). Retrospective study of cytologic features of well-differentiated hepatocellular carcinoma in dogs. *Vet Clin Patholol* 41: 382–390.

44 Masserdotti, C., Rossetti, E., De Lorenzi, D. et al. (2014). Characterization of cytoplasmic hyaline bodies in a hepatocellular carcinoma of a dog. *Res Vet Sci* 96: 143–146.

45 Burton, I.R., Limpus, K., Thompson, K.G. et al. (2005). Ectopic hepatocellular carcinoma in a dog. *N Z Vet J* 53: 465–467.

46 Boland, L., Lindsay, S., Brunel, L. et al. (2017). Caecocolic intussusception associated with a caecal polyp and concurrent hepatocellular carcinoma in a cat. *JFMS Open Rep* 3: 1–6.

47 Stockhaus C, van den Ingh T, Rothuizen J, E Teske A multistep approach in the cytologic evaluation of liver biopsy samples of dogs with hepatic diseases. *Vet Pathol* 2004;41:461–470.

48 Loynachan, A.T., Bolin, D.C., Hong, C.B., and Poonacha, K.B. (2007). Three equine cases of mixed hepatoblastoma with teratoid features. *Vet Pathol* 44: 211–214.

49 Gold, J.R., Warren, A.L., French, T.W., and Stokol, T. (2008). What is your diagnosis: biopsy impression smear of a hepatic mass in a yearling Thoroughbred filly. *Vet Clin Pathol* 37: 339–343.

50 Cullen, J.M. and Stalker, M.J. (2016). Liver and biliary system. In: *Jubb, Kennedy and Palmer's Pathology of Domestic Animals*, 6e (ed. Maxie, M.G.), 258–352. St. Louis, MO: Elsevier.

51 Cullen, J.M. (2017). Tumors of the liver and gallbladder. In: *Tumors in Domestic Animals*, (ed. Meuten D.J.), 5e, 602–631. Ames, IA: Wiley.

52 Shiga, A., Shirota, K., and Enomoto, M. (2001). Combined hepatocellular and cholangiocellular carcinoma in a dog. *J Vet Med Sci* 63: 483–486.

53 Kato, M., Higuchi, T., Orita, Y. et al. (1997). Combined hepatocellular carcinoma and cholangiocarcinoma in a mare. *J Comp Pathol* 116: 409–413.

54 Allen, R.A. and Lisa, J.R. (1949). Combined liver cell and bile duct carcinoma. *Am J Pathol* 25: 647–655.

55 Kamiiee, J., Fueki, K., Amagai, H. et al. (2009). Multicentric myelolipoma in a dog. *J Vet Med Sci* 71: 371–373.

56 Prater, M.R., Bender, H., and Sponenberg, D.P. (1998). Intra-abdominal mass aspirate from an aged dog. *Vet Clin Patholol* 27: 65–66.

57 Cullen, J.M. (2009). Summary of the world small animal association standardization committee guide to classification of liver disease of dogs and cats. *Vet Clin North Am Small Anim Pract* 39: 395–418.

58 Kapatkin, A.S., Mullen, H.S., Matthiesen, D.T., and Patnaik, A.K. (1992). Leiomyosarcoma in dogs: 44 cases (1983–1988). *J Am Vet Med Assoc* 201: 1077–1079.

59 Le Roux, A., Rabillard, M., Gauthier, O. et al. (2010). What's your diagnosis; Liver osteosarcoma. *J Am Vet Med Assoc* 237: 1241–1242.

60 Minkus, G. and Hillemanns, M. (1997). Botryoid-type embryonal rhabdomyosarcoma of liver in a young cat. *Vet Pathol* 34: 618–621.

61 Galafaro, V., Rapisarda, G., Lanteri, G., and Marino, F. (2008). Primary pleomorphic liposarcoma of the liver in a dog. *Pol J Vet Sci* 11: 385–388.

62 Jeraj, K., Yano, B., Osborne, C.A. et al. (1981). Primary hepatic osteosarcoma in a dog. *J Am Vet Med Assoc* 179: 1000–1003.

63 Linton, M., Tong, L., Simon, A. et al. (2016). Hepatic fibrosarcoma incarcerated in a peritoneopericardial diaphragmatic hernia in a cat. *JFMS Open Rep* 2: 2055116916638681.

64 Dhaliwal, R., Johnson, R., and Kitchell, B. (2003). Primary extraskeletal hepatic osteosarcoma in a cat. *J Am Vet Med Assoc* 222: 340–342.

65 Chikata, S., Nakamura, S., Katayama, R. et al. (2006). Primary chondrosarcoma in the liver of a dog. *Vet Pathol* 43: 1033–1036.

66 Caserto, B. and Almes, K. (2012). Pathology in practice: primary hepatic chondroblastic osteosarcoma in a dog. *J Am Vet Med Assoc* 240: 1067–1069.

67 Louwerens, M., London, C.A., Pedersen, N.C., and Lyons, L.A. (2005). Feline lymphoma in the post-feline leukemia virus era. *J Vet Intern Med* 19: 329–335.

68 Gabor, L.J., Malik, R., and Canfield, P.J. (1998). Clinical and anatomical features of lymphosarcoma in 118 cats. *Aust Vet J* 76: 725–732.

69 Cienava, E.A., Barnhart, K.F., Brown, R. et al. (2004). Morphologic, immunohistochemical, and molecular characterization of hepatosplenic T-cell lymphoma in a dog. *Vet Clin Pathol* 33: 105–110.

70 Keller, S.M., Vernau, W., Hodges, J. et al. (2013). Hepatosplenic and hepatocytotrophic T-cell lymphoma: two distinct types of T-Cell lymphoma in dogs. *Vet Pathol* 50: 281–290.

71 Carter, J.E., Tarigo, J.L., Vernau, W. et al. (2008). Erythrophagocytic low-grade extranodal T-cell lymphoma in a cat. *Vet Clin Pathol* 37: 416–421.

72 Fry, M.M., Vernau, W., Pesavento, P.A. et al. (2003). Hepatosplenic lymphoma in a dog. *Vet Pathol* 40: 556–562.

73 Roccabianca, P., Paltrinieri, S., Gallo, E., and Giuliani, A. (2002). Hepatosplenic T-cell lymphoma in a mare. *Vet Pathol* 39: 508–511.

74 Mellor, P.J., Haugland, S., Murphy, S. et al. (2006). Myeloma-related disorders in cats commonly present as extramedullary neoplasms in contrast to myeloma in human patients: 24 cases with clinical follow up. *J Vet Intern Med* 20: 1376–1383.

75 Valli, V.E., Bienzle, D., and Meuten, D.L. (2017). Tumors of the hemolymphatic system. In: *Tumors in Domestic Animals*, 5e, (ed. Meuten D.J.), 203–321. Ames, IA: Wiley.

76 Patnaik, A.K., Lieberman, P.H., Hurvitz, A.I., and Johnson, G.F. (1981). Canine hepatic carcinoids. *Vet Pathol* 18: 445–453.

77 Patnaik, A.K., Newman, S.J., Scase, T. et al. (2005). Canine hepatic neuroendocrine carcinoma: an immunohistochemical and electron microscopic study. *Vet Pathol* 42: 140–146.

78 Kita, C., Yamagami, T., Kinouchi, S. et al. (2014). A feline case of hepatic neuroendocrine carcinoma with gastrin immunoreactivity. *J Vet Med Sci* 76: 887–890.

79 Asakawa, M.G., Cullen, J.M., and Linder, K.E. (2013). Necrolytic migratory erythema associated with a glucagon-producing primary hepatic neuroendocrine carcinoma in a cat. *Vet Dermatol* 24: 466–e110.

80 Boes, K., Zimmerman, K., Saunders, G. et al. (2009). What is your diagnosis? Shoulder mass in a dog with lameness. *Vet Clin Pathol* 38: 511–515.

81 Moore, A.R., Chu, C., Singh, K. et al. (2015). What is your diagnosis? Liver aspirate from a hypoglycemic dog. *Vet Clin Pathol* 44: 463–464.

82 Adle, R. and Wilson, D.W. (1995). Biliary cystadenoma of cats. *Vet Pathol* 32: 415–418.

83 Moon, S.J., Kim, J.W., Sur, J.H. et al. (2011). Biliary cystadenoma in a Maltese dog: clinical and diagnostic findings. *J Vet Med Sci* 73: 1677–1679.

84 Hayes, H.M., Morin, M.M., and Rubenstein, D.A. (1983). Canine biliary carcinoma: epidemiological comparisons with man. *J Comp Path* 93: 99–103.

85 Patnaik, A.K., Hurvitz, A.I., Lieberman, P.H., and Johnson, G.F. (1981). Canine bile duct carcinoma. *Vet Pathol* 18: 439–444.

86 Andrade, R.L.F.S., Dantas, A.F.M., Pimental, L.A. et al. (2012). *Platynosomum fastosum*-induced cholangiocarcinomas in cats. *Vet Parasitol* 190: 277–280.

87 Wong, D., Hepworth, K., Yaeger, M. et al. (2015). Imaging diagnosis-hypoglycemia associated with cholangiocarcinoma and peritoneal carcinomatosis in a horse. *Vet Radiol Ultrasound* 56: E9–E12.

88 Lawrence, H.J., Erb, H.N., and Harvey, H.J. (1994). Nonlymphomatous hepatobiliary masses in cats: 41 cases (1972–1991). *Vet Surg* 23: 365–368.

89 Sugimoto, S., Matsubayashi, H., Kimura, H. et al. (2015). Diagnosis of bile duct cancer by bile cytology: usefulness of post-brushing biliary lavage fluid. *Endosc Int Open* 3: E323–E328.

90 Nagata, N., Shibata, S., Sakai, H. et al. (2015). Gallbladder lymphoma in a miniature dachshund. *J Vet Med Sci* 77: 117–121.

91 Bhandal, J., Head, L.L., Francis, D.A. et al. (2009). Use of color flow Doppler ultrasonography to diagnose a bleeding neuroendocrine tumor in the gallbladder of a dog. *J Am Vet Med Assoc* 235: 1326–1329.

92 Birettoni, F., Porciello, R., Caivano, D. et al. (2008). Primary neuroendocrine carcinoma of the gallbladder in a dog. *Vet Res Commun* 32: S239–S242.

93 Bahr, K.L., Sharkey, L.C., Murakami, T., and Feeney, D.A. (2013). Accuracy of US-guided FNA of focal liver lesions in dogs: 140 cases (2005–2008). *J Am Anim Hosp Assoc* 49: 190–196.

94 Masserdotti, C. and Bertazzolo, W. (2016). Cytologic features of hepatic fibrosis in dogs: a retrospective study on 22 cases. *Vet Clin Pathol* 45: 361–367.

95 Baxter, K.J., Hill, R.C., Parfitt, S.L. et al. (2012). Gastrointestinal small-cell lymphoma with gall bladder involvement in a cat. *J Feline Med Surg* 14: 267–271.

96 Geigy, C.A., Dandrieux, J., Miclard, J. et al. (2010). Extranodal B-cell lymphoma in the urinary bladder with cytological evidence of concurrent involvement of the gall bladder in a cat. *J Sm Anim Pract* 51: 280–287.

36

Pancreas

Leslie C. Sharkey and Sarah Crain

Introduction

Clinical signs of pancreatic disease overlap with disorders of other abdominal organs, compounded by the potential for bystander pathology based on regional anatomy.[1] Diagnosis is based on integrated interpretation of history, clinical signs, laboratory testing, and imaging. Despite an increasing array of testing available to assess the pancreas that is beyond the scope of this chapter to evaluate in detail, definitive diagnosis of pancreatic disease remains challenging, particularly for chronic inflammatory conditions. Ultrasound is often used to evaluate the pancreas; however, limitations include the overlapping appearance of different conditions, lack of sensitivity, and inter-operator variation.[2] Computed tomography and magnetic resonance imaging (MRI) show more promise, but microscopy is still required for diagnosis.[3] Although microscopic evaluation of the pancreas was historically avoided due to concerns about potential complications, an increasing body of evidence suggests that cytology can be a safe and effective diagnostic tool, particularly in dogs and cats.[4–6] Due to patchy distribution of pancreatic lesions,[7] normal fine-needle aspirate (FNA) results do not exclude disease. However, aspirate results demonstrating neoplasia or infectious agents are considered highly specific.[7,8]

Collection

Indications

Indications for FNA of the pancreas are usually based on clinical and imaging findings. Nodules or mass-like effects on or adjacent to the pancreas identified on ultrasound promote aspiration of the pancreas to evaluate for the presence of neoplasia. Nodular hyperplasia can appear as multifocal pancreatic nodules and manifest similar clinical presentation as neoplasms, so it is important to differentiate between these conditions microscopically.[9–12] Findings consistent with pancreatitis such as organomegaly, altered echogenicity, mesenteric hyperechogenicity, and peritoneal fluid can also prompt sampling in some cases.[5,13]

Methods

FNA samples are typically collected using a 20 or 22 G, 1.5 in. hypodermic or spinal needle and a 3–6 mL syringe with ethylenediaminetetraacetic acid (EDTA). Some authors advocate smaller 25 G needles to minimize trauma.[1] Using ultrasound guidance, the needle is directed into lesions and sampled by "woodpeckering" (fenestration of) the lesion and/or aspirating back on the syringe.[5,6,14] Several samples should be collected, ideally from different locations to ensure representation of lesions. The use of laparoscopy for gross examination and collection of histopathology samples is considered safe and useful in dogs and cats.[15–17] This technique could also facilitate collection of cytology samples, either by FNA or preparation of impression smears from biopsy tissue.

Overall, the diagnostic yield for ultrasound-guided aspirates is similar to or slightly lower than for FNA of other intra-abdominal organs.[14,18] Diagnostic yields are reported between 67 and 73.5% and appear to be lower in normal pancreata due to poor exfoliation.[5,6,19–21] Intraoperative aspirates and impression smears from biopsy samples of normal pancreatic tissue were more likely to be of diagnostic quality.[19]

Safety

Several human and veterinary studies have demonstrated the safety of ultrasound-guided pancreatic FNA. In a study of 92 dogs, no adverse effects after pancreatic aspiration

Veterinary Cytology, First Edition. Edited by Leslie C. Sharkey, M. Judith Radin, and Davis Seelig.

were noted in the records of 87 (92.6%). Six of the seven dogs with complications had additional diagnostic procedures performed concurrently, and all had significant comorbidities.[6] This study also reported no complications in seven dogs having surgical biopsy of the pancreas. A case–control study of cats with suspected pancreatic disease and ultrasonographic abnormalities of the pancreas did not demonstrate any increased risk of complications up to 48 hours after pancreatic FNA compared with control cats not undergoing aspiration.[5] Aspiration and surgical biopsy sampling of 27 healthy Beagles did not result in increased serum pancreatic lipase immunoreactivity; however, some dogs had increased trypsin-like immunoreactivity after surgical biopsy but not aspiration.[19] A study of healthy Beagles demonstrated the safety of transgastric and transduodenal endoscopic ultrasound-guided sampling.[21] Human studies document similarly low rates of complications.[8] For comparison, a retrospective study of surgical biopsy of the pancreas primarily using the suture fracture technique in 24 dogs and 19 cats reported complications in 7 dogs and 3 cats, including vomiting, cranial abdominal pain, nausea, anorexia, and lethargy, supporting that FNA may have fewer clinical sequelae.[22]

Normal Tissue Architecture and Cytology

The pancreas is composed of acinar tissue arranged in lobules separated by a fine stromal tissue that also supports the pancreatic ducts draining the acini. The endocrine component of the pancreas (1–2%) occurs as islets interspersed within the exocrine tissue. Regulation of exocrine pancreatic function is by hormones originating in the gut mucosa, by products of the endocrine pancreas distributed through an insulo-acinar portal system, and by the autonomic and enteric nervous systems.[23] Although morphologically homogeneous, islet cells include five cell types, with insulin and amylin-producing β-cells predominating. Other islet cells include α-cells that produce glucagon, somatostatin-producing δ-cells, ghrelin-producing ε-cells and pancreatic polypeptide (PP) cells that produce PP and adrenomedullin.[23]

Cytology samples from normal pancreatic tissue tend to be of low cellularity, consisting of scattered clusters of mature acinar epithelial cells characterized by light blue cytoplasm filled with fine pink to red granules, a single round to oval nucleus, stippled chromatin, and a single round prominent nucleolus (Figure 36.1).[4,21] Blood, proteinaceous fluid, broken cells, free zymogen granules, and mesothelial cells can be present in the background.[1,6] Other cellular elements of the pancreas are not commonly reported in aspirates of normal tissue. Depending on sampling, occasional smears can contain cells from regional organs such as the liver, spleen, or gastrointestinal tract.[4] Rarely, splenic tissue can occur within the pancreas (see section on hyperplasia below), or ectopic acinar pancreatic tissue is observed in other abdominal organs.[23]

Conditions of the Exocrine Pancreas Diagnosed by Cytology

Hyperplasia

Nodular hyperplasia of the exocrine component of the pancreas is common, particularly in older dogs and cats.[22–24] Ductal hyperplasia also can occur.[23] A study of 101 consecutive canine necropsies revealed nodular hyperplasia in 80%, correlating with age and occurring in dogs without evidence of other lesions including inflammation.[24] Imaging can be helpful in distinguishing nodular hyperplasia from neoplasia. Hyperplastic nodules tend to be multiple and smaller (<2 cm) rather than single and/or larger lesions, but there is overlap, and microscopy is required for definitive diagnosis.[10,24] Adequate cytology/histopathology correlation studies are not available to definitively characterize cytology of nodular hyperplasia. Anecdotally, nodular hyperplasia is characterized by normal acinar cell morphology or by mild atypia, including cytoplasmic basophilia and mild anisocytosis and anisokaryosis (Figure 36.2).[4–6]

Ectopic splenic tissue has been identified rarely as solitary or a few small (usually <2 cm) masses in the pancreas and are likely due to developmental variation.[25] Cytology has not been reported, but, based on histology, should resemble samples from normal splenic tissue.

Cysts

Cystic pancreatic lesions are most often pseudocysts lined by fibrous connective tissue rather than true epithelial-lined cysts.[23,26] Pseudocysts up to several centimeters in diameter have been reported. Aspiration generally reveals a low cellularity fluid, with mild neutrophilic inflammation reported in some animals.[26,27] Measurement of fluid amylase and lipase activities demonstrates higher concentrations than serum, suggesting communication with pancreatic ducts.[26,27]

Necrosis

Pancreatic necrosis is often used interchangeably with pancreatitis in the clinical literature, although it may technically be the inciting pathological event, preceding an

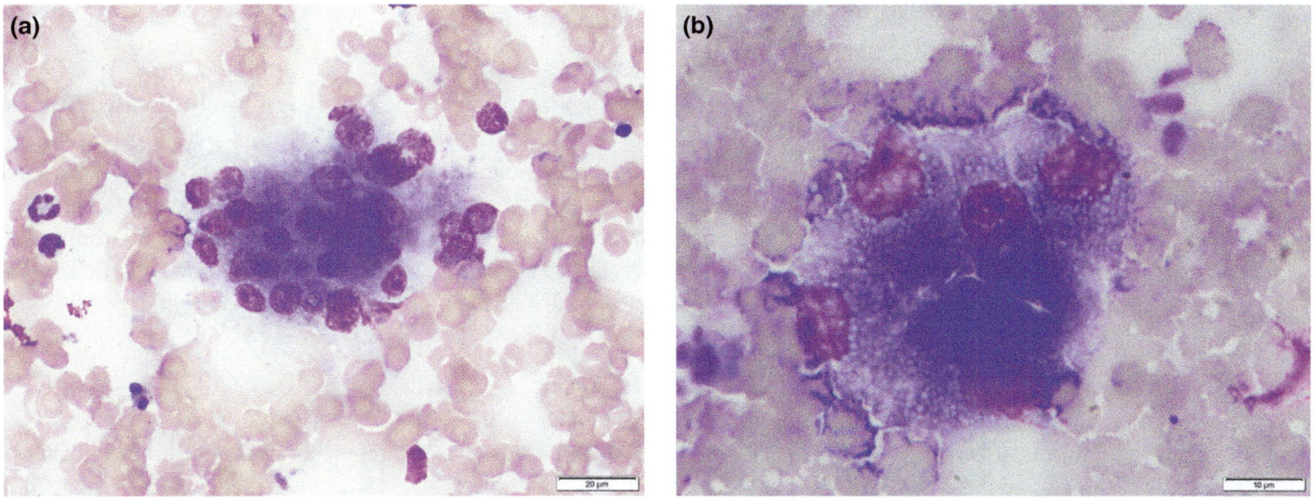

Figure 36.1 (a) A cluster of normal canine pancreatic exocrine epithelial cells characterized by a moderate amount of amphophilic granular cytoplasm and single round to oval nuclei with one prominent nucleolus. (b) Similar cells at higher magnification (Wright Giemsa).

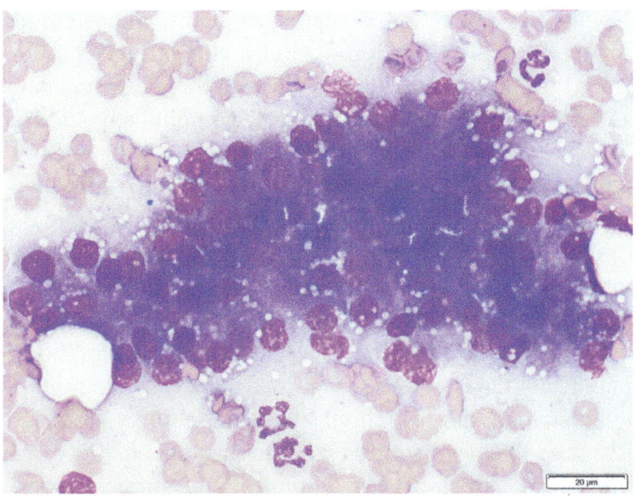

Figure 36.2 A cluster of hyperplastic canine pancreatic exocrine cells. Morphology is similar to normal cells; however, this is a larger cluster. Cells display some clear vacuoles, slightly increased cytoplasmic basophilia, and focally increased nuclear to cytoplasmic ratio and anisokaryosis (Wright Giemsa).

inflammatory reaction.[23] Metabolic, nutritional, toxic, and hypoxia/reperfusion etiologies have been proposed.[23] Zinc toxicosis is a cause of pancreatic necrosis, although the hemolytic effects may overshadow the pancreatic pathology at presentation.[28,29] Asparaginase has also been implicated as a cause of pancreatic necrosis,[30] with subsequent necrosis and inflammation of peripancreatic fat.[23] Anecdotally, necrosis appears cytologically as amorphous basophilic debris.[4,6] A potentially unique finding is relatively frequent dystrophic mineralization associated with saponification of adipose, which is reflected cytologically as colorless refractile round crystalline material.[6]

Inflammation

As noted above, pancreatic necrosis is thought to be an important contributing event in the clinical presentation of pancreatitis. Pancreatitis is often classified as either acute or chronic, based on clinical presentation and severity (acute worse than chronic) and histologic pattern of inflammation, which is rarely determined antemortem.[1,23,31] Acute pancreatitis is characterized by suppurative inflammation, edema, necrosis, and mineralization. Features of chronic pancreatitis might be harder to appreciate cytologically than the acute changes and include fibrosis, acinar loss, and a mixed or mononuclear inflammatory infiltrate.[32,33] Most cases of pancreatitis are nonseptic.[23] A challenge to diagnosis is the randomly discrete nature of foci of pancreatic inflammation.[32,34] A histologic grading scheme for nonneoplastic lesions of the canine exocrine pancreas has been proposed that incorporates neutrophilic and lymphocytic inflammation, pancreatic and fat necrosis, edema, fibrosis, atrophy, and hyperplastic nodules.[35] Out of 101 consecutive canine pancreata evaluated on necropsy, 93 contained inflammatory lesions.[35]

Granulomatous pancreatic inflammation is uncommon and to our knowledge has been reported once in pancreatic aspirates associated with infection in small animals.[36] However, infections such as *Heterobilharzia americana* are associated with granulomatous changes in canine pancreatic biopsies and should be considered when granulomatous inflammation is present cytologically.[37–39] Clinical signs associated with trematode infection are typically present (diarrhea, weight loss, anorexia), along with lesions in the small intestine and liver.[38] Rarely, other infections such as *Toxoplasma gondii* and systemic fungal infections can be found in the pancreas but are typically associated with significant disease in organs other than the pancreas and gastrointestinal tract.[36,40,41]

Pancreatitis

There are no large-scale definitive studies on the cytologic diagnosis of pancreatitis, and some findings associated with chronic pancreatitis such as atrophy and fibrosis are likely to be difficult to assess cytologically.[34,42,43,44] It has been suggested that pancreatic aspirates are more likely to be performed when neoplasia is a differential diagnosis, which is supported by a recent study demonstrating that cats undergoing the procedure were more likely to have nodular or mass lesions.[4,5] Anecdotally, pancreatitis in small animals is described cytologically as consisting of inflammatory cells (most often degenerate or nondegenerate neutrophils, lymphocytes occasionally in cats), cellular and necrotic debris, lipid, mineralization, and normal to hyperplastic exocrine pancreatic cells occurring individually or in clusters (Figure 36.3).[4–6] Very limited cytology/histopathology correlation data suggest good correlation between techniques for the diagnosis of inflammatory disease.[5,6]

Pancreatic Abscess

There are infrequent reports of pancreatic abscesses in dogs and cats. These are often sterile and the sequela of pancreatitis; however, some are septic.[23,44,45] In one canine study, only 2/15 pancreatic cultures were positive for growth; however, in a small number of cases, culture of abdominal fluid was positive when the pancreatic culture was negative, suggesting a septic process despite a negative pancreatic culture.[45] Pancreatic cytology was not specifically evaluated. Cytology has been reported in the diagnosis of both sterile and septic pancreatic abscesses in cats.[46–48] A sterile abscess histologically diagnosed with severe necrotizing suppurative pancreatitis in one cat was characterized cytologically by neutrophilic and mononuclear inflammation, tissue degeneration and necrosis, and possible saponification of fat.[46] Other reports of feline pancreatic abscess cytology describe neutrophilic inflammation with Gram-positive cocci that cultured as *Staphylococcus aureus*.[47] Aspirates from a diabetic cat revealed degenerate neutrophils but no observed organisms with cytology; however, *Escherichia coli* was recovered using culture.[48]

Neoplasia

Benign

Benign neoplasia of the pancreas is rarely reported in dogs and cats, and cytologic descriptions are not available. Exocrine pancreatic adenomas appear to be most common, although even with histology, they can be confused with nodular hyperplasia.[11,23] An acinar cell cystadenoma was recently reported in a cat; however, cytologic features were not described.[49] Ductal adenomas are possible.[50]

Malignant

Epithelial

Acinar carcinomas are reported most commonly, although ductular carcinomas also are described. One review article suggests that poorly differentiated tumors should be easy to diagnose cytologically based on typical cytologic criteria of malignancy, but more difficulty is expected in distinguishing well differentiated variants from reactive hyperplasia or adenomas.[4] A retrospective study of eight cases of histologically diagnosed feline pancreatic carcinoma noted a wide age range (4–20 years), frequent comorbidities (including diabetes mellitus), and a clinical presentation similar to acute pancreatitis.[11] Three of these cats had pancreatic FNA performed; one sample was nondiagnostic and two were considered diagnostic for pancreatic adenocarcinoma; however, the cytologic features were not described. In two other studies, a total of four cats had pancreatic aspirates that were diagnostic for exocrine pancreatic carcinoma and histologically confirmed, but again, no cytologic descriptions were included.[5,51] Another relatively large retrospective study of feline exocrine pancreatic carcinoma included 34 cases, with 18 diagnosed only by cytology without histologic confirmation; cytologic features were not described.[20] The diagnosis of exocrine pancreatic carcinoma in dogs using FNA or imprints of surgical biopsy samples has been documented, but similar to cats, no cytologic features were included in the report.[51] A large retrospective study of pancreatic cytology in the dog reported concordance of cytologic and histologic diagnosis in two cases of exocrine pancreatic carcinoma (Figure 36.4).[6] The diagnostic criteria described were standard criteria of malignancy; however, the authors noted that mild to moderate cytologic atypia in the presence of inflammation was interpreted to be most likely reactive, while marked atypia was considered more suggestive for malignancy. Hyalinizing pancreatic adenocarcinoma has been reported in six dogs and histologically characterized by the presence of homogeneous extracellular eosinophilic material within tubular lumina and the stroma; cytology was not described.[52] Two cases of acinar cell carcinoma in horses

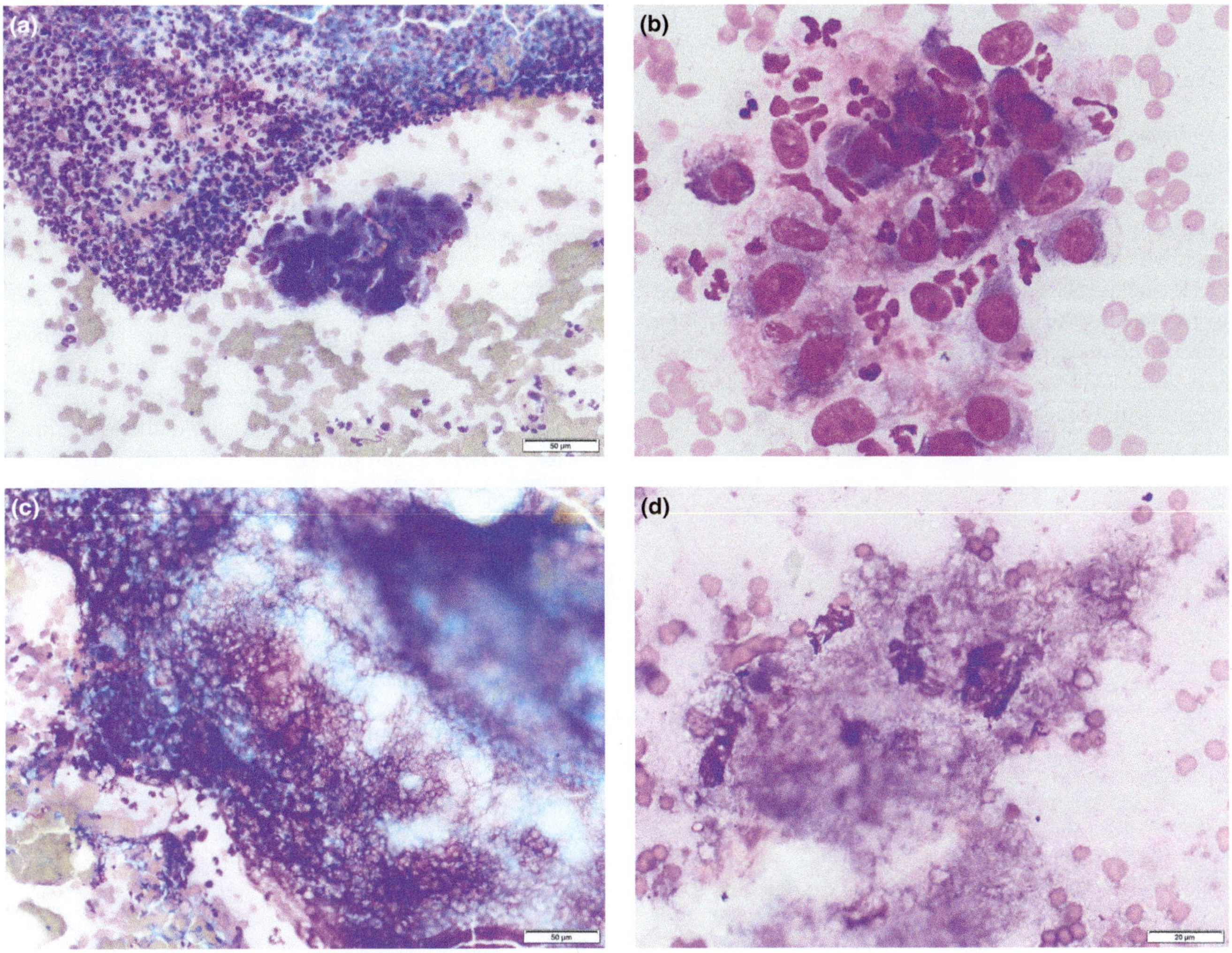

Figure 36.3 (a) A cluster of reactive pancreatic exocrine cells adjacent to a mass of neutrophils in a case of canine pancreatitis. (b) Higher magnification image of neutrophils interspersed with exocrine pancreatic cells and pink extracellular material (500× oil immersion). (c) Mineralized debris and inflammatory cells. (d) Degenerating cells with mineral (Wright Giemsa).

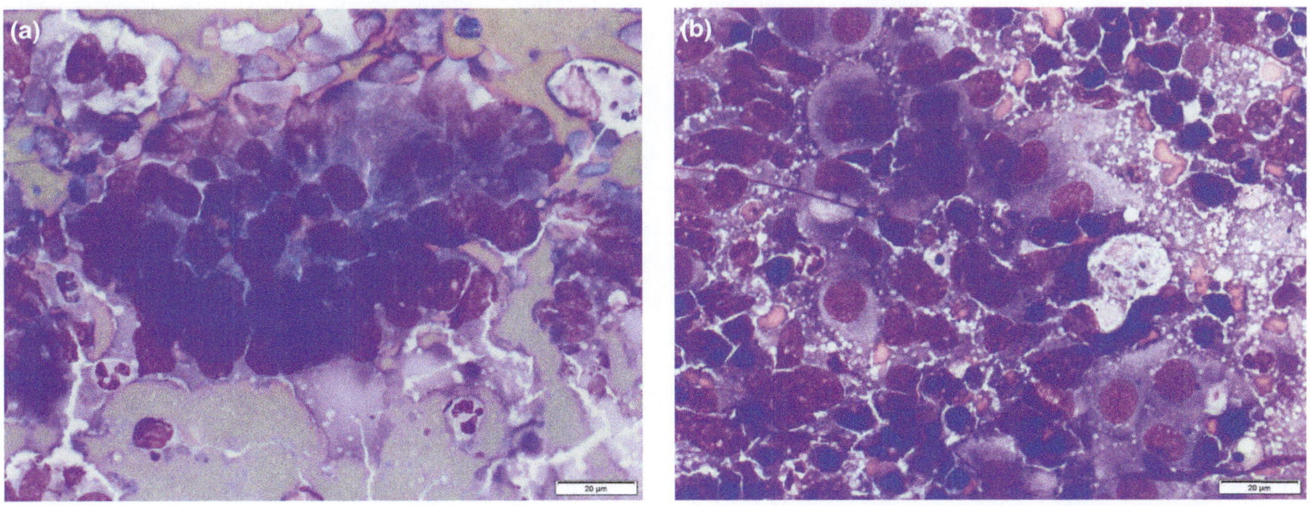

Figure 36.4 Histologically confirmed canine pancreatic carcinomas. (a) The cohesive cluster of exocrine cells is disorganized and characterized by moderate anisokaryosis and nuclear crowding. Blood and macrophages are present in the background. (b) A more anaplastic tumor has less cohesive epithelial cells that lack characteristics definitive for exocrine pancreatic origin. Degenerating cells and macrophages are seen in the background (Wright Giemsa).

have been reported with histologic features similar to other species;[53] presumably cytology would be as well.

Mesenchymal

Primary sarcomas of the pancreas appear to be extremely rare, and cytologic descriptions could not be identified in the literature other than a single case in a large canine retrospective characterized by typical features such as spindloid to stellate cells with moderately abundant vacuolated basophilic cytoplasm and oval to elongated nuclei.[6] The histologic diagnosis was liposarcoma (Figure 36.5a and b). There is a single case report in a cat of a pancreatic carcinosarcoma with metastases of the mesenchymal component to the uterus, omentum, and diaphragm.[54]

Round Cell

Lymphoma of the pancreas has been reported, often as part a multisystemic process.[5,6,55]

Conditions of the Endocrine Pancreas Diagnosed by Cytology

Because the endocrine component of the pancreas is such a small fraction of the organ, cytology is not sufficiently sensitive to characterize nonneoplastic lesions; thus the literature is quite limited. There are reports of increased lymphocytes in the islets associated with diabetes mellitus in cats.[56] Based on the pathogenesis of feline diabetes, it

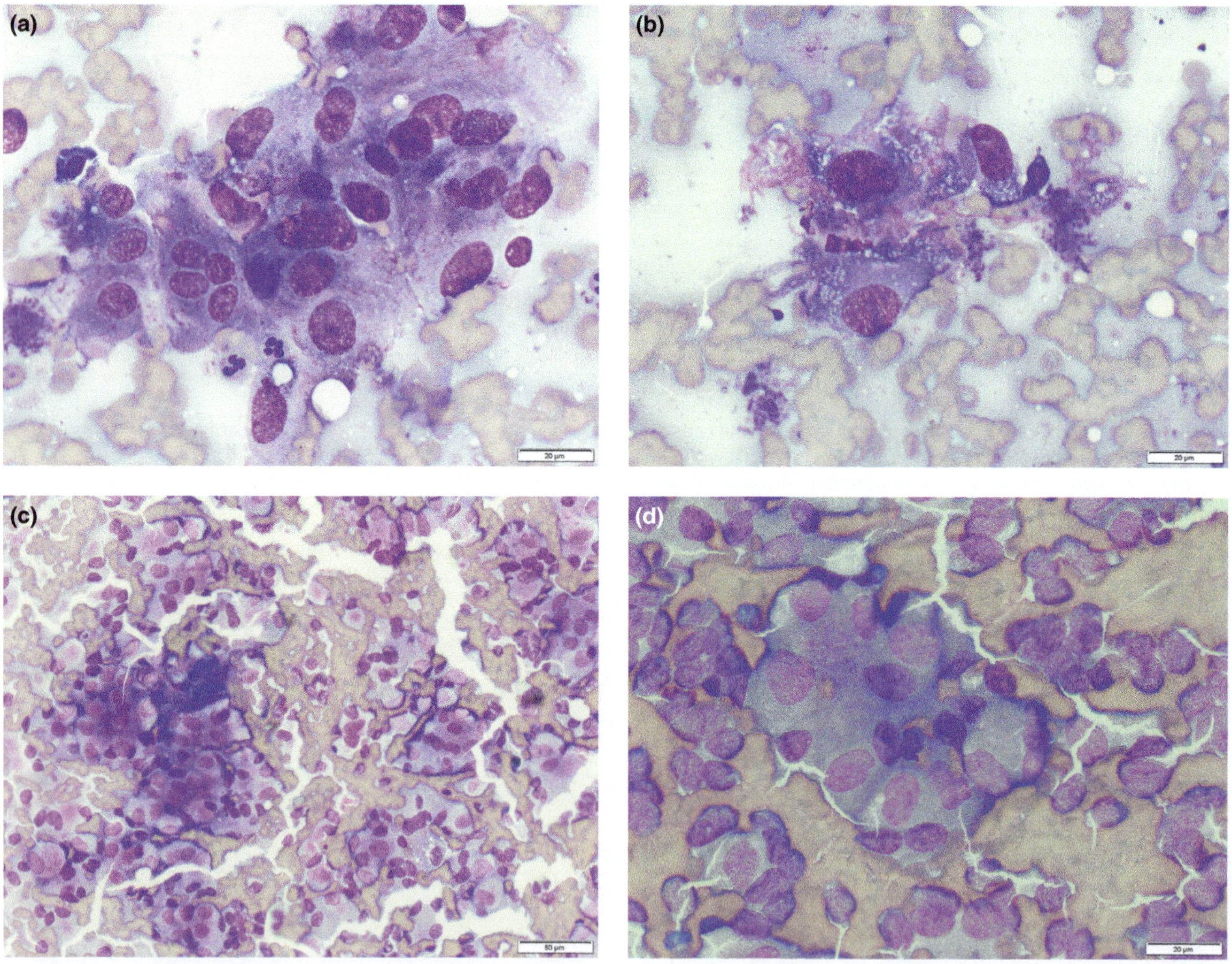

Figure 36.5 (a) A histologically confirmed liposarcoma in the pancreas of a dog has features characteristic of a sarcoma including indistinct cell margins and nuclear pleomorphism. (b) A higher magnification of the same liposarcoma as in (a). (c) Aspirate of a canine insulinoma exhibits high cellularity, many broken cells, and scattered clusters of relatively uniform cells. (d) Higher magnification of the insulinoma in (c). Cells are cuboidal to polyhedral with a moderate amount of pale blue cytoplasm and single oval to angular nuclei. They exhibit few cytologic criteria of malignancy (Wright Giemsa).

was hypothesized that islets of diabetic cats would contain increased amyloid; however, one study failed to find an increase compared with controls.[56]

Neoplasia

Insulinoma is the most common endocrine pancreatic malignancy in dogs and cats.[57] Metastasis to the liver and lymph nodes is common. Clinical suspicion is based on clinical signs, profound and refractory hypoglycemia, and imaging, although masses are often small.[57] Cytologic features are well described as a neuroendocrine appearance characterized by many free nuclei and individualized or packeted cells with scant to moderate pale basophilic cytoplasm that sometimes contains fine clear vacuoles or fine eosinophilic granules and single round to oval nuclei (Figure 36.5c and d).[4,57,58] Cytologic atypia is usually minimal, and biological behavior is best determined histologically and clinically. Microscopically, they are usually distinct from well-differentiated exocrine pancreatic tumors; however, there can be overlap between endocrine and exocrine neoplasms if islet cells are more cohesive or if acinar cells are poorly granular.[4] One case of osseous metaplasia in an insulinoma in a dog is described.[58] While insulinomas are the most common islet cell neoplasm, tumors can originate from other islet cells but have a similar cytologic appearance.[59] Clinical signs and special stains or measurement of serum hormones can be performed to distinguish the cell of origin.

References

1 Mansfield, C. (2013). Practical interpretation and application of exocrine pancreatic testing in small animals. *Vet Clin North Am Small Anim Pract* 43: 1241–1260.

2 Larson, M.M. (2016). Ultrasound imaging of the hepatobiliary system and pancreas. *Vet Clin North Am Small Anim Pract* 46: 453–480.

3 Marolf, A.J. (2016). Computed tomography and MRI of the hepatobiliary system and pancreas. *Vet Clin North Am Small Anim Pract* 46: 481–497.

4 Bjorneby, J.M. and Kari, S. (2002). Cytology of the pancreas. *Vet Clin North Am Small Anim Pract* 32: 1293–1312.

5 Crain, S.K., Sharkey, L.C., Cordner, A.P. et al. (2015). Safety of ultrasound-guided fine-needle aspiration of the feline pancreas: a case control study. *J Feline Med Surg* 17: 858–863.

6 Cordner, A.P., Sharkey, L.C., Armstrong, P.J., and KD, M.A. (2015). Cytologic findings and diagnostic yield in 92 dogs undergoing fine-needle aspiration in the pancreas. *J Vet Diagn Invest* 27: 236–240.

7 Xenoulis, P.G. (2008). Current concepts in feline pancreatitis. *Top Comp Anim Med* 23: 185–192.

8 Binek, J., Spieler, P., Hurlimann, R. et al. (1995). Ultrasound-guided fine-needle aspiration of abdominal masses: Accuracy and short-term complications. *Eur J Ultrasound* 2: 199–203.

9 Hecht, S. and Henry, G. (2007). Sonographic evaluation of the normal and abnormal pancreas. *Clin Tech Small Anim Pract* 22: 115–121.

10 Hecht, S., Penninck, D.G., and Keating, J.H. (2007). Imaging findings in pancreatic neoplasia and nodular hyperplasia in 19 cats. *Vet Radiol Ultrasound* 48: 45–50.

11 Seaman, R.L. (2004). Exocrine pancreatic neoplasia in the cat: a case series. *J Am Anim Hosp Assoc* 40: 238–245.

12 Lamb, C.R., Simpson, K.W., Boswood, A., and Matthewman, L.A. (1995). Ultrasonography of pancreatic neoplasia in the dog: a retrospective review of 16 cases. *Vet Rec* 137: 65–68.

13 Kook, P.H., Kohler, N., Hartnack, S. et al. (2014). Agreement of serum spec cPL with the 1,2-o-dilauryl-rac-glycero glutaric acid (6′-methylresorufin) ester (DGGR) lipase assay and with pancreatic ultrasonography in dogs with suspected pancreatitis. *J Vet Intern Med* 28: 863–870.

14 Bonfanti, U., Bussadori, C., Zatelli, A. et al. (2004). Percutaneous fine-needle biopsy of deep thoracic and abdominal masses in dogs and cats. *J Small Anim Pract* 45: 191–198.

15 Cosford, K.L., Shmon, C.L., Myers, S.L. et al. (2010). Prospective evaluation of laparoscopic pancreatic biopsies in 11 healthy cats. *J Vet Intern Med* 24: 104–113.

16 Webb, C.B. and Trott, C. (2008). Laparoscopic diagnosis of pancreatic disease in dogs and cats. *J Vet Intern Med* 22: 1263–1266.

17 Kim, H., Oh, Y., Choi, J. et al. (2014). Use of laparoscopy for diagnosing experimentally induced acute pancreatitis in dogs. *J Vet Sci* 15: 551–556.

18 Wypji, J.M. (2011). Getting to the point: Indications for fine-needle aspiration of internal organs and bone. *Top Comp Anim Med* 26: 77–85.

19 Cordner, A.P., Armstrong, P.J., Newman, S.J. et al. (2010). Effect of pancreatic tissue sampling on serum pancreatic enzyme levels in clinically healthy dogs. *J Vet Diagn Invest* 22: 702–707.

20 Linderman, M.J., Brodsky, E.M., de Lorimer, L.-P. et al. (2013). Feline exocrine pancreatic carcinoma: a

retrospective study of 34 cases. *Vet Comp Oncol* 11: 208–218.

21 Kook, P.H., Baloi, P., Ruetten, M. et al. (2012). Feasibility and safety of endoscopic ultrasound-guided fine needle aspiration of the pancreas in dogs. *J Vet Intern Med* 26: 513–517.

22 Pratschke, K.M., Ryan, J., McAlinden, A., and McLauchlan, G. (2015). Pancreatic surgical biopsy in 24 dogs and 19 cats: postoperative complications and clinical relevance of histologic findings. *J Small Anim Pract* 56: 60–66.

23 Jubb, K.V.F. and Stent, A.W. (2016). Pancreas. In: *Pathology of Domestic Animals*, (ed. Maxie, M.G.), 6e, vol. 2, 353–375. St Louis, MO: Elsevier.

24 Newman, S.J., Steiner, J.M., Woosley, K. et al. (2005). Correlation of age and incidence of pancreatic exocrine nodular hyperplasia in the dog. *Vet Pathol* 42: 510–513.

25 Ramirez, G.A., Altimira, J., Garcia-Gonzalez, B., and Vilafranca, M. (2013). Intrapancreatic ectopic splenic tissue in dogs and cats. *J Comp Path* 148: 361–364.

26 Branter, E.M. and Viviano, K.R. (2010). Multiple recurrent pancreatic cysts with associated pancreatic inflammation and atrophy in a cat. *J Feline Med Surg* 12: 822–827.

27 VanEnkevort, B.A., O'Brien, R.T., and Young, K.M. (1999). Pancreatic pseudocysts in 4 dogs and 2 cats: ultrasonographic and clinicopathologic findings. *J Vet Intern Med* 13: 309–313.

28 Blundel, R. and Adam, F. (2012). Haemolytic anaemia and acute pancreatitis associated with zinc toxicosis in a dog. *Vet Rec* 172: 17–19.

29 Mikszewski, J.S., Saunders, H.M., and Hess, R.S. (2003). Zinc-associated acute pancreatitis in a dog. *J Small Anim Pract* 44: 177–180.

30 Schleis, S.E., Rizzo, S.A., Phillips, J.C., and LeBlanc, A.K. (2011). Asparaginase-associated pancreatitis in a dog. *Can Vet J* 52: 1009–1012.

31 Ferreri, J.A., Hardam, E., Kimmerl, S.E. et al. (2003). Clinical differentiation of acute necrotizing from chronic nonsuppurative pancreatitis in cats: 63 cases (1996–2001). *J Am Vet Med Assoc* 223: 469–474.

32 Newman, S.J., Steiner, J., Woosley, K. et al. (2004). Localization of pancreatic inflammation and necrosis in dogs. *J Vet Intern Med* 18: 488–493.

33 Watson, P. (2015). Pancreatitis in dogs and cats: definitions and pathophysiology. *J Small Anim Pract* 56: 3–12.

34 De Cock, H.E.V., Forman, M.A., Farver, T.B., and Marks, S.L. (2007). Prevalence and histopathologic characteristics of pancreatitis in cats. *Vet Pathol* 44: 39–49.

35 Newman, S.J., Steiner, J.M., Woosley, K. et al. (2006). Histologic assessment and grading of the exocrine pancreas in the dog. *J Vet Diagn Invest* 18: 115–118.

36 Tangeman, L., Davignon, D., Patel, R., and Littman, M. (2015). Abdominal cryptococcosis in two dogs: diagnosis and medical management. *J Am Anim Hosp Assoc* 51: 107–113.

37 Le Donne, V., McGovern, A., Fletcher, M., and Grasperge, B.J. (2016). Cytologic diagnosis of *Heterobilharzia americana* infection in a liver aspirate from a dog. *Vet Pathol* 53: 633–636.

38 Rodriguez, J.Y., Lewis, B.C., and Snowden, K.F. (2014). Distribution and characterization of *Heterobilharzia americana* in dogs in Texas. *Vet Parasitol* 203: 35–42.

39 Rodriguez, J.Y., Camp, J.W., Lenz, S.D. et al. (2016). Identification of *Heterobilharzia americana* infection in a dog residing in Indiana with no history of travel. *J Am Vet Med Assoc* 248: 827–830.

40 Nassise, M.P., van Ee, R.T., and Wright, B. (1985). Ocular changes in a cat with disseminated blastomycosis. *J Am Vet Med Assoc* 187: 629–631.

41 Dubey, J.P. and Carpenter, J.L. (1993). Histologically confirmed clinical toxoplasmosis in cats: 100 cases (1952–1990). *J Am Vet Med Assoc* 203: 1556–1566.

42 Watson, P.J., Archer, J., Roulois, A.J. et al. (2010). Observational study of 14 cases of chronic pancreatitis in dogs. *Vet Rec* 167: 968–976.

43 Bostrom, B.M., Xenoulis, P.G., Newman, S.J. et al. (2013). Chronic pancreatitis in dogs: a retrospective study of clinical clinicopathological, and histopathological findings in 61 cases. *Vet J* 195: 73–79.

44 Johnson, M.D. and Mann, F.A. (2006). Treatment for pancreatic abscesses via comentalization with abdominal closure versus open peritoneal drainage in dogs: 15 cases (1994–2004). *J Am Vet Med Assoc* 228: 397–402.

45 Anderson, J.R., Cornell, K.K., Parnell, N.K., and Salisbury, S.K. (2008). Pancreatic abscesses in 36 dogs: a retrospective analysis of prognostic indicators. *J Am Anim Hosp Assoc* 44: 171–179.

46 Son, T.T., Thompson, L., Serrano, S., and Seshadri, R. (2010). Surgical intervention in the management of severe acute pancreatitis in cats: 8 cases (2003–2007). *J Vet Emerg Crit Care* 20: 426–435.

47 Nemoto, Y., Haraguchi, T., Shimokawa Miyama, T. et al. (2017). Pancreatic abscess in a cat due to *Staphylococcus aureus* infection. *J Vet Med Sci* 79: 1146–1150.

48 Lee, M., Kang, J.H., Chang, D. et al. (2015). Pancreatic abscess in a cat with diabetes mellitus. *J Am Anim Hosp Assoc* 51: 180–184.

49 Yoshimura, H., Matsuda, Y., Kawamoto, Y. et al. (2013). Acinar cell cystadenoma of the pancreas in a cat. *J Comp Pathol* 149: 225–228.

50 Munday, J.S., Löhr, C.V., and Kiupel, M. (2017). Tumors of the alimentary tract. In: *Tumors in Domestic Animals*, (ed. Meuten, D.J.), 5e, 499–601. Ames, IA: Wiley-Blackwell.

51 Bennett, P.F., Hahn, K.A., Toal, R.L., and Legendre, A.M. (2001). Ultrasonographic and cytopathological diagnosis of exocrine pancreatic carcinoma in the dog and cat. *J Am Anim Hosp Assoc* 37: 466–473.

52 Dannis, M.M., O'Brien, T.D., Wayne, T. et al. (2008). Hyalinizing pancreatic adenocarcinoma in six dogs. *Vet Pathol* 45: 475–483.

53 De Brot, S., Junge, H., and Hilbe, M. (2014). Acinar cell carcinoma of exocrine pancreas in two horses. *J Comp Path* 150: 388–392.

54 Yamamoto, R., Suzuki, K., Uchida, K. et al. (2012). Pancreatic carcinosarcoma in a cat. *J Comp Path* 147: 223–226.

55 Takeuchi, Y., Takahashi, M., Tsuboi, M. et al. (2012). Intestinal T-cell lymphoma with severe hypereosinophilic syndrome in a cat. *J Vet Med Sci* 74: 1057–1062.

56 Zini, E., Lunardi, F., Zanetti, R. et al. (2016). Endocrine pancreas in cats with diabetes mellitus. *Vet Pathol* 53: 136–144.

57 Goutal, C.M., Brugmann, B.L., and Ryan, K.A. (2012). Insulinoma in dogs: a review. *J Am Anim Hosp Assoc* 48: 151–163.

58 Pieczarka, E.M., Russell, D.S., Santangelo, K.S. et al. (2014). Osseous metaplasia within a canine insulinoma. *Vet Clin Pathol* 43: 89–93.

59 Cruz Cardona, J.A., Wamsley, H.L., Farina, L.L., and Kiupel, M. (2010). Metastatic pancreatic polypeptide-secreting islet cell tumor in a dog. *Vet Clin Pathol* 39: 371–376.

60 Watson, P.J., Roulois, A.S.A., Scase, T. et al. (2007). Prevalence and breed distribution of chronic pancreatitis at post-mortem examination in first-opinion dogs. *J Small Anim Pract* 48: 609–618.

Part X

Urinary Tract

37

Kidney

Camille A. McAloney and Leslie C. Sharkey

Introduction

Although urinalysis and biochemical indicators are useful for assessing renal function, they are not specific to the etiology of disease in many cases and lack sensitivity. As with other tissues, microscopic evaluation of renal tissue aids in obtaining a specific diagnosis and can be prognostic. While there is an extensive literature describing the histopathology of kidney disease, the literature describing renal cytology is much more limited.

Collection

Indications

Renal cytology is typically pursued after identification of kidney masses, renomegaly, or altered echogenicity on ultrasound, suggesting an infiltrative process.[1] Retrospective studies of dogs and cats support that masses and altered echotexture were commonly observed ultrasonographically in animals undergoing renal fine-needle aspiration (FNA).[2,3] Some pathologic processes affecting the kidney that are presumed to be ineffectively assessed by cytology include poorly exfoliative lesions such as fibrosis and those requiring assessment of architectural changes for diagnosis, including congenital abnormalities such as renal dysplasia and glomerular disease.[1] Although some sources caution against sampling renal abscesses because of the potential risk of secondary peritonitis, there are reports of cytologic diagnosis.[4,5]

Methods

Needles that are 1.5 in. long and 21–27 G are typically used for renal FNA, with larger bore needles generally yielding more cellular samples.[1,6,7] Renal cytology samples are usually collected using ultrasound guidance, although sampling with computed tomography has been described.[1,6,7] Anecdotally, the left kidney is sampled more often than the right because of the proximity of the right kidney to the bowels and pancreas. However, the authors could not identify primary literature that confirmed that sampling the right kidney actually increases the risk of damaging or aspirating nearby organs. When focal lesions are present, it is recommended to take samples from both the center and periphery to increase the likelihood of obtaining a diagnostic sample due to potential variation within mass.[1] Air-dried samples are typically stained using a Romanowsky stain such as Wright Giemsa. Other stains such as Gram and periodic acid-Schiff are occasionally used.

In dogs and cats, renal FNA was shown to have a diagnostic yield of 68–72% in retrospective studies, compared with 95–96% and 77–98% for canine and feline liver aspirates, respectively, and 74% for the canine pancreas.[2,3,8,9] A retrospective study of renal aspiration in dogs demonstrated that unclear corticomedullary distinction, pelvic dilation, an infiltrative or nodular appearance, and the presence of a mass or masses on ultrasound were associated with higher diagnostic yield.[2] In a similar feline paper, kidneys with subcapsular renal infiltrate, diffuse renal enlargement without pelvic dilation, and infiltrative/nodular appearance were more likely to generate diagnostic cytology samples.[3] Studies on renal cytology in horses could not be identified in the literature beyond rare case reports.

Safety

Anecdotally, a common reason for selecting cytology over biopsy is a perception of increased safety, in addition to more rapid availability of results. One large-scale multi-institutional retrospective study of 283 dogs and 65 cats reported complications in 13.4% of dogs and 18.5% of cats

Veterinary Cytology, First Edition. Edited by Leslie C. Sharkey, M. Judith Radin, and Davis Seelig.

undergoing renal biopsy.[10] Over 85% of samples were considered of acceptable quality, which is higher than the diagnostic yield of cytology samples.[2,3,10] Severe hemorrhage was the most common complication of renal biopsy in that study; bleeding was slightly more common in animals with abnormal coagulation profiles but also occurred in cats with normal coagulation test results.[10] Complications of renal cytology specifically have not been systematically reported, but hemorrhage is anecdotally the most common. It is worth noting that the most common indication for renal biopsy in dogs was proteinuria, while cats were most often biopsied for chronic kidney disease (CKD), masses, or renomegaly.[10] Differences between populations undergoing biopsy and cytology could influence reported complications and frequency. Seeding of tumor cells along the sampling track has been described in cases of transitional cell carcinoma.[11,12] A large-scale multicenter study of renal biopsies in horses reported a complication rate of 11%, but only 3% of required treatment.[13] The most common complications were hemorrhage or signs of colic, and fatality was reported in only 0.7% of cases. Samples were of sufficient quality for diagnosis in 94% of cases; however, surgical biopsy diagnosis had only fair agreement (72%) with postmortem findings. Complications were more common in horses with a diagnosis of neoplasia and those with low urine specific gravity. The most common diagnoses were tubulointerstitial disease, glomerular disease, and tubular disease. Neoplasia was uncommon.

Normal Structure and Cytology

The kidney is divided into the cortex, medulla, and pelvis. The cortex is composed of blood vessels, glomeruli, and the proximal and distal tubules, as well as a portion of the collecting duct. The tubules appear as winding hollow tubes composed of renal tubular epithelial cells that vary in shape from cuboidal to nearly columnar. Glomeruli are composed of a tuft of capillaries within Bowman's capsule. Bowman's capsule consists of a parietal layer of simple squamous cells and a visceral layer of podocytes, which appear histologically as epithelial cells. Within Bowman's capsule and surrounding the glomerulus is the mesangium. Combined, the glomerulus, mesangium, and Bowman's capsule form the renal corpuscle. On one end of the renal corpuscle, a urinary pole occurs where the parietal layer of Bowman's capsule joins the proximal tubule of the nephron, while at the vascular pole, the arterioles of the glomerulus enter and leave the renal corpuscle and abut the macula densa of the distal tubule.[14]

The medulla contains many blood vessels, the descending and ascending limbs of the tubules, the loop of Henle, and a portion of the collecting duct. Collecting ducts contain two types of cells: principal (light) cells that are cuboidal and stain palely eosinophilic and intercalated (dark) cells that are often columnar and stain darkly eosinophilic. The renal pelvis is an empty space and beginning of the ureters. The most central layer of the pelvis is composed of transitional epithelial cells, followed by the lamina propria (sans muscularis mucosae) and the tunica muscularis.[14]

In FNAs of normal kidneys, renal tubular epithelial cells are the primary cell type observed.[15] Renal epithelial cells exfoliate as individual cells, small clusters, and intact renal tubular fragments. Fragments are straight or curved structures composed of tightly adhered round to columnar epithelial cells (Figure 37.1a and b).[16] Individual epithelial cells are round to polygonal and have abundant basophilic cytoplasm, with minimal anisocytosis.[15] In cats the cytoplasm often contains variable numbers of clear relatively uniform lipid vacuoles, while in dogs the cytoplasm typically contains few vacuoles.[2,3,16] Round nuclei are often pericentric with stippled chromatin and one round, small nucleolus; minimal anisokaryosis is seen.[15] Dark blue, indistinct to granular cytoplasmic granules in renal tubular cells has been described[1] and in humans indicate the tubular cells originate from the ascending loop of Henle or distal tubules.[15] Care should be taken not to confuse these cells for well-differentiated melanocytes.

Glomeruli are rarely seen but when present appear as round to lobulated multilayered clusters of basophilic cells with round to oval nuclei (Figure 37.1c and d). It is difficult to distinguish the individual cells composing a glomerulus, but the cells generally display minimal anisocytosis and anisokaryosis.[15,16] Blood contamination is common; numbers of leukocytes must be assessed in the context of peripheral leukocyte numbers.[15]

Conditions Diagnosed by Cytology

Hyperplasia, Degeneration, and Necrosis

Cytologic assessment of hyperplasia is largely restricted to the tubular component of the kidneys. Numerous underlying stimuli include trauma, acute kidney injury, early- to mid-stage CKD, inflammation, and neoplasia. The cytologic characteristics of hyperplasia include mild to marked anisocytosis, and anisokaryosis, increased nuclear to cytoplasm ratio (N:C), and increased numbers of nucleoli[1–3]; however, robust cytology/histopathology correlation data is lacking. One retrospective study of dogs describes overlap in the cytologic features of reactive epithelial hyperplasia and carcinoma leading to false-positive and false-negative cytologic diagnoses compared with histopathology;

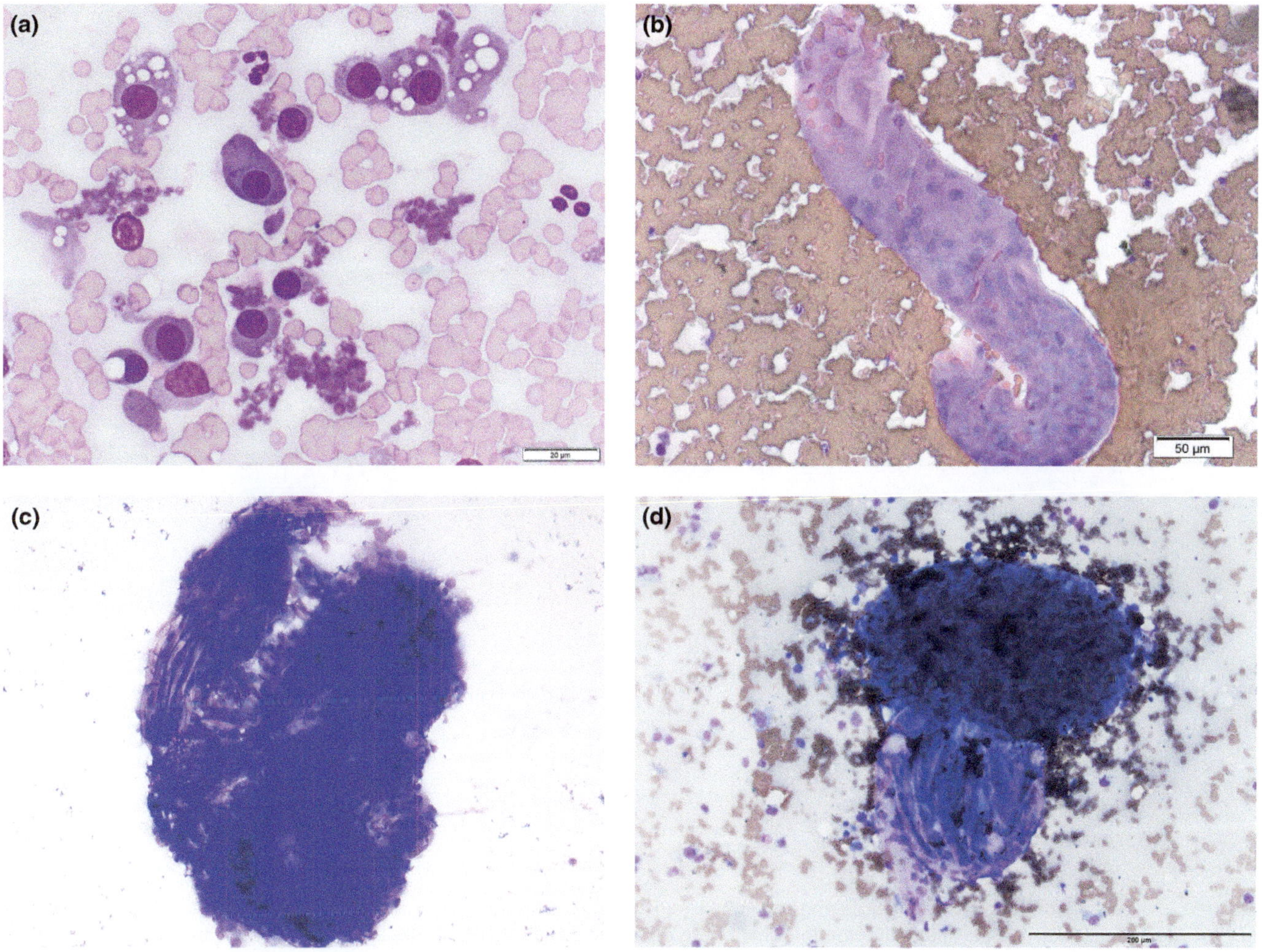

Figure 37.1 Normal renal tubular cells in dogs and cats. (a) Individualized renal epithelial tubular cells from a cat. The cells are round to polygonal with abundant basophilic cytoplasm and a pericentric nucleus with finely stippled chromatin and a round, faint nucleolus. Few dark blue indistinct cytoplasmic granules are seen, which are of no clinical significance. Many of the epithelial cells have variable numbers of lipid vacuoles. Neutrophils consistent with peripheral blood origin are present in the background (Wright Giemsa, 500×). (b) Renal epithelial tubular cells from a dog. The cells have exfoliated as an intact renal tubular fragment. They appear similar to feline epithelial cells, but without cytoplasmic vacuoles (Wright Giemsa, 200×). (c) Glomerulus and capillary tuft from a cat. The capillaries are seen as wispy pink structures that connect to a large, lobulated, multilayered cluster of basophilic cells. The cells display minimal atypia (Wright Giemsa, 200×). (d) Glomerulus from a dog (Wright Giemsa).

however, the presence of a mass lesion on imaging in combination with moderate to marked cytologic atypia was strongly suggestive for carcinoma (Figure 37.2).[2] Anecdotally, the authors have observed similar difficulties in cats, but insufficient cases with definitive histologic diagnoses were available for systematic evaluation (Figure 37.3).

Typical morphologic criteria of tissue degeneration and necrosis have been applied to the cytologic evaluation of renal tissue including poorly preserved cells and amorphous basophilic debris.[2,3] Damage to tubular cells can cause the formation of casts, which can be detected microscopically in some FNAs[14] and during the sediment exam of a complete urinalysis (see Chapter 39).[15] Acute renal injury, often due to ischemia or exposure to nephrotoxins, tends to result in formation of cellular to granular casts, while waxy casts are often present with CKD.[17]

Neoplasia

Benign

Renal adenomas are rare in dogs and cats but more common in horses, often occurring as solitary incidental lesions of <2 cm diameter with minimal cellular atypia.[17] Renal cystadenoma was reported in a domestic short-haired

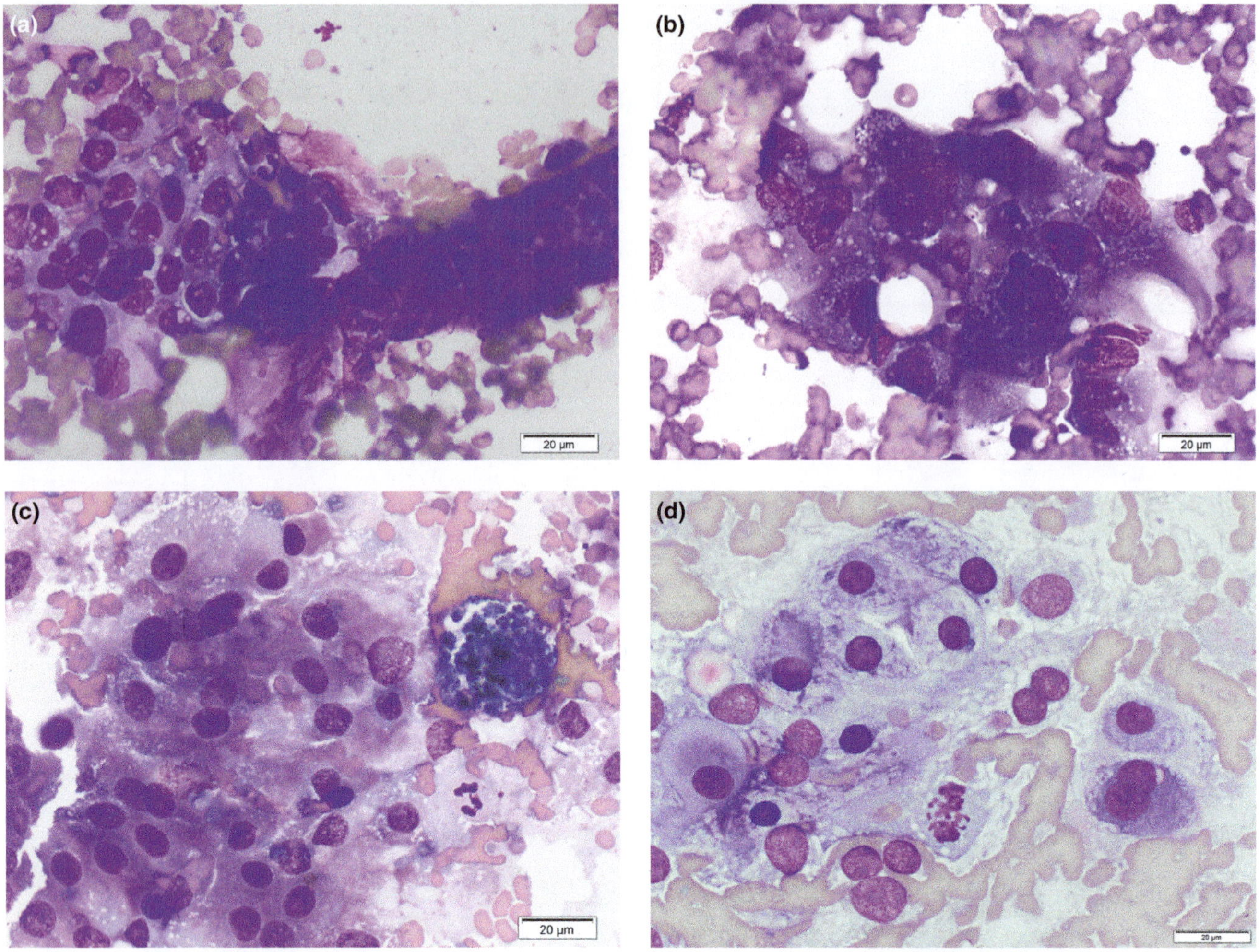

Figure 37.2 Comparison of renal hyperplasia and carcinoma. (a) Hyperplasia of renal epithelial cells in a dog. The cells display mild anisocytosis and anisokaryosis with lacy chromatin. Some of the cells exfoliated as a renal tubule (Wright Giemsa, 500×). (b) Hyperplasia of renal epithelial cells from a dog. These cells display moderate to marked anisocytosis and anisokaryosis and prominent nucleoli (Wright Giemsa, 500×. *Source:* Reprinted with permission from McAloney et al.[2]) (c) Renal carcinoma in a dog. The cells maintain some degree of organization, display mild to moderate anisocytosis and anisokaryosis, and have inconspicuous nucleoli. The hemosiderin-laden macrophage is consistent with evidence of previous hemorrhage (Wright Giemsa, 500×). (d) Renal carcinoma in a dog. The cells display marked anisocytosis and anisokaryosis with multinucleation and a bizarre mitotic figure. A single normal renal epithelial cell is present (Wright Giemsa, 500×. *Source:* Reprinted with permission from McAloney et al.[2]).

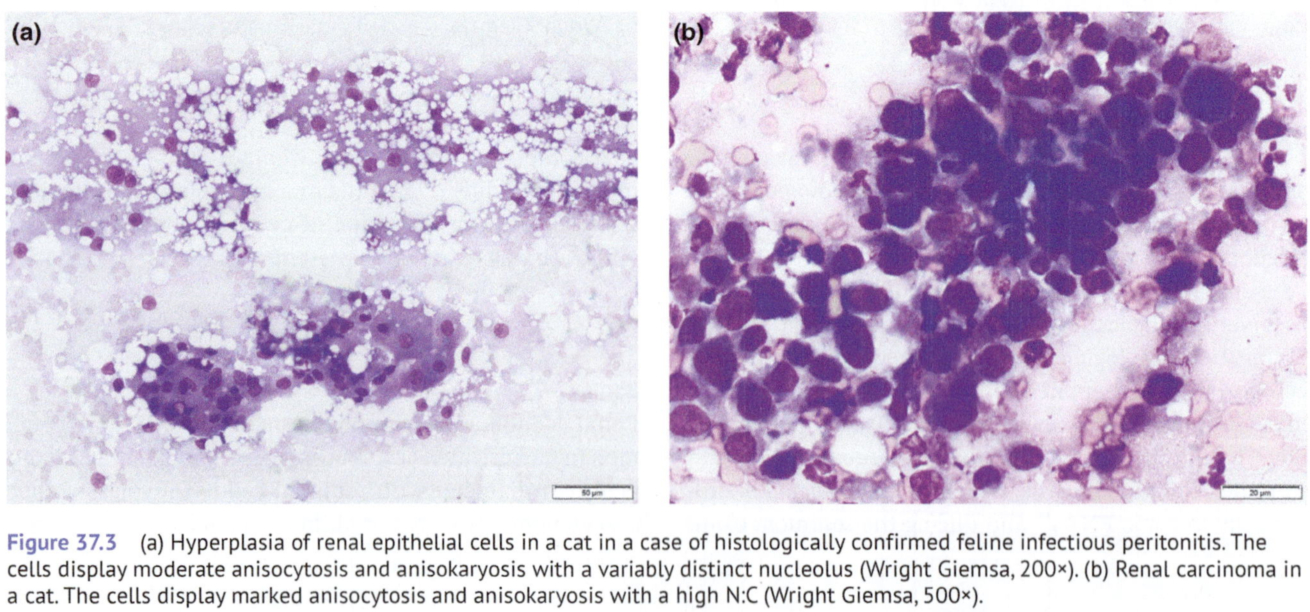

Figure 37.3 (a) Hyperplasia of renal epithelial cells in a cat in a case of histologically confirmed feline infectious peritonitis. The cells display moderate anisocytosis and anisokaryosis with a variably distinct nucleolus (Wright Giemsa, 200×). (b) Renal carcinoma in a cat. The cells display marked anisocytosis and anisokaryosis with a high N:C (Wright Giemsa, 500×).

feline.[18] A complex cystic structure of the left kidney was observed ultrasonographically, and cyst fluid contained 400 nucleated cells/μL, most of which were macrophages (70%) with fewer mature lymphocytes (30%), scattered neutrophils, and clusters of basilar epithelial cells. Cytology of an oncocytoma of the right kidney in a domestic shorthaired cat was of moderate cellularity, consisting of individualized cells and papillary sheets and clusters of oncocytes characterized by moderate to abundant densely staining cytoplasm with a single round nucleus and indistinct nucleoli.[19]

Malignant

Most malignant tumors of the kidney originate outside the organ, and renal involvement is by direct extension or hematogenous and lymphatic metastasis.[17,20] One retrospective study of primary renal neoplasia in 82 dogs described 49 carcinomas, 28 sarcomas (predominantly hemangiosarcoma), and 5 nephroblastomas.[21] In cats, approximately 75% of primary renal tumors were epithelial, and the remainder mesenchymal.[20] In contrast, a retrospective study of renal neoplasia in the horse described a predominance of primary tumors, including nine renal carcinomas and four renal adenomas.[22] Metastatic tumors included lymphoma, melanoma, and hemangiosarcoma. Other studies have reported primary renal carcinoma in the horse; however, cytologic features have not been described.[23,24]

Carcinoma

As previously described, a single study suggests that the cytologic characteristics of epithelial hyperplasia and renal carcinoma overlap in the dog; however, integrating the data with imaging studies might help refine the diagnosis (Figures 37.2 and 37.3).[2] Specifically, moderate to marked anisocytosis, anisokaryosis, and high N:C can characterize both reactive hyperplasia and carcinoma. There are several histologic subtypes of renal carcinoma (solid, tubular, papillary, cystic, clear cell); however, the biological behavior is often aggregated because of insufficient information of how subtype impacts prognosis.[20] Likewise, systematic study of cytologic features is not available. A case of renal carcinoma with hyaline globules was characterized cytologically by a high cellularity, consisting of many sheets of epithelial cells with pale basophilic cytoplasm, rare clear vacuoles, and indistinct cytoplasmic margins.[25] Single round to oval nuclei with stippled chromatin contained indistinct nucleoli, and anisocytosis and anisokaryosis were mild to moderate with rare binucleation.[25] Another case of renal carcinoma in a dog with paraneoplastic leukocytosis was characterized cytologically by high cellularity, consisting of large clusters of round to polyhedral cells with distinct cytoplasmic margins and a moderate amount of vacuolated basophilic cytoplasm.[26] Nuclei were round to oval with somewhat prominent nucleoli. Mild inflammation and hematoidin were also described. Transitional cell carcinomas also occur in the kidney, generally arising in the pelvis, but they are unusual.[20]

Sarcoma

Hemangiosarcoma in the kidney is often metastatic, and classic cytologic features are described in Chapter 28. Primary renal hemangiosarcoma is rare, and reports suggest slower progression than other visceral manifestations of this malignancy in dogs (Figure 37.4).[27] An epithelioid hemangiosarcoma of the prostate, testis, kidney, and other organs presented cytologically as aggregates of highly anaplastic cells occurring singly or in aggregates.[28] Cells had distinct margins, cytoplasmic vacuolization, 1–3 nuclei, and bizarre nucleoli. They were initially interpreted to potentially be epithelial and of prostatic origin; however, immunohistochemistry was positive for von Willebrand factor and negative for cytokeratin, supporting a diagnosis of epithelioid hemangiosarcoma.[28] Immunocytochemical techniques for cytokeratin and vimentin have recently been reported for the dog and might be helpful in similar cases.[29]

Although not renal, a primary ureteral giant cell sarcoma was described in a Pomeranian dog with a mass and left-sided hydronephrosis.[30]

Round Cell Tumor

Most round cell tumors of the kidney are considered metastatic.[17] Much of the literature on the cytology of round cell tumors of the kidney describes lymphoma, which is the most common renal neoplasm of cats (Figure 37.5). General references suggest that cytologic evaluation of kidney tissue for lymphoma is a common indication and that diagnostic accuracy is high.[1,31] There is limited cytology/histopathology correlation data for renal lymphoma in the literature, although one canine study and one feline study describe small numbers of cases that would support this.[2,3] The canine study also used polymerase chain reaction for antigen receptor rearrangement (PARR) as a reference test in conjunction with histopathology.[2] The authors describe problems retrieving DNA from archived renal cytology samples and identified one sample that was diagnostic for lymphoma by cytology and histopathology, but negative using PARR, suggesting a false-negative result.[2] B-cell lymphoma with aberrant CD3 expression was identified in the kidney of a cat; cytology consisted of a population of pleomorphic round cells with one to three prominent nucleoli, dense chromatin, and markedly basophilic cytoplasm occasionally with vacuoles.[32]

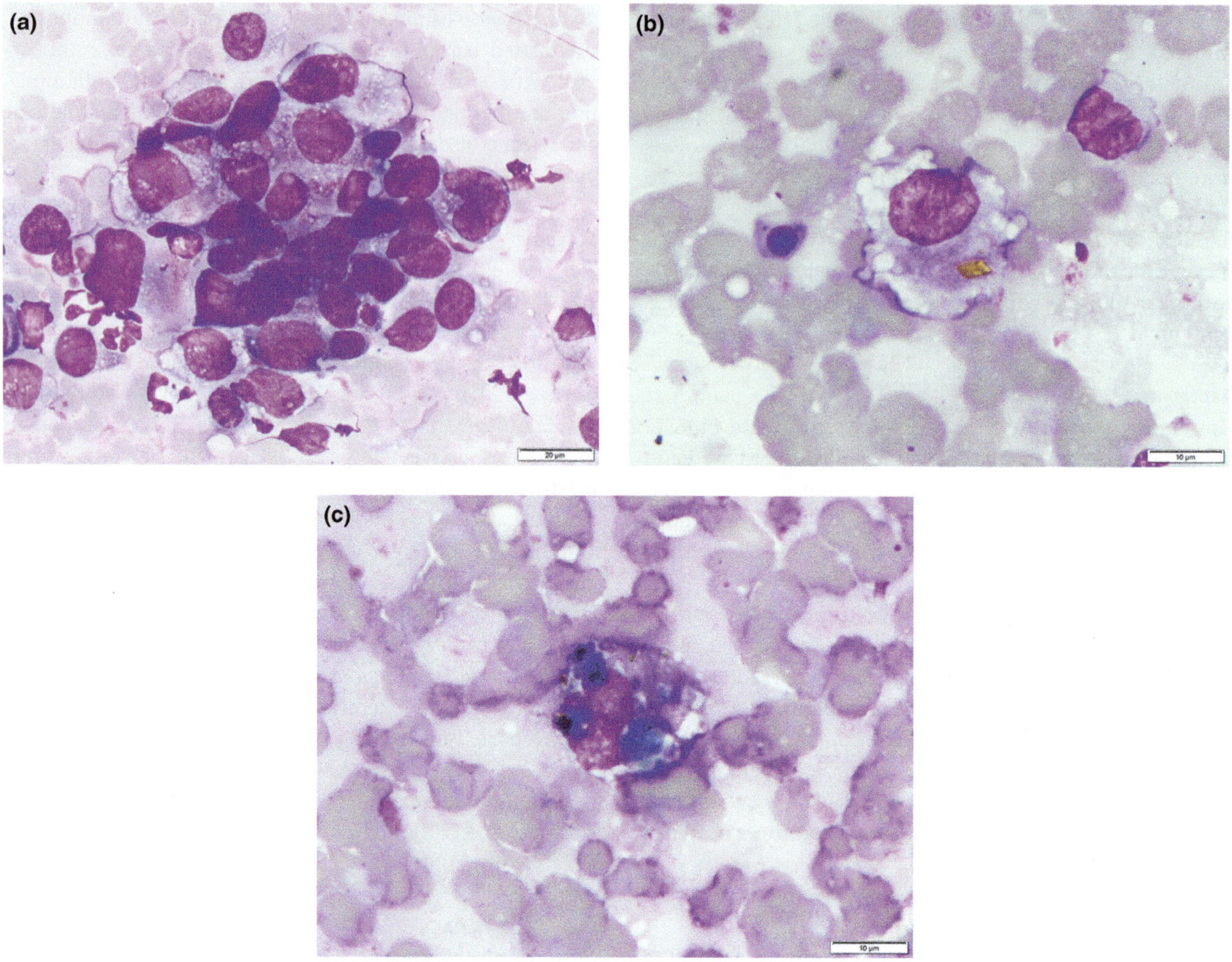

Figure 37.4 Metastatic hemangiosarcoma in a dog. (a) An aggregate of mesenchymal cells. The cells display moderate anisocytosis, marked anisokaryosis, and multiple variably sized nucleoli. Neutrophils (consistent with blood leukocytes) are present in the background (Wright Giemsa, 500×) (b) The presence of a hematoidin crystal within a macrophage (center) indicates previous hemorrhage, likely from the hemangiosarcoma. The nucleated red blood cell (metarubricyte) is due to concurrent extramedullary hematopoiesis, which occasionally occurs in the kidney (Wright Giemsa, 1000×). (c) The presence of hemosiderin (globular blue-black material) and hematoidin crystals within the macrophage indicate previous hemorrhage (Wright Giemsa, 1000×).

Nephroblastoma

These are embryonal tumors that occur uncommonly in domestic animals, and cytology is rarely described despite the fact that it can be diagnostic. In one canine case, cytology samples were described as markedly cellular and consisting of a population of atypical large round cells with some aggregation and extracellular matrix.[33] Round cells were characterized by scant to moderate amounts of basophilic cytoplasm that was frequently mildly vacuolated and single round to oval nuclei that occasionally had irregular nuclear margins. Cell cohesion, absence of cytoplasmic fragments, and matrix were considered to be features that differentiated the cells from lymphoma.[33]

Inflammation

Infectious

As with other tissues, cytology can be used as a method for rapid screening for infectious disease. Although cytology is rarely performed to screen for viral etiologies, one study evaluated the feasibility of screening for feline infectious peritonitis in the kidney by identification of normal cellular elements with mixed inflammation.[6] The authors concluded this technique had low sensitivity (approximately 40%). Diagnosis of renal abscesses in six cats was described with all aspirates containing many neutrophils, and organisms were identified in 5/6 cases,

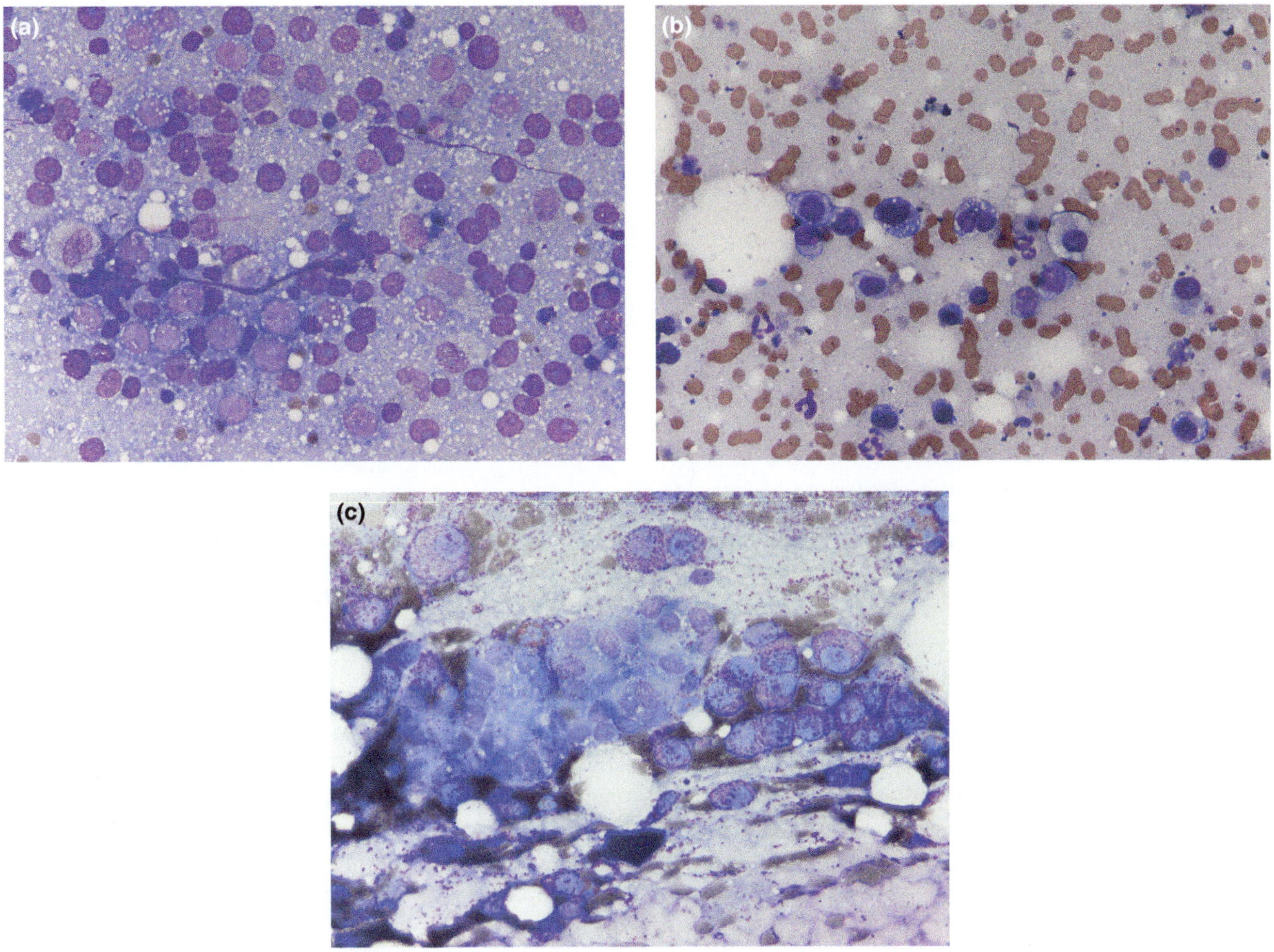

Figure 37.5 Renal round cell tumors. (a) Renal lymphoma in a cat. The majority of cells are large lymphocytes, many of which are broken. Intact cells have a high N:C and a large, faint nucleolus. No normal renal structures are seen (Wright Giemsa, 500×). (b) Renal lymphoma in a cat. The neoplastic cells are round with a variable amount of deeply basophilic cytoplasm that often contains clear vacuoles, a round eccentrically placed nucleus, smooth chromatin, and a single large, round, faint nucleolus. When the cells have a moderate N:C, they appear similar to individualized renal tubular epithelial cells (Wright Giemsa, 500×). (c) Renal mast cell tumor with eosinophilic inflammation in a Shar Pei dog. Numerous poorly granulated mast cells and occasional well-differentiated eosinophils are present. The renal epithelial cells display minimal atypia. The pink hyaline background with occasional windrowing of cells is of unknown significance (Wright Giemsa, 500×).

corresponding to the culture results (4 *Escherichia coli* and 1 group G *Streptococcus* sp.). Mycotic infections of the kidney can be identified cytologically, including *Histoplasma*, *Cryptococcus*, and others.[1] Typically, organisms are noted with mixed inflammation (see Chapter 3 for the details of cytologic identification of common fungal pathogens). Although the availability of urine fungal antigen testing can partially supplant cytology, rapid turnaround and the potential for negative urine antigen test results as previously described in a cat with renal histoplasmosis suggest a continuing role for cytology.[34] Systemic *Exophiala jeanselmei* infection was detected by renal cytology in a cat.[35] Smears collected from an enlarged and irregular left kidney revealed renal tubular epithelial cells, neutrophils, macrophages, and many fungal hyphae. Urine culture was negative; however, fungal culture of kidney tissue revealed phaeohyphomycosis.

Halicephalobus gingivalis infection is a systemic infection occurring in both horses and people.[36] Characteristic nematode larvae can be identified in kidney cytology samples along with granulomatous inflammation (Figure 37.6); larvae can also be present in urine.[36]

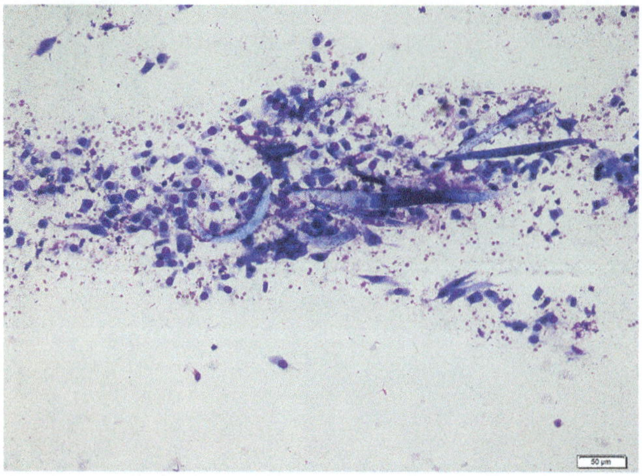

Figure 37.6 *Halicephalobus gingivalis* infection in a 14-year-old horse with multifocal granulomatous nephritis. The smear shows nematode larvae admixed with numerous renal tubule epithelial cells, macrophages, fibroblasts, and cell debris (Diff-Quik. *Source:* Image courtesy of Marian Taulescu).

Noninfectious

When cytologic findings involve inflammatory cell infiltrate without the presence of infectious agents, the specific type of inflammation (suppurative vs. mixed) is categorized identically to infectious inflammatory lesions. However, it is vitally important to remember that failure to identify infectious agents does not exclude infection. Most inflammatory kidney diseases require histopathology for diagnosis.

Renal toxicoses that have been described cytologically include calcium oxalate (due to ethylene glycol toxicosis)[16] and melamine and cyanuric acid (due to ingestion of contaminated pet food).[16,37] Calcium oxalate crystals are clear and oblong with ragged to sharply demarcated edges. These crystals are refractile and polarize under polarized light. Melamine and cyanuric acid crystals are pale green to yellow gold and round to dumbbell shaped. These crystals can be mistaken for calcium carbonate or smooth ammonium biurate, so careful attention to clinical signs and history is vital. Analytical methods can be used to confirm melamine and cyanuric toxicity by testing urine, serum, or milk.[37] See Chapter 39 for more information on crystals of the urinary tract.

Conclusion

Renal cytology is a rapid, minimally invasive means of assessing the kidney for the presence of variety of pathologies. The information obtained from renal FNAs can often guide further diagnostics, if not providing a diagnosis outright. Pathologies that are readily assessed by renal FNA and cytology include but are not limited to necrosis, mesenchymal neoplasia, round cell neoplasia, nephroblastomas, infection, cystic lesions, and crystals. At least one study has documented difficulty in differentiating epithelial neoplasia and hyperplasia and the utility of using imaging findings to inform the diagnosis. In all cases, clinicians should consider the entire clinical picture when interpreting cytopathology. There are numerous aspects of renal cytology that remain to be studied, including safety and cytology/histopathology correlation for hyperplasia, various carcinomas, lymphoma, and others.

References

1 Borjesson, D.L. (2003). Renal cytology. *Vet Clin North Am Small Anim Pract* 33: 119–134.

2 McAloney, C.A., Sharkey, L.C., Feeney, D.A. et al. (2018). Evaluation of the diagnostic utility of cytologic examination of renal fine-needle aspirates from dogs and the use of ultrasonographic features to inform cytologic diagnosis. *J Am Vet Med Assoc* 252: 1247–1256.

3 McAloney, C.A., Sharkey, L.C., Feeney, D.A., and Seelig, D.M. (2018). Diagnostic utility of renal fine-needle aspirate cytology and ultrasound in the cat. *J Feline Med Surg* 20: 544–553.

4 Murgia, D. (2014). Investigation of parenchymal abdominal organ disease in cats. *J Feline Med Surg* 16: 216–230.

5 Faucher, M.R., Theron, M.L., and Reynolds, B.S. (2017). Renal abscesses in cats: six cases. *J Feline Med Surg* 19: 484–492.

6 Giordano, A., Paltrinieri, S., Bertazzolo, W. et al. (2005). Sensitivity of Tru-cut and fine-needle aspiration biopsies of the liver and kidney for diagnosis of feline infectious peritonitis. *Vet Clin Pathol* 34: 368–374.

7 Taylor, A.J., Lara-Garcia, A., and Benigni, L. (2014). Ultrasound characteristics of canine renal lymphoma. *Vet Radiol Ultrasound* 55: 441–446.

8 Weiss, D.J. and Moritz, A. (2002). Liver cytology. *Vet Clin North Am Small Anim Pract* 32: 1267–1291.

9 Cordner, A.P., Sharkey, L.C., Armstrong, P.J., and KD, M.A. (2015). Cytologic findings and diagnostic yield in 92 dogs undergoing fine-needle aspiration of the pancreas. *J Vet Diagn Invest* 27: 236–240.

10 Vaden, S.L., Levine, J.F., Lees, G.E. et al. (2005). Renal biopsy: a retrospective study of methods and complications in 283 dogs and 65 cats. *J Vet Intern Med* 19: 794–801.

11 Nyland, T.G., Wallack, S.T., and Wisner, E.R. (2002). Needle-tract implantation following US-guided fine-needle aspiration biopsy of transitional cell carcinoma of the bladder, urethra, and prostate. *Vet Radiol Ultrasound* 41: 50–53.

12 Vignoli, M., Rossi, F., Chierici, C. et al. (2007). Needle tract implantation after fine needle aspiration biopsy (FNAB) of transitional cell carcinoma of the urinary bladder and adenocarcinoma of the lung. *Schweiz Arch Tierheilkd* 149: 314–318.

13 Tyner, G.A., Nolen-Walston, R.D., Hall, T. et al. (2011). A multicenter retrospective study of 151 renal biopsies in horses. *J Vet Intern Med* 25: 532–539.

14 Maxie, G. (2016). *Jubb, Kennedy & Palmer's Pathology of Domestic Animals*, 6e, vol. 2, 376–464. St. Louis, MO: Elsevier.

15 Valenciano, A.C. and Cowell, R.L. (2014). *Cowell and Tyler's Diagnostic Cytology and Hematology of the Dog and Cat*, 4e, 387–430. St. Louis, MO: Elsevier.

16 Raskin, R.E. and Meyer, D.J. (2016). *Canine and Feline Cytology: A Color Atlas and Interpretation Guide*, 3e, 284–312. St. Louis, MO: Elsevier.

17 Cianciolo, R.E. and Mohr, F.C. (2016). Urinary system. In: *Jubb, Kennedy, and Palmer's Pathology of Domestic Animals*, (ed. Maxie M.G.), 6e, 376–464. St. Louis, MO: Elsevier.

18 Mosenco, A.S., Culp, W.T.N., Johnson, V. et al. (2008). Renal cystadenoma in a domestic shorthair cat. *J Feline Med Surg* 10: 102–105.

19 Lee, S., Choi, H.J., Lee, H.B. et al. (2017). Renal oncocytoma in a cat with chronic renal failure. *JFMS Open Rep* 3: 2055116917693491.

20 Meuten, D.J. and Meuten, T.L.K. (2017). Tumors of the urinary system. In: *Tumors in Domestic Animals*, (ed. Meuten D.J.), 5e, 632–688. Ames, IA: Wiley Blackwell.

21 Bryan, J.N., Henry, C.J., Turnquist, S.E. et al. (2006). Primary renal neoplasia of dogs. *J Vet Intern Med* 20: 1155–1160.

22 Vienenkötter, J., Suidak, K., Stallenberger, L., and Herden, C. (2017). Renal neoplasia in horses: a retrospective study. *Tierärztliche Praxis Großtiere* 45: 290–295.

23 Brown, P.J. and Holt, P.E. (1985). Primary renal cell carcinoma in four horses. *Equine Vet J* 17: 473–477.

24 Haschek, W.M., King, J.M., and Tennant, B.C. (1981). Primary renal cell carcinoma in two horses. *J Am Vet Med Assoc* 179: 992–994.

25 Collicut, N.B., Garner, B.C., Brown, C.A., and Camus, M.S. (2013). What is your diagnosis? Renal mass in a dog. *Vet Clin Pathol* 42: 389–390.

26 Petterino, C., Luzio, E., Baracchini, L. et al. (2011). Paraneoplastic leukocytosis in a dog with a renal carcinoma. *Vet Clin Pathol* 40: 89–94.

27 Locke, J.E. and Barber, L.G. (2006). Comparative aspects and clinical outcomes of canine renal hemangiosarcoma. *J Vet Intern Med* 20: 962–967.

28 Shor, S., Helfand, S.C., Gorman, E., and Lohr, C.V. (2009). Diagnostic exercise: epithelioid hemangiosarcoma mimicking metastatic prostatic neoplasia in a dog. *Vet Pathol* 46: 548–552.

29 Sawa, M., Inoue, M., Yabuki, A. et al. (2017). Rapid immunocytochemistry for the detection of cytokeratin and vimentin: assessment of its diagnostic value in neoplastic diseases of dogs. *Vet Clin Pathol* 46: 172–178.

30 Rigas, J.D., Smith, T.J., Gorman, M.E. et al. (2012). Primary ureteral giant cell sarcoma in a Pomeranian. *Vet Clin Pathol* 41: 141–146.

31 Monaghan, K., Nolan, B., and Labato, M. (2012). Feline acute kidney injury: approach to diagnosis, treatment, and prognosis. *J Feline Med Surg* 14: 785–793.

32 Granum, L., Gorman, E., Ruaux, C., and Vernau, W. (2015). Biphenotypic B-cell lymphoma in 2 cats. *Vet Clin Pathol* 44: 320–325.

33 Michael, H.T., Sharkey, L.C., Kovi, R.C. et al. (2013). Pathology in practice. Renal nephroblastoma in a young dog. *J Am Vet Med Assoc* 15: 471–473.

34 Jarchow, A. and Hanzlicek, A. (2015). Antigenemia without antigenuria in a cat with histoplasmosis. *JFMS Open Rep* 1: 2055116915618422.

35 Helms, S.R. and McLeod, C.G. (2000). Systemic *Exophiala jeanselmei* infection in a cat. *J Am Vet Med Assoc* 217: 1858–1861.

36 Taulescu, M.A., Ionică, A.M., Diugan, E. et al. (2016). First report of fatal systemic *Halicephalobus gingivalis* infection in two Lipizzaner horses from Romania: clinical, pathological, and molecular characterization. *Parasitol Res* 115: 1097–1103.

37 Puschner, B. and Reimschuessel, R. (2011). Toxicosis caused by melamine and cyanuric acid in dogs and cast: uncovering the mystery and subsequent global implications. *Clin Lab Med* 31: 181–199.

38

Urinary Bladder

Joyce S. Knoll and Mary Anna Labato

Introduction

Many disorders of the urinary bladder have a similar clinical presentation of hematuria, pollakiuria and/or stranguria, and incontinence. Ultrasound, contrast radiography, and cystoscopy can be essential for identifying the presence of bladder lesions. Cytology preparations of these lesions are most useful for diagnosis of transitional cell carcinoma (TCC); finding epithelial cells with multiple criteria of malignancy can provide a diagnosis without the need for more invasive techniques.

Collection

Indications

When evaluation of urine sediment fails to identify the cause of the clinical signs, or if atypical cells are noted in the sediment, further evaluation of the urinary bladder is warranted.

Methods

There are several methods to obtain urinary bladder origin cells for evaluation, including urine sediment (see Chapter 39), traumatic urethral catheterization, percutaneous fine-needle aspiration (FNA), and cystoscopy. The least invasive is a free catch voided sample, but it is also the least accurate for assessing the bladder, especially when there is a concern for neoplasia.[1] Cells in urine will deteriorate over time, losing essential morphologic features.[2] While the presence of atypical cells can suggest a diagnosis of neoplasia, the location of the tumor (e.g. bladder, urethra, prostate) cannot be determined. Because of variable rates of tumor exfoliation, negative results are inconclusive. One study found that urine cytology successfully diagnosed only approximately 30% of TCCs.[1]

Collection of a sample directly from the bladder, either via percutaneous FNA or cystoscopy, can increase cellularity and optimize essential morphologic features, increasing the likelihood of a diagnosis.[1] Traumatic catheterization and suction techniques can be performed blindly,[3] via ultrasound guidance,[4–6] or using the instrument channel of the cystoscope. Depending upon the size of the patient, a 3, 5, or larger (8,10) French red rubber catheter is advanced retrograde along the urethra into the bladder. After emptying the bladder of urine, the catheter is directed into the lesion. Ultrasound guidance will help bring the tip of the catheter with side ports into the mass. The plunger of the syringe is rapidly withdrawn three to five times, and then, while maintaining negative pressure, the catheter is quickly withdrawn from the urethra. The sample is placed in saline, while the process is repeated three to four times. Samples can be used for cytology or histopathology. When using cystoscopy, the sample is obtained using a syringe attached to the channel port. Brush cytology is another option. The brush can be advanced through the working channel of a cystoscope or advanced retrograde along the urethra. Traumatic suction biopsies have been performed using a cystoscope, but more often direct visualization facilitates collection using a cytology brush or a biopsy instrument (Figure 38.1). Percutaneous FNA of the bladder wall or mass is ideally performed with ultrasound assistance. Smears should be air-dried and stained with a Romanowsky stain such as Diff-Quik or Wright stain. While a Sedi-Stain wet mount may be useful for diagnosis of inflammatory disease, this type of preparation is not recommended when neoplasia is suspected.

Veterinary Cytology, First Edition. Edited by Leslie C. Sharkey, M. Judith Radin, and Davis Seelig.

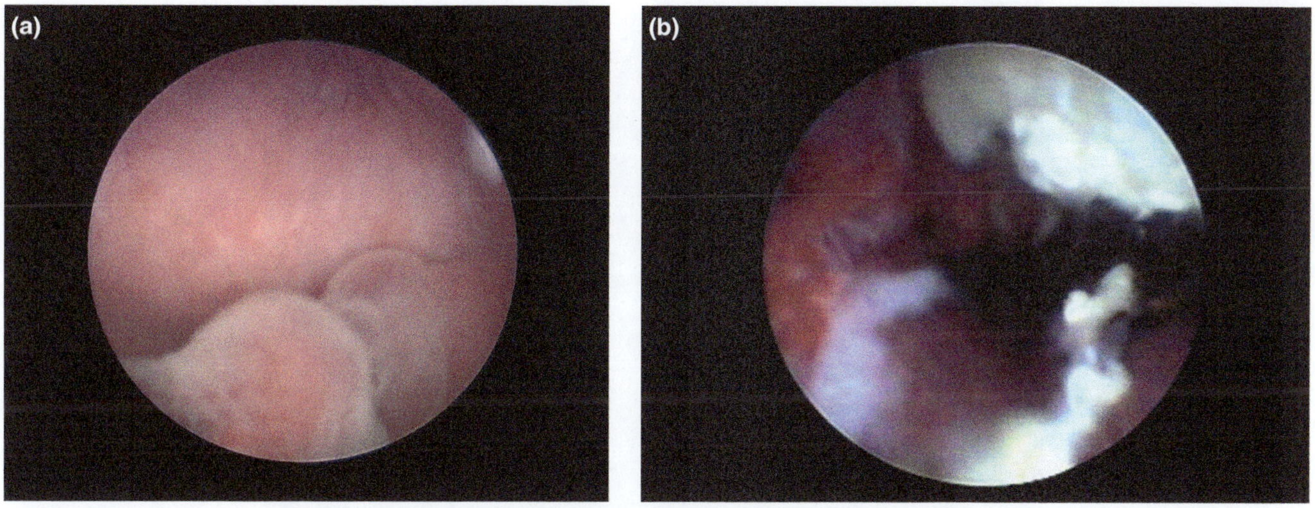

Figure 38.1 Cystoscopic images of bladder lesions. While these images illustrate some typical gross features of benign versus neoplastic lesions, tissue sampling (cytology or biopsy) is still needed to confirm the diagnosis. (a) Cystoscopic image of an inflammatory polyp. Note the smooth and somewhat cystic appearance of the lesion. This lesion is typical of polyps and helps to distinguish this from a TCC. Cytology samples can be obtained via cytology brush or biopsy forceps. (b) Cystoscopic image of TCC. The fluffy irregular surface helps to distinguish this from a polyp or papilloma.

Safety

Common complications are typically mild and include hemorrhage (gross and microscopic), stranguria and dysuria. Bladder or urethral rupture is a very rare complication of collection by traumatic catheterization and is most likely to occur if the catheter or cystoscope is in an area with very friable or necrotic tissue. Surgery will be needed to close a tear in the bladder. If the tear involves the urethra, it can usually be treated with an indwelling urinary catheter for a minimum of a week of healing.

Seeding of TCC has been reported following percutaneous FNA or even cystocentesis (Figure 38.2), but the incidence of this complication appears to be low.[7–11] Cutaneous metastases are more often caused by tumor cell "spilling" during a surgical procedure to remove or debulk the tumor, with one study reporting abdominal wall lesions in 10.2% (18/177) of those dogs who had undergone cystotomy, compared with an incidence of only 1.6% (6/367) in dogs without a history of cystotomy.[12] Incontinence and tumor seeding of urine scalded skin can be another important cause of cutaneous lesions, especially ones around the prepuce and vulva.[13] Whatever the cause, once TCC becomes established in the skin, response to treatment is poor, and owners often elect euthanasia due to a perceived poor quality of life.[12,13] Therefore, although tumor seeding by FNA may be uncommon, this method of collection should only be used if other methods fail to obtain a diagnostic specimen.

With all techniques, a nondiagnostic sample due to insufficient cellularity or a high proportion of broken cells is an unfavorable possibility. The presence of lubricant or ultrasound gel in samples collected by catheter or ultrasound-guided techniques, respectively, can obscure cellular morphology and absorb the stain, resulting in inadequate staining of cells.

Normal Tissue Architecture and Cytology

The urinary bladder lumen is lined by a stratified epithelium, consisting of three to six layers of transitional epithelial cells that provide a barrier against injurious substances and pathogens. Because these cells are unique to the urinary tract, they are also known as urothelium. However, in this chapter, the more common term transitional epithelium will be used. The epithelium has three functionally distinct layers: one apical row of umbrella cells, several layers of intermediate cells (number varies by species), and a single row of proliferative basal cells. The barrier function is largely achieved through umbrella cell specializations,[14] including tight junctions, lateral membrane interdigitations, an apical glycan layer, and a unique apical membrane containing the transmembrane protein uroplakin.[15] Large changes in urine volume are accommodated through umbrella cells altering their apical surface area by dynamic apical membrane exocytosis/endocytosis. Distention of the bladder is facilitated by fusion of cytoplasmic vesicles with the cell's apical surface.[16,17] Uroplakins are highly specific for mammalian

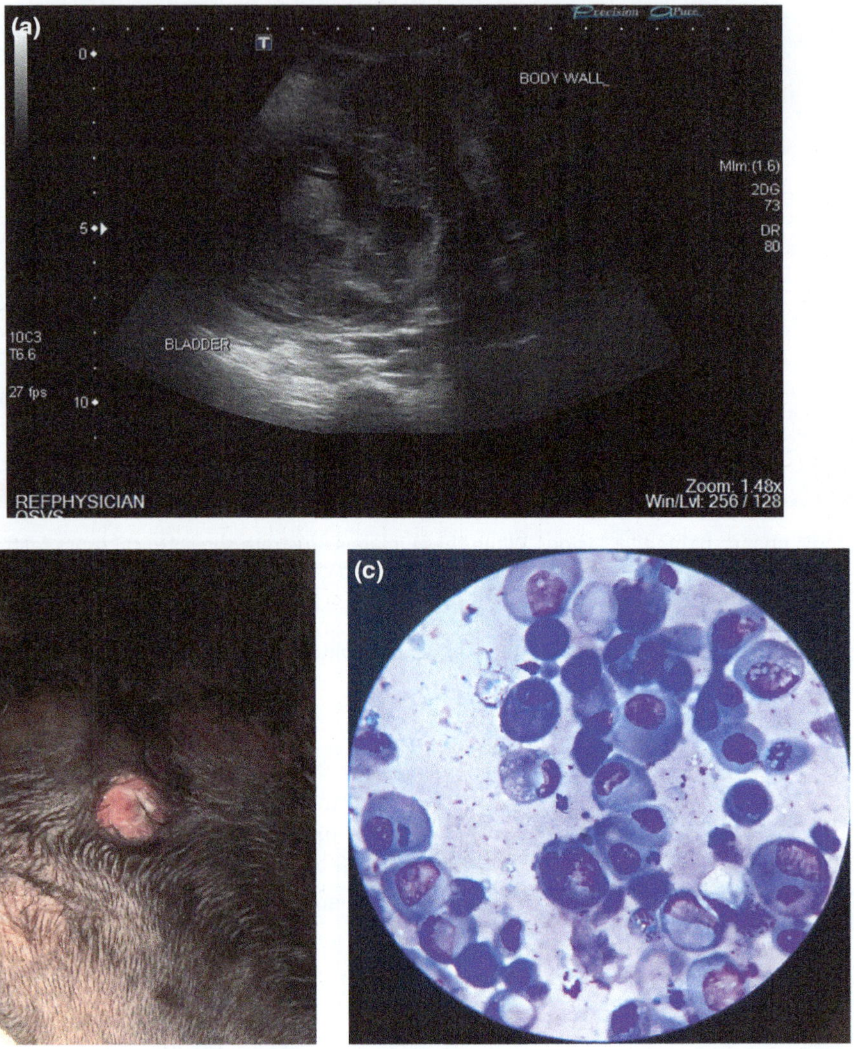

Figure 38.2 Images from a 10-year-old Labrador retriever diagnosed with TCC and cutaneous metastasis. (a) Ultrasound of bladder. Note the large, broad-based, irregularly shaped mass extending into the bladder lumen. The bladder wall is diffusely thickened. In the near field, there is a poorly echogenic mass (2.5 cm) extending from the bladder into the ventral body wall. (b) Ulcerated, cutaneous lesion. Following cystocentesis for recurrent urinary tract infections, this dog developed bilateral lesions on the ventral abdomen over the region of the bladder. (c) Impression smear of the cutaneous lesion is consistent with TCC. While a number of these cells appear individualized, many are loosely cohesive, forming small clusters. The cells are round with a moderate amount of basophilic cytoplasm, sometimes containing some small, pale cytoplasmic vacuoles, and they exhibit moderate anisocytosis and anisokaryosis. While some of the nuclei are poorly preserved and pyknotic, the better preserved cells have nuclei that are irregularly round to reniform with coarse chromatin and occasionally a large nucleolus. Few cells are binucleated (Diff-Quik, 1000×. *Source:* Images courtesy of Andrew Adezio).

transitional epithelium and facilitate epithelial stabilization during bladder distention. A dense capillary plexus in the lamina propria removes any substances that penetrate through the transitional epithelium, explaining the frequency of hematuria in bladder disease. The layers of the smooth muscle forming the detrusor muscle have a spiral orientation around the bladder in a way that facilitates complete expulsion of urine from the lumen.

Cytology of a healthy bladder should contain few cells, although in the authors' experience, their numbers can be higher in samples collected by suction or transurethral catheterization due to traumatic sloughing. The cells are round, oval, or pear shaped, with a moderate amount of lightly basophilic cytoplasm and well-defined cell margins. They vary considerably in size, with a cell diameter from 9 to 40 µm, perhaps reflecting their origins from different layers of the transitional epithelium (Figure 38.3a).[18,19] Nuclei

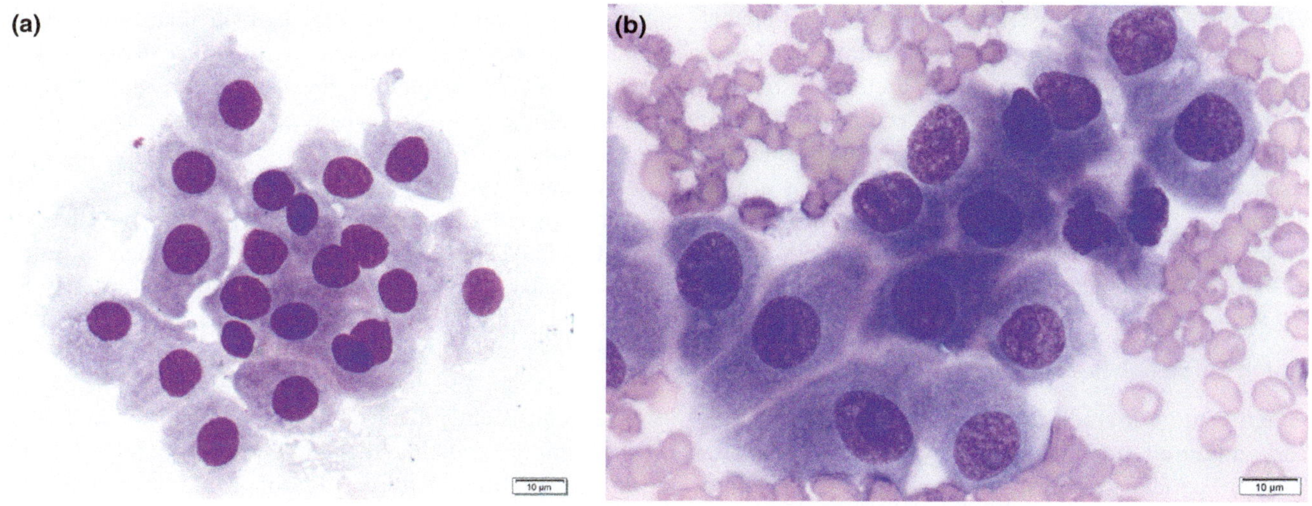

Figure 38.3 Cytologic appearance of normal and hyperplastic transitional epithelium. (a) This cluster of normal transitional cells was collected from a thickened bladder wall by cystoscope and cytology brush. The cells are irregularly round to polygonal with a moderate amount of slightly grainy, lightly basophilic cytoplasm. The nuclei are round with a coarse chromatin pattern and lack visible nucleoli. Note the binucleated cell in the bottom of the cluster. The cells show mild anisocytosis and anisokaryosis (Wright stain) (b) This cluster of hyperplastic transitional epithelial cells was collected from an inflammatory polyp from a 9-year-old Labrador retriever with a history of uroliths. The cells have grainy, moderately basophilic cytoplasm. Their nuclei are round with a coarse chromatin pattern and a single prominent nucleolus. The cells show moderate anisocytosis and mild anisokaryosis (Wright stain).

are round to oval and either eccentrically or centrally located, with coarse chromatin and sometimes one or two small nucleoli. Binucleated and occasional multinucleated cells can be seen.[2] Few inflammatory cells should be found unless the sample has blood contamination.

Hyperplasia

Transitional cell hyperplasia, sometimes accompanied by inflammation and hemorrhage, can be caused by mechanical trauma (e.g. prolonged indwelling catheterization, uroliths), chronic inflammation, and treatment with cytotoxic chemicals.[20] These conditions will increase the number of transitional cells in the urine.[2] They can be found as solitary cells, loosely cohesive clusters, small clusters, or occasionally in large sheets (Figure 38.3b).[21] Cells can exhibit relatively mild atypia that includes increased cytoplasmic basophilia, decreased nuclear to cytoplasmic ratio (N:C), coarsely clumped chromatin, or sometimes a prominent nucleolus. Bland morphologic features should be interpreted with caution since it can be difficult to distinguish transitional cell hyperplasia from benign epithelial tumors or low-grade TCC. Furthermore, epithelial tumors can be associated with concurrent inflammation, infections, and the potential for hyperplastic changes, introducing a diagnostic dilemma. With ultrasonography, transitional cell hyperplasia will look similar to wall thickening associated with inflammation.

Neoplasia

Bladder tumors are most often diagnosed in dogs, comprising <1% of all tumors.[22] Bladder tumors are less common in cats, perhaps due to low renal excretion of cocarcinogenic tryptophan metabolites,[23] and rarely reported in horses.[22] Survey radiographs are not typically useful for identifying neoplasia of the bladder wall,[24] although radiographs can be useful for detecting metastatic disease in the lungs or osteolytic lesions in bones (pelvis, sacral bones, and vertebral bodies).[1] Positive and/or double contract cystography can demonstrate intraluminal filling defects. Abdominal ultrasound is the imaging method of choice for identification of urinary bladder tumors, and lesions 3 mm or greater can often be detected if the bladder is distended with urine or injected saline.[24] Ultrasound also can be used to assess regional lymph node involvement. Neoplasia of the bladder wall is generally characterized by focal mural thickening or an intraluminal mass.[24] However, echotexture is variable, and it is generally not possible to determine tumor type by imaging. Blood clots can be mistaken for neoplastic masses, but clots are often moveable and lack the internal blood flow typical of most neoplastic masses.[25]

With more invasive tumors, including TCC,[26] lymphoma,[27] and fibrosarcomas,[28] hydroureter and hydronephrosis are common complications secondary to ureteral obstruction. Cystoscopic visualization, if available, with either cytology or biopsy (ideally both), is the preferred diagnostic technique to determine the tumor type. Cytology is a quick screening test and can provide a definitive diagnosis. If cytology is equivocal, formalin-fixed tissue can be submitted to further characterize the lesion.

Benign Epithelial Tumors

Benign tumors include transitional cell polyps, papillomas, and, rarely, adenomas. Grossly, benign lesions often consist of papillary projections of transitional epithelium, and ultrasound reveals polypoid to pedunculated masses, most often arising from the cranioventral, or less often, the craniodorsal bladder mucosa.[29] Histologically, benign lesions are characterized by the presence and width of a stalk (papilloma and polyp) and the formation of glands in the lamina propria (adenoma). Cytology cannot distinguish benign tumors from hyperplasia or distinguish between these three distinct benign epithelial lesions, but it can help exclude non-epithelial tumors. The transitional cells in these lesions show minimal cellular pleomorphism, distinguishing them from TCC. Typical findings include variably sized, well-organized sheets of transitional cells with mild anisocytosis, a relatively high N:C, variable cytoplasmic basophilia, uniform nuclei, often with a coarse chromatin pattern, and occasional binucleated cells.[21,30] Aspirates from polyps can include a mixture of inflammatory cells.

Malignant Epithelial Tumors of the Bladder

Approximately 90% of the tumors in dogs, cats, and horses are epithelial in origin, and most are malignant.[22] TCC (urothelial carcinoma) accounts for at least 75% of the canine bladder tumors and 90% in cats.[22]

Transitional Cell Carcinoma

In animals, TCCs are locally invasive and very frequently metastasize, primarily to the internal iliac and sublumbar lymph nodes and commonly to the lung, abdominal organs such as liver and spleen,[31] and bone, especially lumbar vertebrae.[1,32,33] The incidence of skeletal lesions ranges from 8 to 14%,[1,32,33] and these are important to identify with imaging since bone pain can reduce quality of life, leading to euthanasia.[33] An eight-year-old castrated male Hound mix with TCC had metastasis to multiple joints.[34] Several reports suggest a slight predisposition in female dogs[35–37] and small breeds such as the Shetland Sheepdog, and Beagle.[1,36] The Scottish Terrier has an 18-fold increased risk compared with mixed breed dogs.[37] Other risk factors include obesity and exposure to older-generation flea control products, herbicides, and pesticides.[38]

Although cytology or biopsy is needed to confirm the tumor type, there are several sonographic features that suggest TCC. These tumors usually appear as single or multiple sessile, irregularly shaped intraluminal masses of variable echogenicity (Figure 38.2a). In dogs, TCC most often involves the trigone or dorsal wall, which helps distinguish them from benign epithelial tumors.[39] The trigone is less consistently involved in cats, with only about half of the tumors occurring there.[40] TCCs frequently have an abrupt transition between the tumor and normal bladder mucosa, although this demarcation can be less obvious in the highly infiltrative TCC.[26] Because these tumors are often invasive, they can affect all layers of the urinary bladder.[25] Diffuse infiltration of the bladder wall instead of the formation of a distinct mass is also possible with TCC, which can be interpreted as inflammatory cystitis. By contrast, polyps typically have a narrow base of attachment to the bladder wall.[39] TCCs are often highly vascular, as seen with color Doppler.

TCCs in most domestic animals are high grade tumors,[41] with strong criteria of malignancy, and it is therefore often possible to make a diagnosis cytologically. One report found that prostatic or urethral wash was diagnostic in 10 of 13 (77%) dogs, while FNA was diagnostic in 20 of 22 dogs (91%).[1] This diagnosis can be made by finding large, round to polygonal, markedly pleomorphic cells both individually and in variably sized clusters.[30,31] Cells typically show marked anisocytosis and anisokaryosis, with a variable to low N:C due to a low to moderate amount of variably basophilic cytoplasm. Nuclear chromatin is coarse with single to multiple variably sized round to irregular nucleoli. Binucleation, multinucleation, and mitotic figures can be present.[30,31] When inflammation is present, a greater level of pleomorphism is needed to distinguish TCC from transitional cell hyperplasia, since inflammation can induce some cellular atypia.[30] Some of the neoplastic cells can contain one or more characteristic large cytoplasmic vacuoles, ranging from 2 to 6 μm and containing finely stippled, pale-pink to magenta material (Figure 38.4).[31,42] These inclusions have been described for TCCs in humans and are known as Melamed-Wolinska bodies.[29] These inclusions can be seen in normal or neoplastic transitional cells;[43] similar appearing vesicles have occasionally been seen in human pulmonary carcinoma cells,[44] and there are anecdotal reports of similar inclusions in the mesothelium. These vesicles in transitional cells are PAS positive and will stain for uroplakin.

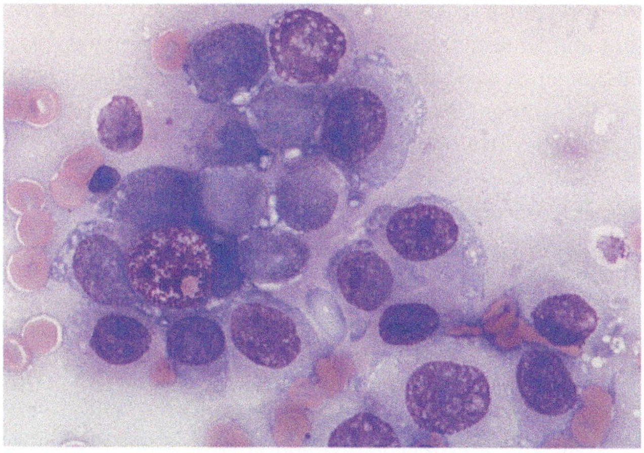

Figure 38.4 TCC from an 11-year-old Labrador retriever who presented for stranguria and pollakiuria and had been previously treated for recurrent urinary tract infections. The sample was collected by traumatic catheterization and suction. The neoplastic urothelial cells are loosely cohesive and pleomorphic, exhibiting significant anisocytosis and anisokaryosis. Nucleoli vary in number, size, and shape. One cell has a large vacuole filled with coarse pink material (resembling a Melamed-Wolinska body) that displaces the nucleus to one side of the cell. When present, this type of inclusion is characteristic of a TCC (Wright stain, 500×).

In humans, finding cells with these distinctive inclusions in a sample from a lymph node, body cavity effusion, or bone lesion warrants evaluation of the urinary tract and prostate for the presence of a TCC.[43] Clear vacuoles, displacing the nucleus and producing a signet ring appearance can also be seen but are less specific for TCC.

Recommendations for grading TCC as low or high grade are most applicable to histologic specimens, which can better assess mitotic index and tissue invasion.[22] It is important to note that cytology is best suited for identifying high grade TCC, since these manifest the most atypia. It is not possible to distinguish the less common low-grade TCC from a papilloma or hyperplastic lesion using cytology, especially in the presence of inflammation.

In the absence of a definitive histologic diagnosis, immunostaining for uroplakin III (UP III) can help confirm transitional cell origin and is especially useful to identify potential metastatic lesions in lymph node, skin, or bone. Commercial antibodies are suitable for histologic or cytologic preparations. UP III staining has been used to identify urothelial tumors and metastases in dogs, cows, and cats.[13,34,45,46] UP III is a terminal differentiation product of normal transitional epithelium, and staining is uneven within a TCC, with as few as 5% positive cells.[47] UP III expression can be lost in some high grade TCCs, reducing the negative predictive value of this stain.[48] Cytokeratin 7 (CK7) will also stain transitional epithelium and is more sensitive, with more intense staining, but is less specific and also labels non-urothelial cells, making it less useful for identification of metastatic lesions.[48] Although the mere presence of either UP III or CK7 cannot be used to distinguish neoplastic transitional epithelium from normal or hyperplastic tissue, an association has been shown between the grade of TCC and the immunohistologic staining patterns for these two markers.[46] In the normal transitional epithelium of higher mammals (e.g. humans, dogs, cattle) UP III and CK7 expression are restricted to the superficial umbrella cells;[47] this pattern persists in urothelial polyps and cases of polypoid cystitis.[46] By contrast, the majority of TCC had randomly distributed patchy immunoreactivity for UP III and CK7.[46] One recent immunohistochemical study found that TCC had significantly lower levels of p63, a homolog of the p53 tumor suppressor gene and cell adherence protein β-catenin.[49] TCC also had higher levels of proliferation marker Ki67 than seen in normal bladder urothelium or with polypoid cystitis. Low p63 expression was significantly related to the presence of vessel invasion and metastasis and has potential as a marker of TCC prognosis.[49]

Several urine tests have been promoted for early diagnosis of TCC, and details about these tests can be found in Chapter 39. The veterinary bladder tumor-associated antigen test (V-BTA; Cortland, NY, USA) is a noninvasive way to exclude TCC, but is not recommended due to a high rate of false positive results.[50–52] A newly developed test, which identifies a mutation in the canine BRAF gene, the CADET BRAF Mutation Detection Assay (Sentinel Biomedical, Raleigh, NC, USA) holds promise.[53]

Squamous Cell Carcinoma

Squamous cell carcinoma is the most commonly reported type of bladder tumor in horses but is occasionally reported in dogs and cats.[22,54,55] These tumors likely arise from a population of squamous cells identified in the trigone of the canine bladder or foci of squamous epithelium in the equine bladder, or as a sequela of squamous metaplasia of transitional epithelium.[2,22] Cytologic features are similar to those reported in other locations (Chapters 12, 19, 20, 21, and 30). Samples consist of a population of large round to polygonal pleomorphic squamous cells, with scant to abundant variably keratinized cytoplasm, often with perinuclear vacuolization. Squamous cells can be tadpole to spindloid. Asynchronous maturation of the cytoplasm and nucleus is characteristic. Areas of squamous metaplasia can also occur within TCC,[22] which might lead to a misdiagnosis of a squamous cell carcinoma, if this region was the only region sampled.

Mesenchymal Tumors

Primary mesenchymal tumors have been reported in dogs, cats, and occasionally in horses. Mesenchymal cells are unlikely to freely exfoliate into a cavity, so samples usually must be collected directly from mass lesions. Most mesenchymal tumors are cytologically similar, characterized by oval to spindloid cells that exfoliate individually or in small, loose aggregates. Cytoplasm is scant to moderate in amount, lightly to moderately basophilic, and sometimes contains small, clear punctate vacuoles. Cell margins can be poorly defined.

Leiomyoma and Leiomyosarcoma

Leiomyomas and leiomyosarcomas arise from smooth muscle in the bladder wall, with few reports in dogs and cats,[22] goats,[56,57] and a horse.[58] Three dogs had masses in the cranial to middle urinary bladder.[59] Smooth muscle tumors are suggested ultrasonographically by a smoothly marginated hypoechoic or heterogeneous intraluminal mass.[59] Unlike TCC, blood flow is not always visualized.[59] An intraluminal filling defect can be present.[59] Expression of desmin or smooth muscle actin by immunohistochemistry can help distinguish these tumors from fibromas or fibrosarcomas.

Fibroma and Fibrosarcoma

Fibrosarcoma is an uncommon bladder tumor in dogs and cats, with histologic and cytologic features similar to those found in more typical primary locations. Malignant variants tend to show greater pleomorphism compared with their benign counterparts, but histopathology is required for definitive diagnosis (Chapter 16). In the dog, fibrosarcoma in the urinary bladder is thought to have poor prognosis due to diffuse invasive growth and a high rate of metastasis.[35,60–62] While malignant bladder neoplasms usually occur in middle aged to older dogs,[35] fibrosarcoma was reported in the bladder of an 18-month-old Bassett hound[61] and a 14-month-old Gos d'Atura Catala.[62] These tumors might be less aggressive in cats, although, to date, there have been only two reported cases.[28,63]

Fibromas have been reported in the bladders of dogs, but not cats. They are described as single and well demarcated, sometimes forming a distinct polyp with a narrow stalk. They are composed of uniform fusiform cells with abundant stroma.[64] Because aggregates of neutrophils and eosinophils are common in these lesions, there is some controversy about whether these might actually be inflammatory fibrous polyps (i.e. eosinophilic cystitis), rather than benign neoplasms.[65,66] Regardless of how these lesions are classified, the cytologic presence of eosinophils suggests a benign lesion. Neutrophils are more difficult to interpret since fibrosarcomas often have superficial ulceration and/or secondary infection, with overlying hyperplastic transitional epithelium. Even cystoscopic biopsies can be misleading if they capture the superficial ulceration and miss deeper components of the lesion.

Hemangiosarcoma

Hemangiomas and hemangiosarcomas are uncommon in most species, with few reports of primary hemangiosarcomas in the canine bladders.[67–71] Metastatic hemangiosarcomas have been reported in horses.[72,73]

Botryoid Rhabdomyosarcoma

This variant of embryonal rhabdomyosarcoma is uncommon, but most often reported in bladders of young dogs (1–2 years of age)[60,74–79] and one 2-year-old filly.[80] Basset hounds and large breed dogs, particularly St. Bernards, are overrepresented with female predisposition (2 : 1).[22] Tumors usually occur at the trigone as botryoid masses projecting into the bladder lumen, which can be seen on imaging. Hypertrophic osteopathy has occasionally been associated with these bladder tumors in dogs.[81] Embryonal rhabdomyosarcomas recapitulate myogenesis; the botryoid variant has a distinctive histologic appearance than can be evident cytologically.[82] Tumors consist of spindle shaped or stellate cells with abundant basophilic cytoplasm and oval nuclei with coarse chromatin and prominent nucleoli. Large multinucleated cells with linearly arranged nuclei (strap cells) are intermixed. Some strap cells have cross striations extending the width of the cell. Low numbers of myotubes, forming relatively well-differentiated narrow muscle fibers can be present. These structures are more easily appreciated histologically, especially with phosphotungstic acid hematoxylin staining. Identification of strap cells and striations in a cytology preparation is diagnostic. Immunohistochemical staining for sarcomeric actin and myoglobin can help distinguish these tumors from other mesenchymal tumors.[83]

Round Cell Tumors

Lymphoma

Lymphoma has rarely been reported in the bladder of dogs, cats, and a horse.[84] While primary bladder lymphoma can occur, it usually accompanies generalized disease.[27,85–87] Lymphoma can arise in any part of the urinary bladder wall, presenting as variable echogenicity wall thickening or a mural mass with a smooth mucosal surface. There is often a long transition zone between the tumor and normal bladder wall, similar to smooth muscle tumors and consistent with infiltration of the mucosal and submucosal layers.[27,39] In some cases, lymphoma will invade adjacent

tissues through the bladder serosa, sometimes causing urinary tract rupture.[27] Lymphoma is cytologically suggested by large numbers of intermediate to large lymphocytes (Chapter 27) in urine sediment or an FNA of the bladder wall.[27,88] On routine urinalysis, large lymphocytes may be indistinguishable from other leukocytes when looking at an unstained wet mount. Preparation of an air-dried smear of sediment for cytologic examination may be necessary to identify the neoplastic lymphocytes.[88] Immunohistochemistry or flow cytometry can facilitate subclassification (Chapter 27).

Histiocytic Sarcoma

There is one report of a histiocytic sarcoma involving the bladder of a 1-year-old, male-neutered cocker spaniel.[89] Immunohistochemical staining (CD18+, CD3−, CD79a−, cytokeratin−, SMA−, and S100−) of a poorly differentiated round cell tumor confirmed the diagnosis. There was no evidence of regional lymph node involvement or distant metastasis, suggesting that this was a solitary (primary) tumor rather than a metastatic lesion.

Miscellaneous Tumors

There is one report of a peripheral nerve sheath tumor arising in the dorsal wall of a cat's urinary bladder and extending into the lumen.[90] Ultrasonography revealed a well-marginated, vascular mass of mixed echogenicity. Metastatic chemodectoma and ganglioneuroma have been reported.[91,92]

Inflammatory Conditions of the Bladder

Cystitis is common in dogs and cats and is often, but not always, due to a bacterial infection. Imaging can be unremarkable in early or mild cases. But in chronic and more severe cases, abdominal ultrasound or double contrast cystography can demonstrate diffuse thickening and irregularity of the urinary bladder wall, especially in the cranioventral portion of the bladder. The bladder wall might have decreased echogenicity, with a smooth outline of the mucosal surface and a gradual transition from edematous to normal mucosa.[24]

Noninfectious Cystitis

Feline Idiopathic Cystitis

While a variety of conditions can cause lower urinary tract disease in cats, the exact cause is unknown in most nonobstructed cats, leading to a diagnosis of feline idiopathic cystitis (FIC).[93] Cats diagnosed with FIC have a variety of clinical presentations, including urethral obstruction or nonobstructive disease with either an acute self-limiting episode or more chronic disease, sometimes with frequently recurring episodes.[93] While the underlying cause is unknown, studies suggest multiple potential causes of FIC including local bladder abnormalities (e.g. decreased glycosaminoglans[94,95] and increased epithelium permeability[96,97]), stress-related neuroendocrine changes (e.g. increased plasma catecholamines[98,99] and increased concentration of corticotropin-releasing factor in the cerebrospinal fluid[98]), and environmental factors contributing to stress and/or reduced voiding frequency and increased urine concentration.[93] Ultrasound shows a thickened bladder wall from edema and hemorrhage due to vasodilation of submucosal vessels. Significant mononuclear or neutrophilic infiltrate is absent, although increased numbers of mast cells have been observed in the bladder of cats with FIC.[100–102] It has been suggested that mast cell activation could be a by-product of the stress response associated with this disorder.[101,103] These histologic changes are reflected in the urinalysis that often shows hematuria, sometimes with small clusters of mildly atypical (hyperplastic) transitional cells.[30] Cytology and biopsy are not usually indicated in these cases. Since FIC is a diagnosis of exclusion, urinalysis, survey radiographs, quantitative urine culture, and abdominal ultrasound are warranted to exclude urolithiasis, urinary tract infection, and anatomic defects such as ectopic ureter.

Drug-Induced Cystitis

There is widespread awareness of the role of cyclophosphamide as a cause of sterile hemorrhagic cystitis (SHC) in people, dogs, and cats.[104] SHC is characterized by lower urinary tract signs (hematuria, stranguria, and pollakiuria) in the absence of urinary tract infection. Acrolein, a cyclophosphamide breakdown product, causes submucosal edema and hemorrhage, along with necrosis and fibrosis of the bladder epithelium.[105,106] SHC from oral cyclophosphamide appears to primarily cause a delayed toxicity resulting from high cumulative doses.[106] In dogs, the incidence of SHC following oral administration of the maximum-tolerated dose of cyclophosphamide as an undivided treatment has been estimated at 9–15%.[107,108] One study found no cases of SHC in 57 dogs given a maximum-tolerated dose of cyclophosphamide orally, divided over three days.[109] When a metronomic dosing protocol was used (i.e. daily or every other day administration of cyclophosphamide at much lower than the maximum-tolerated dose), almost 25% of dogs (16/65) developed SHC within 7–686 days (median of 110 days), based on development of hematuria.[105] The majority of these dogs (10/16) did not develop clinical signs of stranguria or pollakiuria.[105]

An apparent drug-induced cystitis following prolonged oral administration of phenylbutazone was reported in a 15-year-old Quarter Horse gelding and a 26-year-old Thoroughbred gelding with hematuria.[110] Cystoscopy showed ulceration and hemorrhage of the urinary bladder, with no evidence of uroliths. Although a definitive diagnosis was not made, hematuria and proteinuria resolved after discontinuation of phenylbutazone treatment and administration of synthetic prostaglandins.

Drug-induced cystitis associated with other drugs might be underreported. There is no specific histologic feature distinguishing drug-induced from interstitial cystitis; therefore the diagnosis is based on a high index of suspicion and a careful drug history. In people, drug-induced cystitis has been reported with several different nonsteroidal anti-inflammatory drugs (e.g. tiaprofenic acid, ketoprofen, diclofenac, and naproxen), and allopurinol.[111]

Polypoid Cystitis

Chronic inflammation in the urinary bladder can cause epithelial and stromal proliferation and polyp formation. Polyps consist of proliferative epithelium surrounding inflamed, hemorrhagic, connective tissue stroma. The bladder mucosa can form folds or villous mucosal projections that sonographically present as pedunculated masses (Figure 38.5).[29,112] Bladder wall samples contain variable numbers of inflammatory cells, ranging from predominantly lymphoplasmacytic to neutrophilic.[112] Mildly atypical hyperplastic transitional cells can be present. Polypoid cystitis is suggested when consistent cytologic and imaging findings are present. Some canine cases have been associated with cystic calculi, and concurrent bacterial infection is common.[112] Eosinophilic polypoid cystitis might be a variant of polypoid cystitis.[112,113]

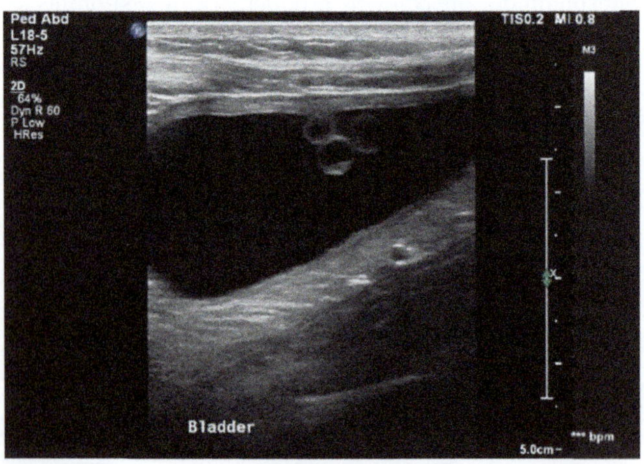

Figure 38.5 Ultrasound of urinary bladder with polypoid cystitis. The circular anechoic structures projecting into the bladder were reported as cystic polyps on histopathology.

Polypoid cystitis usually develops in the cranial ventral bladder wall, whereas TCCs more commonly arise from the bladder neck. It is impossible to distinguish polyps from low-grade TCC with complete confidence by gross or cytologic evaluation; histopathology is required.

Follicular Cystitis

Follicular cystitis is characterized by the formation of numerous lymphoid follicles in the lamina propria of the trigonal region of the bladder, and, in humans, likely results from repeated urinary tract infection. It has been reported in dogs associated with mild bladder wall thickening rather than mass lesions.[114,115] Follicular cystitis is cytologically distinguished from chronic cystitis by a prominent lymphocytosis including cells representing germinal centers of lymphoid follicles. Mildly atypical epithelial cells from the overlying hyperplastic urothelium can be seen. Follicular cystitis is distinguished from lymphoma by a more heterogeneous lymphoid population similar to a reactive lymph node.[114]

Infectious Cystitis

Canine Distemper Virus Infection

Cytoplasmic viral inclusions can be found within the urothelium of the bladder approximately 8–10 days after infection with canine distemper virus, during the acute respiratory phase of infection, sometimes before significant clinical signs.[116] These appear as variably sized, irregularly round, oval, or irregularly shaped eosinophilic inclusions (see Chapter 19 for images).

Bacterial Infections

Bacteria are a common cause of cystitis in dogs and cats, and diagnosis does not generally require imaging or sample collection for either cytology or histopathologic evaluation aside from urinalysis. Mildly atypical transitional cells may be found in a urinalysis due to secondary hyperplastic changes.[30] However, there are a few less common forms of urinary tract infection that warrant comment.

Emphysematous cystitis is an uncommon complication of infection of the urinary bladder by gas-producing microorganisms. A diagnosis is usually possible using survey radiographs, where variably sized gas opacities are associated with the bladder wall (and possibly the lumen). With ultrasound, the gas inclusions appear as hyperechoic areas with distal reverberation artifacts.[25] Care must be taken to distinguish these pathologic gas accumulations from intraluminal gas introduced during cystocentesis, catheterization, or endoscopy; this can be accomplished by repositioning the dog. While free luminal gas will move with a change in patient position, gas within the wall remains static. Reported bacterial isolates include *Escherichia coli*, *Enterococcus* spp., *Klebsiella pneumoniae*, *Proteus mirabilis*, *Streptococcus* spp., with *Actinomyces* spp., and *Enterococcus* spp. always part of a mixed infection with gas-producing bacterial species.[117] Most dogs with emphysematous cystitis have a predisposing condition such as diabetes mellitus, neurologic disease, or adrenal disease.[117]

Encrusting cystitis is an uncommon type of urinary tract infection, occasionally caused by urease producing bacteria. Urease activity leads to the formation of excessive ammonia, urine alkalization, and ammonium magnesium phosphate (struvite) deposition on the bladder mucosa. This type of cystitis is most often caused by *Corynebacterium urealyticum*, an aerobic, Gram-positive bacillus that has potent urease activity and strongly adheres to transitional epithelium.[118,119] This form of cystitis also has been reported secondary to *Corynebacterium matruchotii* infection in a horse,[120] and *Staphylococcus pseudintermedius* infection in dog.[121]

Ulcerative cystitis has been reported as a sequela of urine retention in horses with pelvic abscessation and adhesions,[122] and in horses with bladder paresis secondary to ingestion of sorghum-type plants.[123] Hydrocyanic acid, the toxic chemical found in sorghums, appears to be responsible for axon degeneration and demyelination, with subsequent bladder paresis and posterior ataxia. Some of these horses developed irregular polypoid masses that projected into the bladder lumen.

Conclusion

Diseases of the bladder result in nonspecific lower urinary tract signs including hematuria, pollakiuria, and/or dysuria. Imaging techniques, such as cystoscopy and abdominal ultrasound, help to identify ulceration and new growths in the urinary bladder, but do not allow the different types of tumor to be distinguished. Because there is overlap in the imaging appearance of various bladder/urethral tumor types and tumors and inflammatory conditions, biopsy is often necessary for a definitive diagnosis. However, cytology can be useful for diagnosis of TCC, mesenchymal tumors, and lymphoma, potentially eliminating the need for more invasive techniques. Although urinary tract infections do not typically require cytology or biopsy for a diagnosis, it is important to remember that TCCs will often be associated with secondary bacterial infections, and so recurrent infections may warrant diagnostic imaging and tissue sampling for cytologic or histologic assessment.

References

1 Norris, A.M., Laing, E.J., Valli, V.E.O. et al. (1992). Canine bladder and urethral tumors: a retrospective study of 115 cases (1980–1985). *J Vet Intern Med* 6: 145–153.

2 Batamuzi, E.K. and Kristensen, F. (1995). Diagnostic importance of urothelial cells of the dog and cat. *J Small Anim Pract* 36: 17–21.

3 Nyland, T., Wallack, S., and Wisner, E. (2004). Needle-tract implantation following US-guided fine-needle aspiration biopsy of transitional cell carcinoma of the bladder, urethra, and prostate. *Vet Radiol Ultrasound* 43: 50–53.

4 Melhoff, T. and Osborne, C. (1977). Catheter biopsy of the urethra, urinary bladder, and prostate gland. In: *Current Veterinary Therapy*, (ed. Kirk, R.), vol. VII. Philadelphia, PA: W.B. Saunders, 1173–1175.

5 Hager, D.A., Nyland, T.G., and Fisher, P. (1985). Ultrasound-guided biopsy of the canine liver, kidney and prostate. *Vet Radiol* 26: 82–88.

6 Lamb, C.R., Trower, N.D., and Gregory, S.P. (1996). Ultrasound-guided catheter biopsy of the lower urinary tract: technique and results in 12 dogs. *J Small Anim Pract* 37: 413–416.

7 Lopez, J. and Norman, B.C. (2014). Ultrasound-guided urinary bladder biopsy through a urinary catheter in a bitch. *J Am Anim Hosp Assoc* 50: 414–416.

8 Fry, M.M. (2011). Cytology of the urinary tract and prostate. In: *Nephrology and Urology of Small Animals*, (eds. Bartges, J., and Polzin, D.J.), Hoboken, NJ: Wiley-Blackwell.

9 Knapp, D.W., Ramos-Vara, J.A., Moore, G.E. et al. (2014). Urinary bladder cancer in dogs, a naturally occurring model for cancer biology and drug development. *ILAR J* 55: 100–118.

10 Vap, L.M. and Shropshire, S.B. (2017). Urine cytology: collection, film preparation, and evaluation. *Vet Clin North Am Small Anim Pract* 47: 135–149.

11 Vignoli, M., Rossi, F., Chierci, C. et al. (2007). Needle tract implantation after fine needle aspiration biopsy (FNAB) of transitional cell carcinoma of the urinary bladder and adenocarcinoma of the lung. *Schweiz Arch Tierheilkd* 49: 314–318.

12 Higuchi, T., Burcham, G., Childress, M.O. et al. (2013). Characterization and treatment of transitional cell carcinoma of the abdominal wall in dogs: 24 cases (1985–2010). *J Am Vet Med Assoc* 242: 499–506.

13 Reed, L.T., Knapp, D.W., and Miller, M.A. (2012). Cutaneous metastasis of transitional cell carcinoma in 12 dogs. *Vet Pathol* 50: 676–681.
14 Khandelwal, P., Abraham, S.N., and Apodaca, G. (2009). Cell biology and physiology of the uroepithelium. *Am J Physiol Ren Physiol* 297: F1477–F1501.
15 Kreplak, L., Wang, H., Aebi, U., and Kong, X.-P. (2007). Atomic force microscopy of mammalian urothelial surface. *J Mol Biol* 374: 365–373.
16 Lewis, S.A. and de Moura, J.L. (1982). Incorporation of cytoplasmic vesicles into apical membrane of mammalian urinary bladder epithelium. *Nature* 297: 685–688.
17 Truschel, S.T., Wang, E., Ruiz, W.G. et al. (2002). Stretch-regulated exocytosis/endocytosis in bladder umbrella cells. *Mol Biol Cell* 13: 830–846.
18 Bibbo, M. and Kern, W.H. (2015). Urinary tract. In: *Comprehensive Cytopathology*, (ed. Bibbo, M., and Wilbur, D.C.), 3e, 409–437. Amsterdam: Elsevier.
19 Osborne, C.A. and Steven, J.S. (1981). *Handbook of Canine and Feline Urinalysis*, 145. St Louis, MO: Ralston Purina.
20 Gopinath, C. and Mowat, V. (2014). *Urinary Bladder Atlas of Toxicologic Pathology*, 126–128. New York: Springer.
21 Borjesson, D.L. and DeJong, K. (2015). Urinary tract. In: *Canine and Feline Cytology: A Color Atlas and Interpretation Guide*, (ed. Raskin, R.E. and Meyer, D.J.), 3e, 284–294. St Louis, MO: Elsevier.
22 Meuten, D.J. and Meuten, T.L.K. (2016). Tumors of the urinary system. In: *Tumors in Domestic Animals*, (ed. Meuten, D.J.), 5e, 632–688. Ames, IA: Iowa State Press.
23 Beatty, J.A., Martin, P., Kendall, K., and Malik, R. (1999). Haematuria in a geriatric cat. *Aust Vet J* 77 (160): 166–167.
24 Leveille, R. (1998). Ultrasonography of urinary bladder disorders. *Vet Clin North Am Small Anim Pract* 28: 799–821.
25 Widmer, W.R., Biller, D.S., and Adams, L.G. (2004). Ultrasonography of the urinary tract in small animals. *J Am Vet Med Assoc* 225: 46–54.
26 Leveille, R., Biller, D.S., Partington, B.P., and Miyabayashi, T. (1992). Sonographic investigation of transitional cell carcinoma of the urinary bladder in small animals. *Vet Radiol Ultrasound* 33: 103–107.
27 Benigni, L., Lamb, C.R., and Corzo-Menendez, N. (2006). Lymphoma affecting the urinary bladder in three dogs and a cat. *Vet Radiol Ultrasound* 47: 592–596.
28 Greci, V., Rocchi, P.M., Sontuoso, A.F. et al. (2017). Primary fibrosarcoma of the urinary bladder in a cat: follow-up after incomplete surgical excision. *JFMS Open Rep* 3: 2055116917714881.
29 Takiguchi, M. and Inaba, M. (2005). Diagnostic ultrasound of polypoid cystitis in dogs. *J Vet Med Sci* 67: 57–61.
30 Weeden, A.L. and Wamsley, H.L. (2015). Atypical transitional epithelial cells. *Clinician's Brief*, 83–88.
31 Valli, V.E., Norris, A., Jacobs, R.M. et al. (1995). Pathology of canine bladder and urethral cancer and correlation with tumour progression and survival. *J Comp Pathol* 113: 113–130.
32 Webb, K., Stowe, D., DeVanna, J., and Neel, J. (2015). Pathology in practice. Transitional cell carcinoma. *J Am Vet Med Assoc* 247: 1249–1251.
33 Charney, V.A., Miller, M.A., Heng, H.G. et al. (2017). Skeletal metastasis of canine urothelial carcinoma: pathologic and computed tomographic features. *Vet Pathol* 54: 380–386.
34 Colledge, S.L., Raskin, R.E., Messick, J.B. et al. (2013). Multiple joint metastasis of a transitional cell carcinoma in a dog. *Vet Clin Pathol* 42: 216–220.
35 Hayes, H. (1976). Canine bladder cancer: epidemiologic features. *Am J Epidemiol* 104: 673–677.
36 Burnie, A.G. and Weaver, A.D. (1983). Urinary bladder neoplasia in the dog: a review of seventy cases. *J Small Anim Pract* 24: 129–143.
37 Knapp, D.W., Glickman, N.W., DeNicola, D.B. et al. (2000). Naturally occurring canine transitional cell carcinoma of the urinary bladder. A relevant model of human invasive bladder cancer. *Urol Oncol* 5: 47–49.
38 Glickman, L., Raghavan, M., Knapp, D. et al. (2004). Herbicide exposure and the risk of transitional cell carcinoma of the urinary bladder in Scottish terriers. *J Am Vet Med Assoc* 224: 1290–1297.
39 Hecht, S. (2015). Diagnostic imaging of lower urinary tract disease. *Vet Clin North Am Small Anim Pract* 45: 639–663.
40 Wilson, H.M., Chun, R., Larson, V.S. et al. (2007). Clinical signs, treatments, and outcome in cats with transitional cell carcinoma of the urinary bladder: 20 cases. *J Am Vet Med Assoc* 231: 101–106.
41 Mutsaers, A.J., Widmer, W.R., and Knapp, D.W. (2003). Canine transitional cell carcinoma. *J Vet Intern Med* 17: 136–144.
42 LeBlanc, C., Roberts, C., Bauer, R., and Ryan, K.A. (2004). Firm rib mass aspirate from a dog. *Vet Clin Pathol* 33: 253–256.
43 Ayra, P., Khalbuss, W.E., Monaco, S.E., and Pantanowitz, L. (2012). Melamed-Wolinska bodies. *Diagn Cytopathol* 40: 150–151.
44 Renshaw, A.A., Madge, R., and Granter, S.R. (1997). Intracytoplasmic eosinophilic inclusions (Melamed-Wolinska bodies) association with metastatic transitional cell carcinoma in pleural fluid. *Acta Cytol* 41: 995–998.
45 Carvalho, T., Naydan, D., Nunes, T. et al. (2009). Immunohistochemical evaluation of vascular urinary bladder tumors from cows with enzootic hematuria. *Vet Pathol* 46: 211–221.

46 Sledge, D.J., Patrick, D.J., Fitzgerald, S.D. et al. (2015). Differences in expression of uroplakin III, cytokeratin 7, and cyclooxygenase-2 in canine proliferative urothelial lesions of the urinary bladder. *Vet Pathol* 52: 74–82.

47 Wu, X.-R., Kong, X.-P., Pellicer, A. et al. (2009). Uroplakins in urothelial biology, function, and disease. *Kidney Int* 75: 1153–1165.

48 Ramos-Vara, J.A., Miller, M.A., Boucher, M. et al. (2003). Immunohistochemical detection of uroplakin III, cytokeratin 7 and cytokeratin 20 in canine urothelial tumors. *Vet Pathol* 40: 55–62.

49 Hanazono, K., Nishimori, T., Fukumoto, S. et al. (2016). Immunohistochemical expression of p63, Ki67 and β-catenin in canine transitional cell carcinoma and polypoid cystitis of the urinary bladder. *Vet Comp Oncol* 14: 263–269.

50 Borjesson, D.L., Christopher, M.M., and Ling, G.V. (1999). Detection of canine transitional cell carcinoma using a bladder tumor antigen urine dipstick test. *Vet Clin Pathol* 28: 33–38.

51 Billet J-P, H.G., Moore, A.H., and Holt, P.E. (2002). Evaluation of a bladder tumor antigen test for the diagnosis of lower urinary tract malignancies in dogs. *Am J Vet Res* 63: 370–373.

52 Henry, C.J., Tyler, J.W., McEntee, M.C. et al. (2003). Evaluation of a bladder tumor antigen test as a screening test for transitional cell carcinoma of the lower urinary tract in dogs. *Am J Vet Res* 64: 1017–1020.

53 Mochizuki, H., Shapiro, S.G., and Breen, M. (2015). Detection of BRAF mutation in urine DNA as a molecular diagnostic for canine urothelial and prostatic carcinoma. *PLoS One* 10: e0144170.

54 Fischer, A.T., Spier, S., Carlson, G.P., and Hackett, R.P. (1985). Neoplasia of the equine bladder as a cause of hematuria. *J Am Vet Med Assoc* 186: 1294–1296.

55 Traub-Dagartz, J.L. (1998). Urinary tract neoplasia. *Vet Clin North Am Equine Pract* 14: 495–504.

56 Lairmore, M.D., Knight, A.P., and DeMartini, J.C. (1987). Three primary neoplasms in a goat: hepatocellular carcinoma, pheochromocytoma and leiomyoma. *J Comp Pathol* 97: 267–271.

57 Timurkaan, N., Yener, Z., and Yuksel, H. (2001). Leiomyoma of the urinary bladder in a goat. *Aust Vet J* 79: 708–709.

58 Hurcombe, S.D., Slovis, N.M., Kohn, C.W., and Oglesbee, M. (2008). Poorly differentiated leiomyosarcoma of the urogenital tract in a horse. *J Am Vet Med Assoc* 233: 1908–1912.

59 Heng, H.G., Lowry, J.E., Boston, S. et al. (2006). Smooth muscle neoplasia of the urinary bladder wall in three dogs. *Vet Radiol Ultrasound* 47: 83–86.

60 Osborne, C.A., Low, D.G., Perman, V., and Barnes, D.M. (1968). Neoplasms of the canine and feline urinary bladder: incidence, etiologic factors, occurrence and pathologic features. *Am J Vet Res* 29: 2041–2053.

61 Schiller, A.G., Maksic, D., Beamer, P.D., and Albrecht, A.D. (1958). Fibrosarcoma of the urinary bladder in the dog. *J Am Vet Med Assoc* 133: 594–598.

62 Olausson, A., Stieger, S.M., Loefgren, S., and Gillingstam, M. (2005). A urinary bladder fibrosarcoma in a young dog. *Vet Radiol Ultrasound* 46: 135–138.

63 Capasso, A., Raiano, V., Sontuoso, A.F. et al. (2015). Fibrosarcoma of the urinary bladder in a cat. *JFMS Open Rep* 1: 1–6.

64 Esplin, D.G. (1987). Urinary bladder fibromas in dogs: 51 cases (1981–1985). *J Am Vet Med Assoc* 190: 440–444.

65 Gelberg, H.B. (2010). Urinary bladder mass in a dog. *Vet Pathol* 47: 181–184.

66 Fuentealba, I.C. and Illanes, O.G. (2000). Eosinophilic cystitis in 3 dogs. *Can Vet J* 41: 130–131.

67 Brown, N.O., Patnaik, A.K., and MacEwen, E.G. (1985). Canine hemangiosarcoma: retrospective analysis of 104 cases. *J Am Vet Med Assoc* 186: 56–58.

68 Martinez, S.A. and Schulman, A.J. (1988). Hemangiosarcoma of the urinary bladder in a dog. *J Am Vet Med Assoc* 192: 655–656.

69 Srebernik, N. and Appleby, E.C. (1991). Breed prevalence and sites of haemangioma and haemangiosarcoma in dogs. *Vet Rec* 129: 408–409.

70 Liptak, J.M., Dernell, W.S., and Withrow, S.J. (2004). Haemangiosarcoma of the urinary bladder in a dog. *Aust Vet J* 82: 215–217.

71 Sebastiani, V., Romanelli, G., and Zausa, F. (2009). Haemangiosarcoma of the urinary bladder in a dog. *Veterinaria (Cremona)* 23: 47–51.

72 Schumacher, J., Schumacher, J., and Schmit, D. (2002). Macroscopic haematuria of horses. *Equine Vet Educ* 14: 201–210.

73 Schumacher, J. (2007). Hematuria and pigmenturia of horses. *Vet Clin North Am Equine Pract* 23: 655–675.

74 Stamps, P. and Harris, D.L. (1968). Botyroid rhabdomyosarcoma of the urinary bladder of a dog. *J Am Vet Med Assoc* 153: 1064–1068.

75 Kelly, D.E. (1973). Rhabdomyosarcoma of the urinary bladder in dogs. *Vet Pathol* 10: 375–384.

76 Halliwell, W.H. and Ackerman, N. (1974). Botyroid rhabdomyosarcoma of the urinary bladder and hypertrophic osteoarthropathy in a young dog. *J Am Vet Med Assoc* 165: 911–913.

77 Pletcher, J.M. and Dalton, L. (1981). Botyroid rhabdomyosarcoma in the urinary bladder of a dog. *Vet Pathol* 18: 695–697.

78 Andreasen, C.B., White, M.R., Swayne, D.E., and Graves, G.N. (1988). Desmin as a marker for canine botryoid rhabdomyosarcoma. *J Comp Pathol* 98: 23–29.

79 Bae, I.-H., Kim, Y., Pakhrin, B. et al. (2007). Genitourinary rhabdomyosarcoma with systemic metastasis in a young dog. *Vet Pathol* 44: 518–520.

80 Turnquist, S.E., Pace, L.W., Keegan, K. et al. (1993). Botryoid rhabdomyosarcoma of the urinary bladder in a filly. *J Vet Diagn Invest* 5: 451–453.

81 Brody, R.S. (1971). Hypertrophic osteoarthropathy in the dog: a clinicopathologic survey of 60 cases. *J Am Vet Med Assoc* 159: 1242–1256.

82 Alleman, A.R. and Senior, D.R. (1991). What is your diagnosis? Bladder mass from an 11-month old dog. *Vet Clin Pathol* 20: 44–50.

83 Caserto, B.G. (2013). A comparative review of canine and human rhabdomyosarcoma with emphasis on classification and pathogenesis. *Vet Pathol* 55: 806–826.

84 Sweeney, R.W., Hamir, A.N., and Fisher, R.R. (1991). Lymphosarcoma with urinary bladder infiltration in a horse. *J Am Vet Med Assoc* 199: 1177–1178.

85 Maiolino, P. and DeVico, G. (2000). Primary epitheliotropic T-cell lymphoma of the urinary bladder in a dog. *Vet Pathol* 37: 184–186.

86 Bennett, S.L., Holland, J.A., and Meehan, M.C. (2003). Mural lymphoma associated with the urinary bladder of a cat. *Aust Vet Pract* 33: 155–159.

87 Kessler, M., Kandel-Tschiederer, B., Pfleghaar, S., and Tassani-Prell, M. (2008). Primary malignant lymphoma of the urinary bladder in a dog: long term remission following treatment with radiation and chemotherapy. *Schweiz Arch Tierheilkd* 150: 565–569.

88 Geigy, C.A., Dandrieux, J., Miclard, J. et al. (2010). B-cell lymphoma in the urinary bladder with cytological evidence of concurrent involvement of the gall bladder in a cat. *J Small Anim Pract* 51: 280–287.

89 Amores-Fuster, I., Elliott, J.W., Freeman, A.I., and Blackwood, L. (2011). Histiocytic sarcoma of the urinary bladder in a dog. *J Small Anim Pract* 52: 665.

90 Pavia, P.R., Havig, M.E., Donovan, T.A., and Craft, D. (2012). Malignant peripheral nerve sheath tumour of the urinary bladder in a cat. *J Small Anim Pract* 53: 245–248.

91 Patnaik, A.K., Lord, P.F., and Liu, S.K. (1974). Chemodectoma of the urinary bladder in a dog. *J Am Vet Med Assoc* 164: 797–800.

92 Sakai, H., Yonemaru, K., Takeda, M. et al. (2011). Ganglioneuroma in the urinary bladder of a dog. *J Vet Med Sci* 73: 801–803.

93 Forrester, S.D. and Towell, T.L. (2015). Feline idiopathic cystitis. *Vet Clin N Am Small Anim Pract* 45: 783–806.

94 Buffington, C.A., Blaisdell, J.L., Binns, S.P. Jr., and Woodworth, B.E. (1996). Decreased urine glycosaminoglycan excretion in cats with interstitial cystitis. *J Urol* 155: 1801–1804.

95 Pereira, D.A., Aguiar, J.A., Hagiwara, M.K., and Michelacci, Y.M. (2004). Changes in cat urinary glycosaminoglycans with age and in feline urologic syndrome. *Biochim Biophys Acta* 1672: 1–11.

96 Lavelle, J.P., Meyers, S.A., Ruiz, W.G. et al. (2000). Urothelial pathophysiological changes in feline interstitial cystitis: a human model. *Am J Physiol Ren Physiol* 278: F540–F553.

97 Birder, L.A., Wolf-Johnston, A., Buffington, C.A. et al. (2005). Altered inducible nitric oxide synthase expression and nitric oxide production in the bladder of cats with feline interstitial cystitis. *J Urol* 173: 625–629.

98 Westropp, J.L. and Buffington, C.A. (2003). Cerebrospinal fluid corticotrophin releasing factor and catecholamine concentrations in healthy cats and cats with interstitial cystitis. *Proceedings Research Insights into Interstitial Cystitis*. Alexandria, VA.

99 Buffington, C.A., Teng, B., and Somogyi, G.T. (2002). Norepinephrine content and adrenoceptor function in the bladder of cats with feline interstitial cystitis. *J Urol* 167: 1876–1880.

100 Hostutler, R.A., Chew, D.J., and DiBartola, S.P. (2005). Recent concepts in feline lower urinary tract disease. *Vet Clin North Am Small Anim Pract* 35: 147–170.

101 Sant, G.R., Kempuraj, D., Marchand, J.E., and Theoharides, T.C. (2007). The mast cell in interstitial cystitis: role in pathophysiology and pathogenesis. *Urology* 69: 34–40.

102 Buffington, C.A.T. (2011). Idiopathic cystitis in domestic cats: beyond the lower urinary tract. *J Vet Intern Med* 25: 784–796.

103 Buffington, C.A.T., Chew, D.J., and Woodworth, B.E. (1997). Animal model of human disease: feline interstitial cystitis. *Comp Path Bull* 29: 3–6.

104 Crow, S.E., Theilen, G.H., Madewell, B.R. et al. (1977). Cyclophosphamide-induced cystitis in the dog and cat. *J Am Vet Med Assoc* 171: 259–262.

105 Gaeta, R., Brown, D., Cohen, R., and Sorenmo, K. (2012). Risk factors for development of sterile haemorrhagic cystitis in canine lymphoma patients receiving oral cyclophosphamide: a case–control study. *Vet Comp Oncol* 12: 277–286.

106 Harper, A. and Blackwood, L. (2017). Toxicity of metronomic cyclophosphamide chemotherapy in a UK population of cancer-bearing dogs: a retrospective study. *J Small Anim Pract* 58: 227–230.

107 Garrett, L.D., Thamm, D.H., Chun, R. et al. (2002). Evaluation of a 6-month chemotherapy protocol with no maintenance therapy for dogs with lymphoma. *J Vet Intern Med* 16: 704–709.

108 Charney, S.C., Bergman, P.J., Hohenhaus, A.E., and JA, M.K. (2003). Risk factors for sterile hemorrhagic cystitis in dogs with lymphoma receiving cyclophosphamide with or without concurrent administration of furosemide: 216 cases (1990–1996). *J Am Vet Med Assoc* 222: 1388–1393.

109 Best, M.P. and Fry, D.R. (2013). Incidence of sterile hemorrhagic cystitis in dogs receiving cyclophosphamide orally for three days without concurrent furosemide as part of a chemotherapeutic treatment for lymphoma: 57 cases (2007–2012). *J Am Vet Med Assoc* 243: 1025–1029.

110 Aleman, M. and Nieto, J.E. (2011). Ulcerative cystitis associated with phenylbutazone administration in two horses. *J Am Vet Med Assoc* 239: 499–503.

111 Bramble, F.J. and Morley, R. (1997). Drug-induced cystitis: the need for vigilance. *Br J Urol* 79: 3–7.

112 Martinez, I., Mattoon, J.S., Eaton, K.A. et al. (2003). Polypoid cystitis in 17 dogs (1978–2001). *J Vet Intern Med* 17: 499–509.

113 Ozaki, K., Nakahara, Y., and Narama, I. (2008). Polypoid eosinophilic cystitis with pseudosarcomatous proliferative tissue in a dog. *J Vet Med Sci* 70: 289–291.

114 Zaharopoulos, P. (2002). Cytologic manifestations of cystitis follicularis in urine specimens. *Diagn Cytopathol* 27: 205–209.

115 Sul, R.M., Hammond, G., and Pratschke, K. (2014). Follicular cystitis in a dog. *Vet Rec Case Rep* 2: e000106.

116 Henderson, S.E., Clark, E.S., Stromberg, P.C. et al. (2015). Pathology in practice. Canine morbillivirus infection. *J Am Vet Med Assoc* 247: 1375–1377.

117 Merkel, L.K., Lulich, J., Polzin, D. et al. (2017). Clinicopathologic and microbiologic findings associated with emphysematous cystitis in 27 dogs. *J Am Anim Hosp Assoc* 53: 313–320.

118 Nl, B., Westropp, J.L., Jang, S.S., and Ling, G.V. (2005). *Corynebacterium urealyticum* urinary tract infection in dogs and cats: 7 cases (1996–2003). *J Am Vet Med Assoc* 10: 1676–1680.

119 Raab, O., Beraud, R., Tefft, K.M., and Muckle, C.A. (2015). Successful treatment of *Corynebacterium urealyticum* encrusting cystitis with systemic and intravesical antimicrobial therapy. *Can Vet J* 56: 471–475.

120 Saulez, M.N., Cebra, C.K., Heidel, J.R. et al. (2005). Encrusted cystitis secondary to *Corynebacterium matruchotii* infection in a horse. *J Am Vet Med Assoc* 226: 246–248, 220.

121 Biegen, V.R., Slusser, P.G., Fischetti, A.J., and Geist, M.R. (2013). Successful treatment of encrusted cystitis associated with *Staphylococcus pseudintermedius* infection in the urinary bladder of a dog. *J Am Vet Med Assoc* 242: 798–802.

122 Squinas, S.C. and Britton, A.P. (2013). An unusual case of urinary retention and ulcerative cystitis in a horse, sequelae of pelvic abscessation and adhesions. *Can Vet J* 54: 690–692.

123 Adams, L.G., Dollahite, J.W., and Romane, W.M. (1969). Cystitis and ataxia associated with sorghum ingestion by horses. *J Am Vet Med Assoc* 155: 518–524.

39

Urine Cytology

Nicole M. Weinstein

Introduction

Microscopic evaluation of urine sediment is a commonly used diagnostic tool in veterinary practices and laboratories. Examination of unstained urine sediment to quantify a variety of formed elements is a standard component of the urinalysis, while examination of stained urine specimens (urine cytology) is often reserved for specific specimen types or clinical presentations. Evaluation of unstained sediment is more advantageous in some instances, including assessing numbers of erythrocytes and leukocytes as this quantification is easily standardized given established urinalysis protocols.[1–3] Also, some structures, such as hyaline, waxy, or granular casts, which can clearly be identified on unstained sediment preparations, are difficult to appreciate on cytology smears. Crystalluria is readily apparent on unstained sediments (Figure 39.1a). Staining sediment samples may preserve sediment smears with interesting crystalluria. While evaluation of unstained urine sediment does allow for identification of epithelial cells, leukocytes, and infectious agents, cytologic evaluation of dried and stained urine samples is recommended for the most accurate characterization of these formed elements (Figure 39.1b–d). Urine cytology is a logical extension of the microscopic sediment evaluation in routine urinalysis when more detailed evaluation of the cellular elements is needed or when infection is suspected. For this chapter, urine cytology and evaluation of unstained urine sediment will be approached as complementary but distinct diagnostic techniques, with a focus on the utility and known limitations of stained urine sample evaluation.

Indications and Collection Methods

Indications

Urine cytology is a method for identifying and diagnosing a spectrum of urinary tract disease and some systemic diseases that supplements traditional urine sediment evaluation. It can be useful in any animal with signs of lower urinary tract pathology. In patients with a bacterial urinary tract infection, a commonly diagnosed condition, confirmation, and more detailed characterization is provided by evaluation of routinely stained and/or Gram-stained slides (Figure 39.2).[4] Evaluation of stained urine samples can be useful for investigation of bladder masses or urethral abnormalities. In some cases, diagnosis via urine cytology can avoid more invasive and costly procedures such as fine-needle aspiration or biopsy of the urinary bladder (see Chapter 38).

Collection Methods

Collection methods are identical to those for routine urinalysis, including free catch, catheterization, and cystocentesis. Traumatic catheterization of urethral and/or urinary bladder masses, another method used to diagnose lower urinary tract disease, is covered in Chapter 38. This is useful in poorly exfoliative masses or when cell preservation is poor.

Free Catch

The advantages of free catch samples are frequently overlooked. For dogs at least, ease of collection is obvious. First morning samples, although often preferred for assessment

Veterinary Cytology, First Edition. Edited by Leslie C. Sharkey, M. Judith Radin, and Davis Seelig.

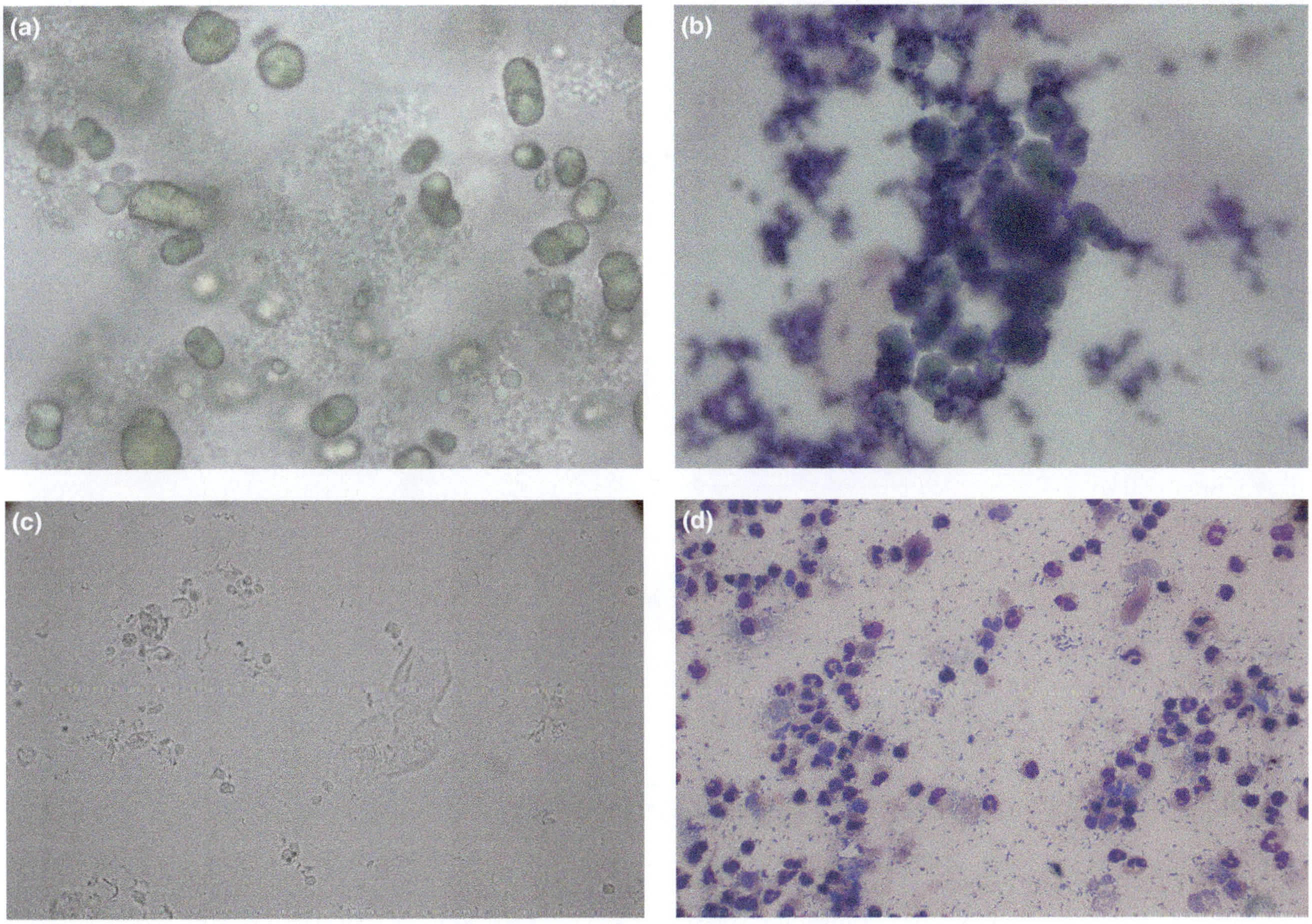

Figure 39.1 Comparison of unstained versus stained urine sediment. (a) Preparation with calcium phosphate carbonate crystalluria and many bacterial cocci (Unstained, 1000×). (b) Same urine sample as (a) but stained (modified Wright Giemsa, 1000×. *Source:* Images (a) and (b) courtesy of Reema Patel). (c) Leukocytes and bacterial rods with few squamous epithelial cells in urine sediment from a dog with a urinary tract infection (Unstained, 400×). (d) Same case as in (c) with more easily visualized bacteria and neutrophils (Wright Giemsa, 500×).

of urine specific gravity, might not be ideal for cytology samples because cells degrade in urine overnight. Free catch samples sometimes contain exfoliated cells from urethral masses, and the risk of seeding neoplastic epithelial cells from transcutaneous aspiration of a bladder mass is avoided.[5] There are infrequent reports that local spread also can occur from direct implantation of a urine-scalded epidermis.[5,6] Free catch samples do introduce potential contamination from the distal urethra, genital tract, or skin, which could influence interpretation of findings.

Catheterization

Assessing cellularity from catheterized samples should be done with caution. There can be cytologic overlap between squamous and some urothelial cells, and indwelling catheters or stents can cause hyperplasia and dysplasia to both squamous and urothelial populations.

Cystocentesis

Cystocentesis is often described as the preferred urine collection method, especially in cases where sterility is preferred. While this method limits introduction of bacteria and urethral squamous epithelial cells to the sample, neoplastic cells from masses located within the urethra are unlikely to be detected. There is also the concern for seeding of transitional cell carcinoma when neoplastic cells are present in urine.[5] While the risk of iatrogenic bleeding increases with cystocentesis, blood contamination does not preclude accurate cytologic evaluation.

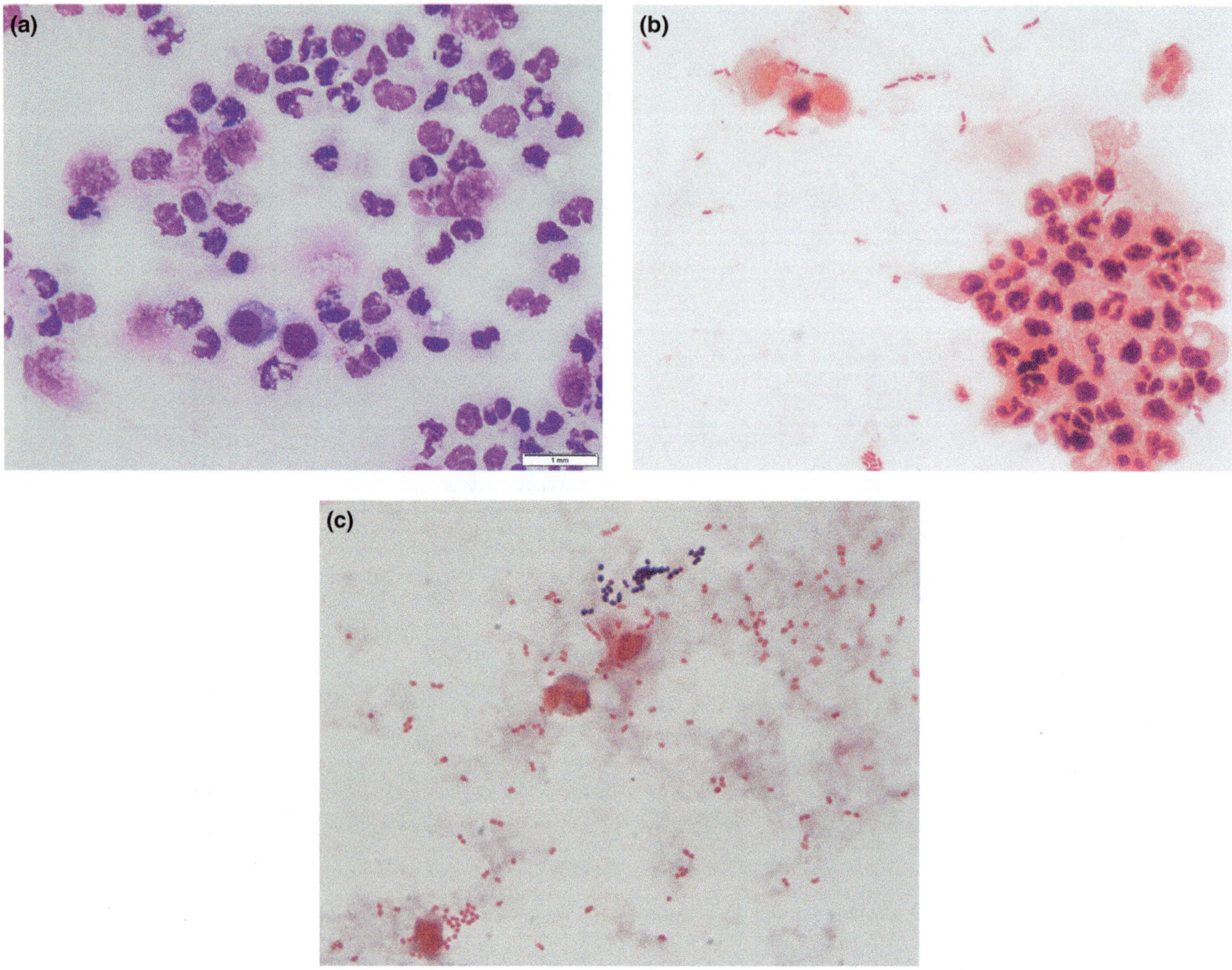

Figure 39.2 Bacterial urinary tract infection. (a) Numerous variably well-preserved and some degenerate neutrophils with intracellular bacterial rods (Wright Giemsa, 1000×). (b) Aggregate of neutrophils and frequent extracellular Gram-negative bacterial rods (Gram stain, 1000×). (c) Variable staining of bacterial cocci on a Gram stain (Gram stain, 1000×).

Slide Preparation

There is no standardized approach to urine cytology slide preparation in veterinary medicine. Cytologic evaluation of urine samples most often involves concentrating the specimen, either through preparation of urine sediment and/or cytocentrifugation of the specimen. The volume required can be estimated from evaluating specimen cellularity by examination of a direct wet prep. Care must be taken to maintain cell integrity.

Direct smears can be useful for high cellularity samples, especially if there is significant hematuria or many inflammatory and/or epithelial cells. Sediment smear slides can increase the cellularity of examined specimens and enhance the diagnostic quality. If the equipment is available, cytospin preparations maximize cell recovery and preservation. Samples with numerous erythrocytes due to hematuria or iatrogenic blood contamination are not ideal for this method. Diagnostic laboratories typically utilize specialized instruments for preparation of cytospin-centrifuged slides, but slides of similar quality can be prepared using a less conventional method incorporating a salad spinner.[7]

Romanowsky stains are preferred for the evaluation of dried urine specimens. The use of Sedi-Stain (BD Sedi-Stain™, BD Biosciences, San Jose, CA, USA) is intended for wet sediment preparation rather than dried preparation. In samples with suspected or proven bacteriuria, Gram staining of urine can assist in general classification of rods versus cocci. In human medicine, grading schemes are used to characterize epithelial cell atypia as neoplastic or not. These are based heavily on nuclear morphology, so the use of monolayer liquid-based cytology methods and Papanicolaou staining is common.[8] Papanicolaou staining enhances visualization of the nuclear membrane and chromatin, important components of grading schemes for routine cytopathology in people.[8] It does require specialized sample handling and sample preparation as well as a multistep stain protocol. Papanicolaou staining of cytology specimens in veterinary medicine has yet to gain significant traction for diagnostic purposes. A few reports describe the methodology involved with routine and rapid protocols, including some detail on cytologic findings. None emphasize urine cytology or differentiation of benign versus malignant urinary tract conditions similar to the grading system used in human cytopathology.[9–11]

Normal Tissue Architecture and Cytology

Normal microanatomy of the urinary bladder and urethra is covered in Chapter 38. Squamous and urothelial (transitional) epithelial cells comprise the majority of epithelial cells identified in urine cytology and urine sediment samples. Both can be present in otherwise normal urine samples, with greater numbers of squamous epithelial cells expected with catheterized and some free catch samples.

Urothelial Cells

Urothelial (transitional) epithelial cells are highly variable in size, shape, and even in number of nuclei.[12,13] In human pathology, urothelial cells are divided into (i) deep urothelial cells, which include basal and intermediate cells; (ii) larger and sometimes multinucleated superficial (umbrella) cells; and (iii) columnar epithelial cells.[13] In dogs, the term “ordinary” transitional epithelial cells have been used for deep and superficial cells.[12,13] Ordinary transitional/urothelial epithelial cells line the proximal and mid-urethra, urinary bladder, parts of the ureter, renal pelvis, and calyces.[12,13] Deeper cells are typically smaller, ranging from small and cuboidal to somewhat larger and ovoid with a centrally located round, finely granular to coarse nucleus, and indistinct nucleoli; cytoplasm is small to moderate in volume with occasional fine vacuoles.[13] Superficial cells are larger, similar in size to mature squamous epithelial cells, with abundant cytoplasm and a moderately sized nucleus, but multiple nuclei are described.[13] Caudate cells primarily line the ureters, renal pelvis, and calcyces.[12] Caudate transitional cells are often more elongate and columnar with an offset, small round nucleus and more elongated, slightly tapering cytoplasm opposite from the nucleus.[12,13] Normal variation in morphology reflects different cell populations and should not be mistaken for pleomorphism suggestive of neoplasia (Figure 39.3a–c).

Squamous Epithelial Cells

Squamous epithelial cells line the distal urethra and portions of the trigone as well as the vagina.[12] Squamous epithelial cells are polygonal with a small round condensed nucleus. Occasional cells display a slightly larger nucleus with more open chromatin, resembling transitional cells.[12] Cytoplasm is pale blue with angular borders, and cells often appear to fold.[12] Squamous epithelial cells can be numerous in catheterized urine samples and in some free catch samples (Figure 39.3d).

Renal Tubular Epithelial Cells

Renal tubular epithelial cells are not expected in urine sediment or cytology, and their presence has been associated with renal tubular injury and death.[14] Renal tubular epithelial cells are cuboidal to slightly columnar with a round, dense nucleus and a small amount of basophilic cytoplasm (Chapter 37). With tubular injury, cellular, granular, and waxy casts can be seen in unstained urine sediment. Formed cells reflect sloughing of individual or entire cellular casts.

Conditions Diagnosed by Urine Cytology

Epithelial Cell Hyperplasia, Dysplasia, and Neoplasia

Epithelial cells can be a normal and frequent finding in urine sediment and urine cytology even in patients without urinary tract disease. Both squamous epithelial cells and urothelial cells can be present, with numbers of each influenced by underlying urinary tract conditions and collection method and slide preparation techniques.[13,15,16] There can be notable variability in urothelial cell size, nuclear size, and even numbers of nuclei, which must be kept in mind when evaluating urine cytology.[12,13] There is some morphologic overlap between superficial urothelial cells and squamous epithelial cells due to their larger sizes, which can lead to difficulty in definitively differentiating one from another.[12,13] Morphologic variability of epithelial cells also results from contact with urine, collection technique, time from urine collection to slide preparation,

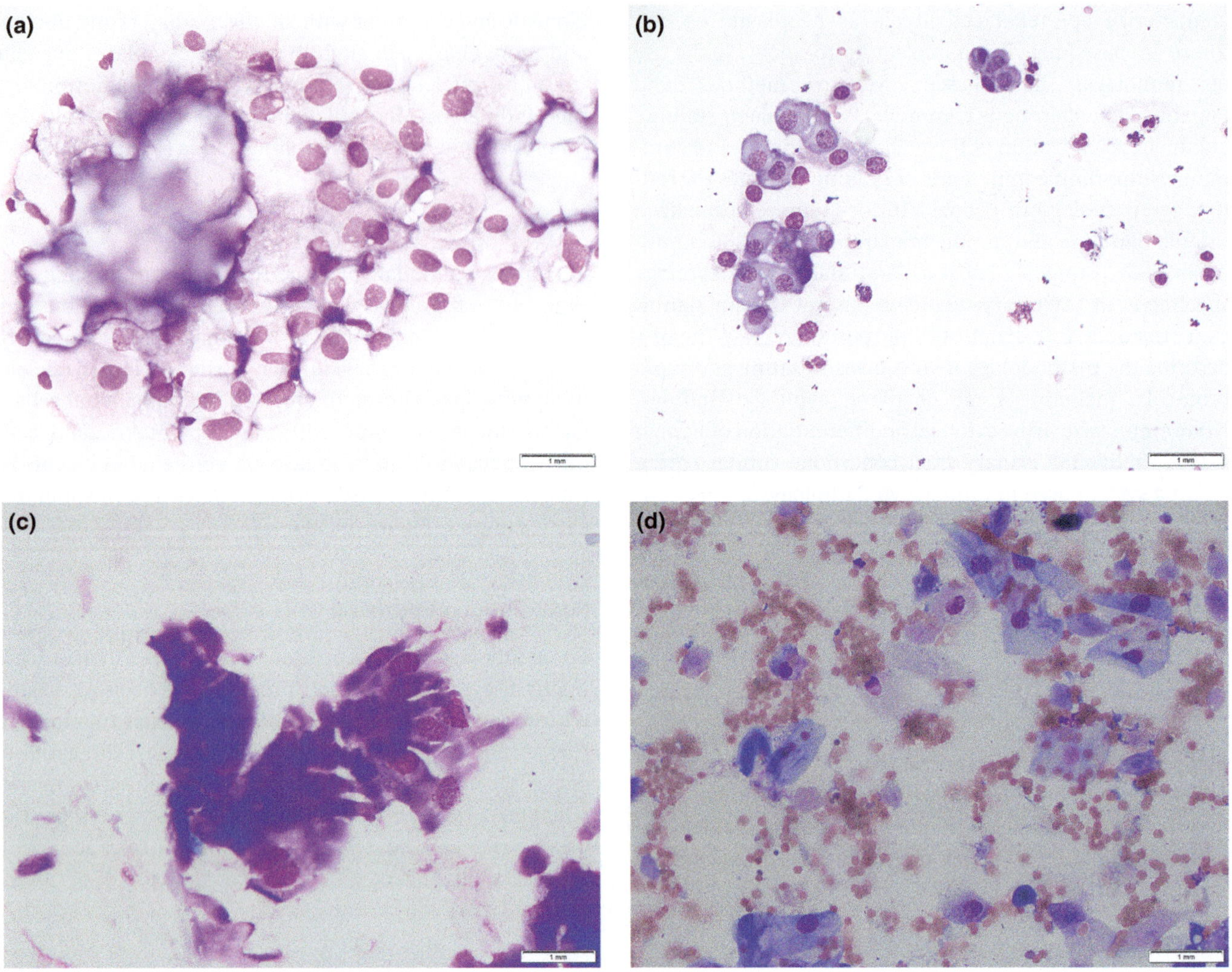

Figure 39.3 Different epithelial cell types present in urine. (a) Superficial urothelial cells in a dog with cystinuria and cystine stones (Wright Giemsa, 500×). (b) Urothelial hyperplasia in a dog with bacterial urinary tract infection and neutrophilic inflammation. Cells consistent with intermediate and few basal urothelial cells are seen (Wright Giemsa, 500×). (c) Caudate urothelial cells from a dog with hypertension (Wright Giemsa, 1000×). (d) Squamous epithelial cells and hematuria from a female dog with pollakiuria, stranguria, and hematuria due to bladder stones (Wright Giemsa, 500×).

method of slide preparation, and concurrent urinary tract disease.

Degradation of epithelial cells following exposure to urine is common and can significantly hinder cytologic evaluation and negatively impact accuracy of diagnosis.[16] Changes secondary to urine exposure, sometimes termed "urine scalding" include nuclear swelling and disintegration, cytoplasmic vacuolization, and the appearance of cytoplasmic granulation (Figure 39.4a).[12] Routine Romanowsky stains likely do not allow for consistent differentiation of nuclear degeneration versus irregularities secondary to malignant transformation.[13,17,18] In the face of nuclear disruption secondary to urine scalding, only well-preserved epithelial cells should be assessed. This can require repeat sample collection and careful attention to sample processing.

Epithelial cell hyperplasia resulting from inflammation and chronic irritation can increase numbers of epithelial cells in urine (Figure 39.4b). This is commonly due to urinary tract infection, uroliths, an indwelling urinary catheter, a urethral stent, or epithelial or nonepithelial neoplasia.[13] Ultrasonographic findings sometimes include thickened areas in the urethra and/or bladder as a result of inflammation or physical irritation, and these can prompt urine cytology evaluation. Epithelial cell numbers and/or atypia in urine samples should be interpreted with caution in any animal with a potential cause for inflammation. As urothelial cells readily exfoliate, increased numbers do not

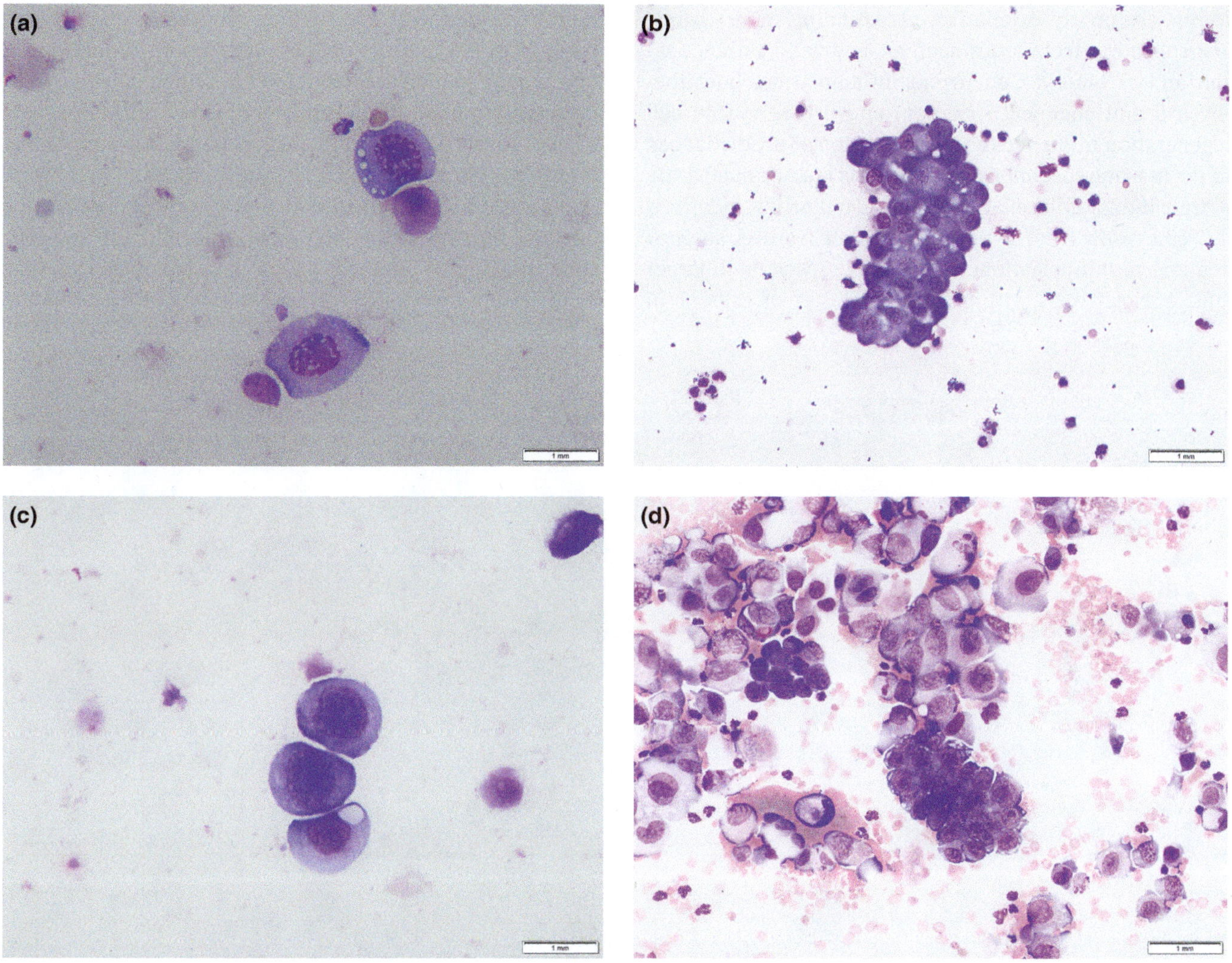

Figure 39.4 Atypical epithelial cell morphology in urine. (a) Nuclear degradation resulting in swollen nuclei in "urine-scalded" urothelial cells (Wright Giemsa, 1000×). (b) A cluster of epithelial cells with an increased N:C in a dog with a urinary tract infection (Wright Giemsa, 500×). (c) Urine from a 12-year-old female spayed Chihuahua with incidental bladder wall thickening and no lower urinary tract signs. Urine cytology was suspicious for carcinoma given the high N:C in several cells, mitotic figures (not pictured), and lack of inflammation. BRAF mutation was detected supporting urothelial neoplasia (Wright Giemsa, 1000×). (d) Urine from a dog with urothelial carcinoma. Nuclear atypia characterized by a markedly increased N:C, two- to threefold variation in nuclear size, occasional bi- and multinucleation, and prominent, large nucleoli in the neoplastic urothelial cells (Wright Giemsa, 500×).

necessarily reflect neoplasia. Fragments of urothelial cells, sometimes referred to as papillary clusters, can be seen secondary to routine or traumatic catheterization or the presence of uroliths.[13] In human medicine, the presence of papillary clusters even without atypia in a spontaneously voided sample in the absence of uroliths warrants additional evaluation for neoplasia.[13] There is known overlap between hyperplasia-induced dysplasia and morphologic changes associated with neoplastic urothelium. Both can be characterized by increased cell size and anisocytosis, an increased nuclear to cytoplasm ratio (N:C), coarse chromatin, and prominent nucleoli.[13] As areas adjacent to urothelial cell carcinoma can become hyperplastic, it can be difficult to definitively differentiate hyperplastic from neoplastic cells in complex lesions (Figure 39.4c and d).

Diagnosis of Transitional Cell Carcinoma (Urothelial Carcinoma)

Overlap in the ultrasound findings between benign and malignant lesions of the urinary tract prevents definitive diagnosis by imaging alone. Even in some urine cytology specimens, differentiation is challenging. Some mass lesions are poorly exfoliative, necessitating more aggressive collection techniques such as traumatic catheterization and/or biopsy. Concurrent inflammation, infection, physical and chemical irritation, and urine-induced cell degeneration influence the interpretation of urothelial cell atypia in urine specimens. Anisocytosis is a normal feature of transitional epithelial cells and a uniformly increased N:C can result from hyperplasia. Other features such as frequent multinucleation; a high N:C, especially in larger cells; anisokaryosis within a single cluster of cells or in multinucleated cells; immature chromatin; prominent, large, multiple, and/or angular nucleoli; and/or mitotic figures would all increase suspicion for malignancy in a well-preserved sample. High numbers of these cells, especially in the absence of confounding hyperplasia, support an interpretation of carcinoma (Figure 39.5). Some consideration should be given to epithelial cell numbers in both the unstained urine sediment preparation and the cytology slide preparation method. Cytospin samples can be misleading in more cellular specimens because differentiation

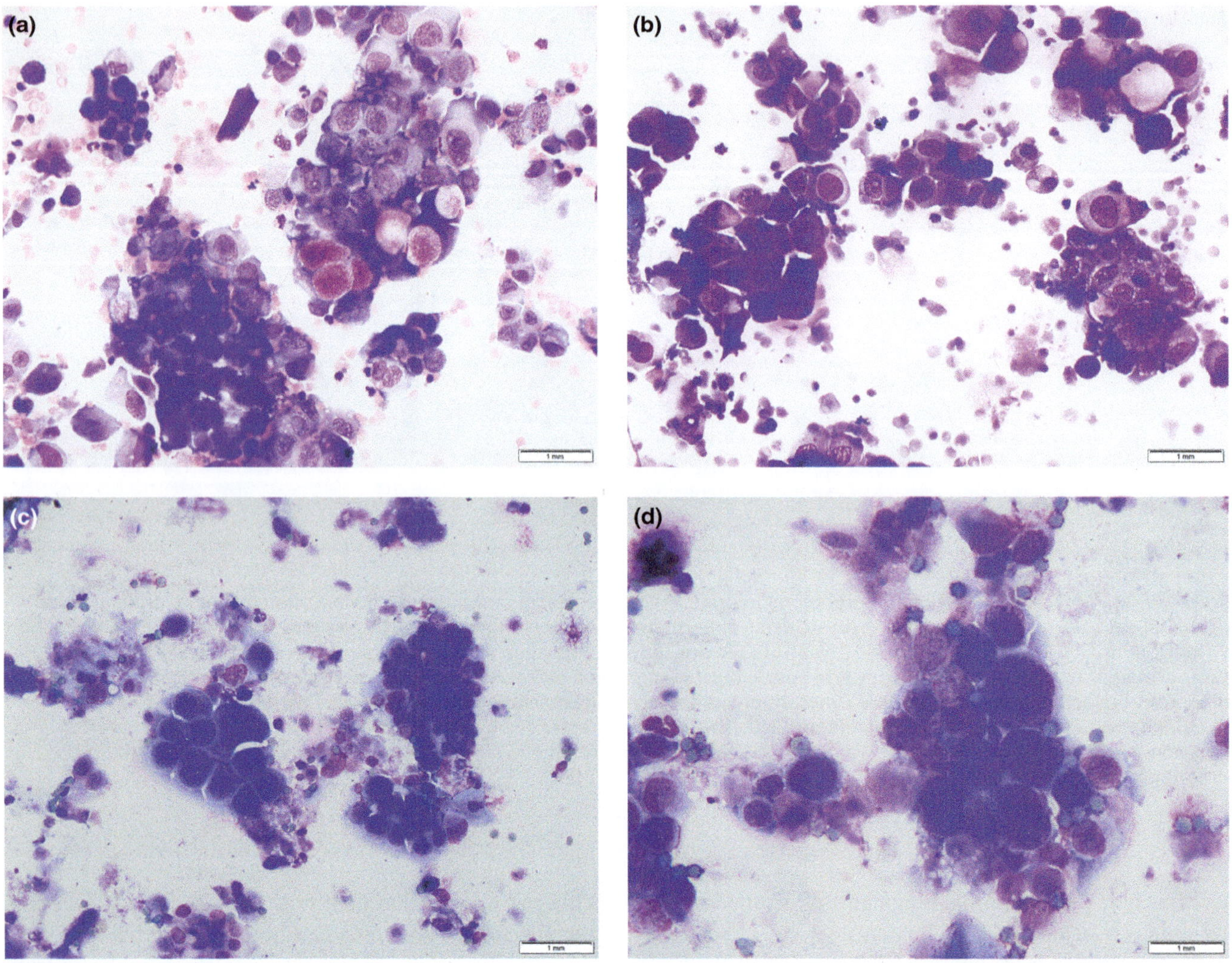

Figure 39.5 Urothelial carcinoma in free catch urine samples. (a) Clusters of neoplastic urothelial cells with characteristic pink, cytoplasmic inclusions from a dog with a mass extending from the trigone into the urethra (Wright Giemsa, 500×). (b) Same case as in (a) (Diff-Quik, 500×). (c) Carcinoma, presumptive urothelial, in an 8-year-old female spayed Dachshund with metastatic carcinoma to bone. Abdominal ultrasound revealed bladder thickening but no distinct mass. Urine cytology was performed to look for a primary site, and hematuria and moderate numbers of epithelial cells were observed in the urine sediment. Epithelial cells exhibit moderate to marked anisokaryosis with a four- to fivefold variation in cell size. Cells have a large nucleus that sometimes occupies 80–90% of the cell volume, even in very large cells. Cytoplasmic inclusions were not identified. Urine testing was negative for the BRAF mutation (Wright Giemsa, 500×). (d) Same case as in (c). The high N:C, binucleation in cells with a high N:C, and nucleoli that are visible, dark, and prominent support interpretation of malignancy (Wright Giemsa, 1000×).

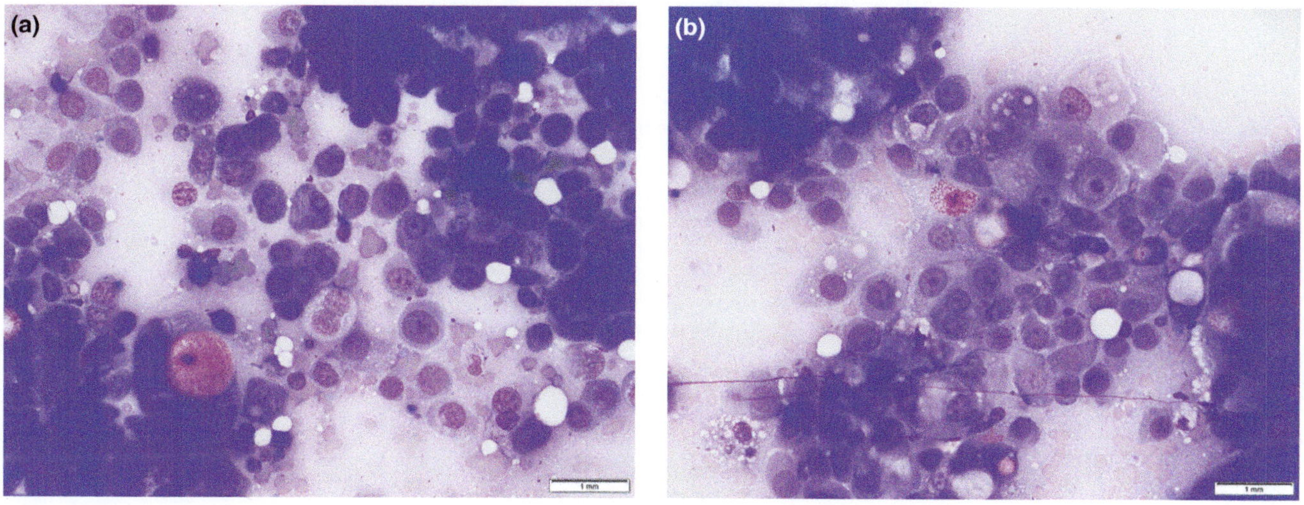

Figure 39.6 (a and b) Aspirate of a cutaneous mass on the ventral abdomen of an adult dog. Given the prior diagnosis of urothelial carcinoma in the urine, seeding from aspiration was considered likely. Cells are individualized and in clusters. Individualized epithelial cells appear discrete to sometimes slightly fusiform, which can be misleading. The individualized appearance and variable shape may be more common in tissue aspirates of metastatic urothelial carcinoma. Cells display marked anisocytosis and anisokaryosis, high N:C, and frequent bi- and multinucleation. The nuclei have immature, stippled to coarsely stippled chromatin with prominent, large, dark purple nucleoli. Characteristic magenta cytoplasmic inclusions support an interpretation of urothelial carcinoma in this skin mass (Wright Giemsa, 500×).

of true cell clusters from cells that are pushed together due to preparation techniques can be challenging. Some urothelial cells contain a characteristic pink to dark pink and variably sized, round to ovoid cytoplasmic inclusion resembling a Melamed-Wolinska body (Figures 39.5a and 39.6).[19] These are not pathognomonic for malignancy, and similar-appearing cytoplasmic inclusions are sometimes seen in other cell types. See Chapter 38 for additional details.

A cytologic grading system for differentiating hyperplastic from neoplastic urothelium in urine samples has not been established in veterinary medicine. In human cytopathology, both low- and high-grade urothelial carcinomas are seen, with the latter being more similar to what is described clinically in dogs and cats with transitional cell carcinoma.[8,20–22] There are defined grading criteria and a consensus group, The Paris System (TPS), devoted to the standardization of urinary cytology in human medicine.[17,18] Some morphologic features that are considered definitive for the diagnosis of high-grade urothelial carcinoma on urine cytology are highlighted only with Papanicolaou stain, which emphasizes nuclear features more characteristic of neoplasia. Criteria established by TPS include identification of the following in at least five cells: (i) a high N:C where the nucleus occupies at least 70% of the cytoplasm (assigned a ratio of 0.7), (ii) moderate to severe hyperchromasia, (iii) markedly irregular nuclear borders, and (iv) coarse, clumpy chromatin.[17] Some papers demonstrate that a ratio of >0.5, determined by digital imaging and computerized analysis, is predictive of high-grade transitional cell carcinoma.[23] Even with defined criteria, definitive diagnosis is not always possible, and TPS includes categories which reflect the ambiguity of diagnosis.[17]

A relatively new commercially available test to diagnosis transitional cell carcinoma is the CADET℠ BRAF Mutation Detection Assay (Sentinel Biomedical, Raleigh, NC, USA). This assay identifies tumor cells carrying a specific mutation in the BRAF gene in dogs.[24–26] Reported sensitivity is 85% and results are not affected by hematuria or bacteria, which are often concurrently present in dogs with transitional cell carcinoma.[24,27] This test is not used in cats.[24] In some dogs with confirmed transitional cell carcinoma where the test is negative, other unidentified genetic mutations are likely contributory.

Round Cell Neoplasia

Neoplastic lymphoid cells are occasionally present in urine of animals with lymphoma involving the urinary tract (Figure 39.7). Diagnosis is based on finding many intermediate and/or large lymphoid cells, similar to diagnosis of lymphoma at other sites.[28,29] The presence of numerous small lymphocytes can reflect chyle within the urine

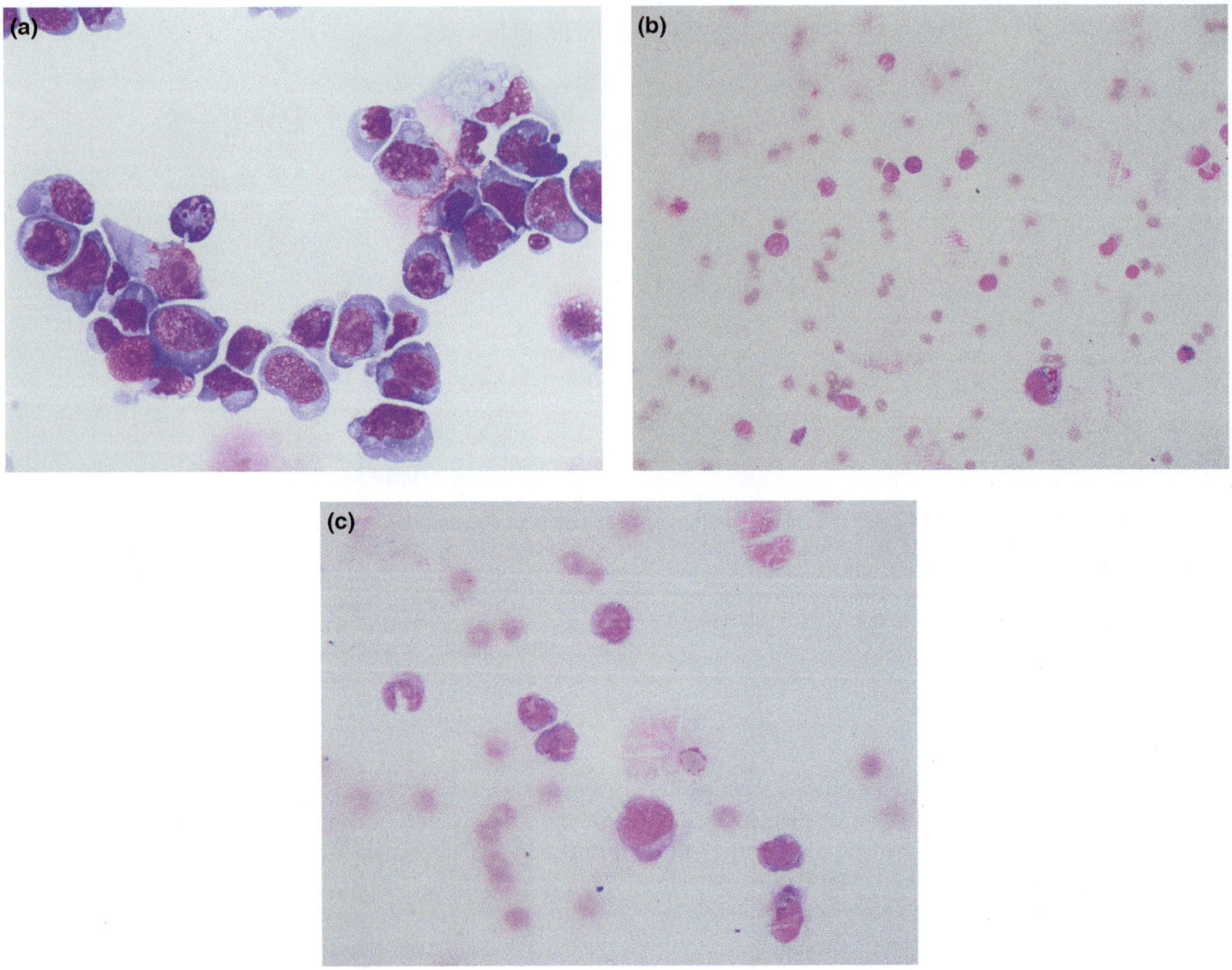

Figure 39.7 Lymphoma detected in the urine from two different dogs. (a) Large neoplastic lymphoid cells in free catch urine from a 10-year-old male castrated Brittany Spaniel who presented in acute renal failure. Cells are characterized by moderate amounts of glassy basophilic cytoplasm and round to oval to pleomorphic nuclei with stippled chromatin. Autopsy revealed T-cell lymphoma limited to the kidneys and local lymph nodes (Wright Giemsa, 1000×). (b) Large lymphoid cells, blood, and one binucleated urothelial cell with a pink cytoplasmic inclusion (lower right) (Wright Giemsa, 500×). (c) Same case as in (b) (Wright Giemsa, 1000×).

(chyluria) rather than lymphoma. This unusual phenomenon is only described in human medicine, primarily associated with filarial infection; a white urine color and elevated urine triglyceride level would be expected.[30]

Hematuria

Hematuria is a relatively common clinical complaint.[31,32] Both macroscopic and microscopic causes of hematuria should be investigated, some of which can be identified via urine cytology. Although some conditions causing hematuria are not amenable to microscopic diagnosis using urine samples, other diseases can be readily identified in urine sediment. Causes of hematuria that are identified, or sometimes excluded, via cytologic evaluation of stained urine in patients include bacterial, parasitic, fungal, or algal infections; some types of bladder or lower urinary tract neoplasia such as transitional cell carcinoma or lymphoma; and inflammatory conditions such as eosinophilic cystitis in dogs or idiopathic cystitis in cats.[31–39] Other causes of hematuria are not microscopically apparent. These include poorly exfoliative benign or malignant renal or bladder neoplasia, uroliths, some types of prostatic disease, structural or congenital abnormalities, some forms of familial glomerular disease, trauma, and hemostatic disorders.[31,32,39–44]

Inflammation

Urinary tract inflammation has many causes, including primary processes or secondary to underlying infection, neoplasia, or physical trauma. While neutrophils often predominate, macrophages, lymphocytes, plasma cells, and eosinophils also can be seen depending on the underlying cause (Figure 39.8). Urine can cause degradation of any cell in urine, including leukocytes; this can hinder accurate characterization of inflammation. Bacterial infection can also cause degenerative changes in neutrophils with resulting nuclear swelling (Figure 39.8a).

Evidence of inflammation should prompt investigation for underlying infection. Neoplasia, chemical irritation, physical trauma from indwelling catheters, stents, uroliths, trauma, and idiopathic cystitis can all have associated inflammation and should be considered in the absence of an obvious infectious etiology. Eosinophilic inflammation, although an uncommon finding, can occur secondary to infectious etiologies, such as parasitic disease, fungal infection, and algal infection, as well as neoplasia, including carcinoma, lymphoma, and fibroma. Eosinophilic cystitis, an infrequently reported diagnosis in veterinary medicine,

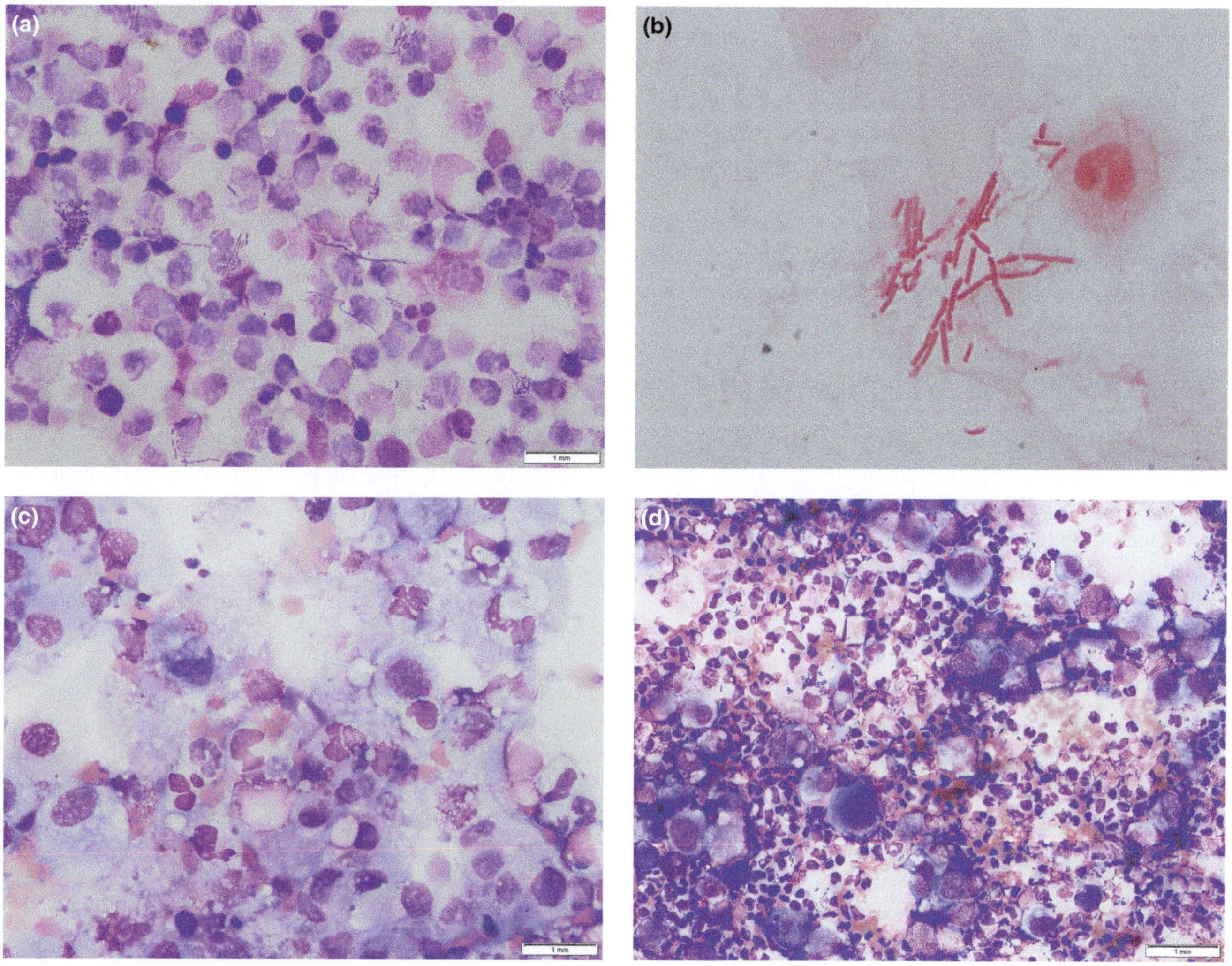

Figure 39.8 Inflammation in urine. (a) Degenerate neutrophils and bacterial rods in a free catch sample of urine from dog with pollakiuria (Wright Giemsa, 1000×). (b) Gram-negative bacterial rods and a squamous epithelial cell (Gram stain, 1000×). (c) Mixed inflammation with neutrophils, macrophages, and eosinophils in a dog with stranguria. A bladder mass was identified histologically as mixed inflammation (Wright Giemsa, 1000×). (d) Neutrophilic inflammation in a dog with urothelial carcinoma, concurrent infection with bacterial rods, calcium oxalate dihydrate crystalluria, and hematuria (Wright Giemsa, 500×).

is poorly understood and sometimes without an obvious cause.[36] In some reports, it has been associated with urolithiasis and chronic urinary tract infection.[36] Inflammation in urine may not be representative of bladder inflammation, depending on the degree and underlying cause (Figure 39.8c). Chapter 38 addresses specific inflammatory diseases of the bladder.

Infection

Bacterial Infection

Bacterial urinary tract infection is a frequent differential diagnosis when evaluating urine in dogs and cats but is very uncommon in horses.[45] Common bacterial isolates in dogs include *Escherichia coli*, *Staphylococcus* spp., and *Enterococcus* spp.[46–48] *Enterococcus* spp. and *E. coli* are the most common isolates in cats.[47,49,50] Bacterial urinary tract infections are both under- and overdiagnosed using routine urine sediment evaluation, depending on patient clinical signs, collection method, sediment findings, and technical skill of the microscopist.[51] Positive results for bacteriuria by routine urinalysis correlate poorly with subsequent urine culture results.[51–54] Incorrect interpretation of sediment findings by veterinary staff can result in misdiagnosis of a urinary tract infection. Lipid droplets, cell debris, contaminants, and some crystals can be mistakenly identified as bacterial agents on unstained urine sediment smears. Contaminated stain used for either wet or dried urine preparations can be a source of bacteria and lead to erroneous interpretation, especially in practices where stain sets are shared for use with fecal and/or ear specimens. According to several studies, cytologic evaluation of dried urine sediment can improve accurate diagnosis of bacterial urinary tract infections (Figures 39.1c and d and 39.8a).[4,51–53] Gram-stained slides can further enhance bacterial identification and facilitate initial antimicrobial selection (Figure 39.8b).[4,51] Gram stain has limitations in the evaluation of other cell types, so there is benefit to performing both stains on urine cytology smears given the potential for complex pathogenesis of urinary tract disease. Performing Gram staining does require some experience to obtain optimally stained smears. It should also be noted that the morphology and Gram staining characteristics of bacteria can be influenced by bacterial degradation within cells or urine and previous treatment with antimicrobials. Most often, damage to bacterial walls can cause Gram-positive organisms to appear Gram negative in some parts of the smears (Figure 39.2c).

Fungal Infection

Fungal organisms identified in urine can represent normal urogenital flora, environmental contamination, lower urinary tract fungal infection, or systemic fungal disease. Urine cytology can confirm the presence of fungal agents and occasionally help differentiate local from systemic infection. The majority of reports of urinary tract manifestations of systemic fungal disease are from dogs with fewer from cats; local yeast overgrowth is seen in both dogs and cats.[37,38,55–59]

Candida sp.

Candida sp. can be a component of the normal flora of the urogenital tract, and occasional organisms observed in free catch samples can represent fecal contamination.[60] Large numbers or identification in cystocentesis samples would support an interpretation of overgrowth or infection.[37,57,58] *Candida albicans* is the most common *Candida* sp. identified, but urinary tract candidiasis includes other species.[37,58,61] Lower urinary tract candidiasis is often a complication of other pathology involving the urinary tract or be treatment related.[37,58] Urinary tract and non-urinary tract neoplasia, non-fungal urinary tract disease, indwelling urinary catheters, aciduria, diabetes mellitus, and treatment with systemic antibiotics or corticosteroids can alter normal host defenses and increase the risk of *Candida* spp. urinary tract infection.[37,57,58] Localized *Candida* sp. infections predominate, but disseminated infection can result from patient risk factor or organism virulence factors.[61,62]

Candida sp. are ovoid, 2–4 μm diameter, lack internal structure, and stain dark blue–purple with Romanowsky stains.[63] Budding is frequently noted, and the presence of pseudohyphae further supports an interpretation of candidiasis.[63] Some morphologic overlap exists between *Candida* sp. organisms and lipid droplets, the latter remaining unstained in cytologic preparations and existing in a different plain of focus than cells in unstained sediment slides (Figure 39.9).

Systemic Mycosis

Urine cytology, and even urine sediment evaluation, can support the diagnosis of systemic fungal infection in some animals with renal and/or prostatic involvement (Figure 39.10). The presence of fungal hyphae in samples collected using sterile technique, particularly in the presence of concurrent inflammation, supports fungal infection with an opportunistic fungal agent, such as aspergillosis or other saprophytic fungus.[55,56,64–66] In addition to *Aspergillus* sp. infections, saprophytic agents described include *Penicillium* sp., *Westerdykella* sp., *Paecilomyces* sp., *Chrysosporium* sp., and others; prognosis is variable, depending on host immunocompetence, fungal virulence factors, and response to therapy.[56,65,66] Renal involvement is common.[56,64–66] Hyphal morphology is not sufficient for speciation, so fungal culture at a reference laboratory is

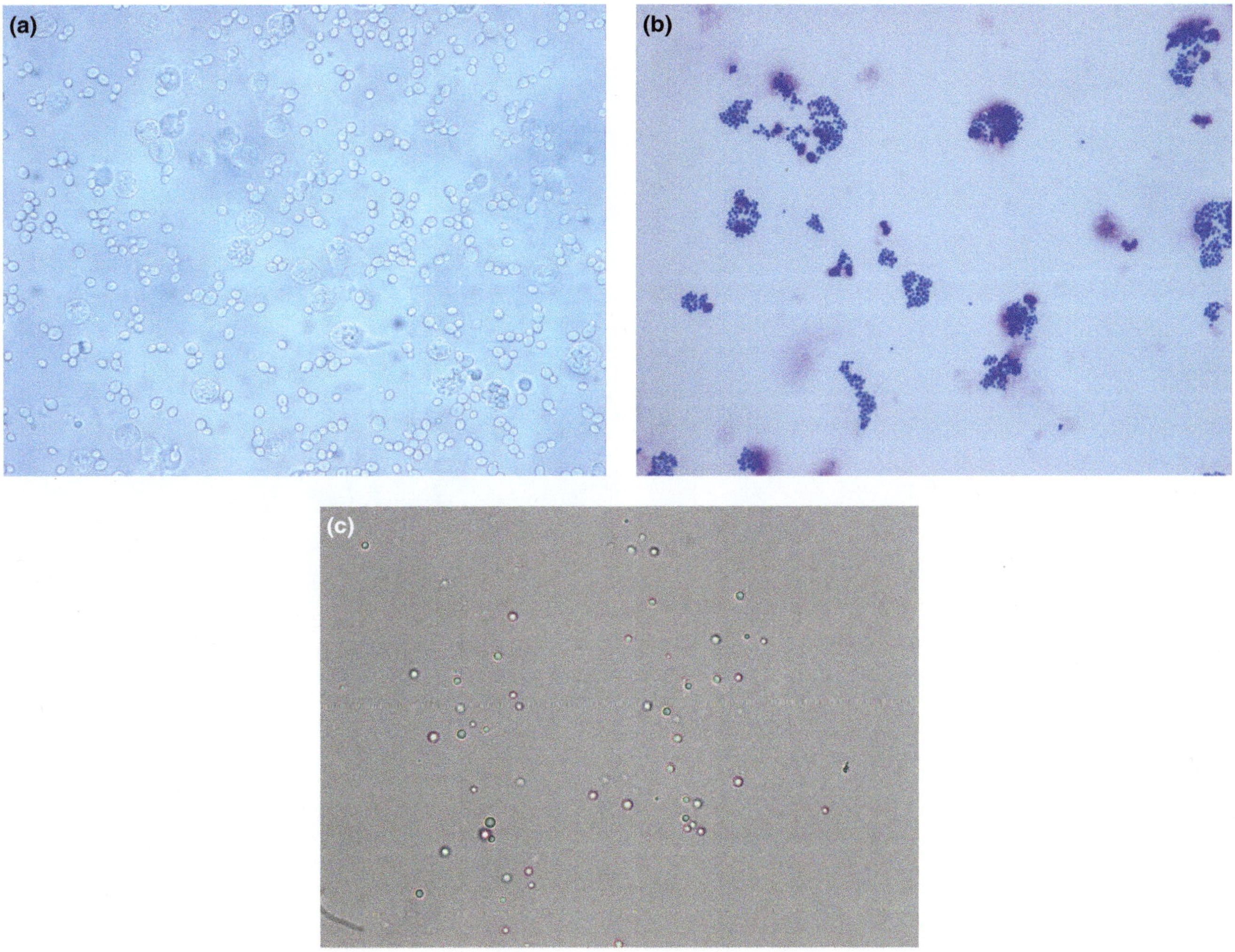

Figure 39.9 Candidiasis in the urine from a cat with poorly controlled diabetes mellitus. (a) Numerous budding yeast organisms and many neutrophils in urine (Unstained, 400×). (b) *Candida* sp. yeast is round to ovoid, 2–4 μm, and darkly basophilic and exhibits frequent budding. These can be extracellular and present within leukocytes (Wright Giemsa, 200×). (c) Free lipid in urine can have overlapping appearance with small yeast organisms in unstained urine sediment. Lipid sits in a different focal plane than formed elements such as leukocytes and organisms and should not take up stain (Unstained, 400×).

necessary for specific identification. In patients where disseminated fungal disease is a differential, microscopic urine evaluation and urine fungal culture should be routine given the frequent incidence of visible hyphal agents.[56] Owing to the slow growth of some fungi, urine cytology can offer a more immediate, if not preliminary, answer to whether or not there is fungal infection. Chapter 3 contains more information on the cytologic diagnosis of fungal disease.

Infrequently, yeast of *Blastomyces* or *Cryptococcus* species have been described in urine from infected animals (Figure 39.11).[67–69] Prostate, rather than renal involvement, is a likely source for *B. dermatitidis* in urine.[70] Urinary tract cryptococcal infection has been described as a component of both local and systemic cryptococcosis in cats. Renal involvement was part of systemic infection and ultimately the cause of the cryptococcuria.[68,69] Recognition of fungal disease in urine is also significant for the protection of laboratory staff working with cultures. The utility of urine in the diagnosis of systemic fungal disease more recently involves antigen detection, specifically for histoplasmosis, blastomycosis, and aspergillosis.[71–73] Urine cytology, especially for differentiating a saprophytic, hyphal fungus from a dimorphic fungus, would be a useful adjunct tool.

The presence of *Cyniclomyces guttulatus* yeast in the urine of dogs is uncommon.[74] It has been described in

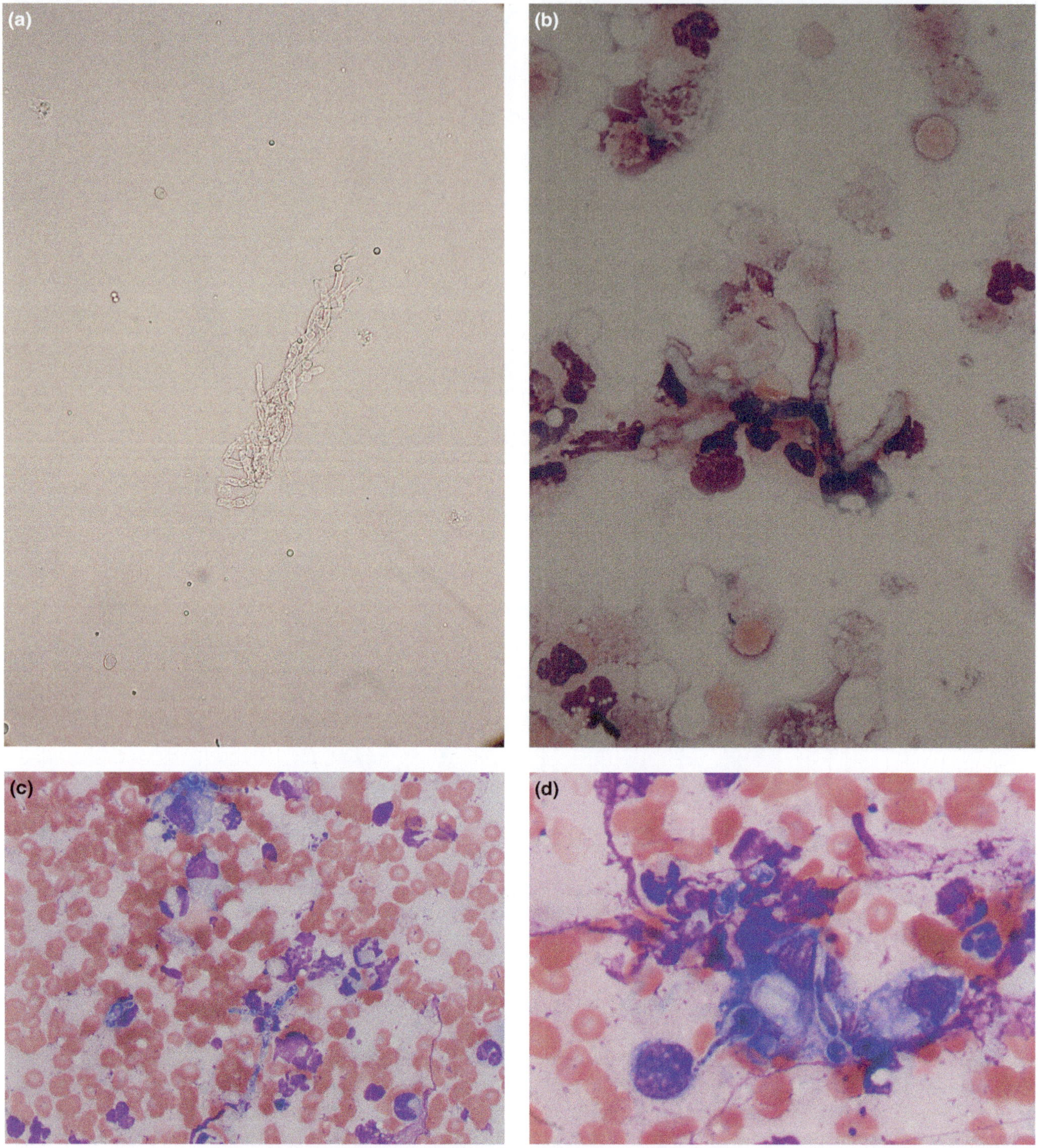

Figure 39.10 Systemic aspergillosis in a dog that developed lytic bone lesions and renal azotemia following immunosuppressive therapy for suspected steroid responsive meningitis. The dog was euthanized following imaging. Culture results later identified *Aspergillus* sp. (a) A group of fungal hyphae in urine obtained via cystocentesis (Unstained sediment, 400×). (b) Branching, septate fungal hyphae in urine with hematuria and pyuria. Hyphae vary from darkly basophilic with a thin, poorly staining wall to minimally staining. The lack of staining may reflect nonviable hyphae (Wright Giemsa, 1000×). (c and d) Fungal hyphae and mixed inflammation in computed tomography-guided aspirates of the kidney (c) and bone (d) from the same dog. Morphology of saprophytic fungi in tissue can be highly variable and shared between different fungal agents. Culture is required for specific identification of fungal organism (Wright Giemsa, (c) 500×, (d) 1000×).

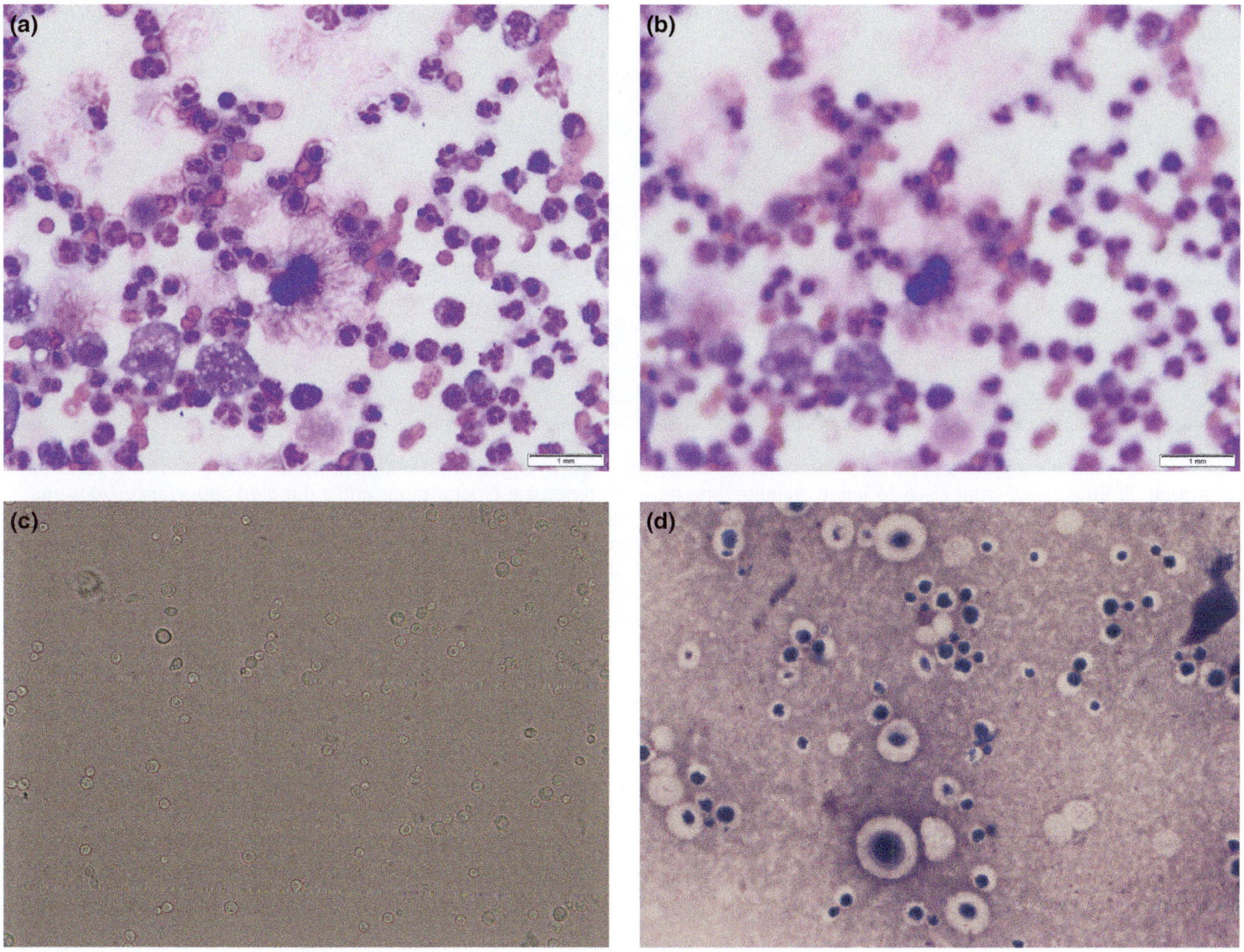

Figure 39.11 Systemic fungal disease. (a) Free catch urine from a middle-aged castrated male Weimaraner with significant weight loss and prostatomegaly. Image is focused on leukocytes surrounding a budding *Blastomyces dermatitidis* yeast (Wright Giemsa, 1000×). (b) Same as in (a) but focused on the yeast, which is darkly basophilic, one to two times the size of a neutrophil, with a double-contoured wall and broad-based budding (Wright Giemsa, 1000×). (c) Urine from a 12-year-old female spayed domestic short hair cat with renal azotemia and weight loss. Numerous circular budding yeasts are observed in the urine sediment (Unstained, 500×). (d) Same urine as in (c). Variably sized basophilic yeast with a negatively staining capsule of variable thickness and rare narrow-based budding are consistent with *Cryptococcus* sp. (modified Wright Giemsa, 500×. *Source:* Images (c) and (d) courtesy of Laura Brandt).

samples obtained via cystocentesis, but contamination in these cases was suspected rather than true infection given the absence of inflammation.[74] It is important not to confuse this elongated yeast with saprophytic fungal agents. See Chapter 33 for more information and morphology of *C. guttulatus*.

Parasites

Two primary parasitic infections can be identified in urine (Figure 39.12). Ova from the giant kidney worm, *D. renale*, can be present in the urine from infected dogs, who often present with hematuria but without azotemia.[75,76] *C. plica* (syn. *P. plica*), the bladder worm, is a lower urinary tract parasite causing disease in both dogs and cats.[34,77–79] Clinical signs can include pollakiuria and dysuria from cystitis and pigmenturia from hematuria.[34,77] Nematode larvae, fragments of adult stages, and/or ova can be present in urine.[34,77]

Other Infectious Etiologies

Other infectious agents can be identified in urine samples from patients with local or systemic infectious diseases. In some dogs with protothecosis, thecal structures can be identified in urine samples.[80] See Chapters 32 and 33 for further information about protothecosis.

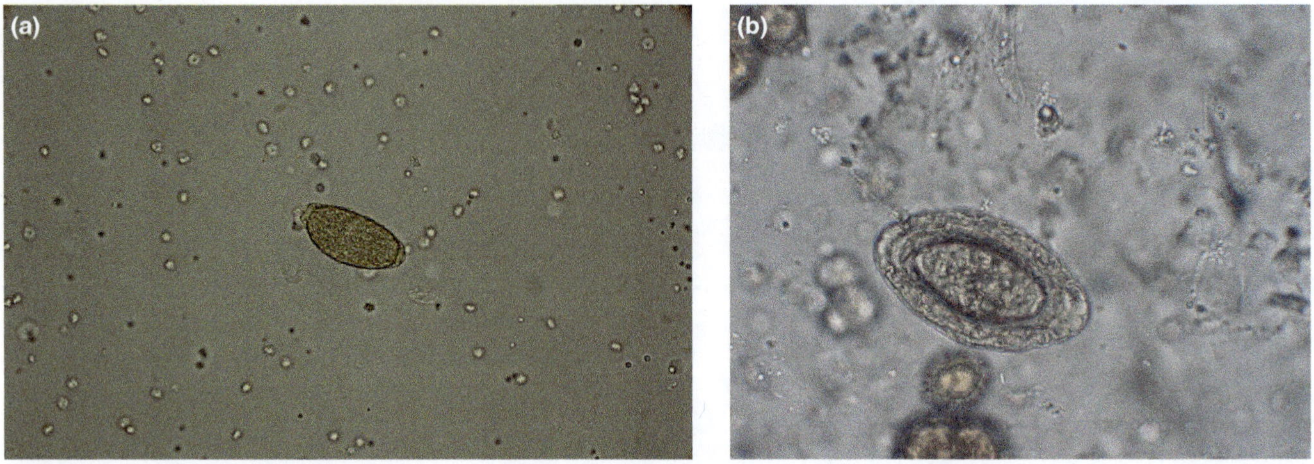

Figure 39.12 Parasitic agents. (a) *Pearsonema plica* (formerly *Capillaria plica*) egg in urine sediment from a young dog with pollakiuria and stranguria. Eggs range from 25 to 65 μm in diameter and have asymmetrical bipolar plugs and a dimpled appearance. Dogs and cats can present with lower urinary tract signs, (pollakiuria and stranguria), and hematuria is often present. Mature threadlike, white to pale yellow worms and/or large eggs can be seen following ingestion of earthworms, the intermediate host (Unstained, 100×. *Source:* Image courtesy of Katie Boes). (b) *Dioctophyma renale* egg in urine from a Maned wolf. Giant kidney worm eggs range from 45 to 75 μm, are unembryonated, and are yellow–brown in unstained sediments. Ingestion of earthworms, raw fish, or amphibians can result infection. Flank pain and hematuria are common (Unstained, 1000×. *Source:* Image courtesy of Tom Nolan).

Conclusions

Urine cytology offers several advantages over microscopic evaluation of unstained urine sediment. For accurate diagnosis, skill for both slide preparation and evaluation is required, and accuracy can be hindered by poorly exfoliative lesions, poor cell preservation, and current processes confounding interpretation. Urine cytology can confirm and better characterize bacterial urinary tract infections and local and systemic fungal and other infectious conditions. Although not always a definitive diagnostic test for urothelial cell carcinoma, owing to inherent variability in urothelial cells, morphologic overlap with hyperplasia, and the caustic nature of urine, it can be definitive in some patients.

References

1 Reine, N.J. and Langston, C.E. (2005). Urinalysis interpretation: how to squeeze out the maximum information from a small sample. *Clin Tech Small Anim Pract* 20: 2–10.

2 Ko, D.-H., Ji, M., Kim, S. et al. (2016). An approach to standardization of urine sediment analysis via suggestion of a common manual protocol. *Scand J Clin Lab Invest* 76: 256–263.

3 O'Neil, E., Burton, S., Horney, B., and MacKenzie, A. (2013). Comparison of white and red blood cell estimates in urine sediment with hemocytometer and automated counts in dogs and cats. *Vet Clin Pathol* 42: 78–84.

4 Way, L.I., Sullivan, L.A., Johnson, V., and Morley, P.S. (2013). Comparison of routine urinalysis and urine Gram stain for detection of bacteriuria in dogs. *J Vet Emerg Crit Care* 23: 23–28.

5 Nyland, T.G., Wallack, S.T., and Wisner, E.R. (2002). Needle-tract implantation following us-guided fine-needle aspiration biopsy of transitional cell carcinoma of the bladder, urethra, and prostate. *Vet Radiol Ultrasound* 43: 50–53.

6 Reed, L.T., Knapp, D.W., and Miller, M.A. (2013). Cutaneous metastasis of transitional cell carcinoma in 12 dogs. *Vet Pathol* 50: 676–681.

7 Marcos, R., Santos, M., Marrinhas, C. et al. (2016). Cytocentrifuge preparation in veterinary cytology: a quick, simple, and affordable manual method to concentrate low cellularity fluids. *Vet Clin Pathol* 45: 725–731.

8 Thiryayi, S.A. and Rana, D.N. (2012). Urine cytopathology: challenges, pitfalls, and mimics. *Diagn Cytopathol* 40: 1019–1034.

9 Sawa, M., Yabuki, A., Miyoshi, N. et al. (2012). Rapid-air-dry Papanicolaou stain in canine and feline tumor cytology: a quantitative comparison with the Giemsa stain. *J Vet Med Sci* 74: 1133–1138.

10 Jörundsson, E., Lumsden, J.H., and Jacobs, R.M. (1999). Rapid staining techniques in cytopathology: a review and

comparison of modified protocols for hematoxylin and eosin, Papanicolaou and Romanowsky stains. *Vet Clin Pathol* 28: 100–108.

11 Pérez, C.C., Rodríguez, I., Dorado, J., and Hidalgo, M. (2005). Use of ultrafast Papanicolaou stain for exfoliative vaginal cytology in bitches. *Vet Rec* 156: 648–650.

12 Batamuzi, E.K. and Kristensen, F. (1995). Diagnostic importance of urothelial cells of the dog and cat. *J Small Anim Pract* 36: 17–21.

13 DeMay, R. (2007). *Practical Principals of Cytopathology*, 95–114. Chicago, IL: American Society for Clinical Pathology Press.

14 Falkenö, U., Tvedten, H.W., and Spångberg, C. (2014). What is your diagnosis? Urine sediment changes in a dog with hemorrhagic shock and disseminated intravascular coagulation after pyometra surgery. *Vet Clin Pathol* 43: 463–464.

15 Brimo, F., Vollmer, R.T., Case, B. et al. (2009). Accuracy of urine cytology and the significance of an atypical category. *Am J Clin Pathol* 132: 785–793.

16 Vap, L.M. and Shropshire, S.B. (2017). Urine cytology. *Vet Clin North Am Small Anim Pract* 47: 135–149.

17 VandenBussche, C.J. (2016). A review of the Paris system for reporting urinary cytology. *Cytopathology* 27: 153–156.

18 Barkan, G.A., Wojcik, E.M., Nayar, R. et al. (2016). The Paris system for reporting urinary cytology: the quest to develop a standardized terminology. *Acta Cytol* 60: 185–197.

19 Ayra, P., Khalbuss, W.E., Monaco, S.E., and Pantanowitz, L. (2012). Melamed-Wolinska bodies. *Diagn Cytopathol* 40: 150–151.

20 Wilson, H.M., Chun, R., Larson, V.S. et al. (2007). Clinical signs, treatments, and outcome in cats with transitional cell carcinoma of the urinary bladder: 20 cases (1990–2004). *J Am Vet Med Assoc* 231: 101–106.

21 Mutsaers, A.J., Widmer, W.R., and Knapp, D.W. (2003). Canine transitional cell carcinoma. *J Vet Intern Med* 17: 136–144.

22 Knapp, D.W., Ramos-Vara, J.A., Moore, G.E. et al. (2014). Urinary bladder cancer in dogs, a naturally occurring model for cancer biology and drug development. *ILAR J* 55: 100–118.

23 Hang, J.-F., Charu, V., Zhang, M.L., and CJ, V.B. (2017). Digital image analysis supports a nuclear-to-cytoplasmic ratio cutoff value of 0.5 for atypical urothelial cells. *Cancer Cytopathol* 125: 710–716.

24 Sentinel Biomedical (2018). CADET BRAF MUTATION DETECTION ASSAY. https://www.sentinelbiomedical.com/wp-content/uploads/CADET-BRAF-BROCHURE-DIAGNOSIS-MONITORING.pdf. Accessed: 01-January-2020.

25 Decker, B., Parker, H.G., Dhawan, D. et al. (2015). Homologous mutation to human BRAF V600E is common in naturally occurring canine bladder cancer: evidence for a relevant model system and urine-based diagnostic test. *Mol Cancer Res* 13: 993–1002.

26 Mochizuki, H., Shapiro, S.G., and Breen, M. (2015). Detection of BRAF mutation in urine DNA as a molecular diagnostic for canine urothelial and prostatic carcinoma. *PLoS One* 10: e0144170.

27 Budreckis, D.M., Byrne, B.A., Pollard, R.E. et al. (2015). Bacterial urinary tract infections associated with transitional cell carcinoma in dogs. *J Vet Intern Med* 29: 828–833.

28 Benigni, L., Lamb, C.R., Corzo-Menendez, N. et al. (2006). Lymphoma affecting the urinary bladder in three dogs and a cat. *Vet Radiol Ultrasound* 47: 592–596.

29 Geigy, C.A., Dandrieux, J., Miclard, J. et al. (2010). Extranodal B-cell lymphoma in the urinary bladder with cytological evidence of concurrent involvement of the gall bladder in a cat. *J Small Anim Pract* 51: 280–287.

30 Vera, M., Molano, A., and Rodriguez, P. (2010). Turbid white urine. *Clin Kidney J* 3: 45–47.

31 Adamama-Moraitou, K., Pardali, D., Prassinos, N. et al. (2017). Evaluation of dogs with macroscopic haematuria: a retrospective study of 162 cases (2003–2010). *N Z Vet J* 65: 204–208.

32 Forrester, S.D. (2004). Diagnostic approach to hematuria in dogs and cats. *Vet Clin North Am Small Anim Pract* 34: 849–866.

33 Merkel, L.K., Lulich, J., Polzin, D. et al. (2017). Clinicopathologic and microbiologic findings associated with emphysematous cystitis in 27 dogs. *J Am Anim Hosp Assoc* 53: 313–320.

34 Basso, W., Spänhauer, Z., Arnold, S., and Deplazes, P. (2014). *Capillaria plica* (syn. *Pearsonema plica*) infection in a dog with chronic pollakiuria: challenges in the diagnosis and treatment. *Paramed Int* 63: 140–142.

35 Nakagawa, T.L.D.R., Bracarense, A.P.F.R.L., dos Reis, A.C.F. et al. (2007). Giant kidney worm (*Dioctophyma renale*) infections in dogs from northern Paraná, Brazil. *Vet Parasitol* 145: 366–370.

36 Ozaki, K., Nakahara, Y., and Narama, I. (2008). Polypoid eosinophilic cystitis with pseudosarcomatous proliferative tissue in a dog. *J Vet Med Sci* 70: 289–291.

37 Jin, Y. and Lin, D. (2005). Fungal urinary tract infections in the dog and cat: a retrospective study (2001–2004). *J Am Anim Hosp Assoc* 41: 373–381.

38 Taylor, A.R., Barr, J.W., Hokamp, J.A. et al. (2012). Cytologic diagnosis of disseminated histoplasmosis in the wall of the urinary bladder of a cat. *J Am Anim Hosp Assoc* 48: 203–208.

39 Defauw, P.A., Van de Maele, I., Duchateau, L. et al. (2011). Risk factors and clinical presentation of cats with feline idiopathic cystitis. *J Feline Med Surg* 13: 967–975.

40 Bryan, J.N., Henry, C.J., Turnquist, S.E. et al. (2006). Primary renal neoplasia of dogs. *J Vet Intern Med* 20: 1155–1160.

41 Furman, E., Hooijberg, E.H., Leidinger, E. et al. (2015). Hereditary xanthinuria and urolithiasis in a domestic shorthair cat. *Comp Clin Pathol* 24: 1325–1329.

42 Adin, C.A., Chew, D.J., Heng, H.G. et al. (2011). Bladder inversion and secondary hematuria in a 6-month-old domestic shorthair cat. *J Am Vet Med Assoc* 239: 370–373.

43 White, J.D., Norris, J.M., Bosward, K.L. et al. (2008). Persistent haematuria and proteinuria due to glomerular disease in related Abyssinian cats. *J Feline Med Surg* 10: 219–229.

44 Tasker, S., Mackin, A.J., and Day, M.J. (1999). Primary immune-mediated thrombocytopenia in a cat. *J Small Anim Pract* 40: 127–131.

45 Frye, M.A. (2006). Pathophysiology, diagnosis, and management of urinary tract infection in horses. *Vet Clin North Am Equine Pract* 22: 497–517.

46 Wong, C., Epstein, S.E., and Westropp, J.L. (2015). Antimicrobial susceptibility patterns in urinary tract infections in dogs (2010–2013). *J Vet Intern Med* 29: 1045–1052.

47 KuKanich, K.S. and Lubbers, B.V. (2015). Review of enterococci isolated from canine and feline urine specimens from 2006 to 2011. *J Am Anim Hosp Assoc* 51: 148–154.

48 Windahl, U., Holst, B.S., Nyman, A. et al. (2014). Characterization of bacterial growth and antimicrobial susceptibility patterns in canine urinary tract infections. *BMC Vet Res* 10: 217.

49 Litster, A., Moss, S., Platell, J., and Trott, D.J. (2009). Occult bacterial lower urinary tract infections in cats-urinalysis and culture findings. *Vet Microbiol* 136: 130–134.

50 Puchot, M.L., Cook, A.K., and Pohlit, C. (2017). Subclinical bacteriuria in cats: prevalence, findings on contemporaneous urinalyses and clinical risk factors. *J Feline Med Surg* 19: 1238–1244.

51 O'Neil, E., Horney, B., Burton, S. et al. (2013). Comparison of wet-mount, Wright-Giemsa and Gram-stained urine sediment for predicting bacteriuria in dogs and cats. *Can Vet J* 54: 1061–1066.

52 Swenson, C.L., Boisvert, A.M., Kruger, J.M., and Gibbons-Burgener, S.N. (2004). Evaluation of modified Wright-staining of urine sediment as a method for accurate detection of bacteriuria in dogs. *J Am Vet Med Assoc* 224: 1282–1289.

53 Swenson, C.L., Boisvert, A.M., Gibbons-Burgener, S.N., and Kruger, J.M. (2011). Evaluation of modified Wright-staining of dried urinary sediment as a method for accurate detection of bacteriuria in cats. *Vet Clin Pathol* 40: 256–264.

54 McGhie, J.A., Stayt, J., and Hosgood, G.L. (2014). Prevalence of bacteriuria in dogs without clinical signs of urinary tract infection presenting for elective surgical procedures. *Aust Vet J* 92: 33–37.

55 Taylor, A.R., Young, B.D., Levine, G.J. et al. (2015). Clinical features and magnetic resonance imaging findings in 7 dogs with central nervous system aspergillosis. *J Vet Intern Med* 29: 1556–1563.

56 Watt, P.R., Robins, G.M., Galloway, A.M., and O'Boyle, D.A. (1995). Disseminated opportunistic fungal disease in dogs: 10 cases (1982–1990). *J Am Vet Med Assoc* 207: 67–70.

57 Lulich, J.P. and Osborne, C.A. (1996). Fungal infections of the feline lower urinary tract. *Vet Clin North Am Small Anim Pract* 26: 309–315.

58 Pressler, B.M., Vaden, S.L., Lane, I.F. et al. (2003). *Candida* spp. urinary tract infections in 13 dogs and seven cats: predisposing factors, treatment, and outcome. *J Am Anim Hosp Assoc* 39: 263–270.

59 Hartmann, K., Lloret, A., Pennisi, M.G. et al. (2013). Aspergillosis in cats. *J Feline Med Surg* 15: 605–610.

60 Brito, E.H., Fontenelle, R.O., Brilhante, R.S. et al. (2009). The anatomical distribution and antimicrobial susceptibility of yeast species isolated from healthy dogs. *Vet J* 182: 320–326.

61 Fisher, J.F., Kavanagh, K., Sobel, J.D. et al. (2011). Candida urinary tract infection: pathogenesis. *Clin Infect Dis* 52 (Suppl 6): S437–S451.

62 Heseltine, J.C., Panciera, D.L., and Saunders, G.K. (2003). Systemic candidiasis in a dog. *J Am Vet Med Assoc* 223: 821–824, 810.

63 Pressler, B.M. (2012). Candidiasis and rhodotorulosis. In: *Infectious Diseases of the Dog and Cat*, 4e, 666–672. St. Louis, MO: Elsevier.

64 Schultz, R.M., Johnson, E.G., Wisner, E.R. et al. (2008). Clinicopathologic and diagnostic imaging characteristics of systemic aspergillosis in 30 dogs. *J Vet Intern Med* 22: 851–859.

65 Tappin, S.W., Ferrandis, I., Jakovljevic, S. et al. (2012). Successful treatment of bilateral Paecilomyces pyelonephritis in a German shepherd dog. *J Small Anim Pract* 53: 657–660.

66 Armentano, R.A., Cooke, K.L., and Wickes, B.L. (2013). Disseminated mycotic infection caused by Westerdykella species in a German Shepherd dog. *J Am Vet Med Assoc* 242: 381–387.

67 Shull, R.M., Hayden, D.W., and Johnston, G.R. (1977). Urogenital blastomycosis in a dog. *J Am Vet Med Assoc* 171: 730–735.

68 Brandt, L.E. and Blauvelt, M.M. (2010). What is your diagnosis? Urine sediment from a southern California cat with weight loss. *Vet Clin Pathol* 39: 517–518.

69 Chapman, T.L. and Kirk, S.E. (2008). An isolated cryptococcal urinary tract infection in a cat. *J Am Anim Hosp Assoc* 44: 262–265.

70 Totten, A.K., Ridgway, M.D., and Sauberli, D.S. (2011). *Blastomyces dermatitidis* prostatic and testicular infection in eight dogs (1992–2005). *J Am Anim Hosp Assoc* 47: 413–418.

71 Garcia, R.S., Wheat, L.J., Cook, A.K. et al. (2012). Sensitivity and specificity of a blood and urine galactomannan antigen assay for diagnosis of systemic aspergillosis in dogs. *J Vet Intern Med* 26: 911–919.

72 Spector, D., Legendre, A.M., Wheat, J. et al. (2008). Antigen and antibody testing for the diagnosis of blastomycosis in dogs. *J Vet Intern Med* 22: 839–843.

73 Cook, A.K., Cunningham, L.Y., Cowell, A.K., and Wheat, L.J. (2012). Clinical evaluation of urine *Histoplasma capsulatum* antigen measurement in cats with suspected disseminated histoplasmosis. *J Feline Med Surg* 14: 512–515.

74 Winston, J.A., Piperisova, I., Neel, J., and Gookin, J.L. (2016). *Cyniclomyces guttulatus* infection in dogs: 19 cases (2006–2013). *J Am Anim Hosp Assoc* 52: 42–51.

75 Ferreira, V.L., Medeiros, F.P., July, J.R., and Raso, T.F. (2010). *Dioctophyma renale* in a dog: clinical diagnosis and surgical treatment. *Vet Parasitol* 168: 151–155.

76 Mesquita, L.R., Rahal, S.C., Faria, L.G. et al. (2014). Pre- and post-operative evaluations of eight dogs following right nephrectomy due to *Dioctophyma renale*. *Vet Q* 34: 167–171.

77 Rossi, M., Messina, N., Ariti, G. et al. (2011). Symptomatic *Capillaria plica* infection in a young European cat. *J Feline Med Surg* 13: 793–795.

78 Bédard, C., Desnoyers, M., Lavallée, M.-C., and Poirier, D. (2002). Capillaria in the bladder of an adult cat. *Can Vet J* 43: 973–974.

79 Mariacher, A., Millanta, F., Guidi, G., and Perrucci, S. (2016). Urinary capillariosis in six dogs from Italy. *Open Vet J* 6: 84–88.

80 Stenner, V.J., Mackay, B., King, T. et al. (2007). Protothecosis in 17 Australian dogs and a review of the canine literature. *Med Mycol* 45: 249–266.

Part XI

Reproductive Tract

40

Testes, Ovaries, and Prostate

Francisco de Oliveira Conrado, and Sally E. Henderson

Testes

Introduction

Indications for testicular cytology include poor semen quality, infertility, orchitis or epididymitis, testicular masses, and assessment of lesions appreciated on ultrasound or grossly apparent.

Collection

Indication for fine-needle aspiration (FNA) of testes is unilateral or bilateral enlargement, and cytologic evaluation can help differentiate between inflammatory, neoplastic, or degenerative conditions.[1,2] Enlargement of the epididymis, with or without concurrent testicular enlargement, may prompt FNA. Atrophied or degenerate testicles are small and firm (Figure 40.1), and FNAs of these conditions are usually not fruitful. Semen evaluation may also provide valuable information (Chapter 41). FNA of the testicles can be useful for the evaluation of male infertility[3] and is nearly the only suitable way to evaluate sperm production and testicular pathology in male cats, as sperm collection in this species is difficult.[4]

FNAs are performed with or without sedation or general anesthesia, particularly for intra-abdominal or inguinal cryptorchid testicles and with or without ultrasound guidance. Sedation may not be required in already painful cases such as orchitis.[5] Collection by capillary action using a 21 or 22 G needle without applied negative pressure is preferred due to cellular fragility.[2] For the same reason, slide preparation of the aspirated sample should be done with minimal applied force. A smaller diameter needle (29 G) can be used in cats.[6] Impression smears from surgical biopsies or surgically excised testicles can provide good quality samples.

Quality and cellularity of testicular FNAs depend on underlying pathology, area sampled, and aggressiveness of collection technique (e.g. with or without concurrent suction). Sensitivity of cytologic evaluation of different testicular tumors is reportedly high (>88%) with 100% specificity for the diagnosis of testicular neoplasia compared with histopathology.[2] Approximately 10% of the FNAs from one study in stallions yielded nondiagnostic, hemodilute samples.[7]

Possible complications of testicular FNA are parenchymal damage that directly disrupts spermatogenesis or adhesions that hamper testicular thermoregulation,[8] along with minimal scrotal swelling and erythema, with possible hemorrhage and necrosis identified histologically.[5,6] Complications related to testicular FNA are rare in men, with long-term effects on sperm output reported.[9] Testicular biopsies do not appear to have long-term effects on sperm output in boars, bulls, rams, or stallions.[7,10] In dogs, FNA is considered safe with no effects on libido or semen quality, even among dogs submitted to repeated collections for long periods of time.[3,11,12] Following aspiration, clinical and ultrasonographic appearance of the testis is unchanged, although hemorrhage can be detected for up to a week after collections in dogs and cats.[4,13,14] FNA can induce production of antisperm antibodies (ASA) due to disruption of the blood–testis barrier. However, testicular biopsy induced only transient ASAs in dogs, with negligible long-term effects.[8] In stallions, aspiration should be performed on the craniolateral quarter of the testicle, to avoid damaging the lateral testicular artery.[7]

Normal Histologic Architecture and Cytology

The testes are complex tubular glands with both exocrine (spermatogenesis) and endocrine (hormone production) functions. They are suspended within the scrotum in the *tunica vaginalis* and are enclosed in a dense connective tissue capsule called the *tunica albuginea*. The vascular layer in the *tunica albuginea* is superficial in dogs and deep in

Veterinary Cytology, First Edition. Edited by Leslie C. Sharkey, M. Judith Radin, and Davis Seelig.

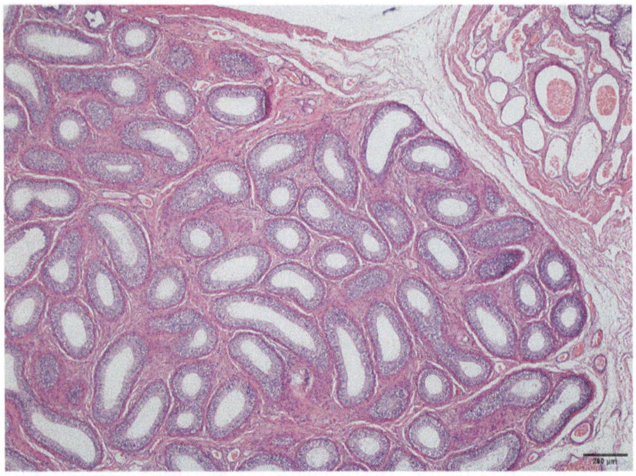

Figure 40.1 Atrophied testicle from a 5-year-old Chihuahua with attached epididymis and pampiniform plexus. The spermatic tubules have decreased cell volume and limited cell activity, with minimal sperm production. The epididymis is unremarkable and contains only small numbers of sperm (hematoxylin & eosin).

stallions, occasionally containing smooth muscle fibers in the latter. The *tunica albuginea* is continuous with the mediastinum, surrounding the *rete testis*, which is extratesticular in the stallion. The testicle lobules are composed of convoluted seminiferous tubules, lined by specialized, stratified epithelium containing two major cell types: the Sertoli cells, which provide physical support for developing sperm, and the spermatogenic cells. The interstitium between the seminiferous tubules contains connective tissue, blood and lymphatic vessels, and Leydig (interstitial) cells. The latter are responsible for producing testicular androgens under influence of luteinizing hormone (LH). Leydig cells are also known to produce estrogen in the boar. The overall architecture of the feline testicle was found to be age-independent between 1 and 6 years of age.[15]

Cytologically, a pleomorphic population is typically seen, including spermatozoa and cellular precursors (i.e. spermatogonia, spermatocytes, and spermatids), Sertoli cells, Leydig cells, and mesenchymal cells (Figure 40.2).[16] Abundant lysed nuclei and streaming nuclear material are usually retrieved with testicular FNAs, and a fair amount of blood contamination is expected, along with some mucus-like fluid.[6,16] Spermatogonia are difficult to recognize and appear as intermediate-sized round cells that contain an oval nucleus with occasional semilunar chromatin pattern. The cytoplasm is scant and stains lighter than that of more mature cells.[7] Spermatocytes are the largest of the spermatozoa precursors and appear as round, occasionally multinucleated cells with a round nucleus and coarse chromatin pattern that varies with stage of meiosis.[16] Spermatids are the most common of the precursors. Early-staged spermatids are slightly smaller than spermatocytes and contain a variable amount of pale basophilic cytoplasm with one to multiple perinuclear colorless vacuoles. Spermatids have a round or oval nucleus, are frequently multinucleated, and often contain one single, inconspicuous nucleolus. Late-staged spermatids contain a characteristic elongated nucleus with clumped, condensed chromatin. Mature spermatozoa are small cells with a small, condensed, oval nucleus, and a long, thin tail. No spermatozoa are identified in testes and epididymis of cats younger than 6 months.[6] Multinucleated spermatids and spermatocytes can be present in normal testicles, and mitotic figures are frequently observed. Sertoli cells are round to oval, with variably distinct cytoplasmic borders, abundant pale basophilic cytoplasm, and a round, eccentric nucleus with finely stippled chromatin and a single round, prominent nucleolus. Sertoli cells frequently appear poorly preserved or partially lysed.[7] Leydig cells are rare and can be arranged in variably sized sheets. These cells are round with abundant pale basophilic cytoplasm that frequently contains several discrete, variably sized vacuoles. Rare spindle-shaped mesenchymal cells are seen that appear individualized, with scant, pale basophilic, wispy cytoplasm and a centrally placed nucleus with finely stippled chromatin.

Conditions Diagnosed by Cytology

Neoplasia

Primary testicular tumors account for up to 90% of all tumors affecting the canine male genitalia.[17,18] Overall, the testes are the second most common location for tumor development in intact male dogs. The major types of testicular tumor are sex cord-stromal tumors, germ cell tumors, and mixed germ cell–sex cord-stromal tumors. Occurrence of two concurrent distinct testicular neoplasms is relatively common in the dog, particularly in cryptorchid animals, with the frequency reported as 20–40%.[19,20] Epithelial tumors rarely develop from the epithelial surfaces of the testes and include *rete* adenomas and carcinomas. The most frequent canine testicular tumors are Sertoli cell tumors (SCTs), interstitial cell tumors (ICTs), and seminomas, which occur with similar frequency.[17,19,21] While ICTs account for half of the testicular tumors in one study,[22] these constitute less than 10% of neoplasms reported in two separate studies where seminomas predominated,[23,24] suggesting population differences in tumor frequencies. Certain dog breeds seem to have an increased risk of developing primary testicular tumors, including Maltese, Poodle, Boxer, German Shepherd, Afghan Hound, and Weimaraner.[18] Collies and Shetland Sheepdogs were five times more likely to have testicular tumors in one

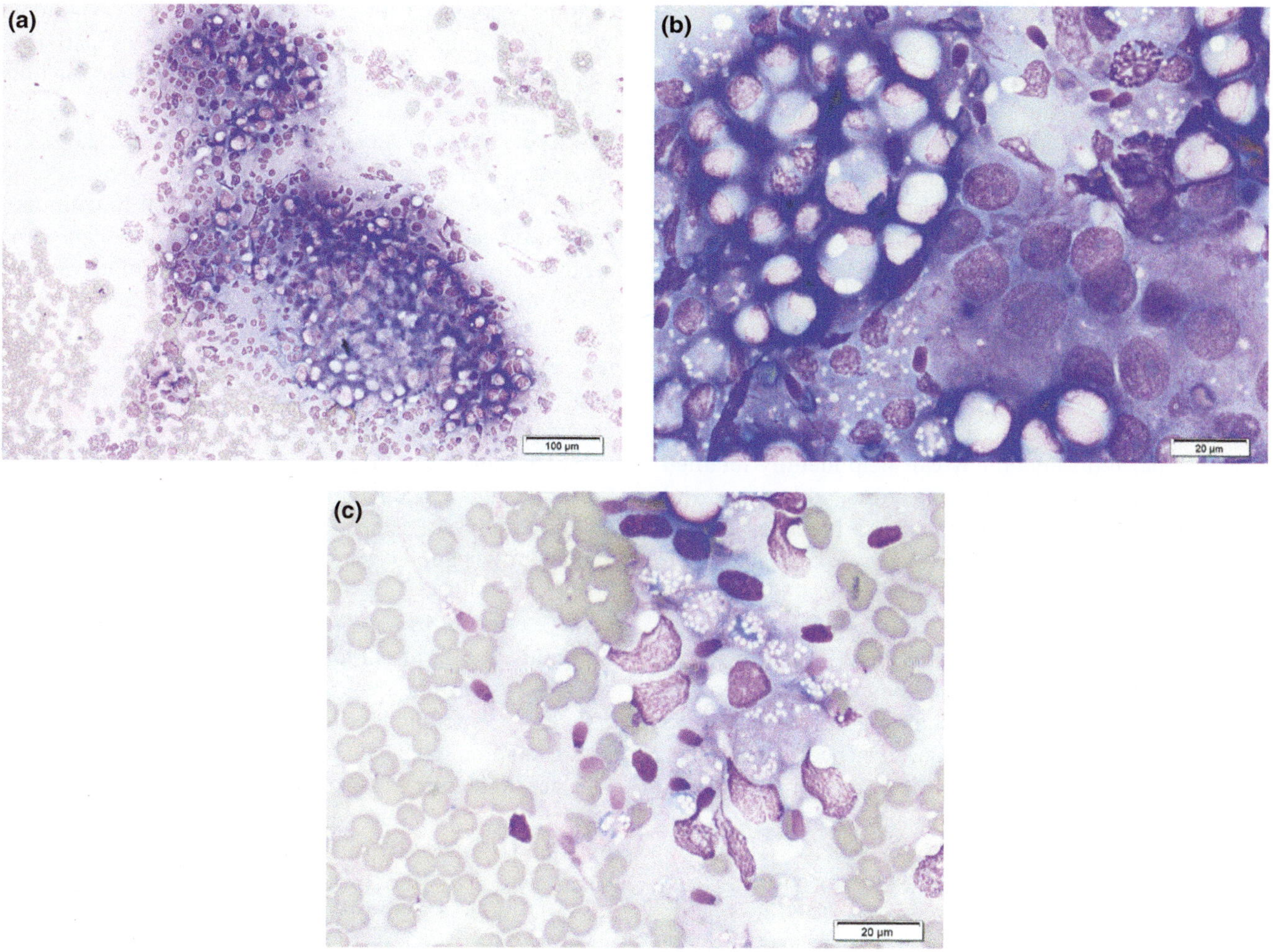

Figure 40.2 Normal canine testicle. (a) A variety of different cell populations, including germ cells in different stages of maturation (spermatogonia, spermatocytes, and spermatids). (b) A mixture of germ cells, Sertoli cells with a prominent single nucleolus, and several spermatozoa. (c) Detail of mixed cells and mature spermatozoa (Wright's. *Source:* Images courtesy of Leslie Sharkey).

study.[21] Most testicular tumors are identified in middle-aged to older dogs and are rarely reported before the age of 6 years.[18,25] However, there is no significant correlation between age and tumor development or type.[18] ICTs are the most common tumors (>50%) identified in clinically normal testes (i.e. no signs of testicular tumor, feminization, or cryptorchidism).[22,26] This suggests that ICTs may develop slowly and are not identified until large enough to draw attention during older age.[18]

Testicular tumors are rare in stallions. Germ cell tumors including seminomas and teratomas are most common, whereas SCTs and ICTs occur less frequently.[1] Testicular tumors are rare in cats,[20,27–29] so information regarding biologic behavior and frequency is scarce.

Cryptorchid testes are 14 times more likely to develop a tumor than scrotal testes in the dog,[17,23] and all tumors have been reported, although ICTs with much lower frequency.[18] In stallions, cryptorchidism is a risk factor for the development of ICTs.[30] The contralateral testis has increased risk of developing neoplasms, even if located in the scrotum.[31] Canine testicular tumorigenesis is poorly understood, and it appears unlikely that the insulin-like growth factor (IGF) system or cyclins D1, D2, and E (cell cycle regulators) are important for tumor maintenance and growth in the dog testes.[32,33] Vascular endothelial growth factor (VEGF) and cyclin A expression may be associated with the development of canine seminomas.[32,34] Upregulation of peroxisome proliferator-activated receptors is reported in canine testicular tumors in comparison with normal testicular tissue.[35] Since cryptorchidism is associated with testicular tumors, toy dog breeds may be at high risk for testicular neoplasia given the more frequent occurrence of cryptorchidism in these breeds.[25] Failure of testicle descent is twice as frequent on the right than on the left,[25,36] and incidence of testicular neoplasia is approximately twice as high in dogs with inguinal testicles than abdominal cryptorchids.[25] Testicular tumors can occur in neutered males and presumably arise from embryologic testicular remnants, ectopic testicular tissue (e.g. polyorchidism), or transplanted tissue (from previous surgery or trauma).[37] Metastases are observed in a low number of cases, and orchiectomy with or without adjunct chemotherapy or radiation therapy is often curative for localized tumors. Some authors, however, recommend orchiectomy at the earliest opportunity with high ligation of the spermatic cord to minimize the risk of metastasis.[38]

Abdominal ultrasonography can help identify retained testicles, including internal architecture and location, and assess lymph nodes and other organs for possible metastasis. The ultrasonographic appearance of testicular neoplasms is variable and does not allow for definitive distinction of tumor types, but ultrasonography can be used to locate testicular masses for biopsy[39] or non-palpable tumors.[40] Testicular ultrasound can help differentiate between neoplastic and nonneoplastic disorders such as inflammation, testicular torsion, degeneration/atrophy, and herniation.[41]

Sertoli Cell Tumors

SCTs are a sex cord-stromal tumor that arises from the sustentacular cells of seminiferous tubules. They frequently occur in the testicles of older dogs or retained testicles in cryptorchid animals[17] and present as testicular enlargement. Dogs with SCTs frequently exhibit feminization due to estrogen production by the neoplasm, a finding that has not been reported in cats.[27,42] Clinical signs of feminization syndrome include bilateral alopecia, hyperpigmentation, gynecomastia, galactorrhea, and penile atrophy. Estradiol-17β concentration is not always increased, suggesting that other forms of estrogen and/or estrogen-like substances produced by the tumor and decreased testosterone/estradiol ratio can trigger signs of feminization.[43,44] Bone marrow hypoplasia occurs in approximately 15% of dogs with SCTs and signs of feminization[45]; however, the exact mechanism of myelotoxicity and hematopoietic stem cell death is uncertain. Bone marrow hypoplasia can be fatal, and clinical signs include hemorrhage secondary to thrombocytopenia, persistent non-regenerative anemia, and infections due to neutropenia. Metastatic SCTs are infrequent, and primary sites of metastasis include lymph nodes (iliac, sublumbar, and pelvic), peritoneum, and other abdominal organs.[46] In the horse, metastases from malignant SCTs are reported in the kidneys, liver, lung, and diaphragm,[47] with near effacement of the hepatic parenchyma by a malignant SCT reported in a 13-year-old cryptorchid Morgan gelding.[48] Hypertrophic osteoarthropathy is reported in a dog with a SCT that metastasized to the lung and kidneys.[49]

SCTs are typically very firm, nodular, or lobulated, with a white-gray cut surface, and are greasy on palpation.[20,50] Histologically, SCTs are composed of round to columnar cells arranged individually and in distinct palisading arrangements.[2,51] Cytologically, the cells exhibit variable sizes and shapes. The abundant pale basophilic cytoplasm frequently contains several discrete, variably sized, colorless vacuoles (Figure 40.3). The large, round, or oval nucleus is paracentral to eccentric and has finely stippled chromatin with one to multiple, round or oval, prominent nucleoli. Call–Exner bodies are small, bright eosinophilic, fluid-filled spaces surrounded by cells that can occasionally be seen in SCTs and stain positive with Periodic acid–Schiff (PAS) (Figure 40.4).[52,53]

Germ Cell Neoplasms

Seminoma is a germ cell tumor that rarely produces clinical signs by itself, and the right testicle is more commonly affected.[54] Comorbidities such as prostatitis, prostatic hyperplasia, and/or perianal gland neoplasms are reported. Unilateral testicular enlargement is the most common clinical sign in dogs, and rare cases of bilateral seminomas are reported in stallions.[55] Tumors are locally invasive and can become very large prior to diagnosis. Despite a malignant histological appearance, these tumors usually are benign. However, among the three most common testicular tumors, seminomas are the most likely to metastasize.[20] Reported sites for metastasis include lymph nodes (inguinal, iliac, and sublumbar), lungs, and abdominal and thoracic organs.[1,38,56] Metastases affecting the bone, skin, eyes, and brain are reported.[57–59] Metastatic disease is more frequent in horses than dogs,[1,60,61] and reports of seminomas in stallions regularly describe sudden enlargement of the testis, attributed to rapid cellular division characteristic of germ cells.[1] A rare case of renal metastasis is reported in a stallion.[62] Cryptorchidism predisposes to development of seminomas, and one case of seminoma in a hermaphrodite bitch is reported.[63]

Seminomas are homogeneous, soft and bulging, occasionally lobulated, and cream-colored on the cut surface.[20,50] Cytologically, seminomas appear as a variably cellular, monomorphic population of round, discrete cells with a variable amount of medium basophilic, finely stippled cytoplasm that occasionally exhibits a perinuclear clearing (Figure 40.5). The round or oval nucleus is paracentral to eccentric and has coarse to clumped chromatin with one to multiple, round or oval, prominent nucleoli that vary in size. Binucleation and multinucleation are common. Mitotic figures are frequently observed, along

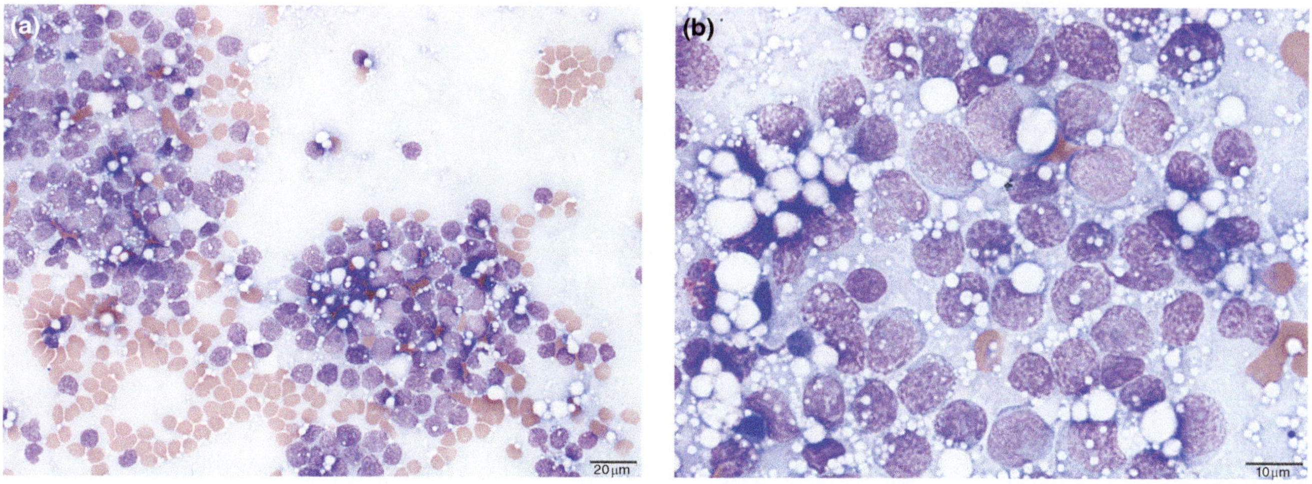

Figure 40.3 Sertoli cell tumor in an undescended left inguinal testicle from a 7-year-old Great Dane. (a) Cells are arranged in variably sized, poorly cohesive clusters, as well as individualized throughout the preparation. Many cells are lysed. (b) Round to oval tumor cells have a scant to moderate amount of pale to medium basophilic cytoplasm with discrete colorless vacuoles. The nucleus contains finely to coarsely stippled chromatin, and one to three, round or oval, ill-defined nucleoli. Overall anisocytosis and anisokaryosis are mild to moderate, and the N:C is moderate to high. Histopathologic evaluation confirmed the diagnosis and contralateral testicular degeneration/atrophy (Wright–Giemsa).

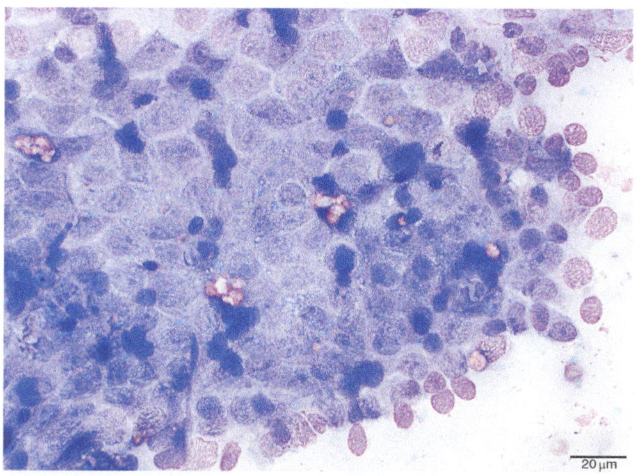

Figure 40.4 Sertoli cell tumor in a dog. Small amounts of amorphous, bright eosinophilic material, presumably Call–Exner bodies, are associated with aggregates of neoplastic Sertoli cells (Wright–Giemsa).

with a dense, variably eosinophilic background and a heterogeneous lymphoid infiltrate (predominantly $CD8^+$ T lymphocytes).[2,64]

Teratomas arise from totipotential primordial germ cells and contain more than one germinal layer, with cells in various stages of maturation. Testicular teratomas are reported in stallions[65] and rarely in the dog and cat.[28] They occur in young, cryptorchid stallions, suggesting that these are congenital neoplasms and, presumably, inhibit the normal descent of the testis.[66,67] Teratomas can be unilateral or bilateral and contain a multitude of different mature tissues (e.g. bone, cartilage, haired skin, fat).[28] Teratocarcinomas are composed of both mature and primitive germ cell tissue (Figure 40.6). A case of teratocarcinoma is reported to arise from a severely enlarged cryptorchid testicle from a 1.5-year-old horse, with metastasis to the liver and diaphragm.[68]

Embryonal carcinoma is a rare testicular neoplasm that arises from poorly differentiated embryonal epithelium of uncertain origin. A single case of metastatic embryonal carcinoma is reported in a 7-year-old Standardbred stallion.[69] This tumor can be difficult to distinguish from other poorly differentiated neoplasms. Diagnosis of embryonal carcinoma is based on the histopathologic and ultrastructural appearance, along with immunohistochemical staining for alpha-fetoprotein, a protein normally synthesized by the fetal liver and yolk sac.[69] Embryonal carcinoma in a calf expressed placental alkaline phosphatase (PLAP), cytokeratin, and carcinoembryonic antigen as well as alpha-fetoprotein on immunohistochemistry (IHC).[70]

Interstitial Cell Tumors

These are sex cord-stromal tumors composed of Leydig cells, the androgen-producing cells of the testicle. ICTs rarely produce testicular enlargement and are often incidental necropsy findings. They rarely are associated with feminization[71] but are reported to produce testosterone and may predispose to prostatic disease or perianal gland tumors.[20,72] The vast majority of these tumors are benign, although metastases to the skeletal musculature of the left hind leg[73] and the skin[74] are described in dogs.

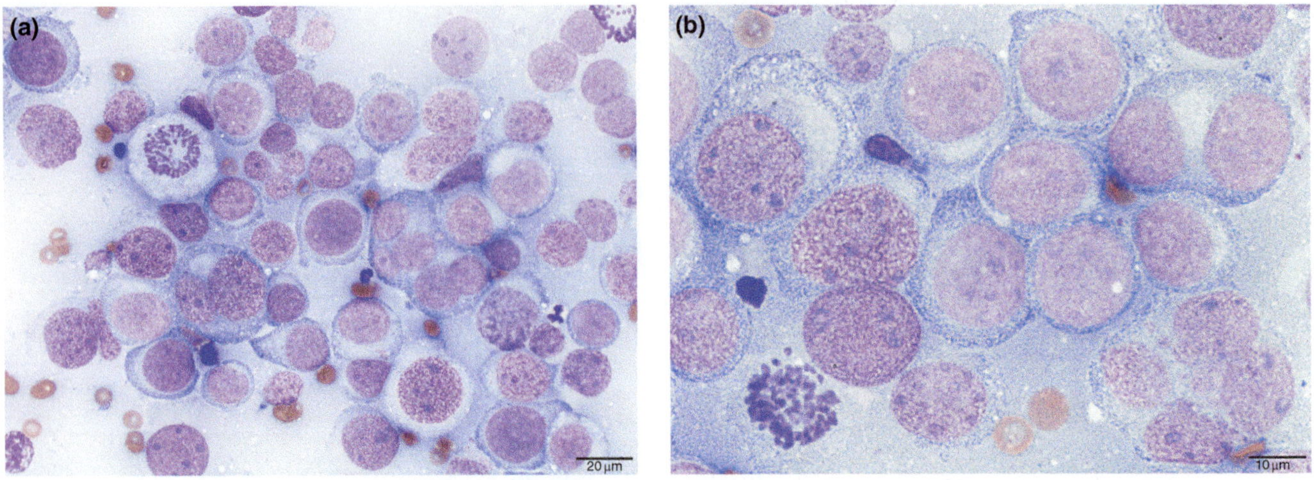

Figure 40.5 Seminoma in an enlarged testicle from a 12-year-old Golden Retriever. The dog presented for obstipation and inappetence. Metastases were found in multiple enlarged intra-abdominal lymph nodes. (a) Discrete round cells exhibit medium to deeply basophilic, finely stippled cytoplasm that often contains a paranuclear clear zone or a perinuclear clearing. Binucleated and multinucleated cells and mitotic figures are common. (b) Nuclei have coarsely stippled chromatin and multiple, prominent nucleoli that vary in size (Wright–Giemsa).

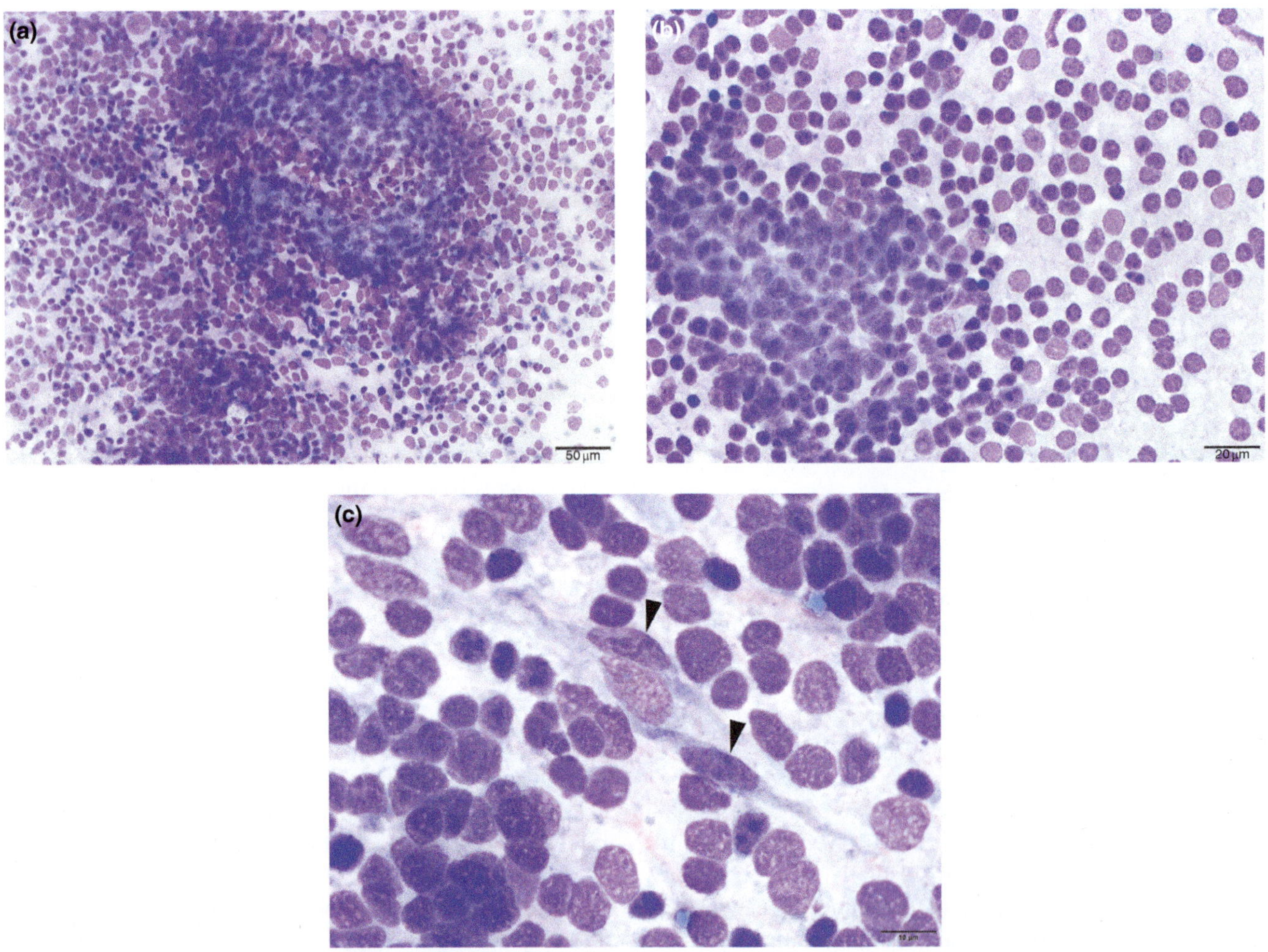

Figure 40.6 Malignant teratoma from an 8-month-old Arabian colt. (a and b) Small, round, germ-like cells predominate and are arranged individually, in variably sized palisading rows and clusters. Occasional pattern is consistent with rosette/acinar formations. (c) A second population of mesenchymal cells found individually throughout the preparation (arrowheads). These cells have indistinct cytoplasmic borders, with a moderate amount of pale basophilic, wispy cytoplasm (Quick Stain. *Source:* Image photographed by author from glass slide provided by Seth Chapman and presented at the 2007 ASVCP case review session).

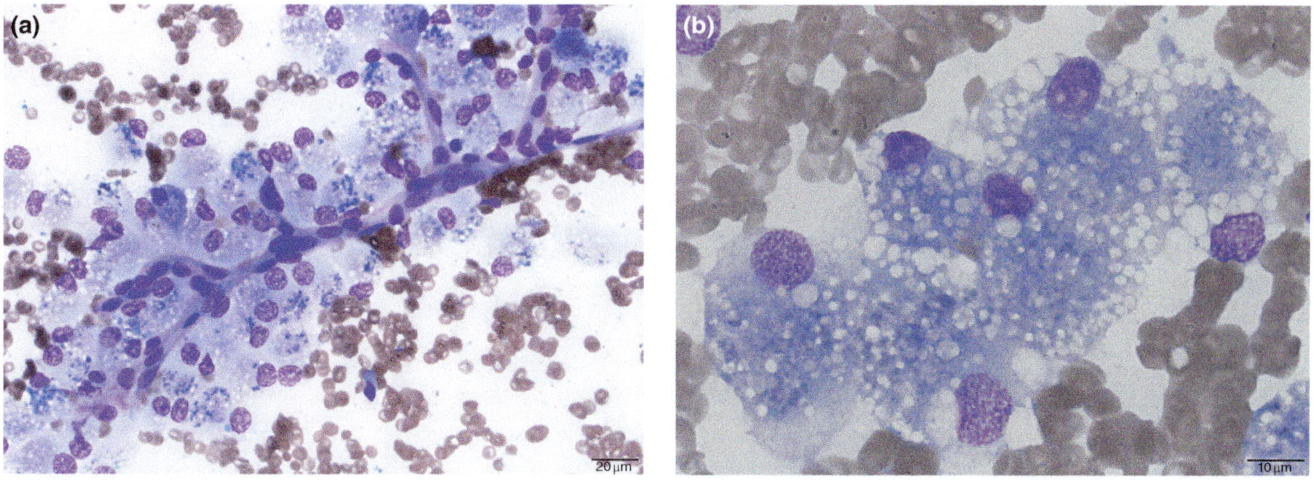

Figure 40.7 Interstitial (Leydig) cell tumor. Aspirate from a 2.0-cm mass within the left testicle of a 12-year-old mixed-breed dog. (a) Cells are found individually or in small sheets associated with intact capillaries. (b) Cellular characteristics include a moderate to abundant amount of pale to medium basophilic cytoplasm with numerous colorless vacuoles and/or a variable amount of bluish-black granular pigment, consistent with lipofuscin. The nucleus is paracentral to eccentric with coarse chromatin and a single small, round, distinct nucleolus (Wright–Giemsa).

ICTs are soft, bulging, with a yellow-brown cut surface, and often contain fluid-filled cysts.[20,50] Cytologically, ICTs yield variably cellular samples with cells arranged in variably sized cohesive clusters that are frequently admixed with intact capillaries (Figure 40.7).[2,51] Cells are pleomorphic, oval, or columnar to spindle-shaped, with variably indistinct cytoplasmic borders. The abundant, pale to medium basophilic cytoplasm contains numerous variably distinct colorless vacuoles and/or, less frequently, a fine, bluish-black cytoplasmic granulation consistent with lipofuscin.[2,31] The round or oval nucleus is small to intermediate-sized, has finely to coarsely stippled chromatin, and occasionally contains one or two, round or oval, variably sized nucleoli. Membrane-bound intranuclear inclusions are a distinguishing cytologic feature of ICTs.[2,75] Cytologic evidence of necrosis and hemorrhage are common.

Mixed Tumors

Mixed tumors are divided into two groups: gonadoblastomas and mixed germ cell–sex cord-stromal tumors.[76] Mixed germ cell–sex cord-stromal tumors include neoplastic elements derived from both the germ cell and sex cord-stromal elements within a single tumor (Figure 40.8) and are rare entities, particularly in the horse.[61] IHC for neuron-specific enolase (NSE), desmin, and vimentin is useful for distinguishing the two separate cell populations.[46,76] Sertoli cells are positive for both NSE and desmin, whereas germ cells are typically negative. Other IHC panels have been investigated, with different immunostaining patterns observed, suggesting that both neoplastic Sertoli cells and germ cells have a dedifferentiated phenotype.[77] Mineralization, Call–Exner bodies, and interstitial cells are not usually encountered in these neoplasms.[78] The biologic behavior of these tumors may be different from single-type tumors, in that they do not induce feminization and are usually benign.[46]

Gonadoblastomas are mixed tumors that contain germ cell (seminoma-like) and sex cord-stromal (Sertoli/granulosa-like) elements, with immature-looking sex cord-stromal cells. Gonadoblastomas are extremely rare in dogs.[79] Histologically, these typically benign tumors exhibit a jigsaw arrangement, with Sertoli-like cells arranged in a pseudopalisading pattern with surrounding germ cells. Call–Exner bodies were identified in one dog.[80] In horses, gonadoblastoma tumor cells form nests containing mineralized foci (presumably derived from Call–Exner bodies) and can contain foci of interstitial cells.[78] In humans, gonadoblastomas occur in genetic females with abnormal external genitalia and gonads.[46] A case of bilateral gonadoblastomas is reported in a 10-year-old male dog with mixed gonadal dysgenesis.[81]

Other Testicular Neoplasms

Hemangiomas, hemangiosarcomas, lipomas, granulosa cell tumors, sarcomas, lymphomas, Schwannomas, and a rare *rete testis* mucinous carcinoma are described.[24,82,83] A leiomyoma of the *tunica vaginalis* with concurrent hydrocele and testicular atrophy in a dog[84] and a leiomyoma of the *tunica albuginea* in a horse are reported.[85] An 11-month-old stallion had bilateral leiomyosarcomas in the abdominal testes.[86] Mesotheliomas of the *tunica vaginalis* are reported in two dogs, with immunohistochemical

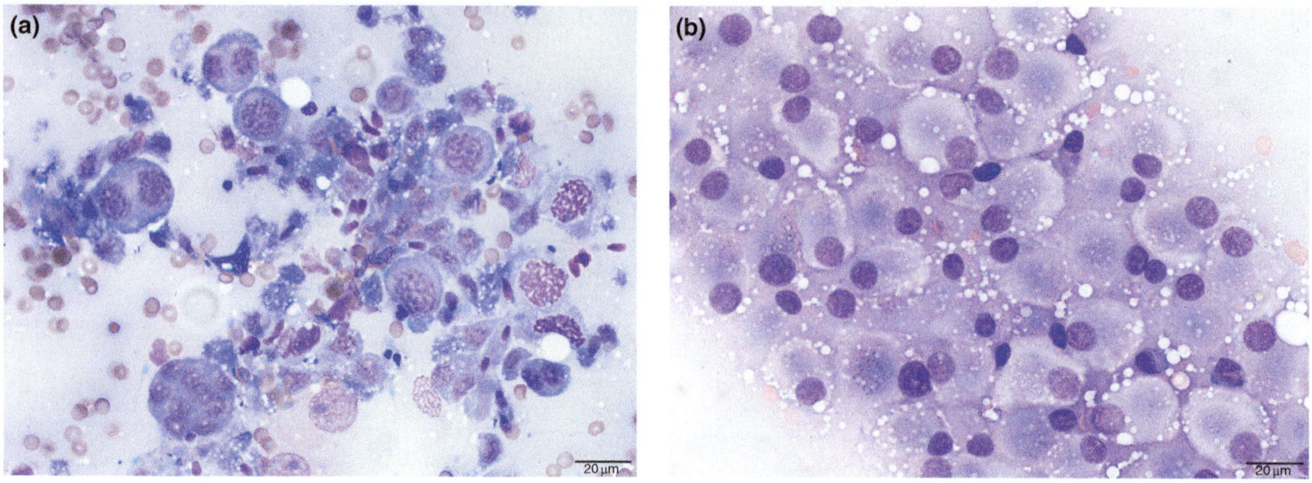

Figure 40.8 Mixed germ cell–sex cord-stromal tumor in the testicle of a dog. (a) Germ cell component, with discrete seminoma-like cells predominating. (b) Interstitial (Leydig) cell component, with cells arranged in loosely cohesive sheets or aggregates (Wright–Giemsa).

confirmation for one of the cases. Both dogs died three to four months after diagnosis with recurrence and metastasis.[87,88] One case of multiple mast cell tumors confined to the testicular capsule is reported in a dog.[89]

Metastases to the testes are rare. Metastasis or testicular involvement is reported with canine lymphoma, mast cell tumor, lymphangiosarcoma, gastrointestinal adenocarcinomas, and rarely in dogs with hemangiosarcoma.[20,24,90,91]

Inflammation

Infectious

Orchitis is an uncommon condition that has similar cytomorphology as inflammation elsewhere. It occurs less frequently than epididymitis, although both conditions often occur concurrently.[31] The inflammatory pattern will depend on the underlying etiology, but non-degenerate to variably degenerate neutrophils tend to predominate in acute cases, and phagocytosis of sperm can be observed (Figure 40.9). A definitive etiologic agent can be identified by cytology, although histopathology, microbiology techniques, or molecular methods are usually required for confirmation or exact diagnosis.

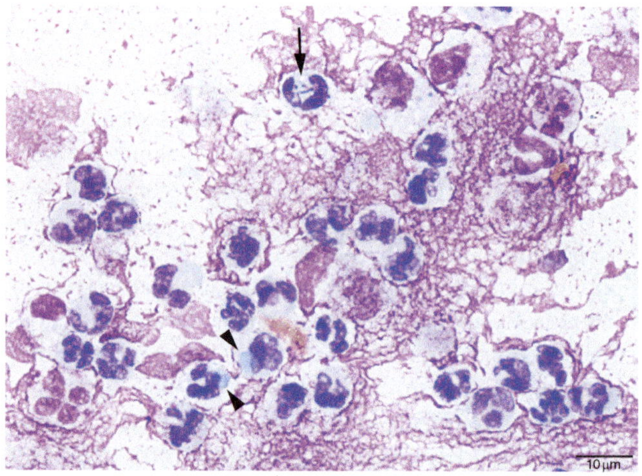

Figure 40.9 Septic orchitis and epididymitis in the right testicle from a 1-year-old American Pit Bull Terrier. *Serratia marcescens* was cultured from the urine and testicular aspirate. Infection was presumed to have ascended from the bladder. Non-degenerate to markedly degenerate neutrophils predominate. Neutrophils occasionally contain a few pleomorphic thin and plump bacilli (arrow) and/or phagocytized sperm heads (arrowheads) (Wright–Giemsa).

Infection with Gram-negative bacteria is frequent, presumably via ascending infection, hematogenous route, or local spread from epididymitis.[31] The most common etiologic agents in canine orchitis or epididymitis are *Brucella canis*, *Pseudomonas* spp., *Escherichia coli*, and *Proteus* spp.[92] *B. canis* infections are rarely apparent, and bacteriological isolation of the microorganism is necessary for a definitive diagnosis.[92] Blastomycosis is occasionally identified on cytology or histology,[93] although severe pyogranulomatous inflammation with multinucleated giant cells can be observed cytologically even in the absence of identifiable *Blastomyces dermatitidis* organisms.[94] Orchitis associated with canine distemper can present with characteristic intracytoplasmic or intranuclear viral inclusions, particularly within Sertoli cells.[95] Other rare etiologies for canine orchitis/epididymitis such as *Mycoplasma* spp. or *Ricketssia* spp. are reported.[41,96] Dogs with leishmaniasis can present with inflammation of the testes,[97] resulting in parasite shedding into the semen.[98] Orchitis or epididymitis are uncommon in cats, and reported etiologic agents include Coronavirus[99] and *Sporothrix schenckii*.[100]

Noninfectious

Sperm Granulomas Any injury that exposes spermatozoa to the interstitial tissue results in severe, typically granulomatous inflammation. Infiltration by lymphocytes and production of ASAs are reported.[101] Development of sperm granulomas is associated with a variety of underlying conditions including congenital (e.g. epididymal and ductal abnormalities) and acquired (e.g. trauma, infection, and surgery, including vasectomies) causes.[102–105] Cytologically, a mixed inflammatory population is noted.[105]

Other

Cystic structures such as hematoceles and hydroceles form from the accumulation of blood or ascites fluid within the cavity formed by the *tunica vaginalis*. Hydroceles are reported with testicular neoplasia or inflammation, ascites, or post-castration in geldings.[106] Cytologically, hydroceles appear as acellular preparations against a pale to densely basophilic proteinaceous background. Hematoceles exhibit evidence of acute and chronic hemorrhage (i.e. erythrophagocytic and hemosiderin-laden macrophages, hematoidin crystals) with variable amounts of blood and large numbers of neutrophils.[107] FNA from a spermatocele in a 2-year-old azoospermic dog is described as hemorrhagic fluid with abundant nonmotile spermatozoa.[108] A spermatocele with concurrent inflammatory, infiltrates and fibrosis is also referred to as a sperm granuloma.

Germ cell degeneration and depletion can result from direct injury to the testes or from disrupted hormonal regulation. Reported causes of testicular atrophy/degeneration include heat, fever, epididymitis, orchitis, scrotal dermatitis or edema, poor health status, hormonal imbalances, drugs (including chemotherapy), and systemic inflammatory diseases.[109] Germ cells are particularly sensitive, whereas Sertoli cells are relatively resistant.[31] Cytologic preparations from an injured testicle can yield numerous Sertoli cells and spermatogonia, with an overall paucity of other cell types. The formation of multinucleated spermatid giant cells and phagocytosis of spermatozoa by Sertoli cells can be observed.[31]

Testicular degeneration and atrophy are usually diagnosed clinically, evidenced by testes that are reduced in size after puberty. It is a common condition in dogs, particularly in older animals. Specific causes of testicular degeneration are numerous and include infection, neoplasia, toxic injury, and nutritional disorders. Spermatogenic arrest at one or more stages of the spermatogenic cycle is identified in the initial stages. In the final stages of testicular degeneration, Sertoli cells are the single lining cells that remain, until they disappear themselves.[31] Variable amounts of mineralized material can be observed. With severe degenerative change, it may become difficult to obtain sufficient material for cytologic evaluation.[3]

Testicular FNA in oligozoospermic or azoospermic cases can display a variety of different cytologic patterns: Sertoli cell-only syndrome, hypospermatogenesis, maturative disturbances, or normal spermatogenesis. Large numbers of mature spermatozoa in azoospermic or severely oligozoospermic dogs indicates complete or partial obstruction, while a complete absence of mature spermatozoa suggests congenital testicular damage.[12]

Advanced Diagnostic Techniques

Testicular neoplasms, particularly poorly differentiated tumors, can be difficult to differentiate cytologically. However, when signalment, clinical signs, and cytomorphologic findings are evaluated in context, a definitive diagnosis is generally achievable. Laboratory tests, including hormonal concentrations can help differentiate between testicular neoplasms. Both SCTs and ICTs can cause increased estrogen production leading to signs of feminization. SCTs have considerable inhibin-like immunoreactivity, resulting in a reduction in follicle-stimulating hormone (FSH) concentrations.[110] Increased estradiol-17β concentration, decreased testosterone levels, and decreased testosterone/estradiol ratios are also useful in the diagnosis of SCTs.[43] Anti-Müllerian hormone (AMH) is expressed by Sertoli cells, and dogs with SCTs or mixed tumors containing SCTs had AMH concentrations higher than 22 ng/mL,[111] making it a useful biomarker for canine SCTs.[112] In stallions, AMH expression is detected in SCTs, but not in seminomas or teratomas.[113]

A broad summary of IHC of canine testicular tumors is present on Table 40.1. IHC is not well established for equine testicular tumors, as only a small number of studies have been done.[121] ICTs produce inhibins and 3β-hydroxysteroid dehydrogenases[122] and express LH receptors,[123] which allow differentiation from other testicular neoplasms. Canine SCTs and ICTs are strongly positive for transcription factor GATA-4, whereas seminomas are negative.[124] Calretinin expression was detected in all canine SCTs, ICTs, and seminomas with a cytoplasmic and nuclear pattern of cellular distribution.[125] Sex-determining region Y box9 gene (SOX9) is expressed in canine SCTs and is absent in ICTs.[126]

Testicular germ cell tumors can be further classified as classic and spermatocytic seminomas or intratubular germ cell neoplasia of undifferentiated origin (IGCNU) based on IHC.[127,128] A study using PLAP immunostaining and PAS staining for the further classification of canine seminomas into classic seminomas (PLAP+/PAS+) and spermatocytic seminomas (PLAP−/PAS−) found a correlation between classic seminomas and tumor angiogenesis, suggesting a more aggressive behavior to this subtype.[129] Canine

Table 40.1 Summary of select immunohistochemistry markers for the most commonly reported canine testicular tumors.[37,77,114–120]

	VIM	DES	CK	INH-α	AMH	cKIT	NSE	PLAP	GATA-4	PGP9.5	S100	MEL-A	E-CAD
SCTs	+	±	±	+	+	−	±	±	+	−	±	±	+
ICTs	+	−	−	+	−	+	−	−	±	−	±	+	−
SEMs	±	±	−	±	−	±	±	±	−	+	−	−	±

AMH, anti-Müllerian hormone; CK, cytokeratin; DES, desmin; E-CAD, E-cadherin; GATA-4, transcription factor GATA-4; INH-α, inhibin-α; MEL-A, melanin-A; NSE, neuron-specific enolase; PLAL, placental alkaline phosphatase; PPGP.5, protein gene product 9.5; VIM, vimentin.
+ indicates positive staining, ± variable staining, − negative staining.

seminomas are predominantly of the spermatocytic type, and SCTs and ICTs concomitant with seminomas appears frequent.[54] Classic seminomas express c-KIT protein (CD117).[114] Some cases of spermatocytic seminomas may originate from germinal cell stages in which the expression of the c-KIT protein has not been downgraded.[130]

Ovaries

Introduction

Cytologic evaluation is a valuable tool in the diagnosis of canine ovarian tumors and cysts,[5] with high diagnostic accuracy.[131] Rare conditions, such as oophoritis also can be diagnosed via cytology in dogs and cats. Ovarian remnant syndrome is one of the most common conditions associated with the ovaries and can usually be diagnosed clinically without the use of ovarian cytology.[132] Indications for the use of transvaginal ovarian biopsies in the mare include abnormal ovarian consistency, inconclusive hormonal findings, abnormal ultrasonographic echotexture, behavioral or estrous cycle irregularities, and investigation of possible neoplastic disease.[133]

Collection

FNAs are collected by ultrasound-guided percutaneous aspiration or intraoperatively during exploratory laparotomy, while tissues collected for surgical biopsy are used for impression smears.[131] Blind FNAs can be performed if the ovarian lesion consists of a large space-occupying mass. Specific information on recovery rate and complications are scant, although some authors do not recommend transabdominal FNAs due to risk of tumor seeding.[134] Cytologic examination of abdominal effusions is reported as useful for rapid diagnosis of ovarian tumors.[135,136] Ovarian biopsies can be collected transvaginally in mares, although most reports describe collection of core biopsies for histopathologic evaluation. Mares require sedation, but usually tolerate the procedure without complications.[133]

Normal Histologic Architecture and Cytology

The ovaries are divided into the outer cortex and inner medulla, which are reversed in the mature mare. The ovarian surface is covered by low cuboidal, germinal epithelium. Immediately beneath this surface epithelium is a layer of connective tissue called the *tunica albuginea*. The cortex contains follicles in various stages of development and *corpora lutea*, embedded in a loose connective tissue stroma. Ova develop within the follicles (primordial, primary, secondary, and tertiary), which contain an oocyte surrounded by specialized epithelial cells (called granulosa cells from the primary follicle forward). With the growth of the follicle, the surrounding stromal cells differentiate into several layers of spindle-shaped theca cells. The canine ovaries have specific channels lined by cuboidal epithelium that can be continuous with the surface epithelium, called subsurface epithelial structures (SES). The medulla contains connective tissue, nerves, large blood and lymphatic vessels, and is continuous with the mesovarium. The *rete ovarii*, the female homologue of the *rete testis*, are short channels lined by cuboidal epithelium within the medullary zone. These complex structures go through many changes induced by the estrous cycle, age, and steroid hormone environment.[137]

FNAs of normal ovaries yield variable amounts of blood and nucleated cells embedded in a pale to densely basophilic, proteinaceous background with abundant free, nonstaining lipid, occasional lakes of amorphous, basophilic mucinous material, and rare pink amorphous structures consistent with the *corpus albicans*. Depending on the stage of the estrous cycle, variable numbers of adipocytes, fibroblasts, granulosa cells, leukocytes, immature round cells, and luteal cells are found.[138] Luteal cells are only observed during diestrus and are large, oval to polygonal, with variably distinct cytoplasmic borders. Cytoplasm is abundant, amphophilic to densely basophilic, with occasional multiple discrete colorless vacuoles that vary in size. From early to late diestrus, leuteal cells exhibit less anisocytosis and anisokaryosis and have bleb-like cytoplasmic projections. The finely stippled nuclear chromatin becomes coarse, often containing one or two, round or oval, prominent nucleoli. Conversely, morphology of granulosa and spindle-shaped cells is not linked to the estrous cycle. Granulosa cells are frequently arranged in variably sized, loosely cohesive aggregates, or occasionally in a concentric pattern consistent with acinar formations. These cells are round or oval with variably distinct cytoplasmic borders. The scant, pale basophilic cytoplasm occasionally forms a wispy projection and rarely contains a few small, discrete, colorless vacuoles. The round or oval nucleus is variably placed, has finely stippled chromatin, and sometimes contains variably distinct nucleoli. Round, individualized immature cells are noted, and these have discrete cytoplasmic borders, a high nuclear to cytoplasmic ratio (N:C), and a small amount of pale basophilic cytoplasm that typically contains several punctate, colorless vacuoles. The round or oval nucleus is centrally placed, has finely stippled chromatin, and frequently contains multiple small, inconspicuous nucleoli. These immature cells are not observed during anestrus.[138]

Conditions Diagnosed by Cytology

Neoplasia

Ovarian tumors are rare, accounting for 0.5–6.3% of all canine tumors and 0.7–3.6% of all feline tumors.[20,134,139] Ovarian tumors may be infrequent because the majority of dogs and cats are spayed at an early age and underreported as ovaries are not routinely inspected unless grossly abnormal.[140] The most common ovarian tumors are epithelial and sex cord-stromal tumors with germ cell and mesenchymal tumors rarely occurring. Clinical signs are usually related to space-occupying masses or neoplastic effusion.[136] Colic is a frequent presenting sign in mares with large ovarian tumors.[141] Canine ovarian tumors can actively produce estrogen and/or progesterone and incite secondary clinical signs such as persistent estrus, endometrial hyperplasia, pyometra, endocrine alopecia, and bone marrow hypoplasia/aplasia.[142] Breed predispositions are not well defined, though Poodles, Boston Terriers, Yorkshire Terriers, German Shepherds, and Boxers appear overrepresented.[131,135,143]

Epithelial Neoplasms

These tumors arise from the epithelial surfaces of the ovary and include adenomas, carcinomas, and their cystic counterparts. They account for nearly half of canine ovarian tumors.[20,135,143] Adenocarcinomas are the most common ovarian neoplasms in the bitch.[143] They typically originate from the SES and frequently metastasize to the abdominal cavity, omentum, intra-abdominal organs, and lymph nodes.[143] Neoplastic effusions are common with canine ovarian tumors.[136] Feline epithelial neoplasms are extremely uncommon.[144]

In the mare, epithelial tumors are uncommon and arise from the surface epithelium of the ovary or from the *rete ovarii* and rarely metastasize. Evaluation of peritoneal fluid in mares with adenocarcinomas may be useful, as neoplastic cells can exfoliate into the fluid.[145] Although most tumors are unilateral, bilateral tumors are reported, and contralateral ovarian cysts may occur. A ruptured bilateral ovarian adenocarcinoma is reported in a mare with colic and concurrent hemoabdomen.[141] One case of paraneoplastic hypercalcemia with a serous papillary adenocarcinoma is described in a dog,[146] and hypertrophic osteopathy was seen secondary to metastatic ovarian adenocarcinoma in a mare.[147]

Cytologically, adenocarcinomas exfoliate in variably sized cohesive sheets that can form papillary projections, and cells are occasionally arranged in concentric patterns, consistent with acinar formations.[51] Cells are oval to polygonal with variably distinct cytoplasmic borders and a variable amount of pale to medium basophilic cytoplasm that occasionally contains multiple discrete, colorless vacuoles that vary in size (Figure 40.10). Large cytoplasmic vacuoles can displace the nucleus, producing a signet ring appearance.[131,146] The round or oval nucleus is paracentral to eccentric and has finely stippled to coarse chromatin with one to multiple, variably distinct nucleoli. Psammoma bodies (laminated, rounded mineralized structures surrounded by neoplastic cells) are reported in a bilateral ovarian papillary cystic adenocarcinoma in a dog.[148] Neoplastic effusions from primary ovarian carcinomas are common and contain exfoliated monomorphic cells with similar appearance as the primary masses.[136,148,149]

Sex Cord-Stromal Neoplasms

These include granulosa cell tumors, luteomas (interstitial cell tumors), thecomas, and Sertoli–Leydig cell tumors.[150] They arise from the ovarian gonadal stroma and have the capacity of secreting steroid hormones. Granulosa cell tumors account for nearly half of canine ovarian neoplasms and usually affect middle-aged to older dogs. Canine granulosa cell tumors are mostly benign, with a 20% chance of metastatic disease.[134,143] It is the most common sex cord-stromal tumor in cats, and the majority are malignant.[20,144] Granulosa cell tumor is the most common ovarian tumor in the mare[141] and almost invariably benign.[151,152] In mares, contralateral ovarian atrophy is associated with increased AMH production and suppression of FSH effects on follicular development.[152,153] Granulosa cell tumors have a classic ultrasonographic appearance in the mare, referred to as a "cluster of grapes," accompanied by a small, inactive contralateral ovary.[133,152]

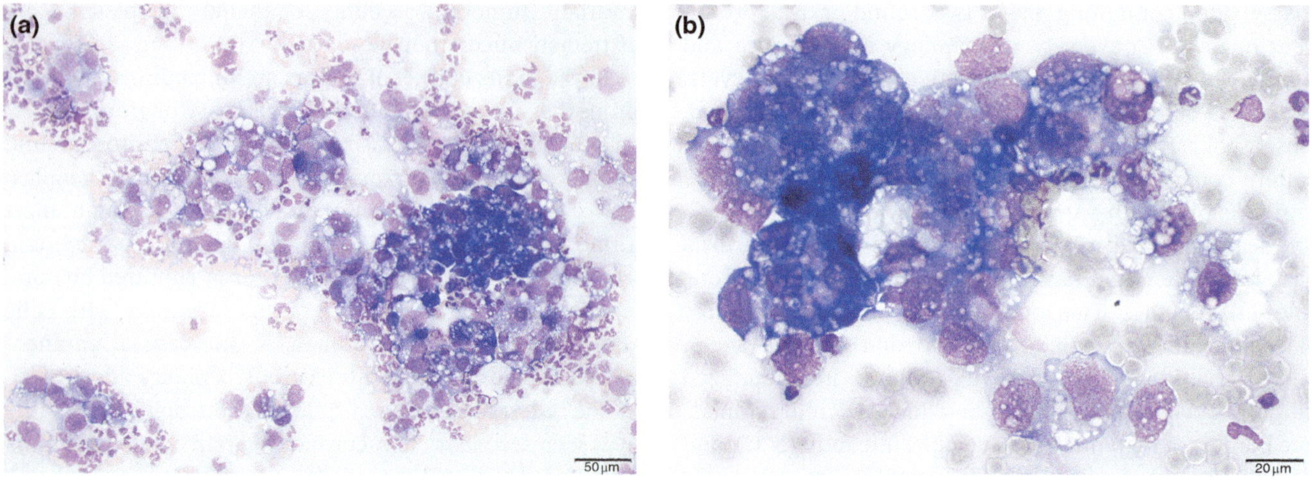

Figure 40.10 Anaplastic ovarian carcinoma. Abdominal effusion from a 19-month-old, female, Doberman Pinscher with a large mixed echogenic intra-abdominal mass and metastatic disease. (a) Moderately to occasionally markedly atypical epithelial cells are arranged in variably sized cohesive sheets. Mixed inflammatory cells are present in the background. (b) Cellular characteristics of the carcinoma include variably distinct cytoplasmic borders and a moderate amount of medium to deeply basophilic cytoplasm that frequently contains several, variably distinct, colorless vacuoles that vary in size. The round or oval nucleus has finely to coarsely stippled chromatin and one to multiple nucleoli (Wright–Giemsa. *Source:* Image photographed by author from glass slide provided by Ruth Houseright and presented at the 2014 ASVCP case review session).

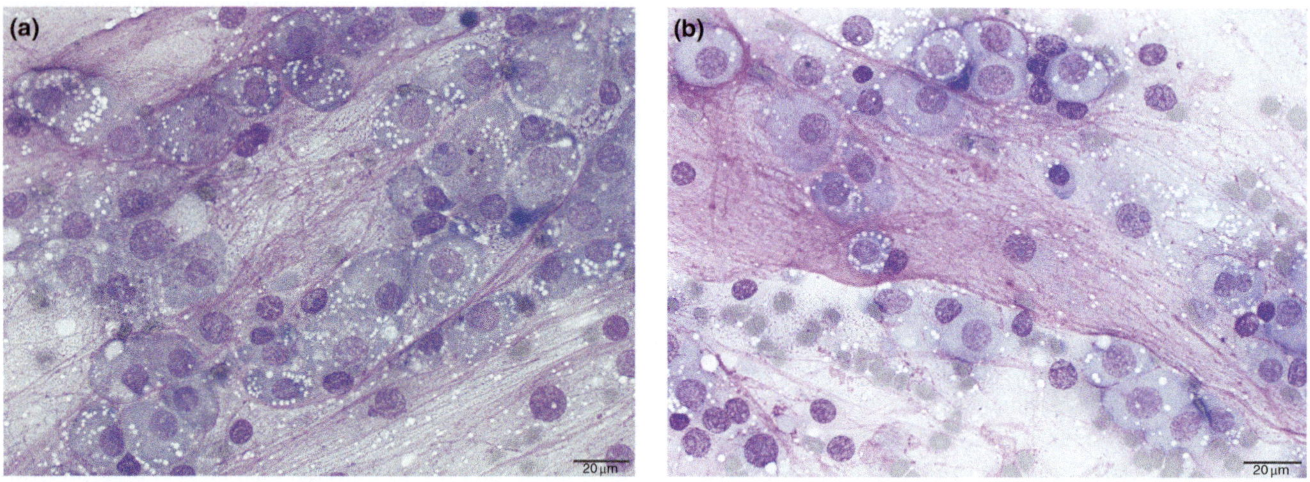

Figure 40.11 Granulosa cell tumor. Impression smear of a large ovarian mass from a 4-year-old English Bulldog. (a) The cells are round to polygonal and found individualized and in variably sized clusters. The basophilic cytoplasm is moderate to abundant in amount, with discrete, colorless vacuoles, and occasionally fine purple granules. The round nucleus contains finely to coarsely stippled chromatin and a single to multiple prominent nucleoli. (b) The cells are often admixed with abundant bright eosinophilic, amorphous to streaming material (Wright–Giemsa. *Source:* Image photographed by author from glass slide provided by Kaikhushroo Banajee and presented at the 2012 ASVCP case review session).

Many granulosa cell tumors produce AMH, estrogens, androgens, and/or inhibin. Mares can exhibit signs of anestrus with inhibin-producing neoplasms, nymphomania, or stallion-like behavior with estrogen and androgen-producing tumors, respectively.[141,154] Prolonged estrus and pyometra can occur in the dog.[155] Granulosa cell tumors arising from incompletely excised ovarian tissue during ovariohysterectomy are reported.[156]

Cytologically, granulosa cell tumors are variably cellular. Cells exfoliate individualized or in variably sized loose clusters that are occasionally concentrically arranged around Call–Exner bodies. Granulosa cells are oval to polygonal with variably indistinct cytoplasmic borders. Cytoplasm is scant to moderate in amount, lightly basophilic, and frequently contains a few, discrete, colorless vacuoles that vary in size (Figure 40.11). The round or oval nucleus is paracentral to eccentric, has coarsely stippled chromatin, and one to multiple, round or oval, ill-defined nucleoli.[131] Some granulosa cell tumors in the bitch and mare may resemble SCTs of the testes. Cells resembling theca cells and collagen-producing fibroblasts are frequent and may outnumber granulosa cells. Extensive luteinization can occur.[156]

Thecomas and luteomas are considered benign. Feline luteomas exfoliate large, oval to polygonal cells that are individualized or arranged in variably sized loose clusters and resemble the cells found in the normal interstitial glands of the feline ovary.[157] Cytoplasm is medium basophilic and moderate to abundant in amount, with several discrete, lipid-filled vacuoles that vary in size and/or infrequent small purple granules. The round or oval nucleus is central to paracentral and has coarsely stippled chromatin with small, prominent nucleoli.[157] Thecomas are composed of oval or spindle-shaped cells with abundant amounts of highly vacuolated, lipid-rich cytoplasm. The nucleus is round to pleomorphic, often containing large, prominent nucleoli.[158] Special stains for lipid (e.g. Sudan Black, Oil Red O) may help differentiate thecomas from fibromas or other mesenchymal tumors.

Sertoli–Leydig cell tumors are not fully characterized in the dog, seldom recognized, and classified as granulosa cell tumors by most pathologists. One case is reported in a 6-year-old cat.[159] These tumors exhibit a wider range of histologic patterns and cell types than do most ovarian neoplasms and often contain heterologous elements mimicking teratoma or teratocarcinomas.[160] Histopathologic evaluation and recognition of the different subtypes is important as these tumors can present with retiform patterns similar to papillary adenocarcinomas or contain lipid, similar to luteal cell tumors. These tumors are commonly bilateral, and metastasis is described in one dog.[150,160]

Germ Cell Neoplasms

These tumors include dysgerminomas, embryonal carcinomas, teratomas, and teratocarcinomas.[161] Dysgerminomas and teratomas together account for roughly 10% of all canine ovarian tumors[162] and are rarely seen in cats. In the mare, they are reported as the second most frequent ovarian neoplasms after granulosa-theca cell tumors.[163] Cysts in the contralateral ovary and uterine abnormalities are common in dogs.[162] Despite high mitotic activity and cytologic criteria of malignancy, the majority of dysgerminomas are clinically benign. Metastases to either regional lymph nodes and/or adjacent intra-abdominal organs are reported in up to 20% of canine cases.[20] In a case of malignant dysgerminoma in an 18-year-old mare, metastases were identified in the retroperitoneal tissue and lymph nodes.[164] Mares with disseminated germ cell neoplasms may exhibit hypertrophic osteopathy.[165]

Cytologically, dysgerminomas are composed of large, pleomorphic cells with variably distinct to discrete cytoplasmic borders and a variable amount of pale to medium basophilic cytoplasm that occasionally contains a small amount of pinkish, granular material.[131] The round or oval nucleus is paracentral to eccentric and has finely to coarsely stippled chromatin. Prominent nucleoli are multiple, round, oval or angular, and variable in size. Binucleated or multinucleated cells and mitotic figures are common. Overall anisocytosis and anisokaryosis are typically marked. A heterogeneous lymphoid infiltrate is frequently observed.[131,142]

Teratomas are composed of any combination of at least two types of embryonic germ layers (i.e. ectoderm, including neuroepithelium, mesoderm, and endoderm). Cytologically, they may be composed of a variety of mature cell types, including adipocytes, osteocytes, chondrocytes, and squamous epithelial cells with abundant necrotic debris in the background.[131] Histopathology is ultimately required for a definitive diagnosis.[166] Teratomas are hormonally inactive and usually do not affect the estrous cycle in the mare.[163,166] However, tumor growth can cause abdominal pain, pressure symptoms, and adhesions to the surrounding structures, indirectly affecting fertility.[163] Teratocarcinomas are extremely rare[162] and, on cytology, comprise atypical, immature cells with frequent mitotic figures.[161] Necrosis with accompanying pyogranulomatous inflammation, sebaceous-like epithelial cells, keratinized debris, and mature keratinocytes also can be seen.[131,161,167] Any component can become malignant, and distant metastasis and/or carcinomatosis are common in teratocarcinomas.[20]

Mesenchymal Ovarian Tumors

Mesenchymal tumors are rare in the dog and include hemangiosarcoma,[135] leiomyoma[168] and rhabdomyosarcoma.[169] Ovarian fibromas and leiomyomas have similar appearance as in other tissues and may be difficult to distinguish from thecomas. A primary fibroleiomyoma is described in a pregnant mare.[170]

Other Ovarian Neoplasms

A bilateral ovarian mixed malignant Müllerian tumor composed of variably admixed malignant epithelial and nonepithelial elements is reported in a dog.[171] A congenital hamartoma is described in a mare.[172] Vascular hamartomas are blood-filled spaces with proliferation of blood vessels lined by mature endothelial cells that look cytologically indistinguishable from vascular neoplasms (e.g. hemangiomas). They are usually incidental findings in the mare, cow, and sow and extremely rare in other species.[155]

Reported metastases of different neoplasms to the ovaries include mammary carcinomas, particularly inflammatory forms,[173] pancreatic and intestinal carcinomas, melanomas, and transmissible venereal tumors.[20] Lymphomas may be diagnosed within the ovarian tissue but are usually present concurrently in lymphoid organs.[20,144]

Inflammatory

Oophoritis is rare in domestic animals, and the ovarian response to inflammation is not well understood. The observation of neutrophilic and lymphocytic inflammation in bacterial and viral infections, respectively, indicates that this tissue responds similarly to infectious organisms as other organs.[155] Oophoritis caused by infectious organisms is rarely diagnosed in domestic animals. Bacterial oophoritis is reported in dogs and cats, and ascending infection from the uterus is the proposed pathologic mechanism.[174] Ovarian abscesses usually are unilateral in the mare, and ultrasonography is the most accurate diagnostic tool to differentiate an abscess from other ovarian conditions, as they usually exhibit a homogeneous hyperechoic appearance surrounded by a thick wall.[166] Bacterial perioophoritis is occasionally found in dogs and cats, and it must be differentiated from feline infectious peritonitis (FIP) granulomas in affected cats.[155] Bacterial oophoritis should produce suppurative inflammation.

Other

Intraovarian or paraovarian cysts are common in bitches, queens, and mares and can be confused with cystic neoplasms. Intraovarian cysts most commonly include cystic *rete ovarii* and cystic SESs in dogs.[155] Cysts of the *rete ovarii* are relatively common in dogs and cats, and cysts of the surface epithelium are most common in the mare.[155] Cytologically, ovarian cysts usually have low cellularity with occasional, variably vacuolated macrophages and variable amounts of blood on a pale to densely basophilic, proteinaceous background. Histologic examination of ovarian cysts provides distinction between follicular cysts and cysts arising in the *rete ovarii*, SESs, or paraovarian. However, clinical significance is minimal unless there is disruption of ovarian architecture, and ovarian cysts are usually found incidentally during ultrasound or surgery.[175] A report of cytologic preparations of ovarian cystic fluid from a 24-year-old Quarter Horse mare contained several round, pale to deeply basophilic, partially to completely ciliated structures, consistent with detached ciliary tufts (ciliary/ciliated bodies), and the authors urged the importance of recognizing these structures that could be mistaken for ciliated parasites.[176]

Ovarian hematomas are common in mares and are presumed a consequence of excessive hemorrhage in the follicular cavity following ovulation.[177,178] In rare cases, the hemorrhage can be extensive enough to cause hemoperitoneum,[155] although they usually regress by the next ovulation without affecting cycle length.

Rare cases of hermaphroditism and bilateral ovotestes are reported in dogs.[179,180] The ovaries contained tubular tissue lined by Sertoli-like cells within the medullary zones, with no germ cells appreciated.

Advanced Diagnostic Techniques

A summary of IHC markers is presented in Table 40.2. Useful IHC markers to differentiate ovarian tumors are cytokeratin 7, inhibin-α, and Hector Battifora mesothelial epitope-1 (HBME-1). Epithelial tumors are positive for cytokeratin 7 and HBME-1, while thecomas and granulosa cell tumors are positive for inhibin-α.[181,183] Canine granulosa cells are also positive for vimentin, S100, inhibin-α, and endothelin-1.[137,184] Equine granulosa cell tumors express vimentin, glutathione S-transferase α (GST-α), and c-erbB-2 oncoprotein (cerb). Expression is much lower in malignant tumors than in benign tumors, suggesting that this IHC panel may provide an indication of malignancy in equine granulosa cell neoplasms.[182] Carcinomas are often immunoreactive for cytokeratin, desmin, vimentin, cyclooxygenase-2, and endothelin-1 but usually negative for inhibin-α.[46,137,185] A canine bilateral retiform Sertoli–Leydig cell tumor was positive for inhibin-α, while epithelial membrane antigen was negative.[150]

Determination of serum AMH concentrations can be used to monitor granulosa cell tumors. Serum AMH is higher in mares with granulosa cell tumors than in

Table 40.2 Summary of select immunohistochemistry markers for the most commonly reported canine ovarian tumors.[46,137,181,182]

	VIM	DES	CK	INH-α	S100	END-1
Epithelial	±	+	+	–	±	+
Granulosa cell tumors	+	–	±	+	+	+
Dysgerminomas	+	–	–	–	–	NA

CK, cytokeratin; DES, desmin; END-1, endothelin-1; INH-α, inhibin-α; VIM, vimentin.
+ indicates positive staining, ± variable staining, – negative staining, NA not assessed.

cyclic or pregnant mares and decreases after tumor removal.[153] Inhibin or testosterone concentrations are less consistent.[186]

Prostate

Introduction

Disorders of the prostate affect approximately 2.8% of male dogs and are extremely rare in other species.[95,187,188] However, 75.6% of dogs that died of diseases unrelated to the prostate had evidence of prostatic disease on necropsy.[189] The most common prostatic disorders include benign prostatic hyperplasia (BPH), prostatitis, prostatic abscesses, prostatic and paraprostatic cysts, and neoplasia.[109,187,190] The mean age of onset of prostatic disease in dogs is 8.9 years,[190] and Doberman pinschers are reported to have a higher incidence of prostate disease. Prevalence of BPH and prostatic neoplasia increases with age, but prostatitis is not influenced by age.[189] Clinical signs of prostatic disorders overlap; therefore, accurate diagnosis requires thorough evaluation, including historical assessment, physical exam, digital rectal exam (DRE), abdominal radiography and ultrasound, and evaluation of prostatic fluid, FNAs, and/or histopathology.[191,192]

Collection

Indications

Clinical signs of prostatic disease are common in male dogs, especially those over 6 years of age.[191] Signs suggestive of prostatic disease include ribbon or tapered stools, tenesmus, lower urinary signs (stranguria and hematuria), preputial or urethral discharge, and locomotor difficulty.[190,191] Poor semen quality, infertility, and recurrent urinary tract infections also warrant investigation of the prostate.[5] On DRE, a normal prostate is smooth, symmetrical, and pain free.[191] DRE has a high specificity (75%) and positive predictive value (87%) but has a low sensitivity (53%) and negative predictive value (34%) for detecting prostatic disease.[189] Ultrasound is recommended for all dogs with prostatic disease, as it can detect abnormalities unapparent on physical exam, identify additional lesions, and be used for guidance when performing percutaneous biopsy or FNA.[5,193,194] With ultrasound, inflammation, hyperplasia, and neoplasia are associated with a loss of gland homogeneity and focal to multifocal areas of hyperechoic and/or hypoechoic tissue, whereas prostatic cysts and abscesses are associated with anechoic or hypoechoic areas, respectively.[5,191,195]

Methods

Transabdominal ultrasound guidance is preferred for obtaining FNAs.[5,196] Perirectal and rectal aspiration techniques are also described.[191] The area is surgically prepared, and a sterile sleeve is placed over the ultrasound probe. A sterile 21-G needle is visualized as it passes into the prostate, and negative pressure is applied several times by syringe. More than one sample should be taken, especially if multifocal lesions are present.[5,197] Aspiration of any significant amount of fluid is abnormal; normal prostatic fluid is minimal, light yellow to translucent, and resembles urine.[191] Obtaining a diagnostic sample by FNA is successful approximately 50% of the time in dogs.[198]

Prostatic massage and wash is recommended for suspected prostatitis or abscessation.[199] The patient is sedated, the bladder catheterized aseptically, and urine removed. The bladder is rinsed several times with 10–20 mL saline, and the last rinse is kept as a pre-massage sample. The catheter is retracted to the prostatic urethra. The prostate is vigorously massaged for 1–2 minutes, followed by slow injection of 10 mL of saline, which is aspirated back as a post-massage sample. Pre- and post-massage samples are compared in order to localize the disease process to the urinary bladder or prostate.[5,191,197,199] Because interpretation of prostatic fluid cytology is complicated by dilution, centrifugation and examination of the pellet is recommended.[5] Normal post-massage samples typically contain a few erythrocytes and urothelial cells.[197] Inflammation in prostatic fluid is >80% correlated with inflammation identified histologically.[5,191,197] Cytologic samples obtained by catheterization frequently contain a mixed population of urothelial cells, which can complicate diagnosis of neoplasia or squamous metaplasia.[200]

Of the three ejaculation fluid fractions, the third is very specific to the prostate. Occasional erythrocytes, leukocytes, and squamous epithelial cells are seen in the normal dog. Large numbers of erythrocytes can indicate recent hemorrhage, whereas a coffee ground appearance indicates chronic hemorrhage.[191] Numerous leukocytes occur with inflammation, and bacteria engulfed by leukocytes indicate a septic process.[201] Since bacterial flora are normal in the distal urinary tract, culture from ejaculate should be interpreted cautiously. Infection is indicated by heavy growth or pure culture of Gram-negative bacteria or when there is ≥2 log 10 of one or more bacterial species in prostatic fluid over the number of colonies of the same species in the paired urethral specimens.[201]

Histopathology is the gold standard for evaluation of the prostate. Histopathology is warranted when less invasive tests do not give a diagnosis, therapy is ineffective, or to give a definitive diagnosis of prostatic adenocarcinoma as biopsy has greater diagnostic accuracy than FNA.[5,191]

Prostatic histology is diagnostic in approximately 66.7% of cases.[5] Cytology can be advantageous over histopathology: it is less invasive, turnaround time is shorter, multiple samples can be obtained, and it is more sensitive for the detection of sepsis.[200] Overall, cytologic diagnosis agrees with histologic diagnosis approximately 80% of the time.[200,202] The reasons for discordant results include poor cellularity when fibrotic tissue is aspirated, dysplasia misinterpreted as neoplasia, and/or failure to obtain representative samples from all lesions when more than one disease process is present.[200]

Safety

The major contraindication to FNA or biopsy is prostatic abscessation or bacterial prostatitis, where seeding of the needle tract and secondary peritonitis is a concern.[191,199] However, in a study of 13 dogs with either prostatic abscesses or cysts, no complications followed percutaneous drainage.[196] Hematuria and/or hemospermia,[5] usually of less than four days duration, has been described after FNA and tru-cut needle or wedge biopsy.[5,198] Dissemination of neoplastic cells along the needle tract has been reported for transitional cell carcinoma (TCC) of the bladder, urethra, and prostate in dogs.[203] Urethral catheterization to obtain a cytologic diagnosis of TCC is recommended whenever possible; however, if the urethra cannot be catheterized, percutaneous FNA should still be performed, as accurate diagnosis outweighs the rare chance of needle-tract implantation.[203] Induction of urinary tract infections following improper procedure for prostatic wash and massage is possible,[197] and priapism following manual ejaculation is reported.[5]

Normal Tissue Architecture and Cytology

The prostate is a bilobed, oval to spherical exocrine gland that encircles the proximal urethra and consists of a dorsal and ventral sulcus surrounded by smooth muscle and connective tissue.[204] In the dog, the dorsal sulcus and caudal element of the gland can be identified with DRE.[191,193] It contributes fluid to the first and third fractions of ejaculate.[193] The glandular portion of the prostate has a compound tubuloalveolar structure with a discontinuous basal layer. The prostatic stroma is composed of smooth muscle cells and fibroblasts in a collagenous matrix along with capillaries, lymphatics, and nerves.[204] In intact dogs, prostatic acini contain luminal tall columnar to cuboidal secretory epithelial cells; however, after castration, the prostate epithelium regresses, and the remaining tubules contain cells showing a ductal phenotype.[204,205] In the stallion, the prostate has well-defined small to medium pockets of prostatic fluid that increase in size with sexual stimulation.[206] The prostate in geldings is less apparent and lacks fluid-filled spaces.[207]

Cytologically, epithelial cells are cuboidal to columnar and uniform in appearance. Cells have a low to moderate N:C, a round to slightly oval nucleus, coarse chromatin, and frequently a single small round nucleolus. The cytoplasm is basophilic and occasionally vacuolated.[199]

Conditions of the Prostate Diagnosed by Cytology

Hyperplasia

BPH is a spontaneous disease of intact male dogs. BPH occurs in more than 80% of dogs over 5 years of age and in greater than 95% by 9 years of age; however, most will not develop clinical signs.[189,191,208] There is no breed predisposition.[209] BPH also is described in the bull.[95] BPH is associated with dihydrotestosterone stimulation of growth and secretion of prostatic epithelial cells.[210] The increase in size is primarily a diffuse increase[211]; nodular hyperplasia is rare.[95] Hyperplasia develops between sexual maturity and 4 years of age, progressing from diffuse glandular to diffuse complex BPH by 6 years of age. At this point, the gland is cystic and atrophied, giving it a honeycombed appearance, with periglandular chronic inflammation composed of lymphocytes and large mononuclear cells.[191,204]

Definitive diagnosis of BPH requires histopathology, but a presumptive diagnosis can be made based on history, physical exam, and cytology.[191] Hemorrhage is the most frequent abnormal finding in semen and prostatic fluid washes. Peripheral blood leukocyte counts are typically normal; lymphopenia and/or eosinopenia can be seen.[198,212] On DRE, lateral radiographs, and ultrasound, the prostate is uniformly enlarged.[208] Ultrasound demonstrates loss of gland homogeneity and focal to multifocal areas of hyperechoic and/or hypoechoic tissue.[5,191,195] Cytologically, uniform cuboidal to columnar cells similar to normal epithelial cells are seen; however, cells can have a more moderate N:C. The cells are regularly arranged with distinct cell margins, exhibiting a honeycomb pattern (Figure 40.12). Inflammatory cells, if present, are few in number.[51,199] As canine BPH is commonly associated with other conditions, including abscessation, cysts, and neoplasia, it is prudent to obtain multiple samples from a gland where clinical signs or examination are not entirely consistent with BPH.[193,200]

Neoplasia

Benign

Benign tumors are rare. A single case report describes a dog with a mass involving only the left lobe of prostate and compatible with nodular hyperplasia or benign adenoma

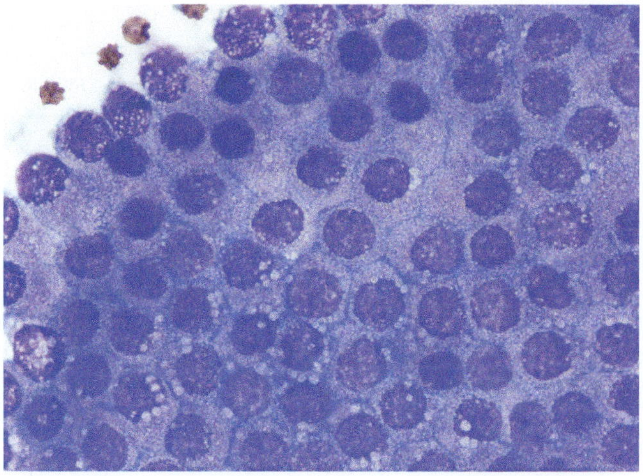

Figure 40.12 BPH in a dog. Uniform cuboidal hyperplastic epithelial cells exhibit a honeycomb pattern characteristic of BPH. Cells are similar to normal prostatic epithelial cells but with a more moderate N:C. Nuclei are round with coarse chromatin and often one small round nucleolus. Cells have moderate amounts of basophilic cytoplasm that occasionally contains variable numbers of small clear vacuoles (Wright–Giemsa, 500×. *Source:* Image courtesy of Nina Zitzer).

with smooth muscle proliferation; surgical resection and castration were curative.[213] Leiomyomas of the canine prostate are rarely reported.[214] An obstructive prostatic cystadenoma was described in a gelding.[206]

Malignant

Epithelial Prostate cancer is rare in domestic animals but highly aggressive.[204] It accounts for 5–7% of prostatic disease in dogs and has a prevalence of 0.2–0.6% based on necropsy studies.[191,215] The age at diagnosis ranges from 5 to 17 years (median 10 years),[190,193,216] which is older than dogs with other prostatic diseases (8.4 years).[187] Most dogs are medium-sized to large breed,[216] with increased risk in Bouvier des Flandres.[187] Only a few cases are reported in cats,[217,218] and there is one report in a gelding[206] and in an old Rhesus macaque.[204]

Unlike in people, most canine tumors do not respond to androgen depletion.[193] Castration does not appear protective, as neutered dogs have similar or greater prevalence when compared with intact males,[187,191,204,219,220] and the most common prostatic disease in castrated dogs is carcinoma.[190] The risk associated with neutering is highest for TCC.[219] Mean age is not different between castrated and intact dogs[187]; however, prevalence of pulmonary metastasis may be higher in castrated dogs.[215]

Adenocarcinoma, TCC, and undifferentiated carcinoma are most common.[187,191] TCC involves the prostate in approximately 30% of urogenital cases.[221] Squamous cell carcinoma (SCC) also is described in the canine prostate.[109] However, the majority of canine tumors exhibit intratumoral heterogeneity and are poorly differentiated,[95,216] with poorly differentiated carcinomas more common in castrated dogs.[191] The cell of origin in canine prostate cancer is unknown.[204] Studies suggest that the origin may be the prostatic collecting ducts, which have expression patterns of both prostatic epithelial and urothelial cells,[222,223] including positive staining for uroplakin III.[222,224] Furthermore, prostatic intraepithelial neoplasia (PIN) is observed in a high percentage of older male dogs, with and without prostatic adenocarcinoma, suggesting that PIN may be a precursor to adenocarcinoma.[193,225]

Prostate carcinoma often is not diagnosed until clinical signs are present, and by this time, local or regional metastasis is likely.[191] Prevalence of metastasis may be as high as 80%.[193] Metastatic sites include the lungs, regional lymph nodes, liver, urethra, spleen, colon, rectum, urinary bladder, bone, heart, kidneys, distant lymph nodes, and adrenal glands.[215,216,226,227] Skeletal metastasis, predominately in lumbar vertebrae and pelvis,[193,215,216] is common, especially in young dogs.[216,228] Clinical signs secondary to bone metastasis may be the only initial signs.[193,229] Prostatic TCC has shorter survival time and distant metastasis by the time of diagnosis than other urogenital TCCs.[221] Multiple joint metastases were reported in a dog with primary prostatic TCC.[224]

Hematuria, proteinuria, and pyuria are frequent; however, atypical cells in the urine sediment suggestive of epithelial neoplasia are uncommon, resulting in frequent false negative results.[197,198,215] Peripheral blood leukocyte counts typically are normal.[198] On DRE, the prostate is irregular, asymmetric, enlarged, and sometimes painful. A palpable prostate in an old castrated male raises strong suspicion for neoplasia.[191] Radiographic findings include prostatomegaly, mineralization, regional lymphadenopathy, and evidence of metastasis.[191,193] Hypertrophic osteopathy is reported.[95] Ultrasound findings include focal to diffuse hyperechoic areas, mineralization, and loss of normal contour.[191,193,215] Neutered dogs with prostatic mineralization are likely to have prostatic neoplasia (84% sensitivity and 100% specificity). However, prostatomegaly and mineralization in intact dogs also occurs with paraprostatic cysts, BPH, or prostatitis.[230]

FNA with or without ultrasound-guided placement is diagnostic for prostatic carcinoma in about 80% of affected dogs.[193] Definitive diagnosis requires histologic confirmation and may require the use of immunohistochemical stains (Table 40.3). Neoplastic glands can have foci of BPH, cystic glandular dilatation, and suppurative and lymphoplasmacytic inflammation[204]; therefore, multiple aspirates are recommended to avoid an incorrect diagnosis.

Table 40.3 Summary of select immunohistochemistry markers for commonly reported canine prostatic tumors.[223,231–233]

	CK	VIM	DES	α-SMA	CK7	PAP	UPIII	FVIII RA
Prostatic adenocarcinoma	+	–	–	–	±[a]	+	NA	NA
Transitional cell carcinoma	+	–	–	–	+	–	+	NA
Sarcomatoid carcinoma	+	+	–	–	–	–	NA	NA
Leiomyosarcoma	–	+	+	+	–	–	NA	NA
Hemangiosarcoma	–	+	NA	NA	NA	NA	NA	+

CK, cytokeratin; CK7, cytokeratin 7; DES, desmin; FVIII RA, factor VIII-related antigen; PAP, prostatic acid phosphatase; α-SMA, α-smooth muscle actin; UPIII, uroplakin III; VIM, vimentin.

+ indicates positive staining, ± variable staining, – negative staining, NA not assessed.

[a] Cytokeratin 7 is expressed by normal canine urothelium and periurethral prostatic ducts.[232] It is reported to be negative in adenocarcinoma and positive in transitional cell carcinoma in some sources[231,232] but positive in both adenocarcinoma and TCC in other sources.[223]

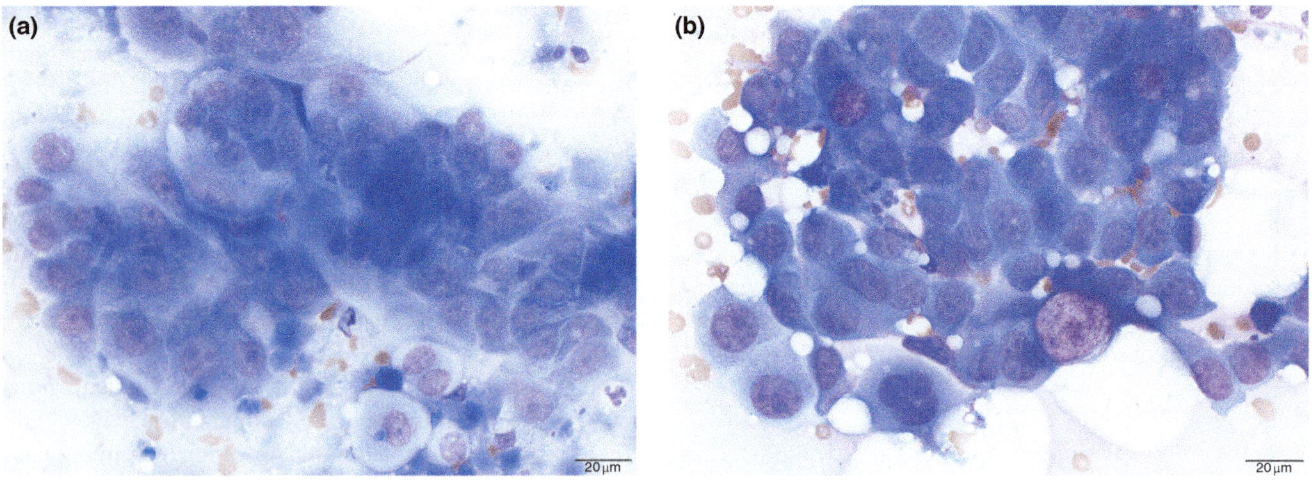

Figure 40.13 (a) Prostatic adenocarcinoma from a dog. Clusters of round to oval to polygonal epithelial cells with marked anisocytosis and anisokaryosis. The N:C is variable but often high. Nuclei are round to oval with stippled chromatin and one to multiple variably sized and shaped prominent nucleoli. Cells contain scant to moderate amounts of moderately basophilic cytoplasm. Binucleate and multinucleated cells are present (Wright–Giemsa). (b) Prostatic transitional cell carcinoma (TCC) from a dog. Clusters of polygonal epithelial cells arranged in sheets display moderate anisocytosis and anisokaryosis with a high N:C. Nuclei are round to oval with stippled chromatin and one to multiple, variably sized, round prominent nucleoli. Cells contain moderate amounts of moderately basophilic cytoplasm. Rare cells contain a large vacuole with finely stippled granular azurophilic material thought to be characteristic of TCC (resembling Melamed-Wolinska bodies); however, similar granular inclusions have been described in histologically confirmed adenocarcinomas. Prostatic adenocarcinoma and TCC can appear similar and may require histology with special immunohistochemical stains to differentiate (Wright–Giemsa).

Cytologically, prostatic adenocarcinoma is composed of individualized or clusters of polygonal epithelial cells demonstrating mild to marked anisokaryosis and anisocytosis with a variable, often high, N:C (Figure 40.13a).[199,234] Nuclei are round to oval with multiple variably sized and shaped nucleoli. Cytoplasm is deeply basophilic and variably vacuolated, occasionally giving a signet ring appearance. Mitoses are common and may be abnormal. Mild inflammation and chronic hemorrhage can be seen in the background.[199,234] Prostatic adenocarcinoma and TCC can be difficult to distinguish cytologically. In one study, sheets of cells with prominent intracytoplasmic red, granular inclusions were identified as TCC on cytology and were concordant with histopathology, suggesting that cytology can be used to accurately differentiate TCC from adenocarcinoma (Figure 40.13b).[200] However, features of both adenocarcinoma and TCC can occur in sections from one tumor,[200,224] and cytoplasmic vacuoles containing finely to coarsely stippled azurophilic material have been described in histologically confirmed adenocarcinomas.[234]

Clinical signs, imaging findings, metastatic rate, and prognosis of prostatic adenocarcinoma in cats are similar to dogs.[217,218] Prostatic adenocarcinoma was described in one gelding and consisted of proliferating acini of monomorphic cuboidal cells strongly positive for cytokeratin markers.[206] The horse originally presented for hematuria and was ultimately euthanized following poor response to treatment.[206]

Sarcomatoid carcinoma is rarely reported but has a high metastatic rate in dogs. Cytologically, there are large, loosely cohesive, atypical spindle cells with indistinct cell borders and moderate to abundant homogenous basophilic cytoplasm.[231] Round to oval paracentral or eccentric nuclei have fine to moderately stippled chromatin and one to three small, round nucleoli. Multinucleated cells and mitotic figures can be observed. Histologically, there are bundles of neoplastic spindle cells, rare pseudoacinar structures, and signet rings. Neoplastic cells co-express cytokeratin and vimentin.[231] Sarcomatoid carcinoma was reported in a 12-year-old male neutered mixed-breed cat. Unlike the aggressive nature described in dogs, the cat was successfully treated with surgery.[235]

Mesenchymal Mesenchymal tumors are rare. Hemangiosarcoma is reported most frequently.[214] Hematuria is common.[236] Cytologically, prostatic hemangiosarcoma is similar to other sites, with atypical polyhedral to spindle-shaped cells predominating. Cells have round to oval nuclei with prominent nucleoli, moderate amounts of cytoplasm, and rare vacuolization.[236] Mitosis, necrosis, hemorrhage, and suppurative inflammation are common, and extensive metastasis is described.[237] Other differentials include fibrosarcoma, leiomyosarcoma, rhabdomyosarcoma, malignant fibrous histiocytoma, malignant mesenchymoma, and osteosarcoma.[95,204,223,231] Prostatic leiomyosarcoma is rare but aggressive with widespread metastasis. Histologically, interlacing fascicles of neoplastic spindle cells are interspersed with sheets of haphazardly arrayed tumor cells, and there can be intense interstitial infiltrates of lymphocytes and plasma cells.[214]

Round Cell Lymphoma with prostate as the primary site is reported.[223,238] FNAs and histology are needed for definitive diagnosis, as DRE and ultrasound findings are nonspecific.[238]

Metastasis to Prostate Metastasis of tumors to the prostate are described for hemangiosarcoma,[237] histiocytic sarcoma,[239] and intestinal lymphoma.[240] Although lymphoma often is disseminated, the prostate is not routinely examined.[95]

Inflammation

Infectious

Bacterial prostatitis is common in intact dogs and may follow an acute or chronic course with variable clinical signs.[190] Prostatitis is rare in bulls, boars, stallions, rams, bucks, and tomcats but, if present, has a similar range of changes as in the dog.[95,241] Clinical and subclinical prostatitis are uncommon in castrated dogs, and castration may speed resolution of infection.[189,241–243] The prostate has mechanisms to protect against infection, but when compromised by other conditions such as BPH or cysts, prostatitis can occur,[191] typically due to ascent of normal aerobic urethral bacteria into the prostate gland.[193]

Acute Prostatitis Acute prostatitis primarily affects mature intact male dogs.[244] *E. coli* is the most common isolate in dogs, followed by *Staphylococcus aureus*, *Klebsiella* spp., *Proteus mirabilis*, *Mycoplasma canis*, *Pseudomonas aeruginosa*, *Enterobacter* spp., *Streptococcus* spp., *Pasteurella* spp., and *Haemophilus* spp.[190,197,244] *B. canis* can infect the canine prostate but is more commonly associated with epididymal and testicular infection. However, *B. canis* serology is indicated in dogs with prostatitis.[193] *B. canis* infection in the prostate is extensive but lobular in distribution, with fibrosis, atrophy, and interstitial lymphocytic inflammation.[95] Although uncommon, prostatitis can be caused by fungal organisms, including *B. dermatitidis*, *Cryptococcus neoformans*, and *Coccidioides immitis*, due to hematogenous spread, urethral ascent, or penetration through the scrotum and descent from the testes to the prostate.[191,193] Histologically, prostatic architecture may be obscured by granulomatous inflammation with many yeasts identified. Mineralization may or may not be present.[245] Primary prostatic pythiosis was reported in a castrated male Irish Setter.[246] Infection with *Leishmania* spp. can cause prostatitis, although less commonly in the prostate compared with other tissues.[98,247] Cytologically, mild chronic macrophagic and plasma cell prostatitis with intracytoplasmic amastigotes is described.[248]

Dogs often present with signs of systemic disease, including anorexia, fever, depression, vomiting, caudal abdominal pain, stiff or stilted gait, pollakiuria, and/or preputial discharge.[191] Functional urethral obstruction due to urethral spasm secondary to bacterial prostatitis is reported.[249] A mature neutrophilia, commonly with a left shift, and a mild nonregenerative anemia of inflammatory disease can be present, along with hematuria, proteinuria, pyuria, and bacteruria.[193,199] The prostate is often painful on palpation and normal to slightly enlarged. Edema of the scrotum, prepuce, and hind limbs can occur.[193] Radiographs may show prostatomegaly and rarely intraprostatic mineralization. On ultrasound, there is a diffuse increase in echodensity, which becomes more pronounced over time. On cytology, neutrophils predominate and range from non-degenerate to markedly degenerate with engulfed bacteria and bacteria free in the background (Figure 40.14a). Leukophagia, erythrophagia, and hemosiderin-laden macrophages also can be observed. Prostatic epithelial cells typically have normal morphology in acute prostatitis.[191,197,199] FNA of an infected prostate or abscess should be avoided when possible to prevent bacterial seeding of the needle tract.[193,196]

Chronic Prostatitis Chronic prostatitis often presents with no or vague signs. Most common signs include urinary tract infection or urethral discharge.[191] Infertility or deceased libido can be seen in the intact dog.[193] Affected dogs are usually older and often have concurrent BPH and cysts.[95] On DRE, the prostate gland is normally contoured and nonpainful. Pyuria is frequent, and peripheral blood leukocyte counts are typically normal.[198] Suppurative inflammation in semen and prostatic wash fluid is the most common finding,[5,197,198] and, histologically, inflammation may be segmental or multifocal and coalescing. Focal squamous metaplasia can occur and be mistaken for PIN.[95,199] Prostatic fluid cytology and culture are generally well-correlated with histology, but tissue culture may be more accurate in detecting infection.[5] Bacterial culture of semen is sensitive but not specific due to false positive results from urethral contamination.[198]

Abscessation Abscessation can be a sequela to chronic prostatitis, with cavities of purulent fluid found within the parenchyma.[201] Clinical signs vary depending on the size of the abscess and whether the infection becomes systemic. Peripheral leukocytosis, a left shift, and toxic neutrophils can occur.[198] On DRE, the prostate may or may not be enlarged and/or painful.[201] Ultrasound is the most reliable noninvasive tool for differentiating prostatitis from an abscess.[195] Cytology is similar to chronic prostatitis, and squamous metaplasia of prostatic epithelium can be seen.[199] Histopathology and culture are required for definitive diagnosis and exclusion of concurrent neoplasia.[195,250] With walled off abscesses or chronic infections, culture of prostatic fluid can lead to false negative results.[201] A prostatic abscess due to *E. coli* is described in a neutered cat.[195]

Noninfectious

Cysts Prostatic cysts form when canaliculi become obstructed, leading to accumulation of prostatic fluid.[191,197] Cysts can be within the parenchyma of the prostate, referred to as retention cysts, or paraprostatic, typically craniolateral to the prostate.[191,193] They are often associated with BPH but can be seen with other prostatic diseases or be congenital in dogs.[95,191] Cysts are described in cats,[251] in ferrets with proliferative adrenal lesions,[252] and in normal geldings without prostatomegaly.[207] Mean age in dogs is 8.0 years.[193] Clinical signs are nonexistent or referable to concurrent BPH or to physical displacement of abdominal viscera, especially with paraprostatic cysts.[193,253] In one study, prostatic cysts were culture positive in 42% of dogs, and urine culture was positively correlated with cyst culture in 80% of dogs.[254]

Prostatic cysts are typically diagnosed via ultrasound, appearing as anechoic areas in or around the prostate.[191,195] Small cysts may not alter the contour of the prostate, making them difficult to detect with DRE or radiography.[191,193] Paraprostatic cysts can be mineralized.[253] Cytologically, cysts have low cellularity with predominately large, vacuolated, and phagocytic macrophages in a proteinaceous background (Figure 40.14b).[255] Macrophages can have a moth-eaten appearance due to cytoplasmic vacuoles that overlie the nucleus.[255] Prostatic epithelial cells have normal morphology or demonstrate squamous metaplasia.[199]

Other Squamous metaplasia in the prostate (Figure 40.14c) can be observed in dogs with Sertoli cell tumor or following administration of estrogens, in swine exposed to estrogenic mycotoxins and in ferrets with proliferative adrenal lesions.[95,252] Prostatic calculi are extremely rare in dogs and have been reported in sheep.[95]

Advanced Diagnostic Techniques

Canine prostate specific esterase (CPSE) is the major secretory product of the canine prostate. Serum CPSE was significantly higher in dogs with prostatic lesions than in normal dogs, but did not differentiate BPH, bacterial prostatitis, or prostatic carcinoma.[256] CPSE serum concentration greater than 50 ng/mL in asymptomatic dogs was associated with ultrasonographic alterations and increased prostatic size.[257] Prostate specific antigen (PSA) was not detected in canine serum, and prostatic acid phosphatase (PAP) was not different between normal dogs and those with prostatic disease.[256]

Numerous immunohistochemical biomarkers of canine prostate cancer have been investigated. PSA is commonly used to identify tissues of prostatic origin[258]; however, in one study, PSA was only positive in 40% of canine prostate cancer tissues. In contrast, uroplakin III was positive in 85% of samples.[222] While studies have found differences in the expression of various other markers, including estrogen receptor,[259] angiogenic markers,[260] and cyclooxygenase-1 and -2,[261,262] between normal, hyperplastic, and neoplastic tissues, further work needs to be done to fully establish the diagnostic, prognostic, and therapeutic significance of these markers.[263–265]

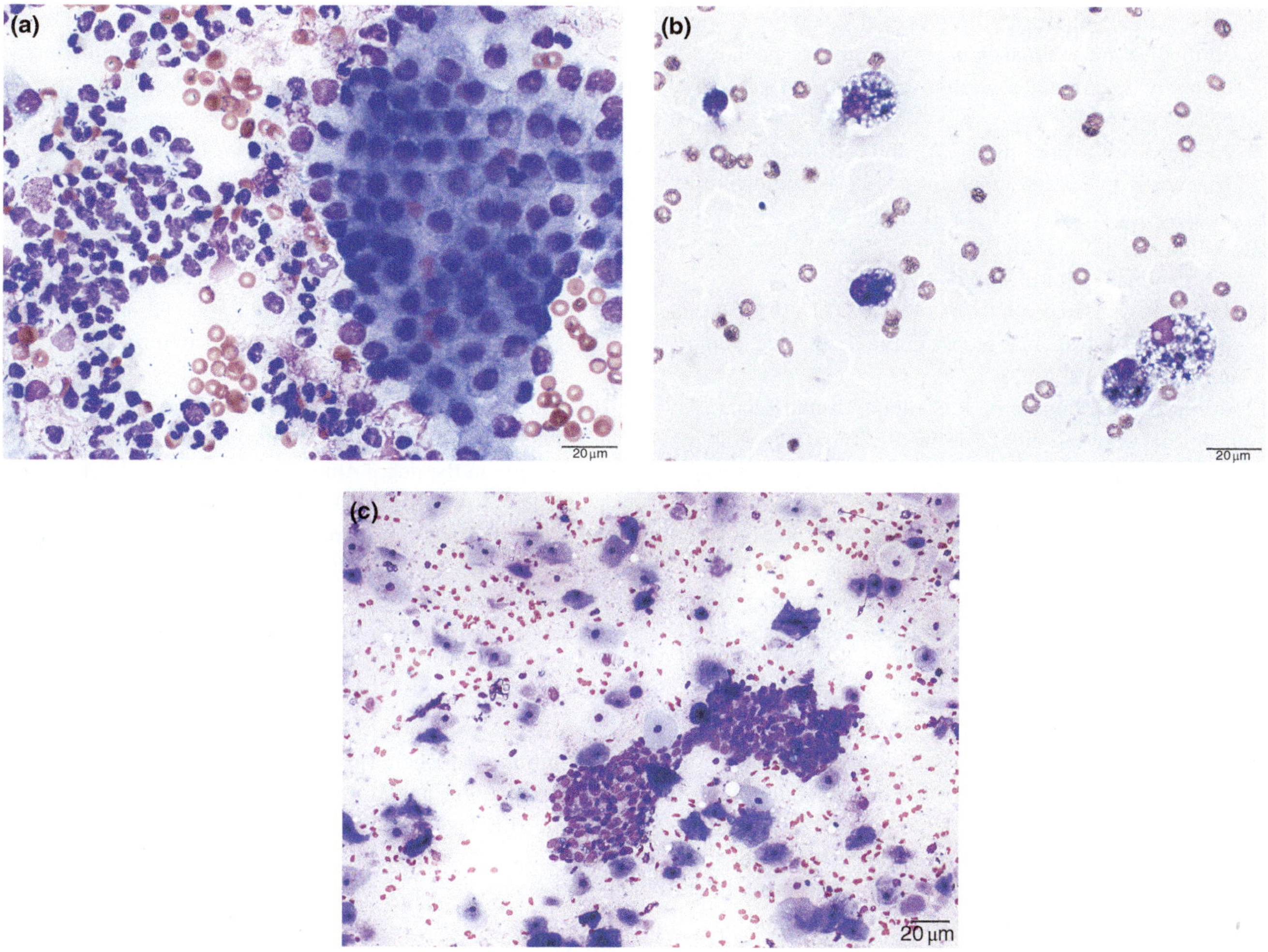

Figure 40.14 (a) Septic prostatitis in a dog. Non-degenerate to degenerate neutrophils predominate with occasional macrophages and streaming nuclear debris in the background. Intracellular and extracellular short rod-shaped bacteria are present, and culture was positive for *E. coli*. Prostatic epithelial cells (right) have a normal morphology (Wright–Giemsa). (b) Prostatic cyst in a dog. Cellularity is minimal in a lightly eosinophilic proteinaceous background with numerous erythrocytes. Rare to occasional vacuolated macrophages contain blue-green pigment, compatible with hemosiderin and evidence of hemorrhage (Wright–Giemsa). (c) Squamous metaplasia in a dog. Numerous oval to polyhedral squamous epithelial cells are present, characterized by a low N:C, small round nuclei with condensed chromatin, and abundant lightly basophilic cytoplasm. A cluster of hyperplastic prostatic epithelial cells are in the center (Wright–Giemsa, 100×).

References

1 Brinsko, S.P. (1998). Neoplasia of the male reproductive tract. *Vet Clin North Am Equine Pract* 14: 517–533.

2 Masserdotti, C., Bonfanti, U., De Lorenzi, D. et al. (2005). Cytologic features of testicular tumours in dog. *J Vet Med A Physiol Pathol Clin Med* 52: 339–346.

3 Dahlbom, M., Mäkinen, A., and Suominen, J. (1997). Testicular fine needle aspiration cytology as a diagnostic tool in dog infertility. *J Small Anim Pract* 38: 506–512.

4 Gouletsou, P.G., Galatos, A.D., Sideri, A.I., and Kostoulas, P. (2012). Impact of fine needle aspiration (FNA) and of the number of punctures on the feline testis: clinical, gross anatomy and histological assessment. *Theriogenology* 78: 172–181.

5 Kustritz, M.V.R. (2006). Collection of tissue and culture samples from the canine reproductive tract. *Theriogenology* 66: 567–574.

6 Leme, D.P., Visacre, E., Castro, V.B., and Lopes, M.D. (2018). Testicular cytology by fine needle aspiration in domestic cats. *Theriogenology* 106: 46–52.

7 Leme, D.P. and Papa, F.O. (2000). Cytological identification and quantification of testicular cell types using fine needle aspiration in horses. *Equine Vet J* 32: 444–446.

8 Attia, K.A., Zaki, A.A., Eilts, B.E. et al. (2000). Anti-sperm antibodies and seminal characteristic after testicular biopsy or epididymal aspiration in dogs. *Theriogenology* 53: 1355–1563.

9 Al-Jitawi, S.A., Al-Ramahi, S.A., and Hakooz, B.A. (1997). Diagnostic role of testicular fine needle aspiration biopsy in male infertility. *Acta Cytol* 41: 1705–1708.

10 Galina, C.S. (1971). An evaluation of testicular biopsy in farm animals. *Vet Rec* 88: 628–631.

11 James, R.W., Heywood, R., and Fowler, D.J. (1979). Serial percutaneous testicular biopsy in the Beagle dog. *J Small Anim Pract* 20: 219–228.

12 Romagnoli, S., Bonaccini, P., Stelletta, C. et al. (2009). Clinical use of testicular fine needle aspiration cytology in oligozoospermic and azoospermic dogs. *Reprod Domest Anim* 44: 329–333.

13 Gouletsou, P.G., Galatos, A.D., Leontides, L.S., and Sideri, A.I. (2010). Impact of fine or large needle aspiration on the dog's testis: in vitro ultrasonographic, bacteriological, gross anatomy and histological assessment. *Theriogenology* 74: 1604–1614.

14 Gouletsou, P.G., Galatos, A.D., Leontides, L.S., and Sideri, A.I. (2011). Impact of fine- or large-needle aspiration on canine testes: clinical, in vivo ultrasonographic and seminological assessment. *Reprod Domest Anim* 46: 712–719.

15 Diagone, K.V., Feliciano, M.A., Pacheco, M.R., and Vicente, W.R. (2012). Histology and morphometry of the testes of adult domestic cats (*Felis catus*). *J Feline Med Surg* 14: 124–130.

16 Santos, M., Marcos, R., and Caniatti, M. (2010). Cytologic study of normal canine testis. *Theriogenology* 73: 208–214.

17 Hayes, H.M. and Pendergrass, T.W. (1976). Canine testicular tumors: epidemiologic features of 410 dogs. *Int J Cancer* 18: 482–487.

18 Liao, A.T., Chu, P.Y., Yeh, L.S. et al. (2009). A 12-year retrospective study of canine testicular tumors. *J Vet Med Sci* 71: 919–923.

19 Santos, R.L., Silva, C.M., Ribeiro, A.F.C., and Serakides, R. (2000). Testicular tumors in dogs: frequency and age distribution. *Arq Bras Med Vet Zootec* 52: 25–26.

20 McEntee, M.C. (2002). Reproductive oncology. *Clin Tech Small Anim Pract* 17: 133–149.

21 Nødtvedt, A., Gamlem, H., Gunnes, G. et al. (2011). Breed differences in the proportional morbidity of testicular tumours and distribution of histopathologic types in a population-based canine cancer registry. *Vet Comp Oncol* 9: 45–54.

22 Grieco, V., Riccardi, E., Greppi, G.F. et al. (2008). Canine testicular tumours: a study on 232 dogs. *J Comp Pathol* 138: 86–89.

23 Ortega-Pacheco, A., Rodríguez-Buenfil, J.C., Segura-Correa, J.C. et al. (2006). Pathological conditions of the reproductive organs of male stray dogs in the tropics: prevalence, risk factors, morphological findings and testosterone concentrations. *Reprod Domest Anim* 41: 429–437.

24 D'Angelo, A.R., Vita, S., Marruchella, G., and Di Francesco, G. (2012). Canine testicular tumours: a retrospective investigation in Abruzzo and Molise, Italy. *Vet Ital* 48: 329–333, 335–339.

25 Reif, J.S., Maguire, T.G., Kenney, R.M., and Brodey, R.S. (1979). A cohort study of canine testicular neoplasia. *J Am Vet Med Assoc* 175: 719–723.

26 Lipowitz, A.J., Schwartz, A., Wilson, G.P., and Ebert, J.W. (1973). Testicular neoplasms and concomitant clinical changes in the dog. *J Am Vet Med Assoc* 163: 1364–1368.

27 Miller, M.A., Hartnett, S.E., and Ramos-Vara, J.A. (2007). Interstitial cell tumor and Sertoli cell tumor in the testis of a cat. *Vet Pathol* 44: 394–397.

28 Miyoshi, N., Yasuda, N., Kamimura, Y. et al. (2001). Teratoma in a feline unilateral cryptorchid testis. *Vet Pathol* 38: 729–730.

29 Asproni, P., Millanta, F., Lorenzi, D., and Poli, A. (2013). A Leydig cell tumour in a cat: histological and immunohistochemical findings. *Case Rep Vet Med*: 1–3.

30 Gelberg, H.B. and McEntee, K. (1987). Equine testicular interstitial cell tumors. *Vet Pathol* 24: 231–234.

31 Foster, R.A. (2017). Male reproductive system. In: *Pathologic Basis of Veterinary Disease*, 6e (ed. J.F. Zachary), 1194–1222. St. Louis, MO: Elsevier.

32 Murakami, Y., Tateyama, S., Uchida, K., and Yamaguchi, R. (2001). Immunohistochemical analysis of cyclins in canine normal testes and testicular tumors. *J Vet Med Sci* 63: 909–912.

33 Peters, M.A., Mol, J.A., van Wolferen, M.E. et al. (2003). Expression of the insulin-like growth factor (IGF) system and steroidogenic enzymes in canine testis tumors. *Reprod Biol Endocrinol* 1: 22–29.

34 Restucci, B., Maiolino, P., Paciello, O. et al. (2003). Evaluation of angiogenesis in canine seminomas by quantitative immunohistochemistry. *J Comp Pathol* 128: 252–259.

35 Sozmen, M., Kabak, Y.B., Gulbahar, M.Y. et al. (2013). Immunohistochemical characterization of peroxisome proliferator-activated receptors in canine normal testis and testicular tumours. *J Comp Pathol* 149: 10–18.

36 Cox, V.S., Wallace, L.J., and Jessen, C.R. (1978). An anatomic and genetic study of canine cryptorchidism. *Teratology* 18: 233–240.

37 Doxsee, A.L., Yager, J.A., Best, S.J., and Foster, R.A. (2006). Extratesticular interstitial and Sertoli cell tumors in previously neutered dogs and cats: a report of 17 cases. *Can Vet J* 47: 763–766.

38 Tennant, B. and Kelly, D.F. (1992). Malignant seminoma with gross metastases in a dog. *J Small Anim Pract* 33: 242–246.

39 Johnston, G.R., Feeney, D.A., Johnston, S.D., and O'Brien, T.D. (1991). Ultrasonographic features of testicular neoplasia in dogs: 16 cases (1980–1988). *J Am Vet Med Assoc* 198: 1779–1784.

40 England, G.C. (1995). Ultrasonographic diagnosis of non-palpable Sertoli cell tumours in infertile dogs. *J Small Anim Pract* 36: 476–480.

41 Ober, C.P., Spaulding, K., Breitschwerdt, E.B. et al. (2004). Orchitis in two dogs with Rocky Mountain spotted fever. *Vet Radiol Ultrasound* 45: 458–465.

42 Benazzi, C., Sarli, G., and Brunetti, B. (2004). Sertoli cell tumour in a cat. *J Vet Med A Physiol Pathol Clin Med* 51: 124–126.

43 Mischke, R., Meurer, D., Hoppen, H.O. et al. (2002). Blood plasma concentrations of oestradiol-17beta, testosterone and testosterone/oestradiol ratio in dogs with neoplastic and degenerative testicular diseases. *Res Vet Sci* 73: 267–272.

44 Withers, S.S., Lawson, C.M., Burton, A.G. et al. (2016). Management of an invasive and metastatic Sertoli cell tumor with associated myelotoxicosis in a dog. *Can Vet J* 57: 299–304.

45 Sanpera, N., Masot, N., Janer, M. et al. (2002). Oestrogen-induced bone marrow aplasia in a dog with a Sertoli cell tumour. *J Small Anim Pract* 43: 365–369.

46 Agnew, D.W. and MacLachlan, N.J. (2017). Tumors of the genital systems. In: *Tumors in Domestic Animals*, 5e (ed. D.J. Meuten), 689–722. Ames, IA: Wiley.

47 Duncan, R.B. (1998). Malignant Sertoli cell tumour in a horse. *Equine Vet J* 30: 355–357.

48 Pratt, S.M., Stacy, B.A., Whitcomb, M.B. et al. (2003). Malignant Sertoli cell tumor in the retained abdominal testis of a unilaterally cryptorchid horse. *J Am Vet Med Assoc* 222: 486–490.

49 Barrand, K.R. and Scudamore, C.L. (2001). Canine hypertrophic osteoarthropathy associated with a malignant Sertoli cell tumour. *J Small Anim Pract* 42: 143–145.

50 Ciaputa, R., Nowak, M., Kiełbowicz, M. et al. (2012). Seminoma, Sertolioma, and Leydigoma in dogs: clinical and morphological correlations. *Bull Vet Inst Pulawy* 56: 361–367.

51 Masserdotti, C. (2006). Architectural patterns in cytology: correlation with histology. *Vet Clin Pathol* 35: 388–396.

52 Bazzo, R., Sarli, G., Mandrioli, L., and Marcato, P.S. (2002). Sertoli cell tumour with Call-Exner-like bodies in a dog. *J Vet Med A Physiol Pathol Clin Med* 49: 535–537.

53 Masserdotti, C., De Lorenzi, D., and Gasparotto, L. (2008). Cytologic detection of Call-Exner bodies in Sertoli cell tumors from 2 dogs. *Vet Clin Pathol* 37: 112–114.

54 Bush, J.M., Gardiner, D.W., Palmer, J.S. et al. (2011). Testicular germ cell tumours in dogs are predominantly of spermatocytic seminoma type and are frequently associated with somatic cell tumours. *Int J Androl* 34 (4 Pt 2): 288–295.

55 Govaere, J., Ducatelle, R., Hoogewijs, M. et al. (2010). Case of bilateral seminoma in a trotter stallion. *Reprod Domest Anim* 45: 537–539.

56 Dhaliwal, R.S., Kitchell, B.E., Knight, B.L., and Schmidt, B.R. (1999). Treatment of aggressive testicular tumors in four dogs. *J Am Anim Hosp Assoc* 35: 311–318.

57 HogenEsch, H., Whiteley, H.E., Vicini, D.S., and Helper, L.C. (1987). Seminoma with metastases in the eyes and the brain in a dog. *Vet Pathol* 24: 278–280.

58 Takiguchi, M., Iida, T., Kudo, T., and Hashimoto, A. (2001). Malignant seminoma with systemic metastases in a dog. *J Small Anim Pract* 42: 360–362.

59 Dugat, D.R., Medici, E.L., Rochat, M.C. et al. (2015). An unusual case of metastatic seminoma in a dog. *J Am Anim Hosp Assoc* 51: 401–406.

60 Trigo, F.J., Miller, R.A., and Torbeck, R.L. (1984). Metastatic equine seminoma: report of two cases. *Vet Pathol* 21: 259–260.

61 Brito, L.F., Engiles, J.B., Turner, R.M. et al. (2009). Bilateral testicular mixed germ cell-sex cord-stromal tumours in a stallion. *Reprod Domest Anim* 44: 846–851.

62 De Lange, V., Chiers, K., Lefère, L. et al. (2015). Malignant seminoma in two unilaterally cryptorchid stallions. *Reprod Domest Anim* 50: 510–513.

63 Thomas, T.N., Olson, P.N., and Hoopes, P.J. (1986). Lateral hermaphroditism and seminoma in a dog. *J Am Vet Med Assoc* 189: 1596–1597.

64 Grieco, V., Rondena, M., Romussi, S. et al. (2004). Immunohistochemical characterization of the leucocytic infiltrate associated with canine seminomas. *J Comp Pathol* 130: 278–284.

65 Arighi, M., Singh, A., Bosu, W.T., and Horney, F.D. (1987). Histology of the normal and retained equine testis. *Acta Anat* 129: 127–130.

66 Cotchin, E. (1977). A general survey of tumours in the horse. *Equine Vet J* 9: 16–21.

67 Pollock, P.J., Prendergast, M., Callanan, J.J., and Skelly, C. (2002). Testicular teratoma in a three-day-old thoroughbred foal. *Vet Rec* 150: 348–350.

68 Shaw, D.P. and Roth, J.E. (1986). Testicular teratocarcinoma in a horse. *Vet Pathol* 23: 327–328.

69 Valentine, B.A. and Weinstock, D. (1986). Metastatic testicular embryonal carcinoma in a horse. *Vet Pathol* 23: 92–96.

70 Aihara, N., Yamamoto, N., Takagi, T., and Une, Y. (2011). Embryonal carcinoma in the abdominal cavity of a male calf. *J Vet Diagn Invest* 23: 598–602.

71 Suess, R.P. Jr., Barr, S.C., Sacre, B.J., and French, T.W. (1992). Bone marrow hypoplasia in a feminized dog with an interstitial cell tumor. *J Am Vet Med Assoc* 200: 1346–1348.

72 Tucker, A.R. and Smith, J.R. (2008). Prostatic squamous metaplasia in a cat with interstitial cell neoplasia in a retained testis. *Vet Pathol* 45: 905–909.

73 Togni, A., Rütten, M., Bley, C.R., and Hurter, K. (2015). Metastasized Leydig cell tumor in a dog. *Schweiz Arch Tierheilkd* 157: 111–115.

74 Canadas, A., Romão, P., and Gärtner, F. (2016). Multiple cutaneous metastasis of a malignant leydig cell tumour in a dog. *J Comp Pathol* 155: 181–184.

75 Sanford, S.E., Miller, R.B., and Hoover, D.M. (1987). A light and electron microscopical study of intranuclear cytoplasmic invaginations in interstitial cell tumours of dogs. *J Comp Pathol* 97: 629–635.

76 Patnaik, A.K. and Mostofi, F.K. (1993). A clinicopathologic, histologic, and immunohistochemical study of mixed germ cell-stromal tumors of the testis in 16 dogs. *Vet Pathol* 30: 287–295.

77 Banco, B., Giudice, C., Ghisleni, G. et al. (2015). Immunohistochemical study of mixed germ cell sex cord stromal tumours in 13 canine testes. *J Comp Pathol* 152: 182–187.

78 Cullen, J.M., Whiteside, J., Umstead, J.A., and Whitacre, M.D. (1987). A mixed germ cell-sex cord-stromal neoplasm of the testis in a stallion. *Vet Pathol* 24: 575–577.

79 Dzimira, S., Nizanski, W., Ochota, M., and Madej, J.A. (2015). Histopathological pattern of gonads in cases of sex abnormalities in dogs: an attempt of morphological evaluation involving potential for neoplasia. *Pathol Res Pract* 211: 772–775.

80 Turk, J.R., Turk, M.A., and Gallina, A.M. (1981). A canine testicular tumor resembling gonadoblastoma. *Vet Pathol* 18: 201–207.

81 Reis-Filho, J.S., Ricardo, S., Gärtner, F., and Madej, J.A. (2004). Bilateral gonadoblastomas in a dog with mixed gonadal dysgenesis. *J Comp Pathol* 130: 229–233.

82 Rothwell, T.L., Papadimitriou, J.M., Xu, F.N., and Middleton, D.J. (1986). Schwannoma in the testis of a dog. *Vet Pathol* 23: 629–631.

83 Radi, Z.A., Miller, D.L., and Hines, M.E. 2nd (2004). Rete testis mucinous adenocarcinoma in a dog. *Vet Pathol* 41: 75–78.

84 Patnaik, A.K. and Liu, S.K. (1975). Leiomyoma of the tunica vaginalis in a dog. *Cornell Vet* 65: 228–231.

85 Johnson, R.C. and Steinberg, H. (1989). Leiomyoma of the tunica albuginea in a horse. *J Comp Pathol* 100: 465–468.

86 Allison, N. and Moeller, R.B. Jr. (1999). Bilateral testicular leiomyosarcoma in a stallion. *J Vet Diagn Invest* 11: 179–182.

87 Cihak, R.W., Roen, D.R., and Klaassen, J. (1986). Malignant mesothelioma of the tunica vaginalis in a dog. *J Comp Pathol* 96: 459–462.

88 Vascellari, M., Carminato, A., Camali, G. et al. (2011). Malignant mesothelioma of the tunica vaginalis testis in a dog: histological and immunohistochemical characterization. *J Vet Diagn Invest* 23: 135–139.

89 Oikonomidis, I.L., Tsouloufi, T.K., Brellou, G.D. et al. (2015). A case of multiple bilateral testicular capsule mast cell tumours in a dog. *J Biol Regul Homeost Agents* 29: 417–421.

90 Esplin, D.G. and Wilson, S.R. (1998). Gastrointestinal adenocarcinomas metastatic to the testes and associated structures in three dogs. *J Am Anim Hosp Assoc* 34: 287–290.

91 Sagartz, J.E., Lairmore, M.D., Haines, D. et al. (1996). Lymphangiosarcoma in a young dog. *Vet Pathol* 33: 353–356.

92 Wanke, M.M. (2004). Canine brucellosis. *Anim Reprod Sci* 82–83: 195–207.

93 Reilly, T.J., Calcutt, M.J., Wennerdahl, L.A. et al. (2014). Isolation of *Aureimonas altamirensis*, a *Brucella canis*-like bacterium, from an edematous canine testicle. *J Vet Diagn Invest* 26: 795–798.

94 Totten, A.K., Ridgway, M.D., and Sauberli, D.S. (2011). Blastomyces dermatitidis prostatic and testicular infection in eight dogs (1992–2005). *J Am Anim Hosp Assoc* 47: 413–418.

95 Foster, R.A. (2016). Male genital system. In: *Jubb, Kennedy, and Palmer's Pathology of Domestic Animals*, 6e (ed. M.G. Maxie), 465–510. St. Louis, MO: Elsevier.

96 L'Abee-Lund, T.M., Heiene, R., Friis, N.F. et al. (2003). Mycoplasma canis and urogenital disease in dogs in Norway. *Vet Rec* 153: 231–235.

97 Manna, L., Paciello, O., Morte, R.D., and Gravino, A.E. (2012). Detection of *Leishmania* parasites in the testis of a dog affected by orchitis: case report. *Parasit Vectors* 5: 216.

98 Diniz, S.A., Melo, M.S., Borges, A.M. et al. (2005). Genital lesions associated with visceral leishmaniasis and shedding of *Leishmania* sp. in the semen of naturally infected dogs. *Vet Pathol* 42: 650–658.

99 Sigurdardóttir, O.G., Kolbjørnsen, O., and Lutz, H. (2001). Orchitis in a cat associated with coronavirus infection. *J Comp Pathol* 124: 219–222.

100 Schubach, T.M., de Oliveira Schubach, A., dos Reis, R.S. et al. (2002). *Sporothrix schenckii* isolated from domestic cats with and without sporotrichosis in Rio de Janeiro, Brazil. *Mycopathologia* 153: 83–86.

101 Kawakami, E., Koga, H., Hori, T., and Tsutsui, T. (2003). Sperm granuloma and sperm agglutination in a dog with asthenozoospermia. *J Vet Med Sci* 65: 409–412.

102 Althouse, G.C., Evans, L.E., and Hopkins, S.M. (1993). Episodic scrotal mutilation with concurrent bilateral sperm granuloma in a dog. *J Am Vet Med Assoc* 202: 776–778.

103 Mayenco Aguirre, A.M., García Fernandez, P., and Sanchez Muela, M. (1996). Sperm granuloma in the dog: complication of vasectomy. *J Small Anim Pract* 37: 392–393.

104 Batista-Arteaga, M., Santana, M., Lozano, O. et al. (2011). Bilateral epididymal sperm granulomas following urethrostomy in a German Shepherd dog. *Reprod Domest Anim* 46: 731–733.

105 Pérez-Marín, C.C., López, R., Domínguez, J.M., and Zafra, R. (2006). Clinical and pathological findings in testis, epididymis, deferens duct and prostate following vasectomy in a dog. *Reprod Domest Anim* 41: 169–174.

106 Colbourne, C.M., Adkins, A.R., and Yovich, J.V. (1996). Hydrocele formation after castration in 3 geldings. *Aust Vet J* 73: 156–157.

107 Gygax, A.P., Donawick, W.J., and Gledhill, B.L. (1973). Haematocoele in a stallion and recovery of fertility following unilateral castration. *Equine Vet J* 5: 128–130.

108 Hesser, A.C. and Davidson, A.P. (2015). Spermatocele in a South African Boerboel dog. *Top Companion Anim Med* 30: 28–30.

109 Foster, R.A. (2012). Common lesions in the male reproductive tract of cats and dogs. *Vet Clin North Am Small Anim Pract* 42: 527–545.

110 Peters, M.A., de Jong, F.H., Teerds, K.J. et al. (2000). Ageing, testicular tumours and the pituitary-testis axis in dogs. *J Endocrinol* 166: 153–161.

111 Holst, B.S. and Dreimanis, U. (2015). Anti-Müllerian hormone: a potentially useful biomarker for the diagnosis of canine Sertoli cell tumours. *BMC Vet Res* 11: 166.

112 Ano, H., Hidaka, Y., and Katamoto, H. (2014). Evaluation of anti-Müllerian hormone in a dog with a Sertoli cell tumour. *Vet Dermatol* 25: 142–145.

113 Ball, B.A., Conley, A.J., Grundy, S.A. et al. (2008). Expression of anti-Müllerian hormone (AMH) in the equine testis. *Theriogenology* 69: 624–631.

114 Grieco, V., Banco, B., Giudice, C. et al. (2010). Immunohistochemical expression of the KIT protein (CD117) in normal and neoplastic canine testes. *J Comp Pathol* 142: 213–217.

115 Owston, M.A. and Ramos-Vara, J.A. (2007). Histologic and immunohistochemical characterization of a testicular mixed germ cell sex cord-stromal tumor and a leydig cell tumor in a dog. *Vet Pathol* 44: 936–943.

116 Yu, C.H., Hwang, D.N., Yhee, J.Y. et al. (2009). Comparative immunohistochemical characterization of canine seminomas and Sertoli cell tumors. *J Vet Sci* 10: 1–7.

117 Banco, B., Giudice, C., Veronesi, M.C. et al. (2010). An immunohistochemical study of normal and neoplastic canine sertoli cells. *J Comp Pathol* 143: 239–247.

118 Ramos-Vara, J.A., Beissenherz, M.E., Miller, M.A. et al. (2001). Immunoreactivity of A103, an antibody to Melan A, in canine steroid-producing tissues and their tumors. *J Vet Diagn Invest* 13: 328–332.

119 Banco, B., Veronesi, M.C., Giudice, C. et al. (2012). Immunohistochemical evaluation of the expression of anti-Müllerian hormone in mature, immature and neoplastic canine Sertoli cells. *J Comp Pathol* 146: 18–23.

120 Hara, S., Morita, R., Shiraki, A. et al. (2014). Expression of protein gene product 9.5 and Sal-like protein 4 in canine seminomas. *J Comp Pathol* 151: 10–18.

121 Zanghì, A., Catone, G., Marino, G. et al. (2004). Malignant mixed sex cord-stromal tumour in a stallion. *Reprod Domest Anim* 39: 376–379.

122 Taniyama, H., Hirayama, K., Nakada, K. et al. (2001). Immunohistochemical detection of inhibin-α, -βB, and -βA chains and 3β-hydroxysteroid dehydrogenase in canine testicular tumors and normal testes. *Vet Pathol* 38: 661–666.

123 Peters, M.A., Teerds, K.J., van der Gaag, I. et al. (2001). Use of antibodies against LH receptor, 3beta-hydroxysteroid dehydrogenase and vimentin to characterize different types of testicular tumour in dogs. *Reproduction* 121: 287–296.

124 Ramos-Vara, J.A. and Miller, M.A. (2009). Immunohistochemical evaluation of GATA-4 in canine testicular tumors. *Vet Pathol* 46: 893–896.

125 Radi, Z.A. and Miller, D.L. (2005). Immunohistochemical expression of calretinin in canine testicular tumours and normal canine testicular tissue. *Res Vet Sci* 79: 125–129.

126 Banco, B., Palmieri, C., Sironi, G. et al. (2016). Immunohistochemical expression of SOX9 protein in immature, mature, and neoplastic canine Sertoli cells. *Theriogenology* 85: 1408–1414.

127 Grieco, V., Riccardi, E., Rondena, M. et al. (2007). Classical and spermatocytic seminoma in the dog: histochemical and immunohistochemical findings. *J Comp Pathol* 137: 41–46.

128 Hohšteter, M., Artuković, B., Severin, K. et al. (2014). Canine testicular tumors: two types of seminomas can be differentiated by immunohistochemistry. *BMC Vet Res* 10: 169.

129 Kim, J.H., Yu, C.H., Yhee, J.Y. et al. (2010). Canine classical seminoma: a specific malignant type with human classifications is highly correlated with tumor angiogenesis. *BMC Cancer* 10: 243.

130 Thorvaldsen, T.E., Nødtvedt, A., Grotmol, T., and Gunnes, G. (2012). Morphological and immunohistochemical characterisation of seminomas in Norwegian dogs. *Acta Vet Scand* 54: 52.

131 Bertazzolo, W., Dell'Orco, M., Bonfanti, U. et al. (2004). Cytological features of canine ovarian tumours: a retrospective study of 19 cases. *J Small Anim Pract* 45: 539–545.

132 Ball, R.L., Birchard, S.J., May, L.R. et al. (2010). Ovarian remnant syndrome in dogs and cats: 21 cases (2000–2007). *J Am Vet Med Assoc* 236: 548–553.

133 Amorim, M.D., Nairn, D., Manning, S. et al. (2016). Evaluation of diagnostic utility, safety considerations, and effect on fertility of transvaginal ultrasound-guided ovarian biopsy in mares. *Theriogenology* 85: 1030–1036.

134 Saba, C.F. and Lawrence, J.A. (2013). Tumors of the female reproductive system. In: *Withrow & MacEwen's Small Animal Clinical Oncology*, 4e (eds. S.J. Withrow, D.M. Vail and R.L. Page), 532–537. St. Louis, MO: Elsevier.

135 Sforna, M., Brachelente, C., Lepri, E., and Mechelli, L. (2003). Canine ovarian tumours: a retrospective study of 49 cases. *Vet Res Commun* 27 (1): 359–361.

136 Bertazzolo, W., Bonfanti, U., Mazzotti, S., and Gelain, M.E. (2012). Cytologic features and diagnostic accuracy of analysis of effusions for detection of ovarian carcinoma in dogs. *Vet Clin Pathol* 41: 127–132.

137 Akihara, Y., Shimoyama, Y., Kawasako, K. et al. (2007). Histological and immunohistochemical evaluation of canine ovary. *Reprod Domest Anim* 42: 495–501.

138 Piseddu, E., Masserdotti, C., Milesi, C., and Solano-Gallego, L. (2012). Cytologic features of normal canine ovaries in different stages of estrus with histologic comparison. *Vet Clin Pathol* 41: 396–404.

139 Gelberg, H.B. and McEntee, K. (1985). Feline ovarian neoplasms. *Vet Pathol* 22: 572–576.

140 Sapierzyński, R., Malicka, E., Bielecki, W. et al. (2007). Tumors of the urogenital system in dogs and cats. Retrospective review of 138 cases. *Pol J Vet Sci* 10: 97–103.

141 Pauwels, F.E., Wigley, S.J., Munday, J.S., and Roe, W.D. (2012). Bilateral ovarian adenocarcinoma in a mare causing haemoperitoneum and colic. *N Z Vet J* 60: 198–202.

142 Brazzell, J.L. and Borjesson, D.L. (2006). Intra-abdominal mass aspirate from an alopecic dog. *Vet Clin Pathol* 35: 259–262.

143 Patnaik, A.K. and Greenlee, P.G. (1987). Canine ovarian neoplasms: a clinicopathologic study of 71 cases, including histology of 12 granulosa cell tumors. *Vet Pathol* 24: 509–514.

144 Stein, B.S. (1981). Tumors of the feline genital tract. *J Am Anim Hosp Assoc* 17: 1022–1025.

145 Morris, D.D., Acland, H.M., and Hodge, T.G. (1985). Pleural effusion secondary to metastasis of an ovarian adenocarcinoma in a horse. *J Am Vet Med Assoc* 187: 272–274.

146 Hori, Y., Uechi, M., Kanakubo, K. et al. (2006). Canine ovarian serous papillary adenocarcinoma with neoplastic hypercalcemia. *J Vet Med Sci* 68: 979–982.

147 Browne, N.S., Scarratt, W.K., and Robertson, J. (2016). Hypertrophic osteopathy secondary to metastatic ovarian adenocarcinoma in a mare. *Can Vet J* 57: 1237–1241.

148 Petterino, C., Modesto, P., and Ratto, A. (2010). A bilateral ovarian psammomatous papillary cystic adenocarcinoma in a German Shepherd bitch. *Comp Clin Pathol* 19: 389–395.

149 Salgado, B.S., Monteiro, L.N., Grandi, F. et al. (2012). What is your diagnosis? Ascites fluid from a dog with abdominal distension. *Vet Clin Pathol* 41: 605–606.

150 Gómez-Laguna, J., Millán, Y., Reymundo, C. et al. (2008). Bilateral retiform Sertoli–Leydig cell tumour in a bitch. Alpha-inhibin and epithelial membrane antigen as useful tools for differential diagnosis. *J Comp Pathol* 139: 137–140.

151 Patrick, D.J., Kiupel, M., Gerber, V., and Carr, E.A. (2003). Malignant granulosa-theca cell tumor in a two-year-old Miniature Horse. *J Vet Diagn Invest* 15: 60–63.

152 McCue, P.M., Roser, J.F., Munro, C.J. et al. (2006). Granulosa cell tumors of the equine ovary. *Vet Clin North Am Equine Pract* 22: 799–817.

153 Almeida, J., Ball, B.A., Conley, A.J. et al. (2011). Biological and clinical significance of anti-Müllerian hormone determination in blood serum of the mare. *Theriogenology* 76: 1393–1403.

154 Crabtree, J. (2011). Review of seven cases of granulosa cell tumour of the equine ovary. *Vet Rec* 169: 251.

155 Foster, R.A. (2017). Female reproductive system and mammae. In: *Pathologic Basis of Veterinary Disease*, 6e (ed. J.F. Zachary), 1147–1193. St. Louis, MO: Elsevier.

156 Sivacolundhu, R.K., O'Hara, A.J., and Read, R.A. (2001). Granulosa cell tumour in two spayed bitches. *Aust Vet J* 79: 173–176.

157 Choi, U.S., Seo, K.W., Oh, S.Y. et al. (2005). Intra-abdominal mass aspirate from a cat in heat. *Vet Clin Pathol* 34: 275–277.

158 Cellio, L.M. and Degner, D.A. (2000). Testosterone-producing thecoma in a female cat. *J Am Anim Hosp Assoc* 36: 323–325.

159 Hofmann, W., Arbiter, D., and Scheele, D. (1980). Sex cord stromal tumor of the cat: so-called androblastoma with Sertoli–Leydig cell pattern. *Vet Pathol* 17: 508–513.

160 Patnaik, A.K., Saigo, P.E., Lieberman, P.H., and Greenlee, P.G. (1988). Morphology of canine ovarian Sertoli–Leydig cell neoplasms. A report of 12 cases. *Cancer* 62: 577–584.

161 Gorman, M.E., Bildfell, R., and Séguin, B. (2010). What is your diagnosis? Peritoneal fluid from a 1-year-old female German Shepherd dog. Malignant teratoma. *Vet Clin Pathol* 39: 393–394.

162 Greenlee, P.G. and Patnaik, A.K. (1985). Canine ovarian tumors of germ cell origin. *Vet Pathol* 22: 117–122.

163 Catone, G., Marino, G., Mancuso, R., and Zanghì, A. (2004). Clinicopathological features of an equine ovarian teratoma. *Reprod Domest Anim* 39: 65–69.

164 Gehlen, H., Haist, V., Baumgartner, W., and Klug, E. (2006). Malignant dysgerminoma in an 18-year-old Warmblood mare. *J Equine Vet Sci* 26: 23–26.

165 McLennan, M.W. and Kelly, W.R. (1977). Hypertrophic osteopathy and dysgerminoma in a mare. *Aust Vet J* 53: 144–146.

166 Lefebvre, R., Theoret, C., Doré, M. et al. (2005). Ovarian teratoma and endometritis in a mare. *Can Vet J* 46: 1029–1033.

167 Basaraba, R.J., Kraft, S.L., Andrews, G.A. et al. (1998). An ovarian teratoma in a cat. *Vet Pathol* 35: 141–144.

168 Pecile, A., Groppetti, D., Grieco, V. et al. (2017). Asymptomatic unilateral ovarian leiomyoma in a German Shepherd bitch. *Maced Vet Rev* 40: 97–101.

169 Boeloni, J.N., Reis, A.M., Nascimento, E.F. et al. (2012). Primary ovarian rhabdomyosarcoma in a dog. *J Comp Pathol* 147: 455–459.

170 Carstanjen, B., Schönert, S., Heblinski, N., and Gruber, A.D. (2009). Primary unilateral fibroleiomyoma of the ovary in a pregnant mare: a case report. *Reprod Domest Anim* 44: 952–957.

171 Antuofermo, E., Cocco, R., Borzacchiello, G. et al. (2009). Bilateral ovarian malignant mixed Müllerian tumor in a dog. *Vet Pathol* 46: 453–456.

172 Rhyan, J.C., D'Andrea, G.H., and Smith, L.S. (1981). Congenital ovarian vascular hamartoma in a horse. *Vet Pathol* 18: 131.

173 Clemente, M., Pérez-Alenza, M.D., and Peña, L. (2010). Metastasis of canine inflammatory versus non-inflammatory mammary tumours. *J Comp Pathol* 143: 157–163.

174 Van Israel, N., Kirby, B.M., and Munro, E.A. (2002). Septic peritonitis secondary to unilateral pyometra and ovarian bursal abscessation in a dog. *J Small Anim Pract* 43: 452–455.

175 Ortega-Pacheco, A., Gutiérrez-Blanco, E., and Jiménez-Coello, M. (2012). Common lesions in the female reproductive tract of dogs and cats. *Vet Clin North Am Small Anim Pract* 42: 547–559.

176 Rigas, J.D., Montilla, H.J., Tornquist, S.J. et al. (2012). What is your diagnosis? Equine ovarian cyst fluid. *Vet Clin Pathol* 41: 435–436.

177 Bosu, W.T., Van Camp, S.C., Miller, R.B. et al. (1982). Ovarian disorders: clinical and morphological observations in 30 mares. *Can Vet J* 23: 6–14.

178 Curtin, D.J. (2003). Ovarian hematoma in an 11-year-old Thoroughbred-Hanovarian mare. *Can Vet J* 44: 589–591.

179 Kobayashi, K., Fujiwara, T., Adachi, T. et al. (2007). Bilateral ovotestes in a female Beagle dog. *J Toxicol Pathol* 20: 111–115.

180 Pérez-Gutiérrez, J.F., Monteagudo, L.V., Rodríguez-Bertos, A. et al. (2015). Bilateral ovotestes in a 78, XX SRY-negative Beagle dog. *J Am Anim Hosp Assoc* 51: 267–271.

181 Riccardi, E., Grieco, V., Verganti, S., and Finazzi, M. (2007). Immunohistochemical diagnosis of canine ovarian epithelial and granulosa cell tumors. *J Vet Diagn Invest* 19: 431–435.

182 Ellenberger, C., Bartmann, C.P., Hoppen, H.O. et al. (2007). Histomorphological and immunohistochemical characterization of equine granulosa cell tumours. *J Comp Pathol* 136: 167–176.

183 Banco, B., Antuofermo, E., Borzacchiello, G. et al. (2011). Canine ovarian tumors: an immunohistochemical study with HBME-1 antibody. *J Vet Diagn Invest* 23: 977–981.

184 Borzacchiello, G., Mogavero, S., Tortorella, G. et al. (2010). Expression of endothelin-1 and endothelin receptor A in canine ovarian tumours. *Reprod Domest Anim* 45: e465–e468.

185 Pelkey, T.J., Frierson, H.F. Jr., Mills, S.E., and Stoler, M.H. (1998). The diagnostic utility of inhibin staining in ovarian neoplasms. *Int J Gynecol Pathol* 17: 97–105.

186 Ball, B.A., Almeida, J., and Conley, A.J. (2013). Determination of serum anti-Müllerian hormone concentrations for the diagnosis of granulosa-cell tumours in mares. *Equine Vet J* 45: 199–203.

187 Teske, E., Naan, E.C., van Dijk, E.M. et al. (2002). Canine prostate carcinoma: epidemiological evidence of an increased risk in castrated dogs. *Mol Cell Endocrinol* 197: 251–255.

188 Mordecai, A., Liptak, J.M., Hofstede, T. et al. (2008). Prostatic abscess in a neutered cat. *J Am Anim Hosp Assoc* 44: 90–94.

189 Mukaratirwa, S. and Chitura, T. (2007). Canine subclinical prostatic disease: histological prevalence and validity of digital rectal examination as a screening test. *J S Afr Vet Assoc* 78: 66–68.

190 Krawiec, D.R. and Heflin, D. (1992). Study of prostatic diseases in dogs: 177 cases (1981–1986). *J Am Vet Med Assoc* 200: 1119–1122.

191 Smith, J. (2008). Canine prostatic disease: a review of anatomy, pathology, diagnosis, and treatment. *Theriogenology* 70: 375–383.

192 Troisi, A., Orlandi, R., Bargellini, P. et al. (2015). Contrast-enhanced ultrasonographic characteristics of the diseased canine prostate gland. *Theriogenology* 84: 1423–1430.

193 Johnston, S.D., Kamolpatana, K., Root-Kustritz, M.V., and Johnston, G.R. (2000). Prostatic disorders in the dog. *Anim Reprod Sci* 60–61: 405–415.

194 Mantziaras, G., Alonge, S., Faustini, M., and Luvoni, G.C. (2017). Assessment of the age for a preventive ultrasonographic examination of the prostate in the dog. *Theriogenology* 100: 114–119.

195 Feeney, D.A., Johnston, G.R., Klausner, J.S. et al. (1987). Canine prostatic disease-comparison of radiographic appearance with morphologic and microbiologic findings: 30 cases (1981–1985). *J Am Vet Med Assoc* 190: 1018–1026.

196 Boland, L.E., Hardie, R.J., Gregory, S.P., and Lamb, C.R. (2003). Ultrasound-guided percutaneous drainage as the primary treatment for prostatic abscesses and cysts in dogs. *J Am Anim Hosp Assoc* 39: 151–159.

197 Barsanti, J.A. and Finco, D.R. (1986). Canine prostatic diseases. *Vet Clin North Am Small Anim Pract* 16: 587–599.

198 Barsanti, J.A. and Finco, D.R. (1984). Evaluation of techniques for diagnosis of canine prostatic diseases. *J Am Vet Med Assoc* 185: 198–200.

199 Wright, P.J. and Parry, B.W. (1989). Cytology of the canine reproductive system. *Vet Clin North Am Small Anim Pract* 19: 851–874.

200 Powe, J.R., Canfield, P.J., and Martin, P.A. (2004). Evaluation of the cytologic diagnosis of canine prostatic disorders. *Vet Clin Pathol* 33: 150–154.

201 Ling, G.V., Branam, J.E., Ruby, A.L., and Johnson, D.L. (1983). Canine prostatic fluid: techniques of collection, quantitative bacterial culture, and interpretation of results. *J Am Vet Med Assoc* 183: 201–206.

202 Thrall, M.A., Olson, P.N., and Freemyer, F.G. (1985). Cytologic diagnosis of canine prostatic disease. *J Am Anim Hosp Assoc* 21: 95–102.

203 Nyland, T.G., Wallack, S.T., and Wisner, E.R. (2002). Needle-tract implantation following us-guided fine-needle aspiration biopsy of transitional cell carcinoma of the bladder, urethra, and prostate. *Vet Radiol Ultrasound* 43: 50–53.

204 Leroy, B.E. and Northrup, N. (2009). Prostate cancer in dogs: comparative and clinical aspects. *Vet J* 180: 149–162.

205 Lai, C.L., van den Ham, R., van Leenders, G. et al. (2008). Comparative characterization of the canine normal prostate in intact and castrated animals. *Prostate* 68: 498–507.

206 Knobbe, M., Levine, D., Habacker, P. et al. (2012). Prostatic masses in geldings: two cases. *J Equine Vet Sci* 32: 628–633.

207 Schnobrich, M.R., Turner, R.O., Belcher, C.N., and Slack, J. (2016). Transrectal ultrasonographic characterization of the accessory sex glands, pelvic urethra, and ureters in normal geldings. *Theriogenology* 85: 186–192.

208 Gobello, C., Castex, G., and Corrada, Y. (2002). Serum and seminal markers in the diagnosis of disorders of the genital tract of the dog: a mini-review. *Theriogenology* 57: 1285–1291.

209 Aquino-Cortez, A., Pinheiro, B.Q., Silva, H. et al. (2017). Serum testosterone, sperm quality, cytological, physicochemical and biochemical characteristics of the prostatic fraction of dogs with prostatomegaly. *Reprod Domest Anim* 52: 998–1003.

210 Krakowski, L., Wachocka, A., Brodzki, P. et al. (2015). Sperm quality and selected biochemical parameters of seminal fluid in dogs with benign prostatic hyperplasia. *Anim Reprod Sci* 160: 120–125.

211 Lowseth, L.A., Gerlach, R.F., Gillett, N.A., and Muggenburg, B.A. (1990). Age-related changes in the prostate and testes of the beagle dog. *Vet Pathol* 27: 347–353.

212 Das, M.R., Patra, R.C., Das, R.K. et al. (2017). Hemato-biochemical alterations and urinalysis in dogs suffering from benign prostatic hyperplasia. *Vet World* 10: 331–335.

213 Gilson, S.D., Miller, R.T., Hardie, E.M., and Spaulding, K.A. (1992). Unusual prostatic mass in a dog. *J Am Vet Med Assoc* 200: 702–704.

214 Hayden, D.W., Klausner, J.S., and Waters, D.J. (1999). Prostatic leiomyosarcoma in a dog. *J Vet Diagn Invest* 11: 283–286.

215 Bell, F.W., Klausner, J.S., Hayden, D.W. et al. (1991). Clinical and pathologic features of prostatic adenocarcinoma in sexually intact and castrated dogs: 31 cases (1970–1987). *J Am Vet Med Assoc* 199: 1623–1630.

216 Cornell, K.K., Bostwick, D.G., Cooley, D.M. et al. (2000). Clinical and pathologic aspects of spontaneous canine prostate carcinoma: a retrospective analysis of 76 cases. *Prostate* 45: 173–183.

217 Caney, S.M., Holt, P.E., Day, M.J. et al. (1998). Prostatic carcinoma in two cats. *J Small Anim Pract* 39: 140–143.

218 Tursi, M., Costa, T., Valenza, F., and Aresu, L. (2008). Adenocarcinoma of the disseminated prostate in a cat. *J Feline Med Surg* 10: 600–602.

219 Bryan, J.N., Keeler, M.R., Henry, C.J. et al. (2007). A population study of neutering status as a risk factor for canine prostate cancer. *Prostate* 67: 1174–1181.

220 Obradovich, J., Walshaw, R., and Goullaud, E. (1987). The influence of castration on the development of prostatic carcinoma in the dog. 43 cases (1978–1985). *J Vet Intern Med* 1: 183–187.

221 Mutsaers, A.J., Widmer, W.R., and Knapp, D.W. (2003). Canine transitional cell carcinoma. *J Vet Intern Med* 17: 136–144.

222 Lai, C.L., van den Ham, R., van Leenders, G. et al. (2008). Histopathological and immunohistochemical characterization of canine prostate cancer. *Prostate* 68: 477–488.

223 LeRoy, B.E., Nadella, M.V., Toribio, R.E. et al. (2004). Canine prostate carcinomas express markers of urothelial and prostatic differentiation. *Vet Pathol* 41: 131–140.

224 Colledge, S.L., Raskin, R.E., Messick, J.B. et al. (2013). Multiple joint metastasis of a transitional cell carcinoma in a dog. *Vet Clin Pathol* 42: 216–220.

225 Waters, D.J. and Bostwick, D.G. (1997). Prostatic intraepithelial neoplasia occurs spontaneously in the canine prostate. *J Urol* 157: 713–716.

226 Schkeeper, A.E., Foss, K., and Drost, W.T. (2013). What is your diagnosis? Prostate neoplasm with metastases to bone. *J Am Vet Med Assoc* 243: 483–485.

227 Labelle, P. and De Cock, H.E. (2005). Metastatic tumors to the adrenal glands in domestic animals. *Vet Pathol* 42: 52–58.

228 Waters, D.J., Hayden, D.W., Bell, F.W. et al. (1998). Skeletal metastases in dogs with prostate carcinoma. *Vet Radiol Ultrasound* 39: 240.

229 Cooley, D.M. and Waters, D.J. (1998). Skeletal metastasis as the initial clinical manifestation of metastatic carcinoma in 19 dogs. *J Vet Intern Med* 12: 288–293.

230 Bradbury, C.A., Westropp, J.L., and Pollard, R.E. (2009). Relationship between prostatomegaly, prostatic mineralization, and cytologic diagnosis. *Vet Radiol Ultrasound* 50: 167–171.

231 Pinto da Cunha, N., Ghisleni, G., Romussi, S., and Caniatti, M. (2007). Prostatic sarcomatoid carcinoma in a dog: cytologic and immunohistochemical findings. *Vet Clin Pathol* 36: 368–372.

232 Steinberg, J. (2008). Immunochemistry of prostatic carcinoma. *Vet Clin Pathol* 37: 143.

233 Fujii, Y., Tsuchiya, T., Morita, R. et al. (2013). Tumour endothelial marker-1 is expressed in canine haemangiopericytomas. *J Comp Pathol* 149: 172–181.

234 LeBlanc, C.J., Roberts, C.S., Bauer, R.W., and Ryan, K.A. (2004). Firm rib mass aspirate from a dog. *Vet Clin Pathol* 33: 253–256.

235 Zambelli, D., Cunto, M., Raccagni, R. et al. (2010). Successful surgical treatment of a prostatic biphasic tumour (sarcomatoid carcinoma) in a cat. *J Feline Med Surg* 12: 161–165.

236 Della Santa, D., Dandrieux, J., Psalla, D. et al. (2008). Primary prostatic haemangiosarcoma causing severe haematuria in a dog. *J Small Anim Pract* 49: 249–251.

237 Hayden, D.W., Bartges, J.W., Bell, F.W., and Klausner, J.S. (1992). Prostatic hemangiosarcoma in a dog: clinical and pathologic findings. *J Vet Diagn Invest* 4: 209–211.

238 Winter, M.D., Locke, J.E., and Penninck, D.G. (2006). Imaging diagnosis: urinary obstruction secondary to prostatic lymphoma in a young dog. *Vet Radiol Ultrasound* 47: 597–601.

239 Dias Pereira, P., Santos, M., Montenegro, L., and Faustino, A.M. (2006). A femorotibial joint swelling with popliteal lymph node enlargement in a Rottweiler. *Vet Clin Pathol* 35: 335–338.

240 Assin, R., Baldi, A., Citro, G., and Spugnini, E.P. (2008). Prostate as sole unusual recurrence site of lymphoma in a dog. *In Vivo* 22: 755–757.

241 Roura, X., Camps-Palau, M.A., Lloret, A. et al. (2002). Bacterial prostatitis in a cat. *J Vet Intern Med* 16: 593–597.

242 Cowan, L.A., Barsanti, J.A., Crowell, W., and Brown, J. (1991). Effects of castration on chronic bacterial prostatitis in dogs. *J Am Vet Med Assoc* 199: 346–350.

243 Mullen, H.S., Mathiesen, D.T., and Scavelli, T.D. (1990). Results of surgery and postoperative complications in 92 dogs treated for prostatic abscessation by a multiple Penrose drain technique. *J Am Anim Hosp Assoc* 26: 369–379.

244 Oluoch, A.O., Kim, C.H., Weisiger, R.M. et al. (2001). Nonenteric *Escherichia coli* isolates from dogs: 674 cases (1990–1998). *J Am Vet Med Assoc* 218: 381–384.

245 Reed, L.T., Balog, K.A., Boes, K.M. et al. (2010). Pathology in practice. Granulomatous pneumonia, prostatitis and uveitis with intralesional yeasts consistent with Blastomyces. *J Am Vet Med Assoc* 236: 411–413.

246 Jaeger, G.H., Rotstein, D.S., and Law, J.M. (2002). Prostatic pythiosis in a dog. *J Vet Intern Med* 16: 598–602.

247 Carvalho Junior, C.G., Teixeira Neto, R.G., Lopes, V.V. et al. (2017). Parasitism and inflammation in ear skin and in genital tissues of symptomatic and asymptomatic male dogs with visceral leishmaniasis. *Parasitol Res* 116: 987–995.

248 Mir, F., Fontaine, E., Reyes-Gomez, E. et al. (2012). Subclinical leishmaniasis associated with infertility and chronic prostatitis in a dog. *J Small Anim Pract* 53: 419–422.

249 Lane, I.F., Fischer, J.R., Miller, E. et al. (2000). Functional urethral obstruction in 3 dogs: clinical and urethral pressure profile findings. *J Vet Intern Med* 14: 43–49.

250 Rohleder, J.J. and Jones, J.C. (2002). Emphysematous prostatitis and carcinoma in a dog. *J Am Anim Hosp Assoc* 38: 478–481.

251 Newell, S.M., Mahaffey, M.B., Binhazim, A., and Greene, C.E. (1992). Paraprostatic cyst in a cat. *J Small Anim Pract* 33: 399–401.

252 Coleman, G.D., Chavez, M.A., and Williams, B.H. (1998). Cystic prostatic disease associated with adrenocortical lesions in the ferret (*Mustela putorius furo*). *Vet Pathol* 35: 547–549.

253 Head, L.L. and Francis, D.A. (2002). Mineralized paraprostatic cyst as a potential contributing factor in the development of perineal hernias in a dog. *J Am Vet Med Assoc* 221: 533–535, 500.

254 Black, G.M., Ling, G.V., Nyland, T.G., and Baker, T. (1998). Prevalence of prostatic cysts in adult, large-breed dogs. *J Am Anim Hosp Assoc* 34: 177–180.

255 Solano-Gallego, L. and Masserdotti, C. (2016). Reproductive system. In: *Canine and Feline Cytology: A Color Atlas and Interpretation Guide*, 3e (eds. R.E. Raskin and D.J. Meyer), 313–352. St. Louis, MO: Elsevier.

256 Bell, F.W., Klausner, J.S., Hayden, D.W. et al. (1995). Evaluation of serum and seminal plasma markers in the diagnosis of canine prostatic disorders. *J Vet Intern Med* 9: 149–153.

257 Alonge, S., Melandri, M., Leoci, R. et al. (2018). Canine prostate specific esterase (CPSE) as an useful biomarker in preventive screening programme of canine prostate: CPSE threshold value assessment and its correlation with ultrasonographic prostatic abnormalities in asymptomatic dogs. *Reprod Domest Anim* 53: 359–364.

258 Ramos-Vara, J.A., Avery, P.R., and Avery, A.C. (2016). Advanced diagnostic techniques. In: *Canine and Feline Cytology: A Color Atlas and Interpretation Guide*, 3e (eds. R.E. Raskin and D.J. Meyer), 453–494. St. Louis, MO: Elsevier.

259 Grieco, V., Riccardi, E., Rondena, M. et al. (2006). The distribution of oestrogen receptors in normal, hyperplastic and neoplastic canine prostate, as demonstrated immunohistochemically. *J Comp Pathol* 135: 11–16.

260 Palmieri, C. (2015). Immunohistochemical expression of angiogenic factors by neoplastic epithelial cells is associated with canine prostatic carcinogenesis. *Vet Pathol* 52: 607–613.

261 Sorenmo, K.U., Goldschmidt, M.H., Shofer, F.S. et al. (2004). Evaluation of cyclooxygenase-1 and cyclooxygenase-2 expression and the effect of cyclooxygenase inhibitors in canine prostatic carcinoma. *Vet Comp Oncol* 2: 13–23.

262 L'Eplattenier, H.F., Lai, C.L., van den Ham, R. et al. (2007). Regulation of COX-2 expression in canine prostate carcinoma: increased COX-2 expression is not related to inflammation. *J Vet Intern Med* 21: 776–782.

263 Hood, G., Laufer-Amorim, R., Fonseca-Alves, C.E. et al. (2016). Overexpression of ephrin A3 receptor in canine prostatic carcinoma. *J Comp Pathol* 154: 180–185.

264 Palmieri, C. and Riccardi, E. (2013). Immunohistochemical expression of HOXA-13 in normal, hyperplastic and neoplastic canine prostatic tissue. *J Comp Pathol* 149: 417–423.

265 Lai, C.L., L'Eplattenier, H., van den Ham, R. et al. (2008). Androgen receptor CAG repeat polymorphisms in canine prostate cancer. *J Vet Intern Med* 22: 1380–1384.

41

Evaluation of Semen

Scott Madill and Margaret V. Root Kustritz

Introduction

This chapter focuses on the standard laboratory examination of bovine, canine, and equine semen. The examination is useful tool for identifying likely subfertile males, for screening ejaculates prior to processing at artificial insemination centers, and as a method for initial investigation of infertility. While a major goal of the breeding industry is to have a laboratory test, or group of tests, that would accurately predict the fertility of the male or his semen when used in the field, this remains largely unmet.[1,2] Some studies have identified significant correlations between semen characteristics and fertility,[3–15] but others have identified no or limited correlation.[16–20] Reasons for this include the complexity of spermatozoal function, the myriad of outside influences on fertility, variations in test performance, and the difficulty in obtaining accurate and precise fertility data.[1,2]

Semen Collection

Descriptions of semen collection from the bull using an artificial vagina (AV)[21–23] and electroejaculation,[24–26] the dog by manual stimulation[27–29] and the stallion using AV[30] can be found in the works referenced. Ideally, examination of several collections is made due to normal within-animal variation of semen parameters over time.[12,15,31–34] Samples of frozen or cooled semen sent for evaluation should be shipped and stored at the appropriate temperature. For frozen semen, repeatability studies recommend two to three straws be evaluated from each batch.[34,35] Following thawing and drying, the sealed end of the straw is cut, and contents expelled into a warm vial by pushing the cotton manufacturer's plug through. This gives a more accurate representation of the content than cutting both ends and allowing gravity drainage.[36]

Spermatozoal Structure and Function

Spermatozoa of traditional livestock and companion species are fairly similar in size and shape (Figure 41.1). The spermatozoon consists of a head, connecting piece (neck), midpiece, principal piece, and end piece. For clinical descriptions, it is common to use tail as the collective term for the principal piece and end piece. The head is flattened, and the proximal part of the nucleus is covered by the acrosome. The midpiece is thicker than the principal piece due to the helically arranged mitochondria. Surrounding the entire spermatozoon is the plasma membrane, which is structurally modified for specialized tasks depending on the region it overlies.[37,38] In order to reach the site of fertilization in the oviduct, sperm must display linear progressive motility and normal morphology and plasma membrane architecture.[39–41]

Semen Evaluation

The standard semen evaluation is composed of assessment of color and opacity, volume, pH, motility, concentration/total number, and morphology. Initial examination should occur within five minutes of collection, and the semen should be protected from rapid changes in temperature during that time.[42,43] Glassware and slides should be clean and warm, and any fluids used for extension are kept in an incubator at 35–37 °C.[44] Once the gross examination and volume are obtained, the sample is gently but thoroughly mixed, and a small aliquot is removed for further analysis.

Color and Opacity

Normal semen is white to off-white, and opacity largely depends on spermatozoal concentration,[26,45] so bull

Veterinary Cytology, First Edition. Edited by Leslie C. Sharkey, M. Judith Radin, and Davis Seelig.

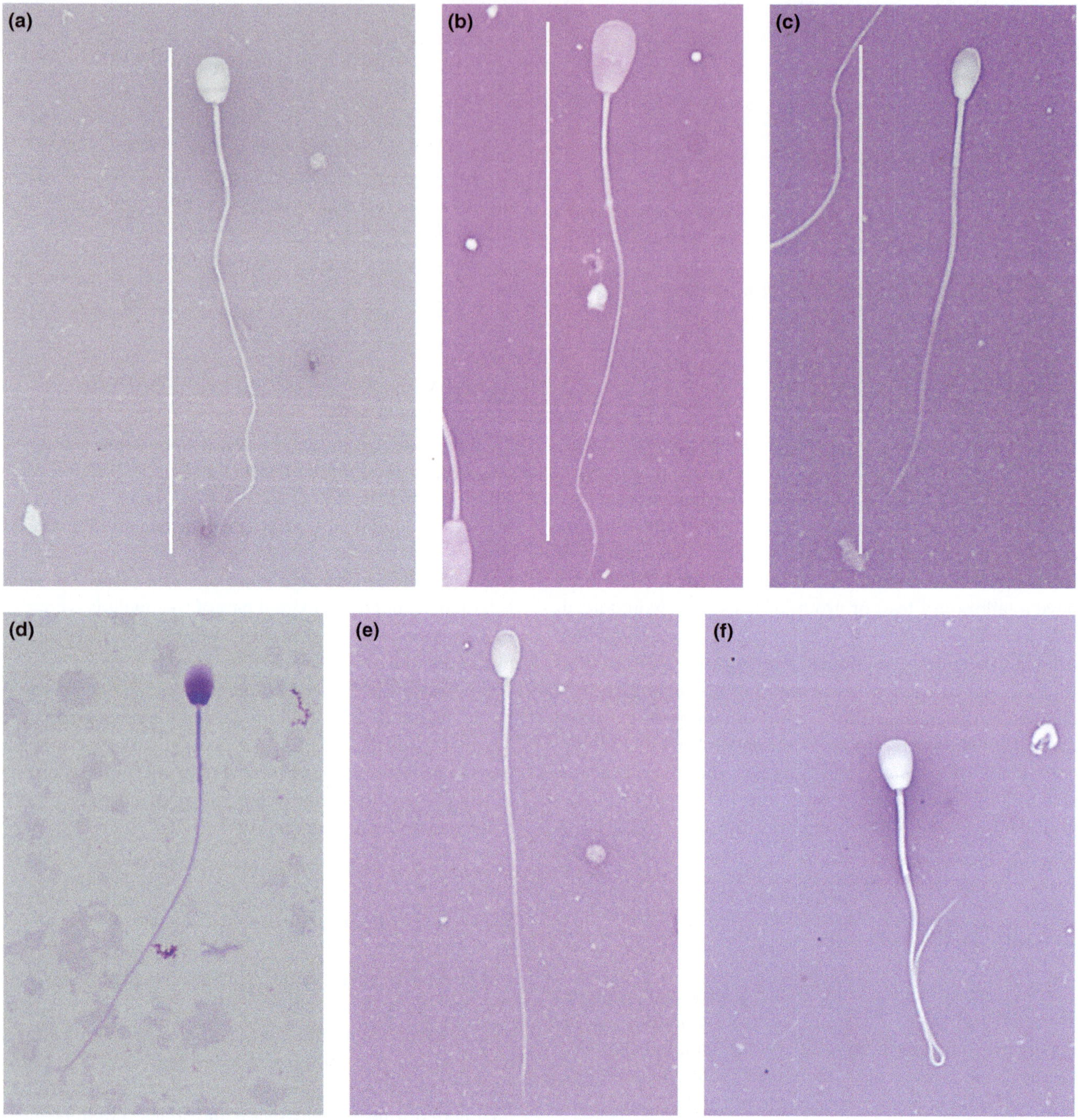

Figure 41.1 Normal spermatozoa from different species. Bars on (a–c) 80 µm for size comparison. (a) Dog. (b) Bull. (c) Stallion. (d) Dog. (e) Spermatozoa from a stallion exhibiting normal abaxial implantation and associated head asymmetry. (f) Dog with principal piece folding artifact from smearing (Eosin Nigrosin stain for all except (d) which is DiffQuik®, 1000×).

semen is more opaque than that of the other species.[42] Bull semen may be yellow as a normal variation due to high riboflavin content without affecting quality.[46,47] In other instances yellow discoloration is indicative of urine contamination.[27,43]

Volume

Volume is measured in a graduated collection tube, volumetric cylinder, or by weight.[44] The measurement in stallions is taken after the gel portion has been removed by filtration.[42,43] Volume usually means little but is necessary for calculating the total number of spermatozoa in the ejaculate.[48] Ejaculate volumes in dogs range from 1 to 30 mL,[49] in bulls from 2 to 15 mL with an average of 5–6 mL,[50] and in stallions from 30 to 300 mL with an average of 50–60 mL.[51]

pH

Measurement of pH is part of the full evaluation[42,49] but in most cases is of limited utility.[48] Elevations may indicate urine contamination in the bull and stallion or the presence of inflammation.[42] Testing should be performed within 10 minutes of ejaculation.[42] Normal values are 6.8–7.7 in the bull,[52,53] 6.1–7.0 in the dog,[49,54] and 7.2–7.6 in the stallion.[33,42]

Motility

Phase-contrast microscopes with a heated stage are preferred for motility estimation.[26,43,44,55] If using a light microscope, the condenser diaphragm is closed, or the condenser lowered to enhance visibility of the sperm.[26]

Gross Motility

Gross motility relies on both rapid progressive motility and high spermatozoal concentration and is only assessed in ruminants.[26] It is occasionally observed in canine semen due to the rapid motility of that species.[56] A drop of neat semen is placed on a slide and examined under 40× magnification without a coverslip. The sample is graded very good if there are rapid swirls, good if there are slow swirls, fair if there are no swirls but obvious individual cell motion, and poor if there is little or no individual motion.[26]

Individual Motility

Estimates of individual motility are made on coverslipped samples at 100× to 400× magnification.[27,43,44] Total motility refers to spermatozoa having any kind of motion except drifting with fluid flow, while progressively motile spermatozoa have purposeful forward motion in a linear direction or large arc. The latter is the parameter most used in reports and calculations.[43] At a magnification of 100× to 200×, a normally progressive canine spermatozoon should traverse the field of view in 2–3 seconds.[57] Warmed microscope stages are recommended as the motility percentage and speed are affected by the temperature of the sample.[58–60]

To improve accuracy and precision, standard techniques should be employed. Neat semen, especially with concentrated samples, is often too dense for assessment of motility, though it is frequently used in the dog.[27] Subjective assessment of motility is correlated to sample concentration, with higher concentration resulting in higher motility estimates[43]. Estimate repeatability is also better on diluted samples than neat semen.[34] For these reasons semen is usually diluted prior to final motility assessment; however, examining a drop of neat semen first acts as a control to ensure diluents used did not adversely affect motility patterns. Ideally, if sample concentration can be obtained in a timely manner, it guides dilution so that an appropriate and consistent sperm concentration for examination is obtained; 25 million/mL is recommended for examination of equine sperm.[43,61] For dilution, warm, species appropriate extenders or simple salt solutions such as phosphate-buffered saline, 2.9% sodium citrate and 0.9% sodium chloride can be used,[44,55,56] with highest motility obtained between 250 and 300 mOsm.[62]

The coverslipped sample needs to be deep enough to permit freedom of spermatozoal movement but shallow enough to keep them within the focal plane. The World Health Organization standard is 20 μm, achieved by placing a 10 μL drop of sperm on the slide and using a 22 × 22 mm coverslip.[63] Bull semen trials resulted in a recommendation of 15 μm, equating to a 7 μL drop for the 22 × 22 mm coverslip.[64] Shallower samples may be needed when assessing frozen-thawed semen due to extender lipid droplets and other debris decreasing visibility of spermatozoa.[65] Motility estimates are artificially increased adjacent to air bubbles, so care in placing the coverslip is needed.[65,66]

The World Health Organization recommends estimation is made on 5–10 fields at least 5 mm from the edge of the coverslip and assessing at least 200 spermatozoa to increase precision.[63] The National Association of Animal Breeders has a similar recommendation at least 2 mm from the coverslip edge.[44,65] Estimates taken from the center of the coverslip overestimate motility, while those taken at the edge underestimate it because placement of the coverslip causes fluid flow toward the edges, moving immotile sperm to those regions, whereas the most motile sperm swim against the current.[64] The most representative results are obtained using fields centered approximately one third of the way in from the edge of the coverslip.[64] Using a systematic approach by deciding whether the motility is less than or greater than 50% and then sequentially narrowing the range in which the value lies is recommended with final estimates made in 5–10% increments.[44]

Typical Findings

The minimum standard for progressive motility for bull sperm on the Society for Theriogenology (SFT) breeding soundness examination (BSE) is 30%, a low standard chosen to reflect adverse conditions of field examinations.[67] The mean progressive motility estimates in various studies were 51.6–75.5% for bulls,[68–72] 79.3–91% for apparently fertile dogs where the expected minimum is 70%,[49,73–76] and 49–67.8% for stallions.[12,77–79]

Concentration and Total Number

Spermatozoal concentration can be determined by direct or indirect methods, and the main techniques along with their strengths and weaknesses have been reviewed.[80] Recommended reference methods are hemocytometer, NucleoCounter®, and flow cytometry.[80]

Most methods require use of a small aliquot, which is then considerably diluted.[80] To ensure accurate, repeatable results, it is essential that the ejaculate be well mixed before the aliquot is taken,[58,81] pipettes are calibrated, and accurate technique is used.[80,82] Due to the viscosity of semen, the use of positive displacement pipettes is recommended.[83–85] When air displacement pipettes are used, a reverse pipetting technique is preferable,[80] or the tip should be flushed several times in the diluent to remove remaining semen.[84,85] Commercial blood dilution systems are convenient but have not been formally validated for use with semen.[80]

Hemocytometer

This technique can be used on any species, on specimens diluted in extenders that are not optically clear, and on those contaminated by other cell types and debris.[86] Precision is increased as more sperm are counted,[63] so dilution ratio may need adjusting. A typical ratio for canine and equine semen is 1 : 100, whereas for bull semen 1 : 200 is often used. The improved Neubauer is the standard for semen counts, giving more repeatable results than other types.[83] Details of methodology for performing hemocytometer counts can be found in referenced material.[63,80,86–88]

Disposable gridded counting chambers also can be used, but these are usually shallower (e.g. 20 µm) and are prone to uneven distribution of spermatozoa when loaded by capillary action. This Segre–Silberberg effect needs to be compensated for when using these chambers, and correction factors are supplied by manufacturers.[80,89]

NucleoCounter®

The NucleoCounter® (Chemometec, Allerod, Denmark) is a system that measures concentration and provides information on spermatozoal viability by assessing membrane integrity. Mixing the sample with a detergent permeabilizes the spermatozoa, which then pass through a cassette coated with propidium iodide (PI). The DNA takes up the stain, and spermatozoa are counted on an integrated fluorescence microscope.[80] For concentration, the technique has been validated as accurate and precise with equine[90] and bull[91] semen. The method is not affected by debris or opaque extenders, and image analysis algorithms differentiate other cells.[80] Comparison with a non-permeabilized sample gives membrane integrity information.

Spectrophotometer

A calibrated spectrophotometer provides rapid, repeatable, and accurate results. They are unreliable with specimens containing debris, lipid droplets, or other cells and cannot be used with samples diluted in extenders that are not optically clear.[92,93] Due to differences in ejaculate concentration, spermatozoal size, and seminal plasma constituents, the calibration curves and dilution ratios are species specific.[80] Following dilution, the test sample is well mixed, and the absorbance read immediately since the spermatozoa will rapidly settle if testing is delayed, resulting in errors.[94]

Flow Cytometry

Since flow cytometry assesses large numbers of cells quickly, it is a very precise method of assessing spermatozoal concentration.[80] The technique is prone to overestimation of spermatozoal concentration particularly if the semen contains significant debris or leukocytes, and it will also be affected by agglutination.[80,95,96] It is important that the sample be directly evaluated under a microscope to identify these potential sources of error.[80]

Comparison of Techniques

Correlations between techniques are typically high with *r* values of 0.91–0.98,[80,90,97–99] in part because in comparative studies they are often not independent as one may have calibrated the other or provided initial dilution information.[94] Within sample repeatability is generally best with flow cytometry (CV 2.3–2.95%)[90,94,100] followed by the NucleoCounter® (CV 3.1–3.17),[90,100] spectrophotometers (CV 3.0–6.2),[94,98] and hemocytometer (CV 6.69–9.6).[90,94,98] Precision of the hemocytometer is significantly better at high spermatozoal concentrations.[101,102]

Typical Concentrations and Total Spermatozoa Counts

Concentration is not assessed in routine bull BSEs using electroejaculation since full ejaculates are not collected. Canine semen concentration depends on how much prostatic fraction is included, and total spermatozoa in the ejaculate (concentration × volume) is the meaningful measure.[27] For bulls the mean reported concentrations range from 1.2 to 1.7×10^9/mL[72,103,104] and total spermatozoa in the ejaculate from 7.57 to 11.4×10^9.[72,103,105] The total spermatozoa per ejaculate in normal male dogs ranges from 300 to 2000×10^6.[49] Spermatozoal output in dogs is related to testicular size, which is associated with body size,[9,106,107] and very small dogs not achieving the above minimum should produce at least 22 million sperm/kg.[108] In the stallion concentration is inversely proportional to volume and ranges from 50 to 800×10^6/mL, with total spermatozoa in the ejaculate from 1 to 20×10^9.[51]

Morphology

Spermatozoal morphology is assessed using bright field microscopy on stained smears or by phase contrast or differential interference contrast (DIC) on wet preparations. The examination should be carried out at a magnification of at least 1000× under oil immersion in order to adequately evaluate the spermatozoa.[109]

A minimum of 100 spermatozoa are evaluated.[26,49,110] This will be adequate in an animal clearly surpassing or failing a threshold percentage of normal cells but will not give the necessary precision when an animal is near the threshold, when infrequent abnormalities are being assessed, or in cases open to legal dispute. The exact number needed can be calculated based on desired precision, and 300–500 per slide may be necessary.[26,111,112]

Phase Contrast and DIC

Semen is usually fixed in buffered formol saline[42,113] or glutaraldehyde in phosphate-buffered saline.[112,114] Having the fixative solution isosmolar avoids induction of artifactual bent or coiled tails.[115] Once fixed, the spermatozoal morphology is stable,[42,116] and resuspension by moderate shaking does not induce an increase in detached heads.[117] To avoid overlapping cells the ratio of semen to fixative depends on spermatozoal concentration and ranges from 1 : 1 to 1 : 100.[15,113,115,118,119] Thin preparations aid in cells lying flat for examination, and a 5 μL drop on a slide with a 22 × 22 mm coverslip is appropriate.[115] Avoiding lateral movement when placing the coverslip prevents an increase in detached heads.[112] Cells are allowed to settle for up to 15 minutes prior to examination.[120] Care is needed to ensure that angled heads are not counted as having an abnormality.[120]

Stained Samples

A variety of stains are suitable for examination of spermatozoa, the two most commonly employed in North America are eosin–nigrosin (EN) and the rapid Wright–Giemsa stains.[88]

EN is the standard stain for ruminants and is frequently used on other species.[26,55,115] The eosin is a vital stain that penetrates and stains dead or damaged cells, while the nigrosin is present as background.[109,121–123] Both stained and unstained cells are included when determining morphology. Using warmed stain and slides, a drop each of stain and semen are placed on one end of the slide and mixed. Another slide is used to draw the smear down in the same technique as creating a blood smear.[55,109] The smearing slide is often used to make another slide without replenishing in order to create a thinner sample. The slides are dried rapidly to prevent formation of midpiece and tail artifacts as the stain is often hypotonic.[109,124] When using EN it is useful to make an unstained smear for later staining by Wright–Giemsa to enable accurate identification of other cell types such as inflammatory cells that are difficult to accurately identify on EN.

Rapid Wright–Giemsa stains are commonly used for canine spermatozoa and are also applied to other species.[27,125] A smear is made by placing a drop of semen on a slide and drawing it down with another angled slide. An alternate technique that does not increase artifacts is to sandwich the drop between the two slides and then slide them apart lengthwise.[126] The smear is dried and then sequentially moved through the fixative and stain as for a blood smear, except that the time in each solution is lengthened to five minutes.[27,127] When used with equine semen, staining quality was considered superior with 30 minutes in each solution.[125]

Assessing Morphology

Slides are examined in a systematic pattern to ensure sperm is not counted more than once. For slides stained with EN, the artifactual increases in midpiece abnormalities, and detached heads are more prevalent at the end of the slide where spermatozoa and stain were mixed, so this area is avoided.[112] Spermatozoa are recorded as normal or as having various abnormalities. Normal spermatozoa are symmetrical when viewed lying flat except that abaxial attachment of the tail is normal in the horse, and such sperm also can have an asymmetric head where the lateral aspect is less curved on the side of midpiece attachment.[42]

Comprehensive images of abnormal spermatozoal morphology are available for the bull[128] and stallion.[129] Abnormal spermatozoa (Figures 41.2–41.6) often have more than a single defect. When the primary aim is to establish percent normal, such as in a routine BSE, it is useful to only record one defect per spermatozoon, usually what is considered the most severe, deleterious, or the most proximal one.[42,79,130] For clinical infertility cases and monitoring effects of experimental manipulation, a

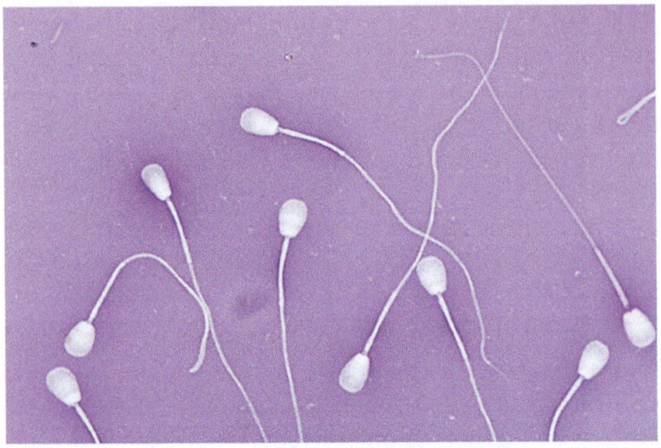

Figure 41.2 Canine sperm from a single ejaculate showing head pleomorphism. All sperm would be considered to be within the normal range except for the cell third from left, which most clinicians would classify as microcephalic (Eosin Nigrosin, 1000×).

more accurate picture is captured by enumerating all abnormalities present on each spermatozoon with a method that tracks the total number of spermatozoa examined, so percent normal cells can be determined.[115,120,131,132]

Abnormalities can be recorded specifically or can be lumped into various categories based on location on the cell, proposed site of origination during the life of the spermatozoon, or anticipated effect on fertility. Recording each abnormality is useful when investigating infertility or monitoring recovery from disease, whereas lumping is more expedient when the main aim is finding percent normal cells such as in a routine BSE. In the primary–secondary system, abnormalities arising during spermatogenesis are considered primary, while those that arise after the spermatozoon has left the testicle are considered secondary.[133] The secondary category is now often divided so that secondary abnormalities are those arising during spermatozoal maturation in the epididymis, and tertiary abnormalities are those due to handling errors during or after collection.[134] Problems arise because the origin of some defects is unknown, while others may have multiple origins. In the major–minor system, defects known to have a deleterious effect on fertility are classified as major, while those that have no known effect are minor.[135] The true fertility effects of some defects are not known, and most change with prevalence. Another classification system also based on fertility divides spermatozoal defects into compensable and uncompensable.[136] A compensable defect prevents the spermatozoa from ever initiating fertilization. In such cases increasing total number of spermatozoa inseminated improves fertility as there are increased numbers of normal spermatozoa deposited, thus increasing fertilization rate. An uncompensable defect allows the abnormal spermatozoa to initiate fertilization and trigger the block to polyspermy, but the resulting embryo is nonviable. In this case increasing total spermatozoa number does nothing for fertility since the ratio of normal and abnormal spermatozoa stays the same and both can fertilize the oocyte. Most obvious head, midpiece, and tail abnormalities are compensable, whereas a DNA defect in the nucleus of an otherwise normal appearing sperm is uncompensable.[136]

Typical Levels

The passing threshold for normal morphology on the SFT bull BSE is 70%,[67] and typical mean values for percent normal are 75.1–83.7%.[4,70,137–139] Semen from normal dogs should contain over 80% normal spermatozoa,[49] though one study found a significant threshold for fertility occurred at 60%.[75] Mean values in apparently fertile dogs range from 78 to 91%.[10,73,76,140] In stallions mean values for normal sperm range from 46 to 61%.[12,77,78,141]

Technique Artifacts

Preparation of stained slides causes artifactual loss of cytoplasmic droplets[112,115,116,118,120] and an increase in detached heads[112,115,120] compared with wet preparations examined with phase or DIC. EN also can result in increased midpiece reflexes and tail abnormalities,[112,120,124] probably due to hypotonicity of the stain.[26,124]

Agreement and Repeatability by Evaluators

There is generally good agreement in percentage of sperm assessed as normal,[127,142] but 10% variation occurred in an equine comparison.[115] Cytoplasmic droplets show good and head abnormalities poor agreement between evaluators, while there are variable results for midpiece and tail defects.[115,127,142] Studies on human spermatozoa show intra-technician variation of 2.8% and inter-technician variation of 5.6%.[101] While training programs decrease variation and increase accuracy of semen evaluation,[143] the effected improvement wanes in six to nine months.[144]

Other Cells

Semen can contain premature germ cells (spermatocytes, spermatids), leukocytes, erythrocytes, and epithelial cells from either the surface of the penis or prepuce, urethra, or accessory sex glands.[48,133] A Wright–Giemsa or similar stain should be used for identification.[42] Premature germ cells are considered rare except in cases of testicular degeneration.[133]

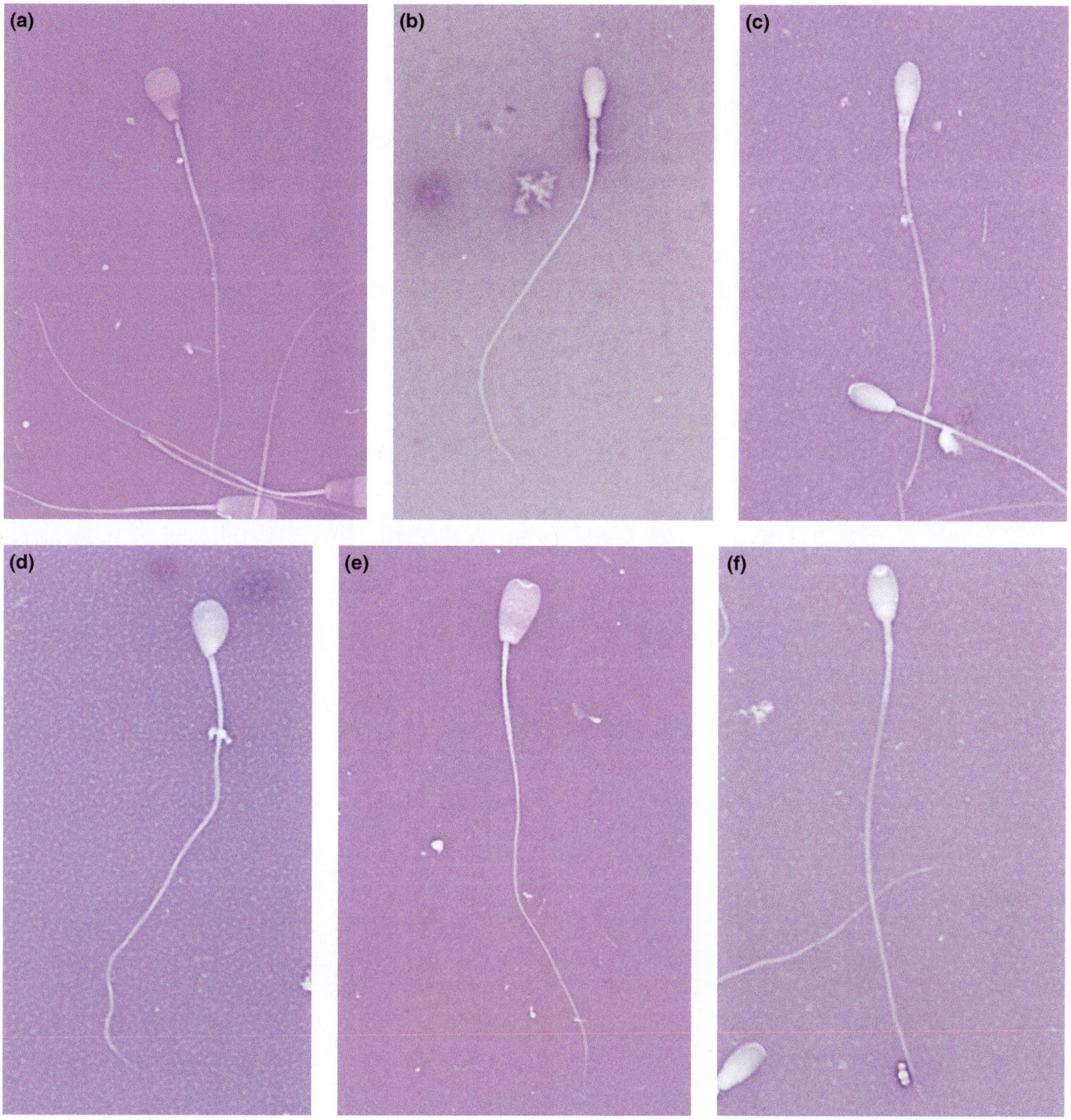

Figure 41.3 Head abnormalities. (a) Pyriform head (bull). (b) Pyriform head (stallion). (c) Pyriform head (stallion). (d) Asymmetric pyriform head (dog). (e) Knobbed acrosome (bull). (f) Knobbed acrosome, beaded form (stallion) (Eosin Nigrosin, 1000×).

Large numbers of inflammatory cells suggest reproductive tract infections, but some can also be found in ejaculates from apparently normal males. An average of 0.35–0.43/high power field (400×) were found in 90% of bull ejaculates.[145] Normal canine semen had 2–4/high power field[140] or 2×10^6/mL.[146] Presence of inflammatory cells in canine semen is neither sensitive nor specific for presence of infection.[147] Leukocytes are generally rare or present in low numbers in stallion ejaculates[148] and were found at a mean of 0.129×10^6/mL in fertile stallions.[149] If only present occasionally, neutrophils in dismount samples collected after natural breeding are considered an indication of

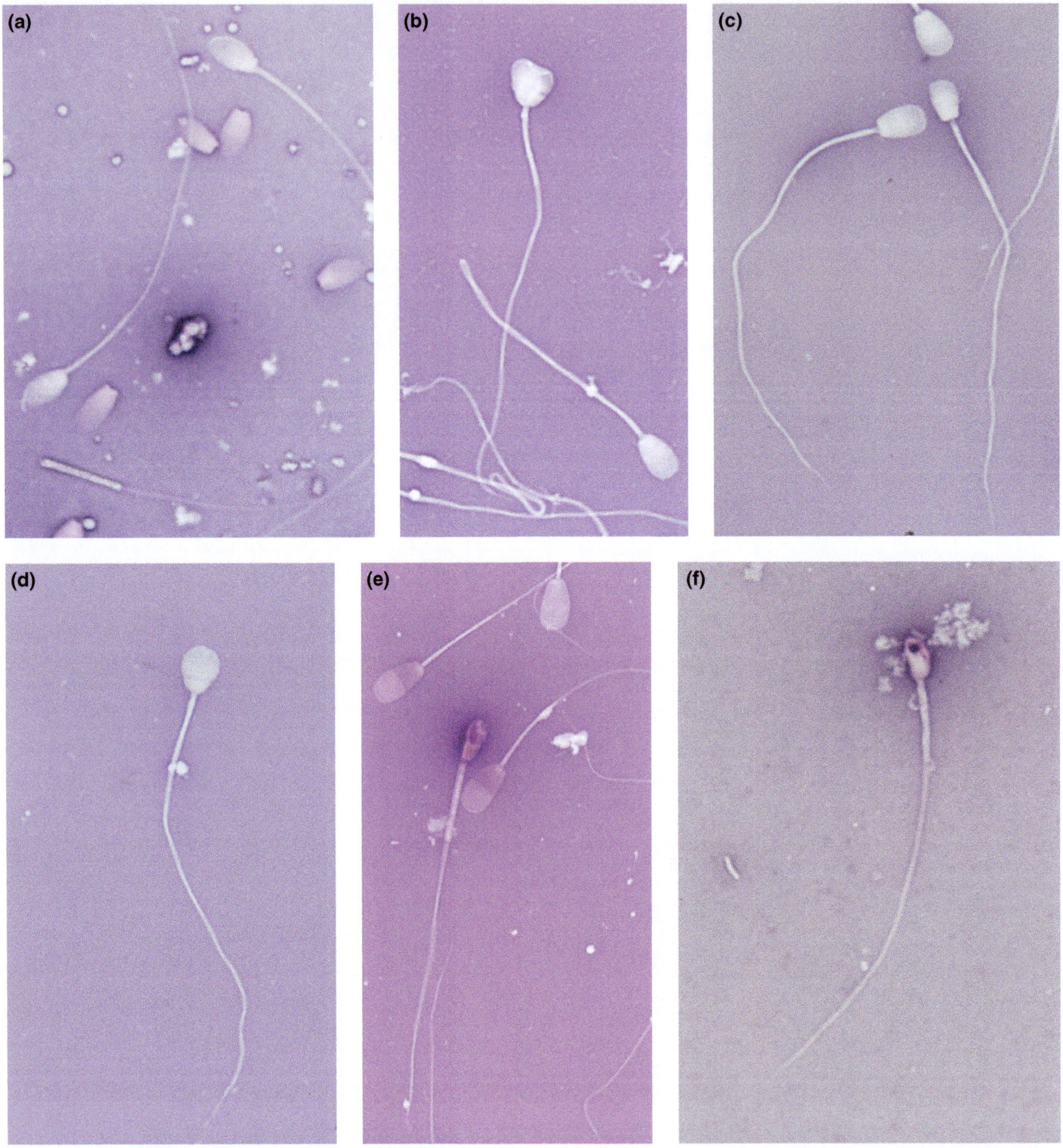

Figure 41.4 Head abnormalities. (a) Detached heads (stallion). (b) Macrocephalic head with abnormal shape and acrosome folding (dog). (c) Microcephalic head with normal comparison (dog). (d) Microcephalic head with rounded shape (dog). (e) Microcephalic head with nuclear vacuole (bull). (f) Microcephalic with nuclear vacuole (stallion) (Eosin Nigrosin, 1000×).

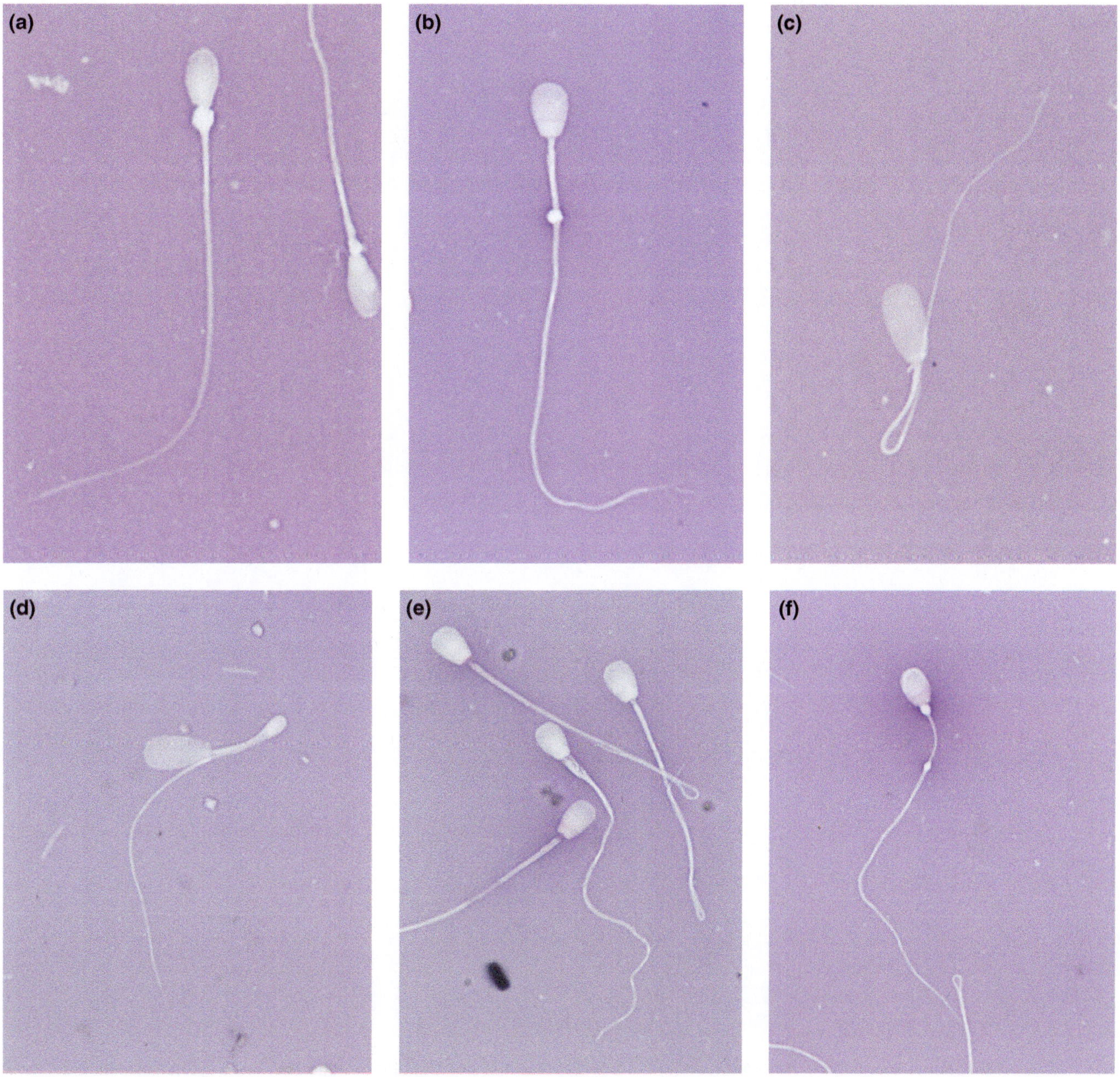

Figure 41.5 Midpiece abnormalities. (a) Proximal cytoplasmic droplet (stallion). (b) Distal cytoplasmic droplet (dog). (c) Distal midpiece reflex (bull). (d) Distal midpiece reflex with retained cytoplasmic droplet (bull). (e) Thickened midpiece with disrupted fibers (dog). (f) Segmental aplasia of mitochondrial sheath (dog) (Eosin Nigrosin, 1000×).

endometritis in the mare rather than infection of the stallion.[150,151] Some[145,149] but not all[152,153] have found a correlation between increased leukocytes and percent abnormal spermatozoa. In these cases macrophages may be increased,[145] and the abnormal spermatozoa appear to be attracting the macrophages that likely have a normal role in their removal.[145,154]

Epithelial cells are found in bull semen at approximately 1 per 1000 spermatozoa for AV collections.[133] In normal canine collections, a few prostatic cells are present in the third fraction, but often there are none.[155]

Medusa forms are detached tufted apices of epithelial cells from the efferent ducts and may be found at 1 per 10 000 sperm in bulls and slightly more in stallions.[133]

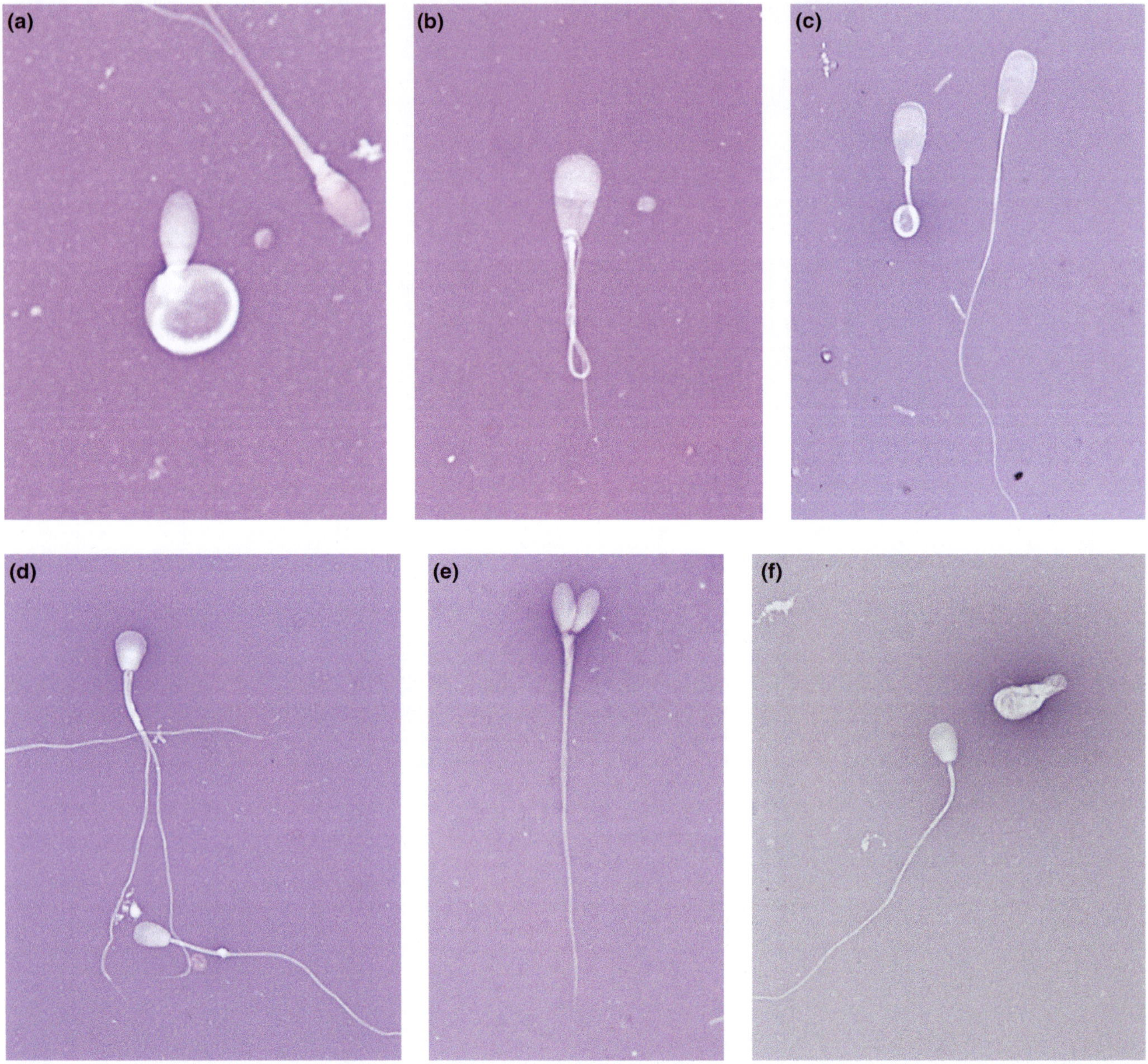

Figure 41.6 Principal piece and other abnormalities. (a) Coiled midpiece and principal piece within retained cytoplasm (stallion). (b) Double folded principal piece (bull). (c) Coiled principal piece (bull). (d) Macrocephalic head with double tail (dog). (e) Double head (stallion). (f) Teratoid (dog) (Eosin Nigrosin, 1000×).

Plasma Membrane Integrity: Live–Dead Counts

This technique is generally not performed during canine and equine examinations and is no longer a formal part of the SFT bull BSE. On EN-stained slides spermatozoa not taking up stain are considered viable while nonviable spermatozoa stain red.[121–123] The percent live is assessed by counting 200 spermatozoa.[63,123] Samples made with cold stain or hypotonic solutions can cause an artifactual increase in staining[156–158] as will glycerol concentration over 4% if used in freezing extenders,[159] whereas egg yolk extender decreased staining by 3%.[157] Stained slides should be read within 20 minutes in extremely humid conditions as uptake of stain may increase dramatically after this time.[42,160] Percent unstained spermatozoa is correlated with motility and normal morphology[161–163] and viability as assessed by PI fluorescent staining, but EN gives higher estimate of viability than PI by approximately 12–16%.[158,163]

Factors Affecting the Results of the Standard Semen Examination

Effects During Semen Collection

Water, soap, or disinfectant residues in collection equipment will decrease motility[30,42,140] as do excessive contact with latex AV liners,[45,164–167] urine contamination,[55,168–172] and even non-spermicidal lubricants.[173–175] Exposure to temperatures above 50 °C[176–178] and rapid cooling to below 15–20 °C[179] both decrease motility. The latter may induce cold shock,[179] evidenced by development of a bend at the junction of the midpiece and principal piece causing the spermatozoa to swim backwards or in tight circles.[180] Canine spermatozoa are more resistant to both heat and cold shock than those of other species.[179,181]

Frequency of Ejaculation

In general terms, more frequent ejaculation will give samples with fewer spermatozoa and improvement in motility and morphology over a celibate animal,[45,107,182,183] but once on a regular collection schedule, these latter improvements are not significant.[31,182] Following prolonged inactivity, a low percentage of bulls and stallions can experience abnormal spermatozoal accumulation and, though initially oligospermic, once blockages are cleared, will ejaculate large numbers of spermatozoa with poor motility and a high percentage of detached heads.[184,185] An increase in detached acrosomes may also occur with prolonged abstinence.[133] A notable commonality of peripubertal males is the presence of a large percentage of proximal cytoplasmic droplets, which rapidly declines with maturity.[119,186–190]

Disease

With all species, diseases of the reproductive tract resulting in orchitis, epididymitis, or testicular degeneration will affect semen parameters.[56,191,192] For example semen from dogs infected with brucellosis has increases in abnormal spermatozoa, increased leukocytes, spermatozoal agglutination, and decreased motility.[191] Animals with testicular degeneration have fewer total spermatozoa, decreased motility, and increased percentage of cells with abnormal morphology.[78,192] Inbreeding causes significant but small deleterious effects on spermatozoal output, motility, and morphology.[193–195] Specific defects of the spermatozoal head, acrosome, connecting piece, midpiece, and principal piece also can be directly inherited,[196] and consistent presence of a defect at a constant level should raise suspicion.[197]

Common insults to the testicle are those associated with heat and stress. While cells at each stage of spermatogenesis can be damaged, the cells most sensitive are the spermatocytes and spermatids.[198] With variations depending on degree and duration, the changes apparent in semen following a discreet episode of elevated temperature or stress follow a similar pattern.[130,199–202] In the first week, there may be no apparent change or a decrease in motility and concentration but little effect on morphology. This has led to the concept that spermatozoa in the epididymis are resistant to the effects of stressors. There is accumulating evidence that while this is true, even normal appearing spermatozoa may be functionally impaired by heat stress,[132] have increased DNA instability,[203,204] and are less able to support normal embryonic development.[198,205,206] After the first week, motility declines further, and there are increases in morphologic abnormalities as cells that were spermatids at the time of the insult appear. These include increases in distal droplets, proximal droplets, detached heads, and midpiece abnormalities including reflex bends by two to three weeks. Nuclear vacuolation and onset of pyriform head appear at approximately 2.5 weeks followed by acrosomal defects and in some cases severe midpiece disruption. Many spermatozoa will have more than one abnormality and recovery often takes six to eight weeks in these controlled experimental situations with short-duration stressors. There is considerable individual variation in response including effects on volume, concentration, and total spermatozoal output.[130,199–202] Scrotal warming in dogs decreased motility within 5 days, with a decline to 0 by 10 days, while the first morphological abnormalities to appear were reflex bent tails and detached heads.[56]

Advanced Techniques

Electron Microscopy

Both scanning and transmission electron microscopy are useful for defining defects in spermatozoal ultrastructure but are not performed routinely.[207–210]

Computer-Assisted Sperm Analysis (CASA)

These systems provide objective data on spermatozoal motility patterns and velocity, concentration estimates, and, with recent models, head and tail morphometry and morphology and cell viability using fluorescent staining.[89] Results are very dependent on appropriate settings for accurate spermatozoal identification, which vary with species, extenders, and any debris present in the sample.[89] Results also vary depending on the chamber used,[59,211] spermatozoal concentration assessed,[59,212] duration of analysis,[213] frame rate,[212] and chamber temperature.[213] Results from one system are not identical to those obtained on another.[89] CASA and visual assessment of motility show good correlation,[5,212,214] while correlations between single CASA parameters and fertility are variable.[5,9,12,215] Motility data is useful for research studies but considered unlikely to provide better information than visual assessment for culling potentially subfertile animals[89]; CASA systems are not currently recommended for concentration estimates. While correlations with other methods were high, CASA counts were inaccurate compared with hemocytometer.[59,212,214] If used, the accuracy and precision of counts are improved by immobilizing sperm, using only the central long axis of disposable chambers and applying appropriate Segre–Silberberg correction factors.[80,89]

Hypo-Osmotic Swelling Test

Sperm with intact functional membranes will take up water in hypo-osmotic conditions, and this is visible as swelling or curling of the tail.[216] Solutions of 50–150 mOsm are used for testing with incubation for 30–60 minutes at 37 °C. Cells are examined as a wet preparation under phase contrast and percent sperm with affected tails counted.[216–218] Unlike supravital stains, which assess membrane damage or death, the hypo-osmotic swelling test assesses functional capability.[158,216] Correlations with motility are higher than those with normal morphology, which are higher than those for EN or fluorescent staining though the latter are variable.[158,216,219,220]

Flow Cytometry Using Fluorescent Stains

While tests using fluorescent stains can be conducted with an appropriate microscope, use of flow cytometry removes subjectivity and permits many more cells to be rapidly assessed, increasing accuracy and precision of the results. The variety of probes available and their uses have been reviewed in detail.[5,221–223] Assessments include plasma membrane integrity, mitochondrial status and activity, capacitation status and patterns of membrane reorganization, acrosomal status, oxidative stress, and apoptotic changes.[5,221–223]

DNA Integrity

Determination of DNA integrity is particularly useful in animals with poor fertility that have apparently normal spermatozoa on standard examinations of motility and morphology.[224] The most commonly used test is the sperm chromatin structure assay (SCSA®, SCSA Diagnostics, Inc., Brookings, SD, USA), which determines spermatozoal susceptibility to developing DNA strand breaks following exposure to acidic conditions.[225] Fluorescence is detected by flow cytometry, and results are reported as a DNA fragmentation index.[225] Increased DNA fragmentation index is negatively associated with fertility.[13,226–228]

Morphometry

Image analysis systems allow detection of subtle variations of spermatozoal head size and shape that are difficult to determine by subjective analysis.[229] Measurement variations due to fixation and staining methods,[230–233] power of the objective lens, and sample concentration[234] occur because of effects on ability to accurately digitize individual spermatozoa.[235] Application has identified spermatozoal subpopulations[229,236,237] with associations to DNA fragmentation[237,238] and fertility.[238–240] Correlation between percent normal spermatozoa assessed by morphometry and subjectively were $r = 0.65–0.87$, with morphometry assessing 3.6–9.4% lower normal morphology.[234]

Conclusion

With all these advances it remains true that no single assay can reliably predict the fertility of a semen sample or male. Using regression models, multiple parameters can be incorporated, and correlations to fertility with $r^2 = 0.24–1.0$ have been obtained.[5,241,242] Interestingly, traditional tests such as subjectively assessed morphology and motility can be an integral part of these models with the addition of one or two newer tests taking their correlation with fertility >0.9.[5,241]

References

1 Amann, R.P. (1989). Can the fertility potential of a seminal sample be predicted accurately? *J Androl* 10: 89–98.

2 Mocé, E. and Graham, J.K. (2008). In vitro evaluation of sperm quality. *Anim Reprod Sci* 105: 104–118.

3 Martin, J.L. (1990). Sperm abnormalities and field fertility. Technical Conference on Artificial Insemination and Reproduction 13: 63–66.

4 Al-Makhzoomi, A., Lundeheim, N., Håård, M., and Rodríguez-Martínez, H. (2008). Sperm morphology and

fertility of progeny-tested AI dairy bulls in Sweden. *Theriogenology* 70: 682–691.
5 Gillan, L., Kroetsch, T., Maxwell, W.M.C., and Evans, G. (2008). Assessment of in vitro sperm characteristics in relation to fertility in dairy bulls. *Anim Reprod Sci* 103: 201–214.
6 Holroyd, R.G., Doogan, V.J., De Faveri, J. et al. (2002). Bull selection and use in northern Australia 4. Calf output and predictors of fertility of bulls in multiple-sire herds. *Anim Reprod Sci* 71: 67–79.
7 Wiltbank, J.N. and Parish, N.R. (1986). Pregnancy rate in cows and heifers bred to bulls selected for semen quality. *Theriogenology* 25: 779–783.
8 Mickelsen, W.D., Memon, M.A., Anderson, P.B., and Freeman, D.A. (1993). The relationship of semen quality to pregnancy rate and litter size following artificial insemination in the bitch. *Theriogenology* 39: 553–560.
9 Rijsselaere, T., Maes, D., Hoflack, G. et al. (2007). Effect of body weight, age and breeding history on canine sperm quality parameters measured by the Hamilton-Thorne analyzer. *Reprod Domest Anim* 42: 143–148.
10 Domoslawska, A., Zdunczyk, S., Nizanski, W., and Janowski, T. (2013). Assessment of semen quality in infertile dogs using computer-assisted sperm analysis by the Hamilton-Thorne semen analyser. *Bull Vet Inst Pulawy* 57: 429–432.
11 Linde-Forsberg, C. and Forsberg, M. (1989). Fertility in dogs in relation to semen quality and the time and site of insemination with fresh and frozen semen. *J Reprod Fertil Suppl* 39: 299–310.
12 Jasko, D.J., Little, T.V., Lein, D.H., and Foote, R.H. (1992). Comparison of spermatozoal movement and semen characteristics with fertility in stallions: 64 cases (1987–1988). *J Am Vet Med Assoc* 200: 979–985.
13 Morrell, J.M., Johannisson, A., Dalin, A.-M. et al. (2008). Sperm morphology and chromatin integrity in Swedish warmblood stallions and their relationship to pregnancy rates. *Acta Vet Scand* 50: 2.
14 Samper, J.C., Hellander, J.C., and Crabo, B.G. (1991). Relationship between the fertility of fresh and frozen stallion semen and semen quality. *J Reprod Fertil Suppl* 44: 107–114.
15 Love, C.C., Varner, D.D., and Thompson, J.A. (2000). Intra- and inter-stallion variation in sperm morphology and their relationship with fertility. *J Reprod Fertil Suppl* 56: 93–100.
16 Pace, M.M., Sullivan, J.J., Elliott, F.I. et al. (1981). Effects of thawing temperature, number of spermatozoa and spermatozoal quality on fertility of bovine spermatozoa packaged in.5-ml French straws. *J Anim Sci* 53: 693–701.
17 Makarechian, M. and Farid, A. (1985). The relationship between breeding soundness evaluation and fertility of beef bulls under group mating at pasture. *Theriogenology* 23: 887–898.
18 Farin, P.W., Chenoweth, P.J., Mateos, E.R., and Pexton, J.E. (1982). Beef bulls mated to estrus synchronized heifers: single- vs multi-sire breeding groups. *Theriogenology* 17: 365–372.
19 Waldner, C.L., Kennedy, R.I., and Palmer, C.W. (2010). A description of the findings from bull breeding soundness evaluations and their association with pregnancy outcomes in a study of western Canadian beef herds. *Theriogenology* 74: 871–883.
20 Nie, G.J., Wenzel, J.G.W., and Johnson, K.E. (2002). Comparison of pregnancy outcome in mares among methods used to evaluate and select spermatozoa for insemination. *Anim Reprod Sci* 69: 211–222.
21 Ax, R.L., Dally, M.R., Didion, B.A. et al. (2000). Artificial insemination. In: *Reproduction in Farm Animals*, 7e (eds. B. Hafez and E.S.E. Hafez), 376–389. Philadelphia, PA: Lippincott Williams & Wilkins.
22 Larson, L.L. (1986). Examination of the reproductive system of the bull. In: *Current Therapy in Theriogenology*, 2e (eds. D.A. Morrow, T. Caruthers and H.E. Pazak), 101–116. Philadelphia, PA: W.B. Saunders.
23 Schenk, J.L. (1998). Bull semen collection procedures. Technical Conference on Artificial Insemination and Reproduction 17: 48–58.
24 Ball, L. and Furman, J.W. (1972). Electroejaculation of the bull. *Bovine Pract* 7: 46–48.
25 Palmer, C.W. (2005). Welfare aspects of theriogenology: investigating alternatives to electroejaculation in bulls. *Theriogenology* 64: 469–479.
26 Barth, A.D. (2007). Evaluation of potential breeding soundness of the bull. In: *Current Therapy in Large Animal Theriogenology*, 2e (eds. R.S. Youngquist and W.R. Threlfall), 228–240. St. Louis, MO: W.B. Saunders.
27 Johnston, S.D., Root Kustriz, M.V., and Olson, P.N. (eds.) (2001). Semen collection, evaluation and preservation. In: *Canine and Feline Theriogenology*, 287–306. Philadelphia, PA: W.B. Saunders.
28 Kutzler, M.A. (2005). Semen collection in the dog. *Theriogenology* 64: 747–754.
29 Feldman, E.C. and Nelson, R.W. (eds.) (2004). Clinical and diagnostic evaluation of the male reproductive tract. In: *Canine and Feline Endocrinology and Reproduction*, 930–952. St Louis, MO: W.B. Saunders.
30 Hurtgen, J.P. (2000). Semen Collection in Stallions. In: *Equine Breeding Management and Artificial Insemination* (ed. J.C. Samper), 81–90. Philadelphia, PA: W.B. Saunders.
31 Mathevon, M., Buhr, M.M., and Dekkers, J.C.M. (1998). Environmental, management, and genetic factors

affecting semen production in Holstein bulls. *J Dairy Sci* 81: 3321–3330.

32 Söderquist, L., Janson, L., Håård, M., and Einarsson, S. (1996). Influence of season, age, breed and some other factors on the variation in sperm morphological abnormalities of Swedish dairy A.I. bulls. *Anim Reprod Sci* 44: 91–98.

33 Pattie, W.A. and Dowsett, K.F. (1982). The repeatability of seminal characteristics of stallions. *J Reprod Fertil Suppl* 32: 9–13.

34 Rousset, H., Chanteloube, P., Magistrini, M., and Palmer, E. (1987). Assessment of fertility and semen evaluations of stallions. *J Reprod Fertil Suppl* 35: 25–31.

35 Barth, A.D. (1989). Evaluation of frozen bovine semen. *Proc Soc Theriogenol*: 92–99.

36 Brito, L.F.C. (2010). Variations in laboratory semen evaluation procedures and testing. Technical Conference on Artificial Insemination & Reproduction 23: 61–67.

37 Varner, D.D. and Johnson, L. (2007). From a sperm's eye view: revisiting our perception of this intriguing cell. *Proc Am Assoc Equine Pract* 53: 104–177.

38 Toshimori, K. and Eddy, E.M. (2015). The spermatozoon. In: *Knobil and Neill's Physiology of Reproduction* (eds. T.M. Plant, A.J. Zeleznik, D.F. Albertini, et al.), 99–148. Amsterdam: Academic Press.

39 Krzanowska, H. (1974). The passage of abnormal spermatozoa through the uterutubal junction of the mouse. *J Reprod Fertil* 38: 81–90.

40 Rath, D., Schuberth, H.J., Coy, P., and Taylor, U. (2008). Sperm interactions from insemination to fertilization. *Reprod Domest Anim* 43 (5): 2–11.

41 Suarez, S. (2015). Gamete and zygote transport. In: *Knobil and Neill's Physiology of Reproduction* (eds. T.M. Plant, A.J. Zeleznik, D.F. Albertini, et al.), 197–232. Amsterdam: Academic Press.

42 Kenney, R.M., Hurtgen, J.P., Pierson, R. et al. (1983). Clinical evaluation of the stallion. *J Soc Theriogenol* 9: 1–100.

43 Jasko, D.J. (1992). Evaluation of stallion semen. *Vet Clin North Am Equine Pract* 8: 129–148.

44 Brito, L., Beckman, B., Cardwell, B. et al. (2012). NAAB-CSS semen quality control program minimum guidelines. Technical Conference on Artificial Insemination and Reproduction 24: 37–41.

45 Boucher, J.H., Foote, R.H., and Kirk, R.W. (1958). The evaluation of semen quality in the dog and the effects of frequency of ejaculation upon semen quality, libido, and depletion of sperm reserves. *Cornell Vet* 48: 67–86.

46 White, I.G. and Lincoln, G.J. (1960). The yellow pigmentation of bull semen and its content of riboflavin, niacin, thiamine and related compounds. *Biochem J* 76: 301–306.

47 Kanchan and Matharoo, J.S. (2015). Effect of semen color on seminal characteristics in cattle bulls. *Indian J Anim Res* 49: 146–147.

48 Root Kustritz, M.V. (2007). The value of canine semen evaluation for practitioners. *Theriogenology* 68: 329–337.

49 Johnston, S.D. (1991). Performing a complete canine semen evaluation in a small animal hospital. *Vet Clin North Am Small Anim Pract* 21: 545–551.

50 Peters, A.R. and PJH, B. (eds.) (1995). Control of reproductive function in the male. In: *Reproduction in Cattle*, 62–74. Oxford: Blackwell Science.

51 Lopate, C., LeBlanc, M., and Knottenbelt, D. (2003). The stallion. In: *Equine Stud Farm Medicine and Surgery* (ed. D.C. Knottenbelt), 43–112. Edinburgh: W.B. Saunders.

52 Davis, H.P. and Williams, N.K. (1939). Evaluating bovine semen. I. Influence of number of ejaculates upon various physical and chemical characteristics and the relationship between those factors. *J Anim Sci* 32: 232–242.

53 Alexander, F.C.M., Zemjanis, R., Graham, E.F., and Schmehl, M.L. (1971). Semen characteristics and chemistry from bulls before and after seminal vesiculectomy and after vasectomy. *J Dairy Sci* 54: 1530–1535.

54 Bartlett, D.J. (1962). Studies on dog semen II. Biochemical characteristics. *Reprod Fertil* 3: 190–205.

55 Ball, L., Ott, R.S., Mortimer, R.G. et al. (1983). Manual for breeding soundness examination of bulls. *J Soc Theriogenol* 12: 5–65.

56 Johnston, S.D., Larsen, R.E., and Olson, P.S. (1982). Society for theriogenology manual for canine. *Theriogenology*: 51–109.

57 Threlfall, W. (2003). Semen collection and evaluation. In: *The Practical Veterinarian: Small Animal Theriogenology* (ed. M.V. Root Kustritz), 97–123. St. Louis, MO: Butterworth-Heinemann.

58 Bane, A. (1952). A study on the technique of hemocytometric determination of sperm motility and sperm concentration in bull semen. *Cornell Vet* 42: 518–530.

59 Iguer-Ouada, M. and Verstegen, J.P. (2001). Evaluation of the "Hamilton-Thorn computer-based automated system" for dog semen analysis. *Theriogenology* 55: 733–749.

60 Amann, R.P. (1987). Computerized evaluation of stallion spermatozoa. *Proc Am Assoc Equine Pract* 33: 453–473.

61 Varner, D.D. (2008). Developments in stallion semen evaluation. *Theriogenology* 70: 448–462.

62 Liu, Z. and Foote, R.H. (1998). Bull sperm motility and membrane integrity in media of varying osmolality. *J Dairy Sci* 81: 1868–1873.

63 World Health Organization (2010). *WHO Laboratory Manual for the Examination and Processing of Human Semen*, 5e, 17–102. Geneva: World Health Organization.

64 Nöthling, J.O. and dos Santos, I.P. (2012). Which fields under a coverslip should one assess to estimate sperm motility? *Theriogenology* 77: 1686–1697.

65 Parks, J.E. and Krieger, K.E. (2012). Subjective evaluation of bull sperm motility. Technical Conference on Artificial Insemination and Reproduction 24: 173–177.

66 Graham, E.F., Schmel, M.K.L., and Nelson, D.S. (1980). Problems with laboratory assays. Technical Conference on Artificial Insemination and Reproduction 8: 59–66.

67 Chenoweth, P.J. (1993). A new bull breeding soundness evaluation form. *Proc Soc Theriogenol*: 63–70.

68 Lasley, J.F. (1951). Spermatozoan motility as a measure of semen quality. *J Anim Sci* 10: 211–218.

69 Fitzpatrick, L.A., Fordyce, G., McGowan, M.R. et al. (2002). Bull selection and use in northern Australia. Part 2. Semen traits. *Anim Reprod Sci* 71: 39–49.

70 Ellis, R.W., Rupp, G.P., Chenoweth, P.J. et al. (2005). Fertility of yearling beef bulls during mating. *Theriogenology* 64: 657–678.

71 Hoflack, G., Van Soom, A., Maes, D. et al. (2006). Breeding soundness and libido examination of Belgian blue and Holstein Friesian artificial insemination bulls in Belgium and the Netherlands. *Theriogenology* 66: 207–216.

72 Seidel, G.E. and Foote, R.H. (1969). Influence of semen collection interval and tactile stimuli on semen quality and sperm output in bulls. *J Dairy Sci* 52: 1074–1079.

73 England, G.C. and Allen, W.E. (1989). Seminal characteristics and fertility in dogs. *Vet Rec* 125: 399.

74 Gunay, U., Polat, U., Gunes, N. et al. (2003). The effects of short-interval ejaculation on semen quality and some biochemical parameters in dogs. *Rev Méd Vét* 154: 459–462.

75 Oettlé, E.E. (1993). Sperm morphology and fertility in the dog. *J Reprod Fertil Suppl* 47: 257–260.

76 Wong, W.T. and Dhaliwal, G.K. (1985). Observations on semen quality of dogs in the tropics. *Vet Rec* 116: 313–314.

77 Paccamonti, D.L., Buiten, A.V., Parlevliet, J.M., and Colenbrander, B. (1999). Reproductive parameters or miniature stallions. *Theriogenology* 51: 1343–1349.

78 Pickett, B.W., Voss, J.L., Bowen, R.A. et al. (1987). Seminal characteristics and total scrotal width (T.S.W.) of normal and abnormal stallions. *Proc Am Assoc Equine Pract* 33: 487–518.

79 Parlevliet, J.M., Kemp, B., and Collebrander, B. (1994). Reproductive characteristics and semen quality in maiden Dutch warmblood stallions. *J Reprod Fertil* 101: 183–187.

80 Brito, L.F.C., Althouse, G.C., Aurich, C. et al. (2016). Andrology laboratory review: evaluation of sperm concentration. *Theriogenology* 85: 1507–1527.

81 Belding, D.L. (1934). Fertility in the male II. Technic of the spermatozoa count. *Am J Obstet Gynecol* 27: 25–31.

82 Freund, M. and Carol, B. (1964). Factors affecting haemocytometer counts of sperm concentration in human semen. *J Reprod Fertil* 8: 149–155.

83 Mahmound, A.M.A., Depoorter, B., Piens, N., and Comhaire, F.H. (1997). The performance of 10 different methods for the estimation of sperm concentration. *Fertil Steril* 68: 340–345.

84 Mortimer, D., Shu, M.A., and Tan, R. (1986). Standardization and quality control of sperm concentration and sperm motility counts in semen analysis. *Hum Reprod* 1: 299–303.

85 Mortimer, D., Shu, M.A., Tan, R., and Mortimer, S.T. (1989). A technical note on diluting semen for the haemocytometric determination of sperm concentration. *Hum Reprod* 4: 166–168.

86 Vanderwall, D.K. (2008). Counting spermatozoa with a hemacytometer. *J Equine Vet Sci* 28: 244–246.

87 Brazil, C., Swan, S.H., Drobnis, E.Z. et al. (2004). Standardized methods for semen evaluation in a multicenter research study. *J Androl* 25: 635–644.

88 Lorton, S.P. (2014). Evaluation of semen in the andrology laboratory. In: *Animal Andrology: Theories and Applications* (ed. P.J. Chenoweth), 100–143. Wallingford: CAB International.

89 Amann, R.P. and Waberski, D. (2014). Computer-assisted sperm analysis (CASA): capabilities and potential developments. *Theriogenology* 81: 5–17.

90 Comerford, K.L., Love, C.C., Brinsko, S.P. et al. (2008). Validation of a commercially available fluorescence-based instrument to evaluate stallion spermatozoal concentration. *Proc Am Assoc Equine Pract* 54: 367–368.

91 Anzar, M., Kroetsch, T., and Buhr, M.M. (2009). Comparison of different methods of assessment of sperm concentration and membrane integrity with bull semen. *J Androl* 30: 661–668.

92 Salisbury, G.W., Beck, G.H., Elliott, I., and Willett, E.L. (1943). Rapid methods for estimating the number of spermatozoa in bull semen. *J Dairy Sci* 26: 69–78.

93 Emik, L.O. and Sidwell, G.M. (1947). Factors affecting the estimation of concentration of sperm in ram's semen by the photoelectrometric method. *J Anim Sci* 6: 467–475.

94 Prathalingham, N.S., Holt, W.W., Revell, S.G. et al. (2006). Precision and accuracy of six different methods to determine sperm concentration. *J Androl* 27: 257–262.

95 Lu, J.-C., Chen, F., Xu, H.-R. et al. (2007). Is flow cytometry really adapted to the determination of sperm concentration? *Scand J Clin Lab Invest* 67: 394–401.

96 Petrunkina, A.M. and Harrison, R.A.P. (2010). Systematic misestimation of cell subpopulations by flow cytometry: a mathematical analysis. *Theriogenology* 73: 839–847.

97 Haag, F.M. (1959). Determination of the approximate sperm concentration of horse semen with the aid of a spectrophotometer. *J Am Vet Med Assoc* 34: 314–316.

98 Rigby, S.L., Varner, D.D., Thompson, J.A. et al. (2001). Measurement of sperm concentration in ejaculates using photometric or direct sperm enumeration techniques. *Proc Am Assoc Equine Pract* 47: 236–238.

99 Foote, R.H. and Boucher, J.H. (1964). A comparison of several photoelectric procedures for estimating sperm concentration in dog semen. *Am J Vet Res* 25: 558–560.

100 Hansen, C., Vermeiden, T., Vermeiden, J.P.W. et al. (2006). Comparison of FACSCount AF system, improved Neubauer hemocytometer, Corning 254 photometer, SpermVision, UltiMate and Nucleocounter SP-100 for determination of sperm concentration of boar semen. *Theriogenology* 66: 2188–2194.

101 Cooper, T.G., Neuwinger, J., Bahrs, S., and Nieschlag, E. (1992). Internal quality control of semen analysis. *Fertil Steril* 58: 172–178.

102 Christensen, P., Stryhn, H., and Hansen, C. (2005). Discrepancies in the determination of sperm concentration using Burker-Turk, Thoma and Makler counting chambers. *Theriogenology* 63: 992–1003.

103 Brito, L.F.C., Silva, A.E.D.F., Rodrigues, L.H. et al. (2002). Effects of environmental factors, age and genotype on sperm production and semen quality in Bos indicus and Bos taurus AI bulls in Brazil. *Anim Reprod Sci* 70: 181–190.

104 Persson, Y., Strid, G., Håård, M., and Söderquist, L. (2007). Comparison of semen samples collected from beef bulls by transrectal massage or artificial vagina. *Vet Rec* 161: 662–663.

105 Everett, R.W. and Bean, B. (1982). Environmental influences on semen output. *J Dairy Sci* 65: 1303–1310.

106 Amann, R.P. (1986). Reproductive physiology and endocrinology of the dog. In: *Current Therapy in Theriogenology*, 2e (eds. D.A. Morrow, T. Caruthers and H.E. Pazak), 532–538. Philadelphia, PA: W.B. Saunders.

107 Olar, T.T., Amann, R.P., and Pickett, B.W. (1983). Relationships among testicular size, daily sperm production and output of spermatozoa, and extragonadal spermatozoal reserves of the dog. *Biol Reprod* 29: 1114–1120.

108 Johnston, S.D., Root Kustriz, M.V., and Olson, P.N. (eds.) (2001). Clinical Approach to infertility in the male dog. In: *Canine and Feline Theriogenology*, 370–387. Philadelphia, PA: W.B. Saunders.

109 Barth, A.D. and Oko, R.J. (eds.) (1989). Preparation of semen for morphological examination. In: *Abnormal Morphology of Bovine Spermatozoa*, 8–18. Ames, IA: Iowa State University Press.

110 Salisbury, G.W. and Mercier, E. (1945). The reliability of estimates of the proportion of morphologically abnormal spermatozoa in bull semen. *J Anim Sci* 4: 174–178.

111 Kuster, C.E., Singer, R.S., and Althouse, G.C. (2004). Determining sample size for the morphological assessment of sperm. *Theriogenology* 61: 691–703.

112 Harasymowycz, J., Ball, L., and Seidel, G.E. (1976). Evaluation of bovine spermatozoal morphologic features after staining or fixation. *Am J Vet Res* 37: 1053–1057.

113 Hancock, J.L. (1956). The morphology of boar spermatozoa. *J R Microsc Soc* 76: 84–97.

114 Johnson, L., Berndtson, W.E., and Pickett, B.W. (1976). An improved method for evaluating acrosomes of bovine spermatozoa. *J Anim Sci* 42: 951–954.

115 Brito, L.F.C., Greene, L.M., Kelleman, A. et al. (2011). Effect of method and clinician on stallion sperm morphology evaluation. *Theriogenology* 76: 745–750.

116 Sekoni, V.O., Gustafsson, B.K., and Mather, E.C. (1981). Influence of wet fixation, staining techniques, and storage time on bull sperm morphology. *Nord Vet Med* 33: 161–166.

117 Mercier, E. and Salisbury, G.W. (1947). Effect of techniques of preparing semen smears for staining on the morphology of bull spermatozoa. *J Anim Sci* 6: 60–66.

118 Sprecher, D.J. and Coe, P.H. (1996). Differences in bull spermiograms using eosin-nigrosin stain, Feulgen stain, and phase contrast microscopy methods. *Theriogenology* 45: 757–764.

119 Arteaga, A., Baracaldo, M., and Barth, A.D. (2001). The proportion of beef bulls in western Canada with mature spermiograms at 11 to 15 months of age. *Can Vet J* 42: 783–787.

120 Freneau, G.E., Chenoweth, P.J., Ellis, R., and Rupp, G. (2010). Sperm morphology of beef bulls evaluated by two different methods. *Anim Reprod Sci* 118: 176–181.

121 Blom, E. (1950). A one minute live-dead sperm stain by means of eosin-nigrosin. *Fertil Steril* 1: 176–177.

122 Mayer, D.T., Squiers, C.D., Bogart, R., and Oloufa, M.M. (1951). The technique for characterizing mammalian spermatozoa as dead or living by differential staining. *J Anim Sci* 10: 226–235.

123 Campbell, R.C., Hancock, J.L., and Rosthchild, L. (1953). Counting live and dead bull spermatozoa. *J Exp Biol* 30: 44–49.

124 Johnson, C., Jacobs, J., and Walker, R. (1991). Diagnosis and control of Brucella canis in kennel situations. Morphology-stain induced spermatozoal abnormalities. *Proc Soc Theriogenol*: 236–239.

125 Pozor, M.A., Zambrano, G.L., Runcan, E. et al. (2012). Usefulness of dip quick stain in evaluating sperm

morphology in stallions. *Proc Am Assoc Equine Pract* 58: 506–510.
126 Salisbury, G.W., Willett, E.L., and Seligman, J. (1942). The effect of the method of making semen smears upon the number of morphologically abnormal spermatozoa. *J Anim Sci* 1: 199–205.
127 Root Kustritz, M.V., Olson, P.N., Johnston, S.D., and Root, T.K. (1998). The effects of stains and investigators on assessment of morphology of canine spermatozoa. *J Am Anim Hosp Assoc* 34: 348–352.
128 Barth, A.D. and Oko, R.J. (eds.) (1989). Photomicrographic features of bovine sperm cell abnormalities. In: *Abnormal Morphology of Bovine Spermatozoa*, 89–129. Ames, IA: Iowa State University Press.
129 Brito, L.F.C. (2007). Evaluation of stallion sperm morphology. *Clin Tech Equine Pract* 6: 249–264.
130 Campos, J.R., Breheny, P., Araujo, R.R. et al. (2014). Semen quality of stallions challenged with the Kentucky 84 strain of equine arteritis virus. *Theriogenology* 82: 1068–1079.
131 Card, C.E. (2005). Cellular associations and the differential spermiogram: making sense of stallion spermatozoal morphology. *Theriogenology* 64: 558–567.
132 Vogler, C.J., Saacke, R.G., Bame, J.H. et al. (1991). Effects of scrotal insulation on viability characteristics of cryopreserved bovine semen. *J Dairy Sci* 74: 3827–3835.
133 Blom, E. (1950). Interpretation of spermatic cytology in bulls. *Fertil Steril* 1: 223–230.
134 Dott, H.M. (1975). Morphology of stallion spermatozoa. *J Reprod Fertil Suppl* 23: 41–46.
135 Blom, E. (1973). The ultrastructure of some characteristic sperm defects and a proposal for a new classification of the bull spermiogram. *Nord Vet Med* 25: 383–391.
136 Saacke, R.G. (2008). Sperm morphology: its relevance to compensable and uncompensable traits in semen. *Theriogenology* 70: 473–478.
137 Bruner, K.A., McCraw, R.L., Whitacre, M.D. et al. (1995). Breeding soundness examination of 1,952 yearling beef bulls in North Carolina. *Theriogenology* 44: 129–145.
138 Chenoweth, P.J., Farin, P.W., Mateos, E.R. et al. (1984). Breeding soundness and sex drive by breed and age in beef bulls used for natural mating. *Theriogenology* 22: 341–349.
139 Hancock, A.S., Younis, P.J., Beggs, D.S. et al. (2016). An assessment of dairy herd bulls in southern Australia: 1. Management practices and bull breeding soundness evaluations. *J Dairy Sci* 99: 9983–9997.
140 Stockner, P.K. and Bardwick, C. (1991). The relationship of semen parameters to fertility in the dog. *Canine Pract* 16: 15–23.
141 Jasko, D.J., Lein, D.H., and Foote, R.H. (1990). Determination of the relationship between sperm morphologic classifications and fertility in stallions: 66 cases (1987–1988). *J Am Vet Med Assoc* 197: 389–394.
142 Baker, H.W.G. and Clarke, G.N. (1987). Sperm morphology: consistency of assessment of the same sperm by different observers. *Clin Reprod Fertil* 5: 37–43.
143 Björndahl, L., Barratt, C.L.R., Fraser, L.R. et al. (2002). ESHRE basic semen analysis courses 1995–1999: immediate beneficial effects of standardized training. *Hum Reprod* 17: 1299–1305.
144 Franken, D.R. and Kruger, T.F. (2006). Lessons learned from a sperm morphology quality control programme. *Andrologia* 38: 225–229.
145 Zart, A.L., Jurgielewicz, V.C., and Fernandes, C.E. (2014). Seminal leucocytary profile in beef bulls. *Reprod Domest Anim* 49: 719–724.
146 Meyers-Wallen, V.N. (1991). Clinical approach to infertile male dogs with sperm in the ejaculate. *Vet Clin North Am Small Anim Pract* 21: 609–633.
147 Root Kustritz, M.V., Johnston, S.D., Olson, P.N., and Lindeman, C.J. (2005). Relationship between inflammatory cytology of canine seminal fluid and significant aerobic bacterial, anaerobic bacterial or mycoplasma cultures of canine seminal fluid: 95 cases (1987–2000). *Theriogenology* 64: 1333–1339.
148 Malmgren, L., Engvall, E.O., Engvall, A., and Albihn, A. (1998). Aerobic bacterial flora of semen and stallion reproductive tract and its relation to fertility under field conditions. *Acta Vet Scand* 39: 173–182.
149 Waheed, M.M., Ghoneim, I.M., and Abdou, M.S.S. (2015). Morphometric characteristics of spermatozoa in the Arabian horse with regard to season, age, sperm concentration and fertility. *J Equine Vet Sci* 35: 244–249.
150 Blanchard, T.L., Thompson, J.A., Brinsko, S.P. et al. (2010). Some factors associated with fertility of Thoroughbred stallions. *J Equine Vet Sci* 30: 407–418.
151 Gunn, A.J. and Brooks, V.J. (2011). Neutrophil prevalence in dismount semen samples of Thoroughbred stallions. *Clin Theriogenol* 3: 477–481.
152 Specher, D.J., Coe, P.H., and Walker, R.D. (1999). Relationships among seminal culture, seminal white blood cells and the percentage of primary sperm abnormalities in bulls evaluated prior to the breeding season. *Theriogenology* 51: 1197–1206.
153 Sutovsky, P., Plummer, W., Baska, K. et al. (2007). Relative levels of semen platelet activating factor-receptor (PAFr) and ubiquitin in yearling bulls with a

high content of semen white blood cells: implications for breeding soundness evaluation. *J Androl* 28: 92–108.
154 Tomlinson, M.J., White, A., Barratt, C.L. et al. (1992). The removal of morphologically abnormal sperm forms by phagocytes: a positive role for seminal leukocytes. *Hum Reprod* 7: 517–522.
155 Olson, P.N. (1989). Exfoliative cytology of the canine reproductive tract. *Proc Soc Theriogenol*: 259–276.
156 Hancock, J.L. (1951). A staining technique for the study of temperature-shock in semen. *Nature* 167: 323–324.
157 Swanson, E.W. and Bearden, H.J. (1951). An eosin-nigrosin stain for differentiating live and dead bovine spermatozoa. *J Anim Sci* 10: 981–987.
158 Brito, L.F.C., Barth, A.D., Bilodeau-Goeseels, S. et al. (2003). Comparison of methods to evaluate the plasmalemma of bovine sperm and their relationship with in vitro fertilization rate. *Theriogenology* 60: 1539–1551.
159 Mixner, J.P. and Saroff, J. (1954). Interference by glycerol with differential staining of bull spermatozoa. *J Dairy Sci* 37: 662 abstract.
160 Berg, B.W. and Merilan, C.P. (1983). Humidity resistant live-dead stain for spermatozoa. *Theriogenology* 19: 259–262.
161 England, G.C. and Plummer, J.M. (1993). Hypo-osmotic swelling of dog spermatozoa. *J Reprod Fertil Suppl* 47: 261–270.
162 Barth, A.D. and Waldner, C.L. (2002). Factors affecting breeding soundness classification of beef bulls examined at the Western College of Veterinary Medicine. *Can Vet J* 43: 274–284.
163 Johansson, C.S., Matsson, F.C., Lehn-Jensen, H. et al. (2008). Equine spermatozoa viability comparing the nucleocounter SP-100 and the eosin-nigrosin stain. *Anim Reprod Sci* 107: 325–326.
164 Flick, D.L. and Merilan, C.P. (1988). Toxicity of artificial vaginal liners for bovine spermatozoa. *Theriogenology* 29: 1207–1213.
165 England, G.C. and Allen, W.E. (1992). Factors affecting the viability of canine spermatozoa I. Potential influences during processing for artificial insemination. *Theriogenology* 37: 363–371.
166 Merilan, C.P. and Loch, W.E. (1987). The effect of artificial vagina liners on livability of stallion spermatozoa. *J Equine Vet Sci* 7: 226–228.
167 Althouse, G.C., Ko, J.C., Hopkins, S.M., and Evans, L.E. (1991). Effect of latex and vinyl examination gloves on canine spermatozoal motility. *J Am Vet Med Assoc* 199: 227–229.
168 Griggers, S., Paccamonti, D.L., Thompson, R.A., and Eilts, B.E. (2001). The effects of pH, osmolarity and urine contamination on equine spermatozoal motility. *Theriogenology* 56: 613–622.
169 Makler, A., David, R., Blumenfeld, Z., and Better, O.S. (1981). Factors affecting sperm motility. VII. Sperm viability as affected by change of pH and osmolarity of semen and urine specimens. *Fertil Steril* 36: 507–511.
170 Guthrie, H.D., Liu, J., and Crister, J.K. (2002). Osmotic tolerance limits and effects of cryoprotectants on motility of bovine spermatozoa. *Biol Reprod* 67: x1811–1816.
171 Contri, A., Gloria, A., Robbe, D. et al. (2013). Kinematic study on the effect of pH on bull sperm function. *Anim Reprod Sci* 136: 252–259.
172 Santos, I.P., Cunha, I.C.N., and Melo, E.J.T. (2011). Effects of urine and NaCl solutions of different osmolarities on canine sperm. *Anim Reprod* 8: 73–76.
173 Froman, D.P. and Amann, R.P. (1983). Inhibition of motility of bovine, canine and equine spermatozoa by artificial vagina lubricants. *Theriogenology* 20: 357–361.
174 Duoos, L., Troedsson, M.H.T., Alghamdi, A.S. et al. (2002). The importance of osmotic pressure for the quality of fresh, cooled and cryopreserved equine spermatozoa. *Theriogenology* 58: 261–264.
175 Limone, L.E., Shaughnessy, D.W., Gómez-Ibáñez, S. et al. (2002). The effect of artificial vaginal lubricants on stallion sperm motion measures and semen pH during cooled storage. *Theriogenology* 55: 333–336.
176 Cooper, W.L. (1979). The effect of rapid temperature changes on oxygen uptake by and motility of stallion spermatozoa. *Proc Soc Theriogenol*: 10–16.
177 Hillman, R.B., Olar, T.T., Squires, E.L., and Pickett, B.W. (1980). Temperature of the artificial vagina and its effect on seminal quality and behavioral characteristics of stallions. *J Am Vet Med Assoc* 177: 720–722.
178 Macmillan, K.L., Hafs, H.D., Desjardins, C., and Kirton, K.T. (1966). Some semen characteristics in dairy bulls ejaculated with artificial vaginas at varying temperatures. *J Dairy Sci* 49: 1132–1133.
179 Watson, P.F. (1981). The effects of cold shock on sperm cell membranes. In: *Effects of Low Temperatures on Biological Membranes* (eds. G.J. Morris and A. Clarke), 189–218. London: Academic Press.
180 Devireddy, R.V. (2013). Biopreservation: heat/mass transfer challenges and biochemical/genetic adaptations in biological systems. *Heat Transfer Res* 44: 245–272.
181 Wales, R.G. and White, I.G. (1959). The susceptibility of spermatozoa to temperature shock. *J Endocrinol* 19: 211–220.
182 Hafs, H.D., Hoyt, R.S., and Bratton, R.W. (1959). Libido, sperm characteristics, sperm output, and fertility of mature dairy bulls ejaculated daily or weekly for thirty-two weeks. *J Dairy Sci* 42: 626–636.

183 Sullivan, J.J. and Pickett, B.W. (1975). Influence of ejaculation frequency of stallions on characteristics of semen and output of spermatozoa. *J Reprod Fertil Suppl* 23: 29–34.

184 Barth, A.D. (2007). Sperm accumulation in the ampullae and cauda epididymides of bulls. *Anim Reprod Sci* 102: 238–246.

185 Love, C.C., Riera, F.L., Oristaglio, R.M. et al. (1992). Sperm occluded (plugged) ampullae in the stallion. *Proc Soc Theriogenol*: 117–127.

186 Madrid, N., Ott, R.S., Rao Veeramachaneni, D.N. et al. (1988). Scrotal circumference, seminal characteristics, and testicular lesions of yearling Angus bulls. *Am J Vet Res* 49: 579–585.

187 Cole, P.H. (1999). Associations among age, scrotal circumference, and proportion of morphologically normal spermatozoa in young beef bulls during an initial breeding soundness examination. *J Am Vet Med Assoc* 214: 1664–1667.

188 Johnson, K.R., Dewey, C.E., Bobo, J.K. et al. (1998). Prevalence of morphologic defects in spermatozoa from beef bulls. *J Am Vet Med Assoc* 213: 1468–1471.

189 Takeishi, M., Toyoshima, T., Ryo, T. et al. (1975). Studies on reproduction in the dog. VI: sexual maturity in male beagles. *Bull Coll Agric Vet Med Nihon Univ* 32: 213–223.

190 Naden, J., Amann, R.P., and Squires, E.L. (1990). Testicular growth, hormone concentrations, seminal characteristics and sexual behavior in stallions. *J Reprod Fertil* 88: 167–176.

191 George, L.W., Duncan, J.R., and Carmichael, L.E. (1979). Semen examination in dogs with canine brucellosis. *Am J Vet Res* 40: 1589–1595.

192 Câmara, L.B.R.M., Maiorino, F.C., Silva Júnior, V.A. et al. (2014). Canine testicular disorders and their influence on sperm morphology. *Anim Reprod* 11: 32–36.

193 Wildt, D.E., Baas, E.J., Chakraborty, P.K. et al. (1982). Influence of inbreeding on reproductive performance, ejaculate quality and testicular volume in the dog. *Theriogenology* 17: 445–452.

194 Marti, C. (2004). Inbreeding and semen quality. Technical Conference on Artificial Insemination and Reproduction 20: 85–91.

195 van Eldik, P., van der Waaij, E.H., Ducro, B. et al. (2006). Possible negative effects of inbreeding on semen quality in Shetland pony stallions. *Theriogenology* 65: 1159–1170.

196 Chenoweth, P.J. (2005). Genetic sperm defects. *Theriogenology* 64: 457–468.

197 Johnson, W.H. (1997). The importance to bull fertility of morphologically abnormal sperm. *Vet Clin North Am Food Anim Pract* 13: 255–270.

198 Setchell, B.P. (1998). The Parkes lecture. Heat and the testis. *J Reprod Fertil* 114: 179–194.

199 Skinner, J.D. and Louw, G.N. (1966). Heat stress and spermatogenesis in *Bos indicus* and *Bos taurus* cattle. *J Appl Physiol* 21: 1784–1790.

200 Freidman, R., Scott, M., Heath, S.E. et al. (1991). The effects of increase testicular temperature on spermatogenesis in the stallion. *J Reprod Fertil Suppl* 44: 127–134.

201 Vogler, C.J., Bame, J.H., DeJarnette, J.M. et al. (1993). Effects of elevated testicular temperature on morphology characteristics of ejaculated spermatozoa in the bovine. *Theriogenology* 40: 1207–1219.

202 Barth, A.D. and Bowman, P.A. (1994). The sequential appearance of sperm abnormalities after scrotal insulation or dexamethasone treatment in bulls. *Can Vet J* 35: 93–102.

203 Karabinus, D.S., Vogler, C.J., Saacke, R.G., and Evenson, D.P. (1997). Chromatin structural changes in sperm after scrotal insulation of Holstein bulls. *J Androl* 18: 549–555.

204 Love, C.C. and Kenney, R.M. (1999). Scrotal heat stress induces altered sperm chromatin structure associated with a decrease in protamine disulfide bonding in the stallion. *Biol Reprod* 60: 615–620.

205 Zhu, B. and Setchell, B.P. (2004). Effects of paternal heat stress on the in vivo development of preimplantation embryos in the mouse. *Reprod Nutr Dev* 44: 617–629.

206 Zhu, B., Walker, S.K., Oakey, H. et al. (2004). Effect of paternal heat stress on the development in vitro of preimplantation embryos in the mouse. *Andrologia* 36: 384–394.

207 Larsen, R.E. and Chenoweth, P.J. (1990). Diadem/crater defects in spermatozoa from two related Angus bulls. *Mol Reprod Dev* 25: 87–96.

208 Barth, A.D. (1986). The knobbed acrosome defect in beef bulls. *Can Vet J* 27: 379–384.

209 Plummer, J.M., Watson, P.F., and Allen, W.E. (1987). A spermatozoal midpiece abnormality associated with infertility in a Llasa Apso dog. *J Small Anim Pract* 28: 743–751.

210 Veeramachaneni, D.N.R., Moeller, C.L., and Sawyer, H.R. (2006). Sperm morphology in stallions: ultrastructure as a functional and diagnostic tool. *Vet Clin North Am Equine Pract* 22: 683–692.

211 Lenz, R.W., Kjelland, M.E., VonderHaar, K. et al. (2011). A comparison of bovine seminal quality assessments using different viewing chambers with a computer-assisted semen analyzer. *J Anim Sci* 89: 383–388.

212 Rijsselaere, T., Van Soom, A., Maes, D., and de Kruif, A. (2003). Effect of technical settings on canine semen

motility parameters measured by the Hamilton-Thorne analyzer. *Theriogenology* 60: 1553–1568.

213 Smith, S.C. and England, G.C. (2001). Effect of technical settings and semen handling upon motility characteristics of dog spermatozoa measured using computer-aided sperm analysis. *J Reprod Fertil Suppl* 57: 151–159.

214 Komori, K., Tsujimura, A., Ishijima, S. et al. (2006). Comparative study of sperm motility analysis system and conventional microscopic semen analysis. *Reprod Med Biol* 5: 195–200.

215 Farrell, P.B., Presicce, G.A., Brockett, C.C., and Foote, R.H. (1998). Quantification of bull sperm characteristics measured by computer-assisted sperm analysis (CASA) and the relationship to fertility. *Theriogenology* 49: 871–879.

216 Jeyendran, R.S., Van der Ven, H.H., Perez-Pelaez, M. et al. (1984). Development of an assay to assess the functional integrity of the human sperm membrane and its relationship to other semen characteristics. *J Reprod Fertil* 70: 219–228.

217 Kumi-Diaka, J. (1993). Subjecting canine semen to the hypo-osmotic test. *Theriogenology* 39: 1279–1289.

218 Nie, G.J. and Wenzel, J.G.W. (2001). Adaptation of the hypoosmotic swelling test to assess functional integrity of stallion spermatozoal plasma membranes. *Theriogenology* 55: 1005–1018.

219 Neild, D., Chaves, G., Flores, M. et al. (1999). Hypoosmotic test in equine spermatozoa. *Theriogenology* 51: 721–727.

220 Correa, J.R. and Zavos, P.M. (1994). The hypoosmotic swelling test: its employment as an assay to evaluate the functional integrity of the frozen-thawed bovine sperm membrane. *Theriogenology* 42: 351–360.

221 Hossain, M.S., Johannisson, A., Wallgren, M. et al. (2011). Flow cytometry for the assessment of animal sperm integrity and functionality: state of the art. *Asian J Androl* 13: 406–419.

222 Niżański, W., Partyka, A., and Rijsselaere, T. (2012). Use of fluorescent stainings and flow cytometry for canine semen assessment. *Reprod Domest Anim* 47 (6): 215–221.

223 Peña, F.J., Ortega Ferrusola, C., and Martín Muñoz, P. (2016). New flow cytometry approaches in equine andrology. *Theriogenology* 86: 366–372.

224 Love, C.C. (2005). The sperm chromatin structure assay: a review of clinical applications. *Anim Reprod Sci* 89: 39–45.

225 Evenson, D.P. (2016). The sperm chromatin structure assay (SCSA®) and other sperm DNA fragmentation tests for evaluation of sperm nuclear DNA integrity as related to fertility. *Anim Reprod Sci* 169: 56–75.

226 Kenney, R.M., Evenson, D.P., Garcia, M.C., and Love, C.C. (1995). Relationships between sperm chromatin structure, motility, and morphology of ejaculated sperm, and seasonal pregnancy rate. *Biol Reprod Monogr* 1: 647–653.

227 Ballachey, B.E., Hohenboken, W.D., and Evenson, D.P. (1987). Heterogeneity of sperm nuclear chromatin structure and its relationship to bull fertility. *Biol Reprod* 36: 915–925.

228 Ballachey, B.E., Evenson, D.P., and Saacke, R.G. (1988). The sperm chromatin structure assay relationship with alternate tests of semen quality and heterospermic performance in bulls. *J Androl* 9: 109–115.

229 Hidalgo, M., Rodríguez, I., Dorado, J., and Soler, C. (2008). Morphometric classification of Spanish thoroughbred stallion sperm heads. *Anim Reprod Sci* 103: 374–378.

230 Katz, D.F., Overstreet, J.W., Samuels, S.J. et al. (1986). Morphometric analysis of spermatozoa in the assessment of human male fertility. *J Androl* 7: 203–210.

231 Sancho, M., Pérez-Sánchez, F., Tablado, L. et al. (1998). Computer assisted morphometric analysis of ram sperm heads: evaluation of different fixative techniques. *Theriogenology* 50: 27–37.

232 Ball, B.A. and Mohammed, H.O. (1995). Morphometry of stallion spermatozoa by computer-assisted image analysis. *Theriogenology* 44: 367–377.

233 Banaszewska, D., Czubaszek, M., Walczak-Jędrzejowska, R., and Andraszek, K. (2015). Morphometric dimensions of the stallion sperm head depending on the staining method used. *Bull Vet Inst Pulawy* 59: 263–270.

234 Rijsselaere, T., Van Soom, A., Hoflack, G. et al. (2004). Automated sperm morphometry and morphology analysis of canine semen by the Hamilton-Thorne analyser. *Theriogenology* 63: 1292–1306.

235 Davis, R.O. and Gravance, C.G. (1993). Standardization of specimen preparation, staining, and sampling methods improves automated sperm-head morphometry analysis. *Fertil Steril* 59: 412–417.

236 Rubio-Guillén, J., González, D., Garde, J.J. et al. (2007). Effects of cryopreservation on bull spermatozoa distribution in morphometrically distinct subpopulations. *Reprod Domest Anim* 42: 354–357.

237 Núñez-Martinez, I., Moran, J.M., and Peña, F.J. (2007). Identification of sperm morphometric subpopulations in the canine ejaculate: do they reflect different subpopulations in sperm chromatin integrity? *Zygote* 15: 257–266.

238 Ostermeier, G.C., Sargeant, G.A., Yandell, B.S. et al. (2001). Relationship of bull fertility to sperm nuclear shape. *J Androl* 22: 595–603.

239 Casey, P.J., Gravance, C.G., Davis, R.O. et al. (1997). Morphometric differences in sperm head dimensions of fertile and subfertile stallions. *Theriogenology* 47: 575–582.

240 Maroto-Morales, A., Ramón, M., García-Álvarez, O. et al. (2015). Sperm head phenotype and male fertility in ram semen. *Theriogenology* 84: 1536–1541.

241 Ericsson, S.A., Garner, D.L., Thomas, C.A. et al. (1993). Interrelationships among fluorometric analyses of spermatozoal function, classical semen quality parameters and the fertility of frozen-thawed bovine spermatozoa. *Theriogenology* 39: 1009–1024.

242 Sellem, E., Broekhuijse, M.L.W.J., Chevrier, L. et al. (2015). Use of combinations of in vitro quality assessments to predict fertility of bovine semen. *Theriogenology* 84: 1447–1454.

42

Vaginal Cytology in the Bitch and Queen

Margaret V. Root Kustritz

Introduction

Vaginal cytology is an underused, simple diagnostic tool that, when coupled with a history, physical examination, and other appropriate diagnostics, enhances one's ability to diagnose and treat diseases of the genitourinary tract in female dogs and, to a lesser extent, female cats. Vaginal cytology allows one to assess character of discharge and to assess whether or not the bitch or queen is under the influence of estrogen. Vaginal cytology does not allow one to localize source of discharge, diagnose brucellosis or other infectious diseases, or determine date of ovulation during estrus. Vulvar discharge may be physiologic or pathologic; may arise from the urinary tract, uterus, or vagina; and may be a manifestation of a systemic condition, such as coagulopathy.[1] Details of diagnosis and treatments are not described; the reader is referred to specific theriogenology texts or sites for that information.[2,3]

Collection

In female dogs, collection of vaginal epithelial cells, inflammatory cells, and any discharge in the vaginal vault is done using a non-sterile cotton-tipped applicator, with or without some sort of speculum. While specula are designed for use in bitches, they are rarely used as they are not well tolerated by all bitches. Some bitches will tolerate a large otoscope cone, through which a cotton-tipped applicator can be passed. Flushing of saline into the vaginal vault with collection of fluid containing cells from the vagina also has been described.[4] To collect a sample using solely a cotton-tipped applicator, moisten the applicator with sterile saline or tap water. Introduce it at the dorsal commissure of the vulva and advance it upward at a 45-degree angle for about half of its length. Roll it and pull it straight out. Studies disagree regarding best site from which to collect a sample. Care should be taken not to sample the clitoral fossa, which always contains cornified cells, potentially confusing interpretation.[4,5]

Roll the swab several times against a clean glass slide and allow it to air dry. Care should be taken not to rub the swab against the slide, so as not to break the cells. The slide can be stained with new methylene blue, and Romanowsky stains, like Diff-Quik (Baxter Healthcare Corporation, Miami FL), often are used. Use of Papanicolaou stain is described but rarely used in clinical settings.[6] Cells are examined under 100× to 1000× magnification. If viewed under oil immersion, a cover slip should be applied first if slides are to be saved, as prolonged exposure to immersion oil will distort epithelial cells over time.[4]

Cats have a short vagina with a significant narrowing just cranial to the vulvar lips. To collect a cytology specimen, a moistened, non-sterile cotton-tipped applicator is introduced straight through the vulvar lips, rolled, and pulled straight out. Slides are prepared as in the dog.

Cell Types

Four types of vaginal epithelial cells commonly are identified. Parabasal cells lie against the basement membrane. They are small and round with a prominent nucleus and low cytoplasm/nucleus ratio. This cell type is always present in the canine vagina. Intermediate cells, when present, are superficial to the parabasal cells. Their morphology is similar to that of the parabasal cells, but they are slightly larger overall and have a higher cytoplasm/nucleus ratio. These two cell types commonly are referred to as non-cornified cells. Superficial cells, also sometimes called superficial intermediate cells, form when parabasal cells are induced to divide by elevation in serum estrogen concentration.[7] Superficial cells are large and often irregular in shape, with a high cytoplasm/nucleus ratio. The nucleus of some superficial cells will fail to take up stain. These large, irregular cells with no

Veterinary Cytology, First Edition. Edited by Leslie C. Sharkey, M. Judith Radin, and Davis Seelig.

visible nucleus are anuclear squame cells. Superficial cells and anuclear squames are commonly referred to as cornified cells. Other cell types common on vaginal cytology specimens are polymorphonuclear cells (PMNs or neutrophils), red blood cells (RBCs), and bacteria.

Physiologic Conditions Managed or Diagnosed by Cytology

Breeding Management

Ascertaining the stage of the estrous cycle using vaginal cytology is somewhat subjective. Accuracy is increased by evaluation of the cytology specimen relative to history, physical examination findings, and gross assessment of vulvar discharge and by practice.[8]

Proestrus is the first stage of the canine estrous cycle. This is the follicular stage of the cycle. Estrogen concentrations rise during proestrus and peak at the end of this stage. Serum progesterone and luteinizing hormone (LH) concentrations are low. Vulvar discharge ranging in character from serous to serosanguinous is present. On vaginal cytology, RBCs can be present throughout proestrus. PMNs are present early in proestrus but disappear as estrus nears and the vaginal epithelium thickens.[9] Lymphocytes may rarely be seen. Early in proestrus, the vaginal epithelial cell population is heterogeneous, with great variation in size and shape of cells and their nuclei (Figure 42.1). The vaginal epithelial cell population gradually changes from completely non-cornified to completely cornified over this stage of the cycle (Figure 42.2).[10] On average, cornification is complete about two days before estrogen peaks and about four days before estrus begins.[11]

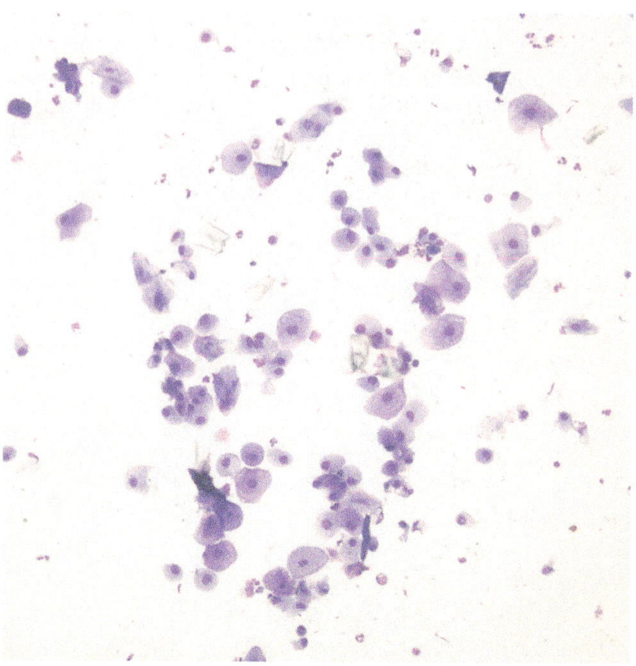

Figure 42.1 Early proestrous canine vaginal cytology (Wright's stain, 400×).

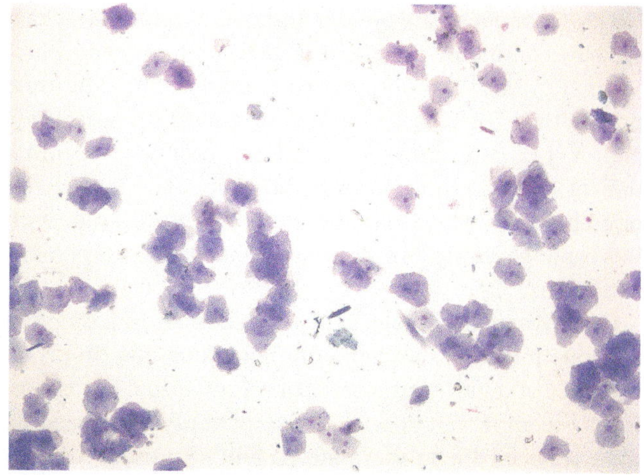

Figure 42.2 Mid to late proestrous canine vaginal cytology (Wright's stain, 400×).

Estrogen concentrations fall at the beginning of estrus. Decreasing estrogen, along with a preovulatory rise in progesterone, is necessary for the appearance of breeding behaviors in the bitch and presumably elicits the LH surge. In the average bitch, a surge of LH is released from the pituitary on or about the first day of estrus and causes ovulation of a primary oocyte two days later. After ovulation, corpora lutea (CLs) form, and progesterone production begins. During estrus, or standing heat, the vulvar discharge can become straw colored but can range from serous to serosanguinous in a normal bitch. The vaginal epithelial cell population is completely cornified throughout estrus, with greater than 50% of the cells anuclear squames (Figure 42.3).

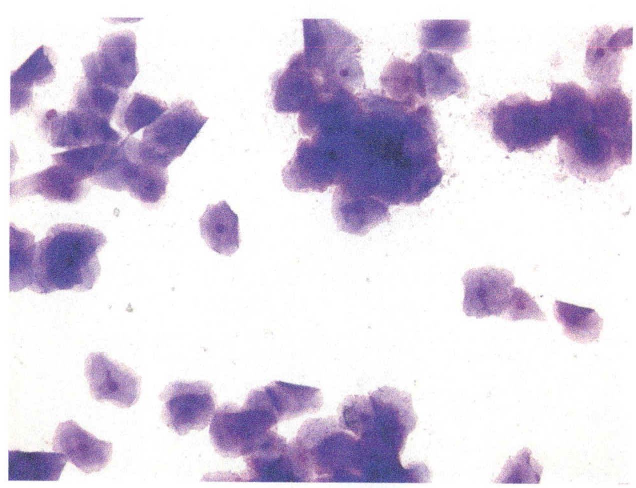

Figure 42.3 Estrous vaginal canine cytology (Wright's stain, 400×).

No PMNs or debris are present. Intra- and extracellular bacteria are commonly present. RBCs may or may not be seen.[4] Vaginal cytology cannot be used to predict ovulation time prospectively; that is best done using serum progesterone and/or LH concentrations.[12,13] Retrospective determination of ovulation date may be possible, as vaginal cytology changes abruptly as the bitch enters diestrus, with this change fairly consistently occurring six days after ovulation.[14]

Use of vaginal cytology to identify spermatozoa is not an accurate indicator of whether or not copulation occurred. Presence of intact spermatozoa or spermatozoal heads confirms breeding, but absence does not verify that breeding did not occur. Intact spermatozoa will be present for only hours after breeding.[15] Spermatozoal heads were identified in about 65% of vaginal cytology specimens collected from bitches one day after breeding.[16]

Diestrus is the luteal phase of the cycle and occurs in all bitches, regardless of breeding or pregnancy status. Small amounts of mucoid vulvar discharge can be present. On the first day of diestrus, the vaginal epithelial cell population abruptly shifts to complete non-cornification. Numerous PMNs can be present, and metestrum cells (non-cornified cells containing leukocytes) and/or foam cells (non-cornified cells containing vacuoles) can be present early in diestrus (Figure 42.4). By mid-diestrus, cytology is characterized by the presence of non-cornified vaginal epithelial cells, occasional PMNs, and some mucoid debris.[10]

Anestrus is a period of reproductive quiescence. Vaginal cytology reveals only a scant number of single cells or small groups of cells, all of which are non-cornified (Figure 42.5).[10]

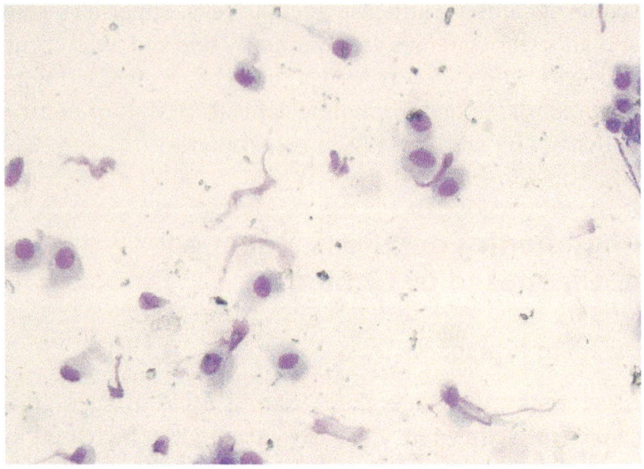

Figure 42.5 Anestrus vaginal canine cytology (Wright's stain, 400×).

Vaginal cytology also can be used to demonstrate stage of the estrous cycle in queens.[17–19] Changes are similar to those described for the bitch. Proestrus is rarely identified cytologically in queens as the first indications of estrus are behavioral and usually are not demonstrated by the queen until she is in cytologic estrus. In estrus, queens are less likely than bitches to demonstrate complete cornification of the vaginal epithelial cells and exfoliate fewer cells. Examples of predominantly cornified and predominantly non-cornified vaginal cytology from queens are described below (see Ovarian Remnant Syndrome Figures 42.6 and 42.7). Some queens do not show behavioral estrus and serial vaginal cytology can help identify estrus. In one study, cats with minimal behavioral signs of estrus were successfully bred using cytology alone.[20]

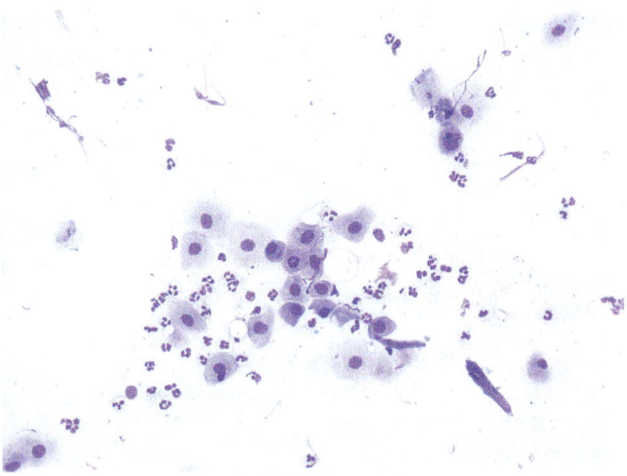

Figure 42.4 Diestrous vaginal canine cytology (Wright's stain, 400×).

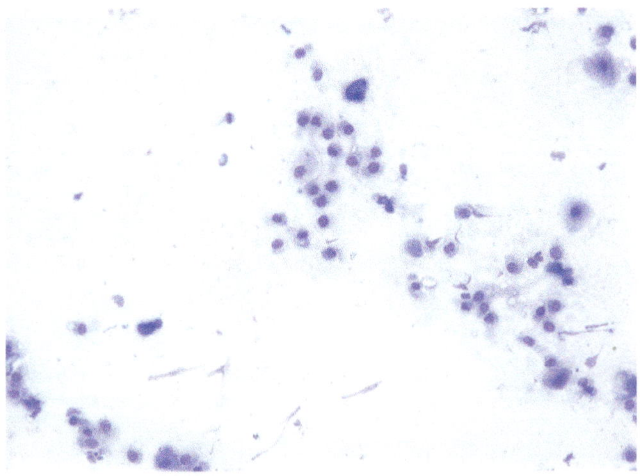

Figure 42.6 Non-cornified feline vaginal cytology (Wright's stain, 400×).

Postpartum

Lochia is the normal postpartum discharge of the bitch. It may be present for up to three weeks after parturition. The discharge varies in color from green to black to red and should decrease in volume over time.[21] It should not be frankly hemorrhagic nor be foul smelling. All vaginal epithelial cells should be non-cornified, and the number of PMNs and bacteria present should not be excessive.

Queens are reported to have a serosanguinous discharge for two to six days. The amount produced is scant, and the queen removes it through normal grooming. RBCs are reported to constitute 75–80% and PMNs 15–20% of cells postpartum, and both diminish to 0 and 1%, respectively, over 20–25 days.[22,23] One study found superficial cells increase to 70% after day 5 postpartum, suggesting an influence of estrogen.[23]

Pathologic Conditions Associated with Cornified Vaginal Epithelium

Ovarian Remnant Syndrome

Ovarian remnant syndrome is the appearance of estrous behavior in previously ovariectomized dogs and cats. The syndrome is more common in cats than in dogs. In cats, vaginal cytology specimens should be collected when the owner perceives the cat to be showing signs of behavioral estrus, including lordosis and repetitive vocalization. Cornified vaginal epithelial cells indicate elevated serum concentrations of estrogen and likely the presence of functional ovarian follicular tissue (Figures 42.6 and 42.7).[24–26] Ovarian remnant tissue can be present at one or both ovarian pedicles or, rarely, elsewhere in the abdomen. Identification of remnants during abdominal exploratory is facilitated by the presence of follicles or CLs, the latter induced to form from follicular tissue by administration of gonadotropin-releasing hormone (GnRH; 25 μg/cat IM).[27]

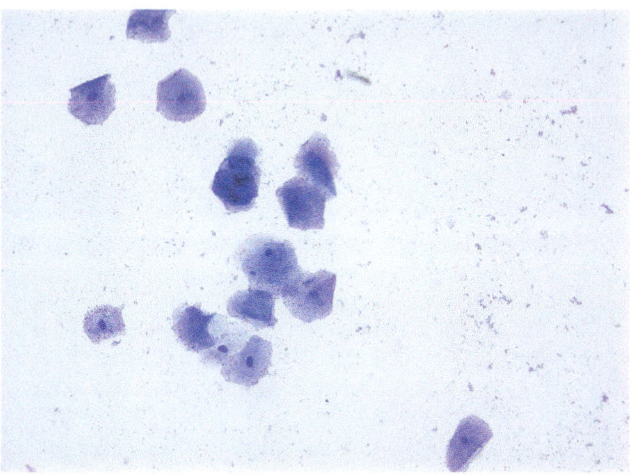

Figure 42.7 Cornified feline vaginal cytology (Wright's stain, 400×).

Ovarian Follicular Cysts

This is an uncommon disorder in bitches and queens. It is most common in young bitches and middle-aged to older queens. Combined length of proestrus and estrus in affected bitches is greater than six weeks, with typical vulvar discharge and behavioral changes. In queens, it may be difficult to identify prolonged signs of estrus as these changes are behavioral and not physical. Vaginal epithelial cells are completely cornified and may appear ragged. PMNs are not present. Bacteria may be visible, adhered to the surface of the epithelial cells.[15] Treatment is by ovariohysterectomy or induction of ovulation (GnRH; 50 μg/dog IM or 25 μg/cat IM).[27,28]

Ovarian Neoplasia

Ovarian tumors are uncommon in bitches and extremely uncommon in queens, most often occurring in older animals (see Chapter 40).[27,28] Granulosa cell tumor is most commonly described, with changes referable to hormone production by the tumor. Combined length of proestrus and estrus in affected bitches is greater than six weeks, with typical vulvar discharge and behavioral changes. In queens, it may be difficult to identify prolonged signs of estrus as these changes are behavioral. Vaginal epithelial cells are completely cornified and may appear ragged. PMNs are not present. Bacteria may be visible, adhered to the surface of the epithelial cells.[28] The ovary usually is grossly enlarged, may be palpable per abdomen, and is visible using ultrasound.

Pathologic Conditions Associated with Non-cornified Vaginal Epithelium and Hemorrhagic Vulvar Discharge

Subinvolution of Placental Sites

Subinvolution of placental sites (SIPS) is an uncommon disorder in dogs. SIPS is most common in young bitches after whelping their first litter. The bitch appears normal, but postpartum discharge continues beyond three weeks. This is a noninflammatory discharge. RBCs usually are present. All vaginal epithelial cells are non-cornified. Trophoblastic cells with abundant, vacuolated cytoplasm can be shed from the endometrium.[29–32] Diagnosis requires collection of samples from the uterus, and so is more commonly done by excluding metritis and brucellosis. Most cases are self-resolving.

Neoplasia of the Genital Tract

Neoplasia of the genital tract is uncommon (see Chapter 43). Masses may or may not be visible. Perineal swelling can occur. The discharge usually is hemorrhagic with no foul odor. Many RBCs and occasional PMNs are present, and vaginal epithelial cells are non-cornified.[17] Finding of neoplastic cells on vaginal smears is uncommon. Tumors that have been observed with vaginal cytology in dogs include transmissible venereal tumor, transitional cell carcinoma, and squamous cell carcinoma.[31,33–35] Leiomyoma is the most common genital tumor and occurs in aged intact or spayed bitches with finding of atypical mesenchymal cells rarely reported.[36]

Coagulopathies and Blood Parasites

Vulvar discharge associated with coagulopathy may occur in intact or spayed bitches of any age. Reported causes include hereditary (von Willebrand's disease, Factor VII deficiency) and acquired (anticoagulant rodenticide toxicity) coagulopathies.[37–39] Babesiosis and ehrlichiosis are reported to be associated with sanguinous vulvar discharge.[1] Dogs present with a frankly hemorrhagic discharge that often waxes and wanes in volume. The microscopic appearance is of peripheral blood. All vaginal epithelial cells are non-cornified.

Pathologic Conditions Associated with Non-cornified Vaginal Epithelium and Mucoid or Mucopurulent Vulvar Discharge

Metritis

Metritis occurs in postpartum bitches and, rarely, in postpartum queens. Often there is a history of dystocia or retained fetuses or placentas. The vulvar discharge is purulent and foul smelling. This is an inflammatory discharge, with full fields of degenerate PMNs. All vaginal epithelial cells are non-cornified.[32] Diagnosis is straightforward based on the history of recent parturition and presence of purulent vulvar discharge.

Pyometra

Pyometra occurs during or after diestrus and is most common in aged, nulliparous bitches and queens. Animals with closed-cervix pyometra do not have vulvar discharge. Bitches and queens with open-cervix pyometra may or may not show signs of systemic disease (anorexia, polyuria, and polydipsia). The vulvar discharge is purulent and foul smelling, often with the appearance of cream of tomato soup. This is an inflammatory discharge, with full fields of degenerate PMNs. All vaginal epithelial cells are non-cornified.[37] Most bitches and queens also will have an elevated total white blood cell count with a left shift. Diagnosis is by demonstration of uterine enlargement due to accumulation of intrauterine fluid.

Vaginitis

This can occur in prepubertal bitches ("puppy" vaginitis) or in spayed, adult bitches. Puppies rarely show evidence of vaginitis, other than sticky discharge gluing together their vulvar lips. Adult dogs may show evidence of vulvar licking and perivulvar dermatitis. The occasional bitch will have traumatized her perivulvar region. The discharge may be scant, mucoid, and sticky (puppy vaginitis), or can vary from mucoid to purulent with tremendous variation in amount present (adult-onset vaginitis). The discharge rarely is bloody. Cytology varies from mucoid (lacking neutrophils) to purulent.[40] Nuclear streaming and proteinaceous debris often are present. Lymphocytes and macrophages can be seen with chronic vaginitis.[31] Vaginal epithelial cells all are non-cornified (Figure 42.8). If cornified cells are present, especially if the discharge appears bloody, ovarian remnant syndrome should be considered.[41]

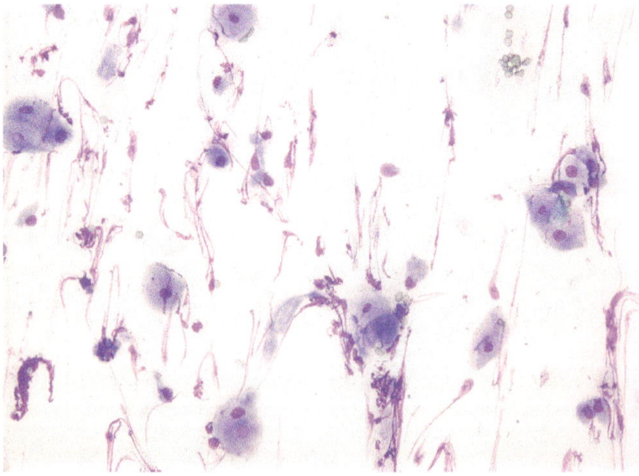

Figure 42.8 Vaginal cytology from a dog with vaginitis (Wright's stain, 400×).

Puppy vaginitis is diagnosed on inspection and usually resolves spontaneously. Adult-onset vaginitis is diagnosed by vaginoscopy and investigation for underlying urinary tract disease or vaginal anatomic anomalies.

Brucellosis

Canine brucellosis usually presents as late-term abortion. Bitches also may present with persistent vulvar discharge that varies from mucopurulent to purulent and may be blood-tinged. All vaginal epithelial cells are non-cornified.[42] Brucellosis is reportable and has zoonotic potential. The rapid slide agglutination test (RSAT) is a good screening test for suspect cases. Animals that test negative are free of infection, provided testing is performed 8–12 weeks after exposure and the animal has not received antibiotics. Animals positive with the RSAT should have the result verified by agarose gel immunodiffusion (AGID) or PCR testing.

References

1 Root Kustritz, M.V. (2006). Collection of tissue and culture samples from the canine reproductive tract. *Theriogenology* 66: 567–574.

2 Root Kustritz, M.V. (2010). Clinical Canine and Feline Reproduction: Evidence-Based Answers. Ames, IA: Wiley-Blackwell.

3 Root Kustritz, M.V. (2016). Books and articles. https://sites.google.com/a/umn.edu/margaret-v-peggy-root-kustritz/home (accessed 9 May 2016).

4 Johnston, S.D., Root Kustritz, M.V., and Olson, P.N. (eds.) (2001). Vaginal cytology. In: Canine and Feline Theriogenology, 32–40. New York, NY: W.B. Saunders.

5 Hiemstra, M., Schaefers-Okkens, A.C., Teske, E., and Kooistra, H.S. (2001). The reliability of vaginal cytology in determining the optimal mating time in the bitch. *Tijdschr Diergeneeskd* 126: 685–689.

6 Perez, C.C., Rodriguez, I., Dorado, J., and Hidalgo, M. (2005). Use of ultrafast Papanicolaou stain for exfoliative vaginal cytology in bitches. *Vet Rec* 156: 648–650.

7 Bell, E.T., Christie, D.W., and Younglai, E.V. (1971). Plasma oestrogen levels during the canine oestrous cycle. *J Endocrinol* 51: 225–226.

8 Moxon, R., Copley, D., and England, G.C.W. (2010). Quality assurance of canine vaginal cytology: a preliminary study. *Theriogenology* 74: 479–485.

9 Groppetti, D., Pecile, A., Barbero, C., and Martino, P.A. (2012). Vaginal bacterial flora and cytology in proestrous bitches: role on fertility. *Theriogenology* 77: 1549–1556.

10 Groppetti, D., Aralla, M., Bronzo, V. et al. (2015). Periovulatory time in the bitch; what's new to know? Comparison between ovarian histology and clinical features. *Anim Reprod Sci* 152: 108–116.

11 Concannon, P.W. (2011). Reproductive cycles of the domestic bitch. *Anim Reprod Sci* 124: 200–210.

12 Holst, P.A. and Phemister, R.D. (1975). Temporal sequence of events in the estrous cycle of the bitch. *Am J Vet Res* 36: 705–706.

13 Bouchard, G.F., Solorzano, N., Concannon, P.W. et al. (1991). Determination of ovulation time in bitches based on teasing, vaginal cytology, and ELISA for progesterone. *Theriogenology* 35: 603–611.

14 Holst, P.A. and Phemister, R.D. (1974). Onset of diestrus in the beagle bitch: definition and significance. *Am J Vet Res* 35: 401–406.

15 Whitacre, M.D., Yates, D.J., VanCamp, S.D., and Meuten, D.J. (1992). Detection of intravaginal spermatozoa after natural mating in the bitch. *Vet Clin Pathol* 21: 85–87.

16 Olson, P.N. (1989). Exfoliative cytology of the canine reproductive tract. *Proceedings of the Annual Meeting of the Society for Theriogenology*, Coeur d'Alene, ID (29–30 September 1989).

17 Mills, J.N., Valli, V.E., and Lumsden, J.H. (1979). Cyclical changes of vaginal cytology in the cat. *Can Vet J* 20: 95–101.

18 Kanca, H., Karakas, K., Dalgic, M.A. et al. (2014). Vaginal cytology after induction of ovulation in the queen: comparison of postoestrus and dioestrus. *Aus Vet J* 92: 65–70.

19 Shille, V.M., Lundström, K.E., and Stabenfeldt, G.H. (1979). Follicular function in the domestic cat as determined by estradiol-17 beta concentrations in plasma: relation to estrous behavior and cornification of exfoliated vaginal epithelium. *Biol Reprod* 21: 953–963.

20 Root, M.V., Johnston, S.D., and Olson, P.N. (1995). Estrous length, pregnancy rate, gestation and parturition lengths, litter size, and pre-weaning mortality in the domestic cat. *J Am Anim Hosp Assoc* 31: 429–433.

21 Johnston, S.D., Root Kustritz, M.V., and Olson, P.N. (eds.) (2001). Canine parturition: eutocia and dystocia. In: Canine and Feline Theriogenology, 105–128. New York, NY: W.B. Saunders.

22 Blanco, P.G., Rodríguez, R., Batista, P.R. et al. (2015). Bidimensional and Doppler ultrasonographic evaluation of postpartum uterine involution in the queen. *Theriogenology* 84: 82–85.

23 Sendag, S., Alan, M., Eski, F. et al. (2016). Postpartum uterus involution observed by real-time ultrasound scanning and vaginal cytology in Van cats. *J Feline Med Surg* 18: 954–958.

24 Miller, D.M. (1995). Ovarian remnant syndrome in dogs and cats: 46 cases (1988–1992). *J Vet Diagn Invest* 7: 572–574.

25 Wallace, M.S. (1991). The ovarian remnant syndrome in the bitch and queen. *Vet Clin North Am Small Anim Pract* 21: 501–507.

26 Demirel, M.A. and Acar, D.B. (2012). Ovarian remnant syndrome and uterine stump pyometra in three queens. *J Feline Med Surg* 14: 913–918.

27 Johnston, S.D., Root Kustritz, M.V., and Olson, P.N. (eds.) (2001). Disorders of the feline ovaries. In: Canine and Feline Theriogenology, 453–462. New York, NY: W.B. Saunders.

28 Johnston, S.D., Root Kustritz, M.V., and Olson, P.N. (eds.) (2001). Disorders of the canine ovary. In: Canine and Feline Theriogenology, 193–205. New York, NY: W.B. Saunders.

29 Sontas, H.B., Stelletta, C., Milani, C. et al. (2011). Full recovery of subinvolution of placental sites in an American Staffordshire terrier bitch. *J Small Anim Pract* 52: 42–45.

30 Dickie, M.B. and Arbeiter, K. (1993). Diagnosis and therapy of the subinvolution of placental sites in the bitch. *J Reprod Fertil Suppl* 47: 471–475.

31 Olson, P.N., Thrall, M.A., Wykes, P.M. et al. (1984). Vaginal cytology. I. A useful tool for staging the canine estrous cycle. II. Its use in diagnosing canine reproductive disorders. *Compend Contin Educ Dent* 6: 288–390.

32 Orfanou, D.C., Ververidis, H.N., Boscos, C.M., and Fthenakis, G.C. (2010). Post-partum pathological conditions in the bitch-part II. *Eur J Compan Anim Pract* 20: 119–135.

33 Johnston, S.D., Root Kustritz, M.V., and Olson, P.N. (eds.) (2001). Disorders of the canine vagina, vestibule, and vulva. In: Canine and Feline Theriogenology, 225–242. New York, NY: W.B. Saunders.

34 Erünal-Maral, N., Findik, N., and Aslan, S. (2000). Use of exfoliative cytology for diagnosis of transmissible venereal tumour and controlling the recovery period in the bitch. *Dtsch Tierarztl Wochenschr* 107: 175–180.

35 Magne, M.L., Hoopes, P.J., Kainer, R.A. et al. (1985). Urinary tract carcinomas involving the canine vagina and vestibule. *J Am Anim Hosp Assoc* 216: 767–772.

36 Ozmen, O., Haligur, M., and Kocamuftuoglu, M. (2008). Clinocopathologic and immunohistochemical findings of multiple genital leiomyomas and mammary adenocarcinomas in a bitch. *Reprod Domest Anim* 43: 377–381.

37 Johnston, S.D., Root Kustritz, M.V., and Olson, P.N. (eds.) (2001). Disorders of the canine uterus and uterine tubes (oviducts). In: Canine and Feline Theriogenology, 206–224. New York, NY: W.B. Saunders.

38 Hamilton, H., Olsen, P.N., and Jonas, L. (1985). Von Willebrand's disease manifested by hemorrhage from the reproductive tract: two case reports. *J Am Anim Hosp Assoc* 21: 637–641.

39 Wheeler, S.L., Weingand, K.W., Thrall, M.A. et al. (1984). Persistent uterine and vaginal hemorrhage in a beagle with factor VII deficiency. *J Am Vet Med Assoc* 185: 447–448.

40 Root Kustritz, M.V. (2008). Vaginitis in dogs: a simple approach to a complex condition. *Vet Med* 103: 562–567.

41 Johnson, C.A. (1991). Diagnosis and treatment of chronic vaginitis in the bitch. *Vet Clin North Am Small Anim Pract* 21: 523–531.

42 Root Kustritz, M.V. (2005). Pregnancy diagnosis and abnormalities of pregnancy in the dog. *Theriogenology* 64: 755–765.

43

Uterine Cytology

Paula M. Krimer and Doris M. Miller

Introduction

Uterine cytology is most commonly used as part of a routine reproductive health examination, breeding soundness examination, or in cases of infertility. The endometrium is evaluated for evidence of infection on cytology, while histological examination is necessary for grading that includes degenerative changes such as fibrosis.

Sample Collection

Cytology techniques for evaluating the endometrium include impression smears from endometrial biopsies, brushings, swabs, and transcervical uterine lavage. The choice of technique depends on circumstance, species, and practical considerations based on environment, i.e. clinical or a field setting. In cattle, lavage is more commonly performed, while swabs are more common in horses, dogs, and cats. All techniques are reported in camelids though lavage is preferred.[1] Aspiration is generally limited to evaluation of suspected uterine tumors. Sampling of pregnant animals is avoided.

Lavage yields large, cohesive endometrial nests and can be more representative of uterine conditions as a larger area is sampled.[2,3] Relative to swabs and brushing, more time and effort is required to produce a cytological sample, and aspiration during lavage can lead to uterine collapse and reduced cellularity.[2,4] Brushing can disrupt morphology, induce hemorrhage, and be contraindicated in bitches during diestrus because of potential inducement of cystic endometrial hyperplasia (CEH) and endometritis.[5] Swabs are most easily collected in a field setting but can cause more cellular distortion than brushing.[4,6] Regardless of collection technique, transrectal or transabdominal ultrasonography is first performed to detect intrauterine fluid which has been associated with the presence of inflammatory cells and pathogenic bacteria.[7] Ultrasonography also evaluates endometrial thickness, uterine cysts, and fibrosis.

To prevent infection and ensure accurate culture, the perineal area should be thoroughly cleaned and sterile materials used. Smaller animals, including alpacas, require vaginoscopy to accurately introduce swabs, pipettes, or catheters through the cervix.[1] Double-guarded swabs and brushes are recommended to maintain sterility and reduce contamination by lubricants.[3,8] After a swab or brush sheath is introduced into uterus, the sampling end is pushed forward and rolled against the uterine walls for approximately 15–60 seconds before retraction into the double protective sheath.[4,9–11] To avoid ultrasound gel from contaminating the sample, slides should be prepared with degloved, clean hands or given to a technician for preparation. The use of sterile slides is recommended so swabs can be placed in transport media for culture after preparation of the cytologic sample. Swabs and cytobrush samples should be gently rolled onto slides without overlap.

Lavage techniques are performed with or without expansion of the uterus with air or CO_2.[2,9] A variable volume of warmed sterile lactated Ringer's or sterile phosphate-buffered 0.9% saline (PBS) is inserted into the uterus via a sterile insemination catheter or other pipette. Reported volumes include approximately 2 mL/kg in bitches,[12] 20–250 mL (commonly 60 or 150 mL) in mares,[3,4,9] and 20 mL[13] (up to 600 mL)[14] in cows. A double-guarded lavage technique has been described in horses.[15] The uterus is gently massaged by abdominal or transrectal palpation, and fluid gently aspirated as the pipette is retracted. In dogs, 25–33% of the infused volume is recovered, 10–58% in horses, and 10–40% in cows.[3,12,13,16] Fluid is directly smeared or centrifuged for cytological examination. Centrifugation time and force is reported from 200 to 1500g for 5–15 minutes.[2–4] The supernatant is mostly discarded and the pellet resuspended in remaining fluid for slide preparation. Cytospins also can be prepared. As with all

Veterinary Cytology, First Edition. Edited by Leslie C. Sharkey, M. Judith Radin, and Davis Seelig.

low-protein fluids, rapid processing is critical to prevent cell degradation.

In horses, reported sensitivities for detecting inflammation vary from 0% in swabs to 80% for lavage, but studies vary tremendously with percentage of neutrophils considered necessary to diagnose inflammation and counting technique.[15,17–20] Brush techniques are generally preferred over swabs or lavage as they yield more endometrial cells and greater proportions of neutrophils for overall greater diagnostic quality.[6,10,15,20,21] Brushing produces fewer deformed cells than swabs but can contain more red blood cells.[6,10,21] Cytology does not always correlate with endometrial biopsies for subclinical endometritis because it does not evaluate the deeper levels of the stratum compactum and correlation is highest during estrus.[19] Anestrus smears are less cellular than diestrus or estrus, though this difference is not present in endometrial biopsies.[19] Cytobrushing samples are more cellular than those made from endometrial biopsies during estrus and diestrus, but not anestrus.[19]

In cattle, cytobrushing and lavage are commonly used and show substantial agreement.[13,22,23] Cytobrush has higher overall precision than lavage, while lavage yields higher cell counts and better sensitivity for diagnosing inflammation.[13,24] Due to delays in slide preparation and fluid handling procedures with lavage, cytobrush better preserves cellular morphology and is more precise.[13,23] Correlation between different pathologists for neutrophil percentage evaluation on smears is high with R^2 values over 0.80.[8,22,25] Inter-operator variability may be higher for cytobrush than lavage samples.[8,13,26] Agreement between neutrophil percentage or vaginal mucous evaluation and presence of bacterial pathogens is inconsistent.[25,26] Lavage may also have therapeutic benefits by reducing the proportion of neutrophils in subsequent lavages.[14] A study in dairy cows evaluated cytology tape to prepare slides from sedimented lavage fluid and found more intact cells and less blood contamination than cytobrushing.[27]

Slides are stained with rapid stains such as Diff-Quik®, or traditional Wright–Giemsa stains.[3,27] There is no consensus on methodology for slide evaluation. The two main techniques for quantifying inflammation are either a differential of 100, 200, or 300 nucleated cells at 400× magnification (40× objective) or evaluation of all nucleated cells in 10 fields at 1000× magnification.[3,8,23] In lavage samples, evaluation of neutrophils per 1000× oil immersion field (OIF) may be more sensitive than neutrophil percentage.[3,20] Epithelial cells (both intact and degenerate), neutrophils, and lymphocytes are most commonly identified, with occasional plasma cells, non-vacuolated or vacuolated macrophages, siderophages, eosinophils, and rarely mast cells seen. Number of erythrocytes is noted and used to subjectively evaluate blood contamination.

Routine aerobic bacterial culture is recommended as part of reproductive evaluation in all species. With uterine lavage, a separate fluid aliquot should be submitted in a tube without additives. Samples for culture should be kept refrigerated and immediately shipped to the laboratory.

Ultrasound-guided fine-needle aspiration can be performed for solid uterine masses and cystic structures but is not commonly used. Unless the gastrointestinal tract is inadvertently penetrated, complications are not expected unless accidentally aspirating infectious lesions.[28,29] Slides are prepared as with other fine-needle aspirates.

Normal Cytology and Histology

Histology is useful in identifying chronic infiltrative endometrial inflammation, infertility, and ability to carry a fetus to term, while cytology is more helpful to detect active inflammation.[18,30] Agreement between histology and cytology is fair for diagnosis of inflammation in horses; cytology has a sensitivity of 53–80% when histology is used as the gold standard outside anestrus.[15,18,19,31] When comparing transcervical and full-thickness biopsies in dogs, both techniques have similar sensitivity for identifying CEH, inflammation, and fibrosis.[32]

The uterine wall is composed of seven interrelated components that are considered in equine endometrial biopsy evaluations (uterine lumen, endometrial epithelial interface, superficial stroma/stratum compactum, glands, stroma, vessels, and myometrium) (Figure 43.1).[33,34] Presence of neutrophils in the stratum compactum

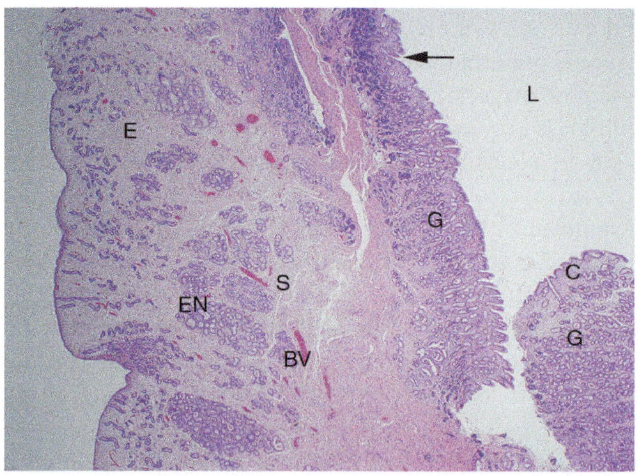

Figure 43.1 Equine endometrial biopsy (Grade IIA) without inflammation. Uterine layers include lumen (L), endometrial epithelial interface (arrow), superficial stroma/stratum compactum (C), uterine glands (G), supporting stroma (S), and blood vessels (BV). Note edema (E) and endometrial nest formation (EN) (hematoxylin & eosin, 20×.)

indicates chronic endometritis.[33,34] In horses, biopsies are scored according to a modified Kenney–Doig standard (category I, IIA, IIB, or III) based on fibrosis, glandular atrophy, inflammatory infiltrates, and lymphatic ectasia.[33–35] The technique for bovine endometrial biopsy has been described but not used routinely.[36,37] If performed appropriately, biopsy is safe and reliable for assessing postpartum uterine health.[36,37]

Two common techniques used to detect endometrial lesions in dogs are wedge biopsy taken during laparotomy or transcervical biopsy (TCB) using fiberoptics.[32,38] Wedge biopsy and laparotomy have the advantages of gross observation of the uterus and ovaries, selecting the sampling site, and a full thickness sample of uterine wall.[30,32,38] Acute and chronic endometritis can be detected by TCB if the lesions are diffuse.[32] In a comparison of transcervical and full-thickness biopsies in dogs, both techniques had similar sensitivity for identifying CEH, inflammation, and fibrosis.[32] Presently, there is no standard grading system for the canine endometrial biopsy.[39]

Endometrial changes occur with reproductive phase, and cytologic findings correlate well with histological findings.[2] A standard for cytological examination does not exist, varying on cell types evaluated, microscope magnification, and the number of fields or cells evaluated. In all species, slide background is evaluated for mucin, damaged epithelial cells, and extracellular organisms. Mucous strands are often found and may be more common during estrus. Thin palely basophilic mucous is typical, while the formation of darker strings or clumps suggests abnormalities. The proportion of debris is noted; in horses this is scored from 1 to 4 in quartiles (1 is less than 25% up to 4 for >75%).[11] With equine lavage samples, increased debris is associated with positive culture; in one study 50% of flushes with positive culture results had moderate or heavy debris on cytology, while only 26% of samples without microorganisms had debris.[20] Ultrasound gel is often present, appearing as brightly eosinophilic granular material, and can cover the slide, preventing accurate evaluation (Figure 43.2). Ruptured cells can be caused by centrifugation in lavage samples, aggressive brushing, or inappropriate slide preparation technique.[20]

Cytology samples will contain varied numbers of endometrial cells, as well as small mature lymphocytes, neutrophils, monocytes/macrophages, erythrocytes, and squamous cells. A minimum of 100 intact cells, or up to 500 cells, can be counted at 400–1000× magnification to calculate cell percentages of all nucleated cell types, including endometrial cells.[11,13,16] Alternatively the number of leukocytes can be averaged in 10 OIF, in which case the most inflamed areas of the slide should be evaluated.[8,13] A small amount of blood contamination can be present, especially with swabs and cytobrushing. Presence of intracellular and extracellular organisms should be noted.

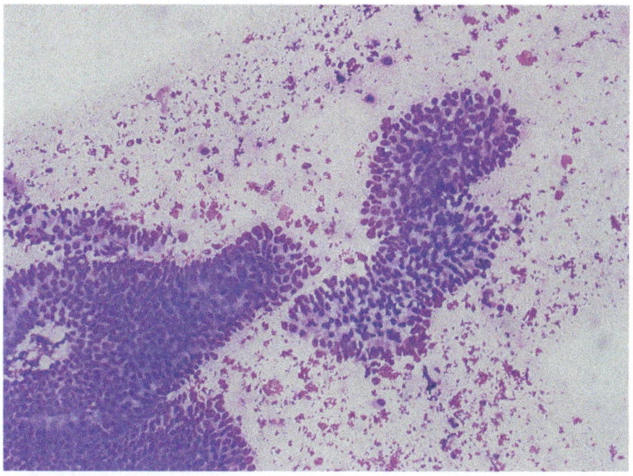

Figure 43.2 Equine endometrial swab. Large cohesive clusters of normal endometrium with palisading. Cells are cuboidal to columnar with small uniform nuclei and variable amounts of pale cytoplasm. Note abundant ultrasound gel in the background (Wright–Giemsa, 200×.)

Endometrial cells are cuboidal to columnar, varying with reproductive stage in dogs, and are sometimes ciliated in horses. They appear individually or in cohesive nests with palisading, or grapelike clusters (Figure 43.2). In dogs, epithelium is cuboidal during proestrus and estrus, growing more columnar during diestrus, with the tallest columnar shape during anestrus (Figure 43.3a–i).[2,40] Luminal and glandular epithelium cannot be readily differentiated on cytology.[40] Cytoplasm is pale with indistinct borders and infrequently contains mucin globules. In dogs, cytoplasm becomes more vacuolated in late diestrus and early anestrus (Figure 43.3f–i).[2] Nuclei are central to basilar with fine stippled, aggregated chromatin and infrequent single small round nucleolus. Degenerate endometrial cells are most common from middle/late diestrus through middle anestrus of healthy dogs and in all cases of uterine pathology, while naked nuclei are more common in proestrus and early diestrus.[2,40] Degenerate cells have pyknotic nuclei and variably vacuolated cytoplasm. With lavage, endometrial exfoliation during proestrus, early diestrus, and late anestrus is higher than in prepubertal dogs or during estrus.[2] Using computer morphometry on lavage samples in dogs, endometrial nuclear cell size is smallest during late diestrus, largest in late anestrus, and most round during estrus and early diestrus.[2] The presence of anucleate squamous vaginal epithelial cells indicates contamination or improper collection.

A normal finding in ewes is marked melanin deposits that impart a black appearance on gross examination

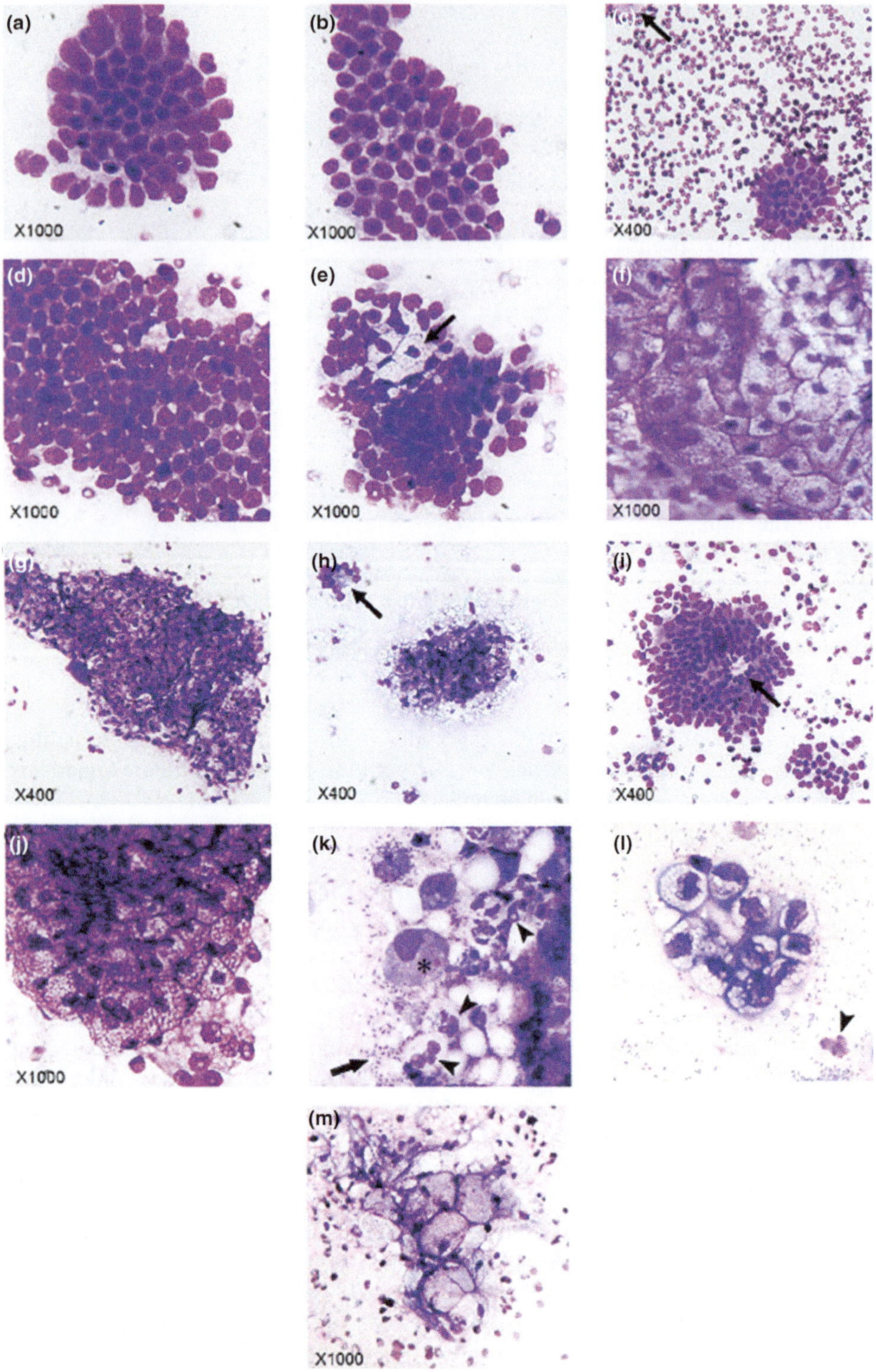

Figure 43.3 Canine uterine cytology. (a) Prepubertal bitch. A large cluster of cohesive endometrial epithelial cells with uniformly stained nuclei and scant cytoplasm. (b) Proestrus. A large cluster of normal endometrial epithelial cells with a high nucleus/cytoplasm ratio. (c) Estrus. A cluster of endometrial cells with regularly shaped nuclei and uniformly stained cytoplasm. Many erythrocytes and a vaginal/cervical cell (arrow) are in the background. (d) Early diestrus. A large cluster of normal-appearing endometrial epithelial cells. Nuclei are regularly shaped with a stippled chromatin pattern. (e) Middle diestrus. A cell (arrow) has a pyknotic nucleus and vacuolated cytoplasm within a cluster of normal-appearing cells. (f) Late diestrus. Endometrial epithelial cells are enlarged. Characteristic features in this stage include cytoplasmic lipid droplets giving the cell a typical "foamy aspect" and pyknotic nuclei. (g) Early anestrus. A degenerated endometrial epithelial cell group with marked nuclear pyknosis and vacuolated cytoplasm. (h) Middle anestrus. A small group of normal endometrial epithelial cells (arrow) and a larger degenerated endometrial epithelial cell group in the same field. (i) Late anestrus. A large group of endometrial epithelial cells exhibiting a glandular appearance with open central lumen (arrow). (j) Cystic endometrial hyperplasia. A cluster of degenerated endometrial epithelial cells with cytoplasmic droplets and pyknotic nuclei. (k) Pyometra. Neutrophils (arrowheads) characterize this condition. Both intracellular and extracellular (arrow) bacteria are observed. Occasional macrophages are present (*). (l) Uterine stump. Degenerated endometrial epithelial cells surrounded extracellular bacteria. A neutrophil is indicated by an arrowhead. (m) Subinvolution of placental sites (SIPS). Giant trophoblast-like cells are detected in uterine smears after parturition in a case of delayed uterine involution (Hemaquick; (a, b, d–f, and j–m) at 1000×; (c and g–i) at 400×. *Source:* With permission from Ref. [2].)

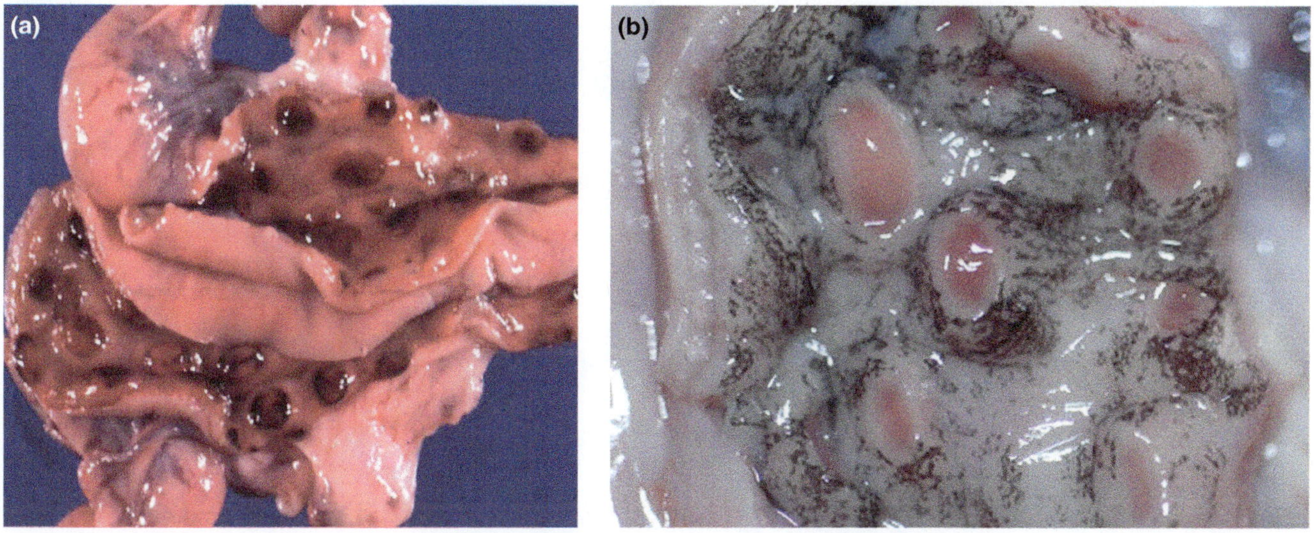

Figure 43.4 Ewe. (a) Opened uterus. Note melanin pigment in the multifocal red to black raised caruncles on the endometrial surface. (b) Opened uterus. Deposition of melanin pigment in the intercaruncular spaces of the endometrium.

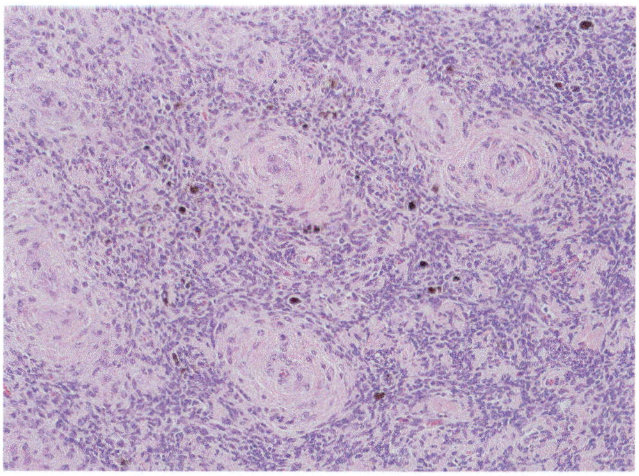

Figure 43.5 Ewe. Scattered melanophages are present in the caruncle stroma (hematoxylin & eosin, 200×. *Source:* With permission from Ref. [41].)

(Figure 43.4) and scattered melanophages on histopathology (Figure 43.5).[41,42] Infrequently, uterine melanin is an incidental finding in llamas and alpacas (personal observation, DMM).

In dogs, low numbers of neutrophils can be present during most stages except anestrus, with highest numbers in proestrus and estrus (Table 43.1).[2,40] Small mature lymphocytes predominate in anestrus into proestrus but also are present in all types of uterine pathology apart from CEH.[2,40] Eosinophils are present in some normal bitches during proestrus and estrus.[2] Macrophages will increase during early anestrus and are present postpartum and into late anestrus with fewer found in diestrus.[2,40] They can be difficult to distinguish from degenerate epithelial cells.[40] Macrophages can contain hemosiderin and other erythroid breakdown products in postpartum samples. Plasma cells are mostly present during late anestrus.[2] Intrauterine bacteria can be observed in proestrus, estrus, and late anestrus, with 100% of samples in diestrus expected to contain organisms in dogs. In one study, 62.5% of cultured canine uterine samples grew bacteria, and vaginal and uterine organisms did not coincide.[43] Bacterial species cultured from normal uterine biopsies in dogs include coagulase negative *Staphylococcus* spp., *Staphylococcus pseudintermedius*, *Micrococcus* spp., *Bacillus* spp., *Corynebacterium* spp., beta hemolytic *Escherichia coli*, and alpha and beta hemolytic *Streptococcus* spp.[43]

In normal mares, lymphocytes are occasionally seen, and neutrophils should rarely be present, but there is no consensus on methods and thresholds to diagnose inflammation.[11] When averaging leukocytes/10 OIF, ≤2 neutrophils/OIF is generally considered normal. When determined as a percent of nucleated cells, <0.5% or up to 5% neutrophils may be normal.[11,44] Studies vary whether brushing or lavage has higher sensitivity using each counting technique.[6,20,21] In healthy horses that are not bred, up to 5% neutrophils are present up to 96 hours after ovulation with <1 bacterium noted in 30 OIF.[11] Up to 1 bacterium in 10 OIF can be seen in bred mares.[11] Bacterial culture should be negative.[11] Hypersegmentation of neutrophils is thought to suggest chronic ongoing inflammation. Macrophages are most common during spring and fall transitions and in winter anestrus. Eosinophils in the mare are considered abnormal and suggestive for pneumovagina.[45]

Table 43.1 Summary of canine uterine cytology.

	Proestrus	Estrus	Diestrus	Anestrus	CEH	Pyometra	Uterine stump	SIPS
Endometrium	Large nests, regular nuclei, high nuclear to cytoplasmic ratio	Fewer nests	Fewest nests. Cytoplasm is foamy with degenerate nuclei	Large nests. Early anestrus: foamy cytoplasm. Late anestrus: rounder cells, scant cytoplasm	Few nests, often cytoplasmic vacuolation	Rare nests	Few nests	Few nests
Degenerate cells	Few	Few	Some, more late diestrus	Frequent early anestrus, few late anestrus	Some	Few	Few	Frequent
Neutrophils	10/OIF	<5/OIF	<5/OIF	<3/OIF	<3/OIF	Many	Many	<3/OIF
Lymphocytes	1/OIF	<0.1/OIF	<0.1/OIF (late diestrus)	<2/OIF	0%	<5/OIF	<2/OIF	<5/OIF
Plasma cells	0	0	0	1/OIF (late anestrus)	0	<2/OIF	<2/OIF	<1/OIF
Macrophages	0	0	<5/OIF (late diestrus)	<2/OIF	0	<2/OIF	<2/OIF	<2/OIF
Eosinophils	<1/OIF	<1/OIF	0	0	0	0	0	<1/OIF
Intracellular bacteria	Rare	Rare	None			Many	Few	Few
Extracellular bacteria	Rare	Rare	None			Many	Few	Few
Other					Amorphous material	Necrotic material	Necrotic material	

OIF, oil immersion field or 1000× magnification; CEH, cystic endometrial hyperplasia; SIPS, subinvolution of placental sites.

Hyperplastic Lesions

Hyperplastic lesions are difficult to diagnose cytologically and normally require histological evaluation to identify.

Cystic Endometrial Hyperplasia (CEH)

CEH in dogs is part of a progressive spectrum of conditions that include mucometra, hematometra, hydrometra, and pyometra and is traditionally referred to as the CEH–pyometra complex.[46,47] CEH can occur alone or with inflammation and is a predisposing factor for the other uterine conditions, though these diseases also occur without CEH.[41,48–50] Hematometra, caused by excessive hemorrhage into the uterine lumen, clinically presents with anemia and hemorrhagic vaginal discharge that can be mistaken for estrus.[47]

CEH occurs with increased and sustained progesterone levels during the luteal phase and can be found in healthy dogs without clinical signs.[49,51,52] Progesterone causes increased proliferation and secretory activity of endometrial glands, as well as decreased contractility of the myometrium and tighter cervical closure.[48] Experimentally induced canine CEH regressed after withdrawal of progesterone.[51] Likewise, prolonged exposure to progestins is associated with endometrial hyperplasia in felids.[53] CEH can lead to implantation failure and is an important differential for infertility in bitches.[54] Uterine expression of progesterone and estrogen receptors is increased.[49] Natural uterine irritants such as bacteria or embryos may contribute to increased uterine expression of progesterone receptors.[51] Anovulatory follicular ovarian cysts predispose to CEH as can some ovarian tumors such as granulosa cell tumors, ovarian adenomas, and adenocarcinoma.[30,55,56] Cystic hyperplasia with squamous metaplasia has been reported in association with an ovarian dysgerminoma in a dog.[57] The risk of CEH increases with age in both dogs and cats.[58] Cervical atresia is a rare cause of mucometra that has been reported in a cat.[59]

Endometrial hyperplasia is common in rabbits[60] and miniature pigs.[61] In rabbits, it presents with a serosanguinous vaginal discharge, can result in mucometra or hydrometra, can occur in rabbits under a year of age, and can occur simultaneously with uterine adenocarcinoma.[60] Sows with polycystic ovaries can develop endometrial mucosal hyperplasia.[62] Cytological findings have not been reported.[60] Endometrial hyperplasia and cervical polyps have been diagnosed in some nonhuman primates.[63–65] In these species, CEH is associated with increasing age, decreased length of menstruation, endometriosis, and decreased parity but not adenomyosis, weight, cesarean sections, or stillbirths.[63] Simple endometrial hyperplasia is documented in rhesus monkeys (*Macaca mulatta*) after exposure to estradiol.[66] CEH has been reported in rhinoceroses (*Ceratotherium simum simum*, *Ceratotherium simum cottoni*) where it is more common in nonparous females and can result in mucometra.[67] It appears common in Asian (*Elephas maximus*) and African (*Loxodonta africana*) elephants, often with endometrial polyps, and increases with age and nonparous animals.[68] Endometrial hyperplasia with chronic endometritis is described in a chinchilla (*Chinchilla lanigera*).[69] Hydrometra was documented in a ferret.[70] Case reports of endometrial hyperplasia are published for a variety of exotic and domestic species.[71–73]

Cystic glands produce watery to mucoid sterile fluid that accumulates in the lumen and enlarges the uterine horns.[46,74] If the fluid remains sterile, hydrometra or mucometra is present, clinical signs are often absent, and endometritis is not present.[49] A cystic honeycomb appearance of the uterine wall is sometimes identified on ultrasound.[47] Histologically, CEH is characterized by irregularly cystic, hyperplastic endometrial glands of differing sizes and shapes lined by attenuated to tall finely vacuolated luteal epithelium (Figure 43.6). Fluid is watery to viscous, transparent to cloudy, and clear to yellow or brown, depending on hemorrhage and endometrial sloughing.[59] Leukocytes should be absent if the fluid is sterile. Vacuolated degenerate epithelial cells and amorphous material on cytology is typical of CEH (Figure 43.3j).[2]

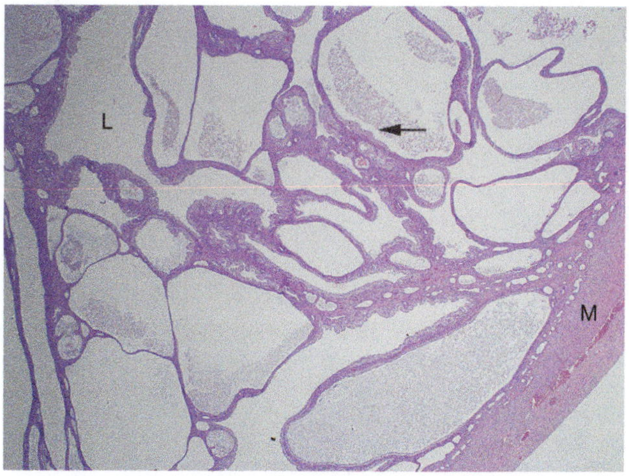

Figure 43.6 Dog with cystic endometrial hyperplasia. Note large dilated cystic endometrial glands often lined by tall finely vacuolated luteal epithelium (arrow). Myometrium (M). Uterine lumen (L) (hematoxylin & eosin, 20×.)

Pseudo-Placentational Endometrial Hyperplasia (PEH)

PEH in dogs, or focal endometrial hyperplasia of pseudopregnancy, occurs during diestrus with a corpus luteum, under the influence of progesterone, but endometrial glands do not become cystic.[46,51,75,76] Histologically, endometrial glands resemble normal pregnancy placentation sites with thin villous folds of endometrial glands that are fused and distended, termed deciduoma (Figure 43.7). Coagulative necrosis can occur, producing amorphous debris without inflammation. Uterine fluid is grossly cloudy and may be green-tinged.[76] Cytology yields amorphous basophilic material without inflammatory cells or bacteria.[76]

Endometrial Polyps

Endometrial polyps are occasionally found in mature bitches and queens. Unless obstructing the uterine lumen, polyps are not clinically significant, though they have been associated with pyometra, focal or diffuse CEH, and uterine torsion (Figure 43.8).[77,78] Most polyps in dogs and cats are solitary and small, arising in areas of interstitial fibrosis. Reported sizes in dogs vary from 0.6 to 25 cm.[77,79] Polyps have a fibrous core covered by a polypoid surface of hyperplastic to cystic endometrial epithelium that projects into the uterine lumen and can ulcerate.[39,79] Polyps can be visible by vaginoscopy if they prolapse through the cervix, while larger masses can be palpated or visualized on radiographs.[77] Polyps are not considered preneoplastic.[79] Polyps are reported in horses,[80] captive African hedgehogs,[81] and elephants.[68]

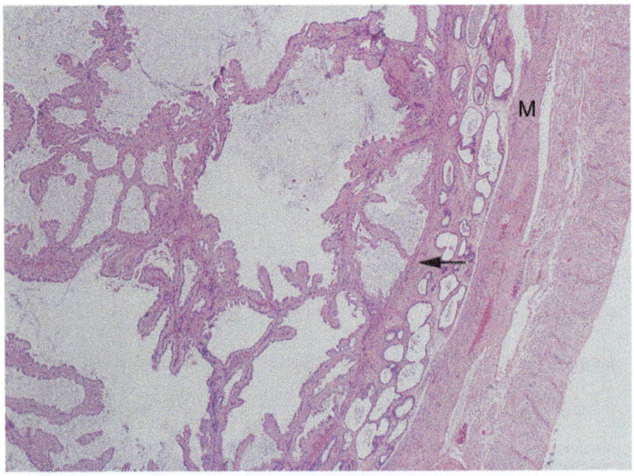

Figure 43.7 Dog. Pseudo-placentational endometrial hyperplasia. Multiple luminal cystic endometrial spaces filled with mucous. Note band of connective tissue (arrow) above dilated deeper endometrial glands over the myometrium (M) (hematoxylin & eosin, 40×.)

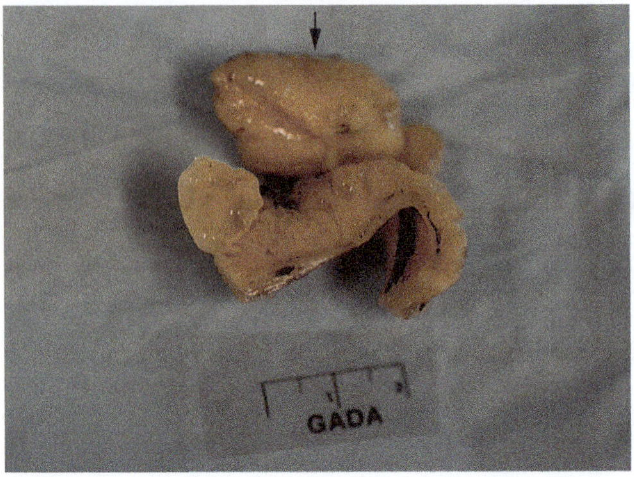

Figure 43.8 Cat. Longitudinal section of uterine horn with cystic endometrial hyperplasia and endometrial polyp (arrow). Note multiple variably sized fluid-filled endometrial cysts distributed throughout the endometrium.

Adenomyosis

Adenomyosis is a condition of unknown pathogenesis in which ectopic endometrial tissue is present in the myometrial layers of the uterus.[39,82] It is often seen in older animals and has been reported in the uterine cervix in dogs or in areas of uterine rupture in cases of pyometra.[66,82–84] Endometrial glands grow into the myometrium, can become cystic, and weaken the uterine wall.[39] Cysts are lined by endometrial cells that flatten as secretions accumulate.[83] A mucoid, hemorrhagic, or suppurative vulvar discharge can be present with degenerate neutrophils and pleomorphic epithelial cells due to endometritis.[83,84] Adenomyosis is rarely reported in sheep where it is associated with endometrial hyperplasia.[85] It is relatively common in miniature pigs with a reported rate of 26.5%.[61] Adenomyosis is described in an orangutan (*Pongo abelii/pygmaeus*).[86]

Serosal Inclusion Cysts

Serosal inclusion cysts are an incidental finding in older bitches. These putatively form after rapid postpartum involution results in mesothelium folds on the uterine external surface or after a cesarean section.[87] They have a thin wall and can create grapelike clusters on the uterine serosal surface. Cytology of the cystic fluid is usually acellular with low-protein content.[87] They are rare in cats.[88]

Glandular Atrophy

Equine endometriosis is a disease of progressive irreversible glandular degeneration in older mares characterized by periglandular fibrosis, endometrial atrophy, lymphangiectasia, and variable inflammation.[76] Equine endometriosis is not the same condition as endometriosis in humans and nonhuman primates and requires histology for confirmation.[41,89]

Subinvolution of Placental Sites (SIPS)

SIPS in bitches are nonhealing areas of necrosis, hemorrhage, glandular distention, and mild inflammation that is thought to be caused by postpartum continuation of trophoblasts (Figure 43.9).[39,90] Uterine fluid appears viscous and dark brown. Lavage yields neutrophils, blood, foamy macrophages, plasma cells, trophoblast-like cells, and occasionally eosinophils (Figure 43.3m).[2,39,90]

Developmental Lesions

Developmental anomalies are uncommon; reported rates are 0.09% in queens and 0.05% in bitches.[91] These include single-horned uterus, segmental agenesis, and horn hypoplasia (Figure 43.10).[91] Mesonephric duct remnants in the uterine wall, especially the proximal uterine horns, can present as small cysts in the mesometrium,[82,92] and paramesonephric (Müllerian) ducts also occur.[82] In sheep, the rate of congenital malformation is 0–0.19% with left horn aplasia most common.[41] Paramesonephric duct aplasia in ewes is reported with concurrent hydrosalpinx where uterine tubes are filled with abundant, clear, acellular to poorly cellular fluid.[41] If infected, a purulent exudate is found.[41] Other abnormalities include uterus didelphys (double uterus, cervix, and cranial vagina), cervical duplication, and incomplete closure of the uterine horn with direct communication to the peritoneal cavity.[41] Cytology is not a useful diagnostic test; gross examination and histology are necessary for diagnosis.

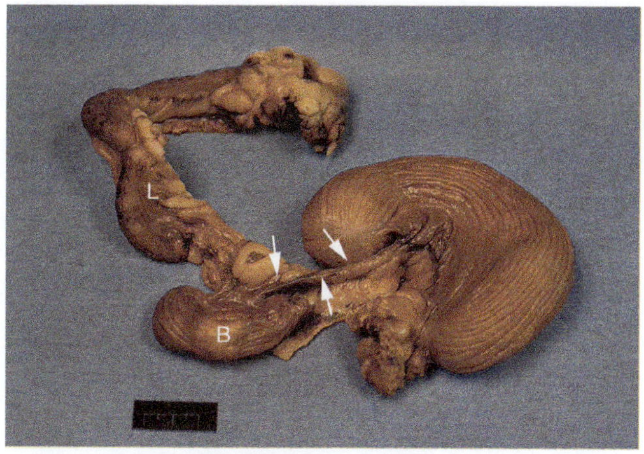

Figure 43.10 Dog. Unilateral segmental uterine aplasia with hydrometra. The right uterine horn is dilated proximal to the thin line of tissue (arrows) attaching the uterine horn to the body of the uterus (B) and left horn (L).

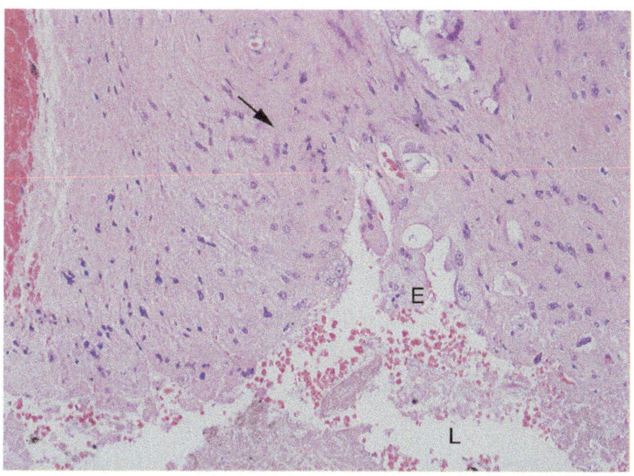

Figure 43.9 Dog. Subinvolution of placental site. Note luminal (L) erythrocytes and necrotic sloughed debris over the finely vacuolated surface epithelium (E) and decidual cells (arrow) of the pedunculated endometrium (hematoxylin & eosin, 200×.)

Traumatic Lesions

Uterine torsion is life-threatening for both dam and fetus, and most commonly presents in mid-pregnancy to late pregnancy. It is more frequent in ruminants, camelids, and horses but is reported in dogs, cats, and buffaloes.[93] An increased risk in multiparous animals is noted in multiple species.[94–97] In cattle, up to 30% of attended dystocias are caused by uterine torsion, while the reported rate in horses is 5–10%.[96–98] Increased blood lactate concentration is a predictor of negative outcomes including uterine necrosis and decreased survival in cows.[99] In camelids, uterine torsion is the second most common cause of dystocia at 23.4% and is the most common cause of cesarean sections in alpacas and llamas.[100] In dogs, uterine torsion accounts for approximately 1% of dystocias, associated with endometrial polyps and CEH in nongravid animals.[101–103] Preferred diagnostic tests are ultrasound for small animals and rectal palpation for large animals. Cytological sampling is not recommended. On histology, there is transmural necrosis and hemorrhage (Figure 43.11).

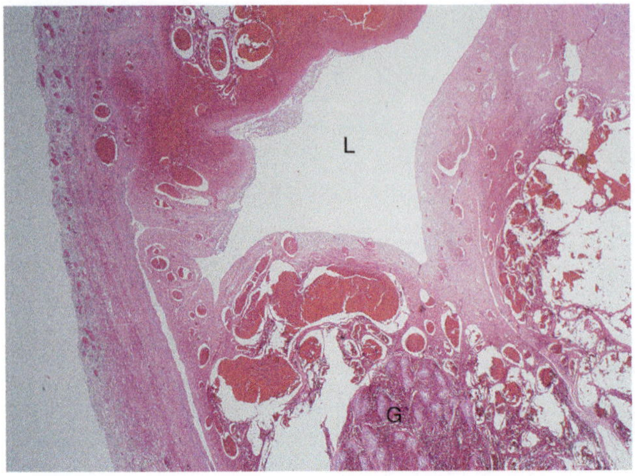

Figure 43.11 Dog. Uterine torsion. Transmural necrosis and hemorrhage. Note diffuse congested vessels, hemorrhage, and degenerate endometrial glands (G). Uterine lumen (L) (hematoxylin & eosin, 20×.)

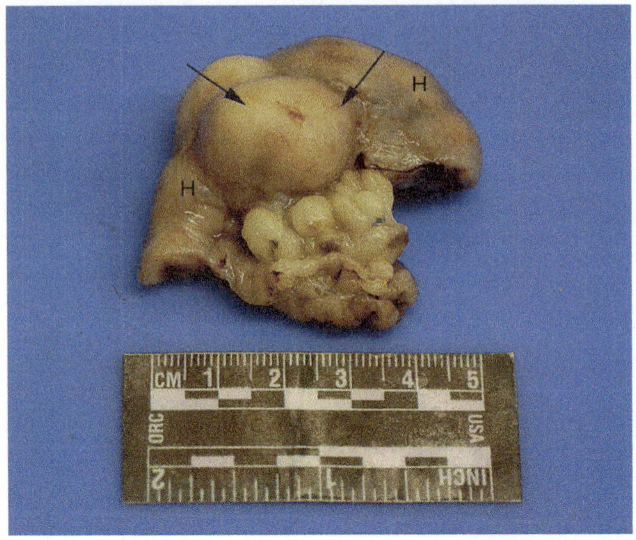

Figure 43.12 Dog. Leiomyoma (arrows) in the uterus. The round firm pale mass was present in and distorting the wall of the right uterine horn (H).

Neoplasia

Uterine neoplasia is uncommon, and the frequency and predominant tumor type vary by species. In dogs only 0.4% of neoplasms originate in the uterus and 0.29% in cats.[104–106] Cytology is rarely diagnostic, and reports of cytologic appearance are few.

Benign Tumors

Leiomyoma

The most common uterine tumors in most species apart from rabbits and cows are leiomyomas and fibroleiomyomas. Dogs and cats frequently do not have clinical signs until tumors are large enough to become space occupying, but can present with vaginal discharge, altered estrus cycle, stranguria, constipation, abdominal distension, weight loss, and pyometra.[104,107] In dogs, leiomyomas can occur concurrently with other reproductive abnormalities including mammary tumors, ovarian follicular cystic tumors, and CEH.[107,108] A mutation in the Birt–Hogg–Dube (DHB) gene in German shepherds has been associated with multiple uterine leiomyomas, bilateral renal cystadenomas, and nodular dermatofibrosis.[109,110] It is important to note that tumors can arise in uterine stumps.[107] In guinea pigs, leiomyomas are associated with ovarian cystadenomas.[104,111] Leiomyomas are documented in a variety of domestic and exotic species.[41,60,61,64,67,106,111–123] In a colony of gray short-tailed opossums (*Monodelphis domestica*), the rate of leiomyoma was 5.5% and was the most common neoplasm after pituitary adenomas.[123] Uterine leiomyoma was reported in 64% of aged Baltic gray seals (*Halichoerus grypus*) in the 1990s, putatively associated with organochlorines and reduced fertility.[124,125] Increased risk of leiomyoma is associated with non-parity and prolonged barren periods in numerous species.[67,116–118,120] Leiomyomas are round, firm nodules that protrude from the serosal surface or uterine lumen (Figure 43.12). They are composed of interlacing bundles of smooth muscle fibers with minimal atypia and low mitotic rate. On immunohistochemistry, they are positive for desmin and smooth muscle actin and negative for S-100.[104]

Fibromas

Fibromas are uncommon and reported in dogs,[82] cats,[126] sheep,[41] pigs,[115] and miniature pigs.[61] Variably ciliated regular tubular epithelium covers mature fibrous tissue.[82] Adenomyomas have stratified cuboidal to columnar endometrium with interwoven smooth muscle bundles.[82]

Uterine Adenomas

Adenomas are reported in rabbits,[127] dogs,[82,128] miniature pigs,[61] swine,[115] and cynomolgus monkeys.[64] They are composed solely of proliferating regularly arranged columnar endometrial cells surrounding an empty lumen on thin stalks of connective tissue. In one canine report, a papillary adenocarcinoma had similar morphology to an adenoma and was differentiated by clinical course rather than morphological characteristics.[82]

Malignant Tumors

Endometrial Adenocarcinomas

Endometrial adenocarcinomas are rare except in rabbits and cattle.[60,106,112,129] Representing 3.9% of all diagnosed tumors, uterine carcinomas were the only reported uterine

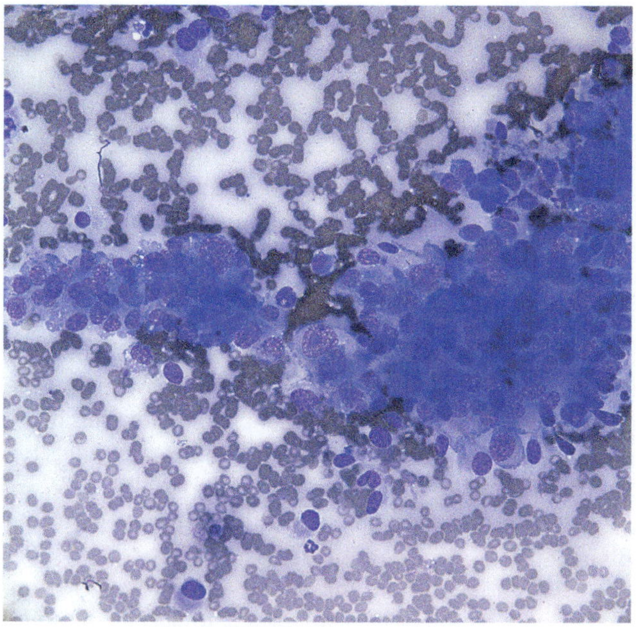

Figure 43.13 Dog. Adenocarcinoma involving the uterine stump characterized by clustered epithelial cells with moderate anisocytosis, anisokaryosis, and prominent variably sized nucleoli (Diff-Quik, 400×. *Source:* Image courtesy of Ulsoo Choi).

tumor in an abattoir study of 1370 tumors submitted from 17 million cattle over a 5-year period.[130] Studies report 17–60% of female rabbits diagnosed with uterine adenocarcinoma, sometimes in both horns.[60,106,129] Most does were over 3 years of age. Endometrial hyperplasia is often a concurrent finding in does, while mammary gland changes, serosanguinous vaginal discharge, and hematuria are typical.[60,112] Cytology of uterine fluid from a rabbit with uterine adenocarcinoma, stained with hematoxylin and eosin stain, exhibited mainly uniform epithelial cells with some pyknotic or degenerate nuclei, some neutrophils, and erythrocytes.[131] Adenocarcinomas metastasize, especially to lung; metastatic uterine tumors are the most common pulmonary neoplasia in slaughtered abattoir cattle.[129,130] Uterine adenocarcinomas are described in dogs including a 10-month-old Golden Retriever puppy and one in the uterine stump of a spayed dog.[132–136] Cytological description in dogs is inconsistent. One report noted tightly clustered epithelial cells of mixed morphology with moderate to abundant amounts of basophilic variably vacuolated cytoplasm, moderate anisokaryosis, dispersed to reticular chromatin, and one or two prominent nucleoli.[136] Another described cells with a higher N:C ratio, occasional small vacuoles, marked anisokaryosis, but similar nuclear features (Figure 43.13).[135] Adenocarcinomas are reported in cats, including in animals less than a year of age,[104,107,137,138] and metastases are described.[139] Adenocarcinomas are also reported in a variety of domestic[41,61,140–143] and exotic species.[117,118,144–153] On histology, anaplastic epithelium forms

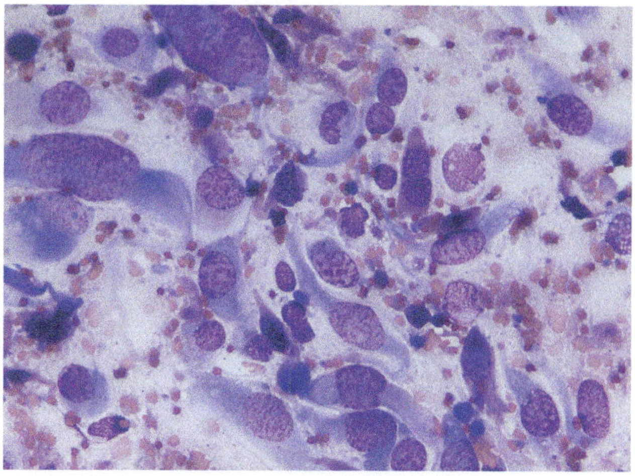

Figure 43.14 Goat. Leiomyosarcoma. Numerous spindle cells with marked anisocytosis and anisokaryosis, scant tapered cytoplasm, oval nuclei, and disrupted chromatin with several prominent nucleoli varying in size and shape (Wright–Giemsa, 500×. *Source:* Image courtesy of Mary White.)

nests and cords in a fibrous connective tissue stroma, invading the myometrium. Tumors are positive for cytokeratins and sometimes estrogen receptors by immunohistochemistry.[104,137]

Leiomyosarcoma

Leiomyosarcomas are rare in most species, and sometimes pyometra is present. Reports include cats,[104,139] dogs,[108] rabbits,[60] miniature pigs,[61] sheep,[41] goat,[142] jaguar (*Panthera onca*),[154] and chimpanzees.[117] One survey of miniature pigs undergoing routine hysterectomy found a leiomyosarcoma rate of 21%,[61] while a larger study found 24% out of 34 examined histological lesions were leiomyosarcoma.[114] Cytologically, they have spindled cells with more anisocytosis and anisokaryosis than benign tumors, loose chromatin, and several prominent nucleoli (Figure 43.14).

Lymphoma

Uterine infiltration by neoplastic lymphocytes is reported in 38–51% of cattle with lymphoma, often with concurrent positive bovine leukemia virus serology.[155] Uterine granular T-cell lymphoma was typed as gamma/delta in a 4-year-old Holstein cow without circulating atypical lymphocytes or peripheral lymphadenopathy but nodal effacement.[156] Uterine lymphoma was characterized as B cell in five dogs,[157,158] but a T-cell phenotype is described in cats.[159,160] Uterine lymphoma is reported in ewes and a horse.[41,161]

Miscellaneous Tumors

Rarely reported tumors include hemangiosarcoma in dogs and sheep[41]; rhabdomyosarcoma in a dog[162]; hemangioma and carcinosarcoma in rabbits and cats[60,112,126,163];

squamous cell carcinoma in rabbits,[60,112] baboons,[164] a cat (uterine remnant),[165] and an ewe (cervix)[166]; choriocarcinoma-like tumor in a pot-bellied pig and rabbit[167,168]; and adenosarcoma (mixed Müllerian tumor) in cats.[104,126] Granulosa cell tumors metastatic to the uterus are reported in dogs.[82]

Inflammatory Lesions

Uterine inflammation is common, and cytology is a useful tool for diagnosis. Uterine inflammation is classified by tissue layers involved, etiology, and timing of the inflammation. Milder inflammation involving the mucosal surface but not extending beyond the stratum spongiosum is termed endometritis. Endometritis can be subclinical with minimal clinical signs and without changes in leukograms or other inflammatory markers, or can be associated with mating, parturition, or an infectious agent with variable discharge and other signs. Metritis is a severe infection associated with the postpartum period, affecting the mucosa and myometrial layers. Uterine inflammation for any reason can lead to infertility. Significant clinical differences exist between domestic species, and each is presented in its own section.

Horses

Endometritis in mares is common after foaling or mating.[11,169] Uterine involution after foaling reduces bacterial populations.[170] Delayed clearance of uterine contents after bacterial introduction contributes to infections and is associated with increased progesterone, suboptimal myometrial function, pendulous uterus, and stretched broad ligament.[171–173] In healthy mares, streptococci inoculated into the uterus are cleared within 12 hours, and neutrophils are present for several days after infection is cleared.[3,11,174] Similarly, after insemination, healthy mares clear spermatozoa, bacteria, and neutrophils within 48 hours.[11,175] Suppression of the uterine inflammatory response by seminal plasma might contribute to the development of endometritis.[11]

Inflammatory cells are not always found on cytology when pathogenic bacteria are identified by culture, especially *E. coli* and other coliforms when compared with streptococcal infections.[10,15,17,20,176] Sensitivity of cytology to detect neutrophilic inflammation varies from 0% for swabs to 80% for lavage, but reports vary tremendously with counting methodology and normal neutrophil threshold.[11,15,17–20] Part of this variation may reflect culture of contaminants (false positives)[15] and lack of understanding of normal uterine microbiome or indicate cytology is not always useful for detection of endometritis caused by certain pathogens.

The diagnosis of inflammation by brushing better correlates with culture of known pathogens, especially *E. coli* and beta hemolytic *Streptococci* than other techniques.[10,15] When inflammation is localized or cultures have been negative, lavage may be more useful than swabs or brushing in detecting endometritis.[20,176] A double-guarded low-volume uterine lavage may have fewer false-positive cultures than previously reported lavage techniques. Centrifugation of lavage fluid at both 200 and 600g yields suitable cytological specimens.[6,15,20]

Evaluation of the background debris is important. A cloudy lavage containing increased mucoid material is typically found with bacterial infections, especially *E. coli* and other coliforms, even when neutrophil numbers are not increased.[15,18,20,176]

The definition of mild, moderate, and severe inflammation is variable.[3,15,21] It is important to specify sampling technique as lavage, and swab samples are less likely to contain endometrial cells than brushings. In swab samples, >2% neutrophils has been reported as inflammation, while a 0.5% threshold is generally considered inflammatory with cytobrushing.[19,44,177] Swabs are more sensitive, but cytobrushing is more specific in detecting inflammation.[19] Following breeding, 5–15% neutrophils indicates mild, 15–30% moderate, and >30% marked inflammation by swab.[11] Detecting inflammation, cytology is most sensitive during estrus, less sensitive in diestrus, and least sensitive during anestrus, due in part to overall lower cellularity in anestrus samples.[19] Free and phagocytosed bacteria should be noted and described (cocci, rods, or coccobacilli). Gram stain can be used; Gram-negative cocci are generally not considered pathogens.[11]

Eosinophils, plasma cells, and macrophages are seen with chronic inflammation or resolving infection. With chronic endometritis, neutrophils are present in the uterine lumen, while predominantly mononuclear cells and rare neutrophils are present in the lamina propria.[169] Macrophages can contain hemosiderin and other erythroid breakdown products in samples collected soon postpartum.

Eosinophils are associated with pneumovagina as well as fungal disease.[33–35,45] Yeast and fungal hyphae are usually extracellular with accompanying neutrophilic to lymphoplasmacytic inflammation (Figure 43.15).[20,178,179] Yeast appears oval with a clear distinct halo and can be present without inflammatory cells.[178,179] *Candida*, *Aspergillus*, and *Mucor* spp. are most commonly implicated with *Actinomyces*, *Fusarium*, and *Cryptococcus* spp. less common.[4,180,181] While yeast are readily visualized with cytology, period acid-Schiff or Gomori's methenamine silver

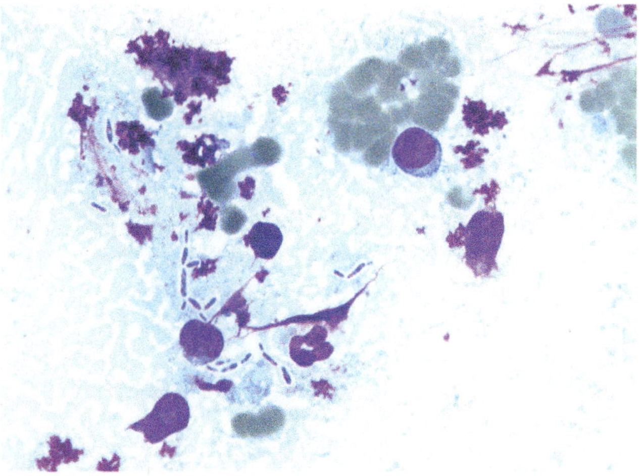

Figure 43.15 Horse. Uterine swab. Fungal infection with *Candida guilliermondii*. Extracellular elongated oval hyphal structures with irregular branching and a distinct halo. Neutrophilic and lymphocytic inflammation was seen (Wright-Giemsa stain. 1000×. *Source:* Image courtesy of Judith Radin.)

stains may be needed for recognition of fungal hyphae on histology. Fungal organisms can be slow or difficult to culture; therefore polymerase chain reaction (PCR) with or without genetic sequencing may help with identification, though PCR does not allow determination of susceptibility to antifungal treatment.[180,181] Diluents and uterine fluid do not appear to inhibit PCR amplification.[180]

Cattle

Though the uterus is sterile during pregnancy, bacterial infections are expected immediately postpartum until approximately 28–35 days postpartum.[50,182,183] Infections are most commonly caused by *E. coli*, *Trueperella pyogenes*, *Fusobacterium necrophorum*, and *Prevotella* spp.[184–186] Uterine infections have a negative economic impact through delayed ovulation, lower conception rates, and lower milk yields.[22,187–191] Cattle may suffer long-term fertility impairment after infections have resolved.[192,193]

Milder bacterial infection can cause superficial endometrial inflammation not extending past the stratum spongiosum.[194] Though neutrophils can be found on cytology,[23] these infections do not result in clinical signs and are termed subclinical endometritis. Infections >21 days postpartum with a mucopurulent vaginal discharge are termed clinical endometritis.[22,185,188] The reported prevalence of clinical and subclinical endometritis varies by diagnostic method, time of collection relative to parturition, and demographic differences including environmental factors such as housing and bedding.[13,26,195,196] Studies on dairy cows suggest subclinical endometritis 4–8 weeks postpartum is very common, with reported rates between 5 and 74%.[13,22,23,186,197] Clinical endometritis is present in 10–27% of dairy cattle,[186,187] and cows with delayed involution may be at increased risk.[198] Inflammation can persist despite inability to culture organisms.[22] The percentage of neutrophils required to diagnose subclinical endometritis is not established, varies by counting technique (counting up to 500 nucleated cells or counting inflammatory cells in 10 OIF),[8] and is impacted by time of collection postpartum.[26] One publication proposed >18% neutrophils in lavage samples collected 21–33 days postpartum, or >10% neutrophils at 34–47 days to diagnose subclinical endometritis.[185] Alternatively, >5% at 18–62 days postpartum and >8% at 21–41 days postpartum also are published.[8,25,26,185] Uterine aspiration may yield a higher inflammatory cell count than uterine swabs for subacute and chronic endometritis.[199] Relative to biopsy, cytology has a sensitivity of 78.6% and specificity of 95.8% for diagnosing subclinical endometritis.[200]

To determine an endometritis clinical score, vaginal mucus is evaluated for color, volume of fluid, and odor.[184] This technique is rapid, is inexpensive, and correlates fairly well with lavage cytology at 28 days postpartum (kappa = 0.29); however, the correlation decreases with time.[25] The preferred method for diagnosis of endometritis remains uterine cytology.[13,23,25] Reagent test strips that test for leukocyte esterase, protein, and pH are not superior to conventional cytology to diagnose endometritis, although correlating with endometritis (sensitivity, 86%; specificity, 41.7%) when >6.7% neutrophils are present on cytobrushing.[16,196,201]

Clinical metritis is defined by transmural inflammation affecting the endometrium, submucosa, muscularis, and serosa.[194] Cows have enlarged uteri and purulent to mucopurulent vulvar discharge with cytological neutrophilic endometritis.[185] This condition is more common with dystocia, delayed uterine involution, retained fetal membranes, hypocalcaemia, twins, or stillbirth.[202] Puerperal metritis is characterized by fever, dullness, and reduced milk production.[203,204] Reported rates of metritis in dairy cattle range from 18.5[205] to 40%.[202,206]

Sheep

Metritis, endometritis, and CEH are reported in ewes and strongly correlate with ovarian cysts and ovarobursal adhesions.[41,42] In one abattoir study, endometritis affected 2.3% of ewes, metritis affected 0.5%, and CEH affected 0.2%.[207] Rumen metabolism of phytoestrogen-rich legumes into estrogenic compounds triggers CEH leading to uterine cysts, hydrometra, pyometra, and uterine prolapse.[41,208,209] Hydrometra and mucometra can occur secondary to artificial insemination and estrus synchronization, presumably due to hormonal influences and possibly mechanical irritation.[41] Acute metritis and pyometra are uncommon and usually caused by *E. coli*. A green-yellow purulent exudate with sloughed epithelium is the typical cytological finding.[85]

Infectious agents causing chronic endometritis in sheep include *Corynebacterium pyogenes*, *E. coli*, *Streptococcus* spp., *Staphylococcus aureus*, *Mycoplasma agalactiae var. bovis*, *Chlamydia abortus*, and *Chlamydia psittaci*.[41] With chlamydial infection, the initial mild purulent response is eventually replaced by a chronic lymphoplasmacytic infiltrate characterized by lymphoid follicles and fibrosis.[210] The cystic stage of the dog and cat tapeworm *Taenia hydatigena* can cause fluid-filled serosal cysts containing a single scolex and can calcify into firm nodules.[41]

Camelids

Uterine infections in alpacas, llamas, and camels are associated with overbreeding, early embryonic death, and postpartum complications.[1,211,212] As camels and alpacas accept being bred even when not fertile, a pre-breeding examination to confirm an active follicle is recommended to reduce unnecessary breeding that can lead to local trauma or infection and impair fertility.[1] Camelids have a diverse normal bacterial flora that complicates investigations of chronic endometritis; however, agents causing endometritis are similar to mares and cows with *E. coli* predominating.[1,213] *T. pyogenes*, *S. aureus*, *Pseudomonas aeruginosa*, *Klebsiella pneumoniae*, *Streptococcus zooepidemicus*, and β-hemolytic streptococcus are also linked to infertility.[211,213] Fungal infections with *Aspergillus* and *Mucor* spp. are reported.[1]

Cytology is useful for distinguishing acute from chronic endometritis. Acute endometritis is characterized predominantly by neutrophils with few small lymphocytes and plasma cells.[1] Chronic endometritis is mostly lymphocytic with variable proportions of plasma cells, macrophages, eosinophils, and mast cells.[1] Hemosiderin-laden macrophages can be present with uterine hemorrhage following parturition or embryonic loss. A histological grading scheme for camelids has been proposed.[1]

Complete uterine involution is expected by 15 days postpartum in llamas and alpacas and 25 days in camels; delayed involution suggests infection.[1] Pyometra is most often a postpartum complication with increased risk associated with vaginal or cervical adhesions.[1]

Dogs and Cats

Chronic endometritis in dogs and cats is subclinical, can cause infertility, and can be a sequela of dystocia, retained placenta, or mummified fetus.[46] It appears less common than in large animals.[12] In dogs, over 70% of cases are bacterial, likely from contaminating vaginal flora.[12] Evaluation for endometritis should be performed during early anestrus when progesterone decreases and the endometrium becomes less sensitive to irritation.[12] Histology is helpful as luminal inflammatory cells are not always present on cytology. Lymphocytes, plasma cells, fibroblasts, neutrophils, or macrophages are found on both cytology and histology (Figure 43.16).[12,39] Fibrosis is variably present.[39] Eosinophilic infiltrates are most common with fetal loss.[214]

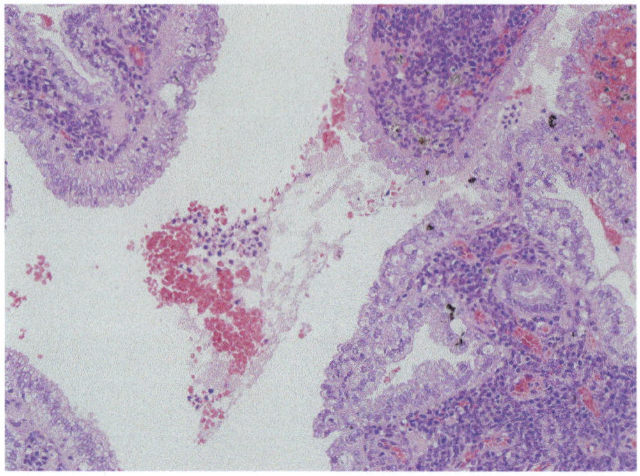

Figure 43.16 Dog. Chronic endometritis. Note luminal contents including numerous neutrophils, erythrocytes, and cellular debris. There is diffuse plasmacytic interstitial infiltrate in the endometrium. The uterine luminal epithelium is markedly hyperplastic (hematoxylin & eosin, 200×.)

Pyometra

Pyometra develops because of infection by opportunistic vaginal bacteria, often in association with CEH and/or endometritis in dogs. Controversy exists between the traditional concept of the CEH–pyometra complex that holds that hyperplasia is a precursor to infection and a newer theory that holds that subclinical endometrial mechanical irritation or bacterial endometritis initiates CEH.[48,49,215] In the latter theory, if the initiating irritation is sterile (e.g. endometrial polyp or artificial insemination), mucometra results and the condition should be considered a CEH–mucometra syndrome, while if bacteria are the stimulus for CEH, an endometritis–pyometra syndrome is present with secondary CEH.[48] Mucometra, hydrometra, and pyometra can be present without CEH.[48,49,215]

Pyometra is up to 10 times more common in nulliparous than multiparous dogs.[75] In wild canids, the number of barren years is associated with pyometra and CEH.[216] Studies suggest 15–24% of intact female dogs will develop pyometra in their lifetime.[215,217] Compared with dogs with mucometra or CEH, dogs with pyometra are clinically more depressed, have a more pronounced leukocytosis with neutrophilia and left shift, and have higher concentrations of cholesterol, albumin, and C-reactive protein.[38,218] With an open cervix, drainage of the uterine contents occurs, and a hemorrhagic to mucopurulent discharge with an unpleasant odor is present.[46] Systemic signs of illness are more severe with a closed cervix and include lethargy, depression, polyuria, polydipsia, anorexia, vomiting, diarrhea and in severe cases dehydration, septicemia, and shock.[46] The most common bacterial isolate is *E. coli*, which can cause endotoxin release and septic shock, though *S. aureus*, *Streptococcus* spp., *Pseudomonas* spp., and *Proteus* spp. are also reported.[39,48,218–220] The genetic profile of endometrium from dogs with open or closed pyometra found those with prior exogenous progesterone treatment had a specific molecular profile that differed from dogs without prior progesterone exposure, suggesting different etiologies.[221] Dogs treated with progesterone had higher expression of S100A8, S100A9, and S100A12 genes; these are associated with inflammatory cytokines including tumor necrosis factor, interleukin (IL)-6, IL-1β, and IL-8.[221] Cyclooxygenase-2 and lactotransferrin genes also were overexpressed.[221] Interestingly, gene expression did not differ between open and closed pyometra.[221]

As induced ovulators, queens have less exposure to endogenous progesterone, so overall incidence of pyometra is low.[46,74] Pyometra develops most often after an unsuccessful breeding rather than in conjunction with CEH.[46,74] Pyometra usually occurs one to four weeks after estrus and is associated with exposure to endogenous or experimentally administered progesterone.[46,74] There are isolated reports of pyometra during the follicular phase of the reproductive cycle in queens.[74,222] Estrogen stimulation plays a larger role in the development of pyometra in cats where frequent repeated heat cycles without pregnancy permit an estrogen-stimulated increase in uterine progesterone receptors and cervical dilation that may permit the entry of vaginal bacteria.[74,222] Corpus luteum are present in 40–70% of cases.[74] Bacteria not only are predominantly *E. coli* but also include species of *Streptococcus*, *Staphylococcus*, *Klebsiella*, *Pseudomonas*, *Proteus*, *Moraxella*, and *Pasteurella*.[74]

Cytologic examination of vaginal discharge is the most expedient way to diagnose pyometra. Ultrasonography is helpful in distinguishing CEH–pyometra complex conditions and to exclude pregnancy.[47] Transabdominal aspiration is not recommended to avoid uterine rupture and peritonitis. Variably degenerate neutrophils with intracellular and extracellular bacteria are expected.

Acute Metritis

Acute metritis is most common in dogs and cats in the first week postpartum from opportunistic bacterial infection through a dilated cervix. Animals often have signs of systemic illness including fever, puppy/kitten neglect, decreased milk production, lethargy, and anorexia. Infection involves the mucosa and myometrium; affected animals usually have an odorous vaginal discharge and can become septicemic. *E. coli* is the most common culprit, but *Proteus* spp., *Streptococcus* spp., and *Staphylococcus* spp. have all been isolated.[39] Ultrasound and radiographs can confirm retained fetus or placenta that predisposes to acute metritis. Histologically, the superficial endometrium has a neutrophilic infiltrate with accompanying subepithelial vascular congestion and edema. Neutrophils migrate into the lumen and are present in uterine lavage or swabs. Dogs with embryonic resorption have serous hemorrhagic uterine fluid with a high leukocyte count that is predominantly neutrophilic.[30]

Artificial Insemination

Artificial insemination causes mild uterine neutrophilic infiltration in dogs.[223] In bitches, neutrophils averaged 2.75% of all cells prior to insemination compared with 3.55% neutrophils 12 hours after insemination.[190] Another study found a pre-breeding average of 5.9% neutrophils and post-insemination average of 10.2%.[223,224] Use of extender for sperm preservation more than doubled the infiltrate to 7.8% neutrophils.[224]

References

1 Tibary, A. and Anouassi, A. (2001). Uterine infections in Camelidae. *Vet Sci Tomorrow* 3: 1–12.

2 Groppetti, D., Pecile, A., Arrighi, S. et al. (2010). Endometrial cytology and computerized morphometric analysis of epithelial nuclei: a useful tool for reproductive diagnosis in the bitch. *Theriogenology* 73: 927–941.

3 Katila, T. (2016). Evaluation of diagnostic methods in equine endometritis. *Reprod Biol* 16: 189–196.

4 Ferris, R.A. (2016). Endometritis: diagnostic tools for infectious endometritis. *Vet Clin North Am Equine Pract* 32: 481–498.

5 Watts, J.R., Wright, P.J., Lee, C.S., and Whithear, K.G. (1997). New techniques using transcervical uterine cannulation for the diagnosis of uterine disorders in bitches. *J Reprod Fertil Suppl* 51: 283–293.

6 Bohn, A.A., Ferris, R.A., and McCue, P.M. (2014). Comparison of equine endometrial cytology samples

collected with uterine swab, uterine brush, and low-volume lavage from healthy mares. *Vet Clin Pathol* 43: 594–600.

7 McKinnon, A.O., Squires, E.L., Harrison, L.A. et al. (1988). Ultrasonographic studies on the reproductive tract of mares after parturition: effect of involution and uterine fluid on pregnancy rates in mares with normal and delayed first postpartum ovulatory cycles. *J Am Vet Med Assoc* 192: 350–353.

8 Melcher, Y., Prunner, I., and Drillich, M. (2014). Degree of variation and reproducibility of different methods for the diagnosis of subclinical endometritis. *Theriogenology* 82: 57–63.

9 Ball, B.A., Shin, S.J., Patten, V.H. et al. (1988). Use of a low-volume uterine flush for microbiologic and cytologic examination of the mare's endometrium. *Theriogenology* 29: 1269–1283.

10 Walter, J., Neuberg, K.P., Failing, K., and Wehrend, A. (2012). Cytological diagnosis of endometritis in the mare: investigations of sampling techniques and relation to bacteriological results. *Anim Reprod Sci* 132: 178–186.

11 Card, C. (2005). Post-breeding inflammation and endometrial cytology in mares. *Theriogenology* 64: 580–588.

12 Fontaine, E., Levy, X., Grellet, A. et al. (2009). Diagnosis of endometritis in the bitch: a new approach. *Reprod Domest Anim* 44 (Suppl 2): 196–199.

13 Barlund, C.S., Carruthers, T.D., Waldner, C.L. et al. (2008). A comparison of diagnostic techniques for postpartum endometritis in dairy cattle. *Theriogenology* 69: 714–723.

14 Dini, P., Farhoodi, M., Hostens, M. et al. (2015). Effect of uterine lavage on neutrophil counts in postpartum dairy cows. *Anim Reprod Sci* 158: 25–30.

15 Christoffersen, M., Brandis, L., Samuelsson, J. et al. (2015). Diagnostic double-guarded low-volume uterine lavage in mares. *Theriogenology* 83: 222–227.

16 Cheong, S.H., Nydam, D.V., Galvao, K.N. et al. (2012). Use of reagent test strips for diagnosis of endometritis in dairy cows. *Theriogenology* 77: 858–864.

17 Overbeck, W., Witte, T.S., and Heuwieser, W. (2011). Comparison of three diagnostic methods to identify subclinical endometritis in mares. *Theriogenology* 75: 1311–1318.

18 Nielsen, J.M., Nielsen, F.H., and Petersen, M.R. (2012). Diagnosis of equine endometritis-microbiology, cytology and histology of endometrial biopsies and the correlation to fertility. *Pferdeheilkunde* 28: 8–13.

19 Kozdrowski, R., Sikora, M., Buczkowska, J. et al. (2015). Effects of cycle stage and sampling procedure on interpretation of endometrial cytology in mares. *Anim Reprod Sci* 154: 56–62.

20 LeBlanc, M.M., Magsig, J., and Stromberg, A.J. (2007). Use of a low-volume uterine flush for diagnosing endometritis in chronically infertile mares. *Theriogenology* 68: 403–412.

21 Cocchia, N., Paciello, O., Auletta, L. et al. (2012). Comparison of the cytobrush, cottonswab, and low-volume uterine flush techniques to evaluate endometrial cytology for diagnosing endometritis in chronically infertile mares. *Theriogenology* 77: 89–98.

22 Gilbert, R.O., Shin, S.T., Guard, C.L. et al. (2005). Prevalence of endometritis and its effects on reproductive performance of dairy cows. *Theriogenology* 64: 1879–1888.

23 Kasimanickam, R., Duffield, T.F., Foster, R.A. et al. (2004). Endometrial cytology and ultrasonography for the detection of subclinical endometritis in postpartum dairy cows. *Theriogenology* 62: 9–23.

24 Thome, H.E., de Arruda, R.P., de Oliveira, B.M. et al. (2016). Uterine lavage is efficient to recover endometrial cytology sample and does not interfere with fertility rate after artificial insemination in cows. *Theriogenology* 85: 1549–1554.

25 McDougall, S., Hussein, H., Aberdein, D. et al. (2011). Relationships between cytology, bacteriology and vaginal discharge scores and reproductive performance in dairy cattle. *Theriogenology* 76: 229–240.

26 de Boer, M.W., LeBlanc, S.J., Dubuc, J. et al. (2014). Invited review: systematic review of diagnostic tests for reproductive-tract infection and inflammation in dairy cows. *J Dairy Sci* 97: 3983–3999.

27 Pascottini, O.B., Dini, P., Hostens, M. et al. (2015). A novel cytologic sampling technique to diagnose subclinical endometritis and comparison of staining methods for endometrial cytology samples in dairy cows. *Theriogenology* 84: 1438–1446.

28 Glinska-Suchocka, K., Jankowski, M., Kubiak, K. et al. (2013). Fine needle biopsy of abdominal organs in dogs – indications, contraindications and performance technique. *Pol J Vet Sci* 16: 835–842.

29 Barr, F. (1995). Percutaneous biopsy of abdominal organs under ultrasound guidance. *J Small Anim Pract* 36: 105–113.

30 Mir, F., Fontaine, E., Albaric, O. et al. (2013). Findings in uterine biopsies obtained by laparotomy from bitches with unexplained infertility or pregnancy loss: an observational study. *Theriogenology* 79: 312–322.

31 Buczkowska, J., Kozdrowski, R., Nowak, M. et al. (2014). Comparison of the biopsy and cytobrush techniques for diagnosis of subclinical endometritis in mares. *Reprod Biol Endocrinol* 12: 27.

32 Christensen, B.W., Schlafer, D.H., Agnew, D.W. et al. (2012). Diagnostic value of transcervical endometrial

biopsies in domestic dogs compared with full-thickness uterine sections. *Reprod Domest Anim* 47 (Suppl 6): 342–346.

33 Kenney, R.M. (1978). Cyclic and pathologic changes of the mare endometrium as detected by biopsy, with a note on early embryonic death. *J Am Vet Med Assoc* 172: 241–262.

34 Kenney, R.M. and Doig, P.A. (1986). Equine endometrial biopsy. In: *Current Therapy in Theriogenology: Diagnosis, Treatment, and Prevention of Reproductive Diseases in Small and Large Animals*, 2e (ed. D.A. Morrow). Philadelphia, PA: W.B. Saunders; 723–729 pages.

35 Snider, T.A., Sepoy, C., and Holyoak, G.R. (2011). Equine endometrial biopsy reviewed: observation, interpretation, and application of histopathologic data. *Theriogenology* 75: 1567–1581.

36 Bonnett, B.N., Miller, R.B., Etherington, W.G. et al. (1991). Endometrial biopsy in Holstein-Friesian dairy cows. I. Technique, histological criteria and results. *Can J Vet Res* 55: 155–161.

37 Chapwanya, A., Meade, K.G., Narciandi, F. et al. (2010). Endometrial biopsy: a valuable clinical and research tool in bovine reproduction. *Theriogenology* 73: 988–994.

38 Hagman, R. (2014). Diagnostic and prognostic markers for uterine diseases in dogs. *Reprod Domest Anim* 49 (Suppl 2): 16–20.

39 Schlafer, D.H. (2012). Diseases of the canine uterus. *Reprod Domest Anim* 47 (Suppl 6): 318–322.

40 Watts, J.R., Wright, P.J., and Lee, C.S. (1998). Endometrial cytology of the normal bitch throughout the reproductive cycle. *J Small Anim Pract* 39: 2–9.

41 Palmieri, C., Schiavi, E., and Della Salda, L. (2011). Congenital and acquired pathology of ovary and tubular genital organs in ewes: a review. *Theriogenology* 75: 393–410.

42 Regassa, F., Mengesha, D., Dargie, M., and Tolosa, T. (2009). Abattoir evidence on association between uterine and ovarian abnormalities in Ethiopian highland ewes. *Anim Reprod Sci* 111: 384–390.

43 Maksimovic, A., Maksimovic, Z., Filipovic, S. et al. (2012). Vaginal and uterine bacteria of healthy bitches during different stages of their reproductive cycle. *Vet Rec* 171: 375.

44 Ricketts, S.W. and Mackintosh, M.E. (1987). Role of anaerobic bacteria in equine endometritis. *J Reprod Fertil Suppl* 35: 343–351.

45 Slusher, S.H., Freeman, K.P., and Roszel, J.F. (1984). Eosinophils in equine uterine cytology and histology specimens. *J Am Vet Med Assoc* 184: 665–670.

46 Ortega-Pacheco, A., Gutierrez-Blanco, E., and Jimenez-Coello, M. (2012). Common lesions in the female reproductive tract of dogs and cats. *Vet Clin North Am Small Anim Pract* 42: 547–559.

47 Troxel, M.T., Cornetta, A.M., Pastor, K.F. et al. (2002). Severe hematometra in a dog with cystic endometrial hyperplasia/pyometra complex. *J Am Anim Hosp Assoc* 38: 85–89.

48 Verstegen, J., Dhaliwal, G., and Verstegen-Onclin, K. (2008). Mucometra, cystic endometrial hyperplasia, and pyometra in the bitch: advances in treatment and assessment of future reproductive success. *Theriogenology* 70: 364–374.

49 De Bosschere, H., Ducatelle, R., and Tshamala, M. (2002). Is mechanically induced cystic endometrial hyperplasia (CEH) a suitable model for study of spontaneously occurring CEH in the uterus of the bitch? *Reprod Domest Anim* 37: 152–157.

50 Hussain, A.M., Daniel, R.C., and O'Boyle, D. (1990). Postpartum uterine flora following normal and abnormal puerperium in cows. *Theriogenology* 34: 291–302.

51 Chen, Y.M., Lee, C.S., and Wright, P.J. (2006). The roles of progestagen and uterine irritant in the maintenance of cystic endometrial hyperplasia in the canine uterus. *Theriogenology* 66: 1537–1544.

52 Pretzer, S.D. (2008). Clinical presentation of canine pyometra and mucometra: a review. *Theriogenology* 70: 359–363.

53 Munson, L., Gardner, A., Mason, R.J. et al. (2002). Endometrial hyperplasia and mineralization in zoo felids treated with melengestrol acetate contraceptives. *Vet Pathol* 39: 419–427.

54 Freshman, J.L. (1991). Clinical approach to infertility in the cycling bitch. *Vet Clin North Am Small Anim Pract* 21: 427–435.

55 Fayrer-Hosken, R.A., Durham, D.H., Allen, S. et al. (1992). Follicular cystic ovaries and cystic endometrial hyperplasia in a bitch. *J Am Vet Med Assoc* 201: 107–108.

56 Patnaik, A.K. and Greenlee, P.G. (1987). Canine ovarian neoplasms: a clinicopathologic study of 71 cases, including histology of 12 granulosa cell tumors. *Vet Pathol* 24: 509–514.

57 Brazzell, J.L. and Borjesson, D.L. (2006). Intra-abdominal mass aspirate from an alopecic dog. *Vet Clin Pathol* 35: 259–262.

58 Dow, C. (1959). The cystic hyperplasia-pyometra complex in the bitch. *J Comp Pathol* 69: 237–250.

59 Batista-Arteaga, M., Santana, M., Espinosa-de-los-Monteros, A. et al. (2012). Exuberant mucometra associated with atresia of the cervix in a queen. *Reprod Domest Anim* 47: e71–e74.

60 Kunzel, F., Grinninger, P., Shibly, S. et al. (2015). Uterine disorders in 50 pet rabbits. *J Am Anim Hosp Assoc* 51: 8–14.

61 Ilha, M.R., Newman, S.J., van Amstel, S. et al. (2010). Uterine lesions in 32 female miniature pet pigs. *Vet Pathol* 47: 1071–1075.

62 Szulanczyk, K. (2009). Histological changes within ovarian cortex, oviductal and uterine mucosa in case of ovarian cysts presence in sows. *Folia Histochem Cytobiol* 47: 99–103.

63 Bennett, M.W., Dick, E.J. Jr., Schlabritz-Loutsevitch, N.E. et al. (2009). Endometrial and cervical polyps in 22 baboons (*Papio* sp.), 5 cynomolgus macaques (*Macaca fascicularis*) and one marmoset (*Callithrix jacchus*). *J Med Primatol* 38: 257–262.

64 Kaspareit, J., Friderichs-Gromoll, S., Buse, E., and Habermann, G. (2007). Spontaneous neoplasms observed in cynomolgus monkeys (*Macaca fascicularis*) during a 15-year period. *Exp Toxicol Pathol* 59: 163–169.

65 Arifin, E., Shively, C.A., Register, T.C., and Cline, J.M. (2008). Polycystic ovary syndrome with endometrial hyperplasia in a cynomolgus monkey (*Macaca fascicularis*). *Vet Pathol* 45: 512–515.

66 Baskin, G.B., Smith, S.M., and Marx, P.A. (2002). Endometrial hyperplasia, polyps, and adenomyosis associated with unopposed estrogen in rhesus monkeys (*Macaca mulatta*). *Vet Pathol* 39: 572–575.

67 Hermes, R., Hildebrandt, T.B., Walzer, C. et al. (2006). The effect of long non-reproductive periods on the genital health in captive female white rhinoceroses (*Ceratotherium simum simum, C.s. cottoni*). *Theriogenology* 65: 1492–1515.

68 Agnew, D.W., Munson, L., and Ramsay, E.C. (2004). Cystic endometrial hyperplasia in elephants. *Vet Pathol* 41: 179–183.

69 Granson, H., Carr, A., Parker, D., and Davies, J.L. (2011). Cystic endometrial hyperplasia and chronic endometritis in a chinchilla. *J Am Vet Med Assoc* 239: 233–236.

70 Jekl, V., Hauptman, K., Jeklova, E. et al. (2006). Hydrometra in a ferret-case report. *Vet Clin North Am Exot Anim Pract* 9: 695–700.

71 Napier, J.E., Caron, S., Reavill, D.R. et al. (2009). Proliferative endometrial lesions in a group of Seba's short-tailed bats (*Carollia perspicillata*). *J Zoo Wildl Med* 40: 437–444.

72 Schulman, M.L., Kirberger, R.M., Tordiffe, A.S. et al. (2015). Ultrasonographic and laparoscopic evaluation of the reproductive tract in older captive female cheetahs (*Acinonyx jubatus*). *Theriogenology* 84: 1611–1619.

73 Radi, Z.A. (2005). Endometritis and cystic endometrial hyperplasia in a goat. *J Vet Diagn Invest* 17: 393–395.

74 Agudelo, C.F. (2005). Cystic endometrial hyperplasia-pyometra complex in cats. A review. *Vet Q* 27: 173–182.

75 Schlafer, D.H. and Gifford, A.T. (2008). Cystic endometrial hyperplasia, pseudo-placentational endometrial hyperplasia, and other cystic conditions of the canine and feline uterus. *Theriogenology* 70: 349–358.

76 Sato, Y. (2011). Pseudo-placentational endometrial hyperplasia in a dog. *J Vet Diagn Invest* 23: 1071–1074.

77 Marino, G., Barna, A., Rizzo, S. et al. (2013). Endometrial polyps in the bitch: a retrospective study of 21 cases. *J Comp Pathol* 149: 410–416.

78 Gumber, S., Springer, N., and Wakamatsu, N. (2010). Uterine endometrial polyp with severe hemorrhage and cystic endometrial hyperplasia-pyometra complex in a dog. *J Vet Diagn Invest* 22: 455–458.

79 Gelberg, H.B. and McEntee, K. (1984). Hyperplastic endometrial polyps in the dog and cat. *Vet Pathol* 21: 570–573.

80 Yamini, B. and Borg, L. (1994). Endometrial polyps and endometritis in a thoroughbred filly. *J Vet Diagn Invest* 6: 496–498.

81 Mikaelian, I., Reavill, D.R., and Practice, A. (2004). Spontaneous proliferative lesions and tumors of the uterus of captive African hedgehogs (*Atelerix albiventris*). *J Zoo Wildl Med* 35: 216–220.

82 Gelberg, H.B. and McEntee, K. (1986). Pathology of the canine and feline uterine tube. *Vet Pathol* 23: 770–775.

83 Tamada, H., Kawate, N., Inaba, T. et al. (2005). Adenomyosis with severe inflammation in the uterine cervix in a dog. *Can Vet J* 46: 333–334.

84 Stocklin-Gautschi, N.M., Guscetti, F., Reichler, I.M. et al. (2001). Identification of focal adenomyosis as a uterine lesion in two dogs. *J Small Anim Pract* 42: 413–416.

85 Dawood, K.E. (2010). Pathological abnormalities of the reproductive tracts of ewes in Basra, Iraq. *Vet Rec* 166: 205–207.

86 Graham, K.J., Hulst, F.A., Vogelnest, L. et al. (2009). Uterine adenomyosis in an orang-utan (*Pongo abelii/pygmaeus*). *Aust Vet J* 87: 66–69.

87 Arnold, S., Hubler, M., Hauser, B. et al. (1996). Uterine serosal inclusion cysts in a bitch. *J Small Anim Pract* 37: 235–237.

88 Godfrey, D.R. and Silkstone, M.A. (1998). Uterine serosal inclusion cysts in a cat. *Vet Rec* 142: 673.

89 Hanada, M., Maeda, Y., and Oikawa, M.A. (2014). Histopathological characteristics of endometrosis in thoroughbred mares in Japan: results from 50 necropsy cases. *J Equine Sci* 25: 45–52.

90 Orfanou, D.C., Ververidis, H.N., Pourlis, A. et al. (2009). Post-partum involution of the canine uterus: gross anatomical and histological features. *Reprod Domest Anim* 44 (2): 152–155.

91 McIntyre, R.L., Levy, J.K., Roberts, J.F., and Reep, R.L. (2010). Developmental uterine anomalies in cats and dogs undergoing elective ovariohysterectomy. *J Am Vet Med Assoc* 237: 542–546.

92 Bartel, C., Berghold, P., and Walter, I. (2011). Ectopic endometrial tissue in mesonephric duct remnants in bitches. *Reprod Domest Anim* 46: 950–956.

93 Hussein, H.A. (2013). Validation of color Doppler ultrasonography for evaluating the uterine blood flow and perfusion during late normal pregnancy and uterine torsion in buffaloes. *Theriogenology* 79: 1045–1053.

94 Ali, A., Derar, D., Tharwat, M. et al. (2016). Dystocia in dromedary camels: prevalence, forms, risks and hematobiochemical changes. *Anim Reprod Sci* 170: 149–156.

95 Anderson, D.E. (2009). Uterine torsion and cesarean section in llamas and alpacas. *Vet Clin North Am Food Anim Pract* 25: 523–538.

96 Mock, T., Hehenberger, E., Steiner, A. et al. (2015). Uterine torsion in Brown Swiss cattle: retrospective analysis from an alpine practice in Switzerland. *Vet Rec* 177: 152.

97 Yorke, E.H., Caldwell, F.J., and Johnson, A.K. (2012). Uterine torsion in mares. *Compend Contin Educ Vet* 34: E2.

98 Aubry, P., Warnick, L.D., DesCoteaux, L., and Bouchard, E. (2008). A study of 55 field cases of uterine torsion in dairy cattle. *Can Vet J* 49: 366–372.

99 Murakami, T., Nakao, S., Sato, Y. et al. (2017). Blood lactate concentration as diagnostic predictors of uterine necrosis and its outcome in dairy cows with uterine torsion. *J Vet Med Sci* 79: 513–516.

100 Miller, B.A., Brounts, S.H., Anderson, D.E., and Devine, E. (2013). Cesarean section in alpacas and llamas: 34 cases (1997–2010). *J Am Vet Med Assoc* 242: 670–674.

101 Darvelid, A.W. and Linde-Forsberg, C. (1994). Dystocia in the bitch: a retrospective study of 182 cases. *J Small Anim Pract* 35: 402–407.

102 Barrand, K.R. (2009). Unilateral uterine torsion associated with haematometra and cystic endometrial hyperplasia in a bitch. *Vet Rec* 164: 19–20.

103 Chambers, B., Laksito, M., Long, F., and Yates, G. (2011). Unilateral uterine torsion secondary to an inflammatory endometrial polyp in the bitch. *Aust Vet J* 89: 380–384.

104 Miller, M.A., Ramos-Vara, J.A., Dickerson, M.F. et al. (2003). Uterine neoplasia in 13 cats. *J Vet Diagn Invest* 15: 515–522.

105 Brodey, R.S. and Roszel, J.F. (1967). Neoplasms of the canine uterus, vagina, and vulva: a clinicopathologic survey of 90 cases. *J Am Vet Med Assoc* 151: 1294–1307.

106 Cotchin, E. (1964). Spontaneous uterine cancer in animals. *Br J Cancer* 18: 209–227.

107 Saba, C.F. and Lawrence, J.A. (2013). Tumors of the female reproductive system. In: *Withrow and MacEwen's Small Animal Clinical Oncology*, 5e (eds. S.J. Withrow, D.M. Vail and R.L. Page), 532–537. Saint Louis, MO: W.B. Saunders.

108 Tsioli, V.G., Gouletsou, P.G., Loukopoulos, P. et al. (2011). Uterine leiomyosarcoma and pyometra in a dog. *J Small Anim Pract* 52: 121–124.

109 Lingaas, F., Comstock, K.E., Kirkness, E.F. et al. (2003). A mutation in the canine BHD gene is associated with hereditary multifocal renal cystadenocarcinoma and nodular dermatofibrosis in the German Shepherd dog. *Hum Mol Genet* 12: 3043–3053.

110 Lium, B. and Moe, L. (1985). Hereditary multifocal renal cystadenocarcinomas and nodular dermatofibrosis in the German Shepherd dog: macroscopic and histopathologic changes. *Vet Pathol* 22: 447–455.

111 Pilny, A. (2014). Ovarian cystic disease in guinea pigs. *Vet Clin North Am Exot Anim Pract* 17: 69–75.

112 Walter, B., Poth, T., Bohmer, E. et al. (2010). Uterine disorders in 59 rabbits. *Vet Rec* 166: 230–233.

113 Munday, J.S. and Stedman, N.L. (2002). Uterine leiomyomas in two Vietnamese pot-bellied pigs (*Sus scrofa*). *Vet Pathol* 39: 580–583.

114 Cypher, E., Videla, R., Pierce, R. et al. (2017). Clinical prevalence and associated intraoperative surgical complications of reproductive tract lesions in pot-bellied pigs undergoing ovariohysterectomy: 298 cases (2006–2016). *Vet Rec* 181: 685.

115 Akkermans, J.P. and van Beusekom, W.J. (1984). Tumors and tumor-like lesions in the genitalia of sows. *Vet Q* 6: 90–96.

116 Field, K.J., Griffith, J.W., and Lang, C.M. (1989). Spontaneous reproductive tract leiomyomas in aged guinea-pigs. *J Comp Pathol* 101: 287–294.

117 Lowenstine, L.J., McManamon, R., and Terio, K.A. (2016). Comparative pathology of aging great apes: bonobos, chimpanzees, gorillas, and orangutans. *Vet Pathol* 53: 250–276.

118 Smith, L.N., Rotstein, D.S., Ball, R.L. et al. (2015). Reproductive neoplasms in wild and long-term captive female Florida manatees (*Trichechus manatus latirostris*). *J Zoo Wildl Med* 46: 895–903.

119 Van Bressem, M.F., Van Waerebeek, K., Siebert, U. et al. (2000). Genital diseases in the peruvian dusky dolphin (*Lagenorhynchus obscurus*). *J Comp Pathol* 122: 266–277.

120 Munson, L. (1993). Diseases of captive cheetahs (*Acinonyx jubatus*): results of the cheetah research council pathology survey, 1989–1992. *Zoo Biol* 12: 105–124.

121 Junginger, J., Hansmann, F., Herder, V. et al. (2015). Pathology in captive wild felids at German zoological gardens. *PLoS One* 10: e0130573.

122 Done, L.B., Deem, S.L., and Fiorello, C.V. (2007). Surgical and medical management of a uterine spindle

cell tumor in an African hedgehog (*Atelerix albiventris*). *J Zoo Wildl Med* 38: 601–603.
123 Hubbard, G.B., Mahaney, M.C., Gleiser, C.A. et al. (1997). Spontaneous pathology of the gray short-tailed opossum (*Monodelphis domestica*). *Lab Anim Sci* 47: 19–26.
124 Bredhult, C., Backlin, B.M., Bignert, A., and Olovsson, M. (2008). Study of the relation between the incidence of uterine leiomyomas and the concentrations of PCB and DDT in Baltic gray seals. *Reprod Toxicol* 25: 247–255.
125 Backlin, B.M., Eriksson, L., and Olovsson, M. (2003). Histology of uterine leiomyoma and occurrence in relation to reproductive activity in the Baltic gray seal (*Halichoerus grypus*). *Vet Pathol* 40: 175–180.
126 Papparella, S. and Roperto, F. (1984). Spontaneous uterine tumors in three cats. *Vet Pathol* 21: 257–258.
127 Chambers, J.K., Uchida, K., Ise, K., and Nakayama, H. (2014). Cystic rete ovarii and uterine tube adenoma in a rabbit. *J Vet Med Sci* 76: 909–912.
128 Marino, G., Quartuccio, M., Cristarella, S. et al. (2007). Adenoma of the uterine tube in the bitch: two case reports. *Vet Res Commun* 31 (Suppl 1): 173–175.
129 Elsinghorst, T.A., Timmermans, H.J., and Hendriks, H.G. (1984). Comparative pathology of endometrial carcinoma. *Vet Q* 6: 200–208.
130 Dukes, T.W., Bundza, A., and Corner, A.H. (1982). Bovine neoplasms encountered in Canadian slaughterhouses: a summary. *Can Vet J* 23: 28–30.
131 Sommerville, L.M. (1998). Treatment of a uterine adenocarcinoma in a domestic rabbit by ovariohysterectomy. *Vet Rec* 142: 550–551.
132 Pires, M.A., Seixas, F., Palmeira, C., and Payan-Carreira, R. (2010). Histopathologic and immunohistochemical exam in one case of canine endometrial adenocarcinoma. *Reprod Domest Anim* 45: 545–549.
133 Pena, F.J., Gines, J.A., Duque, J. et al. (2006). Endometrial adenocarcinoma and mucometra in a 6-year-old Alaska Malamute dog. *Reprod Domest Anim* 41: 189–190.
134 Cave, T.A., Hine, R., Howie, F. et al. (2002). Uterine carcinoma in a 10-month-old Golden Retriever. *J Small Anim Pract* 43: 133–135.
135 Choi, U.S. (2013). A case of uterine adenocarcinoma in a spayed female dog. *Korean J Clin Vet Med* 30: 53–56.
136 Hyang Mi, C., Hyun Wook, K., Hye Jin, K. et al. (2011). A case of canine uterine adenocarcinoma with negative estrogen and progesterone receptor expression. *J Vet Clin* 28: 303–306.
137 Gil da Costa, R.M., Santos, M., Amorim, I. et al. (2009). An immunohistochemical study of feline endometrial adenocarcinoma. *J Comp Pathol* 140: 254–259.
138 Payan-Carreira, R., Saraiva, A.L., Santos, T. et al. (2013). Feline endometrial adenocarcinoma in females <1 year old: a description of four cases. *Reprod Domest Anim* 48: e70–e77.
139 Cooper, T.K., Ronnett, B.M., Ruben, D.S., and Zink, M.C. (2006). Uterine myxoid leiomyosarcoma with widespread metastases in a cat. *Vet Pathol* 43: 552–556.
140 Harmon, B.G., Munday, J.S., and Crane, M.M. (2004). Diffuse cystic endometrial hyperplasia and metastatic endometrial adenocarcinoma in a vietnamese pot-bellied pig (*Sus scrofa*). *J Vet Diagn Invest* 16: 587–589.
141 Cannon, C.Z., Godfrey, V.L., King-Herbert, A., and Nielsen, J.N. (2009). Metastatic uterine adenocarcinoma in an 8-year-old gilt. *J Am Assoc Lab Anim Sci* 48: 795–800.
142 Dockweiler, J.C., Cossic, B., McDonough, S.P. et al. (2017). Tumor collision of uterine adenocarcinoma and leiomyosarcoma in a goat. *J Vet Diagn Invest* 29: 696–699.
143 Klopfleisch, R., van der Grinten, E., and Gruber, A.D. (2009). Metastatic uterine adenocarcinoma and hepatic lipomatosis in a llama (*Lama glama*). *J Vet Diagn Invest* 21: 280–282.
144 Thompson, R., Armien, A.G., Rasmussen, J.M., and Wolf, T.M. (2014). Uterine adenocarcinoma in a Przewalski's wild horse (*Equus ferus przewalskii*). *J Zoo Wildl Med* 45: 441–445.
145 Duncan, C., Powers, J., Davis, T., and Spraker, T. (2007). Abomasal and uterine adenocarcinomas with ovarian metastasis in a captive elk (*Cervus elaphus nelsoni*). *J Vet Diagn Invest* 19: 560–563.
146 Robert, N. and Posthaus, H. (1999). Uterine adenocarcinoma in a captive sika deer. *J Wildl Dis* 35: 141–144.
147 Wilson, M., Hermes, R., Bainbridge, J., and Bassett, H. (2010). A case of metastatic uterine adenocarcinoma in a southern white rhinoceros (*Ceratotherium simum simum*). *J Zoo Wildl Med* 41: 111–114.
148 Lair, S., De Guise, S., and Martineau, D. (1998). Uterine adenocarcinoma with abdominal carcinomatosis in a beluga whale. *J Wildl Dis* 34: 373–376.
149 Sanchez, J., Kuba, L., Beron-Vera, B. et al. (2002). Uterine adenocarcinoma with generalised metastasis in a bottlenose dolphin *Tursiops truncatus* from northern Patagonia, Argentina. *Dis Aquat Org* 48: 155–159.
150 Linnehan, R.M., Edwards, J.L., and Edwards, J.L. (1991). Endometrial adenocarcinoma in a Bengal Tiger (*Panthera tigris bengalensis*) implanted with melengestrol acetate. *J Zoo Wildl Med* 22: 130–134.
151 Chittick, E., Rotstein, D., Brown, T., and Wolfe, B. (2001). Pyometra and uterine adenocarcinoma in a

melengestrol acetate-implanted captive coati (*Nasua nasua*). *J Zoo Wildl Med* 32: 245–251.
152 Olias, P., Schulz, E., Ehlers, B. et al. (2012). Metastatic endocervical adenocarcinoma in a western lowland gorilla (*Gorilla g. gorilla*): no evidence of virus-induced carcinogenesis. *J Med Primatol* 41: 142–146.
153 Stringer, E.M., De Voe, R.S., Valea, F. et al. (2010). Medical and surgical management of reproductive neoplasia in two western lowland gorillas (*Gorilla gorilla gorilla*). *J Med Primatol* 39: 328–335.
154 Frazier, K.S., Hines, M.E., Ruiz, C. et al. (1994). Immunohistochemical differentiation of multiple metastatic neoplasia in a jaguar (*Panthera onca*). *J Zoo Wildl Med* 25: 286–293.
155 Burton, A.J., Nydam, D.V., Long, E.D., and Divers, T.J. (2010). Signalment and clinical complaints initiating hospital admission, methods of diagnosis, and pathological findings associated with bovine lymphosarcoma (112 cases). *J Vet Intern Med* 24: 960–964.
156 Tanaka, H., Takai, H., Sato, K. et al. (2003). Nodal, uterine and meningeal gamma(delta) T-cell lymphomas in cattle. *J Vet Med A Physiol Pathol Clin Med* 50: 447–451.
157 Ko, J.S., Kim, H.J., Han, S., and Do, S.H. (2013). Primary lymphoma of the uterine horn in a Lhasa Apso dog. *Ir Vet J* 66: 24.
158 Novotny, L., Taylor, F., Claxton, K. et al. (2017). Uterine B-cell lymphoma in two dogs: a case report. *Acta Vet Brno* 86: 195–198.
159 Azakami, D., Onozawa, E., Miyabe, M. et al. (2016). Primary T-cell high-grade lymphoma of the feline uterus. *J Vet Med Sci* 78: 913–916.
160 Conversy, B., Freulon, A.L., and Graille, M. (2017). Focal uterine T-cell lymphoma in an ovariectomized cat. *J Am Vet Med Assoc* 251: 1059–1063.
161 Canisso, I.F., Pinn, T.L., Gerdin, J.A. et al. (2013). B-cell multicentric lymphoma as a probable cause of abortion in a Quarter horse broodmare. *Can Vet J* 54: 288–291.
162 Bae, I.H., Kim, Y., Pakhrin, B. et al. (2007). Genitourinary rhabdomyosarcoma with systemic metastasis in a young dog. *Vet Pathol* 44: 518–520.
163 Fukui, K. and Matsuda, H. (1983). Uterine haemangioma in a cat. *Vet Rec* 113: 375.
164 Haddad, J.L., Dick, E.J. Jr., Guardado-Mendoza, R., and Hubbard, G.B. (2009). Spontaneous squamous cell carcinomas in 13 baboons, a first report in a spider monkey, and a review of the non-human primate literature. *J Med Primatol* 38: 175–186.
165 Hayashi, A., Tanaka, H., Tajima, T. et al. (2013). A spayed female cat with squamous cell carcinoma in the uterine remnant. *J Vet Med Sci* 75: 391–393.
166 Ferrer, L.M., Lacasta, D., Ramos, J.J. et al. (2011). Squamous cell carcinoma of the vagina and cervix in sheep: case report. *Acta Vet Hung* 59: 123–127.
167 Hirata, A., Miyazaki, A., Sakai, H. et al. (2014). Choriocarcinoma-like tumor in a potbellied pig (*Sus scrofa*). *J Vet Diagn Invest* 26: 163–166.
168 Kaufmann-Bart, M. and Fischer, I. (2008). Choriocarcinoma with metastasis in a rabbit (*Oryctolagus cuniculi*). *Vet Pathol* 45: 77–79.
169 Causey, R.C. (2006). Making sense of equine uterine infections: the many faces of physical clearance. *Vet J* 172: 405–421.
170 Gygax, A.P., Ganjam, V.K., and Kenney, R.M. (1979). Clinical, microbiological and histological changes associated with uterine involution in the mare. *J Reprod Fertil Suppl* 27: 571–578.
171 Evans, M.J., Hamer, J.M., Gason, L.M. et al. (1986). Clearance of bacteria and non-antigenic markers following intra-uterine inoculation into maiden mares: effect of steroid hormone environment. *Theriogenology* 26: 37–50.
172 LeBlanc, M.M., Neuwirth, L., Jones, L. et al. (1998). Differences in uterine position of reproductively normal mares and those with delayed uterine clearance detected by scintigraphy. *Theriogenology* 50: 49–54.
173 Troedsson, M.H., Liu, I.K., Ing, M. et al. (1993). Multiple site electromyography recordings of uterine activity following an intrauterine bacterial challenge in mares susceptible and resistant to chronic uterine infection. *J Reprod Fertil* 99: 307–313.
174 Williamson, P., Munyua, S., Martin, R., and Penhale, W.J. (1987). Dynamics of the acute uterine response to infection, endotoxin infusion and physical manipulation of the reproductive tract in the mare. *J Reprod Fertil Suppl* 35: 317–325.
175 Katila, T., Lock, T.F., and Smith, A.R. (1984). Uterine changes and fertility of mares after an induced streptococcal endometritis. *Proceedings of 10th International Congress on Animal Reproduction and Artificial Insemination*, Urbana-Champaign, IL (10–14 June 1984); III: 452a.
176 LeBlanc, M.M. and Causey, R.C. (2009). Clinical and subclinical endometritis in the mare: both threats to fertility. *Reprod Domest Anim* 44 (Suppl 3): 10–22.
177 Leblanc, M.M. (2011). Uterine cytology. In: *Equine Reproduction*, 2e (eds. A.O. McKinnon, E.L. Squires, W.E. Vaala and D.D. Varner), 1922–1928. Oxford: Wiley-Blackwell.
178 Goldman, E.E., Grindem, C.B., McDorman, K.S., and Van Camp, S. (1998). Uterine fluid from a mare. *Vet Clin Pathol* 27: 15.

179 Lu, K.G. and Morresey, P.R. (2006). Reproductive tract infections in horses. *Vet Clin North Am Equine Pract* 22: 519–552.

180 Ferris, R.A., Dern, K., Veir, J.K. et al. (2013). Development of a broad-range quantitative polymerase chain reaction assay to detect and identify fungal DNA in equine endometrial samples. *Am J Vet Res* 74: 161–165.

181 Beltaire, K.A., Cheong, S.H., and Coutinho da Silva, M.A. (2012). Retrospective study on equine uterine fungal isolates and antifungal susceptibility patterns (1999–2011). *Equine Vet J Suppl* 43: 84–87.

182 Hussain, A.M. (1989). Bovine uterine defense mechanisms: a review. *Zentralbl Veterinarmed B* 36: 641–651.

183 Hussain, A.M. and Daniel, R.C. (1991). Bovine endometritis: current and future alternative therapy. *Zentralbl Veterinarmed A* 38: 641–651.

184 Williams, E.J., Fischer, D.P., Pfeiffer, D.U. et al. (2005). Clinical evaluation of postpartum vaginal mucus reflects uterine bacterial infection and the immune response in cattle. *Theriogenology* 63: 102–117.

185 Sheldon, I.M., Lewis, G.S., LeBlanc, S., and Gilbert, R.O. (2006). Defining postpartum uterine disease in cattle. *Theriogenology* 65: 1516–1530.

186 Prunner, I., Pothmann, H., Wagener, K. et al. (2014). Dynamics of bacteriologic and cytologic changes in the uterus of postpartum dairy cows. *Theriogenology* 82: 1316–1322.

187 Borsberry, S. and Dobson, H. (1989). Periparturient diseases and their effect on reproductive performance in five dairy herds. *Vet Rec* 124: 217–219.

188 LeBlanc, S.J., Duffield, T.F., Leslie, K.E. et al. (2002). Defining and diagnosing postpartum clinical endometritis and its impact on reproductive performance in dairy cows. *J Dairy Sci* 85: 2223–2236.

189 Gobikrushanth, M., Salehi, R., Ambrose, D.J., and Colazo, M.G. (2016). Categorization of endometritis and its association with ovarian follicular growth and ovulation, reproductive performance, dry matter intake, and milk yield in dairy cattle. *Theriogenology* 86: 1842–1849.

190 Krogh, M.A. and Enevoldsen, C. (2014). Evaluation of effects of metritis management in a complex dairy herd health management program. *J Dairy Sci* 97: 552–561.

191 Sheldon, I.M., Noakes, D.E., Rycroft, A.N. et al. (2002). Influence of uterine bacterial contamination after parturition on ovarian dominant follicle selection and follicle growth and function in cattle. *Reproduction* 123: 837–845.

192 Plontzke, J., Madoz, L.V., De la Sota, R.L. et al. (2010). Subclinical endometritis and its impact on reproductive performance in grazing dairy cattle in Argentina. *Anim Reprod Sci* 122: 52–57.

193 Potter, T.J., Guitian, J., Fishwick, J. et al. (2010). Risk factors for clinical endometritis in postpartum dairy cattle. *Theriogenology* 74: 127–134.

194 Bondurant, R.H. (1999). Inflammation in the bovine female reproductive tract. *J Anim Sci* 77 (Suppl 2): 101–110.

195 Noakes, D.E., Wallace, L., and Smith, G.R. (1991). Bacterial flora of the uterus of cows after calving on two hygienically contrasting farms. *Vet Rec* 128: 440–442.

196 Cheong, S.H., Nydam, D.V., Galvao, K.N. et al. (2011). Cow-level and herd-level risk factors for subclinical endometritis in lactating Holstein cows. *J Dairy Sci* 94: 762–770.

197 Gautam, G., Nakao, T., Yusuf, M., and Koike, K. (2009). Prevalence of endometritis during the postpartum period and its impact on subsequent reproductive performance in two Japanese dairy herds. *Anim Reprod Sci* 116: 175–187.

198 Sheldon, I.M. and Noakes, D.E. (1998). Comparison of three treatments for bovine endometritis. *Vet Rec* 142: 575–579.

199 Ahmadi, M.R., Tafti, A.K., Nazifi, S. et al. (2005). The comparative evaluation of uterine and cervical mucosa cytology with endometrial histopathology in cows. *Comp Clin Pathol* 14: 90–94.

200 Moscuzza, C., Alvarez, G., Gutierrez, B. et al. (2015). Endometrial cytology as a diagnostic tool for subclinical endometritis in beef heifers. *Turk J Vet Anim Sci* 39: 34–41.

201 Couto, G.B., Vaillancourt, D.H., and Lefebvre, R.C. (2013). Comparison of a leukocyte esterase test with endometrial cytology for diagnosis of subclinical endometritis in postpartum dairy cows. *Theriogenology* 79: 103–107.

202 Giuliodori, M.J., Magnasco, R.P., Becu-Villalobos, D. et al. (2013). Metritis in dairy cows: risk factors and reproductive performance. *J Dairy Sci* 96: 3621–3631.

203 Sheldon, I.M. and Dobson, H. (2004). Postpartum uterine health in cattle. *Anim Reprod Sci* 82–83: 295–306.

204 Horowitz, G.L. (2008). *Defining, Establishing, and Verifying Reference Intervals in the Clinical Laboratory: Approved Guideline*, 3e. Wayne, PA: Clinical and Laboratory Standards Institute.

205 Drillich, M., Beetz, O., Pfutzner, A. et al. (2001). Evaluation of a systemic antibiotic treatment of toxic puerperal metritis in dairy cows. *J Dairy Sci* 84: 2010–2017.

206 Markusfeld, O. (1987). Periparturient traits in seven high dairy herds. Incidence rates, association with parity, and interrelationships among traits. *J Dairy Sci* 70: 158–166.

207 Alosta, R.A., Vaughan, L., and Collins, J.D. (1998). An abattoir survey of ovine reproductive tracts in Ireland. *Theriogenology* 50: 457–464.

208 Cantero, A., Sancha, J.L., Flores, J.M. et al. (1996). Histopathological changes in the reproductive organs of Manchego ewes grazing on lucerne. *Zentralbl Veterinarmed A* 43: 325–330.

209 Adams, N.R. (1973). Relationship between uterine cysts and ovarian activity in Western Australian ewes. *Aust Vet J* 49: 176.

210 Tomlinson, L., Barker, I.K., Foster, R.A. et al. (2000). Naturally occurring lesions of the uterine tube in sheep and serologic evidence of exposure to *Chlamydophila abortus*. *Can J Vet Res* 64: 229–231.

211 Ali, A., Derar, R., Al-Sobayil, F. et al. (2015). A retrospective study on clinical findings of 7300 cases (2007–2014) of barren female dromedaries. *Theriogenology* 84: 452–456.

212 Powers, B.E., Johnson, L.W., Linton, L.B. et al. (1990). Endometrial biopsy technique and uterine pathologic findings in llamas. *J Am Vet Med Assoc* 197: 1157–1162.

213 Mshelia, G.D., Okpaje, G., Voltaire, Y.A., and Egwu, G.O. (2014). Comparative studies on genital infections and antimicrobial susceptibility patterns of isolates from camels (*Camelus dromedarius*) and cows (*Bos indicus*) in Maiduguri, north-eastern Nigeria. *Springerplus* 3: 91.

214 Gifford, A.T., Scarlett, J.M., and Schlafer, D.H. (2014). Histopathologic findings in uterine biopsy samples from subfertile bitches: 399 cases (1990–2005). *J Am Vet Med Assoc* 244: 180–186.

215 Fukuda, S. (2001). Incidence of pyometra in colony-raised beagle dogs. *Exp Anim* 50: 325–329.

216 Asa, C.S., Bauman, K.L., Devery, S. et al. (2014). Factors associated with uterine endometrial hyperplasia and pyometra in wild canids: implications for fertility. *Zoo Biol* 33: 8–19.

217 Egenvall, A., Hagman, R., Bonnett, B.N. et al. (2001). Breed risk of pyometra in insured dogs in Sweden. *J Vet Intern Med* 15: 530–538.

218 Enginler, S.O., Ates, A., Diren Sigirci, B. et al. (2014). Measurement of C-reactive protein and prostaglandin F2alpha metabolite concentrations in differentiation of canine pyometra and cystic endometrial hyperplasia/mucometra. *Reprod Domest Anim* 49: 641–647.

219 Fransson, B., Lagerstedt, A.S., Hellmen, E., and Jonsson, P. (1997). Bacteriological findings, blood chemistry profile and plasma endotoxin levels in bitches with pyometra or other uterine diseases. *Zentralbl Veterinarmed A* 44: 417–426.

220 Mateus, L., Henriques, S., Merino, C. et al. (2013). Virulence genotypes of *Escherichia coli* canine isolates from pyometra, cystitis and fecal origin. *Vet Microbiol* 166: 590–594.

221 Voorwald, F.A., Marchi, F.A., Villacis, R.A. et al. (2015). Molecular expression profile reveals potential biomarkers and therapeutic targets in canine endometrial lesions. *PLoS One* 10: e0133894.

222 von Reitzenstein, M., Archbald, L.F., and Newell, S.M. (2000). Theriogenology question of the month. Pyometra, hydrometra, or mucometra. *J Am Vet Med Assoc* 216: 1221–1223.

223 England, G.C., Russo, M., and Freeman, S.L. (2013). The bitch uterine response to semen deposition and its modification by male accessory gland secretions. *Vet J* 195: 179–184.

224 Ribeiro, A.P., Vicente, W.R., Apparicio, M. et al. (2006). Uterine leucocyte infiltration after artificial insemination in bitches. *Theriogenology* 66: 1462–1464.

44

Mammary Gland

Natalie Hoepp

Introduction

Canine and feline mammary glands are composed of paired, subcutaneous, compound tubuloalveolar glands, suspected to be modified sweat glands. Glands are composed of ductular and glandular (lobular) epithelium, myoepithelium, and surrounding stroma with connective tissue septa. Canines have five pairs, while felines typically have four, but some individual variation exists. They are arranged in tandem along the ventral abdomen from the cranial thorax to the inguinal region and designated cranial thoracic, caudal thoracic, cranial abdominal, caudal abdominal, and inguinal. Mare mammary glands are of similar composition and include four individual glands that are inguinal, within the udder, and paired (larger cranial gland, smaller caudal gland), with division by a midline septum. Mares, like cats, can also have variation in the number of glands present, some having six. Mammary masses are common in female dogs and cats and include neoplastic, hyperplastic, dysplastic, cystic, and inflammatory lesions that originate within the mammary tissue, are associated with metastasis of non-mammary neoplasms, or arise from surrounding skin. Differentiating cutaneous masses from primary mammary neoplasia, or in cats, hyperplasia versus neoplasia, is often an initial goal of fine-needle aspiration and cytologic evaluation. In the mare, fine-needle aspirate and evaluation of milk secretions are performed to differentiate mastitis from neoplasia. Mammary neoplasms in dogs frequently involve a heterogeneous cellular and matrix composition, with elements of mesenchymal and epithelial proliferation, stroma, matrix (that can be myxoid, chondroid, or osseous), inflammation, and surrounding fluid accumulation with macrophages. Multiple mammary masses are often present in dogs, with 50–60% presenting with more than one neoplastic type.[1] Additionally, gross appearance, clinical history (signalment, reproductive status), cytologic appearance, histologic diagnosis, and biologic behavior are all important determinants of malignant potential and therapeutic intervention. In feline and equine patients, mammary tumors tend to be homogenous and malignant, with the majority being carcinomas, specifically adenocarcinomas, thus simplifying microscopic evaluation of fine-needle aspirate samples when compared with dogs.[2–6]

Mammary tumor incidence increases significantly in bitches who remain sexually intact or are spayed following the second estrus, and similarly, queens have an increased risk associated with delayed ovariohysterectomy.[3,7,8] This is due to hormone-driven development of mammary neoplasia in both species. The complex cellular composition of the mammary gland, susceptibility to hormonal influence, and variety of lesions encountered often necessitate biopsy with evaluation of tumor architecture and assessment of local stromal and lymphovascular invasiveness to determine final diagnosis and expected biologic behavior. Initial cytologic examination can provide useful differential diagnostic information to aid in determining additional testing and treatment planning, including collection of local or regional lymph node samples for staging prior to surgical intervention. Preliminary staging samples can be collected at the same time and submitted with mammary mass aspirates for greater diagnostic efficiency.

Collection

Collection of fine-needle aspirate samples from mammary neoplasms is similar to other cutaneous masses and has been thoroughly reviewed elsewhere (see Chapter 1).[9,10] Additionally, evaluation of mammary discharge can be performed and may yield sufficient cellularity for assessment of inflammation, as in mastitis,

Veterinary Cytology, First Edition. Edited by Leslie C. Sharkey, M. Judith Radin, and Davis Seelig.

or underlying neoplasia.[11] In canine mammary neoplasms, lesion heterogeneity warrants collection from more than one area of the mass to provide a representative sample.[12] Insertion of a 20–25 G needle, removal without exiting the skin and redirecting several times in a "woodpecker" method, are recommended, taking with care not to cause unnecessary hemorrhage and hemodilution of samples. Use of a smaller needle is recommended if the mass appears vascular or erythematous and likely to lead to hemorrhagic samples. A syringe with air drawn into it is attached to the needle, and the sample is gently expelled onto slides and spread with a coverslip or spreader slide. This method can be adjusted depending on clinician preference, gross appearance of the mass, and patient tolerance of sample acquisition, particularly in patients with surrounding areas of edema and inflammation. In canine patients, multiple masses with different cytologic composition are often present, necessitating evaluation of each mass individually for appropriate interpretation. Following preparation of slides, the sample is allowed to air-dry completely, without fixation by heat or fixative. Unstained, air-dried samples are preferred for submission to reference laboratories. Ensuring that samples have dried completely prior to transport avoids artifact changes, such as hemoglobin crystallization and cell disruption that can occur when slides are exposed to cold temperatures during air travel or winter months. Additionally, formalin-fixed tissue should be submitted separately to avoid formalin artifact, which may still occur due to formalin vapors despite tightly sealed biopsy containers being placed in plastic bags (see Chapter 50). Samples submitted to reference laboratories should include individually labeled slides, pertinent clinical information, signalment, reproductive status, and gross lesion descriptions.

Normal Cytologic Appearance

Normal mammary tissue does not exfoliate well, and fine-needle aspirate samples often lack cellularity; nonetheless, low numbers of ductular epithelial cells can be present.[13] Few vacuolated macrophages, neutrophils, lymphocytes, and uniform mesenchymal cells also can be seen depending on location aspirated and presence of secretory material. Exfoliated glandular secretory epithelium is uncommon and appears as cohesive clusters of round to polygonal cells with moderate amounts of basophilic to amphophilic cytoplasm and central round nuclei with coarsely stippled to condensed chromatin and indistinct nucleoli. Ductular epithelial cells have a higher nuclear to cytoplasmic ratio (N:C) with a more cuboidal appearance when intact and also lack atypia in the absence of hyperplasia or neoplasia. Evaluation of mammary secretions also is performed. In normal patients, secretory product is a combination of basophilic globular milk proteins, a homogenous basophilic proteinaceous background, lipid, low numbers of vacuolated macrophages, and a few lymphocytes and neutrophils.

Feline Mammary Hyperplasia and Neoplasia

Hyperplasia, Benign Tumors, and Mastitis

In cats, mammary neoplasms are the third most common tumor type and are almost exclusively seen in mature females, often with queens greater than 10 years of age.[14] Mammary neoplasia is rarely reported in males.[14] Malignant tumors are common, and simple carcinomas, of various subtypes, are most prevalent and often demonstrate lymphatic or vascular invasion.[8,14] Of the benign mammary proliferations in cats, fibroepithelial hyperplasia (also called fibroadenomatous hyperplasia, fibroadenomatous change, and feline mammary hypertrophy) is most common. Benign discrete adenomatous lesions (simple, complex, and fibroadenomas) and local areas of lobular, ductular, and fibrocystic hyperplasia also occur.[14] Cysts are rare in cats, and fibrocystic disease can be difficult to differentiate from the more common lobular hyperplasia in cats.[14,15] Adenomatous lesions are expected to have a similar cytologic appearance to adenomas in other locations, with a uniform population of round to slightly polygonal glandular epithelial cells lacking criteria of malignancy, while fibroepithelial hyperplasia has a distinct microscopic appearance (Figure 44.1) that includes epithelial cells, mesenchymal cells, and pink wispy matrix.[16,17] The mesenchymal cells are fusiform with scant to moderate amounts of basophilic cytoplasm, have round to ovoid nuclei with stippled chromatin and small nucleoli, and exhibit mild to moderate anisocytosis and anisokaryosis. The epithelial cells are associated with hyperplastic ductal epithelium, similar to ductal adenoma, and are expected to appear cytologically similar. The epithelial cells are seen in dense clusters, are round to polygonal, and often have indistinct cell borders. They have a scant to moderate amount of basophilic cytoplasm and round central nuclei with coarsely stippled to condensed chromatin and indistinct nucleoli. Overall, anisocytosis and anisokaryosis are mild, with more moderate variation possible.

Fibroepithelial hyperplasia is known to be progesterone dependent, with progesterone receptors demonstrated on

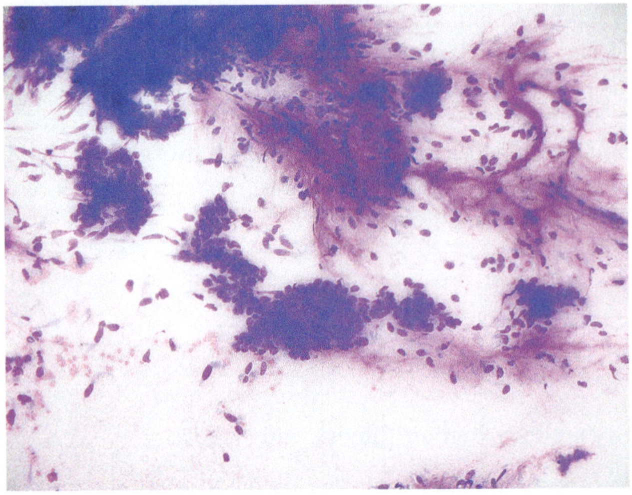

Figure 44.1 Fine-needle aspirate of fibroepithelial hyperplasia from a 10-month-old, nonpregnant female, domestic shorthair cat with acute onset of mammary gland swelling and multiple glands affected. The sample includes intact and disrupted mildly pleomorphic fusiform mesenchymal cells with aggregates of pink matrix and fragments of capillary endothelium (Wright's stain, 200×).

epithelial cells.[18–20] Fibroepithelial hyperplasia is primarily seen in young pregnant or actively cycling queens due to endogenous progesterone but also can occur in both male and female cats exposed to exogenous compounds containing progestins with or without estrogen combination (e.g. megestrol acetate).[21] Ovariohysterectomy or removal of exposure to hormone containing compounds should result in resolution. This condition has also been reported in male cats with and without known exposure to exogenous progesterone or evidence of reproductive neoplasia. Additional hormonal influence and interplay is suspected as part of the pathogenesis.[16,22] Clinical history is an important feature for evaluation of fine-needle aspirate samples from cats with suspected fibroepithelial hyperplasia, as this typically affects multiple glands and causes diffuse enlargement. This finding, combined with cytologic appearance (Figure 44.1) and microscopic exclusion of mastitis as a differential diagnosis, is often sufficient to obtain a presumptive diagnosis without the need for biopsy.

Mastitis in post-parturient queens is uncommon and occurs less frequently than in dogs. Mastitis may be septic, which is more common, or non-septic (associated with milk stasis). Bacterial infection can be ascending or hematogenous in origin and include bacterial isolates of *Escherichia coli*, *Staphylococcus* spp., or *Streptococcus* spp.[23,24] Mastitis can be localized or diffuse, involving one or multiple glands, with mild to systemic clinical signs, and lesions can include areas of necrosis and gangrene.[23,25] The cytologic appearance of milk or secretions is as expected for septic neutrophilic inflammation, with a predominance of degenerate neutrophils and lesser numbers of macrophages, foam cells (vacuolated epithelial cells resembling macrophages), and other leukocytes. Culture is warranted regardless of the presence or absence of bacteria on cytology, as most feline mastitis cases are associated with ascending bacterial infection, with *E. coli* being a frequent pathogen.

Malignant Mammary Tumors

With feline mammary neoplasms, determination of inflammatory or cutaneous versus neoplastic lesions is more likely to be the primary goal of cytologic examination, rather than determination of malignancy. Feline mammary neoplasms are commonly malignant, with histopathology required for confirmation prior to surgery. Chain mastectomy is the likely clinical sequel in feline mammary neoplasia, necessitating definitive diagnosis prior to radical surgery since prognosis may be poor regardless.

Malignant mammary tumors in the cat are often simple carcinomas and adenocarcinomas, with adenocarcinomas being more frequent.[3,14,26] Several histologic subtypes are described, including solid, tubulopapillary, and anaplastic. These tumors tend to be invasive, with infiltration of surrounding tissue and vessels, rapid growth, and metastasis. Noninvasive tumors (in situ) can occur but are uncommon.[5,8,14,27] The actual incidence of mammary neoplasia in cats is uncertain, as recent epidemiologic studies are lacking and literature sources often refer to a review of veterinary tumor types within two California counties that was reported in 1968.[28] In this reference, mammary tumors are reported to be the third most common neoplasm of cats, following cutaneous neoplasia and lymphoma, with an incidence of 17% of all neoplasms in queens. Additionally, spay and neuter practices vary between Europe and the United States, as well as geographically within the United States and among feline subpopulations, including purebred cats, which likely affect incidence rates. The cytologic appearance of feline mammary carcinomas has been described and are similar to carcinomas and adenocarcinomas in other locations, with cohesive clusters of rounded epithelial cells that have central to eccentric round nuclei, moderate amounts of cytoplasm with or without vacuolation, moderate to marked anisocytosis and anisokaryosis, and mitotic figures (Figures 44.2 and 44.3).[5,29,30] Areas of necrosis, inflammation, and fibrous stroma also can be present (Figures 44.4 and 44.5). While criteria of malignancy are expected in feline mammary carcinomas allowing for

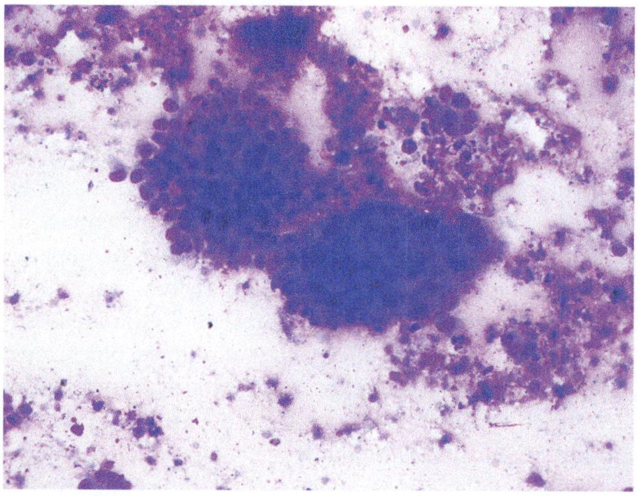

Figure 44.2 Fine-needle aspirate of a simple tubulopapillary mammary adenocarcinoma with necrosis and mixed inflammation from a 16-year-old, spayed female, domestic shorthair cat. She was spayed at an early age (not specified). In this field, cellular pleomorphism is limited, overlapping with adenomatous lesions (Wright's stain, 200×).

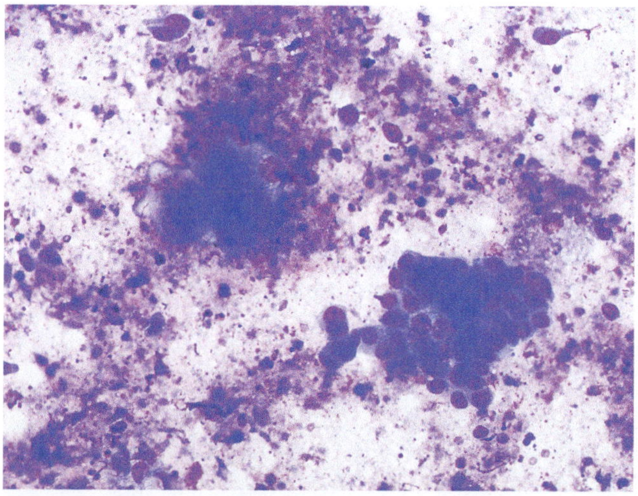

Figure 44.3 Fine-needle aspirate from the same patient in Figure 44.2. There is greater cellular atypia and more criteria of malignancy. These features may not be consistent throughout the epithelial population (Wright's stain, 200×).

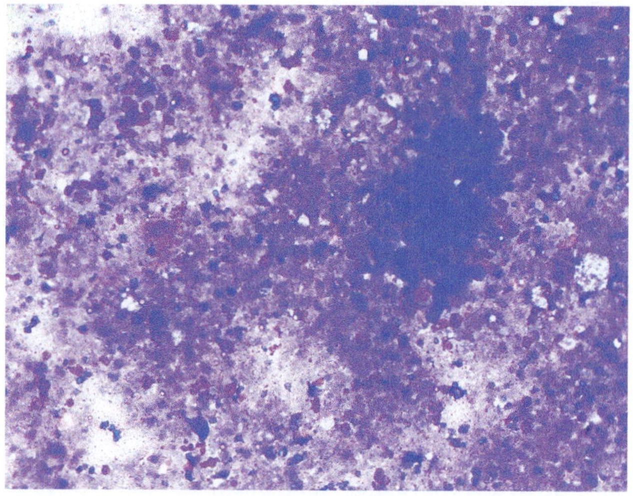

Figure 44.4 Fine-needle aspirate of a carcinoma from a 15-year-old spayed female domestic shorthair cat. The aspirate sample consists primarily of necrosis with lysed cells. Grossly, the mass was 3.0 × 1.5 cm, subcutaneous, and located in the caudal mammary gland per submission for cytologic exam, but was described as 2.5 × 2.0 cm, red, raised, and hairless in line with the mammary chain per biopsy submission. Mammary gland ductal origin was suspected, but cutaneous adnexal origin was not excluded by histopathologic examination (Wright's stain, 200×).

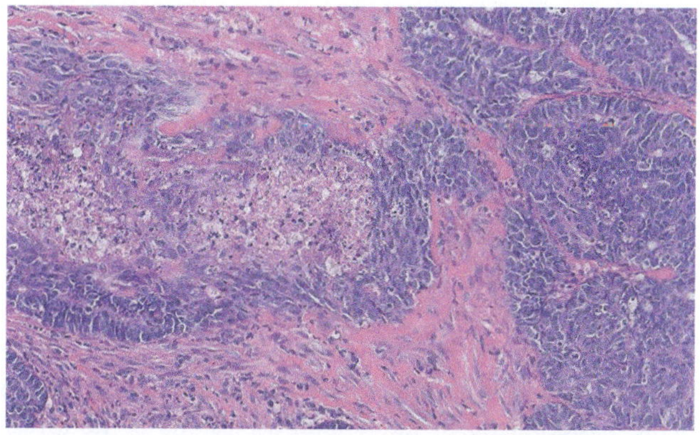

Figure 44.5 Biopsy sample from the same patient in Figure 44.4, demonstrating a central area of necrosis and inflammation that correlates with the appearance of the aspirate cytology. The necrotic area is surrounded by epithelial proliferation within fibrous stroma (hematoxylin & eosin, 400×).

initial suspicion of carcinoma and potential diagnosis based on cytology alone, the cytologic appearance has not been adequately compared with histopathologic findings in cats to allow for comparative conclusions regarding malignancy.[1] Also, some tumor types, including adenocarcinomas, can have limited criteria of malignancy and appear similar on cytology to adenomas (Figure 44.2). Given that most feline mammary neoplasms are histologically malignant and with tumor size being an important prognostic indicator,[4] biopsy is indicated and, depending on clinician preference and clinical suspicion, could be submitted postoperatively with the presumption of malignancy.[31]

Canine Mammary Hyperplasia and Neoplasia

Canine mammary masses represent a diverse group of hyperplastic, dysplastic, neoplastic, cystic, and inflammatory lesions, with combinations of these features, and simple to complex cellular and matrix composition. These features create a challenge for cytologic interpretation of this tumor type in dogs. With appropriate whole case evaluation, cytologic examination can be a useful initial diagnostic tool that is relatively noninvasive, often can be performed without sedation, and can be easily combined with local lymph node evaluation for preliminary staging purposes. In dogs, the majority of tumors will originate in the fourth (caudal abdominal) and fifth (inguinal) glands, potentially due to increased glandular tissue in these locations.[32] Unlike in feline patients, mature female dogs are equally likely to have benign or malignant mammary masses, with prevalence being roughly equivalent in most studies and anecdotally. Often dogs have more than one mass, and each mass can represent a different tumor type and malignant potential, depending on classification and evaluation of invasiveness. Several mammary neoplasia classification systems have been proposed for dogs. These include overlap of major categories with modifications of nomenclature based on increased understanding of biologic behavior, histogenesis, molecular markers, and descriptive characteristics.[14,33–37] For consistency, the classification proposed by Goldschmidt et al.[33] will be referenced and encompasses previously proposed systems. Emerging molecular markers are addressed separately at the end of this chapter and likely will be incorporated into future classification systems.

Hyperplasia, Dysplasia, and Mastitis

Hyperplasia of mammary epithelium is a normal physiologic response to pregnancy and lactation. The primary epithelial components of the canine mammary gland are ductular, lobular, and myoepithelial, with the former two being hyperplastic in adenomatous lesions of nonpregnant animals and the latter also proliferating in both benign and malignant complex tumor types. Ductular epithelium is simple cuboidal to columnar. Lobular epithelium (epithelium associated with clusters of alveoli creating lobules within the gland) is similarly cuboidal when not in a secretory phase, but varies in morphology with milk production. Vacuolated lobular epithelial cells can be seen in mammary secretions, appearing similar to macrophages, and have been referred to as "foam cells." Myoepithelium is associated with both cell types, often found between the epithelium and basement membrane. Masses due to hyperplasia and dysplasia can be discrete, adjacent to malignancy, or seen as a cellular continuum of malignant transformation, adding to the heterogeneity of mammary masses that are aspirated or collected for biopsy.[33,38]

Benign hyperplastic/dysplastic lesions include duct ectasia, which may have a cystic component, lobular hyperplasia/adenosis (regular, with secretory activity, with fibrosis, or with atypia), epitheliosis, papillomatosis, fibroadenomatous change, and gynecomastia.[33] On cytologic examination, these hyperplastic changes are expected to appear similar to benign neoplasms because they encompass the same cellular populations, including ductular, lobular, and myoepithelial cells. In some cases, a mesenchymal, inflammatory, or cystic component is present. Cystic areas and fluid accumulation are often noted on microscopic examination of mammary neoplasms or in areas of duct ectasia. Cytologically, this appears as a proteinaceous fluid background with an inflammatory cell population predominated by vacuolated macrophages containing phagocytosed cellular and secretory material (Figure 44.6). Neutrophilic inflammation can be seen, particularly if the mass has been traumatized by the patient or has keratinaceous material associated with squamous metaplasia that incites inflammation. Cholesterol crystals can also be present. These cytologic features can coincide with areas of necrosis as well.

Canine mastitis has overlapping clinical and cytologic features with mastitis in the cat and horse, but with a few species-specific variations. Similar to the queen, most canine cases occur during post-parturient lactation or pseudopregnancy as a result of ascending bacterial infection, often with *Staphylococcus pseudintermedius*. In the dog, mastitis can be acute or chronic, involve systemic signs (fever, enlarged painful glands), or be suspected based on neonatal puppies exhibiting failure to thrive, though bacteria isolated from mastitic glands do not

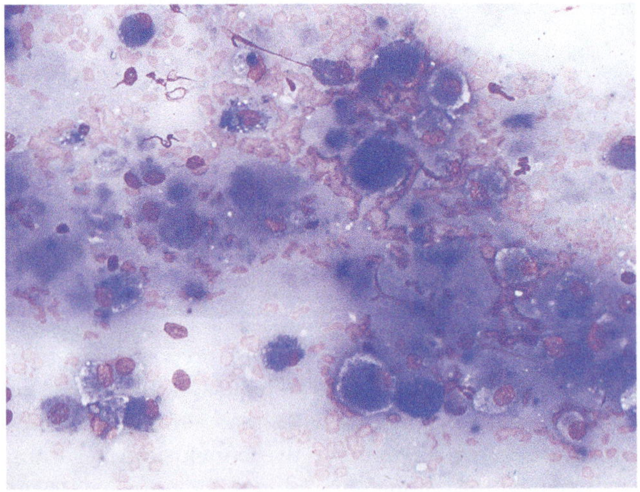

Figure 44.6 Secretory material from a canine benign mixed mammary tumor that includes macrophages containing phagocytosed blue-gray proteinaceous material, with darker aggregates that may be hemosiderin. This background appearance can be present in aspirates of a variety of mammary lesions (Wright's stain, 500×).

necessarily correlate with isolates from septic puppies.[39] As with other species, mastitis may be focal in a single gland, diffuse, or affect more than one gland. Hematogenous origin for infection is possible but uncommon, and as with cats, necrosis and ulceration of the overlying skin can occur, a feature not expected in the mare. Evaluation of milk secretions for evidence of neutrophilic inflammation, exfoliating neoplasia, or visible bacteria can be performed, followed by culture and sensitivity.[11]

Benign Tumors

Benign tumors in dogs include adenomas (simple, intraductal papillary, ductal, fibroadenoma, complex), fibroadenoma, myoepithelioma, and benign mixed tumor. Benign tumors tend to be small, firm, and well circumscribed compared with their more invasive, nodular, and inflammatory malignant counterparts. Most canine mammary tumors, whether benign or malignant, are mixed.[40] The "mixed" or "compound" terminology used within histopathologic classification schemes references the presence of osseous or chondroid metaplasia. The exception to this is malignant mixed mammary tumor, or carcinosarcoma, which is deemed a mixed tumor because it includes both malignant epithelial and malignant mesenchymal cell populations. Mixed tumors are different than "complex" tumor types. Complex tumors, including the complex adenoma, exhibit proliferation of two epithelial cell populations (epithelial, myoepithelial). While this includes benign complex adenomas, complex tumors that are malignant include proliferation of malignant epithelial and benign myoepithelial populations. Myoepithelial cells can be differentiated from epithelial cells by immunohistochemical analysis with expected combined expression of p63, smooth muscle actin, and vimentin.[35]

Canine benign mixed mammary tumors are common. These are composed of epithelial cells, myoepithelial cells, mesenchymal cells, and stroma or matrix. In addition, cells associated with bone formation, such as osteoclasts and osteoblasts, as well as hematopoietic precursors from medullary spaces or extramedullary hematopoiesis within the mammary tissue have been described.[41,42] True extramedullary hematopoiesis is rare, and the presence of these cell types is more likely attributed to homing to areas of osseous metaplasia.[41,42] Bone formation is by endochondral ossification of cartilage, potentially formed by myoepithelial cells, stromal connective tissue, or epithelial metaplasia (Figures 44.7 and 44.8). Myoepithelial cells are suspected to contribute to mesenchymal differentiation.[33] On cytologic examination, the epithelial component includes cohesive clusters, often densely packed, of uniform round to polygonal epithelial cells with scant to

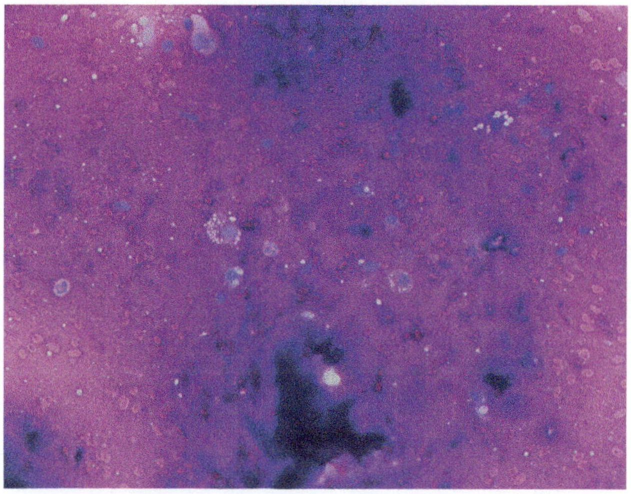

Figure 44.7 Fine-needle aspirate of an ossified area within a benign mixed mammary tumor from a 5-year-old female pregnant Scottish terrier dog. The 1.0 cm mass was located near the fourth right mammary gland. Chondroblasts or osteoblasts are embedded in a chondroid matrix (Wright stain, 200×).

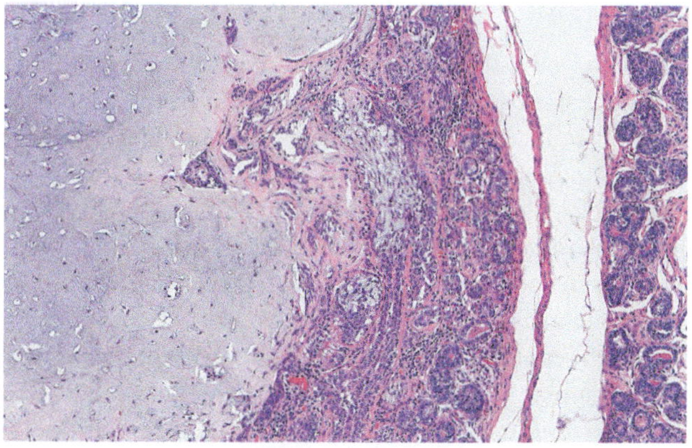

Figure 44.8 Biopsy sample from the same patient in Figure 44.7 showing homogeneous pale blue bone formation (left) adjacent to tubular epithelial cells arranged within fibrovascular stroma (hematoxylin & eosin, 200×).

moderate amounts of basophilic cytoplasm and round central nuclei with condensed to coarsely stippled chromatin and indistinct nucleoli. While the epithelial cells are expected to be uniform, atypia may be present in benign lesions (e.g. adenomas with atypical cells). Areas of benign proliferation can be adjacent to malignancy, and malignant tumors can lack pleomorphism, necessitating evaluation of the epithelial population in the context of the total microscopic appearance, gross lesion description, and case history (Figure 44.9).[13,33,40] On cytology, small aggregates of slender uniform spindloid cells are seen and can originate from myoepithelium or fibrous stroma.[14,29] The myoepithelial component has been described as having mesenchymal features, including the presence of small, dark-staining

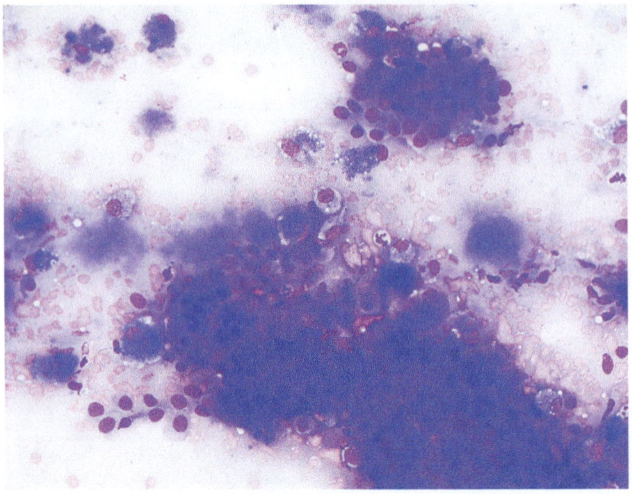

Figure 44.9 Fine-needle aspirate of a benign mixed mammary tumor from an 8-year-old female Yorkshire terrier dog with a 1.0 cm gritty irregular mass medial to the third nipple on the left mammary chain. Cytologic features include a uniform epithelial population with high N:C, a background of secretory material, and increased macrophages (Wright's stain, 500×).

free nuclei or cells with scant cytoplasm; however, cytologic appearance of myoepithelial cells overlaps with that of both productive and local stromal mesenchymal cells making this distinction problematic.[13,30,40,42–44] A mildly to moderately pleomorphic mesenchymal cell population with admixed pink matrix or evidence of osteoid or chondroid are the additional two elements necessary to suggest a mixed neoplasm. The mesenchymal cells can appear fusiform with scant basophilic attenuated cytoplasm or exhibit greater atypia, with plump fusiform to stellate cells with moderate amounts of cytoplasm, ovoid nuclei, and finely stippled chromatin with 1–3 small nucleoli.

Malignant Tumors

Mammary carcinomas in dogs include the following: carcinoma in situ; carcinoma of simple, tubular, tubulopapillary, cystic papillary, cribriform, micropapillary invasive, or solid types; comedocarcinoma; anaplastic; mixed; complex; and carcinoma arising in a complex adenoma or benign mixed tumor. Squamous cell carcinoma and special carcinoma variants, such as spindle cell, lipid-rich, and mucinous, are possible but uncommon.[33] The cytologic appearance correlates with previously described mammary carcinomas, with moderate epithelial pleomorphism and demonstration of criteria of malignancy (Figures 44.10 and 44.11). As the histopathologic subtypes imply, each tumor type can include additional findings, such as cystic areas, or, in the case of comedocarcinoma, necrotic cellular material and deteriorated leukocytes.[11,13,40]

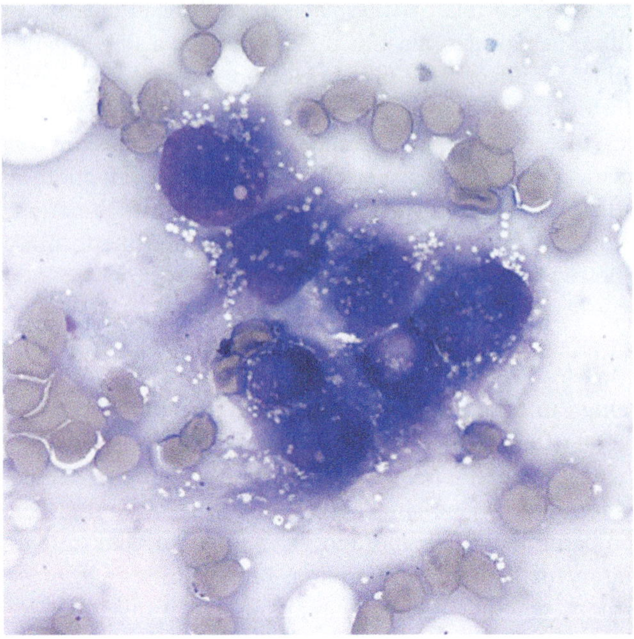

Figure 44.10 Fine-needle aspirate of the right inguinal lymph node from a 12-year-old female German Shepherd dog taken for staging of mammary carcinoma. No lymphoid tissue is present, and the cell population includes low numbers of cohesive-appearing neoplastic cells exhibiting anisokaryosis and prominent nucleoli (Wright's stain, 1000×).

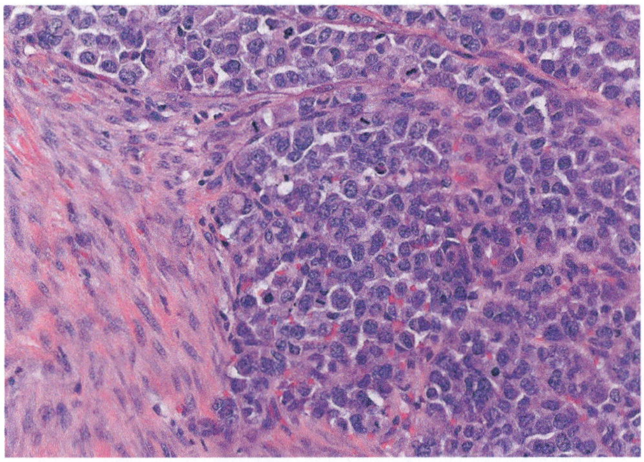

Figure 44.11 Biopsy of a firm, 6.0 in. diameter, fusiform, mass located on the right mid mammary chain from the same patient in Figure 44.10. Histopathologic diagnosis is carcinoma, solid subtype, multifocal, grade III with lymphatic invasion. The karyomegaly and atypia present on fine-needle aspirate of the suspected lymph node mirror the nuclear features seen on biopsy, which also includes frequent mitoses and areas of necrosis and inflammation (not pictured) (hematoxylin & eosin, 400×).

Canine inflammatory mammary carcinoma is described as being one of the most malignant types of mammary neoplasia, similar to human inflammatory breast carcinoma. It is rare and includes clinical features such as edema, pain, warmth, and more diffuse gross appearance that can be mistaken for an infectious inflammatory process, such as mastitis or dermatitis.[8,33,45–47] Several histopathologic types have been described, and histologic confirmation of this type of carcinoma includes the invasion and blockage of dermal lymphatics with neoplastic emboli, leading to severe edema.[33]

Squamous epithelial characteristics and keratinization can be present with squamous metaplasia, squamous cell carcinoma arising from mammary ductal epithelium, adenosquamous carcinoma or in lesions where cutaneous squamous cell carcinoma is located adjacent to or invading mammary tissue.[33] Mammary squamous cell carcinomas that arise from areas of squamous metaplasia are more invasive and aggressive than squamous cell carcinoma arising from local cutaneous tissue.[48] Acantholytic squamous cell carcinoma, a rare form associated with sun exposure in humans, has also been reported as a mammary mass in a dog.[49] The cytologic appearance of squamous cell carcinoma shows better correlation with histologic diagnosis than other mammary tumor types.[40,50] This is likely associated with uniformity in appearance despite location, lack of matrix or other components, and common presence of an associated inflammatory population. The squamous cells are large and polygonal and have a spectrum of nuclear and cytoplasmic maturation with dyssynchrony between nuclear and cytoplasmic features. The cells are keratinized and have homogenous medium blue cytoplasm that often includes punctate vacuolation, including perinuclear vacuoles, and distinct cell borders. Cells often exhibit decreased cohesion and appear individually. The nuclei are round to ovoid and vary from small with condensed chromatin to medium in size with reticulate chromatin. Nucleoli are often limited or small. Moderate to marked anisocytosis and anisokaryosis are often described. In some forms, pleomorphism includes cells with abundant clear cytoplasm and signet ring forms. Emperipolesis also is observed. Distinguishing carcinoma from similarly appearing squamous metaplasia and dysplastic changes can be difficult in the presence of inflammation, but interpretation tends to be reliable, particularly if an inflammatory response is limited or lacking.

Mesenchymal tumors include extraskeletal osteosarcoma (the most common mesenchymal neoplasm of the canine mammary gland), chondrosarcoma, fibrosarcoma, and hemangiosarcoma, among others.[33] Carcinosarcoma, or malignant mixed mammary tumor, also includes a malignant mesenchymal component and often presents as carcinoma and osteosarcoma.[33] While the cytologic appearance of these lesions is similar to descriptions for other locations, the presence of cartilage and bone formation, as well as proliferative stromal and mesenchymal elements in tumors that arise from the mammary gland, complicates cytologic diagnosis. Osteosarcoma has a distinct cytologic appearance, with pleomorphic plasmacytoid osteoblasts exhibiting criteria of malignancy and low numbers of osteoclasts. Reactive and proliferative bone can be very difficult to differentiate from osteosarcoma in the absence of histologic architecture, particularly when tumor location and clinical findings are not initially suggestive of osteosarcoma. Aspiration of osseous metaplasia could be mistaken for being representative of the lesion as a whole, leading to misdiagnosis. Chondrosarcoma and the presence of chondroid formation present a similar problem, but of the two tumor types, osteosarcoma is more common in this location and would raise greater index of suspicion. Hemangiosarcoma can be cutaneous or arise directly from the mammary gland. Aspirates include atypical mesenchymal cells that exhibit with moderate to marked anisocytosis and anisokaryosis. Cells have moderate to abundant basophilic cytoplasm, with or without cytoplasmic vacuolation, and round to plump ovoid or irregular nuclei. This neoplasm can appear similar to other sarcomas, necessitating biopsy for definitive diagnosis. In general, if aspirate samples from a mammary neoplasm include pleomorphic mesenchymal cells but lack other elements of mammary tumors, such as epithelial proliferation, fluid accumulation with histiocytic inflammation, neutrophilic inflammation, or matrix production, greater consideration of a primary sarcoma is warranted.

Correlation of Cytologic and Histologic Diagnosis in Canine Mammary Neoplasia

The accuracy of fine-needle aspiration cytology for diagnosis of canine mammary neoplasia, as well as comparisons of cytologic diagnosis to histopathologic diagnosis, has shown a broad range in sensitivity and specificity, in part owing to different study designs and goals. Depending on study design, inconclusive samples with fluid accumulation and inflammation are common and can be accounted for in different manners or not included in statistical analysis, further complicating determination of cytologic diagnostic accuracy. Overall, most recent studies report better sensitivity and specificity for cytologic determination of canine mammary malignancy than that originally reported by Allen et al.[13] Based on ten cytologic grading criteria with evaluation by two cytopathologists, diagnostic sensitivity for accurately diagnosing malignancy was 25 and 17%, but this analysis classified poorly diagnostic samples and inconclusive results as incorrect diagnoses, and excluding these samples increased diagnostic accuracy.[13] The limitations of that study were well defined by the authors and likely improved subsequent study designs.[13] Recent studies report cytologic sensitivity as high as 88.6–96.2% with 100% specificity for diagnosing canine mammary malignancy, but sensitivity declined to 60.7% when inadequate or suspicious samples were excluded in one study.[12,30,40,51,52] In another study, the effect of nondiagnostic samples on cytologic accuracy was not evaluated, and these samples were only excluded for comparison of histologic versus cytologic diagnosis.[30,40] Determination of malignancy can often be achieved by cytologic examination, but this does not necessarily reflect biologic behavior, clinical outcome, or final determination of tumor subtype, creating a challenge for comparison with histopathologic examination, which has the advantage of tissue architecture and ability to evaluate infiltrative tendency and lymphatic and vascular invasion. Additionally, determination of histopathologic grade has historically included variations on criteria with prognostic features that cannot be readily correlated among studies or with clinical outcomes.[53]

Canine mammary tumors that exhibit moderate to marked cytologic criteria of malignancy, including anisokaryosis, prominent nucleoli, and atypical mitotic figures, which are consistent within the cellular elements of a single population within the sample, are likely to correlate with a histopathologic diagnosis of malignant neoplasia, but there is potential for cellular atypia associated with benign lesions to be misinterpreted (e.g. ductal adenoma with atypical cells). Carcinomas that lack significant criteria of malignancy are the greater challenge, with the potential to be incorrectly diagnosed as benign adenomatous lesions, while being infiltrative or invasive and thus having a poorer prognosis. For these reasons, biopsy remains the preferred diagnostic tool for final diagnosis and assessment of malignant potential in canine mammary neoplasms.

Equine Mammary Gland Cytology

Mastitis

Mastitis in lactating mares tends to occur in the months following weaning of a foal, rather than in the periparturient period typical of dogs and cats. Differentiating mastitis from neoplasia in mature non-lactating mares with udder enlargement and pain can include cytologic and histopathologic evaluation of the lesion. Ulceration is a clinical feature that has primarily been described with carcinoma/adenocarcinoma, and draining tracts or ulcerated areas are not an expected feature of mastitis in horses, aiding clinical interpretation.[54,55] As with dogs, mammary secretions can be evaluated for the presence of neutrophilic inflammation, bacteria, or exfoliating atypical cells suggestive of underlying neoplasia. The absence of bacteria with a limited neutrophilic component does not exclude subclinical mastitis, warranting culture.

Neoplasia

In horses, mammary neoplasia is primarily a disease of mature mares and includes primary tumors (adenocarcinoma, carcinoma, rarely adenoma), masses associated with the overlying skin (melanoma of gray horses, sarcoid, squamous cell carcinoma), and metastatic lesions. The majority of mammary tumors are adenocarcinomas, and clinical features include mammary gland enlargement, pain on palpation, discharge, ulceration, and failure to respond to antimicrobial therapy instituted for suspected mastitis.[6] Fine-needle aspirate of an equine mammary carcinoma has been described as having clusters of pleomorphic rounded epithelial cells with occasional prominent nucleoli,[55] while adenocarcinoma (papillary ductal) has been described with overlapping features (clusters of rounded pleomorphic epithelial cells), but with greater nuclear and nucleolar atypia.[56] The cytologic appearance mirrors mammary carcinoma in cats and dogs. Surgical excision of the affected gland is the treatment of choice, but prognosis is guarded due to high incidence of metastasis to additional glands and inguinal lymph nodes.[6]

Advanced Diagnostic Techniques

Canine and feline mammary neoplasia have comparative features that overlap with human breast cancer, leading to research into molecular markers to allow for more thorough and specific characterization of tumor type and expected behavior. Molecular tools for evaluation include gene expression profiling, immunohistochemistry, and immunocytochemistry, with the latter two being most accessible. A thorough review of the molecular carcinogenesis of canine mammary neoplasia with consideration of molecular markers that have been recently evaluated, including comparative features, is provided elsewhere.[57] Currently, there is some challenge in preserving samples for evaluation of genetic material, with RNA quickly degrading and DNA in paraffin-embedded formalin-fixed tissue having degraded, small fragments that are not easily amplified.[53] Techniques for DNA extraction from formalin-fixed tissue have improved and would allow for evaluation of larger groups utilizing archived tissue, but even with standardized preparation, the samples themselves can be problematic due to variation in sectioning, storage, and formalin pH, among other factors.[53]

The hormone-influenced nature of mammary cancer has warranted evaluation of hormone receptor expression via gene expression profiling as well as immunohistochemistry. Human breast cancer has been categorized into five molecular subtypes using expression of the estrogen receptor (ER), progesterone receptor (PR), and human epidermal growth factor receptor 2 (HER-2).[58] Analysis of a combination of the histologic grading system provided by Goldschmidt et al.[33] and the five molecular subtypes of human breast cancer with consideration of known prognostic features in human breast cancer has been done with canine mammary tumors.[35] In this study, histologic classification, histologic grade, and lymphatic invasion were all related to molecular subtype.[35] The luminal A subtype (ER positive, HER-2 negative) was the most common for canine mammary carcinoma, and positive ER expression (luminal A and luminal B subtypes) was associated with a lower histologic grade and lower likelihood of lymphatic invasion.[35] The basal-like subtype (ER negative, HER-2 negative) was more likely to be classified as histologic grade III and have lymphatic invasion. Luminal subtypes (ER positive) are known to have a better prognosis in human breast cancer, and low ER expression is associated with poor prognosis in dogs.[35,59–62] Studies evaluating the relationship of HER-2 expression and prognosis present mixed results.[35,61,62]

Literature review with evaluation of molecular markers (HER-2, ER, PR, and others) in context of gross and histologic parameters, tumor grade (adapted from human breast cancer grading system but not including lymphovascular invasion), and proliferation markers (Ki67, AgNOR, PCNA) has been performed in cats.[4] In this review, the majority of feline mammary tumors are reported to be ER negative and lack HER-2 overexpression, suggesting more aggressive behavior similar to human triple negative tumors.[4] This author's review of the literature also demonstrated prognostic challenges related to lack of consensus on classification of feline mammary tumors, limited significant data on survival due to retrospective nature of previous studies, and necessity of standard classification against which to compare molecular markers in feline patients.[4,63,64]

A small study of mammary tumors from mares found that 3/7 cases stained positive for the ER, suggesting similarities to dogs and cats.[65]

While immunohistochemistry is available in most veterinary pathology laboratories, variation in immunohistochemistry protocols and evaluation systems creates limitations for comparison of studies. Standardization of protocols, as has been done with HER-2 immunohistochemistry testing for human breast cancer, is needed.[66] Continued comparative research with standardization of procedures, testing protocols, and classification is the goal for molecular characterization of companion animal mammary tumors, which may ultimately lead to progression in treatment approaches and useful correlates for human breast cancer research models.

References

1 Solano-Gallego, L. and Masserdotti, C. (2016). Reproductive system. In: *Canine and Feline Cytology* (eds. R.E. Raskin and D.J. Meyer), 313–352. St. Louis, MO: Elsevier.

2 Giminez, F., Hecht, S., Craig, L.E., and Legendre, A.M. (2010). Early detection, aggressive therapy. Optimizing the management of feline mammary masses. *J Feline Med Surg* 12: 214–224.

3 Hayes, H.M.J., Milne, K.L., and Mandell, C.P. (1981). Epidemiological features of feline mammary carcinoma. *Vet Rec* 108: 476–479.

4 Zappulli, V., Rasotto, R., Caliari, D. et al. (2014). Prognostic evaluation of feline mammary carcinomas: a review of the literature. *Vet Pathol* 52: 46–60.

5 Amorim, F.V., Souza, H.J.M., Ferreira, A.M.R., and Fonseca, A.B. (2006). Clinical, cytological and histopathological evaluation of mammary masses in cats from Rio de Janeiro, Brazil. *J Feline Med Surg* 8: 379–388.

6 Snyder, J.R. and Maher, O. (2011). Mammary neoplasia. In: *Equine Reproduction*, 2e (eds. A.O. McKinnon, E.L. Squires, W.E. Vaala and D.D. Varner). Oxford: Wiley-Blackwell.

7 Overley, B., Shofer, F.S., Goldschmidt, M.H. et al. (2005). Association between ovarihysterectomy and feline mammary carcinoma. *J Vet Intern Med* 19: 560–563.

8 Sorenmo, K.U., Worley, D.R., and Goldschmidt, M.H. (2012). Tumors of the mammary gland. In: *Withrow MacEwen's Small Animal Clinical Oncology*, 5e (eds. S.J. Withrow, D.M. Vail and R.L. Page), 538–556. St. Louis, MO: Elsevier/Saunders.

9 Meyer, D.J. (2016). The acquisition and management of cytology specimens. In: *Canine and Feline Cytology* (eds. R.E. Raskin and D.J. Meyer), 1–15. St. Louis, MO: Elsevier.

10 Meinkoth, J.H., Cowell, R.L., Tyler, R.D., and DB, D.N. (2014). Sample collection and preparation. In: *Diagnostic Cytology and Hematology of the Dog and Cat*, 4e (eds. A.C. Valenciano and R.L. Cowell), 1–19. St. Louis, MO: Elsevier.

11 Cassali, G.D., Monteiro, L.N., Gamba Cde, O. et al. (2015). Cytologic analysis of the mammary papillar discharge in a canine micropapillary carcinoma. *Vet Clin Pathol* 44: 448–451.

12 Simon, D., Schoenrock, D., Nolte, I. et al. (2009). Cytologic examination of fine-needle aspirates from

mammary gland tumors in the dog: diagnostic accuracy with comparison to histopathology and association with postoperative outcome. *Vet Clin Pathol* 38: 521–528.

13 Allen, S.W., Prasse, K.W., and Mahaffey, E.A. (1986). Cytologic differentiation of benign from malignant canine mammary tumors. *Vet Pathol* 23: 649–655.

14 Misdorp, W. (2002). Tumors of the mammary gland. In: *Tumors in Domestic Animals* (ed. D.J. Meuten), 575–606. Ames, IA: Iowa State Press.

15 Manesh, J.Y.Y., Shafiee, R., Pedram, B. et al. (2014). Improving the diagnosis, treatment, and biology patterns of feline mammary intraepithelial lesions: a potential model for human breast masses with evidence from epidemiologic and cytohistopathologic studies. *Tumor Biol* 35: 12109–12117.

16 Leidinger, E., Hooijberg, E., Sick, K. et al. (2011). Fibroepithelial hyperplasia in an entire male cat: cytologic and histopathological features. *Tierarztl Prax Ausg K Kleintiere Heimtiere* 39: 198–202.

17 Mesher, C.I. (1997). What is your diagnosis? Subcutaneous nodule from a 14-month-old cat. *Vet Clin Pathol* 26: 4.

18 Hayden, D.W., Johnson, K.H., and Ghobrial, H.K. (1983). Ultrastructure of feline mammary hypertrophy. *Vet Pathol* 20: 254–264.

19 Rutteman, G.R., Blankenstein, M., and Minke, J. (1991). Steroid receptors in mammary tumours of the cat. *Acta Endocrinol* 125: 32–37.

20 Martín De Las Mulas, J., Millán, Y., Bautista, M.J. et al. (2000). Oestrogen and progesterone receptors in feline fibroadenomatous change: an immunohistochemical study. *Res Vet Sci* 68: 15–21.

21 MacDougall, L.D. (2003). Mammary fibroadenomatous hyperplasia in a young cat attributed to treatment with megestrol acetate. *Can Vet J* 44: 227–229.

22 Görlinger, S., Kooistra, H.S., van den Broek, A., and Okkens, A.C. (2002). Treatment of fibroadenomatous hyperplasia in cats with aglépristone. *J Vet Intern Med* 16: 710–713.

23 Jutkowitz, L.A. (2005). Reproductive emergencies. *Vet Clin North Am Small Anim Pract* 35: 397–420.

24 Wiebe, V.J. and Howard, J.P. (2009). Pharmacologic advances in canine and feline reproduction. *Top Companion Anim Med* 24: 71–99.

25 Wilson, C.R. (2013). Feline gangrenous mastitis. *Can Vet J* 54: 292–294.

26 MacEwen, E.G., Hayes, A.A., Harvey, H.J. et al. (1984). Prognostic factors for feline mammary tumors. *J Am Vet Med Assoc* 185: 201–204.

27 Brown, N.O., Hayes, A.A., and Mooney, S. (1985). Feline mammary tumors. *Vet Clin North Am Small Anim Pract* 15: 513–520.

28 Dorn, C.R., Taylor, D.O.N., Frye, F.L., and Hibbard, H.H. (1968). Survey of animal neoplasms in Alameda and Contra Costa counties, California. I. Methodology and description of cases. *J Natl Cancer Inst* 40: 295–305.

29 Allison, R.W. (2014). Subcutaneous glandular tissue: mammary, salivary, thyroid, and parathyroid. In: *Diagnostic Cytology and Hematology of the Dog and Cat*, 4e (eds. A.C. Valenciano and R.L. Cowell), 110–117. St. Louis, MO: Elsevier.

30 Sontas, B., Yüzbaşıoğlu Öztürk, G., Toydemir, T. et al. (2012). Fine-needle aspiration biopsy of canine mammary gland tumours: a comparison between cytology and histopathology. *Reprod Domest Anim* 47: 125–130.

31 Viste, J.R., Myers, S.L., Singh, B., and Simko, E. (2002). Feline mammary adenocarcinoma: tumor size as a prognostic indicator. *Can Vet J* 43: 33–37.

32 Sorenmo, K.U. (2003). Canine mammary gland tumors. *Vet Clin North Am Small Anim Pract* 33: 573–596.

33 Goldschmidt, M., Peña, L., Rasotto, R., and Farhadi, M. (2011). Classification and grading of canine mammary tumors. *Vet Pathol* 48: 117–131.

34 Rivera, P. and von Euler, H. (2011). Molecular biological aspects on canine and human mammary tumors. *Vet Pathol* 48: 132–146.

35 Im, K.S., Kim, N.H., Lim, H.Y. et al. (2014). Analysis of a new histological and molecular-based classification of canine mammary neoplasia. *Vet Pathol* 51: 549–559.

36 Misdorp, W., Cotchin, E., Hampe, J.F. et al. (1973). Canine malignant mammary tumors. 3. Special types of carcinomas, malignant mixed tumors. *Vet Pathol* 10: 241–256.

37 Misdorp, W., Cotchin, E., Hampe, J.F. et al. (1972). Canine malignant mammary tumours II. Adenocarcinomas, solid carcinomas and spindle cell carcinomas. *Vet Pathol* 9: 447–470.

38 Sorenmo, K.U., Kristiansen, V.M., Cofone, M.A. et al. (2009). Canine mammary gland tumours; a histological continuum from benign to malignant; clinical and histopathological evidence. *Vet Comp Oncol* 7: 162–172.

39 Schäfer-Somi, S., Spergser, J., Breitenfellner, J., and Aurich, J.E. (2003). Bacteriological status of canine milk and septicaemia in neonatal puppies: a retrospective study. *J Veterinary Med Ser B* 50: 343–346.

40 Cassali, G.D., Gobbi, H., Malm, C., and Schmitt, F.C. (2007). Evaluation of accuracy of fine needle aspiration cytology for diagnosis of canine mammary tumours: comparative features with human tumours. *Cytopathology* 18: 191–196.

41 Grandi, F., Colodel, M.M., Monteiro, L.N. et al. (2010). Extramedullary hematopoiesis in a case of benign mixed mammary tumor in a female dog: cytological and histopathological assessment. *BMC Vet Res* 6: 45.

42 Fernandes, P.J., Guyer, C., and Modiano, J.F. (1998). Mammary mass aspirate from a Yorkshire Terrier. *Vet Clin Pathol* 27: 1–3.

43 Tyler, R., Cowell, R., and Meinkoth, J. (1989). Cutaneous and subcutaneous lesions: masses, cysts, ulcers, and fistulous tracts. In: *Diagnostic Cytology of the Dog and Cat* (eds. R.L. Cowell and R.D. Tyler), 22–46. Goleta, GA: American Veterinary Publications.

44 DeMay, R. (1996). Breast. In: *The Art and Science of Cytopathology, Aspiration Cytology*, 847–893. Chicago, IL: American Society of Clinical Pathology.

45 Clemente, M., Pérez-Alenza, M.D., Illera, J.C., and Peña, L. (2010). Histological, immunohistological, and ultrastructural description of vasculogenic mimicry in canine mammary cancer. *Vet Pathol* 47: 265–274.

46 Marconato, L., Romanelli, G., Stefanello, D. et al. (2009). Prognostic factors for dogs with mammary inflammatory carcinoma: 43 cases (2003–2008). *J Am Vet Med Assoc* 235: 967–972.

47 Pérez, M.D., Tabanera, E., and Peña, L. (2001). Inflammatory mammary carcinoma in dogs: 33 cases (1995–1999). *J Am Vet Med Assoc* 219: 1110–1114.

48 Ginn, P.E., Mansell, J.E.K., and Rakich, P.M. (2007). Skin and appendages. In: *Jubb, Kennedy & Palmer's Pathology of Domestic Animals* (ed. M.G. Maxie), 748–751. New York: Elsevier/Saunders.

49 Asakawa, M.G., Lewis, S.M., Buckles, E.L., and Stokol, T. (2015). What is your diagnosis? Cutaneous mass in a dog. *Vet Clin Pathol* 44: 607–608.

50 Griffiths, G.L., Lumsden, J.H., and Valli, V.E.O. (1984). Fine needle aspiration cytology and histologic correlation in canine tumors. *Vet Clin Pathol* 13: 13–17.

51 Haziroglu, R., Yardimci, B., Aslan, S., and Schmitt, F.C. (2010). Cytological evaluation of canine mammary tumours with fine needle aspiration biopsy technique. *Rev Med Vet* 161: 212–218.

52 Hellmén, E. and Lindgren, A. (1989). The accuracy of cytology in diagnosis and DNA analysis of canine mammary tumours. *J Comp Pathol* 101: 443–450.

53 Matos, A.J.F., Baptista, C.S., Gärtner, M.F., and Rutteman, G.R. (2012). Prognostic studies of canine and feline mammary tumours: the need for standardized procedures. *Vet J* 193: 24–31.

54 Seahorn, T.L., Hall, G., Brumbaugh, G.W. et al. (1992). Mammary adenocarcinoma in four mares. *J Am Vet Med Assoc* 200: 1675–1677.

55 Prendergast, M., Bassett, H., and Larkin, H.A. (1999). Mammary carcinoma in three mares. *Vet Rec* 144: 731–732.

56 Reppas, G.P., McClintock, S.A., Canfield, P.J., and Watson, G.F. (1996). Papillary ductal adenocarcinoma in the mammary glands of two horses. *Vet Rec* 138: 518–519.

57 Klopfleisch, R., von Euler, H., Sarli, G. et al. (2011). Molecular carcinogenesis of canine mammary tumors: news from an old disease. *Vet Pathol* 48: 98–116.

58 Sorlie, T., Tibshirani, R., Parker, J. et al. (2003). Repeated observation of breast tumor subtypes in independent gene expression data sets. *Proc Natl Acad Sci U S A* 100: 8418–8423.

59 Chang, C.-C., Tsai, M.-H., Liao, J.-W. et al. (2009). Evaluation of hormone receptor expression for use in predicting survival of female dogs with malignant mammary gland tumors. *J Am Vet Med Assoc* 235: 391–396.

60 Hsu, W.L., Huang, H.M., Liao, J.W. et al. (2009). Increased survival in dogs with malignant mammary tumours overexpressing HER-2 protein and detection of a silent single nucleotide polymorphism in the canine HER-2 gene. *Vet J* 180: 116–123.

61 Nieto, A., Peña, L., Pérez-Alenza, M.D. et al. (2000). Immunohistologic detection of estrogen receptor alpha in canine mammary tumors: clinical and pathologic associations and prognostic significance. *Vet Pathol* 37: 239–247.

62 Martín De Las Mulas, J., Ordás, J., Millán, Y. et al. (2003). Oncogene HER-2 in canine mammary gland carcinomas: an immunohistochemical and chromogenic in situ hybridization study. *Breast Cancer Res Treat* 80: 363–367.

63 Burrai, G.P., Mohammed, S.I., Miller, M.A. et al. (2010). Spontaneous feline mammary intraepithelial lesions as a model for human estrogen receptor- and progesterone receptor-negative breast lesions. *BMC Cancer* 10: 156.

64 Wiese, D.A., Thaiwong, T., Yuzbasiyan-Gurkan, V., and Kiupel, M. (2013). Feline mammary basal-like adenocarcinomas: a potential model for human triple-negative breast cancer (TNBC) with basal-like subtype. *BMC Cancer* 13: 403.

65 Hughes, K., Scase, T.J., and Foote, A.K. (2015). Estrogen receptor and signal transducer and activator of transcription 3 expression in equine mammary tumors. *Vet Pathol* 52: 631–634.

66 Peña, L., Gama, A., Goldschmidt, M.H. et al. (2014). Canine mammary tumors: a review and consensus of standard guidelines on epithelial and myoepithelial phenotype markers, HER2, and hormone receptor assessment using immunohistochemistry. *Vet Pathol* 51: 127–145.

Part XII

Endocrine

45

Thyroid and Parathyroid Glands

M. Judith Radin and Maxey L. Wellman

Introduction

Diseases of the thyroid and parathyroid glands are often assessed by biochemical and endocrine testing. However, when a mass lesion is present in the laryngeal region or along the trachea, cytology can be helpful in determining if the mass is thyroid or parathyroid in origin or if it derives from another tissue. Because both thyroid and parathyroid glandular tissue can be located anywhere from the base of the tongue through the mediastinum, cytology also can prove useful in identifying accessory tissue or neoplasms that originate in an ectopic location.

Collection

Indications

Thyroid Gland

Clinical signs referable to a space-occupying lesion in the area of the larynx often prompt evaluation of the thyroid gland. Signs include dyspnea, coughing, dysphagia, and change in voice.[1–4] In horses, esophageal obstruction (choke) or abnormal movement of the head and neck when ridden can be evident.[3,4] Because ectopic thyroid masses can arise in the heart, patients can present for pericardial effusion, signs of cardiac insufficiency, and exercise intolerance.[5–9] In cats, clinical signs of hyperthyroidism, such as weight loss, polyphagia, polydipsia, polyuria, unkempt or greasy pelage, and increased serum thyroxine (T4) concentrations often prompt further evaluation,[10] whereas dogs rarely exhibit clinical signs associated with functional thyroid masses.[2] Thyroid masses typically are palpable in both dogs and cats. Additional physical examination findings in cats can include tachycardia and hypertension.

Parathyroid Glands

Clinical signs of hyperparathyroidism are indications for assessment of the parathyroid glands. Primary hyperparathyroidism (PHP) is characterized by persistent hypercalcemia, high ionized calcium, variable (often normal to decreased) phosphorus, normal to increased parathyroid hormone (PTH), and undetectable PTH-related protein (PTH-rp).[11–14] Clinical signs include polyuria, polydipsia, dysuria, urolithiasis, gastrointestinal signs, weakness, and lethargy.[15] Palpation, ultrasonography, or scintigraphy can detect parathyroid enlargement or the presence of masses.[14,16]

Methods

Fine needle aspiration (FNA) is commonly used to evaluate cervical masses, and the technique is similar to that described for other tissues (see Chapter 1). Nodules are sampled by FNA using 22–25 G needles with or without a 6–12 mL syringe.[10,17,18] Ultrasound can be used to determine the size and demarcation of the lesion, and the presence of cystic areas or mineralization, and to guide needle positioning.[18] Pressure over the aspiration site is used to prevent bleeding because the lesions often are very vascular.[10,17]

FNA with or without ultrasound is the primary presurgical modality for evaluating thyroid lesions in people. Studies examining the diagnostic accuracy and causes of nondiagnostic samples indicate that the primary reasons for nondiagnostic samples include aspiration of cystic lesions resulting in low cellularity samples, and inadequate operator expertise affecting selection of region to aspirate or quality of preparation.[19–21] Diagnostic accuracy improved from 76% using free-hand FNA to 88% with ultrasound guidance.[22]

Veterinary Cytology, First Edition. Edited by Leslie C. Sharkey, M. Judith Radin, and Davis Seelig.

Similar studies are scarce in veterinary literature. In a study of 12 dogs with cervical masses, a positive or suspect diagnosis of thyroid malignancy was obtained in 11 of 12 cases (92%), with one false negative.[17] One to two repeat aspirates were needed to obtain a positive diagnosis in 6/12 dogs because the initial samples consisted of blood, likely due to hematomas in the thyroid gland. In another study, FNAs were considered diagnostic in only 47% of thyroid aspirates from 26 dogs.[1] In this study, nondiagnostic samples were due to hemodilution, cell fragility, or low cellularity. A study of 10 dogs with enlarged thyroids found only 10% inadequate samples, which may reflect the benefit of ultrasound guidance.[18] Another study correctly classified 4/4 thyroid carcinomas in dogs and cats in agreement with histology.[23]

Safety and Complications

Hemorrhage is the primary complication of FNA, due to the vascular nature of the glandular tissue and neoplasms, as well as proximity to large blood vessels in the neck.[17] Hemorrhage typically is mild and controlled by gentle pressure.

Normal Architecture and Cytology

Thyroid Gland

The thyroid gland is bilobed and located lateral to the trachea, just caudal to the larynx. Histologically, the thyroid gland consists of follicles with associated blood vessels and stroma. Follicular cells (thyrocytes) originate from the pharyngeal plate and line the follicles. They concentrate iodine, produce colloid (thyroglobulin), and secrete thyroxine in response to thyroid stimulating hormone (TSH). Follicular cells are cuboidal to columnar, and histologic morphology varies with glandular activity and stimulus by TSH.[24] Thyroid C-cells are interspersed within the follicle wall or in between follicles, sometimes forming aggregates (C-cell complexes) along blood vessels. C-cells migrate from the ultimobranchial body and are neural crest in origin. C-cells secrete calcitonin, which lowers serum calcium concentrations in response to hypercalcemia. Because of embryologic development, accessory thyroid tissue may be found from the tongue base to the diaphragm in dogs[6,25–27] and cats.[28–30] This extra-thyroidal accessory tissue can contain functioning follicles, permitting detection using sodium pertechnetate scintigraphy.[31–33] Ectopic tissue typically lacks C-cells.

FNA of normal thyroid gland yields variably intact follicular cells, blood, and pink to light blue amorphous material considered to be colloid (Figure 45.1a).[34] C-cells usually are not seen in FNA from normal thyroid gland. Follicular cells often exfoliate in clusters and can form acinar-like structures. Follicular cells have a single round nucleus with coarse chromatin and occasional nucleoli. Because of cellular fragility, bare nuclei are frequent. The basophilic cytoplasm is moderate to abundant, and cytoplasmic borders can be indistinct. The cytoplasm occasionally contains dark blue-black granules, which are thought to be tyrosine, a nonessential amino acid that forms the backbone of thyroglobulin (Figure 45.1b and c).[17,34,35]

Parathyroid Glands

The parathyroid glands arise from the third and fourth pharyngeal pouches. There usually are four main parathyroid glands; however, the number can be variable, and ectopic tissue can occur throughout the neck to the mediastinum.[16,24,36,37] In dogs and cats, two external parathyroid glands are located at the cranial pole of the thyroid gland and can be superficial to the capsule, just under the capsule, or embedded in the thyroid parenchyma. The two internal parathyroid glands are located within the caudal pole of the thyroid gland. In horses, the two upper parathyroid glands are found outside the capsule of the cranial pole of the thyroid gland.[36] The lower parathyroid glands can be located along the trachea from the bicarotid trunk to and sometimes embedded in the thymus.

The primary cell of the normal parathyroid gland is the chief (principal) cell, which synthesizes and secretes PTH in response to low serum calcium. Published cytological descriptions of normal parathyroid glands are lacking. Cytologically, there are dense clusters and ribbons of cells with indistinct cytoplasmic borders (Figure 45.1d and e). Nuclei are round and uniform with coarse chromatin and occasional nucleoli. The cytoplasm is scant and lightly basophilic with occasional fine black granules. Histologically, chief cells are cuboidal to polyhedral with scant eosinophilic to basophilic cytoplasm and a central round nucleus.[24,36] Lipofuscin granules and lipid vacuoles can be seen in the cytoplasm. Oxyphil cells are found in low numbers scattered throughout the parathyroid glands and sometimes occur in small clusters. Oxyphil cells are characterized by abundant, lightly eosinophilic cytoplasm. The function of oxyphil cells is unknown and may represent an aging change in chief cells as numbers increase in older animals.

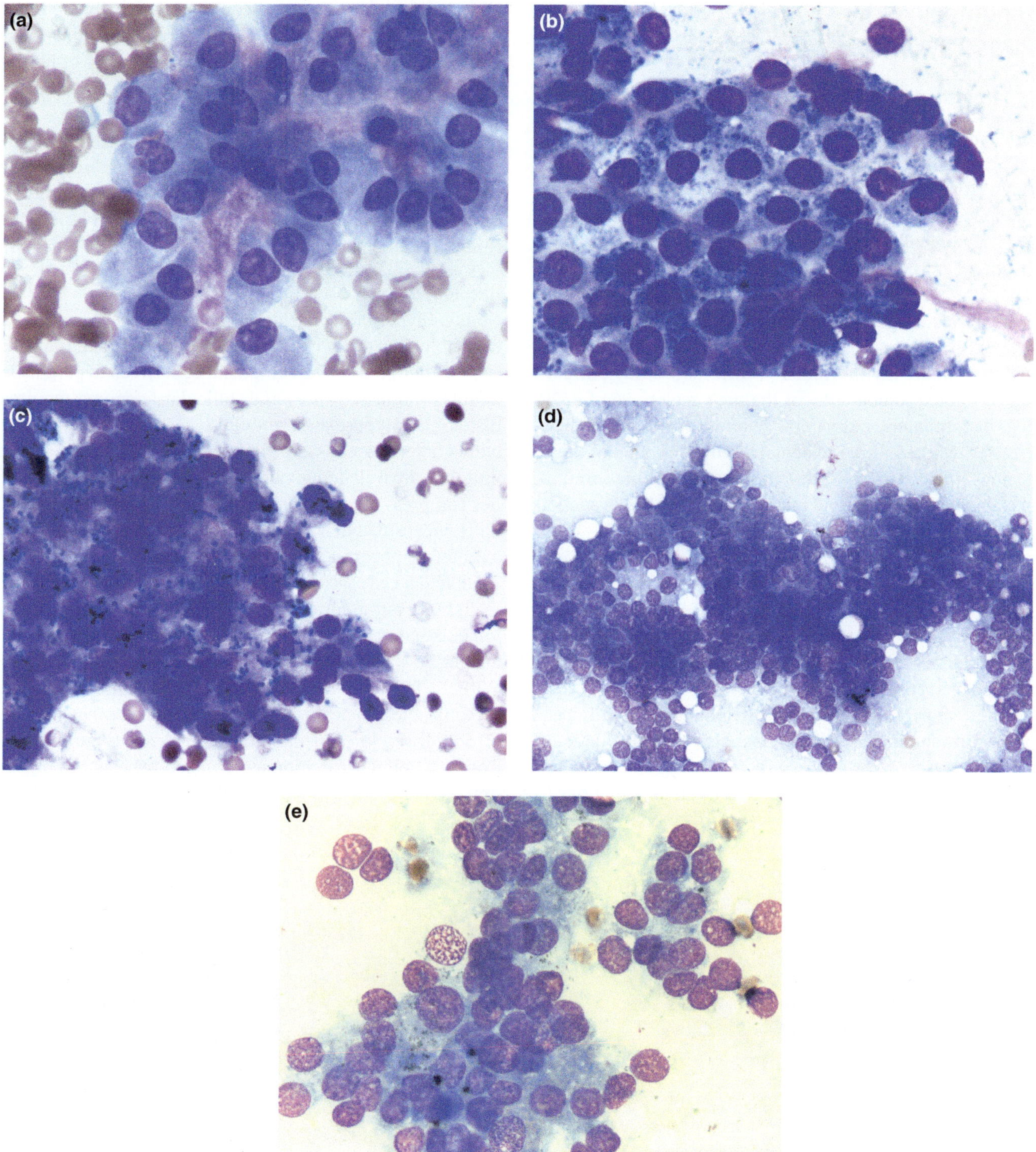

Figure 45.1 (a) Aspirate of a well-differentiated thyroid follicular carcinoma from a 10-year-old Boxer dog. Acinar-like formations of uniform cells are associated with pink extracellular material that is compatible with colloid (Wright–Giemsa, 1000×). (b) Aspirate of a thyroid mass from an 8-year-old cat showing clinical signs of hyperthyroidism with a serum T4 concentration of 23.0 μg/dL (reference interval = 1.0–5.0 μg/dL). Numerous, variably sized dark blue granules in the cytoplasm are thought to be tyrosine, a component of thyroglobulin (Wright–Giemsa, 1000×). (c) Aspirate of a thyroid mass from a 25-year-old Arabian stallion showing similar dark blue granules (Wright–Giemsa, 1000×). (d) Impression smear of normal parathyroid gland from a dog. Cells form dense clusters and ribbons with ill-defined cytoplasmic borders. The nuclei are round and uniform with coarse chromatin and occasional nucleoli. The cytoplasm is scant and lightly basophilic (Wright–Giemsa, 500×). (e) Higher magnification of (d). Note the fine, black cytoplasmic granules in a few cells (Wright–Giemsa, 1000×).

Conditions of the Thyroid Gland Diagnosed by Cytology

Hyperplasia, Adenoma, and Carcinoma

Incidence

Enlargement of or masses involving the thyroid gland result from hyperplasia (goiter) or neoplasia. In dogs, the incidence of thyroid neoplasia is 1–4%, and approximately 90% of clinically apparent masses are carcinomas.[2,38,39] Staging and histologic classification schemes are reported.[10,40,41] Metastasis is common at the time of initial presentation and frequently occurs in the lung prior to the regional lymph nodes, due to vascular invasion of the cranial and caudal thyroid veins.[24,38] In a large study evaluating computed tomography of the neck region, 96 of 4520 dogs had unilateral or bilateral thyroid tumors (prevalence, 2.12%).[39] Masses were incidental discoveries in 34 of these 96 dogs (incidentalomas) despite 24 tumors being carcinomas. A rate of 15% thyroid incidentaloma with 22% adenocarcinomas was observed in another study.[42] Older dogs (>9–10 years of age) are more likely to be affected, but there is no sex predilection.[2,38,39] Some studies suggest that Beagles, Golden Retrievers, Boxers, and Siberian Huskies are at increased risk.[38,39,43] Although adenomas are often an incidental finding, they can be associated with hypothyroidism or space-occupying effects if they are large.[10,38,44,45]

Older cats are often affected by nodular thyroid hyperplasia or adenoma, with approximately 3% incidence of carcinoma.[10,29,33,46] Carcinomas frequently metastasize, with regional lymph nodes preferential to the lungs.[47] Hyperplasia, adenomas, and carcinomas usually are functional, resulting in clinical hyperthyroidism. Functional ectopic thyroid tissue has been reported in 4–21% of hyperthyroid cats, contributing to unresolved hyperthyroidism following thyroidectomy.[29,32,33,46]

Nodular lesions of the thyroid gland occur commonly in older horses with rates ranging from 30 to 60% and reaching as high as 75% after 20 years of age.[48–50] The majority of these lesions are adenomas or nodular hyperplasia with carcinomas being relatively uncommon.

Histology

Nodular hyperplasia, adenoma, and carcinoma can develop from follicular cells residing in the thyroid gland and in ectopic thyroid tissue. Distinguishing between hyperplastic nodules (nodular goiter) and follicular adenoma requires histology.[24] Hyperplastic nodules consist of follicular cells with a heterogeneous appearance of the follicles, are often multiple, are well demarcated but not encapsulated, and do not compress adjacent tissue. Adenomas are fully or partially encapsulated, compress the adjacent tissue, and have a uniform appearance of the follicular cells.

Follicular cell carcinomas have several histologic variants, including well-differentiated (follicular, compact cellular, follicular-compact cellular, papillary), poorly differentiated, anaplastic (undifferentiated), and carcinosarcoma.[2,24,41] With the follicular variant, cuboidal to columnar cells form recognizable follicles of varying shape and size. The volume of colloid varies and can be mineralized (Figure 45.2). Compact cellular carcinomas form solid sheets of polyhedral cells with scant or absent follicle formation and colloid

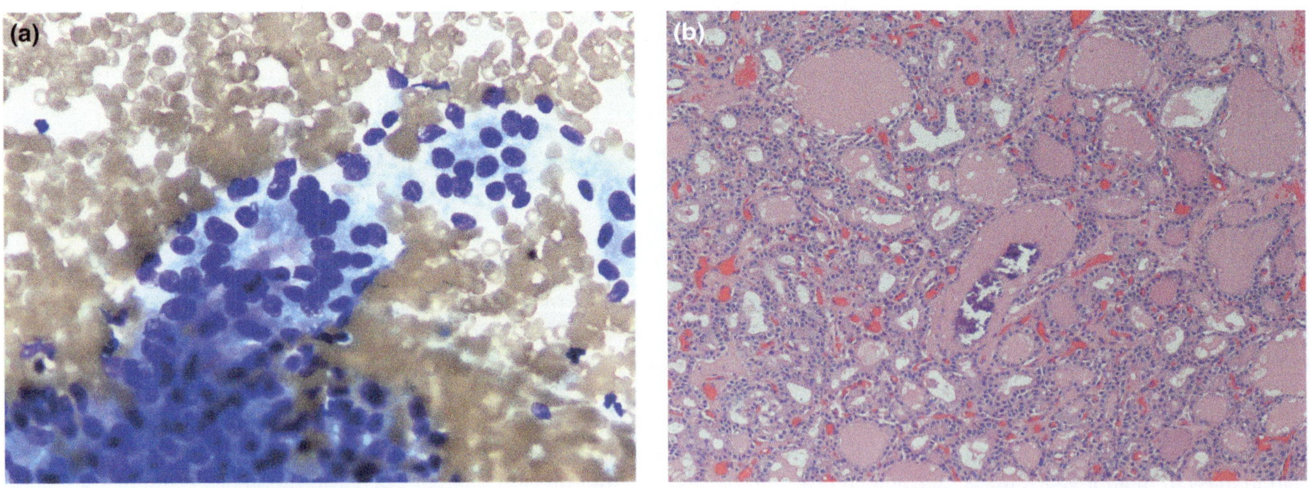

Figure 45.2 Well-differentiated thyroid follicular carcinoma from an 11-year-old Golden Retriever dog. (a) On cytology, the cells form sheets and occasionally acinar like structures with minimal anisocytosis and anisokaryosis. Nuclei are round with coarse chromatin, and cytoplasm is scant and lightly basophilic (Wright–Giemsa, 500×). (b) The malignant epithelial cells are arranged in tubular and follicular structures. Colloid (the extracellular pink material) is present, and mineralization (the dark purple material in a pool of colloid in the center) can be seen (hematoxylin & eosin, 100×).

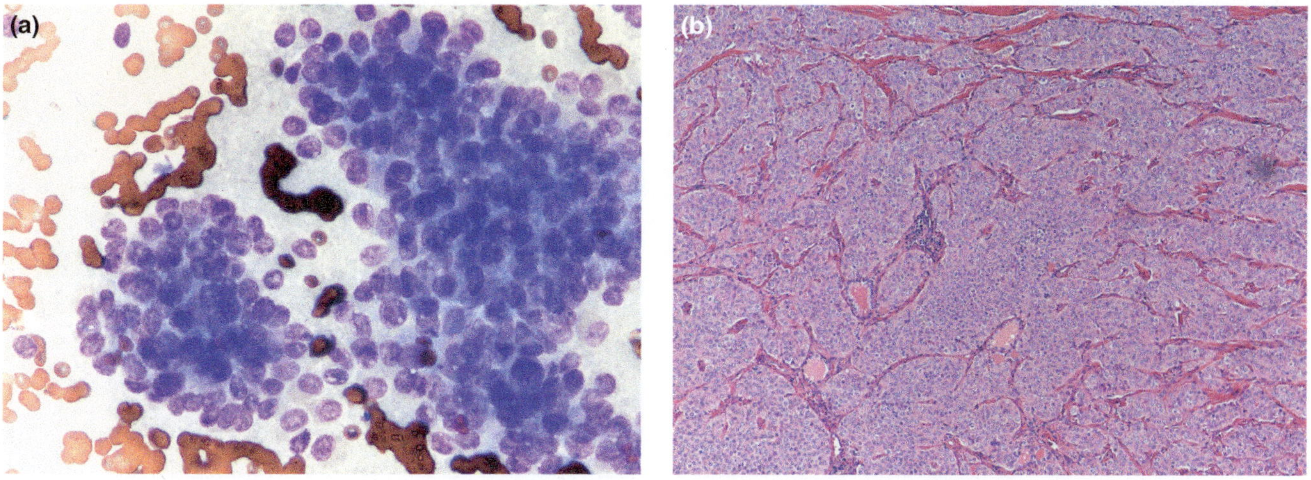

Figure 45.3 Compact (solid) follicular thyroid carcinoma from a 6-year-old, male Golden Retriever dog. (a) The cells form sheets and tightly arranged clusters with variably distinct cytoplasmic borders. Nuclei are round with stippled to coarse chromatin and one to several nucleoli. Cytoplasm is blue-gray, but granules are lacking in this case. Anisokaryosis and anisocytosis are minimal (Wright–Giemsa, 500×). (b) Cells form solid sheet surrounded by a moderate fibrovascular stroma. Rare follicles are present within the tumor. Despite the uniform cellular appearance, this tumor exhibited evidence of malignancy with vascular invasion (not shown) (hematoxylin & eosin, 100×).

secretion (Figure 45.3). Follicular-compact cellular carcinomas exhibit a mix of colloid-secreting follicles and solid sheets of cells. This is the most common carcinoma morphology in dogs[24] and cats.[47] Papillary carcinomas are cystic with papillary projections of neoplastic cells into the cystic space. Carcinosarcomas (malignant mixed thyroid tumors) are rare and consist of malignant follicular cells and malignant mesenchymal cells.

Tumors arising from C-cells include adenomas and medullary (parafollicular) carcinomas.[24] Histologically, C-cell adenomas compress adjacent tissue, have a thin connective tissue capsule, and may encompass normal follicles or have residual pools of colloid within the sheets of cells. Adenomas can exhibit neuroendocrine packeting. The neoplastic C-cells have moderate to abundant cytoplasm, coarsely clumped chromatin, and a single nucleolus. Medullary carcinomas are often multinodular and efface the thyroid gland (Figure 45.4). The cells are polygonal to spindle shaped with an oval nucleus. The distinction between C-cell tumors and compact cellular carcinomas of follicular origin can be difficult and may require immunohistochemistry.

Cytology

Most authors suggest that it is not possible to distinguish follicular hyperplasia, adenoma, and adenocarcinoma or exclude C-cell adenoma or medullary carcinoma based on cytology.[27,34] There are no case series directly comparing aspirates from these different entities. Several cytological descriptions of follicular adenomas in cats appear similar to normal thyroid gland.[34,35]

The cytology of FNAs of carcinomas of follicular cell origin in dogs has been described.[1,8,17,34,35,51] These typically contain clusters or sheets of round to polygonal cells with variably distinct cytoplasmic borders (Figures 45.2 and 45.3). Acinar arrangements can be seen.[8] Cells tend to be fragile, and abundant bare nuclei are often present. The background is often bloody,[1,17] and hemosiderin-laden and erythrophagocytic macrophages are sometimes present.[8] Nuclei are round to oval with clumped chromatin and one to multiple nucleoli.[17,34,35] While some carcinomas may exhibit mild atypia, characteristics considered suggestive for malignancy include nuclear pleomorphism, occasional macronuclei, nuclear hyperchromasia, and prominent, multiple, variably sized nucleoli.[8,17,34] Cytoplasm is moderate in amount and blue-gray to basophilic. When present, dark blue-black cytoplasmic granules, presumably tyrosine, are thought to be useful in determining follicular cell origin.[17,34,35] Variable amounts of pink to blue staining amorphous material, suggestive for colloid, can be seen extracellularly and sometimes within cells. Cytologic features of ectopic thyroid follicular carcinomas are similar to tumors found within the thyroid gland.[8,51] FNAs of a follicular compact cellular carcinoma and a thyroid adenocarcinoma from two horses exhibited similar cytologic characteristics, including the presence of colloid[52] and cytoplasmic granules.[53] Anisocytosis and anisokaryosis were moderate to marked.

A histologically confirmed carcinosarcoma of the thyroid gland was described in a dog.[54] Two cell populations

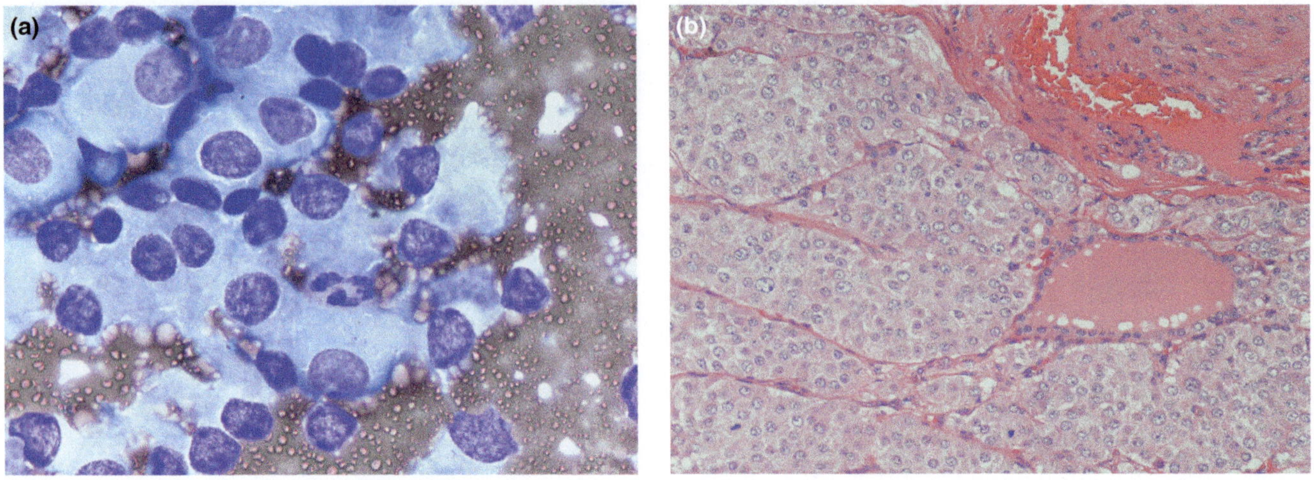

Figure 45.4 Medullary (C cell) carcinoma from a 6-year-old, spayed female Labrador Retriever dog. (a) The cytology is characterized by clusters of cells. Nuclei are round with stippled chromatin and one to two prominent nucleoli. Cytoplasm is scant to moderate in amount and gray-blue in color. Cytoplasmic borders are variably distinct (Wright–Giemsa, 500×). (b) Packets of neoplastic C cells are surrounded by a scant fibrovascular stroma. Similar to the FNA, cells exhibit moderate anisokaryosis and have a single round nucleus with one to two prominent nucleoli. One entrapped follicle with colloid is seen (hematoxylin & eosin, 200×).

were present on FNA cytology. One population consisted of clusters of cells that occasionally appeared to form acini. These cells had small round nuclei with condensed chromatin and exhibited mild to moderate anisocytosis. Neither colloid nor blue-black cytoplasmic granules were seen. The second population consisted of large spindle cells that exhibited moderate to marked anisokaryosis. Cytoplasm was basophilic. Nuclei were round to oval with clumped chromatin and multiple large, prominent nucleoli.

Cytology of C-cell medullary carcinomas has been described.[34,35,55] Cells are arranged in clusters occasionally manifesting acinar-like or rosette arrangement (Figure 45.4). The cells are round to polygonal, and cytoplasmic borders are often distinct. Nuclei are round to oval, eccentric, with coarse chromatin and prominent nucleoli. Occasional binucleated and multinucleated cells and rare nuclear pseudoinclusions are seen.[34,55] Nuclear pseudoinclusions are a protrusion of cytoplasm into the nucleus that is delineated by the invaginated nuclear membrane and are considered common in papillary thyroid carcinoma and uncommon in medullary and parathyroid tumors in people.[56] Cytoplasm varies in amount and is eosinophilic and finely granular. While colloid may be present, blue-black cytoplasmic granules are absent.[35]

Cystic Lesions

Cystic ectopic thyroid tissue from the base of the tongue of a cat consisted of proteinaceous fluid (32 g/L), resulting in a pale eosinophilic background and lacking cells on cytology.[57] Histopathology and clinical outcome were consistent with non-neoplastic ectopic thyroid tissue.

Thyroglossal duct remnants can become cystic or neoplastic. Thyroglossal duct cysts are reported in dogs[58–60] and cats.[61,62] Histologically, these cysts are lined with flat to cuboidal epithelium with associated thyroid follicular tissue. Aspiration of fluid from a thyroglossal duct cyst in a dog revealed sterile, noninflammatory serosanguinous fluid[60] and an acellular transudate in a cat.[61] Thyroglossal duct carcinomas are either papillary carcinomas or squamous cell carcinomas. Fluid from a thyroglossal duct carcinoma in a cat was of low cellularity with evidence of chronic hemorrhage.[63]

Inflammatory Lesions

Lymphocytic thyroiditis can be congenital or acquired. It is usually associated with thyroid hypoplasia and subsequent hypothyroidism in dogs.[45,64,65] Reports of cytologic appearance of these lesions are lacking, most likely because diagnosis is by clinical signs and endocrine assays supporting a diagnosis of hypothyroidism. Incidence of thyroid tumors was higher in Beagle dogs with hypothyroidism secondary to lymphocytic thyroiditis (54.5%) compared with euthyroid dogs (22.8%).[44]

Conditions of the Parathyroid Glands Diagnosed by Cytology

Hyperplasia, Adenoma, and Carcinoma

Incidence

Enlargement or masses of the parathyroid glands can result from hyperplasia, adenoma, or carcinoma, and all can be associated with clinical signs of PHP. Dogs with PHP are often over 10 years of age, and Keeshonds, Siberian Huskies, and Golden Retrievers are overrepresented.[11,13,14] Keeshonds have a hereditary predisposition to develop adenomas.[66] Solitary adenomas are most common, followed by single or multiple hyperplastic nodules (adenomatous hyperplasia) with carcinomas being relatively uncommon. In a study of 21 dogs with PHP, 20 masses were adenomas, and one was a carcinoma,[11] whereas in a second study, 19 histologically evaluated samples consisted of 14 adenomas, 2 carcinomas, and 3 cases of hyperplastic parathyroid tissue.[14] In another study, six dogs with PHP had multinodular adenomatous hyperplasia.[13] With PHP, the unaffected parathyroid glands are atrophied, whereas in dogs with secondary hyperparathyroidism, parathyroid glands exhibit diffuse hyperplasia of all four glands.[24,67–69]

Similar to dogs, the majority of lesions in cats are parathyroid adenomas with fewer instances of hyperplasia and carcinomas,[70–76] all of which can be associated with clinical signs of PHP. Cats are middle age to older, and Siamese are overrepresented.

Functional parathyroid adenomas are rarely reported in horses.[77–80] Diffuse hyperplasia of the parathyroid glands occurs in secondary hyperparathyroidism.[36,81]

Histology

Histologically, single or multiple hyperplastic nodules are poorly demarcated, lack a capsule, and compress adjacent parenchyma.[24] Diffuse hyperplasia is more likely to occur with renal or nutritional secondary hyperparathyroidism. Hyperplastic chief cells are morphologically uniform with condensed nuclear chromatin with increased amounts of eosinophilic cytoplasm. Histologically, it may be difficult to distinguish hyperplastic nodules from adenomas. Adenomas are encapsulated and compress both the normal parathyroid parenchyma and the adjacent thyroid gland (Figure 45.5). Neoplastic chief cells have a moderate amount of eosinophilic cytoplasm and occasional karyomegaly. Some adenomas exhibit oxyphil cell or water clear cell morphology. Because these tumors are functional, C-cell hyperplasia can occur in the thyroid gland. Carcinomas in dogs and cats are characterized by neoplastic cells that exhibit pleomorphism and invade outside the capsule of the gland. In cats, these tumors can become cystic.

Cytology

There are few cytologic descriptions of parathyroid hyperplasia or neoplasia, which may reflect the small size of many of these nodules, with some as small as 2.0 mm.[82] It likely would be difficult to distinguish hyperplasia and adenoma from normal parathyroid tissue on cytology (Figures 45.1d, e and 45.5). Cytology from a dog with a histologic diagnosis of diffuse hyperplasia exhibited sheets of cells with round nuclei with one to several nucleoli and occasional karyomegaly.[83] Cytoplasm had variably distinct cytoplasmic borders, was scant to moderate in amount, and was basophilic. No cytoplasmic granules were noted. Adenomas were described as clusters of benign appearing

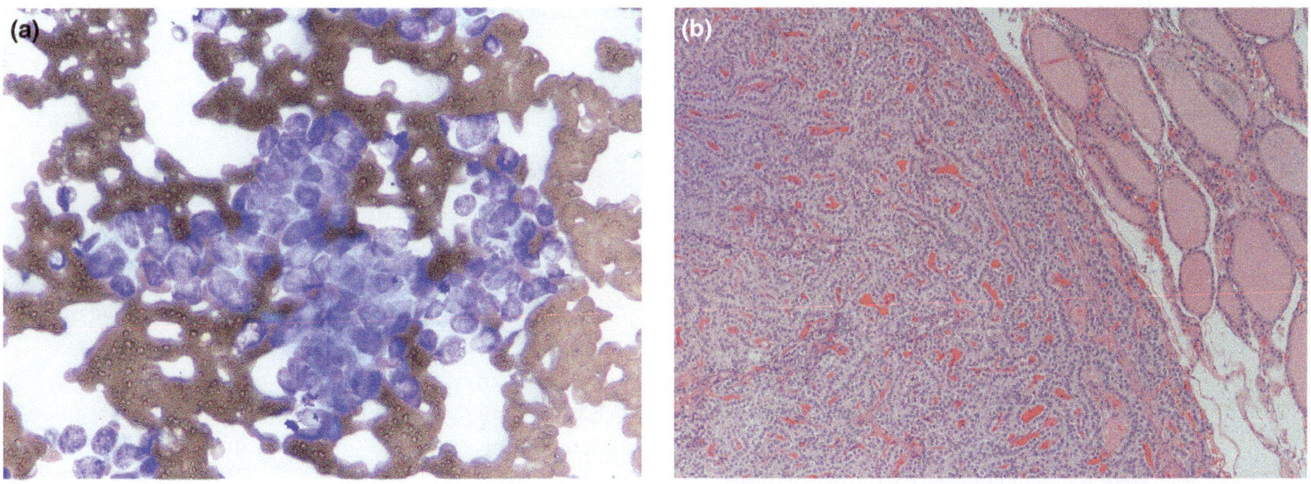

Figure 45.5 Parathyroid adenoma from an 11-year-old, castrated male Greyhound. The dog had persistent hypercalcemia with a total calcium of 13.1 mg/dL (reference interval = 9.3–11.6), an ionized calcium of 6.2 mg/dL (reference interval = 4.9–5.8), PTH of 1.1 pmol/L (reference interval = 0.5–5.8), and PTH-rp of 0 pmol/L (reference interval < 1.0). (a) The FNA is characterized by dense clusters and cords of uniform cells with minimal anisokaryosis and indistinct cytoplasmic borders. Nuclei are round with coarse to stippled chromatin and occasional, indistinct nucleoli. Cytoplasm is pale blue. Note the similarity to normal parathyroid in Figure 45.1d and e (Wright–Giemsa, 500×). (b) The parathyroid adenoma on the left is well demarcated, and the cells form cords with a thin fibrovascular stroma. Similar to the cytology, the cells exhibit mild atypia. Thyroid follicles with abundant eosinophilic colloid are seen on the right (hematoxylin & eosin, 200×).

epithelial cells in a cat[68] and consistent with neuroendocrine tumor in a horse.[80] An adenocarcinoma in a dog was characterized by numerous free nuclei and a diffuse blue background.[35,84] The cells formed clusters and acinar-like arrangements, suggestive for a neuroendocrine pattern. Nuclei were round to oval with clumped chromatin and occasional nucleoli. Occasional cells contained dark black granules or eosinophilic needle-like inclusions in the cytoplasm. A cystic carcinoma from cat was characterized by clusters of cells with round nuclei, coarse chromatin, and one to several nucleoli.[76] Occasional macronuclei and mitotic figures were seen. Cytoplasm was basophilic with occasional, small purple granules.

Advanced Diagnostic Techniques

Thyroid Gland

Differentiation of medullary (C-cell) carcinoma from follicular carcinomas, especially compact cellular variants, frequently requires immunohistochemistry. Follicular carcinomas are positive for thyroglobulin, whereas medullary carcinomas are positive for calcitonin.[85–89] Staining for thyroid transcription factor 1 (TTF1) and Pax8 is usually positive in follicular tumors but with less sensitivity than thyroglobulin.[90] C-cell tumors stain positively for napsin A and for neuroendocrine markers such as neuron specific enolase and chromogranin A.[90,91]

A few studies have examined various biomarkers for usefulness in predicting metastasis and clinical outcome. Ki-67 labeling index was negatively associated with time to metastasis for both follicular and medullary tumors in dogs.[2] E-cadherin staining was not associated with outcome in that study.

Parathyroid Glands

Normal canine chief cells stain positively for PTH by immunohistochemistry; however, adenomas and hyperplastic parathyroid tissue can show variable staining intensity and patterns. Gröne et al. reported 2 of 3 adenomas as positive for PTH.[92] While normal chief cells and inactive chief cells adjacent to parathyroid nodules exhibit perinuclear staining, primary nodular and secondary diffuse hyperplasia exhibit diffuse cytoplasmic staining with variable perinuclear positivity.[68] In adenomas, regions of diffuse cytoplasmic staining and perinuclear staining were observed. Although normal parathyroid chief cells express chromogranin A, only 3 of 7 parathyroid adenomas stained positive for chromogranin A in one study.[91]

Conclusion

FNA can be used to identify cervical masses as thyroid or parathyroid in origin and is useful when ectopic tissue or tumors occur. Distinguishing between hyperplasia, adenoma, and carcinoma is often not possible with FNA, and histopathology with immunohistochemistry is often needed for definitive diagnosis. While inflammatory lesions of the thyroid gland occur, they are rarely evaluated by aspiration.

References

1 Harari, J., Patterson, J.S., and Rosenthal, R.C. (1986). Clinical and pathologic features of thyroid tumors in 26 dogs. *J Am Vet Med Assoc* 188: 1160–1164.

2 Campos, M., Ducatelle, R., Rutteman, G. et al. (2014). Clinical, pathologic, and immunohistochemical prognostic factors in dogs with thyroid carcinoma. *J Vet Intern Med* 28: 1805–1813.

3 Troillet, A., Böttcher, D., Brehm, W., and Scharner, D. (2016). Retrospective evaluation of hemithyroidectomy in 14 horses. *Vet Surg* 45: 949–954.

4 Marcatili, M., Voss, S.J., and Pollock, P.J. (2018). Standing thyroidectomy in 10 horses. *Vet Surg* 47: 86–92.

5 Almes, K.M., Heaney, A.M., and Andrews, G.A. (2008). Intracardiac ectopic thyroid carcinosarcoma in a dog. *Vet Pathol* 45: 500–504.

6 Liptak, J.M., Kamstock, D.A., Dernell, W.S. et al. (2008). Cranial mediastinal carcinomas in nine dogs. *Vet Comp Oncol* 6: 19–30.

7 Di Palma, S., Lombard, C., Kappeler, A. et al. (2010). Intracardiac ectopic thyroid adenoma in a dog. *Vet Rec* 167: 709–710.

8 Boes, K., Messick, J., Green, H. et al. (2010). What is your diagnosis? Impression smear from an intracardiac mass in a dog. *Vet Clin Pathol* 39: 119–120.

9 Rajagopalan, V., Jesty, S.A., Craig, L.E., and Gompf, R. (2013). Comparison of presumptive echocardiographic and definitive diagnoses of cardiac tumors in dogs. *J Vet Intern Med* 27: 1092–1096.

10 Barber, L.G. (2007). Thyroid tumors in dogs and cats. *Vet Clin North Am Small Anim Pract* 37: 755–773.

11 Berger, B. and Feldman, E.C. (1987). Primary hyperparathyroidism in dogs: 21 cases (1976–1986). *J Am Vet Med Assoc* 191: 350–356.

12 Rosol, T.J., Nagode, L.A., Couto, C.G. et al. (1992). Parathyroid hormone (PTH)-related protein, PTH, and

1,25-dihydroxyvitamin D in dogs with cancer-associated hypercalcemia. *Endocrinology* 131: 1157–1164.

13 DeVries, S.E., Feldman, E.C., Nelson, R.W., and Kennedy, P.C. (1993). Primary parathyroid gland hyperplasia in dogs: six cases (1982–1991). *J Am Vet Med Assoc* 202: 1132–1136.

14 Gear, R.N., Neiger, R., Skelly, B.J., and Herrtage, M.E. (2005). Primary hyperparathyroidism in 29 dogs: diagnosis, treatment, outcome and associated renal failure. *J Small Anim Pract* 46: 10–16.

15 Feldman, E.C., Hoar, B., Pollard, R., and Nelson, R.W. (2005). Pretreatment clinical and laboratory findings in dogs with primary hyperparathyroidism: 210 cases (1987–2004). *J Am Vet Med Assoc* 227: 756–761.

16 Wisner, E.R. and Nyland, T.G. (1998). Ultrasonography of the thyroid and parathyroid glands. *Vet Clin North Am Small Anim Pract* 28: 973–991.

17 Thompson, E.J., Stirtzinger, T., and Lumsden, J.H. (1980). Fine needle aspiration cytology in the diagnosis of canine thyroid carcinoma. *Can Vet J* 21: 186–188.

18 Georgescu, G. (2008). Fine needle aspiration cytology (FNAC) as a method of diagnosis in the dog thyroid diseases. *Bull Vet Med* 65: 9–11.

19 Ali, S.Z. and Cibas, E. (2010). *The Bethesda System for Reporting Thyroid Cytopathology: Definitions, Criteria and Explanatory Notes*, vol. 171. New York: Springer.

20 Cross, P., Chandra, A., Giles, T. et al. (2016). *Guidance on the Reporting of Thyroid Cytology Specimens*, 1–22. London: Royal College of Pathologists.

21 Poller, D.N., Baloch, Z.W., Fadda, G. et al. (2016). Thyroid FNA: new classifications and new interpretations. *Cancer Cytopathol* 124: 457–466.

22 Krishnappa, P., Ramakrishnappa, S., and Kulkarni, M.H. (2013). Comparison of free hand versus ultrasound-guided fine needle aspiration of thyroid with histopathological correlation. *J Environ Pathol Toxicol Oncol* 32: 149–155.

23 Ménard, M., Fontaine, M., and Morin, M. (1986). Fine needle aspiration biopsy of malignant tumors in dogs and cats: a report of 102 cases. *Can Vet J* 27: 504–510.

24 Rosol, T.J. and Gröne, A. (2016). Endocrine glands. In: *Jubb, Kennedy, and Palmer's Pathology of Domestic Animals* (ed. M.G. Maxie), 291–336. St. Louis: Elsevier.

25 Stephens, L.C., Saunders, W.J., and Jaenke, R.S. (1982). Ectopic thyroid carcinoma with metastases in a beagle dog. *Vet Pathol* 19: 669–675.

26 Constantino-Casas, P., Rodriguez-Martinez, H.A., and Gutiérrez Díaz-Ceballos, M.E. (1996). A case report and review: the gross, histological and immunohistochemical characteristics of a carcinoma of ectopic thyroid in a dog. *Br Vet J* 152: 669–672.

27 Broome, M.R., Peterson, M.E., and Walker, J.R. (2014). Clinical features and treatment outcomes of 41 dogs with sublingual ectopic thyroid neoplasia. *J Vet Intern Med* 28: 1560–1568.

28 Noxon, J.O., Thornqburg, L.P., DiMender, M.J., and Jones, B.D. (1983). An adenoma in ectopic thyroid tissue causing hyperthyroidism in a cat. *J Am Anim Hosp Assoc* 19: 369–372.

29 Swalec, K.M. and Birchard, S.J. (1990). Recurrence of hyperthyroidism after thyroidectomy in cats. *J Am Anim Hosp Assoc* 26: 433–437.

30 Patnaik, A.K., Peterson, M.E., and Hidgon, A. (2000). Ectopic lingual thyroid tissue in a cat. *J Feline Med Surg* 2: 143–146.

31 Kameda, Y. (1972). Accessory thyroid glands of the dog around the intrapericardial aorta. *Arch Histol Jpn* 34: 375–391.

32 Harvey, A.M., Hibbert, A., Barrett, E.L. et al. (2009). Scintigraphic findings in 120 hyperthyroid cats. *J Feline Med Surg* 11: 96–106.

33 Peterson, M.E. and Broome, M.R. (2015). Thyroid scintigraphy findings in 2096 cats with hyperthyroidism. *Vet Radiol Ultrasound* 56: 84–95.

34 Bertazzolo, W. (2014). Cytological examination of the endocrine glands. In: *Manual of Diagnostic Cytology of the Dog and Cat*, 1e (ed. J. Dunn), 195–203. Chichester, West Sussex: Wiley.

35 Choi, U.S. and Arndt, T. (2016). Endocrine/Neuroendocrine system. In: *Canine and Feline Cytology. A Color Atlas and Interpretation Guide*, 3e (eds. R.E. Raskin and D.J. Meyer), 430–438. St. Louis: Elsevier.

36 Krook, L. and Lowe, J.E. (1964). Nutritional secondary hyperparathyroidism in the horse, with a description of the normal anatomy of the normal equine parathyroid gland. *Pathol Vet* 1: 1–98.

37 Patnaik, A.K., MacEwen, E.G., Erlandson, R.A. et al. (1978). Mediastinal parathyroid adenocarcinoma in a dog. *Vet Pathol* 15: 55–63.

38 Wucherer, K.L. and Wilke, V. (2010). Thyroid cancer in dogs: an update based on 638 cases (1995–2005). *J Am Anim Hosp Assoc* 46: 249–254.

39 Bertolini, G., Drigo, M., Angeloni, L., and Caldin, M. (2017). Incidental and nonincidental canine thyroid tumors assessed by multidetector row computed tomography: a single-centre cross sectional study in 4520 dogs. *Vet Radiol Ultrasound* 58: 304–314.

40 Owen, L.N. (1980). *TNM Classification of Tumours in Domestic Animals*, 51–52. Geneva: World Health Organization.

41 Kiupel, M., Capen, C., Miller, M., and Smedley, R. (2008). *Histological Classification of the Endocrine System of Domestic Animals*, WHO International

Histological Classification of Tumors of Domestic Animals, 25–39. Washington, DC: Armed Forces Institute of Pathology.
42 Pollard, R.E., Bohannon, L.K., and Feldman, E.C. (2015). Prevalence of incidental thyroid nodules in ultrasound studies of dogs with hypercalcemia (2008–2013). *Vet Radiol Ultrasound* 56: 63–77.
43 Liptak, J.M. (2007). Canine thyroid carcinoma. *Clin Tech Small Anim Pract* 22: 75–81.
44 Benjamin, S.A., Stephens, L.C., Hamilton, B.F. et al. (1996). Associations between lymphocytic thyroiditis, hypothyroidism, and thyroid neoplasia in beagles. *Vet Pathol* 33: 486–494.
45 Mooney, C.T. (2011). Canine hypothyroidism: a review of aetiology and diagnosis. *N Z Vet J* 59: 105–114.
46 Forrest, L.J., Baty, C.J., Metcalf, M.R., and Thrall, D.E. (1996). Feline hyperthyroidism: efficacy of treatment using volumetric analysis for radioiodine dose calculation. *Vet Radiol Ultrasound* 37: 141–145.
47 Turrel, J.M., Feldman, E.C., Nelson, R.W., and Cain, G.R. (1988). Thyroid carcinoma causing hyperthyroidism in cats: 14 cases (1981–1986). *J Am Vet Med Assoc* 193: 359–364.
48 Schlotthauer, C.F. (1931). The incidence and types of disease of the thyroid gland of adult horses. *J Am Vet Med Assoc* 78: 211–218.
49 Dalefield, R.R. and Palmer, D.N. (1994). The frequent occurrence of thyroid tumours in aged horses. *J Comp Pathol* 110: 57–64.
50 Ueki, H., Kowatari, T., Oyamada, T. et al. (2004). Non-functional C-cell adenoma in aged horses. *J Comp Pathol* 131: 157–165.
51 Leissinger, M.K., Del Piero, F., Kawabata, A. et al. (2015). Pathology in practice. Mediastinal thyroid follicular carcinoma and adrenal carcinoma. *J Am Vet Med Assoc* 246: 303–305.
52 Froment, R., Allano, M., Chiasson, A. et al. (2016). Pathology in practice. *J Am Vet Med Assoc* 248: 1355–1357.
53 Ramirez, S., McClure, J.J., Moore, R.M. et al. (1998). Hyperthyroidism associated with a thyroid adenocarcinoma in a 21-year-old gelding. *J Vet Intern Med* 12: 475–477.
54 Fernandez, N.J., Clark, E.G., and Larson, V.S. (2008). What is your diagnosis? Ventral neck mass in a dog. *Vet Clin Pathol* 37: 447–451.
55 Bertazzolo, W., Giudice, C., Dell'Orco, M., and Caniatti, M. (2003). Paratracheal cervical mass in a dog. *Vet Clin Pathol* 32: 209–212.
56 Ip, Y.T., Dias Filho, M.A., and Chan, J.K. (2010). Nuclear inclusions and pseudoinclusions: friends or foes of the surgical pathologist? *Int J Surg Pathol* 18: 465–481.
57 Reed, T.P., Brisson, B.A., and Schutt, L.K. (2011). Cystic ectopic lingual thyroid tissue in a male cat. *J Am Vet Med Assoc* 239: 981–984.
58 Harkema, J.R., King, R.R., and Hahn, F.F. (1984). Carcinoma of thyroglossal duct cysts: a case report and review of the literature. *J Am Anim Hosp Assoc* 20: 319–324.
59 Dallman, M.J. and Johnson, E.O. (1986). Thyroglossal duct cyst in a dog. *J Am Anim Hosp Assoc* 22: 839–841.
60 McCally, R.E., Kim, S.E., Bacon, N.J. et al. (2012). Surgical management of a subepiglottic thyroglossal duct cyst in a dog. *J Am Anim Hosp Assoc* 48: 198–202.
61 Giles, J.T. III, Rochat, M.C., and Snider, T.A. (2007). Surgical management of a thyroglossal duct cyst in a cat. *J Am Vet Med Assoc* 230: 686–689.
62 Lynn, A., Dockins, J.M., Kuehn, N.F. et al. (2009). Caudal mediastinal thyroglossal duct cyst in a cat. *J Small Anim Pract* 50: 147–150.
63 Moorer, J.D., Breshears, M.A., and Dugat, D.R. (2016). Thyroglossal duct carcinoma in a cat. *J Am Anim Hosp Assoc* 52: 251–255.
64 Graham, P.A., Nachreiner, R.F., Refsal, K.R., and Provencher-Bolliger, A.L. (2001). Lymphocytic thyroiditis. *Vet Clin North Am Small Anim Pract* 31: 915–933.
65 Bojanić, K., Acke, E., and Jones, B.R. (2011). Congenital hypothyroidism of dogs and cats: a review. *N Z Vet J* 59: 115–122.
66 Goldstein, R.E., Atwater, D.Z., Cazolli, D.M. et al. (2007). Inheritance, mode of inheritance, and candidate genes for primary hyperparathyroidism in Keeshonden. *J Vet Intern Med* 21: 199–203.
67 Watson, A.D. and Canfield, P.J. (1979). Renal failure, hyperparathyroidism and hypercalcaemia in a dog. *Aust Vet J* 55: 177–180.
68 van Vonderen, I.K., Kooistra, H.S., Peeters, M.E. et al. (2003). Parathyroid hormone immunohistochemistry in dogs with primary and secondary hyperparathyroidism: the question of adenoma and primary hyperplasia. *J Comp Pathol* 129: 61–69.
69 Stillion, J.R. and Ritt, M.G. (2009). Renal secondary hyperparathyroidism in dogs. *Compend Contin Educ Vet* 31: E8.
70 Kallet, A.J., Richter, K.P., Feldman, E.C., and Brum, D.E. (1991). Primary hyperparathyroidism in cats: seven cases (1984–1989). *J Am Vet Med Assoc* 199: 1767–1771.
71 Marquez, G.A., Klausner, J.S., and Osborne, C.A. (1995). Calcium oxalate urolithiasis in a cat with a functional parathyroid adenocarcinoma. *J Am Vet Med Assoc* 206: 817–819.
72 den Hertog, E., Goossens, M.M.C., van der Linde-Sipman, J.S., and Kooistra, H.S. (1997). Primary hyperparathyroidism in two cats. *Vet Q* 19: 81–84.

73 Sueda, M.T. and Stefanacci, J.D. (2000). Ultrasound evaluation of the parathyroid glands in two hypercalcemic cats. *Vet Radiol Ultrasound* 41: 448–451.

74 Kaplan, E. (2002). Primary hyperparathyroidism and concurrent hyperthyroidism in a cat. *Can Vet J* 43: 117–119.

75 Cavana, P., Vittone, V., Capucchio, M.T., and Farca, A.M. (2006). Parathyroid adenocarcinoma in a nephropathic Persian cat. *J Feline Med Surg* 8: 340–344.

76 Faucher, M.R., Freiche, V., Bongrand, Y., and German, A.J. (2014). Primary hyperparathyroidism caused by a parathyroid carcinoma in a 16-year-old male neutered cat with concurrent chronic kidney disease. *Vet Q* 34: 37–40.

77 Bienfet, V., Dewaele, A., Van Essche, R. et al. (1964). Un trouble parathyroidien primaire? Un cas d'osteofibrose chez le poney Shetland par adenome parathyroidien. Guerison par ablation chirurgicale. *Ann Med Vet* 108: 252–256.

78 Peauroi, J.R., Fisher, D.J., Mohr, F.C., and Vivrette, S.L. (1998). Primary hyperparathyroidism caused by a functional parathyroid adenoma in a horse. *J Am Vet Med Assoc* 212: 1915–1918.

79 Wong, D., Sponseller, B., Miles, K. et al. (2004). Failure of technetium Tc 99m sestamibi scanning to detect abnormal parathyroid tissue in a horse and a mule with primary hyperparathyroidism. *J Vet Intern Med* 18: 589–593.

80 Tomlinson, J.E., Johnson, A.L., Ross, M.W. et al. (2014). Successful detection and removal of a functional parathyroid adenoma in a pony using technetium Tc 99m sestamibi scintigraphy. *J Vet Intern Med* 28: 687–692.

81 Benders, N.A., Junker, K., Wensing, T. et al. (2001). Diagnosis of secondary hyperparathyroidism in a pony using intact parathyroid hormone radioimmunoassay. *Vet Rec* 149: 185–187.

82 Luyre, J.C. and Behrend, E.N. (2001). Endocrine tumors. *Vet Clin North Am Small Anim Pract* 31: 1083–1110.

83 Diaconu, I.V., Bucur, E.O., and Tihulca, C.R. (2008). Histopathological and histochemical aspects in a case of dog hyperparathyroidism. *Lucrări Stiintifice Medicină Veterinară* 41: 608–618.

84 Ramaiah, S.K., Alleman, A.R., Hanel, R., and Uhl, E. (2001). A mass in the ventral neck of a hypercalcemic dog. *Vet Clin Pathol* 30: 177–179.

85 Moore, F.M., Kledzik, G.S., Wolf, H.J., and RA, D.L. (1984). Thyroglobulin and calcitonin immunoreactivity in canine carcinomas. *Vet Pathol* 21: 168–173.

86 Leblanc, B., Paulus, G., Andreu, M., and Bonnet, M.C. (1990). Immunocytochemistry of thyroid C-cell complexes in dogs. *Vet Pathol* 27: 445–452.

87 Leblanc, B., Parodi, A.L., Lagadic, M. et al. (1991). Immunocytochemistry of canine thyroid tumors. *Vet Pathol* 28: 370–380.

88 Patnaik, A.K. and Lieberman, P.H. (1991). Gross, histologic, cytochemical and immunocytochemical study of medullary thyroid carcinoma in sixteen dogs. *Vet Pathol* 28: 223–233.

89 Ramos-Vara, J.A., Miller, M.A., Johnson, G.C., and Pace, L.W. (2002). Immunohistochemical detection of thyroid transcription factor-1, thyroglobulin, and calcitonin in canine normal, hyperplastic, and neoplastic thyroid gland. *Vet Pathol* 39: 480–487.

90 Ramos-Vara, J.A., Frank, C.B., DuSold, D., and Miller, M.A. (2016). Immunohistochemical detection of Pax8 and Napsin A in canine thyroid tumours: comparison with thyroglobulin, calcitonin and thyroid transcription factor 1. *J Comp Pathol* 155: 286–298.

91 Doss, J.C., Gröne, A., Capen, C.C., and Rosol, T.J. (1998). Immunohistochemical localization of chromogranin A in endocrine tissue and endocrine tumors of dogs. *Vet Pathol* 35: 312–315.

92 Gröne, A., Werkmeister, J.R., Steinmeyer, C.L. et al. (1994). Parathyroid hormone related protein in normal and neoplastic canine tissues: immunohistochemical localization and biochemical extraction. *Vet Pathol* 31: 308–315.

46

Adrenal Gland

Walter Bertazzolo

Collection

Cytologic examination of adrenal glands in companion animal practice is limited to some neoplastic proliferations. Other disorders (e.g. atrophy, inflammation, degenerative diseases, functional abnormalities) cannot be adequately investigated by cytology and require different diagnostic approaches (histopathology, serum biochemistry, hormonal testing, etc.) to achieve a definitive diagnosis. Moreover, some adrenal tumors are not easily investigated by cytology since they are often too small to be sampled (e.g. diffuse cortical hyperplasia, small adenomas).[1]

Adrenal cytology might be indicated when an adrenal mass is detected by diagnostic imaging. In fact, with the advent and widespread use of advanced diagnostic techniques such as ultrasonography, computed tomography (CT), and magnetic resonance imaging (MRI), the detection of adrenal tumors has markedly increased in human and veterinary medicine.[2] Some tumors can be associated with functional disorders (hypo- or hypersecretion of related hormones), space-occupying effects (e.g. vena cava invasion), and distant metastases, but often they are found incidentally during abdominal diagnostic imaging, without related symptoms. In these latter cases, the term "adrenal incidentaloma" is used to define these masses.[2] In the human literature, several authors have proposed guidelines to manage adrenal incidentalomas, in order to reduce unnecessary investigation, decrease medical expenses, and reduce risk associated with some of these techniques (e.g. risk associated with biopsy and radiation exposure due to frequent CT scans).[3–5] These guidelines have been recently adapted to small animal veterinary practice.[2]

Fine needle aspiration (FNA) cytology may be routinely performed using ultrasound- or CT-guided techniques. Needle sizes between 21 and 25 G are preferable to larger needles, although studies evaluating risks related to FNA of adrenal tumors are lacking in the literature. Since percutaneous imaging-guided FNA of adrenals are reported to have up to 28% of nondiagnostic samples and up to 12% of adverse events in humans, a novel endoscopic ultrasound-guided FNA technique has been developed in human medicine.[6–11] Using endoscopic ultrasound-guided FNA, several intra-abdominal, mediastinal, and pelvic organs can be sampled, including adrenals.[12] This technique is considered extremely safe, but its main disadvantage is that only the left adrenal gland can be sampled regularly in humans.[11,13] On the other hand, it has a very high recovery rate, with 100% of adequate samples collected in some studies.[13,14] Endoscopic ultrasound-guided FNA has not been extensively used and studied in veterinary patients, and published data on this matter are lacking.

In humans, FNA of adrenal tumors is considered a valuable tool for diagnosing primary adrenocortical cancer and adrenal metastases by some authors, with accuracy rates close to 100%.[9,15–17] The accuracy of 19-G Tru-Cut biopsy was comparable or even worse than cytology in a human study and did not seem to add significant advantages over endoscopic ultrasound-guided FNA cytology.[18]

However, a couple of major concerns have been raised by other authors against the use of cytology in assessing adrenal masses in practice. Firstly, some complications have been described after FNA biopsy of adrenal tumors, and this risk should be taken into account and evaluated in every individual case. If a pheochromocytoma cannot be excluded, FNA is discouraged by some authors since potential severe and even fatal side effects could arise in the event of a catecholamine-producing tumor being incidentally biopsied (e.g. pain, uncontrolled hemorrhage, severe hypertensive crisis due to sudden release of catecholamine).[19] Single case reports of severe complications have been reported sporadically in human medicine,[20–22] including abscess formation after an FNA,[23] but studies evaluating the risk of this procedure are not available in veterinary species. In a study on

Veterinary Cytology, First Edition. Edited by Leslie C. Sharkey, M. Judith Radin, and Davis Seelig.

canine and feline adrenal tumor cytology on 24 cases, 6 samples were performed by ultrasound-guided FNA (all adrenocortical tumors) and 4 samples by intraoperative FNA (2 adrenocortical tumors and 2 malignant pheochromocytomas).[24] No adverse effects were reported in this study. Since cytological distinction between adrenocortical tumor and pheochromocytoma is quite easy even for an inexperienced cytologist, a possible alternative to avoid percutaneous FNA is to perform intraoperative FNA or make imprints from biopsies immediately after the surgical removal of the neoplasm. A prompt diagnosis may reduce the risks associated with aspiration of a catecholamine-producing tumor and could give immediate information, assisting clinicians in better managing the case while awaiting for the final histological diagnosis.

The second major concern regards the actual usefulness of cytologic results in the clinical management of an adrenal tumor.[25] In humans, adrenal tumors are primarily defined by their appearance on advanced diagnostic imaging, their growth behavior, and their possible hormonal activity.[3–5] Cytology is suggested only when hormonal testing is nondiagnostic, when malignancy is suspected (in particular due to metastatic cancer), and only if pheochromocytoma is excluded by measuring catecholamine metabolites in urine.[3–5,26] The main criticism regarding the use of adrenal fine needle biopsy is that cytologic findings usually do not change the management of the tumor and cannot discriminate between benign and malignant primary adrenal tumors.[5,25] On the contrary, cytology is strongly recommended in cases of suspected adrenal metastases in humans.[4]

A study on adrenalectomy in dogs showed that the perioperative death risk seems to be associated with adrenal hemorrhage, which in turn is associated with tumor size (i.e. large tumors have a higher risk of rupture).[27] Based on these findings, preoperative needle aspiration cytology of large tumors might not be advisable, and intraoperative needle biopsy or, more easily, imprint from the removed tumor could reduce the risk of perioperative complications and possibly death.

A point in favor of FNA cytology of adrenal masses is that results could aid clinicians with perioperative management of adrenal tumors. The presurgical treatment of patients bearing pheochromocytomas with phenoxybenzamine seems to decrease the mortality rate in dogs.[28] Since the cytological diagnosis of pheochromocytoma is quite simple (see section "Primary Neoplasia"), intraoperative cytology could represent a rapid and easy method to correctly address an adrenal tumor and to decide if phenoxybenzamine is needed during surgery, in cases where a pheochromocytoma is diagnosed.[29]

Normal Histological Architecture and Normal Cytology

The adrenals are two small symmetrical endocrine glands located near each kidney and beside the caudal vena cava and abdominal aorta. These glands are histologically composed of two distinct areas: an external cortical layer surrounding an internal medulla. These two regions have different embryologic origin and different functional activity. The cells of the adrenal cortex are of mesodermal origin. The cortex is composed of steroid secreting cells and is subdivided into three different zones: the external zona glomerulosa, the zona fasciculata in the middle, and the inner zona reticularis. These three layers produce different hormones. Aldosterone is produced in the zona glomerulosa. Cortisol, other corticosteroids, and sex hormones are produced in the zona fasciculata and zona reticularis. Moreover, the cells of the cortex (mainly in the fasciculata and reticularis) are under the control of the hypothalamic-hypophyseal axis through the adrenocorticotropic hormone (ACTH).[30,31]

The medulla is composed of neuroendocrine cells of ectodermal origin, which produce catecholamines (epinephrine and norepinephrine). These cells function as postganglionic modified neurons that release catecholamines in response to sympathetic stimulation.[30,31]

Since adrenal glands are typically sampled in the case of increased size or neoformation, normal cytology has not been described in detail. However, normal cytology could be suggested by well-differentiated tumor or hyperplasia of the corresponding region. Cortical cells have the typical appearance of steroid-producing endocrine cells (e.g. similar to the Leydig cells of the testicle) that include a low nuclear to cytoplasmic ratio (N:C), an abundant slightly basophilic cytoplasm containing lipid vacuoles, and a round central to paracentral nucleus. Cells from the medulla have a typical neuroendocrine appearance, characterized by a high N:C, scant lightly basophilic cytoplasm, and a round central to eccentric nucleus.[1]

Adrenal Gland Diseases and Corresponding Cytological Findings

Adrenal glands can be affected by several disorders, including inflammation (adrenalitis), infection, hyperplasia (e.g. cortical hyperplasia due to an ACTH-producing pituitary tumor), hypoplasia (e.g. cortical hypoplasia causing Addison's disease), cysts, primary neoplasia, and metastatic neoplasia. Among these conditions, cytology has been proved useful only in the case of infective adrenalitis and primary or metastatic tumor in humans and animals.

Adrenalitis

Adrenal tissues can be affected by several kinds of inflammatory diseases. Idiopathic immune-mediated disorders are associated with lymphoplasmacytic or lymphocytic inflammation leading to atrophy and loss of cortical secretory cells, causing adrenocortical insufficiency (Addison's disease). Most of the infiltrating lymphocytes were CD3 positive T cells in one study, supporting the hypothesis of an immune-mediated destruction of secretory cortical cells.[32] The diagnosis of this condition is based on hormonal testing (e.g. ACTH stimulation test) rather than cytology, since an adrenal cytologic sampling is not possible in case of adrenocortical atrophy.

Infectious agents (bacteria, fungi, and protozoa) can reach the adrenals mainly by the hematogenous route causing suppurative to granulomatous adrenalitis.[31,32] In humans, several case reports and case series have described adrenal infection due to bacteria, including those caused by tubercular mycobacteria,[33,34] and fungi, in particular *Blastomyces* spp., *Cryptococcus* spp., *Histoplasma* spp., *Paracoccidioides* spp., and *Pneumocystis carinii*. Some of these infections have been diagnosed by cytology, with microorganisms being evident in cytological samples.[35–45] Similar reports are lacking in the veterinary literature.

Primary Neoplasia

Adrenal tumors are reported to be quite common in dogs and relatively uncommon in cats.[19] Primary adrenal tumors can arise from the different regions of the adrenal gland. Neoplastic proliferations of the cortical layer are classified as adrenal adenoma or adrenal carcinoma, depending on their biologic behavior. Adrenal medullary tumors are called pheochromocytomas, are classified as neuroendocrine tumors, and can be either benign or malignant. Extra-adrenal pheochromocytomas rarely occur, are usually near large thoracic and abdominal vessels, and are called chromaffin paragangliomas. Many primary adrenal tumors are functionally active in dogs and cats and can secrete an inappropriate amount of one or more hormones causing related clinical syndromes. Primary adrenocortical tumors usually cause hyperadrenocorticism in dogs and hyperadrenocorticism or hyperaldosteronism in cats (Cohn's syndrome).[30,46] Pheochromocytomas can secrete catecholamines and consequently cause clinical symptoms such as hypertension, tachycardia, and tachypnea, or they can have a mass effect on surrounding tissue. About 50% of pheochromocytomas are incidentally discovered and without evident clinical signs.[47] Clinical findings and laboratory tests are often useful in accurately addressing the origin of many adrenal masses. Hormonal testing such as the low-dose desamethazone suppression test, urinary cortisol to creatinine ratio, ACTH stimulation tests, and endogenous ACTH concentration coupled with diagnostic imaging is routinely used to support a diagnosis of adrenal-dependent hyperadrenocorticism. Primary hyperaldosteronism of cats, which is characterized by systemic hypertension, severe hypokalemia causing muscular weakness, and the presence of an adrenal mass, can be confirmed by a high plasma aldosterone concentration and the plasma aldosterone to renin ratio.[46]

In dogs with a clinical suspicion of pheochromocytoma, the measurement of catecholamine metabolites in urine or plasma may be used as a screening test.[48] In a canine study, the measurement of plasma-free normetanephrine has shown promising results in differentiating dogs with pheochromocytoma from healthy dogs, dogs with adrenocortical tumors, and dogs with non-adrenal illness.[49] Plasma-free normetanephrine showed a higher accuracy than free metanephrine in this study. However, these catecholamine metabolites were measured using liquid chromatography–tandem spectrometry, an advanced technology that is not widely available in veterinary laboratories. Serum inhibin is another promising marker for discriminating adrenocortical tumors from pheochromocytoma. Inhibin is produced mainly by gonadostromal cells (granulosa cells and Sertoli cells) and by adrenocortical cells. In a recent study, dogs with pheochromocytoma had very low inhibin concentration compared with dogs with adrenocortical tumors, although the interpretation of inhibin concentration could be confusing in intact dogs.[50]

Many adrenal "incidentalomas" are clinically silent, do not produce significant amounts of hormones or produce unusual hormones, and are therefore difficult to classify. The definitive morphologic classification of adrenal tumors is based on histological features and requires invasive surgery with biopsy. Cytology can offer a minimally invasive diagnostic alternative in some selected cases, even if a conservative approach consisting of periodic monitoring with diagnostic imaging may be suitable for small nonfunctional incidentalomas.[2]

Based on the author's experience, the distinction between adrenocortical tumors and pheochromocytoma is quite straightforward on cytology.[24] Pheochromocytomas show the usual cytological features of other neuroendocrine tumors, such as pancreatic islet cell tumors, C-cell carcinomas of the thyroid gland, parathyroid tumors, and chemodectomas (Figure 46.1). Samples are usually characterized by numerous uniform naked nuclei on a slightly basophilic granular background. This may be due to cellular membrane

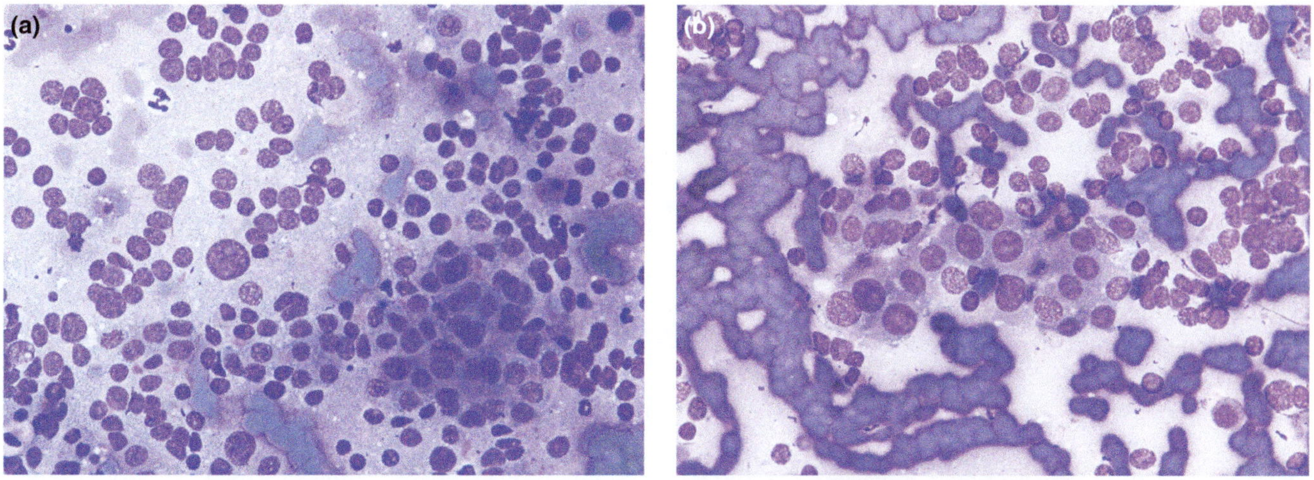

Figure 46.1 Pheochromocytoma from a dog that evidenced metastasis. (a) Many naked nuclei, often arranged in rows or rosette-like structures, are scattered on a basophilic background. A single intact round cell is seen in the upper right. (b) More intact and cohesive cells are evident in this image (May-Grunwald-Giemsa, 400×).

fragility coupled with a nuclear membrane resistance to the trauma caused by sampling and smearing. Thc basophilic background is the result of the release of the cytoplasmic contents. Cells and nuclei are sometimes arranged in rows or in a "rosette-like" pattern. Nuclei appear round to oval, usually with mild anisokaryosis, fine to reticular chromatin, and inconsistent nucleoli. Rare intact cells sometimes have a plasma cell-like appearance, with a moderate amount of basophilic cytoplasm and a paracentral to eccentric nucleus. Cells can be single to slightly cohesive in small clusters. The resulting N:C is high. Cellular atypia is not associated with the clinical behavior.[1]

Adrenocortical tumors are characterized by aggregates of polygonal to rounded cells, with a low N:C, abundant basophilic and often microvacuolated cytoplasm, round eccentric nuclei with coarse chromatin, and small nucleoli (Figure 46.2). Evidence of extramedullary hematopoiesis can be seen in aspirates from adrenocortical neoplasms (Figure 46.3), including megakaryocytes, erythroid, and myeloid precursors.[1,24] Extramedullary hematopoiesis has been more commonly reported in adrenocortical adenomas than carcinomas.[51,52]

A perivascular cellular arrangement can be observed in both adrenocortical tumors and pheochromocytoma, and therefore this feature cannot be used to differentiate these tumors. Unfortunately, cytology cannot be used to define the biologic behavior of adrenal neoplasms, and the same is true for the histological appearance of primary adrenal tumors. Only microscopic or macroscopic assessment of invasiveness into adjacent tissue and metastasis should be considered reliable indicators of malignancy.[1,51] A specific proliferative index of cell cycle (the nuclear protein Ki-67) has been used as a marker of malignancy for adrenocortical tumors but is used only on histologic samples.[51] The differential diagnostic cytological features of primary adrenal tumors are summarized in Table 46.1.

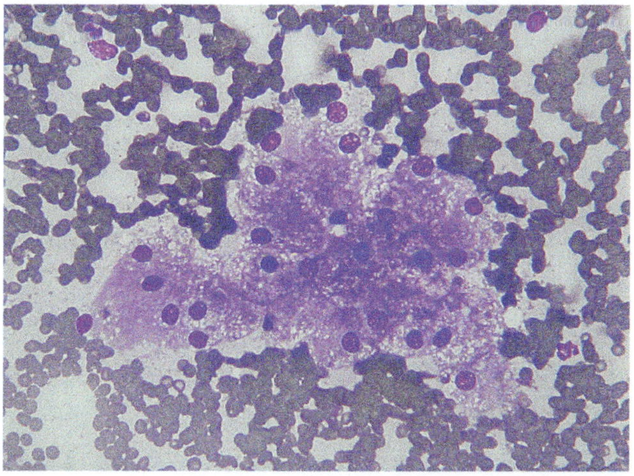

Figure 46.2 Adrenocortical adenoma in a cat with Cohn's syndrome. Clusters of cohesive cells have abundant basophilic and vacuolized cytoplasm (May-Grunwald-Giemsa, 400×).

Other rare primary adrenal gland tumors include neuroblastoma, ganglioneuroma, myelolipoma, and schwannoma.[31,53] Neuroblastomas and ganglioneuroma arise from the medulla, whereas myelolipoma arises from the cortex but may extend into the medulla.[31,52] Neuroblastoma occurs rarely in young dogs. On cytological examination, cells from this tumor may resemble small lymphocytes and sometimes aggregate in clusters or nests with a pseudoacinar arrangement. Histology and immunohistochemistry are needed for a definitive diagnosis.[1,6,52] Ganglioneuroma and schwannoma have been described only by histology and cytological reports are lacking. Myelolipomas are composed of a mixture of well-differentiated adipose tissue and hematopoietic tissue and can occur in spleen, liver, and rarely adrenal glands. Rare cases of adrenal myelolipoma have been diagnosed by cytology in humans[54,55] and are characterized by adipocytes with a mixture of hematopoietic precursors. Finally, a unique case of extra-ovarian granulosa cell tumor of the adrenal gland was diagnosed by cytology in a woman and was confirmed after surgery.[56]

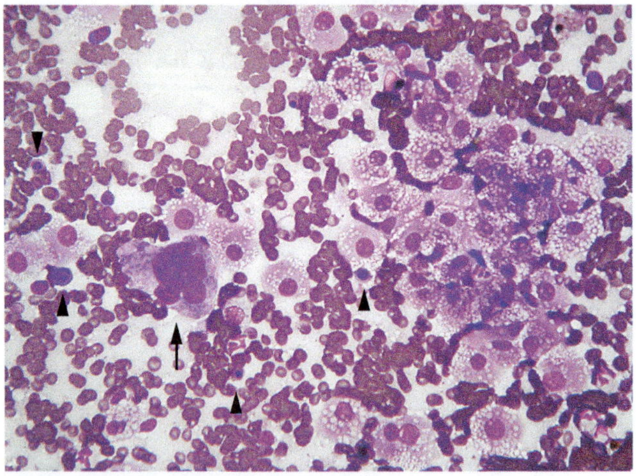

Figure 46.3 Adrenocortical neoplasia in a dog. Extramedullary hematopoiesis is represented by a megakaryocyte (arrow) and some erythroid precursors (arrowhead) (May-Grunwald-Giemsa, 400×).

Metastatic Adrenal Neoplasia

Several case reports and case series in human medicine have documented the ability of cytology to detect metastases and hematopoietic neoplasia involving the adrenal glands, including melanoma,[7,57] histiocytic sarcoma,[58] carcinomas,[7,59,60] liposarcoma,[61] cancer of unknown primary origin,[62] and different subtypes of lymphoma.[7,63,64] In some cases, the neoplastic involvement may be responsible for adrenal insufficiency.[65,66]

Although adrenal metastases seem to be somewhat common in animals based on pathologic data,[65] reports of cytology used to detect and diagnose metastases are not available in veterinary literature. Carcinomas, hemangiosarcoma, and melanoma are the most commonly reported tumors metastatic to the adrenal gland in domestic species.[65]

Adrenal Cysts

Cysts affecting the adrenals are not uncommon in humans and can be endothelial, epithelial, pseudocysts, and parasitic in origin.[67] Up to 7% of adrenal cysts are reported to be malignant, but the usefulness of cytology in such cases is anticipated to be poor in addressing the cyst type and possible malignancy.[68] An adrenal cyst was reported in a ferret.[69]

Table 46.1 Cytological features of adrenocortical tumors and pheochromocytomas.

	Adrenocortical tumors	Pheochromocytomas
General architecture	Many intact cells, singly or in cohesive clusters, with distinct cellular borders Perivascular arrangement possible	Many uniform naked nuclei, often located in a finely granular and basophilic background; rare intact round and plasmacytoid cells Perivascular arrangement possible Sometimes cells or free nuclei arranged in rows or rosette-like structures
N:C	Low	High
Cytoplasm	Basophilic and markedly vacuolated (small to medium-sized clear vacuoles)	Pale blue, finely granular
Nucleus	Round to oval, central to paracentral with coarse or condensed chromatin	Round to oval, with fine to reticular chromatin
Nucleoli	Indistinct to prominent	Indistinct
Other features	Extramedullary hematopoiesis sometimes seen	

References

1 Choi, U.S. and Arndt, T. (2016). Endocrine/Neuroendocrine system. In: *Canine and Feline Cytology: A Color Atlas and Interpretation Guide*, 3e (eds. R.E. Raskin and D.J. Meyer), 430–452. St. Louis: Elsevier.

2 Reusch, C.E. (2015). Pheochromocytoma and multiple endocrine neoplasia. In: *Canine and Feline Endocrinology*, 4e (eds. E.C. Feldman, R.W. Nelson, C.E. Reusch and J.C.R. Scott-Moncrieff), 521–554. St. Louis: Elsevier/Saunders.

3 Gopan, T., Remer, E., and Hamrahian, A.H. (2006). Evaluation and managing adrenal incidentalomas. *Cleve Clin J Med* 73 (6): 561–568.

4 Cowood, T.J., Hunt, P.J., O'Shea, D. et al. (2009). Recommended evaluation of adrenal incidentaloma is costly, has high false-positive rates and confers a risk of fatal cancer that is similar to the risk of the adrenal lesion becoming malignant: time for a rethink? *Eur J Endocrinol* 161: 513–527.

5 Niemann, L.K. (2012). Approach to a patient with adrenal incidentaloma. *J Clin Endocrinol Metab* 95: 4106–4113.

6 Wadih, G.E., Nance, K.V., and Silverman, J.F. (1992). Fine-needle aspiration cytology of the adrenal gland. Fifty biopsies in 48 patients. *Arch Pathol Lab Med* 116: 841–846.

7 Saboorian, M.H., Katz, R.L., and Charnsangavej, C. (1995). Fine needle aspiration cytology of primary and metastatic lesions of the adrenal gland. A series of 188 biopsies with radiologic correlation. *Acta Cytol* 39: 843–851.

8 de Agustín, P., López-Ríos, F., Alberti, N., and Pérez-Barrios, A. (1999). Fine-needle aspiration biopsy of the adrenal glands: a ten-year experience. *Diagn Cytopathol* 21: 92–97.

9 Jhala, N.C., Jhala, D., Eloubeidi, M.A. et al. (2004). Endoscopic ultrasound-guided fine needle-aspiration biopsy of the adrenal glands. *Cancer* 102: 308–314.

10 Martinez, M., LeBlanc, J., Al-Haddad, M. et al. (2014). Role of endoscopic ultrasound fine-needle aspiration evaluating adrenal gland enlargement or mass. *World J Nephrol* 3: 92–100.

11 Puri, R., Thandassery, R.B., Choudhary, N.S. et al. (2015). Endoscopic ultrasound-guided fine-needle aspiration of the adrenal glands: analysis of 21 patients. *Clin Endosc* 48: 165–170.

12 Jhala, N.C., Eltoum, I.A., Eloubeidi, M.A. et al. (2007). Providing on-site diagnosis of malignancy on endoscopic-ultrasound-guided fine-needle aspirates: should it be done? *Ann Diagn Pathol* 11: 176–181.

13 Eloubeidi, M.A., Black, K.R., Tamhane, A. et al. (2010). A large single-center experience of EUS-guided FNA of the left and right adrenal glands: diagnostic utility and impact on patient management. *Gastrointest Endosc* 71: 745–753.

14 Stelow, E.B., Debol, S.M., Stanley, M.W. et al. (2005). Sampling of the adrenal glands by endoscopic ultrasound-guided fine-needle aspiration. *Diagn Cytopathol* 33: 26–30.

15 Fassina, A.S., Borsato, S., and Fedeli, U. (2000). Fine needle aspiration cytology (FNAC) of adrenal masses. *Cytopathology* 11: 302–311.

16 Lumachi, F., Borsato, S., Tregnaghi, A. et al. (2003). CT-scan, MRI and image-guided FNA cytology of incidental adrenal masses. *Eur J Surg Oncol* 29: 689–692.

17 Lumachi, F., Borsato, S., Tregnaghi, A. et al. (2007). High risk of malignancy in patient with incidentally discovered adrenal masses: accuracy of adrenal imaging and image-guided fine-needle aspiration cytology. *Tumori* 93: 268–274.

18 Varadarajulu, S., Fraig, M., Schmulewitz, N. et al. (2004). Comparison of EUS-guided 19-gauge Trucut needle biopsy with EUS-guided fine-needle aspiration. *Endoscopy* 36: 397–401.

19 Bailey, D.B. and Page, R.L. (2007). Tumors of the endocrine system. In: *Withrow & MacEwen's Small Animal Clinical Oncology*, 4e (eds. S.J. Withrow, D.M. Vail and R.L. Page), 583–609. St. Louis: Saunders Elsevier.

20 McCorkell, S.J. and Niles, N.L. (1985). Fine-needle aspiration of catecholamine-producing adrenal masses: a possible fatal mistake. *Am J Roentgenol* 145: 113–114.

21 Casola, G., Nicolet, V., van Sonnembreg, E. et al. (1986). Unsuspected pheochromocytoma: risk of blood-pressure alterations during percutaneous adrenal biopsy. *Radiology* 159: 733–735.

22 de Vries, A.C. and Poley, J.W. (2014). Hypertensive crisis after endoscopic ultrasound-guided fine-needle aspiration of the right adrenal gland. *Endoscopy* 46: 447–448.

23 Masmiquel, L., Hernandez-Pascual, C., Simo, R., and Mesa, J. (1993). Adrenal abscess as a complication of adrenal fine-needle biopsy. *Am J Med* 95: 244–245.

24 Bertazzolo, W., Didier, M., Gelain, M.E. et al. (2014). Accuracy of cytology in distinguishing adrenocortical tumors from pheochromocytoma in companion animals. *Vet Clin Pathol* 43: 453–459.

25 Quayle, F.J., Spitler, J.A., Pierce, R.A. et al. (2007). Needle biopsy of incidentally discovered adrenal masses is rarely informative and potentially hazardous. *Surgery* 142: 497–502.

26 Anagnostic, P., Karagiannis, A., Tziomalos, K. et al. (2009). Adrenal incidentaloma: a diagnostic challenge. *Hormones* 8: 163–184.

27 Lang, J.M., Schertel, E., Kennedy, S. et al. (2011). Elective and emergency surgical management of adrenal gland tumors: 60 cases (1999–2006). *J Am Anim Hosp Assoc* 47: 428–435.

28 Herrera, M.A., Kass, M.P.H., Pascoe, K.P.J. et al. (2008). Predictive factors and the effect of phenoxybenzamine on outcome in dogs undergoing adrenalectomy for pheochromocytoma. *J Vet Intern Med* 22: 1333–1339.

29 Shidham, V.B. and Galindo, L.M. (1999). Pheochromocytoma. Cytologic findings on intraoperative scrape smears in five cases. *Acta Cytol* 43: 207–213.

30 Feldman, E.C. and Nelson, R.W. (eds.) (2004). The adrenal gland. In: *Canine and Feline Endocrinology and Reproduction*, 3e, 251–484. Philadelphia: W.B. Saunders.

31 La Perle, K.M.D. and Capen, C.C. (2007). Endocrine system. In: *Pathologic Basis of Veterinary Disease*, 4e, 693–742. St. Louis: Mosby Elsevier.

32 Frank, C.B., Valentin, S.Y., Scott-Moncrieff, J.C.R., and Miller, M.A. (2013). Correlation of inflammation with adrenocortical atrophy in canine adrenalitis. *J Comp Pathol* 149: 268–279.

33 Buxi, T.B., Vohra, R.B., Sujatha et al. (1992). CT in adrenal enlargement due to tuberculosis: a review of literature with five new cases. *Clin Imaging* 16: 102–108.

34 Rajasekharan, C., Ajithkumar, S., Anto, V., and Parvathy, R. (2013). Extrapulmonary disseminated tuberculosis with tuberculous adrenalitis: a stitch in time saves nine. *BMJ Case Rep* pii: bcr2012008011.

35 Takeishita, A., Nazakawa, H., Akiyama, H. et al. (1992). Disseminated cryptococcosis presenting with adrenal insufficiency and meningitis: resistant to prolonged antifungal therapy but responding to bilater adrenalectomy. *Intern Med* 31: 1401–1405.

36 Rimondi, A.P., Bianchini, E., Barucchello, G., and Panzavolta, R. (1995). Addison's disease caused by adrenal blastomycosis: a case report with fine needle aspiration (FNA) cytology. *Cytopathology* 6: 277–279.

37 Deodhare, S. and Sapp, M. (1997). Adrenal histoplasmosis: diagnosis by fine-needle aspiration biopsy. *Diagn Cytopathol* 17: 42–44.

38 Agarwal, J., Agarwal, G., Ayyagari, A. et al. (2001). Isolated *Pneumocystis carinii* infection of adrenal glands causing Addison's disease in a non-immunocompromised adult. *Endocr Pathol* 12: 87–91.

39 Kumar, N., Singh, S., and Govil, S. (2003). Adrenal histoplasmosis: clinical presentation and imaging features in nine cases. *Abdom Imaging* 28: 703–708.

40 Azhar, J.K., Jacqueline, H.S.G., Tony, L.K.H. et al. (2011). Bilateral adrenal histoplasmosis: endoscopic ultrasound-guided fine needle aspiration as a method of diagnosis and assessment. *Med J Malaysia* 66: 504–506.

41 Colaiacovo, R., Ganc, R.L., Leone, A.C. et al. (2011). Diagnosis of left adrenal paracoccidioidomycosis by endoscopic ultrasound fine needle aspiration. *Endoscopy* 43: 236–237.

42 Jaiswal, S., Vij, M., Chand, G. et al. (2011). Diagnosis of adrenal histoplasmosis by fine needle aspiration cytology: an analysis based on five cases. *Cytopathology* 22: 323–328.

43 Matsuda, Y., Kawate, H., Okishige, Y. et al. (2011). Successful management of cryptococcosis of the bilateral adrenal glands and liver by unilateral adrenalectomy with antifungal agents: a case report. *BMC Infect Dis* 11: 340.

44 Ahuja, A., Mathur, S.R., Iyer, V.K. et al. (2012). Histoplasmosis presenting as bilateral adrenal masses: cytomorphological diagnosis of three cases. *Diagn Cytopathol* 40: 729–731.

45 Rana, C., Kumari, N., and Krishnani, N. (2011). Adrenal histoplasmosis: a diagnosis on fine needle aspiration cytology. *Diagn Cytopathol* 39: 438–442.

46 Djajadiningrat-Laanen, S., Galac, S., and Kooistra, H. (2011). Primary hyperaldosteronism: expanding the diagnostic net. *J Feline Med Surg* 13: 641–650.

47 Barthez, P.Y., Marks, S.L., Woo, J. et al. (1997). Pheochromocytoma in dogs: 61 cases (1984–1995). *J Vet Intern Med* 11: 272–278.

48 Quante, S., Boretti, F.S., Kook, P.H. et al. (2010). Urinary catecholamine and metanephrine to creatinine ratios in dogs with hyperadrenocorticism or pheochromocytoma, and in healthy dogs. *J Vet Intern Med* 24: 1093–1097.

49 Gostelow, R., Bridger, N., and Syme, H.M. (2013). Plasma-free metanephrine and free normetanephrine measurement for the diagnosis of pheochromocytoma in dogs. *J Vet Intern Med* 27: 83–90.

50 Brömel, C., Nelson, R.W., Feldman, E.C. et al. (2013). Serum inhibin concentration in dogs with adrenal gland disease and healthy dogs. *J Vet Intern Med* 27: 76–82.

51 Labelle, P., Kyles, A.E., Farver, T.B., and De Cock, H.E. (2004). Indicators of malignancy of canine adrenocortical tumors: histopathology and proliferation index. *Vet Pathol* 41: 490–497.

52 Wills, T.B. and Haldorson, G.J. (2014). The adrenal gland. In: *Cowell and Tyler's Diagnostic Cytology and Hematology of the Dog and the Cat*, 4e (eds. A.C. Valenciano and R.L. Cowell), 527–531. St. Louis: Elsevier.

53 Jakowski, J.D., Wakely, P.E. Jr., and Jimenez, R.E. (2008). An uncommon type of adrenal incidentaloma: a case report of a schwannoma of the adrenal medulla with cytological, histological, and ultrastructural correlation. *Ann Diagn Pathol* 12: 356–361.

54 Settakorn, J., Sirivanichai, C., Rangdaeng, S., and Chaiwun, B. (1999). Fine-needle aspiration cytology of adrenal myelolipoma: case report and review of the literature. *Diagn Cytopathol* 21: 409–412.

55 Hasan, M., Siddiqui, F., and Al-Ajmi, M. (2008). FNA diagnosis of adrenal myelolipoma: a rare entity. *Diagn Cytopathol* 36: 925–926.

56 Hameed, A. and Coleman, R.L. (2000). Fine-needle aspiration cytology of primary granulosa cell tumor of the adrenal gland: a case report. *Diagn Cytopathol* 22: 107–109.

57 Bang, J.Y., Hebert-Magee, S., and Varadarajulu, S. (2011). Diagnosis of bilateral adrenal metastases secondary to malignant melanoma by EUS-guided FNA. *Am J Gastroenterol* 106: 1862–1863.

58 Singh, C., Schmechel, S.C., Cioc, A.M. et al. (2014). Hemophagocytosis in an adrenal aspirate: histiocytic sarcoma. *Diagn Cytopathol* 42: 863–867.

59 Dusenbery, D. and Dekker, A. (1996). Needle biopsy of the adrenal gland: retrospective review of 54 cases. *Diagn Cytopathol* 14: 126–134.

60 Schuurbiers, O.C., Tournoy, K.G., Schoppers, H.J. et al. (2011). EUS-FNA for the detection of left adrenal metastasis in patients with lung cancer. *Lung Cancer* 73: 310–305.

61 McCutcheon, J., Irvine, A., and Derias, N.W. (1995). Metastatic liposarcoma in the adrenal gland: report of two cases diagnosed by fine-needle aspiration. *Diagn Cytopathol* 13: 330–332.

62 Lee, J.E., Evans, D.B., Hickey, R.C. et al. (1998). Unknown primary cancer presenting as an adrenal mass: frequency and implications for diagnostic evaluation of adrenal incidentalomas. *Surgery* 124: 1115–1122.

63 Cavanna, L., Civardi, G., Vallisa, D., and Bertè, R. (1999). Primary adrenal non-Hodgkin's lymphoma associated with autoimmune hemolytic anemia: a case diagnosed by ultrasound-guided fine needle biopsy. *Ann Ital Med Int* 14: 298–301.

64 Tumino, S., Leotta, M.L., Branciforte, G. et al. (2003). Bilateral adrenal non-Hodgkin lymphoma type B. *J Endocrinol Investig* 26: 1120–1123.

65 Labelle, P. and De Cock, H.E.V. (2005). Metastatic tumors to the adrenal glands in domestic animals. *Vet Pathol* 42: 52–58.

66 Askarian, F. and Xu, D. (2006). Adrenal enlargement and insufficiency: a common presentation of intravascular large B-cell lymphoma. *Am J Hematol* 81: 411–413.

67 Wedmid, A. and Palese, M. (2010). Diagnosis and treatment of the adrenal cyst. *Curr Urol Rep* 11: 44–50.

68 Schmid, H., Mussack, T., Wörnle, M. et al. (2005). Clinical management of large adrenal cystic lesions. *Int Urol Nephrol* 37: 767–771.

69 Besso, J.G., Tidwell, A.S., and Gliatto, J.M. (2000). Retrospective review of the ultrasonographic features of adrenal lesions in 21 ferrets. *Vet Radiol Ultrasound* 41: 345–352.

Part XIII

Central Nervous System

47

Central Nervous System Neoplasia in the Dog and Cat

Diana Schwartz, William Vernau, and Karen M. Vernau

Sample Collection and Preparation

Suspicion of neoplasia based on clinical presentation and imaging findings is the primary indication for collection of central nervous system (CNS) biopsy samples. The utility of needle biopsy for diagnosis of inflammatory conditions has been described;[1] however, if possible, less invasive initial approaches, such as cerebrospinal fluid (CSF) analysis, are preferred. CSF analysis may aid in the diagnosis of CNS neoplasia; however, findings are frequently nonspecific, and exfoliated tumor cells are uncommonly reported. Comprehensive studies to determine the incidence of neoplastic cells in CSF of dogs and cats with primary, nonhemic, CNS tumors are lacking. Tumor location has been shown to be an important predictor of neoplastic cell exfoliation into CSF of humans, with lesions involving the leptomeninges and/or ventricular system associated with more frequent identification of neoplastic cells in CSF specimens.[2] Biopsy samples can be collected surgically following craniotomy or laminectomy; however, a number of less invasive techniques have been developed including computed tomography (CT)-guided stereotactic,[3–5] magnetic resonance imaging (MRI)-guided stereotactic[6] or free hand,[1] ultrasound-guided free hand,[7] and endoscopically[8] collected biopsies. Samples are typically collected via needle biopsy, but fine needle aspiration (FNA), true cut,[9] and pinch biopsies[8] have also been described.

Reported diagnostic yields for CT guided stereotactic needle biopsy range from 91 to 95%.[3,4] Accuracy of CT-guided and MRI-guided biopsies was similar[6]; however, reported disadvantages of MRI over CT included decreased spatial resolution, increased cost, prolonged anesthetic periods, and the inability to confirm needle placement prior to biopsy for frame-based systems.[10] Limitations of the other biopsy collection systems include low diagnostic recovery and inability to sample deeper lesions.[7,8] Comparison of true-cut biopsies and FNA of CNS lesions from cadaver specimens confirmed adequate tissue recovery with both methods, but true-cut biopsies were concordant with necropsy findings in 90% of cases versus 60% concordance with FNA samples.[9]

Complication rates for needle biopsy collection systems range from 12 to 27%.[3,4] The most significant and potentially fatal complications arose from increased intracranial pressure secondary to hemorrhage or edema.[3,4,10] Exacerbation of preexisting neurologic deficits and development or progression of seizures have been reported, which may resolve over time and with additional medical interventions.[3,4] Other complications include epistaxis,[3] subcutaneous emphysema,[5] and cardiac arrhythmias.[4]

Samples of biopsy material from the CNS can be prepared using a touch impression technique and a smear, also called squash or crush technique. These techniques are ideal for use with needle biopsy systems because they require only very small pieces of tissue, allowing for maximum preservation of remaining collected tissue for routine fixation and paraffin embedding or fresh frozen sectioning. Care must be taken not to apply excessive pressure during smear preparation, which can result in cell rupture, as well as use of an appropriately small piece of tissue to avoid smears that are too thick for useful cytological interpretation.[10] In one study, diagnostic accuracy of impression and smear techniques were similar, 55 and 48% respectively.[11] In other studies, cytologic diagnosis from squash/smear preparations of samples collected intraoperatively or from necropsy specimens had complete agreement with the histologic diagnosis in 76–80% of cases.[10,12] An additional 14% of samples in one study were classified as partially correct in that the cytologic diagnosis was not fully specific, the lineage or degree of malignancy was only partially correct, or mixed lesions were not correctly identified as such.[12] The smear technique has the greatest reported diagnostic yield and is currently the most prevalent method of CNS sample preparation in both veterinary and human medicine.[10–12]

Veterinary Cytology, First Edition. Edited by Leslie C. Sharkey, M. Judith Radin, and Davis Seelig.

Multiple rapid staining techniques have been described with diagnostic accuracy largely dependent on the familiarity of the cytopathologist with the stain in use. Classically, smear preparations have been wet fixed with alcohol and stained with hematoxylin and eosin (H&E), toluidine blue, Giemsa, or Papanicolaou's stain. These preparations allow for improved visualization of nerve and glial cell processes but must be quickly (wet) fixed once made to avoid air-drying artifact (nuclear distortion and poor stain uptake).[10] For air-dried smears, Romanowsky-type stains (modified Wright, May-Grunwald-Giemsa), new methylene blue and toluidine blue have all been reported to produce excellent cytoplasmic and nuclear staining and superior evaluation of inflammatory cell populations compared with H&E.[11,12]

Normal Histologic Architecture and Cytology

Samples from different areas of the CNS may have a very different appearance, and detailed characterization of the normal cytological appearance of various regions of the brain in veterinary species has not been performed, but is presumed to be similar to that observed in human CNS tissues. Cells of the CNS can be broadly divided into either neuroectodermal or mesenchymal origin. Glial cells, neurons, and ependymocytes comprise the major neuroectodermal cell populations, while meninges, microglia, and endothelial cells represent the major mesenchymal component (Figure 47.1).

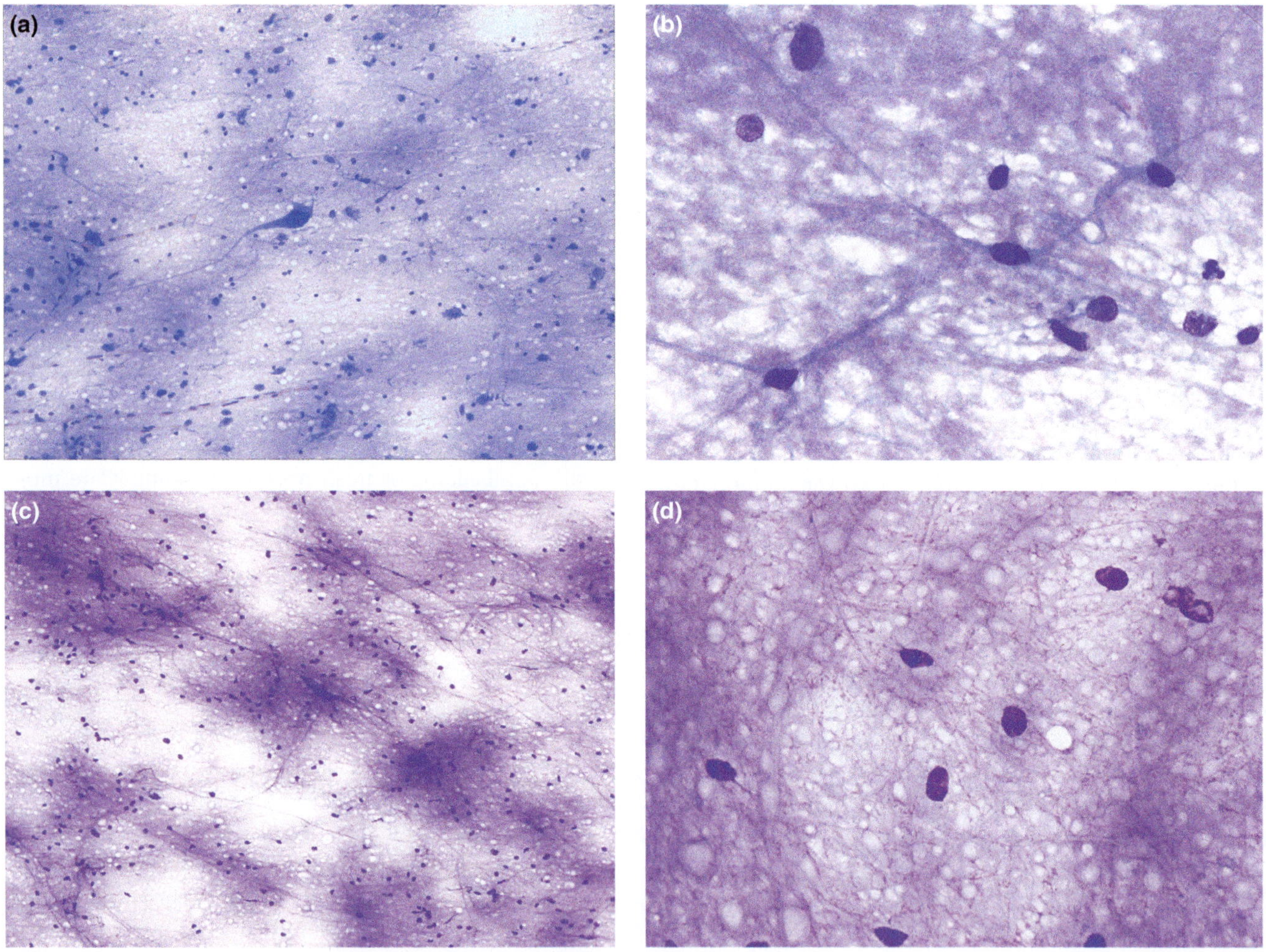

Figure 47.1 Normal canine brain tissue. (a) Temporal gray matter with a neuron (large caudate cell) in the center, many scattered glial cells, and a few fine capillaries. The fibrillar blue background is neuropil (Wright Giemsa, 100×). (b) Temporal gray matter. Astrocytes have ovoid nuclei with long, branching basophilic cytoplasmic processes (Wright Giemsa, 500×). (c) Cerebral white matter. Glial cells are admixed with white matter/myelin, which appears as a pink to purple, coarsely vacuolated to foamy background (Wright Giemsa, 100×). (d) Cerebral white matter/myelin clearly demonstrating the pink to purple vacuolated background (Wright Giemsa, 500×).

The morphology of neurons is highly variable throughout the CNS, but in general, neuron soma (cell bodies) are large, often with a large nucleus and a prominent single nucleolus. Neurons may also contain Nissl substance (aggregates of rough endoplasmic reticulum).[13] Neurons vary dramatically in size, with the smallest in the granular layer of the cerebellum (4–5 μm in diameter) and the largest, up to 100 μm in diameter, in the ventral horn of the spinal cord.[14]

Glial cells represent the greatest cellular component of the CNS and are almost 10-fold higher in numbers than neurons. Astrocytes are the most prominent of the glial cells and play an essential role in maintenance and function of neurons, the blood–brain barrier, and cellular signaling.[15] Astrocytes frequently proliferate around sites of nerve cell injury, and reactive astrocytes must sometimes be distinguished from neoplastic cells, especially in samples from a more peripheral area of a tumor. Astrocytes are ovoid to spindloid and have a small amount of pale basophilic cytoplasm with variable numbers of cytoplasmic processes, which appear as thin, often clear or negatively staining filamentous structures with Romanowsky-type stains. They have oval nuclei with fine chromatin and inconspicuous nucleoli and often appear as naked nuclei.[14] Oligodendrocytes are the second major population of glial cells. CNS myelin is formed from wrapping of oligodendrocyte cell membranes around nerve axons; as such they are most numerous in CNS white matter. Oligodendrocytes are round to oval with a small amount of pale basophilic cytoplasm with variable degrees of fine vacuolation. Nuclei are round with dense hyperchromatic chromatin and inapparent nucleoli.[15]

Microglia are the resident phagocytes and are derived from primitive embryonic yolk sac macrophages that colonize the CNS early in embryogenesis.[16–21] Bone marrow-derived macrophages also can colonize the postnatal brain and differentiate into microglia but only under nonphysiologic conditions associated with disruption of the blood–brain barrier and inflammatory cytokine production.[22] Morphologically, microglia are small ovoid to spindloid cells with scant pale cytoplasm and dense round nuclei. Microglia are especially prominent perivascularly.[14] The immunophenotype of microglia has some species specific variation. Generally speaking microglia can be distinguished from other macrophages and monocytes by low to absent CD45 expression in combination with more typical strong CD11b and CD18 expression.[23]

Ependymocytes are ciliated cells that line the ventricles of the brain and central canal of the spinal cord.[15] They are large polygonal to cuboidal cells with abundant pale purple cytoplasm and frequently many fine azurophilic cytoplasmic granules. Nuclei are round to oval with finely granular chromatin and inapparent nucleoli. Cilia are not typically observed in cytology preparations. Modified ependymal cells make up the choroid plexus, which is the major site of CSF production.[15]

The cells of the CNS are embedded within neuropil, a matrix of neuronal and glial cell processes. Neuropil appears as fluffy to finely fibrillar pale blue-purple material with Romanowsky stains and pale pink on H&E.[14] Overlaying the CNS are three layers of meninges. The innermost pia mater is essentially adherent to the CNS parenchyma. CSF circulates from the ventricular system to the subarachnoid space between the pia mater and the arachnoid membrane, which together comprise the leptomeninges. The dura mater is the outermost layer of the meninges and is adherent to the calvarium but separated from the vertebral bodies by the epidural space.[15]

Neoplasia

Primary tumors of the CNS can be classified into three major categories: neuroectodermal, meningeal/mesenchymal, and hemic. Distant metastatic lesions or direct invasion by aggressive local tumors can secondarily involve the CNS as well. CSF analysis may aid in the diagnosis of CNS neoplasia as alluded to earlier. Normal cells of the leptomeninges, choroid plexus, and ependyma may exfoliate into CSF and must be distinguished from neoplastic cell populations on the basis of frequency and morphology.[2] Identification of cell types in CSF samples can be facilitated through use of an immunocytochemical panel to distinguish leukocytes from ependymal, choroid plexus, or astrocytic cells (Tables 47.1 and 47.2).

Table 47.1 Immunocytochemistry panel for identifying tumor cells in canine and feline CSF.

	Immunophenotype			
Cell type	**CD45**	**CK**	**GFAP**	**Olig2**
Leukocytes	+	–	–	–
Ependymocytes and Choroid plexus cells	–	+	+	–
Astrocytes	–	–	+	–
Oligodendrocytes	–	–	±	+
Metastatic carcinoma cells	–	+	–	–

CK, cytokeratin; GFAP, glial fibrillary acid protein; Olig2, oligodendrocyte transcription factor 2.

Table 47.2 Immunophenotype of Canine and Feline CNS Tumors.[a]

Tumor	Immunophenotype							Other	Additional tests/other
	GFAP	Olig2	CK	Vimentin	SYN	NeuN	NFP		
Astrocytoma	+			+				+ S-100, Nestin	Processes refractile with H&E', may also stain with toluidine blue
Oligodendroglioma	±	+						± DCX + PDGFRα	CSF: cells may exfoliate
Ependymoma	+		±	+				− E-Cadherin	
Choroid plexus papilloma/ Carcinoma	±		±	±				+ E-Cadherin + β-Catenin	CSF: cells may exfoliate CSF TP <80 mg/dL = papilloma or carcinoma CSF TP >80 mg/dL = carcinoma only
Meningioma				+				± S-100	
Gangliocytoma/Ganglioma/ Neurocytoma	±				±	±	±		
Primitive Neuroectodermal tumors/ medulloblastoma	±		±	±	±			± NSE, S-100	May be negative for all conventional markers
Spinal nephroblastoma	−		+	+				+S-100, WT-1	
Granular cell tumor			−	±	−			+ Ubiquitin ± S-100	PAS positive, variably diastase resistant

CK, cytokeratin; DCX, doublecortin; GFAP, glial fibrillary acid protein; H&E, hematoxylin and eosin stain; NFP, neurofilament protein; NSE, neuron-specific enolase; NeuN, neuron-specific nuclear protein; Olig2, oligodendrocyte transcription factor 2; PAS, periodic acid Schiff stain; PDGFRα, platelet-derived growth factor alpha-receptor; SYN, synaptophysin; TP, total protein; WT-1, Wilm's tumor antigen.

[a] The majority of immunophenotyping of canine and feline CNS tumors has been done on formalin-fixed tissues. Reported staining characteristics may not necessarily completely correlate when applied to air-dried cytologic preparations.

Neuroectodermal Tumors

Tumors of neuroectodermal origin are intra-axial and involve the CNS parenchyma. They usually have a soft to gelatinous texture that smears easily to produce even, highly cellular cytological preparations.[12] Vascular proliferation is a prominent feature, in part as a result of increased expression of vascular endothelial growth factor (VEGF) by neoplastic cells. While increased VEGF expression has been observed in many primary CNS tumors, the highest levels have been reported in gliomas.[24] Increased VEGF expression also correlated to higher tumor grade with increased density of VEGF receptors (VEGF-R) observed in the microvasculature of these tumors, suggestive of paracrine signaling.[24,25] Increased VEGF and VEGF-R expression is frequently associated with necrotic lesions but can be identified in tumor cells preceding the appearance of histologically evident necrosis, suggesting the evolution of specific tumor clones with increased angiogenic activity in addition to a response to environmental factors such as regional ischemia.[24,25] Gliomas in both humans and dogs also have been shown to overexpress a variety of tyrosine kinase growth factor receptors including epidermal growth factor receptor (EGFR), platelet-derived growth factor alpha-receptor (PDGFRα), and insulin-like growth factor binding protein 2 (IGFBP2), further supporting the role of autocrine or paracrine production of growth factors in the pathogenesis of gliomas.[26]

Gliomas are the most common of the neuroectodermal tumors in dogs, with brachycephalic breeds (especially Boston Terrier and Boxer dogs) markedly overrepresented.[10,27–29] Gliomas have a propensity for younger individuals, although dogs and cats of all ages may be affected.[30,31] Histologic grading schemes have been largely adopted from human pathology and applied to CNS tumors in animals,[32] despite a paucity of information correlating tumor grade with biologic behavior in veterinary species. In the following sections, histologic grading schemes described reflect the recommendations of the World Health Organization international histological classification of tumors in domestic animals (WHO) in cooperation with the American Registry of Pathology and the Armed Forces Institute of Pathology.

Astrocytoma

Astrocytomas are typically solitary masses that most commonly arise in the brain, more specifically within the white matter of the telencephalon and diencephalon (forebrain).[28] High-grade astrocytomas, also called glioblastoma multiforme (GBM), have also been reported in the caudal brain stem and can be more diffusely invasive along white matter tracts.[33] Estimated incidence of astrocytomas in dogs range from 17 to 28% of all primary brain tumors.[28,30]

Astrocytomas in animals are classified histologically as low, intermediate, and high grade. Tumor grade is largely dependent on the degree of differentiation, with low-grade tumors being characterized by lower cellularity, good cellular differentiation, minimal invasiveness, and absent mitotic activity. Fibrillary, protoplasmic, and gemistocytic subtypes are considered low grade. Intermediate grade tumors, designated anaplastic astrocytomas, are hypercellular with increased cellular and nuclear atypia, observable mitotic activity and occasional multinucleated tumor cells. High-grade astrocytomas, called GBM, are characterized by regions of necrosis, endothelial proliferation, and marked invasiveness into adjacent parenchyma.[28,33]

Cytologically, astrocytomas are of moderate to high cellularity, often with extensive, fine branching capillaries (Figure 47.2). Tumor cells are typically observed along the margins of these blood vessels, sometimes in a pseudopalisading arrangement. Cells are oval to spindloid, with scant pale cytoplasm and numerous, thin, elongated, clear cytoplasmic processes (Romanowsky stain). On alcohol-fixed H&E stained smears, these astrocyte processes appear as an extensive network of pale eosinophilic fibrillary structures, which are refractile with phase contrast,[10,28] and blue with toluidine blue.[11] Nuclei are typically oval to elongated with finely stippled chromatin and inconspicuous nucleoli. Nuclear to cytoplasmic ratios (N:C) are moderate to high; anisocytosis and anisokaryosis are typically low. The tumor cells of anaplastic astrocytomas and GBM (intermediate and high-grade astrocytomas) may appear more round to polygonal and can be confused with poorly differentiated carcinomas.[12]

Immunophenotypically, astrocytomas are characterized by cytoplasmic expression of glial fibrillary acid protein (GFAP) and S-100.[28,34] The more poorly differentiated tumor cells in high-grade astrocytoma/GBM display inconsistent GFAP expression but are reliably vimentin positive, and coexpression of these two markers can help confirm astrocyte origin in more anaplastic lesions.[28] Astrocytomas often express EGFR with higher expression reported in high-grade tumors.[26] High-grade astrocytomas/GBM are also reportedly positive for nestin, an intermediate filament involved in axonal growth.[34]

Oligodendroglioma

Oligodendrogliomas are the second most common glioma in dogs, up to 15–20% of all intracranial neoplasms.[15,30,35] These tumors present typically as solitary masses, most often within the forebrain white matter. In dogs, oligodendrogliomas are more likely to arise adjacent to, and protruding into, the lateral ventricles than astrocytomas and have been less commonly reported within the ventricles

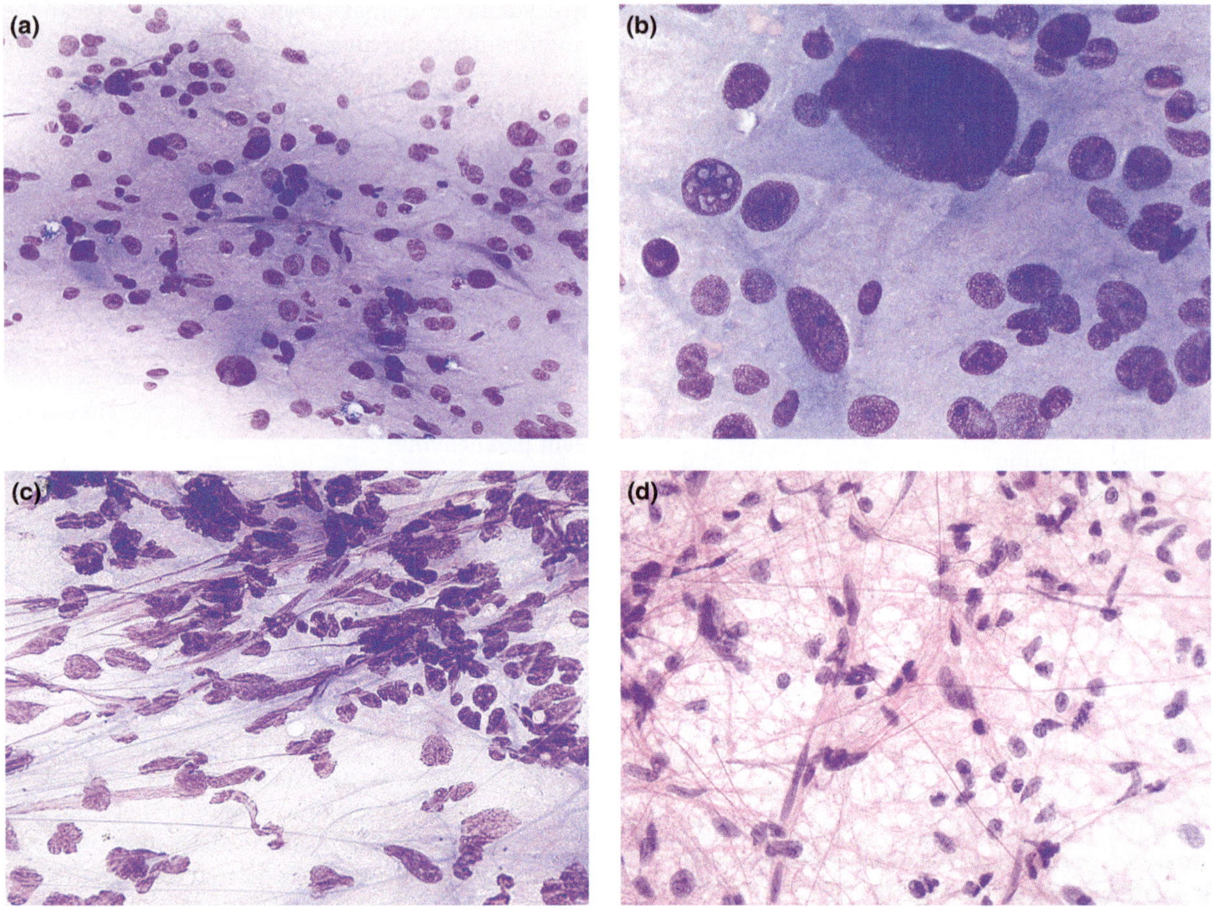

Figure 47.2 Canine astrocytoma. (a) High-grade astrocytoma, also called glioblastoma multiforme. Note the high cellularity and the long, basophilic cytoplasmic processes compatible with astrocytic origin, in concert with clear cytologic criteria of malignancy (Wright Giemsa, 200×). (b) High-grade astrocytoma with many cytologic features of malignancy including karyomegaly, marked anisocytosis and anisokaryosis, finely dispersed to irregularly clumped chromatin, and multiple, prominent nucleoli (Wright Giemsa, 500×). (c) Astrocytomas have numerous fine basophilic cytoplasmic processes streaming and crisscrossing throughout the background (Wright Giemsa, 500×). (d) Astrocyte cell processes are more clearly delineated with a wet fixed hematoxylin and eosin stain (400×).

and the spinal cord or as multiple discrete masses throughout the CNS.[30,32,36] Oligodendrogliomas are uncommon in cats, with only intracranial masses reported.[37] While tumors have been noted within the cerebral hemispheres, the distribution of lesions in cats appears to be less restricted, with lesions also reported in the midbrain and cerebellum, and adjacent to the fourth ventricles.[37]

Histologically oligodendrogliomas are classified as benign or malignant (anaplastic). In addition to increased cellularity and pleomorphism, anaplastic oligodendrogliomas are characterized by prominent proliferation of glomeruloid vessels, which may appear as tortuous capillary fragments in smear preparations. Additional features associated with malignant oligodendrogliomas include necrosis and/or meningeal infiltration.[32]

Cytologic preparations of oligodendrogliomas are typically highly cellular with a distinct background of abundant pink, stippled to fibrillar, mucinous matrix (Figure 47.3). Capillary fragments are often observed and, in contrast to astrocytomas, are typically free of attached tumor cells. Cells are individual, round to ovoid with a low to moderate amount of pale blue cytoplasm that often contains punctate vacuoles. Nuclei are round, central to eccentric, and with fine, granular, immature appearing chromatin and inconspicuous nucleoli. Anisocytosis and anisokaryosis are typically low to moderate. Few mitotic figures and reactive astrocytes may also be observed.[10] In cats, neoplastic oligodendrocytes have been observed in CSF cytocentrifuge preparations, with or without an inflammatory pleocytosis or increased protein concentration.[37]

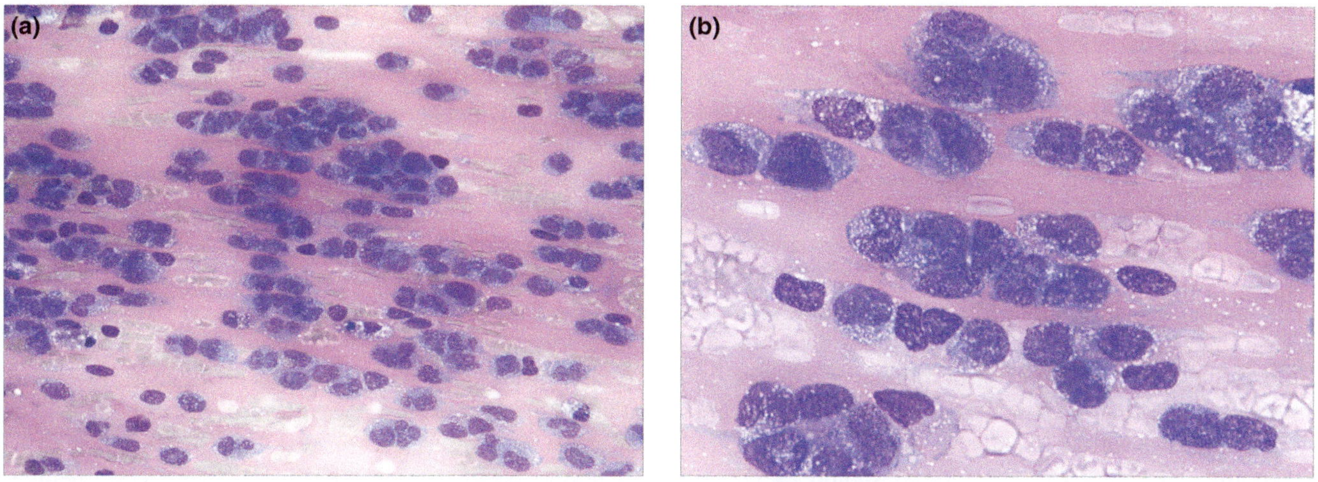

Figure 47.3 Canine oligodendroglioma. (a) Note the dense mucinous pink background typical of oligodendroglioma that frequently results in windrowing of cells (Wright Giemsa, 250×). (b) Cells are relatively uniform and round to ovoid with high N:C ratios, finely granular chromatin, inapparent or small nucleoli, and a small volume of blue, often finely vacuolated cytoplasm (Wright Giemsa, 600×).

Oligodendrocyte transcription factor (Olig2) is a sensitive marker for oligodendrogliomas, with 75–100% of tumors having strong nuclear immunoreactivity in formalin-fixed paraffin-embedded tissues.[36,38] Doublecortin (DCX) expression, a microtubule-associated protein seen in developing neurons, has also been reported in oligodendrogliomas.[34] Anaplastic oligodendrogliomas are consistently immunoreactive for PDGFRα and often also express IGFBP2.[26]

Mixed Glioma (Oligoastrocytoma)

Mixed gliomas are defined by the presence of at least 25% of either glial types, which may be intermixed or geographically distinct. Mixed gliomas can be well differentiated or anaplastic (malignant).[32] Foci of mineralization are reported.[10] Mixed gliomas appear rare in dogs and cats, with few reports in the veterinary literature.[30,39]

Gliomatosis cerebri, widespread infiltration of the brain and spinal cord by neoplastic glial cells with minimal disruption of adjacent parenchyma, has been uncommonly reported in dogs.[32,38,40] In humans, gliomatosis cerebri is divided into two types, with Type I characterized by diffuse infiltration of multiple CNS divisions and Type II defined as the concurrent presence of a discrete mass lesion.[38] While this classification scheme has not been formally adopted in veterinary medicine, both manifestations of gliomatosis cerebri have been described.[38] Lesions are typically bilateral in dogs and involve both gray matter and white matter tracts, often adjacent to ventricles and pia mater.[38,40] While the histogenesis of gliomatosis cerebri is not fully defined, in humans the majority of cases are presumed to be astrocytic in origin on the basis of cell morphology and GFAP positivity, with fewer reports of both oligodendrocytic and mixed cell populations.[38,40] In contrast, results of immunohistochemical studies in dogs suggest predominantly an oligodendrocyte origin with all lesions in multiple small case series showing positive Olig2 nuclear reactivity and negative GFAP cytoplasmic immunoreactivity, in putative neoplastic cells.[38,40] Possible microglial and leukocytic origins were also assessed immunohistochemically, and in all cases neoplastic cells did not express CD18, CD45, CD3, or CD79a, excluding these origins.[40]

Ependymal Tumors

Ependymal tumors are relatively uncommon in animals but have been more frequently reported in cats compared with dogs.[31,32,41] Ependymomas are expansile, slow-growing mass lesions and are predominantly located supratentorially, associated with the ventricular system (especially the third and lateral ventricles) in the brain and the central canal of the spinal cord.[31,41] Extraventricular ependymomas have been rarely described in cats, associated with the neocortex and subarachnoid space.[41]

Histologically ependymomas are classified as benign or anaplastic (malignant), with anaplastic tumors having increased mitotic rates, cellular atypia, and evidence of parenchymal infiltration.[32] Multiple different histologic variants have been reported and include classic, papillary, tanycytic, and clear cell; however, the prognostic significance of these subtypes in animals has yet to be determined.[32,41,42] Tumors can be associated with areas of necrosis and mineralization with cholesterol clefts and hemorrhage.[41]

Cytologic preparations are highly cellular, often with prominent vasculature. Tumor cells are observed in sheets and may be adherent in a perpendicular arrangement to capillaries (Figure 47.4). Pseudorosettes are a prominent feature. Cells are oval to elongate with well-defined margins. Nuclei are central to eccentric, round to oval, and with finely stippled chromatin and inconspicuous nucleoli. Eccentric nuclei may be especially prominent in cats.[10] Cilia are uncommonly reported.[32]

Differential diagnoses for ependymomas include choroid plexus tumors and metastatic carcinomas. Papillary ependymomas have a glial rather than fibrovascular core as observed in choroid plexus tumors. Ependymomas are typically GFAP positive, E-cadherin negative, and largely cytokeratin (CK) negative. Carcinomas should be GFAP negative and strongly CK positive, and choroid plexus tumors have variable GFAP expression but are E-cadherin positive.[10,41,43]

Choroid Plexus Tumors

Choroid plexus tumors account for approximately 7–10% of primary brain tumors in dogs[30,44] and have been sporadically reported in cats.[31] These tumors arise from the epithelium of the choroid plexus, typically forming discrete mass lesions associated with the ventricular system of the brain and spinal cord, particularly the fourth ventricles.[44] While metastasis outside of the CNS has not been reported in veterinary species, the majority of cases metastasize to the subarachnoid space, and disseminated intracranial lesions have also been described.[44]

Choroid plexus tumors have been divided into benign (papillomas) and malignant (carcinomas) categories

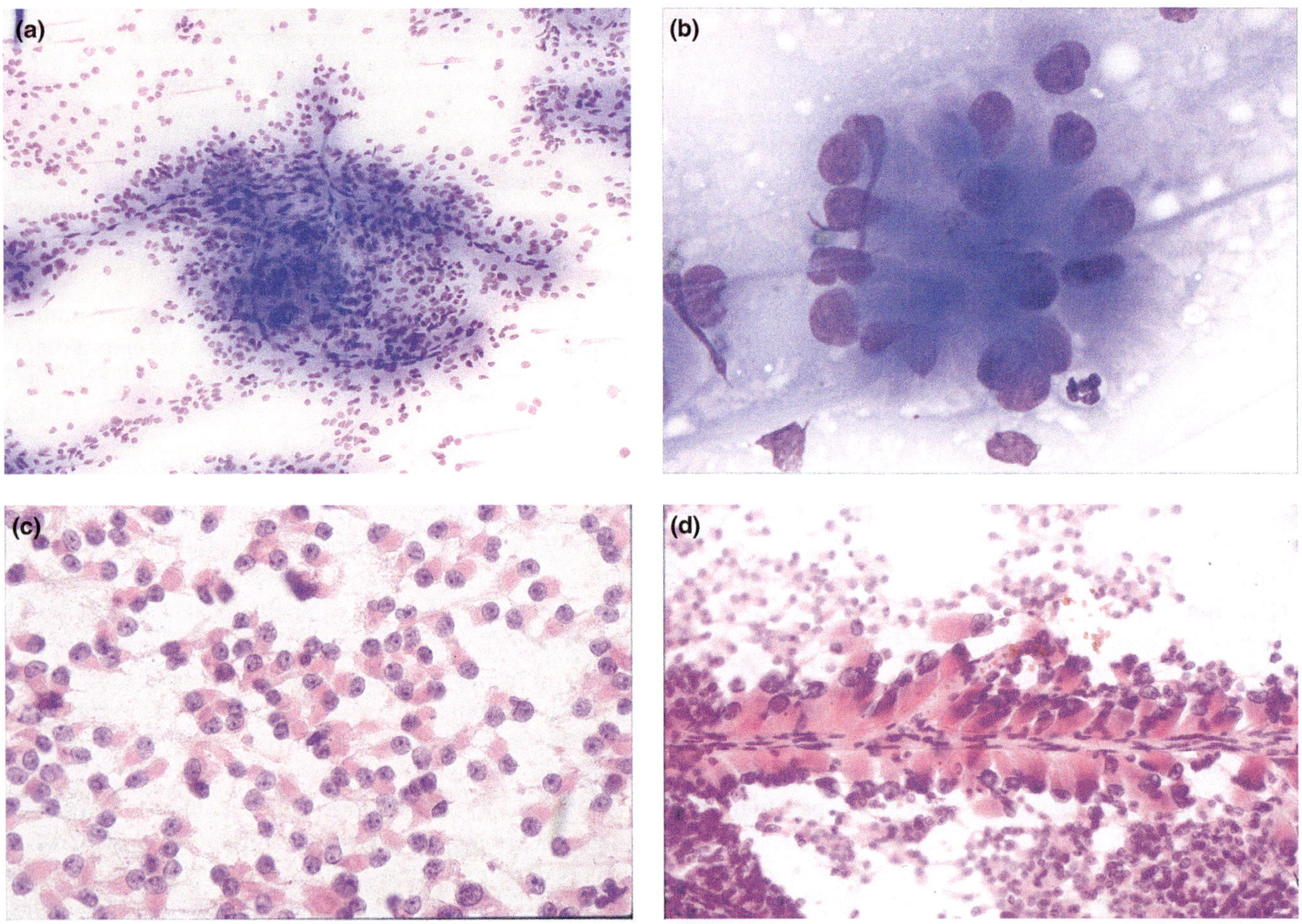

Figure 47.4 Feline ependymoma. (a) Note the arrangement of cells palisading along prominent branching capillaries (Wright Giemsa, 100×). (b) Rosettes can be observed in ependymomas (Wright Giemsa, 600×). (c) Individual cells in ependymomas are oval to cuboidal to columnar, with central to basal nuclei (Wet fixed hematoxylin and eosin stain, 200×). (d) Prominent palisading of tumor cells occurs along vasculature (Wet fixed hematoxylin and eosin stain, 200×).

histologically, solely on the degree of cellular atypia.[32] Additional proposed criteria of malignancy include the presence of metastases within the ventricles and along the neuraxis, thereby including well-differentiated but biologically aggressive choroid plexus tumors as carcinomas. However, this recommendation has not been universally applied in the veterinary literature.[32,43,44] Choroid plexus carcinomas appear more common than papillomas in dogs.[43,44]

Cytologic preparations are highly cellular with abundant branching blood vessels (Figure 47.5). Neoplastic cells are round, polygonal, or columnar and may be arranged in sheets or radiating patterns often adherent to associated vasculature. Cells have abundant cytoplasm with round to oval, sometimes basilar nuclei. Marked anisokaryosis has been reported in carcinomas. Scattered foci of mineralization can be observed.[10]

Exfoliated neoplastic cells, usually in small clusters or picket fence-type arrangements, have been observed in the CSF of dogs with choroid plexus tumors and may be more commonly seen in carcinomas.[44,45] Additionally, the CSF protein concentration has been found to be discriminatory between benign and malignant choroid plexus tumors in dogs. All papillomas had a CSF protein concentration <80 mg/dL. CSF protein concentrations >80 mg/dL only occurred with choroid plexus carcinomas, although some carcinomas did have <80 mg/dL protein.[44]

The immunohistochemical staining characteristics of choroid plexus tumors vary by report with variable CK,

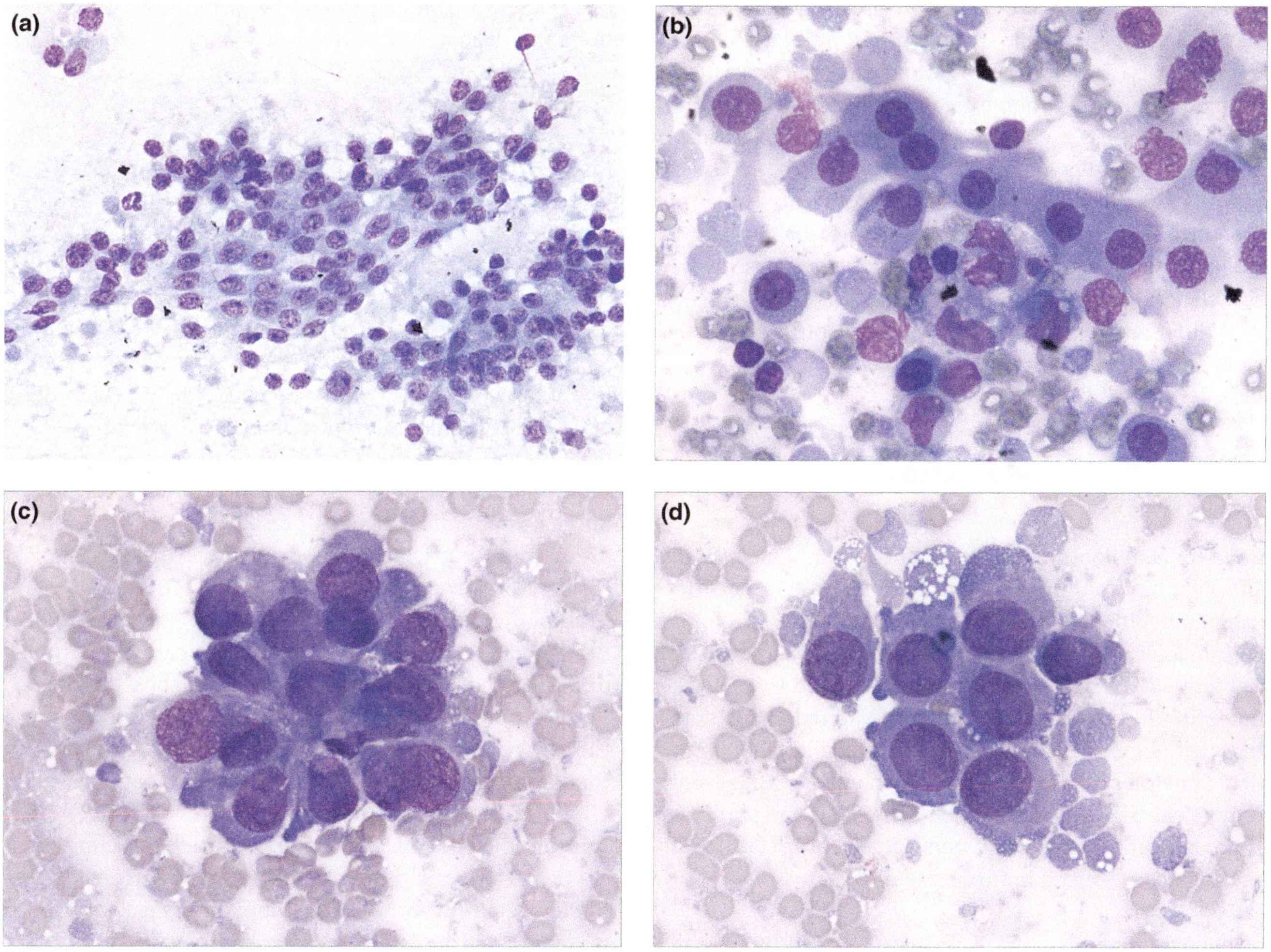

Figure 47.5 Canine choroid plexus tumors. (a) Choroid plexus papilloma exhibits uniform rafts of polygonal to fish-scale like cells. There is minimal anisocytosis and anisokaryosis (Wright Giemsa, 100×). (b) Choroid plexus carcinoma displays increased anisokaryosis compared with a choroid plexus papilloma. Neoplastic cells can sometimes be present in picket fence-type formations (Wright Giemsa, 600×). (c) Choroid plexus carcinoma. Neoplastic cells are round, polygonal, or columnar and may be arranged in sheets and clusters. Carcinomas have moderate to marked anisokaryosis and can have prominent nucleoli (Wright Giemsa, 600×). (d) Choroid plexus carcinoma. Neoplastic cells can exhibit prominent cytoplasmic blebbing (Wright Giemsa, 600×).

vimentin, and GFAP expression.[10,32,34,43,45,46] It has been postulated that the observed focal GFAP positivity sometimes described in choroid plexus tumors may represent associated reactive astrocytosis, although glial differentiation of tumor cells is also possible.[43,45] Choroid plexus tumors express E-cadherin and β-catenin and often have aberrant cytoplasmic and/or nuclear expression of these proteins, compared with the membranous positivity observed in normal choroid plexus tissue.[43] Aberrant E-cadherin and β-catenin expression did not correlate with a histologic diagnosis of malignancy.[43]

Neuronal/Neuronal-Glial Tumors

Tumors with neuronal differentiation are rarely reported in dogs and include neurocytoma, gangliocytoma, and ganglioglioma. These are typically slow-growing mass lesions that arise in the brain or spinal cord of young to middle-aged animals (four months to seven years) and consist of a population of well-differentiated neurons (neurocytoma, gangliocytoma), which may be admixed with neoplastic glial cells (ganglioglioma).[47–49] Neurocytomas appear to have a predilection for the ventricular system.[47] Histologically, tumor cells are reported to be variable in size, often with Nissl substance, and sometimes display binucleation. Mineral deposits have been described.[48–50] Well-differentiated neuronal elements express neurofilament protein,[48,50] neuron-specific enolase (NSE), and synaptophysin.[47,49]

Embryonal/Primitive Neuroectodermal Tumors (PNET)

Embryonal tumors are uncommon neoplasms that typically affect young to mature dogs and cats and arise from germinal neuroepithelial cells.[10,30,32,51,52] They share a similar morphologic appearance to the so called "small round blue cell tumors."[53] These lesions are characterized by a population of uniform, small to medium size, round to polygonal cells, with high N:C ratios and deeply basophilic cytoplasm, that can easily be mistaken for lymphoma.[51,54] Embryonal tumors can arise throughout the body; however, particular emphasis on embryonal tumors largely restricted to the CNS will be described in further detail below.

Medulloblastoma

Medulloblastoma is infrequently reported in dogs and cats but is the most common PNET in these species.[51,52,55] The histogenesis is not entirely clear, but these tumors are thought to arise from the external granular layer of the cerebellum and may display variable and mixed glial and neuronal differentiation.[52,56] Enhanced telomerase and KIT receptor tyrosine kinase activity may play a role in the pathogenesis of medulloblastoma in dogs.[56] Tumors are most commonly observed in the cerebellar vermis and cerebellar hemispheres but can infiltrate the adjacent medulla, spinal cord, and meninges.[51,52,55,56] Exfoliated tumor cells have been reported in CSF.[51] Histologically, neoplastic cells are arranged in sheets, cords, and rosettes surrounding pools of pale eosinophilic fibrillary material.[51] Cytologically, most cells are round but also can appear polygonal to ovoid. Nuclei are typically round but can have some membrane irregularity, and have fine, granular chromatin. Cells have high N:C ratios and frequent, often atypical, mitotic figures.[10,51] Variable results of immunohistochemical studies have been reported. Medulloblastomas are described as being positive for vimentin,[52,56] GFAP,[52,55] S-100,[52] synaptophysin,[56] CK,[56] and NSE.[55,56] Tumors can also be negative for all conventional markers, reflecting their lack of differentiation.[51]

Spinal Nephroblastoma

Few case series and case reports of spinal nephroblastoma in dogs exist. This tumor has also been referred to by a variety of other terms including thoracolumbar spinal tumor of young dogs, embryonal nephroma, and Wilm's tumor.[57,58] Nephroblastomas arise from the primitive metanephric blastema, which ultimately differentiates to form the epithelial and stromal elements of the kidney. Stem cells of the metanephric blastema that do not differentiate into elements of the kidney ultimately undergo apoptosis. Spinal nephroblastomas arise when these stem cells persist and become trapped in the dura during fetal development.[58] Tumors are typically solitary, intradural, and extramedullary masses present at the T9-L3 regions of the spinal cord and are associated with clinical signs of spinal cord compression. Multifocal, metastatic, and intramedullary spinal nephroblastomas have rarely been described.[58] Histologically and cytologically, nephroblastomas are characterized by tumors composed of two to three different cell populations, including stromal, epithelial, and undifferentiated elements.[57,58] Notably, epithelial components may be arranged in papillae, acini, glomeruli, tubules and pseudorosettes (Figure 47.6).[57] Immunohistochemically, the epithelial component expresses CK and S-100, often with concurrent positive nuclear staining of Wilm's tumor antigen (WT-1). The mesenchymal and blastemal components are vimentin positive.[57,58]

Neuroblastoma (Olfactory, Cerebral), Pineoblastoma, Spongioblastoma, Ependymoblastoma

Characterization of other PNETs in veterinary medicine is largely limited to few case reports and case series.

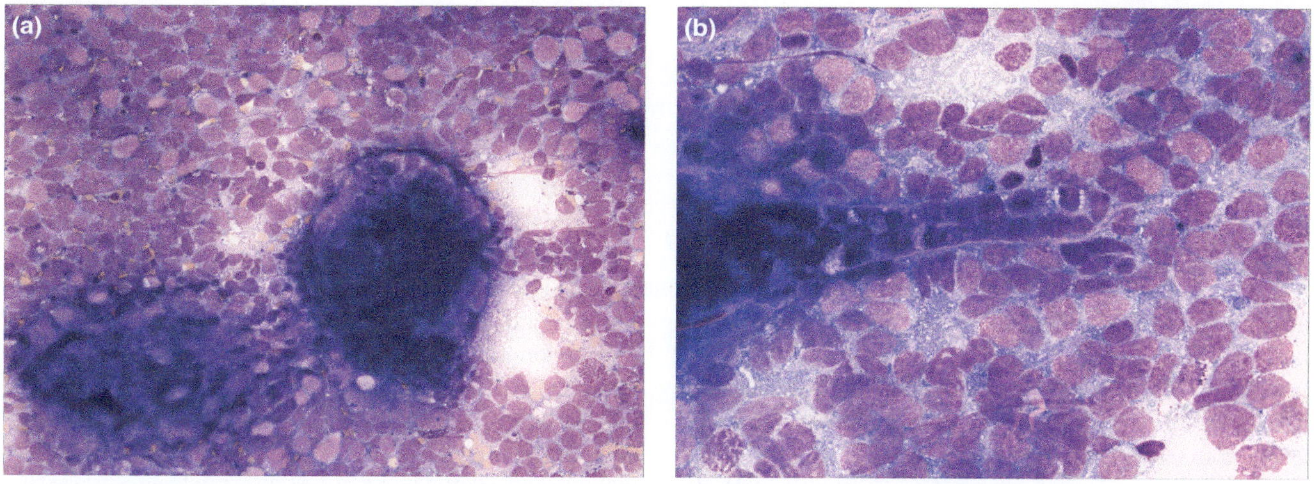

Figure 47.6 Canine spinal nephroblastoma. (a) The tumor is highly cellular, consisting predominantly of undifferentiated round cells (blasts) but forming glomerulus-like structures in some areas (center, bottom left) (Wright Giemsa, 200×). (b) The undifferentiated round cells (blasts) have high N:C ratios; finely stippled, immature chromatin; and variably prominent nucleoli. In addition to glomerulus-like structures, tubule formation may also be present (center) (Wright Giemsa, 400×).

Histological and cytological classification can be challenging as theses tumors may lack distinguishing architectural and cytomorphologic features.[59] Neoplastic cells can have variable immunoreactivity to vimentin,[54,59] S-100,[54] GFAP,[59] CK,[59] NSE,[54,59,60] synaptophysin,[47,50,60] and microtubule-associated protein-2 (MAP-2). Neoplastic cells may be negative for all conventional markers, reflecting their primitive origins.

Meningeal/Mesenchymal Tumors

Meningeal and mesenchymal tumors of the CNS are typically extra-axial lesions. They have a varied composition ranging from soft to firm and gritty, which often results in unevenly clumped, highly cellular smear preparations.[10,12] VEGF expression is documented in canine meningiomas. Increased VEGF expression is a positive predictor of tumor recurrence and is associated with decreased survival.[61] That being said, hypoxia appears to be a primary stimulus for increased VEGF expression, with the most pronounced increases observed in tumors with widespread necrosis.[61] Additionally, progesterone influences tumor progression. Progesterone receptors (PR) have been identified in both canine and feline meningiomas. Decreased PR expression is associated with lesions that have a higher proliferative index and more aggressive histologic phenotype.[62]

Meningioma

Meningiomas are the most common primary CNS tumor in dogs and cats, accounting for 22.3–59% of canine and feline brain tumors.[30,61–66] Meningiomas are typically slow-growing discrete masses with broad dural attachments.[32] Intracranial meningiomas are most common and usually arise from cells of the arachnoid meninges.[64] In dogs, intracranial meningiomas are typically solitary, located within the telencephalon.[30] Spinal meningiomas are most common cranially to C3, followed by the lumbar segments.[67] In a retrospective study of 160 cats, intracranial meningiomas were mostly supratentorial, with up to 17.2% of individuals having multiple discrete meningiomas of the same type.[31,65] In cats, meningiomas are often associated with the tela choroidea of the third ventricle.[31,32] Cats are more likely to have multiple intracranial neoplasms of different types, compared with dogs.[30,31]

Histologically, there are many different subtypes of meningiomas in dogs, the majority of which have benign biologic behavior, the space occupying effects notwithstanding. As in other CNS tumors of animals, grading of meningiomas has not been fully correlated to clinical behavior. Histologically, meningiomas are divided into either benign or anaplastic (malignant) categories.[32] Anaplastic malignant meningiomas are associated with increased mitotic index, invasiveness, necrosis, and metastasis.[32,65] More recently, the human WHO tumor grading scheme has been applied to canine meningiomas in an effort to include additional histologic subtypes and provide improved prognostic information.[65] Canine meningiomas typically have mixtures of different histologic patterns with tumors classified by the dominant pattern observed. Grade 1 (benign) meningiomas include meningothelial and transitional (most commonly) as well as microcystic, psammomatous, and angiomatous subtypes.

Grade 2 meningiomas are characterized by increased mitotic activity, cellular atypia, necrosis, and patternless growth and include atypical and chordoid subtypes. The prevalence of Grade 2 meningiomas may be higher in dogs than humans (>40% vs. 8%),[66] although recent revision of the human WHO scheme has resulted in increased diagnosis of Grade 2 meningiomas (20–35%) in people. In humans, Grade 2 meningiomas may grow faster or recur more quickly following excision than Grade 1 meningiomas.[68] Grade 3 (anaplastic/malignant) meningiomas have the highest mitotic rate and cytologic features of malignancy. Tissue invasiveness was not included in the veterinary WHO grading scheme but is more commonly observed in canine meningiomas compared with feline.[65] Feline meningiomas are more uniform in their morphology, the majority of which have a fibrous/spindloid phenotype often associated with foci of calcification, necrosis, and cholesterol crystals.[10]

Smear preparations from meningiomas are typically highly cellular and are often associated with branching capillaries, although to a lesser extent than gliomas (Figures 47.7 and 47.8). Cells are arranged in variably sized cohesive aggregates, with fewer interspersed individual cells, and are round to elongated with polygonal to wispy cytoplasm. Nuclei are also round to elongated and usually fairly uniform, with finely stippled chromatin and single, small prominent nucleoli. Intranuclear pseudoinclusions (cytoplasmic invaginations) can be observed, most commonly associated with the meningothelial subtype. Additionally, nuclei may have a central longitudinal fold. Transitional subtypes often have distinctive whorls.

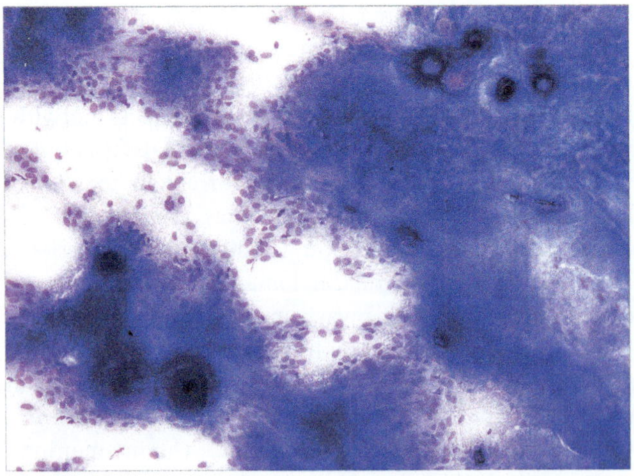

Figure 47.7 Canine psammomatous meningioma. Note the frequent, variably sized, mineralized structures (psammoma bodies) often surrounded by whorls of spindle cells (Wright Giemsa, 100×).

Psammoma bodies are observed in psammomatous subtypes.[10] Abundant background pink extracellular matrix material is present in chordoid subtypes in humans,[69] and similar findings have been observed in cytology preparations from canine chordoid meningiomas (Figure 47.8d, Authors' observation).

Meningiomas can typically be reliably identified via morphology alone, and ancillary tests (e.g. immunochemistry, CSF analysis) are generally nonspecific.[10,64] Peripheral nerve sheath tumors (PNST) are a primary differential for meningioma, especially in the case of cervical spinal cord lesions. In these circumstances, S-100 expression in the neoplastic cell population can help identify PNST and exclude meningioma, although meningiomas can sometimes express S-100.[12]

Hemic Tumors

Lymphoma

Primary lymphomas of the CNS are relatively uncommon in dogs and cats, accounting for 4% all intracranial tumors in dogs.[30] CNS involvement is most often metastasis of multicentric lymphoma, and lymphoma was the most common secondary CNS tumor reported in a series of cats.[31,70–72] In contrast to humans, primary CNS lymphoma in small animals appears to be predominantly of T cell origin,[71] although in a recent case series in dogs, the only primary CNS lymphoma identified was a diffuse large B-cell lymphoma (DLBCL) in the cervical spinal cord.[72] It appears that neuroanatomic localization of metastatic CNS lymphoma corresponds to specific WHO lymphoma subtype in dogs, with perivascular, periventricular, and pituitary involvement over represented in B-cell lymphomas, most notably DLBCL. Peripheral nervous system infiltration, typically of spinal nerves and nerve roots, was most often observed with peripheral T-cell lymphoma, although less commonly this pattern was also noted in dogs with DLBCL.[72] In cats, feline leukemia virus has been associated with the development of CNS lymphoma, particularly in the thoracic segments of the spinal cord.[73–76] Neoplastic lymphocytes can often be observed in CSF, but their absence does not preclude the diagnosis.[30,70,72,76] The magnitude of neoplastic pleocytosis present in CSF analysis is directly related to the degree of meningeal and periventricular infiltration by neoplastic lymphocytes.[72] Intravascular lymphoma is a rare multisystemic lymphoma that appears to have a predilection for the CNS and has been reported in dogs and cats.[77,78] Neoplastic lymphocytes localize to small- and medium-sized arteries and veins throughout the CNS and other tissues, resulting in microthrombosis and parenchymal injury. In a small case series

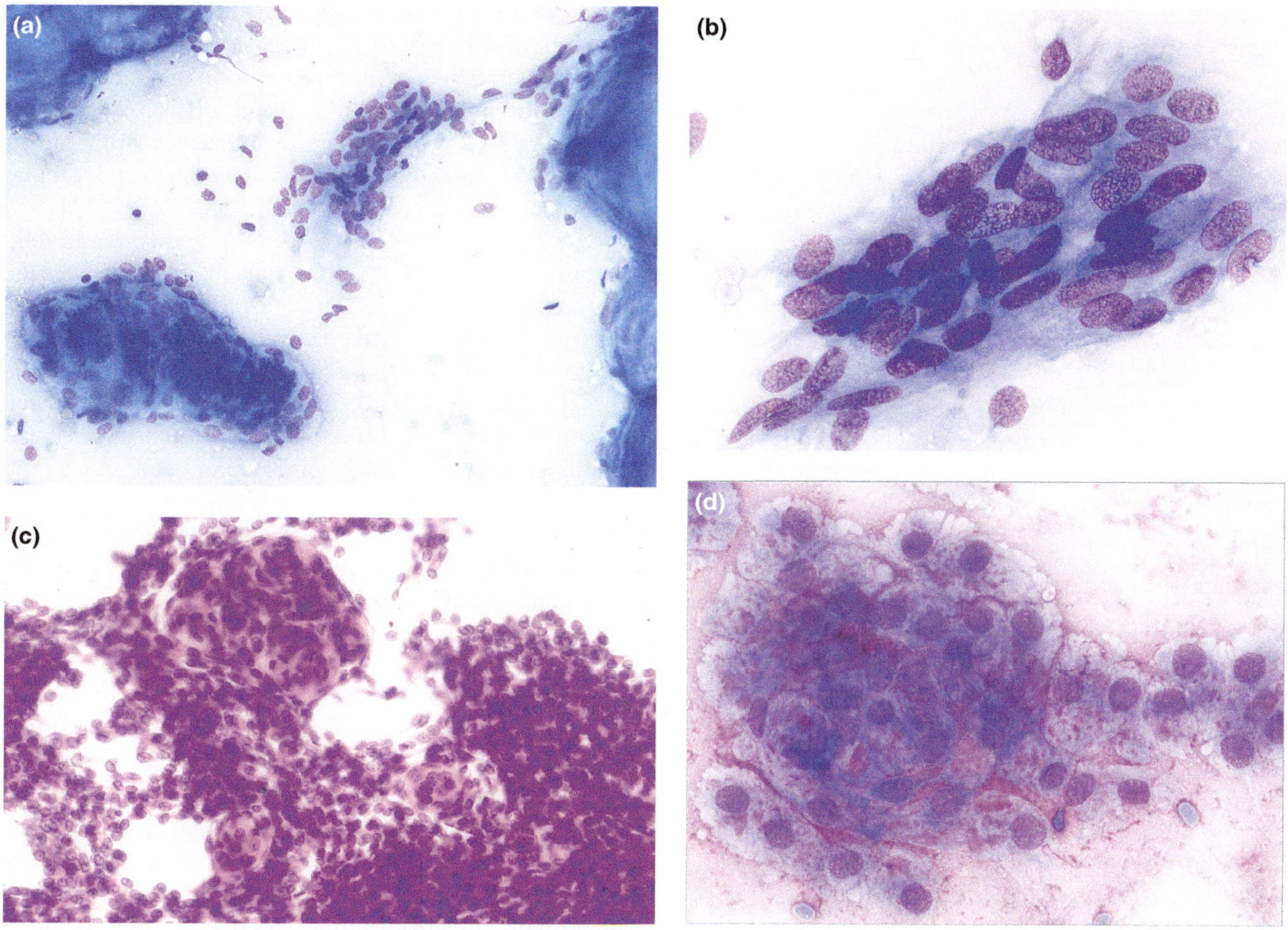

Figure 47.8 Meningiomas. (a) Feline meningiomas usually have a fibrous texture resulting in variably cellular and clumped preparations of spindle cells arranged in aggregates (upper center) and sometimes whorls (Wright Giemsa, 200×). (b) Canine transitional meningioma consists of relatively uniform spindloid cells with oval to elongate nuclei. Note the nuclear membrane invagination (lower right hand corner of the smear) (Wright Giemsa, 500×). (c) Canine meningioma. Note the prominent whorled arrangement of cells (top center) (Wet fixed hematoxylin and eosin stain, 200×). (d) Canine chordoid meningioma. This meningioma type is characterized by prominent mucoid to fibrillary, bright pink, extracellular material that is also often intercalated between cells. Cells often have more abundant cytoplasm than is typically observed in other meningioma subtypes and can be more round to oval in shape (Wright Giemsa, 400×).

of 17 dogs with intravascular lymphoma, the majority were either T cell or non-T non-B cell, although one B cell was reported.[72,77] Again, this is in contrast to people where a B-cell origin predominates in intravascular lymphoma. Ancillary diagnostic tests for primary or secondary CNS lymphoma are similar to those that have been described elsewhere (Chapter 27).[79]

Histiocytic Sarcoma

Histiocytic sarcoma can involve the CNS either as part of disseminated disease or as the primary site of involvement in dogs and rarely in cats.[70,80–83] The entire neuraxis can be affected with a predominance of solitary extra-axial lesions in the meninges overlying the brain, whereas spinal lesions can be both intradural and extramedullary or intramedullary. Less commonly, multifocal nodular masses or diffuse meningeal and nerve root involvement is reported.[80,81,84] Although Bernese Mountain dogs, Retrievers (Golden, Labrador, Flat-coated), and Rottweiler dogs have a greater risk for developing histiocytic sarcoma, this risk does not appear to extend to primary CNS histiocytic sarcoma. In two small case series, Pembroke Welsh Corgi dogs appear to be at increased risk for primary CNS histiocytic sarcoma, while secondary CNS involvement of systemic histiocytic sarcoma has been observed only in Retrievers.[80,83] Neoplastic cells can be present in CSF; however, their absence does not preclude the diagnosis.[30,80,81] Neoplastic interstitial dendritic cells express CD1 and CD11c, detectable in cytologic preparations (CSF or aspirates of masses) and fresh frozen tissue.[81,84]

Infiltrating Leukemia

Involvement of the CNS by infiltrating acute lymphoblastic and myeloid leukemias has been reported rarely in dogs and cats.[85–87] Lesions typically manifest as diffuse infiltration of the dura mater and leptomeninges in the brain and spinal cord.[85–87] A report of a single dog documented infiltration of cranial nerves and spinal ganglia as well.[86] Atypical hemic blast cells were observed in CSF in most cases.[85–87] Meningeal metastasis of acute leukemias is not uncommon in people and may be underreported in dogs and cats, possibly due to euthanasia at the time of diagnosis or limited diagnostic work-up and staging.[85]

Miscellaneous Tumors

Many other tumors may involve the CNS in dogs and cats. The primary CNS lesions in this group are uncommonly sampled antemortem either due to their location (e.g. skull base tumors) or apparent rarity in these species. A variety of locally invasive and metastatic lesions may also involve the CNS. Briefly, some features of other more notable CNS tumors will be described.

Tumors of the Sellar and Suprasellar Regions

This category encompasses a variety of different neoplasms that arise near the base of the skull, at or adjacent to the region of the pituitary fossa. Tumors that arise in this location include meningiomas, pituitary adenomas/carcinomas, craniopharyngiomas, and germ cell tumors, among others.

In a small case series of dogs, pituitary tumors were one of the most common skull base tumors reported, second only to meningiomas.[88] Pituitary adenomas are more common than carcinomas and may be functional if arising from the adrenocorticotropic hormone (ACTH) producing corticotrophs. Functional pituitary tumors are associated with the development of pituitary dependent hyperadrenocorticism. Microadenomas (<5 mm in diameter) are most common and typically arise from the pars distalis and to a lesser extent the pars intermedia of the pituitary.[89,90] Macroadenomas (both functional and inactive) are most often associated with neurologic deficits due to compression and infiltration of adjacent neural parenchyma.[89] Pituitary carcinomas are classified by the presence of either cerebrospinal or systemic metastasis, as macroadenomas also can be invasive into surrounding soft tissue and boney structures.[89] Functional pituitary adenomas (both micro- and macroadenomas) have strong ACTH immunoreactivity.[89] Cytologic features of pituitary neoplasms in dogs and cats have not been described. Histologic features include polygonal to spindloid cells arranged in solid or sinusoidal patterns with minimal cellular pleomorphism and a low mitotic rate. Carcinomas are distinguished primarily by local invasiveness but may also have increased cellular atypia and mitotic rate.[32]

Craniopharyngiomas have been rarely reported in dogs and cats and arise from Rathke's pouch, the embryonic tissue that gives rise to the anterior pituitary. Tumors typically are benign expansile masses; however, variants with aggressive regional infiltration have been reported.[91] While the cytologic appearance of these tumors has not been described, histologically they are composed of a mixed epithelial component, which forms small acini, ducts, and cysts, as well as a mesenchymal component composed of dense bundles of spindle cells.[91] Epithelial components express CK, while mesenchymal components are vimentin and alpha-smooth muscle actin positive.[91]

Germ cell tumors most commonly arise from the gonads but have been uncommonly reported in the CNS of dogs,[92,93] presumably as a manifestation of the extensive, sometimes misplaced, migration of germ cells during embryogenesis.[92] Germ cell tumors typically present as large extramedullary masses at the ventral midline of the brain[92] and rarely also arise in the spinal cord.[93] Tumors are typically locally invasive; however, intracranial metastasis has rarely been reported in dogs.[92] Germ cell tumors in humans are divided into seven different categories: germinoma, teratoma, embryonal carcinoma, choriocarcinoma, yolk sac tumor, gonadoblastoma, and mixed tumors. Most canine tumors are consistent with the mixed tumor type, having components of both germinoma and teratoma.[94] While the cytomorphology of CNS germ cell tumors has not been described in veterinary species, histologically, these tumors consist of a variable mixture of three different cell populations including large round cells in small clusters (germinomatous-type), large hepatoid cells that are sometimes vacuolated, and cuboidal to columnar epithelial cells that sometimes have squamous differentiation.[93] Immunohistochemically the hepatoid and epithelial cell types are reportedly strongly CK positive.[93] All three cell types are variably but diffusely alpha-fetoprotein positive with strongest staining observed in hepatoid-type cells.[92,93] In humans, germinomas often express placental alkaline phosphatase, which was not observed in a small case series of dogs, possibly due to lack of antibody cross reactivity in this species.[92]

Granular Cell Tumors

Granular cell tumors (GCTs) comprise a heterogeneous group that occur infrequently within the CNS of dogs and cats, as well as within a variety of extraneural tissues, especially the oral cavity.[95–98] The histogenesis of these tumors remains unclear, and it is likely that GCTs consist of a variety of different lineages that share a common morphology.[98] In humans as well as in dogs, extracranial GCTs have been hypothesized to have a neural crest tissue origin, more specifically Schwann cells of the peripheral nervous system. The cell type of origin of intracranial GCT is unknown, but in some cases GCTs appear to arise from the meninges.[97–100] These tumors are typically expansile compressive masses that can infiltrate adjacent tissue but rarely metastasize.[97,98,100] GCTs typically produce highly cellular smear or aspirate preparations that are composed of a population of discrete to cohesive large round to polygonal cells. Cells contain abundant cytoplasmic granules, which vary in shape from coarse to fine, and in color, with both a glassy pale basophilic[97] or metachromatic to eosinophilic[99] appearance reported. Nuclei are typically small and round with clumped chromatin and inapparent nucleoli. N:C ratios are low, and anisocytosis and anisokaryosis are mild to moderate.[99] The ultrastructural features of the cytoplasmic granules of GCTs suggest a lysosomal and/or autophagosomal origin.[98,100] Positive staining of GCT granules for microtubule-associated protein light chain 3 (LC3), P62, and ubiquitin also support an autophagolyosomal origin.[99,100] On routine cytochemical staining, the granules are reliably periodic acid–Schiff positive that is variably diastase resistant.[97–99] The immunophenotype of GCTs varies in the literature although most are cytoplasmic vimentin positive and are CK and synaptophysin negative.[97,98,100]

Pineal Tumors (Pineocytoma/Papillary Tumor of the Pineal Region)

Primary pineal tumors are extremely rare in animals.[101] Tumors arising in the location of the pineal gland may represent true pineocytomas, arising from the endocrine cells of the pineal gland, or papillary tumors of the pineal region, arising from a combination of the pineocytes and/or the specialized ependymal cells of the subcommisural organ.[101] Pineal tumors are expansile mass lesions that can result in compressive hydrocephalus given the anatomic location.[101] Cytologic descriptions of these tumors are lacking in veterinary medicine. Histologically, pseudorosettes and lobules of cohesive polygonal cells are described in one canine case report.[101] Many melanin-laden cells were interpreted as an incidental finding given the presence of melanin in normal pineal glands of dogs.[101] Human pineal tumors have consistent CK and NSE immunoreactivity, which was also observed in the canine case report.[101]

Metastatic Tumors and Local Extension of Regional Tumors

Metastatic tumors to the CNS have historically been less commonly reported in dogs and cats than in humans[32]; however, up to 65% of intracranial tumors in dogs in a large case series were reportedly secondary lesions.[102] As therapies for animals with neoplasia are increasingly employed, resulting in longer life spans and more progressed clinical disease course, the reported incidence of metastatic CNS lesions may increase in dogs and cats.

The most common metastatic CNS tumor in dogs is hemangiosarcoma, which accounted for 49 of 117 cases, followed by lymphoma, metastatic carcinoma, histiocytic sarcoma, and melanoma.[102] Most metastatic lesions were identified in the cerebrum, followed by the cerebellum and diencephalon, with 28% of cases having multiple CNS metastases on necropsy examination.[102] In dogs with intracranial metastasis, 76–80% had concurrent pulmonary metastatic lesions.[102] In a large feline case series, 5.6% of intracranial lesions were reported as metastatic lesions, with lymphoma most commonly identified, followed by metastatic carcinoma, and less commonly sarcomas.[31] Antemortem diagnosis of metastatic carcinoma to the leptomeninges following identification of neoplastic cells in CSF has been reported in a dog.[103]

Local extension of regional tumors into CNS tissue is less commonly reported than metastatic lesions and includes nasal tumors (adenocarcinomas and sarcomas), multilobular tumor of bone, osteosarcomas, chondrosarcomas, and hemic tumors (histiocytic sarcoma, lymphoma).[31,88,102]

References

1 Flegel, T., Oevermann, A., Oechtering, G., and Matiasek, K. (2012). Diagnostic yield and adverse effects of MRI-guided free-hand brain biopsies through a mini-burr hole in dogs with encephalitis. *J Vet Intern Med* 26: 969–976.

2 Vernau, W., Vernau, K.A., and Bailey, C.S. (2008). Cerebrospinal fluid. In: *Clinical Biochemistry of Domestic Animals*, 6e (eds. J.J. Kaneko, J.W. Harvey and M. Bruss), 769–820. Amsterdam; Boston: Academic Press/Elsevier.

3 Koblik, P.D., LeCouteur, R.A., Higgins, R.J. et al. (1999). CT-guided brain biopsy using a modified Pelorus Mark III stereotactic system: experience with 50 dogs. *Vet Radiol Ultrasound* 40: 434–440.

4 Moissonnier, P., Blot, S., Devauchelle, P. et al. (2002). Stereotactic CT-guided brain biopsy in the dog. *J Small Anim Pract* 43: 115–123.

5 Troxel, M.T. and Vite, C.H. (2008). CT-guided stereotactic brain biopsy using the Kopf stereotactic system. *Vet Radiol Ultrasound* 49: 438–443.

6 Chen, A.V., Wininger, F.A., Frey, S. et al. (2012). Description and validation of a magnetic resonance imaging-guided stereotactic brain biopsy device in the dog. *Vet Radiol Ultrasound* 53: 150–156.

7 Thomas, W.B., Sorjonen, D.C., Hudson, J.A., and Cox, N.R. (1993). Ultrasound-guided brain biopsy in dogs. *Am J Vet Res* 54: 1942–1947.

8 Klopp, L.S. and Ridgway, M. (2009). Use of an endoscope in minimally invasive lesion biopsy and removal within the skull and cranial vault in two dogs and one cat. *J Am Vet Med Assoc* 234: 1573–1577.

9 Platt, S.R., Alleman, A.R., Lanz, O.I., and Chrisman, C.L. (2002). Comparison of fine-needle aspiration and surgical-tissue biopsy in the diagnosis of canine brain tumors. *Vet Surg* 31: 65–69.

10 Vernau, K.M., Higgins, R.J., Bollen, A.W. et al. (2001). Primary canine and feline nervous system tumors: intraoperative diagnosis using the smear technique. *Vet Pathol* 38: 47–57.

11 Long, S.N., Anderson, T.J., Long, F.H., and Johnston, P.E. (2002). Evaluation of rapid staining techniques for cytologic diagnosis of intracranial lesions. *Am J Vet Res* 63: 381–386.

12 De Lorenzi, D., Mandara, M.T., Tranquillo, M. et al. (2006). Squash-prep cytology in the diagnosis of canine and feline nervous system lesions: a study of 42 cases. *Vet Clin Pathol* 35: 208–214.

13 Garman, R.H. (2011). Histology of the central nervous system. *Toxicol Pathol* 39: 22–35.

14 DeMay, R.M. (1996). *The Art & Science of Cytopathology*. Chicago: ASCP Press.

15 Vandevelde, M., Higgins, R.J., and Oevermann, A. (2012). *Veterinary Neuropathology: Essentials of Theory and Practice*, 200. Ames, IA: Wiley-Blackwell.

16 Davalos, D., Grutzendler, J., Yang, G. et al. (2005). ATP mediates rapid microglial response to local brain injury in vivo. *Nat Neurosci* 8: 752–758.

17 Nimmerjahn, A., Kirchhoff, F., and Helmchen, F. (2005). Resting microglial cells are highly dynamic surveillants of brain parenchyma in vivo. *Science* 308: 1314–1318.

18 Ginhoux, F., Greter, M., Leboeuf, M. et al. (2010). Fate mapping analysis reveals that adult microglia derive from primitive macrophages. *Science* 330: 841–845.

19 Ginhoux, F., Lim, S., Hoeffel, G. et al. (2013). Origin and differentiation of microglia. *Front Cell Neurosci* 7: 45.

20 Kierdorf, K., Erny, D., Goldmann, T. et al. (2013). Microglia emerge from erythromyeloid precursors via Pu.1- and Irf8-dependent pathways. *Nat Neurosci* 16: 273–280.

21 Kierdorf, K. and Prinz, M. (2013). Factors regulating microglia activation. *Front Cell Neurosci* 7: 44.

22 Ginhoux, F. and Prinz, M. (2015). Origin of microglia: current concepts and past controversies. *Cold Spring Harb Perspect Biol* 7: a020537.

23 Stein, V.M., Czub, M., Hansen, R. et al. (2004). Characterization of canine microglial cells isolated ex vivo. *Vet Immunol Immunopathol* 99: 73–85.

24 Rossmeisl, J.H., Duncan, R.B., Huckle, W.R., and Troy, G.C. (2007). Expression of vascular endothelial growth factor in tumors and plasma from dogs with primary intracranial neoplasms. *Am J Vet Res* 68: 1239–1245.

25 Chan, A.S., Leung, S.Y., Wong, M.P. et al. (1998). Expression of vascular endothelial growth factor and its receptors in the anaplastic progression of astrocytoma, oligodendroglioma, and ependymoma. *Am J Surg Pathol* 22: 816–826.

26 Higgins, R.J., Dickinson, P.J., LeCouteur, R.A. et al. (2010). Spontaneous canine gliomas: overexpression of EGFR, PDGFRalpha and IGFBP2 demonstrated by tissue microarray immunophenotyping. *J Neuro-Oncol* 98: 49–55.

27 Summers, B.A., Cummings, J.F., and DeLahunta, A. (1995). *Veterinary Neuropathology*, 527. St. Louis, MO: Mosby.

28 Stoica, G., Levine, J., Wolff, J., and Murphy, K. (2011). Canine astrocytic tumors: a comparative review. *Vet Pathol* 48: 266–275.

29 Fernandez, F.R., Grindem, C.B., Brown, T.T. Jr. et al. (1997). Cytologic and histologic feature of a poorly differentiated glioma in a dog. *Vet Clin Pathol* 26: 182–186.

30 Snyder, J.M., Shofer, F.S., Van Winkle, T.J., and Massicotte, C. (2006). Canine intracranial primary neoplasia: 173 cases (1986–2003). *J Vet Intern Med* 20: 669–675.

31 Troxel, M.T., Vite, C.H., Van Winkle, T.J. et al. (2003). Feline intracranial neoplasia: retrospective review of 160 cases (1985–2001). *J Vet Intern Med* 17: 850–859.

32 Koestner, A., Armed Forces Institute of Pathology (U.S.), American Registry of Pathology et al. (1999). *Histological Classification of Tumors of the Nervous System of Domestic Animals*, 71. Washington, DC: Armed Forces Institute of Pathology in cooperation with the American Registry of Pathology and the World Health Organization Collaborating Center for Worldwide Reference on Comparative Oncology.

33 Lipsitz, D., Higgins, R.J., Kortz, G.D. et al. (2003). Glioblastoma multiforme: clinical findings, magnetic resonance imaging, and pathology in five dogs. *Vet Pathol* 40: 659–669.

34 Ide, T., Uchida, K., Kikuta, F. et al. (2010). Immunohistochemical characterization of canine neuroepithelial tumors. *Vet Pathol* 47: 741–750.

35 Johnson, G.C., Coates, J.R., and Wininger, F. (2014). Diagnostic immunohistochemistry of canine and feline intracalvarial tumors in the age of brain biopsies. *Vet Pathol* 51: 146–160.

36 Rissi, D.R., Levine, J.M., Eden, K.B. et al. (2015). Cerebral oligodendroglioma mimicking intraventricular neoplasia in three dogs. *J Vet Diagn Invest* 27: 396–400.

37 Dickinson, P.J., Keel, M.K., Higgins, R.J. et al. (2000). Clinical and pathologic features of oligodendrogliomas in two cats. *Vet Pathol* 37: 160–167.

38 Bentley, R.T., Burcham, G.N., Heng, H.G. et al. (2014). A comparison of clinical, magnetic resonance imaging and pathological findings in dogs with gliomatosis cerebri, focusing on cases with minimal magnetic resonance imaging changes. *Vet Comp Oncol* 14: 318–330.

39 Walmsley, G.L., Chandler, K., Davies, E.S. et al. (2009). Multi-focal cerebral oligoastrocytoma in a puppy. *J Small Anim Pract* 50: 435–439.

40 Porter, B., de Lahunta, A., and Summers, B. (2003). Gliomatosis cerebri in six dogs. *Vet Pathol* 40: 97–102.

41 Woolford, L., de Lahunta, A., Baiker, K. et al. (2013). Ventricular and extraventricular ependymal tumors in 18 cats. *Vet Pathol* 50: 243–251.

42 Traslavina, R.P., Kent, M.S., Mohr, F.C. et al. (2013). Clear cell ependymoma in a dog. *J Comp Pathol* 149: 53–56.

43 Nentwig, A., Higgins, R.J., Francey, T. et al. (2012). Aberrant E-cadherin, beta-catenin, and glial fibrillary acidic protein (GFAP) expression in canine choroid plexus tumors. *J Vet Diagn Invest* 24: 14–22.

44 Westworth, D.R., Dickinson, P.J., Vernau, W. et al. (2008). Choroid plexus tumors in 56 dogs (1985–2007). *J Vet Intern Med* 22: 1157–1165.

45 Pastorello, A., Constantino-Casas, F., and Archer, J. (2010). Choroid plexus carcinoma cells in the cerebrospinal fluid of a Staffordshire Bull Terrier. *Vet Clin Pathol* 39: 505–510.

46 Hirose, N., Uchida, K., Matsunaga, S. et al. (2015). Expression of cell adhesion molecules in canine choroid plexus tumors. *J Vet Med Sci* 77: 255–259.

47 Rossmeisl, J.H. Jr., Pineyro, P., Sponenberg, D.P. et al. (2012). Clinicopathologic features of intracranial central neurocytomas in 2 dogs. *J Vet Intern Med* 26: 186–191.

48 Uchida, K., Nakayama, H., Endo, Y. et al. (2003). Ganglioglioma in the thalamus of a puppy. *J Vet Med Sci* 65: 113–115.

49 Huisinga, M., Henrich, M., Frese, K. et al. (2008). Extraventricular neurocytoma of the spinal cord in a dog. *Vet Pathol* 45: 63–66.

50 Kuwamura, M., Kotera, T., Yamate, J. et al. (2004). Cerebral ganglioneuroblastoma in a golden retriever dog. *Vet Pathol* 41: 282–284.

51 Thompson, C.A., Russell, K.E., Levine, J.M., and Weeks, B.R. (2003). Cerebrospinal fluid from a dog with neurologic collapse. *Vet Clin Pathol* 32: 143–146.

52 Steinberg, H. and Galbreath, E.J. (1998). Cerebellar medulloblastoma with multiple differentiation in a dog. *Vet Pathol* 35: 543–546.

53 Rajwanshi, A., Srinivas, R., and Upasana, G. (2009). Malignant small round cell tumors. *J Cytol* 26 (1): 10.

54 Choi, U.S., Philippe, L., Alleman, A.R. et al. (2012). Cytologic and immunohistochemical characterization of a primitive neuroectodermal tumor in the brain of a dog. *Vet Clin Pathol* 41: 153–157.

55 Kitagawa, M., Koie, H., Kanayamat, K., and Sakai, T. (2003). Medulloblastoma in a cat: clinical and MRI findings. *J Small Anim Pract* 44: 139–142.

56 Mandrioli, L., Biserni, R., Panarese, S. et al. (2011). Immunohistochemical profiling and telomerase activity of a canine medulloblastoma. *Vet Pathol* 48: 814–816.

57 De Lorenzi, D., Baroni, M., and Mandara, M.T. (2007). A true "triphasic" pattern: thoracolumbar spinal tumor in a young dog. *Vet Clin Pathol* 36: 200–203.

58 Brewer, D.M., Cerda-Gonzalez, S., Dewey, C.W. et al. (2011). Spinal cord nephroblastoma in dogs: 11 cases (1985–2007). *J Am Vet Med Assoc* 238: 618–624.

59 Headley, S.A., Koljonen, M., Gomes, L.A., and Sukura, A. (2009). Central primitive neuroectodermal tumour with ependymal differentiation in a dog. *J Comp Pathol* 140: 80–83.

60 Brosinski, K., Janik, D., Polkinghorne, A. et al. (2012). Olfactory neuroblastoma in dogs and cats: a histological and immunohistochemical analysis. *J Comp Pathol* 146: 152–159.

61 Platt, S.R., Scase, T.J., Adams, V. et al. (2006). Vascular endothelial growth factor expression in canine intracranial meningiomas and association with patient survival. *J Vet Intern Med* 20: 663–668.

62 Mandara, M.T., Ricci, G., Rinaldi, L. et al. (2002). Immunohistochemical identification and image analysis quantification of oestrogen and progesterone receptors in canine and feline meningioma. *J Comp Pathol* 127: 214–218.

63 Zimmerman, K.L., Bender, H.S., Boon, G.D. et al. (2000). A comparison of the cytologic and histologic features of meningiomas in four dogs. *Vet Clin Pathol* 29: 29–34.

64 Dickinson, P.J., Sturges, B.K., Kass, P.H., and LeCouteur, R.A. (2006). Characteristics of cisternal cerebrospinal

fluid associated with intracranial meningiomas in dogs: 56 cases (1985–2004). *J Am Vet Med Assoc* 228: 564–567.

65 Motta, L., Mandara, M.T., and Skerritt, G.C. (2012). Canine and feline intracranial meningiomas: an updated review. *Vet J* 192: 153–165.

66 Sturges, B.K., Dickinson, P.J., Bollen, A.W. et al. (2008). Magnetic resonance imaging and histological classification of intracranial meningiomas in 112 dogs. *J Vet Intern Med* 22: 586–595.

67 Petersen, S.A., Sturges, B.K., Dickinson, P.J. et al. (2008). Canine intraspinal meningiomas: imaging features, histopathologic classification, and long-term outcome in 34 dogs. *J Vet Intern Med* 22: 946–953.

68 Rogers, L., Barani, I., Chamberlain, M. et al. (2015). Meningiomas: knowledge base, treatment outcomes, and uncertainties. A RANO review. *J Neurosurg* 122: 4–23.

69 Di Ieva, A., Laiq, S., Nejad, R. et al. (2015). Chordoid meningiomas: incidence and clinicopathological features of a case series over 18 years. *Neuropathology* 35: 137–147.

70 Marioni-Henry, K., Van Winkle, T.J., Smith, S.H., and Vite, C.H. (2008). Tumors affecting the spinal cord of cats: 85 cases (1980–2005). *J Am Vet Med Assoc* 232: 237–243.

71 Kim, N.H., Ciesielski, T., Kim, J.H. et al. (2012). Primary central nervous system B-cell lymphoma in a young dog. *Can Vet J* 53: 559–564.

72 Siso, S., Marco-Salazar, P., Moore, P.F. et al. (2017). Canine nervous system lymphoma subtypes display characteristic neuroanatomical patterns. *Vet Pathol* 54: 53–60.

73 Nakamoto, Y., Ozawa, T., Uchida, K. et al. (2009). Primary intra-axial B-cell lymphoma in a cat. *J Vet Med Sci* 71: 207–210.

74 Guil-Luna, S., Carrasco, L., Gomez-Laguna, J. et al. (2013). Primary central nervous system T-cell lymphoma mimicking meningoencephalomyelitis in a cat. *Can Vet J* 54: 602–605.

75 Morita, T., Kondo, H., Okamoto, M. et al. (2009). Periventricular spread of primary central nervous system T-cell lymphoma in a cat. *J Comp Pathol* 140: 54–58.

76 Lane, S.B., Kornegay, J.N., Duncan, J.R., and Oliver, J.E. Jr. (1994). Feline spinal lymphosarcoma: a retrospective evaluation of 23 cats. *J Vet Intern Med* 8: 99–104.

77 McDonough, S.P., Van Winkle, T.J., Valentine, B.A. et al. (2002). Clinicopathological and immunophenotypical features of canine intravascular lymphoma (malignant angioendotheliomatosis). *J Comp Pathol* 126: 277–288.

78 Lapointe, J.M., Higgins, R.J., Kortz, G.D. et al. (1997). Intravascular malignant T-cell lymphoma (malignant angioendotheliomatosis) in a cat. *Vet Pathol* 34: 247–250.

79 Keller, S.M., Vernau, W., and Moore, P.F. (2016). Clonality testing in veterinary medicine: a review with diagnostic guidelines. *Vet Pathol* 53: 711–725.

80 Mariani, C.L., Jennings, M.K., Olby, N.J. et al. (2015). Histiocytic sarcoma with central nervous system involvement in dogs: 19 cases (2006–2012). *J Vet Intern Med* 29: 607–613.

81 Tzipory, L., Vernau, K.M., Sturges, B.K. et al. (2009). Antemortem diagnosis of localized central nervous system histiocytic sarcoma in 2 dogs. *J Vet Intern Med* 23: 369–374.

82 Ide, T., Uchida, K., Tamura, S., and Nakayama, H. (2010). Histiocytic sarcoma in the brain of a cat. *J Vet Med Sci* 72: 99–102.

83 Ide, T., Uchida, K., Kagawa, Y. et al. (2011). Pathological and immunohistochemical features of subdural histiocytic sarcomas in 15 dogs. *J Vet Diagn Invest* 23: 127–132.

84 Cluzel, C., Aboulmali, A.A., Dugas, S. et al. (2016). Diffuse leptomeningeal histiocytic sarcoma in the cerebrospinal fluid of 2 dogs. *Vet Clin Pathol* 45: 184–190.

85 Vernau, K.M., Terio, K.A., LeCouteur, R.A. et al. (2000). Acute B-cell lymphoblastic leukemia with meningeal metastasis causing primary neurologic dysfunction in a dog. *J Vet Intern Med* 14: 110–115.

86 Christopher, M.M., Metz, A.L., Klausner, J. et al. (1986). Acute myelomonocytic leukemia with neurologic manifestations in the dog. *Vet Pathol* 23: 140–147.

87 Morozumi, M., Sasaki, N., Oyama, Y. et al. (1993). Computed tomography and magnetic resonance findings of meningeal syndrome in a leukemic cat. *J Vet Med Sci* 55: 1035–1037.

88 Rissi, D.R. (2015). A retrospective study of skull base neoplasia in 42 dogs. *J Vet Diagn Invest* 27: 743–748.

89 Gestier, S., Cook, R.W., Agnew, W., and Kiupel, M. (2012). Silent pituitary corticotroph carcinoma in a young dog. *J Comp Pathol* 146: 327–331.

90 Attia, M.A. (1980). Cytological study on pituitary adenomas in senile untreated beagle bitches. *Arch Toxicol* 46: 287–293.

91 Nagata, T., Nakayama, H., Uchida, K. et al. (2005). Two cases of feline malignant craniopharyngioma. *Vet Pathol* 42: 663–665.

92 Valentine, B.A., Summers, B.A., de Lahunta, A. et al. (1988). Suprasellar germ cell tumors in the dog: a report of five cases and review of the literature. *Acta Neuropathol* 76: 94–100.

93 Ferreira, A.J., Peleteiro, M.C., Carvalho, T. et al. (2003). Mixed germ cell tumour of the spinal cord in a young dog. *J Small Anim Pract* 44: 81–84.

94 Brooks, A.N., Brooks, K.N., and Oglesbee, M.J. (2012). A suprasellar germ cell tumor in a 16-month-old Wagyu heifer calf. *J Vet Diagn Invest* 24: 587–590.

95 Higgins, R.J., LeCouteur, R.A., Vernau, K.M. et al. (2001). Granular cell tumor of the canine central nervous system: two cases. *Vet Pathol* 38: 620–627.

96 Mandara, M.T., Ricci, G., and Sforna, M. (2006). A cerebral granular cell tumor in a cat. *Vet Pathol* 43: 797–800.

97 Barnhart, K.F., Edwards, J.F., and Storts, R.W. (2001). Symptomatic granular cell tumor involving the pituitary gland in a dog: a case report and review of the literature. *Vet Pathol* 38: 332–336.

98 Patnaik, A.K. (1993). Histologic and immunohistochemical studies of granular cell tumors in seven dogs, three cats, one horse, and one bird. *Vet Pathol* 30: 176–185.

99 Sharkey, L.C., McDonnell, J.J., and Alroy, J. (2004). Cytology of a mass on the meningeal surface of the left brain in a dog. *Vet Clin Pathol* 33: 111–114.

100 Suzuki, S., Uchida, K., Harada, T. et al. (2015). The origin and role of autophagy in the formation of cytoplasmic granules in canine lingual granular cell tumors. *Vet Pathol* 52: 456–464.

101 Williams, J.M., Michal, U., Botteron, C. et al. (2009). Papillary tumor of the pineal region of a dog. *J Vet Diagn Invest* 21: 910–914.

102 Snyder, J.M., Lipitz, L., Skorupski, K.A. et al. (2008). Secondary intracranial neoplasia in the dog: 177 cases (1986–2003). *J Vet Intern Med* 22: 172–177.

103 Behling-Kelly, E., Petersen, S., Muthuswamy, A. et al. (2010). Neoplastic pleocytosis in a dog with metastatic mammary carcinoma and meningeal carcinomatosis. *Vet Clin Pathol* 39: 247–252.

48

Cerebrospinal Fluid Analysis in the Dog and Cat

Marlyn S. Whitney and Joan Ripley Coates

Introduction

Cerebrospinal fluid (CSF) analysis is a common procedure in the diagnosis of central nervous system (CNS) disease. It is simple and inexpensive and, though rarely diagnostic by itself, is often useful in concert with other diagnostic testing. In addition to or instead of CSF analysis, examination of aspirates or imprints of CNS lesions can be diagnostically useful.

Contraindications and Complications

Collection of CSF is contraindicated with known trauma or intoxication[1–3] or when clinical signs or imaging suggest increased intracranial pressure.[2–4] Contraindications for anesthesia also preclude CSF collection.[1,2,4,5] A study of 23 animals described the clinicopathologic features of brain herniation; in 7 animals (4 dogs, 2 cats, and 1 horse), it was preceded by anesthesia, CSF collection, or both.[4] Complications of CSF collection, such as brainstem injury,[6] spinal cord injury,[7] hematomyelia,[8] subarachnoid hemorrhage,[9] and meningitis[10] can occur.

Indications

CSF analysis sometimes identifies specific etiologic agents or neoplastic cells.[5,11–18] Normal CSF findings exclude many disorders.[1,2,11,19] Beyond these instances, CSF analysis has diagnostic limitations. In a retrospective study of 256 dogs with concurrent CSF analysis and magnetic resonance imaging (MRI), CSF analysis resulted in a specific etiologic diagnosis only 2% of the time.[11] Some CNS disorders, such as congenital malformations, metabolic disorders, toxicities, and nutritional disorders are unlikely to cause CSF abnormalities. With obvious MRI findings such as intervertebral disc herniation (IVDH) or vertebral malformation/instability, CSF analysis may be unnecessary.[11] Nonetheless, CSF analysis remains useful in combination with cross-sectional imaging,[11,20,21] serology, culture, polymerase chain reaction (PCR) testing and detection of various biomarkers.[21]

Collection and Handling of CSF

For dogs and cats, CSF samples are most commonly collected from the subarachnoid space at the cerebellomedullary cistern (CM), but collection from the lower lumbar subarachnoid space is more suitable in some instances.[1–3,19,21] A study of 158 samples from 145 dogs with focal, noninflammatory myelopathy showed that abnormal CSF analysis was more likely if collected from the lumbar region caudal to the lesion.[22]

Ideally, CSF specimens should be processed within 30 minutes, primarily due to rapid deterioration of cell morphology.[19] Cell counts can decrease due to cell lysis.[23] Results of 2 studies suggest that while analysis should take place as soon as possible, a delay of 4–8 (and possibly as long as 12) hours is unlikely to alter diagnostic interpretation, especially if the CSF protein concentration (PROT) is >50 mg/dL.[24,25] The total nucleated cell count (TNCC) is less likely than the leukocyte differential count (LDIF) to be adversely affected by a delay. If immediate analysis (within 30–60 minutes) is not possible, the sample should be divided into an unaltered aliquot for the TNCC and PROT, and a second aliquot to which 20% fetal calf serum or 10% autologous serum has been added to preserve the LDIF and morphologic evaluation.[24,25] Hetastarch can be used 1 : 1 as a preservative, though fetal calf serum better stabilized mononuclear cells. Hetastarch has the advantage of not affecting protein concentration, obviating the need to divide small samples into two aliquots.[24] Formalin is no longer recommended as a CSF preservative, as it alters cell morphology.[26]

Veterinary Cytology, First Edition. Edited by Leslie C. Sharkey, M. Judith Radin, and Davis Seelig.

Components of Routine CSF Analysis

Routine CSF analysis usually includes gross evaluation (color and clarity), PROT, TNCC, LDIF, and cytologic evaluation of a stained slide preparation.

Gross Evaluation

Normal CSF is colorless and clear. With pathology, CSF may be turbid, discolored, or both. Turbidity can result from the presence of cells, bacteria, or fat. Turbidity occurs when at least 200 WBC/μL or 700 RBC/μL are present,[3] or when a total of at least 500 cells/μL are present.[14] Pink to red discoloration occurs with pathologic hemorrhage or iatrogenic blood contamination. Yellow to orange discoloration (xanthochromia) occurs with lysis of erythrocytes present as a result of pathologic hemorrhage.[2]

Microprotein Concentration

The origin of PROT in CSF is detailed elsewhere.[27] Albumin makes up approximately 80–90% of PROT in normal CSF. The Pandy and Nonne–Apelt semiquantitative tests for the presence of globulins are generally negative in normal CSF but may be useful for screening.[2,28] Most clinical pathology laboratories now use quantitative means of determining PROT.[28] Because PROT is normally very low, sensitive microprotein methodologies must be used. In a prospective study of 53 dogs with and without neurologic disease, PROT was significantly higher at lumbar versus CM sites.[29]

PROT in health has often been stated to be <25–30 mg/dL with CM collection and <45 mg/dL with lumbar collection.[1,2,12] However, results vary with the microprotein detection method used. These include turbidimetric methods, the trichloroacetic acid method, and dye-binding methods using Ponceau S red, Coomassie Brilliant Blue, or pyrogallol red-molybdate binding.[28] Dye-binding methods are considered most accurate.[30–32] Reference intervals (RI) for canine PROT as measured by three methodologies were determined using an indirect *a posteriori* method. Turbidimetric (using benzethonium chloride as the precipitating agent) and pyrogallol red-molybdate methods were shown to be in excellent agreement, and a RI of 8–35 mg/dL was derived. A Coomassie blue dye-binding assay resulted in higher values and a RI of 17–55 mg/dL.[28]

Ideally, each laboratory performing CSF analysis should establish its own RI, reflecting the use of its specific equipment, methodology, and reagents and deriving an appropriate range for the population of animals from which the bulk of its samples originate. However, collecting CSF from sufficient numbers of non-diseased patients to derive a RI is problematic, especially for smaller laboratories.[28,33] Laboratories may need to use transference validation of a RI adopted from another source, or generation of common RIs with contributions from several laboratories serving similar animal populations.[33]

Disorders that alter the blood–brain barrier (BBB) and/or production of immunoglobulins and other proteins within the CNS can increase PROT.[1,2,19,27,28] PROT may be increased in the absence of cytologic abnormalities, referred to as albuminocytologic dissociation or, sometimes, cytoalbuminologic dissociation. Causes include increased permeability of the BBB, local necrosis, interruption of normal CSF flow and absorption, and intrathecal globulin production.[2,12,34–36] Various calculated values have been advocated in relation to CSF protein analysis. The albumin quotient (AQ) = (CSF albumin/serum albumin) × 100. Elevations suggest an altered BBB.[12] The IgG index = (CSF IgG/serum IgG) × (serum albumin/CSF albumin), with an increase suggesting increased intrathecal IgG production. Diagnostic utility of such calculations has varied between studies.[37,38] An increased IgG index is typical for infectious inflammatory diseases, whereas animals with noninflammatory diseases usually have a normal IgG index. The IgG index may be useful for detecting inflammatory disease in dogs without CSF pleocytosis.[38]

Alterations in the electrophoretic patterns of CSF proteins suggested categories of disease in some studies.[12,39–41] High-resolution protein electrophoresis of paired CSF and serum samples in 6 healthy controls and 94 dogs with a variety of neurologic diseases revealed a strong linear correlation between PROT and AQ, suggesting increased PROT indicates BBB dysfunction, but electrophoretograms were not characteristic of a particular disease.[39] Testing paired serum and CSF samples for immunoglobulins yielded varied results for confirming suspected diseases.[2,42,43]

Cell Counts

The RI for TNCC has been reported to be <6 cells/μL for dogs[3,12] and <8 cells/μL for cats.[3,5,12] TNCC counts of <5 or 6 cells/μL have been considered normal for dogs.[1,2] A 1970 study of 58 dogs produced a range of 0–5, but only 12 of the dogs were clinically healthy.[44] A frequently cited 1954 study[45] gave a range of 0–24 with a mean of 6 for 50 dogs, but the source of dogs was unclear and some appeared to be from earlier studies with little detail provided. A 1977 study of CM samples produced a range of 0–8[46] from a colony of 9 related beagle dogs, and a 1974 study[47] reported a range of 1–10.3 using CM samples from 20 clinically healthy dogs from unstated sources. Several studies, all using dogs from unstated sources except as noted otherwise below, suggest lower counts in healthy dogs.[3,4,48–52] CM CSF samples from 50 clinically and histopathologically normal mongrel dogs of varying age and sex resulted in a RI of 0–2 cells/μL.[48] A study of 31 clinically and histopathologically normal dogs of varying breed and sex resulted in a range of 0–4 cells/μL for both CM and lumbar samples, with the mean for lumbar samples being significantly lower; 26 of the 31 CM samples and 30 of the 31 lumbar samples had 0–2 cells/μL.[34] A study of CM CSF from 25 dogs of various breeds, most of which were from a breeding unit but some of which were dogs brought in for treatment of non-neurologic disease and a few of which were dogs brought for necropsy reported <1.2 cells/μL.[49] Samples (CM) from 71 clinically normal dogs of 15 breeds, resulted in the finding of 37 acellular samples and 34 samples with varying numbers of RBCs but no nucleated cells.[50] A later paper from the same author reported finding WBCs in only 2 CM samples from 71 clinically normal dogs; 1 dog had 2 and another had 3 WBC/μL, with both samples containing 1000–2000 RBC/μL. Samples with higher numbers of RBCs contained no WBCs. The two samples that did contain WBCs were colony dogs from which CSF has been obtained weekly for the previous month.[51] Samples (CM) from 10 clinically normal mixed breed dogs resulted in a TNCC of 0.3 ± 0.7.[52] A study of CM CSF from 33 clinically and histopathologically normal cats gave a range of 0–2 cells/μL, with 30 cats having no cells present.[53] In light of some studies cited above, all of which employed manual counts, a range of 0–2 cells/μL for normal dogs and cats has been advocated.[32]

Manual counting using a hemocytometer has been the gold standard for RBC counts and TNCC in CSF specimens in veterinary laboratories, though manual counting is prone to imprecision.[54,55] Automated cell counting via the ADVIA 120 hematology instrument (Siemens, Tarrytown, NY) offers a separate CSF assay shown to have a high correlation to manual methods for WBC, RBC, and differential cell counts on human specimens.[54] Canine samples showed good correlation for total WBC and RBC counts, but only moderate correlation for the LDIF.[55] The ADVIA 2120 demonstrated precision that was equivalent to or only slightly higher than that of manual methods for the TNCC and RBC count. Limitations were noted regarding the LDIF when the TNCC was low, especially in regard to monocytes. For samples with moderate to severe pleocytosis (defined by the authors as 30–1747 cells/μL), leukocytes were correctly classified. Unless test volume is high, reagent costs for automated cell counts may be prohibitive, and a sample volume of 300 μL is required.[56]

Likely owing to the variability regarding what has been considered the "normal" TNCC for canine and feline CSF, the choice of different "normal" cutoff points for TNCC in various research studies evaluating dogs and cats with neurologic disease has likely contributed some degree of arbitrariness to the classification of "normal" versus "slightly abnormal" TNCC in CSF.

Slide Preparation and Cytology

Cytology is used to determine the LDIF and to identify abnormal cell morphology and presence of etiologic agents, neoplastic cells, evidence of hemorrhage, etc. Unless the TNCC is markedly increased, fluid concentration is necessary for the preparation of slides. Sedimentation techniques have been described and can be used if a specimen cannot be immediately sent to a laboratory. Large clinical pathology laboratories commonly prepare CSF slides using a cytocentrifuge.[2] Even when the TNCC is within normal limits, evaluation of slide preparations may be diagnostically useful.[1,2,21,57] In a prospective study of 145 dogs with suspected neurologic disease, 24.5% of low cellularity CSF specimens (defined as <8 cells/μL) were cytologically abnormal on cytocentrifuge concentrated slide preparations.[57] A study of 61 cats with CNS disease indicated the LDIF is often abnormal when the TNCC count is within the RI (defined as <2 cells/μL).[58,59] Cell morphology was considered better on cytocentrifuge versus sedimentation preparations, but the greater numbers of cells on sedimentation preparations were thought by the authors to more likely yield accurate LDIFs.[58,59] Cell yield and LDIF on cytocentrifuge preparations is imprecise, based on a study wherein 10 concurrent replicate cytocentrifuge concentrated slide preparations were made from CSF collected from 60 dogs used for other terminal studies. Probability based on linear regression showed that one slide preparation is sufficient to identify samples with >3% neutrophils, but the unknowable true percentage in a sample that appears to have 3% neutrophils could be anywhere from 1 to 7%. The study also compared manual with calibrated pipetting techniques, with both resulting in an average 31% coefficient of variation for total cell yield. The manual technique resulted in a nearly 10-fold increase in the number of foamy macrophages, suggesting that sample handling can create a foamy appearance in macrophages.[60] Mononuclear cells deteriorate most rapidly in CSF, possibly also contributing to technique-related variability in the LDIF.[24,60] Cytocentrifugation can alter the appearance of mononuclear cells as compared with sedimentation techniques.[61,62] There is controversy regarding the identity of specific mononuclear cells that appear lymphoid with sedimentation techniques but are more commonly classified as indeterminate mononuclear cells using slides prepared by cytocentrifugation.[57,63] Immunophenotyping of cells in CSF would likely yield more objective cell classification than does microscopic analysis.[63]

The majority of cells present in normal CSF are mononuclear cells: small lymphocytes and monocytoid cells.[1–3,5,12,21,53] Small lymphocytes[5] or monocytic cells[48] predominate in dogs, whereas monocytes usually predominate in cats.[3,5,53] There is disagreement regarding the percentage of neutrophils considered normal.[12,13,52,53,57,60,64] Some authors suggest that any neutrophils are abnormal.[13,57] Prospective studies have indicated a wide range of neutrophil percentages in healthy dogs,[48,52,60,64,65] though higher ranges sometimes appear to be due to outliers or blood contamination. Using cytocentrifuge preparations from research dogs, RBC-free samples from 23 healthy dogs had a mean of 4.8 ± 2.8% neutrophils (range 0–42),[64] and 39 low TNCC (<5 WBC/μL) samples had a mean of 1.4 ± 3.7% (range 0–23).[60] Means of 1 ± 2 and 2 ± 6% neutrophils were derived from 20 sediment and 22 cytocentrifuge preparations of low RBC content samples, respectively, from healthy cats.[53] Using cytocentrifuge slides, a 3% neutrophil count may represent a true neutrophil percentage of 1–7%.[60] Eosinophils are rare in the CSF of healthy dogs and cats and when present may be the result of blood contamination.[12,53] Incidental findings include occasional surface epithelial cells (leptomeningeal lining cells, choroid plexus cells, and ependymal cells).[5,21,66]

Pleocytosis is the term applied to an increased TNCC in CSF and is further defined by the predominating cell type(s): neutrophilic, eosinophilic, mononuclear, or mixed. Seemingly arbitrarily, some references classify pleocytosis as mild if the TNCC/μL is 6–50 (5 or less considered normal), moderate if 51–500 or 1000, and marked if >500 or >1000.[2,12,15]

Sample Quality

Blood Contamination

Studies of the effects of blood contamination on CSF parameters give variable information.[22,51,67] Together, these studies suggest the TNCC is likely reliable with contamination up to 5000 RBC/μL, though when the RBC count is >500/μL, the LDIF for neutrophils is unreliable, eosinophils can be present, and small to moderate PROT elevations can be artifactual. Blood contamination is more likely to alter LDIF in samples with a low TNCC (<5 cells/μL). Activated macrophages and/or reactive lymphocytes provoked suspicion of CNS abnormalities regardless of blood contamination, but a more recent study of uncontaminated CSF from healthy dogs indicated sample handling can create foamy macrophages.[60]

Additional Contaminants

Contrast agents used for myelography can alter CSF findings, likely by causing mild inflammation.[12] Metrizamide,[52,65,68–70] ioversol,[70] and iopamidol[65,71] have been noted to cause mild increases in CSF PROT and TNCC, though in one study, it was unclear whether the increases were due to the use of iopamidol or to experimental compression of the spinal cord.[71] In another study, the PROT increase was believed due to repeated sampling.[52] In a double crossover study comparing iohexol and iotrolan in 6 dogs, PROT was increased at 24 hours (but not at 3, 7, or 14 days) post injection with iohexol; no TNCC increase was seen with either agent at any sampling time.[72] Another study of iohexol in eight healthy dogs found increased PROT at 24 and 48 hours relative to pre-myelography values; though there was no increase in TNCC, neutrophils increased in proportion relative to small mononuclear cells.[73] Increases in CSF albumin and IgG 24 hours after intrathecal metrizamide administration to 9 dogs as compared with 2 control dogs not receiving metrizamide resolved by 5 days, suggesting transient leakage across the blood-CSF barrier. There were no changes in test dogs relative to control dogs at three hours post injection.[69]

Though repeated sampling has been thought to possibly increase TPROT[52] and/or TNCC,[74] CM puncture and withdrawal of 1 mL of CSF with saline replacement from 20 adult beagle dogs for 10 consecutive days appeared to have little effect on protein and cell content, except for 1 dog that developed meningitis.[10] Repeated cisternal CSF collection via an implanted cannula from 8 unanesthetized mongrel cats over 24 days caused no alterations in TPROT (TNCC not reported).[75]

Collection-associated contaminants seen in CSF samples include myelin-like material, neurons, and neuropil.[76,77] Hematopoietic precursors may arise from vertebral marrow puncture[78] or from sites of extramedullary hematopoiesis.[79] In a retrospective study, myelin-like material was observed in 20 of 98 dogs with neurologic disease. It was observed more often in lumbar CSF and in dogs of less than 10 kg.[76] Larger amounts were present in dogs with IVDH; there was no association with outcome. Owing to its association with sampling site and body weight, the authors concluded that presence of myelin is most often an artifact of collection and anatomy.[76]

CSF in Various Neurologic Disorders

Table 48.1 summarizes typical CSF findings in various CNS disorders.

Table 48.1 Summary of CSF analysis in disease.

Disease	Appearance	WBC/μL[a]	Characteristic pleocytosis[b]	Protein (mg/dL)
Infectious inflammatory				
Bacterial[80]	Clear to turbid	Mild to marked increase	Neutrophilic and/or Monocytic	Increased, usually >100
Viral[15,58,81–83]	Clear	Normal or mild to marked increase	Lymphocytic Mononuclear Mixed with mononuclear cells, neutrophils, rarely eosinophils Neutrophilic with feline infectious peritonitis (FIP)	Increased, usually <100; FIP >100
Fungal[15,84–88]	Clear to turbid	Mild to marked increase	Neutrophilic Mononuclear Eosinophils sometimes (Cryptococcus) Capsid or yeast sometimes seen	Increased, variable
Protozoal[15,81,88–93]	Clear	Mild to marked increase	Mononuclear Mixed with monocytes, lymphocytes, neutrophils, rarely eosinophils Eosinophilic sometimes Tachyzoites sometimes seen	Increased, usually >100
Rickettsial[94]	Clear	Mild to moderate increase	Lymphocytic Mixed Morulae sometimes seen	Increased, usually <100
Algal[95–97]	Clear to xanthochromic	Marked increase	Eosinophilic Mixed with mononuclear cells, lymphocytes, neutrophils Organisms sometimes seen	Increased, usually >100
Parasitic[88,98]	Clear to xanthochromic	Variable increase	Mixed Mononuclear Eosinophilic sometimes	Increased, usually >100
Noninfectious inflammatory				
Meningoencephalitis of Unknown Origin[81,99]	Clear to turbid	Mild to marked increase	Mononuclear Lymphocytic Mixed with neutrophils	Increased, variable
Steroid responsive meningitis arteritis[81,100–102]	Clear to xanthochromic	Moderate to marked increase	Neutrophilic Monocytic when chronic	Increased, usually >100
Eosinophilic meningoencephalitis[88,103,104]	Clear	Moderate to marked increase	Eosinophilic >50–90%	Increased, variable
Neoplasia				
CNS neoplasia[11,13,16,17,59,105–111]	Clear	Normal to moderate increase; Sometimes marked increase	Mononuclear Neutrophilic (meningioma caudal fossa) Tumor cells if mass is adjacent to CSF space (ependymoma, choroid plexus, glioma, histiocytic sarcoma, and lymphoma)	Normal to variable increase; usually >100 with choroid plexus carcinoma

Table 48.1 (Continued)

Disease	Appearance	WBC/µL[a]	Characteristic pleocytosis[b]	Protein (mg/dL)
Miscellaneous CNS disorders				
Intervertebral disc herniation[112,113]	Clear to xanthochromic	Mild to moderate increase	Lymphocytic (chronic) Neutrophilic (acute) Mixed	Increased, usually <100
Spinal cord trauma[114]	Clear to xanthochromic	Normal to mild increased	RBCs Mixed with neutrophils, lymphocytes, monocytes; macrophages	Increased, usually <100
Caudal cervical spondylomyelopathy[115]	Clear	Normal	Normal	Normal
Discospondylitis[116]	Clear	Normal to mild increased	Neutrophilic Lymphocytic Mixed	Normal to increased, usually <100
Empyema[117]	Clear	Normal to mild increase	Neutrophilic	Normal to increased, usually <100
Idiopathic epilepsy[118]	Clear	Normal to mild increase	Mononuclear	Normal, increased, usually <100
Fibrocartilaginous embolism[119–122]	Clear to xanthochromic	Normal or mild to moderate increase	Neutrophilic Mixed	Normal, increased, usually <100
Acute noncompressive nucleus pulposus extrusion[123]	Clear	Normal to mild increase	Neutrophilic Mixed	Normal, increased, usually <100
Cerebrovascular accident[98,124–127]	Clear to xanthochromic	Normal to mild increase	Neutrophilic Mononuclear	Normal, increased, usually <100

[a] Pleocytosis classifications are arbitrarily defined as mild = <50 cells/µL; moderate = 51–500 cells/µL and severe >500 cells/µL.[12]
[b] Neutrophilic >70% neutrophils; Eosinophilic >10–20% eosinophils; Mononuclear >70% lymphocytes, monocytes, macrophages or plasma cells.[1]

Infectious and Noninfectious CNS Inflammation

CSF analysis is considered the most useful test for CNS inflammatory disease,[1,11,81,129] though pleocytosis is not always observed and, when present, is of variable degree.[11] CNS inflammation is often categorized as “infectious” or “noninfectious,” but making the distinction is problematic. Organisms found in CSF are well illustrated in recent cytology atlases.[1,2,19] Infection is still possible when no organisms are seen, and such cases cannot be properly diagnosed using CSF findings alone.[11,81] Combining CSF findings with cross-sectional imaging, histopathology, and/or other ancillary testing is often required to determine the cause of inflammatory disorders, and sometimes a cause is not determined.[11,81,99,129–131] When organisms are not found, bacterial or fungal culture or virus isolation in CSF can be useful.[21] All viral diseases must stay in the differential when mononuclear pleocytosis is present and no other cause is found.[81] Serology and PCR testing can be helpful.[1,128]

In a retrospective study of 62 cats with clinical signs of CNS disease and CSF findings indicating inflammation, a presumptive diagnosis based on a combination of clinical signs, clinicopathologic data, and ancillary diagnostic tests was made in 63%.[15] CSF findings used alone were useful only for diagnosis of feline infectious peritonitis (FIP), cryptococcosis, lymphoma, and trauma. The type of inflammatory pattern was helpful only in cats with lymphoma, all of which had mononuclear inflammation. Mixed inflammation was the most common pattern at 48.8% of cases, but this pattern was of little aid in diagnosis.[15] In a combined retrospective and prospective study of 27 cats with postmortem diagnosed inflammatory disease, more than 75% were diagnosed with viral or suspected viral disease.[58] FIP was the cause in half of those cases, and no specific virus was identified for the other half.

Even when bacterial CNS infection is present, bacteria may not be seen on CSF cytology, and culture is often negative.[2,80,132,133] Nonetheless, a retrospective study of dogs with bacterial meningoencephalomyelitis confirmed at necropsy indicated CSF analysis is the most consistent test for finding an abnormality and that in combination with a thorough clinical workup can provide a strong index of diagnostic suspicion.[80] Another retrospective study indicated bacterial encephalitis is highly probable based on marked neutrophilic pleocytosis and a rapidly declining clinical course.[81]

In addition to the above, many other case reports and case series reports detail CSF findings in infectious diseases such as rabies,[82] canine distemper,[83] cryptococcosis,[84] coccidioidomycosis,[85] aspergillosis,[86] neosporosis,[89–93] granulocytic ehrlichiosis,[94] protothecosis,[95–97] and cuterebriasis.[98] A review paper covers diagnosis of several fungal diseases that may affect the CNS (Figure 48.1).[87]

CSF eosinophilia (TNCC >3 cells/μL with >20% eosinophils) can occur in a variety of infectious and noninfectious conditions.[88,103,134] In a retrospective study of CSF from 23 dogs, an etiologic agent was found on necropsy in four (*Cryptococcus* in two, *Baylisascaris* and *Neospora* in one each). Three dogs had acute IVDH; the remaining 16 had idiopathic meningoencephalomyelitis.[88] In another case series (11–5500 cells/μL, 21–98% eosinophils), two dogs had protozoal infection and six cases remained idiopathic.[103] Eosinophils have been reported in CSF with *Angiostrongylus* infection, protothecosis, canine distemper virus, rabies, bacterial encephalitis, and toxoplasmosis, though sometimes not in large enough percentages to constitute eosinophilic pleocytosis.[88] In another canine case series, eosinophils were seen in a variety of conditions, but there was no correlation with pathologic findings and were thought in some cases to have reflected peripheral eosinophilia.[134] Idiopathic eosinophilic meningoencephalitis was described in Rottweiler dogs.[104]

Recently, the term meningoencephalomyelitis of unknown origin (MUO) has been used when clinical presentation, CSF analysis, and/or MRI findings indicate inflammation, but a known infectious etiology is not identified and definitive histopathology is lacking.[11,99,130,135,136] MUO incorporates all subtypes of noninfectious inflammatory brain disease, except steroid responsive meningitis arteritis (SRMA), which involves primarily the meninges.[130] Such disorders described in dogs include granulomatous meningoencephalomyelitis (GME); necrotizing encephalitis (NE) of small breed dogs, with the latter encompassing necrotizing meningoencephalitis (NME); and necrotizing leukoencephalitis (NLE).[1,2,130] MUO likely has a multifactorial pathogenesis, including genetic and immune-mediated factors.[130,136]

Review of 457 published cases of canine noninfectious inflammatory disease for which histopathologic findings were available revealed considerable variability and overlap in CSF findings between the disorders diagnosed.[99] TNCC varied widely and was often normal (0–5 cells/μL).[99] Cross-sectional imaging combined with the CSF LDIF can narrow the differential list.[11,129,136] In several case studies of dogs with GME, most affected dogs had a mild to moderate lymphocytic or mixed pleocytosis, with some having a neutrophilic predominance (Figure 48.2). PROT was variably elevated.[137–140] Some dogs with focal signs had a normal TNCC.[138] In one case series, CSF electrophoresis indicated intrathecal production of immunoglobulin in dogs with a chronic course and disruption of the BBB in those with a short survival time.[139] When used along with signalment and neurologic examination, CSF analysis is considered a good indicator of GME, though it

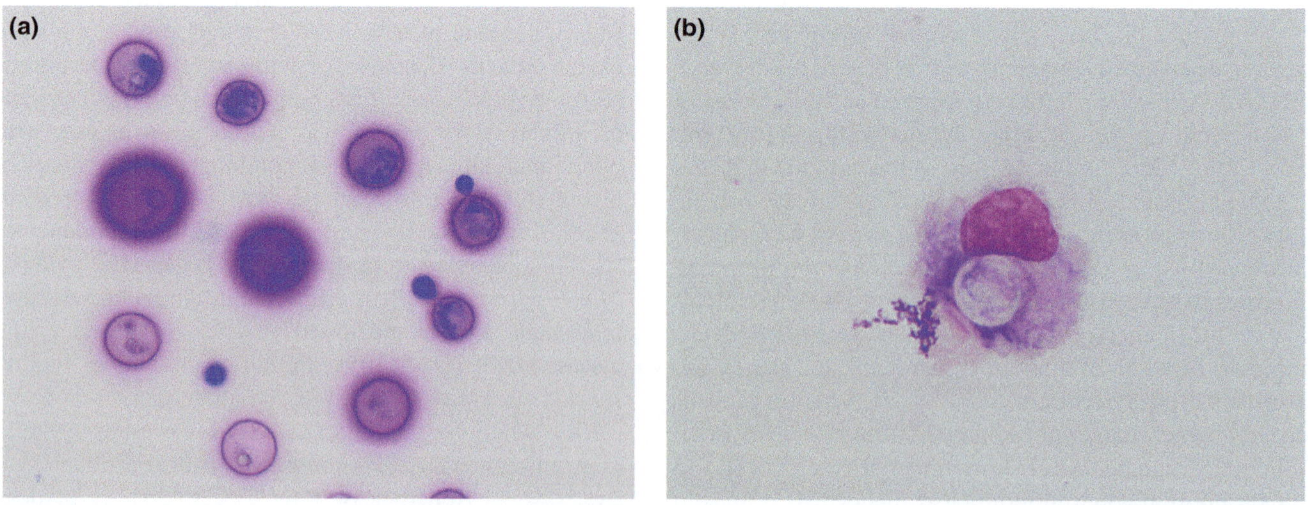

Figure 48.1 *Cryptococcus* spp. in the CSF from a dog. (a) Two organisms exhibit narrow-based budding (on right) (New methylene blue, 1000×). (b) Large mononuclear cell with a phagocytized yeast (Wright giemsa, 1000×. *Source:* Images courtesy of Leslie Sharkey).

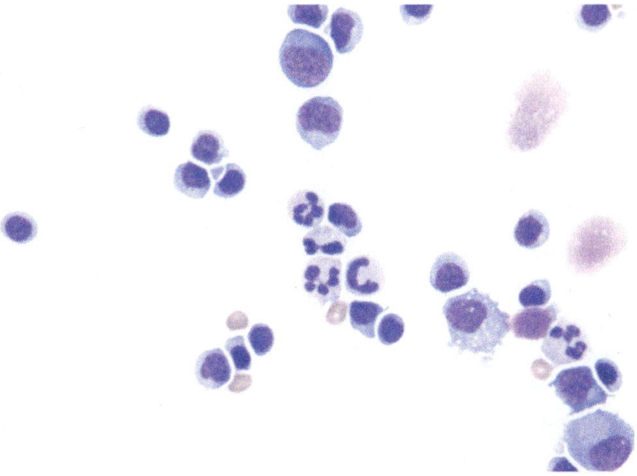

Figure 48.2 Mixed pleocytosis from an eight-year-old, spayed female, Bichon mix breed dog with inflammatory brain disease consistent with GME. The fluid was characterized as clear and colorless with a TNCC of 1218/μL and PROT of 140 mg/dL. MRI revealed multifocal brain lesions in the cerebrum, thalamus, pons, and medulla with concurrent meningeal and right optic nerve enhancement (Wright giemsa, 500×. *Source:* Image courtesy of Leslie Sharkey).

must be differentiated from other inflammatory CNS disorders.[137,139]

NE is characterized as NME or NLE.[136] Historically referred to as Pug dog encephalitis (Figure 48.3), it has now been reported in many toy breeds including the Pug,[1,2,136,141,142] Maltese Terrier,[2,136,143] Chihuahua,[136,144] Yorkshire Terrier,[2,136,145–148] Pekingese,[136,149] West Highland White Terrier,[136,150] French Bulldog,[151] Papillion, Shih Tzu, Coton de Tulear, and Brussels Griffon.[152] It is typically described as a rapidly progressive and fatal inflammatory CNS disorder affecting young dogs (6 months to 7 years at

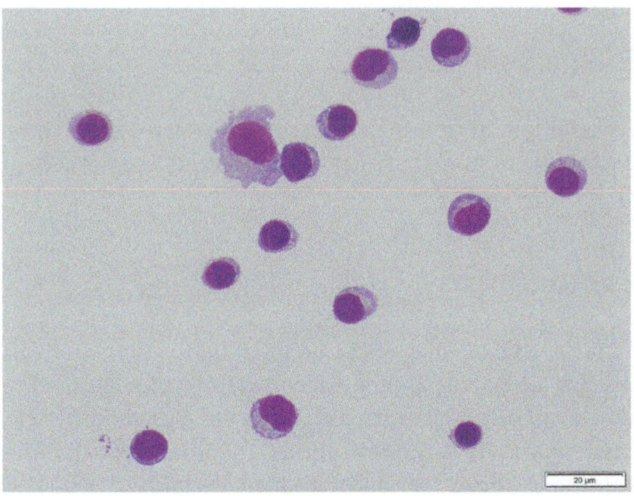

Figure 48.3 Lymphocytic pleocytosis from a Pug dog with "Pug dog encephalitis" or necrotizing encephalitis. TNCC was 501/μL (Wright Giemsa. *Source:* Image courtesy of Daniel Heinrich).

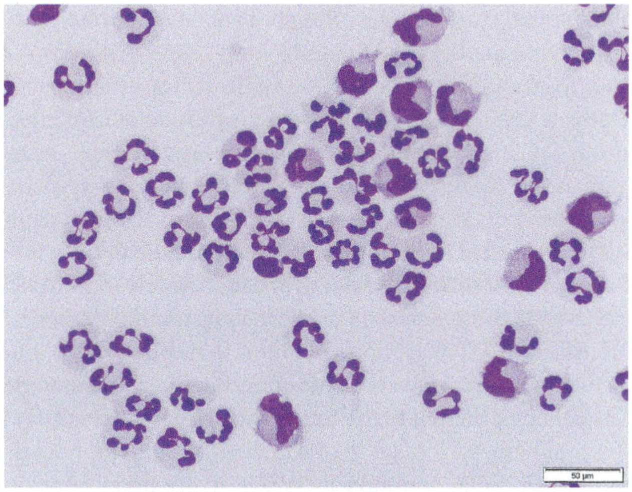

Figure 48.4 Neutrophilic pleocytosis from a dog with SRMA. The TNCC was 3277/μL with 74% neutrophils (Wright Giemsa. *Source:* Image courtesy of Daniel Heinrich).

age of onset with mean of 20 months). Histopathologically, it is characterized by nonsuppurative inflammation of the meninges and brain with extension into the subcortical and deep cortical white matter and mild to severe cerebrocortical necrosis with or without cavitation.[136,152] In a study of 14 pugs, CSF analysis revealed a pleocytosis of varying severity (mean 120 cells/μL), which was lymphocytic (66%), mononuclear (17%), or mixed (17%), with a mean PROT of 88.4 mg/dL.[142]

SRMA is an idiopathic aseptic suppurative steroid responsive inflammatory CNS disease usually affecting young to middle age dogs (Figure 48.4). It is characterized by fever, cervical pain, hyperesthesia, paresis, and an elevated PROT and TNCC (usually >500 cells/μL), often with >75% neutrophils.[2,12,100,153,154] Boxers, Bernese Mountain Dogs, Beagles, Weimaraners, and Nova Scotia Duck Tolling Retrievers are overrepresented, though any dog breed can be affected.[154] Histopathology of affected dogs reveals a meningeal polyarteritis.[153] Though neutrophils usually predominate in the CSF in the acute form of the disease, in the protracted form, a mononuclear or mixed-cell pleocytosis is usually present.[101] In both forms, high levels of IgA have been shown to be produced both systemically and intrathecally.[101,155] Many case series and case reports have contributed to the characterization of SRMA.[100–102,153,155–170]

Miscellaneous Disorders

A retrospective study of 506 dogs with IVDH indicated that TNCC, RBC count, PROT, and percent neutrophils are correlated with the severity and duration of injury, but the results did not appear useful for differentiating IVDH from other spinal cord diseases.[112] A study of 54 nonambulatory dogs[171] and another of 31 dogs lacking deep nociception[172] due to thoracolumbar IVDH indicated a relationship between severity of injury and the magnitude of CSF alterations. A high monocyte percentage and a high macrophage to monocyte ratio were predictive of a negative outcome.[171,172] A study of 118 samples from 107 dogs with IVDH suggested neutrophils may predominate in the acute stages or with severe disease, with a mononuclear or mixed pleocytosis more common in more long-standing cases.[173] Increased PROT was more common than pleocytosis, but CSF alterations were most pronounced when the sample was collected caudal to the lesion by lumbar subarachnoid space puncture.[173] A study of 423 dogs found lymphocytic pleocytosis to be common in IVDH, likely more often in chronic rather than acute cases and possibly due to an immune response to herniated disc material.[113]

Case reports and case series have detailed CSF findings associated with naturally occurring spinal cord trauma,[114] caudal cervical spondylomyelopathy,[115] discospondylitis,[116] spinal empyema,[117] idiopathic epilepsy,[118] fibrocartilaginous embolism,[119–122] acute noncompressive nucleus pulposus extrusion,[123] and cerebrovascular accident.[98,124–127]

Neoplasia

Primary and secondary intracranial neoplasia is well described and illustrated in cytology atlases and Chapter 47.[1,2,19] Neoplastic cells are only occasionally found via CSF cytology. The likelihood of finding neoplastic cells in CSF depends on the location of the neoplasm.[2]

CSF analysis is not usually diagnostic for a specific type of neoplasm. The TNCC and PROT are often moderately elevated but may be either normal or markedly elevated.[105] In a retrospective study of 53 dogs with primary brain tumors that had CSF analysis, 9.4% had normal CSF findings, with normal CSF most commonly occurring in dogs with deeply seated astrocytomas and oligodendrogliomas. The most common abnormality was increased PROT, and the least common was an increased TNCC. The CSF of dogs with meningiomas differed from that of other neoplasms in having high TNCCs with a predominance of neutrophils, but this is correlated with necrosis or neutrophilic infiltration of the tumor.[106] A retrospective study of 56 dogs with meningiomas concluded that neutrophilic pleocytosis (especially with a TNCC >50 cells/μL) is not typical of this neoplasm, though meningiomas located in the caudal cranial fossa were significantly more likely to have an increased TNCC than those located within the middle or rostral portions. There was no significant correlation between neutrophilic pleocytosis and the presence of necrosis within the tumor. No CSF abnormalities were present in 16%.[13] Retrospective study of CSF analysis in 51 dogs with intracranial primary neoplasms found no abnormalities in 10%, an increased TNCC in 58%, and albuminocytologic dissociation in 30%. The most common cytologic abnormality was mixed cell pleocytosis, though other types of pleocytosis were seen. Atypical or neoplastic cells were seen in two of six dogs with CNS lymphoma. It was concluded that CSF cytology might be helpful for diagnosing CNS lymphoma, but the inflammatory nature of the CSF in many patients with primary intracranial neoplasia may prevent neoplasia being distinguished from other causes of CNS inflammation.[16] A retrospective study of MRI findings for 40 dogs included CSF analysis findings for 16 dogs, with results similar to the above study.[107] MRI findings suggestive of lymphoma should be confirmed by cytology or histopathology.[108] Case reports have described neoplastic cells of histiocytic origin within CSF.[109,110]

CSF analysis on 25 dogs with choroid plexus tumors (7 with papilloma and 18 with carcinoma) showed all had increased PROT (>25 mg/dL), with significantly larger increases in the carcinomas; only carcinomas had a PROT of >80 mg/dL. All papillomas and 50% of carcinomas had elevated TNCCs (>5 cells/μL). Both tumor types often had a mixed cell pleocytosis. It was concluded that CSF analysis and MRI findings can help differentiate between choroid plexus papilloma and carcinoma.[17]

CSF findings in cats with intracranial neoplasia are similar to findings reported for dogs. In a retrospective study of 28 cases of feline intracranial neoplasia confirmed by biopsy or necropsy, albuminocytologic dissociation was noted in 8 cats (28.6%). PROT ranged from 16 to 427 mg/dL (RI of <25 mg/dL). The remaining 20 cats (71.4%) had varied increases in TNCC (defined as >5 cells/μL), with a range of 0–162.[111]

Biomarkers in CSF

In addition to routine testing, numerous studies have explored the utility of measuring various biomarkers in CSF (Table 48.2).[114,174–191]

Conclusions

While a valuable diagnostic aid in animals with neurologic disease, CSF analysis alone does not often provide a definitive diagnosis as abnormal findings are often nonspecific. Infectious versus noninfectious inflammatory diseases can be difficult to differentiate. Diagnostic value is increased by combining CSF analysis with clinical presentation, cross-sectional imaging, and other ancillary diagnostic techniques.

Table 48.2 CNS disease-associated biomarkers evaluated in CSF and blood.

Biomarker	Source	Diagnostic applications
NSE	Cytoplasm of neurons, oligodendrocytes, and neuroendocrine cells; thrombocytes; erythrocytes	Detects neuronal damage and degeneration but lacks specificity. Diagnostic utility undetermined Higher concentrations seen in CSF in dogs with GM1 gangliosidosis and CNS inflammation.[174,175]
MBP	Produced by oligodendrocytes	Marker of white matter disease Acute SCI in dogs: >3 ng/mL in CSF indicates poor prognosis with 78% sensitivity, 76% specificity.[176–178] Successful long-term outcome predicted when creatine kinase activity is <38 U/L and MBP <3 ng/mL in CSF.[179] Indicates diagnosis of DM but increase is not disease specific.[180]
GFAP and anti-GFAP autoantibodies	Intermediate filament in astrocytes	Evaluates the blood brain barrier. Helpful in diagnosis of inflammation but lacks specificity in differential diagnosis. For diagnosis of myelomalacia: blood levels are 75% sensitive; 97% specific.[181] Necrotizing meningoencephalitis (Pugs): >0.1 ng/mL in serum is 67% sensitive, 100% specific[182]; anti-GFAP autoantibodies in CSF are 91% sensitive, 73% specific.[183]
c-tau	Protein associated with microtubule structures localized in axons	Plegic dogs with IVDH: >41.3 pg/mL in CSF predicts an unsuccessful outcome with 86% sensitivity, 83% specificity.[184]
pNF-H	Major cytoskeletal component of axons	Paraplegic dogs with absent nociception: pNF-H >1590 pg/mL in blood is 34.8% sensitive, 100% specific in predicting prognosis for recovering ambulation.[185] Diagnosis of DM: pNF-H > 20.25 ng/mL in CSF is 80.4% sensitive, 93.6%.[186]
MMP-9; MMP-2	Endopeptidases that degrade extracellular matrix as part of tissue remodeling	Detectable in paraplegic dogs with IVDH[187] Detectable in CSF of dogs with brain tumors but not correlated with malignancy.[188,189]
Acute Phase Proteins (CRP, Hp)	CRP results from endothelial damage; Hp inhibits neutrophil chemotaxis	Dogs with IVDH: Concentrations of CRP and Hp in CSF are significantly higher in dogs with severe injury; but no correlation with 42 day motor outcome.[190]
Cytokines and Chemokines	Reflect innate and adaptive immune responses	Dogs with IVDH: In CSF, IL-8 is significantly higher with SCI and negatively correlated with duration of SCI; MCP-1 and KC-like protein are negatively associated with 42-day post injury outcome.[114]
PLA2, LTC4, PGE2	Arachidonic acid metabolites	Mediators of secondary spinal cord injury Dogs with IVDH: Concentrations of PLA2 and PGE2 were higher and LTC4 lower in CSF; PGE2 was positively associated with severity of SCI and poor recovery.[191]

CNS, central nervous system; CRP, C-reactive protein; CSF, cerebrospinal fluid; c-tau, cleaved-tau; DM, degenerative myelopathy; GFAP, glial fibrillary acidic protein; Hp, haptoglobin; IL, interleukin; IVDH, intervertebral disc herniation; KC-like, keratinocyte chemotactic-like; LTC4, leukotriene C4; MBP, myelin basic protein; MCP-1, monocyte chemotactic protein-1; MMP, matrix-metalloproteases; NSE, neuron-specific enolase; PGE2, prostaglandin E2; PLA2, phospholipase A2; pNF-H, phosphorylated neurofilament heavy; SCI, spinal cord injury.

References

1 Cook, J.R. and Levine, G.J. (2014). Cerebrospinal fluid and central nervous system cytology. In: *Cowell and Tyler's Diagnostic Cytology and Hematology of the Dog and Cat*, 4e (eds. A.C. Valenciano and R.L. Cowell), 222–243. St. Louis: Elsevier.

2 De Lorenzi, D. and Mandara, M.T. (2016). The central nervous system. In: *Canine and Feline Cytology: A Color Atlas and Interpretation Guide*, 3e (eds. R.E. Raskin and D.J. Meyer), 369–407. St. Louis: Elsevier.

3 Parent, J.M. and Rand, J.S. (1994). Cerebrospinal fluid collection and analysis. In: *Consultations in Feline Internal Medicine*, 2e (ed. J.R. August), 385–392. Philadelphia: W.B. Saunders.

4 Kornegay, J.N., Oliver, J.E., and Gorgacz, E.J. (1983). Clinicopathologic features of bran herniation in animals. *J Am Vet Med Assoc* 82: 1111–1116.

5 Cook, J.R. and DeNicola, D.B. (1988). Cerebrospinal fluid. *Vet Clin North Am Small Anim Pract* 18: 475–499.

6 Feliu-Pascual, A.L., Garosi, L., Dennis, R., and Platt, S. (2008). Iatrogenic brain stem injury during cerebellomedullary cistern puncture. *Vet Radiol Ultrasound* 49: 467–471.

7 Kishimoto, M., Yamada, K., Kobayashi, Y. et al. (2004). Spinal cord effects from lumbar myelographic injection technique in the dog. *J Vet Med Sci* 66: 67–69.

8 Platt, S.R., Dennis, R., Murphy, K., and Stefani, A. (2005). Hematomyelia secondary to lumbar cerebrospinal fluid acquisition in a dog. *Vet Radiol Ultrasound* 46: 467–471.

9 Packer, R.A., Bergman, R.L., Coates, J.R. et al. (2007). Intracranial subarachnoid hemorrhage following lumbar myelography in two dogs. *Vet Radiol Ultrasound* 48: 323–327.

10 Heywood, R., Osborne, B.E., and Street, A.E. (1973). The effect of repeated cisternal puncture and withdrawal of cerebro-spinal fluid in the dog. *Lab Anim* 7: 85–87.

11 Bohn, A.A., Wills, T.B., West, C.L. et al. (2006). Cerebrospinal fluid analysis and magnetic resonance imaging in the diagnosis of neurologic disease in dogs: a retrospective study. *Vet Clin Pathol* 35: 315–320.

12 Chrisman, C.L. (1992). Cerebrospinal fluid analysis. *Vet Clin North Am Small Anim Pract* 22: 781–810.

13 Dickinson, P.J., Sturges, B.K., Kass, P.H., and RA, L.C. (2006). Characteristics of cisternal cerebrospinal fluid associated with intracranial meningiomas in dogs: 56 cases (1985–2004). *J Am Vet Med Assoc* 228: 564–567.

14 Fenner WR. Diseases of the brain. Stephen J. Ettinger, Edward C. Feldman *Textbook of Veterinary Internal Medicine*, 5. Philadelphia: W.B. Saunders 2000;552–602.

15 Singh, M., Foster, D.J., Child, G., and Lamb, W.A. (2005). Inflammatory cerebrospinal fluid analysis in cats: clinical diagnosis and outcome. *J Feline Med Surg* 7: 77–93.

16 Snyder, J.M., Shofer, F.S., Van Winkle, T.J., and Massicotte, C. (2006). Canine intracranial primary neoplasia: 173 cases (1986–2003). *J Vet Intern Med* 20: 669–675.

17 Westworth, D.R., Dickinson, P.J., Vernau, W. et al. (2008). Choroid plexus tumors in 56 dogs (1985–2007). *J Vet Intern Med* 22: 1157–1165.

18 Zimmermann, K.L., Bender, H.S., Boon, G.D. et al. (2000). A comparison of the cytologic and histologic features of meningiomas in four dogs. *Vet Clin Pathol* 29: 29–34.

19 Baker, R. and Lumsden, J.H. (eds.) (2000). Cerebrospinal fluid. In: *Color Atlas of Cytology of the Dog and Cat*, 95–105. St. Louis: Mosby.

20 Bush, W.W., Barr, C.S., Darrin, E.W. et al. (2002). Results of cerebrospinal fluid analysis, neurological examination findings and age at the onset of seizures as predictors for results of magnetic resonance imaging of the brain in dogs examined because of seizures: 115 cases (1992–2000). *J Am Vet Med Assoc* 220: 781–784.

21 Di Terlizzi, R. and Platt, S.R. (2009). The function, composition and analysis of cerebrospinal fluid in companion animals: Part II – Analysis. *Vet J* 180: 15–32.

22 Thomson, C.E., Kornegay, J.N., and Stevens, J.B. (1990). Analysis of cerebrospinal fluid from the cerebellomedullary and lumbar cisterns of dogs with focal neurologic disease: 145 cases (1985–1987). *J Am Vet Med Assoc* 196: 1841–1844.

23 Steele, R.W., Marmer, D.J., O'Brien, M.D. et al. (1986). Leukocyte survival in cerebrospinal fluid. *J Clin Microbiol* 23: 965–966.

24 Fry, M.M., Vernau, W., Kass, P.H., and Vernau, K.M. (2006). Effects of time, initial composition, and stabilizing agents on the results of canine cerebrospinal fluid analysis. *Vet Clin Pathol* 35: 72–77.

25 Bienzle, D., McDonnell, J.J., and Stanton, J.B. (2000). Analysis of cerebrospinal fluid from dogs and cats after 24 and 48 hours of storage. *J Am Vet Med Assoc* 216: 1761–1764.

26 Wamsley, H. (2012). Clinical pathology. In: *British Small Animal Veterinary Association Manual of Canine and Feline Neurology*, 4e (eds. S.R. Platt and N.J. Olby), 36–58. Gloucester: BVSA.

27 Coates, J.R. (2000). Cerebrospinal proteins. In: *Schalm's Veterinary Hematology*, 5e (eds. B.F. Feldman, J.G. Zinkl and N.C. Jain), 917–924. Philadelphia: Lippincott, Williams and Wilkins.

28 Riond, B., Steffen, F., Schmied, O. et al. (2014). Total protein measurement in canine cerebrospinal fluid: agreement between a turbidimetric assay and 2 dye-binding methods and determination of reference intervals using an indirect a posteriori method. *Vet Clin Pathol* 43: 78–88.

29 Hurtt, A.E. and Smith, M.O. (1997). Effects of iatrogenic blood contamination on results of cerebrospinal fluid analysis in clinically normal dogs and dogs with neurologic disease. *J Am Vet Med Assoc* 211: 866–867.

30 Marshall, T. and Williams, K.M. (2000). Protein determination in cerebrospinal fluid by protein dye-binding assay. *Br J Biomed Sci* 57: 281–286.

31 Pesce, M.A. and Strand, C.S. (1973). A new micromethod for determination of protein in cerebrospinal fluid and urine. *Clin Chem* 19: 1265–1267.

32 Vernau, W., Vernau, K., and Bailey, C.S. (2008). Cerebrospinal fluid. In: *Clinical Biochemistry of Domestic Animals*, 6e (eds. J.J. Kaneko, J.W. Harvey and M.L. Bruss), 769–819. Boston: Academic Press.

33 Friedrichs, K.R., Harr, K.L., Freeman, K.P. et al. (2012). ASVCP reference interval guidelines: determination of de novo reference intervals in veterinary species and other related topics. *Vet Clin Pathol* 41: 441–453.

34 Bailey, C.S. and Higgins, R.J. (1985). Comparison of total white blood cell count and total protein content of lumbar and cisternal cerebrospinal fluid of healthy dogs. *Am J Vet Res* 46: 1162–1165.

35 Reiber, H. (1994). Flow rate of cerebrospinal fluid (CSF): a concept common to normal blood-CSF barrier function and to dysfunction in neurological diseases. *J Neurol Sci* 122: 189–203.

36 Carmichael, N. (1998). Nervous system. In: *Manual of Small Animal Clinical Pathology* (eds. M.G. Davidson, R.W. Else and J.H. Lumsden), 235–240. Cheltenham: British Small Animal Veterinary Association.

37 Steinberg, T.A., Boettcher, I.C., Matiasek, K. et al. (2008). Use of albumin quotient and IgG index to differentiate blood- vs brain-derived proteins in the cerebrospinal fluid of cats with feline infectious peritonitis. *Vet Clin Pathol* 37: 207–216.

38 Tipold, A., Pfister, H., and Vandevelde, M. (1993). Determination of the IgG index for the detection of intrathecal immunoglobulin synthesis in dogs using an ELISA. *Res Vet Sci* 54: 40–44.

39 Behr, S., Trumel, C., Cauzinille, L. et al. (2006). High resolution protein electrophoresis of 100 paired canine cerebrospinal fluid and serum. *J Vet Intern Med* 657: 657–662.

40 Sorjonen, D.C. (1987). Total protein, albumin quota, and electrophoretic patterns in cerebrospinal fluid of dogs with central nervous system disorders. *Am J Vet Res* 48: 301–305.

41 Sorjonen, D.C., Golden, D.L., Levesque, D.C. et al. (1991). Cerebrospinal fluid protein electrophoresis: a clinical evaluation of a previously reported diagnostic technique. *Prog Vet Neurol* 2: 261–268.

42 Boettcher, I.C., Steinberg, T., and Matiasek, K. (2007). Use of anti-coronavirus antibody testing of cerebrospinal fluid for diagnosis of feline infectious peritonitis involving the central nervous system. *J Am Vet Med Assoc* 230: 199–206.

43 Maiolini, A., Carlson, R., Schwartz, M. et al. (2012). Determination of immunoglobulin A concentrations in the serum and cerebrospinal fluid of dogs: an estimation of its diagnostic value in canine steroid-responsive meningitis-arteritis. *Vet J* 191: 219–224.

44 Slesinger, S. and Hrazdira, C.L. (1970). Untersuchungen der zerebrospinalflüssigkeit von hunden und pferden. *Zentrabl Veterinarmed A* 17: 338–350.

45 Fankhauser, H. (1954). De liquor cerebrospinalis in der veterinarmedizin. *Zentrabl Veterinarmed A* 1: 136–159.

46 Jordan, J.E. (1977). Normal laboratory values in beagle dogs of twelve to eighteen months of age. *Am J Vet Res* 38: 509–513.

47 Schmidt, U. and Hübner, S. (1974). Zytomorphologische untersuchungen der cerebrospinalflüssigkeit von gesuden hunden und in 7 fallen nach auftrenen von zns-störungen. *Zentrabl Veterinarmed A* 21: 157–164.

48 Jamison, E.M. and Lumsden, J.H. (1988). Cerebrospinal fluid analysis in the dog: methodology and interpretation. *Semin Vet Med (Small Anim)* 3: 122–132.

49 Croft, P.G. (1955). Biochemistry of the cerebrospinal fluid of the dog. *Vet Rec* 67: 872–876.

50 Wilson, J.W. (1976). Canine cerebrospinal fluid: normal composition. *Minn Vet* 16: 25–26.

51 Wilson, J.W. and Stevens, J.B. (1977). Effects of blood contamination on cerebrospinal fluid analysis. *J Am Vet Med Assoc* 171: 256–258.

52 Carakostas, M.C., Gossett, K.A., Watters, J.W., and PS, M.W. (1983). Effects of metrizamide myelography on cerebrospinal fluid analysis in the dog. *Vet Radiol* 24: 267–270.

53 Rand, J.S., Parent, J., Jacobs, R., and Percy, D. (1990). Reference intervals for feline cerebrospinal fluid: cell counts and cytologic features. *Am J Vet Res* 51: 1044–1048.

54 Aune, M.W. and Sandburg, S. (1984). Electronic counting of spinal fluid cells. *Am J Clin Pathol* 81: 506–511.

55 Ruotsala, K., Poma, R., da Costa, R.C., and Bienzle, D. (2008). Evaluation of the Advia 120 CSF assay for analysis of canine cerebrospinal fluid. *Vet Clin Pathol* 37: 242–248.

56 Becker, M., Bauer, N., and Moritz, A. (2008). Automated flow cytometric cell count and differentiation of canine cerebrospinal fluid cells using the ADVIA 2120. *Vet Clin Pathol* 37: 344–352.

57 Christopher, M.M., Perman, V., and Hardy, R.M. (1988). Reassessment of cytologic values in canine cerebrospinal fluid by use of cytocentrifugation. *J Am Vet Med Assoc* 192: 1726–1729.

58 Rand, J.S., Parent, J., Percy, D., and Jacobs, R. (1994). Clinical, cerebrospinal fluid and histological data from twenty-seven cats with primary inflammatory disease of the central nervous system. *Can Vet J* 35: 103–110.

59 Rand, J.S., Parent, J., Percy, D., and Jacobs, R. (1994). Clinical, cerebrospinal fluid and histological data from thirty-four cats with primary noninflammatory disease of the central nervous system. *Can Vet J* 35: 174–181.

60 Krimer, P.M., Haley, A.C., Harvey, S.B., and Schatzberg, S.J. (2016). Evaluation of cytospin precision in low cellularity canine cerebrospinal fluid. *J Vet Diagn Invest* 28: 158–164.

61 Jamison, E.M. (1992). A study of cerebrospinal fluid in dogs with central nervous system disease. Thesis. Guelph, ON: University of Guelph.

62 Sornäs, R. (1971). Transformation of mononuclear cells in cerebrospinal fluid. *Acta Cytol* 5: 545–551.

63 Duque, C., Parent, J., and Bienzle, D. (2002). The immunophenotype of blood and cerebrospinal fluid mononuclear cells in dogs. *J Vet Intern Med* 16: 714–719.
64 Krakowka, S., Fenner, W., and Miele, J.A. (1981). Quantitative determination of serum origin cerebrospinal fluid proteins in the dog. *J Am Vet Res* 42: 1975–1977.
65 Widmer, W.R., DeNicola, D.B., Blevins, W.E. et al. (1992). Cerebrospinal fluid changes after iopamidol and metrizamide myelography in clinically normal dogs. *Am J Vet Res* 53: 396–401.
66 Wessmann, A., Volk, H.A., Chandler, K. et al. (2010). Significance of surface epithelial cells in canine cerebrospinal fluid and relationship to central nervous system disease. *Vet Clin Pathol* 39: 358–364.
67 Doyle, C. and Solano-Gallego, L. (2009). Cytologic interpretation of canine cerebrospinal fluid samples with low total nucleated cell concentration, with and without blood contamination. *Vet Clin Pathol* 38: 392–396.
68 Widmer, W.R., Blevins, W.E., Cantwell, H.D. et al. (1990). Cerebrospinal fluid response following metrizamide myelography in normal dogs: effects of routine myelography and postmyelographic removal of contrast medium. *Vet Clin Pathol* 19: 66–76.
69 Johnson, G.C., Fuciu, D.M., Fenner, W.R., and Krakowka, S. (1985). Transient leakage across the blood-cerebrospinal fluid barrier after intrathecal metrizamide administration to dogs. *Am J Vet Res* 46: 1303–1308.
70 Sarmento, L.V.C., Tudury, E.A., Teixeira, M.N. et al. (2002). Myelography in normal dogs with ioversol contrast medium. Cerebrospinal fluid and anatomohistopathological results. *Cienc. Rural* 32: 427–432.
71 Nagpal, J.S. and Dhablania, D.C. (1997). Cerebrospinal fluid changes following spinal cord compression with special reference to iopamidol myelography in dogs. *Indian Vet J* 74: 965–968.
72 van Bree, H., van Rijssen, B., and van Ham, L. (1991). Comparison of nonionic contrast agents iohexol and iotrolan for cisternal myelography in dogs. *Am J Vet Res* 52: 926–933.
73 Rigueira, F.d.L., APB, B., ME, B. et al. (2006). Physical, chemical and cytological characteristics of cerebrospinal fluid in dogs submitted to myelography with iohexol. *Veterinária Notícias* 12: 97–102.
74 Oftedal, S.-I. (1973). Meningeal reactions to water-soluble contrast media in cats. *Acta Radiol* 335 (Suppl): 153–160.
75 Yaksh, T.L., Fedele, L.A., and Yamamura, H.I. (1973). Effects of repeated withdrawal of cerebrospinal fluid by cisternal puncture on cisternal protein levels in the unanesthetized cat. *Physiol Behav* 10: 149–151.
76 Zabolotsky, S.M., Vernau, K.M., Kass, P.H., and Vernau, W. (2010). Prevalence and significance of extracellular myelin-like material in canine cerebrospinal fluid. *Vet Clin Pathol* 39: 90–95.
77 Fallin, C.W., Raskin, R.E., and Harvey, J.W. (1996). Cytologic identification of neural tissue in the cerebrospinal fluid of two dogs. *Vet Clin Pathol* 25: 127–129.
78 Christopher, M.M. (1992). Bone marrow contamination of canine cerebrospinal fluid. *Vet Clin Pathol* 21: 95–98.
79 Bienzle, D., Kwiecien, J.M., and Parent, J.M. (1995). Extramedullary hematopoiesis in the choroid plexus of five dogs. *Vet Pathol* 32: 437–440.
80 Radaelli, S.T. and Platt, S.R. (2002). Bacterial meningoencephalomyelitis in dogs: a retrospective study of 23 cases (1990–1999). *J Vet Intern Med* 16: 159–163.
81 Tipold, A. (1995). Diagnosis of inflammatory and infectious diseases of the central nervous system in dogs: a retrospective study. *J Vet Intern Med* 9: 304–314.
82 Barnes, H.L., Chrisman, C.L., Farina, L., and Detrisac, C.J. (2003). Clinical evaluation of rabies virus meningoencephalomyelitis in a dog. *J Am Anim Hosp Assoc* 39: 547–550.
83 Sorjonen, D.C., Cox, N.R., and Swango, L.J. (1989). Electrophoretic determination of albumin and gamma globulin concentrations in the cerebrospinal fluid of dogs with encephalomyelitis attributable to canine distemper virus infection: 13 cases (1980–1987). *J Am Vet Med Assoc* 195: 977–980.
84 Sykes, J.E., Sturges, B.K., Cannon, M.S. et al. (2010). Clinical signs, imaging features, neuropathology, and outcome in cats and dogs with central nervous system cryptococcosis from California. *J Vet Intern Med* 24: 1427–1438.
85 Bentley, R.T., Heng, H.G., Thompson, C. et al. (2015). Magnetic resonance imaging features and outcome for solitary central nervous system *Coccidioides* granulomas in 11 dogs and cats. *Vet Radiol Ultrasound* 56: 520–530.
86 Taylor, A.R., Young, B.D., Levine, G.J. et al. (2015). Clinical features and magnetic resonance imaging findings in 7 dogs with central nervous system aspergillosis. *J Vet Intern Med* 29: 1556–1563.
87 Lavely, J. and Lipsitz, D. (2005). Fungal infections of the central nervous system in the dog and cat. *Clin Tech Small Anim Pract* 20: 212–219.
88 Windsor, R.C., Sturgis, B.K., Vernau, K.M., and Vernau, W. (2009). Cerebrospinal fluid eosinophilia in dogs. *J Vet Intern Med* 23: 275–281.
89 Cuddon, P., Lin, D.S., Bowman, D.D. et al. (1992). *Neospora caninum* infection in English Springer Spaniel littermates. Diagnostic evaluation and organism isolation. *J Vet Intern Med* 6: 325–332.
90 Garosi, L., Dawson, A., Couturier, J. et al. (2010). Necrotizing cerebellitis and cerebellar atrophy caused by

Neospora caninum infection: magnetic resonance imaging and clinicopathologic findings in seven dogs. *J Vet Intern Med* 24: 571–578.

91 Gaitero, L., Anor, S., Montoliu, P. et al. (2006). Detection of *Neospora caninum* tachyzoites in canine cerebrospinal fluid. *J Vet Intern Med* 20: 410–414.

92 Barber, J.S., Payne-Johnson, C.E., and Trees, A.J. (1996). Distribution of *Neospora caninum* within the central nervous system and other tissues of six dogs with clinical neosporosis. *J Small Anim Pract* 37: 568–574.

93 Parzefall, B., Driver, C.J., Benigni, L., and Davies, E. (2014). Magnetic resonance imaging characteristics in four dogs with central nervous system neosporosis. *Vet Radiol Ultrasound* 55: 539–546.

94 Maretzki, C.H., Fisher, D.J., and Greene, C.E. (1994). Granulocytic ehrlichiosis and meningitis in a dog. *J Am Vet Med Assoc* 205: 1554–1556.

95 Tyler, D.E., Lorenz, M.D., Blue, J.L. et al. (1980). Disseminated protothecosis with central nervous system involvement in a dog. *J Am Vet Med Assoc* 176: 987–993.

96 Gupta, A., Gumber, S., Bauer, R.W., and Royal, A.B. (2011). What is your diagnosis? Cerebrospinal fluid from a dog. Eosinophilic pleocytosis due to protothecosis. *Vet Clin Pathol* 40: 105–106.

97 Lane, L.V., Meinkoth, J.H., Brunker, J. et al. (2012). Disseminated protothecosis diagnosed by evaluation of CSF in a dog. *Vet Clin Pathol* 41: 147–152.

98 Glass, E.N., Cornetta, A.M., de Lahunta, A. et al. (1998). Clinical and clinicopathologic features in 11 cats with *Cuterebra* larvae myiasis of the central nervous system. *J Vet Intern Med* 12: 365–368.

99 Granger, N., Smith, P.M., and Jeffery, N.D. (2010). Clinical findings and treatment of non-infectious meningoencephalomyelitis in dogs: a systematic review of 457 published cases from 1962–2008. *Vet J* 184: 290–297.

100 Tipold, A. and Jaggy, A. (1994). Steroid responsive meningitis-arteritis in dogs: long-term study of 32 cases. *J Small Anim Pract* 35: 311–316.

101 Cizinauskas, S., Jaggy, A., and Tipold, A. (2000). Long-term treatment of dogs with steroid-responsive meningitis-arteritis: clinical, laboratory and therapeutic results. *J Small Anim Pract* 41: 295–301.

102 Lowrie, M., Penderis, J., McLaughlin, M. et al. (2009). Steroid responsive meningitis-arteritis: a prospective study of potential disease markers, prednisolone treatment, and long-term outcome in 20 dogs (2006–2008). *J Vet Intern Med* 23: 862–870.

103 Smith-Maxie, L.L., Parent, J.P., Rand, J. et al. (1989). Cerebrospinal fluid analysis and clinical outcome of eight dogs with eosinophilic meningoencephalomyelitis. *J Vet Intern Med* 3: 167–174.

104 Bennett, P.F., Allan, F.J., Guilford, W.G. et al. (1997). Idiopathic eosinophilic meningoencephalitis in Rottweiler dogs: three cases (1992–1997). *Aust Vet J* 75: 786–789.

105 Dickinson, P.J. (2014). Advances in diagnostic and treatment modalities for intracranial tumors. *J Vet Intern Med* 28: 1165–1185.

106 Bailey, C.S. and Higgins, R.J. (1986). Characteristics of the cerebrospinal fluid associated with primary brain tumors in the dog: a retrospective study. *J Am Vet Med Assoc* 188: 414–417.

107 Rodenas, S., Pumarola, M., Gaitero, L. et al. (2011). Magnetic imaging findings in 40 dogs with histologically confirmed intracranial tumours. *Vet J* 187: 85–91.

108 Palus, V., Volk, H.A., Lamb, C.R. et al. (2012). MRI features of CNS lymphoma in dogs and cats. *Vet Radiol Ultrasound* 53: 44–49.

109 Zimmerman, K., Almy, F., Carter, L. et al. (2006). Cerebrospinal fluid from a 10-year-old dog with a single seizure episode. *Vet Clin Pathol* 35: 127–131.

110 Tzipory, L., Vernau, K.M., Sturges, B.K. et al. (2009). Antemortem diagnosis of localized central nervous system histiocytic sarcoma in 2 dogs. *J Vet Intern Med* 23: 369–374.

111 Troxel, M.T., Vite, C.H., Van Winkle, T.J. et al. (2003). Feline intracranial neoplasia: retrospective review of 160 cases (1985–2001). *J Vet Intern Med* 17: 850–859.

112 Levine, G.J., Cook, J.R., Kerwin, S.C. et al. (2014). Relationships between cerebrospinal fluid characteristics, injury, severity and functional outcome in dogs with and without intervertebral disk herniation. *Vet Clin Pathol* 43: 437–446.

113 Windsor, R.C., Vernau, K.M., Sturges, B.K. et al. (2008). Lumbar cerebrospinal fluid in dogs with type I intervertebral disc herniation. *J Vet Intern Med* 22: 954–960.

114 Taylor, A.R., Welsh, C.J., Young, C. et al. (2014). Cerebrospinal fluid inflammatory cytokines and chemokines in naturally occurring canine spinal cord injury. *J Neurotrauma* 31: 1561–1569.

115 Martin-Vaquero, P., da Costa, R.C., Moore, S.A. et al. (2014). Cytokine concentrations in the cerebrospinal fluid of Great Danes with cervical spondylomyelopathy. *J Vet Intern Med* 28: 1268–1274.

116 Harris, J.M., Chen, A.V., Tucker, R.L., and Mattoon, J.S. (2013). Clinical features and magnetic resonance imaging characteristics of diskospondylitis in dogs: 23 cases (1997–2010). *J Am Vet Med Assoc* 242: 359–365.

117 Lavely, J.A., Vernau, K.M., Vernau, W. et al. (2006). Spinal epidural empyema in seven dogs. *Vet Surg* 35: 176–185.

118 Goncalves, R., Anderson, T.J., Innocent, G., and Penderis, J. (2010). Effect of seizures on cerebrospinal fluid analysis in dogs with idiopathic epilepsy. *Vet Rec* 166: 497–498.

119 Mikszewski, J.S., Van Winkle, T.J., and Troxel, M.T. (2006). Fibrocartilaginous embolic myelopathy in five cats. *J Am Anim Hosp Assoc* 42: 226–233.

120 Theobald, A., Volk, H.A., Dennis, R. et al. (2013). Clinical outcome in 19 cats with clinical and magnetic resonance imaging diagnosis of ischaemic myelopathy (2000–2011). *J Feline Med Surg* 15: 132–141.

121 De Risio, L., Adams, V., Dennis, R. et al. (2007). Magnetic resonance imaging findings and clinical associations in 52 dogs with suspected ischemic myelopathy. *J Vet Intern Med* 21: 1290–1298.

122 Bartholomew, K.A., Stover, K.E., Olby, N.J., and Moore, S.A. (2016). Clinical characteristics of canine fibrocartilaginous embolic myelopathy (FCE): a systematic review of 393 cases (1973–2013). *Vet Rec* 179: 650.

123 De Risio, L., Adams, V., Dennis, R., and FJ, M.C. (2009). Association of clinical and magnetic resonance imaging findings with outcome in dogs with presumptive acute noncompressive nucleus pulposus extrusion: 42 cases (2000–2007). *J Am Vet Med Assoc* 234: 495–504.

124 Garosi, L., McConnell, J.E., Platt, S.R. et al. (2005). Results of diagnostic investigations and long-term outcome of 33 dogs with brain infarction (2000–2004). *J Vet Intern Med* 19: 725–731.

125 Kent, M., Glass, E.N., Haley, A.C. et al. (2014). Ischemic stroke in Greyhounds: 21 cases (2007–2013). *J Am Vet Med Assoc* 245: 113–117.

126 McConnell, J.F., Garosi, L., and Platt, S.R. (2005). Magnetic resonance imaging findings of presumed cerebellar cerebrovascular accident in twelve dogs. *Vet Radiol Ultrasound* 46: 1–10.

127 Altay, U.M., Skerritt, G.C., Hilbe, M. et al. (2011). Feline cerebrovascular disease: clinical and histopathologic findings in 16 cats. *J Am Anim Hosp Assoc* 47: 89–97.

128 Lorenz, M.D., Coates, J.R., and Kent, M. (eds.) (2011). Confirming a diagnosis. In: *Handbook of Veterinary Neurology*, 5e, 72–92. St. Louis: Elsevier.

129 Lamb, C.R., Croson, P.J., Cappello, R., and Cherubini, G.B. (2005). Magnetic imaging findings in 25 dogs with inflammatory cerebrospinal fluid. *Vet Radiol Ultrasound* 46: 17–22.

130 Coates, J.R. and Jeffery, N.D. (2014). Perspectives on meningoencephalomyelitis of unknown origin. *Vet Clin Small Anim* 44: 1157–1185.

131 Griffin, J.F., Levine, J.M., Levine, G.J., and Fosgate, G.T. (2008). Meningomyelitis in dogs: a retrospective review of 28 cases (1999 to 2007). *J Small Anim Pract* 49: 509–517.

132 Cizinauskas, S., Tipold, A., Fatzer, R. et al. (2001). Streptococcal meningoencephalomyelitis in 3 dogs. *J Vet Intern Med* 15: 157–161.

133 Fenner, W.R. (1998). Central nervous system infections. In: *Infectious Diseases of the Dog and Cat*, 2e (ed. C.E. Greene), 647–657. Philadelphia: W.B. Saunders.

134 Vandevelde, M. and Spano, J.S. (1977). Cerebrospinal fluid cytology in canine neurologic disease. *Am J Vet Res* 38: 1827–1832.

135 Lowrie, M., Smith, P.M., and Garosi, L. (2013). Meningoencephalitis of unknown origin: investigation of prognostic factors and outcome using a standard treatment protocol. *Vet Rec* 172: 527–532.

136 Talarico, L.R. and Schatzberg, S.J. (2010). Idiopathic granulomatous and necrotising inflammatory disorders of the canine central nervous system: a review and future perspectives. *J Small Anim Pract* 51: 138–149.

137 Bailey, C.S. and Higgins, R.J. (1986). Characteristics of the cerebrospinal fluid associated with canine granulomatous meningoencephalomyelitis: a retrospective study. *J Am Vet Med Assoc* 188: 418–421.

138 Munana, K.R. and Luttgen, P.J. (1998). Prognostic factors for dogs with granulomatous meningoencephalomyelitis: 42 cases (1982–1986). *J Am Vet Med Assoc* 212: 1902–1906.

139 Sorjonen, D.C. (1990). Clinical and histopathological features of granulomatous meningoencephalomyelitis in dogs. *J Am Anim Hosp Assoc* 26: 141–147.

140 Thomas, J.B. and Eger, C. (1989). Granulomatous meningoencephalomyelitis in 21 dogs. *J Small Anim Pract* 30: 287–293.

141 Cordy, D.R. and Holliday, T.A. (1989). A necrotizing meningoencephalitis of pug dogs. *Vet Pathol* 26: 191–194.

142 Levine, J.M., Fosgate, G.T., Porter, B. et al. (2008). Epidemiology of necrotizing meningoencephalitis in Pug dogs. *J Vet Intern Med* 22: 961–968.

143 Stalis, I.H., Chadwick, B., Dayrell-Hart, B. et al. (1995). Necrotizing meningoencephalitis of Maltese dogs. *Vet Pathol* 32: 230–235.

144 Higgins, R.J., Dickinson, P.J., Kube, S.A. et al. (2008). Necrotizing meningoencephalitis in five Chihuahua dogs. *Vet Pathol* 45: 336–346.

145 Tipold, A., Fatzer, R., Jaggy, A. et al. (1993). Necrotizing encephalitis in Yorkshire terriers. *J Small Anim Pract* 34: 623–628.

146 Ducote, J.M., Johnson, K.E., Dewey, C.W. et al. (1999). Computed tomography of necrotizing meningoencephalitis in 3 Yorkshire Terriers. *Vet Radiol Ultrasound* 40: 617–621.

147 Jull, B.A., Merryman, J.I., Thomas, W.B., and McArthur, A. (1997). Necrotizing encephalitis in a Yorkshire terrier. *J Am Vet Med Assoc* 211: 1005–1007.

148 Kuwamura, M., Adachi, T., Yamate, J. et al. (2002). Necrotising encephalitis in the Yorkshire terrier: a case report and literature review. *J Small Anim Pract* 43: 459–463.

149 Cantile, C., Chianini, F., Arispici, M., and Fatzer, R. (2001). Necrotizing meningoencephalitis associated with cortical hippocampal hamartia in a Pekingese dog. *Vet Pathol* 38: 119–122.

150 Aresu, L., D'Angelo, A., Zanatta, R. et al. (2007). Canine necrotizing encephalitis associated with anti-glomerular basement membrane glomerulonephritis. *J Comp Pathol* 136: 279–282.

151 Timmann, D., Konar, M., Howard, J., and Vandevelde, M. (1989). Necrotizing encephalitis in a French bulldog. *J Small Anim Pract* 48: 339–342.

152 Cooper, J.J., Schatsberg, S.J., Vernau, K.M. et al. (2014). Necrotizing meningoencephalitis in atypical dog breeds: a case series and literature review. *J Vet Intern Med* 28: 198–203.

153 Behr, S. and Cauzinille, L. (2006). Aseptic suppurative meningitis in juvenile boxer dogs: retrospective study of 12 cases. *J Am Anim Hosp Assoc* 42: 277–282.

154 Tipold, A. and Schatzberg, S.J. (2010). An update on steroid responsive meningitis-arteritis. *J Small Anim Med Surg* 51: 150–154.

155 Burns, J.C., Felsburg, P.J., Wilson, H. et al. (1991). Canine pain syndrome is a model for the study of Kawasaki disease. *Perspect Biol Med* 35: 68–73.

156 Brooks, P.N. (1984). Necrotizing vasculitis in a group of beagles. *Lab Anim* 18: 285–290.

157 Felsburg, P.J., Hogenesch, H., Somberg, R.L. et al. (1992). Immunologic abnormalities in canine juvenile polyarteritis syndrome: a naturally occurring animal model of Kawasaki disease. *Clin Immunol Immunopathol* 65: 110–118.

158 Harcourt, R.A. (1978). Polyarteritis in a colony of beagles. *Vet Rec* 17: 519–522.

159 Hayes, T.J., Roberts, G.K., and Halliwell, W.H. (1989). An idiopathic febrile necrotizing arteritis syndrome of the dog: beagle pain syndrome. *Toxicol Pathol* 17: 129–137.

160 Hoff, E.J. and Vandevelde, M. (1981). Case report: necrotizing vasculitis in the central nervous systems of two dogs. *Vet Pathol* 18: 219–223.

161 Irving, G. and Chrisman, C. (1990). Long-term outcome of five cases of corticosteroid-responsive meningomyelitis. *J Am Anim Hosp Assoc* 28: 324–328.

162 Meric, S.M., Child, G., and Higgins, R.J. (1986). Necrotizing vasculitis of the spinal pachyleptomeningeal arteries in three Bernese mountain dogs littermates. *J Am Anim Hosp Assoc* 22: 459–465.

163 Meric, S.M., Perman, V., and Hardy, R. (1985). Corticosteroid-responsive meningitis in 10 dogs. *J Am Anim Hosp Assoc* 21: 677–684.

164 Poncelet, L. and Balligand, M. (1993). Steroid responsive meningitis in three boxer dogs. *Vet Rec* 132: 361–362.

165 Presthus, J. (1991). Aseptic suppurative meningitis in Bernese mountain dogs. *Eur J Comp Anim Pract* 2: 24–28.

166 Ruben, Z., Deslex, P., and Nash, G. (1989). Spontaneous disseminated panarteritis in laboratory beagle dogs in a toxicity study: a possible genetic predilection. *Toxicol Pathol* 17: 145–152.

167 Russo, E.A., Lees, G.E., and Hall, C.L. (1983). Corticosteroid-responsive aseptic suppurative meningitis in three dogs. *Southwestern Vet* 35: 197–201.

168 Scott-Montcrieff, J.C., Snyder, P.W., and Glickman, L.T. (1992). Systematic necrotizing vasculitis in nine young beagles. *J Am Vet Med Assoc* 201: 1553–1558.

169 Snyder, P.W., Kazacos, E.A., Scott-Moncrieff, J.C. et al. (1995). Pathologic features of naturally occurring juvenile polyarteritis in beagle dogs. *Vet Pathol* 32: 337–345.

170 Stejskal, V., Havu, N., and Malmfors, T. (1982). Necrotizing vasculitis as an immunological complication in a toxicity study. *Arch Toxicol* Suppl 5: 283–286.

171 Srugo, I., Aroch, I., Christopher, M.M. et al. (2011). Association of cerebrospinal fluid analysis findings with clinical signs and outcome in acute nonambulatory thoracolumbar disc disease in dogs. *J Vet Intern Med* 25: 846–855.

172 Chamisha, Y., Aroch, I., Kuzi, S. et al. (2015). The prognostic value of cerebrospinal fluid characteristics in dogs without deep pain perception due to thoracolumbar disc herniation. *Res Vet Sci* 100: 180–196.

173 Thomson, C.E., Kornegay, J.N., and Stevens, J.B. (1989). Canine intervertebral disc disease: changes in the cerebrospinal fluid. *J Small Anim Pract* 30: 685–688.

174 Satoh, H., Yamato, O., Asano, T. et al. (2007). Cerebrospinal fluid biomarkers showing neurodegeneration in dogs with GM1 gangliosidosis: possible use for assessment of a therapeutic regimen. *Brain Res* 1133: 200–208.

175 Nakamura, K., Miyasho, T., Nomura, S. et al. (2012). Proteome analysis of cerebrospinal fluid in healthy beagles and canine encephalitis. *J Vet Med Sci* 74: 751–756.

176 Levine, J.M., Fosgate, G.T., Chen, A.V. et al. (2009). Magnetic resonance imaging findings associated with

neurologic impairment in dogs with acute thoracic and lumbar intervertebral disk herniation. *J Vet Intern Med* 23: 1220–1226.

177 Levine, G.J., Levine, J.M., Witsberger, T.H. et al. (2010). Cerebrospinal fluid myelin basic protein as a prognostic biomarker in dogs with thoracolumbar intervertebral disk herniation. *J Vet Intern Med* 24: 890–896.

178 Ito, D., Matsunaga, S., Jeffrey, N.D. et al. (2005). Prognostic value of magnetic resonance imaging in dogs with paraplegia caused by thoracolumbar intervertebral disk extrusion: 77 cases (2000–2003). *J Am Vet Med Assoc* 227: 1454–1460.

179 Witsberger, T.H., Levine, J.M., Fosgate, G.T. et al. (2012). Associations between cerebrospinal fluid biomarkers and long-term neurologic outcome in dogs with acute intervertebral disk herniation. *J Am Vet Med Assoc* 240: 555–562.

180 Oji, T., Kamishina, H., Cheeseman, J.A., and Clemmons, R.M. (2007). Measurement of myelin basic protein in the cerebrospinal fluid of dogs with degenerative myelopathy. *Vet Clin Pathol* 36: 281–284.

181 Sato, Y., Shimamura, S., Mashita, T. et al. (2013). Serum glial fibrillary acidic protein as a diagnostic biomarker in dogs with progressive myelomalacia. *J Vet Med Sci* 75: 949–953.

182 Miyake, H., Inoue, A., Tanaka, M., and Matsuki, N. (2013). Serum glial fibrillary acidic protein as a specific marker for necrotizing meningoencephalitis in Pug dogs. *J Vet Med Sci* 75: 1543–1545.

183 Toda, Y., Matsuki, N., Shibuya, M. et al. (2007). Glial fibrillary acidic protein (GFAP) and anti-GFAP autoantibody in canine necrotising meningoencephalitis. *Vet Rec* 161: 261–264.

184 Roerig, A., Carlson, R., Tipold, A., and Stein, V.M. (2013). Cerebrospinal fluid tau protein as a biomarker for severity of spinal cord injury in dogs with intervertebral disc herniation. *Vet J* 197: 253–258.

185 Nishida, H., Nakayama, M., Tanaka, H. et al. (2014). Evaluation of serum phosphorylated neurofilament subunit NF-H as a prognostic biomarker in dogs with thoracolumbar intervertebral disc herniation. *Vet Surg* 43: 289–293.

186 Toedebusch, C.M., Bachrach, M., Garcia, V.B. et al. (2017). Cerebrospinal fluid phosphorylated neurofilament heavy as a diagnostic marker of canine degenerative myelopathy. *J Vet Intern Med* 31: 513–520.

187 Levine, J.M., Ruaux, C.G., Bergman, R.L. et al. (2006). Matrix metalloproteinase-9 activity in the cerebrospinal fluid and serum of dogs with acute spinal cord trauma from intervertebral disk disease. *Am J Vet Res* 67: 283–287.

188 Mariani, C.L., Boozer, L.B., Braxton, A.M. et al. (2013). Evaluation of matrix metalloproteinase-2 and -9 in the cerebrospinal fluid of dogs with intracranial tumors. *Am J Vet Res* 74: 122–129.

189 Mandara, M.T., Pavone, S., Mandrioli, L. et al. (2009). Matrix metalloproteinase-2 and metalloproteinase-9 expression in canine and feline meningioma. *Vet Pathol* 46: 836–845.

190 Anderson, K.M., Welsh, C.J., Young, C. et al. Acute phase proteins in cerebrospinal fluid from dogs with naturally-occurring spinal cord injury. *J Neurotrauma* 32: 1658–1665.

191 Russell, R.L., Levine, J.M., Jeffery, N.D. et al. (2016). Arachidonic acid pathway alterations in cerebrospinal fluid of dogs with naturally occurring spinal cord injury. *BMC Neurosci* 17 (1): 31.

49

Cerebrospinal Fluid Analysis in Horses and Large Animals

Eric J. Fish and Joseph J. Bertone

Cerebrospinal Fluid Formation, Functions, and Physiology

Cerebrospinal fluid (CSF) is a plasma ultrafiltrate that undergoes active transport modification and is secreted by the choroid plexus of the ventricles and adjacent ependymal lining cells. After release from the ventricles and ependyma, CSF flows caudally and is reabsorbed by the arachnoid villi.[1] CSF serves several critical physiological functions, including protecting delicate nervous tissue, regulating intracranial pressure (ICP), supplying nutrients and exporting metabolic wastes, and acting as a solvent for neurotransmitters. The rate of CSF formation is relatively stable but does depend on plasma osmotic pressure, rather than plasma hydrostatic pressure. This is why hyperosmolar therapeutic agents are able to reduce CSF production and thus ICP.[1]

Relative to plasma, CSF has higher sodium, chloride, and magnesium, along with lower glucose, potassium, calcium, and protein. CSF protein, in particular, is much lower, with a concentration <1/100th of plasma.[1] The average protein concentration for normal CSF in cattle and small ruminants is <40 and <50 mg/dL in llamas, while in horses the range is a bit higher, with up to 100 mg/dL being potentially normal.[2–4] CSF typically contains very few nucleated cells, with <3/μL in normal llamas, <6/μL in normal horses, and <10/μL in cows and sheep.[2–5] Many drugs and metabolites are excluded from CSF through the action of the blood–brain barrier (BBB).

Evaluation of CSF, in conjunction with diagnostic imaging, is an important part of the neurologic evaluation in equine, bovine, and small ruminant species. While rarely providing a definitive diagnosis in isolation, increases in nucleated cells, shifts in cell populations, elevated protein, identification of infectious organisms and neoplastic cells, and ancillary enzymatic or molecular testing can all support and occasionally confirm the ultimate diagnosis. When performed correctly, CSF sampling is a safe, minimally invasive, rapid, and cost-effective procedure.

Collection

Neurologic dysfunction and neuroanatomic diagnosis must be accurately established prior to CSF collection. This is especially important in horses, where musculoskeletal abnormalities can often be mistaken as primary central nervous system (CNS) disease. Imaging of the appropriate associated structures is warranted when indicated and achievable (e.g. radiography, myelography, scintigraphy, ultrasonography, brain and/or spinal column magnetic resonance imaging, and computed tomography). It is critical to interpret CSF analysis in light of the neurologic imaging findings. CNS imaging may also reveal contraindications to CSF collection, such as abnormalities associated with increased ICP. CSF is typically collected from horses and ruminants via the lumbosacral cistern (LS) or the atlanto-occipital space (AO). Collection from the LS is possible in standing or restrained animals, while collection from the AO typically requires general anesthesia.[6] In general, the risk of blood contamination in collecting CSF is least using the anesthetized AO method (though it can occur if the lateral venous sinus is sampled) than the standing ultrasound-guided dorsal AO method.[6] The LS technique has the greatest risk of blood contamination.[6] The AO method could be contaminated with synovial fluid from the atlanto-occipital joint.[6]

Complications of CSF collection are uncommon with proper technique but may include brain herniation in animals with increased ICP, local hemorrhage, adhesion formation, or infection of the CNS or subcutaneous tissues (this risk is minimized by rigorous aseptic technique).[6] One study showed that repeated CSF sampling by in-dwelling

Veterinary Cytology, First Edition. Edited by Leslie C. Sharkey, M. Judith Radin, and Davis Seelig.

catheter could result in neutrophilic pleocytosis that was self-limiting and resolved within a few days.[7]

Atlanto-Occipital Technique

AO collection is well described and preferred in most cases.[6] The dorsal AO method requires general anesthesia.[6] One should assure that the animals are neurologically stable enough for recovery, and the risk is worth the benefit. This technique is preferred when performing a myelogram since fluid can be collected and dye inserted through the same needle. The CSF can be collected very quickly and often an injectable short acting anesthetic protocol is sufficient when a myelogram is not being performed. Sterile local preparation and clipping is highly recommended. The animal's head is flexed to open a path to the AO space. This is often a flex to 90° with respect to the dorsal area of the neck. This flexes the neck to more than 90° with respect to the cervical spine. A CSF specific needle with stylet and 3.5 in. length is recommended. Samples and the CNS can be contaminated with peripheral blood (or potentially surface debris, squamous cells, or bacteria from skin) if an appropriate needle with stylet is not used.[6] The point of needle insertion is the intersection of the dorsal midline and the cranial edge of the wings of the axis. The needle should be inserted with the bevel directed cranially or caudally to avoid the needle deviating to one side or other. That is one purpose of the square female insertion hub of spinal needles. Slow insertion with multiple checks for fluid are highly recommended to avoid damaging the spinal cord. The insertion will require more pressure as one penetrates the nuchal ligament. A clear pop is often felt when penetrating the cistern through the dura mater, but should not be depended on in lieu of checking depth. In a normal size horse, this occurs at 2–2.5 in. of needle insertion. Fluid should run freely if the needle is inserted properly.

A standing method for lateral AO collection using ultrasound guidance and sedation is described and, in the authors' experience, is applicable in horses that are at high risk for general anesthesia.[8] However, the technique is more equipment and aid dependent.[8] Stocks are highly recommended for restraint and stability of the horse. Heavy sedation and analgesia is essential. The cranial cervical area just caudal to the mandible, dorsal to the wings of the atlas, and ventral to the midline is clipped and surgically prepared. A 10-MHz microconvex transducer oriented dorsoventrally is placed just below the mane and just cranial to the wings of the atlas. The subarachnoid space is visualized and the needle guided to the subarachnoid space. Fluid will often have to gently be aspirated using this technique.[8]

Lumbosacral Technique

The LS procedure is fraught with blood contamination issues, especially when using samples for immunologic analysis. Stocks are advisable, since almost regardless of the drugs used, horses will flinch when puncturing the dura and could become dangerous. Ultrasound guidance may be useful, but most often structural landmarks are used. Clipping and surgical preparation are essential. A 6–8-in. spinal needle with a stylet is used. Local anesthetic is used to make a small surgical blade stab incision into the skin at the point of insertion. This allows the needle to glide more easily and maintain its sharpness. The bevel must be directed caudal or cranial to avoid the needle deviating laterally as it penetrates the muscle layers. A point is identified where the midline bisects a line drawn dorsally from the cranial edge of the palpable tuber coxae. This will be just caudal to the last palpable lumbar dorsal spinous process. An indentation will be felt at this site where the needle should be inserted. The needle is directed slightly more caudally if bone is struck, and the needle should continue to penetrate more deeply, up to approximated 5 in. Often penetration of the dura is indicated with a pop and a reflex reaction by the horse. The needle is inserted until fluid or bone is reencountered. The needle is slightly retracted if no fluid can be collected once striking bone since the needle tip may be embedded. Another technique is to turn the needle slightly to expose the bevel in a direction that may allow fluid collection. Fluid must be aspirated with this technique and rarely comes freely.

Sample Handling and Submission

In large animal species, CSF collection should provide sufficient volume to aliquot approximately 2 mL into multiple tubes, including one to two red top tubes for most accurate protein measurement and microbiological culture and one to two ethylenediaminetetraacetic acid (EDTA)-anticoagulated tubes for best cell morphology and polymerase chain reaction (PCR) assays. Anticoagulant tubes are rarely needed and can alter protein analysis. Collecting multiple (at least three) sequential aliquots before submission for cell counts and cytologic analysis may decrease sample blood contamination.[9]

After collection, samples should be promptly processed as the fluid is hypoosmotic and cell degeneration can begin with 30–60 minutes. If immediate processing is not possible, cell viability can be extended through preservation with autologous serum, fetal calf serum, or hydroxyethyl starch colloid, following by refrigeration at 4 °C.[10–12] CSF preserved in this way is likely stable for at least 4–8 hours, with minimal change in diagnostic accuracy.

Laboratory Analysis of CSF

The complete laboratory evaluation of CSF has multiple parts, including physical evaluation, determination of total nucleated cell (TNCC) and red blood cell (RBC) counts, measurement of protein concentration, and cytologic evaluation. First, the color and turbidity are noted. Normal CSF is clear to pale straw in color, while a pink to red tinge suggests iatrogenic or peracute hemorrhage. Yellow or orange color (xanthochromia) is due to hemoglobin breakdown pigments and typically indicates prior hemorrhage. Increased turbidity is associated with increased TNCC (pleocytosis), although CSF must have an extremely high nucleated cellularity to notice turbidity (>500/μL).[13]

Xanthochromia and increased protein without increased nucleated cells (so-called "albuminocytologic dissociation") can be seen in CSF from animals with traumatic injury, neoplasia, vascular insults, or infectious diseases due to alteration of the BBB.[14] Xanthochromia can also be a normal finding in healthy neonatal foals.[15] Inflammatory proteins such as fibrinogen can result in increased CSF viscosity.[13]

Protein Analysis

Since the miniscule protein found in CSF is too low for typical total protein measurement via refractometer or routine total protein/albumin assays, a microprotein measurement (in mg/dL) via one of several dye-binding methods is performed. Pyrogallol red is the preferred method as it has the highest accuracy and diagnostic performance, but alternative methods include Ponceau S Acid Red, Coomassie Brilliant Blue, and trichloroacetic acid.[16] Other methods for CSF protein analysis include electrophoresis and measurement of immunoglobulin (Ig) fractions. Protein should be measured on a sample free of anticoagulant such as EDTA, as it may positively interfere with the protein measurement.[17]

CSF protein can be increased for a variety of reasons, including hemorrhage (pathologic or iatrogenic), disruption of the BBB, production of immunoglobulins, cytokines, and inflammatory mediators within the thecal space, damaged CNS cells leaking cytosolic proteins, or impaired drainage/resorption of CSF.[14]

Various equations have been developed to provide more useful information about measured CSF protein. The albumin quotient (AQ) is based on the theory that since albumin is not produced within the thecal space in health, increased CSF albumin, in the absence of hemorrhage, indicates dysfunction of the BBB. An AQ > 2.4 suggests disruption of the BBB.[18] In one small experimental study of neuropathogenic equine herpesvirus-1 (EHV-1), the only CSF abnormalities were xanthochromia and increased AQ.[19] The AQ can be calculated as follows:

$$AQ = \left(\text{CSF albumin} / \text{serum albumin}\right) \times 100$$

The IgG index attempts to identify local production of antibody in response to intrathecal antigenic stimulation. It requires measurement of IgA, IgM, and IgG on serum and CSF. The IgG index is calculated as follows:

$$\text{IgG Index} = \left(\text{CSF IgG} / \text{serum IgG}\right) / \left(\text{CSF albumin} / \text{serum albumin}\right)$$

An IgG index > 1.0 suggests CSF production of antibody.[18] However, the clinical utility of these AQ and IgG index values has not been robustly validated in large populations of animals.

Cell Counts

While the performance of several automated analyzers have assessed using CSF from dogs, the accuracy of automated analyzers for analysis of CSF cell counts or differentials have not been evaluated using equine or bovine CSF.[20,21] Because the cell concentration of even highly cellular CSF is at the performance limit for most automated hematology analyzers, a manual count of nucleated cells and erythrocytes should be performed via a hemocytometer.[13]

Once cell counts and protein are obtained, preparation of a concentrated sample for cytologic evaluation should be performed. Direct CSF preparations are almost always too low in cellularity to evaluate without enrichment. There are several specialized cytopathology machines that can create a "cytospin" preparation, and recently, a low-cost adaptation of a commercial kitchen "salad spinner" was shown to prepare suitable smears for cytologic evaluation of low-cellularity fluids, including CSF.[22] Concentrated preparations of CSF should be air-dried and stained with a Romanowsky-type stain. Wet preps of CSF stained with India ink may be useful if fungal organisms such as *Cryptococcus* are suspected.

CSF Patterns in Neurologic Disease

The nucleated cells typically found in normal CSF of most animals, including ruminants and equids, are rare small lymphocytes and monocytes/monocytoid cells.[23] Small, uniform, cuboidal ependymal lining cells from the choroid plexus may rarely exfoliate into CSF. One study showed these cells are comprised of at least four subtypes, with deeply basophilic alpha cells, light-staining beta cells that have cribriform chromatin, gamma cells that contain vesicular clear cytoplasmic inclusions, and Kolmer cells (macrophage-derived).[24] Ribbons of faint gray to pink staining myelin have been anecdotally associated with traumatic injury, although a study of 98 dogs found myelin material was present in 20% of CSF samples, more prevalent in lumbosacral collections, and did not correlate with disease type or clinical outcome, suggesting this may simply be a collection artifact.[25] The presence of hemosiderin and/or erythrophagia by macrophages supports prior hemorrhage, although this can occur within hours of collection and confound interpretation if CSF is not processed immediately. Formulas exist to try and "correct" the TNCC and protein concentrations for the amount of blood present, but these have been shown to be inaccurate in horse and cattle and should not be used.[10,26]

As mentioned previously, various neurologic diseases in large animal species may alter CSF cell and protein concentrations, although it is not unusual to find normal CSF in the face of neurologic disease, and this is highly variable by etiology. Toxic, nutritional, metabolic, and degenerative diseases are commonly associated with unremarkable CSF. One study of 102 cattle with confirmed neurologic disease found that 70% of animals with noninfectious CNS disease had normal CSF, including 100% of cattle with degenerative disease, 75% with toxic/metabolic disease, and 62% with neoplasia.[27] Even in the face of infectious disease, CSF findings may be an insensitive indicator, as demonstrated by one study where up to 27% of horses with confirmed West Nile virus (WNV) infection had normal CSF results, or another where 38.5% of horses with neuroborreliosis had normal CSF.[28,29]

However, there are data to indicate CSF analysis may be a useful screening tool for large animals in some limited contexts, as in a recent study predicting whether recumbent dairy cows had spinal cord lesions or not.[30] In that population, a CSF microprotein of <0.25 g/L (25 mg/dL) had 94% sensitivity and 32% specificity for a normal spinal cord, while a TNCC > 4.5 cells/μL had 50% sensitivity and 100% specificity for spinal cord pathology.[30]

Mononuclear Pleocytosis

In contrast to degenerative, toxic, and metabolic diseases, infectious and inflammatory CNS disease is often characterized by pleocytosis with increased protein concentration. A mononuclear pleocytosis is one of the more common cytologic patterns of inflammatory CSF, with an increase in lymphoid cells and/or monocytoid cells/macrophages. Because lymphocytes and monocytoid cells are the expected inhabitants of large animal CSF in health, diagnosing a mononuclear/lymphocytic pleocytosis requires an increased TNCC, even if the differential percentages and morphology of cells are normal.[23] Lymphocytes may vary in size from typical small "mature" lymphocytes with scant cytoplasm, a high nucleus to cytoplasm ratio and condensed chromatin, to a mix of intermediate and large lymphocytes that may appear "activated" or "reactive" with increased basophilic cytoplasm and looser chromatin. Small lymphocytes should predominate in nonneoplastic conditions.

Subacute to chronic infections classically result in a mononuclear pleocytosis and are reported in association with *Listeria* spp., *Micronema deletrix*, *Borrelia burgdorferi*, WNV, and many other viral encephalitides.[23,27–29,31] Figure 49.1 illustrates a marked mononuclear pleocytosis in a sheep suspected of having caprine arthritis encephalitis virus (CAEV). Equine protozoal myeloencephalitis (EPM) due to *Sarcocystis neurona* (or less commonly, *Neospora hughesi*) can present with a mononuclear pleocytosis, but CSF TNCC and cytologic findings are inconsistent, necessitating other tools to diagnose this common infection (see section "Ancillary Testing").[32] Immune-mediated conditions such as polyneuritis equi can be associated with a mononuclear pleocytosis (particularly lymphocyte-predominant).[33] However, mononuclear pleocytosis is not specific for infectious/inflammatory disease and can occur with a variety of causes of CNS pathology, particularly if there is chronic damage to neural tissue.

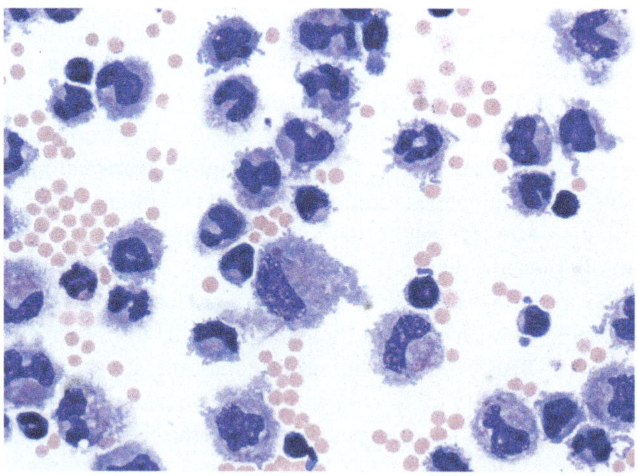

Figure 49.1 CSF from a sheep. The CSF is highly cellular with a TNCC of 363/μL and increased protein of 100.4 mg/dL. There are abundant monocytoid cells and macrophages, comprising 67% of counted cells. There are fewer small lymphocytes and rare non-degenerate neutrophils. Necropsy revealed necrotizing, nonsuppurative leukoencephalitis/leukomyelitis most consistent with lentiviral infection such as CAEV (modified Wright stain, 500×).

Neutrophilic Pleocytosis

Neutrophils are not typically found in large animal CSF in significant numbers, and an increase suggests pathology.[23] Many bacterial illnesses present with marked neutrophilic pleocytosis. A retrospective case series of horses with meningitis or meningoencephalomyelitis found that the median TNCC was 1224/μL with a median neutrophil percentage of 87%.[34] In that study, 65% of cases had degenerate neutrophils on cytology, and 36.4% of CSF samples had visible bacteria.[34] In a retrospective study of 102 cattle, the highest CSF TNCC and neutrophil percentage occurred with neonatal meningitis, with a median TNCC of 2900/μL and median neutrophil percentage of 84%.[27] Older cattle with meningitis, thromboembolic meningoencephalitis, or abscessation had neutrophilic pleocytoses but overall lower median TNCC and a wider range of neutrophil percentage than neonatal meningitis.[27] There are few exceptions to the paradigm of the close association between neutrophilic pleocytosis and bacterial infection, including viral illnesses like eastern equine encephalitis (EEE) and Venezuelan equine encephalitis (VEE), which often present as a mild to moderate neutrophilic pleocytosis, especially early in the disease course (Figure 49.2). Fungal infection with *Cryptococcus* spp. is associated with neutrophilic pleocytosis.[34]

Some infectious agents that are typically thought to result in mononuclear or lymphocyte-predominant pleocytosis, such as Lyme disease, may sometimes present with a neutrophilic or lymphocytic pleocytosis.[29] Additionally, while neurolisteriosis is often considered to exclusively manifest as a mononuclear or mixed pleocytosis in horses and ruminants, in the author's experience, it may on rare occasion present with marked neutrophilic pleocytosis (unpublished observation).[19,35] As such, CSF patterns should be used to support diagnosis, not to definitively exclude differentials.

Eosinophilic Pleocytosis

Eosinophilic pleocytosis in equids and ruminants is typically associated with CNS parasitic infestation. One retrospective study of 20 camelids with CNS nematodiasis found that 95% had increased CSF eosinophils (mean 62% eosinophils) and 90% had increased TNCC (median 21/μL); 90% of cases also had increased CSF RBC and microprotein concentrations.[36] Anecdotally, an eosinophilic pleocytosis is occasionally reported with other infectious diseases, such as fungal or protozoal infections. Figure 49.3 shows CSF from a goat with presumptive meningeal worm infestation. Finally, lack of CSF eosinophilia should not exclude the possibility of CNS parasitism, as *Halicephalobus gingivalis* migration through CNS in a horse was associated with a neutrophilic and lymphocytic pleocytosis.[37] A second report of *H. gingivalis* migration exhibited a monocytoid pleocytosis with rhabditiform nematodes observed in the CSF of that horse.[38]

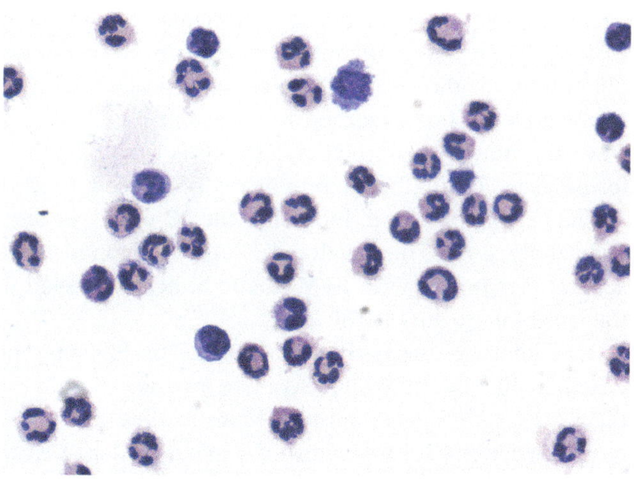

Figure 49.2 CSF from a horse. There is a neutrophilic pleocytosis, with a TNCC of 112/μL, approximately 80% neutrophils, and increased protein of 138.1 mg/dL. Note the non-degenerate morphology of the neutrophils. No infectious organisms are observed. Eastern equine encephalitis (EEE) was confirmed based on positive EEE PCR on brain and spinal cord tissue at necropsy. PCR for equine herpesvirus 1 and 4 and West Nile virus were negative, as was rabies virus by indirect fluorescent antibody (modified Wright stain, 500×).

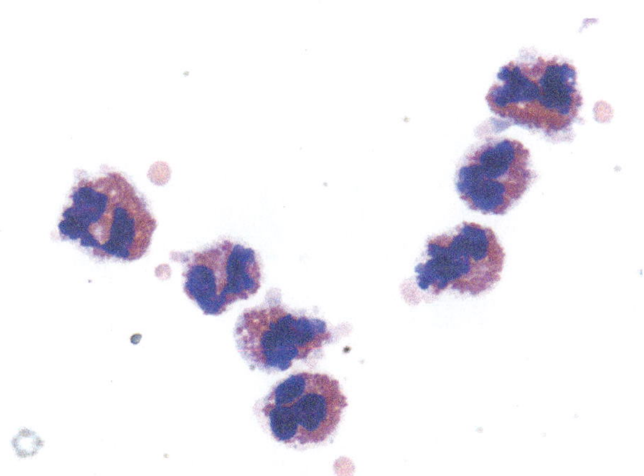

Figure 49.3 CSF from a goat. Marked eosinophilic inflammation is present with a TNCC of 250/μL, protein of 213.1 mg/dL, and approximately 75% eosinophils. Note the rounded to rod-shaped granules that stain burnt orange, typical of ruminant eosinophils. The clinical diagnosis based on neurologic exam, CSF findings, and clinical outcome was CNS nematodiasis, likely due to *Parelaphostrongylus tenuis* (modified Wright stain, 1000×).

Neoplastic Pleocytosis

CNS neoplasia may only result in xanthochromia and/or albuminocytologic dissociation. Neoplastic cells often do not exfoliate into CSF, especially if the mass is extradural or intradural extramedullary. An exception is CNS lymphoma, particularly in bovine patients.[27] Bovine lymphoma is characterized by a variably severe lymphocytic pleocytosis.[27] On occasion, CSF from these cattle include intermediate to large lymphocytes with increased basophilic cytoplasm and pleomorphic nuclei that are often indented, cleaved, or floriform in shape, 12–20 μm in diameter, with dispersed chromatin and variably visible nucleoli (Figure 49.4). Mitotic figures and cytoplasmic fragments (lymphoglandular bodies) may be observed. Unlike small companion animals, other forms of neoplasia are rarely visualized in the CSF of large animal species.

Detection of Etiologic Agents

Various infectious organisms can be visualized on CSF cytology and can provide a preliminary diagnosis, such as "bacterial sepsis" requiring further speciation by culture or PCR, or a definitive diagnosis for characteristic organisms such as *Cryptococcus neoformans*, *Trypanosoma evansi*, and *H. gingivalis*.[34,36,38,39] The diagnostic sensitivity for

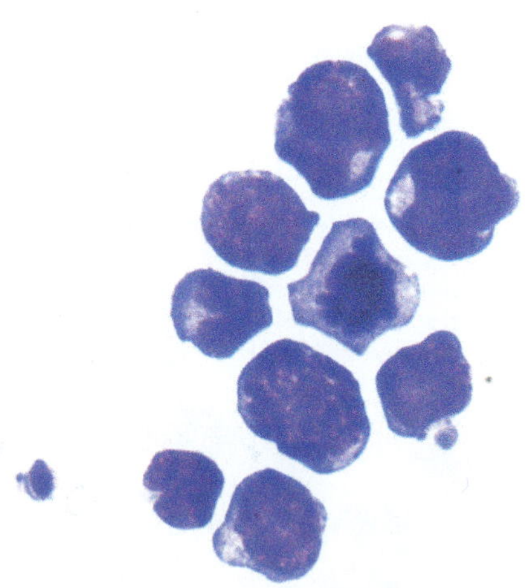

Figure 49.4 CSF from a cow. The TNCC is mildly increased at 36/μL, with a mild increase in protein of 60.9 mg/dL. Seventy-seven percent of the cells are intermediate to large neoplastic lymphocytes. These lymphocytes have scant, deep-blue cytoplasm, pleomorphic nuclei that are sometimes indented or convoluted, and fine chromatin with variably visible nucleoli. A single mitotic figure is visible (center). At necropsy, the spinal cord, heart, omasum, abomasum, left kidney, and multiple lymph nodes were effaced by neoplastic lymphocytes that were immunoreactive to PAX5 but not CD3. The final diagnosis was multicentric B-cell lymphoma (enzootic bovine lymphoma) (modified Wright stain, 1000×).

detection of bacteria in equine CSF ranged from 36.5 to 66.7% in two small studies of meningitis/meningoencephalitis.[34,40] One study in cattle found that the sensitivity of cytology for detecting bacteria ranged from 2/11 (18%) in neonatal meningitis to 3/4 (75%) in older cows with meningitis.[27] Cytologic detection of organisms is useful, because they may be identified even in cases where the CSF cultures are negative.[34]

Ancillary Testing

Infectious Disease Testing

Ancillary testing such as bacterial culture, PCR, and antibody titers can corroborate or confirm the etiologic agent in cases where other CSF findings are merely suggestive of infection. In particular, bacterial culture can provide a specific genus and potentially an organism species/subspecies, along with antimicrobial susceptibility. As such, CSF culture is recommended whenever bacteria are identified or suspected based on cytology. However, not all cases with sepsis will yield a positive culture, as one study in horses found a higher percentage of cases with bacteria visible on cytology (36.5%) than had a positive antemortem CSF bacterial culture (17.4%).[34]

CSF titers can be useful to support a diagnosis of certain infections such as EPM and others. There are a variety of methodologies, including enzyme-linked immunosorbent assay (ELISA) and indirect fluorescent antibody test (IFAT), and their diagnostic performance may vary. Unfortunately, some organisms, such as *S. neurona*, are ubiquitous, leading to high rates of exposure, with as many as 89% of horses seropositive in some populations.[32] One way around this problem is the use of mathematical formulas to correct for the proportion of antibody in CSF versus peripheral blood, including the "C-value" or antibody index (AI). The C-value and AI were found to be accurate for horses with EPM due to *S. neurona*, even in the face of up to 10 000 RBC/μL.[41]

Depending on the pathogen, IgG and/or IgM may be tested. Unlike IgG, IgM should not be produced within the thecal space, and detection of IgM antibodies in the CSF indicates active CNS infection for a given pathogen, such as with M-capture ELISA for WNV.[28]

Western blot (WB) for antigens from organisms such as *N. hughesi* can also be performed on CSF, though the utility of WB in EPM has been questioned based on data that suggests it may lead to overdiagnosis.[32]

PCR assays exist for a number of relevant pathogens, including EHV-1, *N. hughesi*, *S. neurona*, and *B. burgdorferi*.[29,42] A positive PCR in a protected fluid such as CSF is thought to be more specific than antibody titers; however, some PCR assays have low sensitivity.[42] Quantitative or "real-time" PCR allows absolute determination of infectious load in the sample and may minimize the risk of false-positives from transferring amplification products to gel electrophoresis like conventional end-point PCR.[42] Additional factors to consider for PCR include false-negative results due to antimicrobial therapy or inappropriate sample handling.

CSF Electrolytes, Enzymes, and Other Analytes

Various enzymes, electrolytes, and other parameters can be measured in CSF. Decreased CSF glucose concentration has been associated with meningitis in horses.[34] Glucose can be decreased due the presence of bacteria or neutrophils alone. In that study, one horse also had decreased CSF pH and increased lactate, suggesting CNS lactic acidosis within the thecal space due to sepsis.[34] However, CSF glucose should be interpreted in light of age, as it decreases from parturition to 42 days of age.[43]

Aspartate aminotransferase (AST) and creatine kinase (CK) have been measured in CSF of large animal species. Activity for both of these should theoretically be low or absent in normal CSF. Furthermore, the CK-BB isoform is thought to be specific for neurons and can increase with a variety of CNS pathologies, particularly EPM.[44] Unfortunately, artefactual increases in CK are associated with sampling dural/epidural tissue, greatly limiting the diagnostic utility of this enzyme.[45] Lactate dehydrogenase (LDH) enzyme activity and isoform electrophoresis has been shown to differentiate causes of meningitis and CNS neoplasia in people, and the magnitude of enzyme activity may be of prognostic value.[46] LDH enzyme activity has been measured in large animal CSF and normal reference ranges determined for horses, cattle, and llamas, but to the authors' knowledge, there are no published studies demonstrating clinical value.[2–4,14]

CSF is a sequestered and immune-privileged biofluid. As such, residues for metabolites and CNS toxins can occasionally be detected in CSF, even after clearance or degradation in peripheral circulation or tissues. This was demonstrated when a horse suspected of succumbing to idiopathic hyperammonemia was able to be confirmed by elevated CSF levels of ammonia 10 hours after death, long after blood and tissue levels were unsuitable for analysis.[47]

References

1 de Lahunta, A. and Glass, E. (eds.) (2009). Cerebrospinal fluid and hydrocephalus. In: *Veterinary Neuroanatomy and Clinical Neurology*, 3e, 54–65. St. Louis: Elsevier Saunders.

2 Welles, E.G., Tyler, J.W., Sorjonen, D.C., and Whatley, E.M. (1992). Composition and analysis of cerebrospinal fluid in clinically normal adult cattle. *Am J Vet Res* 53: 2050–2057.

3 Welles, E.G., Pugh, D.G., Wenzel, J.G.W., and Sorjonen, D.C. (1994). Composition of cerebrospinal fluid in healthy adult llamas. *Am J Vet Res* 55: 1075–1079.

4 Mayhew, I.G., Whitlock, R.H., and Tasker, J.B. (1977). Equine cerebrospinal fluid: reference values of normal horses. *Am J Vet Res* 38: 1271–1274.

5 Lorenz, M.D., Coates, J.R., and Kent, M. (eds.) (2011). Confirming a diagnosis. In: *Handbook of Veterinary Neurology*, 5e, 81–85. St. Louis: Elsevier Saunders.

6 Johnson, P.J. and Constantinescu, G.M. (2000). Collection of cerebrospinal fluid in horses. *Equine Vet Educ* 12: 7–12.

7 Goehring, L.S., Kessels, B.G.F., Maanen, C. et al. (2006). Evaluation of nephelometry for albumin measurement in serum and cerebrospinal fluid: experiences with an indwelling subarachnoidal catheter system for repetitive cerebrospinal fluid collection in horses. *J Vet Diagn Invest* 18: 251–256.

8 Pease, A., Behan, A., and Bohart, G. (2012). Ultrasound-guided cervical centesis to obtain cerebrospinal fluid in the standing horses. *Vet Radiol* 53: 92–95.

9 Sweeney, C.R. and Russell, G.E. (2000). Differences in total protein concentration, nucleated cell count, and red blood cell count among sequential samples of cerebrospinal fluid from horses. *J Am Vet Med Assoc* 217: 54–57.

10 Fry, M.M., Vernau, W., Kass, P.H., and Vernau, K.M. (2006). Effects of time, initial composition, and stabilizing agents on the results of canine cerebrospinal fluid analysis. *Vet Clin Pathol* 35: 72–77.

11 Bellino, C., Miniscalco, B., Bertone, I. et al. (2015). Analysis of cerebrospinal fluid from cattle with central nervous system disorders after storage for 24 hours with autologous serum. *BMC Vet Res* 11: 201.

12 D'Angelo, A., Miniscalco, B., Bellino, C. et al. (2009). Analysis of cerebrospinal fluid from 20 calves after storage for 24 hours. *Vet Rec* 164: 491–493.

13 Siegel, A. and Walton, R.M. (2014). Cerebrospinal fluid. In: *Equine Clinical Pathology*, 1e (ed. R.M. Walton), 253–269. Ames: Wiley.

14 Mayhew, I.G. (ed.) (2009). Ancillary diagnostic aids. In: *Large Animal Neurology*, 2e, 47–52. Chichester: Wiley.

15 Johnson, P.J. and Constantinescu, G.M. (2000). Analysis of cerebrospinal fluid in horses. *Equine Vet Educ* 12: 13–17.
16 Marshall, T. and Williams, K.M. (2000). Protein determination in cerebrospinal fluid by protein dye-binding assay. *Br J Biomed Sci* 57: 281–286.
17 Di Terlizzi, R. and Platt, S.R. (2009). The function, composition and analysis of cerebrospinal fluid in companion animals: Part II – Analysis. *Vet J* 180: 15–32.
18 Andrews, F.M., Geiser, D.R., Sommardahl, C.S. et al. (1994). Albumin quotient, IgG concentration, and IgG index determinations in cerebrospinal fluid of neonatal foals. *Am J Vet Res* 55: 741–745.
19 Goehring, L.S., van Maanen, C., Berendsen, M. et al. (2010). Experimental infection with neuropathogenic equid herpesvirus type 1 (EHV-1) in adult horses. *Vet J* 186: 180–187.
20 Becker, M., Bauer, N., and Moritz, A. (2008). Automated flow cytometric cell count and differentiation of canine cerebrospinal fluid cells using the ADVIA 2120. *Vet Clin Pathol* 37: 344–352.
21 Ruotsalo, K., Poma, R., Costa, R.C., and Bienzle, D. (2008). Evaluation of the ADVIA 120 for analysis of canine cerebrospinal fluid. *Vet Clin Pathol* 37: 242–248.
22 Marcos, R., Santos, M., Marrinhas, C. et al. (2016). Cytocentrifuge preparation in veterinary cytology: a quick, simple, and affordable manual method to concentrate low cellularity fluids. *Vet Clin Pathol* 45: 725–731.
23 Beech, J. (1983). Cytology of equine cerebrospinal fluid. *Vet Pathol* 20: 553–562.
24 Garma-Avina, A. (2004). Cytology of the normal and abnormal choroid plexi in selected domestic mammals, wildlife species, and man. *J Vet Diagn Invest* 16: 283–292.
25 Zabolotzky, S.M., Vernau, K.M., Kass, P.H., and Vernau, W. (2010). Prevalence and significance of extracellular myelin-like material in canine cerebrospinal fluid. *Vet Clin Pathol* 39: 90–95.
26 Wilson, J.W. and Stevens, J.B. (1977). Effects of blood contamination on cerebrospinal fluid analysis. *J Am Vet Med Assoc* 171: 256–258.
27 Stokol, T., Divers, T.J., Arrigan, J.W., and McDonough, S.P. (2009). Cerebrospinal fluid findings in cattle with central nervous system disorders: a retrospective study of 102 cases (1990–2008). *Vet Clin Pathol* 38: 103–112.
28 Wamsley, H.L., Alleman, A.R., Porter, M.B., and Long, M.T. (2002). Findings in cerebrospinal fluids of horses infected with West Nile virus: 30 cases (2001). *J Am Vet Med Assoc* 221: 1303–1305.
29 Johnstone, L.K., Engiles, J.B., Aceto, H. et al. (2016). Retrospective evaluation of horses diagnosed with neuroborreliosis on postmortem examination: 16 cases (2004–2015). *J Vet Intern Med* 30: 1305–1312.
30 Achard, D., Francoz, D., Grimes, C. et al. (2017). Cerebrospinal fluid analysis in recumbent adult dairy cows with or without spinal cord lesions. *J Vet Intern Med* 31: 940–945.
31 Darien, B.J., Belknap, J., and Nietfeld, J. (1988). Cerebrospinal fluid changes in two horses with central nervous system nematodiasis (*Micronema deletrix*). *J Vet Intern Med* 2: 201–205.
32 Reed, S.M., Furr, M., Howe, D.K. et al. (2016). Equine protozoal myeloencephalitis: an updated consensus statement with a focus on parasite biology, diagnosis, treatment, and prevention. *J Vet Intern Med* 30: 491–502.
33 Aleman, M., Katzman, S.A., Vaughn, B. et al. (2009). Antemortem diagnosis of polyneuritis equi. *J Vet Intern Med* 23: 665–668.
34 Toth, B., Aleman, M., Nogradi, N., and Madigan, J.E. (2012). Meningitis and meningoencephalomyelitis in horses: 28 cases (1985–2010). *J Am Vet Med Assoc* 240: 580–587.
35 Schweizer, G., Ehrensperger, F., Torgerson, P., and Braun, U. (2006). Clinical findings and treatment of 94 cattle presumptively diagnosed with listeriosis. *Vet Rec* 158: 588–592.
36 Bertin, F.R. and Taylor, S.D. (2016). Cerebrospinal nematodiasis in 20 camelids. *J Vet Intern Med* 30: 1390–1395.
37 Adedeji, A.O., Borjesson, D.L., Kozikowski-Nicholas, T.A. et al. (2015). What is your diagnosis? Cerebrospinal fluid from a horse. *Vet Clin Pathol* 44: 171–172.
38 Lepri, E., Beccati, F., Miglio, A. et al. (2017). Pathology in practice. *J Am Vet Med Assoc* 251: 1153–1156.
39 Berlin, D., Loeb, E., and Baneth, G. (2009). Disseminated central nervous system disease caused by *Trypanosoma evansi* in a horse. *Vet Parasitol* 161: 316–319.
40 Viu, J., Monreal, L., Jose-Cunilleras, E. et al. (2012). Clinical findings in 10 foals with bacterial meningoencephalitis. *Equine Vet J* 44: 100–104.
41 Furr, M., Howe, D., Reed, S., and Yeargan, M. (2011). Antibody coefficients for the diagnosis of equine protozoal myeloencephalitis. *J Vet Intern Med* 25: 138–142.
42 Pusterla, N., Madigan, J.E., and Leutenegger, C.M. (2006). Real-time polymerase chain reaction: a novel molecular diagnostic tool for equine infectious diseases. *J Vet Intern Med* 20: 3–12.

43 Furr, M.O. and Bender, H. (1994). Cerebrospinal fluid variables in clinically normal foals from birth to 42 days of age. *Am J Vet Res* 55: 781–789.

44 Furr, M.O. and Tyler, R.D. (1990). Cerebrospinal fluid creatine kinase activity in horses with central nervous system disease: 69 cases (1984–1989). *J Am Vet Med Assoc* 197: 245–248.

45 Jackson, C., de Lahunta, A., Divers, T., and Ainsworth, D. (1996). The diagnostic utility of cerebrospinal fluid creatine kinase activity in the horse. *J Vet Intern Med* 10: 246–251.

46 Houle, J.C., Chen, A.V., Brenna, A.C. et al. (2015). Determination of optimal storage temperature and duration for analysis of total and isoenzyme lactate dehydrogenase activities in canine serum and cerebrospinal fluid. *Vet Clin Pathol* 44: 253–261.

47 Gilliam, L.L., Holbrook, T.C., Dechant, J.E., and Johnson, B.J. (2007). Postmortem diagnosis of idiopathic hyperammonemia in a horse. *Vet Clin Pathol* 36: 196–199.

Part XIV

Fluid Analysis

50

Laboratory Techniques for Fluid Analysis

Linda M. Vap and Wendy S. Sprague

Fluid Analysis Overview

In most healthy animals, serous fluid is present in abdominal, pleural, pericardial, and synovial spaces in sufficient amounts to provide nourishment and lubrication of serosal surfaces. In small animals, this fluid is usually present in limited amounts.[1,2] Horses can have as much as 300 mL of peritoneal fluid in health.[3] Serous fluid is colorless to straw-colored and clear with low cell numbers and protein concentration. Fluid analysis should be performed when an effusion or abnormal fluid accumulation is seen. A basic fluid analysis includes (i) gross appearance of fluid and supernatant, (ii) total nucleated cell count (TNCC), (iii) protein concentration, (iv) differential cell count, and (v) microscopic examination for microorganisms, crystals, and foreign or plant material. Taking into account clinical signs and fluid volume, results from a basic fluid analysis can often identify an underlying etiology for an effusion. Indeed, a rule-based expert system using the C Language Integrated Production System programming language correctly classified 485/508 (95.5%) cavity fluids from animals based on non-microscopic data alone.[4] Synovial and pericardial fluids are often uniquely viscous and hemorrhagic, respectively, requiring slight modifications to testing protocols. Results obtained from basic fluid analyses with ancillary tests, if indicated, can guide the clinician in the identification of underlying etiologies, which will ultimately result in appropriate diagnostic and/or therapeutic decisions. These tests, their utility, availability, and validity are described. Collection techniques are discussed in other chapters, whereas appropriate sample handling and analysis are described here.

Pathophysiology

Serosal cavities include pleural, pericardial, and peritoneal cavities. Parietal walls and organ surfaces within these cavities are covered with a serous membrane consisting of connective tissue and an outer layer of mesothelial cells known as the mesothelium. The mesothelium is composed of flat, cuboidal to squamous cells (approximately 25 μm in diameter) and occurs as a monolayer that is both protective and dynamic. Adjacent cell borders overlap and the luminal surfaces have microvilli.[5] These cells are actively involved in fluid transport, inflammation, coagulation, fibrinolysis, leukocyte migration, antigen presentation, and serosal repair.[6] The mesothelium produces many cytokines, chemokines, and growth factors that promote healing and stimulate or inhibit inflammation in response to a variety of insults.[5–8] It also produces glycosaminoglycans and surfactant (phosphatidylcholine) that facilitate movement between adjacent visceral and parietal surfaces.[7] Healthy mesothelium is thought to protect against tumor implantation by secreting hyaluronan. However, if injured, mesothelial cells likely enhance tumor growth and allow metastasis through intercellular stomata.[5]

Visceral fluid circulation is a balanced process. Fluid leaves tissue capillaries to enter the interstitium, and the fluid is then resorbed from the interstitium by visceral lymphatics. There are differences in how fluid circulates within cavity spaces. For example, peritoneal fluid arises from systemic capillaries. It then crosses parietal mesothelium into peritoneal cavity where it is subsequently resorbed by parietal lymphatics through the parietal mesothelium. The lymphatic pump maintains a small negative pressure within the cavity space. In joint spaces, fluid balance is maintained between synovial capillaries, interstitium (synovial membranes) and subsynovial lymphatics.[2] Fluid passes in either direction through synovial membranes via small fenestrations. Hyaluronan and lubricin, along with lipids and other molecules, minimize friction and wear and tear between joint surfaces. Hyaluronan is a glycosaminoglycan produced by the synovial membrane that contributes to synovial fluid viscosity and ultimately to

Veterinary Cytology, First Edition. Edited by Leslie C. Sharkey, M. Judith Radin, and Davis Seelig.

the challenges associated with *in vitro* testing. Lubricin is a glycoprotein (proteoglycan 4) that provides lubrication and is produced by chondrocytes and lining cells.[9]

An effusion is the accumulation of excess fluid resulting from an imbalance between the amount of fluid that exudes from capillaries and the amount resorbed by lymphatic vessels. Pleural effusions can compress the lungs and impair breathing, whereas peritoneal effusions can induce vomiting, anorexia, and abdominal discomfort; impair diaphragmatic movement; and result in a pendulous abdomen. Pericardial effusions can induce lethargy, fainting, weakness, difficulty breathing, shock, vomiting, and anorexia. Synovial effusions generate joint pain, swelling, and lameness.

Normal pleural and peritoneal fluids are transudates. Transudates are clear, are straw-colored, and contain little protein and few cells. Since a transudate is an ultrafiltrate of plasma, transudates contain concentrations of electrolytes (sodium, potassium, chloride, bicarbonate, calcium, and phosphates) and small molecules (glucose, urea, and creatinine) that are similar to plasma.[3,10] Published reference intervals and interpretive limits for TNCCs, protein content, and cell differentials vary somewhat between species, sample sources, and studies. Mononuclear cells comprise the majority of cells present in a transudate, and these include macrophages, lymphocytes, and occasional mesothelial cells. In small animals, the predominant cell types are mononuclear cells; however, in healthy horses, peritoneal fluid can contain up to 60% neutrophils.[11]

The general pathologic processes that underlay the development of effusions include increased hydrostatic pressure, increased capillary permeability, lymphatic obstruction, and decreased colloidal osmotic pressure. Depending on the underlying pathology, color, clarity, protein concentration, cellularity, and cell differentials can be altered.

Several effusion classification schemes are used in practice.[12,13] All schemes include at least two broad effusion categories: transudates and exudates. Transudates are often further classified according to protein content, with low protein indicating a transudate and high protein considered by some to be a modified transudate. Low-protein transudates have a total protein concentration <2.5 g/dL and a TNCC <1–3000/μL in small animals[12,13] or up to 5000/μL in horses.[14,15] Mean TNCC (2900/μL) and total protein (1.9 g/dL) in apparently healthy periparturient cattle fall into this category.[16] The cells and proteins typically accumulate due to an increase in hydrostatic pressure and/or decreased oncotic pressure within vessels. Causes of increased hydrostatic pressure include congestive heart failure, myocardial degeneration, cardiac hypertrophy, and thrombus formation in the pulmonary vasculature, left auricle of the heart, or distal aorta.[17] Other causes include lymphatic flow blockage secondary to neoplasia involving the anterior mediastinum, thymus, and parietal pleura. Decreased oncotic pressure secondary to severe hypoalbuminemia is caused by cirrhosis, protein-losing enteropathy, nephrotic syndrome, and other etiologies.[12,17]

High-protein transudates are commonly associated with right-sided heart failure and neoplasia[12] as well as caudal vena cava constrictions, gastrointestinal foreign bodies, sterile enteritidis, uroabdomen, splenic venous thromboses, and lymphangiectasia.[18,19] In small animals, the protein concentration is ≥2.5 g/dL with a TNCC < 3–5000/μL, whereas in horses, the protein is similar to small animals, but the TNCC may be as high as 10 000 cells/μL.[14,15] Mean TNCC and total protein in apparently healthy non-periparturient cattle are 12 200/μL and 2.94 g/dL, respectively.[16]

Exudates arise from leaky capillaries during septic or non-septic inflammatory processes and have high-protein concentrations (>3.0 g/dL) and increased TNCC (>3–5000/μL in small animals or >10 000/μL in horses). Differentials for non-septic inflammation include feline infectious peritonitis (FIP), bilious effusion, neoplastic effusion, postoperative irritation, pancreatitis, gastrointestinal foreign body, splenic hematoma with necrosis, lymphangiectasia, uroabdomen, and idiopathic causes. Coagulopathy or trauma can result in hemorrhagic fluid that could occur simultaneously with any of the above conditions.

Utility of Imaging

As several imaging options are available to detect fluid accumulation, deciding which modality to use often depends on the underlying etiology and the effusion location. Ultrasonography is more useful than radiology to examine small volume effusions in large animals, whereas radiography is better for evaluating deep lung lesions.[20] Ultrasonography is also useful for examining pericardial and synovial effusions.[21,22] Computed tomography can be used to assess pericardial effusions,[23] can distinguish pleural effusions from thoracic masses,[24] and can detect migrating grass awns in dogs.[25]

Quality Assurance

Sources of error are commonly categorized into pre-analytical, analytical, and post-analytical testing phases. Pre-analytical procedures involve patient preparation, and sample collection, labeling, and handling. The analytical phase includes the actual testing process, which can involve automated or manual methodologies. The post-analytical testing phase is associated with accuracy of reporting or interpretation of results and is not included in this discussion.

Hiring staff committed to establishing and following a good quality assurance plan reduces error rates. The staff that performs fluid analyses should be familiar with the basic recommendations for instrument operation, be experienced in microscopic evaluation of the sample types in question, and have managerial support to ensure maintenance of a quality assurance program, which includes continuing education about fluid analysis.[26]

Instruments and microscopes should have a maintenance schedule. Instrument performance for fluid analyses should be monitored with sufficient documentation. When problems arise, troubleshooting, corrective actions, and outcomes are described and documented. Pertinent comments should be included in discussions on each specific test.

Standard Operating Procedures (SOP)

Samples submitted for complete fluid analysis arise from a variety of sources (pericardial, pleural, peritoneal, and synovial spaces) and involve similar but not necessarily identical processing. To maintain an appropriate level of consistency and quality, each clinic should have an SOP for fluid analysis in place that addresses most scenarios.[27] At a minimum, the SOP should include appropriate and safe sample collection and handling, standard testing procedures, reference intervals for each species routinely examined, and information on how to report results. When, where, and how to submit samples for further diagnostics or a pathologist's review should be included. Testing procedures include stepwise instructions for each method, including how to make, store, and check the reagent quality, operate equipment, and perform techniques. The following information outlines procedural guidelines for basic fluid analysis. If there is not enough sample to perform a full evaluation, test order prioritization is warranted. In most cases, assessment of color and clarity, direct film preparation, and protein estimation are minimum recommendations. Based on sensitivity, specificity, positive predictive value (PPV), and negative predictive value (NPV), abnormal abdominal fluid color (described as anything other than yellow and transparent), protein concentration, or fluid classification (transudate, modified transudate, or exudate) distinguish surgical from medical cases better than TNCCs in horses with colic.[28]

Basic Equipment and Supplies

Fluid analysis requires minimal additional costs and time investments beyond the staff and equipment costs associated with performing common hematology and biochemistry techniques. Basic equipment needed to assess fluids includes a hemocytometer or automated cell counter to perform a TNCC, a refractometer or in-house chemistry analyzer to obtain protein concentration, microscope slides, a microscope, and a Romanowsky-type stain (quick stains) to assess direct fluid or concentrated fluid films for cells, infectious agents, and foreign material. Concentrating fluid requires a centrifuge and, if possible, a cytocentrifuge. Hyaluronidase is used to counteract viscosity when obtaining cell counts from synovial fluids.[29,30] A mechanism to report and record data using manual reports or laboratory information systems also is needed. Finally, if in-house testing will not be performed, films for microscopic evaluation should be prepared with direct and, if necessary, concentrated fluid. Any pertinent history or data obtained should be included with the fluid and films to support the overall fluid analysis and pathologist's interpretation.

Biosafety

When working in laboratories, standard personnel safety protocols should be established and followed. Since samples might contain zoonotic organisms, testing sites should at least follow Biosafety Level-1 protocol recommendations.[31] These include but are not limited to (i) wearing appropriate personal protective equipment including gloves, eyewear, and laboratory coats; (ii) washing hands thoroughly and frequently; (iii) using appropriate sharps containers for breakable glass containers, slides, pipets, and other items; (iv) prohibiting food and drink in sample collection, preparation, storage, and testing areas; and (v) regular cleaning and decontamination of work surfaces. If there is a high suspicion that samples contain a zoonotic organism, additional protective steps should be taken that include limiting access of unprotected individuals and banning the recapping of needles. In addition, local regulations could require disposal of liquid blood products and contaminated materials in biohazard containers destined for autoclaving.

Pre-Analytical Considerations

Sample Containers

Selection of containers for fluid samples, similar to peripheral blood, varies with the desired testing procedure. Fluid samples for cytologic evaluation should be placed in containers with ethylenediaminetetraacetic acid (EDTA) to preserve the integrity of cellular components, to prevent clot formation, and to test for select biochemical analytes such as glucose or total protein.[32] The tube size should be appropriate for the amount of fluid obtained, and the tube should be at least half-full to avoid falsely high-protein estimates using refractometry, which are caused by excessive EDTA.[33,34] Documenting submitted sample volumes as a fraction of the fluid placed in the collection tube to the overall tube capacity, and type is helpful additional information (e.g. 2.5 mL/5 mL EDTA). This documentation allows tracking of pre-analytical sample collection conditions that could affect result quality, such as underfilled tubes. If sufficient sample volumes of the appropriate type remain after the first tests are completed, additional testing can be performed.

EDTA preserves TNCCs in blood for 24 hours under refrigeration[35] and in synovial fluid for up to 48 hours under refrigeration or at room temperature.[36] Using overnight shipping and avoiding weekends or holidays that might prohibit immediate sample processing by the receiving laboratory helps maintain sample integrity and maximizes the quality of results.

Although EDTA is the preferred anticoagulant for cytological evaluation, cell morphology is only preserved for 6–24 hours, and therefore, films should be prepared as soon as possible after collection.[37,38] Changes due to *in vitro* cellular aging during transport that can affect interpretation are similar to those observed in blood samples and include apoptosis, fragmentation, lysis, and pyknosis.[32] Sample pH, protein content, enzymatic activity, and the presence of bacteria affect the speed over which *in vitro* changes are generated.[39]

Additive-free or heparin tubes might be preferred for biochemical or other testing by the receiving laboratory.[40,41] Serum separator tubes containing gel should not be used as the material in these tubes interferes with biochemical testing.[42] Clotted samples, indicative of blood contamination, are unsuitable for both TNCC and film preparations, but the supernatants can be used for biochemical testing.

Sample collection in heparin tubes prevents clotting and allows for the determination of synovial fluid cell concentrations and mucin clot formation; however, cell morphology is not preserved as with EDTA.[36,38,43,44] Therefore, samples collected in heparin should be processed, and films should be prepared as soon after collection as possible. EDTA inhibits bacterial growth[45] and reduces the strength of mucin clot formation and, therefore, should not be used for culture or the mucin clot test (SE Bush, personal communication, 28 December 2017). For culture, additional fluid should be placed in transport media or a sterile collection tube.

Film Preparation and Staining

Since preservation of cell morphology by EDTA is time-limited, at least two direct films and two concentrated films (if applicable) should be prepared from the native, mixed sample as soon after collection as possible. Smears can be made directly from the needle and syringe or from a well-mixed, non-clotted sample tube (Figure 50.1). With samples that are clear to slightly hazy and are likely to have low cellularity, concentrated samples also should be prepared. Films should be thoroughly air-dried prior to staining or transport to a reference laboratory. The slide(s) should be labeled with the patient identification, sample source, collection date, and whether the film was made from a direct or concentrated sample.[27]

Whether samples are evaluated in-house or shipped to a pathologist for review, one direct or one concentrated sample (or both, depending on cellularity) should be stained and evaluated in-house by qualified staff for quality and to ensure sufficient intact cells are present. The pull or squash technique is used for viscous samples without centrifugation or for sedimented specimens (Figure 50.1). Microscopic evaluation of appropriately made direct films is necessary for estimating cellularity and confirming automated cell counts; however, TNCCs

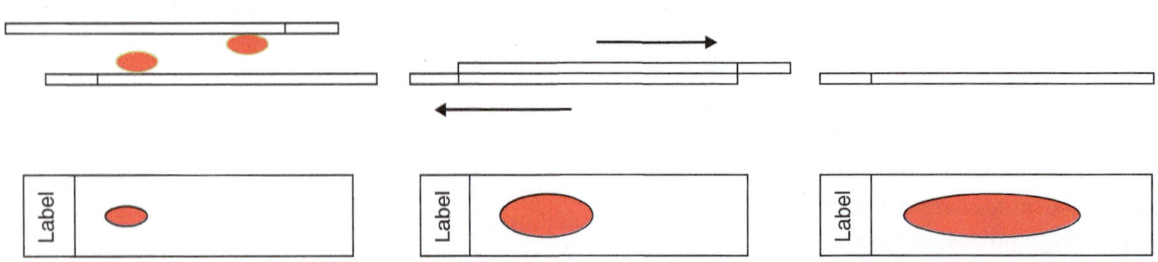

Figure 50.1 Pull/squash film preparation. To make two pull films at once, a drop of thoroughly mixed fluid is applied on each of two clean glass slides near the label end. Hover the slides over each other with sample drops to the inside and labels to opposite ends. Gently lay the top slide onto the bottom slide and allow the material to spread slightly. The slides are quickly pulled apart in parallel but opposite directions. A "squash prep" of flocculent material is made by applying pressure as needed during the spreading phase to obtain a monolayer of cells.

can be overestimated by visual examination.[46] Squash preparations made directly from flocculent material remaining in the sample, such as gut contents, cell aggregates, or organisms, also should be prepared and microscopically examined. Dragging the sample off the end of the slide is a common sequela of films made from large drops of nonviscous fluid. This can result in loss of cells and debris and can adversely impact accurate assessment of cellularity. Broken cells with disrupted nuclear membranes (smudge or basket cells) can be observed when fragile cells are present, excessive centrifugation forces are used, or increased tension and suction between pulled films shred the cells (Figure 50.2).[47]

Films prepared from concentrated samples allow for a more thorough examination of cell populations. Concentrated films from a variety of effusions can be prepared using a cytocentrifuge[47–49]; however, cell recovery can vary, making cell number estimation inaccurate.[50] Cytocentrifugation uses centrifugal force and absorption of excess fluid by a filter to produce sedimentation films of cells from fluids. Manufacturer's instructions should be followed to determine fluid aliquot volumes. One manufacturer (Cytospin™ 3, Thermo Shandon, Waltham, MA, USA) recommends sample volumes of 100–500 μL, depending on the cell concentration; highly concentrated samples may require dilution.[47] A uniform monolayer of flattened cells forms within a small circular area of the slide with minimal damage to the cells and visible nuclear and cytoplasmic details.[47,51] The addition of hyaluronidase to viscous synovial fluids that need cytocentrifugation improves differential counts.[51] It is the authors' experience that hyaluronidase causes large mononuclear cells to become foamy, so direct films should be prepared before treatment.

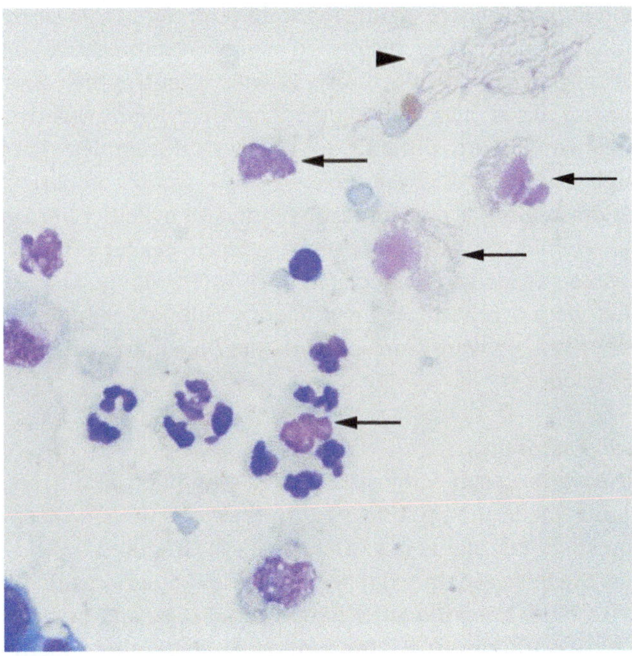

Figure 50.2 Smudge or basket cells are characterized by irregularly shaped and sized, pink-staining globules of disrupted nuclear material that lack cytoplasmic borders. The cell of origin is not usually apparent, so definitive interpretation is not possible. Streaming DNA (arrowhead) can be present. Larger globules (arrows) may be counted as cells by some automated analyzers and should be accounted for in microscopically estimated TNCCs (Wright-Giemsa, 500×).

For tube sedimentation, an aliquot of native, mixed sample is placed in a tube, and a gravitational force of 165–360g (e.g. 1000–1500 rpm in a centrifuge with a radial arm length of 14.6 cm) is applied for 5 minutes to generate a pellet.[52] The sample volume used to form a pellet varies inversely with the cellularity and is commonly based on turbidity of the fluid. The clearer the sample, the more the volume is used to maximize cell retrieval. Depending on sample volume, conical urine tubes or small test tubes can be used. The supernatant is removed, leaving enough liquid to resuspend the pellet. The residual material is gently mixed, and pull films are prepared as described above. In addition to the standard labeling information, "concentrated" or "sedimented" should be indicated on the slide label.

Grossly bloody samples produce a dense background that prohibits the formation of a cell monolayer and obscures the nucleated cell morphology in concentrated preparations. Buffy coat preparations (capillary centrifugation) provide an economical means to concentrate nucleated cells, including low numbers of neoplastic cells.[53–56] For samples collected in EDTA or heparin, plain glass microhematocrit tubes are filled and centrifuged for 3–5 minutes at 1000–1500 rpm.[53,54] The microhematocrit tube is scored and broken at the interface between the packed erythrocytes and the buffy coat. For samples with scant buffy coats, the tube is scored just below the interface (author observation). The edge of a glass slide works well to score the tube at the desired site (author observation). The buffy coat is tapped onto a glass slide, and a pulled film is prepared as described above. The slide label should indicate a "buffy" coat. This method concentrates nucleated cells while minimizing the number of erythrocytes present. Differential cell counts should not be determined from buffy coat preparations. With the buffy coat method, cells are sometimes coated with protein, which can result in poor staining quality. To ameliorate this problem, cells can first be washed. Following tube centrifugation of a sample aliquot for 10 minutes at 1000 rpm, the supernatant is removed, and an equal volume of normal saline is added, followed by with gentle mixing and recentrifugation.[56] The buffy coat is prepared as described above.[56]

Films are air-dried without fixation unless otherwise specified by the receiving laboratory. For thick samples or in locations with high humidity, a small handheld fan or gentle heating can reduce the drying time prior to staining without loss of sample quality.[57]

Unstained and stained films along with the fluid should be shipped to the referral laboratory, allowing for a more thorough evaluation of the pre-analytical conditions. Since some laboratories prefer to use their own stain, at least one unstained direct film should be submitted. If desired, additional films can be made, stained, and retained for education and for reevaluation should a referring laboratory report something previously missed in-house.

Pre-analytical bacterial contamination of slides can occur by exposing slide surfaces to contaminated hands or other dirty surfaces, coughs, or sneezes. “Clean” and “dirty” staining jars should be designated with the latter being reserved for fecal and ear specimens to minimize microbial growth in the stain and subsequent contamination of otherwise sterile specimens. To check for bacterial contamination of stain reagents, a film prepared from a sample known to be free of organisms is stained (e.g. dried drop of sterile saline) and checked for the presence of organisms. When contamination or poor-quality staining is present, jars are cleaned, and the stain is replaced.

Romanowsky Stains

Methanolic-based Romanowsky stains are ideal for cytologic evaluations and preferred by many clinical pathologists (Chapter 2).[58–60] Air-dried films are fixed in methanol, then immersed or flooded with Wright’s or Wright’s-Giemsa stain. Films are subsequently immersed or flooded with buffer, rinsed with water, and air-dried. The buffer–stain combination develops a shiny green layer on the surface when sufficiently mixed.[60] When flooding films on a flat surface, blowing air on the buffer assists with mixing. Specific incubation times vary between stain brands and thicknesses of preparations. Therefore, it is important to consult package inserts or manufacturing technical support, perform staining trials, and adjust timing accordingly. The thiazine basic dyes bind acidic nuclear chromatin and proteins, resulting in a dark purple color. The eosin acidic dyes bind basic proteins, eosinophil and azurophilic granules, and erythrocyte cytoplasm resulting in a pink to red color. Mast cell granules stain variable shades of purple.

Stain precipitates that occur with Romanowsky stains can be mistaken for bacteria. Usually, precipitates are more irregular in shape, size, and arrangement. When focusing up and down, precipitate appears refractile, dark purple, or out of the focal plane. When precipitates interfere with microscopic evaluations, remove immersion oil if present, dip the stained slide once in methanol, and then quickly rinse with water to remove precipitates (author observation) (Figure 50.3).

Quick Stains

Aqueous-based Romanowsky-type quick stains are commonly used in the clinic setting and by some referral laboratories for routine cytologic evaluation. While faster and easier to use than methanol-based stains, users should be aware that these stains may fail to detect mast cell, basophil, or azurophilic granules and can result in poor staining quality.[58]

Gram Stain

Gram stains broadly characterize bacterial organisms as Gram-positive or Gram-negative and can help guide antibiotic selection. Given certain limitations of the Gram stain, methanolic and aqueous Romanowsky-type stains are better at determining if organisms are present in samples, with the exception of *Mycobacteria* spp.[61–63] If organisms are observed in sufficient numbers on a Romanowsky-stained slide, a Gram stain can be performed on another film from the sample to assess bacterial staining characteristics. Gram-positive organisms stain purple, and Gram-negative organisms stain pink to red.[64] Over or under decolorizing results in false Gram-negative or Gram-positive results, respectively. Neutrophils and macrophages also stain pink, making Gram-negative organisms more difficult to observe in samples with high numbers of these cells. A large study comparing Gram staining to culture results found an overall 5% error rate, which was attributed most often to reader errors.[65] Discrepancies were associated with interpreting samples that were overly thick, insufficiently cellular, or improperly fixed, or were from patients previously treated with antibiotics.[65]

Acid-Fast Stain

Mycobacteria spp. are resistant to Romanowsky and Gram stains due to the mycolic acids in their cell walls[66]: therefore, acid-fast stains (e.g. Ziehl-Neelsen) are used.[67] Acid-fast organisms stain red; background and other organisms stain blue. *Nocardia* spp., *Rhodococcus* spp., and cysts of *Cryptosporidium* spp., *Isospora* spp., and other microsporidia are variably acid-fast positive.[68]

Cell Tube Blocks

Cell tube blocks allow submission of fluid samples in formalin (Chapter 8). To make a cell block, plain glass capillary tubes are filled with the sample, sealed with clay, and

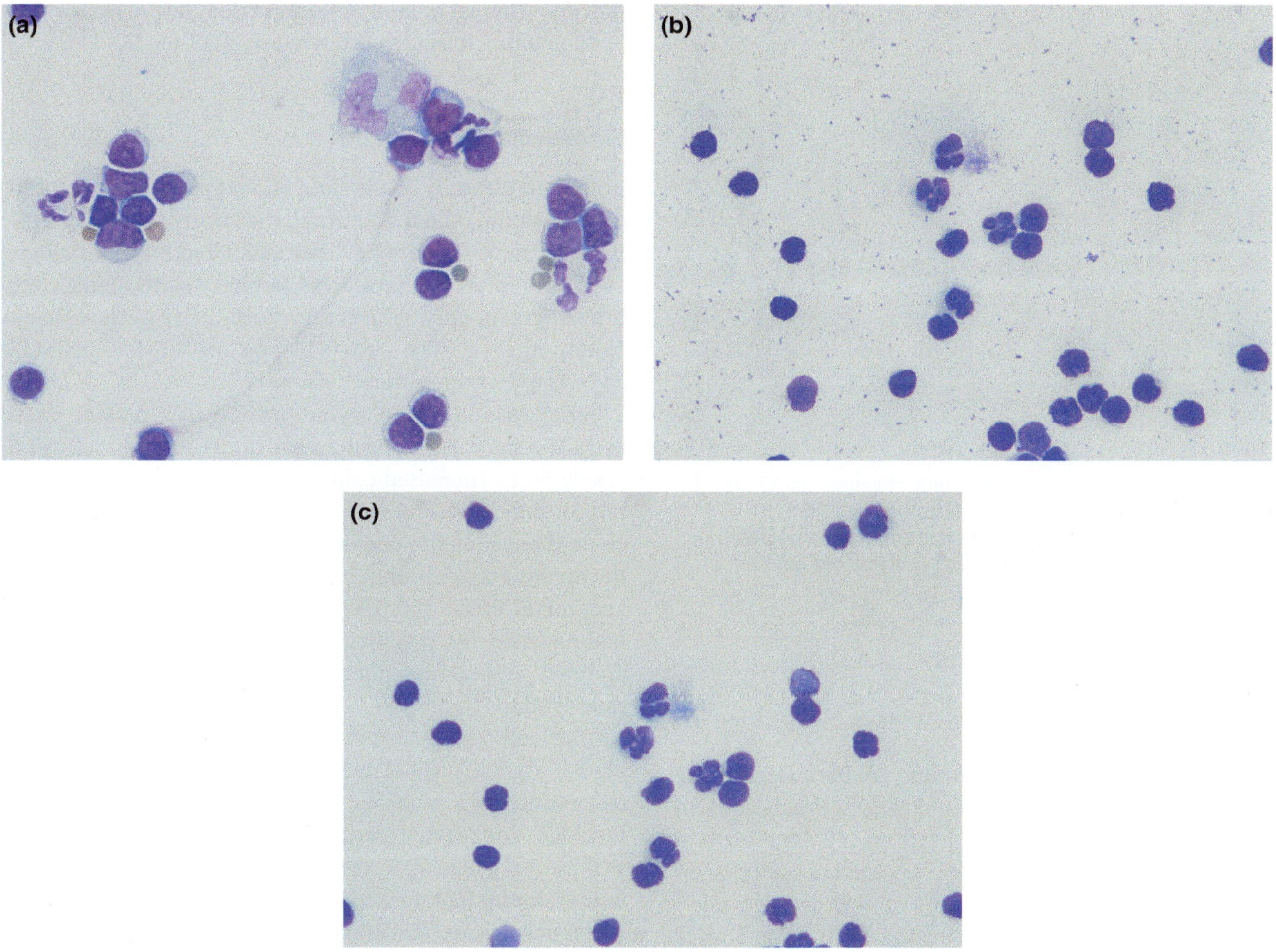

Figure 50.3 (a) Freshly prepared and stained sample of cavity fluid. (b) Aliquot from the same sample heated at 56 °C for 30 minutes. Note the loss of nuclear and cytoplasmic detail after heat exposure and dark purple stain precipitate. (c) The same film as (b) after dipping in methanol once and rinsing with water. The stain precipitates that mimic bacteria are cleared after dipping in methanol (Wright-Giemsa, 1000×).

centrifuged for 5 minutes at 14 500g. Poorly cellular fluids are first concentrated, and the sediment is added to the tube. A high density fluid such as Percoll™ (Sigma, St. Louis, MO, USA) can be added to facilitate separation of cells from the clay. The tube is broken at the supernatant/sediment interface to remove excess fluid and placed in formalin. The fixed sample is extracted from the tube, embedded in paraffin, and processed as for solid tissues.[69] Special procedures, such as histochemistry, immunohistochemistry, and molecular tests can be performed on the tube block similar to other formalin-fixed tissues. This method is particularly useful for samples with low numbers of neoplastic cells within hemorrhagic fluids.[70] Limitations of this method are that the glass tubes are fragile, that xylene-resistant nondrying modeling clay (e.g. Jovi Plastilina, Rubi, Spain) must be used instead of traditional tube clay, and that the fixation requirements result in processing delays of at least 24 hours.

Shipping

Unstained films should be protected from temperature extremes (Figures 50.3 and 50.4), condensation (Figure 50.5), and formalin fumes (Figure 50.6) prior to staining. Unstained slides should not be sent in the same package with containers of formalin-fixed tissue samples as exposure to formalin fumes interferes with staining.[41,71–73] Overnight fluid shipments should be chilled with ice packs that do not directly contact the samples and are insulated from temperature extremes.[74,75]

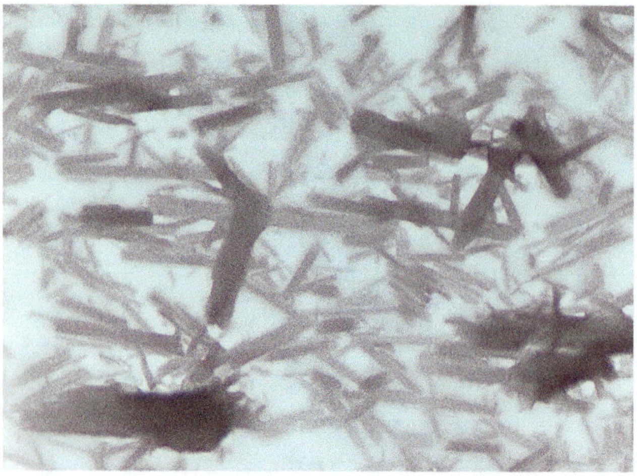

Figure 50.4 Film prepared from a unit of canine packed red cells inappropriately stored under freezing conditions. Crystalized erythrocytes stain the same color as hemoglobin (Wright-Giemsa, 1000×. *Source:* Image courtesy of Camille McAloney).

Analytical Considerations

Volume

In health, body cavity fluid volumes vary between species. Thoracic and peritoneal cavities of large animals contain between 0 and 300 mL,[3,76] while those of dogs contain between 0 and 15 mL.[77] The canine pericardial sac and synovial spaces contain 0.3 and <1.0 mL of fluid, respectively.[77] Effusion volumes should be estimated by imaging and/or measured as collected, and this information is recorded in the medical record. Large volumes indicate a pathologic process, whereas smaller volumes could be normal or due to an inability to access and retrieve all of the fluid.[76]

Gross Evaluation

Color and turbidity of the fluid should be assessed prior to centrifugation, and if abnormal, the supernatant after centrifugation also should be described. Descriptive terms are used for color (e.g. colorless, straw, yellow, pink, red, brown, green, gray, white) and turbidity (e.g. clear, hazy, cloudy, opaque). The terms "bloody" or "chylous" should be reserved for interpretations.

Variations in both color and turbidity can provide clues as to the pathologic mechanism underlying the effusion (Table 50.1). Increased cellularity, lipids, organisms, crystals, or debris will increase turbidity. The intensity of the color change, or the degree of turbidity is proportional to the amount of additional material. In horses with an acute abdominal crisis, fluids with abnormal color and clarity had a sensitivity, specificity, PPV, and NPV of 92, 74, 79, and 89%, respectively, for predicting the need for surgical intervention.[28]

Once cell counts and direct film preparations are completed, a grossly abnormal-appearing fluid warrants centrifugation and supernatant evaluation for color and turbidity. Leukocytes, erythrocytes, and other particulates will form a pellet upon centrifugation. Lipids will remain in the supernatant, maintaining turbidity. Before finalizing the report, gross assessments and microscopic findings should be corroborated. Incongruous results should initiate an investigation to find the discrepancy.

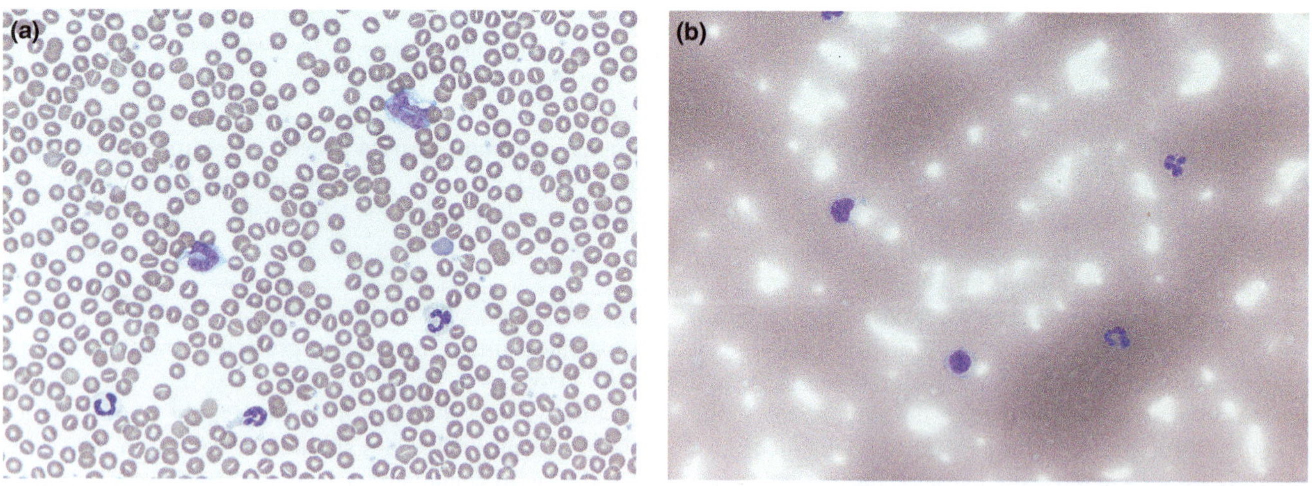

Figure 50.5 Blood films from a dog demonstrating marked hemolysis because of condensation. (a) Film stained after thorough drying at room temperature. (b) Film prepared from the same sample. The unstained film was routinely air-dried at room temperature, but then refrigerated and subsequently warmed to room temperature prior to staining. Note the marked hemolysis of the erythrocytes and loss of cellular detail of the leukocytes (Wright-Giemsa, 400×. *Source:* Images courtesy of Judith Radin).

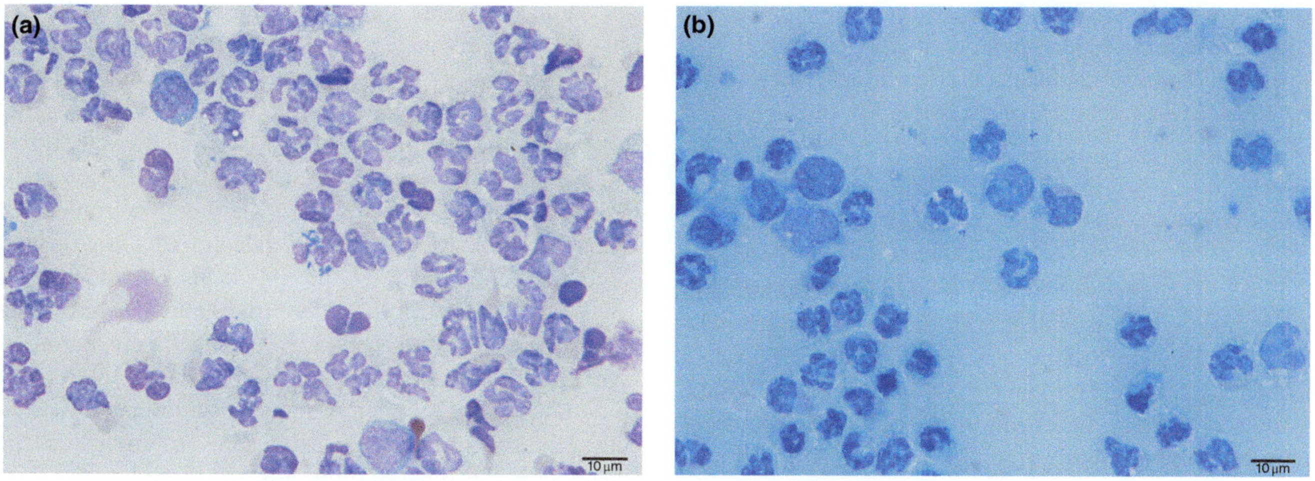

Figure 50.6 Films of septic peritoneal fluid from a dog. (a) This film was routinely air-dried and stained. Note the differential staining of leukocytes and readily apparent intracellular rod-shaped bacteria. (b) Film from the same sample was exposed to formalin fumes prior to staining. Note the monochromatic staining of all cells and less apparent intracellular bacteria (Wright-Giemsa, 1000×).

Table 50.1 Abnormal color and clarity assessments and interpretations.

Color and clarity	Interpretation
Pink to red color Variable turbidity (intact or hemolyzed erythrocytes)	Blood contamination during collection Changes in the appearance during the collection process Samples can clot in a non-additive tube or syringe[78] Platelets can be found microscopically if not fully entrapped in a clot Hemorrhagic effusion Pink/red color present throughout collection Sample does not clot; platelets are absent Microscopic evidence of acute to chronic hemorrhage[79,80] Erythrophagocytosis, hemosiderin-laden macrophages, hematoidin crystals
Straw to yellow, dark yellow Variable turbidity	Bile[81–83]
Gray Hazy to cloudy, turbid Clear supernatant after centrifugation	Neutrophils and/or other inflammatory cells Neoplastic cells
White Cloudy to opaque fluid and supernatant	Chylous effusion
Green, green-brown Variable turbidity	Gut contents[28]
Dark red-brown or brown	Older hemorrhage or devitalized tissues[76]

Protein Determinations

Protein concentrations are reliably estimated with a refractometer or semiquantitated as greater or less than 2.0 g/dL with urine test sticks.[84–86] Lipid and excess EDTA will falsely increase protein estimation by refractometry,[33] while hemolysis impairs instrument scale readings.[33] Protein content of synovial fluid measured by refractometry should be determined before adding hyaluronidase as falsely increased values may occur (author observation). Refractometers should be periodically checked and adjusted to a specific gravity of 1.000 using deionized water. Most scales only allow reading protein concentrations at or above 2.5 g/dL, but values as low as 0.6 g/dL can be derived from the urine specific gravity (USG) conversion table with the Goldberg brand of refractometers.[86] Alternatively, the following regression equation can estimate body fluid protein concentration from a refractometer USG scale (author's formula derived from George and O'Neill[86]):

$$\text{Body fluid protein (g/dL)} = 206.69\ (\text{USG}) - 208.36$$

Biochemical analyses of total protein and albumin concentrations with a calculation for the globulin concentration could be desired in some cases, particularly when evaluating cats for FIP. The IDEXX VetTest 8008 (IDEXX, Westbrook, Maine, USA) can be used to obtain total protein and albumin concentrations in feline effusions, but not albumin/globulin ratios.[87]

Cell Counts

TNCCs obtained from canine pleural and peritoneal cavity effusions are reliable using automated and manual methods.[88] In human fluid samples, automated TNCCs and neutrophil proportions using the Advia 120 flow-based analyzer (Siemens, Tarrytown, NY, USA) compared well with manual methods.[29,30] Mesothelial cells and neoplastic lymphocytes in pleural fluids were counted as leukocytes both manually and by the Advia 120.[30] When used with dog, cat, horse, and alpaca pleural and peritoneal effusions, the Advia 120 with multispecies software sufficiently counted TNCCs down to 1000/μL.[89] The Advia 120 also differentiated nucleated cells, erythrocytes, and platelets to appropriately classify effusions and distinguish neoplastic lymphocytic effusions from those of myelomonocytic origin in dogs.[90] It correctly classified cells in chylous effusions (one dog and one cat) and suppurative effusions in both species.[90] The Sysmex XT-2000iV (Sysmex Europe GmbH, Norderstedt, Germany) provides accurate and precise TNCCs in canine and feline pleural, peritoneal, and pericardial effusions.[91] TNCCs obtained from the Abaxis HM5 impedance automated analyzer (Abaxis, Inc., Union City, CA, USA) compared well with the Advia 120 for canine pleural and peritoneal effusions.[88] Chylous effusions should be run on automated analyzers with caution. In addition to poor precision of nucleated cells counts (31%),[88] lipid contamination with carryover in subsequent analyses can require prolonged cleaning efforts (author observation). Cytologic confirmation is required regardless of the analyzer used, as there are certain limitations with the identification of mesothelial and carcinoma cells.[90,91]

TNCC estimates from direct smears of synovial fluid are unreliable and tend to overestimate cell counts.[46] Sensitivity and specificity for the accurate diagnosis of inflammatory joint diseases ranged from 82–100% to 80–100%, respectively, compared with 0–60% and 20–60% for degenerative joint disease, respectively.[46] TNCCs obtained from equine and canine synovial fluids are reliable by automated impedance-based hematology analyzers such as the scil Vet ABC (scil animal care company, Gurnee, IL, USA), Abaxis HM5, Coulter Electronics ZBI (Counter Electronics, Inc., Hialeah, FL, USA), and Medonic CA620-VET (Boule Medical AB, Stockholm, Sweden).[88,92] Neutrophil differential counts appear reliable in humans but not animals.[29,88] The viscous nature of synovial fluid can compromise automated instrument function. Manual count accuracy can be impaired if diluting solutions containing acetic acid are used[93] or the chamber is overfilled, thereby altering the volume of fluid plated on the hemocytometer. Addition of hyaluronidase to viscous synovial fluid improves the accuracy of automated and manual TNCCs and manual differential cell counts on cytocentrifuged preparations.[29,51,94] One report specifies adding lyophilized hyaluronidase powder (686.6 units/mg, bovine testes type VIII, Sigma-Aldrich, St. Louis, MO, USA) to achieve a final concentration exceeding 250 U/mL.[29] Use of hyaluronidase is not necessary to obtain accurate TNCCs in inflammatory synovial fluids that have low viscosity.[88] Care must be taken to ensure appropriate handling of hyaluronidase as contamination and overgrowth by microorganisms can occur.[95]

TNCCs obtained by manual or automated methods should be routinely verified by comparing results of microscopic observations as part of the quality assurance process. Potential sources of error include misidentified or excluded large cells, clusters of cells counted as one large cell, and particles including yeast or bacteria counted as cells.[96]

Microscopic Evaluation

Microscopic evaluations allow for the differentiation of cell types and identification of malignancies, etiologic agents, and foreign material. If the sample is of low cellularity, concentrated preparations facilitate evaluation. A quality microscope with a 100× oil objective capable of detecting small organisms, e.g. *Mycoplasma* spp., is useful. Films should be evaluated using sequentially higher magnification. Use the low power objectives (4× and 10×) to gain an overall impression of the quality and cellularity of films and to locate other areas of interest, such as sheets or clusters of cells. High dry (40×) and oil (50× and 100×) objectives allow for the evaluation of cell distribution, the performance of differential cell counts, the assessment of cellular detail, and the detection of microorganisms.

Nucleated Cells

Nucleated cells typically present in cavity fluids include neutrophils, lymphocytes (small mononuclear cells), and large mononuclear cells. In freshly obtained samples, neutrophils and lymphocytes resemble those observed in peripheral blood. Neutrophils should be evaluated for evidence of degenerative changes including nuclear swelling and karyolysis, which indicate the presence of bacterial cytotoxins.[14,97] When these changes are observed, a thorough microscopic examination for bacteria and culture are needed. Macrophages and a few mesothelial cells comprise the large mononuclear population. With blood contamination, peripheral blood leukocytes, erythrocytes, and platelets can be present in numbers proportional to the amount of contamination and the peripheral blood cell counts. Eosinophils, plasma cells, and mast cells can be observed in variable numbers.

Mesothelial Cells

Mesothelial cells usually are present in low numbers in cavity fluid; however, increased shedding occurs with irritation. Cytologically, individual mesothelial cells have slightly rounded edges. Mesothelial cell cytoplasm is more deeply basophilic than that of macrophages, and a cytoplasmic "fringe" or corona is often noted, which may reflect the microvilli present on the luminal surface.[6] When present in cohesive sheets, the cells are cuboidal to polygonal with large round nuclei, fine chromatin, and often a single prominent nucleolus. Mesothelial cell clusters occasionally can appear as dense balls that likely denote overlaid sheets of cells. Quiescent cells exhibit minimal anisocytosis and anisokaryosis; however, when activated, mesothelial cells can display marked anisocytosis and anisokaryosis, making them difficult to distinguish from neoplastic cells. Mitotic figures and binucleated cells are occasionally observed since the mesothelium is continually renewing.[5,8] Normal, reactive, and neoplastic mesothelial cells express both mesenchymal intermediate filaments (vimentin and desmin) and epithelial intermediate filaments (cytokeratin).[98] When stimulated, mesothelial cells undergo epithelial or mesothelial to mesenchymal transition.[99,100]

Erythrocytes

Distinguishing blood contamination associated with sample collection technique from acute or chronic hemorrhage is important. Peripheral blood contributes leukocytes in proportion to the amount of blood present and potentially interferes with the interpretation of nucleated cell numbers and distribution. Platelets also might be observed microscopically if the sample is not significantly clotted. One report indicated no significant alteration in interpretation of TNCC or protein concentration with as much as 17% blood contamination in peritoneal fluid from clinically healthy horses.[101] It was suggested that the large volume of peritoneal fluid normally present in horses mitigates by dilution the effects of blood contamination.[101] While the morphology of erythrocytes in effusions is not routinely evaluated, acanthocytes have been observed in cases of hemangiosarcoma in dogs.[102]

Analytical Considerations and Ancillary Testing for Specific Conditions

Hemorrhagic Effusions

True hemorrhage imparts a consistent pink, red, or red-brown coloration throughout the collection process, and the fluid should fail to clot unless contaminated by peripheral or splenic blood.[78] Erythrophagocytosis and hemosiderin-laden macrophages are considered cytologic hallmarks of acute and chronic hemorrhagic effusions, respectively.[103] Erythrophagia can occur *in vitro* within minutes (authors' observation). Hemosiderin is visible approximately three days post-hemorrhage in a mouse model.[79] Hematoidin crystals suggest a chronic hemorrhagic process. Mesothelial cells from a hemorrhagic pericardial effusion in a dog contained fine brown/black granules that positively stained for iron, and the authors suggested that the accumulation of the iron was by absorption rather than erythrophagia.[80] Hemorrhagic pericardial effusions often are associated with neoplasia (Chapter 51). The diagnostic utility of pericardial fluid cytology is approximately 8% and improves to 20% if the fluid hematocrit is <10%.[103,104]

Biliary Effusions

Biliary effusions are more commonly seen in dogs than cats.[105] Rupture of the bile duct releases irritating substances that result in a modified transudate or exudate with protein concentrations typically ≥2.5 g/dL and TNCC between 9000 and 78 000/μL, with predominately neutrophils (84–90%).[105] Bile pigment can be seen in some cases and appears green-gold with Romanowsky stains and green to olive color with Hall's bile stain.[81,82] A few cases of "white bile" peritonitis are reported in dogs. In these cases, the abdominal fluid is characterized by mucinous fibrillary material that is lightly basophilic in color with Wright's-Giemsa stain and positively stains for mucin or mucosubstances with Alcian blue and Meyer's mucicarmine stains.[82] Diagnosis of bile peritonitis, including those effusions associated with "white bile," is aided by measurement of fluid bilirubin concentration that is at least 2.5 times greater than the serum bilirubin concentration.[82,83,105]

Chylous and Non-chylous Effusions in Dogs and Cats

Chylous and non-chylous effusions have a similar milky white to pink appearance.[106] The most useful test to distinguish between chylous and non-chylous effusions is to measure triglyceride concentrations. One study in dogs and cats indicated that triglyceride concentrations >100 mg/dL were 100% sensitive and specific for chylous effusions and those <100 mg/dL were 100% sensitive and specific for non-chylous effusions.[107]

Pancreatitis-Associated Effusions in Dogs

In conjunction with clinical signs, several biochemical assays have been used with peritoneal fluid to improve diagnosis of pancreatitis. Peritoneal fluid amylase activities with cutoff values of 1050 U/L were 71.4% sensitive and 84.2% specific, whereas lipase activities with cutoff values of 500 U/L were 92.9% sensitive and 94.7% specific for the diagnosis of acute pancreatitis.[108,109] A newer peritoneal fluid assay, the pancreas-specific lipase immunoreactivity (cPLI) assay, at cutoff values of 500 µg/L, had a sensitivity of 100% and specificity of 94.7% for the diagnosis of acute pancreatitis, demonstrating a slight improvement over the lipase assay and surpassing fluid amylase.[109]

Acute Colic in Horses

The presence of intestinal ischemia in horses with acute colic increases the probability of fatal outcomes.[110] Measurement of peritoneal fluid lactate has been suggested as an indicator of ischemia. Peritoneal fluid lactate concentration in horses with intestinal ischemia secondary to a strangulating obstruction was increased (mean = 8.45 mmol/L) compared with horses that did not have strangulating obstructions (mean = 2.09 mmol/L).[110] A follow-up study tested the use of a handheld analyzer to measure peritoneal fluid lactate (Accusport analyzer, Boehringer Mannheim, Germany) and presented similar results with odds ratios indicating probabilities of fatal outcomes in horses with acute colic.[111] In horses with strangulating obstructions, 1, 6, 12, and 16 mmol/L of lactate in peritoneal fluid corresponded with probabilities of death at 25, 52, 82, and 92%, respectively. Using the same peritoneal fluid lactate concentrations, horses without strangulating obstructions had lower probabilities of death at 11, 29, 63, and 82%, respectively.[111]

Uroperitoneum

Uroperitoneum is described in dogs, cats, and horses, especially in neonatal foals.[112–115]

In all species, peritoneal fluid–serum creatinine ratios ≥2, are considered diagnostic for uroperitoneum. In two horses with experimentally induced bladder rupture, extreme peritoneal fluid–serum creatinine ratios were found by two hours post bladder rupture in the non-surviving horse.[112]

Neoplastic Effusions

Shedding of tumor cells into cavitary effusions is documented with discrete round cell tumors, carcinomas, and sarcomas.[116] Cytologic detection of malignant tumors in pericardial, peritoneal, or pleural effusions has a sensitivity and specificity of 64 and 99% in dogs and 61 and 100% in cats, respectively.[116] The PPV was 95% for dogs and 100% for cats, with the NPV was 90% for both species.[116] Cytologic detection accuracy was greater for round cell tumors than for carcinomas and sarcomas and might relate to variability in the shedding of tumor cells.[116] In mast cell tumor cases, mast cells and eosinophils exfoliate into effusions in variable proportions.[117–119] Poor staining of granules with aqueous-based Romanowsky stains may hamper diagnoses.[58]

Ancillary testing can be used to improve the diagnostic utility of fluids. For canine and feline lymphoma, stained or unstained effusion films can be evaluated by polymerase chain reaction for antigen receptor rearrangement (PARR) to assess for the presence of a clonal lymphoid population. PARR has been successfully used to characterize clonal lymphocytes in canine blood and in thoracic and peritoneal fluids[120–122]; however, reports on the sensitivity and specificity of PARR analysis on fluids, to our knowledge, have not been published. When sufficient fluid volume is available, immunophenotyping can be performed using flow cytometry[123–125] or immunocytochemistry.[70,126–128]

Mesotheliomas are rare; can produce peritoneal, pleural, pericardial, or bicavitary effusions; and appear epithelioid, fibrous, or biphasic (mixed).[129–131] Mesotheliomas typically are malignant, although benign cases are described.[132] Histopathology usually is required for confirmation given the pleomorphic features associated with reactive mesothelial populations and their resemblance to neoplastic epithelial cells.[133] Microscopic diagnosis of mesothelioma can be aided by identifying co-expression of vimentin and cytokeratin or expression of calretinin using immunocytochemistry or immunohistochemistry.[129,134]

Effusions with Infectious Agents

Septic Effusions

The observation of intracellular bacteria supports septic effusion and is 57–89% accurate for bacterial peritonitis

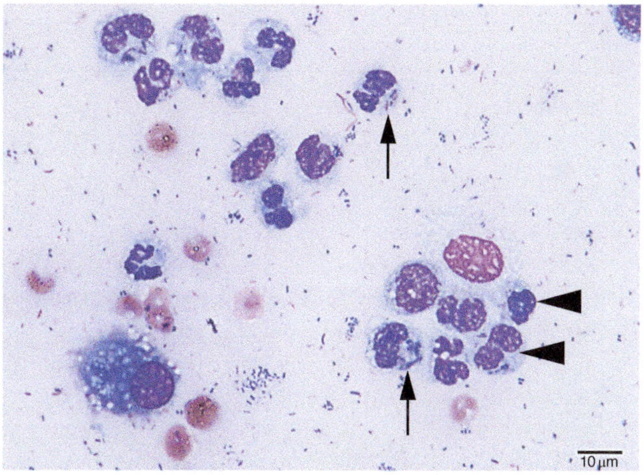

Figure 50.7 Septic inflammation in pleural fluid from a dog. Note degenerate neutrophils (arrowheads) and bacteria of mixed types in the background. Intracellular bacteria (arrows) support a septic process rather than sample contamination provided sample collection and handling utilized best practices (Wright-Giemsa, 1000×. *Source:* Image courtesy of Camille McAloney).

(Figure 50.7).[135] Intra- and extracellular location, size, shape, arrangement, and semiquantitative numbers of bacteria should be recorded. Extracellular bacteria can arise from an infectious process, or they can occur with contamination of fluids or stains (Figure 50.8). Ancillary tests have been evaluated as aids to diagnose septic effusions (Table 50.2). Peritoneal fluid collected anaerobically in heparin is required for pH and lactate determinations and can be used for glucose determination, depending on the instrumentation used.[135–137]

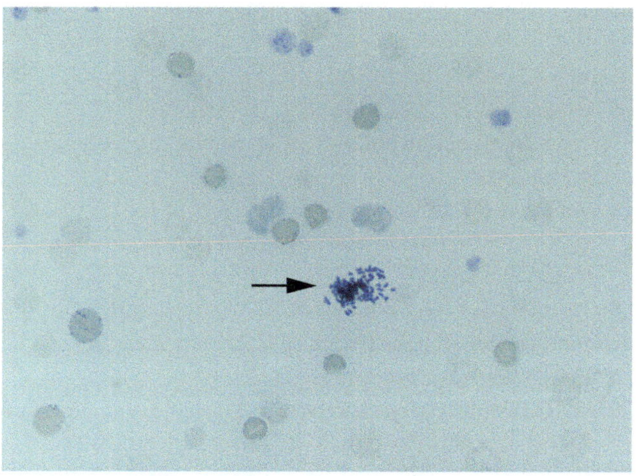

Figure 50.8 Blood film from a cat with colony-like formation of extracellular bacteria due to contamination of the stain (arrow). Several punctate reticulocytes are present in the field (New Methylene Blue, 1000×. *Source:* Image courtesy of Camille McAloney).

Feline Infectious Peritonitis

A variety of analytical tests using cavitary fluids have been evaluated for diagnosis of FIP; however, histopathology remains the gold standard.[138] Direct immunofluorescence for feline coronavirus using cytocentrifuged pleural and peritoneal effusions from infected cats is reportedly 97% reliable (31 of 32 cases) in confirming a diagnosis of FIP, but biopsy and histopathology are needed to exclude false negative results.[139] Unstained films can be stored for up to 7 days at −20 °C prior to testing.

An effusion total protein concentration cutoff of 8.0 g/dL has sensitivity of 55%, specificity of 90%, PPV of 78%, and NPV of 62% for correctly diagnosing FIP, while the serum albumin–globulin ratio has a higher sensitivity (86%) but lower specificity (74%).[140] Rivalta's test subjectively assesses increased gamma globulin and fibrinogen content in FIP effusions and has a sensitivity of 91.3%, specificity of 65.5%, PPV of 58.4%, and NPV of 93.4% for the diagnosis of FIP.[141] Diagnostic utility improved when 2-year-old cats were tested or when cases of lymphoma and bacterial infections were excluded.[140,141] Interpretations of test results using this method are subjective and vary with the individual performing the test.[142] Samples for Rivalta's testing remain stable for up to 21 days at room temperature.

Severe peripheral lymphopenia beginning 2–4 weeks after FIP infection was highly predictive of an adverse disease outcome in 18 cats.[143] Diagnosis of FIP based on immunocytochemistry for feline corona virus in effusion samples has an unacceptably high false-positive rate with sensitivity of 85% and specificity of 72.4%.[144] Possible failure to detect early-stage FIP infection in the control cats with a non-FIP diagnosis but similar appearing effusion was speculated to contribute to the poor specificity in this study.[144] Plasma, serum, or cavitary fluid alpha-1-acid glycoprotein levels >1.5 g/L could discriminate between cats infected with FIP from uninfected cats with similar clinical signs.[145] This test was reported to have a sensitivity of 85% and specificity of 100%.[145]

Fungal Infections

The presence of yeast or hyphal structures on cytology suggests fungal infection, particularly if organisms are intracellular and there is a concurrent appropriate inflammatory response. Culture is warranted when fungal infection is suspected clinically or when organisms cannot be identified by morphology. Etiologic agents reported in effusions include *Paecilomyces*,[146] *Histoplasma*,[147,148] *Blastomyces*,[149,150] and *Candida*.[151] Contaminated stains can result in overgrowth of fungal hyphae, confounding cytologic interpretation.

Table 50.2 Laboratory tests that aid in differentiating septic peritonitis from other causes in horses (H),[136] dogs (D),[135,137] and cats (C).[135,137]

Test (units)	Result	Species	Sensitivity	Specificity	PPV; NPV
Fluid TNCC (cells/μL)	>13 000	D	86%	100%	100%; 92%
	>13 000	C	100%	100%	100%; 100%
Fluid pH	<7.3	H	85.7%	100%	100%; 91.3%
Blood – fluid glucose (mg/dL)	>50	H	80%	95%	NP
	>20	D	100%	100%	100%; 100%
	>20	C	86%	100%	83%; 92%
Fluid fibrinogen (mg/dL)	>200	H	100%	84.2%	NP
Fluid glucose (mg/dL)	<50	D	57%	100%	83%; 83%
Fluid protein (g/dL)	>5	H	73.3%	90.5%	NP
Fluid lactate (mmol/L)	>2.5	D	Diagnostic accuracy: 95%		NP
Blood–fluid lactate (mmol/L)	<–2.0	D	100%	100%	100%; 100%
Fluid–blood lactate ratio	>1	D	Diagnostic accuracy: 90%		NP

NP, not provided; NPV, negative predictive value; PPV, positive predictive value; TNCC, total nucleated cell count.

Synovial Fluids

Synovial fluid contains hyaluronic acid, which imparts viscosity to the fluid and is assessed by the string test or the mucin clot test.[152] Decreased viscosity is suggested when synovial fluid drips like water or forms a string <2cm between the thumb and index finger; this occurs with bacterial infections or hydrarthrosis. The mucin clot test evaluates the strength of the clot that forms after dropping synovial fluid into dilute acetic acid.[153] This method affords little additional value to synovial fluid assessment so may be considered optional.

Conclusion

This chapter has covered analytical techniques for fluid analysis with consideration of pre-analytical and analytical sources of error that can influence the reliability and accuracy of the test results. Based on clinical signs, history, and results of the basic fluid analysis, additional ancillary tests may be warranted to diagnose specific conditions. A more detailed discussion of fluid analysis in different species appears in the following chapters.

References

1. Dempsey, S.M. and Ewing, P.J. (2011). A review of the pathophysiology, classification, and analysis of canine and feline cavitary effusions. *J Am Anim Hosp Assoc* 47: 1–11.
2. Levick, J.R. and McDonald, J.N. (1995). Fluid movement across synovium in healthy joints: role of synovial fluid macromolecules. *Ann Rheum Dis* 54: 417–423.
3. Brownlow, M.A., Hutchins, D.R., and Johnston, K.G. (1981). Reference values for equine peritoneal fluid. *Equine Vet J* 13: 127–130.
4. Hotz, C.S., Templeton, S.J., and Christopher, M.M. (2005). Comparative analysis of expert and machine-learning methods for classification of body cavity effusions in companion animals. *J Vet Diagn Invest* 17: 158–164.
5. Mutsaers, S.E. (2004). The mesothelial cell. *Int J Biochem Cell Biol* 36: 9–16.
6. Mutsaers, S.E. (2002). Mesothelial cells: their structure, function and role in serosal repair. *Respirology* 7: 171–191.
7. Mutsaers, S.E., Birnie, K., Lansley, S. et al. (2015). Mesothelial cells in tissue repair and fibrosis. *Front Pharmacol* 6: 113.
8. Mutsaers, S.E. and Wilkosz, S. (2007). Structure and function of mesothelial cells. *Cancer Treat Res* 134: 1–19.
9. Jay, G.D. and Waller, K.A. (2014). The biology of lubricin: near frictionless joint motion. *Matrix Biol* 39: 17–24.
10. Stockham, S.L. and Scott, M.A. (2008). *Cavitary Effusions: Fundamentals of Veterinary Clinical Pathology*, 831–868. Ames, IA: Backwell Publishing.
11. Brownlow, M.A. (1983). Polymorphonuclear neutrophil leucocytes of peritoneal fluid. *Equine Vet J* 15: 22–24.

12 Bohn, A.A. (2017). Analysis of canine peritoneal fluid analysis. *Vet Clin North Am Small Anim Pract* 47: 123–133.

13 Cowell, R.L., Tyler, R.D., Meinkoth, J.H., and DeNicola, D.B. (eds.) (2008). Effusions: abdominal, thoracic and pericardial. In: *Diagnostic Cytology and Hematology of the Dog and Cat*, 3e. St. Louis, MO: Mosby.

14 DeHeer, H.L., Parry, B.W., and Grindem, C.B. (2002). Pleural fluid. In: *Diagnostic Cytology and Hematology of the Horse*, 2e (eds. R.L. Cowell and R.D. Tyler), 119–126. St. Louis, MO: Mosby.

15 DeHeer, H.L., Parry, B.W., and Grindem, C.B. (2002). Peritoneal fluid. In: *Diagnostic Cytology and Hematology of the Horse*, 2e (eds. R.L. Cowell and R.D. Tyler), 127–162. St. Louis, MO: Mosby.

16 Wilson, A.D., Hirsch, V.M., and Osborne, A.D. (1985). Abdominocentesis in cattle: technique and criteria for diagnosis of peritonitis. *Can Vet J* 26: 74–80.

17 Hayward, A.H. (1968). Thoracic effusions in the cat. *J Small Anim Pract* 9: 75–82.

18 Macintire, D.K., Henderson, R.H., Banfield, C., and Kwapien, R.P. (1995). Budd-Chiari syndrome in a kitten, caused by membranous obstruction of the caudal vena cava. *J Am Anim Hosp Assoc* 31: 484–491.

19 Alleman, A.R. (2003). Abdominal, thoracic, and pericardial effusions. *Vet Clin North Am Small Anim Pract* 33: 89–118.

20 Reef, V.B., Boy, M.G., Reid, C.F., and Elser, A. (1991). Comparison between diagnostic ultrasonography and radiography in the evaluation of horses and cattle with thoracic disease: 56 cases (1984–1985). *J Am Vet Med Assoc* 198: 2112–2118.

21 Kramer, M., Gerwing, M., Hach, V., and Schimke, E. (1997). Sonography of the musculoskeletal system in dogs and cats. *Vet Radiol Ultrasound* 38: 139–149.

22 Raes, E.V., Vanderperren, K., Pille, F., and Saunders, J.H. (2010). Ultrasonographic findings in 100 horses with tarsal region disorders. *Vet J* 186: 201–209.

23 Wong, B.Y., Lee, K.R., and MacArthur, R.I. (1982). Diagnosis of pericardial effusion by computed tomography. *Chest* 81: 177–181.

24 Ohlerth, S. and Scharf, G. (2007). Computed tomography in small animals: basic principles and state of the art applications. *Vet J* 173: 254–271.

25 Schultz, R.M. and Zwingenberger, A. (2008). Radiographic, computed tomographic, and ultrasonographic findings with migrating intrathoracic grass awns in dogs and cats. *Vet Radiol Ultrasound* 49: 249–255.

26 Flatland, B., Freeman, K.P., Vap, L.M., and Harr, K.E. (2013). ASVCP guidelines: quality assurance for point-of-care testing in veterinary medicine. *Vet Clin Pathol* 42: 405–423.

27 Gunn-Christie, R.G. (2012). ASVCP quality assurance guidelines: control of preanalytical, analytical, and postanalytical factors for urinalysis, cytology, and clinical chemistry in veterinary laboratories. *Vet Clin Pathol* 41: 18–26.

28 Matthews, S., Dart, A.J., Reid, S.W. et al. (2002). Predictive values, sensitivity and specificity of abdominal fluid variables in determining the need for surgery in horses with an acute abdominal crisis. *Aust Vet J* 80: 132–136.

29 Froom, P., Diab, A., and Barak, M. (2013). Automated evaluation of synovial and ascitic fluids with the Advia 2120 hematology analyzer. *Am J Clin Pathol* 140: 828–830.

30 Aulesa, C. (2003). Use of the Advia 120 hematology analyzer in the differential cytologic analysis of biological fluids (cerebrospinal, peritoneal, pleural, pericardial, synovial, and others). *Lab Hematol* 9: 214–224.

31 Miller, J.M., Astles, R., Baszler, T. et al. (2012). Guidelines for safe work practices in human and animal medical diagnostic laboratories: recommendations of a CDC-convened, Biosafety Blue Ribbon Panel. *MMWR Suppl* 61: 1–102.

32 Gilor, S. and Gilor, C. (2011). Common laboratory artifacts caused by inappropriate sample collection and transport: how to get the most out of a sample. *Top Companion Anim Med* 26: 109–118.

33 Dubin, S. and Hunt, P. (1978). Effect of anticoagulants and glucose on refractometric estimation of protein in canine and rabbit plasma. *Lab Anim Sci* 28: 541–544.

34 George, J.W. (2001). The usefulness and limitations of hand-held refractometers in veterinary laboratory medicine: an historical and technical review. *Vet Clin Pathol* 30: 201–210.

35 Lippi, G., Salvagno, G.L., Solero, G.P. et al. (2005). Stability of blood cell counts, hematologic parameters and reticulocytes indexes on the Advia A120 hematologic analyzer. *J Lab Clin Med* 146: 333–340.

36 Salinas, M., Rosas, J., Iborra, J. et al. (1997). Comparison of manual and automated cell counts in EDTA preserved synovial fluids: storage has little influence on the results. *Ann Rheum Dis* 56: 622–626.

37 Banfi, G., Salvagno, G.L., and Lippi, G. (2007). The role of ethylenediaminetetraacetic acid (EDTA) as in vitro anticoagulant for diagnostic purposes. *Clin Chem Lab Med* 45: 565–576.

38 Jain, N. (1986). Hematologic techniques. In: *Schalm's Veterinary Hematology*, 4e, vol. 25 (ed. O.W. Schalm). Philadelphia, PA: Lea & Febiger.

39 Sahay, K., Mehendiratta, M., Rehani, S. et al. (2013). Cytological artifacts masquerading interpretation. *J Cytol* 30: 241–246.

40 CLSI (2007). *Analysis of Body Fluids in Clinical Chemistry: Approved Guideline*. Wayne, PA: Clinical Laboratory and Standards Institute.

41 Sharkey, L.C., Dial, S.M., and Matz, M.E. (2007). Maximizing the diagnostic value of cytology in small animal practice. *Vet Clin North Am Small Anim Pract* 37: 351–372.

42 Bowen, R.A. and Remaley, A.T. (2014). Interferences from blood collection tube components on clinical chemistry assays. *Biochem Med (Zagreb)* 24: 31–44.

43 Koolvisoot, A., Rungbanaphan, U., Katchamat, W., and Chinsawangwatanakul, W. (2006). The preservation method and timing on accuracy of manual leukocytes counts in synovial fluid. *J Med Assoc Thail* 89 (Suppl 5): S187–S194.

44 MacWilliams, P.S. and Friedrichs, K.R. (2003). Laboratory evaluation and interpretation of synovial fluid. *Vet Clin North Am Small Anim Pract* 33: 153–178.

45 Finnegan, S. and Percival, S.L. (2015). EDTA: an antimicrobial and antibiofilm agent for use in wound care. *Adv Wound Care* 4: 415–421.

46 Gibson, N.R., Carmichael, S., Li, A. et al. (1999). Value of direct smears of synovial fluid in the diagnosis of canine joint disease. *Vet Rec* 144: 463–465.

47 Sherwood, N. and Cornbleet, J. (1997). Use of the cytospin for hematology and other clinical microscopy specimens. In: *Cytospin 3 Cell Preparation System Operator Guide*, 1-10-1-12. Cheshire, England: ThermoShandon Scientific.

48 Jones, C.D. and Cornbleet, P.J. (1997). Wright-Giemsa cytology of body fluids. *Lab Med* 28: 713–716.

49 Cornbleet, P.J. (1998). Wright-Giemsa cytology of body fluids: criteria for identification of malignant cells. *Lab Med* 29: 26–31.

50 Robb, J., Melello, C., and Odom, C. (1996). Comparison of Cyto-Shuttle(R) and cytocentrifuge as processing methods for nongynecologic cytology specimens. *Diagn Cytopathol* 14: 305–309.

51 Moreno, M.J., Clayburne, G., and Schumacher, H.R. Jr. (2000). Processing of noninflammatory synovial fluids with hyaluronidase for cytospin preparations improves the accuracy of differential counts. *Diagn Cytopathol* 22: 256–258.

52 Meinkoth, J.H., Cowell, R.L., Tyler, R.D. et al. (2014). Sample collection and preparation. In: *Cowell and Tyler's Diagnostic Cytology and Hematology of the Dog and Cat*, 4e (eds. A.C. Valenciano and R.L. Cowell), 1–19. St. Louis, MO: Elsevier.

53 Chu, J.Y. (1979). Buffy-coat smear of bloodstained aspirate and intraperitoneal bleeding. *J Clin Pathol* 32: 198.

54 Piviani, M., Walton, R.M., and Patel, R.T. (2013). Significance of mastocytemia in cats. *Vet Clin Pathol* 42: 4–10.

55 Skeldon, N.C., Gerber, K.L., Wilson, R.J., and Cunnington, S.J. (2010). Mastocytaemia in cats: prevalence, detection and quantification methods, haematological associations and potential implications in 30 cats with mast cell tumours. *J Feline Med Surg* 12: 960–966.

56 Agarwal, P.K. (2009). Cytologic examination of hemorrhagic fluid by capillary centrifugation: a new technique. *Acta Cytol* 53: 527–532.

57 Baig, M., Fathallah, L., Feng, J. et al. (2006). Fast drying of fine needle aspiration slides using a hand held fan: impact on turn around time and staining quality. *CytoJournal* 3: 12.

58 Allison, R.W. and Velguth, K.E. (2010). Appearance of granulated cells in blood films stained by automated aqueous versus methanolic Romanowsky methods. *Vet Clin Pathol* 39: 99–104.

59 Krafts, K.P. and Pambuccian, S.E. (2011). Romanowsky staining in cytopathology: history, advantages and limitations. *Biotech Histochem* 86: 82–93.

60 Woronzoff-Dashkoff, K.K. (2002). The Wright-Giemsa stain: secrets revealed. *Clin Lab Med* 22: 15–23.

61 Woods, G.L. and Walker, D.H. (1996). Detection of infection or infectious agents by use of cytologic and histologic stains. *Clin Microbiol Rev* 9: 382–404.

62 Cowell, R.L., Tyler, R.D., Meinkoth, J.H. et al. (2008). Selected infectious agents. In: *Diagnostic Cytology and Hematology of the Dog and Cat*, 3e (eds. R.L. Cowell, R.D. Tyler, J.H. Meinkoth and D.B. DeNicola), 47. St. Louis, MO: Mosby.

63 Swenson, C.L., Boisvert, A.M., Kruger, J.M., and Gibbons-Burgener, S.N. (2004). Evaluation of modified Wright-staining of urine sediment as a method for accurate detection of bacteriuria in dogs. *J Am Vet Med Assoc* 224: 1282–1289.

64 Harleco Gram Stain Set (2004). *Harleco Gram Stain Set Package Insert*. Gibbstown, NJ: Harleco.

65 Samuel, L.P., Balada-Llasat, J.M., Harrington, A., and Cavagnolo, R. (2016). Multicenter assessment of gram stain error rates. *J Clin Microbiol* 54: 1442–1447.

66 Trifiro, S., Bourgault, A.M., Lebel, F., and René, P. (1990). Ghost mycobacteria on gram stain. *J Clin Microbiol* 28: 146–147.

67 Muricy, E.C.M., Lemes, R.A., Bombarda, S. et al. (2014). Differentiation between *Nocardia* spp. and *Mycobacterium* spp.: critical aspects for bacteriological diagnosis. *Rev Inst Med Trop Sao Paulo* 56: 397–401.

68 Acid Fast Stains (2012). *(Ziehl-Neelsen) Package Insert*. Lexington, KY: Gibson Bioscience.

69 Marcos, R., Santos, M., Marrinhas, C., and Caniatti, M. (2017). Cell tube block: a new technique to produce cell blocks from fluid cytology samples. *Vet Clin Pathol* 46: 195–201.

70 Fernandes, N.C., Guerra, J.M., Ressio, R.A. et al. (2016). Liquid-based cytology and cell block immunocytochemistry in veterinary medicine: comparison with standard cytology for the evaluation of canine lymphoid samples. *Vet Comp Oncol* 14 (Suppl 1): 107–116.

71 Maher, I., Tennant, K.V., and Papasouliotis, K. (2010). Effect of storage time on automated cell count and cytological interpretation of body cavity effusions. *Vet Rec* 167: 519–522.

72 Braun, J.P., Bourges-Abella, N., Geffre, A. et al. (2015). The preanalytic phase in veterinary clinical pathology. *Vet Clin Pathol* 44: 8–25.

73 Martinez, C.R. and Santangelo, K.S. (2017). Preanalytical considerations for joint fluid evaluation. *Vet Clin North Am Small Anim Pract* 47: 111–122.

74 Coakley, W.T. (1987). Hyperthermia effects on the cytoskeleton and on cell morphology. *Symp Soc Exp Biol* 41: 187–211.

75 Culang, D. and Gara-Boivin, C. (2017). What is your diagnosis? Erythrocyte morphology in a cow. *Vet Clin Pathol* 46: 645–646.

76 Swaniwick, R.A. and Wilkinson, J.S. (1976). A clinical evaluation of abdominal paracentesis in the horse. *Aust Vet J* 52: 109–117.

77 Feldman, B.F. and Ruehl, W.W. (1984). Examination of body fluids. *Mod Vet Pract* 65: 295–298.

78 Brockman, D.J., Mongil, C.M., Aronson, L.R., and Brown, D.C. (2000). A practical approach to hemoperitoneum in the dog and cat. *Vet Clin North Am Small Anim Pract* 30: 657–668.

79 Epstein, C.E., Elidemir, O., Colasurdo, G.N., and Fan, L.L. (2001). Time course of hemosiderin production by alveolar macrophages in a murine model. *Chest* 120: 2013–2020.

80 Barger, A. and Riensche, M. (2009). What is your diagnosis? Hemorrhagic effusion in a dog. *Vet Clin Pathol* 38: 529–531.

81 Hall, M.J. (1960). A staining reaction for bilirubin in sections of tissue. *Am J Clin Pathol* 34: 313–316.

82 Owens, S.D., Gossett, R., McElhaney, M.R. et al. (2003). Three cases of canine bile peritonitis with mucinous material in abdominal fluid as the prominent cytologic finding. *Vet Clin Pathol* 32: 114–120.

83 Guillaumin, J., Chanoit, G., Decosne-Junot, C., and Goy-Thollot, I. (2006). Bilothorax following cholecystectomy in a dog. *J Small Anim Pract* 47: 733–736.

84 Rose, A., Funk, D., and Neiger, R. (2016). Comparison of refractometry and biuret assay for measurement of total protein concentration in canine abdominal and pleural fluid specimens. *J Am Vet Med Assoc* 248: 789–794.

85 Braun, J.P., Guelfi, J.F., and Pages, J.P. (2001). Comparison of four methods for determination of total protein concentrations in pleural and peritoneal fluid from dogs. *Am J Vet Res* 62: 294–296.

86 George, J.W. and O'Neill, S.L. (2001). Comparison of refractometer and biuret methods for total protein measurement in body cavity fluids. *Vet Clin Pathol* 30: 16–18.

87 Papasouliotis, K., Murphy, K., Dodkin, S., and Torrance, A.G. (2002). Use of the VetTest 8008 and refractometry for determination of total protein, albumin, and globulin concentrations in feline effusions. *Vet Clin Pathol* 31: 162–166.

88 Brudvig, J.M. and Swenson, C.L. (2015). Total nucleated cell and leukocyte differential counts in canine pleural and peritoneal fluid and equine synovial fluid samples: comparison of automated and manual methods. *Vet Clin Pathol* 44: 570–579.

89 Gorman, M.E., Villarroel, A., Tornquist, S.J. et al. (2009). Comparison between manual and automated total nucleated cell counts using the ADVIA 120 for pleural and peritoneal fluid samples from dogs, cats, horses, and alpacas. *Vet Clin Pathol* 38: 388–391.

90 Bauer, N. and Moritz, A. (2005). Flow cytometric analysis of effusions in dogs and cats with the automated haematology analyser ADVIA 120. *Vet Rec* 156: 674–678.

91 Pinto da Cunha, N., Giordano, A., Caniatti, M., and Paltrinieri, S. (2009). Analytical validation of the Sysmex XT-2000iV for cell counts in canine and feline effusions and concordance with cytologic diagnosis. *Vet Clin Pathol* 38: 230–241.

92 Atilola, M.A., Lumsden, J.H., and Rooke, F. (1986). A comparison of manual and electronic counting for total nucleated cell counts on synovial fluid from canine stifle joints. *Can J Vet Res* 50: 282–284.

93 Pascual, E. and Jovani, V. (2005). Synovial fluid analysis. *Best Pract Res Clin Rheumatol* 19: 371–386.

94 Ekmann, A., Rigdal, M.L., and Grondahl, G. (2010). Automated counting of nucleated cells in equine synovial fluid without and with hyaluronidase pretreatment. *Vet Clin Pathol* 39: 83–89.

95 Robier, C., Stettin, M., and Neubauer, M. (2015). Fungal contamination of hyaluronidase solution mimicking fungal joint infection: a preanalytical pitfall in synovial fluid analysis. *Clin Chem Lab Med* 53: e231–e232.

96 Kim, H.R., Park, B.R., and Lee, M.K. (2008). Effects of bacteria and yeast on WBC counting in three automated hematology counters. *Ann Hematol* 87: 557–562.

97 Valenciano, A.C., Arndt, T.P., and Rizzi, T.E. (2014). Effusions: abdominal, thoracic, and pericardial. In: *Diagnostic Cytology and Hematology of the Dog and Cat,*

4e (eds. A.C. Valenciano and R.L. Cowell), 244–265. St. Louis: Mosby.

98 Przezdziecki, R. and Sapierzynski, R. (2014). Using of immunocytochemistry in differential diagnosis of neoplasms of serosal cavities in dogs. *Pol J Vet Sci* 17: 149–159.

99 Perez-Lozano, M.L., Sandoval, P., Rynne-Vidal, A. et al. (2013). Functional relevance of the switch of VEGF receptors/co-receptors during peritoneal dialysis-induced mesothelial to mesenchymal transition. *PLoS One* 8: e60776.

100 Sandoval, P., Loureiro, J., Gonzalez-Mateo, G. et al. (2010). PPAR-gamma agonist rosiglitazone protects peritoneal membrane from dialysis fluid-induced damage. *Lab Investig* 90: 1517–1532.

101 Malark, J.A., Peyton, L.C., and Galvin, M.J. (1992). Effects of blood contamination on equine peritoneal fluid analysis. *J Am Vet Med Assoc* 201: 1545–1548.

102 Wong, R.W., Gonsalves, M.N., Huber, M.L. et al. (2015). Erythrocyte and biochemical abnormalities as diagnostic markers in dogs with hemangiosarcoma related hemoabdomen. *Vet Surg* 44: 852–857.

103 Berg, R.J., Wingfield, W.E., and Hoopes, P.J. (1985). Idiopathic hemorrhagic pericardial effusion in 8 dogs. *Vet Surg* 14: 46–47.

104 Machida, N., Tanaka, R., Takemura, N. et al. (2004). Development of pericardial mesothelioma in golden retrievers with a long-term history of idiopathic haemorrhagic pericardial effusion. *J Comp Pathol* 131: 166–175.

105 Ludwig, L.L., McLoughlin, M.A., Graves, T.K., and Crisp, M.S. (1997). Surgical treatment of bile peritonitis in 24 dogs and 2 cats: a retrospective study (1987–1994). *Vet Surg* 26: 90–98.

106 Fossum, T.W., Birchard, S.J., and Jacobs, R.M. (1986). Chylothorax in 34 dogs. *J Am Vet Med Assoc* 188: 1315–1318.

107 Waddle, J.R. and Giger, U. (1990). Lipoprotein electrophoresis differentiation of chylous and nonchylous pleural effusions in dogs and cats and its correlation with pleural effusion triglyceride concentration. *Vet Clin Pathol* 19: 80–85.

108 Steiner, J.M. (2003). Diagnosis of pancreatitis. *Vet Clin North Am Small Anim Pract* 33: 1181–1195.

109 Chartier, M.A., Hill, S.L., Sunico, S. et al. (2014). Pancreas-specific lipase concentrations and amylase and lipase activities in the peritoneal fluid of dogs with suspected pancreatitis. *Vet J* 201: 385–389.

110 Latson, K.M., Nieto, J.E., Beldomenico, P.M., and Snyder, J.R. (2005). Evaluation of peritoneal fluid lactate as a marker of intestinal ischaemia in equine colic. *Equine Vet J* 37: 342–346.

111 Delesalle, C., Dewulf, J., Lefebvre, R.A. et al. (2007). Determination of lactate concentrations in blood plasma and peritoneal fluid in horses with colic by an Accusport analyzer. *J Vet Intern Med* 21: 293–301.

112 Genetzky, R.M. and Hagemoser, W.A. (1985). Physical and clinical pathological findings associated with experimentally induced rupture of the equine urinary bladder. *Can Vet J* 26: 391–395.

113 Richardson, D.W. (1985). Urogenital problems in the neonatal foal. *Vet Clin North Am Equine Pract* 1: 179–188.

114 Stafford, J.R. and Bartges, J.W. (2013). A clinical review of pathophysiology, diagnosis, and treatment of uroabdomen in the dog and cat. *J Vet Emerg Crit Care* 23: 216–229.

115 Adams, R., Koterba, A.M., Cudd, T.C., and Baker, W.A. (1988). Exploratory celiotomy for suspected urinary tract disruption in neonatal foals: a review of 18 cases. *Equine Vet J* 20: 13–17.

116 Hirschberger, J., DeNicola, D.B., Hermanns, W. et al. (1999). Sensitivity and specificity of cytologic evaluation in the diagnosis of neoplasia in body fluids from dogs and cats. *Vet Clin Pathol* 28: 142–146.

117 Cowgill, E. and Neel, J. (2003). Pleural fluid from a dog with marked eosinophilia. *Vet Clin Pathol* 32: 147–149.

118 Harris, B.J., Constantino-Casas, F., Archer, J., and Herrtage, M.E. (2013). Loeffler's endocarditis and bicavity eosinophilic effusions in a dog with visceral mast cell tumour and hypereosinophilia. *J Comp Pathol* 149: 429–433.

119 Peaston, A.E. and Griffey, S.M. (1994). Visceral mast cell tumour with eosinophilia and eosinophilic peritoneal and pleural effusions in a cat. *Aust Vet J* 71: 215–217.

120 Thilakaratne, D.N., Mayer, M.N., MacDonald, V.S. et al. (2010). Clonality and phenotyping of canine lymphomas before chemotherapy and during remission using polymerase chain reaction (PCR) on lymph node cytologic smears and peripheral blood. *Can Vet J* 51: 79–84.

121 Burnett, R.C., Vernau, W., Modiano, J.F. et al. (2003). Diagnosis of canine lymphoid neoplasia using clonal rearrangements of antigen receptor genes. *Vet Pathol* 40: 32–41.

122 Rout, E.D., Shank, A.M., Waite, A.H. et al. (2017). Progression of cutaneous plasmacytoma to plasma cell leukemia in a dog. *Vet Clin Pathol* 46: 77–84.

123 Avery, P.R. and Avery, A.C. (2004). Molecular methods to distinguish reactive and neoplastic lymphocyte expansions and their importance in transitional neoplastic states. *Vet Clin Pathol* 33: 196–207.

124 Amati, M., Venco, L., Roccabianca, P. et al. (2014). Pericardial lymphoma in seven cats. *J Feline Med Surg* 16: 507–512.

125 Weiss, D.J. (2002). Application of flow cytometric techniques to veterinary clinical hematology. *Vet Clin Pathol* 31: 72–82.

126 Caniatti, M., Roccabianca, P., Scanziani, E. et al. (1996). Canine lymphoma: immunocytochemical analysis of fine-needle aspiration biopsy. *Vet Pathol* 33: 204–212.

127 Modiano, J.F., Smith, R., Wojcieszyn, J. et al. (1998). The use of cytochemistry, immunophenotyping, flow cytometry, and in vitro differentiation to determine the ontogeny of a canine monoblastic leukemia. *Vet Clin Pathol* 27: 40–49.

128 Priest, H.L., Hume, K.R., Killick, D. et al. (2017). The use, publication and future directions of immunocytochemistry in veterinary medicine: a consensus of the Oncology-Pathology Working Group. *Vet Comp Oncol* 15: 868–880.

129 Stoica, G., Cohen, N., Mendes, O., and Kim, H.T. (2004). Use of immunohistochemical marker calretinin in the diagnosis of a diffuse malignant metastatic mesothelioma in an equine. *J Vet Diagn Invest* 16: 240–243.

130 Schoning, P., Layton, C.E., Fortney, W.D. et al. (1992). Sclerosing peritoneal mesothelioma in a dog evaluated by electron microscopy and immunoperoxidase techniques. *J Vet Diagn Invest* 4: 217–220.

131 Stepien, R.L., Whitley, N.T., and Dubielzig, R.R. (2000). Idiopathic or mesothelioma-related pericardial effusion: clinical findings and survival in 17 dogs studied retrospectively. *J Small Anim Pract* 41: 342–347.

132 Head, K., Cullen, J., Dubielzig, R. et al. (2003). *Histological Classification of Tumors of Alimentary System of Domestic Animals*. WHO Histological Classification of Tumors of Domestic Animals. Washington, DC: Armed Forces Institute of Pathology in Cooperation with the American Registry of Pathology and the World Health Organization Collaborating Center for Worldwide Reference on Comparative Oncology.

133 Hoon-Hanks, L.L., Rout, E.D., Vap, L.M. et al. (2016). Reactive mesothelial hyperplasia associated with chronic peritonitis in a 20-year-old Quarter horse. *Can Vet J* 57: 492–496.

134 Weiss, A.T., da Costa, A.B., and Klopfleisch, R. (2010). Predominantly fibrous malignant mesothelioma in a cat. *Vet Med Int* 2010: 396794.

135 Bonczynski, J.J., Ludwig, L.L., Barton, L.J. et al. (2003). Comparison of peritoneal fluid and peripheral blood pH, bicarbonate, glucose, and lactate concentration as a diagnostic tool for septic peritonitis in dogs and cats. *Vet Surg* 32: 161–166.

136 Van Hoogmoed, L., Rodger, L.D., Spier, S.J. et al. (1999). Evaluation of peritoneal fluid pH, glucose concentration, and lactate dehydrogenase activity for detection of septic peritonitis in horses. *J Am Vet Med Assoc* 214: 1032–1036.

137 Levin, G.M., Bonczynski, J.J., Ludwig, L.L. et al. (2004). Lactate as a diagnostic test for septic peritoneal effusions in dogs and cats. *J Am Anim Hosp Assoc* 40: 364–371.

138 Litster, A.L., Pogranichniy, R., and Lin, T.L. (2013). Diagnostic utility of a direct immunofluorescence test to detect feline coronavirus antigen in macrophages in effusive feline infectious peritonitis. *Vet J* 198: 362–366.

139 Parodi, M.C., Cammarata, G., Paltrinieri, S. et al. (1993). Using direct immunofluorescence to detect coronaviruses in peritoneal and pleural effusions. *J Small Anim Pract* 34: 609–613.

140 Hartmann, K., Binder, C., Hirschberger, J. et al. (2003). Comparison of different tests to diagnose feline infectious peritonitis. *J Vet Intern Med* 17: 781–790.

141 Fischer, Y., Sauter-Louis, C., and Hartmann, K. (2012). Diagnostic accuracy of the Rivalta test for feline infectious peritonitis. *Vet Clin Pathol* 41: 558–567.

142 Fischer, Y., Weber, K., Sauter-Louis, C., and Hartmann, K. (2013). The Rivalta's test as a diagnostic variable in feline effusions: evaluation of optimum reaction and storage conditions. *Tierarztl Prax Ausg K Kleintiere Heimtiere* 41: 297–303.

143 Pedersen, N.C., Eckstrand, C., Liu, H. et al. (2015). Levels of feline infectious peritonitis virus in blood, effusions, and various tissues and the role of lymphopenia in disease outcome following experimental infection. *Vet Microbiol* 175: 157–166.

144 Felten, S., Matiasek, K., Gruendl, S. et al. (2016). Investigation into the utility of an immunocytochemical assay in body cavity effusions for diagnosis of feline infectious peritonitis. *J Feline Med Surg* 19: 410–418.

145 Duthie, S., Eckersall, P.D., Addie, D.D. et al. (1997). Value of alpha 1-acid glycoprotein in the diagnosis of feline infectious peritonitis. *Vet Rec* 141: 299–303.

146 Quance-Fitch, F.J., Schachter, S., and Christopher, M.M. (2002). Pleural effusion in a dog with discospondylitis. *Vet Clin Pathol* 31: 69–71.

147 Kowalewich, N., Hawkins, E.C., Skowronek, A.J., and Clemo, F.A. (1993). Identification of Histoplasma capsulatum organisms in the pleural and peritoneal effusions of a dog. *J Am Vet Med Assoc* 202: 423–426.

148 Mavropoulou, A., Grandi, G., Calvi, L. et al. (2010). Disseminated histoplasmosis in a cat in Europe. *J Small Anim Pract* 51: 176–180.

149 Toribio, R.E., Kohn, C.W., Lawrence, A.E. et al. (1999). Thoracic and abdominal blastomycosis in a horse. *J Am Vet Med Assoc* 214: 1357–1360, 1335.

150 Nielsen, C., Olver, C.S., Schutten, M.M., and Twedt, D.C. (2003). Diagnostic peritoneal lavage for identification of blastomycosis in a dog with peritoneal involvement. *J Am Vet Med Assoc* 223: 1623–1627.

151 Bradford, K., Meinkoth, J., McKeirnen, K., and Love, B. (2013). Candida peritonitis in dogs: report of 5 cases. *Vet Clin Pathol* 42: 227–233.

152 Lemetayer, J. and Taylor, S. (2014). Inflammatory joint disease in cats: diagnostic approach and treatment. *J Feline Med Surg* 16: 547–562.

153 Fernandez, F.R., Grindem, C.B., Lipowitz, A.J. et al. (1983). Synovial fluid analysis: preparation of smears for cytologic examination of canine synovial fluid. *J Am Anim Hosp Assoc* 19: 727–734.

51

Pericardial Fluid

Shelley Burton and Etienne Côté

Introduction

Pericardial effusion fluid is routinely examined because pathologic accumulation in dogs is common.[1–4] It is less common in cats and virtually never causes tamponade in this species.[5–7] It rarely occurs in horses but can cause tamponade.[8–10]

Collection

Sample Collection

Pericardial effusion fluid is collected via pericardiocentesis for cytology and for relief of tamponade when present. Several approaches are described.[11–14] Fluid can be collected into lavender-top tubes (ethylenediaminetetraacetic acid anticoagulant), red-top tubes, sterile tubes for culture, and other tubes for specific tests.[15] Cytologic evaluation allows total nucleated and red blood cell (RBC) counts and permits flow cytometry or polymerase chain reactions (PCR) to be performed. Protein concentrations are determined via refractometry on fluid from lavender-top tubes, as is microscopic examination of stained direct, cytospun, or sediment smears. Fluid in red-top tubes can be analyzed for chemical substances.

Impact of Collection Method on Recovery Rate

Experience suggests that underlying disorders play a greater role in the diagnostic yield of pericardial fluid than does sampling method. Even if it yields a small fluid volume, pericardiocentesis can decrease intrapericardial pressures substantially, which helps patients but makes immediate re-centesis challenging.

Recovery Rate

The decision to perform pericardiocentesis implies that substantial fluid volume has been identified, typically separating the pericardium from the epicardium by >1 cm echocardiographically. While collection of larger volumes allows additional testing, obtaining as little as 1–2 mL allows cell counts, microscopic examination, and protein determination.

Contraindications and Complications

Insufficient pericardial effusion volume, uncontrolled hemostatic disorders, and briskly hemorrhaging cardiac lesions, such as left atrial rupture or hemangiosarcoma, are contraindications. Complications following pericardiocentesis are uncommon and generally mild, affecting 15.2% of dogs within 48 hours and mainly consisting of transient arrhythmias.[16] Similar data are not readily available for cats or horses. Death can occur following pericardiocentesis due to coronary artery laceration,[11] and avoidance of vessels on the left epicardial surface is the main reason pericardiocentesis is performed from the animal's right side.[11,13]

Normal Histologic Architecture and Cytology

The pericardium secures the heart to prevent excessive movement, lubricates the epicardial-pericardial interface, and provides a barrier to extension of infection or neoplasia.[17,18] It consists of an outermost fibrous parietal layer[19] and a delicate inner visceral layer, also called the epicardium.[20,21] The serosal surface of both is a thin monolayer of simple flattened mesothelial cells overlying connective tissue.[15] The pericardial cavity lies between the parietal and visceral layers.[17,21] In healthy dogs, it contains 1–10 mL of

Veterinary Cytology, First Edition. Edited by Leslie C. Sharkey, M. Judith Radin, and Davis Seelig.

serous fluid,[22] a clear, low protein, low cellularity fluid typical of a transudate.[23] Cells include mesothelial cells, lymphocytes, macrophages, and rare non-degenerate neutrophils.

Conditions Diagnosed by Cytology

General

As with other effusions, pericardial fluid is classified using nucleated cell counts and protein concentrations as neoplastic effusions, transudates, modified transudates or exudates,[24] or alternatively as low- or high-protein transudates or exudates (Chapter 50).[23] Fluids with protein concentrations and RBC counts similar to blood are simply classified as hemorrhagic effusions.[23]

Diagnostic Utility

Cytologic evaluation of pericardial fluid only rarely reveals a specific cause.[25,26] In dogs, many pericardial effusions are hemorrhagic irrespective of cause.[26,27] An early study found similar protein concentrations and nucleated cell counts in neoplastic and non-neoplastic effusions in 50 dogs.[28] Cytologic evaluation failed to identify neoplasia in 74% of cases and found a 13% false-positive rate in dogs free of neoplasia.[28] In a later study of 259 dogs, the overall diagnostic utility of cytologic analysis was only 7.7%, but increased to 20.3% in non-hemorrhagic effusions.[27] Despite the generally low diagnostic performance of pericardial fluid cytology, it can be diagnostic in cases of infection or exfoliative lymphoma. Therefore, cytologic examination is justified, particularly if a mass consistent with hemangiosarcoma or a heart-base tumor is not observed echocardiographically and if other features suggest infection or lymphoma.[26]

Differentiating Pathologic and Iatrogenic Hemorrhage

With bloody pericardial fluid, it is important to differentiate previous pathologic hemorrhage from obtaining blood during sampling. In addition to noting if the sample clots (suggesting blood) or not (suggesting effusion), cytologic evaluation helps. Following hemorrhage into a body site, platelets anecdotally are considered to disappear within approximately six hours. Based on equine or human studies, erythrophagocytosis by macrophages takes about one day to become evident,[29] and hemosiderin and possibly hematoidin formation takes two to three days.[30] Therefore, the presence of platelets and absence of erythrophagocytosis, hemosiderin, or hematoidin crystals (Figure 51.1) indicates peracute hemorrhage or iatrogenic blood sampling. Presence of both platelets and erythrophagocytosis or heme breakdown products supports ongoing hemorrhage or past hemorrhage combined with iatrogenic blood sampling.[31]

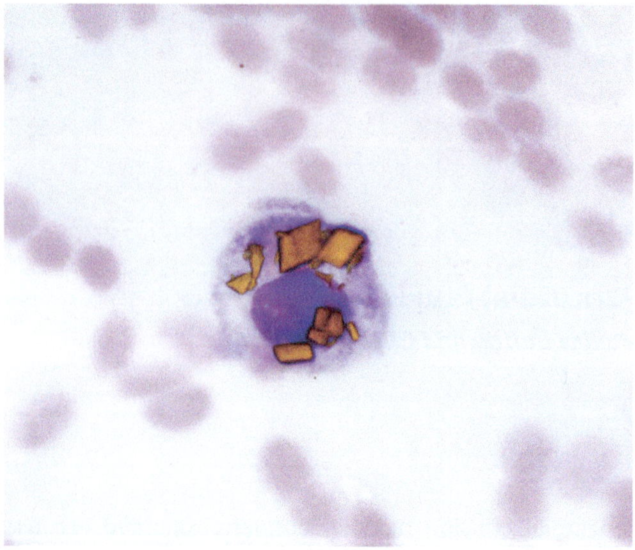

Figure 51.1 Macrophage containing hematoidin crystals in a hemorrhagic pericardial effusion from a dog (Wright-Giemsa, 1000×).

Mesothelial Cell Reactivity

Exfoliation of reactive mesothelial cells into pericardial fluid creates a substantial diagnostic challenge. With chronic effusions, especially if bloody, normally quiescent mesothelial cells proliferate and exfoliate as reactive cells. Cytologic differentiation of reactive mesothelial cells from those exfoliating from a carcinoma or a mesothelioma is difficult[15] to impossible. This is because reactive mesothelial cells (Figure 51.2) can exhibit striking cytomorphologic features mimicking those of malignant cells. Diagnosis is even more difficult when they are in large clusters.[32]

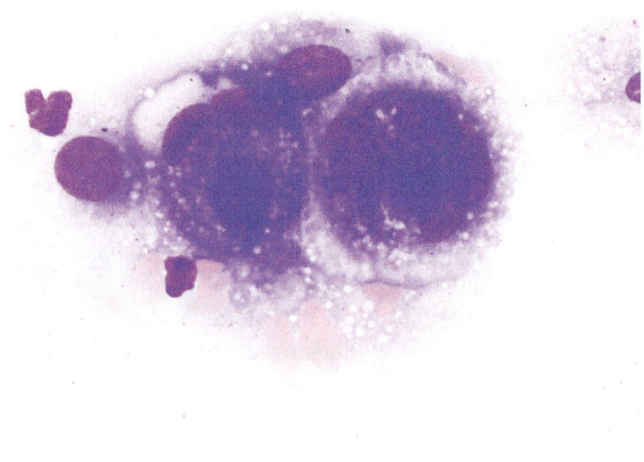

Figure 51.2 Reactive mesothelial cells in a pericardial effusion from a dog (Wright-Giemsa, 1000×).

Histology and sometimes immunohistochemistry (IHC) are typically needed for differentiation.[15,33]

Neoplasia

Benign

Benign pericardial tumors are uncommon in dogs and extremely rare in cats and horses. Lipomas may be the most common type in dogs. Radiographic and ultrasonographic findings, rather than fluid analysis, are distinctive. In reports of pericardial fluid cytology in dogs with cardiac lipomas, adipocytes were absent, and the fluid is described as iatrogenically or pathologically hemorrhagic[34] or reactive.[35]

Malignant

Pericardial effusion in dogs is most commonly due to neoplasia, making up 71% in one study.[4] From most to least frequent, canine tumors causing pericardial effusions are hemangiosarcoma, mesothelioma, and chemodectoma.[4,36,37] Although all can cause bloody effusions, a low fluid RBC makes mesothelioma or chemodectoma more likely. Other helpful considerations are that brachycephalic dogs are predisposed to chemodectoma, that concurrent hemorrhagic pleural and pericardial effusions favor mesothelioma, and that the echocardiographic location of mass lesions is informative. Other types of tumors are only rarely associated with pericardial effusions in dogs and cats. These include ectopic thyroid carcinomas[4], other carcinomas,[27] and lymphoma.[5,6] Although horses develop cardiac lymphoma,[38] reports of concurrent pericardial effusion were not found. Mesotheliomas causing pericardial effusion have occurred; one report in a horse describes the fluid only as serosanguineous.[39]

Hemangiosarcoma

Cardiac hemangiosarcoma represented 57% of canine neoplasms causing pericardial effusion in one study[40] and 69% of all cardiac tumors in another.[37] Thirty-five of 40 dogs with right atrial masses (88%) had hemangiosarcoma as the histologic diagnosis in one case series.[4] Large breed dogs are overrepresented.[37,41] Cardiac hemangiosarcoma has a high metastatic rate by the time of diagnosis.[37,41] These tumors typically are non-exfoliative and cause hemorrhagic pericardial effusions with mesothelial cell reactivity. This makes cytologic differentiation from idiopathic or mesothelioma associated effusions essentially impossible. A working clinical diagnosis of cardiac hemangiosarcoma is based on identifying a right atrial mass in a large breed dog with hemorrhagic pericardial effusion and acute tamponade. Definitive diagnosis is made histologically.

Mesothelioma

Mesothelioma can result in a large volume of pericardial effusion[19] which is typically bloody. It has been considered an uncommon cause of pericardial effusion in animals, but a recent study identified it in about 20% of dogs with neoplasia-associated pericardial effusions.[4] Pericardial involvement can occur in isolation or be combined with pleural or abdominal tumors.[19] Mesothelioma can present as a discrete mass or more often as diffuse infiltration.[4,42] Antemortem diagnosis is challenging. Pericardial effusion cytology typically does not differentiate between mesothelioma and other causes of effusion due to the variable features of reactive mesothelial cells.[28,42] Neoplasia was suspected cytologically in only 2/5 dogs with confirmed mesothelioma in one study.[43] A definitive diagnosis of mesothelioma can be difficult to achieve even histologically, and IHC often is necessary.[4] Cells from mesotheliomas typically express both epithelial cytokeratin and mesenchymal vimentin,[44] allowing differentiation from carcinomas, which typically only express cytokeratin. Several histologic variants of mesotheliomas occur, and one unusual lipid-rich pericardial mesothelioma in a dog was reported.[45] Routine echocardiographic examination does not identify mesotheliomas unless they produce mass lesions.[4,43] Cardiac magnetic resonance imaging can be used when echocardiography is inconclusive.[42]

Chemodectoma

Heart-base chemodectomas make up about 8% of canine cardiac tumors[37] and are found in approximately 10% of dogs with pericardial effusion due to neoplasia.[4,40] Pericardial effusion has been documented in 81% of dogs with heart-base tumors.[46] Brachycephalic breeds are overrepresented, possibly due to chronic hypoxemia.[47] Reports of chemodectomas exfoliating into pericardial fluid are lacking, but it is anticipated that exfoliated cells would resemble those directly aspirated from the tumor.[48]

Lymphoma

Lymphoma is an uncommon cause of pericardial effusion in dogs and cats, affecting only 2 of 164 dogs (1.2%) in 3 studies.[28,40,49] While rare, lymphoma may be the most common tumor causing pericardial effusion in cats. In an older study, 6 of 58 cats necropsied had pericardial effusion associated with neoplasia, with lymphoma accounting for 3 cases.[5] This finding is placed in the context of a historically higher prevalence of feline leukemia virus infection compared with today.[50] Pericardial effusion was described in two of seven cats with pericardial lymphoma; one was a protein-rich transudate and the other a neoplastic effusion.[51] In dogs, pericardial fluid cytology is often diagnostic, with a cytologic diagnosis of lymphoma achieved in 11/12 cases in one study.[52]

Inflammatory

Infectious

Rare case reports of dogs[53–55] and cats[56–58] with pericardial effusion due to bacterial infections exist, typically secondary to migrating foreign bodies.[4,19,59] Fungal infections causing pericardial effusion are even less common.[60–62] *Bartonella* spp. have been associated with pericardial effusions,[63] and although it is uncertain whether or how frequently bartonellosis causes these effusions, fluid culture and PCR may be worthwhile.[15]

Pericardial effusions associated with feline infectious peritonitis (FIP) occur but frequency has varied. In the past, it was listed with heart failure and lymphoma as one of the three most common causes of pericardial effusion in cats.[5] An older study documented FIP in 6/58 necropsied cats with pericardial effusions,[5] but a more recent study of 146 cases of feline pericardial effusion found only 1 cat with suspected FIP.[6] While characteristics of pericardial fluid due to FIP were not described in these studies, it is expected it would be similar to those of other effusions caused by this coronavirus.[64]

Pericardial effusions due to bacterial pericarditis are reported in horses,[9,65] with fluids typically having high numbers of nucleated cells; these are mainly neutrophils which may be degenerate with intracellular bacteria.[9]

Noninfectious

Idiopathic Pericardial Effusion

Idiopathic pericardial effusion refers to a sterile, often hemorrhagic effusion with no evidence of neoplasia, cardiac disease, trauma, infection, foreign bodies, or uremia.[19,66,67] In dogs, it is common and considered second in prevalence only to neoplasia[4,18], representing approximately 20% of pericardial effusions.[4] Males[63] and large breed dogs could be predisposed,[43,67,68] and age varies widely. Effusions typically are bloody and evidence of previous hemorrhage is common, as are reactive mesothelial cells. The ability of mesothelial cells to mimic malignant neoplasia prevents cytologic differentiation of idiopathic pericardial effusions from most neoplastic effusions.[43,67,69,70] Pericardial histology in cases of idiopathic pericardial effusion reveals fibrosis, mild inflammation, hemorrhage, and mesothelial hyperplasia.[66] Uncommon cases of equine idiopathic pericardial effusion have been reported, sometimes causing tamponade, and cytologically characterized by various inflammatory cells.[9,71–73] Fibrinous pericarditis with effusion was seen in three septic foals; the fluid from one was a modified transudate.[74] Fibrinous pericarditis in Kentucky horses was linked to caterpillar exposure, but it was not reported if pericardial effusion was present.[75]

Other Causes of Pericardial Effusion

Cardiac or Renal Disease

Right-sided congestive heart failure and renal disease can be associated with low-protein transudative pericardial effusions[5,40,76] but not tamponade. This is an important distinction because the effusion is not hemodynamically significant and pericardiocentesis is not warranted. Left atrial rupture due to mitral valve myxomatous degeneration is a risk of extreme atrial enlargement.[19,77] Hemorrhage from cardiac rupture following trauma[78,79] or spontaneously from thymic remnants[80] has been documented. Cytologically, these effusions are expected to resemble blood; this has not been specifically reported.

Chylous Effusions

Rare cases of chylous pericardial effusions occur, typically involving large breed dogs.[81,82] One involved a dog initially diagnosed with hemorrhagic idiopathic pericardial effusion that transformed into chylopericardium.[82] In these cases, nucleated cell counts and protein concentrations were consistent with high-protein transudates or exudates, and high triglyceride concentrations were diagnostic of chylous effusions.[83] Nucleated cells were variable proportions of neutrophils, macrophages, lymphocytes, and reactive mesothelial cells.

Miscellaneous

Uncommon causes of pericardial effusion include intrapericardial cysts[84] and hemorrhagic effusions following exposure to anticoagulant rodenticides[85] or penetrating trauma.[86] One case of cholesterol-based pericardial effusion was reported in a dog with hypothyroidism and aortic thromboembolism.[87] The pericardial fluid was characterized by a high cholesterol concentration and cholesterol crystals.

Advanced Diagnostic Techniques

pH

In principle, neoplastic pericardial effusions should have a normal pH, whereas inflammatory fluids could have a low pH due to organic acid production. An early study of pericardial effusions in 51 dogs was consistent with this concept,[88] but the opposite conclusion was reached in a later study.[89] Another study found that pH of pericardial effusions from dogs with idiopathic and neoplastic causes was not different and overlapped in 89% of instances.[25] Overall, it can be concluded that pH is a poor test for differentiating causes of effusion in dogs.

Cardiac Troponin-I

Cardiac troponin-I (cTn-I) is a marker for myocardial damage in dogs.[90,91] Blood concentrations typically are higher in those with pericardial effusion compared with healthy dogs.[92–94] Some studies identified higher blood concentrations in dogs with hemangiosarcoma compared with those with other tumors or non-neoplastic disorders,[92,94] whereas another study did not.[93] Overall, measurement of cTn-I concentrations in pericardial effusion fluid does not appear to improve sensitivity in distinguishing hemangiosarcoma from other causes, or indeed any type of cardiac neoplasia versus non-neoplastic causes.[93] To measure blood cTn-I, samples should be collected prior to pericardiocentesis to avoid confounding results through inadvertent cardiac trauma.[94] Reference intervals for blood cTn-I are instrument-specific,[95] and values can be mildly increased in healthy Greyhounds,[96] Boxers,[97] and dogs with renal disease.[98] While various troponin subtypes are used as cardiac biomarkers in cats[99] and horses,[100,101] investigation into blood or pericardial fluid concentrations in feline or equine patients with pericardial effusion was not found.

Other Biochemical Tests

Evaluation of biochemical analytes in canine pericardial effusions has produced inconclusive results.[25,28,88,89] In one study, pericardial effusion values for lactate, hematocrit, and urea nitrogen were higher, and values for pH, bicarbonate, and chloride were lower, in effusions caused by neoplasia compared non-neoplastic causes.[89] This study also found that the difference between blood and pericardial fluid glucose concentrations was greater in dogs with neoplasia than those without neoplasia.[89] However, the large degree of overlap in values between the two groups limited the value of testing.[89]

Flow Cytometry, PARR and Immunohistochemistry

Additional diagnostic tests include flow cytometry, PCR for analysis of antigen receptor rearrangement (PARR),[15,102] and IHC. Flow cytometry or PARR of pericardial effusion samples can support benign or malignant lymphocyte populations.[15,102] Immunohistochemistry can be performed on pericardial tissue.

References

1 Buchanan, J.W. (1999). Prevalence of cardiovascular disorders. In: *Textbook of Canine and Feline Cardiology*, 2e (eds. P.R. Fox, D. Sisson and N.S. Moïse), 457–470. Philadelphia: W.B. Saunders.

2 Smith, F.W.K. and Rush, J.E. (2000). Diagnosis and treatment of pericardial effusion. In: *Kirk's Current Veterinary Therapy XIII* (ed. J.D. Bonagura), 772–776. St. Louis: Saunders Elsevier.

3 Johnson, M.S., Martin, M., Binns, S., and Day, M.J. (2004). A retrospective study of clinical findings, treatment and outcome in 143 dogs with pericardial effusion. *J Small Anim Pract* 45: 546–552.

4 MacDonald, K.A., Cagney, O., and Magne, M.L. (2009). Echocardiographic and clinicopathologic characterization of pericardial effusion in dogs: 107 cases (1985–2006). *J Am Vet Med Assoc* 235: 1456–1461.

5 Rush, J.E., Keene, B.W., and Fox, P.R. (1990). Pericardial disease in the cat: a retrospective evaluation of 66 cases. *J Am Anim Hosp Assoc* 26: 39–46.

6 Hall, D.J., Shofer, F., Meire, C.K., and Sleeper, M.M. (2007). Pericardial effusion in cats: a retrospective study of clinical findings and outcome in 146 cats. *J Vet Intern Med* 21: 1002–1007.

7 Davidson, B., Paling, A.C., Lahmers, S.L., and Nelson, O.L. (2008). Disease association and clinical assessment of feline pericardial effusion. *J Am Anim Hosp Assoc* 44: 5–9.

8 Robinson, J.A., Marr, C.M., Reef, V.B., and Sweeney, R.W. (1992). Idiopathic, aseptic, effusive, fibrinous, nonconstrictive pericarditis with tamponade in a Standardbred filly. *J Am Vet Med Assoc* 201: 1593–1598.

9 Worth, L.T. and Reef, V.B. (1998). Pericarditis in horses: 18 cases (1986–1995). *J Am Vet Med Assoc* 212: 248–253.

10 Perkins, S.L., Magdesian, K.G., Thomas, W.P., and Spier, S.J. (2004). Pericarditis and pleuritis caused by *Corynebacterium pseudotuberculosis* in a horse. *J Am Vet Med Assoc* 224: 1133–1138.

11 Anderson EL. (2020). Pericardiocentesis. In: *Clinical Veterinary Advisor*, 4e (eds. L. Cohn, Côté, E.), 1150–1151.

12 DeFrancesco, T.C. (2013). Management of cardiac emergencies in small animals. *Vet Clin North Am Small Anim Pract* 43: 817–842.

13 Côté, E. (2015). Pericardiocentesis. In: *Clinical Skills Videos in Veterinary Medicine* (ed. E. Côté). St. Louis: Elsevier.

14 Prošek, R. (2017). Thoracocentesis and pericardiocentesis. In: *Textbook of Veterinary Internal Medicine*, 8e (eds. S.J. Ettinger, E.C. Feldman and E. Côté), 387–389. St. Louis: Elsevier.

15 Dempsey, S.M. and Ewing, P.J. (2011). A review of the pathophysiology, classification and analysis of canine and feline cavitary effusions. *J Am Anim Hosp Assoc* 47: 1–11.

16 Humm, R., Keenaghan-Clark, M.A., and Boag, A.K. (2009). Adverse events associated with pericardiocentesis

in dogs: 85 cases (1999–2006). *J Vet Emerg Crit Care* 19: 352–356.

17 Spodick, D.H. (1997). *The Pericardium: A Comprehensive Textbook*, 1–464. New York: Marcel Dekker.

18 MacDonald, K.A. (2017). Pericardial disease. In: *Textbook of Veterinary Internal Medicine*, 8e (eds. S.J. Ettinger, E.C. Feldman and E. Côté), 1305–1316. St. Louis: Elsevier.

19 Shaw, S.P. and Rush, J.E. (2007). Canine pericardial effusion: pathophysiology and cause. *Compend Contin Educ Pract Vet* 29: 400–404.

20 Holt, J.P. (1970). The normal pericardium. *Am J Cardiol* 26: 455–465.

21 Bezuidenhout, A. (2013). The heart and arteries. In: *Miller's Anatomy of the Dog*, 4e, vol. 428 (eds. H.E. Evans and A. de Lahunta). St. Louis: Elsevier.

22 Santamore, W.P., Constantinescu, M.S., Bogen, D., and Johnston, W.E. (1990). Nonuniform distribution of normal pericardial fluid. *Basic Res Cardiol* 85: 541–549.

23 Stokol, T. (2017). Fluid analysis: thoracic, abdominal, joint. In: *Textbook of Veterinary Internal Medicine*, 8e (eds. S.J. Ettinger, E.C. Feldman and E. Côté), 292–299. St. Louis: Elsevier.

24 Thompson, C.A. and Rebar, A.H. (2016). Body cavity fluids. In: *Canine and Feline Cytology: A Color Atlas and Interpretation Guide*, 3e (eds. R.E. Raskin and D.J. Meyer), 191–219. St. Louis: Elsevier.

25 Fine, D.M., Tobias, A.H., and Jacob, K.A. (2003). Use of pericardial fluid pH to distinguish between idiopathic and neoplastic effusions. *J Vet Intern Med* 17: 525–529.

26 Shaw, S.P. and Rush, J.E. (2007). Canine pericardial effusion: diagnosis, treatment, and prognosis. *Compend Contin Educ Pract Vet* 29: 405–411.

27 Cagle, L.A., Epstein, S.E., Owens, S.D. et al. (2014). Diagnostic yield of cytologic analysis of pericardial effusion in dogs. *J Vet Intern Med* 28: 66–71.

28 Sisson, D., Thomas, W.P., Ruehl, W.W., and Zinkl, J.G. (1984). Diagnostic value of pericardial fluid analysis in the dog. *J Am Vet Med Assoc* 184: 51–55.

29 McKane, S.A. and Slocombe, R.F. (1999). Sequential changes in bronchoalveolar cytology after autologous blood inoculation. *Equine Vet J* 31 (S30): 126–130.

30 Sherman, J.M., Winnie, G., Thomassen, M.J. et al. (1984). Time course of hemosiderin production and clearance by human pulmonary macrophages. *Chest* 86: 409–411.

31 Valenciano, A.C., Arndt, T.P., and Rizzi, T.E. (2014). Effusions: abdominal, thoracic, and pericardial. In: *Cowell and Tyler's Diagnostic Cytology and Hematology of the Dog and Cat*, 4e (eds. A.C. Valenciano and R.L. Cowell), 244–265. St. Louis: Elsevier.

32 Hirschberger, J., DeNicola, D.B., Hermanns, W., and Kraft, W. (1999). Sensitivity and specificity of cytologic evaluation in the diagnosis of neoplasia in body fluids from dogs and cats. *Vet Clin Pathol* 28: 142–146.

33 van Zandwijk, N., Clarke, C., Henderson, D. et al. (2013). Guidelines for the diagnosis and treatment of malignant pleural mesothelioma. *J Thorac Dis* 5: E254–E307.

34 Kolm, U.S., Kleiter, M., Kosztolich, A. et al. (2002). Benign intrapericardial lipoma in a dog. *J Vet Cardiol* 4: 25–29.

35 Brambella, P.G., Roccabianca, P., Locatelli, C. et al. (2006). Primary cardiac lipoma in a dog. *J Vet Intern Med* 20: 691–693.

36 Boddy, K.N., Sleeper, M.M., Sammarco, C.D. et al. (2011). Cardiac magnetic resonance in the differentiation of neoplastic and nonneoplastic pericardial effusion. *J Vet Intern Med* 25: 1003–1009.

37 Ware, W.A. and Hopper, D.L. (1999). Cardiac tumors in dogs: 1982–1995. *J Vet Intern Med* 13: 95–103.

38 Penrose, L.C., Brower, A., Kirk, G. et al. (2012). Primary cardiac lymphoma in a 10-year-old equine gelding. *Vet Rec* 171: 20.

39 Carnine, B.L., Schneider, G., Cook, J.E., and Leipold, H.W. (1977). Pericardial mesothelioma in a horse. *Vet Pathol* 14: 513–515.

40 Berg, R.J. (1984). Pericardial effusion in the dog: a review of 42 cases. *J Am Anim Hosp Assoc* 20: 721–730.

41 Boston, S.E., Higginson, G., and Monteith, G. (2011). Concurrent splenic and right atrial mass at presentation in dogs with hemangiosarcoma: a retrospective study. *J Am Anim Hosp Assoc* 47: 336–341.

42 Gallach, R.C. and Mai, W. (2013). Cardiac MRI findings in a dog with a diffuse pericardial mesothelioma and pericardial effusion. *J Am Anim Hosp Assoc* 49: 398–402.

43 Stepien, R.L., Whitley, N.T., and Dubielzig, R.R. (2000). Idiopathic or mesothelioma-related pericardial effusion: clinical findings and survival in 17 dogs studied retrospectively. *J Small Anim Pract* 41: 342–347.

44 Wallace, K.A., Goldschmidt, M.H., and Patel, R.T. (2015). Converting fluid-based cytologic specimens to histologic specimens for immunohistochemistry. *Vet Clin Pathol* 44: 303–309.

45 Avakian, A., Alroy, J., Rozanski, E. et al. (2008). Lipid-rich pleural mesothelioma in a dog. *J Vet Diagn Invest* 20: 665–667.

46 Vicari, E., Brown, D., Holt, D., and Brockman, D.J. (2001). Survival times and prognostic indicators for dogs with heart-base masses: 25 cases (1986–1999). *J Am Vet Med Assoc* 219: 485–487.

47 Hayes, H.M. (1975). An hypothesis for the aetiology of canine chemoreceptor system neoplasms, based upon an epidemiological study of 73 cases among hospital patients. *J Small Anim Pract* 16: 337–343.

48 Treggiari, E., Pedro, B., Dukes-McEwan, J. et al. (2017). A descriptive review of cardiac tumours in dogs and cats. *Vet Comp Oncol* 15: 273–288.

49 Dunning, D., Monnet, E., Orton, C., and Salman, M.D. (1998). Analysis of prognostic indicators for dogs with pericardial effusion: 46 cases (1985–1996). *J Am Vet Med Assoc* 212: 1279–1280.

50 Sykes, J.E. and Hartmann, K. (2014). Feline leukemia virus infection. In: *Canine and Feline Infectious Diseases* (ed. J.E. Sykes), 224–238. St. Louis: Elsevier.

51 Amanti, M., Venco, L., Roccabianca, P. et al. (2014). Pericardial lymphoma in seven cats. *J Feline Med Surg* 16: 507–512.

52 MacGregor, J.M., Faria, M.L.E., Moore, A.S. et al. (2005). Cardiac lymphoma and pericardial effusion in dogs: 12 cases (1994–2004). *J Am Vet Med Assoc* 227: 1449–1453.

53 Lorenzana, R., Richter, K., Ettinger, S.J. et al. (1984). Infectious pericardial effusion in a dog. *J Am Anim Hosp Assoc* 21: 725–728.

54 Casamian-Sorrosal, D., Fournier, D., Shippam, J. et al. (2008). Septic pericardial effusion associated with pulmonary and pericardial botryomycosis in a dog. *J Small Anim Pract* 49: 655–659.

55 Veloso, G., Franga Manteiga, E., Trehy, M. et al. (2014). Septic pericarditis and myocardial abscess in an English Springer spaniel. *J Vet Cardiol* 16: 39–44.

56 Lobetti, R.G. (2007). Anaerobic bacterial pericardial effusion in a cat. *J S Afr Vet Assoc* 78: 175–177.

57 Wolff, C.A., Fischetti, A.J., and Bond, B.R. (2010). What is your diagnosis? *J Am Vet Med Assoc* 236: 735–736.

58 Majoy, S.B., Sharp, C.R., Dickinson, A.E., and Cunningham, S.M. (2013). Septic pericarditis in a cat with pyometra. *J Vet Emerg Crit Care* 23: 68–76.

59 Aronsohn, L.R. and Gregory, C.R. (1995). Infectious pericardial effusion in five dogs. *Vet Surg* 24: 402–407.

60 Heinritz, C.K., Gilson, S.D., Soderstrom, M.J. et al. (2005). Subtotal pericardectomy and epicardial excision for treatment of coccidioidomycosis-induced effusive-constrictive pericarditis in dogs: 17 cases (1999–2003). *J Am Vet Med Assoc* 227: 435–440.

61 Langlois, D.K., Pelosi, A., and Kruger, J.M. (2013). Successful treatment of intracardiac and intraocular blastomycosis in a dog with combined azole therapy. *J Am Anim Hosp Assoc* 49: 273–280.

62 Ribas, T., Pipe-Martin, H., Kim, K.S. et al. (2015). Fungal myocarditis and pericardial effusion secondary to *Inonotus tropicalis* (phylum *Basidiomycota*) in a dog. *J Vet Cardiol* 17: 142–148.

63 Cherry, N.A., Diniz, P.P.V.P., Maggi, R.G. et al. (2009). Isolation or molecular detection of *Bartonella henselae* and *Bartonella vinsonii* subsp. *berkhoffii* from dogs with idiopathic pericardial effusions. *J Vet Intern Med* 23: 186–189.

64 Kipar, A. and Meli, M.L. (2014). Feline infectious peritonitis: still an enigma? *Vet Pathol* 51: 505–526.

65 Davis, J.L., Gardner, S.Y., Schwabenton, B., and Breuhaus, B.A. (2002). Congestive heart failure in horses: 14 cases (1984–2001). *J Am Vet Med Assoc* 220: 1512–1515.

66 Aronsohn, M.G. and Carpenter, J.L. (1984). Surgical treatment of idiopathic pericardial effusion in the dog: 25 cases (1978–1993). *J Am Anim Hosp Assoc* 35: 521–525.

67 Berg, R.J., Wingfield, W.E., and Hoopes, P.J. (1984). Idiopathic hemorrhagic pericardial effusion in eight dogs. *J Am Vet Med Assoc* 185: 988–992.

68 Gibbs, C., Gaskell, C., Darke, P., and Wotton, P. (1982). Idiopathic pericardial haemorrhage in dogs: a review of fourteen cases. *J Small Anim Pract* 23: 483–500.

69 Day, M.J. and Martin, M.W.S. (2002). Immunohistochemical characterization of the lesions of canine idiopathic pericarditis. *J Small Anim Pract* 43: 382–387.

70 Martin, M.W.S., Green, M.J., Stafford Johnson, M.J. et al. (2006). Idiopathic pericarditis in dogs: no evidence for an immune-mediated aetiology. *J Small Anim Pract* 47: 387–391.

71 Wijnberg, I.D., Vink-Nooteboom, M., and Sloet van oldruitenborgh-Oosterbaan, M.M. (1997). Idiopathic pericardial effusion with tamponade in a Friesian gelding. *Tijdschr Diergeneeskd* 122: 216–219.

72 Freestone, J.R., Thomas, W.P., Carlson, G.P., and Brumbaugh, G.W. (1987). Idiopathic effusive pericarditis with tamponade in the horse. *Equine Vet J* 19: 38–42.

73 Bernard, W., Reef, V.B., Clark, E.S. et al. (1990). Pericarditis in horses: six cases (1982–1986). *J Am Vet Med Assoc* 196: 468–471.

74 Armstrong, S.K., Raidal, S.L., and Hughes, K.J. (2014). Fibrinous pericarditis and pericardial effusion in three neonatal foals. *Aust Vet J* 92: 392–399.

75 Seahorn, J.L., Slovis, N.M., Reimer, J.N. et al. (2003). Case-control study of factors associated with fibrinous pericarditis among horses in central Kentucky during spring 2001. *J Am Vet Med Assoc* 223: 832–838.

76 Madewell, B.R. and Norrdin, R.W. (1975). Renal failure associated with pericardial effusion in a dog. *J Am Vet Med Assoc* 167: 1091–1093.

77 Nakamura, R.K., Tompkins, E., Russell, N.J. et al. (2014). Left atrial rupture secondary to myxomatosus mitral valve disease in 11 dogs. *J Am Anim Hosp Assoc* 50: 405–408.

78 Witt, A., Mathews, K., and Holmberg, D. (2000). Successful management of traumatic right atrial rupture. *J Vet Emerg Crit Care* 1: 85–89.

79 Yamada, K., Sato, F., Horiuchi, N. et al. (2016). Autopsy imaging for cardiac tamponade in a thoroughbred foal. *J Equine Sci* 27: 115–118.

80 Bradley, G.A., Tye, J., Lozano-Alarcon, F. et al. (1992). Hemopericardium in a dog due to hemorrhage originating in a heart base thymic remnant. *J Vet Diagn Invest* 4: 211–212.

81 Boston, S.E., Moens, N.M., and Martin, D.M. (2006). Idiopathic primary chylopericardium in a dog. *J Am Vet Med Assoc* 229: 1930–1933.

82 Groupil, A., Bolliger, C., Lapointe, C. et al. (2012). Embolised mesothelial cells in a tracheobronchial lymph node associated with idiopathic chylopericardium in a dog. *J Small Anim Pract* 53: 664–667.

83 Waddle, J.R. and Giger, U. (1990). Lipoprotein electrophoresis differentiation of chylous and nonchylous pleural effusions in dogs and cats and its correlation with pleural effusion triglyceride concentration. *Vet Clin Pathol* 19: 80–85.

84 Sisson, D., Thomas, W.P., Reed, J. et al. (1993). Intrapericardial cysts in the dog. *J Vet Intern Med* 7: 364–369.

85 Petrus, D. and Henik, R. (1999). Pericardial effusion and cardiac tamponade secondary to brodifacoum toxicosis in a dog. *J Am Vet Med Assoc* 215: 647–648.

86 Elliott, J.M. and Mayhew, P.D. (2011). Diagnostic challenges and treatment options of a suspected pericardial metallic projectile foreign body in a dog. *J Vet Emerg Crit Care* 21: 684–691.

87 MacGregor, J.M., Rozanski, E.A., McCarthy, R.J. et al. (2004). Cholesterol-based pericardial effusion and aortic thromboembolism in a 9 year old mixed breed dog with hypothyroidism. *J Vet Intern Med* 18: 354–358.

88 Edwards, N.J. (1996). The diagnostic value of pericardial fluid pH determination. *J Am Anim Hosp Assoc* 32: 63–67.

89 de Laforcade, A.M., Freeman, L.M., Rozanski, E.A., and Rush, J.E. (2005). Biochemical analysis of pericardial fluid and whole blood in dogs with pericardial effusion. *J Vet Intern Med* 19: 833–836.

90 Oyama, M.A. and Sisson, D.D. (2002). Cardiac troponin-I concentration in dogs with cardiac disease. *J Vet Intern Med* 18: 322–324.

91 Burgener, I.A., Kovacevic, A., Mauldin, G.N., and Lombard, C.W. (2006). Cardiac troponins as indicators of acute myocardial injury in dogs. *J Vet Intern Med* 20: 277–283.

92 Shaw, S.P., Rozanski, E.A., and Rush, J.E. (2004). Cardiac troponins I and T in dogs with pericardial effusion. *J Vet Intern Med* 18: 322–324.

93 Linde, A., Summerfield, N.J., Sleeper, M.M. et al. (2006). Pilot study on cardiac troponin I levels in dogs with pericardial effusion. *J Vet Cardiol* 8: 19–23.

94 Chun, R., Kellihan, H.B., Henik, R.A., and Stepien, R.L. (2010). Comparison of plasma cardiac troponin I concentrations among dogs with cardiac hemangiosarcoma, noncardiac hemangiosarcoma, other neoplasms, and pericardial effusion of nonhemangiosarcoma origin. *J Am Vet Med Assoc* 237: 806–811.

95 Adin, D.B., Oyama, M.A., Sleeper, M.M., and Milner, R.J. (2006). Comparison of canine cardiac troponin I concentrations as determined by 3 analyzers. *J Vet Intern Med* 20: 1136–1142.

96 LaVecchio, D., Marin, L.M., Baumwart, R. et al. (2009). Serum cardiac troponin I concentration in retired racing Greyhounds. *J Vet Intern Med* 23: 87–90.

97 Baumwart, R.D., Orvalho, J., and Meurs, K.M. (2007). Evaluation of serum cardiac troponin I concentrations in Boxers with arrhythmogenic right ventricular cardiomyopathy. *Am J Vet Res* 68: 524–528.

98 Sharkey, L.C., Berzina, I., Ferasin, L. et al. (2009). Evaluation of serum cardiac troponin I concentration in dogs with renal failure. *J Am Vet Med Assoc* 234: 767–770.

99 Herndon, W.E., Rishniw, M., Schrope, D. et al. (2008). Assessment of plasma cardiac troponin I concentration as a means to differentiate cardiac and non-cardiac causes of dyspnea in cats. *J Am Vet Med Assoc* 232: 1261–1264.

100 Van Der Vekens, N., Decloedt, A., Ven, S. et al. (2015). Cardiac troponin I as compared to troponin T for the detection of myocardial damage in horses. *J Vet Intern Med* 29: 348–354.

101 Rossi, T.M., Kavsak, P.A., Maxie, T. et al. (2018). Analytical validation of cardiac troponin I assays in horses. *J Vet Diagn Invest* 30: 226–232.

102 Lana, S.E., Jackson, T.L., Burnett, R.C. et al. (2006). Utility of polymerase chain reaction for analysis of antigen receptor rearrangement in staging and predicting prognosis in dogs with lymphoma. *J Vet Intern Med* 20: 329–334.

52

Abdominal and Thoracic Fluid Analysis in Dogs and Cats

Mary Anna Thrall

Introduction

Dogs and cats normally have a very small amount of fluid in their body cavities, of insufficient quantity to aspirate. Volume of fluid in the thoracic cavity of normal dogs is estimated to be 0.1–0.15 mL/kg.[1,2] Although it is not possible to aspirate adequate fluid for analysis from normal small animals, fluid collected postmortem from the costodiaphragmatic sinus of the pleural space of normal dogs was analyzed. The mean protein concentration was 1.06 g/dL, and the mean total nucleated cell count (TNCC) was 2200/μL. Seventy percent of the cells were mesothelial, 28% were monocytes, and 2% were lymphocytes.[1] A lavage technique in healthy humans allowed the determination of cellular content of normal pleural fluid, which contained a median of 1716 cells/μL, with a median of 75% macrophages, 23% lymphocytes, and 1% mesothelial cells.[2] Effusion develops when the amount of fluid entering the cavity exceeds the amount exiting. The type of effusion depends on the underlying cause. The protein concentration, TNCC, and types of cells present can help determine the cause of fluid accumulation. Determining the type of effusion will provide a differential diagnosis and sometimes a definitive diagnosis.

Normal body cavity fluid is an ultrafiltrate of blood and contains electrolytes, water, and small molecular weight substances such as glucose, with little protein and few cells. The fluid comes from the submesothelial capillaries and enters a body cavity via the submesothelial interstitium. The permeability of capillary endothelium and mesothelium to proteins and cells is normally low. The submesothelial lymphatic system has direct openings to the body cavities located between mesothelial cells, and these are important in reabsorption of fluids, cells, and proteins. The accumulation and removal of fluid depends on hydrostatic and oncotic pressure within the capillaries, increased vascular or mesothelial permeability due to inflammation, or decreased lymphatic absorption. In addition, other types of fluid, such as blood, chyle, bile, or urine, can leak into a body cavity.

Specific causes of pleural and abdominal effusions in dogs and cats include altered oncotic pressure, portal hypertension (PH), heart disease, suppurative or mixed inflammation secondary to infections, feline infectious peritonitis (FIP), neoplasia, hemorrhage, and leakage of chyle, bile, and urine.[3–12] In one study of 106 dogs, severe liver disease and protein-losing enteropathy were the most common causes of low-protein transudates, heart failure was the most common cause of high-protein transudates, and sepsis was the most common cause of exudates.[3] Neoplasia was the most common cause of effusions overall, although the admitting hospital had a large oncology practice that may have skewed results.[3] In older cats, abdominal effusions are usually due to neoplasia, while in younger cats, they are most commonly due to right-sided heart failure.[13] Pleural effusions in dogs and cats are typically bilateral, although only one side can be affected.[8] Bicavitary effusions commonly occur as a result of neoplasia, heart disease, bacterial infections, pancreatitis, and PH.[14] Urothorax with uroabdomen and bilothorax with bile peritonitis are described.[15,16] Combined etiologies are common. For example, inflammation can accompany heart failure, hemorrhage can accompany neoplasia, and neoplasia can result in high-protein transudate formation due to lymphatic or venous obstruction.[17] Neoplasia and heart disease also can result in chylous effusions.[18,19]

Clinical Signs

Clinical signs associated with thoracic effusions include shallow rapid breathing, a preference for sternal recumbency, head and neck extension, restlessness, and sometimes

Veterinary Cytology, First Edition. Edited by Leslie C. Sharkey, M. Judith Radin, and Davis Seelig.

cyanotic mucous membranes. Heart and lung sounds will be muffled, and a fluid line may be percussed. It is often best to remove fluid prior to imaging, since some structures and lesions cannot be seen with fluid present, and the stress of positioning can be fatal.

Animals with abdominal effusions can present with weakness, lethargy, and a pendulous abdomen if a large amount of fluid is present. Animals with effusions due to inflammation often have abdominal pain.[5] Radiographs prior to paracentesis are useful in dogs with a large abdomen to exclude pregnancy, pyometra, a large bladder, or splenic hemangiosarcoma that has not ruptured, all of which are considered by some to be contraindications to paracentesis.

Sample Collection

Body cavity fluids are usually easily aspirated using a 20–22 G needle and 12 mL syringe or a 20–16 G 1½ to 2 in. over the needle catheter. When obtaining abdominal fluid, the site is surgically prepped, and the needle is introduced either on the midline or just to the right of the midline and slightly cranial or caudal to the umbilicus. If omental fat blocks the needle, it should be withdrawn, and another site should be attempted. If fluid is not obtained, a four-quadrant paracentesis can be performed, in which right and left, cranial and caudal quadrants are aspirated as described.[20]

When obtaining thoracic fluid, the seventh or eighth intercostal space is used. Intercostal vessels can be avoided by inserting the needle in the middle of the intercostal space. To decrease the likelihood of lacerating the lung or major blood vessels, an intravenous polyethylene catheter is preferable to a needle. The animal is placed in sternal recumbency or a standing position. Sedation usually is not required and is typically contraindicated in patients with compromised ventilation. Approximately 5–10 mL of fluid should be obtained if possible and placed immediately in ethylenediaminetetraacetic acid (EDTA) to prevent clotting. If biochemical tests will be performed, fluid should be collected in either heparin or a red top tube without anticoagulant. If the presence of bacteria is suspected, fluid should also be collected in culture-transport medium.

Laboratory Evaluation

Physical properties of the fluid are noted, such as volume, color, transparency, clot formation if not in EDTA, and odor. Total protein of thoracic and abdominal fluid is measured using the plasma protein scale of the refractometer. Values correlate well with protein measured using the biuret assay, and the method is more rapid and convenient.[21] Although specific gravity can be measured using the specific gravity scale on the refractometer, it does not provide useful additional information other than as an index of protein content. If the fluid is cloudy due to the presence of cells, total protein determination by refractometry should be performed using the supernatant after the sample has been centrifuged, as the opacity of the sample will interfere with the refractometer reading. However, slide preparation and TNCC should be done prior to centrifugation. TNCC can be determined using either a hemocytometer or an electronic cell counter.

A fresh, direct film of the fluid is prepared using the pull technique (described in Figure 50.1). Films should be made immediately after sample collection, and TNCCs should be performed soon after collection. Cells deteriorate in samples stored at room temperature, particularly in fluids with low protein. Both intracellular bacteria and neoplastic cells can be missed in samples stored at room temperature for 24 hours prior to film preparation.[22]

Sediment preparations should be made on fluids that are clear, rather than opaque, as they likely have low TNCCs.[23] Cells can be concentrated by centrifuging the fluid, pouring off most of the supernatant, and then resuspending the cells in a drop of the effusion by "flicking" the tube with one's finger. Sediment films can then be prepared in the same manner as direct films. Alternately, cytocentrifuges are commercially available that sediment the cells in a small area in the center of the slide. The film is allowed to air-dry and then stained with a Romanowsky stain such as Wright's, Wright-Giemsa, or one of the quick Romanowsky stains.

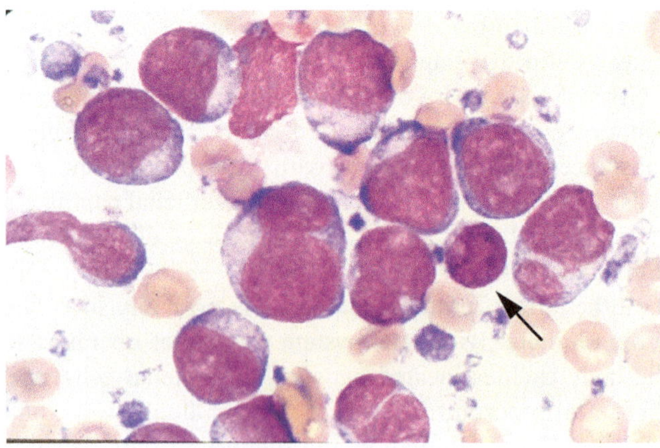

Figure 52.1 Lymphoblasts from thoracic fluid of a dog with mediastinal lymphoma. The cells are large and discrete with high nuclear to cytoplasmic ratio. A small lymphocyte is indicated by the arrow (Wright's stain, 1000×).

Microscopic Examination

The slide is examined at low power (10× objective), then with a 50× or 100× oil objective lens. The predominant cell type is noted, as well as the distribution of other cell types and the presence or absence of microorganisms. The 100× oil objective is often necessary for detection of intracellular bacteria. Most cells seen in effusions are those encountered on blood films or other types of cytologic specimens. Mesothelial cells that line the body cavities are often present.

A cytologic interpretation is based on cell types and concentration. If the TNCC is greater than 3000 cells/μL, the fluid is considered to be an exudate and can be associated with a variety of causes including sepsis, neoplasia, pancreatitis, post-surgery, uroabdomen, biliary disease, foreign bodies, necrosis, and lymphangectasia.[3] If neutrophils markedly predominate, the inflammatory response is considered to be suppurative (purulent or neutrophilic). When large numbers of neutrophils are present, the slide should be carefully examined for bacteria, usually within the cytoplasm of neutrophils. If both neutrophils and macrophages are present in large numbers, inflammation is considered mixed. If macrophages predominate, the inflammation is deemed mononuclear or granulomatous. If eosinophils predominate, the inflammation is eosinophilic, and if lymphocytes predominate, the effusion is classified as a lymphocyte-rich effusion.

Neutrophils

Some authors suggest that neutrophils are the predominant cell type in most abdominal effusions, whether the effusion is a transudate or exudate.[3] In a retrospective study, most transudates (defined as <3000 cells/μL) had ≥50% neutrophils, regardless of protein concentration.[3] In that same study, only 16% of all transudates (low and high protein combined) had less than 30% neutrophils.[3]

Neutrophils are usually well-preserved (nondegenerate) in non-septic inflammatory lesions, appearing much as they do in peripheral blood. As the neutrophils age, the nuclei can become hypersegmented and eventually pyknotic. In septic inflammatory lesions, neutrophils undergo rapid degeneration and eventual rupture. Karyolysis is characterized by nuclear swelling in which the nucleus becomes pink staining and smudged in appearance. Cytoplasm can become more basophilic and vacuolated, but cytoplasmic appearance is relatively unimportant in determining if cells are degenerate. Storage of fluid for several hours at room temperature before preparation of films will also result in degenerate neutrophils.[24] The cytoplasm of neutrophils should be examined for phagocytized bacteria.

Lymphocytes, Immature Lymphocytes, and Plasma Cells

Normal lymphocytes appear much as they do in peripheral blood. Immature lymphocytes and lymphoblasts are typically larger than neutrophils and have a small to moderate amount of cytoplasm, variably shaped nuclei that are usually round to amoeboid, and nucleoli within the nucleus (Figure 52.1). Lymphocyte-rich effusions (>30% lymphocytes) are usually associated with lymphoid neoplasia, thymoma, the presence of chyle, cardiac disease, and enteritis.[3,25] Flow cytometry is useful to differentiate small cell lymphoma from other disorders that result in non-chylous, lymphocyte-rich effusions.[26,27] Plasma cells are similar in size to small lymphocytes, but the nuclear chromatin is more dense, the cytoplasm is blue and abundant, and a perinuclear clear area (Golgi apparatus) is usually apparent. A few plasma cells can be present in effusions resulting from inflammation.

Macrophages

Macrophages in tissue and fluid are derived from blood monocytes. These cells phagocytize cellular debris, foreign material, and certain microorganisms, primarily mycobacteria. Other types of bacteria are less often seen within phagocytic vacuoles of macrophages. Neutrophils, cellular debris, erythrocytes, red blood cell pigments, lipids, and phospholipids are commonly encountered within the cytoplasm of these phagocytic cells. Macrophages range in size from approximately 12–100 μm, have a round to oval nucleus that may contain an apparent nucleolus, can be multinucleated, and have light blue, usually vacuolated cytoplasm.

Eosinophils

Eosinophils in fluids appear similar to eosinophils in peripheral blood and are associated with various causes of effusions, including heart failure; eosinophilic enteritis; allergic hypersensitivity; parasitic diseases; eosinophilic granulomas; collagen necrosis; and neoplasms, including lymphoma and mast cell tumors.[3,28–31] Aging eosinophils in fluids can develop a round, rather than lobed, nucleus (author's observation). Rounding of the nucleus may be part of a mechanism to release intact functional granules, rather than apoptotic death. Human eosinophils have been shown to lyse and release secretion-competent eosinophil granules. Initially, nuclear lobular formation is lost, and following nuclear chromatolysis, plasma membrane lysis liberates DNA that forms weblike extracellular DNA nets and releases free intact eosinophil granules that can be activated.[32]

Mast Cells

Infrequent mast cells can be seen in many types of inflammatory disorders, but if present in high concentrations, mast cell neoplasia should be suspected.[23] Mast cells are round cells with a round to oval nucleus and cytoplasm that contains purple granules. The granules occasionally do not stain well with quick Romanowsky stains such as Diff-Quik®.

Mesothelial Cells

Mesothelial cells that line the peritoneal and pleural cavity tend to proliferate and exfoliate when fluid accumulates in a body cavity. They can appear singly or in small clusters, and the clusters are usually infrequent (Figure 52.2). Mesothelial cells are large (12–30 μm), have light to dark basophilic cytoplasm, and have single or multiple, round to oval nuclei with one or more nucleoli. Cells in mitosis can be seen. The cytoplasmic border may appear to have a pink "fringe" around it. Helpful in differentiating mesothelial cells from carcinoma is the sheer numbers of cells present, as well as the size of the clusters. When carcinoma cells exfoliate, large numbers are usually observed in small to very large clusters.[23]

Microorganisms

Bacteria stain blue with Romanowsky stains and must be distinguished from background protein and stain sediment. They are usually relatively uniform in size and located in the cytoplasm of neutrophils. When in large numbers, they can be both free and phagocytized. Even small numbers of bacteria are significant. If multiple types of bacteria are seen, particularly in large numbers, gastrointestinal rupture should be suspected. Large and acute gastrointestinal ruptures can be difficult to distinguish cytologically from gastrointestinal aspirates, although higher nucleated cell concentrations would be more likely associated with rupture. Clinical signs of sepsis or evidence of severe inflammation in the leukogram (leukopenia, degenerative left shift, etc.) would suggest a rupture. If only one type of organism is identified, alternative sources such as liver, urinary tract, or reproductive tract are more likely.[33] For example, when large Gram-positive, spore-forming rods, suggestive for clostridial organisms, are seen, ruptured liver abscess or liver torsion should be considered (author's observation).[34,35]

Other types of microorganisms, such as fungal organisms, parasites, and protozoa, are rarely seen in body cavity effusions.[36–43] Pathogenic yeasts such as *Coccidioides*, *Blastomyces*, *Histoplasma*, and *Cryptococcus* spp. are associated with systemic infections, are sometimes observed in cavity fluids, and are easy to distinguish cytologically. In contrast, yeast like *Candida* spp. can colonize the abdomen after exposure to gut contents and have a more pleomorphic appearance.[41–43] Fungi and yeast stain blue-black with Gram stain and variably blue to colorless with Romanowsky-type stains.

Toxoplasma gondii tachyzoites can be seen in various tissues when systemic disease is present, including abdominal fluid (Figure 52.3).[44] Tachyzoites can be free or within various cell types, especially macrophages. They usually elicit a mixed inflammatory response. The organisms are blue with a purple nucleus, elongated and curved, and approximately 6 μm in length and 1 μm in width. Cytologically, sarcocystosis appears similar to toxoplasmosis.[30] *Neospora caninum*, another protozoan, also has been identified in abdominal fluid of a dog.[45]

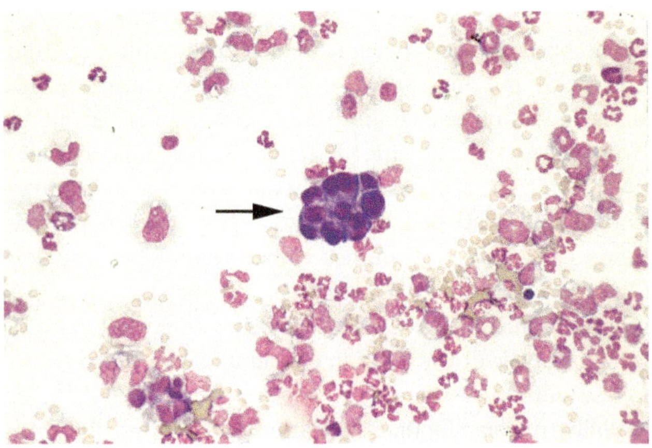

Figure 52.2 A cluster of mesothelial cells is indicated by the arrow. The fluid is inflammatory, as evidenced by numerous neutrophils and macrophages (Wright's stain, 400×).

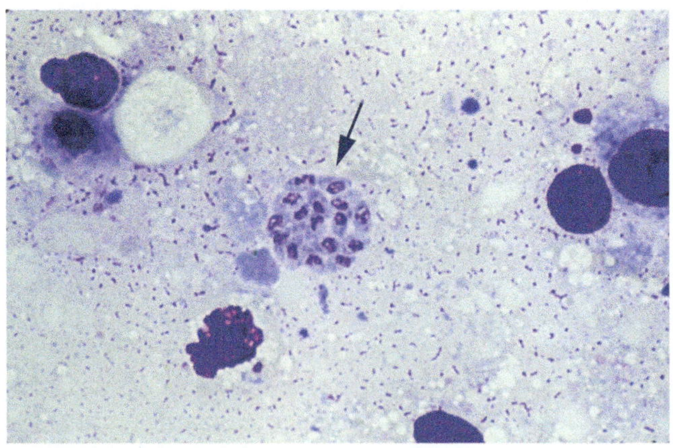

Figure 52.3 A group of *Toxoplasma* organisms (arrow) in abdominal fluid from a cat that also had feline infectious peritonitis. Note the large amount of protein in the background (Wright's stain, 1000×).

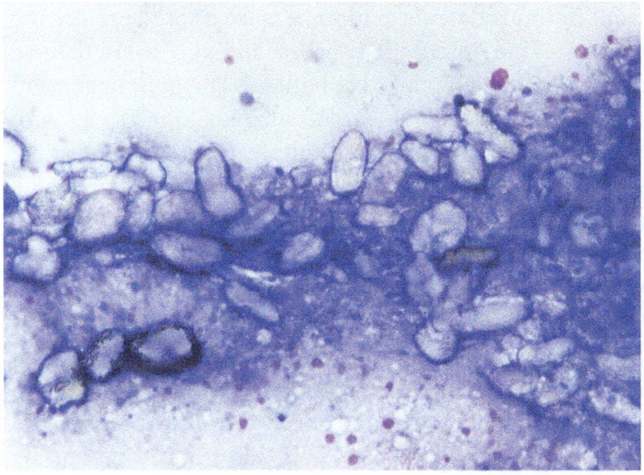

Figure 52.4 Calcareous corpuscles and cestode cellular debris in the abdominal fluid from a dog infected with *Mesocestoides* sp. Calcareous corpuscles are clear to refractile oval structures with occasional laminar appearance (Wright-Giemsa, 500×. *Source:* Image photographed by Judith Radin from glass slide provided by Jocelyn Johnsrude and presented at the 1999 ASVCP case review session).

Peritoneal cestodiasis in dogs caused by *Mesocestoides* spp. can be diagnosed cytologically by the presence of the tapeworm larvae or their remnants, including calcareous corpuscles, organelles specifically found in cestode stromal tissue. Calcareous corpuscles are round to oval, clear to golden brown, 20–30 μm in diameter calcified granules that appear empty or contain concentric rings (Figure 52.4).[40] Peritoneal cestodiasis caused by *Echinococcus* spp. is characterized by the presence of basophilic membrane-like structures that are approximately 60–100 μm wide as well as crystalline calcareous corpuscles.[39]

Classification of Effusions

Effusions are traditionally characterized as transudates or exudates.[12] Transudates are usually the result of decreased oncotic pressure or increased hydrostatic pressure. They typically have low cell and protein concentrations. Albumin in blood is responsible for maintaining oncotic pressure. Increased hydrostatic pressure can be systemic but is usually due to compression or blockage of vasculature and is discussed in more detail below. Effusions in which hypoalbuminemia is a contributing factor usually contain a very small amount of protein that may not be measurable by refractometry (<1.0–2.5 g/dL) and contain very few cells (usually <1000/μL). These are referred to as low-protein or pure transudates. Transudates with more protein are considered high-protein or modified transudates, i.e. modified by the presence of protein and cells.

Exudative effusions are usually the result of increased vascular permeability due to inflammation and contain significant amounts of protein and cells. Effusions caused by neoplasia or leakage of chyle, bile, or urine into the abdominal cavity have variable amounts of protein and cells and can fall into the low-protein transudate, high-protein transudate, or exudate category.

Historically, an effusion was considered a transudate if the protein concentration was less than 3.0 or 3.5 g/dL and the TNCC was less than 5000–7000 cells/μL.[3] Effusions were considered exudates if the protein and TNCCs were greater than those cutoffs.[3,12] This classification scheme can be confusing, because many effusions do not fall unequivocally into either category. For example, exudates due to inflammation can be very cellular but contain less than 3.0 g/dL of protein. Alternatively, effusions resulting from FIP typically contain a large amount of protein but relatively few cells. Effusions caused by neoplasia, or leakage of substances such as urine or chyle, may fall into either category.[46]

These cutoffs unnecessarily complicate the process of fluid analysis. An alternate approach is to categorize fluids as transudates or exudates by simply using a TNCC cutoff of 3000 cells/μL.[3] Transudates can then be further classified into low-protein transudates (<2.5 g/dL) or high-protein transudates (>2.5 g/dL).[3] More important than categorization of fluids as transudates or exudates is the ability to determine the probable cause of the effusion. This can be done based on cytologic findings in addition to the protein and TNCC.

Transudates

Low-Protein Transudates

Low-protein transudates (<2.5 g/dL) in dogs and cats most commonly result from decreased oncotic pressure, a consequence of hypoalbuminemia, or a combination of decreased oncotic pressure and increased hydrostatic pressure, usually pre-sinusoidal PH.[3,47] Hypoalbuminemia can result from inadequate dietary protein intake due to chronic starvation or malnutrition, decreased hepatic albumin synthesis, or increased albumin loss through the intestine (including malabsorption, parasitism, or hemorrhage) or urinary tract (mostly associated with glomerular pathology or hemorrhage). Liver failure/pre-sinusoidal PH and protein-losing enteropathy were the most common causes in one series of cases.[3] Rarely, a massive exudative skin lesion can cause hypoalbuminemia.

In many instances, the effusion protein is below the detectable range of the refractometer. The serum-effusion albumin gradient has been proposed as a way to distinguish transudates from exudates. The serum-effusion gradient is the serum albumin concentration minus the effusion albumin concentration. A gradient of 1.2 or less is considered indicative of a transudate.[48] In humans with transudative abdominal effusions, a serum-effusion albumin gradient of 1.1 or more is considered indicative of PH.[48] In a prospective study of dogs with transudative abdominal effusions, hepatobiliary disease could not be distinguished from other conditions using the serum-effusion albumin gradient.[49]

A serum albumin concentration of 1.5 g/dL or less has been stated as being necessary for formation of a low-protein transudate.[50] However, higher serum albumin concentrations of up to 2.5 g/dL can be present in dogs with low or undetectable amounts of protein in their effusion.[3] It is likely that increased hydrostatic pressure, in addition to decreased oncotic pressure, is also contributing to the effusion formation. It is also likely that some patients with very low serum albumin concentrations (<1.0 g/dL) have artifactually increased serum albumin concentration due to the bromocresol green (BCG) binding to globulins as well as to albumin.[50] It is estimated that the BCG method of measuring albumin, which is commonly used, may overestimate serum albumin by 0.5–0.6 g/dL and perhaps more if the albumin is extremely low.[51]

Low-protein effusions are also seen with prehepatic and pre-sinusoidal PH associated with portal vein hypoplasia, idiopathic hepatic fibrosis, or canine chronic hepatitis resulting in increased resistance in the terminal intrahepatic portal vein tributaries. The serum albumin in 17 dogs with low-protein effusions due to portal vein hypoplasia, hepatic fibrosis, or canine chronic hepatitis ranged from 1.9 to 2.6 g/dL.[47]

High-Protein Transudates

High-protein transudates (modified transudates) are most commonly a result of increased hydrostatic pressure, usually PH.[52,53] PH is the result of increased vascular resistance in the portal circulation, increased portal venous blood flow, or both.[54] It is classified as prehepatic, intrahepatic, or posthepatic. Prehepatic PH results from increased resistance in the extrahepatic portal vein due to obstruction or compression and, as mentioned above, usually results in a low-protein transudate. Congenital or acquired hepatic arteriovenous fistulas cause prehepatic PH because arterial blood flows into the portal venous system. Intrahepatic PH is due to increased resistance in the small portal veins, sinusoids, or small hepatic veins and is further classified as pre-sinusoidal, sinusoidal, or post-sinusoidal. Posthepatic PH is associated with obstruction of the larger hepatic veins, the caudal vena cava, or the right atrium as a result of right heart failure, pericardial disease, mass lesions, or pulmonary hypertension.[54] Most causes of PH result in transudate formation because of pressure driving fluid into the interstitial spaces and the overwhelmed capacity of the regional lymphatics.[54] The protein concentration of the effusion may reflect the anatomic location of PH. Prehepatic and pre-sinusoidal PH increases intestinal lymph formation; the intestinal lymphatic system has a large absorptive capacity resulting in a low-protein effusion.[47] Post-sinusoidal and sinusoidal intrahepatic PH, as well as posthepatic PH, increases hepatic lymph formation, resulting in loss of a high-protein fluid (>2.5 g/dL) through the sinusoidal endothelium. However, if synthesis of albumin is decreased due to severe liver disease, the protein in these effusions may be low. Portal vein pressure is rarely measured in dogs and cats, and the primary presenting abnormality of PH is usually ascites. Other common laboratory abnormalities associated with PH include microcytosis, increased postprandial bile acids, hyperammonemia, and ammonium biurate crystalluria.[54] If liver function is concurrently impaired, hypocholesterolemia and decreased blood urea nitrogen will usually accompany hypoalbuminemia. Hyperbilirubinemia, mild hypoglycemia, and decreased coagulation factors resulting in prolonged clotting times also may be observed.[54]

Cardiogenic pleural effusions in cats are usually protein-rich transudates, and measurement of N-terminal pro-B-type natriuretic peptide (NT-proBNP) has been proposed to differentiate cardiogenic from other causes of protein-rich transudates, although this is somewhat controversial. In one study of 78 cats, the quantitative ELISA performed using plasma and pleural fluid, and the point-of-care (POC) test in plasma but not pleural fluid distinguished cardiac from noncardiac causes of pleural effusion.[55] Others found that the POC test using plasma had a sensitivity of 65.4% and a specificity of 100%.[56] In other words, a negative test result did not exclude cardiac disease, but a positive test result indicated that cardiac disease was likely present.

Exudates

Inflammatory effusions (exudates) form in response to inflammatory mediators that increase capillary permeability. The result is fluid accumulation that contains a large amount of protein and numerous inflammatory cells, usually neutrophils and macrophages, although lymphocytes and eosinophils also can be observed. Inflammation is often the result of bacterial infections, although fungal, yeast, or protozoal infections also produce inflammatory effusions (Figures 52.5 and 52.6).[36–45] Neoplastic effusions can be exudates because of increased vascular permeability, inflammation, or exfoliation of tumor cells into the fluid. Effusions caused by leakage of chyle, bile, or urine can elicit inflammation and fall into the exudate category.[3]

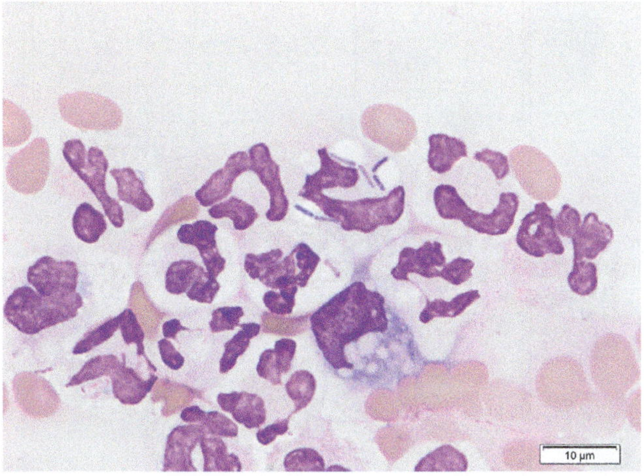

Figure 52.5 Abdominal fluid from a dog with a septic exudate. The TNCC was 27 000/μL, and total protein was 4.7 g/dL. Rod-shaped bacteria have been phagocytized by neutrophils. Neutrophils appear degenerate (Wright's stain, 1000×. *Source:* Image courtesy of Leslie Sharkey).

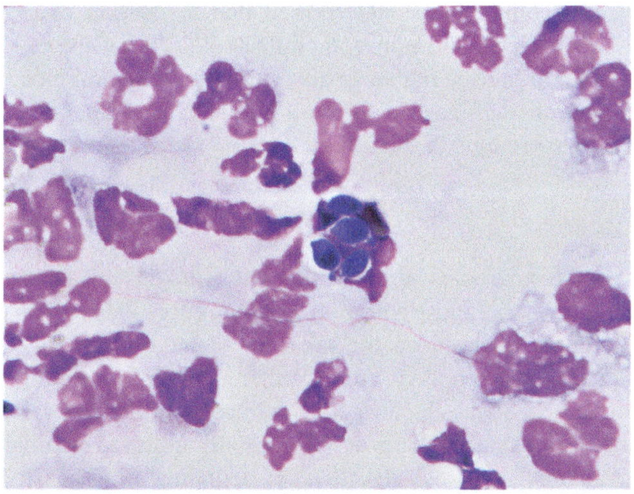

Figure 52.6 Phagocytized yeast with small, narrow buds in abdominal fluid from a dog. *Candida* sp. was cultured (Wright's stain, 1000×. *Source:* Image courtesy of Leslie Sharkey).

Rarely, the leakage of barium from the intestine results in peritonitis or complicates existing bacterial peritonitis (Figure 52.7).[57,58]

Specific Types of Effusions

Peritonitis

Causes of peritonitis include infectious agents such as bacteria, viruses, cestode larvae, and fungal or yeast organisms, as well as noninfectious agents such as sterile foreign bodies and caustic material such as bile or urine.

Bacterial (septic) peritonitis is diagnosed by identification of primarily intracellular bacteria on cytologic examination or a positive culture of properly collected and processed fluid (Figure 52.5). The TNCC is usually quite high in this type of effusion, reported to range from 8 600 to 194 000/μL in one study.[3] The inflammatory response is typically neutrophilic. Protein concentration is usually, but not always, greater than 2.5 g/dL.[3] The most common source of infection is the gastrointestinal tract. Other sources of infection are leakage from the urogenital tract, intra-abdominal abscesses, and the hepatobiliary system.[59] Primary (spontaneous) peritonitis is relatively rare (see below).[59–61] Organisms most commonly cultured from animals with peritonitis are *Escherichia coli*, *Enterococcus*, *Clostridium*, and *Streptococcus* spp.[59] Two or more species of bacteria may be present in some cases.[59,62,63] Although not observed cytologically, *Bartonella henselae* has been identified by enrichment culture and molecular testing of thoracic and peritoneal effusions.[64] The role of *B. henselae* in the pathogenesis of the effusions is unknown, and it is likely an opportunistic infection.[64] Abdominal surgery, the use of ulcerogenic drugs such as corticosteroids or nonsteroidal anti-inflammatory drugs, and perforation of the intestine by foreign bodies or neoplasms allow bacteria originating from the intestine to access the peritoneal cavity.[3]

Primary septic peritonitis, sometimes referred to as spontaneous peritonitis, occurs occasionally in dogs and cats and is defined as an infection of the peritoneal cavity without an identifiable intraperitoneal source of infection or history of penetrating wound.[60,61] The pathophysiology is not well understood, but bacterial translocation across the gastrointestinal tract wall is suspected, since diarrhea is often one of the presenting clinical signs.[60] Failure to detect a source of bacterial leakage during surgery or autopsy and bacterial contamination of the effusion during collection resulting in a positive culture can result in an erroneous diagnosis of primary septic peritonitis.[60]

Clinically, patients with septic peritonitis are categorized into three groups according to the severity of their organ dysfunction. Those without organ dysfunction have a relatively good prognosis, those with dysfunction of only one organ have a moderately good prognosis, and those with multiple organ dysfunction (kidney, liver, and lungs) and concurrent hypotension ("septic shock") have a very poor prognosis.[59] The reported overall mortality rate in small animals with septic peritonitis is variable, ranging from approximately 30–55%, but some are euthanized that might have recovered if treated.[9,61] Cytologic evaluation of effusions in which sepsis is a possibility is probably the only emergency or STAT (from the Latin word statum, meaning *immediately*) cytologic procedure, since antimicrobial

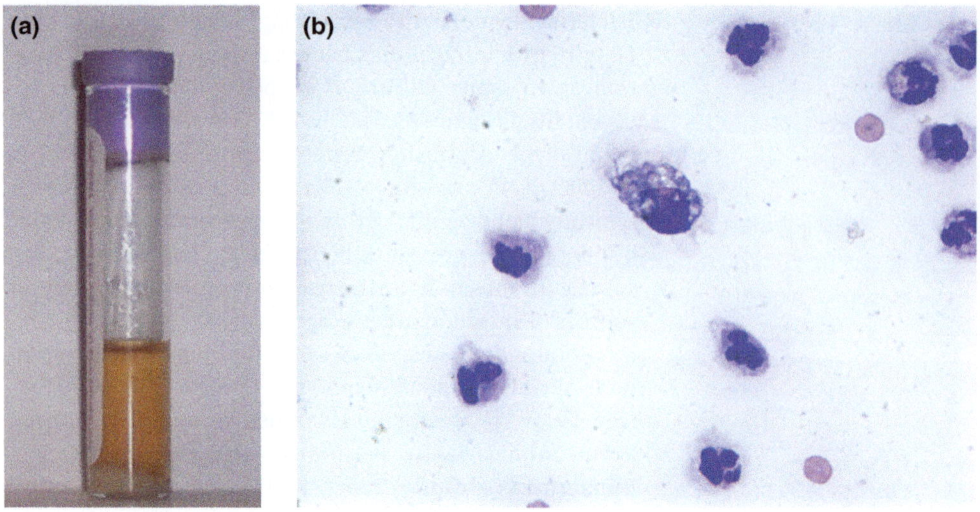

Figure 52.7 Thoracic fluid from a cat. Barium leaked from a ruptured esophagus. (a) Gross appearance of the fluid with barium sedimented to the bottom of the tube. (b) Barium appears as crystalline material that has been phagocytized by a macrophage and several neutrophils and is free in the background (Wright's stain, 500×. *Source:* Image courtesy of Leslie Sharkey).

therapy and surgery to correct the leakage of bacteria when appropriate should be instituted as soon as possible.

The accuracy of peritoneal fluid cytology to detect septic peritonitis is reported to be 57–100% in dogs and cats.[62,63,65] Biochemical analysis of peritoneal fluid, particularly to detect decreased glucose concentrations in the effusion, has been used to suggest sepsis. It is theorized that bacteria and/or neutrophils metabolize the glucose, resulting in the decrease. In one study, a difference between blood glucose and peritoneal fluid glucose was a reliable diagnostic indicator of septic peritoneal effusion in dogs and cats and was more reliable than using peritoneal fluid glucose concentration alone.[65] The peritoneal fluid glucose concentration is subtracted from the blood glucose concentration to determine the blood-to-fluid glucose difference (BFG). The diagnostic accuracy for the BFG when using a cutoff value of ≥20 mg/dL was 100% in dogs and 92% in cats compared with 89 and 100% for cytology, respectively.[65] However, in another study in which a veterinary POC glucometer was used to measure glucose in blood and fluid, the sensitivity using the cutoff of ≥20 mg/dL difference was only 41% with a diagnostic accuracy of 74%.[66] The inherent mild inaccuracy of a POC glucometer likely contributed to this difference in sensitivity.[66]

A blood-to-fluid lactate difference of less than −2.0 mmol/L was 100% specific and sensitive in dogs but was not useful in differentiating septic from nonseptic effusions in cats.[65] In other words, dogs with sepsis had significantly higher lactate concentrations in peritoneal fluid than in blood. Peritoneal effusion pH was lower in cats with septic peritonitis, but not in dogs, and a clinically useful cutoff value in cats could not be determined due to overlap of pH between septic and nonseptic effusions.[65] Potassium concentration may be higher in abdominal fluid than in blood in patients with gastric perforation due to the presence of gastric secretions in the fluid.[67]

Pyothorax

In one retrospective study of thoracic effusions in 81 dogs, pyothorax was most common.[10] A definitive diagnosis of pyothorax is based on the presence of large numbers of neutrophils in thoracic fluid. Bacteria within neutrophils can almost always be found. Protein concentration is variable but usually >2.5 g/dL. Commonly cultured aerobic organisms are *E. coli*, *Pasteurella*, *Actinomyces*, *Nocardia*, *Streptococcus*, *Staphylococcus*, and *Corynebacterium* spp.[10,11,68,69] Numerous anaerobic bacteria can be cultured, and mixed anaerobic bacterial infections are common in cats.[68] Although the source is often not determined, bacteria are thought to enter through a damaged thoracic wall, trachea, bronchi, lung parenchyma, or esophagus. The oral cavity and upper respiratory tract are common sources of microorganisms in pyothorax in dogs and cats.[69] In endemic areas, grass awn migration is a frequent cause of pyothorax in dogs.[70] Parapneumonic spread is thought to be the most common cause in cats.[68] Reported survival rates are approximately 83% in dogs and 62% in cats.[69,71,72] Successful outcome depends on timely diagnosis and treatment. An excellent review of pyothorax in dogs and cats, including diagnosis, treatment, and prognosis, is available.[69]

Feline Infectious Peritonitis (FIP)

FIP is a coronaviral disease that can affect cats of any age but is most common in cats that are 4–36 months old.[73] While some cats have a non-effusive or dry form of FIP, the majority of cats have abdominal, or less commonly, pleural effusion.[74] Most cats also have high serum globulin concentrations, usually a polyclonal gammopathy.[73] The effusion typically has a very high protein content that ranges from 3.5 to 9.8 g/dL, and fluid globulin concentration is consistently higher than albumin concentration.[75] Effusions from cats with FIP usually have a relatively low TNCC (<6000 cells/μL).[23] The high protein and globulin content in the effusion reflects that of the serum and results from leakage of proteins into the effusion due to serositis and vasculitis. The high protein/low TNCC effusion is so characteristic of FIP that it should suggest a presumptive diagnosis. Because of the high protein and the low TNCC, effusions caused by FIP often do not fit into the historical transudate/exudate classification. The fluid is usually straw colored to yellow, is quite viscous, and forms partial clots on standing. The inflammation is usually mixed, with neutrophils predominating. Neutrophils are mildly degenerate to nondegenerate, and a large amount of fine stippled background material representing protein is present (Figure 52.8).

Although the Rivalta test is commonly used to diagnose FIP effusions in Europe, it is rarely performed in the United States. The test was first described by Rivalta in 1885 and was designed to differentiate transudates from exudates.[76] Not only does the high protein content lead to a positive reaction, but high concentrations of fibrinogen and inflammatory mediators play a role.[77] To perform this test, a transparent 10 mL reagent tube is filled with approximately 7–8 mL of distilled water, to which one drop of 98% acetic acid is added and mixed thoroughly. One drop of the effusion fluid is layered on the surface of this solution. If the drop disappears and the solution remains clear, Rivalta's test is negative. If the drop retains its shape, stays attached to the surface or slowly floats down to the bottom of the tube, Rivalta's test is positive. Diseases other than FIP that produce positive Rivalta tests are lymphoma and bacterial peritonitis, which can usually be distinguished by cytologic evaluation of the fluid.[78] In one study, the Rivalta test had a sensitivity of 91.3%, specificity of 65.5%, positive predictive value of 58.4%, and negative predictive value of 93.4% for the diagnosis of FIP.[78] These values improved when cats with lymphoma or bacterial infections were excluded or when only cats less than 2 years of age were considered. Sensitivity, specificity, and positive predictive value of the Rivalta test for the diagnosis of FIP were lower than previously reported except when used in young cats.[78]

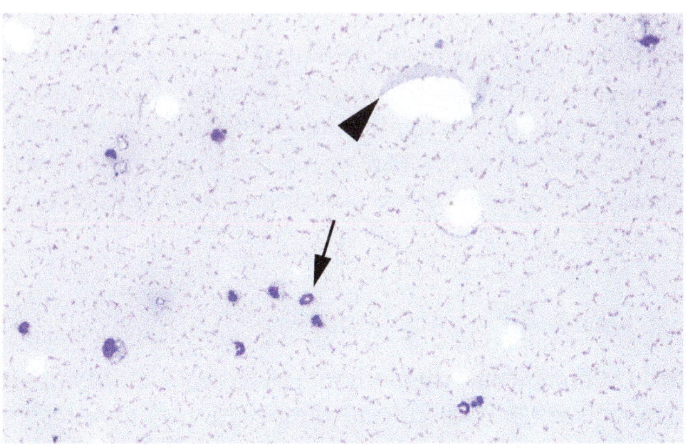

Figure 52.8 Abdominal fluid from a cat with feline infectious peritonitis. Note the relatively few neutrophils present (arrow). The high protein content of the fluid is evidenced by the background amorphous stippled appearance as well as the peeling up of the protein, crescent-shaped areas (arrowhead) (Wright's stain, 400×).

The diagnostic gold standard is still histopathology for visualization of the classic lesions associated with FIP, often in combination with supporting immunohistochemistry for the presence of virus. Molecular tests can be used to help confirm a diagnosis of FIP, such as detection of viral RNA in blood or fluid by reverse transcriptase polymerase chain reaction.[74,79,80] Interpretation of molecular tests are complicated by the presence of healthy coronavirus shedding cats, low numbers of infected macrophages in peritoneal fluid, and molecular overlap of enteric and FIP coronaviruses.[74,79,80] This necessitates use of more than one test, often in conjunction with histopathology, for antemortem diagnosis.

Neoplastic Effusions

Neoplastic effusions can be either transudates or exudates. In one study of 26 neoplastic effusions, three were low-protein transudates, nine were high-protein transudates, and 14 were exudates.[3] The total protein is variable, as is the TNCC. Neoplastic cells can shed into the effusion, particularly if the tumor is epithelial (carcinoma), lymphoid (lymphoma), or less commonly a mast cell tumor or mesothelial tumor (mesothelioma). Sarcomas usually do not exfoliate, although osteosarcoma cells and myxosarcoma cells in pleural effusions are reported.[81,82] In one study of 424 body cavity effusions, malignant tumors were found in 18% of effusions from dogs and 25% of effusions from cats.[83] Approximately 50% of the tumors in both dogs and cats were carcinomas, and approximately 50% of the tumors in cats were discrete cell tumors. The sensitivity of cytologic evaluation for the detection of neoplasia in body cavity effusions was 64% for dogs and 61% for cats.

The specificity was 99% for dogs and 100% for cats.[83] The absence of neoplastic cells in an effusion does not exclude the possibility of neoplasia. In other words, neoplasia can be missed by cytologic evaluation, usually because the tumor is not shedding cells, and neoplasia is rarely falsely diagnosed if the cytologist is experienced.

Neoplastic epithelial cells can be difficult to distinguish from reactive mesothelial cells that are shed from the pleural or peritoneal lining of body cavities. Epithelial origin can be confirmed by immunocytochemical labeling for cytokeratin.[84,85] Epithelial cells are quite variable in size but are usually larger than mesothelial cells. Carcinoma cells typically exhibit numerous criteria of malignancy, including variability in nuclear size, giant nuclei, large atypical nucleoli, numerous cells in mitosis, and nuclear molding (Figure 52.9). Cell cannibalism can be seen in highly malignant tumors.[86] When epithelial cells are present in clusters, they tend to have cell-to-cell association or bridging. Glandular (exocrine) epithelial cells can have moderate to abundant vacuolated cytoplasm. The origin of the carcinoma usually cannot be determined based on cytology of effusions, although a high sensitivity and specificity for diagnosis of ovarian carcinomas has been reported in dogs, due to the characteristic uniform papillary pattern of the cells shed from this tumor.[87] One extremely rare potential complication when aspirating fluid containing carcinoma cells is the seeding of neoplastic cells along the needle tract.[85,88]

Lymphoma is diagnosed by the presence of large immature lymphocytes or lymphoblasts in effusions (Figure 52.1). Mediastinal lymphoma can result in pleural effusion in both dogs and cats. In one series of 42 dogs with mediastinal lymphoma, 45% had pleural effusions.[89] Pleural effusions in dogs with mediastinal lymphoma are usually lymphoblastic and are of T-cell phenotype.[89] Hypercalcemia of malignancy in dogs with mediastinal T-cell lymphoma is common. Of the 42 dogs, 67% were hypercalcemic, with a mean total calcium of 15.5 mg/dL (range from 11.4 to 19.0 mg/dL).[89] In cats, mediastinal lymphoma is more common in younger animals and in Siamese cats, while abdominal lymphoma is more common in older cats.[90] Abdominal lymphoma, most commonly intestinal, can result in abdominal effusions. Gastrointestinal perforation due to intestinal lymphoma in cats occurs occasionally and usually results in a septic suppurative effusion that also contains lymphoblasts.[91] Small cell variants of lymphoma resulting in effusions are difficult to distinguish from nonneoplastic lymphocyte-rich effusions. Flow cytometry can be helpful in these cases.[26]

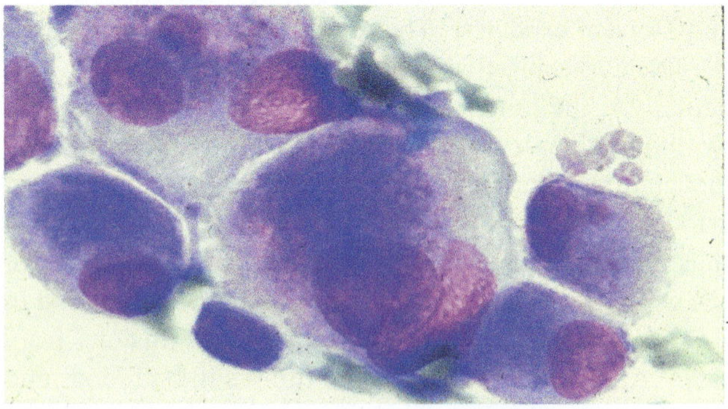

Figure 52.9 A cluster of carcinoma cells in body cavity effusion exhibiting numerous criteria of malignancy, including variable-sized nuclei, nuclear molding, and prominent nucleoli (Wright's stain, 1000×).

Mesotheliomas are rare and can be difficult to distinguish cytologically from carcinomas, especially if they are epitheliod.[92] The presence of a brush border (microvilli) on the neoplastic mesothelial cells may be helpful.[93] Although rare in general, they are the most common papillary tumor in the thorax.[94] The nuclear to cytoplasmic ratio ranges from low to high, and small gray-pink granules have been reported in the cytoplasm.[94] The neoplastic mesothelial cells can appear much like hyperplastic mesothelial cells, or they can appear highly malignant, with multinucleation and multiple large nucleoli. The more highly malignant they are in appearance, the more difficult they are to distinguish from carcinoma cells.[23] Concurrent staining with cytokeratin and vimentin can support a diagnosis of mesothelioma; however, normal and reactive mesothelial cells as well as some carcinomas also can be double labeled.[84,85,92–95] As in humans, mesotheliomas in dogs may be associated with exposure to asbestos.[96]

Biochemical analysis of neoplastic versus nonneoplastic abdominal effusions was evaluated in a relatively small group of dogs (eight with various neoplasms, seven with nonneoplastic effusions).[97] Fluid glucose concentration was significantly lower in dogs with neoplastic effusions, and fluid lactate was significantly higher.[97] However, utility compared with cytology was not evaluated. As stated above, similar findings are observed in septic effusions in dogs that may confound interpretation.[65,66]

Hemoabdomen and Hemothorax

Hemoabdomen and hemothorax are the result of active hemorrhage. The packed cell volume (PCV) or erythrocyte count is used to determine the amount of blood present. Some have defined an effusion as hemorrhagic if the PCV is at least 25% that of the peripheral blood.[98] One study defines a hemorrhagic effusion as containing >500 000 erythrocytes/μL.[3] In hemorrhagic effusions, platelets are rarely observed, and the fluid usually does not clot.

Peripheral blood contamination of the sample is suspected if platelets are observed. Phagocytosis of erythrocytes by macrophages can be seen within a few hours following bleeding. Erythrocyte breakdown products such as hemosiderin and hematoidin are usually observed in macrophages within 72 hours following the onset of hemorrhage and can persist for at least two months.[99] However, erythrophagocytosis also occurs *in vitro* if the sample remains in the tube for several hours before the cytologic preparation is made. The PCV of the fluid can be higher than that of the peripheral blood, since serum is reabsorbed more quickly than erythrocytes. Hemoabdomen in dogs is most commonly associated with trauma, coagulopathy, or neoplasia, usually as a result of vessel erosion, but sometimes as a result of neoplasia-induced disseminated intravascular coagulopathy.[100,101] Hemoabdomen and hemothorax are commonly seen in patients with vitamin K antagonist anticoagulant rodenticide toxicity, resulting in coagulopathy.[102,103]

In 83 dogs with hemoabdomen, the source of hemorrhage was the spleen in 75 (90%).[104] In dogs with nontraumatic hemoabdomen, hemangiosarcoma was found in 63%, splenic hematoma in 27%, splenic torsion in 5%, and neoplasia other than hemangiosarcoma in approximately 5%.[105] In 71 dogs with a splenic mass and hemoabdomen, 50 (70%) had a ruptured hemangiosarcoma.[101] Although acanthocytes can occasionally be seen in hemoabdomen resulting from hemangiosarcoma (Figure 52.10), one report of 40 dogs with hemoabdomen found that acanthocytes in the abdominal fluid were not diagnostically useful in determining if the hemorrhage was secondary to hemangiosarcoma.[106] Hemoabdomen in cats results from trauma, coagulopathy, and neoplasia, most commonly hemangiosarcoma of the spleen.[107]

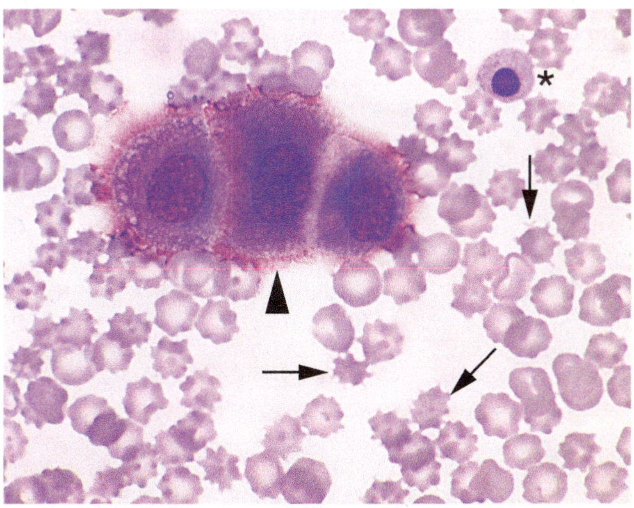

Figure 52.10 Abdominal fluid from a dog with hemoabdomen secondary to ruptured hemangiosarcoma. Note the nucleated erythrocyte (asterisk), acanthocytes (arrows), and cluster of normal-appearing mesothelial cells (arrowhead) (Wright stain, 1000×).

Hemothorax in dogs and cats is most commonly caused by traumatic rupture of blood vessels, coagulopathy, or erosion of vessels by neoplasia, often involving the thoracic wall. The most common presenting signs are tachypnea and lethargy.[108] Extracardiac intrathoracic hemangiosarcoma has been reported to cause spontaneous hemothorax.[109] Lung lobe torsion has also been reported to cause hemothorax in both dogs and cats.[110] Other reported causes in cats include *Dirofilaria immitis* and pulmonary fat embolism secondary to subcutaneous trauma.[111,112] Autologous blood transfusion, using the blood from the thoracic or abdominal cavity as a bridge to hemorrhage control, has been used successfully.[113]

Chylous Effusions

Chylous effusions result from the accumulation of chyle (lymph), usually within the pleural cavity but occasionally in the peritoneal cavity.[114] This occurs due to impaired lymphatic drainage or leakage. The primary lymphatic vessel within the thorax is the thoracic duct, which returns lymph and chyle from the intestines and liver to the venous system at a point where the jugular veins meet the cranial vena cava. Dyspnea and coughing are common presenting clinical signs in patients with chylothorax.[115] The gross appearance of the fluid is typically white and opaque due to the presence of chylomicrons (Figure 52.11). If erythrocytes are present, they will impart a pink color to the fluid. On standing, the lipids may float to the top of the fluid. If the animal is not eating, the fluid may not contain chylomicrons and thus not be white and opaque.

The TNCC of chylous effusions is variable.[23] Initially, almost all cells present are small, normal-appearing lymphocytes. Over time, however, the accumulation of chyle can elicit an inflammatory reaction, and more neutrophils and macrophages are seen. Occasionally very small clear lipid droplets are observed in the background or within neutrophils and macrophages, and these will stain positive with fat stains such as Sudan III. The total protein estimate by refractometry is usually erroneously high due to the opacity of the fluid.

Triglyceride concentration of chylous fluid is greater than in serum or other types of effusions.[116] Although fluid cholesterol:triglyceride ratio of less than one is usually considered very suggestive of chylous effusion, some dogs and cats with non-chylous effusion also have a cholesterol:triglyceride ratio of less than one. Pleural effusions with triglyceride concentrations greater than

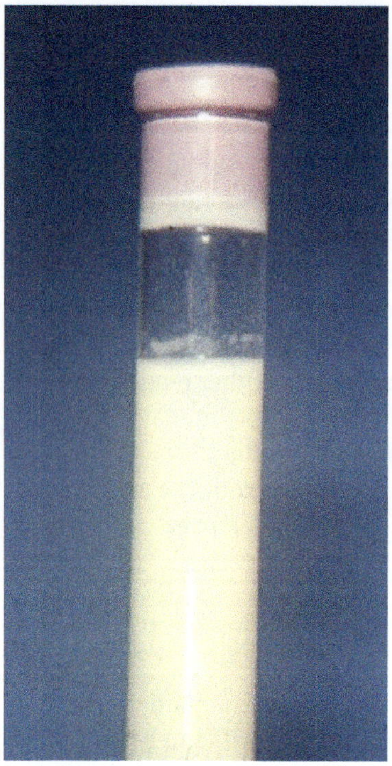

Figure 52.11 Gross appearance of chylous thoracic effusion from a cat.

100 mg/dL are almost always chylous.[117] Fluid triglyceride concentration is the definitive diagnostic test of choice.

Patients with chylothorax can have unilateral effusions, but more commonly the effusion is bilateral.[115] The cause of chylothorax is usually idiopathic, although underlying lung lobe torsion, neoplasia, obstructed vena cava, heart disease, inflammation, and trauma are reported.[18,19,118–122] If lymphoma or carcinoma is the underlying cause, neoplastic cells can be seen in the effusion. Chylothorax is treated either medically or surgically.[8] When treated medically without improvement after four weeks, thoracic duct ligation and pericardiectomy is recommended in order to avoid the complications of constrictive pleuritis and pericarditis.[123,124] Complications following repeated thoracocentesis include bacterial infections, hypoproteinemia, and rarely, electrolyte abnormalities.[125,126] Abdominal chylous effusions can result from a ruptured mesenteric lymphatic or abdominal lymphatic obstruction.[114,127]

Some effusions are sometimes referred to as pseudochylous, because of either their milky appearance or the presence of predominantly lymphocytes in the effusion. Although they have been described in humans, milk-colored effusions that are not chylous are very rare in dogs and cats.[125] Non-chylous fluids that contain predominantly small lymphocytes should be referred to as lymphocyte-rich effusions, rather than pseudochylous effusions.[25] Lymphocyte-rich effusions in cats are usually due to heart disease but may be seen with small cell variants of lymphoma or thymoma.[25]

Bile Peritonitis and Bilothorax

The total protein content and TNCC of biliary effusions are quite variable and somewhat dependent on whether the effusion is sterile or septic. If the effusion is septic, neutrophils will predominate, and bacteria will be present. In acute sterile biliary effusions, macrophages may predominate. The protein content is usually greater than 2.5 g/dL and ranged from 2.9 to 5.6 g/dL in one study.[128] The fluid is usually green to orange in color (Figure 52.12). Bile pigment appears as golden colored to green, somewhat granular pigment that is black in color once it has been phagocytized by macrophages (Figure 52.13). More rarely, only mucinous material that does not stain positive for bilirubin is observed (Figure 52.14); however, the bilirubin concentration of the fluid is still greater than the contemporary serum bilirubin concentration.[128]

The abdominal fluid bilirubin concentration is typically at least twofold greater than that of serum.[129] Rarely, gall bladder rupture and no increase in serum bilirubin can occur, indicating that if gall bladder rupture is suspected, the diagnosis should not be excluded based on a normal serum bilirubin concentration.[130] In those cases, comparison of serum to abdominal fluid bile acid concentrations may be helpful.[130]

Bile peritonitis is usually due to leakage from the biliary tract secondary to trauma, necrotizing cholecystitis, or ruptured gallbladder mucocele.[129,131] The prognosis is better in animals with sterile biliary effusions.[128] Bilothorax rarely occurs in dogs and cats.[8,16,132,133] The diaphragm may be

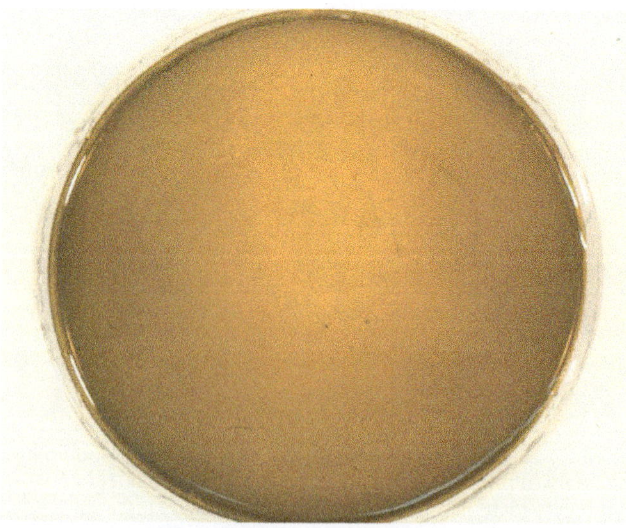

Figure 52.12 Gross appearance of abdominal fluid containing bile from a dog with a ruptured bile duct.

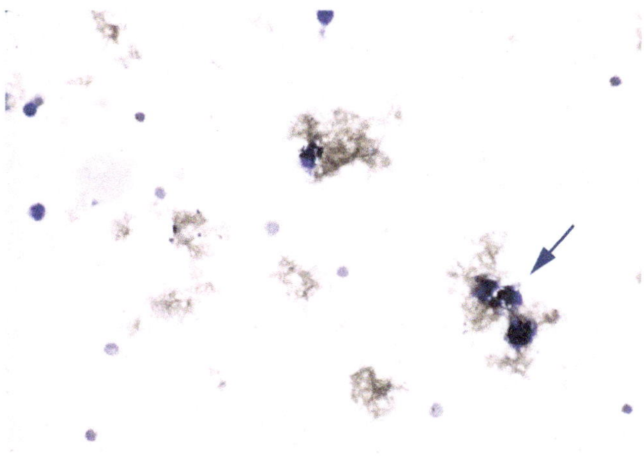

Figure 52.13 Abdominal fluid from a dog with bile peritonitis. The free golden colored amorphous material is representative of bile. When phagocytized by macrophages, it appears black (arrow) (Wright's stain, 200×).

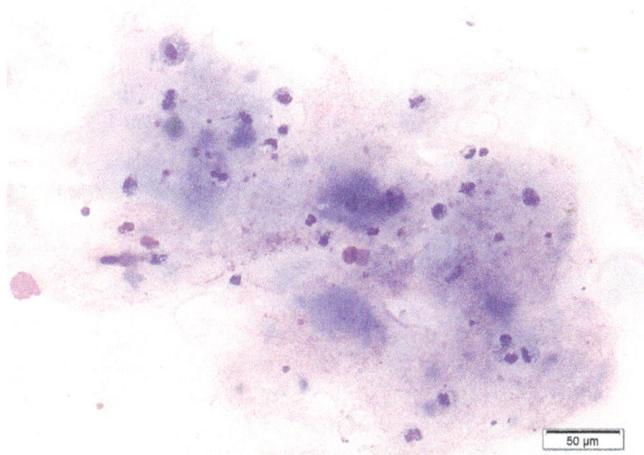

Figure 52.14 Mucinous fibrillar material in clumps and lakes in the abdominal fluid from a dog with bile peritonitis. The fluid is inflammatory with neutrophils and occasional foamy mononuclear cells (Wright's stain. *Source:* Image courtesy of Leslie Sharkey).

ruptured or intact. When intact, it is thought that the bile crosses the diaphragm via lymphatics and subsequently leaks into the pleural space.[8]

Uroabdomen and Urothorax

Leakage of urine from the bladder or urethra is the most common cause of uroabdomen, but leakage from the kidney or ureter can also occur. Trauma is the most common cause, but urinary tract blockage, bladder catheterization or expression, neoplasia, and postoperative leakage are reported.[134,135] Almost all animals recover if the site of leakage is detected and corrected.[134] Traumatic urothorax has also been reported, with extravasation of fluid from the abdominal cavity to the thoracic cavity.[15] Differential diagnosis of bicavitary effusions should include urothorax and uroabdomen.

Protein and TNCC are variable but are usually low unless sepsis accompanies the leakage. In one study, the TNCC ranged from 50 to 6000 cells/µL with neutrophils predominating in all cases, and the total protein ranged from 0.3 to 2.6 g/dL.[3] Rarely, urine crystals can be observed in the fluid. The presence of urine in the abdomen can usually be confirmed by determining the abdominal fluid creatinine concentration to blood creatinine ratio. A ratio of >2 : 1 is predictive of uroabdomen (sensitivity 86%, specificity 100%). In one study, all dogs with uroabdomen had fluid creatinine concentration that was at least four times normal serum creatinine concentrations.[136] Creatinine is used instead of urea because creatinine is a larger molecule that is not absorbed into the blood as quickly as urea. However, over time, animals will become azotemic, and blood creatinine concentrations will increase, making the ratio less diagnostically useful.

An abdominal fluid to blood potassium concentration ratio of >1.4 : 1 is also predictive of uroabdomen, with a sensitivity and specificity of 100% in one study.[136] However, stomach secretions are also high in potassium, and high abdominal fluid potassium concentration with a fluid to blood ratio of greater than 2.67 : 1 has been reported with gastric perforation.[67]

References

1 Miserocchi, G. and Agostoni, E. (1971). Contents of the pleural space. *J Appl Physiol* 30: 208–213.

2 Noppen, M. (2001). Normal volume and cellular contents of pleural fluid. *Curr Opin Pulm Med* 7: 180–182.

3 Bohn, A.A. (2017). Analysis of canine peritoneal fluid analysis. *Vet Clin North Am Small Anim Pract* 47: 123–133.

4 Alleman, A.R. (2003). Abdominal, thoracic and pericardial effusions. *Vet Clin North Am Small Anim Pract* 33: 89–118.

5 Connally, H.E. (2003). Cytology and fluid analysis of the acute abdomen. *Clin Tech Small Anim Pract* 18: 39–44.

6 Davies, C. and Forrester, S.D. (1996). Pleural effusion in cats: 82 cases (1987 to 1995). *J Small Anim Pract* 37: 217–224.

7 Dempsey, S.M. and Ewing, P.J. (2011). A review of the pathophysiology, classification, and analysis of canine and feline cavitary effusions. *J Am Anim Hosp Assoc* 47: 1–11.

8 Epstein, S.E. (2014). Exudative pleural diseases in small animals. *Vet Clin North Am Small Anim Pract* 44: 161–180.

9 Frendin, J. and Obel, N. (1997). Catheter drainage of pleural fluid collections and pneumothorax. *J Small Anim Pract* 38: 237–242.

10 Mellanby, R.J., Villiers, E., and Herrtage, M.E. (2002). Canine pleural and mediastinal effusions: a retrospective study of 81 cases. *J Small Anim Pract* 43: 447–451.

11 Noone, K.E. (1985). Pleural effusions and diseases of the pleura. *Vet Clin North Am Small Anim Pract* 15: 1069–1084.

12 Tyler, R.D. and Cowell, R.L. (1989). Evaluation of pleural and peritoneal effusions. *Vet Clin North Am Small Anim Pract* 19: 743–768.

13 Wright, K.N., Gompf, R.E., and DeNovo, R.C. Jr. (1999). Peritoneal effusion in cats: 65 cases (1981–1997). *J Am Vet Med Assoc* 214: 375–381.

14 Steyn, P.F. and Wittum, T.E. (1993). Radiographic, epidemiologic, and clinical aspects of simultaneous pleural and peritoneal effusions in dogs and cats: 48 cases (1982–1991). *J Am Vet Med Assoc* 202: 307–212.

15 Klainbart, S., Merchav, R., and Ohad, D.G. (2011). Traumatic urothorax in a dog: a case report. *J Small Anim Pract* 52: 544–546.

16 Murgia, D. (2013). A case of combined bilothorax and bile peritonitis secondary to gunshot wounds in a cat. *J Feline Med Surg* 15: 513–516.

17 Christopher, M.M. (1987). Pleural effusions. *Vet Clin North Am Small Anim Pract* 17: 255–270.

18 Peaston, A.E., Church, D.B., Allen, G.S., and Haigh, S. (1990). Combined chylothorax, chylopericardium, and cranial vena cava syndrome in a dog with thymoma. *J Am Vet Med Assoc* 197: 1354–1356.

19 Fossum, T.W., Miller, M.W., Rogers, K.S. et al. (1994). Chylothorax associated with right-sided heart failure in five cats. *J Am Vet Med Assoc* 204: 84–89.

20 Walters, J.M. (2003). Abdominal paracentesis and diagnostic peritoneal lavage. *Clin Tech Small Anim Pract* 18: 32–38.

21 Rose, A., Funk, D., and Neiger, R. (2016). Comparison of refractometry and biuret assay for measurement of total protein concentration in canine abdominal and pleural fluid specimens. *J Am Vet Med Assoc* 248: 789–794.

22 Maher, I., Tennant, K.V., and Papasouliotis, K. (2010). Effect of storage time on automated cell count and cytological interpretation of body cavity effusions. *Vet Rec* 167: 519–522.

23 Rizzi, T.E., Cowell, R.D., and Meinkoth, J.H. (2008). Effusions: abdominal, thoracic, and pericardial. In: *Diagnostic Cytology and Hematology of the Dog and Cat*, 3e (eds. R.L. Cowell, R.D. Tyler, J.H. Meinkoth and D.B. DeNicola), 235–255. St. Louis, MO: Mosby.

24 Meinkoth, J.H., Cowell, R.L., Tyler, R.D. et al. (2008). Sample collection and preparation. In: *Diagnostic Cytology and Hematology of the Dog and Cat*, 3e (eds. R.L. Cowell, R.D. Tyler, J.H. Meinkoth and D.B. DeNicola), 1–19. St. Louis, MO: Mosby.

25 Probo, M., Valenti, V., Venco, L. et al. (2018). Pleural lymphocyte-rich transudates in cats. *J Feline Med Surg* 20: 767–771.

26 Avery, P.R. and Avery, A.C. (2004). Molecular methods to distinguish reactive and neoplastic lymphocyte expansions and their importance in transitional neoplastic states. *Vet Clin Pathol* 33: 196–207.

27 Bode-Lesniewksa, B. (2016). Flow cytometry and effusions in lymphoproliferative processes and other hematologic neoplasias. *Acta Cytol* 60: 354–364.

28 Fossum, T.W., Wellman, M., Relford, R.L., and Slater, M.R. (1993). Eosinophilic pleural or peritoneal effusions in dogs and cats: 14 cases (1986–1992). *J Am Vet Med Assoc* 202: 1873–1876.

29 Harris, B.J., Constantino-Casas, F., and Archer, J. (2013). Loeffler's endocarditis and bicavity eosinophilic effusions in a dog with visceral mast cell tumour and hypereosinophilia. *J Comp Path* 149: 429–433.

30 Allison, R., Williams, P., Lansdowne, J. et al. (2006). Fatal hepatic sarcocystosis in a puppy with eosinophilia and eosinophilic peritoneal effusion. *Vet Clin Pathol* 35: 353–357.

31 Gupta, A., Garber, J., Fowlkes, N. et al. (2013). What is your diagnosis? Abdominal fluid from a dog. *Vet Clin Pathol* 42: 113–114.

32 Ueki, S., Tokunaga, T., Fujieda, S. et al. (2016). Eosinophil ETosis and DNA traps: a new look at eosinophilic inflammation. *Curr Allergy Asthma Rep* 16: 54.

33 Van Israel, N., Kirby, B.M., and Munro, E.A. (2002). Septic peritonitis secondary to unilateral pyometra and ovarian bursal abscessation in a dog. *J Small Anim Pract* 43: 452–455.

34 McKonkey, S., Briggs, C., Solano, M., and Illanes, O. (1997). Liver torsion and associated bacterial peritonitis in a dog. *Can Vet J* 38: 438–439.

35 Farrar, E.T., Washabau, R.J., and Saunders, H.M. (1996). Hepatic abscesses in dogs: 14 cases (1982–1994). *J Am Vet Med Assoc* 208: 243–247.

36 Nielson, C., Olver, C.S., Schutten, M.M., and Twedt, D.C. (2003). Diagnostic peritoneal lavage for identification of blastomycosis in a dog with peritoneal involvement. *J Am Vet Med Assoc* 223: 1623–1627.

37 Kowalewich, N., Hawkins, E.C., Skowronek, A.J., and Clemo, F.A. (1993). Identification of *Histoplasma*

capsulatum organisms in the pleural and peritoneal effusions of a dog. *J Am Vet Med Assoc* 202: 423–426.

38 Schubitz, L.F., Matz, M.E., Noon, T.H. et al. (2001). Constrictive pericarditis secondary to *Coccidioides immitis* infection in a dog. *J Am Vet Med Assoc* 218: 537–540.

39 Brosinski, K., Gutbrod, A., Venzin, C., and Grest, P. (2012). What is your diagnosis? Peritoneal fluid from a dog with abdominal pain. *Vet Clin Pathol* 41: 297–298.

40 Caruso, K.J., James, M.P., Fisher, D. et al. (2003). Cytologic diagnosis of peritoneal cestodiasis in dogs caused by *Mesocestoides* sp. *Vet Clin Pathol* 32: 50–60.

41 Bradford, K., Meinkoth, J., McKeirnen, K., and Love, B. (2013). Candida peritonitis in dogs: report of 5 cases. *Vet Clin Pathol* 42: 227–233.

42 Burgess, H.J. and Gaunt, M.C. (2014). Pathology in practice. *J Am Vet Med Assoc* 245: 1107–1109.

43 Ong, R.K.C., Raisis, A.L., and Swindells, K.L. (2010). Candida albicans peritonitis in a dog. *J Vet Emerg Crit Care* 20: 143–147.

44 Toomey, J.M., Carlisle-Nowak, M.M., Barr, S.C. et al. (1995). Concurrent toxoplasmosis and feline infectious peritonitis in a cat. *J Am Anim Hosp Assoc* 31: 425–428.

45 Holmburg, T.A., Vernau, W., Melli, A.C., and Conrad, P.A. (2006). *Neospora caninum* associated with septic peritonitis in an adult dog. *Vet Clin Pathol* 35: 235–238.

46 Agrawal, V., Doelken, P., and Sahn, S.A. (2008). Pleural fluid analysis in chylous pleural effusion. *Chest* 133: 1436–1441.

47 James, F.E., Knowles, G.W., Mansfield, C.S., and Robertson, I.D. (2008). Ascites due to pre-sinusoidal portal hypertension in dogs: a retrospective analysis of 17 cases. *Aust Vet J* 86: 180–186.

48 Roth, B.J., O'Meara, T.F., and Cragun, W.H. (1990). The serum-albumin gradient in the evaluation of pleural effusions. *Chest* 98: 546–549.

49 Pembleton-Corbett, J.R., Center, S.A., Schermerhorn, T. et al. (2000). Serum-effusion albumin gradient in dogs with transudative abdominal effusion. *J Vet Intern Med* 14: 613–618.

50 Stockam, S.L. and Scott, M.A. (eds.) (2008). Proteins. In: *Fundamentals of Veterinary Clinical Pathology*, 2e, 63–272. Ames, IA: Blackwell Publishing.

51 Brackeen, G.L., Dover, J.S., and Long, C.L. (1989). Serum albumin. Differences in assay specificity. *Nutr Clin Pract* 4: 23–205.

52 Bunch, S.E., Johnson, S.E., and Cullen, J.M. (2001). Idiopathic non-cirrhotic portal hypertension in dogs: 33 cases (1982–1998). *J Am Vet Med Assoc* 218: 392–399.

53 Hunt, G.B., Malik, R., Chapman, B.L. et al. (1993). Ascites and portal hypertension in three young dogs with non-fibrosing liver disease. *J Small Anim Pract* 34: 428–433.

54 Buob, S., Johnston, A.N., and Webster, C.R.L. (2011). Portal hypertension: pathophysiology, diagnosis, and treatment. *J Vet Intern Med* 25: 169–411.

55 Hezzell, M.J., Rush, J.E., Humm, K. et al. (2016). Differentiation of cardiac from noncardiac pleural effusions in cats using second-generation quantitative and point-of-care NT-proBNP measurements. *J Vet Intern Med* 30: 536–542.

56 Harris, A.N., Beatty, S.S., Estrada, A.H. et al. (2017). Investigation of an N-terminal prohormone of brain natriuretic peptide point-of-care ELISA in clinically normal cats and cats with cardiac disease. *J Vet Intern Med* 31: 994–999.

57 Dunbar, M.D. and Alleman, A.R. (2009). A challenging case: abdominal effusion in a dog. Dvm360 Veterinary Medicine.com.

58 Ko, J.J. and Mann, F.A. (2014). Barium peritonitis in small animals. *J Vet Med Sci* 76: 621–628.

59 Dickinson, A.E., Summers, J.F., Wignal, J. et al. (2015). Impact of appropriate empirical antimicrobial therapy on outcome of dogs with septic peritonitis. *J Vet Emerg Crit Care* 25: 152–159.

60 Culp, W.T., Zeldis, T.E., Reese, M.S., and Drobatz, K.J. (2009). Primary bacterial peritonitis in dogs and cats: 24 cases (1990–2006). *J Am Vet Med Assoc* 234: 906–913.

61 Ruthrauf, C.M., Smith, J., and Glerum, L. (2009). Primary bacterial septic peritonitis in cats: 13 cases. *J Am Anim Hosp Assoc* 45: 268–276.

62 Lanz, O.I., Ellison, G.W., Bellah, J.R. et al. (2001). Surgical treatment of septic peritonitis without abdominal drainage in 28 dogs. *J Am Anim Hosp Assoc* 37: 87–92.

63 Mueller, M.G., Ludwig, L.L., and Barton, L.J. (2001). Use of closed suction drains to treat generalized peritonitis in dogs and cats: 40 cases (1997–1999). *J Am Vet Med Assoc* 219: 789–794.

64 Weeden, A.L., Cherry, N.A., Breitschwerdt, E.B. et al. (2017). *Bartonella henselae* in canine cavitary effusions: prevalence, identification, and clinical associations. *Vet Clin Pathol* 46: 326–330.

65 Bonczynski, J.J., Ludwig, L.L., Barton, L.J. et al. (2003). Comparison of peritoneal fluid and peripheral blood pH, bicarbonate, glucose, and lactate concentration as a diagnostic tool for septic peritonitis in dogs and cats. *Vet Surg* 32: 161–166.

66 Koenig, A. and Verlander, L.L. (2015). Usefulness of whole blood, plasma, peritoneal fluid and peritoneal fluid supernatant glucose concentrations obtained by a veterinary point-of-care glucometer to identify septic peritonitis in dogs with peritoneal effusion. *J Am Vet Med Assoc* 247: 1027–1031.

67 Ben Oz, J., Aroch, I., and Segev, G. (2016). Increased ratio of peritoneal effusion-to-serum potassium concentration

in a dog with gastric perforation. *J Vet Emerg Crit Care* 26: 793–797.

68 Barrs, V.R., Allan, G.S., Martin, P. et al. (2005). Feline pyothorax: a retrospective study of 27 cases in Australia. *J Feline Med Surg* 7: 211–222.

69 Stillion, J.R. and Letendre, J.-A. (2015). A clinical review of the pathophysiology, diagnosis, and treatment of pyothorax in dogs and cats. *J Vet Emerg Crit Care* 25: 113–120.

70 Hicks, A., Golland, D., Heller, J. et al. (2016). Epidemiological investigation of grass seed foreign body-related disease in dogs of the Riverina District of rural Australia. *Aust Vet J* 94: 67–75.

71 Demetriou, J.L., Foale, R.D., Ladlow, J. et al. (2002). Canine and feline pyothorax: a retrospective study of 50 cases in the UK and Ireland. *J Small Anim Pract* 43: 388–394.

72 Piek, C.J. and Robben, J.H. (2000). Pyothorax in nine dogs. *Vet Q* 22: 107–111.

73 Pedersen, N.C. (2014). An update on feline infectious peritonitis: diagnostics and therapeutics. *Vet J* 201: 133–141.

74 Kipar, A. and Meli, M.L. (2014). Feline infectious peritonitis: still an enigma? *Vet Pathol* 51: 505–526.

75 Sparkes, A.H., Gruffydd-Jones, T.J., and Harbour, D.A. (1991). Feline infectious peritonitis: a review of clinicopathological changes in 65 cases, and a critical assessment of their diagnostic value. *Vet Rec* 129: 209–212.

76 Berti-Bock, G., Vial, F., Premuda, L., and Rullière, R. (1979). Exudates, transudates and the Rivalta reaction (1895). Current status and historical premises. *Minerva Med* 70: 3573–3580.

77 Sakai, N., Iijima, S., and Shiba, K. (2004). Reinvestigation of clinical value of Rivalta reaction of puncture fluid. *Rinsho Byori* 52: 877–882.

78 Fischer, Y., Sauter-Louis, C., and Hartmann, K. (2012). Diagnostic accuracy of the Rivalta test for feline infectious peritonitis. *Vet Clin Pathol* 41: 558–567.

79 Hartmann, K., Binder, C., Hirshberger, J. et al. (2003). Comparison of different tests to diagnose feline infectious peritonitis. *J Vet Intern Med* 17: 781–290.

80 Stranieri, A., Giordano, A., Paltrinieri, S. et al. (2018). Comparison of the performance of laboratory tests in the diagnosis of feline infectious peritonitis. *J Vet Diagn Invest* 30: 459–463.

81 Mesquita, L., Mortier, J., Ressel, L. et al. (2017). Neoplastic pleural effusion and intrathoracic metastasis of a scapular osteosarcoma in a dog: a multidisciplinary integrated diagnostic approach. *Vet Clin Pathol* 46: 337–343.

82 Sommery, C.C., Borgeat, K.A., Hetzel, U. et al. (2012). Intrathoracic myxosarcoma in a dog. *J Comp Pathol* 147: 199–203.

83 Hirschberger, J., DeNicola, D.B., Hermanns, W., and Kraft, W. (1999). Sensitivity and specificity of cytologic evaluation in diagnosis of neoplasia in body fluids. *Vet Clin Pathol* 28: 142–146.

84 Sawa, M., Yabuki, A., Miyoshi, N. et al. (2012). A simple and rapid immunocytochemical technique for detection of cytokeratin, vimentin, and s-100 protein in veterinary diagnostic cytology. *Res Vet Sci* 93: 1341–1345.

85 Moore, A.R., Coffey, E., Leavell, S.E. et al. (2016). Canine bicavitary carcinomatosis with transient needle tract metastasis diagnosed by multiplex immunocytochemistry. *Vet Clin Pathol* 45: 495–500.

86 Ferreira, F.C., Soares, M.J., Carvalho, S. et al. (2015). Four cases of cell cannibalism in highly malignant feline and canine tumors. *Diagn Pathol* 10: 199.

87 Bertazzolo, W., Bonfanti, U., Mazzotti, S., and Gelain, M.E. (2012). Cytologic features and diagnostic accuracy of analysis of effusions for detection of ovarian carcinoma in dogs. *Vet Clin Pathol* 4: 127–132.

88 Warren-Smith, C.M.R., Roe, K., de la Puerta, B. et al. (2011). Pulmonary adenocarcinoma seeding along a fine needle aspiration tract in a dog. *Vet Rec* 169: 181.

89 Moore, E.L., Vernau, W., Rebhun, R.B. et al. (2018). Patient characteristics, prognostic factors and outcomes of dogs with high-grade primary mediastinal lymphoma. *Vet Comp Oncol* 20: 696–703.

90 Louwerens, M., London, C.A., Pederson, N.C., and Lyons, L.A. (2005). Feline lymphoma in the post–feline leukemia virus era. *J Vet Intern Med* 19: 329–335.

91 Crouze, Z., Phillips, B., Flory, A. et al. (2018). Post-chemotherapy perforation in cats with discrete intermediate- or large-cell gastrointestinal lymphoma. *J Feline Med Surg* 20: 696–703.

92 Przeździecki, R., Czopowicz, M., and Sapierzyński, R. (2015). Cytomorphometry of serosal effusion in dogs. *Pol J Vet Sci* 18: 481–487.

93 Di Tommaso, M., Rocconi, F., Marruchella, G. et al. (2015). Invasive pleural malignant mesothelioma with rib destruction and concurrent osteosarcoma in a dog. *Acta Vet Scand* 57: 85.

94 Sample, S., Webb, J.L., Behr, M., and Shiu, K.B. (2015). What is your diagnosis? Granules galore! *Vet Clin Pathol* 44: 165–166.

95 Przeździecki, R. and Sapierzyński, R. (2014). Using of immunocytochemistry in differential diagnosis of neoplasms of serosal cavities in dogs. *Pol J Vet Sci* 17: 149–159.

96 Harbison, M.L. and Godleski, J.J. (1983). Malignant mesothelioma in urban dogs. *Vet Pathol* 20: 531–540.

97 Nestor, D.D., McCullough, S.M., and Schaeffer, D.J. (2004). Biochemical analysis of neoplastic versus nonneoplastic abdominal effusions in dogs. *J Am Anim Hosp Assoc* 40: 372–375.

98 Prittie, J. and Barton, L. (2004). Hemothorax and sanguinous effusions. In: *Textbook of Respiratory Diseases in Dogs and Cats* (ed. L.G. King), 610–616. St. Louis, MO: W.B. Saunders.

99 Epstein, C.E., Elidemir, O., Colasurdo, G.N. et al. (2001). Time course of hemosiderin production by alveolar macrophages in a murine model. *Chest* 120: 2013–2020.

100 Pintar, J., Breitschwerdt, E.B., Hardie, E.M., and Spaulding, K.A. (2003). Acute nontraumatic hemoabdomen in the dog: a retrospective analysis of 39 cases (1987–2001). *J Am Anim Hosp Assoc* 39: 518–522.

101 Hammond, T.N. and Pesillo-Crosby, S.A. (2008). Prevalence of hemangiosarcoma in anemic dogs with a mass and hemoperitoneum requiring a transfusion: 71 cases (2003–2005). *J Am Vet Med Assoc* 232: 553–558.

102 DuVall, M.D., Murphy, M.J., Ray, A.C., and Reagor, J.C. (1989). Case studies of second-generation anticoagulant rodenticide toxicities in nontarget species. *J Vet Diagn Invest* 1: 66–68.

103 Fitzgerald, S.D., Martinez, J., and Buchweitz, J.P. (2018). An apparent case of brodifacoum toxicosis in a whelping dog. *J Vet Diagn Invest* 30: 169–171.

104 Lux, C.N., Culp, W.T., Mayhew, P.D. et al. (2013). Perioperative outcome in dogs with hemoperitoneum: 83 cases (2005–2010). *J Am Vet Med Assoc* 15: 1385–1391.

105 Aronsohn, M.G., Dubiel, B., Roberts, B., and Powers, B.E. (2009). Prognosis for acute nontraumatic hemoperitoneum in the dog: a retrospective analysis of 60 cases (2003–2006). *J Am Anim Hosp Assoc* 45: 72–77.

106 Wong, R.W., Gonsalves, M.N., Huber, M.L. et al. (2015). Erythrocyte and biochemical abnormalities as diagnostic markers in dogs with hemangiosarcoma related hemoabdomen. *Vet Surg* 44: 852–857.

107 Culp, W.T., Weisse, C., Kellogg, M.E. et al. (2010). Spontaneous hemoperitoneum in cats: 65 cases (1994–2006). *J Am Vet Med Assoc* 236: 978–982.

108 Nakamura, R.K., Rozanski, E.A., and Rush, J.E. (2008). Non-coagulopathic spontaneous hemothorax in dogs. *J Vet Emerg Crit Care* 18: 292–297.

109 Rutherford, L., Stell, A., Smith, K., and Kulendra, N. (2016). Hemothorax in three dogs with intrathoracic extracardiac hemangiosarcoma. *J Am Anim Hosp Assoc* 52: 325–329.

110 Schultz, R.M., Peters, J., and Zwingenbuerger, A. (2009). Radiography, computed tomography and virtual bronchoscopy in four dogs and two cats with lung lobe torsion. *J Small Anim Pract* 50: 360–363.

111 Biasato, I., Tursi, M., Zanet, S. et al. (2017). Pulmonary artery dissection causing hemothorax in a cat: potential role of *Dirofilaria immitis* infection and literature review. *J Vet Cardiol* 19: 82–87.

112 Sierra, E., Rodriguez, F., Herraez, P. et al. (2007). Post-traumatic fat embolism causing haemothorax in a cat. *Vet Rec* 161: 170–172.

113 Higgs, V.A., Rudloff, E., Kirby, R., and Linklater, A.K. (2015). Autologous blood transfusion in dogs with thoracic or abdominal hemorrhage: 25 cases (2007–2012). *J Vet Emerg Crit Care* 25: 731–738.

114 Fossum, T.W., Hay, W.H., Boothe, H.W. et al. (1992). Chylous ascites in three dogs. *J Am Vet Med Assoc* 200: 70–76.

115 Fossum, T.W., Forrester, S.D., Swenson, C. et al. (1991). Chylothorax in cats: 37 cases (1969–1989). *J Am Vet Med Assoc* 198: 672–678.

116 Fossum, T.W., Jacobs, R.M., and Birchard, S.J. (1986). Evaluation of cholesterol and triglyceride concentrations in differentiating chylous and nonchylous pleural effusions in dogs and cats. *J Am Vet Med Assoc* 188: 49–51.

117 Fossum, T.W., Brichard, S.J., and Jacobs, R.M. (1986). Chylothorax in 34 dogs. *J Am Vet Med Assoc* 188: 1315–1318.

118 Waddle, J.R. and Giger, U. (1990). Lipoprotein electrophoresis differentiation of chylous and nonchylous pleural effusions in dogs and its correlation with pleural effusion triglyceride concentration. *Vet Clin Pathol* 19: 80–85.

119 Meadows, R.L., McWilliams, P.S., Dzata, G., and Meinen, J. (1993). Chylothorax associated with cryptococcal mediastinal granuloma in a cat. *Vet Clin Pathol* 22: 109–116.

120 Singh, A. and Brisson, B.A. (2010). Chylothorax associated with thrombosis of the cranial vena cava. *Can Vet J* 51: 847–852.

121 Dixon-Jimenez, A. and Margiocco, M.L. (2011). Infectious endocarditis and chylothorax in a cat. *J Am Anim Hosp Assoc* 47: 121–126.

122 McLane, M.J. and Buote, N.J. (2011). Lung lobe torsion associated with chylothorax in a cat. *J Feline Med Surg* 13: 135–138.

123 Fossum, T.W., Mertens, M.M., Miller, M.W. et al. (2004). Thoracic duct ligation and pericardectomy for treatment of idiopathic chylothorax. *J Vet Intern Med* 18: 307–310.

124 Fossum, T.W., Evering, W.N., Miller, M.W. et al. (1992). Severe bilateral fibrosing pleuritis associated with chronic chylothorax in five cats and two dogs. *J Am Vet Med Assoc* 201: 317–324.

125 Meadows, R.L. and McWilliams, P.S. (1994). Chylous effusions revisited. *Vet Clin Pathol* 23: 54–62.

126 Thompson, M.D. and Carr, A.P. (2002). Hyponatremia and hyperkalemia associated with chylous pleural and peritoneal effusion in a cat. *Can Vet J* 43: 610–613.

127 Savary, K.C., Sellon, R.K., and Law, J.M. (2001). Chylous abdominal effusion in a cat with feline infectious peritonitis. *J Am Anim Hosp Assoc* 37: 35–40.

128 Owens, S.D., Gossett, R., McEkhaney, M.R. et al. (2003). Three cases of canine bile peritonitis with mucinous material in the abdominal fluid as the prominent cytologic finding. *Vet Clin Pathol* 32: 114–120.

129 Ludwig, L.L., McLoughlin, M.A., Graves, T.K., and Crisp, M.S. (1997). Surgical treatment of bile peritonitis in 24 dogs and 2 cats: a retrospective study (1987–1994). *Vet Surg* 26: 90–98.

130 Guess, S.C., Harkin, K.R., and Biller, D.S. (2015). Anicteric gallbladder rupture in dogs: 5 cases (2007–2013). *J Am Vet Med Assoc* 247: 1412–1214.

131 Jaffey, J.A., Graham, A., VanEerde, E. et al. (2018). Gallbladder mucocele: variables associated with outcome and the utility of ultrasonography to identify gallbladder rupture in 219 dogs (2007–2016). *J Vet Intern Med* 32: 195–200.

132 Barnhart, M.D. and Rasmussen, L.M. (1996). Pleural effusion as a complication of extrahepatic biliary tract rupture in a dog. *J Am Anim Hosp Assoc* 32: 409–412.

133 Mullins, R.A., Barandum, M.A., Gallagher, B., and Cuddy, L.C. (2017). Non-iatrogenic traumatic isolated bilothorax in a cat. *JFMS Open Rep* 3: 255116917714871.

134 Grimes, J.A., Fletcher, J.M., and Schmiedt, C.W. (2018). Outcomes in dogs with uroabdomen: 43 cases (2006–2015). *J Am Vet Med Assoc* 252: 92–97.

135 Stafford, J.B. and Bartges, J.W. (2013). A clinical review of pathophysiology, diagnosis, and treatment of uroabdomen in the dog and cat. *J Vet Emerg Crit Care* 23: 216–229.

136 Schmiedt, C., Tobias, K.M., and Otto, C.M. (2001). Evaluation of abdominal fluid: peripheral blood creatinine and potassium ratios for diagnosis of uroperitoneum in dogs. *J Vet Emerg Crit Care* 11: 275–280.

53

Abdominal and Thoracic Fluid Analysis in Horses

Emma Hooijberg and Catriona Lyle

Collection

Collection Techniques

Thoracocentesis

This technique can be performed in the standing horse with minimal restraint. The site for thoracocentesis is best determined using transthoracic ultrasonography to identify the location of pleural fluid and to help avoid inadvertent puncture of vital structures.[1] Alternatively, the technique can be performed "blindly" at the 6th, 7th, or 8th intercostal space, 10–15 cm dorsal to the point of olecranon, avoiding the lateral thoracic vein.[1,2] The mediastinum may be fenestrated so that unilateral fluid collection can be representative of the entire pleural cavity. However, in disease conditions the mediastinum can become obstructed with fibrin, and the two sides of the thorax may be affected differently.[1]

An approximately 10 × 10 cm area is clipped and aseptically prepared. Local anesthetic is infiltrated into the skin, subcutaneous tissue, intercostal muscles, and parietal pleura. An intravenous catheter (e.g. 16 G) or teat cannula is inserted aseptically just cranial to the rib at the selected site to avoid laceration of the intercostal vessels and nerves that run caudal to each rib. If a teat cannula is used, a scalpel blade must first be used to make a stab incision through the skin and muscle to facilitate insertion.

A reasonable amount of steady pressure is required. The dominant hand should be placed on the hub of the catheter/teat cannula with the nondominant hand placed on the catheter/cannula at a predetermined distance to prevent inadvertently placing the catheter/cannula too far into the pleural cavity. Entry into the pleural cavity is recognized by a "popping" sensation or decrease in resistance. If using an intravenous catheter, the needle stylet should be withdrawn into the catheter at this stage.

A three-way stopcock is attached to the catheter/cannula before insertion to prevent aspiration of air and subsequent pneumothorax. A 10–20 mL syringe is connected to the stopcock, and fluid can be aspirated into a syringe and then placed into an EDTA blood collection tube for cytology and protein measurement and into a plain sterile container for microbiology. On removal of the catheter or cannula, a skin suture or staple may be placed.

Abdominocentesis

This technique can be performed in the standing horse with minimal restraint. Transabdominal ultrasonography can be used to locate areas of fluid accumulation and the position of abdominal viscera and therefore to select the site for abdominocentesis.[3] Alternatively, if ultrasonography is not available or no fluid accumulation is identifiable, the most dependent point of the abdomen either on midline or just to the right of midline (to reduce the risk of splenic puncture) is selected for abdominocentesis.[4–6]

An approximately 20 × 20 cm area is clipped and aseptically prepared. The precise site for abdominocentesis should avoid superficial skin vessels to minimize blood contamination of the sample. A needle is inserted at the selected site in an aseptic manner. An 18/19 G 1.5 in. needle is adequate in most horses; however, fatter individuals may necessitate use of a longer needle. The needle is advanced 2–3 mm with rotational movements followed by pauses to observe for appearance of fluid in the hub. If the needle is observed or felt to move against intestine (rasping sensation), it should be withdrawn. Fluid drips slowly or streams out of needle and is collected directly into an EDTA blood collection tube for cytology and protein measurement and into a plain sterile container for microbiology. Additional needles can be placed if no fluid is obtained on the first attempt.

A blunt-ended teat cannula can be used instead of a needle.[4,5,7] In this case, the skin and subcutaneous tissues are infiltrated with a local anesthetic. A stab incision is made through the skin, subcutaneous tissues, and external rectus sheath with a scalpel blade. The cannula is pushed through

Veterinary Cytology, First Edition. Edited by Leslie C. Sharkey, M. Judith Radin, and Davis Seelig.

a 10×10 cm sterile gauze swab before advancing it into the peritoneal cavity to reduce blood contamination of the sample from the skin incision.

Anaerobic fluid retrieval has also been reported with the use of silicon tubing and a three-way stopcock attached to a bitch urinary catheter if measurement of pH, PO_2, PCO_2, HCO_3^-, and Ca^{2+} are required.[8]

Impact of Collection Method

Thoracocentesis

Recovery Rate

In diseased horses (i.e. those with increased pleural fluid), fluid is usually retrieved on the first attempt.[2]

Complications

Complications are rarely reported although mild hemorrhage can occur.[1,2] Mild pneumothorax can occur without clinical signs and resolves quickly as air is resorbed from the pleural space into the pleural veins. In human patients with pneumothorax, approximately 1.25% of the air volume is absorbed daily when patients are breathing atmospheric air.[9] Theoretically, more severe pneumothorax, arrhythmias, cellulitis, and laceration of lung, heart, liver, bowel, intercostal vessels, or lateral thoracic vein are possible. The incidence of these more severe complications is unknown but given the absence of case reports in the literature suggests these are unlikely with proper technique.

Abdominocentesis

Recovery Rate

Retrieval of peritoneal fluid is successful on the first attempt in the majority of horses. Reported success rates on the first attempt range from 60 to 98% using either a needle or a teat cannula.[4,5,7] Fluid is more likely to be retrieved from horses with ultrasonographic evidence of peritoneal fluid.[3]

No effect of technique (needle versus cannula) has been identified on rate of recovery, volume of fluid, time to collect sample (excluding time for local anesthesia), total nucleated cell count (TNCC), differential cell count, or total protein (TP).[5] Red blood cell count (RCC) is lower after needle abdominocentesis than cannula abdominocentesis.[5] Repeated abdominocentesis with a teat cannula has not been shown to affect TNCC, differential cell count, or specific gravity (SG).[5,7,10]

Complications

Blood contamination from vessel penetration is usually seen as a swirl of blood compared with well-mixed, truly serosanguinous fluid. Hemorrhage usually resolves quickly, so a second collection tube should always be available to collect a second non-contaminated sample. Centrifugation of the sample can help in differentiating a blood-contaminated sample (yellow supernatant) from a truly serosanguinous sample (supernatant remains orange/red due to hemolysis) (Figure 53.1).[11] In addition, fresh blood contamination exhibits platelets, whereas blood older than 12 hours has no platelets, and erythrophagocytosis may be evident.[11] Up to 17% blood contamination has been shown not to affect TNCC or TP.[12] Inadvertent splenic puncture occasionally occurs but is not known to cause any significant complications.[6] Fluid retrieved in these cases is likely to have a higher packed cell volume (PCV) than peripheral blood.[6]

Enterocentesis results in collection of dark brown to green malodorous fluid. The needle should be quickly removed. This is a rare complication reported to occur in <4% of attempts.[4] In most cases, this does not lead to any secondary problems but occasionally can result in peritonitis and abdominal wall cellulitis.[3,4,13] In most cases, these complications respond to antimicrobials and hydrotherapy (in the case of cellulitis), but in some instances more extensive bowel laceration or leakage can occur.[4,13]

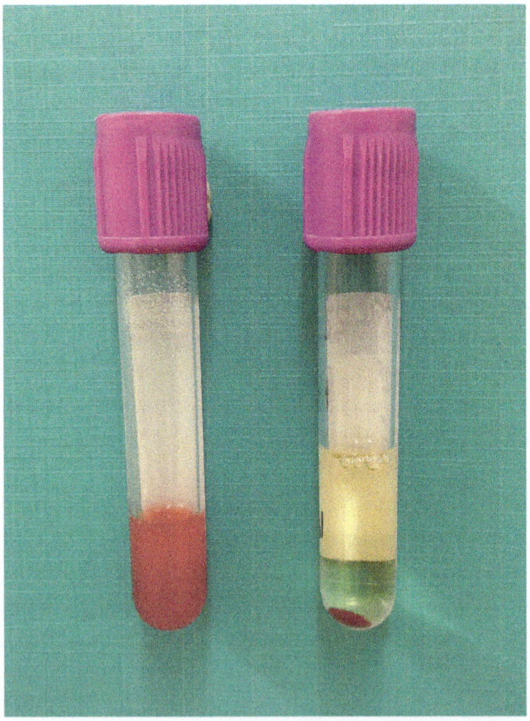

Figure 53.1 Differentiation of blood-contaminated fluid from a truly serosanguinous fluid. (left) Red peritoneal fluid obtained by abdominocentesis. (right) Following centrifugation of the sample, a red cell pellet forms at the bottom of the tube, and the supernatant fluid appears normal. This is consistent with blood contamination during sampling rather than a serosanguinous fluid as no hemolysis has yet occurred to discolor the supernatant fluid.

Enterocentesis does lead to increased TNCC and SG starting at four hours and peaking at two days following enterocentesis.[10] Inadvertent enterocentesis can be diagnostic in cases of sand colic where sand is obtained or felt on abdominocentesis.[14]

No statistically significant association has been identified between either collection method and enterocentesis.[4,5] Increased risks of abdominal wall swelling and omental herniation in foals have been reported with the cannula technique.[5,15]

Normal Cytology

Volume

Healthy horses have small volumes of pleural fluid, around 2–8 mL.[2,16] Normal peritoneal fluid volumes are much higher, ranging from 100 to 300 mL.[6,17]

Appearance

Normal pleural fluid ranges from colorless to light yellow and is clear.[2,16] A red tinge can be seen with blood contamination and is noted at erythrocyte concentrations at and above 50.0×10^9/L.[2] Peritoneal fluid is similarly clear and either colorless, yellow, or orange.[17]

Total Protein, Specific Gravity, and Cellularity

Normal pleural fluid has TP values of up to 47 g/L and SG of 1.008–1.031.[2,16] TNCC ranges from 8.0–12.1×10^9/L with less than 10.0×10^9/L generally considered to be the norm.[2,16] The cell population is dominated by neutrophils (75%), with approximately 20% macrophages, 5% lymphocytes, and occasional eosinophils.[2] The normal RCC has been reported to range from 22.0–540.0×10^9/L.[2]

Peritoneal fluid of healthy adult horses will have TP < 25 g/L and SG in the range of 1.008–1.011.[17–19] Normal reported TNCC is variable with some authors stating $<5.0 \times 10^9$/L as normal and others reporting that up to 10.0×10^9/L is expected.[17–22] The RCC is less than 5.0×10^9/L.[12] Neutrophils make up less than 75% of the normal cell population with proportions of macrophages and lymphocytes in roughly equal amounts; eosinophils are ≤2%.[17] In one study, morphological changes in peritoneal fluid leukocytes in horses with abdominal disease (including those with normal TNCC and TP and without blood contamination) included the presence of band neutrophils and metamyelocytes, Döhle bodies, and fine magenta cytoplasmic granulation of neutrophils. Neutrophils were sometimes seen within sheets of mesothelial cells. Plasma cells and large granular lymphocytes are noted in a small proportion of horses.[18] These findings suggest that a careful cytological examination of fluid should take place even when cellularity is not increased.

Normal equine mesothelial cells appear similar to inactive macrophages in healthy animals, with a pale blue cytoplasm and fine reticular chromatin pattern, and occur singly.[23] Upon activation, they occur in sheets, columns, papilla-like fronds, balls, rosettes, or triads and become large with increased cytoplasmic basophilia, a fuzzy cytoplasmic border and a perinuclear halo. Multinucleation, mitotic figures, and prominent nucleoli are also present.[18,23] "Degenerate" or "transformed" mesothelial cells have been described. These are seen in chronic inflammatory effusions and characterized by cytoplasmic vacuolization, a grey granulated cytoplasm, and coarse chromatin pattern. They were differentiated from macrophages by the presence of a round- to oval-shaped nucleus; however, no other method was used to differentiate the two cell populations.[23] Equine mesothelial cells express pancytokeratin, cytokeratins 8 and 18, calretinin, mesothelin, vimentin, and CD44.[24]

Foals

Two studies found that foals (aged from 13 to 134 days) have lower normal peritoneal fluid TNCC (0.1–1.4×10^9/L[25], mean 1.4×10^9/L with a standard deviation of 1.1×10^9/L[26]) than adult horses. These studies consider a TNCC $> 1.5 \times 10^9$/L or $> 3.0 \times 10^9$/L to be elevated.[25,26] Neutrophils make up less than half the cell population, with mean proportions of nucleated cells reported as 15 and 43% for neutrophils, 22 and 1% for lymphocytes, and 44 and 54% for mononuclear cells.[25,26] Peritoneal fluid TP was <25 g/L, similar to adult equines.[25,26]

Conditions Diagnosed by Cytology

Classification

An effusion is considered to be present if either cavity fluid volumes are increased or there are changes in the TNCC and protein.[27] Effusions in veterinary medicine, including horses, have traditionally been classified as transudates, modified transudates, and exudates based on cellularity and protein concentration.[28,29] Published evidence to support this particular system, particularly the cutoffs for the modified transudate category, is missing.[18,30] An alternative is to classify fluids according to their pathogenesis – transudative or exudative mechanisms or related to specific causes like neoplasia, disruption to lymphatic vessels, hemorrhage, and uroperitoneum – which will be more useful to clinicians.[31,32]

Based on the literature, normal values for adult equine pleural and peritoneal fluids for the purpose of the rest of this chapter will be a TNCC $< 10.0 \times 10^9$/L for both cavities, with TP < 30 g/L for peritoneal and <25 g/L for pleural effusions.[2,16,17]

Transudative Effusions

Transudates occur due to a decrease in oncotic pressure, increase in hydrostatic pressure, or obstruction to drainage via the lymphatic system. However, laboratory characteristics of effusions resulting from these conditions in horses are rarely reported. As equine body cavities contain enough fluid for collection and analysis in health, a fluid with the characteristics of a transudate should be interpreted as pathological only if fluid volumes are increased. Transudative effusions have normal cellularity and variable amounts of protein, depending on the mechanism behind their formation.

Although it is often stated in equine texts that severe hypoproteinemia and thus decreased oncotic pressure cause transudative effusions, no documented cases were found in the literature. Instead, subcutaneous edema appears to be common as a result of hypoproteinemia in horses. Agents like *Lawsonia intracellularis* (equine proliferative enteropathy) and small strongyles (cyathostominosis) cause a severe protein-losing enteropathy with serum albumin levels <20 g/L, but accompanying effusions have not been reported.[33,34] Renal disease is uncommon, and horses with nephropathies develop ventral edema rather than effusion.[35] Hepatic insufficiency does not usually result in hypoproteinemia, due to the long half-life of albumin in horses.[36,37] A transudate in a horse is therefore unlikely to be a result of hypoproteinemia alone.

Portal hypertension can result in both a low- and high-protein peritoneal transudate but appears to be equally uncommon, with detailed published information lacking.[38]

Congestive heart failure (CHF) is rare in horses, and reports detail mostly ventral and pulmonary edema, not effusion.[39–41] Pleural effusion was present in 6 out of 43 horses with CHF, but the nature of the fluid is not further described.[42] Another author suggests that pleural effusions are common with equine CHF but does not provide more details.[43]

Obstruction to lymphatic drainage of fluid that enters the body cavities in normal amounts can lead to accumulation of a protein-poor effusion. The pathogenesis in horses is usually neoplastic (see below).

Exudative Effusions

Exudative effusions occur due to an increase in vascular permeability resulting in egress of proteins and inflammatory cells. Exudates result from infectious or noninfectious causes, like sterile foreign material or neoplasia.

Pleural

Pleuropneumonia has been reported as the most common cause of pleural effusion in Australia and the United States, associated with long-distance transport of horses.[43,44] Most horses with pleuropneumonia have a pleural effusion as a result of pleuritis.[45] The effusion is initially of low cellularity and high TP and with time becomes characterized by high TNCC and TP with >90% degenerate neutrophils.[46–48] Bacteria are seen on cytology in >80% of cases.[46] The infection is usually polymicrobial, with both Gram-positive and Gram-negative aerobes as well as anaerobes (up to 40% of cases) and *Mycoplasma* spp. isolated.[46,48,49] In addition, fluid samples from both sides of the thorax should be submitted as organisms can be different in the two hemithoraces.[46] Both tracheobronchial and pleural fluid from these patients should be concurrently examined and sent for culture as false-negative cultures are possible from both sites.[46,50] *Mycoplasma felis* has been reported as a cause of pleuritis and pleural effusion in horses.[51]

Fungal pneumonia (e.g. *Aspergillus*, *Blastomyces*) can result in low volumes of high cellularity pleural fluid.[52,53]

Pulmonary hydatid cysts due to *Echinococcus* and other metacestodes are usually incidental findings but have been described to cause effusion as a result of rupture. The resulting fluid is reported to have a cellularity of 5.0–80.0 $\times 10^9$/L with 20–80% neutrophils and TP of 50–80 g/L.[52]

Anaplasma phagocytophilum was reported to cause bilateral pleural effusion in two equids.[54] The pathogenesis of fluid formation was suggested to be secondary to vasculitis. Fluid samples had TNCCs $< 8.0 \times 10^9$/L with TP of 20–44 g/L.[54] Morulae were seen in neutrophils in one effusion.

Penetrating wounds to the thorax as well esophageal rupture can result in pleuritis and a septic, high cellularity, exudative effusion.[46,47,55]

Exudative pleural effusions that are not associated with infectious or neoplastic causes are rare.[43,47] The few cases described were related to chronic idiopathic pleuritis or systemic granulomatous disease.[45,56]

Peritoneal

Peritoneal fluid examination, even if an effusion is not present, is a standard tool in the diagnostic evaluation of colic. Fluid findings are rarely specific for certain disorders and reflect the continuum of pathological change occurring in the gastrointestinal tract (GIT). Fluid with normal TNCC, TP, and cell populations should only be interpreted as a pathological transudate if volume is increased. This type of fluid has been reported in cases of impaction, diarrhea, neoplasia, abscessation, and early strangulating lesions but without details of volume.[6,57–59] Fluid with normal TNCC but increased TP can occur with impactions, early infarction and strangulation, and duodenitis–proximal jejunitis.[6,58,60] Once intestinal ischemia, necrosis, or infarction with resulting peritonitis is present, the fluid becomes increasingly orange to red as a result of diapedesis of erythrocytes through damaged intestine.[6,58,61] An increase in the TNCC with a predominance of neutrophils and an increase in TP and turbidity of the fluid occur. When rupture occurs, microorganisms and intestinal contents are additionally seen (Figure 53.2).[58] In peracute cases, the TP and TNCC may not be increased (Figure 53.3). Experimental peritoneal inoculation of horses with *Escherichia coli* and/or *Bacteroides* results in significant increases in TP and TNCC after two and four hours post inoculation, respectively.[62]

Non-GIT causes for exudative peritoneal fluid include ruptures of the urogenital tract, cholangitis, hepatic torsion, intra-abdominal abscesses, and pancreatitis in foals.[57,63–65] Bacteria have been detected cytologically in the peritoneal fluid of 44% of horses with abdominal abscesses.[57] Migrating strongyle larvae may result in peritonitis (Figure 53.4).[66]

Uncomplicated surgery can result in a noninfectious exudate. TNCC of up to 420.0×10^9/L and TP up to 68 g/L were recorded in the peritoneal fluid of ponies after exploratory laparotomy and remained elevated for up to 2 weeks.[67]

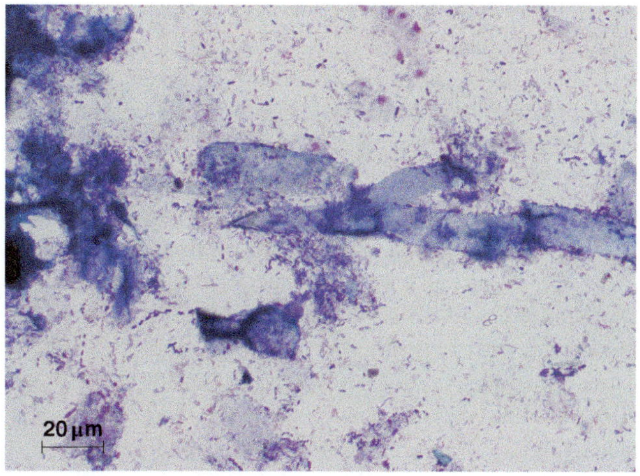

Figure 53.3 Smear of concentrated peritoneal fluid from a stallion with recurrent cecal impaction. Fluid is yellow-brown and turbid with a TNCC of 1.3×10^9/L and TP of 34 g/L. Plant material and numerous extracellular bacteria are seen, while nucleated cells are rare. The interpretation is gastrointestinal content, either due to enterocentesis or peracute rupture. The horse was found on postmortem to have a cecal rupture. Peritoneal fluid collected shortly after gastrointestinal rupture may not show an elevated TNCC and TP (Diff-Quik, 500×).

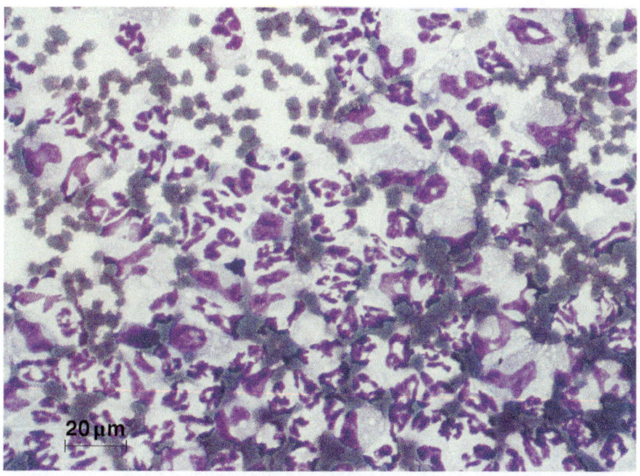

Figure 53.2 Direct smear of peritoneal fluid from an adult gelding presenting with pyrexia and colic three weeks after abdominal surgery for a recurrent nephrosplenic entrapment. During the previous surgery, the entrapment was reduced, and enterotomy was performed at the colonic pelvic flexure to relieve a concurrent impaction. Fluid is orange-red and cloudy with a TNCC of 177.0×10^9/L and TP of 45 g/L. The cell population consists of 60% degenerate neutrophils and 40% highly active macrophages. Phagocytosed bacterial cocci and rods are seen. The interpretation is septic exudative effusion. The horse was euthanized, and severe cecal impaction and rupture with severe serofibrinous peritonitis were found on necropsy. The previous enterotomy site had healed (Diff-Quik, 500×).

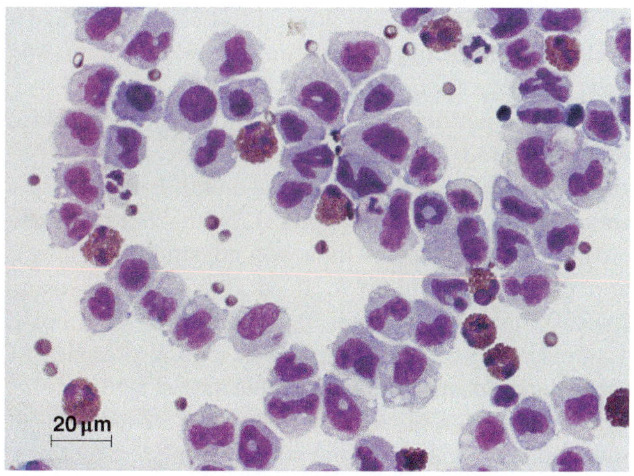

Figure 53.4 Smear of concentrated peritoneal fluid from an adult mare with parasitic thromboembolism due to migrating strongyles. Fluid is dark yellow and turbid with a TNCC of 13.0×10^9/L and TP of 30 g/L. There is a mixed cell population dominated by macrophages (70%) with 20% eosinophils and low numbers of neutrophils and reactive mesothelial cells. The interpretation is exudative effusion with eosinophilic inflammation related to parasitic larval migrans (Diff-Quik, 500×).

Clinical Utility of Peritoneal Fluid Analysis in Colic

Many studies have looked at the information that different peritoneal fluid variables can offer in terms of lesion type, outcome, and whether surgical or medical treatment is necessary.

The appearance of peritoneal fluid has been found to be a very important factor for decision-making and prognosis in colic. The presence of serosanguinous peritoneal fluid or visual hemolysis had a very high specificity (up to 99%) and positive predictive value for the need for surgery in horses presenting with colic in four separate studies.[21,68–70] In terms of prognosis, of 74 horses with severe colic, those with red fluid did not survive, with chances of survival decreasing as color changed from yellow to orange to red.[71] Horses with diaphragmatic hernias and a serosanguinous peritoneal fluid were more likely to die or be euthanized than those with normal appearing fluid, and abnormal color was the only fluid variable that was significantly associated with survival.[72] Serosanguinous or turbid fluid is found to be a predictor of ischemia due to strangulating obstruction.[73] Assessment of color and clarity may therefore be the most important part of peritoneal fluid analysis. Serosanguinous fluid should be differentiated from blood contamination (see sections "Abdominocentesis" and "Complications").

Cell counts, characteristics of the cell population, and evidence of sepsis do not appear helpful in predicting the lesion type, outcome, or need for surgery.[21,68,74] TP of >20 g/L (by refractometry) was found to have a specificity of 86% and sensitivity of 75% for the need for surgery.[21]

Peritoneal fluid glucose <30 mg/dL (1.67 mmol/L) had a specificity of 100% and sensitivity of 67% for discriminating septic from non-septic peritonitis.[75]

Lactate in peritoneal fluid of a group of horses with colic was found to be significantly higher in non-survivors and correlated to non-survival and the presence of a strangulating lesion. No horse with fluid lactate >10 mmol/L survived.[71] In a second study, peritoneal fluid lactate of >4 mmol/L at admission or increasing concentrations, especially if fluid lactate was <4 mmol/L at admission, had high odds ratios for the presence of strangulating obstructions.[76] Fluid lactate of >16 mmol/L corresponded to a probability of death of 92 and 82% in colic horses with and without strangulating obstructions, respectively.[77] Peritoneal fluid lactate must be interpreted together with blood lactate. Healthy horses have a blood to peritoneal fluid lactate ratio of >1.0.[77] Horses with strangulating obstructions were more likely to have a lactate ratio <1.0 than those without strangulation in one study, and 87% of colic horses with a ratio >1.0 survived in another.[73,76]

Neoplasia-Related Effusions

Tumors can cause lymphatic drainage obstruction, hemorrhage, or inflammation, thus resulting in effusions with a range of TNCC and TP that vary from normal to very high. Based on the reports detailed below, TNCC for pleural effusions associated with neoplasia range from $3.0–51.0 \times 10^9$/L and for peritoneal effusions from $0.1–180.0 \times 10^9$/L, TP from <25 to 65 g/L for pleural, and 10–70 g/L for peritoneal fluids. Fluid volumes are not always described. Sensitivity of cytology depends on the location and type of tumor.

Pleural

Neoplasia appears to be the most common cause of pleural effusion in horses in the United Kingdom.[47] Tumors in the mediastinum or pleura are generally associated with a significant volume of effusion, which can be clear, straw-colored, or serosanguinous, with variable TNCC, a mixed cell population, and increased TP.[47,78]

Cytological examination of pleural fluid is considered useful for the diagnosis of neoplasia (Figure 53.5), although data on the diagnostic accuracy of this method is scarce.[47,78] When antemortum pleural fluid from 13 horses with postmortem-confirmed thoracic neoplasia

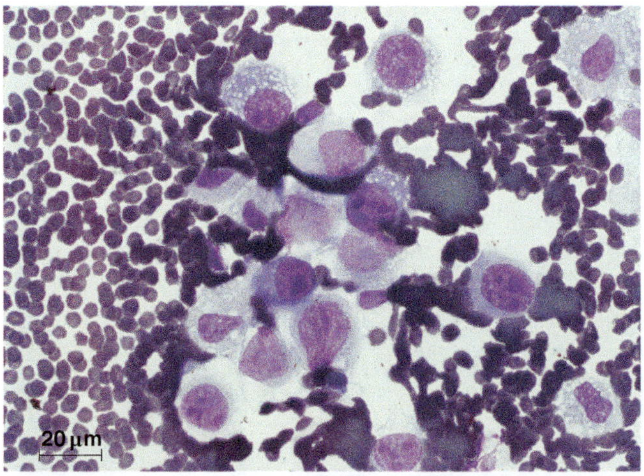

Figure 53.5 Smear of concentrated pleural fluid from a mare with intermittent fever, ataxia, and bilateral pleural effusion. The fluid is red and turbid, with a TNCC of 1.6×10^9/L and TP of 33 g/L. There is a mixed population of non-degenerate neutrophils, active macrophages, and reactive mesothelial cells. There are small, tightly adherent clusters or discretely occurring large cells with a small to medium amount of light blue cytoplasm, often with small clear vacuoles. Nuclei are round to angular, with a coarse chromatin pattern and multiple prominent nucleoli. The interpretation is neoplastic effusion, with differentials of epithelial or histiocytic origin. Following euthanasia, pheochromocytoma with multiple metastatic lesions on the pleural surfaces was diagnosed with histopathology (Diff-Quik, 500×).

was examined, a correct cytologic diagnosis of neoplasia (lymphoid or non-lymphoid) was made in nine samples; four were false negatives.[79]

Primary pulmonary tumors rarely cause effusions. The granular cell tumor is the most common primary lung tumor of horses, but there are no reports of related effusion.[52]

Lymphoma is the most common thoracic tumor of horses, consisting of up to 64% of reported thoracic neoplasms.[16,47,79,80] As it often originates from extra-thoracic sites or is multicentric at diagnosis, lymphoma is considered to be a secondary, not primary, thoracic tumor in the horse.[80,81] Most equine lymphomas are the large T-cell type, and thoracic and mediastinal lymph nodes are usually involved, with the lungs less commonly affected.[79,80,82] Thoracic lymphoma is typically associated with large volumes of fluid, with normal to increased TNCCs and increased TP.[44,47,52,78,82] The fluid may contain a predominance of lymphoid cells with mitoses and bizarre morphology.[44,81] The diagnosis of lymphoma is made on effusion cytology, in up to 80% of cases.[44,78,83] Bilateral sampling is recommended. Immunophenotyping can be performed on the effusion, and flow cytometry findings appear to be consistent with immunohistochemical results.[82] The procedure and available antibodies have been described.[84]

Hemangiosarcoma is the second most common metastatic thoracic neoplasm, involving the lung and pleura. Approximately 20% of cases have a hemorrhagic pleural effusion; the finding of neoplastic cells is rare.[52,85]

Several cases of melanoma causing pleural effusion, usually of low cellularity, have been reported. Melanophages or melanocytes were seen in the fluid in most horses.[86–90]

Squamous cell carcinoma can metastasize to the thorax, originating mostly from the stomach but also from cutaneous, ocular, and oral sites. Pleural effusion, with normal to high cellularity, can be present. Neoplastic squamous cells were identified in the pleural fluid of 4/4 horses with pleural effusion associated with metastatic gastric squamous cell carcinoma.[80,91–93]

Other metastatic tumors that have been documented to cause pleural effusion with neoplastic cells seen on cytology include pancreatic adenocarcinoma, ovarian carcinoma, and fibrosarcoma.[94–96] Metastatic neoplasia in the thorax causing effusion without the presence of malignant cells includes cases of a renal carcinoma, cholangiocellular carcinoma, primitive neuroectodermal tumor, gastric leiomyosarcoma, malignant hepatoblastomas, and a mast cell tumor.[80,97–102]

Peritoneal

Peritoneal effusion cytology is specific but not sensitive for the diagnosis of neoplasia. Abdominal fluid examination leads to a diagnosis in 44% of neoplasms and 20% of abscesses in one study.[103] Repeated samples (mean of 1.45 fluid examinations) were needed to diagnose neoplasia, so examination of multiple samples is important.[103]

Lymphoma is the most common intestinal neoplasm in horses, followed by adenocarcinoma and smooth muscle tumors.[104] Gastric lymphoma on the other hand is rare.[93] Neoplastic lymphoid cells were seen in the peritoneal fluid of 38% of horses with intestinal lymphoma.[104] An eosinophilic (cellularity not given) effusion was reported in a horse with intestinal T-cell lymphoma, suggesting that lymphoma should be included as a differential for effusions of this nature.[105] Disseminated large granular lymphocyte lymphomas have been diagnosed by detecting these cells in peritoneal fluid.[106,107]

Gastric squamous cell carcinoma can result in an effusion, which may be septic if rupture has occurred. Neoplastic squamous cells were detected in peritoneal fluid in approximately 28% of reported cases.[92,93,108]

Reports of other abdominal tumors with the concurrent presence of neoplastic cells in peritoneal fluid include renal carcinoma (3/14 cases), melanoma, and ovarian carcinoma.[86,89,95,109] Intestinal adenocarcinoma can be associated with an exudative effusion, but neoplastic cells were not observed.[104]

Mesothelioma

Mesotheliomas are rare in horses and occur in either or both the pleural and peritoneal cavities.[78,110] These tumors are consistently reported to be associated with large volumes of effusion containing neoplastic mesothelial cells.[78,80,110,111] Cytological features of these cells include mitotic figures, multinucleation, pleomorphism, large cytoplasmic vacuoles, and occurrence in clumps, sheets, or polypoid arrangements of more than 50 cells.[80,111] Lipid-rich and biphasic types are described.[112,113] Biopsy with routine histopathology can be, but is not always, diagnostic.[52,114,115] Immunohistochemistry with calretinin as a marker has been used successfully.[116] Demonstration of mesothelial cell acid mucin by alcian blue staining and intracytoplasmic lipid using oil red O can be helpful.[112,115]

Chylous Effusion

Chylous effusion is caused by an obstruction to lymphatic flow resulting in either distension of lymphatic ducts with subsequent transudation of lymph, or frank rupture.[117] Obstruction can be caused by masses or be functional as a result of increased venous pressure or lymphatic flow.[118] Rupture is rarely caused by trauma.[118] Chylous fluids are opaque and do not clear with centrifugation.[119] Typically, in dogs and cats, fluid triglyceride concentrations are greater than that of serum (>100 mg/dL or 1.13 mmol/L), fluid cholesterol to triglyceride ratio is <1.0, and small lymphocytes predominate on cytology.[118] Chyle may elicit an inflammatory response, in which case neutrophils will predominate.[118,120] Unfortunately, these changes are not consistently investigated in the few equine reports published, and no study has validated similar criteria for horses.

Chyloabdomen is reported in foals with lymphangiectasia and lymphatic rupture due to abdominal abscessation or mesenteric lymphadenomegaly.[117,119–122] Cases in adults are rare; causes include damage to mesenteric lymph vessels due to colonic torsion and tearing of abdominal adhesions and disruption of retroperitoneal lymph vessels post-nephrectomy.[123–125] Effusion TNCC in all these reports varied from very low to increased, with lymphocytes predominating in two cases (reported to be 63–73% of the TNCC) and neutrophils predominating in the others (58–98% of TNCC).

Chylothorax appears rare in horses. Bilateral idiopathic chylothorax was described in a filly; TNCC was 18.0×10^9/L with 84% small lymphocytes.[126] A second foal with idiopathic chylothorax had a bilateral pleural effusion with mildly increased cellularity dominated by neutrophils.[127] A third foal had chylothorax associated with a diaphragmatic hernia characterized by a low cellularity effusion with 74% small lymphocytes; the milky fluid cleared with ether.[128]

Based on these reports, increased numbers of small lymphocytes are not a consistent finding in chylous effusions in horses, similar to dogs and cats.[118] Of the 12 cases described here, 10 had fluid triglyceride concentrations measured, and all had results of >100 mg/dL (1.13 mmol/L), suggesting this may be the most useful test for determining a chylous effusion.

Hemorrhagic Effusions

Laboratory findings, particularly PCV, of hemorrhagic effusions are seldom reported in the literature. An evidence-based approach to defining the cytological characteristics of a hemothorax or hemoperitoneum is therefore difficult. For example, various texts state that PCVs of >3%, >10%, or approaching that of peripheral blood characterize a hemorrhagic effusion in animals but provide no further data or references.[29,32,129] A review of 19 equine cases of hemoperitoneum reported a PCV of 18–39% in the 17 peritoneal fluid samples examined.[130] Hemorrhage should be differentiated from blood contamination, as explained previously.

Causes of hemothorax include trauma, aortic rupture, thoracocentesis, insertion of chest drains, and surgery.[1,131–135]

Causes of hemoperitoneum include trauma, splenic rupture, hepatic torsion, ovarian hematomas, post-parturient uterine artery rupture, idiopathic rupture of other abdominal blood vessels, and mesenteric injury.[63,130,133,136] Up to one quarter of cases were idiopathic in one study.[137]

Neoplasia appears to be an important cause of hemorrhagic effusion in the horse, particularly hemangiosarcoma.[137] As the antemortem rate of hemangiosarcoma diagnosis is low, more effort should be made to check for this tumor in horses with hemothorax or hemoperitoneum.[85] Hemoperitoneum was found in 21% of horses with renal carcinoma and has also been reported with ovarian tumors, melanomas, squamous cell carcinoma, and lymphoma.[104,137]

Coagulopathies rarely result in cavitatory hemorrhage. Reports include hemoperitoneum due to disseminated intravascular coagulation and hemophilia A.[135,137,138]

Uroperitoneum/Urinothorax

Uroperitoneum is well described in neonatal foals with an incidence of 0.2–2.5% due to rupture of the lower urinary tract during parturition.[139] Peritoneal fluid to serum creatinine ratios >2.0 are diagnostic for uroperitoneum, and higher ratios are associated with death.[139] Ratios increase from 2 hours post rupture and start to decline after a further 18 hours.[140] Calcium carbonate crystals may be seen in the abdominal fluid.[141]

A filly with uroperitoneum was reported to have a concurrent urinothorax with a pleural fluid to serum creatinine ratio >1.0.[142] Concurrent pleural effusion not attributed to urinothorax is recognized in foals with uroperitoneum. The pathogenesis of this is unclear but may be related to re-expansion pulmonary edema and/or acute lung injury/acute respiratory distress syndrome following correction of abdominal compartment syndrome.[143,144]

Uroperitoneum may occur as a result of obstructive urethral urolithiasis in adult horses.[145,146]

Other

Cytological examination of fluids may result in findings unrelated to the primary cause of the effusion. For example, oil red O-positive lipid was found within neutrophils and macrophages as well as in the background in the peritoneal fluid of a horse with an exudate secondary to a rectal tear.[147] A filly with pleuropneumonia and resulting bilateral pleural effusion was found incidentally to have carboxymethylcellulose within macrophages in pleural fluid.[148] This was as a result of infusion of the substance during abdominal surgery for an umbilical hematoma. It was thought that the carboxymethylcellulose entered the pleural fluid either from the blood or a small diaphragmatic hernia.

Advanced and Other Diagnostic Techniques

Phosphate, serum amyloid-A, alkaline phosphatase, and lactate dehydrogenase are routine analytes offered by most laboratories and have been investigated in peritoneal fluid of colic horses. Differences were found for different intestinal lesions, but results were not as clinically useful as lactate and glucose.[75,149–152]

Concentrations of peritoneal fluid interleukin-6, transforming growth factor beta, haptoglobin, and myeloperoxidase have been shown to be associated with lesion type in equine colic, but more research into their clinical utility is needed.[152–156]

References

1 Chaffin, M.K. (1999). Thoracocentesis and pleural drainage in horses. *Equine Vet Educ* 11: 106–108.
2 Wagner, A.E. and Bennett, D.G. (1982). Analysis of equine thoracic fluid. *Vet Clin Pathol* 11: 13–17.
3 Beccati, F., Nannarone, S., Gialletti, R. et al. (2014). Evaluation of transabdominal ultrasound as a tool for predicting the success of abdominocentesis in horses. *Vet Rec* 174: 251.
4 Siex, M.T. and Wilson, J.H. (1992). Morbidity associated with abdominocentesis: a prospective study. *Equine Vet J* 24: 23–25.
5 Duesterdieck-Zellmer, K.F., Riehl, J.H., McKenzie, E.C. et al. (2014). Effects of abdominocentesis technique on peritoneal fluid and clinical variables in horses. *Equine Vet Educ* 26: 262–268.
6 Bach, L.G. and Ricketts, S.W. (1974). Paracentesis as an aid to the diagnosis of abdominal disease in the horse. *Equine Vet J* 6: 116–121.
7 Juzwiak, J.S., Ragle, C.A., Brown, C.M. et al. (1991). The effect of repeated abdominocentesis on peritoneal fluid constituents in the horse. *Vet Res Commun* 15: 177–180.
8 Romero, A.E., Nieto, J.E., Dechant, J.E. et al. (2011). Effects of aerobic and anaerobic fluid collection on biochemical analysis of peritoneal fluid in healthy horses and horses with colic. *Vet Surg* 40: 40–45.
9 Chadha, T.S. and Cohn, M.A. (1983). Noninvasive treatment of pneumothorax with oxygen inhalation. *Respiration* 44: 147–152.
10 Schumacher, J., Spano, J.S., and Moll, H.D. (1985). Effects of enterocentesis on peritoneal fluid constituents in the horse. *J Am Vet Med Assoc* 186: 1301–1303.
11 Hardy, J. (2010). Basic procedures in adult equine critical care. In: *Equine Internal Medicine* (eds. S.M. Reed, W.M. Bayly and D.C. Sellon), 258. St. Louis: Saunders/Elsevier.
12 Malark, J.A., Peyton, L.C., and Galvin, M.J. (1992). Effects of blood contamination on equine peritoneal fluid analysis. *J Am Vet Med Assoc* 201: 1545–1548.
13 Tulleners, E.P. (1983). Complications of abdominocentesis in the horse. *J Am Vet Med Assoc* 182: 232–234.
14 Ragle, C.A., Meagher, D.M., Lacroix, C.A., and Honnas, C.M. (1989). Surgical treatment of sand colic. Results in 40 horses. *Vet Surg* 18: 48–51.
15 Cook, V.L. and Hassel, D.M. (2014). Evaluation of the colic in horses: decision for referral. *Vet Clin North Am Equine Pract* 30: 383–398.
16 Mair, T.S. and Sweeney, C.R. (1992). The investigation of pleural effusions in the horse. *Equine Vet Educ* 4: 70–74.
17 Brownlow, M.A., Hutchins, D.R., and Johnston, K.G. (1981). Reference values for equine peritoneal fluid. *Equine Vet J* 13: 127–130.
18 Garma-Avina, A. (1998). Cytology of 100 samples of abdominal fluid from 100 horses with abdominal disease. *Equine Vet J* 30: 435–444.
19 Cohen, N.D., Carter, G.K., Mealey, R.H., and Taylor, T.S. (1995). Medical management of right dorsal colitis in 5 horses: a retrospective study (1987–1993). *J Vet Intern Med* 9: 272–276.
20 Hotz, C.S., Templeton, S.J., and Christopher, M.M. (2005). Comparative analysis of expert and machine-learning methods for classification of body cavity effusions in companion animals. *J Vet Diagn Invest* 17: 158–164.
21 Matthews, S., Dart, A.J., Reid, S.W.J. et al. (2002). Predictive values, sensitivity and specificity of abdominal fluid variables in determining the need for surgery in horses with an acute abdominal crisis. *Aust Vet J* 80: 132–136.
22 Henderson, I.S.F., Mair, T.S., Keen, J.A. et al. (2008). Study of the short- and long-term outcomes of 65 horses with peritonitis. *Vet Rec* 163: 293–297.
23 Brownlow, M.A., Hutchins, D.R., and Johnston, K.G. (1982). Mesothelial cells of peritoneal fluid. *Equine Vet J* 14: 86–88.
24 Lillich, J.D., Ray-Miller, W., Silver, K.S. et al. (2011). Intra-abdominal hyaluronan concentration in peritoneal fluid of horses with sudden signs of severe abdominal pain. *Am J Vet Res* 72: 1666–1673.
25 Grindem, C.B., Fairley, N.M., Uhlinger, C.A., and Crane, S.A. (1990). Peritoneal fluid values from healthy foals. *Equine Vet J* 22: 359–361.

26 Behrens, E., Parraga, M.E., Nassiff, A., and Crane, S.A. (1990). Reference values of peritoneal fluid from healthy foals. *J Equine Vet Sci* 10: 348–352.
27 Walton, R.M. and Southwood, L.L. (2012). Abdominocentesis and peritoneal fluid analysis. In: *Practical Guide to Equine Colic* (ed. L.L. Southwood), 87–98. Ames, IA: Wiley.
28 DeHeer, H.L., Parry, B.W., and Grindem, C.B. (2002). Pleural fluid. In: *Diagnostic Cytology and Hematology of the Horse*, 2e (eds. R.L. Cowell and R.D. Tyler), 107–126. St. Louis, MO: Mosby.
29 DeHeer, H.L., Parry, B.W., and Grindem, C.B. (2002). Peritoneal fluid. In: *Diagnostic Cytology and Hematology of the Horse*, 2e (eds. R.L. Cowell and R.D. Tyler), 127–162. St. Louis, MO: Mosby.
30 Zoia, A. and Drigo, M. (2016). Diagnostic value of Light's criteria and albumin gradient in classifying the pathophysiology of pleural effusion formation in cats. *J Feline Med Surg* 18: 666–672.
31 Lester, S.J., Mollat, W.H., and Bryant, J.E. (2015). Overview of clinical pathology and the horse. *Vet Clin North Am Equine Pract* 31: 247–268.
32 Stockham, S.L. and Scott, M.A. (eds.) (2008). Cavitatory effusions. In: *Fundamentals of Veterinary Clinical Pathology*. Ames, IA: Blackwell.
33 Corning, S. (2009). Equine cyathostomins: a review of biology, clinical significance and therapy. *Parasit Vectors* 2: S1.
34 Pusterla, N. and Gebhart, C. (2009). Equine proliferative enteropathy caused by *Lawsonia intracellularis*. *Equine Vet Educ* 21: 415–419.
35 Schott, H.C. (2007). Chronic renal failure in horses. *Vet Clin North Am Equine Pract* 23: 593–612.
36 Durham, A.E., Newton, J.R., Smith, K.C. et al. (2003). Retrospective analysis of historical, clinical, ultrasonographic, serum biochemical and haematological data in prognostic evaluation of equine liver disease. *Equine Vet J* 35: 542–547.
37 McGorum, B.C., Murphy, D., Love, S., and Milne, E.M. (1999). Clinicopathological features of equine primary hepatic disease: a review of 50 cases. *Vet Rec* 145: 134–139.
38 West, H.J. (1996). Clinical and pathological studies in horses with hepatic disease. *Equine Vet J* 28: 146–156.
39 Davis, J.L., Gardner, S.Y., Schwabenton, B., and Breuhaus, B.A. (2002). Congestive heart failure in horses: 14 cases (1984–2001). *J Am Vet Med Assoc* 220: 1512–1515.
40 Maxson, A.D. and Reef, V.B. (1997). Bacterial endocarditis in horses: ten cases (1984–1995). *Equine Vet J* 29: 394–399.
41 Porter, S.R., Saegerman, C., Van Galen, G. et al. (2008). Vegetative endocarditis in equids (1994–2006). *J Vet Intern Med* 22: 1411–1416.
42 Reef, V.B., Bain, F.T., and Spencer, P.A. (1998). Severe mitral regurgitation in horses: clinical, echocardiographic and pathological findings. *Equine Vet J* 30: 18–27.
43 Sweeney, C.R. (1992). Causes of pleural effusion in the horse. *Equine Vet Educ* 4: 75–77.
44 Smith, B.P. (1977). Pleuritis and pleural effusion in the horse: a study of 37 cases. *J Am Vet Med Assoc* 170: 208–211.
45 Mair, T.S. and Lane, J.G. (1989). Pneumonia, lung abscesses and pleuritis in adult horses: a review of 51 cases. *Equine Vet J* 21: 175–180.
46 Collins, M.B., Hodgson, D.R., and Hutchins, D.R. (1994). Pleural effusion associated with acute and chronic pleuropneumonia and pleuritis secondary to thoracic wounds in horses: 43 cases (1982–1992). *J Am Vet Med Assoc* 205: 1753–1758.
47 Johns, I., Marr, C., Durham, A. et al. (2017). Causes of pleural effusions in horses resident in the UK. *Equine Vet Educ* 29: 144–148.
48 Reuss, S.M. and Giguere, S. (2015). Update on bacterial pneumonia and pleuropneumonia in the adult horse. *Vet Clin North Am Equine Pract* 31: 105–120.
49 Sprayberry, K.A. and Byars, T.D. (1999). Equine pleuropneumonia. *Equine Vet Educ* 11: 290–293.
50 Sweeney, C.R., Holcombe, S.J., Barningham, S.C., and Beech, J. (1991). Aerobic and anaerobic bacterial isolates from horses with pneumonia or pleuropneumonia and antimicrobial susceptibility patterns of the aerobes. *J Am Vet Med Assoc* 198: 839–842.
51 Hoffman, A.M., Baird, J.D., Kloeze, H.J. et al. (1992). Mycoplasma felis pleuritis in two show-jumper horses. *Cornell Vet* 82: 155–162.
52 Davis, E.G. and Rush, B.R. (2013). Diagnostic challenges: equine thoracic neoplasia. *Equine Vet Educ* 25: 96–107.
53 Wilson, J.H., Olson, E.J., Haugen, E.W. et al. (2006). Systemic blastomycosis in a horse. *J Vet Diagn Invest* 18: 615–619.
54 Restifo, M.M., Bedenice, D., Thane, K.E., and Mazan, M.R. (2015). Cavitary effusion associated with *Anaplasma phagocytophilum* infection in 2 equids. *J Vet Intern Med* 29: 732–735.
55 Burbidge, H.M. (1982). Penetrating thoracic wound in a Hackney mare. *Equine Vet J* 14: 94–95.
56 Axon, J.E., Robinson, P., and Lucas, J. (2004). Generalised granulomatous disease in a horse. *Aust Vet J* 82: 48–51.
57 Arnold, C.E. and Chaffin, M.K. (2012). Abdominal abscesses in adult horses: 61 cases (1993–2008). *J Am Vet Med Assoc* 241: 1659–1665.
58 Plummer, A.E., Rakestraw, P.C., Hardy, J., and Lee, R.M. (2007). Outcome of medical and surgical treatment of cecal impaction in horses: 114 cases (1994–2004). *J Am Vet Med Assoc* 231: 1378–1385.

59 Fleming, K. and Mueller, P.O.E. (2011). Ileal impaction in 245 horses: 1995–2007. *Can Vet J* 52: 759–763.
60 Freeman, D.E. (2000). Duodenitis-proximal jejunitis. *Equine Vet Educ* 12: 322–332.
61 Hillyer, M.H. and Wright, C.J. (1997). Peritonitis in the horse. *Equine Vet Educ* 9: 136–142.
62 Mendes, L.C.N., Marques, L.C., Bechara, G.H., and Peiró, J.R. (1999). Experimental peritonitis in horses: peritoneal fluid composition. *Arq Bras Med Vet Zootec* 51: 217–222.
63 Bentz, K.J., Burgess, B.A., Lohmann, K.L., and Shahriar, F. (2009). Hepatic lobe torsion in a horse. *Can Vet J* 50: 283–286.
64 Ollivett, T.L., Divers, T.J., Cushing, T. et al. (2012). Acute pancreatitis in two five-day-old Appaloosa foals. *Equine Vet J Suppl*: 96–99.
65 Taintor, J., Sartin, E.A., Waldridge, B.M., and Schumacher, J. (2006). Acute pancreatitis in a 3-day-old foal. *J Vet Intern Med* 20: 210–212.
66 Dyson, S. (1983). Review of 30 cases of peritonitis in the horse. *Equine Vet J* 15: 25–30.
67 Santschi, E.M., Grindem, C.B., Tate, L.P., and Corbett, W.T. (1988). Peritoneal fluid analysis in ponies after abdominal surgery. *Vet Surg* 17: 6–9.
68 Ducharme, N.G., Pascoe, P.J., Lumsden, J.H., and Ducharme, G.R. (1989). A computer-derived protocol to aid in selecting medical versus surgical treatment of horses with abdominal pain. *Equine Vet J* 21: 447–450.
69 Thoefner, M.B., Ersbøll, B.K., Jansson, N., and Hesselholt, M. (2003). Diagnostic decision rule for support in clinical assessment of the need for surgical intervention in horses with acute abdominal pain. *Can J Vet Res* 67: 20–29.
70 Weimann, C.D., Thoefner, M.B., and Jensen, A.L. (2002). Spectrophotometric assessment of peritoneal fluid haemoglobin in colic horses: an aid to selecting medical vs. surgical treatment. *Equine Vet J* 34: 523–527.
71 Van Den Boom, R., Butler, C.M., and Sloet van Oldruitenborgh-Oosterbaan, M.M. (2010). The usability of peritoneal lactate concentration as a prognostic marker in horses with severe colic admitted to a veterinary teaching hospital. *Equine Vet Educ* 22: 420–425.
72 Hart, S.K. and Brown, J.A. (2009). Diaphragmatic hernia in horses: 44 cases (1986–2006). *J Vet Emerg Crit Care* 19: 357–362.
73 Latson, K.M., Nieto, J.E., Beldomenico, P.M., and Snyder, J.R. (2005). Evaluation of peritoneal fluid lactate as a marker of intestinal ischaemia in equine colic. *Equine Vet J* 37: 342–346.
74 Freden, G.O., Provost, P.J., and Rand, W.M. (1998). Reliability of using results of abdominal fluid analysis to determine treatment and predict lesion type and outcome for horses with colic: 218 cases (1991–1994). *J Am Vet Med Assoc* 213: 1012–1015.
75 Van Hoogmoed, L., Rodger, L.D., Spier, S.J. et al. (1999). Evaluation of peritoneal fluid pH, glucose concentration, and lactate dehydrogenase activity for detection of septic peritonitis in horses. *J Am Vet Med Assoc* 214: 1032–1036.
76 Peloso, J.G. and Cohen, N.D. (2012). Use of serial measurements of peritoneal fluid lactate concentration to identify strangulating intestinal lesions in referred horses with signs of colic. *J Am Vet Med Assoc* 240: 1208–1217.
77 Delesalle, C., Dewulf, J., Lefebvre, R.A. et al. (2007). Determination of lactate concentrations in blood plasma and peritoneal fluid in horses with colic by an accusport analyzer. *J Vet Intern Med* 21: 293–301.
78 Mair, T.S., Rush, B.R., and Tucker, R.L. (2004). Clinical and diagnostic features of thoracic neoplasia in the horse. *Equine Vet Educ* 16: 30–36.
79 Sweeney, C.R. and Gillette, D.M. (1989). Thoracic neoplasia in equids: 35 cases (1967–1987). *J Am Vet Med Assoc* 195: 374–377.
80 Mair, T.S. and Brown, P.J. (1993). Clinical and pathological features of thoracic neoplasia in the horse. *Equine Vet J* 25: 220–223.
81 Mair, T.S., Lane, J.G., and Lucke, V.M. (1985). Clinicopathological features of lymphosarcoma involving the thoracic cavity in the horse. *Equine Vet J* 17: 428–433.
82 Meyer, J., Delay, J., and Bienzle, D. (2006). Clinical, laboratory, and histopathologic features of equine lymphoma. *Vet Pathol* 43: 914–924.
83 Garber, J.L., Reef, V.B., and Reimer, J.M. (1994). Sonographic findings in horses with mediastinal lymphosarcoma: 13 cases (1985–1992). *J Am Vet Med Assoc* 205: 1432–1436.
84 Roberts, M.C. (2008). Equine lymphoma: what are the prospects for cellular differentiation, early diagnosis and intervention strategies? *Equine Vet Educ* 20: 464–466.
85 Southwood, L.L., Schott, H.C. 2nd, Henry, C.J. et al. (2000). Disseminated hemangiosarcoma in the horse: 35 cases. *J Vet Intern Med* 14: 105–109.
86 MacGillivray, K.C., Sweeney, R.W., and Piero, F.D. (2002). Metastatic melanoma in horses. *J Vet Intern Med* 16: 452–456.
87 Metcalfe, L.V.A., O'Brien, P.J., Papakonstantinou, S. et al. (2013). Malignant melanoma in a grey horse: case presentation and review of equine melanoma treatment options. *Ir Vet J* 66: 22–22.
88 Milne, J.C. (1986). Malignant melanomas causing Horner's syndrome in a horse. *Equine Vet J* 18: 74–75.
89 Tarrant, J., Stokol, T., Bartol, J. et al. (2001). Diagnosis of malignant melanoma in a horse from cytology of body cavity fluid and blood. *Equine Vet J* 33: 531–534.
90 Murray, M.J., Cavey, D.M., Feldman, B.F. et al. (1997). Signs of sympathetic denervation associated with a

thoracic melanoma in a horse. *J Vet Intern Med* 11: 199–203.

91 Wrigley, R.H., Gay, C.C., Lording, P., and Haywood, R.N. (1981). Pleural effusion associated with squamous cell carcinoma of the stomach of a horse. *Equine Vet J* 13: 99–102.

92 McKenzie, E.C., Mills, J.N., and Bolton, J.R. (1997). Gastric squamous cell carcinoma in three horses. *Aust Vet J* 75: 480–483.

93 Taylor, S.D., Haldorson, G.J., Vaughan, B., and Pusterla, N. (2009). Gastric neoplasia in horses. *J Vet Intern Med* 23: 1097–1102.

94 Rendle, D.I., Hewetson, M., Barron, R., and Baily, J.E. (2006). Tachypnoea and pleural effusion in a mare with metastatic pancreatic adenocarcinoma. *Vet Rec* 159: 356–359.

95 Morris, D.D., Acland, H.M., and Hodge, T.G. (1985). Pleural effusion secondary to metastasis of an ovarian adenocarcinoma in a horse. *J Am Vet Med Assoc* 187: 272–274.

96 Jorgensen, J.S., Geoly, F.J., Berry, C.R., and Breuhaus, B.A. (1997). Lameness and pleural effusion associated with an aggressive fibrosarcoma in a horse. *J Am Vet Med Assoc* 210: 1328–1331.

97 Facemire, P.R., Facemire, L.M., and Honnold, S.P. (2012). Peripheral primitive neuroectodermal tumor in a two-year-old paint horse. *J Vet Diagn Invest* 24: 794–796.

98 Boy, M.G., Palmer, J.E., Heyer, G., and Hamir, A.N. (1992). Gastric leiomyosarcoma in a horse. *J Am Vet Med Assoc* 200: 1363–1364.

99 Prater, P.E., Patton, C.S., and Held, J.P. (1989). Pleural effusion resulting from malignant hepatoblastoma in a horse. *J Am Vet Med Assoc* 194: 383–385.

100 Axon, J.E., Russell, C.M., Begg, A.P., and Adkins, A.R. (2008). Erythrocytosis and pleural effusion associated with a hepatoblastoma in a Thoroughbred yearling. *Aust Vet J* 86: 329–333.

101 Mueller, P.O., Morris, D.D., Carmichael, K.P. et al. (1992). Antemortem diagnosis of cholangiocellular carcinoma in a horse. *J Am Vet Med Assoc* 201: 899–901.

102 Tan, R.H.H., Crisman, M.V., Clark, S.P. et al. (2007). Multicentric mastocytoma in a horse. *J Vet Intern Med* 21: 340–343.

103 Zicker, S.C., Wilson, W.D., and Medearis, I. (1990). Differentiation between intra-abdominal neoplasms and abscesses in horses, using clinical and laboratory data: 40 cases (1973–1988). *J Am Vet Med Assoc* 196: 1130–1134.

104 Taylor, S.D., Pusterla, N., Vaughan, B. et al. (2006). Intestinal neoplasia in horses. *J Vet Intern Med* 20: 1429–1436.

105 La Perle, K.M.D., Piercy, R.J., Long, J.F., and Blomme, E.A. (1998). Multisystemic, eosinophilic, epitheliotropic disease with intestinal lymphosarcoma in a horse. *Vet Pathol* 35: 144–146.

106 Mastrorilli, C., Cesar, F., Joiner, K. et al. (2015). Disseminated lymphoma with large granular lymphocyte morphology diagnosed in a horse via abdominal fluid and transtracheal wash cytology. *Vet Clin Pathol* 44: 437–441.

107 Grindem, C.B., Roberts, M.C., McEntee, M.F., and Dillman, R.C. (1989). Large granular lymphocyte tumor in a horse. *Vet Pathol* 26: 86–88.

108 Olsen, S. (1992). Squamous cell carcinoma of the equine stomach: a report of five cases. *Vet Rec* 131: 170–173.

109 Wise, L.N., Bryan, J.N., Sellon, D.C. et al. (2009). A retrospective analysis of renal carcinoma in the horse. *J Vet Intern Med* 23: 913–918.

110 Colbourne, C.M., Bolton, J.R., Mills, J.N. et al. (1992). Mesothelioma in horses. *Aust Vet J* 69: 275–278.

111 Kramer, J.W., Nickels, F.A., and Bell, T. (1976). Cytology of diffuse mesothelioma in the thorax of a horse. *Equine Vet J* 8: 81–83.

112 Dobromylskyj, M.J., Copas, V., Durham, A. et al. (2011). Disseminated lipid-rich peritoneal mesothelioma in a horse. *J Vet Diagn Invest* 23: 615–618.

113 Ulrich, R., Eydner, M., Grun, A. et al. (2009). A biphasic malignant mesothelioma of the peritoneum and pleura in a horse. *Dtsch Tierarztl Wochenschr* 116: 186–191.

114 Fry, M.M., Magdesian, K.G., Judy, C.E. et al. (2003). Antemortem diagnosis of equine mesothelioma by pleural biopsy. *Equine Vet J* 35: 723–727.

115 May, J., Fews, D., Tennant, K., and Mair, T. (2016). Diagnostic dichotomy: a question of thoracic mesothelioma. *Equine Vet Educ* 29: 131–137.

116 Stoica, G., Cohen, N., Mendes, O., and Kim, H.T. (2004). Use of immunohistochemical marker calretinin in the diagnosis of a diffuse malignant metastatic mesothelioma in an equine. *J Vet Diagn Invest* 16: 240–243.

117 Clark, E.S., Morris, D.D., Allen, D., and Tyler, D.E. (1988). Lymphocytic enteritis in a filly. *J Am Vet Med Assoc* 193: 1281–1283.

118 Meadows, R.L. and MacWilliams, P.S. (1994). Chylous effusions revisited. *Vet Clin Pathol* 23: 54–62.

119 May, K.A. and Good, M.J. (2007). Congenital lymphangiectasia and chyloperitoneum in a foal. *Equine Vet Educ* 19: 16–18.

120 Cesar, F.B., Johnson, C.R., and Pantaleon, L.G. (2010). Suspected idiopathic intestinal lymphangiectasia in two foals with chylous peritoneal effusion. *Equine Vet Educ* 22: 172–178.

121 Campbell-Beggs, C., Johnson, P., Wilson, D., and Miller, M.A. (1995). Chyloabdomen in a neonatal foal. *Vet Rec* 137: 96–98.

122 Hanselaer, J.R. and Nyland, T.G. (1983). Chyloabdomen and ultrasonographic detection of an intra-abdominal abscess in a foal. *J Am Vet Med Assoc* 183: 1465–1467.

123 Mair, T.S. and Lucke, V.M. (1992). Chyloperitoneum associated with torsion of the large colon in a horse. *Vet Rec* 131: 421.

124 May, K.A., Cheramie, H.S., and Prater, D.A. (1999). Chyloperitoneum and abdominal adhesions in a miniature horse. *J Am Vet Med Assoc* 215: 676–678.

125 Arnold, C.E., Taylor, T., Chaffin, M.K. et al. (2013). Nephrectomy via ventral median celiotomy in equids. *Vet Surg* 42: 275–279.

126 Schumacher, J., Brusie, R., and Spano, J. (1989). Chylothorax in an Arabian filly. *Equine Vet J* 21: 132–134.

127 Scarratt, W.K., Wallace, M.A., Pleasant, R.S. et al. (1997). Chylothorax and meconium impaction in a neonatal colt. *Equine Vet J* 29: 77–79.

128 Mair, T.S., Pearson, H., Waterman, A.E. et al. (1988). Chylothorax associated with a congenital diaphragmatic defect in a foal. *Equine Vet J* 20: 304–306.

129 Dempsey, S.M. and Ewing, P.J. (2011). A review of the pathophysiology, classification, and analysis of canine and feline cavitary effusions. *J Am Anim Hosp Assoc* 47: 1–11.

130 Pusterla, N., Fecteau, M.E., Madigan, J.E. et al. (2005). Acute hemoperitoneum in horses: a review of 19 cases (1992–2003). *J Vet Intern Med* 19: 344–347.

131 Hassel, D.M. (2007). Thoracic trauma in horses. *Vet Clin North Am Equine Pract* 23: 67–80.

132 Schambourg, M.A., Laverty, S., Mullim, S. et al. (2003). Thoracic trauma in foals: post mortem findings. *Equine Vet J* 35: 78–81.

133 Lyle, C.H., Uzal, F.A., McGorum, B.C. et al. (2011). Sudden death in racing Thoroughbred horses: an international multicentre study of post mortem findings. *Equine Vet J* 43: 324–331.

134 Brown, C.M., Kaneene, J.B., and Taylor, R.F. (1988). Sudden and unexpected death in horses and ponies: an analysis of 200 cases. *Equine Vet J* 20: 99–103.

135 Groover, E.S. and Wooldridge, A.A. (2013). Equine haemothorax. *Equine Vet Educ* 25: 536–541.

136 Dyke, T.M. and Friend, S.C.E. (1988). Ruptured splenic haematoma in a mare. *Equine Vet J* 20: 138–140.

137 Dechant, J.E., Nieto, J.E., and Le Jeune, S.S. (2006). Hemoperitoneum in horses: 67 cases (1989–2004). *J Am Vet Med Assoc* 229: 253–258.

138 Henninger, R.W. (1988). Hemophilia A in two related quarter horse colts. *J Am Vet Med Assoc* 193: 91–94.

139 Kablack, K.A., Embertson, R.M., Bernard, W.V. et al. (2000). Uroperitoneum in the hospitalized equine neonate: retrospective study of 31 cases, 1988–1997. *Equine Vet J* 32: 505–508.

140 Genetzky, R.M. and Hagemoser, W.A. (1985). Physical and clinical pathological findings associated with experimentally induced rupture of the equine urinary bladder. *Can Vet J* 26: 391–395.

141 Morley, P.S. and Desnoyers, M. (1992). Diagnosis of ruptured urinary bladder in a foal by the identification of calcium carbonate crystals in the peritoneal fluid. *J Am Vet Med Assoc* 200: 1515–1517.

142 Vander Werf, K.A., Beard, L.A., and McMurphy, R.M. (2010). Urinothorax in a Quarter Horse filly. *Equine Vet Educ* 22: 239–243.

143 Wong, D.M., Leger, L.C., Scarratt, W.K., and Kline, K.A. (2004). Uroperitoneum and pleural effusion in an American Paint filly. *Equine Vet Educ* 16: 290–293.

144 Wilkins, P.A. (2004). Respiratory distress in foals with uroperitoneum: possible mechanisms. *Equine Vet Educ* 16: 293–295.

145 Saam, D. (2001). Urethrolithiasis and nephrolithiasis in a horse. *Can Vet J* 42: 880–883.

146 Gibson, K.T., Trotter, G.W., and Gustafson, S.B. (1992). Conservative management of uroperitoneum in a gelding. *J Am Vet Med Assoc* 200: 1692–1694.

147 Brown, J.S., Johnson, M.C., Sims, W.P. et al. (2011). Oil Red O-positive lipid in peritoneal fluid from a horse with a rectal tear. *Vet Clin Pathol* 40: 265–269.

148 Stokol, T., Gold, J., Johnson, A., and Ainsworth, D. (2008). What is your diagnosis? Pleural fluid from a neonatal Thoroughbred filly with pneumonia. *Vet Clin Pathol* 37: 237–241.

149 Arden, W.A. and Stick, J.A. (1988). Serum and peritoneal fluid phosphate concentrations as predictors of major intestinal injury associated with equine colic. *J Am Vet Med Assoc* 193: 927–931.

150 Saulez, M.N., Cebra, C.K., and Tornquist, S.J. (2004). The diagnostic and prognostic value of alkaline phosphatase activity in serum and peritoneal fluid from horses with acute colic. *J Vet Intern Med* 18: 564–567.

151 Smuts, C., Mills, J., Myles, R., and Gaál, T. (2016). Lactate dehydrogenase activity in abdominal fluid from horses with colic. *J Equine Vet Sci* 36: 58–62.

152 Pihl, T.H., Scheepers, E., Sanz, M. et al. (2015). Influence of disease process and duration on acute phase proteins in serum and peritoneal fluid of horses with colic. *J Vet Intern Med* 29: 651–658.

153 Barton, M.H. and Collates, C. (1999). Tumor necrosis factor and interleukin-6 activity and endotoxin concentration in peritoneal fluid and blood of horses with acute abdominal disease. *J Vet Intern Med* 13: 457–464.

154 Argüelles, D., Casteljins, G., Carmona, J.U. et al. (2010). Peritoneal concentrations of transforming growth factor beta in horses with colic. *Equine Vet J* 42: 451–455.

155 Eurell, T.E., Wilson, D.A., and Baker, G.J. (1993). The effect of exploratory laparotomy on the serum and peritoneal haptoglobin concentrations of the pony. *Can J Vet Res* 57: 42–44.

156 Grulke, S., Franck, T., Gangl, M. et al. (2008). Myeloperoxidase assay in plasma and peritoneal fluid of horses with gastrointestinal disease. *Can J Vet Res* 72: 37–42.

54

Synovial Fluid Analysis of the Dog and Cat

R. Darren Wood and Thomas Gibson

Collection

In dogs and cats, commonly sampled joints include shoulder, stifle, elbow, carpus, and tarsus. Knowledge of the specific joint anatomy and approach is required in order to properly collect the best diagnostic sample while minimizing patient discomfort.[1,2] Equipment includes a sharp needle and a sterile 3 mL syringe. Length of the needle varies with the joint and size of the animal (22- or 23 G 1 in. for dogs, 25 G 5/8-1 in. for smaller dogs and cats). In addition, glass slides for preparation of direct smears, as well as both red top and EDTA (ethylenediaminetetraacetic acid) tubes, should be available. The skin over the joint should be clipped and aseptically prepared.

It is easier to collect sufficient sample required to perform a complete fluid analysis from the shoulder and stifle joints, as these spaces typically have the largest potential space for fluid accumulation.[3] The smaller carpal and tarsal joints typically have a lower volume of fluid. In one feline study, the mean volume of fluid collected could not be measured and was often only one to two drops from stifle and shoulder joints.[4] However, even a drop is sufficient to assess color, clarity, and viscosity, as well as prepare a pull-apart glass slide for estimation of cellularity and differential count.[5] Pathology in a joint that results in effusion often eases sample collection due to increased volume of fluid present.

Care must be taken to sufficiently restrain or immobilize the patient to collect an uncontaminated sample. Use of chemical restraint is common. Excessive movement during the procedure will result in blood contamination and perhaps puncture of the articular cartilage surface, which may result in observation of synoviocytes and damage to the articular surface. Blood contamination dilutes synovial fluid and can make interpretation more difficult because of addition of erythrocytes and leukocytes. If hemorrhage is induced by sampling, platelets may be noted, while erythrophagocytosis, hemosiderin pigment, or hematoidin crystals should be absent. Erythrophagocytosis can occur *in vitro* if the sample remains unexamined for a few hours prior to slide making. Appearance of blood in the syringe after the sample is initially clear is a sure indicator of operator-induced bleeding. Blood contamination can cause the sample to clot, making direct smears more difficult to prepare and interpret. If blood is noted during the collection procedure, it is advisable to place some of the sample in a tube containing EDTA or heparin to prevent clotting. Recent arthrocentesis, even as long ago as three weeks, can complicate interpretation due to induction of inflammation from the sampling procedure.[6]

Physical Characteristics

Physical characteristics such as color and clarity can be noted as soon as the fluid is in the syringe or tube. Synovial fluid should be clear and colorless. Xanthochromia suggests prior hemorrhage, while turbidity is consistent with presence of increased erythrocytes and/or nucleated cells.[5] Once some fluid is expelled from the syringe for slide preparation, a subjective assessment of viscosity can be determined. Synovial fluid should be highly viscous due to presence of hyaluronic acid.[3] When stretched between thumb and index finger, it should form a minimum 2.5 cm string before separating.[7] If viscosity is decreased and the sample seems watery, inflammation, hemorrhage, or other cause for effusion is likely.[5] The mucin clot test is a semiquantitative assessment of viscosity.[7] The mucin clot test is best performed on a sample that is collected into a plain or heparinized tube as EDTA can degrade hyaluronic acid.[8]

Veterinary Cytology, First Edition. Edited by Leslie C. Sharkey, M. Judith Radin, and Davis Seelig.

A rigorous assessment of the additional diagnostic value of the mucin clot test cannot be found.

Cell Counts, Differential, Slide Preparation, and Staining

It is best to make slides immediately after the sample is collected to avoid artifacts and cellular degeneration. Direct smears are the most frequent slide preparation used for examination of synovial fluid. Smears are spread as thinly as possible and dried rapidly. While a sediment smear or cytocentrifuge preparation could be made, these result in very thick samples that will not dry or spread well and can cause clogging within the cytocentrifuge apparatus.[3] Normal synovial fluid is quite dense due to its viscosity, making cell identification challenging due to rounding up artifact. This can be mitigated by addition of hyaluronidase to the sample prior to slide preparation.[9] However, even in the thickest samples, cells can usually be reliably identified near the edges of the smear.

Slides can be stained with any Romanowsky-type stain. It would be unusual to require special stains on a synovial fluid sample except perhaps a Gram stain for bacteria.

Total nucleated cell counts (TNCC) can be determined using a hemocytometer (using oxylate but not acetic acid diluent) or electronic particle counter, or estimated from a direct smear. If automated methods are used, the sample should be pretreated with hyaluronidase to decrease the viscosity.[9] In one study in dogs, manual enumeration from a direct smear resulted in overestimation of counts compared with particle counting.[10] Another more recent study in dogs demonstrated a 78% correct prediction of cellularity as within reference interval, mildly to moderately increased, or markedly increased when estimated from smears, compared with an automated count.[9] A TNCC differential should be performed by classifying a minimum of 100 nucleated cells on the direct smear. This often presents a challenge, particularly in samples with unaltered mucin content, due to the dense nature of the background, which impairs cell spreading (Figure 54.1).

Cellularity of normal synovial fluid in dogs and cats is generally low ($<3.0 \times 10^9$/L for dogs and $<1.0 \times 10^9$/L for cats).[4] Cells consist predominantly of mononuclear cells, which are mostly lymphocytes, macrophages, and synovial cells. Neutrophils are typically less than 5–10% of cells. In a study evaluating 126 synovial fluid samples from cats, the mean cell count was 0.091×10^9/L with 96.4% mononuclear cells and 3.6% neutrophils.[4] The highest cell count in this study was 1.134×10^9/L.

Normal protein values are generally accepted to be less than 25–30 g/L. Protein concentration is better performed using a quantitative biochemical assay. Protein measurement by refractometer often is not performed because of sample viscosity. In one study, a control group of 10 dogs had a mean protein concentration of 14.6 g/L with 0.22 standard deviation, by the Bradford protein method.[11] In the future, more detailed protein assessment may be available using a proteomics approach.[12]

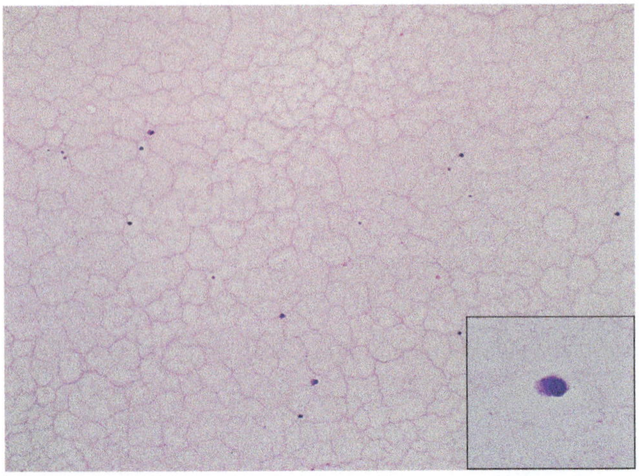

Figure 54.1 Synovial fluid cytology from a healthy dog. Overall cellularity is low, and the background is dense and "pavemented" due to high concentration of hyaluronic acid and glycosaminoglycans. Because of the viscous nature of the fluid and slow drying, cell morphology can be difficult to discern due to minimal spreading on the slide. Inset: Typical mononuclear cell observed in fluid from a healthy animal (Wright's stain, 100×; Inset 400×).

Normal Histologic Architecture and Cytology

Synovial fluid is located in the space contained within a synovial or diarthrodial joint. The bones of these joints are covered with an articular cartilage and capsule. The capsule is composed of an outer fibrous layer and an inner synovial membrane lined by synoviocytes.[13] There are two distinct types of synoviocytes. Type A synoviocytes are derived from bone marrow precursors and exhibit phagocytosis and antigen presentation.[13] Type B synoviocytes are likely of fibroblastic origin and produce hyaluronic acid. Occasionally, synoviocytes of either type can be present in synovial fluid but are indistinguishable from the other mononuclear cells. Additional cell types (neutrophils, erythrocytes) are uncommon unless joint pathology or contamination from the sampling procedure has occurred. Synovial fluid is highly viscous due to production of hyaluronic acid by type B synoviocytes.

Conditions Diagnosed by Cytology

Degenerative Joint Disease/Osteoarthritis

Lameness is a common reason for examination of synovial fluid, and degenerative and osteoarthritic lesions are frequent conditions in dogs and cats. In the hind limb, traumatic injury or degeneration of cruciate ligaments is a frequent cause for lameness and subsequent joint effusion. These are usually chronic lesions, resulting in mononuclear inflammation (Figure 54.2). In a study that experimentally created cranial cruciate ligament rupture (CCLR) in dogs, TNCC ranged from 1.0 to 12.0×10^9/L, and mononuclear cells remained the predominant population, although there was a mild increase in neutrophils in 7/10 dogs.[14] A 2004 study examined synovial fluid from 54 dogs with spontaneous CCLR.[15] They found mildly increased cellularity (maximum TNCC 7.1×10^9/L, mean 2.7×10^9/L) with only a maximum of 5% neutrophils. Using flow cytometry, they documented an increase in both $CD4^+$ and $CD8^+$ T lymphocytes in affected dogs compared with normal dogs. In another study of spontaneous CCLR, the majority of dogs had mild to moderate increase in cellularity with mild increase in protein, and the majority of cells were synoviocytes and macrophages, based on morphology.[16] Only rarely were small lymphocytes noted. This study however did not include flow cytometry to confirm the identity of cell populations. In their 2011 study, Muir et al. reported the immunophenotype of lymphocyte subpopulations in dogs with spontaneous CCLR.[17] While TNCC were not mentioned, proportions of $CD8^+$ and $CD3^+CD4^-CD8^-$ T lymphocytes were increased. Other diseases that can predispose to joint instability or abnormal biomechanics, which can result in mononuclear inflammation, include elbow dysplasia and osteochondritis dissecans.[18]

Neoplasia

Tumors of synovial origin and observation of abnormal cells on cytology are uncommon. The only benign tumor reported in the literature is synovial myxoma, but no cytological findings are mentioned.[13,19] The most common malignant tumor in dogs and cats is histiocytic sarcoma, and neoplastic cells can be observed on cytology (Figure 54.3).[13] Other sarcomas of the joint occur, including various soft tissue sarcomas, but there are no reports describing cells in synovial fluid. Lymphoma with joint involvement is reported, but it is rare to find cells in synovial fluid, despite the periarticular nature of the tumor.[20] Metastatic lesions from carcinomas can occur, and abnormal cells observed in the fluid. There is a case report of transitional cell carcinoma in a dog that metastasized to multiple joints and was readily noted on cytology.[21] Another report described finding neoplastic cells in synovial fluid from a dog with metastatic bronchoalveolar carcinoma.[22]

Inflammatory Disease

Inflammation of the joint space can be due to infectious and noninfectious causes, can range in severity, and affect one or multiple joints. Inflammation is usually characterized by increased cellularity and protein concentration, although with mild disease only the proportion of neutrophils may be increased. Protein concentration can remain elevated for a

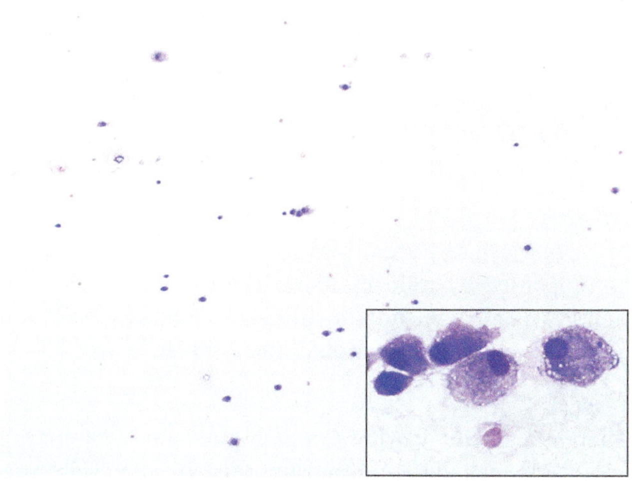

Figure 54.2 Mononuclear inflammation in synovial fluid from a dog. Degenerative joint disease due to trauma, ligament rupture or osteoarthritis results in mild to moderate influx of mononuclear cells. Inset: Mononuclear cells with vacuolated cytoplasm (Wright's stain, 100×; Inset 600×).

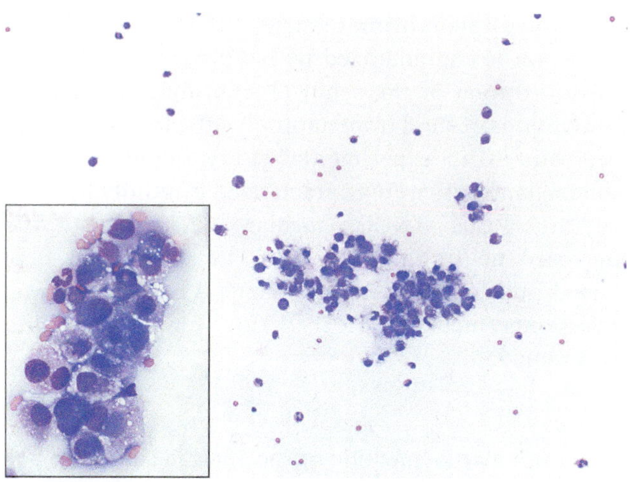

Figure 54.3 Neoplastic cells in synovial fluid from a dog. Overall cellularity is increased with increased proportions of neutrophils and mononuclear cells. Inset: There are large round cells exhibiting criteria of malignancy. Histopathologic diagnosis was histiocytic sarcoma (Wright's stain, 200×; Inset 400×).

longer period of time after decrease in cellularity occurs with resolution of the lesion.[11] Viscosity is frequently reduced, and some hemorrhage may be noted as vascular permeability increases. Compared with immune-mediated disease, infectious causes of arthropathy are uncommon in dogs but may be somewhat more common in cats.

Infectious

Bacteria

Many bacterial agents have been implicated as the cause of joint infection in dogs. Most often, a single joint is affected. In one study of five dogs, *Staphylococcus* spp., *Streptococcus* spp., and *Pasteurella* spp. were isolated.[23] Another study reported the same organisms and additionally *Pseudomonas aeruginosa* and *Bacillus* spp. In this study, TNCC ranged from 10.24 to 362.0×10^9/L, and mean neutrophil percentage was 89%.[24] Yet another study additionally reported infections with *Erysipelothrix rhusiopathiae* and *Enterococcus faecalis*.[25] One study cultured *Bartonella vinsonii* subsp. *berkhoffi* from synovial fluid of a dog with chronic progressive polyarthritis. Fluid was neutrophilic with protein of 56 g/L.[26]

The most common bacterial arthritis in cats is due to *Pastuerella* spp., usually from bites from other cats.[5] Other agents implicated in feline joint sepsis include L-form bacteria, *Escherichia coli*, and group G *Streptococcus* organisms.[5] There is a report of mycoplasma infection (*Mycoplasma gateae*) in a cat causing erosive arthritis.[27] The fluid was turbid, with a protein of 52 g/L and estimated increased cellularity with 86.5% neutrophils and 13.5% mononuclear cells.

Borreliosis or Lyme disease in dogs and cats is caused by *Borrelia burgdorferi* and as part of systemic disease can involve lesions in one or more joints.[13] Histologically, the lesion is characterized by lymphocyte and plasma cell infiltration of the synovial subintima. Cytological descriptions of fluid from naturally affected animals are rare, but in an experimental study, acute infections causing lameness were characterized by mildly to markedly increased TNCC (median 12.7×10^9/L) with increased neutrophils (median 54%).[28] Animals confirmed infected but without lameness had much lower cell counts (median 0.6×10^9/L) and fewer neutrophils (less than 15%).

Viruses

Feline calicivirus infection or vaccination can cause polyarthritis in cats. Synovial fluid exhibits mild to markedly increased cellularity with predominance of mononuclear cells, but neutrophil percentage can be increased.[5] Feline leukemia virus and feline syncytial forming virus are both implicated in inducing inflammatory polyarthritis in cats,[13] but detailed descriptions are lacking.

Rickettsia

Cats infected with *Anaplasma phagocytophilum* and *Ehrlichia canis*-like organisms may develop clinical signs of polyarthritis,[5] which was characterized by increased non-degenerate neutrophils in one case; no organisms were observed in the synovial fluid.[29] The potential for rickettsial infection should be assessed in dogs with neutrophilic polyarthropathy. Although rare, morula have been described in neutrophils in joint fluid from dogs.[30] Organism identification based on serology can be confounded by cross-reactivity between organisms, and PCR suggests the infectious agents are *A. phagocytophilum* and *Ehrlichia ewingii*. In an experimental study where eight dogs were infected with *E. canis*, there was no cytological evidence for inflammation or organisms in any of the samples evaluated.[31] Another report found no serologic evidence for *Rickettsia rickettsiae* or *E. canis* in 44 dogs with neutrophilic polyarthritis.[32] Previously reported cases of morulae in synovial are most likely to have been *A. phagocytophilum* infections.[33,34]

Fungal

Fungal arthritis is uncommon in dogs and cats but can occasionally occur with systemic infection. Possible organisms include *Blastomyces dermatitidis*, *Coccidioides immitis*, *Cryptococcus* spp., and *Histoplasma capsulatum*.[13] Suppurative inflammation is the most common cytological abnormality. In a canine case report, blastomyces organisms were found on cytology of synovial fluid with an estimated cell count $>70 \times 10^9$/L with 77% non-degenerate neutrophils, 23% mononuclear cells, occasional fibroblasts, and occasional multinucleated giant cells.[35]

Protozoa

A study reported 14 dogs with leishmaniasis affecting one or more joints. Mean cellularity was 45×10^9/L, with a mixture of neutrophils and mononuclear cells. Organisms were found in eight dogs.[36] Organisms can be observed within both neutrophils and mononuclear cells.[37]

Parasites

Microfilaria rarely are observed in synovial fluid of dogs, accompanied by mild mononuclear to mixed inflammation.[38,39] These were not thought to be blood origin as there was no blood contamination of the samples.

Yeast

There is a single report of *Candida* infection of a joint in a dog, likely related to immunosuppression from prior intra-articular corticosteroid injections.[40]

Noninfectious

Noninfectious causes of inflammatory joint disease are often categorized by whether or not erosive lesions are present in the articular cartilage.[13] Non-erosive causes are much more common.

Non-erosive

Immune-Mediated Polyarthritis

While it can occur in any breed or age of dog, immune-mediated polyarthritis (IMPA) is most commonly found in young to middle-aged, medium and large breed dogs but also with increased frequency in Cocker Spaniels.[41] IMPA is rare in cats, while reactive polyarthritis is much more common.[5] Type I IMPA (idiopathic) is determined by excluding underlying infectious and erosive diseases.[42] Affected dogs can exhibit reluctance to move, lameness, and possibly swollen joints, fever, and lethargy. Spinal pain due to steroid-responsive meningoencephalitis can be present.[43] Clinical signs are not always evident, and the main finding may be fever of unknown origin. Arthrocentesis is one of the mainstays of diagnosis for this disease, but other conditions that cause neutrophilic inflammation should be excluded as reactive arthropathy can occur secondary to systemic infectious disease. Hocks, carpi, and stifles are most often abnormal and frequently affected bilaterally.[41] Culture should be considered to exclude bacterial involvement. With IMPA, synovial fluid volume tends to be increased, and there is enhanced turbidity and decreased viscosity due to effusion. Color varies from colorless to pale yellow to red.[44] TNCC and protein concentrations are increased, sometimes dramatically, but severity of inflammation is not associated with outcome.[42] Cell counts ranged from 3.7 to 130.0×10^9/L in one study.[42] Another study evaluated synovial fluid total protein concentrations in 24 dogs and found a mean of 32 g/L.[11] Protein concentration remained elevated well after decreased cellularity occurred following therapy.[11] Neutrophils are variably increased to 10–95% and exhibit non-degenerate morphology (Figure 54.4). Breed-associated polyarthritis has been reported as part of systemic autoimmune disease in Akita and Shar-Pei dogs.[13] There is a case report of a cat with presumed immune-mediated, non-erosive, localized arthritis with predominance of eosinophils rather than neutrophils.[45]

Systemic Lupus Erythematosus

Systemic lupus erythematosus (SLE) refers to a constellation of findings that often occur as a result of autoimmunity to various body tissues, resulting in deposition of immune complexes in joint tissues. Antinuclear antibody titers are often elevated.[46] Synovial fluid samples from affected patients can exhibit increased cellularity, protein concentration, and proportion of neutrophils. In some cases, lupus erythematosus (LE) cells and/or "ragocytes" are observed.[47] LE cells are neutrophils that contain opsonized nuclear material that appears as round to irregular pink amorphous material located in the cytoplasm (Figure 54.5). Ragocytes are neutrophils that contain few to many, small irregular dark purple staining intracytoplasmic structures that are considered to be phagocytosed immune complexes or nuclear particles (Figure 54.5). The disease is rare in both dogs and cats.

Erosive

Rheumatoid arthritis is very rare in small animals. In dogs, the stifles, carpi, and digits tend to be affected, often in a symmetrical presentation.[13] In a study of 13 dogs with erosive polyarthritis, only one of four dogs was positive for rheumatoid factor.[48] Eleven of the cases had synovial fluid cytology with a range of estimated cellularity of 4.0–51.0×10^9/L. There was a subjectively higher proportion of

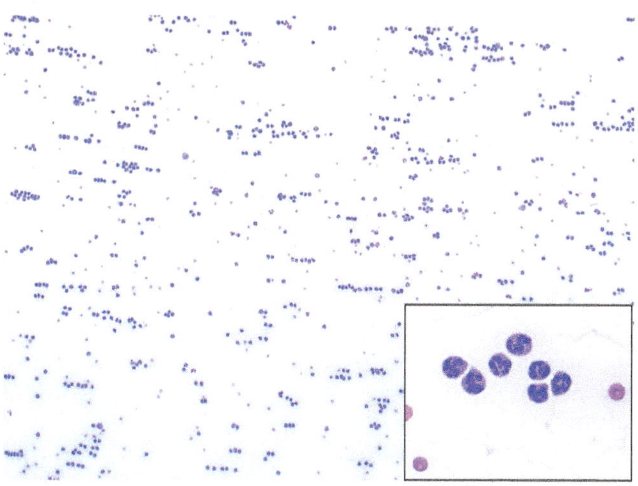

Figure 54.4 Neutrophilic inflammation in synovial fluid from a dog with immune-mediated polyarthritis (IMPA). Neutrophils increase with many inflammatory, infectious, and erosive diseases. Notice the "windrowing" effect of cells. Inset: While the neutrophils are non-degenerate in appearance, culture and sensitivity are still indicated as not all infections will cause cell necrosis (Wright's stain, 100×; Inset 600×).

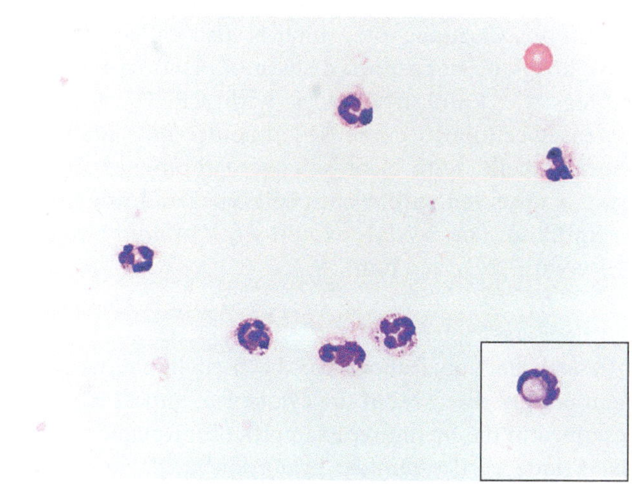

Figure 54.5 Synovial fluid from a dog with systemic lupus erythematosus. Cellularity is increased and comprised mostly of non-degenerate neutrophils. Note that many cells contain dark-staining cytoplasmic inclusions termed "ragocytes" when observed with immune-mediated joint disease. Inset: Lupus erythematosus (LE) cell (Wright's stain, 1000×).

lymphocytes in cases of erosive versus non-erosive disease, and carpal joints were most frequently abnormal.[48]

There are two erosive immune-mediated polyarthritis described in cats: periosteal proliferative polyarthritis and rheumatoid-like arthritis.[5,49] These were formerly grouped together as chronic progressive polyarthritis. In both instances, cytology is characterized by increased cellularity and predominance of non-degenerate neutrophils, while the rheumatoid-like arthritis can exhibit more of a mixed inflammation. *Mycoplasma* infection in cats also rarely results in an erosive arthropathy.[27] Underlying *Mycoplasma* infection is suggested in greyhounds with erosive polyarthritis,[50] although other reports fail to identify a causative agent.[51]

Miscellaneous

Hemarthrosis

Hemarthrosis can be caused by trauma, neoplasia, and hemostatic disorders such as hemophilia, rodenticide toxicosis, Von Willebrand disease, and immune-mediated thrombocytopenia.[52] Blood contamination resulting from the sampling procedure (iatrogenic hemorrhage) needs to be excluded as a cause for blood in the fluid. If pathologic, erythrophagia, and hemosiderin can be noted in macrophages. Samples are discolored red with increased turbidity and mildly increased cellularity and protein concentration.

Crystal Deposition Arthropathy

Uric acid crystal deposition in joint spaces is not reported in dogs and cats, probably because of the high activity of uricase.[13] There are not even definitive cases in Dalmatians that can have much higher uric acid concentrations. Pseudogout, which is also called calcium pyrophosphate deposition disease (CPDD), is reported in dogs.[53,54] Fluid from dogs with CPDD can have increased cellularity composed of neutrophils and mononuclear cells, with clear square to rhomboid shaped crystals observed within both cell types and free in the background. The crystals exhibit weak to mild birefringence with polarized light.[13]

Injections and Implants

Intra-articular medications can be used in the management of joint disease, but the cytological impact is poorly described in the literature. Examples of injectable materials include corticosteroids, hyaluronic acid, antibiotics, autologous serum, platelet-rich plasma, and stem cells. Reports about the effect of these substances on cellularity, proportions of cells, protein concentration, and appearance of foreign material are lacking. In a study evaluating effects of gentamicin sponge implantation in the canine stifle, an increase in neutrophils persisted on cytology as long as 35 days post placement.[55]

Other Diagnostic Techniques and Biomarkers

Culture and PCR

Both aerobic and anaerobic culture should routinely be performed on synovial fluid samples with increased cellularity with predominance of neutrophils, even when organisms are not observed microscopically.

It can be challenging to identify bacteria on cytology when septic arthritis is present and even bacterial culture does not always reliably identify agents responsible for disease. In one study evaluating effectiveness of bacterial culture in dogs with high index of suspicion of bacterial arthritis, only 44% of 36 samples yielded growth.[56] In a study describing seven cases of coxofemoral bacterial arthritis, synovial fluids were grossly turbid and purulent to bloody in appearance, with increased total solids (range 45–64 g/L) and cellularity (range $15–65 \times 10^9$/L).[57] In all cases, neutrophil percentage was >90%, but visible bacteria were only observed in 2/7 samples, while organisms were cultured in 6/7 samples. Agents cultured included *E. coli*, *Staphylococcus intermedius*, and beta-hemolytic *Streptococcus*. No organisms were observed on direct smears 24 hours following experimental injection of bacteria despite neutrophilic inflammation and positive culture results in 18/18 joints. Blood culture medium may provide the best chance to culture organisms from synovial fluid.[58] PCR may provide additional benefit, although some studies don't show much additional value compared with culture and cytology.[24]

Cytokines

Riggio et al. examined cytokine expression in synovial fluid of dogs with various joint diseases including IMPA, septic arthritis, and CCLR.[25] They found increased Toll-like receptor (TLR)2, tumor necrosis factor alpha (TNFα), interleukin (IL)-6, and IL-12 mRNA in all affected samples, compared with synovial fluid from normal dogs. In the samples from septic arthritis patients, expression of TLR2, TLR7, TNFα, and IL-6 was significantly higher compared with other groups. Another study found increased fluid IL-6 concentrations in dogs with osteoarthritis and suppurative arthritis compared with normal dogs.[59] IL-6 was significantly higher in suppurative arthritis.[59]

Biomarkers

There are limited studies evaluating novel biomarkers of disease in synovial fluid of dogs and cats. Matrix metalloproteinase (MMP)-2 and MMP-9 in synovial fluid from 14 dogs with CCLR were compared with 11 non-affected dogs. While MMP-9 was not different from unaffected dogs, MMP-2 was significantly increased in dogs with CCLR.[60] Lactate concentration was significantly higher in synovial fluid from dogs with septic arthritis compared with immune-mediated disease, osteoarthritis, or normal joints, but there was poor correlation with TNCC and protein measurement.[61] To date, most studies evaluating acute phase proteins in synovial fluid, such as C-reactive protein, as markers of underlying disease, have not resulted in conclusive useful results.[62,63] A recent study did suggest a possible role for measuring synovial fluid serum amyloid A to detect early joint disease,[18] but subsequent studies are lacking.

References

1 Clements, D. (2006). Arthrocentesis and synovial fluid analysis in dogs and cats. *In Pract* 28: 256–262.

2 Degner, D. (2014). Arthrocentesis in dogs. *Clinician's Brief*: 69–74.

3 Fernandes, P.J. (2014). Synovial fluid analysis. In: *Cowell and Tyler's Diagnostic Cytology of the Dog and Cat*, 4e (eds. A.C. Valenciano and R.L. Cowell), 195–215. St. Louis, MO: Elsevier Mosby.

4 Pacchiana, P.D., Gilley, R.S., Wallace, L.J. et al. (2004). Absolute and relative cell counts for synovial fluid from clinically normal shoulder and stifle joints in cats. *J Am Vet Med Assoc* 225: 1866–1870.

5 Lemetayer, J. and Taylor, S. (2014). Inflammatory joint disease in cats: diagnostic approach and treatment. *J Feline Med Surg* 16: 547–562.

6 Berg, R.I.M., Sykes, J.E., Kass, P.H., and Vernau, W. (2009). Effect of repeated arthrocentesis on cytologic analysis of synovial fluid in dogs. *J Vet Intern Med* 23: 814–817.

7 MacWilliams, P.S. and Friedrichs, K.R. (2003). Laboratory evaluation and interpretation of synovial fluid. *Vet Clin Small Anim Pract* 33: 153–178.

8 Ogston, A.G. and Sherman, T.F. (1959). Degradation of the hyaluronic acid complex of synovial fluid by proteolytic enzymes and by ethylenediaminetetra-acetic acid. *Biochem J* 72: 301–305.

9 Dusick, A., Young, K.M., and Muir, P. (2014). Relationship between automated total nucleated cell count and enumeration of cells on direct smears of canine synovial fluid. *Vet J* 202: 550–554.

10 Gibson, N.R., Carmichael, S., Li, A. et al. (1999). Value of direct smears of synovial fluid in the diagnosis of canine joint disease. *Vet Rec* 144: 463–465.

11 Murakami, K., Yonezawa, T., and Matsuki, N. (2015). Synovial fluid total protein concentration as a possible marker for canine idiopathic polyarthritis. *J Vet Med Sci* 77: 1715–1717.

12 Garner, B., Kuroki, K., Stoker, A. et al. (2013). Expression of proteins in serum, synovial fluid, synovial membrane, and articular cartilage samples obtained from dogs with stifle joint osteoarthritis secondary to cranial cruciate ligament disease and dogs without stifle joint arthritis. *Am J Vet Res* 74: 386–394.

13 Craig, L.E., Dittmer, K.E., and Thompson, K.G. (2016). Bones and joints. In: *Jubb, Kennedy and Palmer's Pathology of Domestic Animals, Vol 1* (ed. M.G. Maxie), 128–131. St. Louis, MO: Elsevier.

14 Lewis, D., Goring, R., and Parker, R.C.P. (1987). A comparison of diagnostic methods used in the evaluation of early degenerative joint disease in the dog. *J Am Anim Hosp Assoc* 23: 305–315.

15 Faldyna, M., Zatloukal, J., Leva, L. et al. (2004). Lymphocyte subsets in stifle joint synovial fluid of dogs with spontaneous rupture of the cranial cruciate ligament. *Acta Vet Brno* 73: 79–84.

16 Erne, J.B., Goring, R.L., Kennedy, F.A., and Schoenborn, W.C. (2009). Prevalence of lymphoplasmacytic synovitis in dogs with naturally occurring cranial cruciate ligament rupture. *J Am Vet Med Assoc* 235: 386–390.

17 Muir, P., Kelly, J.L., Marvel, S.J. et al. (2011). Lymphocyte populations in joint tissues from dogs with inflammatory stifle arthritis and associated degenerative cranial cruciate ligament rupture. *Vet Surg* 40: 753–761.

18 Kjelgaard-Hansen, M., Christensen, M., Lee, M. et al. (2007). Serum amyloid A isoforms in serum and synovial fluid from spontaneously diseased dogs with joint diseases or other conditions. *Vet Immunol Immunopathol* 117: 296–301.

19 Izawa, T., Tanaka, M., Aoki, M. et al. (2012). Incidental synovial myxoma with extensive intermuscular infiltration in a dog. *J Vet Med Sci* 74: 1631–1633.

20 Lahmers, S.M., Mealey, K.L., Martinez, S.A. et al. (2002). Synovial T-cell lymphoma of the stifle in a dog. *J Am Anim Hosp Assoc* 38: 165–168.

21 Colledge, S.L., Raskin, R.E., Messick, J.B. et al. (2013). Multiple joint metastasis of a transitional cell carcinoma in a dog. *Vet Clin Pathol* 42: 216–220.

22 Meinkoth, J., Rocha, M., and Cowell, R. (1997). Metastatic carcinoma presenting as hind-limb lameness: diagnosis by synovial fluid cytology. *J Am Anim Hosp Assoc* 33: 325–328.
23 Fitch, R.B., Hogan, T.C., and Kudnig, S.T. (2003). Hematogenous septic arthritis in the dog: results of five patients treated nonsurgically with antibiotics. *J Am Anim Hosp Assoc* 39: 563–566.
24 Scharf, V., Lewis, D., Wellehan, J. et al. (2015). Comparison of synovial fluid culture and 16S rRNA PCR in dogs with suspected septic arthritis. *Aust Vet J* 93: 204–207.
25 Riggio, M., Lappin, D., and Bennett, D. (2014). Bacteria and Toll-like receptor and cytokine mRNA expression profiles associated with canine arthritis. *Vet Immunol Immunopathol* 160: 158–166.
26 Diniz, P.P., Wood, M., Maggi, R.G. et al. (2009). Co-isolation of *Bartonella henselae* and *Bartonella vinsonii* subsp. berkhoffii from blood, joint and subcutaneous seroma fluids from two naturally infected dogs. *Vet Microbiol* 138: 368–372.
27 Zeugswetter, F., Hittmair, K., de Arespacohaga, A. et al. (2007). Erosive polyarthritis associated with *Mycoplasma gateae* in a cat. *J Feline Med Surg* 9: 226–231.
28 Straubinger, R., Straubinger, A.F., Härter, L. et al. (1997). *Borrelia burgdorferi* migrates into joint capsules and causes an up-regulation of Interleukin-8 in synovial membranes of dogs experimentally infected with ticks. *Infect Immun* 65: 1273–1285.
29 Breitschwerdt, E., Abrams-Ogg, A.C., Lappin, M.R. et al. (2002). Molecular evidence supporting *Ehrlichia canis*: like infection in cats. *J Vet Intern Med* 16: 642–649.
30 Gieg, J., Rikihisa, Y., and Wellman, M. (2009). Diagnosis of *Ehrlichia ewingii* infection by PCR in a puppy from Ohio. *Vet Clin Pathol* 38: 406–410.
31 Theodorou, K., Leontides, L., Siarkou, V.I. et al. (2015). Synovial fluid cytology in experimental acute canine monocytic ehrlichiosis (*Ehrlichia canis*). *Vet Microbiol* 177: 224–227.
32 Rondeau, M., Walton, R., Bissett, S. et al. (2005). Suppurative, nonseptic polyarthropathy in dogs. *J Vet Intern Med* 19: 654–662.
33 Bellah, J., Shull, R., and Shull Selcer, E. (1986). *Ehrlichia canis*-related polyarthritis in a dog. *J Am Vet Med Assoc* 189: 922–923.
34 Cowell, R., Tyler, R., Clinkenbeard, K., and Meinkoth, J.H. (1988). Ehrlichiosis and polyarthritis in three dogs. *J Am Vet Med Assoc* 192: 1093–1095.
35 Woods, K., Barry, M., and Richardson, D. (2013). Carpal intra-articular blastomycosis in a Labrador retriever. *Can Vet J* 54: 167–170.
36 Marchetti, S.S., Mancianti, F., Guidi, G. et al. (2014). Retrospective study of 14 cases of canine arthritis secondary to *Leishmania* infection. *J Small Anim Pract* 55: 309–313.
37 Santos, M., Marcos, R., Assuncao, M., and Matos, A.J. (2006). Polyarthritis associated with visceral leishmaniasis in a juvenile dog. *Vet Parasitol* 141: 340–344.
38 Hodges, S. and Rishniw, M. (2008). Intraarticular *Dirofilaria immitis* microfilariae in two dogs. *Vet Parasitol* 152: 167–170.
39 Gabriella, S., Giannelli, A., Brianti, E. et al. (2014). Chronic polyarthritis associated to *Cercopithifilaria bainae* infection in a dog. *Vet Parasitol* 205: 401–404.
40 Bufalari, A., Maggio, C., Moretti, G. et al. (2016). Management of *Candida guilliermondii* joint infection in a dog. *Acta Vet Scand* 58: 47–53.
41 Johnson, K.C. and Mackin, A. (2012). Canine immune-mediated polyarthritis. Part 2: Diagnosis and treatment. *J Am Anim Hosp Assoc* 48: 71–82.
42 Clements, D.N., Gear, R.N.A., Tattersall, J. et al. (2004). Type I immune-mediated polyarthritis in dogs: 39 cases (1997–2002). *J Am Vet Med Assoc* 224: 1323–1327.
43 Webb, A.A., Taylor, S.M., and Muir, G.D. (2002). Steroid-responsive meningitis-arteritis in dogs with noninfectious, nonerosive, idiopathic, immune-mediated polyarthritis. *J Vet Intern Med* 16: 269–273.
44 Jacques, D., Cauzinille, L., Bouvy, B., and Dupre, G. (2002). A retrospective study of 40 dogs with polyarthritis. *Vet Surg* 31: 428–434.
45 Silverstein, D., Almy, F., Zinkl, J., and Christopher, M.M. (2000). Idiopathic localized eosinophilic synovitis in a cat. *Vet Clin Pathol* 29: 90–92.
46 Smee, N., Harkin, K., and Wilkerson, M. (2007). Measurement of serum antinuclear antibody titer in dogs with and without systemic lupus erythematosus: 120 cases (1997–2005). *J Am Vet Med Assoc* 230: 1180–1183.
47 Melendez-Lazo, A., Fernandez, M., Solano-Gallego, L., and Pastor, J. (2015). What is your diagnosis? Synovial fluid from a dog. *Vet Clin Pathol* 44: 329–330.
48 Shaughnessy, M., Sample, S., Abicht, C. et al. (2016). Clinical features and pathological joint changes in dogs with erosive immune-mediated polyarthritis: 13 cases (2004–2012). *J Am Vet Med Assoc* 249: 1156–1164.
49 Oohashi, E., Yamada, K., Oohashi, M., and Ueda, J. (2010). Chronic progressive polyarthritis in a female cat. *J Vet Med Sci* 72: 511–514.
50 Barton, M., Ireland, L., Kirschner, J., and Forbes, C. (1985). Isolation of *Mycoplasma spumans* from polyarthritis in a Greyhound. *Aust Vet J* 62: 206–207.

51 Woodard, J., Riser, W., Bloomberg, M. et al. (1991). Erosive polyarthritis in two greyhounds. *J Am Vet Med Assoc* 198: 873–876.
52 Walton, M., Mardell, E., Spoor, M., and Innes, J. (2014). Lameness associated with haemarthrosis as the sole clinical sign of idipathic immune-mediated thrombocytopenia in a dog. *Vet Comp Orthop Traumatol* 27: 491–495.
53 de Haan, J. and Andreasen, C. (1992). Calcium crystal-associated arthropathy (pseudgout) in a dog. *J Am Vet Med Assoc* 200: 943–946.
54 Forsyth, S.F., Thompson, K.G., and Donald, J.J. (2007). Possible pseudogout in two dogs. *J Small Anim Pract* 48: 174–176.
55 Hayes, G., Gibson, T., Moens, N.M. et al. (2016). Intra-articular implantation of gentamicin impregnated collagen sponge causes joint inflammation and impaired renal function in dogs. *Vet Comp Orthop Traumatol* 29: 159–163.
56 Scharf, V.F., Lewis, S.T., Wellehan, J.F. et al. (2015). Retrospective evaluation of the efficacy of isolating bacteria from synovial fluid in dogs with suspected septic arthritis. *Aust Vet J* 93: 200–203.
57 Benzioni, H., Shahar, R., Yudelevitch, S., and Milgram, J. (2008). Bacterial infective arthritis of the coxofemoral joint in dogs with hip dysplasia. *Vet Comp Orthop Traumatol* 21: 262–266.
58 Montgomery, R., Long, I., Milton, J. et al. (1989). Comparison of aerobic culturette, synovial membrane biopsy, and blood culture medium in detection of canine bacterial arthritis. *Vet Surg* 18: 300–303.
59 Hillstrom, A., Bylin, J., Hagman, R. et al. (2016). Measurement of serum C-reactive protein concentration for discriminating between suppurative arthritis and osteoarthritis in dogs. *BMC Vet Res* 12: 240–249.
60 Boland, L., Danger, R., Cabon, Q. et al. (2014). MMP-2 as an early synovial biomarker for cranial cruciate ligament disease in dogs. *Vet Comp Orthop Traumatol* 27: 210–215.
61 Proot, J., de Vicente, F., and Sheahan, D. (2015). Analysis of lactate concentrations in canine synovial fluid. *Vet Comp Orthop Traumatol* 28: 301–305.
62 Boal, S. and Carreira, L. (2015). Serum and synovial fluid C-reactive protein level variations in dogs with degenerative joint disease and their relationships with physiological parameters. *Vet Res Commun* 39: 163–169.
63 Hurter, K., Spreng, D., Rytz, U. et al. (2005). Measurements of C-reactive protein in serum and lactate dehydrogenase in serum and synovial fluid of patients with osteoarthritis. *Vet J* 169: 281–285.

55

Synovial Fluid Analysis of the Horse

R. Darren Wood and Judith Koenig

Collection

Synovial fluid must be collected from an aseptically prepared site (joint/tendon sheath/bursa), or else risk of infection is possible. Familiarity with anatomy is required for proper sampling technique for each specific location.[1] Blood contamination is possible during sample collection. This must be differentiated from pathologic hemorrhage into the joint space (hemarthrosis). Iatrogenic hemorrhage tends to result in a sample that appears clear at the beginning of aspiration and then becomes bloody during the procedure. Microscopically, iatrogenic hemorrhage may result in observation of platelets or clots in the sample, while pathologic hemorrhage will lack these features and can instead include evidence of prior bleeding (erythrophagia and/or iron pigments; Figure 55.1).[2] The sample should be processed quickly, as *in vitro* phagocytosis of erythrocytes can occur with a delay of several hours. Blood contamination can make identification of inflammation challenging, particularly if there is peripheral blood neutrophilia. Attempts have been made to create correction formulas that account for the amount of blood present using concurrent complete blood count values.[3] Because of the possibility of blood contamination, the sample should be placed in an ethylenediaminetetraacetic acid (EDTA) tube to prevent clotting and preserve the sample for cytology. However, if the sample needs to be cultured, a sterile aliquot should be kept aside, put into enrichment broth,[4] and not placed in anticoagulant.

Physical Characteristics

Synovial fluid from healthy horse should be clear, colorless to pale yellow, and highly viscous. If the sample is more turbid or cloudy than clear, this indicates increased cellularity from inflammation. Flecks of material also can be present, which can be observed when inverting the tube.

With acute hemarthrosis, the fluid appears red and turbid, similar to peripheral blood. If prior hemorrhage has occurred, the fluid may be orange-yellow in color (xanthochromic) due to the presence of hemoglobin pigments. The presence of inflammation can result in yellow to orange to red discoloration.

While very thick in consistency due to polymerized hyaluronic acid, synovial fluid does not clot due to the lack of clotting proteins in the fluid.[5] It may become more gelatinous on standing (thixotropy) but can be readily reconstituted by gentle mixing.[2] With either septic or non-septic inflammation, the fluid becomes dilute due to effusion and less viscous due to enzymatic hyaluronic acid degradation. Viscosity can be subjectively assessed when expelling fluid from a needle onto the slide or by stretching it between a thumb and index finger. Microscopically, viscosity is indicated by the appearance of windrowing of cells on the slide (Figure 55.2).

The mucin clot test is a test of hyaluronic acid quantity and quality in a synovial fluid sample. It is performed by adding a defined amount of acetic acid to the fluid, and then subjectively assessing clot formation.[5,6] The clot can be poor with any type of inflammation, because of hyaluronic acid degradation. Therefore, it does not provide additional information for differentiating septic from non-septic processes.

Fluid Analysis

Total nucleated cell counts (TNCC) can be determined using a hemocytometer, automated instrument, or estimated manually from a direct smear. If an automated method is used, the sample should be pretreated with a

Veterinary Cytology, First Edition. Edited by Leslie C. Sharkey, M. Judith Radin, and Davis Seelig.

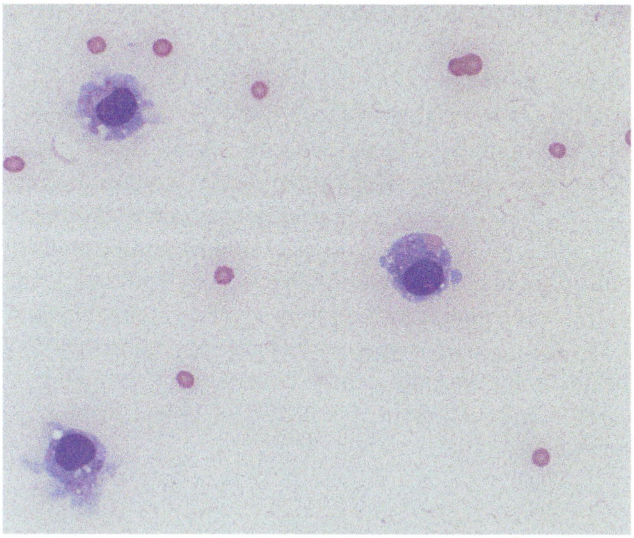

Figure 55.1 Synovial fluid from a 4-year-old quarter horse gelding with synovitis. The mononuclear cell on the right exhibits erythrophagia, with an intact red blood cell located within the cytoplasm. The background is dense and granular due to high concentration of hyaluronic acid and glycosaminoglycans, with occasional extracellular erythrocytes (Wright's stain, 600×).

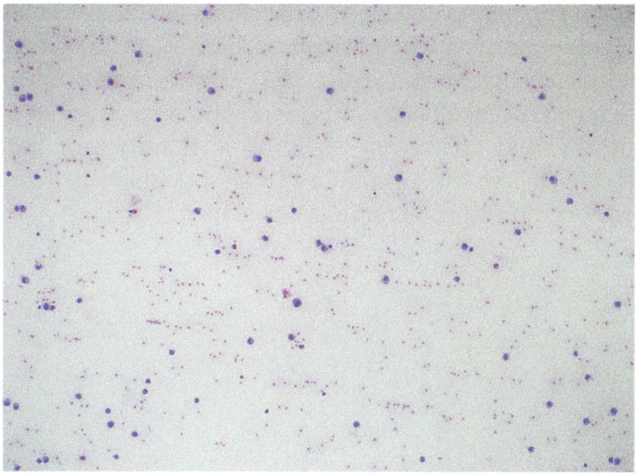

Figure 55.2 Synovial fluid from a horse with synovitis (same as Figure 55.1). At lower magnification, "windrowing" of cells is observed. This tendency to form linear arrangements, particularly with erythrocytes in this image, occurs due to the viscous nature of the sample (Wright's stain, 100×).

small amount of hyaluronidase powder to decrease the viscosity of the sample.[7] Several automated hematology instruments have been shown to effectively enumerate cells in equine synovial fluid, particularly in inflammatory samples with reduced viscosity.[7,8] However, manual methods should be used to assess morphological differentiation of cells.[9] Samples should be stored at 4 °C and be processed and evaluated within 24 hours of collection.[10] If stored beyond this time period and/or at higher temperatures, TNCC can decrease, and cellular morphology becomes compromised.

Cellularity tends to be low in non-diseased fluid. Early studies suggested that TNCC varied between joints sampled but tended to be less than 1.35×10^9/L.[6,11] Mean ± standard deviation (SD) TNCC in middle carpal joints from 12 healthy horses was $0.43 \pm 0.29 \times 10^9$/L.[12] In another study examining various joints from 34 healthy control horses, median TNCC was 0.8×10^9/L (interquartile range 0.7–1.0).[13] Samples from 12 Shetland ponies counted using a hemocytometer resulted in mean ± standard error (SE) TNCC of $0.367 \pm 0.354 \times 10^9$/L.[14] In another 28 healthy horses, the range of TNCC from fetlock joints was $0.002–0.5 \times 10^9$/L as determined by an automated analyzer.[15] Cellularity of fluid collected from tendon sheaths is similar.[16] Fluid from the deep digital flexor tendon sheath in five healthy horses had cell counts $<0.144 \times 10^9$/L.[17]

Protein measurement by refractometer may not be routinely performed on synovial fluid due to the viscous nature of the sample. Protein concentration is better performed using a quantitative biochemical assay. Normal protein values are not commonly reported, but it is generally accepted that values should be less than 25 g/L. In a study of 29 healthy horses, all had total protein concentration <25 g/L when measured by refractometer and a mean of 10.88 g/L when measured by Coomassie blue in 15 of those 29 animals.[18] In another study, mean ± SD protein concentration from 12 healthy horses was 17.8 ± 6.5 g/L.[12] Using the Biuret method in a different group of 15 horses, the mean ± SE of protein measured in fluid obtained from distal interphalangeal joints was 13.0 ± 2.0 g/L.[19] In 34 healthy control horses, as measured by refractometer, median protein concentration was 5.0 g/L (interquartile range 3.0–6.0).[13] In 28 horses, protein concentration range was 6.0–16.0 g/L; however, the method was not reported, and these samples were collected immediately postmortem.[15] Protein concentration will increase after repeated arthrocentesis of healthy joints, with values approaching 35 g/L in some horses.[20]

Direct smears should be prepared from freshly collected fluid, rapidly air-dried, and stained with a Romanowsky-type stain. Low magnification examination is used to assess overall cellularity, contamination with hemorrhage, character of background material, and arrangement of cells. At higher magnification (usually 400–1000×), classification and assessment of cellular morphology (including assessment of degenerative changes in neutrophils) is performed. Samples from healthy horses can be quite dense, and morphology may be best appreciated at the periphery of the sample.

A minimum of 100 nucleated cells should be classified and percentage of each reported. The majority (>90%) of cells tend to be mononuclear with on average less than 10–15% neutrophils.[6,12]

Normal Histology and Cytology

Synovial fluid is located in the space contained within a synovial or diarthrodial joint. The bones of these joints are covered with an articular cartilage and capsule; the latter is composed of an outer fibrous layer and an inner synovial membrane lined by synoviocytes.[21] There are two distinct types of synoviocytes: A and B. Type A synoviocytes are derived from bone marrow precursors and exhibit phagocytosis and antigen presentation.[21] Type B synoviocytes are likely of fibroblastic origin and produce hyaluronic acid. In addition to resident lymphocytes and macrophages, synoviocytes of either type occasionally can be present in synovial fluid but are indistinguishable from the other mononuclear cells (Figure 55.1). Additional cell types (neutrophils, eosinophils, and erythrocytes) are uncommon unless joint pathology or blood contamination from the sampling procedure has occurred. Synovial fluid is highly viscous due to secretion of hyaluronic acid into the fluid matrix by type B synoviocytes. Grossly, it tends to be clear and either colorless or pale yellow. Microscopically, the background is quite dense, granular, and eosinophilic due to the high mucin content and can exhibit protein crescents (Figure 55.3).

Inflammatory Disease

Inflammation of the joint (synovitis), tendon sheath (tenosynovitis), or bursa (bursitis) can occur as a result of infectious and noninfectious causes, can vary in severity, and affect one or multiple sites. Inflammation is typically characterized by increased cellularity and protein concentration, although with mild disease only the proportion of neutrophils may be increased (Figure 55.4). While bacterial culture is the gold standard, it only yields positive results in 31–76% of cases suspected to have septic arthritis.[22–24] The likelihood of septic arthritis is very high if total protein is >40–42 g/L, cell count is >30.0 × 10^9/L, and/or proportion of neutrophils is >80–90%.[22,23,25–27]

Infectious

Bacteria

In both foals and adult horses, the most common causes for septic synovitis are trauma, iatrogenic bacterial infection, or hematogenous seeding of joints, resulting in joint effusion and lameness.[23,28,29] Cytologically, neutrophils tend to be the predominant cell type. Neutrophils can exhibit degenerative changes, which include nuclear swelling, loss of nuclear segmentation, pale staining chromatin, and even cellular lysis (Figure 55.5). Organisms are variably noted, depending on prior antibiotic therapy, sample integrity, and microscopy skills. Even if no agents are observed by cytology or culture a Gram stain should still be performed if suspicion for infection is high.

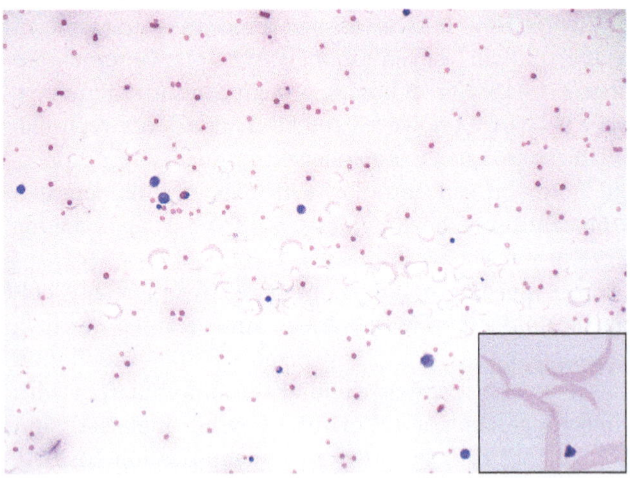

Figure 55.3 Synovial fluid from a 7-year-old Standardbred gelding with lameness. Numerous protein crescents are noted (inset), in addition to low numbers of red blood cells. Occasional neutrophils can originate from blood contamination (Wright's stain, 200×; Inset 400×).

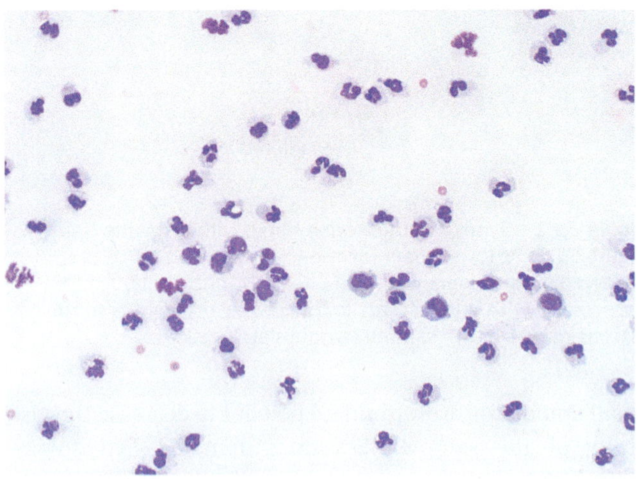

Figure 55.4 Synovial fluid from a 6-day-old Standardbred colt with suspected septic joint. The fluid is yellow and turbid, with cell count of 189.0 × 10^9/L and protein concentration 42 g/L. The majority of cells are neutrophils, some exhibiting degenerative changes, with fewer mononuclear cells. No definitive organisms are observed (Wright's stain, 400×).

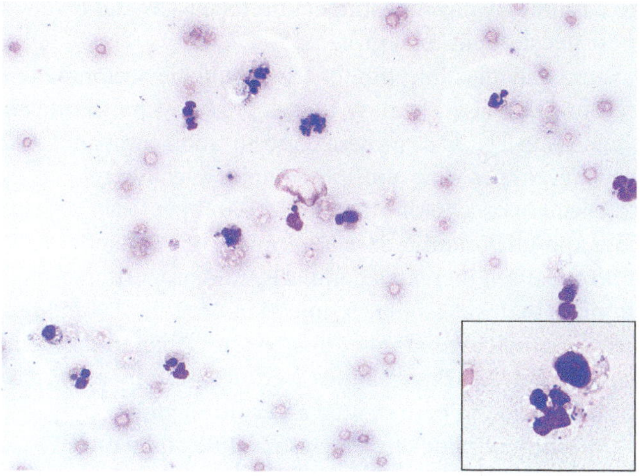

Figure 55.5 Synovial fluid from a 4-day-old Belgian colt with a septic intercarpal joint. The fluid is red and cloudy, with cell count of 12.6×10^9/L and protein concentration of 35 g/L. Most cells are neutrophils with severe degenerative changes and cell lysis. Frequent bacteria are present throughout the background and intracellularly (inset) (Wright's stain, 400×; Inset 1000×).

Joint infections in adult horses can occur following joint injections (iatrogenic) or less commonly, after penetrating traumatic injury.[29] In 15 horses that had received prior intra-articular joint injection of either corticosteroids, hyaluronic acid, glycosaminoglycans, and/or local anesthetics, the range of TNCC was 18.0–258.0 $\times 10^9$/L with median neutrophil percentage of 95% and range of total solids by refractometer of 30–60 g/L.[29] All agents cultured were *Staphylococcus* or *Streptococcus* spp., but there was no mention in how many cases organisms were observed cytologically.

In one study of 48 horses with joint sepsis, the mean TNCC was 45.3×10^9/L with a range of 0.5–152.0 $\times 10^9$/L, and mean protein concentration was 39 g/L with a range of 20–68 g/L.[24] In 26/48 samples, neutrophils were the predominant cell type. Intracellular bacteria were identified microscopically in only 9/48 samples, while bacteria were isolated by culture in 18/48 joints. Cultured agents included *Actinobacillus equuli*, *Staphylococcus aureus*, coagulase-negative *Staphylococcus* spp., *Salmonella* serovar Hadar, *Enterobacter* spp., *Pseudomonas aeruginosa*, and *Streptococcus zooepidemicus*.

In a review of 192 cases of septic arthritis/tenosynovitis, mean TNCC was 76.49×10^9/L (range 1.1–380.0 $\times 10^9$/L), mean percentage neutrophils was 83.7% (range 60–100%), and mean protein concentration was 50 g/L (range 25–98 g/L).[23] Bacteria were only observed cytologically in 24% of cases and detected by culture in 73%. Cultured organisms accounting for 87% of isolates included *Enterobacteriaceae*, *Escherichia coli*, *Staphylococcus* spp., and *Streptococcus* spp.[23] Infection with *Mycobacterium avium* complex was reported in a horse with prior cortisone injections.[30]

In foals, hematogenous spread of bacteria is the most common cause for septic arthritis. In a study of 83 foals with septic arthritis, the mean TNCC was 68.7×10^9/L with a range of 0.56–343.0 $\times 10^9$/L and mean protein concentration of 39 g/L with range of 22–75 g/L.[31] Bacterial culture was successful in 85.7% of samples. The frequency of cytologic detection of bacteria was not reported. The most common isolates included *E. coli*, *A. equuli*, *Staphylococcus epidermidis*, and *Streptococcus* spp. *Klebsiella* spp. were occasionally isolated in this and in other studies.[31,32] Anaerobic infections, such as those caused by *Clostridium septicum*, are reported in foals.[33]

In 150 foals with systemic infection with *Rhodococcus equi*, 25% developed immune-mediated synovitis, while 9% developed septic synovitis.[34] In another study, 17/48 (36%) of infected foals had non-septic synovitis.[35] Immune-mediated polysynovitis also was reported in a horse with *Borrelia burgdorferi* infection.[36] Synovial fluid or tendon sheath fluid samples had cell counts as high as 5.8×10^9/L and protein concentration up to 49 g/L.[36]

Fungi

There is a case report of fungal infection of the metacarpophalangeal joint in a horse that had been previously administered intra-articular steroids.[37] The fluid was red and watery, with TNCC of 19.3×10^9/L and protein concentration of 54 g/L. Neutrophils predominated, no organisms were observed, and bacterial cultures were negative, but fungal culture yielded growth of *Aspergillus fumigatus*. Fungal osteomyelitis of the proximal sesamoid bones was eventually confirmed. Septic arthritis and osteomyelitis caused by *Candida* sp.[38] and *Scedosporium prolificans*[39] has been reported as well.

Noninfectious

It is difficult to find primary literature that documents the cytology of traumatic and degenerative conditions involving equine synovial fluid. Other conditions that have been described in other species, such as systemic lupus erythematosus and rheumatoid arthritis, are rare and poorly documented in horses.

Traumatic Noninfectious Synovitis

In a study with 12 horses with either intra-articular fracture or adjacent soft tissue injury, the range of TNCC was 0.008–9.8 $\times 10^9$/L with protein concentration ranging from 13 to 48 g/L.[15] The proportion of neutrophils present in the samples ranged from 10 to 94%.

Osteoarthritis (OA)

In a study that included 12 horses, median TNCC was 0.388×10^9/L (interquartile range 0.25–0.7) with protein concentration median of 13 g/L (interquartile range 10–24).[13] Proportions of cells were not noted.

Osteochondritis Dissecans (OCD)

In a study with 22 horses, median TNCC was 0.256×10^9/L (interquartile range 0.165–0.5) with protein concentration median of 21 g/L (interquartile range 11–24).[13] Proportions of cells were not noted. In another study examining 23 horses, the range of TNCC was $0.008–1.0 \times 10^9$/L with protein concentration range of 4–24 g/L.[15] Proportions of neutrophils were 4–86%.

Eosinophilic Synovitis

Eosinophilic synovitis occurs rarely in horses. It has been documented following experimental intra-articular injection of bacterial antigen[40] and after intra-articular injection of methylprednisolone acetate.[41] In a recent case report, a horse had effusion of the right tarsocrural joint with increased cellularity of 12.8×10^9/L, and protein of 62 g/L.[42] Seventy-six percent of nucleated cells were eosinophils. Cellularity and protein were decreased by day 21, but there were still 47% eosinophils when a differential was performed.[42] No precipitating cause could be identified.

Systemic Lupus Erythematosus-like Syndrome

A systemic lupus erythematosus-like syndrome has been reported in two horses. In one horse, the diagnosis was based on a positive lupus erythematosus cell preparation and antinuclear antibody titers,[43] while in the other, the diagnosis was based on clinical signs, laboratory testing, and histological findings at postmortem.[44]

Idiopathic Immune-Mediated Polysynovitis

Bacterial culture negative, idiopathic immune-mediated polysynovitis has been reported in horses.[45] From 8 different joints in 3 horses, TNCC ranged from $0.6–6.8 \times 10^9$/L and protein concentration from 16 to 36 g/L. Neutrophil percentage was increased and ranged from 12 to 90%. All horses responded to glucocorticoid therapy.

Intra-articular Injections

Saline lavage of the middle carpal joint in healthy horses resulted in mildly increased protein concentration, TNCC, and percentage of neutrophils up to 28 days after injection.[12] Arthroscopic partial synovectomy resulted in similar changes.[12] In another study, a single injection of 2.5 mL saline in the midcarpal joint of 24 horses resulted in transient increases in TNCC and total protein.[46] Values returned to baseline by day 3 post-injection for TNCC and by day 5 post-injection for total protein.[46]

Intra-articular injection of triamcinolone acetonide in 8 recently exercised healthy horses produced no significant changes in TNCC or protein concentration compared with baseline values with multiple samples over 49 days.[47]

Injection of a combination of sodium pentosan polysulfate and glucosamine in carpal joints of 10 Standardbred horses caused increased cellularity and proportion of neutrophils that was similar to injection of saline.[48] Total protein was increased more in treated joints than in the saline control joints. Abnormalities were resolved by seven days post-injection in both treated and control joints.

Injection of platelet-rich plasma (PRP) increased TNCC (mean 6.4×10^9/L), proportion of neutrophils, and total protein concentration compared with saline injection control for up to four days post-injection.[49] Pre-activation of PRP with bovine thrombin or calcium chloride resulted in even higher TNCC (mean 24.5×10^9/L, and 10.3×10^9/L, respectively).

Injection of allogeneic umbilical cord blood-derived mesenchymal stromal cells (CB-MSCs) as a therapeutic has the potential to stimulate an inflammatory response.[50] In 3 horses that received intra-articular injection of 30 million CB-MSCs, mean (95% confidence interval) for TNCC was 13.1×10^9/L ($7.7–18.5 \times 10^9$/L), and total protein concentration was 33.6 g/L (17.3–65.6), which was higher than saline controls.[50] Values were decreasing but had not returned to pretreatment levels after 72 hours. When administered in conjunction with lipopolysaccharide (LPS), cell count and protein were significantly lower than with LPS injection alone, indicating an immunomodulatory response.

There are rare reports of foreign material observed in joints as a result of injection. Silicon injected into joints appears as clear globules within macrophages and free in the background, associated with a variable inflammatory response in the joint fluid.[51,52]

Hemarthrosis

Hemorrhage into a joint space can occur after trauma, surgery, with coagulopathy, or for unknown reasons. Bleeding will induce synovitis, and erythrophagia and evidence for erythrocyte degradation (i.e. iron pigments) can be noted cytologically. Pathologic hemorrhage must be differentiated from blood contamination during sampling as discussed earlier. In a study reviewing 8 horses with acute and recurrent lameness due to idiopathic hemarthrosis, the median TNCC was 10.0×10^9/L (range $7.4–16.0 \times 10^9$/L), and median protein concentration was 44 g/L (range 40–56).[53]

Other Diagnostic Techniques

Bacterial Culture Versus Polymerase Chain Reaction

While bacterial culture is considered the gold standard for detection of bacterial organisms in synovial fluid, polymerase chain reaction (PCR) assays for detection of these agents may have superior utility and decreased turnaround time for results. In a study evaluating 48 synovial fluid samples from horses with septic synovitis, the relative sensitivity and specificity of reverse transcriptase PCR were 87 and 72%, compared with 56 and 86% for culture.[24] In another study examining 57 septic samples compared with healthy controls and those with aseptic inflammation, 16S rRNA gene PCR was superior to both bacterial culture with either agar or blood culture media.[54] The best sensitivity and specificity occurred when results of both culture and PCR were combined. A disadvantage of PCR is inability to obtain antibiotic sensitivity to choose the most efficacious treatment.

Biomarkers

There are several studies evaluating novel biomarkers of disease in synovial fluid of horses. Many have limited routine use and tend to be used as research tools. Evaluation of biochemical analytes including lactate, glucose, and pH has been used as indicators of joint sepsis, particularly in samples without increased cellularity or protein concentration.[26] Historically, lactate concentration > 4.9 mmol/L, pH < 6.9, and serum-synovial fluid glucose difference >2.2 mmol/L have been suggested to support joint sepsis.[23,27,55] However, in the Dechant study, only one sample had a pH lower than 6.9 and was not a septic fluid.[26] In the majority of samples, lactate concentration was >4.9 mmol/L, and mean glucose concentration was lower in septic samples compared with non-septic samples, but the study was not designed to assess diagnostic utility.[26]

Matrix metalloproteinases two and nine have been used with TNCC for monitoring response to therapy in horses with septic arthritis.[25]

Myeloperoxidase (MPO) activity was measured in synovial fluid of healthy horses and those with septic and non-septic inflammatory disease.[15] MPO activity was significantly higher in septic fluid samples than all other groups evaluated. However, since MPO activity is proportional to neutrophil quantity, an advantage over cytology is unclear.

Acute phase proteins such as serum amyloid A (SAA) have been evaluated as an indicator of inflammation in synovial fluid.[20] An advantage is that SAA does not appear to increase in response to repeated arthrocentesis, as total protein does.[20] Arthroscopic lavage alone also does not seem to increase synovial fluid SAA, whereas TNCC, protein concentration, and proportion of neutrophils did increase from the procedure.[56] Haptoglobin has been measured in synovial fluid and correlated with serum concentration in 12 Shetland ponies with experimentally induced arthritis.[14]

Proteomic analysis on synovial fluid from horses with osteoarthritis and osteochondrosis found altered proteins suggestive of inflammation, coagulation, oxidative injury, and matrix degeneration when compared with the proteome of synovial fluid from healthy horses.[57]

One study suggests using D-dimer concentration in synovial fluid to aid in diagnosis of septic joints, since fibrinolytic activity is often elevated in these samples.[32] D-dimer concentration was also higher in horses with osteoarthritis and osteochondritis dissecans compared with healthy control samples.[13]

A single pilot study used flow cytometry to assess neutrophil viability and mode of cell death to facilitate discernment between septic and non-septic samples.[58] Interestingly, cell viability was greater in septic samples, and more cells died by apoptosis than necrosis, compared with non-septic and healthy samples.

References

1 McIlwraith, C.W., Frisbie, D.D., Kawcak, C.E., and van Weeren, R. (2016). *Joint Disease in the Horse*, 2e. St. Louis, MO: Elsevier.

2 Steel, C.M. (2008). Equine synovial fluid analysis. *Vet Clin North Am Equine Pract* 24: 437–454.

3 Roquet, I., Hendrick, S., and Carmalt, J.L. (2012). The effect of blood contamination on equine synovial fluid analysis. *Vet Comp Orthop Traumatol* 25: 460–465.

4 Dumoulin, M., Pille, F., van den Abeele, A. et al. (2010). Use of blood culture medium enrichment for synoival fluid culture in horses: a comparison of different culture methods. *Equine Vet J* 42: 541–546.

5 Rakich, P.M. and Latimer, K.S. (2011). Cytology. In: *Duncan and Prasse's Veterinary Laboratory Medicine Clinical Pathology*, 5e (ed. K.S. Latimer), 352–353. Ames, IA: Wiley-Blackwell.

6 Van Pelt, R.W. (1962). Properties of equine synovial fluid. *J Am Vet Med Assoc* 141: 1051–1061.
7 Ekmann, A., Rigdal, M., and Grondahl, G. (2010). Automated counting of nucleated cells in equine synovial fluid without and with hyaluronidase pretreatment. *Vet Clin Pathol* 39: 83–89.
8 Brudvig, J. and Swenson, C. (2015). Total nucleated cell and leukocyte differential counts in canine pleural and peritoneal fluid and equine synovial fluid samples: comparison of automated and manual methods. *Vet Clin Pathol* 44: 570–579.
9 Van de Water, E., Oosterlinck, M., Duchateau, L., and Pille, F. (2016). Agreement of manual cell counts and automated counts of the scil Vet abc Plus+ hematology analyzer for analysis of equine synovial fluid. *Res Vet Sci* 106: 62–65.
10 Hughes, K.R.D., Higgins, S., Barron, R. et al. (2017). Effect of storage time and temperature on the results of analysis of synovial and mesothelial fluids. *Equine Vet J* 49: 232–237.
11 Van Pelt, R.W. (1967). Characteristics of normal equine tarsal synovial fluid. *Can J Comp Med Vet Sci* 31: 342–347.
12 Jones, D., Barber, S., and Doige, C. (1993). Synovial fluid and clinical changes after arthroscopic partial synovectomy of the equine middle carpal joint. *Vet Surg* 22: 524–530.
13 Ribera, T., Monreal, L., Delgado, M. et al. (2013). Synovial fluid D-dimer concentration in horses with osteochondritis dissecans and osteoarthritis. *Vet Comp Orthop Traumatol* 26: 54–60.
14 Barrachina, L., Remacha, A., Soler, L. et al. (2016). Acute phase protein haptoglobin as inflammatory marker in serum and synovial fluid in an equine model of arthritis. *Vet Immunol Immunopathol* 182: 74–78.
15 Wauters, J., Pille, F., Martens, A. et al. (2013). Equine myeloperoxidase: a novel biomarker in synovial fluid for the diagnosis of infection. *Equine Vet J* 45: 278–283.
16 Malark, J., Nixon, A., Skinner, K., and Mohammed, H. (1991). Characteristics of digital flexor tendon sheath fluid from clinically normal horses. *Am J Vet Res* 52: 1292–1294.
17 Van Pelt, R.W., Riley, W.F. Jr., and Tillotson, P.J. (1969). Tenosynovitis of the deep digital flexor tendon in horses. *Can Vet J* 10: 235–243.
18 Korenek, N., Andrews, F., Maddux, J. et al. (1992). Determination of total protein concentration and viscosity of synovial fluid from the tibiotarsal joints of horses. *Am J Vet Res* 53: 781–784.
19 Vitanen, M., Bird, J., Makela, O. et al. (2001). Synovial fluid studies in navicular disease. *Res Vet Sci* 71: 201–206.
20 Jacobsen, S., Halling Thomsen, M., and Nanni, S. (2006). Concentrations of serum amyloid A in serum and synovial fluid from healthy horses and horses with joint disease. *Am J Vet Res* 67: 1738–1742.
21 Craig, L.E., Dittmer, K.E., and Thompson, K.G. (2016). Bone and joints. In: *Jubb, Kennedy and Palmer's Pathology of Domestic Animals* (ed. M.G. Maxie), 128–131. St. Louis: Elsevier.
22 Madison, J.B., Sommer, M., and Spencer, P.A. (1991). Relations among synovial membrane histopathologic findings, synovial fluid cytologic findings, and bacterial culture results in horses with suspected infectious arthritis: 64 cases (1979–1987). *J Am Vet Med Assoc* 198: 1655–1661.
23 Schneider, R., Bramlage, L., Moore, R. et al. (1992). A retrospective study of 192 horses affected with septic arthritis/tenosynovitis. *Equine Vet J* 24: 436–442.
24 Elmas, C., Koenig, J., Bienzle, D. et al. (2013). Evaluation of a broad range real-time polymerase chain reaction (RT-PCR) assay for the diagnosis of septic synovitis in horses. *Can J Vet Res* 77: 211–217.
25 Kidd, J., Barr, A., and Tarlton, J. (2007). Use of matrix metalloproteinases 2 and 9 and white blood cell counts in monitoring the treatment and predicting the survival of horses with septic arthritis. *Vet Rec* 161: 329–334.
26 Dechant, J., Symm, W., and Nieto, J. (2011). Comparison of pH, lactate, and glucose analysis of equine synovial fluid using a portable clinical analyzer with a bench-top blood gas analyzer. *Vet Surg* 40: 811–816.
27 Tulamo, R., Bramlage, L., and Gabel, A. (1989). Sequential clinical and synovial fluid changes associated with acute infectious arthritis in the horse. *Equine Vet J* 21: 325–331.
28 Bertone, A.L. (1999). Update on infectious arthritis in horses. *Equine Vet Edu* 11: 143–152.
29 Lapointe, J., Laverty, S., and Lavoie, J. (1992). Septic arthritis in 15 Standardbred racehorses after intra-articular injection. *Equine Vet J* 24: 430–434.
30 Hewes, C., Schneider, R., Baszler, T., and Oaks, J.L. (2005). Septic arthritis and granulomatous synovitis caused by infection with *Mycobacterium avium* complex in a horse. *J Am Vet Med Assoc* 226: 2035–2038.
31 Hepworth-Warren, K., Fulkerson, C., Wang, C. et al. (2015). Bacterial isolates, antimicrobial susceptibility patterns, and factors associated with infection and outcome in foals with septic arthritis: 83 cases (1998–2013). *J Am Vet Med Assoc* 246: 785–793.
32 Ribera, T., Monreal, L., Armengou, L. et al. (2011). Synovial fluid D-dimer concentration in foals with septic joint disease. *J Vet Intern Med* 25: 1113–1117.
33 Kawaguchi, K. and Church, S. (2004). *Clostridium septicum* arthritis in three foals. *Aust Vet J* 82: 612–615.
34 Reuss, S., Chaffin, M., and Cohen, N. (2009). Extrapulmonary disorders associated with *Rhodococcus*

equi infection in foals: 150 cases (1987–2007). *J Am Vet Med Assoc* 235: 855–863.

35 Sweeney, C., Sweeney, R., and Divers, T. (1987). *Rhodococcus equi* pneumonia in 48 foals: response to antimicrobial therapy. *Vet Microbiol* 14: 329–336.

36 Passamonti, F., Veronesi, F., Cappelli, K. et al. (2015). Polysynovitis in a horse due to *Borrelia burgdorferi* sensu infection: case study. *Ann Agric Environ Med* 22: 247–250.

37 Sherman, K., Myhre, G., and Heymann, E. (2006). Fungal osteomyelitis of the axial border of the proximal sesamoid bones in a horse. *J Am Vet Med Assoc* 229: 1607–1611.

38 Madison, J., Reid, B.V., and Raskin, R.E. (1995). Amphotericin B treatment of Candida arthritis in two horses. *J Am Vet Med Assoc* 206: 338–341.

39 Swerczek, T., Donahue, J., and Hunt, R.J. (2001). *Scedosporium prolificans* infection associated with arthritis and osteomyelitis in a horse. *J Am Vet Med Assoc* 218: 1800–1802.

40 Madison, J. and Ziemer, E. (1993). Eosinophilic synovitis following the intra-articular injection of bacterial antigen in horses. *Res Vet Sci* 54: 256–258.

41 Turner, A., Gustafson, S., Zeidner, N. et al. (1990). Acute eosinophilic synovitis in a horse. *Equine Vet J* 22: 215–217.

42 Climent, F., Carmona, J., Cuenca, R., and Prades, M. (2007). Eosinophilic synovitis of the tarsocrural joint in a horse. *Vet Comp Orthop Traumatol* 20: 142–145.

43 Vrins, A. and Feldman, B. (1983). Lupus erythematosus-like syndrome in a horse. *Equine Pract* 5: 18–25.

44 Geor, R., Clark, E., Haines, D., and Napier, P. (1990). Systemic lupus erythematosus in a filly. *J Am Vet Med Assoc* 197: 1489–1492.

45 Pusterla, N., Pratt, S., Magdesian, K., and Carlson, G. (2006). Idiopathic immune-mediated polysynovitis in three horses. *Vet Rec* 159: 13–15.

46 Kawcak, C.E. and McIlwraith, C.W. (2011). Comparison of synovial fluid in middle carpal joints undergoing needle aspiration, infusion with saline, and infusion with a combination of *N*-acetyl-D-glucosamine, hyaluronic acid, and sodium chondroitin sulfate. *J Equine Vet Sci* 31: 155–159.

47 Knych, H., Vidal, M., Chouicha, N. et al. (2017). Cytokine, catabolic enzyme and structural matrix gene expression in synovial fluid following intra-articular administration of triamcinolone acetonide in exercised horses. *Equine Vet J* 49: 107–115.

48 Kwan, C., Bell, R., Koenig, T. et al. (2012). Effects of intra-articular sodium pentosan polysulfate and glucosamine on the cytology, total protein concentration and viscosity of synovial fluid in horses. *Aust Vet J* 90: 315–320.

49 Textor, J. and Tablin, F. (2013). Intra-articular use of a platelet-rich product in normal horses: clinical signs and cytologic responses. *Vet Surg* 42: 499–510.

50 Williams, L., Koenig, J., Black, B. et al. (2016). Equine allogeneic umbilical cord blood derived mesenchymal stromal cells reduce synovial fluid nucleated cell count and induce mild self-limiting inflammation when evaluated in an LPS induced synovitis model. *Equine Vet J* 48: 619–625.

51 Scott, M.A., Tvedten, H.W., and Huang, R.H. (1994). What is your diagnosis? *Vet Clin Pathol* 23: 13–14, 25, 26.

52 Rumbaugh, M.L., Burba, D.J., Tetens, J. et al. (2004). Effects of intra-articular injection of liquid silicone polymer in the equine middle carpal joint. *Proceedings of the 50th Annual Convention of the American Association of Equine Practitioners*, Denver, Colorado (4–8 December 2004).

53 Vallance, S., Lumsden, J., Begg, A., and O'Sullivan, C.B. (2012). Idiopathic haemarthrosis in eight horses. *Aust Vet J* 90: 214–220.

54 Pille, F., Martens, A., Schouls, L. et al. (2007). Broad range 16S rRNA gene PCR compared to bacterial culture to confirm presumed synovial infection in horses. *Vet J* 173: 73–78.

55 Lloyd, K., Stover, S., Pascoe, J., and Adams, P. (1990). Synovial fluid pH, cytologic characteristics, and gentamicin concentration after intra-articular administration of the drug in an experimental model of infectious arthritis in horses. *Am J Vet Res* 51: 1363–1369.

56 Sanchez-Teran, A., Bracamonte, J., Hendrick, S. et al. (2016). Effect of arthroscopic lavage on systemic and synovial fluid serum amyloid A in healthy horses. *Vet Surg* 45: 223–230.

57 Chiaradia, E., Pepe, M., Tartaglia, M. et al. (2012). Gambling on putative biomarkers of osteoarthritis and osteochondrosis by equine synovial fluid proteomics. *J Proteome* 75: 4478–4493.

58 Wauters, J., Martens, A., Pille, F. et al. (2012). Viability and cell death of synovial fluid neutrophils as diagnostic biomarkers in equine infectious joint disease: a pilot study. *Res Vet Sci* 92: 132–137.

Part XV

Species Specific Cytology

56

Exotic Companion Mammals

Courtney Johnson, Kyle Lauren Webb, Jennifer Graham, and Leslie C. Sharkey

Introduction

An increasing number of small mammals are kept as pets. Small size, risk of anesthesia and surgery, and the need to limit expenses make cytology a particularly valuable but often underreported diagnostic technique.[1] Advances in the care of these species such as utilization of imaging, endoscopic, and surgical techniques and the increasing application of specialty-level care will only increase the demand for expertise in the cytology of small mammals.[2–4] This chapter focuses on the cytology of ferrets, hedgehogs, and rodents, including guinea pigs, hamsters, and rats. This does leave some exotic companion mammal species uncovered based on paucity of literature. Relevant material on most of these species in a laboratory setting is addressed in Chapter 66. The cytology literature for small mammals is patchy and dispersed, consisting primarily of case reports and anecdotal observations. Nonetheless, we hope that aggregating the available information will be valuable and spurs research to fill gaps in knowledge. The most complete descriptions of cytology are for lesions of the skin and subcutis, which are frequently sampled.

Sample Collection

Common applications of cytology in exotic companion animal practice include fine-needle aspirates (FNA) from solid masses, cysts, joints, and sinuses. Swabs and scrapings can be taken from the skin, ears, conjunctiva, oropharynx, feces, and freshly cut organ surfaces during necropsy. A 3 or 6 cc syringe with a 22 or 25 G needle is most commonly used in exotic companion mammals for FNA.[5] Manual stabilization of an external mass for aspiration can require sedation or anesthesia in the difficult to restrain exotic mammal. Most patients benefit from administration of preanesthetic agents including sedatives and/or opioid analgesics when internal organs are sampled. Patients can be masked down with isoflurane or sevoflurane if additional immobilization is required. A 22 G butterfly catheter with an attached 12 cc syringe is the preferred method of cavity fluid collection. As many exotic companion mammals with body cavity effusions are depressed, manual restraint can be adequate. For analgesia, local anesthetics including lidocaine can be instilled into a surgically prepared area of needle insertion.

Ferrets

General Information

Domestic ferrets (*Mustela putorius furo*, or the European ferret) are popular pets. Their long narrow shape allows accessibility for fine-needle aspiration of nearly all organs and tissues, and ferret cytology literature is more robust than for other small mammals.[6] Well-established cytologic features of lesions in dogs and cats are usually directly applicable to known diseases of ferrets, so the following sections focus on aspects unique to ferrets.[6]

Skin and Subcutis

Nonneoplastic Conditions

Nonneoplastic conditions in ferrets are far less common than neoplastic ones. Nonneoplastic cutaneous masses in ferrets include hematomas, abscesses, granulomas, hernias, and cysts.[7] Despite the lack of well-developed sweat glands in ferrets,[8] apocrine gland cysts associated with hair follicles have been occasionally reported with smears often being acellular.[6] Bilaterally symmetric, noninflammatory, progressive alopecia, with or without pruritus, is common in ferrets and has been associated with metabolic and endocrine causes not amenable to definitive cytologic diagnosis in many cases. Adrenal neoplasia is often associated

Veterinary Cytology, First Edition. Edited by Leslie C. Sharkey, M. Judith Radin, and Davis Seelig.

with alopecia and pruritus in ferrets. The percentage of cornified preputial epithelial cells collected by preputial lavage was higher in ferrets with adrenocortical disease and correlated with increased serum 17-hydroxyprogesterone concentration but not 17B-estradiol or androstenedione concentrations.[9,10]

The only common viral disease of ferrets known to affect the skin is canine distemper virus (CDV). CDV, a paramyxovirus, causes lesions including generalized erythema, dermatitis, scaling, and severe pruritus, often along with oculonasal discharge. As with dogs, hyperkeratosis of the nasal planum and footpads often occurs with respiratory signs; however, a chin rash might precede these manifestations.[11–13] Antemortem diagnosis is difficult, and cytology is not routinely utilized, other than for immunofluorescent antibody screening on conjunctival, mucosal, and blood smears in the first few days of infection.[11]

Bacterial skin infections, most often a result of bite or puncture wounds, are fairly common and cytologically similar to other species.[6,14] Lumpy jaw (actinomycosis) is rare but can be tentatively diagnosed via cytologic identification of Gram-positive, beaded, filamentous bacteria[6]; however, definitive differentiation from *Nocardia* spp. requires culture. Cutaneous mycobacteriosis can be diagnosed cytologically based on variable numbers of nonstaining intracellular rods (Chapter 3). Multi-organ involvement is common in ferrets, and they are susceptible to various strains of human, avian, bovine, and opportunistic mycobacteria.[6,15]

Ferrets are susceptible to dermatophytosis (*Microsporum canis* or *Trichophyton mentagrophytes*), flea infestation (*Ctenocephalides* spp.), sarcoptic mange (*Sarcoptes scabiei*), otodectic mange (*Otodectes cynotis*), and tick infestation.[16,17] There is some disagreement in the literature regarding the prevalence of dermatophytosis and sarcoptic mange in ferrets; however, young and immunosuppressed animals appear to be predisposed, especially to dermatophytosis.[11,18–22] Dermatophytosis is definitively diagnosed via culture. Ferrets with sarcoptic mange present with either severe, diffuse pruritus, or variable pruritus localized to the feet. Cytologic evaluation of hairs and scrapes from affected skin can be diagnostic; however, false negative results are common (Chapter 11).[11,18,22] *O. cynotis* causes mild to severe otitis and pruritic dermatitis in ferrets.[19] A copious, dark-brown, waxy exudate can be present, with microscopic evaluation frequently revealing many live mites and eggs.[11] Fur mites (*Lynxacarus mustelae*) have also been reported in ferrets often presenting with ulcerative facial lesions; however, the potential for cytologic detection is unclear.[23] Demodectic mange (*Demodex* spp.) is less commonly reported but is occasionally seen in older or immunosuppressed ferrets.[24] Skin scrapings from ferrets with demodicosis can demonstrate nymphs or adult mites (Chapter 11).

Other fungal diseases typically have systemic involvement but will be discussed here since all can have dermal manifestations. These are uncommon in the domestic ferret with similar cytology as in other species (Chapter 3); documented cases of blastomycosis,[25] histoplasmosis,[26,27] coccidioidomycosis[28], and systemic candidiasis with ulcerative skin lesions (*Candida albicans, Candida tropicalis*) are in the literature.[12,28] Cryptococcosis has also been reported, involving neurologic, gastrointestinal, pulmonary, nasal, and cutaneous tissues.[27,29–34] Mucormycosis, *Malassezia* spp., and *Pneumocystis* spp. have also been reported in ferrets, along with an anecdotal case of aspergillosis.[14,35–39] Mucormycosis is caused by the fungus *Absidia corymbifera* (*ramosa*), described only in ferrets in New Zealand.[11,37,40] It occurs concurrently with *O. cynotis* infection, infecting the ears and sometimes causing necrosis of the petrous temporal bone. Cytologic identification of the fungal hyphae from the external ear canal is diagnostic.[20] Ferrets with *O. cynotis* often have *Malassezia* spp. overgrowth identified cytologically as in other species (Chapter 17).[35,36,41] Ferrets have an antigenically and genetically distinct commensal strain of *Pneumocystis carinii*; pathogenicity is restricted to immunosuppressed individuals. Organisms can be identified cytologically on airway samples.[20]

Neoplasia

Most ferrets develop one or more neoplasms between the ages of 3 and 5 years, with up to 20% of ferrets having multiple types.[3,42–47] The three most common neoplasms in ferrets are adrenal tumors, insulinoma, and lymphoma, together comprising over 40% of all ferret neoplasms.[47] Apart from endocrine and hemolymphatic neoplasms, tumors of the skin and subcutis predominate.[48,49]

Round Cell Tumors

Most sources agree that mast cell tumors (MCTs) are the most common cutaneous and subcutaneous neoplasm of ferrets. Ferret MCTs are composed of well-differentiated mast cells (Chapter 13). However, routine metachromatic staining was historically reported to reveal only few cytoplasmic granules and lack of notable eosinophils or collagenolysis.[3,6,45,50,51] In a recent study evaluating the cytological features of 12 cutaneous MCTs in ferrets, mast cell granules were not visualized with modified Wright's stain in any case.[52] When the same samples were stained with toluidine blue and Wright Giemsa, general morphological characteristics were similar to those in other species; however, 83% displayed a marked intracytoplasmic granulation with the remaining cases displaying moderate granulation. Eosinophils and collagenolysis are less common in ferret MCTs than dogs. MCTs in ferrets are often benign, but they can cause local pruritus and resulting traumatization of the lesion.[3,6]

Lymphoma, while the third most common neoplasm overall and the most common neoplasm of young (<1-year-old) ferrets, does not involve the skin as commonly as lymph nodes and other tissues.[3,47,53–55] Cutaneous lymphoma in ferrets is often indicative of disseminated disease.[3,47] Both non-epitheliotrophic and epitheliotrophic lymphoma have been reported in the skin of ferrets with variable clinical presentations. FNA is frequently nondiagnostic except for well-defined skin nodules. Lymphoma should be a differential diagnosis for nonhealing lesions.[6] Cytology of nodules can consist of a monomorphic population of lymphocytes. Large immature morphology is more common in young ferrets and small or mature phenotype in adult ferrets.[6] One study found that epitheliotrophic lymphoma comprised only 1% of 763 cases of cutaneous neoplasia.[3] Interestingly, all cases involved the feet, similar to a case of histologically confirmed epitheliotrophic lymphoma in a ferret.[11]

Epithelial Neoplasms

One retrospective study found that benign sebaceous epitheliomas were equally prevalent to MCT, with each comprising approximately 1/3 of 763 cutaneous neoplasms.[3] Ferret skin contains many sebaceous glands producing secretions that give the ferret its unique odor.[11] Sebaceous epitheliomas with areas of squamous metaplasia or squamous cell carcinoma (SCC) have occasionally been called "basal cell tumors with sebaceous and squamous differentiation," terminology that is now considered incorrect.[43] In addition to sebaceous epitheliomas, other sebaceous gland tumors include sebaceous adenoma, sebaceous ductal adenoma, and sebaceous carcinoma. Cytologic characteristics often mimic those reported in other species with sebaceous epitheliomas uniquely containing reserve cells in addition to mature sebocytes[6,46–48,56]; however, histopathology is required for definitive differentiation of sebaceous tumors.[11] Although basal cell tumors are occasionally reported as common in ferrets (with one source reporting an incidence of 60% of ferret skin tumors),[47] determining their incidence is challenging as they have been confused in the earlier literature with sebaceous epitheliomas.[6,48,56]

In addition to apocrine gland cysts, benign and malignant apocrine gland tumors also occur in ferrets and are typically exfoliative.[6,48,56,57] A few reports of apocrine gland neoplasms of the anal sac, perianal area, prepuce, and tail are available.[58–60] Preputial apocrine adenocarcinomas account for 7% of all ferret cutaneous neoplasms in one study[46] and 2 of 51 total tumors in a second.[50] Differences in the cytology of anal sac apocrine adenocarcinomas between dog and ferrets have been reported. Ferret tumors produce abundant secretory product, and cells have more discrete cytoplasmic margins and can be vacuolated or contain blue granular material.[6,59] Newer reports describe poorly defined cell borders and moderate to marked anisocytosis and anisokaryosis on cytology.[60] Sebaceous gland adenocarcinoma has also been reported in ferrets, although cytologic features have not been well-defined. Other skin tumors of ferrets include sebaceous adenoma, preputial gland tumors (carcinoma, adenoma, adenocarcinoma, and cystadenoma), and SCC.[3,11,50]

SCC represented 1.7% of 763 cutaneous neoplasms in ferrets in one retrospective report.[3] However, SCC of the anal sac, pads, and digits have all been reported in the literature.[61,62] Like other species SCC in ferrets is typically characterized by epithelial cells displaying numerous criteria of malignancy including asynchrony of cytoplasmic and nuclear maturation with concurrent inflammation.[6] Squamous metaplasia and SCC associated with sebaceous tumors has been reported in multiple studies; however, the relationship is unclear.[43,45,63]

While rare overall, both male and female ferrets can be afflicted by mammary gland tumors, including adenomas (simple and complex), adenocarcinomas, and fibroadenomas.[3,47]

Mesenchymal Tumors

Mesenchymal tumors of the ferret skin are described below, but none are well characterized cytologically in this species. Despite being reported by one source as the third most common type of skin tumor in ferrets, cytology of cutaneous hemangiomas has not been well described.[3] Ferrets rarely develop cutaneous hemangiosarcomas.[3] Fibromas and fibrosarcomas, while rare, are more frequently identified in middle-aged to older ferrets.[11] Thirteen reports of dermal leiomyosarcomas are available.[64,65] Piloleiomyosarcomas, a subset of leiomyomas predominantly arising from the arrector pili muscles, are rarely reported in ferrets.[66,67] Two reports of subcutaneous liposarcomas (inguinal and tail base) exist; cytology of one lesion consisted of low numbers of spindle to polygonal cells.[7,68] Dermal and subcutaneous fibrosarcomas are potentially associated with vaccination sites similar to cats, but no cytologic descriptions are available.[69,70]

Fluid Analysis

Effusions are overall uncommon in ferrets, most frequently associated with mediastinal (thymic) lymphoma in young animals.[53] Pleural fluid smears from affected ferrets are typically moderately to highly cellular with a uniform population of large, immature lymphocytes.[6] Eosinophilic effusions can develop in ferrets with heartworm disease, and abdominal effusions occur in adult ferrets with cardiac disease, often displaying cytologic features mirroring those described in other domestic species.[6,71,72] Mesothelioma has been rarely reported in ferrets; as with other species, distinction between reactive and neoplastic mesothelial cells is often challenging cytologically.[46,58] Recently, well-differentiated neoplastic plasma cells were identified in pleural effusion from a ferret with confirmed malignant plasma cell neoplasia of the spleen, liver, lymph nodes, thoracic vertebrae, extradural space, and meninges of the brain.[73] Cells displayed marked anisocytosis and anisokaryosis with round, eccentrically placed nuclei and moderate amounts of deeply basophilic cytoplasm and were also identified in aspirates from the spleen and an iliac lymph node.

Other Systems

Hemolymphatic

Ferrets typically have abundant axillary, inguinal, and popliteal fat, which can be misinterpreted as lymph node enlargement or contaminate lymph node FNAs.[6] Normal mesenteric ferret lymph node cytology samples are moderately to highly cellular, consisting of small mature lymphocytes with scattered medium and large lymphocytes, and small numbers of macrophages, plasma cells, and nondegenerate neutrophils.[74] The most common cause of lymphadenopathy in ferrets is lymphoma.[6] Lymph node involvement is more common in older ferrets with lymphoproliferative disease, and small, well-differentiated lymphocytes are commonly observed in geriatric patients.[6,53] Consequently, a cytologic diagnosis of the lymphocytic form of lymphoma can be difficult early in disease.[6] Lymphoma often involves multiple hematopoietic organs and frequently occurs concurrently with adrenocortical tumors and/or insulinomas.[75,76] SCC can metastasize to lymph nodes and can be identified cytologically in lymph node FNA.[6] A recent report of disseminated plasma cell neoplasia affecting the lymph nodes was also published.[73]

Splenomegaly is common in ferrets and is most often clinically insignificant.[6,77] Extramedullary hematopoiesis is the most common cause of splenomegaly and cytologically appears like other species (Chapter 28). The spleen is commonly infiltrated by neoplastic lymphocytes in ferrets with lymphoma, but diffuse infiltration is required for a confident diagnosis (Figure 56.1).[6] Multifocal malignant plasma cell neoplasia can involve the spleen and can be cytologically characterized by many moderately atypical plasma cells.[73] Splenic myelolipoma has been reported.[43] Mediastinal hemangioma and thymoma have been reported.[43,47]

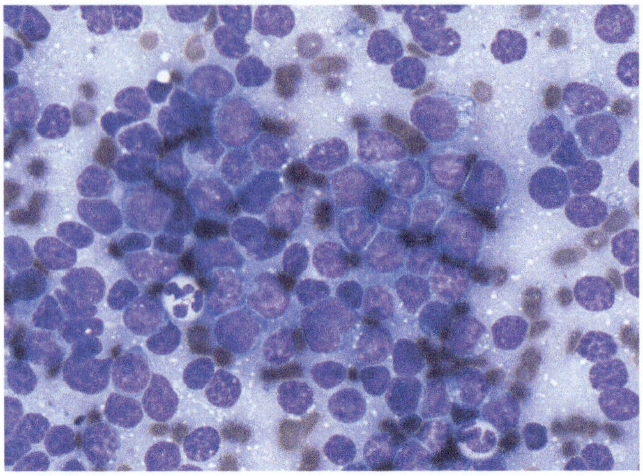

Figure 56.1 Cytology from a ferret (*M. putorius furo*) with splenic lymphoma. Note the predominance of medium to large lymphocytes characterized by scant to moderate amounts of lightly vacuolated basophilic cytoplasm and smooth chromatin. Scattered residual mature lymphocytes are present (Wright-Giemsa, 500×).

Endocrine

Endocrine tumors comprise >50% of all ferret neoplasia.[47] "Adrenocortical disease" is a broad term applied to the production of excessive concentrations of androgenic hormones because of cystic, hyperplastic, or neoplastic changes in the adrenal cortex.[11,63] Male ferrets can present with prostatomegaly, and both sexes can have other clinical signs of adrenal disease, most commonly bilaterally symmetrical, generalized alopecia, and pruritus.[11,78] Other adrenal cortical tumors include leiomyoma, leiomyosarcoma, and spindle cell sarcomas, while pheochromocytoma and neuroblastoma are adrenomedullary tumors.[43,47,79] One study found that 10 of 303 ferrets were affected by two simultaneous adrenal neoplasms, and most were malignant.[43] Another reported 24 cases of intra-abdominal spindle cell neoplasms with vacuolated cells without connection to identifiable organs or tissues.[43] Histologically, neoplastic cells strongly resembled adrenal cortical cells, suggesting a possible ectopic adrenal tissue origin; however, cytology was not performed. Despite the frequency of adrenal disease in ferrets, cytologic evaluation is uncommon because diagnosis is based on history and physical exam, hormonal assays, advanced imaging, and surgery with histopathology.

Thyroid carcinoma has been documented in ferrets.[47] Cytologic findings were described in one case of a rapidly growing mass on the ventral neck of ferret and included high cellularity, hemodilution, and cohesive clusters of cuboidal to polyhedral cells with distinct cell margins that rarely formed acini.[80] Nuclei were round with stippled chromatin and a single large nucleolus. Colloid and tyrosine were not described.

Eye and Ear

Ocular cytology is poorly described in the ferret. Distemper is reported in ferrets, and characteristic inclusions are described histologically, but cytology is not reported.[81] Conjunctival mycobacteriosis was identified on impression cytology in a ferret (Chapter 3).[82] Exudative chorioretinitis with intraretinal *Cryptococcus gattii* was diagnosed in one ferret, and while identified histologically, cryptococcal organisms were also identified in the central nervous system and regional lymph nodes, potentially indicating the diagnostic utility of FNA of regional lymph nodes and cerebrospinal fluid in cases of suspected cryptococcal infection (Chapter 3).[83] Histologically diagnosed case reports of meibomian gland carcinoma, ocular lipoma, basal cell adenocarcinoma of the lacrimal gland, and lacrimal gland adenoma are published.[43,47,83]

Otic cytology is addressed in the skin section. A case report of a histologically diagnosed aural ceruminous gland adenocarcinoma reported concurrent ear mites, mixed bacteria, and yeast identified on presurgical cytology.[84]

Musculoskeletal

Primary tumors of the musculoskeletal system described in ferrets include chordoma, chordosarcoma, osteoma, osteosarcoma, chondrosarcoma, rhabdomyosarcoma, histiocytic sarcoma, intramedullary lumbosacral teratoma, fibrosarcoma, synovial cell sarcoma, leiomyoma, leiomyosarcoma, and piloleiomyosarcoma.[47,49,85–88] Additionally, single cases of a multilobular tumor of the bone originating from the neck and an intraosseous liposarcoma of the mandible have been documented.[89,90] Specific categorization of mesenchymal tumors is rarely possible cytologically; however, cytologic samples from chordomas can contain characteristic clusters of foamy physaliphorous cells in a mucinous background that is considered diagnostic (Figure 56.2).[91–93] Physaliphorous cells are round to polygonal with an abundant amount of eosinophilic cytoplasm, typically obscured by numerous large intracytoplasmic mucoid-laden vacuoles. Nuclei are round to ovoid with coarsely granular chromatin, and cells display moderate anisocytosis and anisokaryosis. Binucleated and multinucleated cells are commonly seen.[91] These tumors originate from the intraosseous remnants of the fetal notochord, occur exclusively in the axial skeleton, and are considered the most common musculoskeletal neoplasm of ferrets, comprising 79% of musculoskeletal neoplasms reviewed in one study and 86% of all bone neoplasms reviewed in another.[88,94,95] While typically found at the tip of the tail, a tail base chordoma, three cases of cervical chordomas, and a thoracic chordoma have been described.[42,93–97] Chordomas are often locally aggressive and have been reported to occasionally undergo both adjacent and distant cutaneous and visceral metastasis.[94,95] On immunohistochemistry, neoplastic chordoma cells express both vimentin and cytokeratin, which can be diagnostic when cytologic and histologic interpretation proves challenging.[91,95,98]

One report highlighted two cases of maxillary osteosarcoma.[43] A report of two ferrets with chondrosarcoma involving the left hock and the right scapula, respectively, describes FNA of the hock mass consisting of atypical mesenchymal cells leading to a preliminary diagnosis of sarcoma.[49] A separate, earlier report described chondrosarcoma of the tails of four ferrets[85]; however, these may have been mischaracterized caudal vertebral chordomas.[88] Benign osteomas originating from flat bones of the skull and ribs are rarely reported in ferrets and typically require histopathology for diagnosis.[88,99]

An invasive histiocytic sarcoma of the lumbar spine and surrounding musculature was characterized cytologically by medium- to large-sized cells containing basophilic cytoplasm, with large eccentric, round-to-oval, partially lobulated nuclei.[87] Multinucleated cells were present. Anisokaryosis, coarse chromatin, and prominent nucleoli were observed.

Rare musculoskeletal round cell tumors have been reported, including plasma cell neoplasia, and a single case of spinal T-cell lymphoma.[100] A recent case series highlighted three cases of malignant plasma cell neoplasia involving the lumbar spine.[73]

Respiratory

Respiratory disease is uncommon in ferrets. Pneumonia is typically caused by viral infection with CDV and/or influenza virus, which have similar clinical presentations.[22] Tracheal wash samples can be collected for cytology and culture when bacterial pneumonia is suspected.[6,101] In the absence of a radiographically distinct pulmonary mass, lung aspiration is usually nondiagnostic, and even with diffuse pulmonary disease, tracheal washes tend to be more diagnostic than aspirates.[6] Respiratory neoplasia is rare and include adenosquamous carcinoma of the trachea, MCT, mesothelioma, pulmonary adenocarcinoma, and a sarcoma arising in the thoracic cavity.[43,47]

Gastrointestinal Tract, Liver, and Pancreas

Salivary gland mucoceles have rarely been reported in ferrets; the zygomatic and molar salivary glands are most commonly affected.[102–108] Aspiration of salivary mucoceles typically reveals viscous fluid with a low cell count and cytologic findings like those in other domestic species.[105] Salivary gland carcinoma is reported to affect ferrets, and a single case of a salivary gland adenoma, diagnosed histologically, was reported in Italy.[43,47]

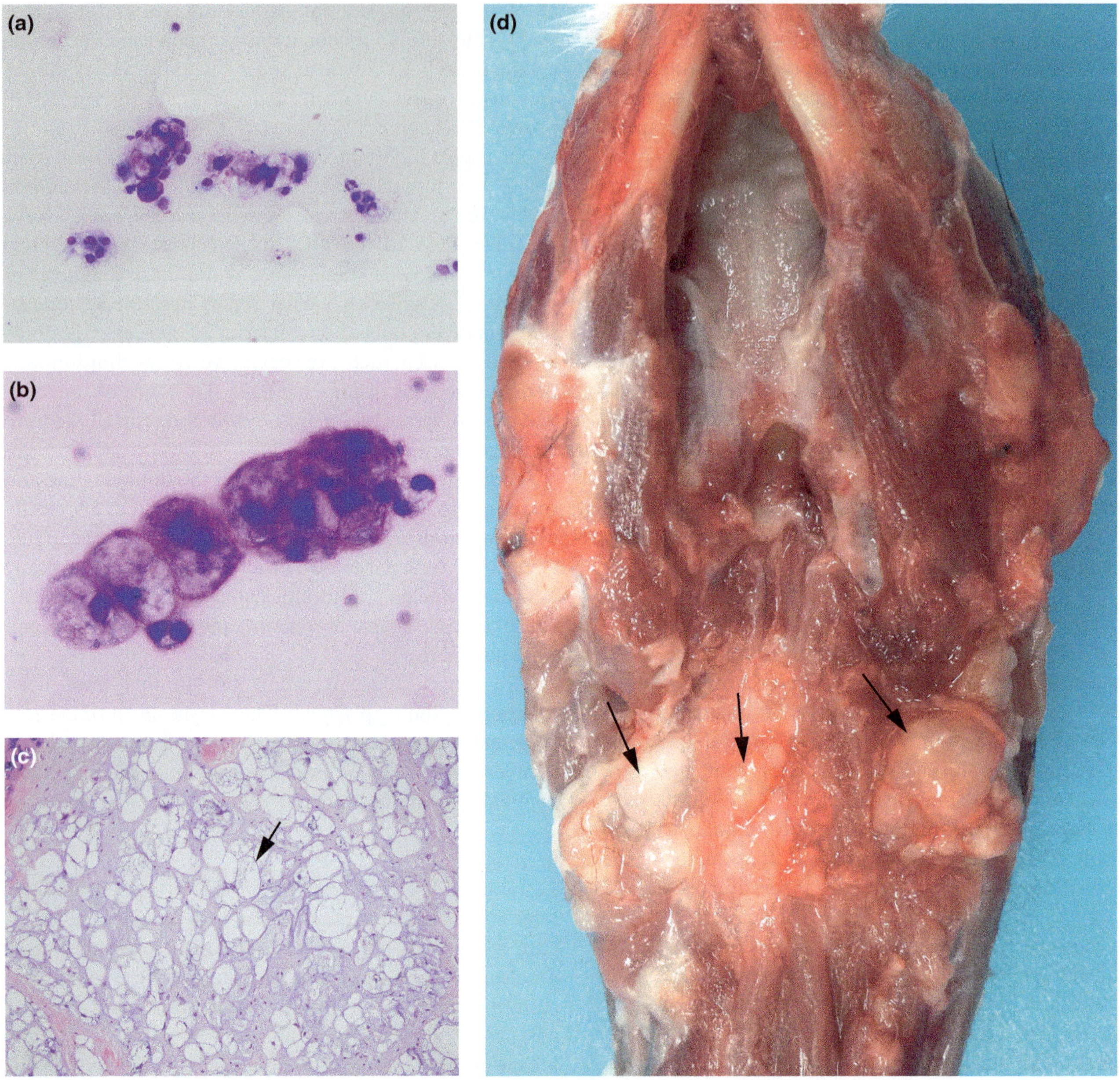

Figure 56.2 Chordoma in a ferret. (a and b) Cytology consists of clusters of round to polyhedral foamy physaliphorous cells characterized by vacuolated amphophilic to eosinophilic cytoplasm. Cells contain one or two small- to medium-sized nuclei. The N:C is moderate with some variability. Anisocytosis and anisokaryosis are moderate (Wright Giemsa stain, (a) 200×, (b) 500×). (c) Histopathology from samples collected at necropsy. Most cells within the field are large neoplastic (physaliferous) cells (arrow) with lightly amphophilic, wispy cytoplasm. These cells are characteristic of chordomas (hematoxylin & eosin, 200×. (d) Gross image at necropsy showing the ventral aspect of head (upper) and neck (lower). The chordoma is a multinodular white to pale tan series of lesions (arrows) at the region of cervical vertebrae. *Source:* Images (c) and (d) courtesy of Nicholas Robinson).

Young ferrets (<6 months of age) are more likely to show clinical signs of diarrhea with *Campylobacter* spp. infection, with organisms potentially detected in Gram-stained feces or through fecal wet mount evaluation (Chapter 33). While *Campylobacter*-induced diarrhea is self-limiting in ferrets, it is zoonotic.[22] *Mycobacterium* spp. have been isolated from the gastrointestinal tract of ferrets, and infection is characterized by a disseminated gastric lesions produced by *Mycobacterium celatum* (type 3).[22] Additional clinical signs (e.g., abdominal lymphadenopathy, hepatomegaly) vary based on the location of the granulomas.[22]

SCC is the most common oral neoplasm of ferrets.[43,47,109] Of the remaining gastrointestinal tract, lymphoma and smooth muscle tumors are most common, with low-grade leiomyosarcomas predominating.[47] Gastric adenocarcinoma and gastric carcinoma have been reported.[43,47] Gastrointestinal stromal cell tumors have been documented in ferrets, but cytologic descriptions are not available.[47]

Nonneoplastic hepatopathies are uncommon in ferrets.[108] The liver is a common site for metastatic neoplasia with lymphoma being the most common and is also affected by a variety of primary, but less common, hepatocellular tumors.[6,47] Other tumors reported to affect the liver and biliary tract in ferrets include biliary cystadenoma, hepatocellular adenoma and carcinoma, peliod hepatocellular carcinoma, cholangiocellular carcinoma, malignant plasma cell neoplasia, hemangiosarcoma, hemangioma, and three cases of undifferentiated round cell neoplasia.[43,47,76] Cytology is poorly characterized but is likely similar to other species.

Insulinomas (pancreatic beta-cell tumors) are common pancreatic neoplasms of ferrets but are not routinely diagnosed cytologically. Other less commonly reported pancreatic neoplasms include exocrine adenocarcinoma and adenoma, other islet cell tumors, and a single case of malignant plasma cell neoplasia.[43,47,76]

Urinary

Urinary pathology in ferrets is rarely reported, and the literature is dominated by neoplastic conditions, though tumors of the urinary tract are overall rare and lack well-established cytologic criteria for diagnosis. Renal carcinoma, adenocarcinoma adenoma, sarcoma, nephroblastoma, and plasma cell neoplasia have been reported,[43,47,76] as well as rare cases of transitional cell carcinoma.[47]

Reproductive

Considering that most ferrets are neutered, the incidence of reproductive disease is not well described. Most neoplasms of the reproductive tract are clinically silent.[47] Cryptorchidism likely increases the risk of testicular neoplasia in male ferrets. Of the neoplasms affecting the reproductive system, tumors of smooth muscle are most common, with low-grade leiomyosarcomas being more common than leiomyomas. In females, these can affect both the ovaries and the uterus. A variety of other tumors can affect the ovary and uterus in ferrets; however, cytologic information is absent throughout the literature (Chapter 40 is a general reference).

Interstitial cell tumors are the most common neoplasm of the ferret testicle, but multiple concurrent neoplasms are reported.[47] Testicular seminomas, Sertoli cell tumors, leiomyosarcomas, mixed germ cell–sex cord-stromal tumors, and peripheral nerve sheath tumors are all reported. Recently, a case of a cystic prostatic lesion associated with adrenal adenocarcinoma and prostatomegaly was published.[110] Fine-needle aspiration and cytology of one of the cystic lesions revealed prostatic squamous metaplasia with neutrophilic inflammation, necrosis, and evidence of chronic hemorrhage. A separate small retrospective study reported that 50% of ferrets presenting with prostatic or paraprostatic cysts exhibited varying degrees of prostatic squamous metaplasia histologically, and in cases where adrenal glands were histologically evaluated, hyperplastic or neoplastic adrenocortical lesions were found.[111] Prostatic adenomas and adenocarcinomas have also been reported.[43,47]

Central Nervous System

Numerous infectious agents have been reported to affect the central nervous system of ferrets, often culminating in meningoencephalitis and/or necrotizing encephalitis. Mucormycosis, candidiasis, cryptococcosis, and CDV are described.[12,30,37]

While neurologic neoplasia of the ferret is uncommon, reported tumors include meningioma, granular cell tumor (prosencephalon), choroid plexus papilloma, melanocytomas, peripheral nerve sheath tumor (Schwannoma), neurofibroma, neurilemmoma, neurofibrosarcoma, ganglioneuroma, and spinal cord lymphoma.[47] Three cases of malignant plasma cell neoplasia affecting the extradural space and meninges have been described.[73]

Hedgehogs

General Information

Hedgehogs are small omnivorous mammals of the subfamily Erinaceinae, in the eulipotyphlan family Erinaceidae. This subfamily comprises 17 species in 5 genera, the best known of which are the European hedgehog (*Erinaceus europaeus*) and the African hedgehog (*Atelerix* spp.). While European hedgehogs are common and widespread, they are a protected species and generally not kept as companion animals. African hedgehogs, on the other hand, are frequently seen in exotic companion mammal practice. Though their taxonomy has become convoluted due to captive cross-breeding of multiple species, most of the literature on pet hedgehogs refers to African pygmy hedgehogs (*Atelerix albiventris*), and this section will follow suit, unless otherwise noted. Unfortunately, pet hedgehogs appear to be predisposed to developing malignant neoplasms, particularly with aging, which figure prominently in the literature describing these animals.[112,113]

Skin and Subcutis

Nonneoplastic Conditions

Microscopic evaluation of skin scrapings can be useful to diagnose ectoparasites in companion hedgehogs. The most important ectoparasite of hedgehogs is the psoroptic mite (*Caparinia* spp.), which aggregate in clusters on the head, dorsum, pinna, and ear canals.[114] *Caparinia tripilis* is especially pathogenic, causing self-trauma and secondary bacterial infection, which can be fatal.[114,115] All stages, from egg to adult, can be identified microscopically based on mite morphology, with specific measurements for all life stages described.[115]

Dermatophytes also frequently affect hedgehogs, and the most common isolate is *Trichophyton erinacei*.[116] Fungal dermatitis is seldom reported in hedgehogs, though there are reports in the literature involving *Paecilomyces variotii* and *Neosartorya hiratsukae*.[117,118] Cytology of the skin and hairs from the margins of the lesion from the hedgehog with *Paecilomyces* infection contained neutrophils and oval structures interpreted as likely conidia.[118] This fungus also has been reported to affect dogs and reptiles, with cats and horses being less susceptible.[118] Scrapings of the squames and quills of hedgehogs affected by *N. hiratsukae* consisted of keratinized epithelial cells and septate hyphae.[118]

Staphylococcal dermatitis has been grossly characterized by well circumscribed hyperkeratosis and alopecia with quills loosely attached to keratin debris. Cytology of exudate scrapings revealed degenerate neutrophils and many intra- and extracellular cocci.[119] Finally, there is one case report of a pemphigus foliaceus-like illness. Microscopic findings resembled pemphigus foliaceus in other species, including mixed neutrophilic and eosinophilic inflammation with acantholytic epithelial cells.[120]

Neoplasia

Neoplasia in hedgehogs is quite frequent, with a reported prevalence of up to 51.5%, and the skin is the most commonly affected organ.[113] Mammary gland adenocarcinoma is the most prevalent neoplasm in hedgehogs overall, though mammary gland carcinoma and mammary papillary adenoma have also been reported. Studies have shown that up to 89% of hedgehog mammary neoplasms are malignant.[113] While histopathology is required for confirmation, cytology can be useful for preliminary evaluation. Previous reports have described multiple cytologic criteria of malignancy, including large epithelial cells with a high nuclear to cytoplasmic ratio (N:C), prominent nucleoli, oval to oblong to bizarrely shaped nuclei, and anisokaryosis.[112,121] Early ovariohysterectomy might be preventive, but further studies are needed. Mammary neoplasms can coexist with concurrent, unrelated tumors, and up to 10% of hedgehogs have more than one tumor type.[113] Hedgehogs can also develop epithelial tumors of the skin, such as sebaceous carcinoma and SCC. Superficial scrapings and tape preparations from cutaneous SCC can be unremarkable; however, deeper FNA can be characterized by the typical features of a keratinizing epithelial malignancy with inflammation (Figure 56.3).[122]

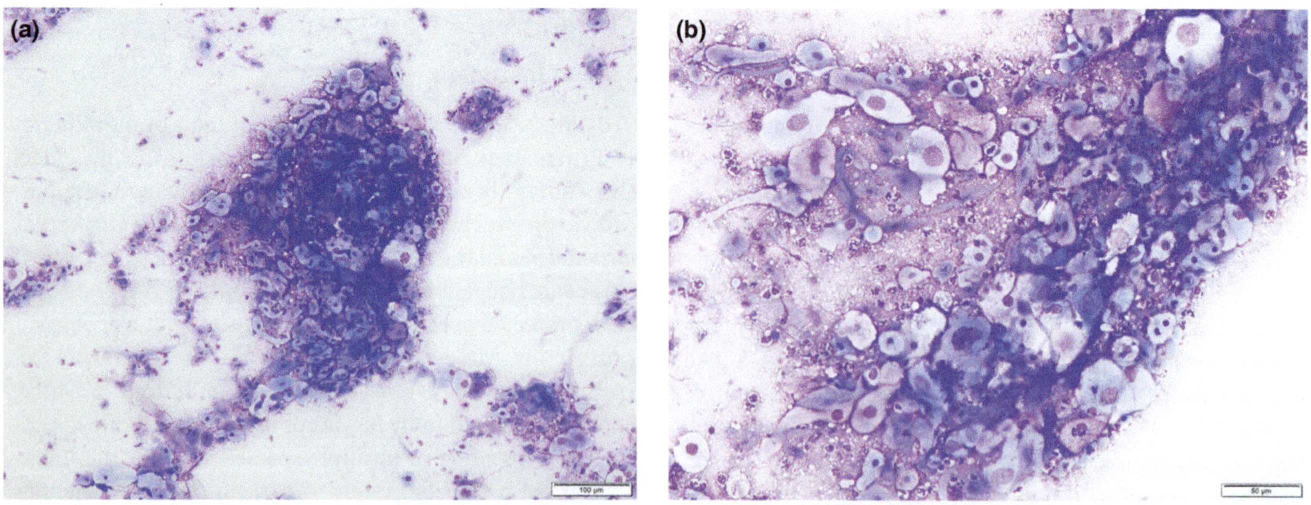

Figure 56.3 (a and b) SCC in a hedgehog. Pictured are variably sized sheets and scattered individualized squamous epithelial cells exhibiting varying maturity and keratinization. Shapes range from round to oval to polygonal. Features of malignancy include retained immature nuclei, variable N:C, anisocytosis, anisokaryosis, and karyomegaly. Neutrophils are scattered among the neoplastic cells, a common finding in SCC (Wright-Giemsa, (a) 100×, (b) 200×. *Source:* Images courtesy of Eric Fish).

Other reported skin tumors in hedgehogs include round cell tumors, such as MCT and plasma cell tumor. MCTs have a similar cytologic appearance to that described in domestic companion animals. In hedgehogs, MCTs have exhibited both benign and malignant biologic behavior, and excision with histopathology is recommended.[113,123,124] Epitheliotrophic T-cell lymphoma has been described in hedgehogs.[125,126] In both cases, animals are presented with signs compatible with dermatitis. In one case, histopathology of a focal lesion that remained after resolution of a secondary pyoderma was diagnostic for lymphoma. In another, FNA of focal skin lesions and histopathology were diagnostic for lymphoma. The cytology consisted of variably sized lymphocytes, mitotic figures, and cytoplasmic fragments.[125]

Mesenchymal tumors of the skin and subcutis include fibrosarcoma, peripheral nerve sheath tumors, myxosarcoma, hemangiosarcoma, extraskeletal osteosarcoma, histiocytic sarcoma, and undifferentiated sarcomas.[113,122,127] Lipomas are also possible.[113] Cytology of these lesions is similar to that described in other species, although an extraskeletal osteosarcoma of the dorsum was cytologically characterized by anaplastic spindloid cells and the initial diagnosis was malignant soft tissue sarcoma.[128] This animal died several months after tumor excision, and necropsy revealed metastatic disease of the lungs, liver, and spleen. Cytology of a peripheral nerve sheath tumor consisted of characteristic moderately atypical spindloid to polygonal mesenchymal cells; however, the smears also contained a moderate number of eosinophils and well-granulated mast cells, so a differential diagnosis of MCT with fibroplasia was also considered.[129]

Fluid Analysis

Diagnostic body cavity fluid analysis is not well described in hedgehogs. Cardiomyopathy is relatively common in this species with a reported incidence of up to 38% and can be associated with pleural effusion and/or ascites.[130] Anecdotally, most of these effusions are modified transudates with low cellularity, predominantly consisting of large mononuclear cells, neutrophils, lymphocytes, plasma cells, and erythrocytes.[112] Large mononuclear cells can contain debris or hemosiderin.[112]

Other Systems

Lymphoid

Lymphoid neoplasia is the second most commonly reported neoplasm of hedgehogs. Lymphoma can also manifest in the gastrointestinal tract or as multicentric lymphoma. Neoplastic cells can be present in the circulation.[113] A retroviral association has been proposed, as two reported cases showed retroviral-like particles on the surface of neoplastic cells via electron microscopy.[131] There is one report of lymphoma with Mott cell differentiation. In this case, cytology of a mesenteric mass revealed large, round cells with a high N:C, deeply basophilic cytoplasm, a peripherally located nucleus, an occasional perinuclear clear zone, and clear granules.[132]

Other Solid Tissues

Nonneoplastic Conditions

There are several non-cutaneous, nonneoplastic conditions of hedgehogs that are amenable to cytologic diagnosis. These include oral and intra-abdominal abscesses, osteomyelitis, suppurative and pyogranulomatous pneumonia, mycobacterial infection, hepatic lipidosis, and splenic extramedullary hematopoiesis. Cytologic appearances are generally like that described in other species.[112]

Hedgehogs can be predisposed to bacterial infection of the oral cavity that can originate from periodontal disease.[112] These can present similarly to oral SCC. Cytologically, these lesions consist of inflammatory cells (neutrophils, foamy macrophages, multinucleated giant cells, plasma cells, and eosinophils), osteoblasts and osteoclasts, and bacteria.[112,133] *Actinomyces naeslundii* infection has been reported to cause mandibular osteomyelitis and cellulitis.[133]

Neoplasia

The third most common neoplasm of companion hedgehogs is oral SCC. These often have a similar cytologic appearance to other species; however, some authors report that nuclear atypia may be very mild and histopathology is generally recommended.[113] These tumors are typically locally invasive, though there are some reports of distant metastasis. Other reported oral lesions include acanthomatous ameloblastoma (formerly acanthomatous epulis) and invasive fibrosarcoma.[134] Other tumors of the hedgehog digestive tract in general include colonic plasmacytoma, gastrointestinal adenocarcinoma, pancreatic exocrine carcinoma, and intestinal neuroendocrine tumor, but these are less common than oral SCC and gastrointestinal lymphoma.[134]

Neoplasms of the endocrine system in hedgehogs include several reports of adrenocortical carcinomas. Pheochromocytomas have rarely been reported.[134] Thyroid neoplasms are seen occasionally and have a neuroendocrine cytologic appearance, similar to other mammals. Reported thyroid neoplasms include follicular adenoma, follicular adenocarcinoma, and C-cell carcinoma.[135] A parathyroid adenoma has also been reported as an incidental finding in a hedgehog with numerous other disease processes, including thyroid follicular adenoma and multicentric skeletal sarcomas.[134] There are also case reports of pituitary adenoma and pancreatic islet cell tumor.[136]

Several reproductive neoplasms have been reported in female hedgehogs, including granulosa cell tumor and teratoma.[121,136] There is also one report of a Sertoli cell tumor in an undescended testicle of a male hedgehog.[133] Other reported tumors include uterine leiomyosarcoma, uterine adenocarcinoma, fibroadenomatous polyp, adenosarcoma, and endometrial stromal sarcoma.[137,138] Again, cytologic appearances are expected to be similar to other domestic species.

Less commonly reported tumors include ocular lesions, such as Meibomian cysts, intraocular hemangioma, acinic cell carcinoma, and lacrimal gland carcinoma.[133] Osteosarcoma, hepatocellular carcinoma, splenic hemangiosarcoma, and transitional cell carcinoma round out reported tumors in hedgehogs.[136,137]

Rodents

General Information

Rodents are the largest order of mammals, with approximately 1500 living rodent species and are native to all continents apart from Antarctica. Many small mammals kept as pets fall into this group, including mice, rats, hamsters, gerbils, chinchillas, and guinea pigs.

Guinea Pigs

Skin and Subcutis

Nonneoplastic Conditions

Cytology has been used to identify ectoparasites of guinea pigs, including the fur mite (*Chirodiscoides caviae*), a species-specific infestation that can be clinical or subclinical.[139] Mites of different developmental stages and eggs can be identified attached to the hair shafts. Both sarcoptic (*Trixacarus caviae*) and demodectic (*Demodex caviae*) mange occur; coinfections are reported, and predisposing factors include chronic disease and poor husbandry.[140,141] Cytologic characteristics are similar to other species (Chapter 11). Dermatophytosis also occurs in guinea pigs, which have been used as animal models for the human disease; however, fungal elements can be difficult to identify (see Chapter 11).[142–144] Pododermatitis (bumblefoot) and abscesses are also relatively common dermatologic conditions that are conducive to cytologic diagnosis, although specific reports describing cytology in guinea pigs are lacking.[144] Anecdotal reports describe the cytology of pododermatitis as pyogranulomatous inflammation often accompanied by bacterial cocci such as *Staphylococcus aureus* and abscesses as composed of suppurative inflammation with mixed bacterial organisms.[143]

Neoplasia

Trichoepitheliomas, trichofolliculomas, and follicular cysts are frequently cited as among the most frequent neoplastic lesions of the guinea pig skin.[1–3,144] Biologic behavior and cytology are similar to other species, with smears characterized by sebum, keratin, basal or sebaceous epithelial cells, and inflammatory cells.[1,2] Lipomas are common as well.[1–3,144] Proliferative mammary gland lesions can occur in both sexes and include cysts, adenomas, cystadenomas, and adenocarcinoma, while lipomas, mastitis, and abscesses are other considerations.[1] Sources vary on the prevalence of benign versus malignant mammary lesions. Many consider them approximately equal or predominantly malignant, and histopathology is recommended for definitive classification.[115] Specific cytologic findings are rarely published.[145] Early ovariohysterectomy is considered preventive.[2]

Melanoma and cutaneous lymphoma have been reported in guinea pigs, although specific cytologic findings are not described.[3,144,146] Soft tissue sarcomas and liposarcomas can occur, and cytology of a subcutaneous fibrosarcoma in a 9-year-old guinea pig consisted of spindloid cells with occasional multinucleated cells.[147] Other sarcomas have been sporadically reported in survey papers, presumably with similar cytologic features as in other species (Chapter 16).[3,144]

Fluid Analysis

The use of diagnostic body cavity fluid analysis does not appear to be well described in companion guinea pigs.

Other Systems

Lymphoid

Cervical lymphadenitis associated with streptococcal infections is infectious in young cavies and in older animals is more often caused by oral trauma or foreign bodies.[1,143,148] Cytologically, these lesions essentially present as abscesses, although anecdotally, bacteria may be difficult to locate.[1,143] Lymphoma is one of the more common malignancies in guinea pigs, often presenting in a multicentric form characterized by large immature lymphoid cells.[1,2,149] Lymph node involvement has also been associated with leukemic manifestations, T-cell epitheliotropic lymphoma, and ocular involvement.[146,149,150]

Other Solid Tissues

Cavies experience infectious keratoconjunctivitis caused by bacteria such as *Streptococcus* spp., *Staphylococcus* spp., and *Chlamydia* spp. with a similar cytologic appearance to other species (see Figure 20.5a for an image of *Chlamydia*).[151]

Other nonneoplastic lesions in cavies that are amenable to cytologic diagnosis include hepatic lipidosis due to similar causes as in other species including a metabolic manifestation of pregnancy toxemia.[2] Ovarian cysts are also common. Neoplastic reproductive conditions in pet guinea pigs have recently been characterized, but unfortunately, cytologic information is lacking.[152] Lesions of the uterine cervix were generally benign, with polyps and hyperplasia predominating. Uterine lining lesions also consisted of polyps and hyperplasia, with a larger number of adenomas and few adenocarcinomas.[152] Leiomyomas of the uterus outnumbered leiomyosarcomas 2 : 1 (Figure 60.21 for cytology image of leiomyoma in a primate). Ovarian teratomas are described.[1,2]

Benign and malignant thyroid tumors are reported in guinea pigs, with benign lesions predominating, and osseous metaplasia occasionally is reported.[1,2,153] As in other species, malignant tumors can be well differentiated, which poses a diagnostic dilemma for cytology. Cytology can be used to distinguish thyroid lesions from other differential diagnoses such as cervical lymphadenitis, lymphoma, and mucocoeles and has been reported to be diagnostic for thyroid adenocarcinoma; however, details were not described.[154]

Insulinomas are reported.[2] Transitional cell carcinomas are described, with anecdotal evidence suggesting similar cytologic features to those in canine tumors (see Chapters 38 and 39).[1]

Rats

Although much of the medical literature on rats (*Rattus norvegicus*) is from laboratory animal populations, these animals are engaging pets, and veterinary care for companion rats is in demand.

Skin and Subcutis

Nonneoplastic Conditions

Like other small mammals, rats are susceptible to a range of ectoparasites. Fur mites (*Radfordia ensifera*) can be identified microscopically on superficial skin scrapes or flea combed hairs; *Demodex* spp. can also occur but is more common in laboratory settings (Chapter 11).[143] Subcutaneous abscesses occur like those described in guinea pigs; *Cuterebra* is an uncommon differential diagnosis.[143] FNA of abscesses should be characterized by suppurative inflammation and possibly bacteria.[1] Dermatophytosis is caused by *T. mentagrophytes* and *Microsporum* spp., although the former is more common and rats are usually asymptomatic[143] (see Chapter 11 for cytologic details).

Neoplasia

Rats are frequently affected by mammary neoplasia, and most are benign mammary fibroadenomas; however, newer reports suggest the percentage may be lower than previously suggested.[1,2,143,154] Tumors are single or multiple and can occur in unexpected locations such as the base of the tail, around the neck, or over the back.[1,2,143,144] They occur in both sexes, can grow rapidly, and frequently ulcerate when large. Anecdotal cytologic description includes poorly cellular samples containing occasional fibroblasts and clusters of well-differentiated glandular epithelial cells; inflammation can be present with ulceration of the mass.[2,3] Early ovariectomy can be preventive.[2]

A specific epithelial tumor reported in rats is the Zymbal gland tumor, arising within sebaceous glands associated with the external ear canal, sometimes induced chemically and occasionally arising as a spontaneous lesion (Figure 56.4).[1,3,145,155] Tumors present as firm, subcutaneous masses ventral to the ear and are often histologically characterized as invasive carcinomas with variable glandular and squamous differentiation, but they appear to be slow to metastasize.[1,2] Cytology of a chemically induced Zymbal gland adenoma was described as consisting of abundant keratin and clusters of minimally atypical basaloid cells with round nuclei and smooth chromatin.[156] One case report documents otitis externa associated with a Zymbal gland adenocarcinoma.[155]

Mesenchymal tumors of pet rats include lipomas and variations of soft tissue sarcoma.[1] Histiocytic sarcoma is considered relatively common in rodents.[1,157] Aspiration of a solitary foot mass on a Sprague–Dawley rat histologically diagnosed as a cutaneous histiocytic sarcoma revealed a mononuclear cell population characterized by moderate amounts of vacuolated basophilic cytoplasm.[157] Nuclei were fairly homogeneous with the exception of occasional cells that exhibited anisokaryosis or multiple variably sized nuclei.

Fluid Analysis

There are few reports of diagnostic fluid analysis in pet rats, and more detail in a laboratory setting is included in Chapter 66. A case report did describe a classic chylous effusion in two rats with dilated cardiomyopathy (see Chapters 50 and 52).[158] Anecdotally, cytology can be performed to investigate thoracic effusions.[1]

Other Systems

The cytology of other solid tissues in pet rats is not well described. Lymphoma occurs in rats, as do reproductive neoplasms, vaginitis, and pyometra, all of which should have cytologic characteristics like those in other species. A spontaneous ameloblastic carcinoma was described in a pet rat, but cytology was not performed.[159]

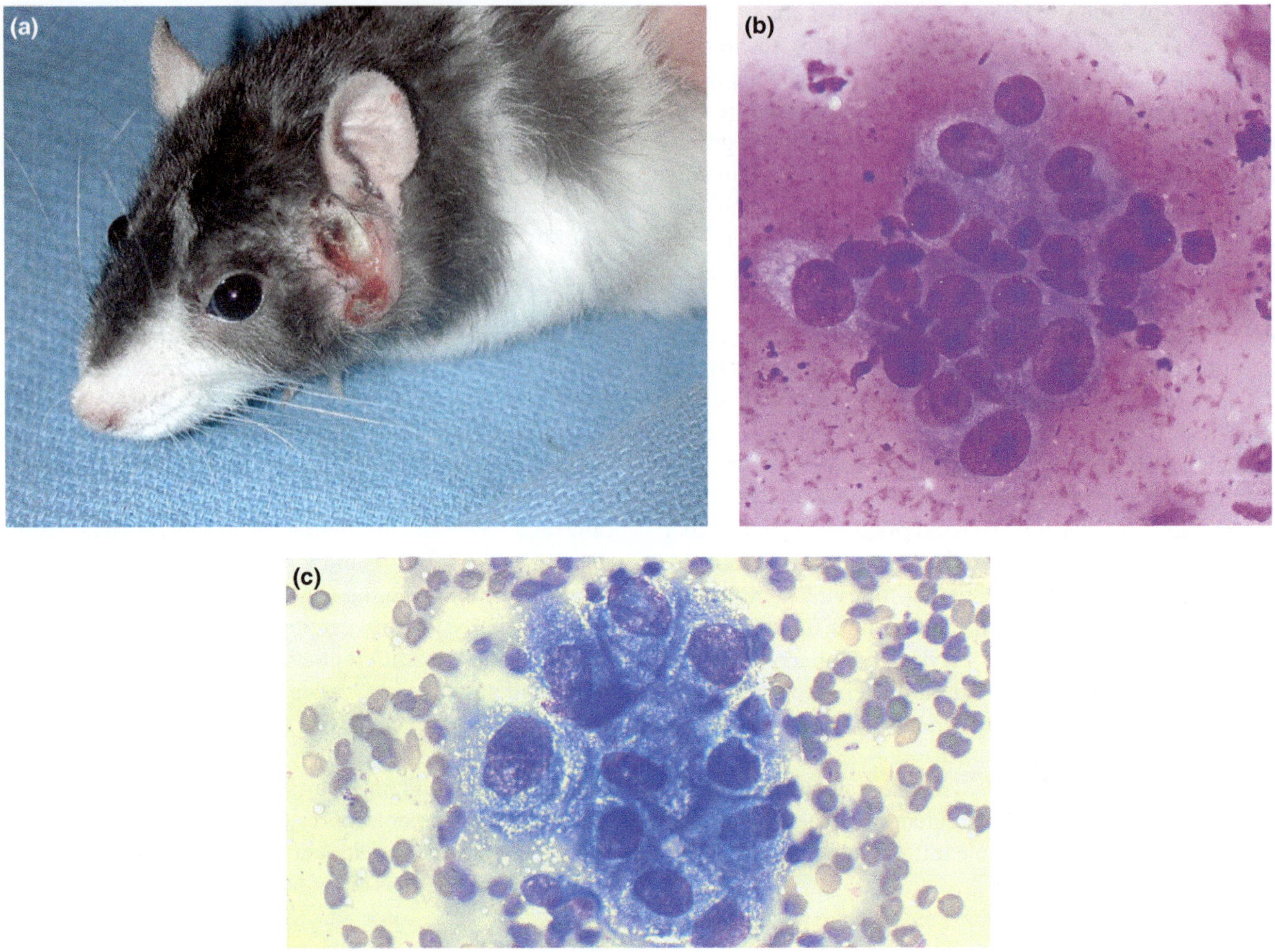

Figure 56.4 (a) Adult rat with nonhealing wound diagnosed as a Zymbal gland tumor. (b and c) Cytology of a Zymbal's gland adenocarcinoma in a rat. Zymbal's gland tumors arise from acinar structures or ductal epithelium and are categorized as adenomas or adenocarcinomas. Here, clusters of neoplastic epithelial cells exhibit round to oval nuclei, one to three prominent nucleoli, coarse chromatin, and a moderate amount of finely vacuolated, basophilic cytoplasm. Features of malignancy include anisocytosis, anisokaryosis, anisonucleoliosis, multinucleation, and high N:C. A marked inflammatory response with fibroplasia and necrosis can be seen in cytology from traumatized or ulcerated tumors (not pictured). Zymbal's gland adenocarcinomas are typically locally invasive with a poor prognosis ((b) Diff Quik, 500×; (c) modified Wright's, 600×. *Source:* Images (b) and (c) courtesy of John Rand).

A relatively unique lesion in rats is the *Taenia taeniaeformis*-induced hepatic neoplasia.[160] Rodents are intermediate hosts for this cestode parasite of cats, although these tumors are relatively unique to rats. Because the larvae localize to the liver, most of the tumors induced by the parasites are locally aggressive hepatic sarcomas that tend to metastasize. The tumor is hypothesized to originate from a host capsule surrounding the larvae. Cytology obtained at necropsy in an affected rat was highly cellular with aggregated and individualized polygonal to plump spindloid cells with finely granular blue cytoplasm, perinuclear clear zones, and oval to indented nuclei with single to multiple prominent nucleoli.[160]

Hamsters and Gerbils

There are five types of hamsters commonly described in the literature including the golden or Syrian hamster (*Mesocricetus auratus*), the Russian or Djungarian hamster (*Phodopus sungorus*), the Roborovski hamster (*Phodopus roborovskii*), Campbell's dwarf hamster (*Phodopus campbelli*), the Chinese hamster (*Cricetulus griseus*), and a single gerbil species, the Mongolian gerbil (*Meriones unguiculatus*). Species can vary in the relative frequency of different conditions, although much of the cytology literature is anecdotal describing single cases of mostly neoplastic lesions.[2] Syrian hamsters have been used extensively in research, generating some literature on spontaneous tumors.[161] Reports suggest that the incidence of neoplasia in Syrian hamsters is lower than Djungarian hamsters with a predominance of hematopoietic tumors such as plasma cell tumors and lymphoma, while Djungarian hamsters have higher rates of neoplasia, most of the skin and subcutis.[161,162]

Skin and Subcutis

Although infrequently reported in the primary literature, cytology can be used to evaluate nonneoplastic cutaneous lesions. The tropical rat mite has been described to infect Syrian hamsters and can be identified cytologically.[163] A young Roborovski hamster presented for multiple firm, subcutaneous masses in all 4 feet. Cytologic examination consisted of mixed macrophages with intracellular cocci and degenerate neutrophils.[164] Histology revealed bacterial pseudomycetoma and bacterial culture identified coagulase positive *Staphylococcus intermedius*. Similar lesions also are reported in Djungarian and dwarf hamsters.[165,166]

The literature describing neoplastic conditions is slightly more robust. One source describes papillomas, SCCs, and atypical fibromas as being among the most common skin tumors in Djungarian hamsters, and MCTs can also occur.[2] Hamster polyomavirus in Syrian hamsters can induce not only papilloma lesions in adult hamsters but also lymphoma under other circumstances (see *Other Systems* below).[167] Syrian hamsters can develop melanomas of their flank organs; these are microscopically similar to tumors in other species.[2] Cutaneous lymphoma has also been described in Syrian hamsters.[168] Case reports of soft tissue sarcomas in hamsters reveal standard cytologic features of these tumors in other species (Chapter 16).[169,170] A report of a subcutaneous extracellular osteosarcoma in a Chinese hamster expressed typical cytologic findings of osteosarcoma, including variably anaplastic, oval to spindloid cells with osteoclasts, and material consistent with osteoid.[171] A study of mammary neoplasia in Djungarian hamsters revealed a slight predominance of adenocarcinomas over adenomas, with a significant number of carcinosarcomas as an unexpected finding; however, cytology was not performed.[161] Anecdotally, cytology and histopathology of hamster mammary tumors appear to have questionable correlation, and biopsy is usually recommended.[2] Cytology of a poorly differentiated non-sebaceous carcinoma of the skin in a Mongolian gerbil was characterized by clusters of moderately to markedly anaplastic epithelial cells characterized by polygonal cells with sparse vacuolated basophilic cytoplasm and ovoid nuclei.[172]

Other Systems

In addition to the epitheliotropic form of lymphoma mentioned above, adult hamsters are susceptible to multicentric lymphoma involving peripheral lymph nodes and visceral organs.[2] Hamster polyomavirus can induce visceral lymphoma in younger hamsters, typically in research colonies, although it has been reported in a pet Syrian hamster.[167] A typical spectrum of reproductive and endocrine tumors has been described in hamsters, but cytology has not been reported.[1,2] An ameloblastoma was histologically diagnosed in a young Syrian hamster, but cytology was not reported.[159]

Conclusions

Cytologic diagnosis of neoplastic cutaneous disease in small mammal species dominates the literature, and in many cases diagnostic features extrapolate from other more common domestic species. Cytologic diagnosis appears to be underutilized in small mammals, and a more robust medical literature in this area would expand diagnostic applications.

References

1 Garner, M.M. (2007). Cytologic diagnosis of diseases of rabbits, guinea pigs, and rodents. *Vet Clin North Am Exot Anim Pract* 10: 25–49.

2 Hocker, S.E., Eshar, D., and Wouda, R.M. (2017). Rodent oncology: diseases, diagnostics, and therapeutics. *Vet Clin North Am Exot Anim Pract* 20: 111–134.

3 Kanfer, S. and Reavill, D.R. (2013). Cutaneous neoplasia in ferrets, rabbits, and guinea pigs. *Vet Clin North Am Exot Anim Pract* 16: 579–598.

4 Divers, S.J. (2010). Exotic mammal diagnostic endoscopy and endosurgery. *Vet Clin North Am Exot Anim Pract* 13: 255–272.

5 Fisher, P. (2015). Using cytology in making exotic companion mammal diagnoses. *Proceedings of the Pacific Veterinary Conference* (June 17-21, Long Beach, CA). https://www.vin.com/doc/?id=6789836.

6 Rakich, P.M. and Latimer, K.S. (2007). Cytologic diagnosis of diseases of ferrets. *Vet Clin North Am Exot Anim Pract* 10: 61–78.

7 D'Ovidio, D., Rossi, G., Melidone, R. et al. (2012). Subcutaneous liposarcoma in a ferret (*Mustela putorius furo*). *J Exot Pet Med* 21: 238–242.

8 Ivey, E. and Morrissey, J. (1999). Ferrets: examination and preventative medicine. *Vet Clin North Am Exot Anim Pract* 2: 471–494.

9 Protain, H.J., Kutzler, M.A., and Valentine, B.A. (2009). Assessment of cytologic evaluation of preputial epithelial cells as a diagnostic test for detection of adrenocortical disease in castrated ferrets. *Am J Vet Res* 70: 619–623.

10 Bakthavatchalu, V., Muthupalani, S., Marini, R.P., and Fox, J.G. (2016). Endocrinopathy and aging in ferrets. *Vet Pathol* 53: 349–365.

11 Kelleher, S.A. (2001). Skin diseases of ferrets. *Vet Clin North Am Exot Anim Pract* 4: 565–572.

12 Mancinelli, E., Meredith, A.L., and Stidworthy, M.F. (2014). Systemic infection due to Candida parapsilosis in a domestic ferret (*Mustela putorius furo*). *J Exot Pet Med* 23: 85–90.

13 Zehnder, A.M., Hawkins, M.G., Koski, M.A. et al. (2008). An unusual presentation of canine distemper virus infection in a domestic ferret (*Mustela putorius furo*). *Vet Dermatol* 19 (4): 232–238.

14 Orcutt, C. (1997). Dermatologic diseases. In: *Ferrets, Rabbits, and Rodents: Clinical Medicine and Surgery*, (ed. Elizabeth V. Hillyer, Katherine E. Quesenberry), 115–125. Philadelphia, PA: W.B. Saunders.

15 Fox, J.G. (1998). Bacterial and mycoplasmal diseases. In: *Biology and Diseases of the Ferret*, (ed. James G. Fox), 2e, 321–354. Baltimore: Williams & Wilkins.

16 Fox, J.G. (1998). Mycotic diseases. In: *Biology and Diseases of the Ferret*, (ed. James G. Fox), 2e, 248–254. Baltimore: Williams & Wilkins.

17 Rosenthal, K. (1994). Ferrets. *Vet Clin North Am Small Anim Pract* 24: 1–23.

18 Chitty, J. and Hendricks, A. (2007). Zoonotic skin disease in small animals. *Comp Anim Pract* 29: 92–97.

19 D'Ovidio, D. and Santoro, D. (2015). Survey of zoonotic dermatoses in client-owned exotic pet mammals in southern Italy. *Zoonoses Public Health* 62: 100–104.

20 Greenacre, C.B. (2003). Fungal diseases of ferrets. *Vet Clin North Am Exot Anim Pract* 6: 435–448.

21 Hagen, K.W. and Gorham, J.R. (1972). Dermatomycoses in fur animals: chinchilla, ferret, mink and rabbit. *Vet Med Small Anim Clin* 67: 43–48.

22 Pignon, C. and Mayer, J. (2011). Zoonoses of ferrets, hedgehogs, and sugar gliders. *Vet Clin North Am Exot Anim Pract* 14: 533–549.

23 Schoemaker, N.J. (1999). Selected dermatologic conditions in exotic pets. *Exot DVM* 1: 5–11.

24 Zewe, C.M., Graham, J., Lam, A.T.H., and Ferrer, L. (2017). Demodicosis in a ferret caused by Demodex canis. *Vet Dermatol* 28: 528–529.

25 Lenhard, A. (1985). Blastomycosis in a ferret. *J Am Vet Med Assoc* 186: 70–72.

26 Levine, N.D., Dunlap, G.I., and Graham, R. (1938). An intracellular parasite encountered in ferret. *Cornell Vet* 28: 249–251.

27 Skulski, G. and Symmers, W.S.T.C. (1954). Actinomycosis and torulosis in the ferret (*Mustela furo* L). *J Comp Pathol* 64: 306–311.

28 Dixon, R.J. (1984). Systemic candidosis in a fitch. *N Z Vet J* 32: 132–133.

29 Eshar, D., Mayer, J., Parry, N.M. et al. (2010). Disseminated, histologically confirmed *Cryptococcus* spp in a domestic ferret. *J Am Vet Med Assoc* 236: 770–774.

30 Greenlee, P.G. and Stephens, E. (1984). Meningeal Cryptococcosis and congestive cardiomyopathy in a ferret. *J Am Vet Med Assoc* 184: 840–841.

31 Hanley, C.S., MacWilliams, P., Giles, S., and Paré, J. (2006). Diagnosis and successful treatment of *Cryptococcus neoformans* variety *grubii* in a domestic ferret. *Can Vet J* 47: 1015–1017.

32 Malik, R., Martin, P., McGill, J. et al. (2000). Successful treatment of invasive nasal Cryptococcosis in a ferret. *Aust Vet J* 78: 158–159.

33 McGill, S., Malik, R., Saul, N. et al. (2009). Cryptococcosis in domestic animals in Western Australia: a retrospective study from 1995–2006. *Med Mycol* 47: 625–639.

34 Morera, N., Juan-Salles, C., Torres, J.M. et al. (2011). *Cryptococcus gattii* infection in a Spanish pet ferret (*Mustela putorius furo*) and asymptomatic carriage in ferrets and humans from its environment. *Med Mycol* 49: 779–784.

35 Fox, J.G. (1998). Mycotic diseases. In: *Biology and Diseases of the Ferret*, 2e, 393–403. Baltimore: Williams & Wilkins.

36 Guillot, J., Gueho, E., Chevrier, G., and Chermette, R. (1997). Epidemiological analysis of *Malassezia pachydermatis* isolates by partial sequencing of the large subunit ribosomal RNA. (ed. James G. Fox), *Res Vet Sci* 62: 22–25.

37 Hiruma, M. and Kume, T. (1984). Mucormycotic meningoencephalitis in a ferret (case report). *Kitasato Arch Exp Med* 57: 67–73.

38 Purcell, K. (1999). Diagnosis and disease. In: *Ferrets: A Guide for Practitioners*, 83–148. Lakewood: AAHA Press.

39 Stokes, D.C., Gigliotti, F., Rehg, J.E. et al. (1987). Experimental *Pneumocystis carinii* pneumonia in the ferret. (ed. Karen Purcell, Susan A. Brown), *Br J Exp Pathol* 68: 267–276.

40 Foil, C.S. (1998). Miscellaneous fungal infections. In: *Infectious Diseases of the Dog and Cat*, 2e, 420–430. Philadelphia, PA: W.B. Saunders.

41 Lloyd, M. (1999). Dermatologic diseases. In: *Ferrets: Health, Husbandry and Diseases*, (ed. Greene, C.E.), 78–87. London: Blackwell Science.

42 Antinoff, N. and Williams, B.H. (2012). Neoplasia. In: *Ferrets, Rabbits, and Rodents: Clinical Medicine and Surgery*, 3e, 103–121. St. Louis, MO: Elsevier.

43 Avallone, G., Forlani, A., Tecilla, M. et al. (2016). Neoplastic diseases in the domestic ferret (Mustela

putorius furo) in Italy: classification and tissue distribution of 865 cases, (ed. Katherine E. Quesenberry, James W. Carpenter), (2000–2010). *BMC Vet Res* 12 (275): 1–8.
44 Fox, J.G., Dangler, C.A., Snyder, S.B. et al. (2000). C-cell carcinoma (medullary thyroid carcinoma) associated with multiple endocrine neoplasms in a ferret (*Mustela putorius furo*). *Vet Pathol* 37: 278–282.
45 Fox, J.G., Muthupalani, S., Kiupel, M., and Williams, B. (2014). Neoplastic diseases. In: *Biology and Diseases of the Ferret*, 3e, 587–626. Ames, IA: Wiley-Blackwell.
46 Brown, S.A. (1997). Neoplasia. In: *Ferrets, Rabbits, and Rodents: Clinical Medicine and Surgery*, (ed. James G. Fox, Robert P. Marini), 99–114. Philadelphia, PA: W.B. Saunders.
47 Schoemaker, N.G. (2017). Ferret oncology: diseases, diagnostics, and therapeutics, (ed. Elizabeth V. Hillyer, Katherine E. Quesenberry), *Vet Clin North Am Exot Anim Pract* 20: 183–208.
48 Li, X. and Fox, J.G. (1998). Neoplastic diseases. In: *Biology and Diseases of the Ferret*, 2e, 405–447. Baltimore: Williams & Wilkins.
49 Maguire, R., Reavill, D.R., Maguire, P., and Jenkins, J.R. (2014). Chondrosarcoma associated with the appendicular skeleton of 2 domestic ferrets, (ed. James G. Fox) *J Exot Pet Med* 23: 165–171.
50 Parker, G.A. and Picut, C.A. (1993). Histopathologic features and post-surgical sequelae of 57 cutaneous neoplasms in ferrets (*Mustela putorius furo* L). *Vet Pathol* 30: 449–504.
51 Stauber, E., Robinette, J., Basaraba, R. et al. (1990). Mast cell tumors in three ferrets. *J Am Vet Med Assoc* 196: 766–767.
52 Vilalta, L., Melendez-Lazo, A., Doria, G. et al. (2016). Clinical, cytological, histological and immunohistochemical features of cutaneous mast cell tumours in ferrets (*Mustela putorius furo*). *J Comp Pathol* 155: 346–355.
53 Erdman, S.E., Brown, S.A., Kawasaki, T.A. et al. (1996). Clinical and pathologic findings in ferrets with lymphoma: 60 cases (1982–1994). *J Am Vet Med Assoc* 208: 1285–1289.
54 Li, X., Fox, J.G., Erdman, S.E., and Aspros, D.G. (1995). Cutaneous lymphoma in a ferret (*Mustela putorius furo*). *Vet Pathol* 32: 55–56.
55 Rosenbaum, M.R., Affolter, V.K., Usborne, A.L., and Beeber, N.L. (1996). Cutaneous epitheliotrophic lymphoma in a ferret. *J Am Vet Med Assoc* 209: 1441–1444.
56 Dillberger, J.E. and Altman, N.H. (1989). Neoplasia in ferrets: eleven cases with a review. *J Comp Pathol* 100: 161–176.
57 Li, X., Fox, J.G., and Padrid, P.A. (1998). Neoplastic diseases in ferrets: 574 cases (1968–1997). *J Am Vet Med Assoc* 212: 1402–1406.
58 Nakata, M., Miwa, Y., Nakayama, H. et al. (2008). Localized radiotherapy for a ferret with possible anal sac apocrine adenocarcinoma. *J Small Anim Pract* 49: 476–478.
59 Pinches, M.D.G., Liebenberg, G., and Stidworthy, M.F. (2008). What is your diagnosis? Preputial mass in a ferret. *Vet Clin Pathol* 37: 443–446.
60 Vilalta, L., Meléndez-Lazo, A., Canturri, A. et al. (2017). Anal sac adenocarcinoma with metastases and hypercalcemia in a ferret (*Mustela putorius furo*). *J Exot Pet Med* 26: 143–149.
61 Muller, S., Puff, C., Thole, M. et al. (2015). Squamous cell carcinoma of the anal sac in a ferret: a case report. *Kleintierpraxis* 60: 646–651.
62 Olsen, G.H., Turk, M.A., and Foil, C.S. (1985). Disseminated cutaneous squamous cell carcinoma in a ferret. *J Am Vet Med Assoc* 186: 702–703.
63 Quesenberry, K. and Carpenter, J.W. (2012). *Ferrets, Rabbits and Rodents: Clinical Medicine and Surgery*, 3e, 86–91. St. Louis, MO: Elsevier.
64 Brunner, S.R., Herron, A.J., and Altman, N.H. (1990). Leiomyosarcoma in a domestic ferret: morphologic and immunocytochemical diagnosis. *Lab Anim Sci* 40: 208–210.
65 Mikaelian, I. and Garner, M.M. (2002). Solitary dermal leiomyosarcomas in 12 ferrets. *J Vet Diagn Invest* 14: 262–265.
66 Mialot, M., Prata, D., Girard-Luc, A. et al. (2010). Multiple progressive piloleiomyomas in a ferret (*Mustela putorius furo*): a case report. *Vet Dermatol* 22: 100–103.
67 Rickman, B.H., Craig, L.E., and Goldschmidt, M.H. (2001). Piloleiomyosarcoma. *Vet Pathol* 38: 710–711.
68 Gardhouse, S., Eshar, D., Fromstein, J., and Smith, D.A. (2013). Diagnosis and successful surgical treatment of an unusual inguinal liposarcoma in a pet ferret (*Mustela putorius furo*). *Can Vet J* 54: 739–742.
69 Munday, J.S., Stedman, N.L., and Richey, L.J. (2003). Histology and immunohistochemistry of seven ferret vaccination-site fibrosarcomas. *Vet Pathol* 40: 288–293.
70 Murray, J. (1998). Vaccine injection-site sarcoma in a ferret. *J Am Vet Med Assoc* 213: 955.
71 Moreland, A.F., Battles, A.H., and Nease, J.H. (1986). Dirofilariasis in a ferret. *J Am Vet Med Assoc* 188: 864.
72 Parrott, T.Y., Greiner, E.C., and Parrott, J.D. (1984). *Dirofilaria immitis* infection in three ferrets. *J Am Vet Med Assoc* 184: 582–583.
73 Clagett, D.O., Johnston, M.S., and Han, S. (2017). Malignant plasma cell neoplasia in ferrets: a review of 6 cases. *J Exot Pet Med* 26: 36–46.
74 Paul-Murphy, J., O'Brien, R.T., Spaeth, A. et al. (1999). Ultrasonography and fine needle aspirate cytology of the mesenteric lymph node in normal domestic ferrets

(*Mustela putorius furo*). *Vet Radiol Ultrasound* 40: 308–309.

75 Ammersbach, M., DeLay, J., Caswell, J.L. et al. (2008). Laboratory findings, histopathology, and immunophenotype of lymphoma in domestic ferrets. *Vet Pathol* 45: 663–673.

76 Sinclair, K.M., Eckstrand, C., Hawkins, M.G., and Moore, P.F. (2016). Epitheliotropic gastrointestinal T-cell lymphoma with concurrent insulinoma and adrenocortical carcinoma in a domestic ferret (*Mustela putorius furo*). *J Exot Pet Med* 25: 34–43.

77 Hillyer, E.V. (1997). Part II. Cardiovascular diseases. In: *Ferrets, Rabbits, and Rodents: Clinical Medicine and Surgery*, 72–73. Philadelphia, PA: W.B. Saunders.

78 Antinoff, N. (1998). Urinary disorders in ferrets. *Semin Avian Exot Pet Med*, (ed. Elizabeth V. Hillyer, Katherine E. Quesenberry),7: 89–92.

79 Miwa, Y., Uchida, K., Nakayama, H., and Asaki, N. (2010). Neuroblastoma of the adrenal gland in a ferret. *J Vet Med Sci* 72: 1229–1232.

80 Wills, T.B., Bohn, A.A., Finch, N.P. et al. (2005). Thyroid follicular adenocarcinoma in a ferret. *Vet Clin Pathol* 34: 405–408.

81 Perpiñán, D., Ramis, A., Tomás, A. et al. (2008). Outbreak of canine distemper in domestic ferrets (*Mustela putorious furo*). *Vet Rec* 163: 246–250.

82 Pollock, C. (2012). Mycobacterial infection in the ferret. *Vet Clin North Am Exot Anim Pract* 15: 121–129.

83 Chambers, J.K., Nakamori, T., Kishimoto, T.E. et al. (2016). Lachrymal gland basal cell adenocarcinoma in a ferret (*Mustela putorius furo*). *J Comp Pathol* 155: 259–262.

84 Fox-Alvarez, W.A., Moreno, A.R., and Bush, J. (2015). Diagnosis and successful surgical removal of an aural ceruminous gland adenocarcinoma in a domestic ferret (*Mustela putorius furo*). *J Exot Pet Med* 24: 350–355.

85 Hendrick, M.J. and Goldschmidt, M.G. (1987). Chondrosarcoma of the tail of ferrets (*Mustela putorius furo*). *Vet Pathol* 24: 272–273.

86 Ohta, G., Kobayshi, M., Yanai, T. et al. (2008). A case of fibrosarcoma on the perivertebral surface of a ferret with hind limb paralysis. *Exp Anim* 57: 397–400.

87 Warschau, M., Hoffmann, M., Dziallas, P. et al. (2017). Invasive histiocytic sarcoma of the lumbar spine in a ferret (*Mustela putorius furo*). *J Small Anim Pract* 58: 115–118.

88 Williams, B.H. and Weiss, C.A. (2004). Neoplasia. In: *Ferrets, Rabbits and Rodents Clinical Medicine and Surgery*, 2e, 91–106. Philadelphia, PA: W.B. Saunders.

89 Fuentealba, C. and Blue-McLendom, A. (1995). Liposarcoma arising from the mandibular bone marrow in a ferret. *Can Vet J* 36: 779–780.

90 Hanley, C.S., Geiger, T., and Frank, P. (2004). What is your diagnosis? Multilobular osteoma (MLO) in a ferret, (ed. Katherine E. Quesenberry, James W. Carpenter), *J Am Vet Med Assoc* 225: 1665–1666.

91 Camus, M.S., Rech, R.R., Choy, F.S. et al. (2009). Pathology in practice. *J Am Vet Med Assoc* 235: 949–951.

92 Roth, L. and Takata, I. (1992). Cytological diagnosis of chordoma of the tail in a ferret. *Vet Clin Pathol* 21: 119–121.

93 Williams, B.H., Eighmy, J.J., Berbert, M.H., and Dunn, D.G. (1993). Cervical chordoma in two ferrets (*Mustela putorius furo*). *Vet Pathol* 30: 204–206.

94 Frohlich, J.R. and Donovan, T.A. (2015). Cervical chordoma in a domestic ferret (*Mustela putorius furo*) with pulmonary metastasis. *J Vet Diagn Invest* 27: 656–659.

95 Munday, J.S., Brown, C.A., and Richey, L.J. (2004). Suspected metastatic coccygeal chordoma in a ferret (*Mustela putorius furo*). *J Vet Diagn Invest* 16: 454–458.

96 Foerster, S.H., Dykes, N., Flanders, J.A., and French, T.W. (2000). What is your diagnosis? Retropharyngeal soft tissue mass in a ferret. *J Am Vet Med Assoc* 216: 665–666.

97 Pye, G.W., Bennett, R.A., Roberts, G.D., and Terrell, S.P. (2000). Thoracic vertebral chordoma in a domestic ferret (*Mustela putorius furo*). *J Zoo Wildl Med* 31: 107–111.

98 Leong, A.S., Wick, M.R., and Swanson, P.E. (1997). The anaplastic round cell tumor. In: *Immunohistology and Electron Microscopy of Anaplastic and Pleomorphic Tumors*, 109–209. Cambridge: Cambridge University Press.

99 Dunn, D.G., Harris, R.K., Meis, J.M., and Sweet, D.E. (1991). A histomorphologic and immunohistochemical study of chordoma in twenty ferrets (*Mustela putorius furo*). *Vet Pathol* 28: 467–473.

100 Hanley, C.S., Wilson, G.H., Frank, P. et al. (2004). T cell lymphoma in the lumbar spine of a domestic ferret (*Mustela putorius furo*). *Vet Rec* 155: 329–332.

101 Rosenthal, K.L. (1997). Respiratory diseases. In: *Ferrets, Rabbits, and Rodents: Clinical Medicine and Surgery*, (ed. Elizabeth V. Hillyer, Katherine E. Quesenberry), vol. 81. Philadelphia, PA: W.B. Saunders.

102 Bauk, L.B. (1985). Salivary mucocele in 2 ferrets. *Mod Vet Pract* 66: 337–339.

103 Fehr, M., Thiele, A., Gerdwilder, A. et al. (2006). Salivary mucocele (Zygomatic gland) in a ferret (*Mustela putorius furo* L.). *Kleintierpraxis* 51: 210–215.

104 Fox, J.G. (1998). Diseases of the gastrointestinal system. In: *Biology and Diseases of the Ferret*, 2e, 274–275. Baltimore: Williams & Wilkins.

105 Hoefer, H.L., Fox, J.G., and Bell, J. (2012). Gastrointestinal diseases. In: *Ferrets, Rabbits, and Rodents: Clinical Medicine and Surgery*, 3e, 27–45. St. Louis, MO: Elsevier.

106 Lightfoot, T., Rubinstein, J., Aiken, S. et al. (2012). Ferrets: soft tissue surgery. In: *Ferrets, Rabbits and Rodents Clinical Medicine and Surgery*, (ed. James G. Fox), 3e, 141–156. St Louis, MO: W.B. Saunders.

107 Miller, P.E. and Picket, J.P. (1989). Zygomatic salivary gland mucocele in a ferret, (ed. Katherine E. Quesenberry, James W. Carpenter), *J Am Vet Med Assoc* 194: 1437–1438.

108 Thas, I. (2012). Acquired salivary mucoceles in two domestic ferrets (*Mustela putorius furo*), (Ed. Katherine E. Quesenberry, James W. Carpenter), *Vet Rec Case Rep* 2: 1–8.

109 Graham, J., Fidel, J., and Mison, M. (2006). Rostral maxillectomy and radiation therapy to manage squamous cell carcinoma in a ferret. *Vet Clin North Am Exot Anim Pract* 9: 701–706.

110 Bau-Gaudreault, L. and Grimes, C.N. (2017). What is your diagnosis? Cystic prostatic lesion in a domestic ferret. *Vet Clin Pathol* 46: 367–368.

111 Coleman, G.D., Chavez, M.A., and Williams, B.H. (1998). Cystic prostatic disease associated with adrenocortical lesions in the ferret (*Mustela putorius furo*). *Vet Pathol* 35: 547–549.

112 Juan-Sallès, C. and Garner, M.M. (2007). Cytologic diagnosis of diseases of hedgehogs. *Vet Clin North Am Exot Anim Pract* 10: 51–59.

113 Heatley, J., Mauldin, G., and Cho, D. (2005). A review of neoplasia in the captive African hedgehog. *Semin Avian Exot Pet Med* 14: 182–192.

114 Demkowska-Kutrzepa, M., Tomczuk, K., Studzińska, M., and Szczepaniak, K. (2014). *Caparinia tripilis* in African hedgehog (*Atelerix albiventris*). *Vet Dermatol* 26: 68–75.

115 Kim, D., Oh, D., Ahn, K., and Shin, S.S. (2012). An outbreak of *Caparinia tripilis* in a colony of African pygmy hedgehogs (*Atelerix albiventris*) from Korea. *Korean J Parasitol* 50: 151–156.

116 Ellis, C. and Mori, M. (2001). Skin diseases of rodents and exotic small mammals. *Vet Clin North Am Exot Anim Pract* 4: 493–542.

117 Han, J. and Na, K. (2008). Dermatitis caused by *Neosartorya hiratsukae* infection in a hedgehog. *J Clin Microbiol* 46: 3119–3123.

118 Han, J. and Na, K. (2010). Cutaneous paecilomycosis caused by *Paecilomyces variotii* in an African pygmy hedgehog (*Atelerix albiventris*). *J Exot Pet Med* 19: 309–312.

119 Han, J., Lee, S., Jang, H. et al. (2011). Isolation of *Staphylococcus* simulans from dermatitis in a captive African pygmy hedgehog. *J Zoo Wildl Med* 42: 277–280.

120 Wack, R. (2000). Pemphigus foliaceus in an African hedgehog. *Proceedings of the 14th Annual North American Veterinary Conference*, Orlando, FL (January 15–19, 2000).

121 Wellehan, J., Southorn, E., Smith, D.A., and Taylor, W.M. (2003). Surgical removal of a mammary adenocarcinoma and a granulosa cell tumor in an African pygmy hedgehog. *Can Vet J* 44: 235–237.

122 Couture, E., Langlois, I., Santamaria-Bouvier, A., and Benoit-Biancamano, M.O. (2015). Cutaneous squamous cell carcinoma in an African pygmy hedgehog (*Atelerix albiventris*). *Can Vet J* 56: 1275–1278.

123 Raymond, J., White, M.R., and Janovitz, E.B. (1997). Malignant mast cell tumor in an African hedgehog (*Atelerix albiventris*). *J Wildl Dis* 33: 140–142.

124 Raymond, J. and Garner, M. (2001). Spontaneous tumours in captive African hedgehogs (*Atelerix albiventris*): a retrospective study. *J Comp Pathol* 124: 128–133.

125 Chung, T., Kim, H., and Choi, U. (2014). Multicentric epitheliotropic T-cell lymphoma in an African hedgehog (*Atelerix albiventris*). *Vet Clin Pathol* 43: 601–604.

126 Spugnini, E., Pagotto, A., Zazzera, F. et al. (2008). Cutaneous T-cell lymphoma in an African hedgehog (*Atelerix albiventris*). *In Vivo* 22: 43–46.

127 Kim, H., Kim, Y.B., Park, J.W. et al. (2010). Recurrent sebaceous carcinoma in an African hedgehog (*Atelerix albiventris*). *J Vet Med Sci* 72: 947–949.

128 Phair, K., Carpenter, J., Marrow, J. et al. (2011). Management of an extraskeletal osteosarcoma in an African hedgehog (*Atelerix albiventris*). *J Exot Pet Med* 20: 151–155.

129 Martin, K. and Johnston, M. (2006). Forelimb amputation for treatment of a peripheral nerve sheath tumor in an African pygmy hedgehog. *J Am Vet Med Assoc* 229: 706–710.

130 Raymond, J. and Garner, M. (2000). Cardiomyopathy in captive African hedgehogs (*Atelerix albiventris*). *J Vet Diagn Invest* 12: 468–472.

131 Raymond, J., Clarke, K., and Schafer, K. (1998). Intestinal lymphosarcoma in captive African hedgehogs. *J Wildl Dis* 34: 801–806.

132 Cazzini, P., Richards, J., Fraser, N. et al. (2017). Abdominal mass in a hedgehog. *ESVCP Conference Proceedings*, London, UK (September 07–09, 2017).

133 Martinez, L.S., Juan-Salles, C., Cucchi-Stefanoni, K., and Garner, M.M. (2005). *Actinomyces naeslundii* infection in an African hedgehog (*Atelerix albiventris*) with mandibular osteomyelitis and cellulitis. *Vet Rec* 157: 450–451.

134 Turner, P.V., Brash, M.L., and Smith, D.A. (2018). Hedgehogs. In: *Pathology of Small Mammal Pets*, 387–416. Hoboken, NJ: Wiley.

135 LaRue, M., Flesner, B., Higbie, C. et al. (2016). Treatment of a thyroid tumor in an African pygmy

hedgehog (*Atelerix albiventris*). *J Exot Pet Med* 25: 226–230.

136 Song, S., Park, N., Jung, S. et al. (2014). Bilateral malignant ovarian teratoma with peritoneal metastasis in a captive African pygmy hedgehog (*Atelerix albiventris*). *J Exot Pet Med* 23: 403–408.

137 Greenacre, C. (2004). Spontaneous tumors of small mammals. *Vet Clin North Am Exot Anim Pract* 7: 627–651.

138 Mikaelian, I. and Reavill, D.R. (2004). Spontaneous proliferative lesions and tumors of the uterus of captive African hedgehogs (*Atelerix albiventris*). *J Zoo Wildl Med* 35: 216–220.

139 D'Ovidio, D. and Santoro, D. (2014). Prevalence of fur mites (*Chirodiscoides caviae*) in pet guinea pigs (*Cavia porcellus*) in southern Italy. *Vet Dermatol* 25: 135–138.

140 Nath, A.J. (2016). Treatment and control of *Trixacarus caviae* infestation in a conventional guinea pig (*Cavia porcellus*) breeding colony. *J Parasit Dis* 40: 1213–1216.

141 Schönfelder, J., Henneveld, K., Schönfelder, A. et al. (2010). Concurrent infestation of *Demodex caviae* and *Chirodiscoides caviae* in a guinea pig. *Tierarztl Prax Ausg K Kleintiere Heimtiere* 38: 28–30.

142 Cambier, L., Heinen, M.P., and Mignon, B. (2017). Relevant animal models in dermatophyte research. *Mycopathologia* 182: 229–240.

143 Hoppman, E. and Barron, H.W. (2007). Topics in medicine and surgery. Rodent dermatology. *J Exot Pet Med* 16: 238–255.

144 White, S.D., Guzman, D.S.M., Paul-Murphy, J., and Hawkins, M.G. (2016). Skin diseases in companion guinea pigs (*Cavia porcellus*): a retrospective study of 293 cases seen at the veterinary medical teaching hospital, University of California at Davis (1990–2015). *Vet Dermatol* 27: 395-e100.

145 Grandi, F., Monteiro, L.N., Marietto-Goncalves, G.A., and Rocha, N.S. (2011). Mammary benign neoplasm diagnosed by fine need aspiration in a guinea pig (*Cavia porcellus*). *Acta Vet Bras* 5: 203–206.

146 Koebrich, S., Grest, P., Favrot, C., and Wilhelm, S. (2010). Epitheliotropic T-cell lymphoma in a guinea pig. *Vet Dermatol* 22: 215–219.

147 Steele, H. (2001). Subcutaneous fibrosarcoma in an aged guinea pig. *Can Vet J* 42: 300–302.

148 Murphy, J.C., Ackerman, J.I., Marini, R.P., and Fox, J.G. (1991). Cervical lymphadenitis in guinea pigs; infection via intact ocular and nasal mucosa by *Streptococcus zooepidemicus*. *Lab Anim Sci* 41: 251–254.

149 McEwan, N.A. and Callanan, J.J. (1003). A needle aspirate as an aid to diagnosis of lymphosarcoma in a guinea pig. *Vet Rec* 133: 218.

150 Allgoewer, I., Ewringmann, A., and Pfleghaar, S. (1999). Lymphosarcoma with conjunctival manifestation in a guinea pig. *Vet Ophthalmol* 2: 117–119.

151 Stik, N.I., Alleman, A.R., and Wellehan, J.F.X. (2005). Conjunctival swab cytology from a guinea pig: it's elementary! *Vet Clin Pathol* 34: 169–171.

152 Laik-Schandelmaier, C., Klopfleisch, R., Schöniger, S. et al. (2017). Spontaneously arising tumours and tumour-like lesions of the cervix and uterus in 83 pet guinea pigs (*Cavia porcellus*). *J Comp Pathol* 156: 339–351.

153 Gibbons, P.M., Garner, M.M., and Kiupel, M. (2012). Morphological and immunohistochemical characterization of spontaneous thyroid gland neoplasms in guinea pigs (*Cavia porcellus*). *Vet Pathol* 50: 334–342.

154 Vergneau-Grosset, C., Keel, M.K., Goldsmith, D. et al. (2016). Description of the prevalence, histologic characteristics, concomitant abnormalities, and outcomes of mammary gland tumors in companion rats (*Rattus norvegicus*): 100 cases (1990–2015). *J Am Vet Med Assoc* 249: 1170–1179.

155 Pucheu-Haston, C.M., Brandão, J., Jones, K.L. et al. (2016). Zymbal gland (auditory sebaceous gland) carcinoma presenting as otitis external in a pet rat (*Rattus norvegicus*). *J Exot Pet Med* 25: 133–138.

156 Grandi, F., Ferreira, I., Rocha, R.M., and Rocha, N.S. (2012). What is your diagnosis? Subcutaneous enlargement near the base of the ear canal in a Sprague-Dawley rat. *Vet Clin Pathol* 41: 160–161.

157 Rosenbaum, M.D., Feirer, M.R., Fox, K., and Kendall, L. (2010). Solitary foot mass on a Sprague-Dawley rat. *Lab Anim* 39: 36–39.

158 Dias, S., Anselmi, C., Casanova, M. et al. (2017). Clinical and pathological findings in 2 rats (*Rattus norvegicus*) with dilated cardiomyopathy. *J Exot Pet Med* 26: 205–212.

159 Murphy, B., Michel, A., LaDouceur, E.B. et al. (2017). Ameloblastoma of the jaw in three species of rodent: a domestic brown rat (*Rattus norvegicus*), Syrian hamster (*Mesocricetus auratus*) and Amargosa vole (*Microtus californicus scirpensis*). *J Comp Pathol* 157: 145–149.

160 Irizarry-Rovira, A.R., Wolf, A., and Bolek, M. (2007). *Taenia taeniaeformis*-induced metastatic hepatic sarcoma in a pet rat (*Rattus norvegicus*). *J Exot Pet Med* 16: 45–48.

161 Yoshimura, H., Kimura-Tsukada, N., Ono, Y. et al. (2015). Characterization of spontaneous mammary tumors in domestic Djungarian hamsters (*Phodopus sungorus*). *Vet Pathol* 52: 1227–1234.

162 Kondo, H., Onuma, M., Shibuya, H., and Sato, T. (2008). Spontaneous tumors in domestic hamsters. *Vet Pathol* 45: 674–680.

163 D'Ovidio, D., Noviello, E., and Santoro, D. (2016). Tropical rat mite (*Ornothonyssus bacoti*) infestation in pet Syrian hamsters (*Mesocricetus auratus*) and their owner. *Vet Dermatol* 28: 255–257.

164 Lee, S.Y., Yoo, J.H., Park, H.M., and Kim, D.Y. (2011). Pathology in practice. Bacterial pseudomycetoma. *J Am Vet Med Assoc* 239: 583–585.

165 Eshar, D., Mayer, J., and Keating, J.H. (2010). Dermatitis in a Siberian hamster (*Phodopus sungorus*). *Lab Anim* 39: 71–73.

166 Martorell, H., Gallifa, N., Donfevila, D. et al. (2006). Bacterial pseudomycetoma in a dwarf hamster *Phodopus sungorus*. *Vet Dermatol* 17: 449–452.

167 Simmons, J.H., Riley, L.K., Franklin, C.L. et al. (2001). Hamster polyoma virus infection in a pet Syrian hamster (*Mesocricetus auratus*). *Vet Pathol* 38: 441–443.

168 Harvey, R.G., Whitbread, T.J., Ferrer, L. et al. (1992). Epidermotropic cutaneous T-cell lymphoma (mycosis fungoides) in Syrian hamsters (*Mesocricetus auratus*). A report of six cases and the demonstration of T-cell specificity. *Vet Dermatol* 3: 13–19.

169 Johnson, J.G. III, Blair, R., Brandão, J. et al. (2014). Atypical fibrosarcoma in the skin of a Roborovski hamster (*Phodopus roborovskii*). *Vet Clin Pathol* 43: 281–284.

170 Snyder, L.A., Linder, K.E., and Neel, J.A. (2007). Malignant peripheral nerve sheath tumor in a hamster. *J Am Assoc Lab Anim Sci* 46: 55–57.

171 Conrado, F.O., Bruno, S.F., and de Alencar, N.X. (2013). What is your diagnosis? Scapular mass in a Chinese hamster. *Vet Clin Pathol* 42: 533–534.

172 Fenton, H., Forzàn, M.J., Desmarchelier, M. et al. (2016). Poorly differentiated cutaneous carcinoma of non-sebaceous origin in a 3 year old Mongolian gerbil (*Meriones unguiculatus*). *Can Vet J* 57: 80–83.

173 DuVal-Hudelson, K.A. (1990). Coccidioidomycosis in three European ferrets. *J Zoo Wildl Med* 21: 353–357.

174 Ropstad, E.O., Leiva, M., Pena, T. et al. (2011). *Cryptococcus gattii* chorioretinitis in a ferret. *Vet Ophthalmol* 14: 262–266.

175 Steinberg, H. (2000). Disseminated T-cell lymphoma in a guinea pig with bilateral ocular involvement. *J Vet Diagn Invest* 12: 459–462.

176 Künzel, F., Hierlmeier, B., Christian, M., and Reifinger, M. (2013). Hyperthyroidism in four guinea pigs: clinical manifestations, diagnosis, and treatment. *J Small Anim Pract* 54: 667–671.

57

Rabbit

Laurie Millward

Introduction

The domesticated rabbit, *Oryctolagus cuniculus*, was derived from the European rabbit and is distinct from wild North American species such as the cottontail rabbit (*Sylvilagus audubonii*) and the jack rabbit (*Lepus* spp.). *O. cuniculus* occurs in commercial, laboratory, shelter, and rescue settings and as pets worldwide. The New Zealand and Dutch breeds are commonly used in laboratory studies. The majority of information published on rabbit pathology is based on laboratory settings. Information on pet rabbits, which are quite different from their laboratory counterpart, is sparse and limited to sporadic case reports. Laboratory rabbits are usually intact, genetically homogeneous, and live one to two years in strictly managed environments, which are sometimes pathogen-free. Differences between laboratory and pet rabbits should be considered when interpreting published data. Cytology can aid in assessing husbandry practices and herd health, improve the quality of medical care, and generate data in research settings (see Chapter 66). Most information on rabbit neoplasia is from spontaneous or induced tumors in laboratory rabbits. Common tissues and procedures used for cytologic assessment are similar to dogs and cats. Where cytology is not described specifically for rabbits, cytologic findings from other species might be extrapolated to rabbits. Light sedation with anxiolytic medication such as midazolam is recommended to reduce anxiety. Rabbits are prone to spinal fractures with improper handling, and safe low-stress handling is required.

Skin and Subcutis

Hyperplasia

Nodular dermal fibrosis occurs as small, firm masses in the skin, usually of the dorsum and flanks. Masses are postulated to arise from previous trauma or as developmental hamartomas; however, the exact cause is unknown. Cytology samples are poorly cellular with rare well-differentiated, individualized mesenchymal cells (fibrocytes) and scant blood in the background.[1] Histopathology reveals epidermal hyperplasia with broad bands of dermal collagen and low numbers of well-differentiated fibrocytes. Adnexal hyperplasia and/or inflammation are rarely noted.[1]

Infectious and Inflammatory Conditions

Inflammation in rabbits can be categorized as heterophilic (vs neutrophilic), eosinophilic, mixed cell, or macrophagic. Rabbit heterophils can be confused with eosinophils. Heterophils are smaller in size (10–15 μm) with smaller cytoplasmic granules than eosinophils. Heterophilic inflammation (>80% heterophils) indicates an acute inflammatory response.[2] Like neutrophils, heterophils can be non-degenerate or degenerate, suggesting a potential bacterial etiology. Eosinophilic inflammation (>10%) can be seen with parasitic infections, hypersensitivity reactions, or allergic responses.[2] Mixed inflammation suggests active established inflammation in response to infectious agents, foreign material, or trauma and is composed of heterophils and mononuclear leukocytes. Macrophagic inflammation (>50% macrophages) is typically associated with chronic processes and foreign body reactions.[2]

Veterinary Cytology, First Edition. Edited by Leslie C. Sharkey, M. Judith Radin, and Davis Seelig.

Sebaceous Adenitis

This presents as a progressive, exfoliative, non-pruritic dermatitis with patchy alopecia. Histology shows orthokeratotic hyperkeratosis, absence of sebaceous glands, and mural lymphocytic folliculitis, but cytology has not been reported. A tape preparation taken from the skin of a rabbit with sebaceous adenitis showed degenerative heterophils with intracellular cocci, suggesting a secondary bacterial infection.[3]

Abscesses

Abscesses are often superficial, encapsulated, and mobile structures in the skin, but can involve deeper tissue and be fixed. They often occur secondary to traumatic injury, hematogenous spread, or pressure sores from poor husbandry. Rabbits develop periapical tooth root abscesses presenting as painful swellings along the cheek, ventral border of the mandible, or zygomatic arch. Cytology consists of blood, degenerate heterophils, and macrophages with fewer plasma cells and lymphocytes (Figure 57.1).[1] Proteinaceous fluid, cellular debris, mineral, and intra- and extracellular bacteria are also seen.[1,4] Intracellular bacteria and a monomorphic bacterial population suggest a septic process rather than bacterial contamination. Rabbit heterophils produce less myeloperoxidase than neutrophils, creating thick inspissated pus that is difficult to drain.[4] A larger gauge needle (18–20) is needed for aspiration. A thick capsule of collagen fibers, fibroblasts, blood vessels, and inflammatory cells is usually present.[5] Central aggregates of eosinophilic material resembling Splendore–Hoeppli phenomenon have been noted in rabbit staphylococcal abscesses.[1] *Pasteurella multocida*, *Staphylococcus* spp., *Pseudomonas* spp., *Proteus* spp., and *Fusiformis* spp. are common isolates.[5–7] Lancing and flushing are rarely curative; surgical removal of the abscess capsule will help prevent reoccurrence. Bacteriology samples are best obtained by swabbing the capsule wall or, ideally, submitting tissue from the capsule.[4]

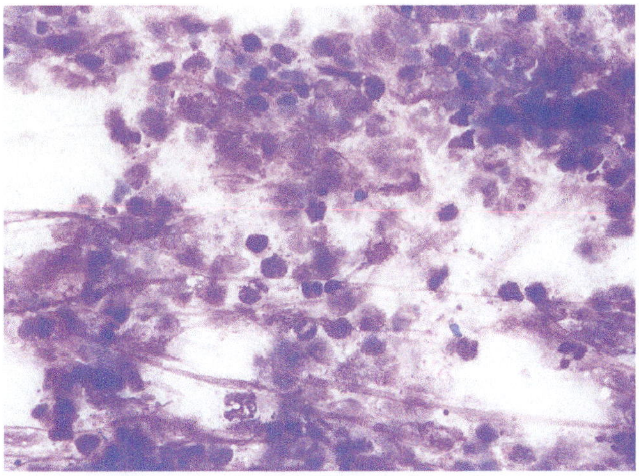

Figure 57.1 Subcutaneous abscess in a rabbit. The sample is highly cellular and primarily consists of heterophils in varying stages of degeneration. Heterophils exhibit marked karyolysis and karyorrhexis. Nuclear streaming, cellular debris, and extracellular bacteria are present in the background (Wright Giemsa, 1000×. *Source:* Image courtesy of Julie Piccione).

Ulcerative Pododermatitis

Ulcerative pododermatitis, or "sore hocks," is an ulcerated and infected lesion on the plantar surface of the metatarsi and tarsi due to avascular necrosis of the feet. It is potentially life-threatening. Septicemia, anorexia, and hemorrhage from erosion of the medial plantar vein and artery can occur. Breeds like the Rex are predisposed due to thin fur. Obesity, poor substrate (wire, concrete, or carpet), arthritis, spondylosis, and excessive moisture predispose. Histology shows acanthosis, hyperkeratosis, and ulceration of the epidermis.[8] Treatment is challenging; osteomyelitis and local joint infections can develop. *Staphylococcus aureus* and *P. multocida* are common isolates.[4]

Mastitis

Mastitis occurs most frequently in intact females and breeding does and less often in pseudopregnant females. Heavy lactation, poor sanitation, injury to the mammary gland, and hormonal influences predispose.[9] Histologic evaluation of mastitis in 204 commercial breeding rabbits described purulent mastitis with variable lymphocytes, macrophages, and plasma cells.[10] Cystic mastitis has been reported to lead to benign neoplasia with progression to mammary adenocarcinoma in laboratory rabbits.[4] All mammary masses should be removed and ovariohysterectomy performed to prevent progression of mastitis to neoplasia.

Rabbit Syphilis

Rabbit syphilis, or treponematosis, is a sexually transmitted disease caused by the spirochete *Treponema paraluis-cuniculi*. It is highly contagious. Vertical transmission can also occur during vaginal delivery in infected does. Clinical signs include red, raised, crusty, hemorrhagic lesions on the mucocutaneous junctions of the mouth, nose, eyes, genitals, or anus. It is suggested that subclinical infections are common.[4] Histology shows epidermal hyperplasia with hyperkeratosis or parakeratosis, erosion and ulceration, microabscesses or vesicle formation, and moderate to severe mixed dermal inflammation.[1,8] Histologic confirmation reveals slender, helical, filamentous spirochetes between epithelial cells in the deeper epidermis and infundibular regions of follicular sheaths.[1] Cytology consists of numerous squamous epithelial cells, non-degenerate to degenerate heterophils, and cellular debris.[1] Special stains such as Warthin–Starry or Steiner silver stains are usually required to visualize organisms cytologically. Dark-field microscopy can be used; wet mount samples are prepared using a scalpel blade or saline-soaked cotton swab to scrape a moistened area of affected skin.[4,8] Giemsa stained samples are prone to false negative results due to loss of the characteristic corkscrew shape of the bacterium during sample preparation.[11] Parenteral penicillin once a week for three weeks is usually curative.

Cutaneous Neoplasia

Cutaneous neoplasms are either viral or nonviral-induced. Intact males appear predisposed to non-viral-induced mesenchymal cutaneous neoplasms.[12,13] Most reports include histologic features and lack cytology descriptions. Additional publications describing the cytologic features of rabbit cutaneous neoplasia are needed.

Epithelial Origin

Shope Papilloma Virus

Shope papilloma virus is a papovavirus most frequent in young Eastern cottontail rabbits, domestic rabbits in large-scale breeding facilities, and European rabbits. It is distinct from oral papilloma virus of rabbits. Lesions commonly occur on haired skin of the face, pinna, or shoulder, appearing as multiple hornlike cutaneous growths.[1,12] Biting arthropods spread the virus. Impression smears are more diagnostic than fine-needle aspirates (FNA) and yield a uniform population of well-differentiated squamous cells with fewer parabasal cells.[1] Rare cells exhibit anisokaryosis and atypia.[1] Histology reveals marked papilliform hyperplasia of the epidermis, a prominent granular cell layer, and occasional koilocytes in the granular layer.[1] Occasionally, viral cytopathic effect is seen, including margination of nuclear chromatin, cytoplasmic clearing, and rare intranuclear inclusion bodies.[12] Some lesions progress to squamous cell carcinoma with subsequent metastasis to the lymph nodes and lungs.[12]

Oral Papilloma Virus

Oral papilloma virus causes solitary papillary growths usually in young rabbits. Lesions occur on nonkeratinized mucous epithelial surfaces (vs haired skin for Shope-induced lesions), most commonly under the tongue. Growths spread by direct contact and transfer of infected epithelial cells. Lesions grow slowly over six to nine months and usually spontaneously regress. Malignant transformation is not reported. Histology reveals small basophilic intranuclear viral inclusions in cells of the stratum spinosum.[8]

Basal Cell Tumor

Basal cell tumor is sometimes reported to be the most common cutaneous neoplasm in the rabbit, although reports in the literature are sparse.[1,14] They are solitary, benign, dermal lesions typically on the trunk or legs. Cytology shows individual or clustered oval to round epithelial cells with scant pale blue cytoplasm, oval to round nuclei, and small nucleoli. Anisokaryosis is mild. Rarely, the cytoplasm contains melanin.[1] Histopathology shows a well-circumscribed, nonencapsulated, intradermal mass containing short cords and small nests of cells resembling normal basal cells of the skin or adnexa (see Chapter 12).[8,14]

Adnexal Neoplasms

Benign adnexal neoplasms include trichoblastoma, trichoepithelioma, pilomatrixoma, tricholemmoma, keratoacanthoma, and sebaceous epithelioma.[1,8,12] They are clinically similar to basal cell tumors but have a laminated core of keratin or a cystic appearance on cut surface. Cytology is similar to basal cell tumors with keratinaceous debris or squamous epithelial cells (see Chapter 12).[1]

Squamous Cell Carcinoma

Squamous cell carcinoma is relatively common in rabbits, reportedly occurring on the skin of the face, ears, feet, subungual area, metatarsus, hind limb, and medial canthus of the eyelid.[1,12] A few invade underlying bone, but metastasis is rare.[8,12] Cytologic features are very similar to squamous cell carcinoma in other species, except that heterophilic inflammation is present instead of neutrophilic (see Chapters 12 and 21).[1]

Mammary Gland Adenocarcinoma

Mammary gland adenocarcinoma is the most frequent mammary gland malignancy in the rabbit, sometimes occurring with uterine adenocarcinoma.[1,15] Cytology consists of individualized or small clusters of neoplastic epithelial cells with variable differentiation. The basophilic cytoplasm is mildly vacuolated. The background contains proteinaceous fluid, mixed inflammatory cells, and blood. Amorphous eosinophilic material can occur in the background, possibly representing an inspissated mammary secretion called corpora amylacea.[1] Cytology can lack sensitivity due to aspiration of cysts and inflammation within the lesions, so histopathology is recommended (see Chapter 44).

Other Epithelial Tumors

Non-viral squamous papilloma occurs on the third eyelid, pinna, and scrotum. Histology shows exophytic, papillated, mildly pleomorphic squamous epithelium without cytopathic effect.[12] Meibomian adenomas rarely occur, consisting histologically of proliferating mature sebocytes and rare reserve cells.[12] Apocrine carcinomas are rare well-demarcated proliferations of cuboidal to columnar cells forming tubules, acini, or cysts in a fibrovascular stroma. Nuclei are basilar with moderate pleomorphism. Mitotic figures and large areas of necrosis can be seen. One report documented recurrence after surgical excision with metastases to skin and liver.[12] A sebaceous carcinoma of the pinna was described as multilobular proliferations of pleomorphic cuboidal to elongated cells effacing the subcutis. Cell borders were indistinct; cytoplasm was amphophilic and variably vacuolated. Scattered mature sebocytes were noted.[12]

Mesenchymal Origin

Non-viral mesenchymal cell tumors are rare, but older male rabbits are reported to be predisposed. Lipomas are common.[12] Cytologic diagnosis of mesenchymal neoplasms can be complicated by poor exfoliation. Malignant mesenchymal neoplasia in rabbits is usually highly locally invasive, and complete surgical excision is rarely achieved. Since rabbit-specific data are sparse, refer to Chapters 12 and 16 for information on specific tumors based on general information from common domestic species.

Myxomatosis

A closely related group of viruses belonging to the *Leporipoxvirus* genus causes myxomatosis in both domestic and wild rabbits. The severity of clinical signs is strain dependent and affected by the genus and species of the infected rabbit. Domesticated rabbits (*Oryctolagus* species) develop more severe disease with high mortality, whereas wild rabbits (*Sylvilagus* species) develop benign skin tumors and serve as reservoirs. Outbreaks among domestic rabbits in California and Oregon were possibly associated with an indigenous brush rabbit (*Sylvilagus bachmani*) reservoir.[8] The virus is spread via direct contact and insect vectors such as mosquitos and rabbit fleas. Lethargy, fever, anorexia, hemorrhage, seizures, and death are noted in severe cases. Infected rabbits surviving the initial infection have dermal masses commonly occurring around body orifices, including the face, eyelids, ears, and periorbital areas that contain mucoid material. Histopathology reveals proliferating undifferentiated mesenchymal cells or "myxoma cells" supported by a mucinous matrix within the dermis.[8] Cytoplasmic viral inclusions can be seen in cells within the epidermis of the lesions.[13] Cytology has not been specifically described.

Shope Fibroma Virus (SFV)

SFV is also a *Leporipoxvirus*. It is endemic in cottontail rabbits in the Eastern United States and occurs sporadically in European rabbits. R. E. Shope first described the tumorigenic virus in 1932.[16] Insect vectors such as mosquitos and fleas spread this virus, with increased incidence in the fall. SFV causes one or several focal dermal fibromas that spontaneously regress in weeks or months. One retrospective study identified the limbs, head, and pinna as most common locations.[12] Fibromas in infected European rabbits resolve within three weeks.[4] Generalized fibromatosis is a more severe and potentially lethal form that can occur in newborns, immunocompromised rabbits, or in rabbits bitten by multiple mosquitos.[4] In large-scale breeding facilities, a respiratory form is caused by aerosolized virus. An ocular manifestation was noted in a rabbit with an enlarging ventral perilimbal mass that was diagnosed as SFV keratitis.[17] Cross-immunity between fibroma virus and myxoma virus occurs in European rabbits.[4]

Shope fibromas are composed of well-circumscribed proliferations of fusiform to polygonal fibroblasts.[18] Cells are highly pleomorphic with abundant eosinophilic cytoplasm. Occasionally, intracytoplasmic eosinophilic inclusion bodies are seen in cells of the epidermis and dermis (Figure 57.2). The mitotic index is high, and there is frequent mixed inflammation. The epidermis is often ulcerated and hyperplastic.[12] Shope fibroma is distinguished from myxoma virus lesions by eosinophilic viral cytoplasmic inclusions in both epithelial cells and fibroblasts, while viral inclusions are only seen in the epidermis with myxoma virus.[13]

Cytology of these lesions is similar to reactive fibroplasia or well-differentiated sarcoma. Cytologic findings of a Shope fibroma on the muzzle included low to moderate cellularity with occasional spindle-shaped cells and rare nonkeratinized squamous epithelial cells.[13] Spindle cells exhibited moderate anisocytosis and anisokaryosis with a moderate amount of basophilic cytoplasm and occasional round to oval eosinophilic 3–5 μm diameter pleomorphic inclusions. Nuclei were round to oval, eccentrically placed, and large (1.5–3 times the diameter of an erythrocyte) with finely stippled chromatin and 1–4 variably sized prominent nucleoli.[13]

Lipoma

Lipomas are soft, subcutaneous, benign proliferations of adipose cells that commonly occur on the trunk, neck, thorax, and hind limbs in rabbits.[1,12] As with other species, a differential diagnosis for a lipoma is aspiration of subcutaneous fat (Chapter 12).

Other Sarcomas

Extraskeletal osteosarcoma is rare; however, there are several reports in rabbits. Osteosarcoma with abdominal organ and cutaneous involvement in a 1-year-old female Polish dwarf pet rabbit was evaluated cytologically.[19] Tissue imprints showed moderate numbers of round to spindloid cells occurring individually and in clusters. Karyomegaly, anisokaryosis, and macronucleoli were present. The cytoplasm was basophilic and occasionally contained clear vacuoles and fine magenta granules interpreted to be osteoid. Occasional multinucleated giant cells were present. A 7-year-old neutered male Rex rabbit

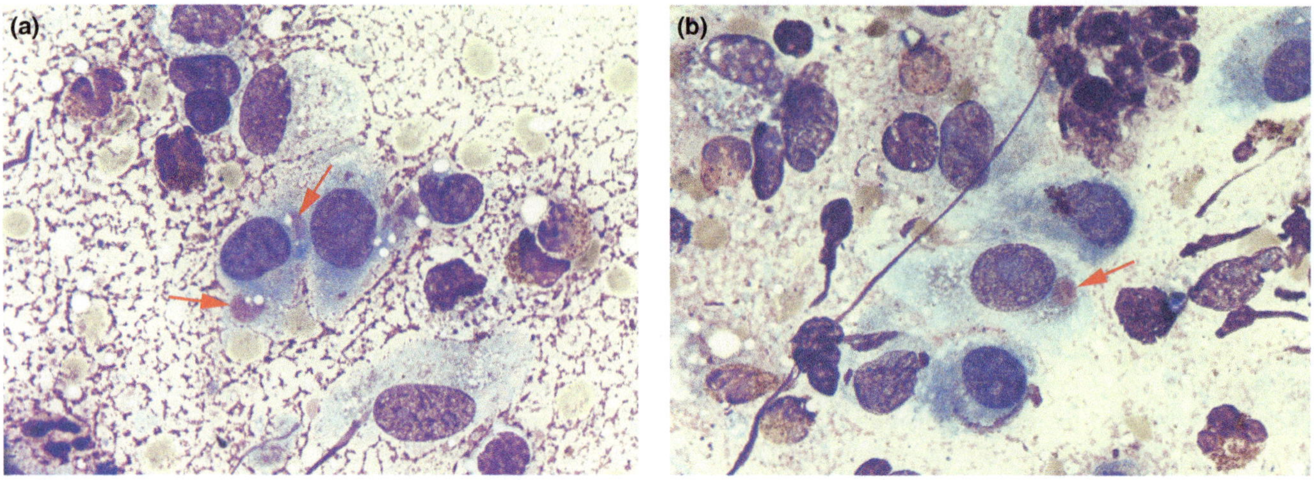

Figure 57.2 Shope fibromatosis in a young rabbit. (a and b) The background contains a moderate number of erythrocytes and a marked amount of eosinophilic granular material consistent with proteinaceous debris. The primary nucleated cell population consists of large, individualized, mesenchymal cells (interpreted as fibroblasts) that vary in shape from round to oval to elongated. These cells have oval to round nuclei with finely granular chromatin and one to several prominent nucleoli of varying shape and size. Bi- and multinucleated cells, satellite nuclei, and mitotic figures can occasionally be seen with these tumors (not shown). The cytoplasm is moderately basophilic and wispy. Occasionally, these mesenchymal cells contain round to oval, smooth to granular, eosinophilic, cytoplasmic viral inclusion bodies. Occasional heterophils, lymphocytes, macrophages, and broken cells are admixed with the mesenchymal cell population (modified Wright's, 1000×. *Source:* Image photographed by author from glass slide provided by Annalisa Hernandez and presented at the 2015 ASVCP case review session).

with a small non-painful lesion on the right upper lip was determined to have fibroblastic osteosarcoma.[20] Another cutaneous osteosarcoma occurred on the flank of an older male rabbit.[12] One leiomyoma on the lip of a 12-year-old male rabbit consisted of proliferating elongated spindle-shaped cells. It was well demarcated and partially encapsulated, with mild cellular pleomorphism and a low mitotic index.[12] Liposarcoma is rare in rabbits; one case describes a myxoid variant with a prominent background of myxoid extracellular ground substance.[12] Myxosarcoma, malignant peripheral nerve sheath tumor, fibrosarcoma, and leiomyosarcoma have been described.[12] Anaplastic sarcoma is documented rarely in middle-aged to older male rabbits on the ventral abdominal skin and axilla.[12] Cutaneous hemangiosarcoma, rhabdomyosarcoma, eosinophilic granulocytic sarcoma, and giant cell sarcoma involving the skin have also been reported (see Chapters 12, 22, and 23).[8,12,21,93]

Cutaneous Lymphoma

Cutaneous lymphoma is rarely reported in rabbits. One 16-year retrospective study analyzing cutaneous neoplasia in 179 pet rabbits in the United States found a single case.[12] It was more frequent in a German survey of pet rabbits with cutaneous neoplasia, which identified the condition in 45/280 cases.[22] A viral etiology was hypothesized to explain geographic variation in incidence; however, a retroviral or herpesviral cause was not found in one small study.[23] Clinically, cutaneous lymphoma has been described as multiple, discrete, dark, raised, nodular cutaneous masses of the mouth, face, and flank.[12,23]

Cytologically, cutaneous lymphoma is characterized by numerous, markedly anaplastic lymphocytes with increased cytoplasmic basophilia, large and sometimes multiple nuclei, multiple nucleoli, multiple occasionally bizarre mitotic figures, and a high nuclear to cytoplasmic ratio (N:C).[1,12,23] The lymphocytes in several reports were highly pleomorphic, with frequent bi- and multinucleated cells, and frequent, sometimes bizarre, mitotic figures. Tumors are diffuse large B-cell lymphomas of either a centroblastic/centrocytic subtype or a T-cell-rich B-cell subtype in contrast to a T-cell predominance for cutaneous lymphoma in other species.[23]

Other Cutaneous Neoplasms

Melanoma

Pet and laboratory rabbits can develop malignant melanoma, with New Zealand White (NZW) rabbits overrepresented.[21] This neoplasm occurs in the skin of the ear pinna, eyelid, head, perivulvar region, scrotum, thigh, and stifle of rabbits. Histologically, epithelioid to spindle-shaped cells are arranged in sheets or packets that efface the dermis. Intraepithelial nests of neoplastic cells have been noted. Nuclei are round to oval with prominent nucleoli. The cytoplasm is amphophilic to gray, contains abundant melanin, and can have multiple small cytoplasmic vacuoles (variant of balloon cell morphology). Anisocytosis and anisokaryosis are marked, and the mitotic index is high. Lymphatic invasion, metastasis, and local recurrence after surgical removal can occur (Figure 57.3).[12]

Two case reports describe amelanotic melanoma.[21,24] A 3.5-year-old intact male double-transgenic NZW laboratory rabbit developed a discrete raised facial mass rostral to the medial canthus of the left eye. The rabbit died approximately four months and two mass removals later. Necropsy revealed multiple metastases in the mandibular lymph nodes, lungs, liver, and adventitial surface of the aorta. Fontana-Masson stain was negative for melanin. A diagnosis of amelanotic melanoma was confirmed with immunohistochemistry yielding positive staining with vimentin and Melanoma-associated antigen recognized by T cells (MART-1) and with transmission electron microscopy demonstrating type II melanosomes[24] (see Chapter 15 for more detail on melanoma).

Hamartomas

Collagenous hamartomas were noted to be the second most common cutaneous growth in pet rabbits in the United States in one retrospective study. They occurred mostly in males in the dermis of the abdomen and thorax. Histologically, dermal nodules contain excessive collagen that blends into the surrounding dermis.[12]

Eye

Infectious and Inflammatory Conditions

The protozoa *Encephalitozoon cuniculi* can cause lens rupture, acute phacoclastic uveitis, and cataract formation.[25] A zonal granulomatous lens-induced uveitis occurs after lens rupture.[26] Histology reveals inflammation focused around the break in the lens capsule. Heterophils with *E. cuniculi* organisms are found in the lens cortex. A ring of fibrous tissue containing lymphocytes and plasma cells surrounds the lens.[27] One report describes using Weber's chromotrope-based stain to cytologically visualize the protozoal spores present in the irrigating solution containing lenticular contents derived from phacoemulsification surgery.[28] A Dwarf Lop rabbit presented with three weeks of unilateral exophthalmos due to a cystic lesion posterior and ventrolateral to the globe.[29] FNA produced 5.5 mL of straw-colored fluid. Exophthalmos recurred, and the cyst was removed. Histology revealed the coenurus of *Taenia serialis*. Cytology did not provide any clues to the parasitic origin of the cyst.[29]

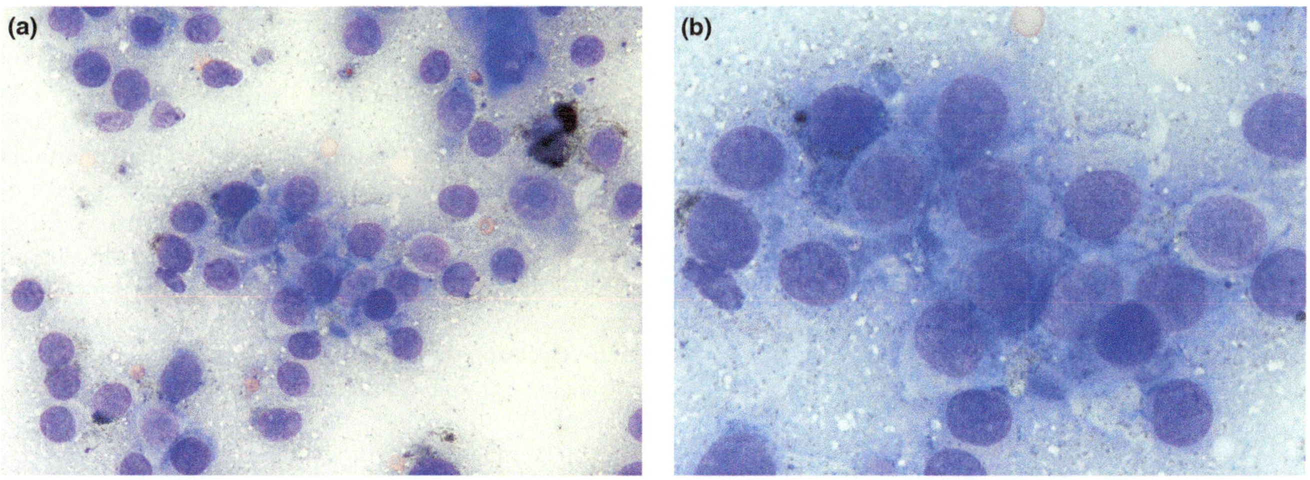

Figure 57.3 Melanoma in an adult rabbit. (a) The sample is highly cellular and consists of neoplastic population of round cells exhibiting mild to moderate anisocytosis and anisokaryosis. The nuclei are round to slightly oval, contain finely stippled chromatin, and contain one to several variably sized and shaped nucleoli. Cell borders are occasionally indistinct. The cytoplasm varies in amount from scant to moderate and exhibits mild to occasionally marked basophilia. A variable number of golden to brownish-black fine cytoplasmic granules compatible with melanin are noted. (b) The sample is highly cellular and consists of neoplastic population of round cells exhibiting mild to moderate anisocytosis and anisokaryosis. The nuclei are round to slightly oval, contain finely stippled chromatin, and contain one to several variably sized and shaped nucleoli. Cell borders are occasionally indistinct. The cytoplasm varies in amount from scant to moderate and exhibits moderate basophilia. (b) A variable number of golden to brownish-black fine cytoplasmic granules compatible with melanin are noted (Wright-Giemsa; a: 200×; b: 500×. *Source:* Images courtesy of Judith Radin).

Neoplasia

Ocular lymphoma is reported in rabbits, sometimes associated with generalized disease.[4] Common locations include the choroid, ciliary body, iris, and anterior chamber.[30] Secondary bilateral uveitis and visible tissue aggregates in the eye can occur.[4]

Two cases of ocular sarcoma in rabbits are described.[31] Both rabbits had a history of chronic inflammation in the eye. Histology revealed invasive proliferation of variably pleomorphic, poorly differentiated spindle cells closely associated with the lens and lens capsular fragments in the eye. Immunohistochemistry of the tumors showed strong diffuse staining for vimentin and negative staining for smooth muscle actin, cytokeratin, S100, and desmin[31] (see Chapters 19, 20, and 21 for more on ocular cytology in other species).

Musculoskeletal

Hyperplastic and Infectious Conditions

Hypertrophic osteopathy was diagnosed in a rabbit with uterine adenocarcinoma and a metastatic lung tumor. A proliferative periosteal lesion was noted in the tarsus and the distal tibia.[8,32]

Osteomyelitis has been documented in rabbits, although cytologic findings have not been published. Common pathogens isolated from osteomyelitis lesions in rabbits include *P. multocida*, *Staphylococcus* spp., and α-hemolytic streptococci.[8,33]

Neoplasia

Although rare, osteosarcoma is the most common skeletal neoplasm in rabbits. It has been reported in both pet and laboratory rabbits in the mandible, ribs, proximal tibia, distal tibia, skull, proximal humerus, and other sites.[8,34–37] Cytology samples are usually highly cellular and consistent with findings in other species (Chapter 23). Osteoblastic, fibroblastic, poorly differentiated, and giant cell types have been reported in rabbits.[20,34,36–38] Metastasis to the lungs, skin, or abdominal organs are reported, but do not always occur.[19,36,37]

Respiratory

Sample Collection

Thorough physical exam, nasal or oropharyngeal culture, cytology, serology, and/or imaging studies aid in accurate diagnosis of rabbit respiratory disease. The cell types of the respiratory tract in healthy rabbits are similar to those in other mammals, and collection methods are similar.[39] General anesthesia with endotracheal tube intubation is often required to reduce stress, to prevent aspiration, and to obtain diagnostic samples. Rhinoscopy is also helpful. Nasal wash samples can yield diagnostic results and are often used when rhinoscopy is not available; the technique is described elsewhere.[2] Nasal swabs can be performed to collect cytology specimens and to submit for culture and sensitivity testing; however, heavy injectable sedation or general anesthesia and intubation are necessary. To prevent contamination of the culture swab, the external nares are cleaned prior to sampling. The nasal mucosa of each nostril is sampled by gently inserting a premoistened cotton swab and lightly rolling the swab along the cavity wall. For abscesses, samples taken from the abscess wall using a premoistened swab will provide most accurate results.[4] Submission of tissue from the abscess wall for culture can be helpful. Cary-Blair medium and Leibovitz medium No. 15 are optimal to transport rabbit nasal swab samples.[40] Samples of *P. multocida* survived for more than 14 days at room temperature.[40]

Bronchoalveolar lavage (BAL) is indicated for chronic coughing, wheezing, dyspnea, respiratory signs unresponsive to standard treatment, abnormal lung sounds, abnormal pulmonary imaging results, suspicion of a respiratory foreign body, or concern for pulmonary neoplasia. BAL fluid can be used to evaluate lung injury in toxicological studies. Various techniques and normal values for BAL have been reported using laboratory rabbits.[41–43] Hawkins et al. used a flexible endoscope and 3 mL of sterile saline solution infused through the biopsy port to obtain a BAL sample. A transient decrease in SpO_2 was noted in some rabbits after the BAL was performed.[43] Rabbits should be recovered in sternal recumbency with supplemental oxygen and careful monitoring until fully recovered. Total nucleated cell counts averaged 400 nucleated cells/μL, similar to healthy dogs and cats and previous rabbit studies.[41,42] Alveolar macrophages were the most common cell. Occasional binucleated and multinucleated macrophages, plasma cells, and reactive lymphocytes were observed without other evidence of inflammation.[43] Rabbit samples appear to contain more erythrocytes and ciliated respiratory epithelial cells than other species.[43] Oropharyngeal contamination was observed in some samples.

Foreign Body

Rabbits with a respiratory foreign body can present with unilateral bloody, mucoid, or purulent nasal discharge.

Rabbits are obligate nasal breathers so hay, seeds, wood chips, hair, or other material can easily become stuck in the nasal cavity. Sometimes, endoscopy is required to visualize and retrieve the foreign body. Cytologic samples are typically composed of a mixed inflammatory cell population.[2] Foreign material may or may not be present along with secondary bacterial infection.

Hyperplasia and Squamous Metaplasia

Chronic irritation or inflammation of the respiratory tract can cause respiratory epithelial cell hyperplasia. Hyperplastic cells have increased N:C, cytoplasmic basophilia, and mild anisokaryosis and anisocytosis. Squamous metaplasia can occur with chronicity and is characterized by numerous squamous epithelial cells present individually and in clusters, increased cytoplasmic basophilia, the absence of inflammatory cells, and little background debris.[2]

Infectious and Inflammatory Conditions

Bacteria cause most rabbit infectious respiratory disease. Importantly, *Bordetella bronchiseptica, P. multocida, Moraxella catarrhalis, Staphylococcus epidermidis*, and *Bacillus* spp. are all normal respiratory tract flora in rabbits. Heterophilic or mixed inflammation with a monomorphic population of intracellular and extracellular bacteria suggests bacterial infection. Intracellular localization of bacteria is a strong indicator of infection rather than sample contamination. Degenerate heterophils may or may not be present. *P. multocida* and *B. bronchiseptica* are the most common causes of upper respiratory infection in rabbits; some infections are opportunistic, associated with immunocompromise. Integration of culture and sensitivity results with clinical signs and cytology is necessary to determine pathogenicity of organisms.

P. multocida infections and outbreaks are common in commercial and laboratory rabbits, usually associated with stress and overcrowding. It is a Gram-negative, bipolar, nonmotile, non-spore-forming coccobacillus. Young animals can develop septicemia, whereas older rabbits can experience a chronic manifestation. *P. multocida* causes rhinitis, conjunctivitis, nasolacrimal duct infection, otitis media, tracheitis, and bronchopneumonia.[4] Infected rabbits can be asymptomatic carriers. Ideally, diagnosis is achieved using a combination of clinical signs, culture, imaging, and/or serology. *B. bronchiseptica* is a small Gram-negative, aerobic, motile, coccobacillus and is another common cause of rhinitis or pneumonia in rabbits. A combination of clinical signs and culture can be used for definitive diagnosis.

Respiratory fungal and viral infections occur rarely. Aspergillosis and *Pneumocystis oryctolagi* pneumonia have been reported.[44,45] Cytologic findings were not described. Myxoma virus has been associated with nasal disease, dyspnea, and acute hemorrhagic pneumonia.[46,47] A fatal herpesvirus affecting mini Rex and crossbred meat rabbits in a commercial rabbitry caused respiratory distress and multifocal pulmonary hemorrhage.[48] No cytologic findings were described in these cases.

Neoplasia

Pulmonary histiocytic sarcoma was reported in an adult male Dutch pet rabbit with sneezing and anorexia.[49] A right dorsal lung mass contained moderate numbers of individualized or aggregated round cells characterized by marked anisocytosis and anisokaryosis. Cell borders were indistinct with a moderate to large amount of cytoplasm containing scattered clear punctate vacuoles. Nuclei were large (5–20 μm diameter) with coarsely stippled chromatin and inconspicuous nucleoli. Occasional binucleated or multinucleated cells and rare mitotic figures were present. Neoplastic cells in histologic sections stained positively with vimentin and negatively for cytokeratin, CD3, and CD79A. CD18 reagents were not available. Based on these findings, a diagnosis of pulmonary histiocytic sarcoma was made. The rabbit was euthanized due to declining clinical condition.[49]

Lymphatic and Thymus

Lymphoma

Lymphoma is the most common neoplasm in juvenile rabbits. A generalized form is most common, involving multiple sites such as lymph nodes, stomach, kidney, liver, skin, oral cavity, and spleen.[1,50] B-cell lymphoma is also described in the Harder's gland of a 22-month-old female pet rabbit presenting with acute unilateral exophthalmos.[51] Lymphoma was also present in mesenteric lymph nodes, cecum, and both kidneys.[51] A 6-year-old pet dwarf rabbit with thymic lymphoma had concurrent chylothorax.[52] Lymphoma in rabbits is often high grade, characterized by marked anaplasia, increased cytoplasmic basophilia, large nuclei with prominent multiple variably shaped and sized nucleoli, a high N:C, and mitoses.[1]

Thymoma

Thymoma is reported to be the most common mediastinal neoplasm in the rabbit; most are benign.[1,53,54] If sufficiently large, they compress the heart and lungs causing dyspnea or exercise intolerance. Bilateral exophthalmos can also occur. Thymic lymphoma and mediastinal abscesses are important differential diagnoses.[52,54,55] Thymomas are classified as lymphocyte predominant, epithelioid, or mixed lymphoepithelial.[1,54] One study reported lymphocyte predominant as the most common form in the rabbit.[54] Cytology can contain clusters of epithelial cells with large nuclei and variable amounts of basophilic cytoplasm along with variable numbers of small and occasionally large lymphocytes.[1,54] A heterogeneous lymphoid population distinguishes thymoma from thymic lymphoma.[54] The absence of metastatic lesions distinguishes thymoma from thymic carcinoma.

Thymic Carcinoma

Thymic carcinoma is rare in rabbits.[56,57] A 5-year-old Chinchilla rabbit presented with transient bilateral exophthalmos and a large cystic cranial mediastinal mass.[56] Cytology showed a predominance of small, mature lymphocytes and 10–20% lymphoblasts. Computed tomography revealed a large hyper-dense mass in the cranial mediastinum. Histology at necropsy showed numerous large, poorly differentiated, neoplastic epithelial cells surrounded by many mature lymphocytes. Similar epithelial cells surrounded by small mature lymphocytes were noted in the kidneys, resulting in a final diagnosis of thymic carcinoma.[56]

Gastrointestinal

Infectious and Inflammatory Conditions

Clostridium spiroforme

Clostridium spiroforme is a large Gram-positive endospore-producing anaerobic bacterium that is not a component of the normal gastrointestinal flora in rabbits. Six- to 12-week-old rabbits are most susceptible due to their immature immune systems and gastrointestinal flora. Adults can become infected with exposure to contaminated food or water, chronic antibiotic treatment, diet change, stress, or improper husbandry. Clinical signs include watery diarrhea, anorexia, lethargy, dehydration, and death within one to two days. Bacteria proliferate in the cecum and produce an iota-like toxin or enterotoxin leading to enterotoxemia.[8,58,59] Fecal Gram stain of the feces can reveal bacteria consistent in size and shape with *C. spiroforme*. The bacteria appear semicircular in shape on fecal smears, instead of a coil or spiral shape observed in culture specimens.[60] Erythrocytes, heterophils, and monocytes can be present.[2]

Proliferative Enteropathy of the Small Intestine

Rabbits are susceptible to small intestinal proliferative enteritis. Clinical signs include watery diarrhea containing mucus and blood, lethargy, dehydration, thickened loops of small intestines, and enlarged mesenteric lymph nodes. The small intestinal mucosa is hyperplastic and inflamed.[61] Curved bacillus-like organisms can be seen in the cytoplasm of the hyperplastic epithelial cells using Warthin–Starry silver stain or electron microscopy.[8,62] Affected rabbit serum was immunohistochemically cross-reactive to *Lawsonia intracellularis* infected porcine tissue.[62]

Saccharomyces spp.

Saccharomyces spp. yeast is present in low numbers in fecal smears from healthy rabbits.[63] Increased numbers might be pathologic. The yeast are large and rod-shaped. Oral antibiotics can increase the number of yeast more than 100-fold in the cecum.[64]

Neoplasia

Rectal Polyps

Rectal polyps occasionally occur in rabbits as fleshy, red growths around the perianal region that can become ulcerated or infected. The etiology is unknown, although they appear similar to viral-induced polyps of other species. Histologically, rectal polyps consist of well-differentiated, hyperplastic, hyperkeratotic squamous epithelium covering inflamed fibrous stroma. Cytology shows a mixed population of well-differentiated squamous epithelial cells, parabasal cells, degenerate heterophils, other mixed leukocytes, and bacteria.[1]

Lymphoma

Lymphoma can occur from the oral cavity to the rectum. It is the most common malignant neoplasm of young rabbits and most are high grade.[30]

Other Neoplasms

Described gastrointestinal neoplasms in rabbits include adenocarcinoma, leiomyoma, and leiomyosarcoma of the stomach and intestines. Papillomas of the sacculus rotundus have also been reported.[59] Cytologic descriptions have not been published.

Hepatobiliary

Sample Collection

Diagnosis of liver disease in rabbits ideally includes a combination of serum biochemical testing, diagnostic imaging, and cytology and/or histopathology. One study evaluated the diagnostic quality of percutaneous ultrasound-guided FNA of the liver and laparoscopically derived liver biopsy specimens from anesthetized rabbits.[65] Liver aspiration was performed using a 22 G needle. A 1.7 mm biopsy forceps and 3.0 mm biopsy forceps were used for the laparoscopic biopsy. Mild bleeding was associated with aspiration. Cytology was considered best for diffuse disease due to the potential for sample bias with focal/multifocal lesions. Larger surgical biopsy samples were considered superior because evaluation of multiple portal triads and central veins was necessary for accurate diagnosis of some infectious and neoplastic diseases.[65] Liver aspiration should be considered to evaluate diffuse liver disease because rabbits are sensitive to general anesthesia.

Infectious and Inflammatory Conditions

Hepatic Coccidiosis

Eimeria stiedae causes hepatic coccidiosis in rabbits and infects biliary epithelial cells. Infected animals have clinical signs ranging from mild inapparent disease to potentially lethal diarrhea. Bile duct expansion and compression can cause marked loss of functional hepatic mass.[66] *E. stiedae* commonly occurs in young rabbits in commercial breeding and rearing farms. Adults can be subclinical carriers. Rabbits become infected by ingesting sporulated oocysts. An impression smear from a liver nodule was highly cellular, consisting of numerous oocysts, hepatocytes, moderately hyperplastic biliary epithelial cells, and few inflammatory cells.[67] A full range of coccidial developmental stages was noted and includes early gametogonous stages, microgametocytes, macrogametocytes, and oocysts (Figure 57.4). Oocysts were oval to ellipsoidal and 30–39 $\times$18–22 µm with flat micropylar ends and smooth bright pink walls that were occasionally wrinkled from processing. Small reactive lymphocytes, plasma cells, and heterophils were present. Minimal hepatocellular vacuolar degeneration and intracellular cholestasis were noted.[67]

Tyzzer's Disease

Clostridium piliforme is the causative agent of Tyzzer's disease, similar to foals. Six- to 12-week-old rabbits are most susceptible; however, infection can occur at any age. Clinical signs include acute profuse watery diarrhea, dehydration, lethargy, and death. The chronic form of the disease causes cachexia, intestinal fibrosis and stenosis, and liver necrosis. Antemortem diagnosis is complicated by the rapid course; however, serology and polymerase chain reaction testing of ileum or liver are available. Cytology has not been described.

Neoplasia

Lymphoma is the most common hepatic neoplasm, and juvenile to young adult rabbits are most often affected. Bile duct carcinoma has been reported; histology is similar to other domestic species. *E. steidae* infection appears similar grossly and is a differential diagnosis.[8] Hepatic hemangiosarcoma is rare. A recent case report describes hepatic and pulmonary hemangiosarcoma in a 5-year-old laboratory NZW rabbit used for production of immunoglobulins. He died acutely, and necropsy showed multiple, pinpoint to 2.5 cm dark red to black, round, fluctuant nodules on the capsular surface and parenchyma of the liver and lungs with hemoabdomen. Histology revealed plump neoplastic spindle cells with poorly defined cytoplasmic borders and scant eosinophilic cytoplasm. Nuclei were large, oval, and often cleaved with finely stippled chromatin and inconspicuous nucleoli. Immunohistochemical staining for von Willebrand factor (VWF) was inconclusive due to background staining from the use of a rabbit polyclonal anti-VWF antibody. Positive staining for platelet endothelial cell adhesion molecule (PECAM or CD31) supported a diagnosis of neoplastic endothelial cells.[68]

Central Nervous System

Cerebrospinal Fluid (CSF)

The cisterna magna is recommended for CSF fluid collection, and the technique is similar to other animals.[4] Reference intervals for CSF parameters have been described: glucose 56–135 mg/dL, WBC count 0–7 cells/mm^3 (up to 20 cells/mm^3 have been noted in healthy rabbits), total protein 16–66 mg/dL, lymphocyte percentage 40–79%, monocyte percentage 21–60%.[4,69,70]

Lymphoma

B-cell lymphoma was described in the spinal cord of a pet rabbit with pelvic limb paralysis.[71] Histologically, large lymphoblasts expanded and effaced the sixth lumbar vertebra and impinged the ventral spinal cord. Lymphoblasts were CD79a positive.

Urinary Tract

Infectious and Inflammatory Conditions

Polypoid Cystitis

Polyps are a differential diagnosis in rabbits with urinary bladder masses or sludge. Two case reports of polypoid cystitis are documented in pet rabbits.[72] The rabbits

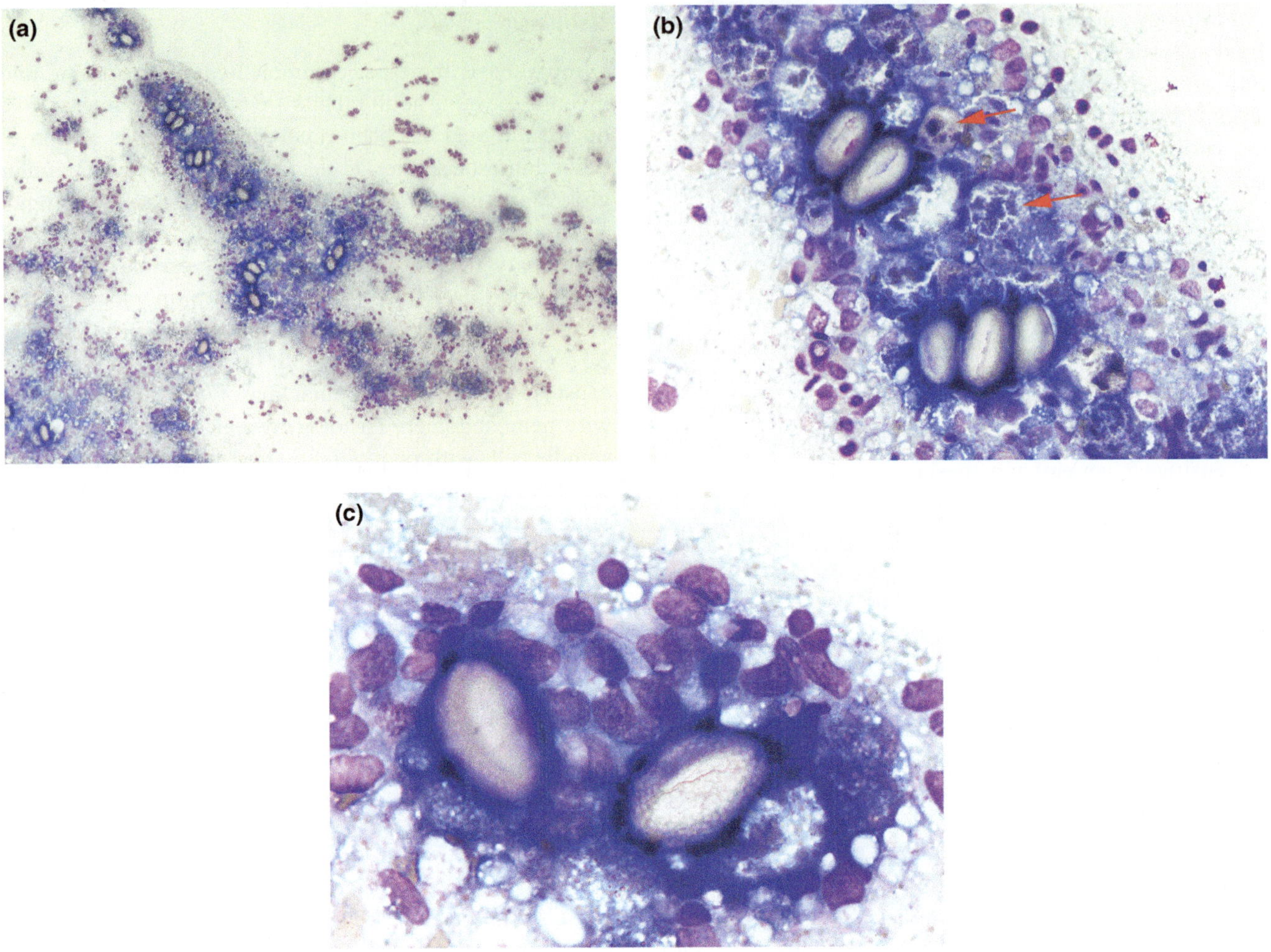

Figure 57.4 *E. stiedae* in the liver of a young rabbit. (a) Liver impression smear is highly cellular. Occasional bare nuclei, clusters of epithelial cells interpreted as bile duct epithelium, leukocytes, and erythrocytes are present. The biliary epithelial cells have oval paracentric nuclei that contain coarsely stippled chromatin. The cytoplasm is scant and lightly basophilic. Rare plasma cells, rare small lymphocytes, and rare heterophils compose the leukocyte population. Admixed within these populations of cells are a high number of extracellular parasitic organisms in varying life stages consistent with *E. stiedae*. Oocysts appear as oval to elliptical individualized structures that measure 30–40 μm in length by 14–20 μm in width. The oocysts have a slightly narrowed anterior end, an indistinct micropyle, and stippled eosinophilic thick wall. (b) Macrogametes in varying stages of development contain eosinophilic to orange granules or basophilic granules (arrows). Oocysts have a stippled eosinophilic thick refractile wall. There are many free nuclei, occasional biliary epithelial cells, cellular debris, and occasional erythrocytes. (c) Higher magnification of oocytes, macrogametes (right) and biliary epithelial cells (Wright-Giemsa, (a) 100×, (b) 500×, (c) 1000×. *Source:* Images photographed by author from glass slide provided by Kristin Loria and presented at the 2013 ASVCP case review session).

presented with anorexia and perineal urine scalding associated with hypercalciuria (urinary bladder sludge) and urinary tract infection. Polypoid cystitis was diagnosed using transurethral cystoscopy and histopathology. Polyps were lined by minimally hyperplastic to attenuated transitional epithelial cells; stalks contained edematous fibrous vascularized tissue and scattered lymphocytes and plasma cells. Chronic inflammation and hyperplasia contributed to the pathogenesis.

Encephalitozoon cuniculi

E. cuniculi infection in rabbits is spread via contact with infected urine and ingestion of infectious spores. Grossly, the kidneys have circumscribed, irregular, pale to tan, depressed foci on the renal cortex surface.[8] Histopathology shows a granulomatous interstitial nephritis.[4,73,74] Chronic infections cause fibrous connective tissue proliferation and collapse of the renal parenchyma.[4] Cytology is not described.

Neoplasia

Embryonal Nephroma

Embryonal nephromas (or nephroblastomas) arise from embryonal blastema. These are often listed as the third most common tumor in rabbits overall, occurring most often in young animals as an incidental finding on necropsy. Secondary erythrocytosis has been reported in rabbits with embryonal nephromas.[75,76] Most are benign and slow growing with little interference with renal function. Metastasis has not been reported, and surgical removal is curative for solitary lesions. Histopathology reveals loose myxomatous mesenchymal tissue that contains epithelium-lined glandular acini resembling tubules or primitive glomeruli. Cytology in other species is described in Chapter 37.

Renal Adenocarcinoma

Renal carcinoma is rare but has been reported in young NZW laboratory rabbits.[77,78] Intra-abdominal masses were identified, and one rabbit had hematuria. Both tumors were associated with the right kidney, and no metastatic disease was identified. Histopathologically, masses were composed of columnar to low cuboidal or spindloid shaped cells that contained eosinophilic cytoplasm and extensive cytoplasmic vacuolization. Acini were observed in one tumor.

Reproductive Tract

Female Reproductive System

Vaginal Cytology

It is important to avoid the vestibule and rima pudenda while obtaining a vaginal smear to prevent sample contamination with debris.[79] This is accomplished using a 15 cm cotton swab to sample the middle part of the vagina through a speculum. The swab is gently rolled over a slide creating a thin air-dried smear. Vaginal cytology was evaluated as a method for selecting does for superovulation.[79] The study used laboratory 5-month-old NZW rabbits receiving hormone injections to induce ovulation, with subsequent artificial insemination. More corpora lutea, oocytes–zygotes, and normal zygotes were found in does with vaginal cytology consisting principally of parabasal and intermediate cells.[79]

Pyometra is sporadically reported in pet rabbits, being more common in industrial breeding does.[10,15,80–82] Vaginal discharge is uncommon.[82] *P. multocida* and *Moraxella bovis* are reported associated with this condition.[83,84]

Uterine Endometrial Venous Aneurysms

Clinically, affected does have an enlarged uterus and will present with hematuria, potentially causing severe anemia. Distinguishing true hematuria from plant porphyrin pigment is done via urinalysis. The uterus contains clotted blood, resembling uterine adenocarcinoma, or polyps. Histopathology shows variably sized, dilated, blood- and fibrin-filled, endometrial-lined vascular spaces within the endometrium.[8] Cytology has not been described.

Cystic Endometrial Hyperplasia

Cystic endometrial hyperplasia is the second most common uterine disorder in pet rabbits.[15,80,82] It can be incidental or associated with behavior changes, serosanguinous vaginal discharge, hematuria, or mammary gland hyperplasia. Cytology reveals significant hyperplasia or dysplasia similar to uterine adenocarcinoma; therefore, histopathology is needed for definitive diagnosis.[1]

Uterine Adenocarcinoma

Uterine adenocarcinoma occurs in nearly 80% of unspayed female rabbits over 3 years of age and is the most common neoplasm of female rabbits.[85] Associated signs include reduced fertility, fetal absorption, abortion, fetal retention, or stillbirth. Bloody vulvar discharge or hematuria are the most common clinical signs. A caudal abdominal mass can be palpated if the tumor has been present ≥6 months.[85] Multiple tumors usually affect both uterine horns.[30] Pyometra, mammary adenocarcinoma, uterine leiomyoma, leiomyosarcomas, squamous cell carcinoma, cystic endometrial hyperplasia, hydrometra, mucometra, and metritis can be concurrent.[15,53,82,85] Uterine adenocarcinoma is slow growing, but metastasis to the peritoneal cavity, lung, bone, brain, and liver occurs.[82,85–87] Seeding of the abdomen with neoplastic cells can occur during FNA.[1] Cytologic interpretation of these lesions must be made cautiously because similar morphologic features are present with cystic endometrial hyperplasia or adenomyosis.[1] Clusters of neoplastic epithelial cells with marked anisocytosis and anisokaryosis, large nucleoli, and mitotic figures can be seen cytologically.[1] Uterine adenocarcinoma can be well-differentiated; thus cytology can be misinterpreted as consistent with a benign process.[8] Ovariohysterectomy can be curative early due to the slow growth of this neoplasm, but all rabbits should be screened for metastases.

Male Reproductive System

There are few reports of testicular tumors in rabbits, possibly because many pet rabbits are neutered and most laboratory rabbits are sacrificed early. Leydig cell tumors are reported to be the most common,[1,88] although seminomas, teratomas, and granular cell tumors are also documented.

Leydig Cell Tumor

Rabbits with Leydig cell (or interstitial cell) tumors have testicular enlargement. Some experience slowly progressive weight loss. Sheets of large polygonal cells that have abundant granular cytoplasm, small oval nuclei, and a single small nucleolus characterize cytology of Leydig cell tumors.[1] Histopathology shows sheets of large polygonal cells containing eosinophilic cytoplasm and eccentric anisokaryotic nuclei with one nucleolus. Binucleate cells can occasionally be found.[85]

Seminoma

A 2-year-old NZW rabbit with an enlarged testicle had a seminoma.[89] Neoplastic cells consisted of sheets of monomorphic, basophilic, polygonal cells that contained scant acidophilic cytoplasm. Nuclei were variably sized, ovoid, and contained hyperchromatic prominent nucleoli. Numerous mitotic figures were present. Although similar cells were present in lesser numbers in the other testicle and the pampiniform plexus, the tumor was considered benign based on biological behavior.[89] Two other reports describe seminomas in pet rabbits with more aggressive behavior.[90,91] A 9-year-old Lionhead rabbit presented with unilateral testicular enlargement and palpable sublumbar lymph nodes.[90] Both the enlarged testicle and nodes were effaced with malignant seminoma cells. The other case describes a 10-year-old mini-lop presenting with bilateral testicular enlargement with the left being larger.[91] Histopathology revealed right gonadal intratubular seminoma and diffuse seminoma of the left.

Testicular Nephroma and Teratoma

A 3-month-old NZW rabbit had an undescended left testicle and a left-sided abdominal mass.[92] The 10 × 10 cm mass was associated with the undescended left testis and was histologically characterized by the presence of cartilage, bone, nerve, muscle, epithelial, and adipose tissue.

Granular Cell Tumor

A granular cell tumor was described in an 8-year-old intact mixed-breed pet rabbit.[88] The left testicle had been progressively enlarging for two months and measured 9 cm on presentation. Impression smears were very cellular, primarily consisting of a monomorphic population of polygonal cells that occurred individually or in dense aggregates in an abundant pink to magenta granular background. Cells had indistinct borders with abundant basophilic cytoplasm and copious pink to magenta granular material that often obscured the nucleus. Nuclei were round to oval with finely stippled chromatin and a single small nucleolus. Histologically, the neoplasm was encapsulated, multilobular, and densely cellular, compressing normal testicular tissue. Sheets of large polygonal cells with abundant granular eosinophilic cytoplasm, round to oval nuclei, fine chromatin, and a singular nucleolus were noted. Anisokaryosis and anisocytosis were moderate, and 0–1 mitotic figures were noted per 40× field. Rare cells contained small clear cytoplasmic vacuoles interpreted to be lipid. Many of the cytologic and histopathologic features noted in this granular cell tumor were similar to those of a Leydig cell tumor, but the presence of secondary lysosomes on electron microscopy and immunohistochemical staining confirmed a diagnosis of granular cell tumor.

Fluid Analysis

Abdominocentesis is rarely performed on pet rabbits and is uncommon in the literature. Mild sedation is recommended, and ultrasound is used for needle placement. After surgical preparation, a 21 or 25 G needle or butterfly needle is inserted on the ventral midline just distal to the umbilicus. The spiral cecum of rabbits occupies a large portion of the peritoneal cavity, and care is required to avoid puncturing it and other parts of the gastrointestinal tract. Analysis of peritoneal fluid is similar to that of dogs and cats.

Conclusion

The popularity of the rabbit as a companion is increasing, and rabbit owners require the same caliber of diagnostic and treatment options available for other companion animals. Rabbits also continue to be an important component of laboratory medicine and the meat industry. To date, most of the literature consists of sporadic case reports of various diseases found in this species. Larger retrospective and prospective studies are rare, and more are required to improve the quality of rabbit medicine. Further analysis and documentation of beneficial diagnostic tests such as cytology and histopathology will add to this body of knowledge to advance our understanding of this species.

References

1 Garner, M.M. (2007). Cytologic diagnosis of diseases of rabbits, guinea pigs, and rodents. *Vet Clin North Am Exot Anim Pract* 10: 25–49.

2 Campbell, T. and Ellis, C. (2007). *Avian and Exotic Animal Hematology and Cytology*, vol. 1. Ames, IA: Blackwell.

3 Kovalik, M., Thoday, K.L., Eatwell, K., and van den Broek, A.H.M. (2012). Successful treatment of idiopathic sebaceous adenitis in a Lionhead rabbit. *J Exot Pet Med* 21: 336–342.

4 Varga, M. (2014). *Textbook of Rabbit Medicine*, 2e. Edinburgh: Elsevier.

5 Chaffee, V.W., James, E.A., and Montali, R.J. (1975). Suppurative mandibular osteomyelitis associated with *Pasteurella multocida* in a rabbit. *Vet Med Small Anim Clin* 70: 1411–1473.

6 Ward, G.S., Crumrine, M.H., and Mattloch, J.R. (1981). Inflammatory exostosis and inflammation associated with *Fusobacterium nucleatum* in a rabbit. *Lab Anim Sci* 31: 459–464.

7 Dominguez, J., Crase, D., and Soave, O. (1975). A case of Pseudomonas osteomyelitis in a rabbit. *Lab Anim Sci* 25: 506.

8 Fudge, A. (2000). *Laboratory Medicine: Avian and Exotic Pets*. Philadelphia, PA: W.B. Saunders.

9 Bergdall, V. and Dysko, R.C. (1994). Metabolic, traumatic, mycotic, and miscellaneous diseases. In: *The Biology of the Laboratory Rabbit*, (eds. Patrick J. Manning, Daniel H. Ringler, Christian E. Newcomer), 2e, 336–355. San Diego, CA: Academic Press.

10 Segura, P., Martinez, J., Peris, B. et al. (2007). Staphylococcal infections in rabbit does on two industrial farms. *Vet Rec* 160: 869–872.

11 Cunliffe-Beamer, T.L. and Fox, R.R. (1981). Venereal spirochetosis of rabbits: description and diagnosis. *Lab Anim Sci* 31: 366–371.

12 von Bomhard, W., Goldschmidt, M.H., Shofer, F.S. et al. (2007). Cutaneous neoplasms in pet rabbits: a retrospective study. *Vet Pathol* 44: 579–588.

13 Dehghanpir, S.D., Canady, L.K., Wakamatsu, N., and Gaunt, S.D. (2016). Subcutaneous nodules on the muzzle of a rabbit. *Vet Clin Pathol* 45: 383–384.

14 Li, X. and Schlafer, D.H. (1992). A spontaneous skin basal cell tumor in a black French minilop rabbit. *Lab Anim Sci* 42: 94–95.

15 Papers, P., Walter, B., Böhmer, E. et al. (2010). Uterine disorders in 59 rabbits. *Vet Rec* 166: 230–233.

16 Shope, R.E. (1932). A transmissible tumor-like condition in rabbits. *J Exp Med* 56: 793–802.

17 Keller, R.L., Hendrix, D.V.H., and Greenacre, C. (2007). Shope fibroma virus keratitis and spontaneous cataracts in a domestic rabbit. *Vet Ophthalmol* 10: 190–195.

18 Strayer, D.S., Cabirac, G., Sell, S., and Leibowitz, J.L. (1983). Malignant rabbit fibroma virus: observations on the culture and histopathologic characteristics of a new virus-induced rabbit tumor. *J Natl Cancer Inst* 71: 91–104.

19 Mazzullo, G., Russo, M., Niutta, P.P., and De Vico, G. (2004). Osteosarcoma with multiple metastases and subcutaneous involvement in a rabbit (*Oryctolagus cuniculus*). *Vet Clin Pathol* 33: 102–104.

20 Renfrew, H., Rest, J.R., and Holden, A.R. (2001). Extraskeletal fibroblastic osteosarcoma in a rabbit (*Oryctolagus cuniculus*). *J Small Anim Pract* 42: 456–458.

21 Hotchkiss, C.E., Norden, H., Collins, B.R., and Ginn, P.E. (1994). Malignant melanoma in two rabbits. *Lab Anim Sci* 44: 377–379.

22 von Bomhard, W., Goldschmidt, M.H., Pfleghaar, S. et al. (2007). Epidemiology and histopathologic findings of skin tumors in pet rabbits in the USA and Germany. *Proceedings of the 25th Annual Meeting of the European Society of Veterinary Pathology*, Munich (August 29–September 01, 2007).

23 Ritter, J.M., Bomhard, W.V., Wise, A.G. et al. (2012). Cutaneous lymphomas in European pet rabbits (*Oryctolagus cuniculus*). *Vet Pathol* 49: 846–851.

24 Zerfas, P.M., Brinster, L.R., Starost, M.F. et al. (2010). Amelanotic melanoma in a New Zealand White rabbit (*Oryctolagus cuniculus*). *Vet Pathol* 47: 977–981.

25 Stiles, J., Didier, E., Ritchie, B. et al. (1997). *Encephalitozoon cuniculi* in the lens of a rabbit with phacoclastic uveitis: confirmation and treatment. *Vet Comp Ophthalmol* 7: 233–238.

26 Peiffer, R.L., Pohm-Thorsen, L., and Corcoran, K. (1994). Models in ophthalmology and vision research. In: *The Biology of the Laboratory Rabbit*, (eds. Patrick J. Manning, Daniel H. Ringler, Christian E. Newcomer), 2e, 410–434. San Diego, CA: Academic Press.

27 Wolfer, J., Grahn, B., Wilcock, B. et al. (1993). Phacoclastic uveitis in the rabbit. *Prog Vet Comp Ophthalmol* 3: 92–97.

28 Felchle, L.M. and Sigler, R.L. (2002). Phacoemulsification for the management of *Encephalitozoon cuniculi*-induced phacoclastic uveitis in a rabbit. *Vet Ophthalmol* 5: 211–215.

29 O'Reilly, A., McCowan, C., Hardman, C., and Stanley, R. (2002). *Taenia serialis* causing exophthalmos in a pet rabbit. *Vet Ophthalmol* 5: 227–230.

30 Weisbroth, S.H. (1994). Neoplastic disease. In: *The Biology of the Laboratory Rabbit*, (eds. Patrick J. Manning, Daniel H. Ringler, Christian E. Newcomer), 2e, 259–292. San Diego, CA: Academic Press.

31 McPherson, L., Newman, S.J., McLean, N. et al. (2009). Intraocular sarcomas in two rabbits. *J Vet Diagn Invest* 21: 547–551.

32 DeSanto, J. (1997). Hypertrophic osteopathy associated with an intrathoracic neoplasm in a rabbit. *J Am Vet Med Assoc* 210: 1322–1323.

33 Yanoff, S.R. (1983). What's your diagnosis? *J Am Vet Med Assoc* 183: 1347–1348.

34 Kondo, H., Ishikawa, M., Maeda, H. et al. (2007). Spontaneous osteosarcoma in a rabbit (*Oryctolagus cuniculus*). *Vet Pathol* 44: 691–694.

35 Walberg, J.A. (1981). Osteogenic sarcoma with metastasis in a rabbit (*Oryctolagus cuniculus*). *Lab Anim Sci* 31: 407–408.

36 Ishikawa, M., Kondo, H., Onuma, M. et al. (2012). Osteoblastic osteosarcoma in a rabbit. *Comp Med* 62: 124–126.

37 Higgins, S., Sanchez-Migallon Guzman, D., Sadar, M.J. et al. (2015). Coxofemoral amputation in a domestic rabbit (*Oryctolagus cuniculus*) with tibiofibular osteoblastic osteosarcoma. *J Exot Pet Med* 24: 455–463.

38 Weiss, A.T. and Muller, K. (2011). Spinal osteolytic osteosarcoma in a pet rabbit. *Vet Rec* 168: 266.

39 Burkhard, M. and Millward, L. (2010). Respiratory tract. In: *Canine and Feline Cytology*, (eds. Rose E. Raskin, Denny J. Meyer), 2e, 123–170. St. Louis, MO: W.B. Saunders/Elsevier.

40 Kawamoto, E., Sawada, T., and Maruyama, T. (1997). Evaluation of transport media for *Pasteurella multocida* isolates from rabbit nasal specimens. *J Clin Microbiol* 35: 1948–1951.

41 Henderson, R.F., Mauderly, J.L., Pickrell, J.A. et al. (1987). Comparative study of bronchoalveolar lavage fluid: effect of species, age, and method of lavage. *Exp Lung Res* 13: 329–342.

42 Mauderly, J.L. (1977). Bronchopulmonary lavage of small laboratory animals. *Lab Anim Sci* 27: 255–261.

43 Hawkins, M.G., Vernau, W., Drazenovich, T.L. et al. (2008). Results of cytologic and microbiologic analysis of bronchoalveolar lavage fluid in New Zealand White rabbits. *Am J Vet Res* 69: 572–578.

44 Dei-Cas, E., Chabe, M., Moukhlis, R. et al. (2006). *Pneumocystis oryctolagi* sp. nov., an uncultured fungus causing pneumonia in rabbits at weaning: review of current knowledge, and description of a new taxon on genotypic, phylogenetic and phenotypic bases. *FEMS Microbiol Rev* 30: 853–871.

45 Schoppler, H. (1919). Pneumonomycosis aspergillina leporis cuniculi. *Zentralbl Bakteriol* 82: 559–564.

46 Kritas, S.K., Dovas, C., Fortomaris, P. et al. (2008). A pathogenic myxoma virus in vaccinated and non-vaccinated commercial rabbits. *Res Vet Sci* 85: 622–624.

47 Marlier, D., Mainil, J., Linde, A., and Vindevogel, H. (2000). Infectious agents associated with rabbit pneumonia: isolation of amyxomatous myxoma virus strains. *Vet J* 159: 171–178.

48 Jin, L., Valentine, B.A., Baker, R.J. et al. (2008). An outbreak of fatal herpesvirus infection in domestic rabbits in Alaska. *Vet Pathol* 45: 369–374.

49 Leissinger, M., Brandão, J., Wakamatsu, N. et al. (2013). Pulmonary histiocytic sarcoma in a rabbit. *Vet Clin Pathol* 42: 364–367.

50 Percy, D.H. and Barthold, S.W. (2007). *Pathology of Laboratory Rodents and Rabbits*, 3e. Ames, IA: Blackwell.

51 Volopich, S., Gruber, A., Hassan, J. et al. (2005). Malignant B-cell lymphoma of the Harder's gland in a rabbit. *Vet Ophthalmol* 8: 259–263.

52 Pilny, A.A. and Reavill, D. (2008). Chylothorax and thymic lymphoma in a pet rabbit (*Oryctolagus cuniculus*). *J Exot Pet Med* 17: 295–299.

53 Green, H. and Strauss, J. (1949). Multiple primary tumors in the rabbit. *Cancer* 2: 673–691.

54 Künzel, F., Hittmair, K.M., Hassan, J. et al. (2012). Thymomas in rabbits: clinical evaluation, diagnosis, and treatment. *J Am Anim Hosp Assoc* 48: 97–104.

55 Franco, K.H. and Cronin, K.L. (2008). What is your diagnosis? Pulmonary abscess in a rabbit. *J Am Vet Med Assoc* 233: 35–36.

56 Wagner, F., Beinecke, A., Fehr, M. et al. (2005). Recurrent bilateral exophthalmos associated with metastatic thymic carcinoma in a pet rabbit. *J Small Anim Pract* 46: 393–397.

57 Orr, J.W. (1939). A malignant tumour of the thymus in a rabbit. *Am J Cancer* 35: 269–274.

58 Deeb, B. (2000). Digestive system and disorders. In: *Manual of Rabbit Medicine and Surgery*, (ed. Paul A. Flecknell), Gloucester: British Small Animal Veterinary Association.

59 Jenkins, J.R. (2004). Gastrointestinal disease. In: *Ferrets, Rabbits, Rodents Clinical Medicine and Surgery*, (ed. Katherine E. Quesenberry, James W. Carpenter), 2e. St. Louis, MO: W.B. Saunders.

60 Carman, R.J. and Borriello, S.P. (1983). Laboratory diagnosis of *Clostridium spiroforme*-mediated diarrhoea (iota enterotoxaemia) of rabbits. *Vet Rec* 113: 184–185.

61 Umemura, T., Tsuchitani, M., Totsuka, M. et al. (1982). Histiocytic enteritis of rabbits. *Vet Pathol* 19: 326–329.

62 Horiuchi, N., Watarai, M., Kobayashi, Y. et al. (2008). Proliferative enteropathy involving *Lawsonia intracellularis* infection in rabbits (*Oryctolagus cuniculus*). *J Vet Med Sci* 70: 389–392.

63 Walberg, J. and Loar, A.S. (2004). Cytology and hematology of small mammals. In: *Ferrets, Rabbits, Rodents Clinical Medicine and Surgery*, (ed. Katherine E. Quesenberry, James W. Carpenter), 2e. St. Louis, MO: W.B. Saunders.

64 Malley, D. (2000). Handling, restraint, and clinical techniques. In: *Manual of Rabbit Medicine and Surgery*, (ed. Paul A. Flecknell), Gloucester: British Small Animal Veterinary Association.

65 Proença, L., Camus, M., Nemeth, N. et al. (2015). Diagnostic quality of percutaneous fine-needle aspirates and laparoscopic biopsy specimens of the liver in rabbits (*Oryctolagus cuniculus*). *J Am Vet Med Assoc* 246: 313–320.

66 Loria, K.O., Beguesse, K.A., Walsh, A., and Sirivelu, M.P. (2017). Pathology in practice. *J Am Vet Med Assoc* 250: 1387–1390.

67 Al-Rukibat, R.K., Irizarry, A.R., Lacey, J.K. et al. (2001). What is your diagnosis? Impression smear of liver tissue from a rabbit. *Vet Clin Pathol* 30: 57–61.

68 Guzman, R.E., Ehrhart, E.J., Wasson, K., and Andrews, J.J. (2000). Primary hepatic hemangiosarcoma with pulmonary metastasis in a New Zealand White rabbit. *J Vet Diagn Invest* 12: 284–286.

69 Kusumi, R.K. and Plouffe, J.F. (1980). Cerebrospinal fluid glucose and protein values in normal rabbits. *Lab Anim* 14: 41–42.

70 Curiel, T.J., Perfect, J.R., and Durack, D.T. (1982). Leukocyte subpopulations in cerebrospinal fluid of normal rabbits. *Lab Anim Sci* 32: 622–624.

71 Reed, S.D., Shaw, S., and Evans, D.E. (2009). Spinal lymphoma and pulmonary filariasis in a pet domestic rabbit (*Oryctolagus cuniculus domesticus*). *J Vet Diagn Invest* 21: 253–256.

72 Di Girolamo, N., Bongiovanni, L., Ferro, S. et al. (2017). Cystoscopic diagnosis of polypoid cystitis in two pet rabbits. *J Am Vet Med Assoc* 251: 84–89.

73 Fuentealba, I.C., Mahoney, N.T., Shadduck, J.A. et al. (1992). Hepatic lesions in rabbits infected with *Encephalitozoon cuniculi* administered per rectum. *Vet Pathol* 29: 536–540.

74 Wesonga, H.O. and Munda, M. (1992). Rabbit encephalitozoonosis in Kenya. *Lab Anim* 26: 219–221.

75 Lipman, N.S., Murphy, J.C., and Newcomer, C.E. (1985). Polycythemia in a New Zealand White rabbit with an embryonal nephroma. *J Am Vet Med Assoc* 187: 1255–1256.

76 Hassan, J., Katic, N., Klang, A. et al. (2012). Treatment of nephroblastoma with polycythaemia by nephrectomy in a rabbit. *Vet Rec* 170: 465.

77 Kaufmann, A.F. and Quist, K.D. (1970). Spontaneous renal carcinoma in a New Zealand white rabbit. *Lab Anim Care* 20: 530–532.

78 Durfee, W.J., Masters, W.G., Montgomery, C.A. et al. (1999). Spontaneous renal cell carcinoma in a New Zealand White rabbit. *Contemp Top Lab Anim Sci* 38: 89–91.

79 Tsiligianni, T., Saratsi, A., Besenfelder, U. et al. (2004). The use of cytological examination of vaginal smears (CEVS) in the selection of rabbits for superovulation. *Theriogenology* 61: 989–995.

80 Saito, K., Nakanishi, M., and Hasegawa, A. (2002). Uterine disorders diagnosed by ventrotomy in 47 rabbits. *J Vet Med Sci* 64: 495–497.

81 Johnson, J.H. and Wolf, A.M. (1993). Ovarian abscesses and pyometra in a domestic rabbit. *J Am Vet Med Assoc* 203: 667–669.

82 Künzel, F., Grinninger, P., Shibly, S. et al. (2015). Uterine disorders in 50 pet rabbits. *J Am Anim Hosp Assoc* 51: 8–14.

83 Hofmann, J.R.J. and Hixson, C.J. (1986). Amyloid A protein deposits in a rabbit with pyometra. *J Am Vet Med Assoc* 189: 1155–1156.

84 Soave, O.A., Dominguez, J., and Doak, R.L. (1977). *Moraxella bovis*-induced metritis and septicemia in a rabbit. *J Am Vet Med Assoc* 171: 972–973.

85 Heatley, J.J. and Smith, A.N. (2004). Spontaneous neoplasms of lagomorphs. *Vet Clin North Am Exot Anim Pract* 7: 561–577.

86 Harkness, J. and Wagner, J. (1995). *The Biology and Medicine of Rabbits and Rodents*, 4e. Philadelphia, PA: Williams and Wilkins.

87 Raftery, A. (1998). Uterine adenocarcinoma in pet rabbits. *Vet Rec* 142: 704.

88 Irizarry-Rovira, A.R., Lennox, A.M., and Ramos-Vara, J.A. (2008). Granular cell tumor in the testis of a rabbit: cytologic, histologic, immunohistochemical, and electron microscopic characterization. *Vet Pathol* 45: 73–77.

89 Anderson, W.I., Car, B.D., Kenny, K., and Schlafer, D.H. (1990). Bilateral testicular seminoma in a New Zealand white rabbit (*Oryctolagus cuniculus*). *Lab Anim Sci* 40: 420–421.

90 Banco, B., Stefanello, D., Giudice, C. et al. (2012). Metastasizing testicular seminoma in a pet rabbit. *J Vet Diagn Invest* 24: 608–611.

91 Alexandre, N., Branco, S., Soares, T.F. et al. (2010). Bilateral testicular seminoma in a rabbit (*Oryctolagus cuniculus*). *J Exot Pet Med* 19: 304–308.

92 Meier, H., Myers, D.D., Fox, R.R., and Laird, C.W. (1970). Occurrence, pathological features, and propagation of gonadal teratomas in inbred mice and in rabbits. *Cancer Res* 30: 30–34.

93 Perkins, S.E., Murphy, J.C., and Alroy, J. (1996). Eosinophil granulocytic sarcoma in a New Zealand white rabbit. *Vet Pathol* 33: 89–91.

58

Cattle

Amy L. Weeden, K. Lisa Hulme-Moir, and Julie Tomlinson

Introduction

Clinical Settings

Cattle are primarily raised for beef and dairy production with some individuals also kept as show animals, pets, rodeo animals, or breeding stock. Herd size, intensity of production, and management practices vary significantly across different geographic locations. In general, emphasis is placed on herd health, but individual cow medicine is still important, particularly with high-value breeding animals.

Applications and Collection Methods

Unless otherwise specified below, clinical applications, collection techniques, and sample handling are similar to those described in other large animal species such as horses.

Body Fluid Samples

Airway Fluid Cytology

This is employed for investigation of bovine respiratory disease. Because infection is the primary concern, samples are often used for bacterial culture or viral diagnostics (e.g. virus isolation, fluorescent antibody testing, polymerase chain reaction). The technique of choice is a matter of opinion and will depend on equipment availability and cost to perform. Techniques described include endoscopically guided bronchoalveolar lavage (BAL), transtracheal wash, or BAL via blind intranasal intubation.[1,2] Sample handling recommendations are similar to the horse (Chapter 26).

Cerebrospinal Fluid (CSF)

As outbreaks of central nervous system (CNS) disease can devastate a herd, it is important to identify or at least categorize the etiology so appropriate management can be employed. Infectious, toxic, metabolic, or nutritional CNS disease is more likely to have an impact at the herd level, as opposed to conditions such as trauma or neoplasia. Lumbosacral (LS) sampling is typically performed as this site requires less restraint and is associated with less risk than atlanto-occipital (AO) collection. Ultrasound can be used to facilitate collection from the AO site.[3] The LS site is accessed midway between L5 and S2, which are the last palpable lumbar and the first palpable sacral dorsal spinous processes, respectively.[4] Calves can be restrained in sternal recumbency with hips flexed, while ambulatory adult cattle are restrained standing in stocks.[4] Local anesthetic should be administered. A 1.5- or 2-in., 19 G spinal needle for calves and a 4-in. 18 G needle for adult cattle should be used.[5]

Abdominal Fluid

Peritoneal fluid can be collected from the right or left cranioventral and caudoventral abdominal quadrants in adult cattle. Midline collection is avoided because puncture of the rumen is likely. Common sites include 5–7 cm cranial and 4 cm medial to the subcutaneous abdominal (milk) vein foramen or 10 cm cranial and 10 cm to the right of the umbilicus.[6,7] Samples also can be obtained from the right or left flanks, cranial to the base of the udder. Due to the frequency of localized peritonitis, the site chosen for abdominocentesis should be selected based on the suspected location of abdominal disease.[8,9] Ultrasound can be used for targeted sampling.[10] Inflammatory or neoplastic effusions can appear heterogeneous on ultrasound, and samples should be obtained from both the sediment and more hypoechoic areas of the effusion.

In adult cattle, abdominocentesis is aseptically performed using 16–18 G, 1.5–3-in. needles, or similar length intravenous or metal teat cannulas. Use of stocks and a tail jack is usually sufficient for restraint. Accidental enterocentesis is more likely when using needles, although this rarely results in complications for the patient.[8] Use of a teat cannula requires local anesthesia and a small stab incision through the skin and muscle fascial layers. Fluid is collected

Veterinary Cytology, First Edition. Edited by Leslie C. Sharkey, M. Judith Radin, and Davis Seelig.

directly into ethylenediaminetetraacetic acid (EDTA) and plain sterile tubes and processed as described for other species. Slides should be made immediately after collection to preserve cell morphology and avoid other *in vitro* changes.

In calves, peritoneal fluid is collected with the animal in left lateral recumbency.[6,11] Unless moribund or severely weakened, sedation is necessary. Sampling should be avoided for at least the first hour after feeding to minimize the risk of accidental abomasal puncture.[12] Abdominocentesis in calves can be performed 4 cm to the right of the midline at the level of the umbilicus, slightly dorsal and caudal to the umbilicus or in the right inguinal area. A technique involving placement of a 14-guage intravenous catheter after local anesthesia and stab incision has been described, which successfully collected up to 1.5 mL of fluid from clinically healthy calves.[11,12]

Pleural and Pericardial Fluid

Thoracocentesis is performed at the 6th or 7th intercostal space, below the suspected fluid line. The height of the fluid line can be located using percussion or ultrasound.[1] If this is not possible, a blind tap can be performed in the 6th intercostal space, just dorsal to the costochondral junction.[13]

Pericardiocentesis is used for the diagnosis of traumatic pericarditis, cardiac lymphoma, and idiopathic hemorrhagic pericarditis and may be used as a palliative treatment.[14–17] Cattle diagnosed with idiopathic hemorrhagic pericarditis have been reported to survive several years after treatment of the pericardial effusion.[14] The procedure is performed under ultrasound guidance at the level of left 5th intercostal space using a 16–18 G, 3.5–5.0-in. spinal needle or a 3-in. teat cannula.[1,18] Using a needle has a higher risk of irritating or lacerating the ventricle, and continuous ECG monitoring is recommended. Unlike a teat cannula, local anesthesia and a stab incision are not required. With both methods, fluid may be collected via gravity or using an administration set and syringe. Pericardial and pleural samples are handled and processed as described for other veterinary species.

Rumen Fluid

Analysis of rumen fluid has not been widely applied to general clinical practice due to the time-consuming nature of sample collection and the need for immediate analysis.[19] It remains a valuable tool for assessing fermentative disorders of the rumen at both the individual and herd level. One of the key challenges of collecting rumen fluid is the avoidance of saliva contamination, which increases fluid pH, a key indicator used for the diagnosis of acute, and subacute rumen acidosis (SARA). Specialized stomach tubes or rumen probes are available to minimize saliva contamination and help direct the tube into the ventral rumen.[19] Selective sampling of the ventrocaudal sack further helps to standardize analysis as pH can vary in different compartments of the rumen.[20] Rumenocentesis through the abdominal wall into the ventrocaudal sack of the rumen is an alternative method of sample collection. Rumenocentesis eliminates the risk of saliva contamination and ensures accurate sampling of the ventrocaudal sack but carries the risk of adverse effects such as abscess formation, hematomas, or localized peritonitis, which occur in up to 5% of cattle.[21] The procedure is performed by placing a 14 G 3-in. needle approximately halfway between the costochondral junction of the last rib and the top of the stifle (approximately 12–15 cm caudal to the last rib). Additional care is required when sampling dry cows because the uterus lies close to the rumen in late gestation.[22] The site is shaved and surgically prepared before the needle is pushed in two movements, first through the abdominal wall and then into the ventral sack of the rumen. The procedure is performed with the animal under physical or chemical restraint, with or without local anesthesia.[21] When using ruminal fluid analysis for the diagnosing and monitoring SARA, both sample timing and the choice of animals to be sampled (number to be sampled in a herd at risk and stage of lactation) are important. Sampling time is dependent on the diet of the herd, and guidelines have been provided by multiple investigators.[22,23]

Analysis of rumen fluid involves a combination of the following: (i) pH measurement, (ii) subjective assessment of color and odor, (ii) direct microscopy of a drop of rumen fluid for protozoa type and activity (Figure 58.1), (iv) Gram

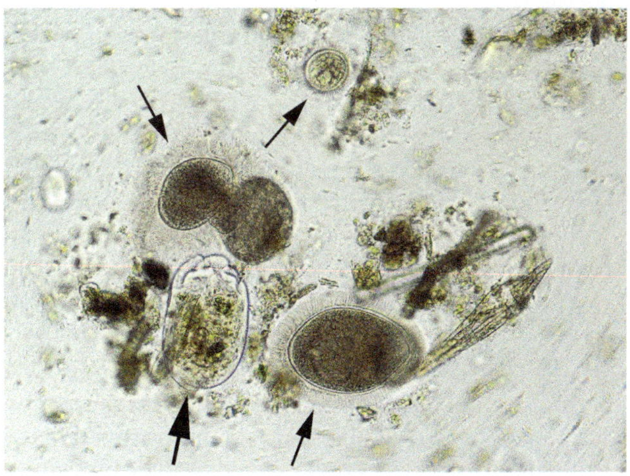

Figure 58.1 Direct examination of rumen fluid. Healthy rumen fluid should contain a mixture of two main types of protozoa. Entodiniomorphs (large black arrow) have cilia on one side of their soma and are medium to large in size. Holotrichs (small black arrows) have many cilia around their entire external surface. Entodiniomorphs are more sensitive to changes in pH and will decrease in number when the rumen pH falls (Unstained, 200×. *Source:* Image courtesy of Judith Radin).

Textbox 58.1 Methylene Blue Reduction Test and Sediment Activity Time Methods

Methylene Blue Reduction Test[24]

1) 0.5 mL of 0.03% methylene blue solution is mixed with 10 mL of fresh rumen fluid, which has been held at body or room temperature.
2) Using a second tube containing rumen fluid only for a comparison, the time to decolorization is measured. This is judged as complete when the majority of the fluid is decolorized. In some cases, a rim of blue can still be present at the surface but is still considered complete if most of the fluid is decolorized.
3) If the rumen fluid contains large amounts of fine particles, it may be sieved/strained before performing the test.
4) The reduction time of normal active rumen fluid collected from cattle on a mixed hay and grain diet is less than three minutes. Cows on mainly hay and a small amount of grain can have a reduction time of three to six minutes.

Sediment Activity Time[24,25]

1) An aliquot of freshly collected rumen fluid is held at body temperature, and the time taken for small particles to settle out and a gray-white foamy layer containing larger fibrous particles to form on the surface is measured.
2) Depending on diet and time after feeding, this takes four to eight minutes to occur in normal active rumen fluid. More rapid sedimentation is seen with inactive fermentation. Sedimentation is delayed with high concentrate pelleted diet or foamy bloat.

Collection of rumen fluid using a stomach tube with only small holes or straining the fluid will affect the formation of the surface layer as large fibrous particles will be excluded.

stain to determine proportion of Gram-negative rods to Gram-positive cocci, (v) methylene blue reduction test, (vi) sedimentation–flotation test, and (vii) measurement of chloride concentration. The pH must be measured immediately on collection and other parameters analyzed within a short time. The methylene blue reduction test and the sedimentation–flotation tests are described in Textbox 58.1.[24,25]

Solid Tissues

Lymphoid Tissue

Assessment of the lymphatic system is generally limited to examination of the lymph nodes that are accessible during a clinical exam. This includes the mandibular, subparotid, retropharyngeal, prescapular, prefemoral, supramammary, and ileofemoral (via rectal palpation) nodes.[26] Due to the bovine's thick skin and lymph node capsule, a stab incision requiring local anesthetic and ultrasound guidance may improve yield from mildly enlarged nodes.[27]

Liver

Liver aspirates can be obtained blindly by passing a 22 G 6-in. needle through an 18 G guide needle that is inserted just cranial to the right 12th rib, approximately two thirds of the way up the rib.[1] The needle should be directed slightly cranially and advanced and withdrawn a number of times into the liver under suction before release of the pressure and withdrawal of the needle. Targeted sampling of specific sites (e.g. abscesses, tumors, gall bladder) can also be performed with ultrasound guidance.[28] A specific technique for the aspiration of bile from the gallbladder for diagnosis of cholecystitis and fascioliasis has been described.[28,29] Aspiration of hepatic abscesses or bile is performed using a 20 G 3.5-in. spinal needle. It is important that the stylet is in place for both insertion and withdrawal from abscesses to minimize contamination of the abdomen.

Cholecystocentesis is usually performed through the right 10th or 11th intercostal space where the gall bladder is most obvious. If sampling is being performed to diagnose fascioliasis, infusion of the gall bladder with 10 mL of isotonic saline followed by immediate re-aspiration is required. The collected sample is refrigerated overnight before the sediment is examined for eggs.

Reproductive

Uterine cytology is a potentially underutilized tool for the diagnosis of subclinical and clinical metritis in cattle (see Chapter 43). These conditions have a significant economic impact due to associated poor reproductive performance. Endometrial cytology samples from cattle can be collected by a guarded cotton swab, uterine lavage, or cytobrush. Results of a comparison study in dairy cattle suggested that the cytobrush technique is a more consistent and reliable method than lavage for evaluation of metritis in postpartum dairy cows.[30] In another study, both swabs and aspirates with plastic uterine pipettes yielded adequate samples for cervical and uterine cytology.[31]

Techniques for semen collection in bulls include the artificial vagina (AV), electroejaculation, and transrectal massage (TRM) of the accessory sexual glands (see Chapter 41). Lower concentrations of spermatozoa and lower percentages of abnormal sperm may be obtained from TRM compared with AV samples, and semen evaluation should be interpreted in context of the collection method.[32]

Conditions Diagnosed by Cytology

Skin and Subcutis

Cytologic techniques can be used to diagnose a similar range of cutaneous conditions as in other species, including dermatophilosis, acariasis, and cutaneous neoplasms.

Infectious and Inflammatory Conditions

Dermatophilosis, also called "rain scald," is a common skin infection caused by *Dermatophilus congolensis* (Figure 58.2). Diagnosis can be made on imprints of crusted tufts of hair by detecting chains of coccoid Gram-positive bacteria arranged in parallel rows ("railroad tracks").[33]

Dermatophytosis occurs commonly in dairy calves or in group housing situations. *Trichophyton verrucosum* is the most common pathogen with fewer instances of *Trichophyton mentagrophytes* and other dermatophytes. Cytologic description of dermatophytosis can be found in Chapter 11. Lesions are similar to those described in other species and are often found on the muzzle, periocular region, ears, neck, and trunk. Diagnosis is often made via clinical signs, dermatophyte culture, potassium hydroxide preparations of material obtained via skin scrapes, or skin biopsies. Scrapings of skin and hair, especially from the margins of the lesions, can be cleared with a 20% potassium hydroxide solution and examined microscopically for the presence of characteristic fungal mycelia and spores (often adherent to hair shafts).[33]

Cattle can become infected with mange mites including *Chorioptes bovis* (Figure 58.3), *Demodex* spp., *Sarcoptes* spp., and *Psoroptes ovis* (see Chapter 11 for more detail). Marked pruritus is typically observed with all except *Demodex*. Diagnosis can be made via skin scrape (deep skin scrapes are required for all except *Chorioptes*). *Sarcoptes* and *Psoroptes* are both reportable diseases in North America.[33]

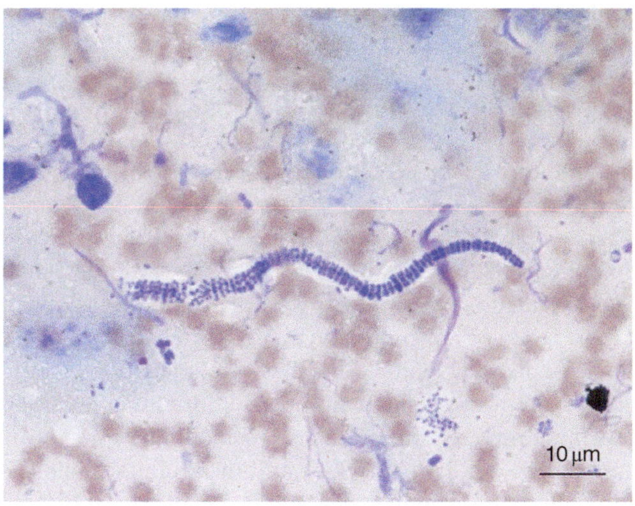

Figure 58.2 Imprint of a crusty lesion on the skin of a cow with dermatophilosis. Parallel chains of coccoid *D. congolensis* bacteria ("railroad track" pattern) are in the center along with keratin, nuclear debris, and other bacteria (Leishman stain. *Source:* Image courtesy of Jenni Donald).

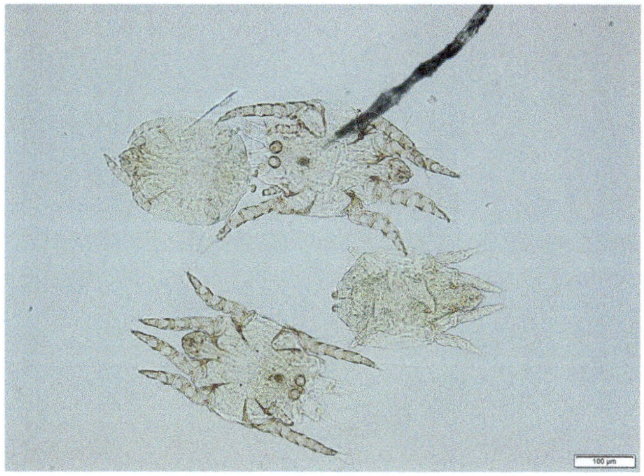

Figure 58.3 Skin scraping from a bovid. *C. bovis* (male and female mites pictured) are approximately 200–300 µm, round, with short, unsegmented stalks bearing the suckers on each leg. Males tend to be larger than females and have copulatory suckers on the posterior end that resemble "eyes" (Unstained. *Source:* Image courtesy of Erin Burton).

Stephanofilaria stilesi is a common cause of filarial dermatitis in cattle in the United States with lesions often located along the ventral midline. Fine-needle aspiration (FNA) may reveal microfilariae and eosinophilic inflammation, although generally histopathology is required for definitive diagnosis.[33] Adults (3–6 mm in length) and microfilariae (50 µm in length) can be found in deep skin scrapings of the lesions. Multiple scrapings may be required. The tissue obtained can be minced, soaked in isotonic saline, and then examined microscopically.[34]

Neoplasia

Cutaneous neoplasms are relatively common in cattle, with lymphoma, fibropapilloma, and squamous cell carcinoma being the three most frequent.[33]

Round Cell Tumors

Cutaneous lymphoma (Figure 58.4) usually occurs in cattle 6–24 months of age is a progressive disease and is not associated with bovine leukemia virus (BLV) infection. Cutaneous lymphoma is characterized by multifocal nodular skin masses that vary from 1 to 10 cm in diameter and sometimes includes lymphadenopathy. Isolated skin tumors also can occur in adult cattle with BLV-associated lymphoma. Similar to other species, FNA can provide a definitive diagnosis.[33,35] One retrospective study revealed

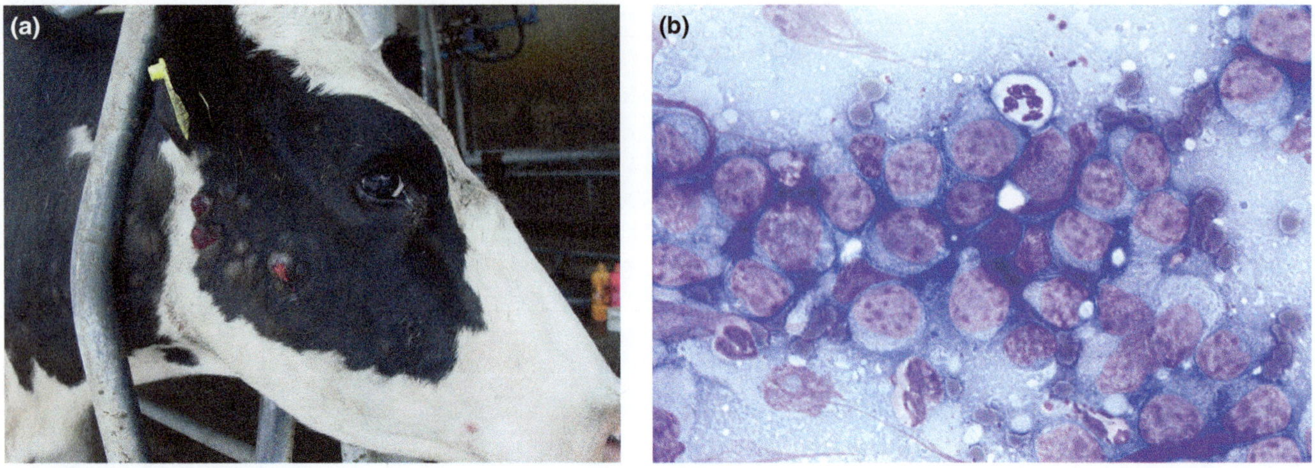

Figure 58.4 Cutaneous lymphoma. (a) Multifocal to coalescing cutaneous nodules over the face and neck of a cow caused by lymphoma. (b) Aspirate cytology from the same case showing monomorphic, intermediate to large immature lymphocytes with coarse chromatin (Diff-Quik, 1000×. *Source:* Images courtesy of Keith Thompson).

the diffuse large cleaved and diffuse large cell subtypes to be predominant, comprising 65.9% of all bovine lymphomas[36] (see Chapter 27 for more information on lymphoma).

Cutaneous melanoma is common in cattle, and the majority (80%) of tumors are benign. Cutaneous melanocytomas predominantly occur in young gray, black, or red cattle.[37] There have been a few reports in the literature of melanomas that have been locally invasive or metastasized to lymph nodes or lungs, but generally surgical excision is successful.[37,38] These tumors are typically heavily pigmented and consist of a mixture of spindloid and epithelioid melanocytes admixed with melanophages.[38] More detail on melanoma can be found in Chapter 15.

Mast cell tumors are uncommon in cattle and have a cytologic appearance similar to other species (see Chapter 13). They generally occur in adult animals as solitary or multiple cutaneous nodules and can metastasize to lymph nodes, lung, liver, spleen, kidney, and muscle.[33,39,40] In a study of 11 cases of mast cell tumors in cattle at slaughter, 3 animals had evidence of metastatic disease.[40]

Epithelial Tumors

Squamous cell carcinoma occurs as a proliferative, often ulcerated lesion at mucocutaneous junctions and on sparsely haired, unpigmented skin including the eyelid, vulva, and pinnae.[37] It also has been reported at branding sites.[41] Cytology can be used to confirm the diagnosis by employing similar criteria as applied in other species, primarily dyssynchrony of nuclear and cytoplasmic maturation in squamous epithelial cells (see Chapters 12 and 21). Significant inflammation is often present in these lesions and can complicate interpretation. Other cutaneous epithelial neoplasms including basal cell tumor, trichoepithelioma, sebaceous adenoma and adenocarcinoma, and apocrine gland carcinoma have rarely been reported in cattle.[37] Cytologic findings would be similar to those described in other species (see Chapter 12).

Mesenchymal Tumors

Fibroma is a common cutaneous tumor in cattle. Other mesenchymal neoplasms including fibrosarcoma, myxoma, myxosarcoma, hemangioma, hemangiosarcoma (Figure 58.5), hemangiopericytoma, lymphangioma, neurofibroma, schwannoma, leiomyosarcoma, lipoma, infiltrating lipoma, and rhabdomyosarcoma have rarely been reported.[37,42–45] More detail can be found on these tumors in Chapters 12 and 16.

Eye

Infectious bovine keratoconjunctivitis is a common, highly contagious disease caused by the blunt-ended Gram-negative bacillus *Moraxella bovis*.[26] Coinfection with *Mycoplasma* spp. and infectious bovine rhinotracheitis virus might predispose to or exacerbate the disease process.[26,46] Cytology of conjunctival scrapings can reveal dysplastic or necrotic epithelium that exfoliates individually rather than in sheets, large numbers of inflammatory cells (predominantly neutrophils and eosinophils with fewer plasma cells and lymphocytes), and intracellular diplobacilli.[47] Puncture wounds, lacerations, or migration of foreign bodies (e.g. grass awns) can lead to orbital cellulitis or retrobulbar abscess. FNA can reveal large numbers of neutrophils with bacterial sepsis. *Trueperella pyogenes* (formerly *Arcanobacterium pyogenes*), a Gram-positive,

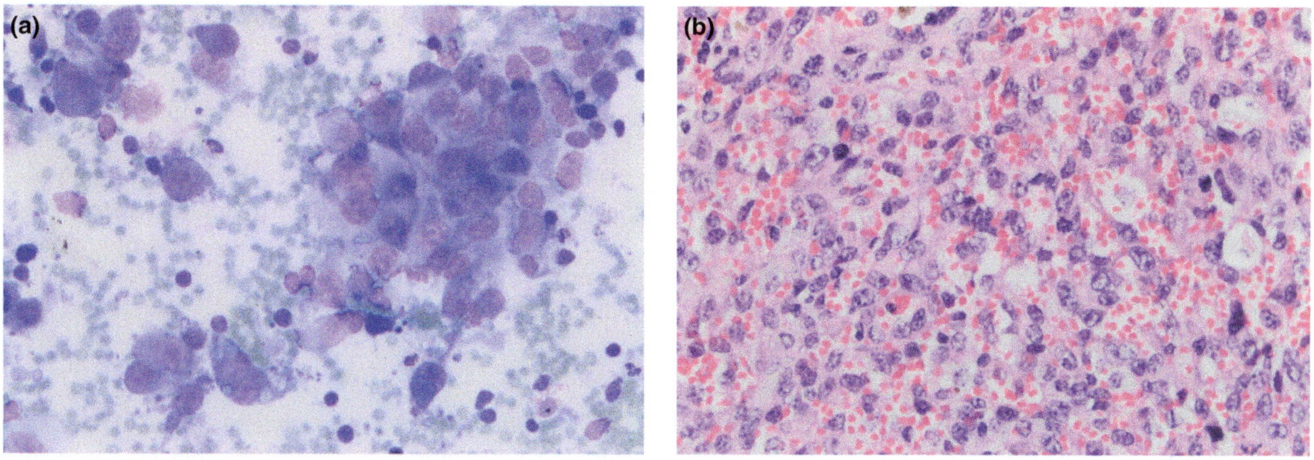

Figure 58.5 Hemangiosarcoma that infiltrated the facial structures of a cow. (a) FNA cytology is characterized by atypical spindle cells found individually or in disorganized clusters within a hemodilute background. The cells have coarse chromatin with multiple prominent nucleoli. Some cells exhibit binucleation or erythrophagia (Leishman stain, 500×). (b) Histopathology of the same lesion demonstrates irregular blood-filled spaces that are lined by pleomorphic spindle cells with a high mitotic rate (hematoxylin & eosin, 500×).

non-spore forming, short rod-shaped bacterium, is a common isolate from orbital abscesses.[33,48]

Ocular squamous cell carcinoma is one of the most common tumors in cattle (Figure 58.6). It typically occurs in cattle ≥5 years old and usually involves the nictitating membrane, medial canthus region, lower eyelid margin, or lateral limbus.[26] Cytology can be useful in diagnosis of early squamous cell carcinoma lesions. One study revealed cytologic and histologic agreement in 90 of 104 cases examined.[26] Changes suggestive of squamous cell carcinoma included condensed chromatin, prominent nucleoli, anisonucleosis, bizarre mitosis, multinucleation, and increased N:C.[49]

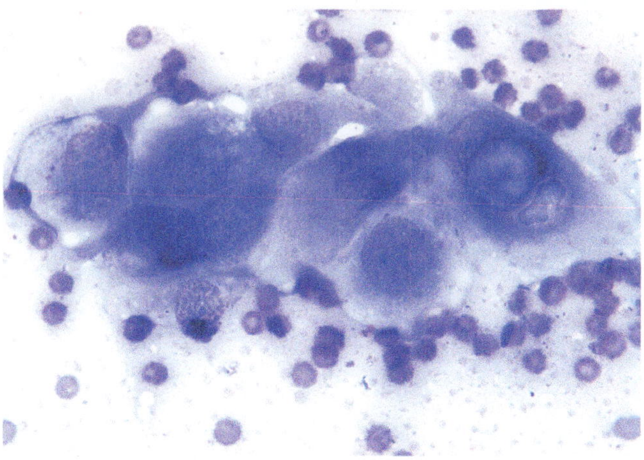

Figure 58.6 Imprint of an ocular squamous cell carcinoma from a cow. A small cluster of atypical squamous cells exhibits variable nuclear to cytoplasmic ratios (N:C) and moderate anisokaryosis. Nuclei contain coarse open chromatin. The cell on the right exhibits emperipolesis; a neutrophil is shown within the cytoplasm of the epithelial cell. This is a common finding in cytology of squamous cell carcinoma (Diff-Quik, 1000×).

Lymphoma is the most common orbital tumor in dairy cattle. Tumors may be unilateral or bilateral and can result in exophthalmos, exposure keratitis, or proptosis. Intraocular invasion is rare, and conjunctival involvement has been reported.[33,50,51] FNA or biopsy may be difficult if the lesion is deep within the orbit. Cytologic evaluation of neoplastic tissue after globe removal may reveal a homogenous lymphoid population.[52]

Musculoskeletal

Synovial fluid evaluation in cattle can be an important component of lameness evaluation. Indications and collection techniques have been recently reviewed.[53] Normal synovial fluid in cattle should contain fewer than 400 leukocytes/mm^3 ($0.4 \times 10^3/\mu L$).[54] Mononuclear cells should predominate with neutrophils comprising <15% of the nucleated cell population in normal joints.[54] A study of repeated arthrocentesis and a single joint lavage in calves demonstrated a transient inflammatory response in the form of increased leukocyte, neutrophil, and monocyte counts; however, four-day sampling intervals did not induce a significant effect.[55] In one retrospective study of cattle with naturally occurring joint disease, those with infectious arthritis had a higher median total protein (TP) concentration, total nucleated cell count (TNCC), neutrophil percentage, and neutrophil count with a lower mononuclear percentage than those with noninfectious arthritis. Conditions in the noninfectious arthritis category included trauma, degenerative joint disease, developmental orthopedic disorders, and periarticular infection. This study reported a very high likelihood for septic arthritis in joint fluids with TP > 4.5 g/dL, TNCC > 25 000 cells/μL, neutrophil count > 20 000 cells/μL, and > 80% neutrophils.[56] Results from a study of experimentally induced septic arthritis in calves support these findings.[57]

Actinomyces bovis is the causative agent of lumpy jaw and results in pyogranulomatous osteomyelitis affecting the mandible or less commonly the maxilla of cattle (Figure 58.7). Characteristic of this infection are pale yellow 1–2 mm sulfur granules containing central Gram-positive filamentous forms with some bacillary and coccoid forms and peripheral club-shaped Gram-negative bodies.[26]

A single case of rhabdomyosarcoma near the stifle of a cow has been reported. Cytologic features included a highly atypical pleomorphic spindle cell population with multinucleated giant cells and a population of small round cells.[45] Muscle origin was confirmed by positive histochemical and immunohistochemical staining with periodic acid Schiff, MyoD1, myoglobin, vimentin, and nonspecific muscle actin. Based on the immunohistochemistry, the round cells were a combination of T lymphocytes and myogenic precursors.[45]

Respiratory

Airway cytology findings in general are nonspecific for causes of airway inflammation, and diagnosis of a particular

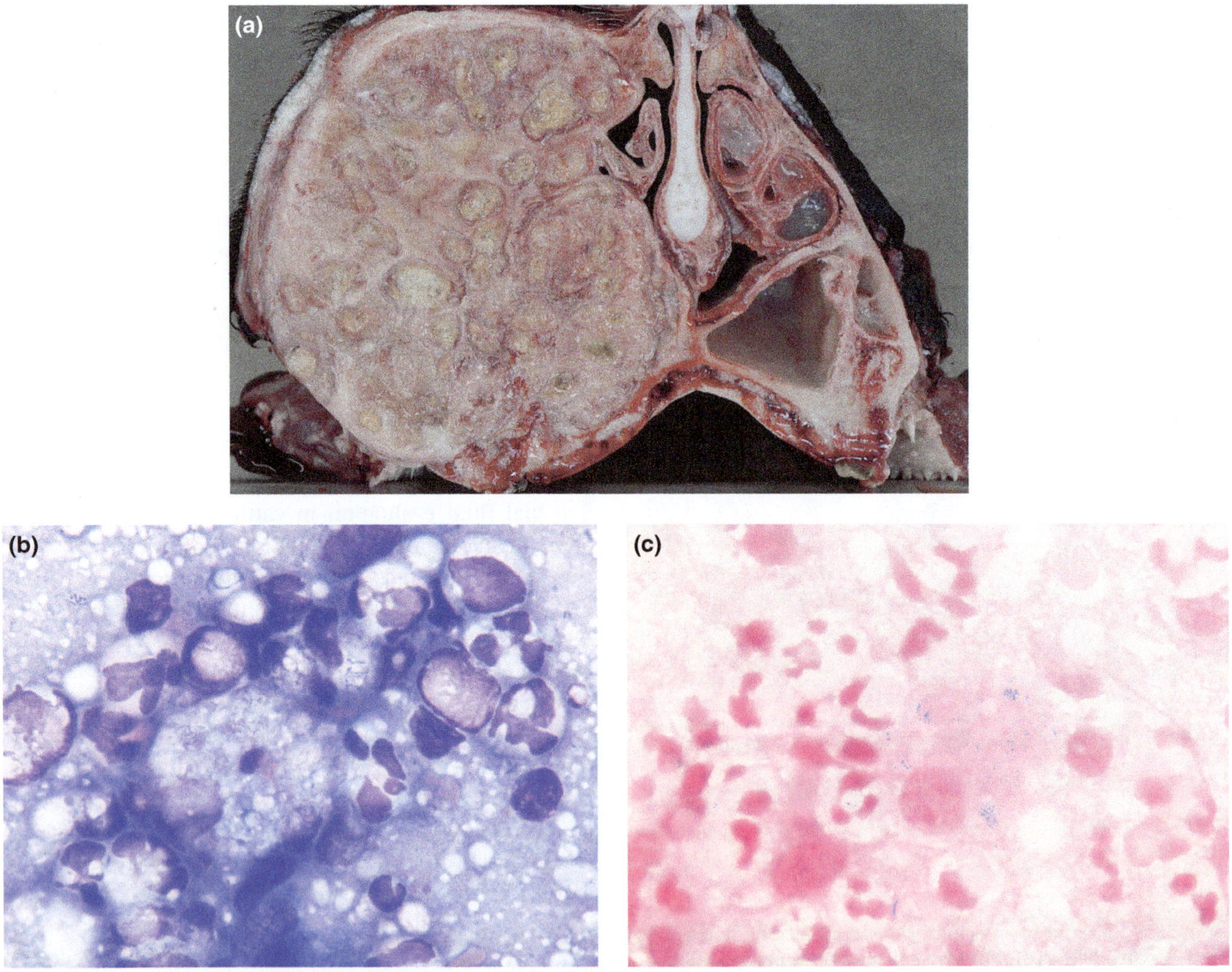

Figure 58.7 *Actinomyces bovis* osteomyelitis lesion from a cow. (a) Gross image of a proliferative bone lesion (lumpy jaw) caused by granulomatous osteomyelitis due to actinomycosis (*Source:* Image courtesy of Richard Irvine). (b) FNA of the lesion shows foamy macrophages and degenerate neutrophils with intracellular and extracellular, variably sized filamentous bacilli (May-Grünwald–Giemsa, 1000×). (c) The bacilli stain Gram-positive within a background of inflammatory cells (Gram stain, 1000×).

agent frequently relies on other means. Selection of animals for respiratory fluid analysis may depend on the expected cause of disease. If virology of the airway sample is an intended part of the diagnostic process, selection of cases in early stages of disease is recommended (e.g. clinical normal except for an elevated rectal temperature) because some methods of virus detection are not accurate in individuals with advanced disease.[2] Note that clinical disease might not correlate with the presence of inflammatory changes on BAL. In a study of feedlot calves, many of the control calves had BAL differential counts compatible with inflammation.[58]

The available literature on airway cytology in cattle primarily involves calves. Differential counts of BAL fluid from normal calves reveal a predominance of macrophages followed by lymphocytes with a lower percentage of neutrophils (<25%) and rare eosinophils (<1%).[59,60] A decreased macrophage to neutrophil ratio is expected with pneumonia.[58,60] Eosinophil and lymphocyte percentages do not differ significantly between normal calves and those with respiratory inflammation.[58,60] A recent study evaluating sensitivity and specificity of BAL fluid cytology and ultrasound for detection of subclinical lung lesions in dairy calves discovered that BAL neutrophil percentages in histologically confirmed completely normal lungs are quite low (median of 1%) and suggested a cut point of >4% to diagnose subclinical respiratory disease.[61] Granulomatous aspiration pneumonia after presumed intratracheal administration of kaolin pectin in a Holstein was characterized by the presence of amorphous basophilic extracellular material, and many small polygonal to irregular clear refractive crystals found extracellular and in macrophages.[62] Immunocytochemistry can be performed on respiratory washes and has been utilized to diagnose bovine respiratory syncytial virus in a calf.[63] As in other species, an increased eosinophil percentage may indicate hypersensitivity or lungworm. Observing *Dictyocaulus viviparus* ova or larvae in a BAL cytology would be diagnostic of infection.

Lymphatic

Lymphadenitis cases reported in the literature include a single case of mesenteric caseous lymphadenitis in a calf in India associated with *Corynebacterium pseudotuberculosis*.[64] Cytology revealed both non-degenerate and degenerate neutrophils with fewer small lymphocytes and bacterial bacilli. Intraneutrophilic bacteria were observed as were the typical Chinese letter-like arrangements.[64] Zygomycotic lymphadenitis was observed over a 12-month period in 194 of 198 California feedlot steers with enlarged lymph nodes (predominantly mesenteric) noted at slaughter (0.04% of total cattle slaughtered).[65] Cytology was not performed, but based on histopathology, anticipated cytologic findings would include granulomatous inflammation with broad, irregularly branching, nonseptate hyphae.[65] *Trypanosoma* spp. were observed in a prescapular lymph node aspirate from a dairy cow in Brazil with severe non-regenerative anemia and leukopenia.[66]

Lymph node cytology can facilitate diagnosis of metastatic neoplasia (e.g. squamous cell carcinoma) or lymphoid neoplasia. Bovine lymphosarcoma (leukosis) is the most common type of neoplasm affecting cattle and is classified into enzootic bovine leukosis (EBL) and sporadic bovine leukosis. The enzootic form typically affects adult cattle and is associated with BLV infection. Peripheral lymphadenopathy is a common clinical manifestation of EBL. In one study, FNA of enlarged peripheral lymph nodes had a sensitivity of 41–53%, specificity of 100%, and a positive predictive value of 100% for EBL; however, specific diagnostic criteria were not described.[27] The sporadic form is much less common, is not associated with BLV infection, typically affects younger animals, and is divided into three main forms. The cutaneous form presents as generalized skin nodules in animals that are 1–3 years of age. The nodules can regress but often recur as generalized lymphoma. The juvenile form typically affects calves <6 months of age and presents as a peripheral lymphadenopathy. The thymic form typically occurs in animals that are 6–24 months of age and presents as a large, firm swelling in the ventral neck region.[67]

Gastrointestinal and Liver

Rumen Fluid Analysis

The characteristics of rumen fluid from healthy cattle and those with various conditions affecting rumen fermentation are provided in Table 58.1. Controversy exists over the exact diagnostic criteria used for diagnosis of SARA, and there is ongoing research to find more accurate methods that can be easily applied in a primary care environment.[22,68,71] Chloride measurement of rumen fluid can be useful in diagnosing decreased pH due to abomasal reflux, keeping in mind the pre-analytical factors influencing results that were discussed in the previous section (see *Collection Method*). Abomasal reflux can be seen with left and right displacement of the abomasum, abomasitis, abomasal lymphoma, vagal indigestion, and peritonitis.[24]

Fecal Smears

Examination of fecal smears stained with Ziehl–Neelsen can be used to diagnose paratuberculosis and cryptosporidiosis.[72,73] A sample is considered positive for paratuberculosis if two groups of three acid-fast *Mycobacteria* are

Table 58.1 Characteristics of rumen fluid in healthy cattle and those with various ruminal disturbances.[24,25,68,69]

	Color[a]	Odor	Viscosity	pH	Protozoa	Bacteria	Methylene blue reduction test (minutes)	Flotation–sedimentation test
Healthy rumen function	Green (pasture) Yellow brown (silage) Light brown to green (concentrate)	Aromatic	Viscous	5.5–7.0	Many large and small protozoa, occasional yeasts[b]	Gram-negative rods predominate	<3	Four to eight minutes
Acute acidosis	Milky green	Sour	Watery	<5.0	None	Gram-positive cocci predominate	>5	No flotation, rapid sedimentation
Subacute rumen acidosis	Slightly milky to brown	Sour	Slightly viscous	5.3–6.2	Many (small protozoa may predominate)	Gram-negative rods predominate	<3	No flotation, rapid sedimentation
Urea toxicity	Dark brown green	Slight ammonia	Variable	>8.0	—	Gram-negative predominate	—	Variable
Inappetence or poor quality diet		Little odor	Watery	>7.0	Decreased numbers		>5	No flotation, rapid sedimentation
Abomasal reflux[c]	Dark brown	Sour/bitter almonds	—	<5.5	—	Gram-negative predominate	—	—

[a] In healthy cattle, color is related to diet, shown in (°).
[b] Large numbers of fungal elements may suggest mycotic rumenitis.[70]
[c] Chloride concentrations >30 mEq/L is consistent with reflux.[25]

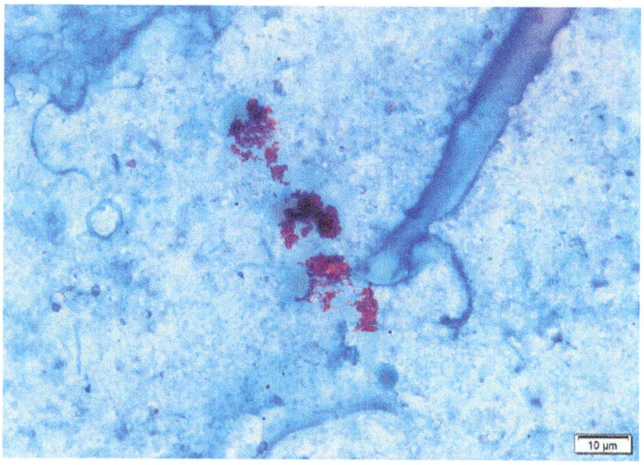

Figure 58.8 Fecal smear demonstrating clusters of acid-fast bacteria, consistent with mycobacterial infection (modified Ziehl–Neelsen, 1000×).

identified in the smear (Figure 58.8). In both diseases, the sensitivity of fecal smear examination is low to moderate compared with other diagnostic tests.[72,74] Yeasts, fungal spores, fat globules, and certain bacteria may be mistaken for cryptosporidia.[75]

Liver

As in other species, FNA can be used to diagnose hepatic lipidosis in cattle, and a grading system for cytology has been proposed.[76] Liver histology is likely more accurate for assessing the degree of lipid retention.[28,77] Ultrasound-guided FNA also can be used to diagnose hepatic abscesses and potentially hepatic neoplasia, which is rare in cattle.[78] A case report described the cytologic features of a liver aspirate from an Aberdeen Angus cow with pyrrolizidine alkaloid toxicosis, which included low cellularity with megalocytes and marked anisokaryosis.[79]

Cholecystocentesis can be performed in cattle with minimal reported adverse effects and has been used to diagnose fascioliasis and cholecystitis.[28] It may be particularly helpful for diagnosis of chronic fascioliasis where fecal samples are negative for fluke eggs. Cytological description of cholecystitis is limited to one case report from a cow with bile duct obstruction due to cholelithiasis and cholangitis.[80] Bile fluid obtained during exploratory laparotomy contained a mixed bacterial population on microscopy. Grossly, collected fluid from cholangitis cases has been described as purulent or mucoid and foul-smelling.[81,82]

Reproductive

Uterine Cytology

Physical exam with vaginal examination and transrectal palpation are typically employed for metritis detection, although a comprehensive approach using cytology with microbiology or ultrasound has been shown to improve accuracy.[83,84] A comparison of bovine uterine histopathology with cervical and endometrial cytology revealed that neutrophil density of cytologic samples from normal cows is significantly lower than those from metritis-affected cows.[31] Inflammation in endometrial cytology samples is often evaluated by calculating neutrophils as a percentage of nucleated cells including epithelial cells. Cutoff values for neutrophil percentage vary across studies with cows being evaluated at different days postpartum. In a recent study of dairy cattle, a cutoff of >6.70% neutrophils on endometrial cytology between 32 and 47 days in milk was associated with reduced odds of pregnancy.[85] A recent study in beef cattle recommended a cutoff of 5.5% for detection of subclinical metritis.[86] Additional information on uterine cytology can be found in Chapter 43.

Semen Evaluation

General information about semen evaluation is covered in Chapter 41. In a large study of Canadian bulls subjected to breeding soundness exam, 17% were deemed unsatisfactory based on sperm morphology alone, which underscores the importance of sperm evaluation.[87] Leukocyte concentration and characterization is not part of a routine breeding soundness exam. Lack of literature on this subject prompted a study of Brazilian beef bulls, which revealed an average seminal leukocyte concentration of 4.73×10^6/mL when collected by AV.[88] In Diff-Quik stained semen smears, up to 1 leukocyte/400× field was considered physiologically normal, while >5 leukocytes/400× field was associated with poor semen quality.[88] Neutrophils and macrophages with altered cell morphology (e.g. cytoplasmic granules, loss of cell contour, and nuclear degeneration) and leukocytes in clusters were observed in semen from unsatisfactory bulls but were absent in satisfactory bulls.[88]

Mammary Gland

Mastitis is the primary focus of mammary evaluation in cattle. Microbiology is the main means of diagnosis as most cases of mastitis involve bacterial agents. Multiple automated differential leukocyte count methods are available for milk with high somatic cell count (SCC) from mastitic cows.[89] A study comparing automated SCC and cytologic polymorphonuclear cell counts found that results correlated well; however, cytology did not improve assessment of bulk tank milk quality (i.e. concentrations of total protein, whey protein, casein, fat, and lactose).[90] In low SCC milk, cytology can be utilized, although flow cytometry techniques have been developed and studied for this purpose.[89,91] Results indicate that flow cytometry performs

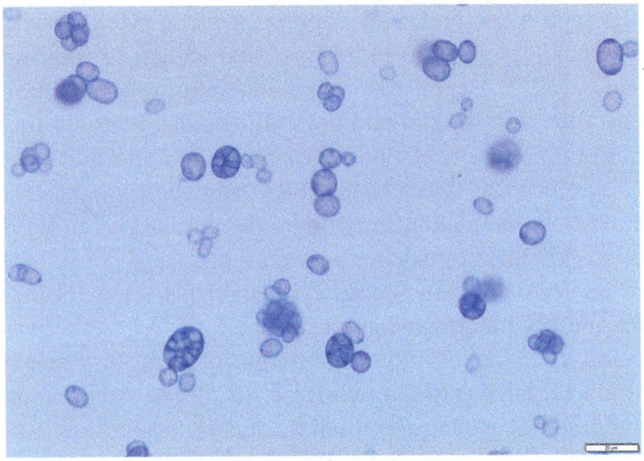

Figure 58.9 Algal mastitis in a cow. This is a new methylene blue-stained preparation from a culture plate. *Prototheca zopfii* was cultured from mastitic milk during a herd outbreak of mastitis. The organisms can be identified on aspirate cytology or cytology of cultured colonies (New Methylene Blue, 500×).

well in comparison with manual cytology methods for diagnosis of mastitis.[91]

Mastitis caused by the algal agent, *Prototheca*, can be diagnosed readily by routine cytology of mammary aspirates.[92] *Prototheca* is also isolated on conventional bacterial culture media, which then be confirmed with cytologic preparations made from cultured colonies (Figure 58.9). *Prototheca* mastitis can spread quickly through a herd; thus, rapid detection by cytologic means can be a valuable tool in outbreak situations.

Central Nervous System

Cytologic examination of the CNS is conducted primarily through evaluation of cerebrospinal fluid (CSF). In a study of clinically normal cattle, CSF protein concentrations were ≤66 mg/dL, and leukocytes were ≤9 cells/μL.[93] As in other species, lymphocytes should be the most numerous cell in the CSF with fewer large mononuclear cells and rare neutrophils (<0.18 cells/μL).[93] In general, infectious CNS diseases result in a higher median TP, erythrocyte concentration, and TNCC than noninfectious conditions, and cases of noninfectious CNS disease are more likely to have a normal CSF (Table 58.2).[94]

With neurologic listeriosis, most cattle will have a histiocytic pleocytosis with a mild increase in protein concentration.[94,95] Neonatal meningitis produces a marked inflammatory response with a predominantly neutrophilic pleocytosis.[94] In a study of neonatal calves with meningitis, the CSF findings included pleocytosis, turbidity, xanthochromia, and a high protein concentration. While acute cases had a neutrophilic pleocytosis, chronic cases had predominantly mononuclear cells.[96] With antibiotic treatment, TNCCs are expected to decrease with a shift from neutrophilic to mononuclear inflammation.[94] CNS abscesses result in highly variable CSF findings that range from no cytologic abnormalities to neutrophilic pleocytosis.[94] Otitis-related meningitis has a variable presentation with normal CSF or a mononuclear or mixed pleocytosis.[94] In cases of thromboembolic meningoencephalitis, results are also variable. Neutrophilic, histiocytic, or lymphocytic pleocytosis is possible, and Gram-negative bacilli may be found on CSF cytology. Abscesses in the vertebral body with associated spinal cord compression or viral disease can result in increased microprotein or a mononuclear pleocytosis.[94]

CSF from cattle with toxic, metabolic, and degenerative disease is often normal, but a mild mononuclear pleocytosis

Table 58.2 Potential causes of various CSF findings in cattle.[5,94–97]

CSF finding	Potential causes
Neutrophilic pleocytosis	Acute neonatal meningitis Thromboembolic meningoencephalitis CNS abscess
Mixed mononuclear or histiocytic pleocytosis	Listeriosis Chronic neonatal meningitis Neonatal meningitis after antibiotic treatment Otitis-related meningitis Thromboembolic meningoencephalitis CNS abscess Vertebral body abscess Viral disease Salt poisoning Polioencephalomalacia Sacral trauma Neoplasia
Lymphocytic pleocytosis	Thromboembolic meningoencephalitis Neoplasia
Mixed pleocytosis	Otitis-related meningitis Neonatal meningitis CNS abscess
Increased microprotein alone	CNS abscess Vertebral body abscess Viral disease Neoplasia
Normal	Otitis-related meningitis CNS abscess Toxin exposure Metabolic disease Degenerative disease Neoplasia

CNS, central nervous system.

can be seen with salt poisoning[94] or polioencephalomalacia.[5,94] CSF from two cases of sacral trauma revealed mild histiocytic pleocytosis, moderately increased protein concentration, and erythrophagia (one of these cases had xanthochromia). Neoplastic conditions can have normal CSF, lymphocytic or histiocytic pleocytosis, or increased microprotein.[94,97]

Peritoneal Fluid

In healthy cattle, up to 5 mL of pale straw-colored fluid can be collected from the peritoneal space although fluid can be unobtainable from some animals.[98,99] Generally TNCC are between 1 and 4×10^9/L and TP < 30 g/L.[6,99,100] However, some individuals may have TNCCs > 6×10^9/L and TP > 30 g/L. Equal numbers of non-degenerate neutrophils and mononuclear cells are usually present with variable numbers of eosinophils.[6,100,101] In one study from Saskatchewan, the mean eosinophil percentage of fluid collected from a herd of healthy nonpregnant dairy cows was 51%.[99] Other studies in Michigan and Kansas also have reported relatively high eosinophil percentages, but other investigators have found eosinophils uncommon (<10%).[6,100–102] The increased eosinophil percentage seen in some regions has been suggested to be due to the presence of *Setaria* spp., a nematode found in the abdomen of cattle in many areas of the United States and in Saskatchewan, Canada.[99,103] The TNCCs in the study from Saskatchewan were also higher than reported by others illustrating the importance of locally derived reference intervals for peritoneal fluid.[99] Mesothelial cells are often seen, particularly in later stages of pregnancy.[101] The volume of peritoneal fluid increases in late pregnancy and becomes pink.[101] This is accompanied by lower TNCC and TP values, presumably due to dilution.[99,104] TNCC > 10×10^9/L with a predominance of neutrophils and eosinophils has been noted in cattle in the first two weeks postparturition.[8]

Significant age differences in the characteristics of peritoneal fluid have been reported between calves and adult cattle. Ideally, peritoneal fluid obtained from calves should be interpreted with age-appropriate reference intervals.[6,11,12] TNCC values for 4–8 week old calves range from 0.2 to 13.5×10^9/L with a mean of approximately 4×10^9/L. Mononuclear cells tend to be present in higher numbers and eosinophils in lower percentages than in adult cattle. TP are generally similar to adult cattle but can be >40 g/L in some instances.

The changes that occur in peritoneal fluid after exploratory laparotomy and omentopexy and surgical correction of left displaced abomasum have been described.[104,105] In one study performed on clinically healthy cows, TNCC did not increase significantly until two days post exploratory laparotomy and omentopexy.[104] The mean TNCC rose from 3 200 cells/μL pre-surgery to 16 336 cells/μL on day 2, and further to 20 542 cells/μL by day 6, the last day of study. In another study of cattle undergoing surgical correction of left displaced abomasum, mean TNCC and neutrophil percentage increased to $>10 \times 10^9$/L and >80%, respectively, by day 1 post-surgery and then slowly fell on day 2 and day 3.[105] In both studies, some individual cows had TNCC between 40 000 and 55 000 cells/μL in the days following surgery. The magnitude of the increase was found to vary with different surgical techniques. Detailed data beyond six days have not been recorded in the literature although one author has noted that TNCC and individual cell counts should gradually fall to within reference intervals by 10–14 days after surgery.[7]

Accidental enterocentesis in adults and abomasal puncture in calves is not uncommon. Enterocentesis or rumenocentesis in adults is recognized by the presence of plant material and a mixture of extracellular bacteria and/or protozoa (Figure 58.10). Provided the sample is examined relatively soon after collection, other cytological features of the fluid should remain unaltered. In other words, TNCC should be low and neutrophils non-degenerate with no phagocytosed bacteria in samples from normal peritoneal fluid or noninflammatory effusions. Plant material and mixed predominantly extracellular bacteria can also be noted with acute gastrointestinal rupture. However, in these cases, neutrophils are markedly degenerate or lysed.[106]

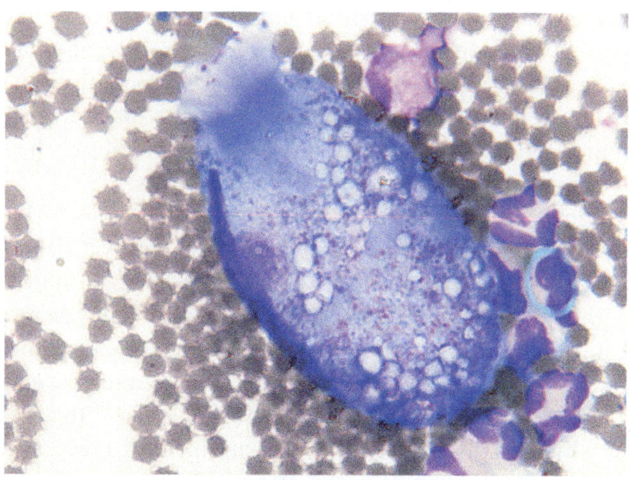

Figure 58.10 Accidental rumenocentesis from a cow. A large entodiniomorph protozoa and a circular fragment of plant material (on right) are present on a cytocentrifuge preparation of peritoneal fluid. Other than mild blood contamination, the sample was otherwise unremarkable (May-Grünwald–Giemsa, 1000×. *Source:* Image courtesy of Ronnie Barron).

The risk of accidental abomasal puncture in calves is increased if sampling is performed within an hour of feeding.[12] Peritoneal fluid contaminated with abomasal contents in calves can be recognized by the presence of large white clots in the fluid and the aroma of digested milk. The pH of the collected fluid is also decreased compared with non-contaminated abdominal fluid, which is normally around pH 7.[1]

Peritonitis

Fluid collected from cattle with peritonitis can vary significantly in gross appearance, TNCC and TP.[9,98–100,107] Although TNCCs > 10×10^9/L are considered most typical of peritonitis, it is not uncommon for very low TNCCs to be observed and for the fluid to appear grossly normal. Consequently, there is significant overlap in TNCC and TP between clinically healthy cattle and those with peritonitis. Microscopic examination for increased neutrophil percentage, degenerative changes, and bacteria is critical for diagnosis.[98] Some authors also advocate the use of biochemical tests such as peritoneal fluid d-dimer concentration as another option to diagnose peritonitis.[108] The neutrophil percentage in cases of peritonitis is usually increased, but this can decrease with chronicity.[101] Localized peritonitis is common in cattle; therefore, a normal peritoneal fluid exam does not exclude the possibility of peritonitis.[7,9,109] Sequential sampling from all four quadrants of the abdomen can be used to minimize the possibility of missing localized peritonitis, and ultrasound can be more effective in identifying fluid pockets.[8,10]

The most frequent cause of peritonitis in cattle is traumatic reticuloperitonitis, but other differentials include perforated abomasal ulcers, postsurgical sepsis, abdominal accidents such as gastrointestinal or reproductive tract perforation, intestinal volvulus, abomasal torsion, and, more rarely, severe enteritis or systemic infections such as pasteurellosis, anthrax, and mycobacteriosis.[9,10,13,98,99,110] When acute gut perforation is present, plant material, squamous epithelial cells, mixed bacteria, highly degenerate neutrophils, and an elevated TP are typically noted. Although traumatic reticuloperitonitis also has a septic component, bacteria are rarely seen in collected fluid, likely due to the chronicity of the disease and the efficiency of cattle in walling off areas of infection.[98] In cases in which sepsis is suspected, measurement of glucose in peritoneal fluid can be useful alongside cytological analysis.[108] In one study low peritoneal fluid glucose concentration was found to be highly predictive of the presence of bacteria and degenerate neutrophils on cytology. Bile peritonitis has rarely been reported in cattle, and fluid can appear grossly hemorrhagic or green cloudy/bilious.[111] Unfortunately the cytologic appearance of the peritoneal fluid in these cases has not been recorded.

Uroperitoneum

Uroperitoneum is most commonly caused by bladder rupture secondary to urolithiasis in male cattle and dystocia in females.[112,113] Other reported causes include rupture of remnant urachus and bladder rupture secondary to compression of the urethra by hematomas or abscesses.[114–116] As with other species, the collected fluid often has a very low protein concentration, and a peritoneal fluid to serum creatinine ratio >2 : 1 is considered diagnostic. The neutrophil percentage is usually increased, and an odor of urine may or may not be noted.[112]

Noninflammatory Effusions

Noninflammatory effusions in cattle can be classified as transudates or modified transudates according to the traditional system used in other animal species.[13,102] Transudates are most often a result of right-sided congestive heart disease or low oncotic pressure. Causes of right-sided congestive heart disease include traumatic reticulopericarditis, valvular endocarditis, cardiac lymphoma, and other cardiomyopathies. Low oncotic pressure is typically a consequence of parasitism, Johne's disease, chronic salmonellosis, starvation, or renal amyloidosis. Modified transudates can be noted with congestive heart disease, chronic abomasal displacement, and portal hypertension due to liver disease.[102] Hemoperitoneum is uncommon in cattle and can be distinguished from iatrogenic blood contamination using the features described in other animal species. Chylous effusions are also rarely reported and are typical of those seen in other species.[117]

Mesothelioma[8,110,118] and lymphoma[16,98] are the most commonly reported neoplastic effusions in cattle although overall the incidence of neoplastic effusions in this species appears low. Rare reports of metastatic squamous cell carcinoma have also been recorded.[13,98] Cattle with mesothelioma tend to have very high volume effusions, and differentiation between reactive and neoplastic mesothelial cells can be challenging as in other species.[10,13,102] Lymphomatous effusions are characterized by a predominance of large atypical lymphocytes.[98]

Pleural Fluid

Pleural fluid from clinically healthy cattle should have a TNCC < 5×10^9/L and TP < 25 g/L.[13,106] Effusions are uncommon but can be noted with right-sided congestive heart disease or profound hypoproteinemia. These are typically transudates and are often accompanied by ascites.[13,15,114] Lymphoma[16,119,120] and mesothelioma[118] have been diagnosed in pleural effusions. Single case reports describe pleural effusion accompanying uroperitoneum secondary to a ruptured urachus,[114] a chylothorax,[117] and a fistulating abomasal ulcer.[109] In the calf presenting with uroperitoneum and pleural effusion, the pleural fluid creatinine to serum creatinine was 2 : 1 suggesting it consisted of urine.[114] The exact mechanism underlying the pleural fluid accumulation was unknown, and direct transfusion across the diaphragm was one suggested mechanism. The fluid obtained from a calf with chylothorax was grossly milky with a TNCC of $17.6 \times 10^3/\mu L$ composed predominantly of small- and medium-sized lymphocytes and lesser numbers of macrophages and non-degenerate neutrophils.[117] The fluid to serum triglyceride ratio was greater than 50 : 1. The abomaso-pleural fistula resulting from an abomasal ulcer produced a pleural fluid that was cloudy yellow and grossly contained plant material.[109] The TNCC was low ($1.1 \times 10^3/\mu L$), and the TP < 25 g/L with degenerate neutrophils and a mixed population of bacteria and yeast was seen on microscopy.

Pericardial Fluid

The most common cause of pericardial effusion is traumatic pericarditis. The gross appearance and foul odor of the collected fluid is generally sufficient for diagnosis although cytologic examination and bacteriology can be used for additional confirmation.[15] Cytologic examination of pericardial fluid can be used to distinguish cardiac lymphoma,[16] which is a common site for lymphoma in BLV endemic areas, from idiopathic hemorrhagic pericarditis.[14,17] Cattle diagnosed with idiopathic hemorrhagic pericarditis can be successfully treated with repeat pericardiocentesis although in one case series of BLV-positive cattle, the animals represented with cardiac lymphoma approximately 100 days to 2.5 years later.[17]

Conclusion

Cytology is infrequently performed in bovine practice. With readily accessible reference material for the practitioner regarding collection, handling, and interpretation, hopefully cytology will be used more frequently. The rapid, inexpensive, and often minimally invasive nature of this diagnostic modality should make it an attractive component of the diagnostic workup. While most cytologic indications are better suited to the individual, important herd level information may be gained through cytologic evaluation as well.

References

1 Bohn, A.A. and Callan, R.J. (2007). Cytology in food animal practice. *Vet Clin North Am Food Anim Pract* 23: 443–479.

2 Caldow, G. (2001). Bronchoalveolar lavage in the investigation of bovine respiratory disease. *In Pract* 23: 41–43.

3 Braun, U., Attiger, J., and Brammertz, C. (2015). Ultrasonographic examination of the spinal cord and collection of cerebrospinal fluid from the atlanto-occipital space in cattle. *BMC Vet Res* 11: 227.

4 Scott, P.R. (1993). Collection and interpretation of cerebrospinal fluid in ruminants. *In Pract* 15: 298–300.

5 Scott, P.R. (1995). The collection and analysis of cerebrospinal fluid as an aid to diagnosis in ruminant neurological disease. *Br Vet J* 151: 603–614.

6 Anderson, D.E., Cornwell, D., Anderson, L.S. et al. (1995). Comparative analyses of peritoneal fluid from calves and adult cattle. *Am J Vet Res* 56: 973–976.

7 Oehme, F.W. (1969). Cytologic examination of the peritoneal fluid in the diagnosis of cattle disease. *J Am Vet Med Assoc* 155: 1923–1927.

8 Kopcha, M. and Schultze, A.E. (1991). Peritoneal fluid. Part II. Abdominocentesis in cattle and interpretation of non-neoplastic samples. *Compend Contin Educ Pract Vet* 13: 703–709.

9 Palmer, J.E. and Whitlock, R.H. (1984). Perforated abomasal ulcers in adult dairy cows. *J Am Vet Med Assoc* 184: 171–174.

10 Braun, U. (2016). Ascites in cattle. *Vet Clin North Am Food Anim Pract* 32: 55–83.

11 Burton, S., Lofstedt, J., Webster, S., and McConkey, S. (1997). Peritoneal fluid values and collection technique in young, normal calves. *Vet Clin Pathol* 26: 38–44.

12 Mendes, L.C.N., Peiró, J.R., Feitosa, F.L.F. et al. (2005). Effect of age and abomasal puncture on peritoneal fluid, hematology, and serum biochemical analyses in young calves. *J Vet Intern Med* 19: 899–904.

13 Whitney, M.S., Roussel, A.J., and Cole, D.J. (1999). Cytology in bovine practice: solid tissue, pleural fluid, and peritoneal fluid specimens. *Vet Med* 94: 277–289.

14 Jesty, S.A., Sweeney, R.W., Dolente, B.A., and Reef, V.B. (2005). Idiopathic pericarditis and cardiac tamponade in two cows. *J Am Vet Assoc* 226: 1555–1558.

15 Braun, U. (2009). Traumatic pericarditis in cattle: clinical, radiographic and ultrasonographic findings. *Vet J* 182: 176–186.

16 Burton, A.J., Nydam, D.V., Long, E., and Divers, T.J. (2010). Signalment and clinical complaints initiating

hospital admission, methods of diagnosis, and pathological findings associated with bovine lymphosarcoma (112 cases). *J Vet Intern Med* 24: 960–964.

17 Peek, S.F., McGuirk, S.M., Gaska, J. et al. (2012). Idiopathic hemorrhagic pericardial effusion as a precursor to epicardial lymphosarcoma in three cows. *J Vet Intern Med* 26: 1069–1072.

18 Buczinski, S., Boulay, G., and DesCôteaux, L. (2011). Repeated pericardiocentesis as palliative treatment for tamponade associated with cardiac lymphoma in a Holstein cow. *Can Vet J* 52: 663–666.

19 Steiner, S., Neidl, A., Kinhart, N. et al. (2015). Randomised prospective study compares efficacy of five different stomach tubes for rumen fluid sampling in dairy cows. *Vet Rec* 176: 50–56.

20 Duffield, T., Plaizier, J.C., Fairfield, A. et al. (2004). Comparison of techniques for measurement of rumen pH in lactating dairy cows. *J Dairy Sci* 87: 59–66.

21 Kleen, J.L., Hooijer, G.A., Rehage, J., and Noordhuizen, J.P. (2004). Rumenocentesis (rumen puncture): a viable instrument in herd health diagnosis. *Dtsch Tieräztl Wschr* 111: 453–484.

22 Nordlund, K.V., Garrett, E.F., and Oetzel, G.R. (1995). Herd-based rumenocentesis: a clinical approach to diagnosis of subacute rumen acidosis. *Compend Contin Educ Pract Vet* 17: S48–S56.

23 Kleen, J.L., Hooijer, G.A., Rehage, J. et al. (2003). Subacute ruminal acidosis (SARA): a review. *J Vet Med A* 50: 406–414.

24 Dirksen, G. and Smith, M.C. (1987). Acquisition and analysis of bovine rumen fluid. *Bovine Pract* 22: 108–116.

25 Belknap, E.B. and Navarre, C.B. (2000). Differentiation of gastrointestinal diseases in adult cattle. *Vet Clin North Am Food Anim Pract* 16: 59–86.

26 Parkinson, T.J., Vermunt, J.J., and Malmo, J. (2010). *Diseases of Cattle in Australasia: A Comprehensive Textbook*, 220–221, 611–612, 616–625. Wellington: VetLearn.

27 Washburn, K.E., Streeter, R.N., Lehenbauer, T.W. et al. (2007). Comparison of core needle biopsy and fine-needle aspiration of enlarged peripheral lymph nodes for antemortem diagnosis of enzootic bovine lymphosarcoma in cattle. *J Am Vet Med Assoc* 230: 228–232.

28 Braun, U. (2009). Ultrasonography of the liver in cattle. *Vet Clin North Am Food Anim Pract* 25: 591–609.

29 Braun, U. and Gerber, D. (1992). Percutaneous ultrasound-guided cholecystocentesis in cows. *Am J Vet Res* 53: 1079–1084.

30 Kasimanickam, R., Duffield, T.F., Foster, R.A. et al. (2005). A comparison of the cytobrush and uterine lavage techniques to evaluate endometrial cytology in clinically normal postpartum dairy cows. *Can Vet J* 46: 255–259.

31 Ahmadi, M.R., Tafti, A.K., Nazifi, S., and Ghaisari, H.R. (2005). The comparative evaluation of uterine and cervical mucosa cytology with endometrial histopathology in cows. *Comp Clin Pathol* 14: 90–94.

32 Sylla, L., Palombi, C., Stradaioli, G. et al. (2015). Effect of semen collection by transrectal massage of accessory sexual glands or artificial vagina on the outcome of breeding soundness examinations of Italian yearling beef bulls. *Theriogenology* 83: 779–785.

33 Divers, T.J. and Peek, S.F. (2008). *Rebhun's Diseases of Dairy Cattle*, 295–323, 561–563. St. Louis: Elsevier.

34 Smith, B.P. (2015). *Large Animal Internal Medicine*, 1210. St. Louis: Elsevier.

35 Loh, C.C. (2007). Atypical presentation of cutaneous T-cell lymphosarcoma in a 19-month-old Holstein heifer. *Can Vet J* 48: 309–311.

36 Vernau, W., Valli, V.E.O., Dukes, T.W. et al. (1992). Classification of 1,198 cases of bovine lymphoma using the National Cancer Institute working formulation for human non-Hodgkin's lymphomas. *Vet Pathol* 29: 183–195.

37 Scott, D.W. and Anderson, W.I. (1992). Bovine cutaneous neoplasms: literature review and retrospective analysis of 62 cases (1978 to 1990). *Compend Contin Educ Pract Vet* 14: 1405–1418.

38 Miller, M.A., Weaver, A.D., Stogsdill, P.L. et al. (1995). Cutaneous melanocytomas in 10 young cattle. *Vet Pathol* 32: 479–484.

39 Genovese, L.M. and Schipp, R.J. (1995). Multiple cutaneous mast cell tumours in a cow. *Aust Vet J* 72: 276–277.

40 Hill, J.E., Langheinrich, K.A., and Kelly, L.C. (1991). Prevalence and location of mast cell tumors in slaughter cattle. *Vet Pathol* 28: 449–450.

41 O'Toole, D. and Fox, J.D. (2003). Chronic hyperplastic and neoplastic cutaneous lesions (Marjolin's ulcer) in hot-brand sites in adult beef cattle. *J Vet Diagn Invest* 15: 64–67.

42 Sartin, E.A., Doran, S.E., Riddell, M.G. et al. (1994). Characterization of naturally occurring cutaneous neurofibromatosis in Holstein cattle: a disorder resembling neurofibromatosis type I in humans. *Am J Pathol* 145: 1168–1174.

43 Ahmadi, N., Oryan, A., Ghane, M., and Daneshbod, Y. (2012). Cutaneous schwannoma in a cow. *Braz J Vet Pathol* 5: 81–85.

44 Priestnall, S.L., De Bellis, F., Bond, R. et al. (2010). Spontaneous regression of congenital cutaneous hemangiomas in a calf. *Vet Pathol* 47: 343–345.

45 Bisby, T.M., Pratt, S.M., Fenton, R.K. et al. (2009). What is your diagnosis? Perifemoral mass in a cow. *Vet Clin Pathol* 38: 343–347.

46 Brown, M.H., Brightman, A.H., Fenwick, B.W., and Rider, M.A. (1998). Infectious bovine keratoconjunctivitis: a review. *J Vet Intern Med* 12: 259–266.

47 Wilcox, G.E. (1970). The aetiology of infectious bovine keratoconjunctivitis in Queensland 1. *Moraxella bovis*. *Aust Vet J* 46: 409–414.

48 Ribeiro, M.G., Risseti, R.M., Bolaños, C.A. et al. (2015). Trueperella pyogenes multispecies infections in domestic animals: a retrospecitve study of 144 cases (2002 to 2012). *Vet Q* 35 (2): 82–87.

49 Hoffman, D., Spradbrow, P.B., and Wilson, B.E. (1978). An evaluation of exfoliative cytology in the diagnosis of bovine ocular squamous cell carcinoma. *J Comp Pathol* 88: 497–504.

50 Gharagozlou, M.J., Hekmati, P., and Ashrafihelan, J. (2007). A clinical and histopathological study of ocular neoplasms in dairy cattle. *Vet Arch* 77: 209–426.

51 Braun, U., Gerspach, C., Previtali, M. et al. (2011). Conjunctival changes in a Swiss Braunvieh heifer with malignant lymphoma. *Schweiz Arch Tierheilkd* 153: 175–178.

52 Fubini, S.L. and Ducharme, N.G. (2017). *Farm Animal Surgery*, 107. St. Louis: Elsevier.

53 Mulon, P.Y., Desrochers, A., and Francoz, D. (2016). Surgical management of septic arthritis. *Vet Clin North Am Food Anim Pract* 32: 777–795.

54 Amrousi, S.E., S., Soliman, M.K., and Youssef, L.B. (1966). Studies on the physiological chemistry of the tibio-tarsal synovial fluid of healthy bovines. *Can J Comp Med Vet Sci* 30: 251–255.

55 Francoz, D., Desrochers, A., and Latouche, J.S. (2007). Effect of repeated arthrocentesis and single joint lavage on cytologic evaluation of synovial fluid in 5 young calves. *Can J Vet Res* 71: 129–134.

56 Rohde, C., Anderson, D.E., Desrochers, A. et al. (2000). Synovial fluid analysis in cattle: a review of 130 cases. *Vet Surg* 29 (4): 341–346.

57 Francoz, D., Desrochers, A., Fecteau, G. et al. (2005). Synovial fluid changes in induced infectious arthritis in calves. *J Vet Intern Med* 19: 336–343.

58 Allen, J.W., Viel, L., and Bateman, K.G. (1992). Cytological findings in bronchoalveolar lavage fluid from feedlot calves: associations with pulmonary microbial flora. *Can J Vet Res* 56: 122–126.

59 Wilkie, B.N. and Markham, R.J. (1981). Bronchoalveolar washing cells and immunoglobulins of clinically normal calves. *Am J Vet Res* 42: 241–243.

60 Lay, J.C., Slauson, D.O., and Castleman, W.L. (1986). Volume-controlled bronchopulmonary lavage of normal and pneumonic calves. *Vet Pathol* 23: 673–680.

61 Ollivett, T.L., Caswell, J.L., and Nydam, D.V. (2015). Thoracic ultrasonography and bronchoalveolar lavage fluid analysis in Holstein calves with subclinical lung lesions. *J Vet Intern Med* 29: 1728–1734.

62 Grimes, C.N., Constant, C., Bau-Gaudreault, L., and Babkine, M. (2016). What is your diagnosis? Bronchoalveolar lavage from a Holstein cow. *Vet Clin Pathol* 45: 387–388.

63 Brazzell, J.L., Kaese, H.J., and Borjesson, D.L. (2006). Bold fusion: transtracheal wash from a Jersey calf. *Vet Clin Pathol* 35: 247–249.

64 Sood, N.K., Sandhu, B.S., Gupta, K. et al. (2012). Mesenteric caseous lymphadenitis in a cow calf caused by *Corynebacterium pseudotuberculosis*: a case report. *Vet Med* 57 (7): 371–375.

65 Ortega, J., Uzal, F.A., Walker, R. et al. (2010). Zygomycotic lymphadenitis in slaughtered feedlot cattle. *Vet Pathol* 47: 108–115.

66 Salgado, B.S., Battaglia, C.T., Stuchi, R.S. et al. (2011). What is your diagnosis? Lymphadenopathy in a cow with severe anemia. *Vet Clin Pathol* 40: 103–104.

67 Nasir, K. (2005). Sporatic juvenile thymic lymphoma in a 6-month-old Holstein heifer. *Can Vet J* 46: 831–833.

68 Enemark, J.M.D. (2009). The monitoring, prevention and treatment of sub-acute ruminal acidosis (SARA): a review. *Vet J* 176: 32–34.

69 Steen, A. (2001). Field study of dairy cows with reduced appetite in early lactation: clinical examinations, blood and rumen fluid analyses. *Acta Vet Scand* 42: 219–228.

70 Alonso, A.N. (1979). Diagnostic analysis of rumen fluid. *Vet Clin North Am Large Anim Pract* 1: 363–376.

71 Plazier, J.C., Krause, D.O., Gozho, G.N., and McBride, B.W. (2009). Subacute ruminal acidosis in diary cows: the physiological causes, incidence and consequences. *Vet J* 176: 21–31.

72 Weber, M.F., Verhoeff, J., van Schaik, G., and van Maanen, C. (2009). Evaluation of Ziehl-Neelsen stained faecal smear and ELISA as tools for surveillance of clinical paratuberculosis in cattle in Netherlands. *Prev Vet Med* 92: 256–266.

73 Chartier, C., Rieux, A., Delafosse, A. et al. (2013). Detection of *Cryptosporidium* oocysts in fresh calf faeces: characteristics of two simple tests and evaluation of a semi-quantitative approach. *Vet J* 198: 148–152.

74 Paul, S., Chandra, D., Tewari, A.K. et al. (2009). Comparative evaluation and economic assessment of coprological diagnostic methods and PCR for detection of *Cryptosporidium* spp. in bovines. *Vet Parasitol* 164: 291–295.

75 Casemore, D.P. (1991). Laboratory methods for diagnosing cryptosporidiosis. *J Clin Pathol* 44: 445–451.

76 Hoff, B., Cote, J., and Steen, A. (1996). Fine needle aspiration and liver cytology: a simple method for

diagnosis and prognosis of fatty liver in cattle. *Bovine Pract* 30: 53–55.

77 Kalaitzakis, E., Roubies, N., Panousis, N. et al. (2007). Clinicopathologic evaluation of hepatic lipidosis in periparturient dairy cattle. *J Vet Intern Med* 21: 835–845.

78 Braun, U., Nuss, K., Soldati, G., and Ossent, P. (2005). Clinical and ultrasonographic findings in four cows with liver tumours. *Vet Rec* 157: 482–484.

79 Emanuelli, M.P., Antoniazzi, A.Q., Cecim, M.S., and Fighera, R.A. (2016). What is your diagnosis? Liver from a cow. *Vet Clin Pathol* 45: 721–722.

80 Cable, C.S., Rebhun, W.C., and Fortier, L.A. (1997). Cholelithiasis and cholecystitis in a dairy cow. *J Am Vet Med Assoc* 211: 899–900.

81 Tulleners, E.P. (1983). Empyema of the gallbladder in a cow. *J Am Vet Med Assoc* 182: 410–412.

82 Braun, U., Götz, M., and Guscetti, F. (1994). Ultrasonographic findings in a cow with extra-hepatic cholestasis and cholangitis. *Schweiz Arch Tierheilkd* 136: 275–279.

83 Westermann, S., Drillich, M., Kaufmann, T. et al. (2010). A clinical approach to determine false positive findings of clinical endometritis by vaginoscopy by the use of uterine bacteriology and cytology in dairy cows. *Theriogenology* 74: 1248–1255.

84 Kasimanickam, R., Duffield, T.F., Foster, R.A. et al. (2004). Endometrial cytology and ultrasonography for the detection of subclinical endometritis in postpartum dairy cows. *Theriogenology* 62: 9–23.

85 Couto, G.B., Vaillancourt, D.H., and Lefebvre, R.C. (2013). Comparison of a leukocyte esterase test with endometrial cytology for diagnosis of subclinical endometritis in postpartum dairy cows. *Theriogenology* 79: 103–107.

86 Moscuzza, C., Álvarez, G., Gutiérrez, B. et al. (2015). Endometrial cytology as a diagnostic tool for subclinical endometritis in beef heifers. *Turk J Vet Anim Sci* 39: 34–41.

87 Menon, A.G., Barkema, H.W., Wilde, R. et al. (2011). Associations between sperm abnormalities, breed, age, and scrotal circumference in beef bulls. *Can J Vet Res* 75: 241–247.

88 Zart, A.L., Jurgielewicz, V.C., and Fernandes, C.E. (2014). Seminal leucocytary profile in beef bulls. *Reprod Domest Anim* 49: 719–724.

89 Dosogne, H., Vangroenweghe, F., Mehrzad, J. et al. (2003). Differential leukocyte count method for bovine low somatic cell count milk. *J Dairy Sci* 86: 828–834.

90 Wickström, E., Persson-Waller, K., Lindmark-Månsson, H. et al. (2009). Relationship between somatic cell count, polymorphonuclear leucocyte count and quality parameters in bovine bulk tank milk. *J Dairy Res* 76: 195–201.

91 Rivas, A.L., Quimby, F.W., Blue, J., and Coksaygan, O. (2001). Longitudinal evaluation of bovine mammary gland health status by somatic cell counting, flow cytometry, and cytology. *J Vet Diagn Invest* 13: 399–407.

92 da Costa, E.O., Ribeiro, M.G., Ribeiro, A.R. et al. (2004). Diagnosis of clinical bovine mastitis by fine needle aspiration followed by staining and scanning electron microscopy in a *Prototheca zopfii* outbreak. *Mycopathologia* 158: 81–85.

93 Welles, E.G., Tyler, J.W., Sorjonen, D.C., and Whatley, E.M. (1992). Composition and analysis of cerebrospinal fluid in clinically normal adult cattle. *Am J Vet Res* 53: 2050–2057.

94 Stokol, T., Divers, T.J., Arrigan, J.W., and McDonough, S.P. (2009). Cerebrospinal fluid findings in cattle with central nervous system disorders: a retrospective study of 102 cases (1990–2008). *Vet Clin Pathol* 38: 103–112.

95 Schweizer, G., Ehrensperger, F., Torgerson, P.R., and Braun, U. (2006). Clinical findings and treatment of 94 cattle presumptively diagnosed with listeriosis. *Vet Rec* 158: 588–592.

96 Green, S.L. and Smith, L.L. (1992). Meningitis in neonatal calves: 32 cases (1983–1990). *J Am Vet Med Assoc* 201: 125–128.

97 Scott, P.R. (1994). Cerebrospinal fluid analysis in the differential diagnosis of spinal cord lesions in ruminants. *In Pract* 16: 301–303.

98 Hirsch, V.M. and Townsend, H.G.G. (1982). Peritoneal fluid analysis in the diagnosis of abdominal disorders in cattle: a retrospective study. *Can Vet J* 23: 348–354.

99 Wilson, A.D., Hirsch, V.M., and Osborne, A.D. (1985). Abdominocentesis in cattle: technique and criteria for diagnosis of peritonitis. *Can Vet J* 26: 74–80.

100 Wittek, T., Grosche, A., Locher, L. et al. (2010). Biochemical constituents of peritoneal fluid in cows. *Vet Rec* 166: 15–19.

101 Oehme, F.W. and Noordsy, J.L. (1970). Examination of peritoneal fluid in differential diagnosis of bovine diseases. *Vet Med* 65: 54–59.

102 Kopcha, M. and Schultze, A.E. (1991). Peritoneal fluid. Part I. Pathophysiology and classification of nonneoplastic effusions. *Compend Contin Educ Pract Vet* 13: 519–525.

103 Becklund, W.W. and Walker, M.L. (1969). Taxonomy, hosts and geographic distribution of the Setaria (hemtoda:filarioidea) in the United States and Canada. *J Parasitol* 55: 359–368.

104 Anderson, D.E., Cornwell, D., St-Jean, G. et al. (1994). Comparison of peritoneal fluid analysis before and after exploratory celiotomy and omentopexy in cattle. *Am J Vet Res* 55: 1633–1637.

105 Wittek, T., Fürll, M., and Grosche, A. (2012). Peritoneal inflammatory response to surgical correction of left displaced abomasum using different techniques. *Vet Rec* 171: 594.

106 Ziemer, E.L. (1989). Cytologic analysis of large-animal body fluids. *Vet Med* 84: 574–583.

107 Hussain, S.A. and Uppal, S.K. (2014). Haemato-biochemical changes and peritoneal fluid cytology in clinical cases of bovine peritonitis. *Indian J Anim Res* 48: 188–193.

108 Wittek, T., Grosche, A., Locher, L.F. et al. (2010). Diagnostic accuracy of d-dimer and other peritoneal fluid analysis measurements in dairy cows with peritonitis. *J Vet Intern Med* 24: 1211–1217.

109 Costa, L.R.R., Gill, M.S., Williams, J. et al. (2002). Abomasal ulceration and abomaso-pleural fistula in an 11-month old beefmaster bull. *Can Vet J* 43: 217–219.

110 Milne, M.H., Mellor, D.J., Barrett, D.C., and Fitzpatrick, J.L. (2001). Observations on ascites in nine cattle. *Vet Rec* 148: 341–344.

111 Braun, U., Schweizer, G., and Pospischil, A. (2005). Clinical and ultrasonographic findings in three cows with ruptured gall bladders. *Vet Rec* 156: 351–353.

112 Braun, U. and Nuss, K. (2015). Uroperitoneum in cattle: ultrasonographic findings, diagnosis and treatment. *Acta Vet Scand* 57: 36.

113 Carr, E.A., Schott, H.C. II, Barrington, G.M., and Parish, S.M. (1993). Ruptured urinary bladder after dystocia in a cow. *J Am Vet Med Assoc* 202: 631–632.

114 Bell, G.J.C., Macrae, A.I., Milne, E.M., and Scott, P.R. (2004). Extensive uroperitoneum and pleural effusion associated with necrotic urachal remnant in a bull calf. *Vet Rec* 154: 508–509.

115 Baxter, G.M., Zamos, D.T., and Mueller, P.O.E. (1992). Uroperitoneum attributable to ruptured urachus in a yearling bull. *J Am Vet Med Assoc* 200: 517–520.

116 Braun, U., Trösch, L., and Sydler, T. (2014). Ruptured urinary bladder attributable to urethral compression by a haematoma after vertebral fracture in a bull. *Acta Vet Scand* 56: 17.

117 Cruz, A.M., Riley, C.B., MacDonald, D.G., and Ferguson, J.G. (1995). Use of mesenteric lymphangiography in a calf with chylothorax and chyloperitoneum. *J Am Vet Med Assoc* 206: 1567–1571.

118 Wolfe, D.F., Carson, R.L., Hudson, R.S. et al. (1991). Mesothelioma in cattle: eight cases (1970–1988). *J Am Vet Med Assoc* 199: 486–491.

119 Alexander, A.N., Constable, P.D., Meier, W.A. et al. (1996). Clinical and immunohistochemical characterization of thymic lymphosarcoma in a heifer. *J Vet Intern Med* 10: 275–278.

120 Angel, K.L., Stott, J., Tyler, J.W., and Groth, A.H. Jr. (1991). Metastatic thymic lymphosarcoma in a calf. *J Am Vet Med Assoc* 198: 1771–1773.

59

Camelids

Susan J. Tornquist, Christopher K. Cebra, and Michala de Linde Henriksen

Introduction

Clinical Settings

New World camelids outside of South America are usually privately owned livestock pets. Herd sizes range from a handful to many hundreds. A few are research animals, and many zoos have small herds. Camelids are kept for commercial fleece production, as show animals, or as breeding stock. Others help maintain pastures or guard sheep, and some are therapy or pack animals. Smaller herds are generally affected by individual animal disorders or problems transferred from neighboring livestock or wildlife. Larger herds can develop endemic problems.

Applications of Cytology and Collection Methods

The most common samples collected are cerebrospinal fluid (CSF) and skin scrapes. In referral settings, peritoneal fluid, joint fluid, lymph node or mass aspirates, and urine sediment examinations are occasionally performed. Corneal swabs, thoracic fluid, bone marrow aspirates, and tracheal or bronchoalveolar lavages (BALs) are also performed if indicated. Unless otherwise noted, sample collection, handling, sources of pre-analytical error, and interpretation are similar to other large animal species (Chapters 49 and 53).

Body Fluid Samples

CSF is usually collected from the lumbosacral space, which is easily palpable in all but the fattest camelids. Compromised camelids may require no sedation and may be easily maintained in sternal recumbency. More vigorous animals are mildly to heavily sedated. Surgical preparation and local anesthesia are required prior to collection. In anesthetized or severely obtunded patients, the sample also can be collected from the atlanto-occipital space.[1]

For abdominocentesis, paramedian collection sites are avoided due to the risk of gastric puncture. A safer alternative is a right lateral paracostal site located 3–4.5 cm caudal to the last costochondral junction.[2] Ultrasonography can identify fluid pockets or proximity of viscera for an alternate site. Sedation and site preparation are similar to the procedure for CSF taps, except local anesthetic is infiltrated into the abdominal muscle layers and a sterile cannula or needle is used instead of a spinal needle. When using a cannula, a scalpel incision through the skin and into the abdominal muscle is necessary, and there are usually one or two distinct tissue pops on introduction of the cannula. Healthy camelids have modest amounts of peritoneal fluid, and collection attempts are often unsuccessful, but sick animals frequently have ascites or peritoneal effusions.

Respiratory Washes

Respiratory tract washes are infrequently performed on camelids, but can yield important diagnostic information in certain cases. Bacterial or fungal pneumonia is the major indication, with lungworms and reactive airway disease being much rarer. Most washes are performed endoscopically, with the scope either free in the trachea or wedged into a bronchus. Camelids have narrow nasal passages, and endoscopy can cause regurgitation of gastric contents, airway obstruction through dorsal displacement of the soft palate, nasal bleeding, or struggling. Thus adequate physical and chemical restraint, efficiency, and a willingness to terminate the procedure are necessary to mitigate risks.[3] After collection, samples are handled similarly to other large animal species (Chapter 26).

Urinalysis

Urinalysis is performed less frequently in camelids than in other species because urine collection is more difficult.[4] The camelid bladder resides partially within the pelvic canal, and the upward slope of their caudoventral

Veterinary Cytology, First Edition. Edited by Leslie C. Sharkey, M. Judith Radin, and Davis Seelig.

abdominal body wall precludes percutaneous collection, unless the bladder is quite distended. Retrograde catheterization in males is difficult because the penis is often still adhered within the prepuce, the urethral diameter is small, and the catheter frequently lodges in the subischial diverticulum before reaching the bladder. It is likewise difficult in females due to the small urethral diameter and the tendency of the catheter to lodge in the suburethral diverticulum. Catheterization attempts usually require moderate to heavy sedation of the patient. Physical or mental stresses do not usually stimulate urination. Patience and free catch collection are often the only recourse. Inflammatory lesions can cause urine dribbling, which aids in collection.

Other Samples

Joint and thoracic fluid collection, lymph nodes aspirates, corneal swabs, and skin scrapes are collected using universal techniques. Joint fluid and corneal swabs are usually collected to diagnose a septic process. Thoracic fluid and lymph node aspirates are collected for septic or neoplastic processes. Skin scrapes may be done for a variety of reasons, with ectoparasites, skin infections, and neoplasms all possibilities. Depending on the procedure, light (e.g. butorphanol) or moderate to heavy sedation may be needed, or even short anesthesia.

Conditions Diagnosed by Cytology

Skin and Subcutis

Skin disorders caused by infectious agents are common in camelids. In a study of 68 alpacas with skin diseases, 22% of the cases were bacterial.[5] Bacterial folliculitis is usually staphylococcal and most often presents as papules, pustules, or crusts on distal hindlegs, ventrum, back, and muzzle. Cytologic evaluation shows neutrophils, often with intracellular bacteria. Eosinophils are uncommon in skin lesions, although they can be associated with insect bite hypersensitivity. *Corynebacterium pseudotuberculosis* can cause solitary or multiple abscesses or nodules that cytologically appear as pyogranulomatous inflammation with Gram-positive, non-spore-forming, rod-shaped organisms sometimes apparent. Dermatophilosis has been reported in camelids in regions with varied climates but typically occurs in wet conditions and is most often diagnosed on impression smears of the underside of the typical crusts or of exudate from a lesion.[6]

Dermatophytoses are the most common fungal skin diseases in camelids and are diagnosed by skin scrapings or examination of hair shafts as in other species. Lesions are most common on the legs, head, and perineum.[7] Other fungal agents reported in dermatitis cases include *Candida* spp., *Coccidioides immitis,* and *Conidiobolus coronatus.*[7–11] Cytologic appearances of *Candida* spp. and *C. immitis* can be found elsewhere in the text. In a granulomatous skin lesion, *Conidiobolus* spp. appeared as 6–12.5 µm round and elongated unstaining hyphae with infrequently septate branching hyphae.[11]

Camelids are often affected by ectoparasites including *Sarcoptes* spp., *Psoroptes* spp., *Chorioptes* spp., sucking and chewing lice, and, less commonly, *Demodex* spp. (Chapter 11).[5,12] Mite infections can be diagnosed by identification of mites on skin scrapings, though negative skin scrapings do not exclude infestation. Sometimes the only cytologic evidence is eosinophilic inflammation. Eosinophilic inflammation has also been observed in a presumed adverse drug reaction, insect bite hypersensitivity, and focal sterile folliculitis along with neutrophilic inflammation.[5] When ectoparasites are suspected, scraping the axillary and interdigital spaces is recommended in addition to sampling the affected areas.

There are several hyperplastic skin diseases of camelids that present as crusting hyperkeratotic lesions with different patterns of distribution.[13] Cytology can help exclude infectious etiologies, but histopathology is required for definitive classification because all are characterized cytologically by increased numbers of normal or hyperplastic mature squamous cells. Hyperplastic conditions include zinc responsive dermatosis that tends to affect lightly haired ventral areas and idiopathic necrolytic neutrophilic hyperkeratotic dermatitis and dermatosis (munge and generalized munge). Munge occurs around the lips, nose, eyes, and ears, with a generalized form primarily affecting young animals.

Neoplastic skin lesions comprised 19% of dermatologic cases in one report[5] and 50% of camelid neoplasms in another.[14] Some are readily diagnosed cytologically. As in other species, mast cell tumors have been reported with typical distinct purple granules in the mast cells and increased numbers of eosinophils.[15] Skin tumors such as trichoepithelioma and cutaneous and subcutaneous lymphoma in camelids have similar cytologic features to other species. Others, including fibropapillomas and fibromas, do not readily exfoliate cells with aspiration, and diagnostic samples are harder to obtain. Fibropapillomas and fibromas have a characteristic gross appearance, and definitive diagnosis is made by histology. These often recur after surgical excision and may not be removed unless they are causing discomfort or becoming irritated or inflamed.

Ear and Eye

Otitis in camelids is less common than in small animals and is suspected based on clinical signs and otoscopic exam and confirmed by cytology of swabs from affected areas or exudate.[6] Implicated bacterial etiologies for otitis externa include *Arcanobacterium pyogenes*, *Staphylococcus* spp., and *Bacillus* spp.[16] The *Psoroptes* mange mite is a known cause and can be seen on swab or scrape.[6] The diagnosis and management of otitis media is complicated by the sigmoid shape of the camelid ear canal and the multicompartmental tympanic bullae.[17]

Ophthalmic diseases are often caused by trauma, infections, or hereditary conditions.[18] The most common conditions benefiting from cytologic evaluation involve the eyelid, conjunctiva, and cornea; however, occasional cases of anterior uveitis are evaluated. Commensal conjunctival flora can cause opportunistic infections of periocular and corneal tissue associated with trauma, stress, or systemic disease.[18] Cytology of blepharitis, conjunctivitis, and corneal ulcerations are therefore important to help define the pathological role of these organisms. Gram-positive bacteria are most commonly cultured from normal alpaca conjunctiva, especially *Staphylococcus xylosus*. *Moraxella ovis* has been found in normal conjunctiva tissue in younger animals.[19] Fungal species are also a common finding in normal llama conjunctiva, with *Aspergillus* spp. being the most common in alpacas.[18] Conjunctivitis is classified as noninfectious, sometimes associated with dust or other irritants, or infectious. Numerous bacteria have been associated with conjunctivitis in camelids, along with the nematode *Thelazia californiensis* and chlamydiae.[20] Young camelids are predisposed to congenital nasolacrimal duct atresia.[20] Moderate to severe mucopurulent discharge associated with secondary infectious rhinocystitis is a sequela amenable to cytologic evaluation, although the underlying cause requires surgical correction.[18,21]

Septic corneal ulceration is common in camelids, often secondary to trauma because of prominent globes and an environment rich in microorganisms.[18,22] Corneal ulcerations can be infected with organisms similar to those in equine corneal lesions.[18,22] Anaerobic bacteria have been identified in 18.8% of alpacas with corneal ulcerations, so cytologic evaluation can be a key method of detection when anaerobic culture is not performed or when growth is poor.[23] A report of 11 cases of fungal keratitis documented that cytologic review of corneal samples was immediately diagnostic in 9/11 cases, facilitating rapid treatment compared with culture (Figure 59.1).[22] Fungal keratitis is most often associated with suppurative inflammation, but pyogranulomatous and mixed neutrophilic/eosinophilic inflammation also are reported. Various fungi have been identified as primary pathogens, although *Aspergillus fumigatus* is common.[17] A case report describing a llama with *Coccidioides posadasii* keratouveitis describes corneal cytology, which consisted of moderate to marked suppurative inflammation with mild macrophagic inflammation, but no organisms were identified.[24] Cytology is used in cases of spontaneous chronic corneal epithelial defects (also known as indolent corneal ulceration) and in calcific band keratopathy to help exclude an infectious component.[18,25,26] Uveitis is caused by trauma or systemic diseases in camelids.[18] Cytology of the aqueous and vitreous humors is not frequently performed due to risk of complications (see Chapter 18), but can be used to screen for ophthalmic involvement in

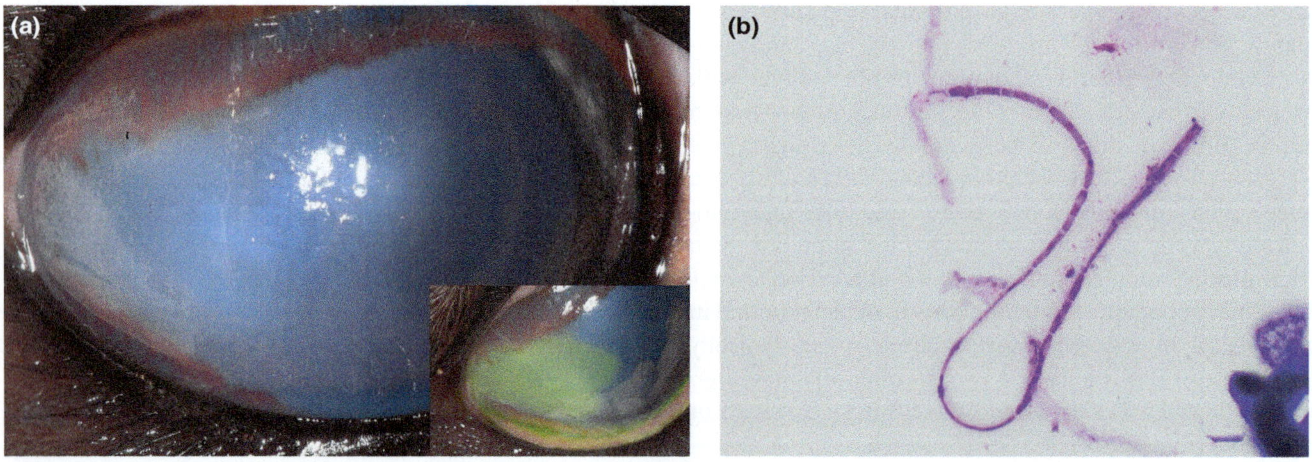

Figure 59.1 Alpaca with fungal ulcerative keratitis. (a) Grossly, there is diffuse corneal edema of the lateral aspect of the cornea with vascularization infiltrating from the dorsal and ventral limbus. The surface of the cornea looks dry and irregular, which can suggest a fungal infection. The inset demonstrates the extent of the corneal ulcer after fluorescein staining. (b) A cytobrush sample of the corneal ulcer found septate fungal hyphae (Wright Giemsa, 500×. *Source:* Image courtesy of Leslie Sharkey).

systemic infections or neoplastic diseases where the blood–aqueous barrier is compromised.[27,28]

Periocular, anterior, and posterior segment neoplasia in camelids is uncommon, and only few cases are reported, including squamous cell carcinoma, epitheliotropic cutaneous lymphoma, and intraocular melanoma.[18,20,29] Cytologically, these appear similar to the same tumors in other species. Fine-needle aspiration from intraocular tumors is not recommended due to risks for complications such as intraocular bleeding and glaucoma.[27] Enucleation followed by histopathology is recommended for these cases.

Musculoskeletal

Evaluation of synovial fluid is an important part of evaluating joint diseases, particularly when a septic cause is suspected. Nucleated cell count, total protein, and differential cell counts have been reported for healthy llamas and alpacas (Table 59.1).[30] While cellular elements are similar to other species, the reference interval for synovial fluid protein concentration is higher in camelids. Bacteria are rarely identified in synovial fluid cytology samples except occasionally in young animals. No specific studies of the diagnostic performance of cytology versus culture of synovial fluid for identification of infectious processes are available in camelids.

Cytologic features of an embryonal rhabdomyosarcoma identified in a shoulder mass in an alpaca included many round to spindloid to stellate cells with discrete borders and vacuolated basophilic cytoplasm.[31] Nuclei were round to ovoid with variable nucleoli; cells exhibited marked anisocytosis and anisokaryosis.[31]

Respiratory

Characteristics of the cell populations have been published for healthy alpaca BAL fluid and llama tracheal wash fluid (Table 59.1).[32,33] Cell types in BAL fluid are reported to be similar to those in horses but with a higher mean percentage of neutrophils. Ciliated columnar airway epithelial cells can be present in BALs due to minor airway trauma during sampling. Eosinophils and mast cells were absent.[33] Tracheal wash fluid from normal llamas contained a predominance of macrophages with few neutrophils and respiratory epithelial cells (Table 59.1).[32]

Bacterial pneumonia and pleuropneumonia can be identified cytologically prior to culture. "Alpaca fever" is caused by *Streptococcus equi* ssp. *zooepidemicus*, is associated with a variety of clinical signs, and is most likely transmitted through respiratory secretions from infected horses and potentially from other infected camelids. Respiratory cytology can also reveal fungal agents including *C. immitis*, *Cryptococcus neoformans, Cryptococcus gattii, Histoplasma capsulatum*, and *Aspergillus* spp. Figure 59.2 shows *C. immitis* in a tracheal wash.

Pleural fluid is relatively scant in normal camelids, but can be obtained when effusions are present. Pleural fluid from clinically healthy llamas has a total nucleated cell count of <1500 cells/μL and a small lymphocyte predominance (Table 59.1).[32] Pulmonary neoplasia has been diag-

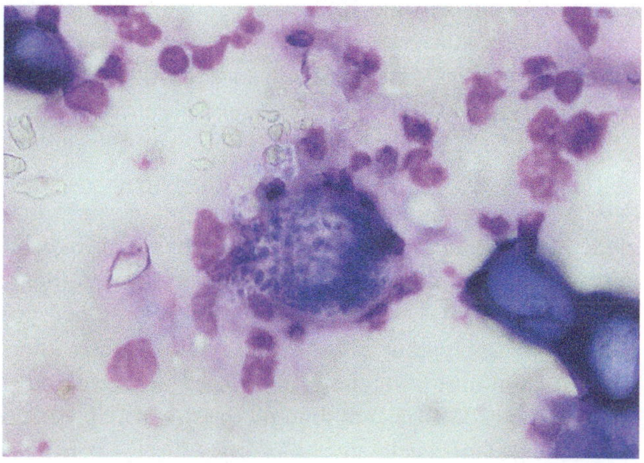

Figure 59.2 *C. immitis* spherule in a tracheal wash from an alpaca (Wright Giemsa, 500×).

Table 59.1 Camelid fluid reference intervals.

Sample	Nucleated cell count (cells/μL)	Total protein	Neutrophils (%)	Large mononuclear cells (%)	Lymphocytes (%)
Abdominal fluid	<3 000	<2.5 g/dL	15–98	2–83	
Pleural fluid	385–768	<2.7 g/dL	0–10	0–20	80–100
Synovial fluid	100–1400	2.0–3.8 g/dL	0–12	4–48	50–96
Cerebrospinal fluid	0–3	31.2–66.8 mg/dL	0–8	4–45	37–92
Bronchoalveolar lavage fluid			0–29	34–83	3–58
Tracheal aspirate			0–40	60–100	0–1

nosed by examination of a pleural fluid sample in a llama.[34] Although the cells appeared individualized and round cytologically, the histologic diagnosis was primary pulmonary carcinoma. A chylous effusion has also been identified in a camelid following thoracic surgery.[3]

Lymph Nodes, Thymus, and Spleen

Lymph node abscesses are the most common inflammatory cause of lymph node enlargement in camelids and are caused by bacteria such as *C. pseudotuberculosis*, which is most often responsible for herd outbreaks, and *Streptococcus zooepidemicus*.[35] Both can be identified in cytologic samples as Gram-positive bacilli and Gram-positive cocci, respectively.

Lymphoma is the most common camelid neoplasm and can be diagnosed cytologically on samples from external lymph nodes and body fluids.[36,37] Although one review suggests that mandibular and inguinal lymph nodes are most often enlarged, most camelid lymphoma is multicentric, with liver, spleen, and internal and external lymph nodes most frequently involved.[15,29,36,38–40] B-cell lymphoma was twice as common as T-cell lymphoma in a report of 12 alpacas and 12 llamas.[39] Some earlier reports of lymphoma may have actually have been a malignant round cell tumor type identified as a primitive malignant round cell tumor (PMRCT) based on lack of staining for lymphoid markers with expression of one or more neural markers (e.g. neuron-specific enolase, synaptophysin, and S-100).[39,41] This tumor type appears to be more common in alpacas, than llamas, and to occur in younger animals on average, though this is based on a relatively low number of reported cases.[39] Distinction between lymphoma and PMRCT probably cannot be made cytologically without the use of immunocytochemistry. Based on their immunophenotype, PMRCTs are thought to arise from pleuripotential neural crest cells.[39,41]

Gastrointestinal, Liver, and Pancreas

Fluid from the first compartment (C1), collected either by tube or percutaneously, can be analyzed in digestive tract disorders. Normal fluid is green to light brown with a pH of 6.4–6.8, although anorexia or salivary fluid contamination can increase pH. Small protozoa and Gram-negative bacteria are present.[42]

Clinically evident hepatic lipidosis affects camelids of all ages and occurs with excessive mobilization of lipids accompanying negative energy balance. Increased serum concentrations of non-esterified fatty acids and beta-hydroxybutyrate can be indicative, along with other serum indicators of hepatocellular damage, cholestasis, and

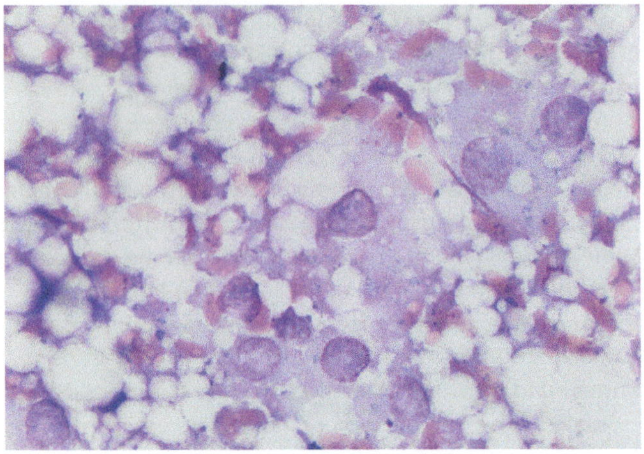

Figure 59.3 Impression smear demonstrating hepatic lipidosis in a llama (Wright Giemsa, 500×).

impaired liver function. Microscopic evaluation of the liver provides a definitive diagnosis, appearing cytologically similar to the feline syndrome (Figure 59.3).[43] Postmortem cytologic evaluation of a liver mass from a llama diagnosed with cholangiocarcinoma revealed cohesive clusters and tubular structures composed of anaplastic cuboidal to columnar cells characterized by multinucleated giant cells, mitotic figures, and inflammation.[44]

Urinary Tract

Urinary tract infection, inflammation, and, rarely, neoplasia, can be detected by examination of urine sediment. Although symptomatic uroliths are somewhat common in male camelids because of their narrow urethra and relatively low urine output, it is uncommon to see crystals in urine samples. When present, crystals include triple phosphate and calcium oxalate but vary with diet and geography.[4]

Reproductive

Uterine cytology is used in conjunction with culture in the diagnostic evaluation of infertility in camelids. Uterine infections are frequently implicated as causes of infertility. If vaginal contamination is avoided, the presence of neutrophils indicates inflammation, and identification of organisms can specify the cause. Bacteria including *Escherichia coli*, *Streptococcus* spp., *Pseudomonas* spp., *Klebsiella* spp., *Actinomyces pyogenes*, and *Staphylococcus* spp. have all been identified, as well as fungal infections with *Aspergillus* spp. and *Mucor* spp.[45,46]

A recent report indicated that fine-needle aspiration and cytologic examination of testicles is a minimally invasive and cost-effective alternative to testicular biopsy for evaluation of testicular cell populations and spermatogenesis in male camelids.[47] Standards for quantitation of cell types in camelids of different ages and breeding activity will be necessary to make this a widely accepted part of breeding soundness examinations.

Central Nervous System

Reference intervals for CSF have been determined for clinically healthy camelids (Table 59.1) with the upper limit for total cell count reported as 3–5 cells/μL and the protein concentration as 31.2–66.8 mg/dL.[16,48] Inflammatory and infectious central nervous system diseases are usually associated with increased cell count and protein concentration in the CSF. In bacterial infection, neutrophils are increased, and organisms can be present or absent with no documented association with degenerate change in cells.[49] With fungal meningitis, including cryptococcosis and disseminated blastomycosis and coccidioidomycosis, organisms have been observed in CSF with neutrophilic inflammation.[50] Viral diseases of the central nervous system can be characterized by normal CSF or increased protein concentration and mononuclear pleocytosis. Serologic testing on CSF is more likely to identify an infectious etiology than cytologic examination. Both greater than 17% eosinophils in the CSF of camelids and >1.5 eosinophils/μL in CSF showed sensitivity and specificity of 85% or greater for *Parelaphostrongylus tenuis* infection in areas of the northeastern United States with endemic white-tailed deer populations (Figure 59.4). Increased CSF protein concentration and monocytic pleocytosis are also characteristic of this infection.[51,52] A PCR assay has been developed for *P. tenuis* and could presumably be performed on CSF for a definitive diagnosis.[53]

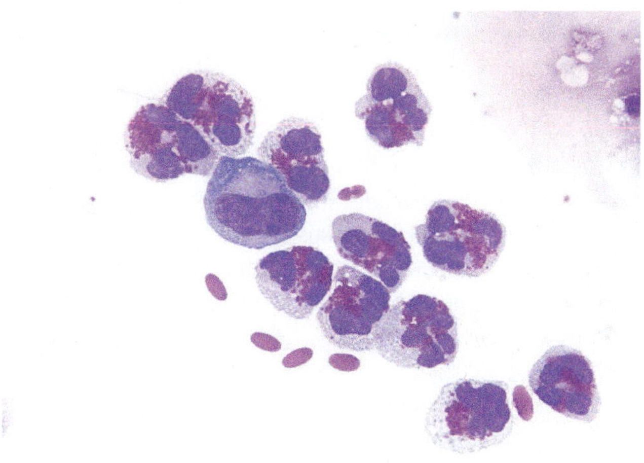

Figure 59.4 Eosinophilic pleocytosis in cerebrospinal fluid from an alpaca with central nervous system *P. tenuis* (Wright Giemsa, 500×. *Source:* Image courtesy of Maxey Wellman).

Approximately 20% of camelids with multicentric lymphoma develop extradural tumor masses close to the lumbosacral space. Cells from these masses can contaminate CSF during collection and can be identified cytologically as large immature mononuclear cells accompanied by an increased protein concentration.[40]

An important rule out for neurologic disease in neonatal camelids is hyperosmolar syndrome, which is characterized by hyperglycemia, hypernatremia, and hyperosmolarity. While no abnormal cytologic findings have been reported in CSF from these cases, biochemical abnormalities including high sodium, high glucose, and high protein have been seen.[54]

Body Cavity Fluid Analysis

Automated total nucleated cell counts appear to be accurate for alpaca abdominal fluid.[55] Cell counts and total protein values for abdominal fluid from clinically healthy alpacas and llamas have been reported (Table 59.1). Higher cell counts and protein concentrations were identified in a small number of healthy animals with only scant fluid volumes. Consequently, these parameters should not be considered highly sensitive for intra-abdominal disease or should be evaluated based on the volume. Organisms can be identified in cases of compromised bowel wall, ruptured gastrointestinal ulcers, urinary bladder rupture, uterine tear, sepsis, intra-abdominal abscesses, traumatic injuries, and post-surgery. A variety of organisms can invade the abdomen through compromised bowel or body wall. *S. zooepidemicus* appears to be the most common cause of hematogenous peritonitis or focal abdominal abscesses beyond the neonatal period (Figure 59.5a).[56,57]

Pancreatic necrosis can be associated with an inflammatory exudate and increased activity of amylase and lipase in the abdominal fluid compared with serum values.[58] As mentioned previously, round cell tumors can be detected by fluid analysis, although advanced diagnostics such as immunohistochemistry may be required for definitive identification of cell lineage (Figure 59.5b).[59]

Conclusion

Cytologic collection and analysis in camelids often has similar indications and applications as in other species. The clinician must be aware of the characteristic shape of camelid erythrocytes and also that their body fluids, like their blood, often contains higher neutrophil numbers than would be found in a typical ruminant. With increasing familiarity with the species and the

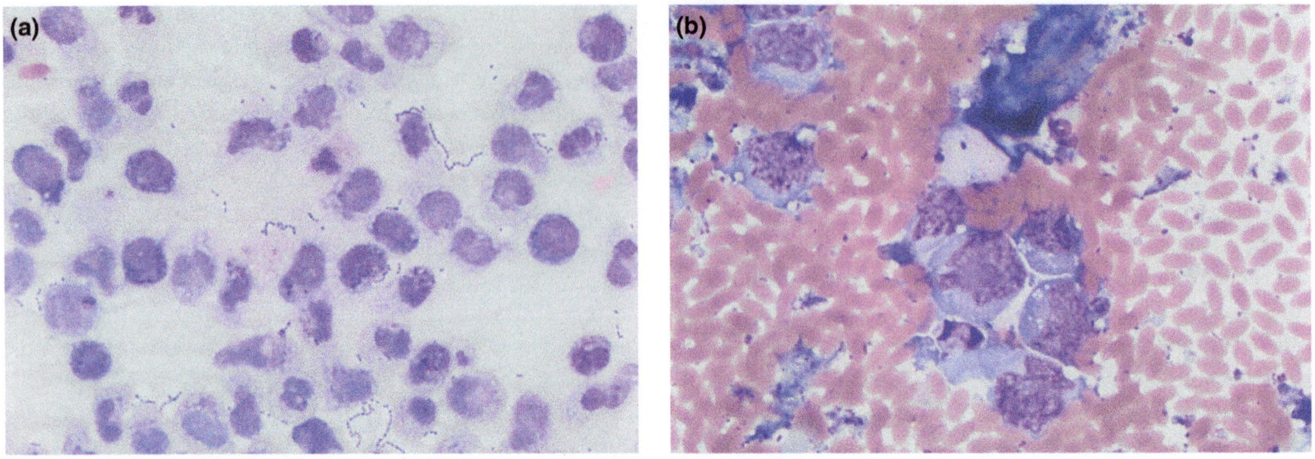

Figure 59.5 (a) Abdominal fluid from an alpaca. *S. zooepidemicus* peritonitis developed following experimental infection by respiratory route (Wright Giemsa, 500×). (b) Abdominal fluid from an alpaca with intestinal lymphoma and a gut rupture showing anaplastic round cells, debris, and a mixed population of extracellular bacteria (Wright Giemsa, 500×).

development of better sampling techniques, submissions that are rare today, such as urine or respiratory tract wash fluids, may become easier to collect and hence more common. Similarly, as our knowledge of the spectrum of camelid diseases advances, newer and more specialized testing is expected to develop.

References

1 Cebra, C. and Gemensky-Metzler, A. (2014). Disorders of the neurologic system and special senses. In: *Llama and Alpaca Care*, (eds. Christopher, C., David E.A., Ahmed, T., Robert J. Van Saun., LaRue W.J.), 438–439. St. Louis, MO: Elsevier.

2 Cebra, C.K., Tornquist, S.J., and Reed, S.K. (2008). Collection and analysis of peritoneal fluid from healthy llamas and alpacas. *J Am Vet Med Assoc* 232: 1357–1361.

3 Cebra, C.K. (2014). Diseases of the respiratory tract. In: *Llama and Alpaca Care*, vol. 434, (eds. Christopher, C., David E.A., Ahmed, T., Robert J. Van Saun., LaRue W.J.). St. Louis, MO: Elsevier.

4 Cebra, C.K. (2014). Diseases of the urinary system. In: *Llama and Alpaca Care*, vol. 465, (eds. Christopher, C., David E.A., Ahmed, T., Robert J. Van Saun., LaRue W.J.). St. Louis, MO: Elsevier.

5 Scott, D.W., Vogel, J.W., Fleis, R.I. et al. (2011). Skin diseases in the alpaca (*Vicugna pacos*): a literature review and retrospective analysis of 68 cases (Cornell University 1997–2006). *Vet Dermatol* 22: 2–16.

6 Sisson, D. and Cebra, C. (2014). Disorders of the skin. In: *Llama and Alpaca Care*, 381, (eds. Christopher, C., David E.A., Ahmed, T., Robert J. Van Saun., LaRue W.J.). St. Louis, MO: Elsevier.

7 Rosychuk, R.A.W. (1994). Llama dermatology. *Vet Clin North Am Food Anim Pract* 10: 228–239.

8 Lamm, C.G., Love, B.C., Rodgers, L.L. et al. (2009). Pathology in practice. Fungal dermatitis in a camel caused by Candida albicans. *J Am Vet Med Assoc*, (eds. Christopher, C., David E.A., Ahmed, T., Robert J. Van Saun., LaRue W.J.), 234: 1013–1015.

9 Fowler, M.E., Pappagianis, D., and Ingram, I. (1992). Coccidioidomycosis in llamas in the United States 19 cases (1981–1989). *J Am Vet Med Assoc* 201: 1609–1614.

10 Moll, H.D., Schumacher, J., and Hoover, T.R. (1992). *Entomophthoramycosis condiobolae* in a llama. *J Am Vet Med Assoc* 200: 969–970.

11 French, R.A. and Ashworth, C.D. (1994). Zygomycosis caused by *Conidiobolus coronatus* in a llama (*Lama glama*). *Vet Pathol* 31: 120–122.

12 Eo, K.Y.H., Kwak, D., Shin, T. et al. (2010). Skin lesions associated with *Demodex* sp. in a llama (*Lama glama*). *J Zoo Wildl Med* 41: 178–180.

13 Charney, V.A., Toth, B., Couetil, L.L. et al. (2012). Pathology in practice: epidermal and follicular infundibular orthokeratosis. *J Am Vet Med Assoc* 243: 1701–1703.

14 Valentine, B.A. and Martin, J.M. (2007). Prevalence of neoplasia in llamas and alpacas (Oregon State University, 2001–2006). *J Vet Diagn Invest* 19: 202–204.

15 Lin, T.Y., Hamber, A., Pentecost, R. et al. (2010). Mast cell tumors in a llama (*Lama glama*). *J Vet Diagn Invest* 22: 808–811.

16 Whitehead, C.E. and Bedenice, D. (2009). Neurologic diseases in llamas and alpacas. *Vet Clin North Am Food Anim Pract* 25: 385–405.

17 Sumer, J.P., Mueller, T., Clapp, K.S. et al. (2012). Modified ear canal ablation and lateral bulla osteotomy for management of otitis media in an alpaca. *Vet Surg* 41: 273–277.

18 Gionfriddo, J.R. (2013). Ophthalmology of new world camelids. In: *Veterinary Ophthalmology*, 2e, 1675–1691. Ames, IA: Wiley-Blackwell.

19 Storms, G., Meersschaert, C., Farnir, S., and Grauwels, M. (2016). Normal bacterial conjunctival flora of the Huacaya alpaca (*Vicugna pacos*). *Vet Ophthalmol* 19: 22–28.

20 Gionfriddo, J.R. (2010). Ophthalmology of South American camelids. *Vet Clin North Am Food Anim Pract*, (eds. Kirk, N.G., Brian C.G., Thomas J.K.), 26: 531–555.

21 Mangan, B.G., Gionfriddo, J.R., and Powell, C.C. (2008). Bilateral nasolacrimal duct atresia in a cria. *Vet Ophthalmol* 11: 49–54.

22 Ledbetter, E.C., Montgomery, K.W., Landry, M.P., and Kice, N.C. (2013). Characterization of fungal keratitis in alpacas: 11 cases (2003–2012). *J Am Vet Med Assoc* 243: 1616–1622.

23 Ledbetter, E.C. and Scarlett, J.M. (2008). Isolation of obligate anaerobic bacteria from ulcerative keratitis in domestic animals. *Vet Ophthalmol* 11: 114–122.

24 Coster, M.E., Ramos-Vara, J.A., Vemulapalli, R. et al. (2010). *Coccidioides posadasii* keratoconjunctivitis in a llama (*Llama glama*). *Vet Ophthalmol* 13: 53–57.

25 Jones, M.L., Gilmour, M.A., and Streeter, R.N. (2007). Use of grid keratotomy in the treatment of indolent corneal ulcers in a llama. *Can Vet J* 48: 416–419.

26 Pucket, J.D., Boileau, M.J., and Sula, M.J. (2014). Calcific band keratopathy in an alpaca. *Vet Ophthalmol* 17: 286–289.

27 Featherstone, H.J. and Heinrich, C.L. (2013). Part 1: The eye examination and diagnostic procedures. In: *Veterinary Ophthalmology*, 2e, (eds. Kirk, N.G., Brian C.G., Thomas J.K.), 533–613. Ames, IA: Wiley-Blackwell.

28 Linn-Pearl, R.N., Powel, R.M., Newman, H.A., and Gould, D.J. (2015). Validity of aqueocentesis as a component of anterior uveitis investigation in dogs and cats. *Vet Ophthalmol* 18: 326–334.

29 Aboellail, T.A. (2013). Pathologic and immunophenotypic characterization of 27 camelid malignant round cell tumors. *J Vet Diagn Invest* 25: 168–172.

30 Waguespack, R.W., Belknap, E.B., Spano, J.S. et al. (2002). Analysis of synovial fluid from clinically normal alpacas and llamas. *Am J Vet Res* 63: 576–578.

31 Goncarovs-Gran, K.O., Frank, C.B., Baird, A.N. et al. (2013). Pathology in practice: Embryonal rhabdomyosarcoma in an alpaca. *J Am Vet Med Assoc* 243: 1113–1115.

32 Gerros, T.C. and Andreasen, C.B. (1999). Analysis of transtracheal aspirates and pleural fluid from clinically healthy llamas (*Lama glama*). *Vet Clin Pathol* 28: 29–32.

33 Pacheco, A.P., Bedenice, D., Mazan, M.R., and Hoffman, A.M. (2012). Respiratory mechanics and results of cytologic examination of bronchoalveolar lavage fluid in healthy adult alpacas. *Am J Vet Res* 73: 146–152.

34 Ramos-Vara, J.A., Loiacono, C.M., Williams, F. 3rd et al. (2004). Pulmonary neoplasia in two llamas (*Lama glama*). *Vet Pathol* 41: 520–523.

35 Cebra, C.K. and Sisson, D. (2014). Diseases of the cardiovascular and hemolymphatic systems. In: *Llama and Alpaca Care*, 415, (eds. Christopher, C., David E.A., Ahmed, T., Robert J. Van Saun., LaRue W.J.). St. Louis, MO: Elsevier.

36 Cebra, C.K., Garry, F.B., Powers, B.E., and Johnson, L.W. (1995). Lymphosarcoma in 10 New World camelids. *J Vet Intern Med* 9: 381–385.

37 Martin, J.M., Valentine, V.A., and Cebra, C.K. (2010). Clinical, ultrasonographic, and laboratory findings in 12 llamas and 12 alpacas with malignant round cell tumors. *Can Vet J* 51: 1379–1382.

38 Fowler, M.E., Gillespie, D., and Harkema, J. (1985). Lymphosarcoma in a llama. *J Am Vet Med Assoc* 187: 1245–1246.

39 Martin, J.M., Valentine, B.A., Cebra, C.K. et al. (2009). Malignant round cell neoplasia in llamas and alpacas. *Vet Pathol* 46: 288–298.

40 Pusterla, N., Colegrove, K.M., Moore, P.F. et al. (2006). Multicentric T-cell lymphosarcoma in an alpaca. *Vet J* 171: 181–185.

41 Sartin, E.A., Crowe, D.R., Whitley, E.M. et al. (2004). Malignant neoplasia in four alpacas. *J Vet Diagn Invest* 16: 226–229.

42 Navarre, C.B., Pugh, D.G., Heath, A.M., and Simpkins, S.A. (1999). Analysis of first gastric compartment fluid collected via percutaneous paracentesis from healthy llamas. *J Am Vet Med Assoc* 214: 812–815.

43 Tornquist, S.J., Van Saun, R.J., Smith, B.B. et al. (1999). Hepatic lipidosis in llamas and alpacas: 31 cases (1991–1997). *J Am Vet Med Assoc* 214: 1368–1372.

44 Taulescu, M.A., Bolfa, P.F., Buiga, R. et al. (2012). Metastatic cholangiocarcinoma in a llama (*Llama glama*). *J Vet Diagn Invest* 24: 986–989.

45 Bildfell, R.J., Lohr, C.V., and Tornquist, S.J. (2012). Diagnostic sampling and gross pathology of New Worldcamelids. *Vet Clin North Am Food Anim Pract* 28: 577–591.

46 Tibary A, Pearson LK., Rodriguez JS, et al. (2002). Uterine infection in camelidae: diagnostic and therapeutic approaches. *Proceedings of the International Camelid Health Conference*, Columbus, OH (March 24–28, 2010), 437–439.

47 Stelletta, C., Juyena, N.S., Salazar, D.P. et al. (2011). Testicular cytology of alpaca: comparison between impressed and smeared slides. *Anim Reprod Sci* 125: 133–137.

48 Welles, E.G., Pugh, D.G., Wenzel, J.G., and Sorjonen, D.C. (1994). Composition of cerebrospinal fluid in healthy adult llamas. *Am J Vet Res* 55: 1075–1079.

49 Frank, N., Couëtil, L.L., and Clarke, K.A. (1998). Listeria monocytogenes and *Escherichia coli* septicemia and meningoencephalitis in a 7 day old llama. *Can Vet J* 39: 100–102.

50 Goodchild, L.M., Dart, A.J., Collins, M.B. et al. (1996). Cryptococcal meningitis in an alpaca. *Aust Vet J* 74: 428–430.

51 Pinn, T.L., Bender, H.S., Stokol, T. et al. (2013). Cerebrospinal fluid eosinophilia is a sensitive and specific test for the diagnosis of *Parelaphostrongylus tenuis* in camelids in the northeastern United States. *J Vet Diagn Invest* 25: 54–60.

52 Bertin, F.R. and Taylor, S.D. (2016). Cerebrospinal nematodiasis in 20 camelids. *J Vet Intern Med* 30: 1390–1395.

53 Dobey, C.L., Grunenwald, C., Newman, S.J. et al. (2014). Retrospective study of central nervous system lesions and association with *Parelaphostrongylus* species by histology and specific nested polymerase chain reaction in domestic camelids and wild ungulates. *J Vet Diagn Invest* 26: 748–754.

54 Cebra, C.K. (2000). Hyperglycemia, hypernatremia, and hyperosmolarity in 6 neonatal llamas and alpacas. *J Am Vet Med Assoc* 217: 1701–1704.

55 Gorman, M.E., Villarroel, A., Tornquist, S.J. et al. (2009). Comparison between manual and automated total nucleated cell counts using the ADVIA 120 for pleural and peritoneal samples from dogs, cats, horses, and alpacas. *Vet Clin Pathol* 38: 388–391.

56 Cebra, C.K., Heidel, J.R., Cebra, M.L. et al. (2000). Pathogenesis of *Streptococcus zooepidemicus* infection after intratracheal inoculation in llamas. *Am J Vet Res* 61: 1525–1529.

57 Hewson, J. and Cebra, C.K. (2001). Peritonitis in a llama caused by *Streptococcus equi* subsp. *Zooepidemicus*. *Can Vet J* 42: 465–467.

58 Pearson, E.G. and Snyder, S.P. (2000). Pancreatic necrosis in New World camelids 11 cases (1990–1998). *J Am Vet Med Assoc* 217: 241–244.

59 Sorensen, N.J. and Allison, R.W. (2015). What is your diagnosis? Abdominal fluid from an adult alpaca. *Vet Clin Pathol* 44: 459–460.

60 Koenig, J., Watrous, B.J., Kaneps, A.J. et al. (2001). Otitis media in a llama. *J Am Vet Med Assoc* 218: 619–623.

60

Nonhuman Primates

Mark A. Suckow, Jodi A. Scholz, and Kirstin F. Barnhart

Introduction

Nonhuman primates (NHP) have played a significant role in major medical advancements related to infectious disease, organ transplantation, pharmacology, aging, and neuroscience. Such work typically involves the careful evaluation of many parameters to answer relevant research questions. Cytology is an important tool in the characterization of animal models and in investigating experimental manipulation. Because of their value and longevity, NHP are often maintained as research subjects for long periods of time. As a result, animals develop either spontaneous or research-associated illness, and cytology is employed as a diagnostic and prognostic tool.

NHP are rarely kept as companion animals due to complex husbandry needs and regulatory prohibitions. The risks of zoonotic disease further challenge the ability to safely maintain NHP for purposes of companionship and fancy. Nonetheless, some are kept as pets or assistance animals and require diagnostic evaluation that includes cytology. NHP are common at zoological parks. Maintaining healthy animals despite a relatively direct interface with the public that poses additional risks to the animals' health and well-being is challenging. The need to demonstrate to the public a high level of health leads to significant expectations for veterinary care. As a result, diagnostic veterinary medicine, including cytology, plays an important role. Animals often live a natural life span; thus geriatric conditions are encountered. Cytological evaluation is additionally complicated by the myriad NHP species encountered in some zoological parks. For some species, a dearth of information regarding what is to be considered normal further complicates the interpretation of samples.

Applications of Cytology in the Clinical Setting

Common Tissues and Organs Sampled

The clinical cytology samples in NHP are similar to other species, including aspirates, cervical scrapings, skin scrapes, impression smears, smears of exudates, and fluid analysis, particularly cerebrospinal or synovial fluids. Vaginal cytology is useful for timed mating in breeding programs. Samples from the proximal-third of the vagina are obtained using a cotton-tipped swab. Semen quality evaluation is used to optimize successful breeding programs; samples are obtained by massage and electroejaculation.[1,2] More details on investigative cytology in research settings can be found in Chapter 66.

Methods of Collection

NHP pose risks of bite and scratch injuries and are usually physically or chemically restrained for sample collection.[3] The most common methods of physical restraint include a squeeze-back cage (research), hand restraint using bite-resistant gloves (leather, stainless steel mesh, or Kevlar®), other personal protective equipment, net entrapment, and restraint chairs after training (research). For chemical restraint, intramuscular ketamine hydrochloride (5–25 mg/kg) is appropriate. Operant conditioning, including positive reinforcement training, can be used to accommodate both rhesus macaques and chimpanzees to in-cage venipuncture.[3,4] The ability to obtain samples without active restraint enhances the well-being of the animals and strengthens the bond between animal and handler. Positive reinforcement training is more typically employed

Veterinary Cytology, First Edition. Edited by Leslie C. Sharkey, M. Judith Radin, and Davis Seelig.

in zoological parks and research situations than with pets. Once properly restrained, cytological sampling from NHP is similar to other species. Emphasis should be on using methods that minimize pain and distress. This includes minimizing restraint time, which is facilitated by careful advanced planning for procedures.

Cytology as a Diagnostic Tool

Cytology is used to assess outcomes in experimental NHP models as described in Chapter 66. In addition, cytology is an important diagnostic tool for the clinical management of individual NHP. For example, fine-needle aspirate (FNA) of the spleen identified toxoplasmosis in a howler monkey with jaundice, weight loss, and hepatosplenomegaly.[5] Morulae of *Ehrlichia chaffeensis* were observed in lymphocytes and monocytes from FNAs of enlarged lymph nodes in ring-tailed and ruffed lemurs experiencing anorexia, fever, and lethargy.[6] Likewise, impression smears have been used to diagnose disease in NHP, such as a cutaneous melanocytoma in a cynomolgus monkey,[7] and leprosy in that same species.[8] As with other species, cytology is often complementary to other diagnostic methods. Observation of specific cell types or microorganisms should be correlated with clinical presentation and other data to establish a definitive diagnosis.

Conditions Evaluated by Cytology

Skin and Subcutis

Impression smears of lesions or FNA of pustules or masses are utilized for cytologic evaluation of the skin and subcutis. Skin scrapes can be useful for ectoparasites.

Inflammatory and Infectious Disease

Histoplasma capsulatum var. *duboisii* is a fungal organism endemic in central and western Africa. Disease has been reported in baboons originating from Africa and in captive-born animals from Texas. Infection typically causes ulcerated nodules in areas of the body most often in contact with the ground (hands, feet, tail, buttocks) and the face.[9–12] The organism is usually abundant in affected tissues, and diagnosis can often be made cytologically. The yeast forms of *H. capsulatum* var. *duboisii* are found inside macrophages or giant cells and are visible as large thick-walled oval structures that demonstrate narrow-base budding, ranging from 7 to 15 μm in size (as opposed to the variety *capsulatum*, which are approximately 3 μm in size). Organisms are best viewed using a fungal stain such as Gomori's methenamine silver, Periodic acid–Schiff, or Gridley stains.[13–15]

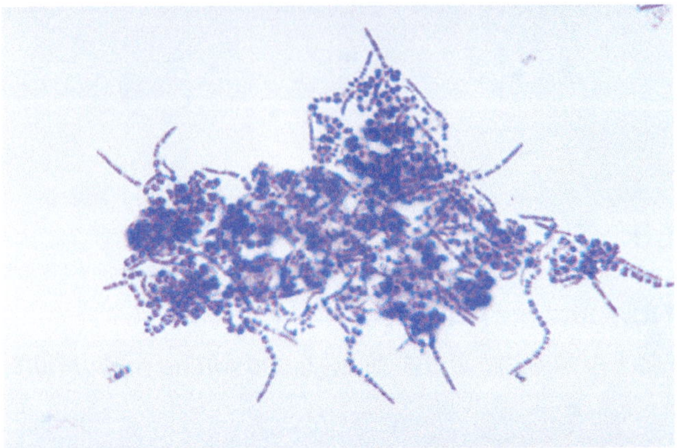

Figure 60.1 *D. congolensis* seen in typical rows of Gram-positive cocci and forming a "railroad track" appearance (Giemsa stain, estimated 1000×. *Source:* Image from the Centers for Disease Control and Prevention's Public Health Image Library, identification #2986).

Dermatophilus congolensis is a Gram-positive, non-acid-fast actinomycete affecting NHP, most notably owl monkeys.[16,17] It causes scaling that progresses to the formation of crusts of dried exudate and matted fur. Diagnosis can be made by cytology of fresh crusts or impression smears of moist lesions. For cytologic examination of the crusts, the sample is minced and placed onto a slide with sterile saline, air-dried, and stained with a Giemsa or Romanowsky stain. The organisms are viewed under oil immersion and appear as bundles or rows of Gram-positive cocci, which can form a "railroad track" appearance, with branching filaments measuring 1–5 μm in diameter (Figure 60.1).[12,16,17]

Nonhuman primates are susceptible to infestation by many ectoparasites including fleas (e.g. *Tunga penetrans*, *Pulex irritans*), lice (primarily Anoplura e.g. *Pedicinus* spp.), mites (e.g. *Sarcoptes scabiei*, *Prosarcoptes pitheci*), and ticks (e.g. *Ixodes* spp.), most of which cause little to no pathology. For a more comprehensive list of ectoparasites that have been reported in NHPs, as well as information regarding morphology, life cycle, and associated lesions, other sources should be consulted.

Hyperplasia and Neoplasia

There are numerous reports of spontaneous mammary hyperplasia and neoplasia in NHP, predominantly in rhesus and cynomolgus macaques, likely reflecting the high frequency of use in biomedical research. Invasive ductular carcinoma is the most commonly reported mammary tumor; less common tumors include ductal carcinoma *in situ* and invasive lobular carcinoma.[18–21] FNA can be an important part of initial clinical workup to assess for signs of malignancy, such as large pleomorphic nuclei, high mitotic index, prominent nucleoli, and amphophilic

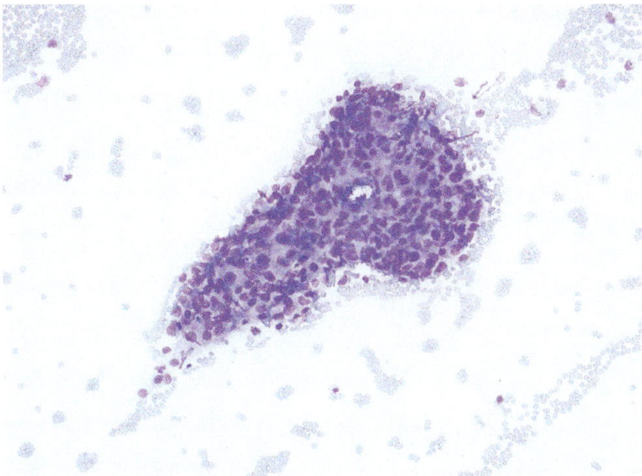

Figure 60.2 Amelanotic melanoma on the digit of a lemur. The neoplasm did not exfoliate well. The aspirate contained small poorly organized aggregates of cells with generally indistinct cytoplasmic margins and moderate anisocytosis. Melanin granules were not identified (modified Wright Giemsa, 200×. *Source:* Image courtesy of Karen Terio, University of Illinois Zoological Pathology Program).

to slightly basophilic cytoplasm; however, definitive diagnosis requires histopathology.[20–22]

Neoplasia affecting the skin and subcutaneous tissues (including the mammary gland) is relatively common in NHP.[12,23,24] FNA can be useful for guiding further diagnostics and prognosis, especially for neoplasms that have characteristic cytology such as epithelial skin tumors.[24] The most commonly reported skin neoplasm in NHP is squamous cell carcinoma.[12,24–26] Other reported tumors of the skin and subcutis include but are not limited to basal cell carcinoma, melanoma (Figure 60.2), melanocytoma, mast cell tumor, hemangioma, hemangiosarcoma, leiomyosarcoma, lipoma, and fibrosarcoma; all have cytological features similar to other species.[7,12,24,25,27]

In the cervical region, palpable subcutaneous masses can originate from the thyroid gland. Thyroid adenomas and cystadenomas have been described infrequently in prosimians, marmosets, tamarins, and macaques.[24,25,28,29] While most reports describe benign adenomas, thyroid adenocarcinomas have been identified rarely (Figure 60.3).[30,31]

Miscellaneous

Calcinosis circumscripta is an uncommon condition resulting in nodular ectopic deposition of semisolid calcium salts in subcutaneous tissues. In NHP, the condition is thought to be a consequence of traumatic injury, possibly associated with microchip implantation.[12,32,33] FNA produces a thick, white fluid, and microscopy reveals small lightly basophilic amorphous mineralized granules. Cells are infrequent but include macrophages and giant cells (Figure 12.12).[33–35] See Chapter 12 for more details on this condition in other species.

Ear and Eye

Cytology of the eye and ear is largely limited to evaluation of discharge. Normal conjunctival cytology of the common marmoset and the Cebus monkey consists of abundant squamous epithelial cells with melanin.[36]

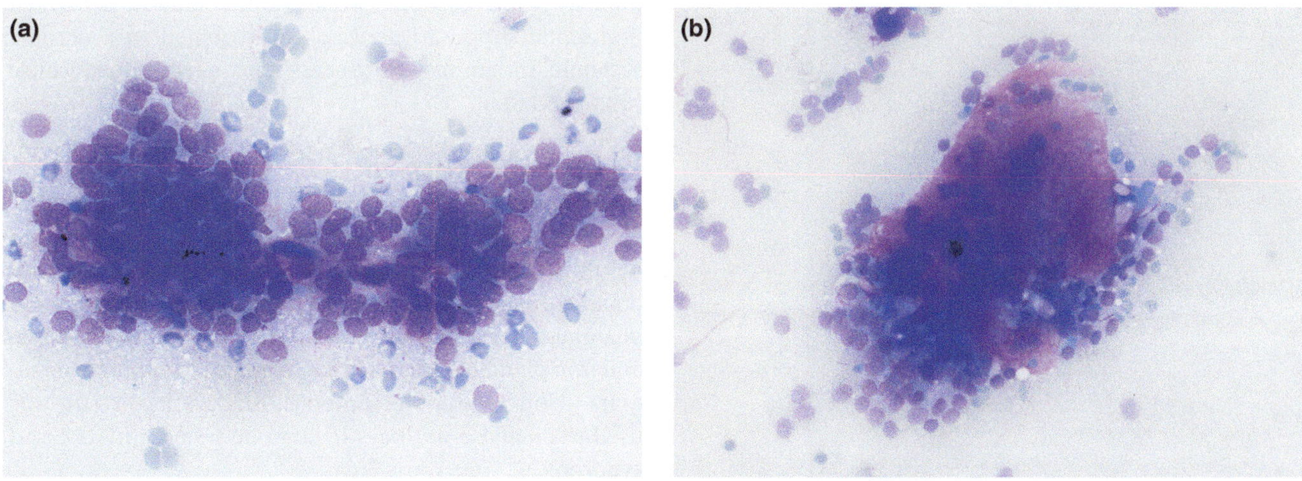

Figure 60.3 Thyroid adenocarcinoma in the ventral cervical region of a Rhesus monkey. (a) A highly cellular sample with multiple clusters of cells that had poorly defined cytoplasmic margins. The nuclei are round and fairly uniform with mild anisokaryosis. (b) The cells did not contain tyrosine granules but were frequently admixed with eosinophilic matrix consistent with colloid. Similar to thyroid neoplasms in other species, thyroid adenocarcinomas frequently display minimal criteria of malignancy (modified Wright Giemsa, 600×. *Source:* Image courtesy of Keeling Center for Comparative Medicine and Research, M. D. Anderson Cancer Center).

Inflammatory and Infectious Disease

Infection with opportunistic bacterial pathogens, particularly *Staphylococcus* spp., can be associated with conjunctivitis and ocular discharge. Infections and inflammation of the ear are unusual in NHP and would likely be associated with traumatic injury. Cytologic examination of ocular and otic discharge should include Gram stain, although bacterial culture is also recommended. Viral infections such as measles virus in both New and Old World species and herpes simplex virus type 1 can cause conjunctivitis in owl and capuchin monkeys,[3] although diagnosis is usually via other methods such as polymerase chain reaction (PCR) of body fluids for the former and of conjunctival swabs for the latter.

Hyperplasia and Neoplasia

Hyperplastic lesions of the eye and ear of NHP are not widely reported. Reports of spontaneous primary tumors involving the eye or ear are rare for NHP. Nonetheless, cytological examination of smears of samples could be used as part of a diagnostic effort in the case of neoplasia.

Musculoskeletal

The cytology literature for these tissues in NHP is scant at this time.

Inflammatory and Infectious Disease

Synovial fluid analysis is rare in NHP. It can be used to diagnose septic (Figure 60.4) and non-septic arthritis. In polyarthropathies with multiple joint effusions, the stifle is typically aspirated due to the relative ease of collection. Arthrocentesis of the stifles of a lowland gorilla and a rhesus monkey with lameness diagnosed pyogenic arthritis, the latter due to infection of the joint with *Streptobacillus moniliformis*, the causative agent of rat bite fever.[37,38] Stifle samples from a small group of cynomolgus monkeys experiencing digital and stifle swelling identified large numbers of neutrophils and monocytes indicative of polyarthritis of undetermined origin.[39] Aspiration of the stifle in a rhesus monkey with multiple swollen joints showed a marked non-septic suppurative response attributed to a chronic systemic inflammatory process of undetermined cause (Figure 60.5).

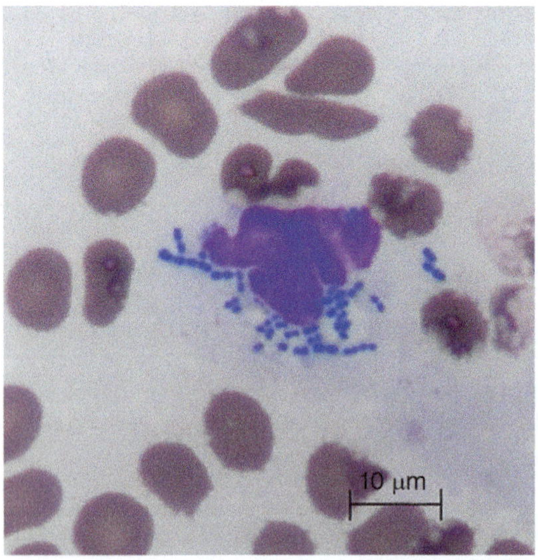

Figure 60.4 Synovial fluid from a swollen and painful stifle from a rhesus monkey. Intracytoplasmic cocci are arranged in pairs or short chains. Aerobic culture of synovial fluid yielded growth of *Streptococcus agalactiae* (modified Wright Giemsa, 1000×. *Source:* Image courtesy of Caroline Zeiss).

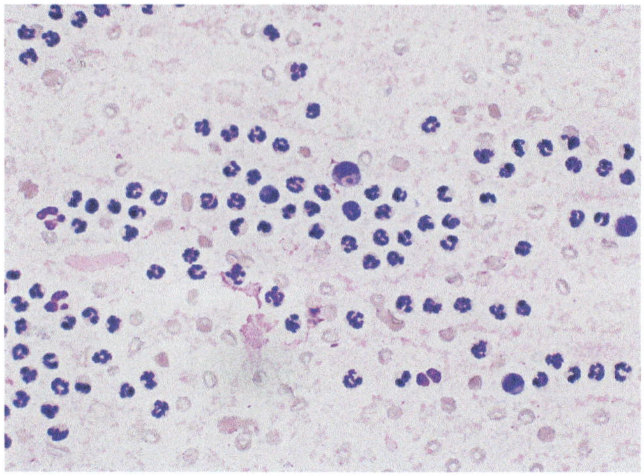

Figure 60.5 Synovial fluid from the stifle of a Rhesus monkey. This animal had multiple swollen joints. The synovial fluid was consistent with non-septic, suppurative inflammation with abundant neutrophils and occasional large mononuclear cells that infrequently displayed phagocytosis. The quality of the mucinous background was poor with no evidence of windrowing (modified Wright Giemsa, 400×. *Source:* Image courtesy of Keeling Center for Comparative Medicine and Research, M. D. Anderson Cancer Center).

Hyperplasia and Neoplasia

Reports of hyperplastic or neoplastic disease of the musculoskeletal system of NHP are rare. Cytological examination of ulnar intramedullary curettage and aspirate samples obtained from a lethargic Geoffroyi's spider monkey with bilateral expansile ulnar deformities revealed erythrocyte- and iron pigment-laden macrophages indicative of a hematoma. Along with other findings, this cytology result was used to diagnose multicystic bone disease (Gorham-Stout syndrome).[40]

Respiratory

Cytologic diagnosis of respiratory pathology can involve nasal flushing for upper airway disease, or transtracheal aspiration or bronchoalveolar lavage (BAL) for lower airway disease. Ultrasound-guided percutaneous FNA of discrete lesions can be performed if the lesion is accessible, and thoracic fluid can also be collected for analysis (see section "Body Cavity Fluid Analysis").[41–47]

BAL can be useful for diagnosis of infectious diseases of the lower airway. Collection techniques and resultant cell counts in normal animals have been described for multiple species of NHP.[41–43,45,46] The predominant cells collected were alveolar macrophages (generally 80% or greater), with the remaining cells composed of lymphocytes, neutrophils, and eosinophils; basophils, goblet cells, and mast cells were variably present in low numbers. A detailed morphological description of cells collected by BAL from cynomolgus macaques was published.[42] The BAL procedure has been demonstrated to result in extravasation of neutrophils from the pulmonary microvasculature into the bronchoalveolar space, with a 48-hour period between lavages required to mitigate additional increases in BAL neutrophil numbers when sequential samples are taken.[42,43]

Inflammatory and Infectious Disease

Primates are susceptible to lung infections. When discrete lesions are accessible percutaneously, diagnosis can sometimes be made cytologically, such as the diagnosis of bacterial pneumonia (Figure 60.6) or pulmonary abscessation. An important differential diagnosis for intrathoracic masses in NHP is *Mycobacterium tuberculosis*. Appropriate precautions are required for animal and sample handling because of zoonotic potential. Mycobacteria are slightly curved or straight rod-shaped bacteria that are negatively staining in routine preparations but clearly visible with acid-fast staining. Another bacteria, *Nocardia*, also stains positive with acid-fast stains, though not as strongly as *Mycobacterium* spp.; *Nocardia* spp. are beaded and branching, making differentiation from *Mycobacterium* spp. relatively straightforward. Cytologic differentiation between these two organisms can be a critical step in early diagnosis, since (i) both bacteria are fastidious and would not be identified using routine culture methods and (ii) antimicrobial and management strategies differ in the treatment or control of disease caused by these organisms.[47] Additional details and images for these organisms are in Chapter 3. *Streptococcus pneumoniae* can cause a severe and potentially fatal pneumonia in both wild and captive chimpanzees and gorillas.[48,49] Many cases have been associated with an initial viral infection, particularly human respiratory syncytial virus in captive animals.[50] *S. pneumoniae* typically causes a purulent bronchopneumonia characterized cytologically by degenerate neutrophils and intracellular cocci (Figure 60.7). Infectious pleural effusion can occur secondary to pneumonia (e.g. *S. pneumoniae*), following infection of adjacent structures such as pleura or pericardium, associated with lymphatic or hematogenous spread, or from direct introduction of organisms (e.g. trauma, surgery).[47]

Fungal infections also occur. A Mandrill baboon (*Mandrillus sphinx*) with a hypoechoic mass in the apical left thorax underwent ultrasound-guided percutaneous aspiration of the mass.[51] Wright's-type stain revealed numerous organisms with large spherical extracellular

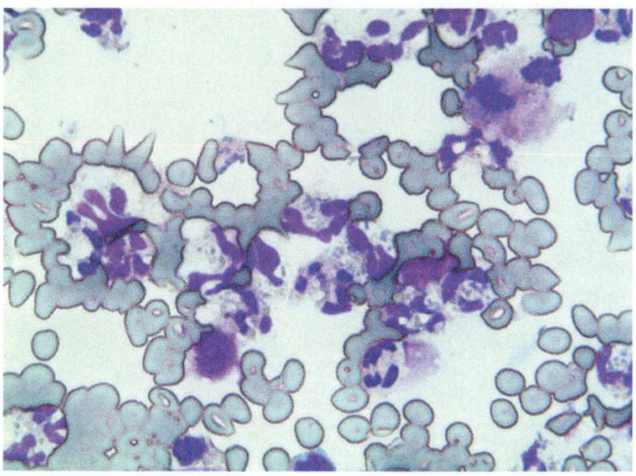

Figure 60.6 BAL sample taken from a male rhesus macaque with pneumonia due to *Streptococcus faecalis*. Samples were collected in 10 mL sterile saline with a bronchoscope and prepared using cytocentrifugation (Wright-Giemsa stain, 400×. *Source:* Image courtesy of Peter Didier).

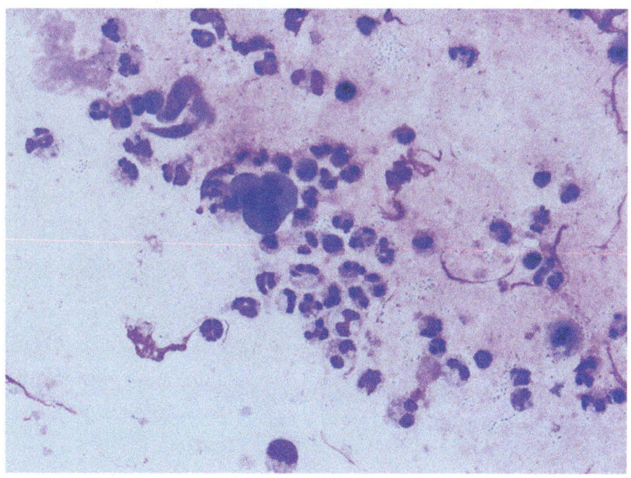

Figure 60.7 Transtracheal wash from a gorilla with septic suppurative inflammation. The sample consists primarily of degenerate neutrophils and small clusters of epithelial cells in a mucinous background. Abundant extracellular cocci appear both singly and in pairs. Cocci were also present within neutrophils (modified Wright Giemsa, 600×. *Source:* Image courtesy of Keeling Center for Comparative Medicine and Research, M. D. Anderson Cancer Center).

structures with double refractile cell wall morphology consistent with *Coccidioides spherules*. Fungal culture confirmed *Coccidioides immitis* (Chapter 3). *Pneumocystis* sp. is a fungal organism that can cause significant pathology in immune-compromised individuals, and fluid collected by BAL can be diagnostic. Staining of BAL fluid contents with stains such as methenamine silver, toluidine blue, or cresyl echt violet reveal characteristic round to oval thick-walled organisms often containing sporozoites (Figure 60.8). Immunohistochemical stains are also available. PCR testing of BAL fluid can be used to confirm the diagnosis.[47,53,54]

Lung mites such as *Pneumonyssus* and *Pneumonyssoides* spp. can be prevalent in wild-caught NHP, although these pathogens have been virtually eliminated from contemporary domestic NHP colonies.[47,54] Disease is usually subclinical, though acariasis can predispose to secondary infections. BAL is useful for antemortem diagnosis. Cytology can reveal a high concentration of eosinophils and/or actual mite specimens. The mites are 500–850 μm long, have a small dorsal plate, and have long legs with small setae and terminal claws. Associated macrophages contain birefringent golden brown to black crystals suspected to be a product of the mite.[41,47,55–57] Eosinophils were reported to comprise 15–36% of cells in BAL fluid from rhesus macaques infected with *Pneumonyssus simicola*, versus 0.5–2.5% in uninfected cynomolgus macaques.[41] Differential diagnoses for eosinophilia in BAL fluid also include eosinophilic bronchitis and asthma.[47]

Neoplasia

Respiratory tract neoplasia is relatively uncommon in NHP. One exception is carcinomas of the oral cavity and upper respiratory tract in common marmosets, which are hypothesized to be associated with an oncogenic viral infection.[24,47] Of the other reported upper respiratory tract tumors, carcinomas of the nasal cavity and nasopharynx appear most common, with sporadic reports of other tumors such as laryngeal adenoma, nasal papillary adenocarcinoma, and fibromyxomatous polyposis of the nasal cavity.[23,24,47] Only rare cases of pulmonary neoplasia have been reported, most notably carcinomas but also including adenomas, adenocarcinomas, and sarcomas.[23,24,47] A spontaneous primary squamous cell carcinoma of the lung was reported in a rhesus macaque.[58] Diagnosis of solid tumors of the respiratory tract is generally made by surgical biopsy

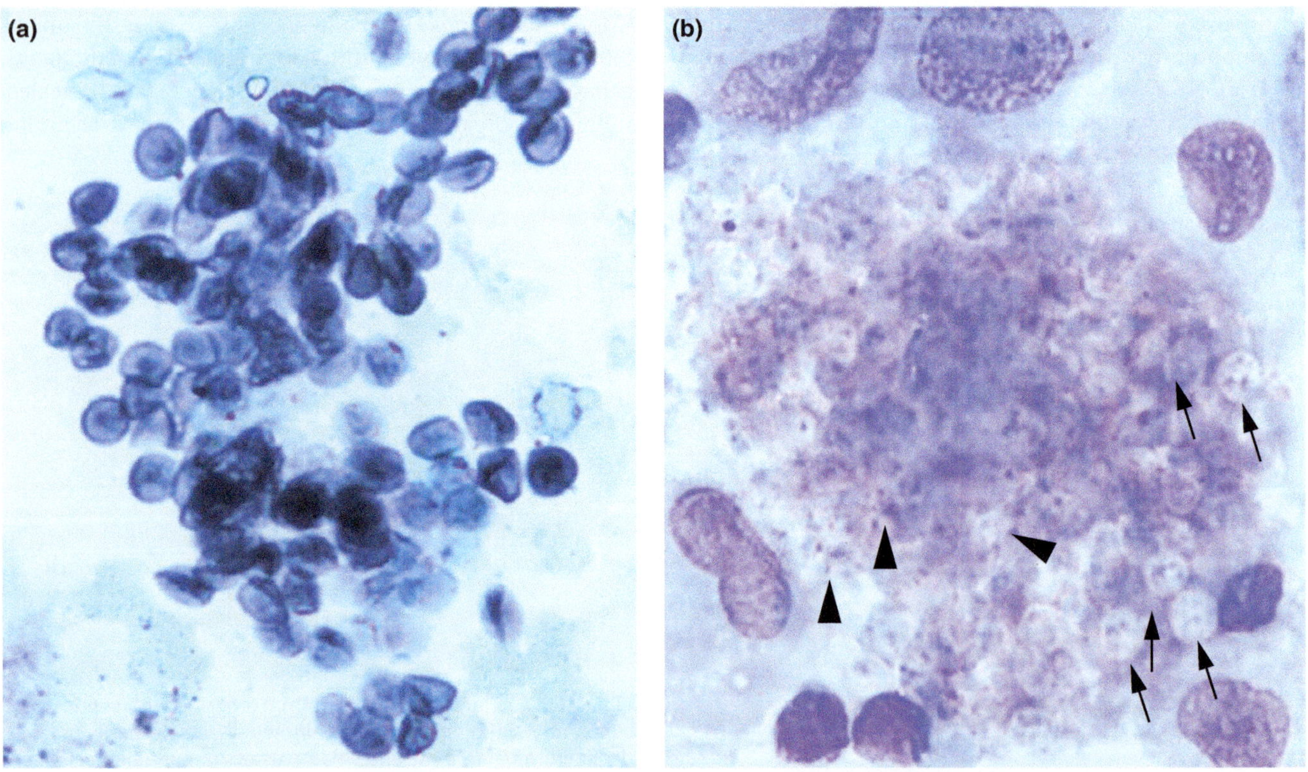

Figure 60.8 BAL fluid samples demonstrating *Pneumocystis* spp. organisms. (a) The cell walls of the round to oval, 4–5 μm cysts are highlighted with this stain. (Gomori methenamine silver stain, 500×) (b) Intracystic bodies are seen at the periphery of the cysts (arrows). Trophic forms are characterized by small nuclei and light blue-gray cytoplasm (arrowheads) (Giemsa stain, 500×. *Source:* Reprinted from Catherinot et al.[52], with permission from Elsevier).

or at the time of necropsy because of difficulty sampling. Pleural fluid analysis can be useful if neoplastic cells are shed into effusion.[47] For example, spontaneous malignant mesothelioma causing pleural effusion was described in a baboon; fluid contained pleomorphic cells with foamy vacuolated cytoplasm and variable numbers of nuclei.[59]

Lymph Nodes, Thymus, and Spleen

Lymph node excisional biopsy or FNA can be performed to evaluate lymphadenopathy or when systemic disease, such as tumor metastasis, is suspected. Sampling of the thymus or spleen typically requires a surgical approach, though ultrasound-guided fine-needle biopsy of the spleen has been described in the chimpanzee and howler monkey.[5,60] For most NHP, the axillary and superficial inguinal lymph nodes are the most accessible for sampling.

Inflammatory and Infectious Disease

Any systemic infection can seed the lymphatic tissues. Lymphoid cytology can be useful in instances where lymphadenopathy suggests involvement of the lymphoid system. Impression smears of the spleen stained with modified Wright's stain demonstrated pyogranulomatous inflammation and fungal organisms consistent with *Blastomyces dermatitidis* in a rhesus monkey.[61] Lymphocyte subsets of lymph node FNAs of the inguinal lymph nodes of rhesus monkeys experimentally infected with simian immunodeficiency virus (SIV) were characterized by flow cytometry.[62]

Hyperplasia and Neoplasia

Hyperplasia of the lymphatic tissues is a general response to a local or systemic inflammatory stimulus (Figure 60.9). Hepatosplenomegaly caused by *Toxoplasma gondii* was diagnosed in a howler monkey using a FNA of the spleen that microscopically demonstrated cysts containing bradyzoites.[5]

Many neoplasms metastasize to lymphatic tissues, and cytology can aid in diagnostic evaluation. Myelolipomas are mesenchymal tumors that contain both mature adipocytes and hematopoietic cells that occur in the spleen, liver, and adrenal gland (Figure 60.10). Myelolipomas appear to have a higher prevalence in Goeldi's monkeys, marmosets, and tamarins than other NHP species and animal species such as dogs, cats, and cattle.[63] Lymphoma has been reported in macaques associated with SIV infection.[64,65] Though a variety of tissues were involved, lymphadenopathy was common, with the mesenteric and thoracic nodes most often affected.[64] Diagnosis is typically made via biopsy or at the time of necropsy; however, ultrasound-guided FNA of enlarged lymph nodes is an option.

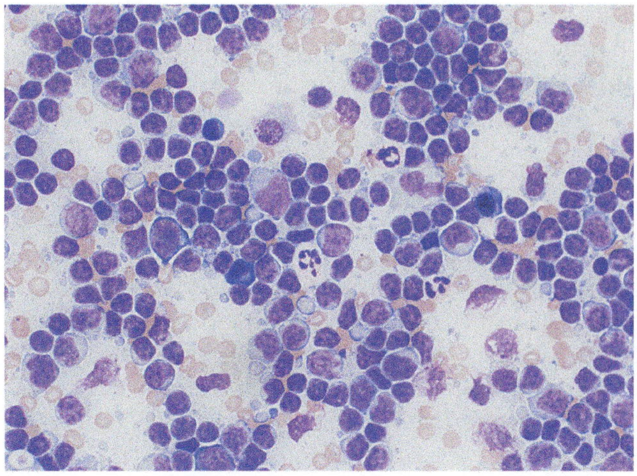

Figure 60.9 Aspirate of a mildly enlarged popliteal lymph node from a Rhesus monkey. The sample consists primarily of small lymphocytes with an expansion of intermediate to large lymphocytes, a small increase in plasma cells, and occasional neutrophils, compatible with hyperplasia. No etiologic agent was identified, and the cause of the hyperplastic response was not determined (modified Wright Giemsa, 600×. *Source:* Image courtesy of Keeling Center for Comparative Medicine and Research, M. D. Anderson Cancer Center).

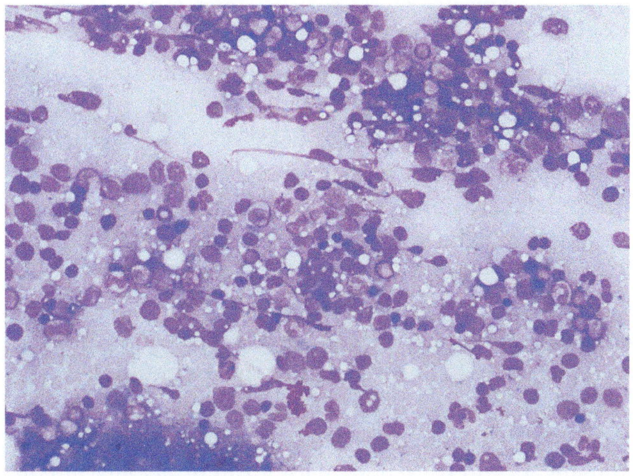

Figure 60.10 Impression smear of a splenic myelolipoma from a Golden lion tamarin. The aspirate was highly cellular with many disrupted cells and intact round cells in a proteinaceous, vacuolated background. The round cell population consisted of abundant myeloid and erythroid precursors (modified Wright Giemsa, 400×. *Source:* Image courtesy of Karen Terio, University of Illinois Zoological Pathology Program).

Few attempts have been made to subclassify lymphoma of nonhuman primates, though a World Health Organization standard was applied to classify lymphoma tissue from Japanese macaques following immunohistochemical staining for cell surface markers such as CD3, CD4, CD8, CD20, and CD30.[66] Though polymerase chain reaction for receptor rearrangement and flow cytometry could offer viable options in this regard, the lack of available reagents requires application of those designed for human testing, with uncertain results.

Gastrointestinal, Liver, Pancreas

While FNA and cytology of masses or lesions in the abdominal cavity is possible, biopsy is more commonly used, since it is more apt to result in a definitive diagnosis and can be performed percutaneously using minimally invasive methods.[24,67] Cytology of biopsy specimen impressions can be useful, particularly for rapid screening in emergent situations.[68] Oral and rectal samples are more readily collected. Lastly, cytology of feces or intestinal contents can aid in the diagnosis of infectious conditions.

Inflammatory and Infectious Disease

For gastrointestinal bacterial disease, culture and PCR are the mainstays of diagnosis. During shigellosis outbreaks, microscopic analysis of feces can be useful while waiting for culture or PCR results. *Shigella* sp. causes toxin-mediated damage to the intestinal mucosa with a resultant infiltration of inflammatory cells. The rod-shaped Gram-negative *Shigella* organisms can be seen on microscopic examination, although this is not a reliable finding due to the presence of a mixed bacterial population and the tendency for low and intermittent shedding. Rather, high numbers of neutrophils (>20/high power field) in a fecal wet mount preparation are highly suggestive of *Shigella* infection.[67]

Blastocystis is a single-cell protozoan commonly found in the intestinal tract of humans and animals, including NHP.[16,69–72] Despite the almost ubiquitous occurrence, it is still unclear whether *Blastocystis* is a pathogen, commensal, or an opportunist.[70,72] *Blastocystis* can be found in multiple forms, including vacuolar, granular, amoeboid, and cyst forms (Figure 60.11).[69,70] The vacuolar form is most common in fecal samples and usually used for diagnosis. It contains a central vacuole, with a rim of cytoplasm containing organelles at the periphery. The granular form is larger, and the central vacuole is filled with granules. The rare amoeboid form has an irregular shape with cytoplasmic projections. The cyst form is smaller than the other forms and has a cyst wall, condensed cytoplasm and many small vacuoles, with a refractile appearance with phase-contrast microscopy.[69,70] Safranin-methylene blue and modified Ziehl–Neelsen are the best stains for identification of *Blastocystis* in fecal smears; modified trichrome staining also works but is less specific.[73]

Helminth parasites in contemporary facilities housing NHP are unusual, though exposure risk should be considered. For an overview of fecal parasitology in NHP, the reader is referred to other resources.[57,74]

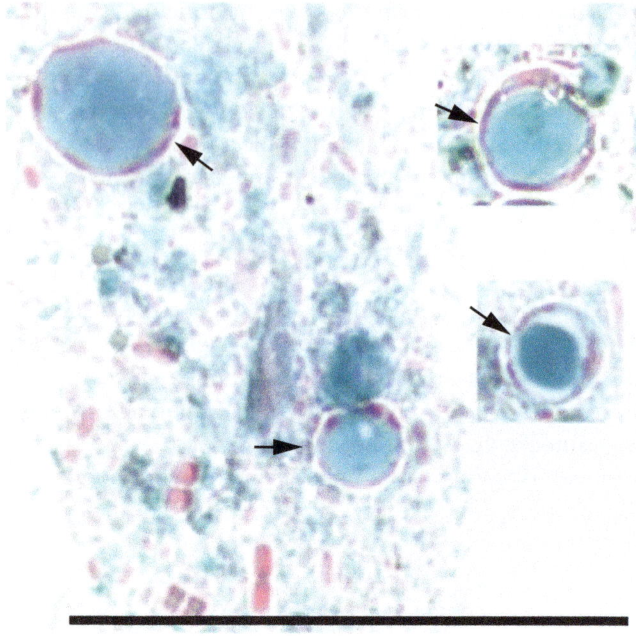

Figure 60.11 Impression smear from the colon of a vervet demonstrating various vacuolar forms of *Blastocystis* (arrows) (Trichrome stain, bar = 50 μm. *Source:* Image courtesy of Carmen Booth).

Secondary amyloidosis occurs in many species of NHP and is often attributed to chronic inflammation. In recent years, a specific form of amyloidosis that manifests primarily as canalicular deposition in the liver has been commonly identified in rhesus breeding colonies.[75]

Neoplasia

The most common oral neoplasm of NHP is squamous cell carcinoma and occurs in the tongue, gingiva, and buccal mucosa (Figure 60.12). Other tumors of the mouth and head amenable to cytology include oral papilloma, ameloblastoma, odontoma, and salivary gland carcinoma (Figure 60.13)[24,67] The cytologic presentations should resemble tumors in other species; however, descriptive reports have not been published for NHP. Chapter 30 presents additional detail on oral cytology in domestic species.

While a full review of gastrointestinal, pancreatic, and hepatic neoplasia in NHP is beyond the scope of this chapter, adenocarcinoma of the small intestine and/or colon is relatively common in some species, particularly callitrichids and macaques.[24,67] In rhesus macaques, adenocarcinomas typically occur at the ileocecal colic junction or in the proximal colon unassociated with polyps or progression from adenoma.[76] These adenocarcinomas frequently demonstrate abundant mucin, and vascular and/or lymphatic invasion is common. The degree of cytologic atypia

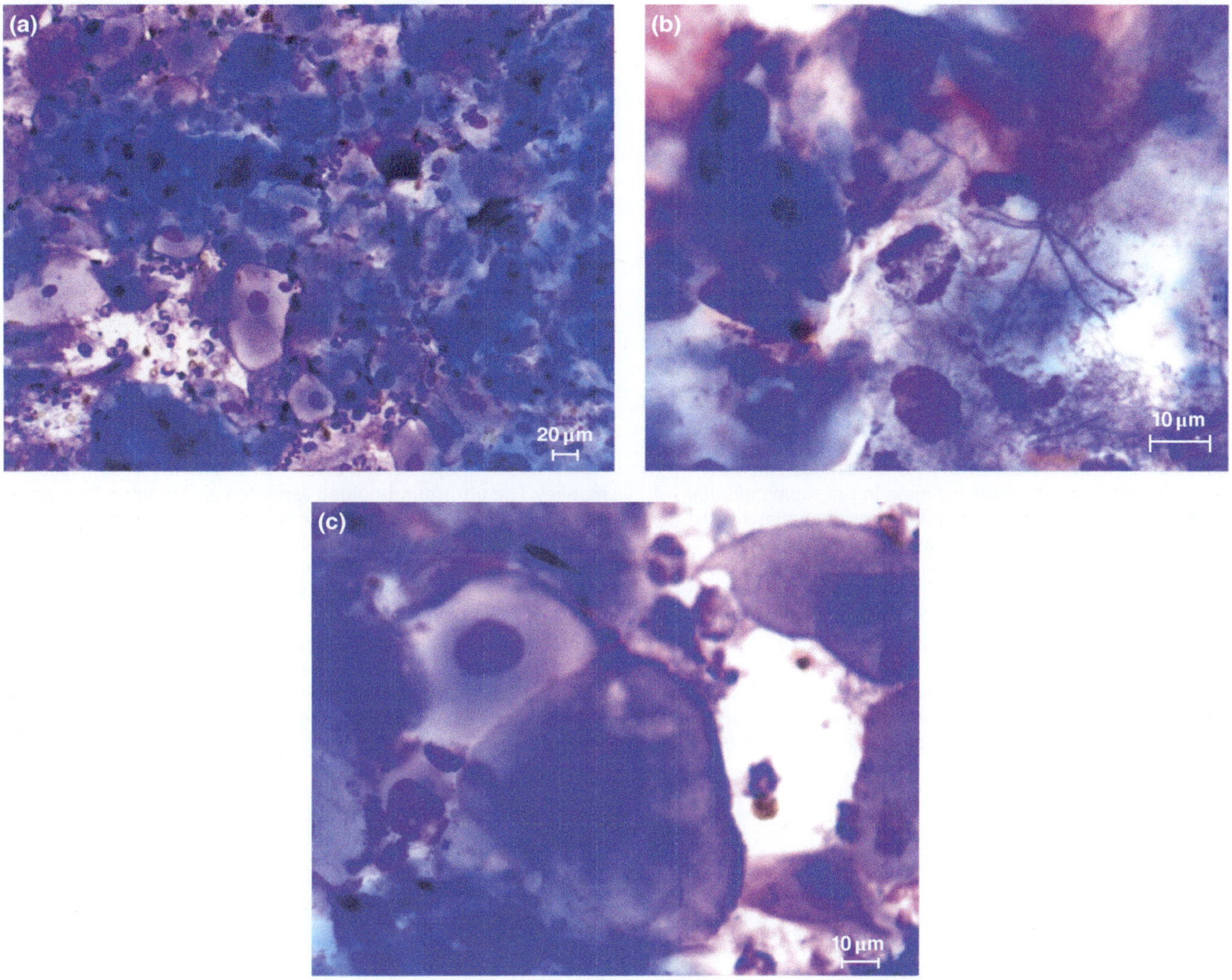

Figure 60.12 Squamous cell carcinoma of the tongue with secondary overgrowth of *Actinomyces* spp. from a rhesus macaque. (a) Exudative cytology revealed squamous epithelial cells and suppurative inflammation. (b) Filamentous branching and curved bacteria are consistent with *Actinomyces* spp., which was confirmed by fungal culture. (c) The squamous epithelial cells exhibited anisocytosis and anisokaryosis (Diff Quik. *Source:* Image courtesy of Caroline Zeiss).

in these tumors is generally high but can vary from a more well-differentiated appearance to marked cellular atypia. Based on correlation with histopathology and clinical signs, this is likely due in part to the stage at which the tumor becomes clinically apparent and the region of the tumor that is sampled by ultrasound-guided aspirates. At the time of diagnosis, the tumors can present as a discrete mass or a widely disseminated neoplasm with carcinomatosis (Figures 60.14 and 60.15).

Urinary Tract

Cytologic assessment of the urinary tract occurs primarily by evaluation of urine. Various collection methods are available and are described in Chapter 66.[77–79] If animals are dehydrated or moribund, urine is aspirated from the bladder during necropsy. Transitional epithelial cell numbers can increase due to postmortem exfoliation, particularly if there is a delay in collection. In the chimpanzee, the outer layer of transitional epithelial cells can resemble the highly vacuolated umbrella cells seen in humans (Figure 60.16).[80]

Inflammatory and Infectious Disease

Bacterial infection of the urinary tract has been described in nonhuman primate species, most commonly coliforms and *Corynebacterium* species.[81] Bacterial culture of urine is considered the reference standard for evaluation in

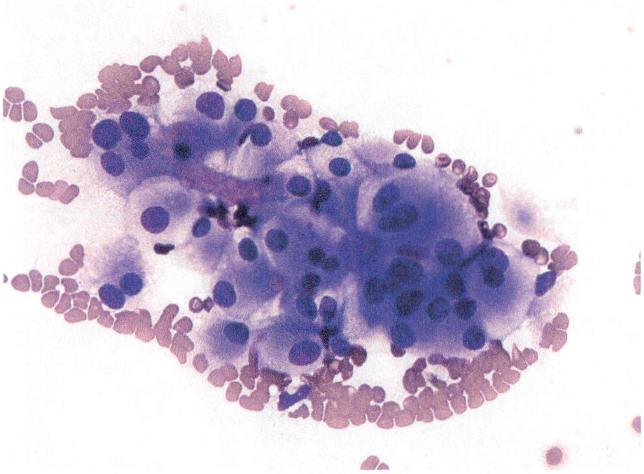

Figure 60.13 Aspirate of salivary gland adenocarcinoma that presented as a subcutaneous mass in the submandibular region of a chimpanzee. This animal was asymptomatic with the exception of the fluid-filled mass located lateral to the larynx. The aspirate consisted of serosanguinous fluid with mild blood contamination. The neoplastic population consisted of round to polygonal cells with variable amounts of basophilic cytoplasm. The cells were frequently clustered and occasionally resembled small acini. Anisocytosis, multinucleation, and atypical nucleoli were consistent features (modified Wright Giemsa, 400×. *Source:* Image courtesy of Keeling Center for Comparative Medicine and Research, M. D. Anderson Cancer Center).

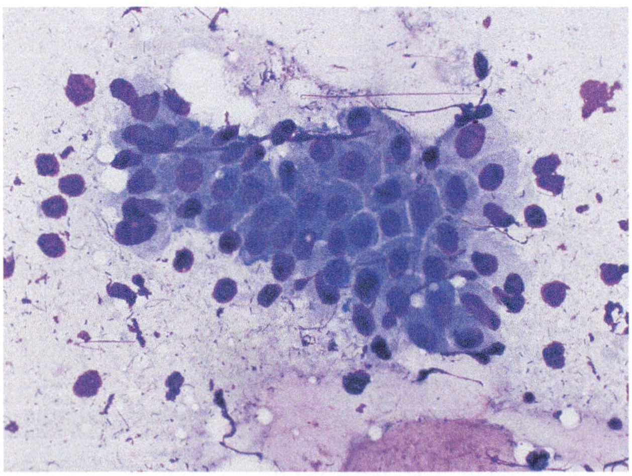

Figure 60.14 Aspirate of a colorectal carcinoma in a Rhesus monkey. The ultrasound-guided aspirate was obtained from a mid-abdominal mass. The sample was highly cellular with abundant clusters of cuboidal to columnar cells on a background consistent with the gastrointestinal tract. The cells displayed mild anisocytosis and anisokaryosis. The nuclei frequently contained 1–2 prominent nucleoli. This tumor displayed much less atypia than the example in Figure 60.16 (modified Wright Giemsa, 600×. *Source:* Image courtesy of Keeling Center for Comparative Medicine and Research, M. D. Anderson Cancer Center).

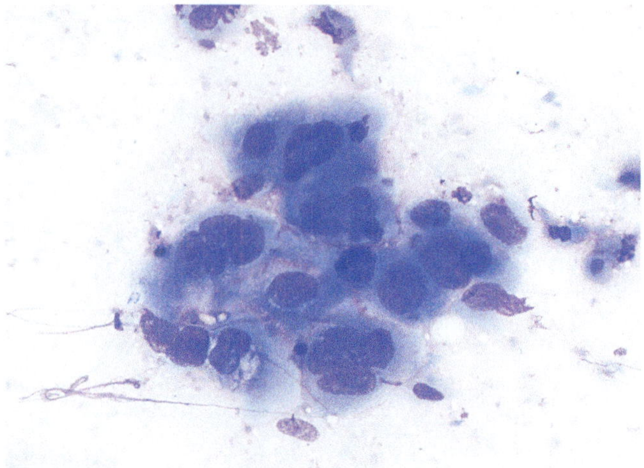

Figure 60.15 Aspirate of a colorectal carcinoma in a Rhesus monkey. The ultrasound-guided aspirate was obtained from a mid-abdominal mass. The sample was moderately cellular. Cells presented both individually and in clusters and displayed marked atypia. The cells contained dark blue cytoplasm with occasional small, irregular vacuoles. They exhibited marked anisocytosis and anisokaryosis, a highly variable nuclear to cytoplasmic ration (N:C) and frequent multinucleation. The nuclei contained multiple atypical nucleoli. A mild neutrophilic response also was present (modified Wright Giemsa, 500×. *Source:* Image courtesy of Keeling Center for Comparative Medicine and Research, M. D. Anderson Cancer Center).

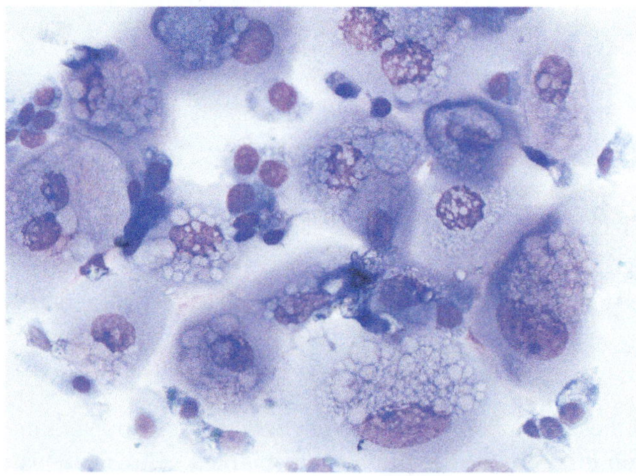

Figure 60.16 Umbrella cells in the urine sediment from a chimpanzee. The urine sample was collected via cystocentesis approximately 30–60 minutes after the time of death. The sample contained abundant large epithelial cells with numerous variably sized cytoplasmic vacuoles. These cells typically contained abundant cytoplasm, but the N:C and the size of the cells was variable. The vacuolated cells are consistent with the outer layer of transitional epithelial cells in the human bladder (termed umbrella cells) and considered a postmortem artifact. A population of smaller epithelial cells with a higher N:C is also present. The bladder was histologically normal (modified Wright Giemsa, 600×. *Source:* Image courtesy of Keeling Center for Comparative Medicine and Research, M. D. Anderson Cancer Center).

cases of suspected infection. Parasitic infections of the urinary tract are rare but reported, with *Schistosoma* species most notably described. While a thorough description of urinary cytology is lacking, these parasites cause inflammatory and proliferative lesions in the urinary tract, resulting in the presence of inflammatory cells, blood and/or epithelial cells, and parasitic ova that are typically ovoid and with a lateral or terminal spine.[82–85] See Chapter 39 for more details.

Hyperplasia and Neoplasia

Although neoplasms of the urinary tract occur, cytologic diagnosis has not been described. See Chapters 37–39 for general information about cytologic diagnosis in common domestic species.

Reproductive

Cytology is used for the diagnosis of pathologic conditions affecting the female reproductive tract and to assess cyclicity. The characteristics of vaginal cytology throughout the menstrual or estrous cycle are described for several primate species and are particularly useful in species without obvious external signs of cyclicity, such as menstruation or sex skin turgescence.[81,86–92] However, even in species that do present external signs of cyclicity, understanding normal cytology is important as a baseline for interpretation (Figure 60.17). A single sample may not provide conclusive information about reproductive status, but serial samples can be very useful. While measurement of serum hormone levels can also be used, the advantages of vaginal cytology include noninvasiveness,

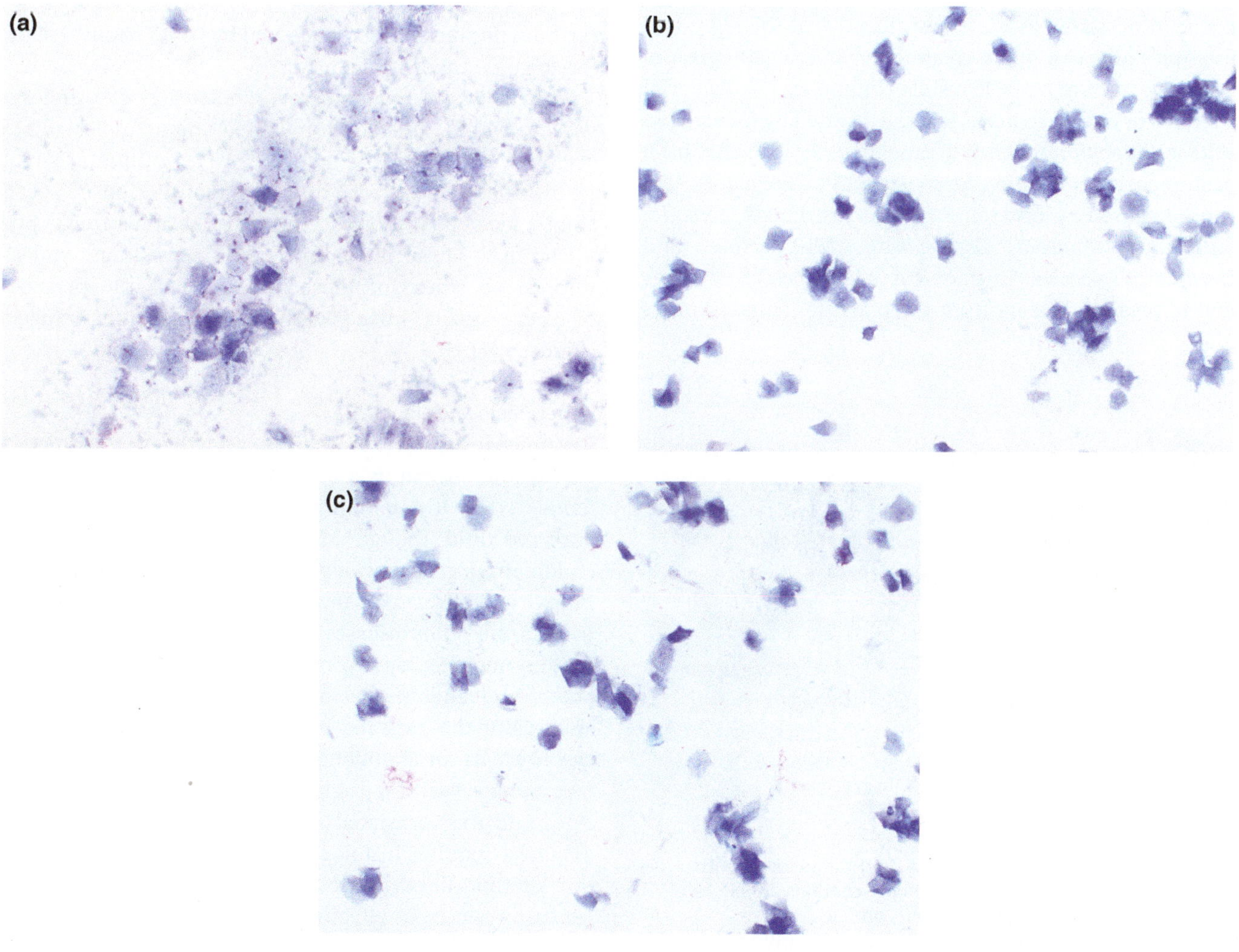

Figure 60.17 Vaginal cytology from a female rhesus macaque throughout the menstrual cycle. (a) Day 2 (menstruation), (b) Day 8, and (c) Day 25 of the menstrual cycle (100×, Diff Quik, 100×. *Source:* Images taken by author from slides shared by Steven Wilson, Department of Comparative Medicine, Yale University School of Medicine).

especially with training to present for vaginal swabbing, and inexpensive point of care testing providing rapid results.[81,92] Papanicolaou staining is recommended, though Romanowsky-type stains also are sufficient.[81] Additional information on cytologic evaluation of estrous cycling in NHP is in Chapter 66.

In both males and females, FNA of abnormal reproductive organs or masses can be performed for structures accessible percutaneously; ultrasound guidance is ideal. However, FNA should not be performed for ovarian tumors because essentially all forms of ovarian neoplasia require surgical excision and puncture could rupture a cystic tumor.[81] Impression smears of excised ovarian tissue may be useful.[93] If lesions are accessible externally, impression smears or brush smears may be rewarding.[94]

Inflammatory and Infectious Disease

Vaginal swabs or washes can provide valuable initial diagnostic information in bacterial infections of the reproductive tract and can guide treatment while awaiting more definitive culture or PCR results (Figure 60.18). Bacterial vaginitis or endometritis is generally caused by *Escherichia coli* or *Staphylococcus* spp., though other bacteria have been reported, including *Mycoplasma*.[81,95] Pregnancy loss can be caused by *Listeria, Streptococcus, E. coli, Yersinia, Salmonella, Shigella, Leptospirosis, Mycoplasma*, and *Ureaplasma* species. In these cases, samples of exudates and impression smears from the placenta, fetus, or other birthing products can be evaluated by Gram or silver staining to guide case management.[81]

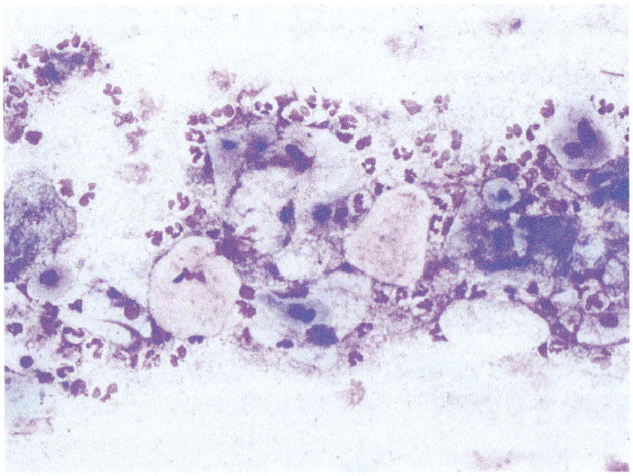

Figure 60.18 Vaginal swab from a Ring-tailed lemur with septic suppurative vaginitis. The sample contains a mixture of superficial keratinized epithelial cells and degenerate neutrophils. Bacteria were seen both intracellularly and extracellularly (modified Wright Giemsa; 400×. *Source:* Image courtesy of Karen Terio, University of Illinois Zoological Pathology Program).

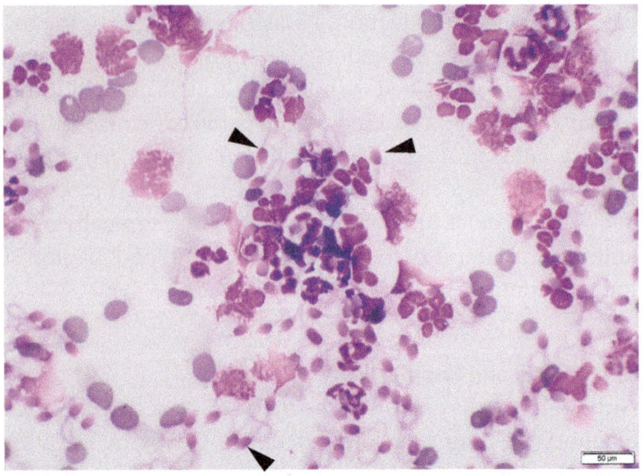

Figure 60.19 Impression smear from a rhesus macaque with a sperm granuloma. Cytological evaluation of these lesions generally reveals the presence of neutrophils, macrophages, and spermatozoa (arrowheads) (Diff Quik. *Source:* Image courtesy of Meghan Connolly and Michael Eckhaus).

Male NHPs in zoo and research settings can undergo vasectomy to prevent unwanted pregnancies when socially housed with females. Sperm granuloma, which is an inflammatory response to accumulation of sperm from a leakage at the vasectomy site, can form as a complication.[96] These often form draining fistulas, and an impression smear of these areas reveals the presence of spermatozoa mixed with occasional macrophages (Figure 60.19).

Hyperplasia and Neoplasia

Endometriosis, or extrauterine growth of endometrial glands and stroma, is a common reproductive disease in female NHP. It commonly causes large cysts filled with dark red fluid, though small dispersed cysts, masses, or endometrial cells enveloped in fatty masses can occur. Biopsy or FNA can be rewarding to distinguish endometriosis from other diseases causing uterine enlargement or tumors such as leiomyoma (Figure 60.20), endometrial polyp, and endometrial decidualization.[81,97–99] Cytologic analysis of the dark red brown fluid from endometriosis cysts reveals an abundance of foamy, hemosiderin-laden macrophages with a background of degenerate erythrocytes and the occasional neutrophil. Although definitive diagnosis requires histology, exploratory surgery or aspiration of fluid-filled masses with subsequent cytology are generally the most effective methods for diagnosing this condition.[81,100]

Papillomavirus-induced lesions occur in the cervix, vagina, and vulva of female macaques, and papillomavirus

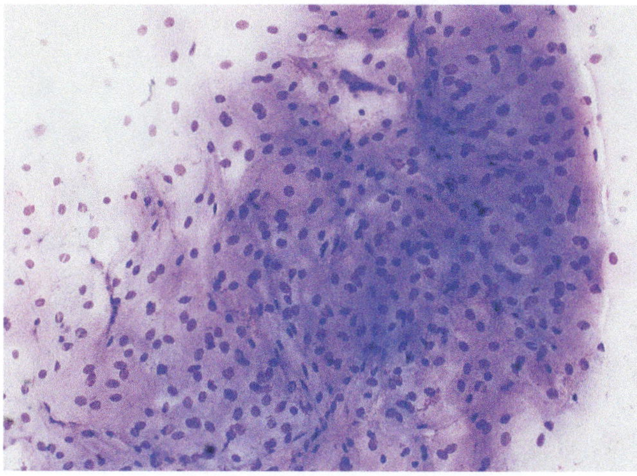

Figure 60.20 Aspirate of a uterine leiomyoma in a chimpanzee. The ultrasound-guided aspirate contained multiple aggregates of well-differentiated mesenchymal cells (modified Wright Giemsa, 200×. *Source:* Image courtesy of Keeling Center for Comparative Medicine and Research, M. D. Anderson Cancer Center).

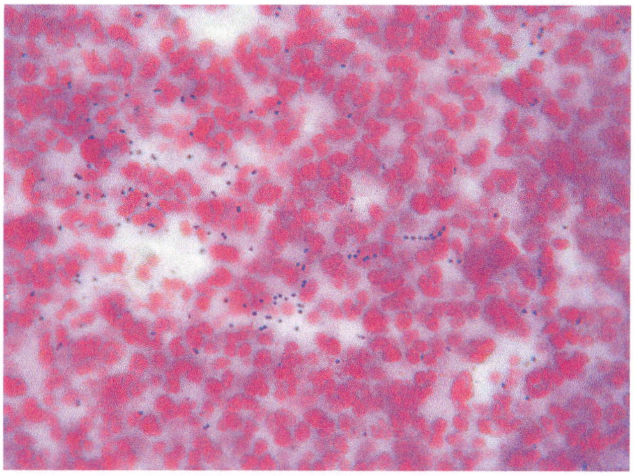

Figure 60.21 Cytospin preparation of CSF. Gram-positive cocci are present in pairs and short chains, suggestive of *S. pneumoniae*. The background consists of neutrophils (Gram stain, 1000×. *Source:* Image courtesy of Yuri E. Amatnieks).

DNA has been isolated from a metastasis of a primary penile neoplasia in a male rhesus macaque.[81,101,102] Cytological exam of cervical mucosal smears from rhesus macaques with evidence of papillomavirus-induced cervical neoplasia revealed atypical epithelial cells that contain large, irregular nuclei with a dense chromatin pattern.[102]

FNA has the potential to facilitate the diagnosis of hyperplastic and neoplastic diseases of the female reproductive tract, but there is little in the literature specifically for NHP at this time. Some of the more commonly reported conditions include adenocarcinoma, leiomyoma, cervical and endometrial polyps, and adenomyosis.[81]

Although reports in the literature are sparse, male NHP can develop testicular neoplasia, including seminomas, adenomas, Leydig cell tumors, and interstitial cell tumors.[81,103] Because this area is easily accessible percutaneously, fine-needle aspiration is a logical choice for initial diagnostics. Chapter 40 provides general information on the cytology of the ovary and testis.

Central Nervous System

Analysis of cerebrospinal fluid (CSF) is a common method for cytologic evaluation of the central nervous system (CNS). CSF can be collected via either the cisternal or lumbosacral locations, though the cisterna magna is sometimes preferred, especially for older animals.[3,77]

Inflammatory and Infectious Disease

Bacterial organisms infect the CNS in NHP, most notably *S. pneumoniae* and *Staphylococcus aureus*.[104] Although definitive diagnosis is made by culture and/or PCR, cytology can facilitate preliminary diagnosis to guide initial therapy. While *S. pneumoniae* and *S. aureus* are both Gram-positive cocci, *S. pneumoniae* occurs in pairs (diplococci) or short chains (Figure 60.21), and *S. aureus* typically forms grapelike clusters.[105] Hematologic findings can suggest bacterial disease when bacteria are not identified.[106,107]

Primates are susceptible to many viral diseases causing CNS pathology. Cytologic examination of CSF can support a viral cause for pathology, since some viruses (measles, poliovirus) can lead to mononuclear pleocytosis in the CSF, including specifically a lymphohistiocytosis.[108,109] Though CSF analysis is rarely definitive, diagnosis relies on viral isolation and identification.

Encephalitozoon cuniculi is a protozoal organism of the CNS in NHP and in rabbits, dogs, and humans. It can cause meningoencephalitis, usually nonsuppurative, though there may be species differences in the inflammatory profile.[110,111] NHP are also susceptible to other parasitic infections that can affect the CNS, including *Baylisascaris* and *Angiostrongylus*. In affected animals, analysis of CSF fluid can reveal eosinophilia, but organisms are generally not observed, and diagnosis is typically made by PCR evaluation or immunohistochemical staining of tissues (kidney, lung, liver, heart, brain, and skeletal muscle).[112]

Neoplasia

Spontaneous tumors of the CNS are rare. Intracranial meningiomas have been reported in a baboon, a collared brown lemur, and a rhesus macaque.[28,113] A high-grade intramedullary tumor of the spine that was most consistent with an ependymoma was described in a rhesus macaque.[114] While published descriptions of neoplastic cells in CSF are lacking, it is expected that CSF cytology may be a useful adjunct to diagnosis, as with other species including humans.[115] FNA and impression smear cytology from surgical biopsy or necropsy samples can be performed, and the cytology of some CNS neoplasms has been described in domestic species (Chapter 47).

Body Cavity Fluid Analysis

Cytological analysis of thoracic or abdominal fluid is a valuable diagnostic tool in NHP. Though few diseases of NHP can be diagnosed solely by fluid analysis, distinctions between inflammatory versus neoplastic causes can often be achieved. Methods similar to those used in other species for percutaneous sampling are also used for NHP. See Chapter 50 for general laboratory techniques for fluid analysis.

Published reference values for NHP body cavity fluid cytology do not generally exist, though samples obtained by laparotomy from adult female rhesus monkeys contained mesothelial cells (54 ± 1.5%), neutrophils (22.4 ± 1.3%), histiocytes (10.2 ± 0.7%), monocytes (7.6 ± 0.5%), lymphocytes (4.8 ± 0.8%), and mast cells (0.8 ± 0.2%).[116] While a number of case reports describe the presence of pleural, pericardial, or abdominal fluids, relatively few include cytological descriptions.

Inflammatory and Infectious Disease

Inflammation in thoracic or abdominal fluid samples suggests infection, though the possibility of sterile inflammation associated with a foreign body or neoplasia should also be considered. *Staphylococcus*, *Streptococcus*, and *Pasteurella* species are often associated with suppurative exudates. Appendicitis in a chimpanzee was accompanied by abdominal effusion characterized mainly by lymphocytes, neutrophils, and monocytes in the absence of observable or cultured microorganisms.[117]

Chylothorax was associated with respiratory compromise and death in a group of rhesus monkeys that had been instrumented with intravenous catheters, though no specific lesion was described to account for the accumulation of chyle.[118]

Gastric dilatation ("bloat") is a condition that occurs in both Old World and New World NHP as the result of rapid gas production in the gastrointestinal tract by clostridial organisms.[3] This is an acute medical emergency requiring removal of the excess gas and fluid. Abdominal effusion results from vascular compromise; lymphocytic effusions have been seen (Figure 60.22). Thoracocentesis of a De Brazza's monkey (*Cercopithecus neglectus*) with echocardiographic evidence of pleural effusion and dilated cardiomyopathy yielded a large volume of serosanguineous fluid characterized cytologically by large numbers of erythrocytes, fewer mesothelial cells, and occasional neutrophils.[119] Cytological evaluation of a transudative thoracic effusion in a squirrel monkey euthanized due to severe dilated cardiomyopathy consisted largely of erythrocytes and fewer white blood cells.[120]

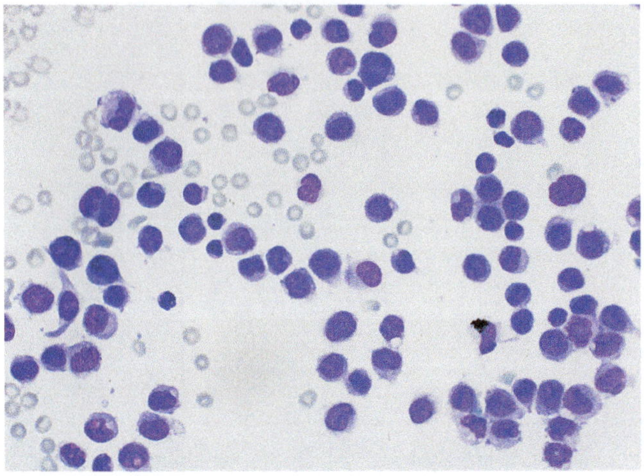

Figure 60.22 Abdominal fluid from Rhesus monkey. This animal presented acutely with abdominal distension due to gastric bloat. At necropsy, an increased amount of pale yellow abdominal fluid was present. The fluid was a modified transudate consisting predominantly of small- to intermediate-sized lymphocytes. No disease processes other than bloat were identified, and the lymphocytic effusion was attributed to compromised vascular flow (modified Wright Giemsa, 600×. *Source:* Image courtesy of Keeling Center for Comparative Medicine and Research, M. D. Anderson Cancer Center).

Neoplasia

Supportive literature is lacking; however, it is reasonable to expect that fluids present in body cavities secondary to neoplasia could provide cytological evidence of disease. Cytological evaluation of abdominal fluid harvested following euthanasia of a severely ill marmoset showed features supporting a diagnosis of biliary carcinoma (Figure 60.23).

Conclusion

Cytology is a useful diagnostic tool for NHP medicine. NHP can be expected to continue to gain focus as important subjects of conservation efforts, zoological specimens, and research subjects. Given the medical needs of the diverse species comprising NHP, diagnostic efforts, including diagnostic cytology, will expand and be reflected in a growing body of literature describing such approaches.

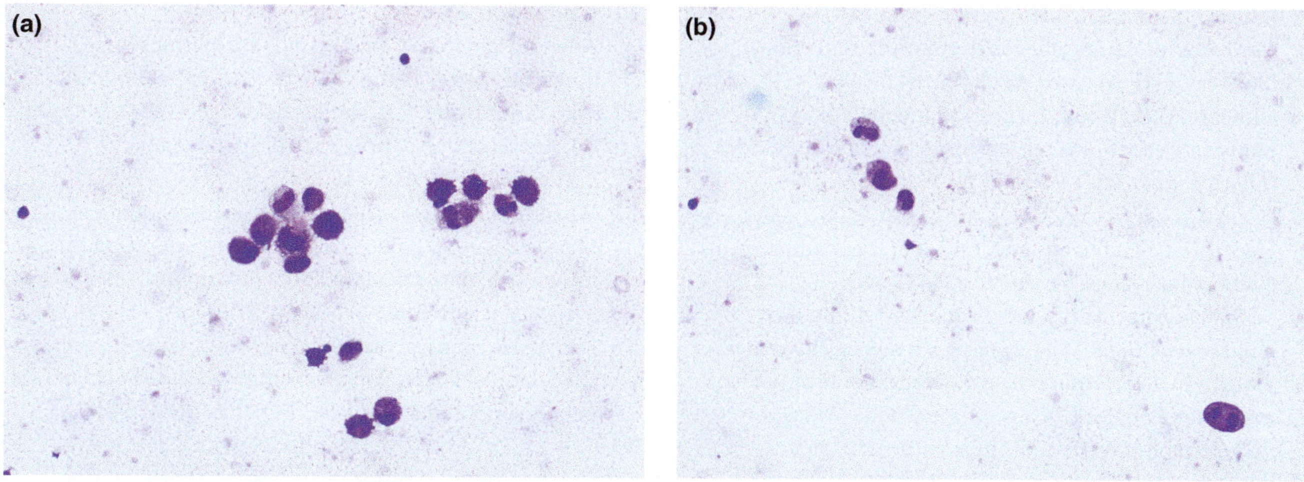

Figure 60.23 Abdominal fluid collected at necropsy from a marmoset with biliary carcinoma. (a) The fluid had low cellularity with a mildly proteinaceous granular background. The neoplastic population consisted of small- to medium-sized cells with a moderate to high N:C. Nuclear features were difficult to discern, and rare binucleated cells were seen. (b) Mitotic figures (lower right) were occasionally identified (modified Wright Giemsa, 400×. *Source:* Images courtesy of Karen Terio, University of Illinois Zoological Pathology Program).

References

1 Bornman, M.S., van Vuuren, M., Meltzer, D.G. et al. (1988). Quality of semen obtained by electroejaculation from chacma baboons (*Papio ursinus*). *J Med Primatol* 17: 57–61.

2 Gould, K.G. and Mann, D.R. (1988). Comparison of electrostimulation methods for semen recovery in the rhesus monkey (*Macaca mulatta*). *J Med Primatol* 17: 95–103.

3 Fortman, J.D., Hewitt, T.A., and Halliday, L.C. (2002). *The Laboratory Nonhuman Primate*, 174–177. Boca Raton, FL: CRC Press.

4 Coleman, K., Pranger, L., Maier, A. et al. (2008). Training rhesus macaques for venipuncture using positive reinforcement techniques: a comparison with chimpanzees. *J Am Assoc Lab Anim Sci* 47: 37–41.

5 Grandi, F., Monteiro, L.N., Salgado, B.S. et al. (2012). What is your diagnosis? Hepatosplenomegaly in a howler monkey (*Alouatta fusca*). *Vet Clin Pathol* 41: 433–434.

6 Williams, C.V., Van Steenhouse, J.L., Bradley, J.M. et al. (2002). Naturally occurring *Ehrlichia chaffeensis* infection in two prosimian primate species: ring-tailed lemurs (*Lemur catta*) and ruffed lemurs (*Varecia variegate*). *Emerg Infect Dis* 8: 1497–1500.

7 Ameri, M., Anderson, W.I., and Orlando, H.M. (2012). Cutaneous melanocytoma in a cynomolgus monkey (*Macaca fascicularis*): cytologic and histologic characteristics. *Comp Clin Pathol* 21: 205–207.

8 Valverde, C.R., Canfield, D., Tarara, R. et al. (1998). Spontaneous leprosy in a wild-caught cynomolgus macaque. *Int J Leprosy* 66: 140–148.

9 Butler, T.M., Gleiser, C.A., Bernal, J.C., and Ajello, L. (1988). Case of disseminated African histoplasmosis in a baboon. *J Med Primatol* 17: 153–161.

10 Butler, T.M. and Hubbard, G.B. (1991). An epizootic of *Histoplasmosis duboisii* (African histoplasmosis) in an American baboon colony. *Lab Anim Sci* 41: 407–410.

11 Gades, N.M. and Marler, R.J. (2009). Pathology in practice. Histoplasmosis. *J Am Vet Med Assoc* 234: 1535–1537.

12 Kramer, J.A. and Bielitzki, J. (2012). Integumentary system diseases of nonhuman primates. In: *Nonhuman Primates in Biomedical Research: Diseases* (eds. C.R. Abee, K. Mansfield, S. Tardif and T. Morris), 563–588. San Diego, CA: Academic Press.

13 Migaki, G., Hubbard, G.B., and Butler, T.M. (1993). *Histoplasma capsulatum* var. *duboisii* infection, Baboon. In: *Nonhuman Primates* (eds. T.C. Jones, U. Mohr and R.D. Hunt), 19–23. Berlin, Heidelberg: Springer.

14 Wheat, L.J. and Kauffman, C.A. (2003). Histoplasmosis. *Infect Dis Clin N Am* 17: 1–19, vii.

15 Aiello, S.E., Moses, M.A., and Allen, D.G. (2016). Histoplasmosis. In: *The Merck Veterinary Manual* (eds. S.E. Aiello and M.A. Moses), 639–640. Kenilworth: Merck & Co, Inc.

16 McClure, H.M., Kaplan, W., Bonner, W.B., and Keeling, M.E. (1971). Dermatophilosis in owl monkeys. *Sabouraudia* 9: 185–190.

17 Fox, J.G., Campbell, L.H., Reed, C. et al. (1973). Dermatophilosis (cutaneous streptothricosis) in owl monkeys. *J Am Vet Med Assoc* 163: 642–644.

18 Hubbard, G.B., Wood, D.H., and Butcher, W.I. (1984). Mammary carcinoma with metastasis in a rhesus monkey (*Macaca mulatta*). *Vet Pathol* 21: 531–533.

19 Wood, C.E., Usborne, A.L., Starost, M.F. et al. (2006). Hyperplastic and neoplastic lesions of the mammary gland in macaques. *Vet Pathol* 43: 471–483.

20 Williams-Fritze, M.J., Carlson Scholz, J.A., Bossuyt, V., and Booth, C.J. (2011). Use of p63, a myoepithelial cell marker, in determining the invasiveness of spontaneous mammary neoplasia in a rhesus macaque (*Macaca mulatta*). *J Am Assoc Lab Anim Sci* 50: 252–257.

21 Beck, A.P., Brooks, A., and Zeiss, C.J. (2014). Invasive ductular carcinoma in 2 rhesus macaques (*Macaca mulatta*). *Comp Med* 64: 314–322.

22 Smith, J.M., Rao, S.S., Stump, K.C. et al. (2005). Mammary ductal carcinoma with comedo pattern in a rhesus macaque. *Contemp Top Lab Anim Sci* 44: 29–33.

23 Beniashvili, D.S. (1989). An overview of the world literature on spontaneous tumors in nonhuman primates. *J Med Primatol* 18: 423–437.

24 Miller, A.D. (2012). Neoplasia and proliferative disorders of nonhuman primates. In: *Nonhuman Primates in Biomedical Research: Diseases* (eds. C.R. Abee, K. Mansfield, S. Tardif and T. Morris), 325–356. San Diego, CA: Academic Press.

25 Kaspareit, J., Friderichs-Gromoll, S., Buse, E., and Habermann, G. (2007). Spontaneous neoplasms observed in cynomolgus monkeys (*Macaca fascicularis*) during a 15-year period. *Expand Tox Pathol* 59: 163–169.

26 Haddad, J.L., Dick, E.J. Jr., Guardado-Mendoza, R., and Hubbard, G.B. (2009). Spontaneous squamous cell carcinomas in 13 baboons, a first report in a spider monkey, and a review of the non-human primate literature. *J Med Primatol* 38: 175–186.

27 Myers, D.D. Jr., Dysko, R.C., Chrisp, C.E., and Decoster, J.L. (2001). Subcutaneous hemangiosarcomas in a rhesus macaque (*Macaca mulatta*). *J Med Primatol* 30: 127–130.

28 Remick, A.K., Van Wetter, A.J., and Williams, C.V. (2009). Neoplasia in prosimians: case series from a captive prosimian population and literature review. *Vet Pathol* 46: 746–772.

29 David, J.M., Dick, E.J. Jr., and Hubbard, G.B. (2009). Spontaneous pathology of the common marmoset (*Callithrix jacchus*) and tamarins (*Saguinus oedipus, Saguinus mystax*). *J Med Primatol* 38: 347–359.

30 Brown, S.L., Anderson, D.C., Dick, E.J. Jr. et al. (2009). Neoplasia in the chimpanzee (*Pan* spp.). *J Med Primatol* 38: 137–144.

31 Williamson, M.E. and Hunt, R.D. (1970). Adenocarcinoma of the thyroid in a marmoset (*Saguinus nigricollis*). *Lab Anim Care* 20: 1139–1141.

32 Line, S.W., Ihrke, P.J., and Prahalada, S. (1984). Calcinosis circumscripta in two rhesus monkeys. *Lab Anim Sci* 34: 616–618.

33 Wachtman, L.M., Pistorio, A.L., Eliades, S., and Mankowski, J.L. (2006). Calcinosis circumscripta in a common marmoset (*Callithrix jacchus jacchus*). *J Am Assoc Lab Anim Sci* 45: 54–57.

34 Marcos, R., Santos, M., Oliveira, J. et al. (2006). Cytochemical detection of calcium in a case of calcinosis circumscripta in a dog. *Vet Clin Pathol* 35: 239–242.

35 Tyler, R.D., Cowell, R.L., and Meinkoth, J.H. (2008). Cutaneous and subcutaneous lesions. In: *Diagnostic Cytology and Hematology of the Dog and Cat* (eds. R.L. Cowell, R.D. Tyler, J.H. Meinkoth and D.B. DeNicola), 78–111. St. Louis, MO: Mosby.

36 Oria, A.P., Pinna, M.H., Almeida, D.S. et al. (2013). Conjunctival flora, Schirmer's tear test, intraocular pressure, and conjunctival cytology in neotropical primates from Salvador, Brazil. *J Med Primatol* 42: 287–292.

37 Neiffer, D.L., Rothschild, B.M., Marks, S.K. et al. (2000). Management of reactive arthritis in a juvenile gorilla (*Gorilla gorilla gorilla*) with long-term sulfasalazine therapy. *J Zoo Wildl Med* 31: 539–551.

38 Valverde, C.R., Lowenstine, L.J., Young, C.E. et al. (2002). Spontaneous rat bite fever in non-human primates: a review of two cases. *J Med Primatol* 31: 345–349.

39 Takei, S. (2013). A case report of spontaneous polyarthritis in cynomolgus monkeys. *J Vet Med Sci* 75: 531–534.

40 Wimsatt, J., Withrow, S.J., Danner, D. et al. (2011). Multicystic bone disease (Gorham-Stout syndrome) in a spider monkey (*Ateles geoffroyi*). *J Med Primatol* 40: 61–70.

41 Kastello, M.D., Emmert, A.D., Denson, R.F., and Kishimoto, R.A. (1979). Recovery of alveolar macrophages from rhesus and cynomolgus macaques by lung lavage. *Am J Vet Res* 40: 271–273.

42 Haley, P.J., Muggenburg, B.A., Rebar, A.H. et al. (1989). Bronchoalveolar lavage cytology in cynomolgus monkeys and identification of cytologic alterations following sequential saline lavage. *Vet Pathol* 26: 265–273.

43 Krombach, F., Fiehl, E., Burkhardt, D., and Rienmueller, R. (1994). Short-term and long-term effects of serial bronchoalveolar lavages in a nonhuman primate model. *Am J Respir Crit Care Med* 150: 153–158.

44 Dysko, R.C. and Hoskins, D.E. (1995). Collection of biological samples and therapy administration. In: *Nonhuman Primates in Biomedical Research: Biology and*

Management (eds. B.T. Bennett, C.R. Abee and R. Henrickson), 270–286. San Diego, CA: Elsevier.

45 Tate, M.K., Rico, P.J., and Roy, C.J. (2004). Comparative study of lung cytologic features in normal rhesus (*Macaca mulatta*), cynomolgus (*Macaca fascicularis*), and African green (*Chlorocebus aethiops*) nonhuman primates by use of bronchoscopy. *Comp Med* 54: 393–396.

46 Singletary, M.L., Phillippi-Falkenstein, K.M., Scanlon, E. et al. (2008). Modification of a common bronchoalveolar technique to enhance sample diagnostic value. *J Am Assoc Lab Anim Sci* 47: 47–51.

47 Lowenstein, L. and Osborn, K. (2012). Respiratory diseases of nonhuman primates. In: *Nonhuman Primates in Biomedical Research: Diseases* (eds. C.R. Abee, K. Mansfield, S. Tardif and T. Morris), 413–482. San Diego, CA: Academic Press.

48 Szentiks, C.A., Kondgen, S., Silinski, S. et al. (2009). Lethal pneumonia in a captive juvenile chimpanzee (*Pan troglodytes*) due to human-transmitted human respiratory syncytial virus (HRSV) and infection with *Streptococcus pneumoniae*. *J Med Primatol* 38: 236–240.

49 Denapaite, D. and Hakenbeck, R. (2011). A new variant of the capsule 3 cluster occurs in *Streptococcus pneumoniae* from deceased wild chimpanzees. *PLoS One* 6: e25119.

50 Unwin, S., Chatterton, J., and Chantrey, J. (2013). Management of severe respiratory tract disease caused by human respiratory syncytial virus and *Streptococcus pneumoniae* in captive chimpanzees (*Pan troglodytes*). *J Zoo Wildl Med* 44: 105–115.

51 Johnson, J.H., Wolf, A.M., Edwards, J.F. et al. (1998). Disseminated coccidioidomycosis in a mandrill baboon (*Mandrillus sphinx*): a case report. *J Zoo Wildl Med* 29: 208–213.

52 Catherinot, E., Lanternier, F., Bougnoux, M.-E. et al. (2010). *Pneumocystis jirovecii* pneumonia. *Infect Dis Clin North Am* 24: 107–138.

53 Board, K.F., Patil, S., Lebedeva, I. et al. (2003). Experimental *Pneumocystis carinii* pneumonia in simian immunodeficiency virus-infected rhesus macaques. *J Infect Dis* 187: 576–588.

54 Saravanan, C., Sasseville, V.G., and Mansfield, K. (2015). Nonhuman primate diseases of relevance in drug development and their impact on the interpretation of study findings. In: *The Nonhuman Primate in Nonclinical Drug Development and Safety Assessment* (eds. E. Schenck, J. Bluemel, S. Korte and G. Weinbauer), 187–213. San Diego, CA: Academic Press.

55 Furman, D.P., Bonasch, H., Springsteen, R. et al. (1974). Studies on the biology of the lung mite, *Pneumonyssus simicola banks* (Acarina: Halarachnidae) and diagnosis of infestation in macaques. *Lab Anim Sci* 24: 622–629.

56 Joseph, B.E., Wilson, D.W., Henrickson, R.V. et al. (1984). Treatment of pulmonary acariasis in rhesus macaques with ivermectin. *Lab Anim Sci* 34: 360–364.

57 Cogswell, F. and Baker, D.G. (2008). Parasites of non-human primates. In: *Flynn's Parasites of Laboratory Animals* (ed. D.G. Baker), 693–743. Ames, IA: Blackwell.

58 Jean, S.M., Morales, P.R., Paul, K., and Garcia, A. (2011). Spontaneous primary squamous cell carcinoma of the lung in a rhesus macaque (*Macaca mulatta*). *J Am Assoc Lab Anim Sci* 50: 404–408.

59 Fortman, J.D., Manaligod, J.R., and Bennet, B.T. (1993). Malignant mesothelioma in an olive baboon (*Papio anubis*). *Lab Anim Sci* 43: 503–505.

60 Eder, G., Harkanyi, Z., and Schaff, Z. (1996). Ultrasound guided spleen biopsy in chimpanzees (*Pan troglodytes*). *Ultrasound Med Biol* 22: 19–24.

61 Wilkinson, L.M., Wallace, J.M., and Cline, J.M. (1999). Disseminated blastomycosis in a rhesus monkey (*Macaca mulatta*). *Vet Pathol* 36: 460–462.

62 Klippert, A., Stolte-Leeb, N., Neumann, B. et al. (2015). Frequencies of lymphoid T-follicular helper cells obtained longitudinally by lymph node fine-needle aspiration correlate significantly with viral load in SIV-infected rhesus monkeys. *J Med Primatol* 44: 253–262.

63 Kleinschmidt, L., Langan, J.N., Warneke, M.R. et al. (2015). Retrospective review of the prevalence of myelolipoma in goeldi's monkeys (*Callimico goeldii*). *J Zoo Wildl Med* 46: 273–278.

64 Terrell, G.B., Gribble, D.H., and Osburn, B.I. (1980). Malignant lymphoma in macaques: a clinicopathologic study of 45 cases. *J Natl Cancer Inst* 64: 561–568.

65 Feichtinger, H., Putkonen, P., Parravicini, C. et al. (1990). Malignant lymphomas in cynomolgus monkeys infected with simian immunodeficiency virus. *Am J Pathol* 137: 1311–1315.

66 Hirata, A., Hashimoto, K., Katoh, Y. et al. (2015). Characterization of spontaneous malignant lymphomas in Japanese macaques (*Macaca fuscata*). *Vet Pathol* 52: 566–572.

67 Brady, A.D. and Carville, A.A.L. (2012). Digestive system diseases of nonhuman primates. In: *Nonhuman Primates in Biomedical Research: Diseases* (eds. C.R. Abee, K. Mansfield, S. Tardif and T. Morris), 590–627. San Diego, CA: Academic Press.

68 Wamsley, H.L., Wellehan, J.F., Harvey, J.W. et al. (2005). Cytologic diagnosis of *Lawsonia intracellularis* proliferative ileitis in a Japanese snow macaque (*Macaca fuscata*). *Vet Clin Pathol* 34: 57–60.

69 Stenzel, D.J. and Boreham, P.F. (1996). *Blastocystis hominis* revisited. *Clin Microbiol Rev* 9: 563–584.

70 Tan, K.S. (2004). Blastocystis in humans and animals: new insights using modern methodologies. *Vet Parasitol* 126: 121–144.

71 Parkar, U., Traub, R.J., Kumar, S. et al. (2007). Direct characterization of Blastocystis from faeces by PCR and evidence of zoonotic potential. *Parasitology* 134: 359–367.

72 Alfellani, M.A., Jacob, A.S., Perea, N.O. et al. (2013). Diversity and distribution of *Blastocystis* sp. subtypes in non-human primates. *Parasitology* 140: 966–971.

73 Khalifa, A.M. (1999). Diagnosis of *Blastocystis hominis* by different staining techniques. *J Egypt Soc Parasitol* 29: 157–165.

74 Strait, K., Else, J.G., and Eberhard, M.L. (2012). Parasitic diseases of nonhuman primates. In: *Nonhuman Primates in Biomedical Research: Diseases* (eds. C.R. Abee, K. Mansfield, S. Tardif and T. Morris), 197–297. San Diego, CA: Academic Press.

75 MacGuire, J.G., Christe, K.L., Yee, J.L. et al. (2009). Serologic evaluation of clinical and subclinical secondary hepatic amyloidosis in rhesus macaques (*Macaca mulatta*). *Comp Med* 59: 168–173.

76 Harbison, C.E., Taheri, F., Knight, H., and Miller, A.D. (2015). Immunohistochemical characterization of large intestinal adenocarcinoma in the rhesus macaque (*Macaca mulatta*). *Vet Pathol* 52: 732–740.

77 Wolf, R.F. and White, G.L. (2012). Clinical techniques used for nonhuman primates. In: *Nonhuman Primates in Biomedical Research: Biology and Management* (eds. C.R. Abee, K. Mansfield, S. Tardif and T. Morris), 323–338. San Diego, CA: Academic Press.

78 Kurien, B.T., Everds, N.E., and Scofield, R.H. (2004). Experimental animal urine collection: a review. *Lab Anim* 38: 333–361.

79 Bloomsmith, M., Neu, K., Franklin, A. et al. (2015). Positive reinforcement methods to train Chimpanzees to cooperate with urine collection. *J Am Assoc Lab Anim Sci* 54: 66–69.

80 Moll, R., Wu, X.R., Lin, J.H. et al. (1995). Uroplakin, specific membrane proteins of urothelial umbrella cells, as histologic markers of metastatic transitional cell carcinomas. *Am J Pathol* 147: 1383–1397.

81 Cline, J.M., Brignolo, L., and Ford, E.W. (2012). Urogenital system. In: *Nonhuman Primates in Biomedical Research: Diseases* (eds. C.R. Abee, K. Mansfield, S. Tardif and T. Morris), 483–562. San Diego, CA: Academic Press.

82 Taylor, M.G., Nelson, G.S., and Andrews, B.J. (1972). A case of natural infection of *S. haematobium* in a Senegalese baboon (*Papio* sp.). *Trans R Soc Trop Med Hyg* 66: 16–17.

83 Sturrock, R.F. (1986). A review of the use of primates in studying human schistosomiasis. *J Med Primatol* 15: 267–279.

84 Jordan, P., Von Lichtenberg, F., and Goatly, K.D. (1967). Experimental schistosomiasis in primates in Tanzania. *Bull World Health Organ* 37: 393–403.

85 Kuntz, R.E., Moore, J.A., and Huang, T.C. (1979). Distribution of egg deposits and gross lesions in nonhuman primates infected with *Schistosoma haematobium* (Iran). *J Med Primatol* 8: 167–178.

86 MacLennan, A.H. and Wynn, R.M. (1971). Menstrual cycle of the baboon. I. Clinical features, vaginal cytology and endometrial histology. *Obstet Gynecol* 38: 350–358.

87 Dukelow, W.R. (1983). The squirrel monkey (*Saimiri sciureus*). In: *Reproduction in New World Primates* (ed. J. Hearn), 151–179. Hingham, MA: MTP Press.

88 Nagle, C.A. and Denari, J.H. (1983). The Cebus monkey (*Cebus apella*). In: *Reproduction in New World Primates* (ed. J. Hearn), 39–67. Hingham, MA: MTP Press.

89 Lohiya, N.K., Sharma, R.S., Puri, C.P. et al. (1988). Reproductive exocrine and endocrine profile of female langur monkeys, *Presbytis entellus*. *J Reprod Fertil* 82: 485–492.

90 Eley, R.M., Tarara, R.P., Worthman, C.M., and Else, J.G. (1989). Reproduction in the vervet monkey (*Cercopithecus aethiops*): III. The menstrual cycle. *Am J Primatol* 17: 1–10.

91 Gluckman, T.L., Walz, S.E., Schultz-Darken, N., and Bolton, I.D. (2004). Cytologic assessment of the vaginal epithelium in the common marmoset (*Callithrix jacchus*): a preliminary new approach to reproductive screening. *Contemp Top Lab Anim Sci* 43: 28–31.

92 Tardif, S., Carville, A., Elmore, D. et al. (2012). Reproduction and breeding of nonhuman primates. In: *Nonhuman Primates in Biomedical Research: Biology and Management* (eds. C.R. Abee, K. Mansfield, S. Tardif and T. Morris), 197–249. San Diego: Academic Press.

93 Irizarry Rovira, A.R., Lynch, S., David, M., and Vara, J.A.R. (2012). Gonadoblastoma in the ovaries of a lesser galago (*Galago senegalensis braccatus*). *J Comp Pathol* 147: 204–248.

94 Harari, A., Wood, C.E., Van Doorslaer, K. et al. (2013). Condylomatous genital lesions in cynomolgus macaques from Mauritius. *Toxicol Pathol* 41: 893–901.

95 Doyle, L., Young, C.L., Jang, S.S., and Hillier, S.L. (1991). Normal vaginal aerobic and anaerobic bacterial flora of the rhesus macaque (*Macaca mulatta*). *J Med Primatol* 20: 409–413.

96 Alexander, N.J. (1981). Primates: their use in research on vasectomy. *Am J Primatol* 1: 167–173.

97 Mattison, J.A., Ottinger, M.A., Powell, D. et al. (2007). Endometriosis: clinical monitoring and treatment procedures in rhesus monkeys. *J Med Primatol* 36: 391–398.

98 Cruzen, C.L., Baum, S.T., and Colman, R.J. (2011). Glucoregulatory function in adult rhesus macaques (*Macaca mulatta*) undergoing treatment with medroxyprogesterone acetate for endometriosis. *J Am Assoc Lab Anim Sci* 50: 921–925.
99 Beck, A.P., Erdelyi, I., and Zeiss, C.J. (2014). Endometrial decidualization and deciduosis in aged rhesus macaques (*Macaca mulatta*). *Comp Med* 64: 148–156.
100 Muth, D.C., McAlexander, M.A., Ostrenga, L.J. et al. (2015). Potential role of cervicovaginal extracellular particles in diagnosis of endometriosis. *BMC Vet Res* 11: 187.
101 Ostrow, R.S., McGlennen, R.C., Shaver, M.K. et al. (1990). A rhesus monkey model for sexual transmission of a papillomavirus isolated from a squamous cell carcinoma. *Proc Natl Acad Sci U S A* 87: 8170–8174.
102 Wood, C.E., Chen, Z., Cline, J.M. et al. (2007). Characterization and experimental transmission of an oncogenic papillomavirus in female macaques. *J Virol* 81: 6339–6345.
103 Yearley, J.H., King, N., Liu, X. et al. (2008). Biphasic malignant testicular sex cord-stromal tumor in a cotton-top tamarin (*Saguinus oedipus*) with review of the literature. *Vet Pathol* 45: 922–927.
104 Gilbert, S.G., Reuhl, K.R., Wong, J.H., and Rice, D.C. (1987). Fatal pneumococcal meningitis in a colony-born monkey (*Macaca fascicularis*). *J Med Primatol* 16: 333–338.
105 Fahey, M.A. and Westmoreland, S.V. (2012). Nervous systems disorders of non-human primates and research models. In: *Nonhuman Primates in Biomedical Research: Diseases*, 734–782. San Diego, CA: Elsevier Academic Press.
106 Lemoy, M.-J.M.F., Lopes, D.A., Reader, J.R. et al. (2012). Meningoencephalitis due to *Listeria monocytogenes* in a pregnant Rhesus macaque (*Macaca mulatta*). *Comp Med* 62: 443–447.
107 Machotka, S.V., Chapple, F.E., and Stookey, J.L. (1975). Cerebral tuberculosis in a rhesus monkey. *J Am Vet Med Assoc* 167: 648–650.
108 Suleman, M.A., Johnson, B.J., Tarara, R. et al. (1984). An outbreak of poliomyelitis caused by poliovirus type I in captive black and white colobus monkeys (*Colobus Abyssinicus Kikuyuensis*) in Kenya. *Trans R Soc Trop Med Hyg* 78: 665–669.
109 Troan, B.V., Perelygina, L., Patrusheva, I. et al. (2007). Naturally transmitted herpesvirus papio-2 infection in a black and white colobus monkey. *J Am Vet Med Assoc* 231: 1878–1883.
110 Zeman, D.H. and Baskin, G.B. (1985). Encephalitozoonosis in squirrel monkeys (*Saimiri sciureus*). *Vet Pathol* 22: 24–31.
111 Juan-Sallés, C., Garner, M.M., Didier, E.S. et al. (2016). Disseminated encephalitozoonosis in captive, juvenile, cotton-top (*Saguinus oedipus*) and neonatal emperor (*Saguinus imperator*) tamarins in North America. *Vet Pathol* 43: 438–446.
112 Carlisle, M.S., Prociv, P., Grennan, J. et al. (1998). Cerebrospinal angiostrongyliasis in five captive tamarins (*Sanguinus* spp). *Aust Vet J* 76: 167–170.
113 Tanaka, T. and Canfield, D.R. (2012). Intracranial meningioma with opthalmoplegia in a rhesus macaque (*Macaca mulatta*). *Comp Med* 62: 439–442.
114 Hanley, P.W., Wilkerson, G.K., Bernacky, B.J. et al. (2013). Spontaneous high-grade glial intramedullary tumor of the spine in a rhesus macaque (*Macaca mulatta*). *J Med Primatol* 42: 158–160.
115 Weston, C.L., Glantz, M.J., and Connor, J.R. (2011). Detection of cancer cells in the cerebrospinal fluid: current methods and future directions. *Fluids Barriers CNS* 8: 14.
116 Davis, R.H., McDonald, J., Kyriazis, G.A., and Schneider, H.P. (1973). The peritoneal fluid cytology of the adult female rhesus monkey. *Experientia* 29: 1242.
117 D'Agostino, J., Isaza, R., Fingland, R. et al. (2007). Acute appendicitis in a chimpanzee (*Pan troglodytes*). *J Med Primatol* 36: 119–123.
118 Olson, L.C. and Anver, M.R. (1979). Chylothorax in rhesus monkeys with intravenous catheters. *Lab Anim Sci* 29: 791–796.
119 Felkai, A., Vogelnest, L., McNabb, S. et al. (2014). Dilated cardiomyopathy in a De Brazza's monkey (*Cercopithecus neglectus*). *J Med Primatol* 43: 209–212.
120 Tolwani, R.J., Waggie, K.S., Green, S.L. et al. (2000). Dilative cardiomyopathy leading to congestive heart failure in a male squirrel monkey (*Saimiri sciureus*). *J Med Primatol* 29: 42–45.

61

Reptiles and Birds

Nicole I. Stacy, Helene Pendl, and Peter M. Wencel

Introduction

Cytology is a simple and rapid baseline diagnostic tool with particular benefit to birds and reptiles, since clinically overt disease in these species is often not evident until advanced stages. The reptiles, more technically called the *Sauropsida*, with over 20 000 extant species, include the *Dinosauria* of which the birds are the only surviving member.[1] For the purpose of discussion in this chapter, they will be referred to as birds and (non-avian) reptiles. Since hemodilution is commonly present in cytologic samples of these species, some unique specific features regarding their blood cells need to be considered.[2] Although reptiles and birds are vastly different from mammals in many aspects of biology and physiology, similar standard principles of cytologic evaluation apply across all species with due consideration of major differences in inflammatory responses, prevalence of certain infectious agents, and frequency and type of certain tumor types by species.

Clinical Settings

Cytology in birds and reptiles is useful in individual care of pet animals as well as group management. Examples of the latter include routine wellness examinations in zoological, research, and commercial collections, and wildlife surveys in field studies. Cytology performed during necropsy in outbreaks involving a group of animals (e.g. zoological collection, wild animal population) represents an invaluable tool for initial diagnostic evaluation that can guide initial treatment and selection of additional diagnostic tests while awaiting results with longer turnaround times, such as histopathology, culture, or molecular testing.

Applications of Cytology and Collection Methods

Cytology samples from reptile and avian patients are frequently collected from external lesions (e.g. from skin, shell, feathers, nares, nasal cavity, less frequently eye), the oral cavity, the avian crop, the cloaca, the coelomic cavity (i.e. effusion), the respiratory tract (e.g. mucus recovered from the endotracheal tube, tracheal wash, bronchoalveolar lavage, biopsies), synovial fluid, urine, and fecal material. Body fluids should be collected into heparin, since it allows handling of small sample volumes for multiple analyses, including culture. Ethylenediaminetetraacetic acid (EDTA) causes hemolysis in some species of reptiles (e.g. chelonian) and birds (e.g. corvids, cranes, ratites) and inhibits bacterial growth, which is contraindicated if a fluid sample is intended for bacterial culture. Body fluids for cytology processing can be collected in EDTA in species in which EDTA is known to not cause hemolysis. Unless otherwise noted, needed equipment, sample collection techniques, sample handling and processing, and sources of pre-analytical error are similar to other species.

External Samples

External lesions are often sampled using a cotton swab, preferably moistened with saline to avoid damaging the mucosa of nares, conjunctiva, oral cavity, or cloaca. Shell lesions can require scraping for exfoliation of cellular material. Although the feather can be fully examined for parasites or other abnormalities under low magnification, the pulp of the feather should be squashed between two slides to obtain sufficient cellular material for cytologic evaluation. Other external lesions are collected as for other species.

Coelomic Cavity

For diagnostic evaluation of the coelomic cavity in reptiles, a coelomic wash can be performed if aspiration does not yield adequate diagnostic material. The coelomic wash or directly collected coelomic fluid should be processed similar to other species with preparation of direct and concentrated smears. Coelomic washes are inappropriate in birds because the air

Veterinary Cytology, First Edition. Edited by Leslie C. Sharkey, M. Judith Radin, and Davis Seelig.

sacs extend extensively into the intestinal peritoneal cavity, and the procedure risks fluid accumulation within the respiratory tract.[3] The coelomic cavity in birds is divided into multiple distinct peritoneal cavity compartments as discussed further in section "Body Cavity Fluids."

Respiratory Tract

Since endoscopy has become more clinically available, washes of the respiratory tract (e.g. nasal, tracheal, avian air sacs) can be performed, in addition to imprints of tissue biopsies.[4–6] Fine-needle aspirates from swellings in the sinuses of birds typically contain abundant cellular material.

Other Samples

Gastrointestinal sampling includes crop washes and swabs in birds and, rarely, gastric and cloacal washes in reptiles. Gastric washes require a tube of appropriate length in snakes given the extended length of their stomachs. Cloacal swabs are used in reptiles and birds, often in conjunction with fecal collection for direct smear evaluation and additional testing as needed. If a cloacal swab does not exfoliate sufficient cellular material, a cloacal wash can be performed in reptiles with due consideration of unique anatomical features in various reptile species. The white portion of cloacal excretions represents urinary waste (urates) in reptiles and birds and should be separated from fecal material for evaluation of both portions. As for other species, tissue imprints from biopsies or samples collected during necropsy from organ parenchyma should be blotted onto clean absorbable tissue before imprinting onto glass slides to remove excess blood. In contrast to tissue imprints, properly performed squash preparations yield samples of higher cellularity and of excellent diagnostic quality, especially for diagnosis of infectious agents. After being expelled onto a slide, the sample is spread gently with a second slide or coverslip. Pressure should be applied with caution to ensure sufficient cell separation with minimal disruption. The sample size should be small enough (1–4 mm^3) to be well distributed on the slide resulting in a blood film-like monolayer with feathered edge.

General Cytologic Categories

Although reptiles and birds are physiologically distinct from mammals, the cytologic evaluation of samples collected from these species follows the universal systematic approach that applies to all other species (Chapter 5). When evaluating cytology samples from this diverse group of animals, it is of utmost importance to consider their unique inflammatory responses and the prevalence of species-specific infectious agents, metabolic disorders, and neoplasms.

Inflammation

Evaluation of inflammatory lesions in reptiles and birds requires basic knowledge of leukocyte morphology in non-mammalian species and consideration of temperature-dependent immune responses in poikilotherm reptile species.[7] The assessment of the type of inflammation provides clues to pathogenesis, possible etiology, and the duration of the process. Since hemodilution is common, differentiation of lymphocytes and thrombocytes can be challenging given the similarity in size and shape. Thrombocytes are often densely clumped in cytologic preparations, which can help in their differentiation from lymphocytes. The main circulating inflammatory cell in many reptiles and birds is the heterophil, which lacks myeloperoxidase and depends both on oxidative and non-oxidative antimicrobial mechanisms.[7,8] In contrast to mammalian neutrophils and avian heterophils that occasionally show degenerative changes reflective of toxic microenvironmental conditions especially with bacterial infections (Figure 61.1), such morphologic changes are infrequently observed in reptiles.[9] Snakes and some lizard species have azurophils that contain peroxidase and are frequently involved in acute inflammatory processes.[10] Azurophils are the second most frequently observed circulating leukocyte type in many snake species.[11] Azurophils are often present

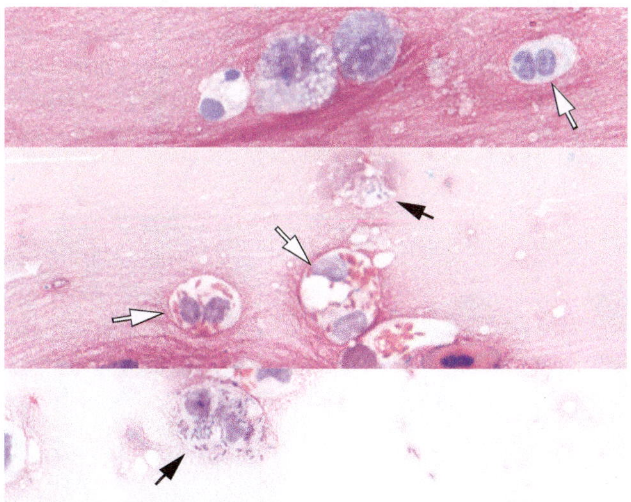

Figure 61.1 Oral swab of a tongue lesion from a grey parrot (*Psittacus erithacus*) illustrating variably degenerative heterophils (white arrows) and phagocytosis of mixed bacilli (black arrows) (Wright–Giemsa, 1000×).

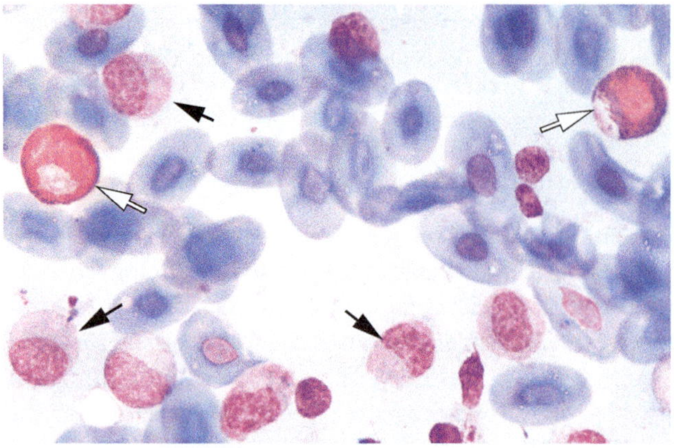

Figure 61.2 Azurophils (black arrows) and heterophils (white arrows) from a skin lesion from an Indian rock python (*Python molurus*). Histopathology confirmed histiocytic and heterophilic cellulitis of unknown etiology (Wright–Giemsa, 1000×).

in cytology samples from these species due to hemodilution and should not be confused with other round cell populations, such as lymphoid neoplasia or poorly cohesive carcinoma (Figure 61.2). Reptile species other than snakes and lizards can have monocytes with similar morphology to azurophils; however, their features are less distinct (e.g. irregular cell shape vs. round spheres in snake azurophils), and they are less frequent. Given the lack of peroxidase staining, these cells are placed in the monocyte category in leukocyte differentials.[12] *Psittaciformes* have eosinophils with granules that stain basophilic instead of eosinophilic, i.e. blue eosinophils (Figure 61.3), which can be difficult to differentiate from basophils cytologically.

Reptilian and avian inflammatory responses are notably distinct from other species and also from each other. Table 61.1 provides an overview of inflammatory responses in reptiles and birds. Reptilian inflammatory responses are generally characterized by formation of granulomas. Heterophils infiltrate the inflammatory site within hours, macrophages follow within a day (Figure 61.4a and b), and subsequent progression into a granuloma develops over a minimum of seven days. This process is thought to be accelerated at higher environmental temperatures.[13] Granulomas are readily identified by histology but not by cytology. A representative cytology sample can provide diagnostic information for the characterization of inflammation based on the presence and proportions of inflammatory cells.

Avian inflammatory lesions are different from reptiles and are illustrated by a classical inflammatory reaction in chicken skin that follows a distinct chronologic pattern regardless of the stimulus.[14] Heterophils and monocytes arrive within 30 minutes to 3 hours after initiation (Figure 61.4c), followed by transient basophil infiltration, which typically peaks between 3 and 6 hours. The influx of basophils can be difficult to assess cytologically because basophils tend to degranulate and/or granules may not fully take up dye in aqueous Romanowsky dip stains, such as Diff-Quik™.[17] Lymphocytes tend to gradually increase beginning at 6 hours, reaching their maximum at about 24 hours and often persisting as the predominate inflammatory cell for the following 2–3 days. The transformation of monocytes into macrophages, epithelioid variants, or giant cells (Figure 61.4d) occurs shortly after migration into the affected tissue, depending on the stimulus. Giant cells, representing fused macrophages, and epithelioid macrophages are prominent in areas of tissue necrosis and Type IV delayed hypersensitivity responses. Histologically, these cells appear by 12 hours after stimulation. Distinct granulomas form by 24–28 hours. Considerable plasma cell response with increased immunoglobulin production is present at day 2–3. In contrast to mammals, eosinophils are not a feature of acute hypersensitivity reactions, but account for 20–30% of the granulocytes in experimentally provoked

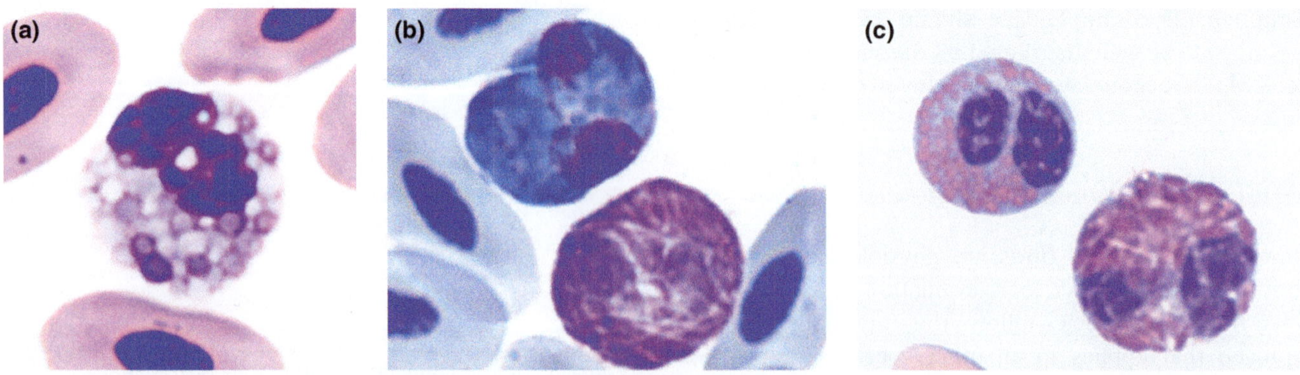

Figure 61.3 Eosinophil and heterophil morphology in avian species. (a) Blue eosinophil from a grey parrot (*Psittacus erithacus*). (b) Eosinophil (top) and heterophil (bottom) from a Palm cockatoo (*Probosciger aterrimus*). (c) Eosinophil (top) and heterophil (bottom) from a domestic chicken (*Gallus gallus domesticus*) (Wright–Giemsa, 1000×).

Table 61.1 Inflammatory responses with cytologic characteristics and potential etiologies in reptiles and birds.[13–16]

Species	Type of inflammation	Cytologic characteristics	Potential etiologies
Reptiles	Heterophilic predominant	Mixed heterophils and macrophages (similar to pyogranulomatous inflammation in mammals)	Extracellular pathogens (especially bacteria), tissue injury, necrosis
	Histiocytic predominant	Predominantly macrophages, often with multinucleated histiocytes	Obligate intracellular pathogens (e.g. *Mycobacterium* sp., *Chlamydia* sp.), fungi
	Chronic (end-stage lesion only recognized by histology)	May include reactive fibroplasia, metaplasia, necrosis, inflammation	Subsequent to heterophilic and/or histiocytic inflammation. Initial type of inflammation often is not possible to identify
	Lymphoplasmacytic	≥50% lymphocytes ± plasma cells	Chronic inflammation, including infectious and noninfectious causes
	Eosinophilic component	Variable % of eosinophils	Parasites, fungi, nonspecific as part of chronic inflammation
Birds	Heterophilic	≥80% heterophils; often accompanied by phagocytosis of pathogens or cellular debris; nuclear degenerative changes possible	Frequently associated with extracellular pathogens (especially bacteria, fungi), trauma, necrosis
	Mixed	Heterophils, macrophages, lymphocytes; most common inflammatory response in birds	Frequently associated with infectious agents such as bacteria, fungi
	Granulomatous	≥50% macrophages; possibly multinucleated giant cells, epithelioid macrophages, heterophils, lymphocytes	Infectious causes: fungi (e.g. *Aspergillus* sp.), *Mycobacterium* sp., *Trichomonas* sp. Noninfectious causes: necrosis, xanthomatosis, foreign bodies, granulation tissue
	Lymphoplasmacytic	≥50% lymphocytes ± plasma cells	Chronic inflammation without major tissue destruction of both infectious and noninfectious origin; hypersensitivity reactions Types II–IV
	Eosinophilic	≥10% eosinophils	Chronic inflammation with delayed hypersensitivity reaction (often associated with dermal, gastrointestinal, respiratory conditions); unreliable for parasitism and immediate hypersensitivity

Type IV hypersensitivity reactions. Fibroblasts appear around day 2, with prominent reactive fibroplasia apparent by days 7–10. Avian disorders presumably associated with at least some component of delayed hypersensitivity include aspergillosis, mycobacteriosis, erysipelas, listeriosis, streptococcosis, and staphylococcosis.[18] Experiments triggering eosinophilia in mammals produce inconsistent results in birds, making eosinophils an unreliable indicator for intestinal parasitism and hypersensitivity reactions.[7,19,20] Clinical and experimental findings suggest that avian eosinophils participate in delayed rather than acute hypersensitivity reactions (Figure 61.5).[15,18,19,21]

It is essential to carefully evaluate inflammatory lesions for infectious agents while considering that recent or current antimicrobial treatment may hinder the identification of microorganisms. Low cellularity samples and washes can fail to be representative of the underlying pathology, and infectious organisms may not exfoliate into a cytology sample. Thus, the absence of an infectious organism in a cytology sample does not exclude infection, especially if clinical findings suggest an infectious process. Furthermore, culture protocols might not be optimized for certain microorganisms, resulting in negative culture despite the cytologic observation of microorganisms. This underscores the diagnostic utility of cytology, and the importance of interpreting clinical findings in context of cytology and culture/sensitivity results in poikilotherm species.[22] Since polymerase chain reaction (PCR) testing has become more readily available and affordable, it may be useful in cases with negative culture or whenever clinically indicated.

Infectious Agents

Inflammatory lesions in response to infection are the most frequent cytodiagnoses in reptile and bird medicine. Cytology often provides a rapid tentative diagnosis, since many microorganisms can be readily identified. Additional

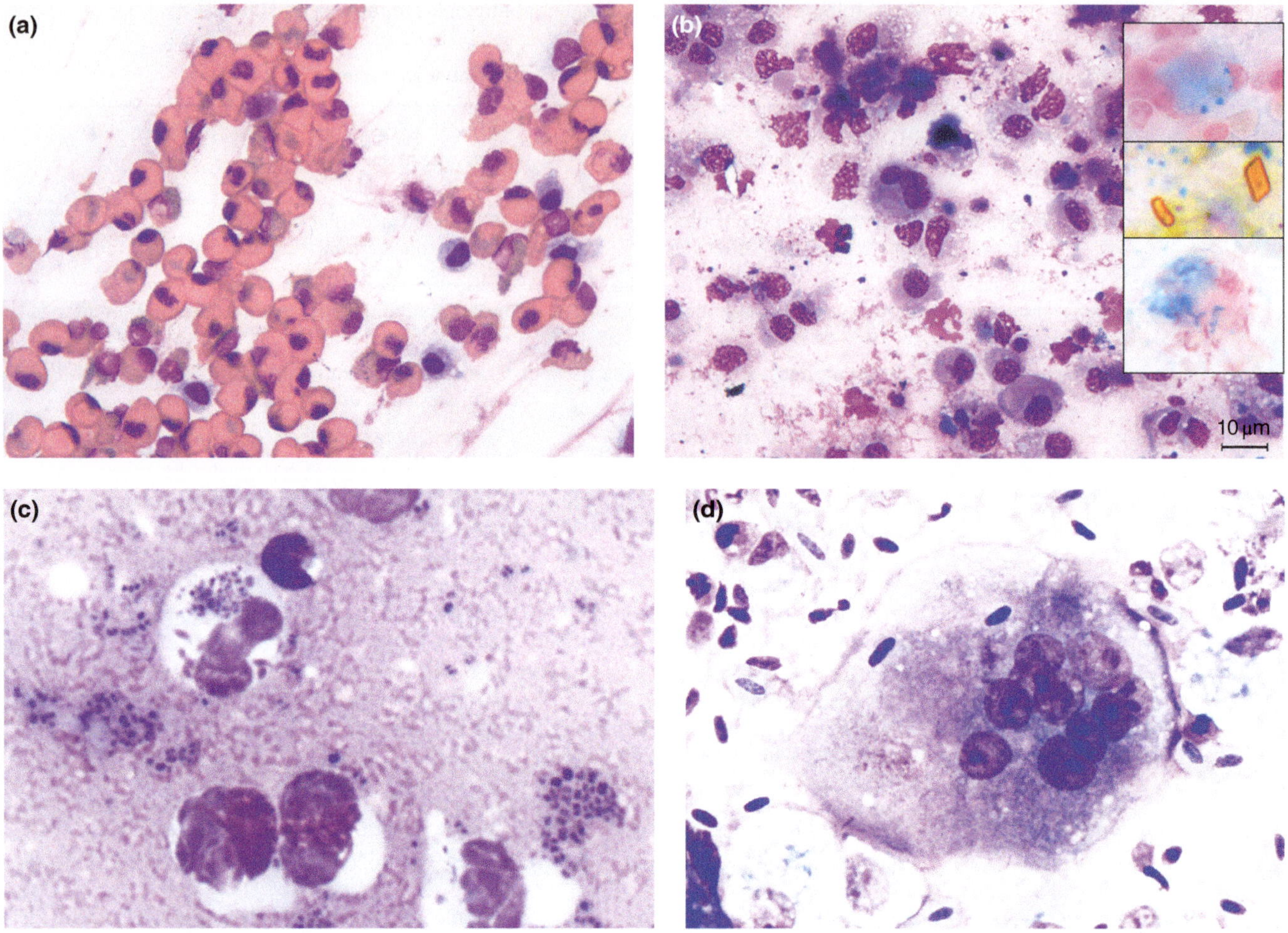

Figure 61.4 (a) Heterophilic inflammation with mild histiocytic component from a fresh knee wound after traumatic injury in a gopher tortoise (*Gopherus polyphemus*) (Wright–Giemsa, 1000×). (b) Cytology of mucus recovered from the endotracheal tube after anesthesia in a Kemp's ridley sea turtle (*Lepidochelys kempii*) demonstrating marked histiocytic inflammation with multinucleated histiocytes and presence of chronic hemorrhage visible as pale to medium basophilic amorphous material suggestive of hemosiderin. Although negative-staining bacilli were not observed cytologically, the type of inflammation warranted further stains for infectious agents (e.g. acid fast) (Wright–Giemsa, 500×). Insets Top: Prussian blue for confirmation of hemosiderin consistent with chronic hemorrhage. Middle: Hematoidin crystals. Bottom: Acid-fast positive bacilli. PCR confirmed *Mycobacterium chelonae* (Inset images, 1000×). (c) Heterophilic keratitis with phagocytosis of cocci and diplococci in a corneal scraping from a peregrine falcon (*Falco peregrinus*). Heterophils exhibit degenerative change (karyolysis) and degranulation (Wright–Giemsa, 1000×). (d) Giant cell of histiocytic origin in an air sac biopsy imprint from a saker falcon (*Falco cherrug*) with *Serratospiculum* sp. infection. The organism is not visible in this image (Diff-Quik, 1000×).

diagnostics, such as culture, parasitologic evaluation, and/or PCR might be necessary for further diagnostic workup or confirmation. See Chapter 3 for more information on the general microbiologic review of cytology samples.

Bacteria

Bacteria are categorized by their morphology and affinity to routine and special stains, such as Romanowsky-type, Gram, and acid fast. For instance, in cytologic skin samples from any aquatic species, considerations for bacteria and/or fungal elements include normal flora, environmental contaminants, or pathogenic organisms. Normal fecal microflora in most species is typically composed of mixed rod-shaped bacteria and possibly low numbers of cocci. Abnormal flora can present as a predominance of a monomorphic organism. The presence of concurrent inflammation and phagocytized organisms are consistent with bacterial infection, which can be primary or secondary. This differentiation is often difficult to make cytologically. *Chlamydia* present as very small, dark blue, pin-point dots that may be observed intracellularly and/or extracellularly (see section "Respiratory Tract"; images also available in Chapter 20).[7] They can be difficult to differentiate from other basophilic staining bacteria of similar size and granular debris by routine Romanowsky-type stains. Since PCR has become readily available, special stains for

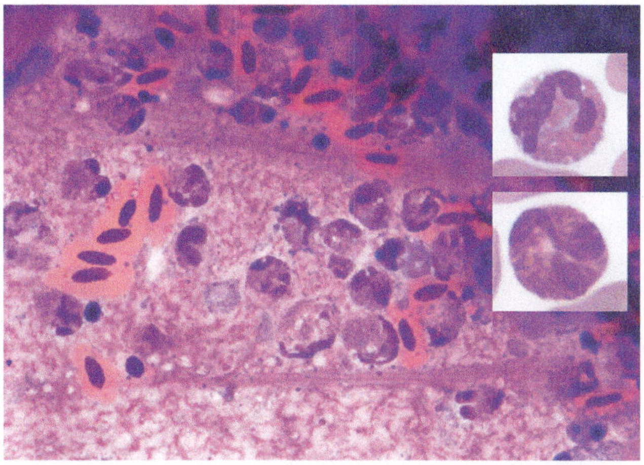

Figure 61.5 Fecal direct smear from a great white pelican (*Pelecanus onocrotalus*) with diarrhea and eosinophilic colitis due to suspected hypersensitivity to bacterial antigens. There is a large amount of mucus and variably sized punctate structures with considerations including cocci and/or mucus. Cultures were persistently positive for *Staphylococcus sciuri* and *Enterococcus* sp. (Diff-Quik, 1000×). Insets are from the peripheral blood film from the same patient. Top: eosinophil. Bottom: heterophil.

visualization of chlamydial stages by cytology, such as Gimenez or Macchiavello stain, are not commonly used.

Viruses

Viral inclusion bodies (IBs) are infrequently identified cytologically in birds and rarely in reptiles. Absence of IBs in cytology samples does not rule out viral infection, as not every virus produces IBs. The presence and quantity of IBs for those that do is inconsistent and depends on the immune status of the host as well as the stage and course of infection. Suspected (e.g. clinically, cytologically) viral infections should be confirmed by molecular diagnostics (e.g. PCR), transmission electron microscopy, and/or, if available, immunohistochemistry (IHC). Highly pathogenic viral strains can result in peracute death before IB formation and is often associated with prominent hemorrhage and necrosis in the affected tissues.[23,24] Cytologic examination of organ squash preparations collected during necropsy are highly recommended in such cases, since this technique produces high-cellularity samples and thus higher diagnostic utility compared with other cytologic preparations. Samples from the five large "red organs" (heart, lung, liver, spleen, and kidney) should be collected at minimum. The cytologic observation of suspicious structures should always be confirmed with other diagnostic means such as PCR, transmission electron microscopy, and/or IHC.

Cytology samples from boas and pythons infected with Arenavirus-associated inclusion body disease (IBD) can contain characteristic pale basophilic intracytoplasmic inclusions in lymphocytes, heterophils, erythrocytes, thrombocytes, and/or tissue cells (Figure 61.6).[25,26] Romanowsky-type stains are mostly sufficient for identification of IBD inclusions; however, hematoxylin and eosin will stain these inclusions bright pink and can facilitate visualization in cytology samples, blood films, and buffy coat smears.[26] Iridoviral inclusions in various blood cells as described in a box turtle and a peninsula ribbon snake can be identified in hemodiluted cytology samples.[27,28]

In birds, intracytoplasmic inclusion bodies (ICIB) are most commonly produced by infections with circoviruses and poxviruses, whereas intranuclear inclusion bodies (INIB) are frequently seen in adenovirus, herpesvirus, and polyomavirus infections.[2,29] The purpose of the following short description is to provide an overview of the most common diseases associated with these viruses. Clinical, cytologic, and pathologic key features are summarized in Table 61.2.

Avian circovirus affects many bird species and is the causative agent of the so-called psittacine beak and feather disease in parrots.[23,30–34] Disease is characterized by hemorrhagic necrotizing inflammatory lesions of skin, appendages, and lymphoid and hematopoietic tissues, such as spleen, bursa, and bone marrow. Depending on host species and viral strain, skin and feather lesions, anemia, or secondary opportunistic infections due to immunosuppression will determine the clinical presentation. Concurrent beak lesions with necrosis and loss of keratin are especially seen in cockatoos.[23] Circovirus ICIBs are infrequently found cytologically, usually within cells of the mononuclear phagocytic system (MPS) of affected organs. They are basophilic to amphophilic botryoid structures that vary in size and number. Large ICIBs can fill and distort the cytoplasm of affected cells (Figure 61.7a and b). This unique morphology presents a challenge in cytologic diagnosis because they can easily be mistaken for translucent, spheroid crystals, or proteinaceous material.

Avian poxviruses are rather species and genus specific with a strong tropism for surface epithelia of skin, respiratory tract, and oropharynx.[23,32–34] Glandular epithelia such as hepatocytes can be affected in systemic disease. Clinical manifestations include cutaneous (dry), mucosal (wet), and systemic–septicemic forms with transitional forms possible. The systemic form mostly affects canaries with up to 100% mortality. Clinical and pathologic key features include hepatosplenomegaly and respiratory disease in the systemic course, whereas dry and wet forms present with nodular to diffuse proliferation of unfeathered skin, skin adnexa, and oropharynx. Hemorrhagic–ulcerative bacterial superinfections are common and can obscure the primary viral etiology. Cytologic characteristics of poxviral infections include proliferation, cytoplasmic ballooning, degeneration of epithelial cells, and presence of pale eosinophilic

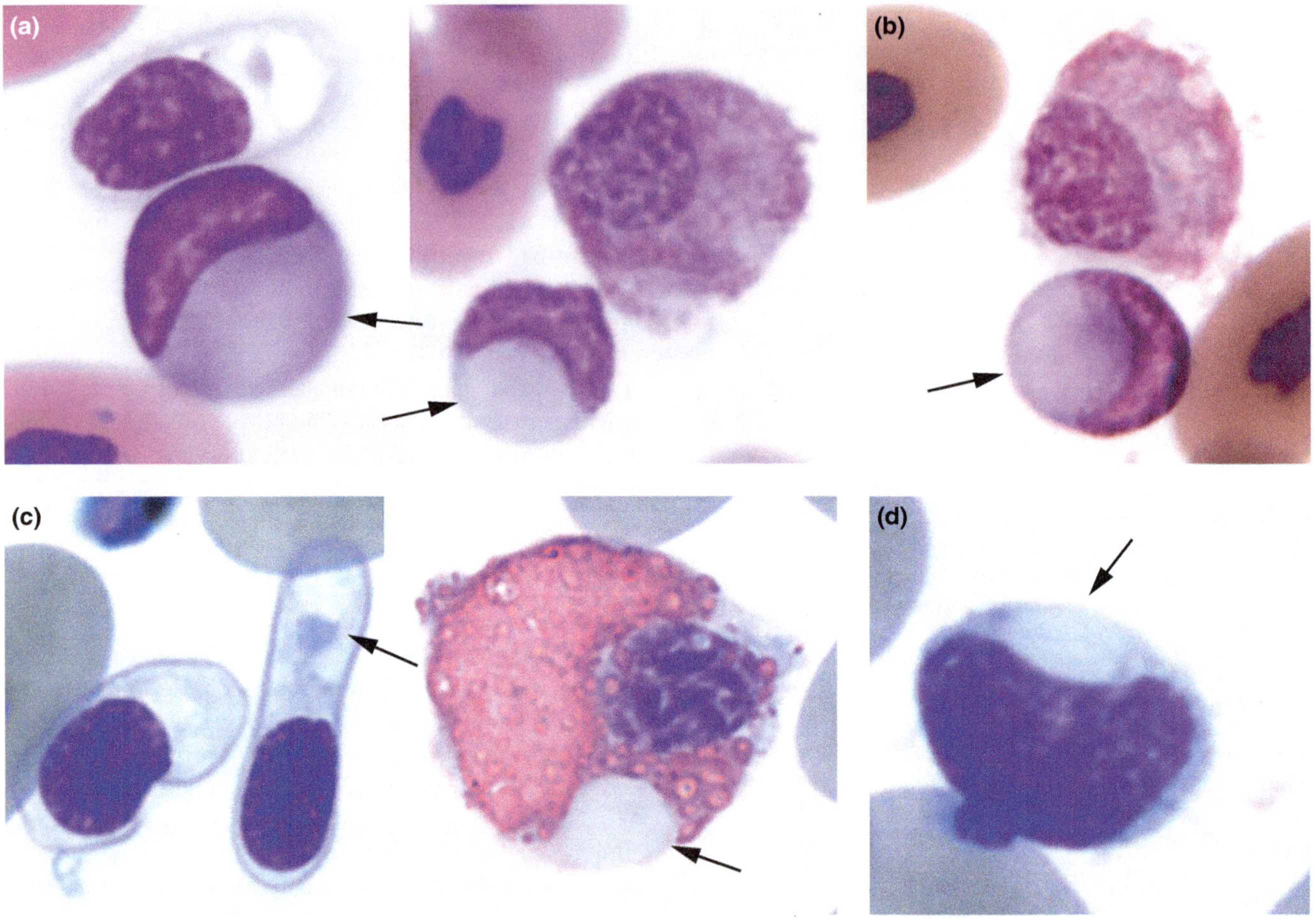

Figure 61.6 Characteristic oval, round, or lentiform, pale basophilic, glassy-appearing intracytoplasmic inclusions of the Arenavirus-associated inclusion body disease (IBD) as indicated by arrows. These pale basophilic, glassy IBD inclusions have been documented in lymphocytes, heterophils, erythrocytes, thrombocytes, and in antemortem tissue liver imprints of boids. (a and b) IBD inclusions in lymphocytes from a ball python (*Python regius*). (c) IBD inclusion in a heterophil (right) and a suspected inclusion in a thrombocyte (left) from a *Boa constrictor*. (d) IBD inclusion in a lymphocyte from the same *B. constrictor* (Wright–Giemsa, 1000×).

ICIBs (Bollinger bodies) (Figure 61.8). Bollinger bodies contain pinkish-grey granular Borrel bodies, which can be visible by cytology or accumulate as clot-like structure in the center of the inclusion.[7,14]

Adenoviruses are prevalent in many bird species worldwide.[23,32–39] Apart from a few primary pathogenic strains, most are subclinical with low pathogenicity. Clinical outbreaks are encountered with adenoviral infection as a cofactor accompanied by conditions causing increased stress and/or immunosuppression. Secondary bacterial infections are common in these scenarios. In a flock situation, the course of an outbreak is acute to peracute (24–48 hours) with rapid spread in juveniles and a moderate (adult) to high (juvenile) mortality. Key findings include septicemic–hemorrhagic enteritis, hepatosplenitis, and serofibrinous polyserositis often with hydropericardium. Bronchitis is only encountered in quail.[23] Characteristic adenoviral INIBs stain basophilic to amphophilic with variable color intensity (Figure 61.9). Size and number of INIBs per nucleus vary from several small to medium bodies in inclusion body hepatitis in chickens and pigeons, to extremely large inclusions in other organs and species. These pan-nuclear single IBs can enlarge and completely fill the nucleus while marginalizing the nucleolus. They are most commonly found in epithelial and lymphoid tissue and can be detected at 100× magnification.

Similar to other species, survival of a herpesvirus infection in birds results in lifelong persistence of the virus in asymptomatic carriers with intermittent shedding during stressful periods.[23,32–34] Typical stressors in flocks include breeding, overcrowding, transport, introduction of new birds, immunosuppressive primary disease, poor nutrition or housing, and adaptation to new environment (e.g. arctic species in temperate climates). Clinical disease predominantly develops in naive companion birds of the flock. The course is often peracute with rapid spread and high

Table 61.2 Overview of cytologic characteristics of viral inclusions in birds.

Virus	Cytologic findings	Clinical and pathologic key findings
Intracytoplasmic inclusion bodies		
Circo	Single or multiple, botryoid, translucent, basophilic to amphophilic inclusions Mostly in macrophages of skin (especially feather pulps) and lymphoid tissue (especially bursa)	Affects many bird species Hemorrhagic necrotizing inflammation of skin, skin adnexa, hematopoietic tissue, and lymphoid tissue Secondary opportunistic infections due to immune suppression Psittacine beak and feather disease (Psittaciformes)
Pox	Pale eosinophilic Bollinger bodies, often with translucent (ring-forms) or granular, pinkish-grey center (Borrel bodies) Proliferation and ballooning degeneration of surface epithelia Epitheliotropic: surface epithelia (especially skin, respiratory tract, oropharynx); less common in glandular epithelia (e.g. hepatocytes in systemic infections)	Cutaneous form (many species): nodular to diffuse proliferation and inflammation of unfeathered skin and adnexa; hemorrhagic–ulcerative bacterial superinfections common Septicemic form (especially in canaries): systemic hemorrhages, tissue necrosis, hyperplasia of respiratory epithelium up to complete obstruction of airways; intracytoplasmic inclusion bodies rare due to peracute course Wet form: nodular to diffuse oropharyngeal proliferation and inflammation with caseous covering; hemorrhagic–ulcerative bacterial superinfections common
Intranuclear inclusion bodies		
Adeno	Basophilic to amphophilic, small to medium-sized IB in liver of *Columbiformes* Extremely large, pan-nuclear, single inclusion body in surface and glandular epithelia of the gastrointestinal, respiratory, and urogenital tracts, serosal layers, or lymphoid tissue in other species	Hemorrhagic necrotizing hepatosplenitis, enteritis, serofibrinous polyserositis, nephritis in *Galliformes*, *Columbiformes*, *Falconiformes*, *Psittaciformes*, *Passeriformes* Hemorrhagic necrotizing bronchitis (only quail)
Herpes	Small, eosinophilic to basophilic inclusion, with or without halo; always one single inclusion body per nucleus Nuclear pyknosis Formation of syncytia, karyomegaly in cytomegalovirus infections of passerines	Hemorrhagic diphtheroid to necrotizing (laryngo-) tracheitis (especially in *Galliformes*, *Psittaciformes*, *Passeriformes*) Pacheco's disease (*Psittaciformes*): hemorrhagic necrotizing hepatosplenitis Duck plague: hemorrhagic diphtheroid to necrotizing enteritis with neurologic signs (especially in *Anseriformes*) Inclusion body hepatitis: hemorrhagic necrotizing hepatosplenitis, oropharyngitis, esophagitis, gastroenteritis, myelonecrosis (especially in *Falconiformes*, *Gruiformes*, *Strigiformes*, *Columbiformes*)
Polyomavirus	Medium-sized to large, light basophilic inclusion associated with chromatin marginalization (hollow nuclei) and karyomegaly In all basic tissue types (epithelial, endothelial, mesenchymal, neural) Most commonly found in the skin, liver, kidney, heart, spleen, cerebellum	Feather dystrophy is a key finding Budgie fledgling disease: also called French molt, or feather duster syndrome in *Melopsittacus undulatus*; coinfection with circovirus possible Non-budgerigar polyomavirus infection: hepatosplenitis, polyserositis, nephritis, myocarditis, enteritis, encephalitis (*Psittaciformes*, *Passeriformes*, *Anseriformes*, *Falconiformes*, *Columbiformes*, *Phasianiformes*, *Galliformes*, *Struthioniformes*) Peracute hemorrhagic–septicemic course in pre-weaned chicks with varying degrees of aforementioned lesions

mortality. Tissue tropism varies among viral genera and susceptible hosts. Species of the genus *Iltovirus* cause hemorrhagic, necrotizing, diphtheroid (laryngo-) tracheitis in *Galliformes*, *Psittaciformes*, and *Passeriformes*.[40–42] Psittacine herpesvirus 1 is the etiologic agent of Pacheco's disease, which causes peracute hemorrhagic necrotizing hepatosplenitis in parrots.[43,44] Duck plague is characterized by diphtheroid to necrotizing enteritis associated with neurologic signs in *Anseriformes*.[45] Other herpesviruses have a predilection for the gastrointestinal tract (GIT), lymphoid, and hematopoietic tissues and cause hemorrhagic necrotizing hepatosplenitis, gastroenteritis, and myelonecrosis in many bird species such as *Falconiformes, Gruiformes, Strigiformes, and Columbiformes*. Cytologically, the small,

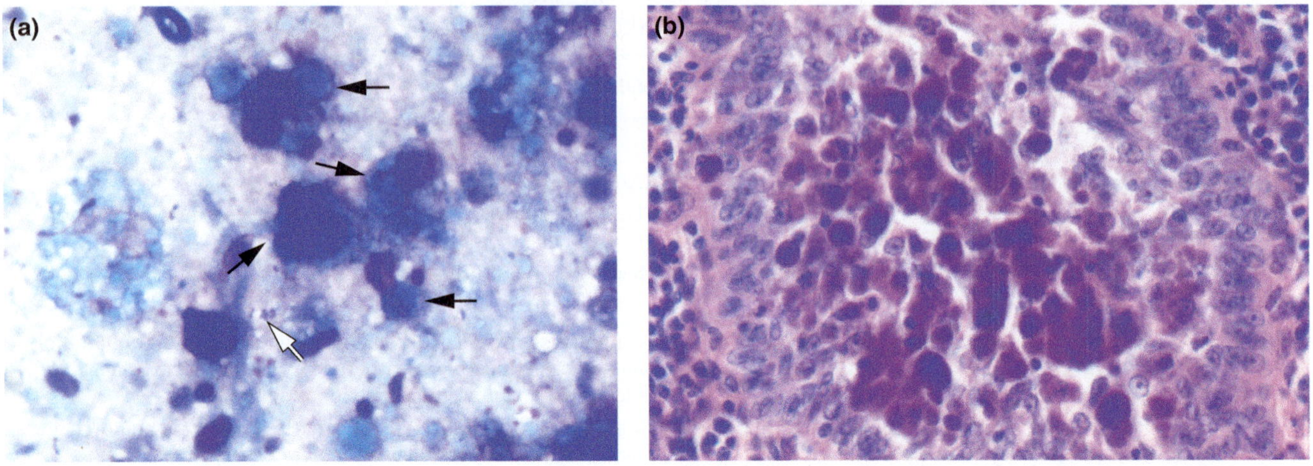

Figure 61.7 (a) Pigeon circovirus in a racing pigeon (*Columba livia*). Multiple bluish intracytoplasmic circovirus inclusions are visible in mononuclear cells (black arrows), and small coccobacilli are seen in the background (white arrow). Note the size and globular shape of circovirus inclusions, which are often described as botryoid, as well as their translucency resembling crystalline structures. Multiple free inclusions likely originating from ruptured cells are visible (Diff-Quik, 1000×). (b) Histology of the bursa of Fabricius from a grey parrot (*Psittacus erithacus*) demonstrating numerous large basophilic to amphophilic, botryoid ICIBs in medullary reticuloendothelial cells of a bursal follicle with concurrent lymphoid necrosis. Circovirus infection was confirmed by PCR (hematoxylin & eosin, 400×.)

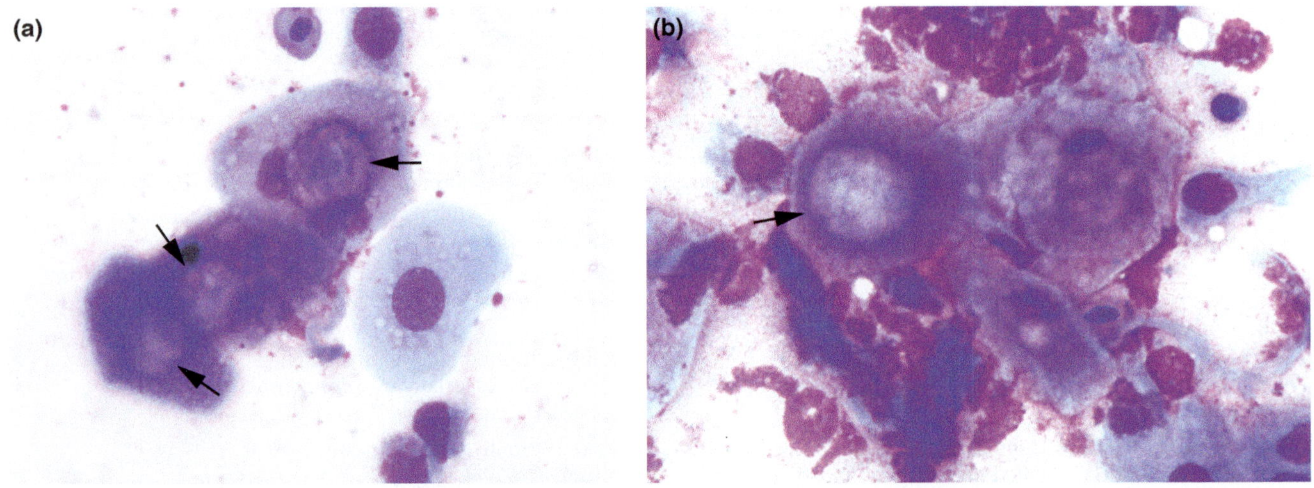

Figure 61.8 (a and b) Conjunctival swab from a bald eagle (*Haliaeetus leucocephalus*) that presented with typical dry pox lesions around the head. Both images show oval to polygonal squamous epithelial cells and poorly preserved presumptive mucosal epithelial cells. Large distinct intracytoplasmic poxvirus inclusions (Bollinger bodies, arrows) are seen in the squamous epithelial cells. PCR confirmed poxvirus (Diff-Quik, 1000×).

single eosinophilic to basophilic INIBs with or without halo are highly suggestive of herpesvirus, especially if associated with nuclear pyknosis and formation of syncytia (Figure 61.10). Karyomegaly with very large INIBs can be present in cytomegalovirus infections of passerines.[46]

Avian polyomavirus has been reported in various avian hosts with clinical manifestations and IB formation most commonly seen in parrots and finches.[23,32–34,47–49] The clinical course is typically acute to peracute with rapid spread and high mortality. Key clinical features consist of nonspecific apathy with varying degrees of septicemic–hemorrhagic, hepatorenal, neurologic, and dermal changes. Feather dysplasia and loss seems to be restricted to psittacine species and is the primary clinical sign in budgerigars, which lead to common names such as "budgie fledgling disease," "French moult," or "feather dusters." Differentiation from circovirus infection is challenging to achieve macroscopically and coinfections with both viruses do occur. Epithelial, endothelial, mesenchymal, and neuroectodermal tissues can be infected by polyomavirus and typically present with karyomegaly and light basophilic to amphophilic, medium sized to large INIBs, which fill the entire nucleus and displace the nucleolus laterally toward the nuclear membrane (Figure 61.9). Chromatin

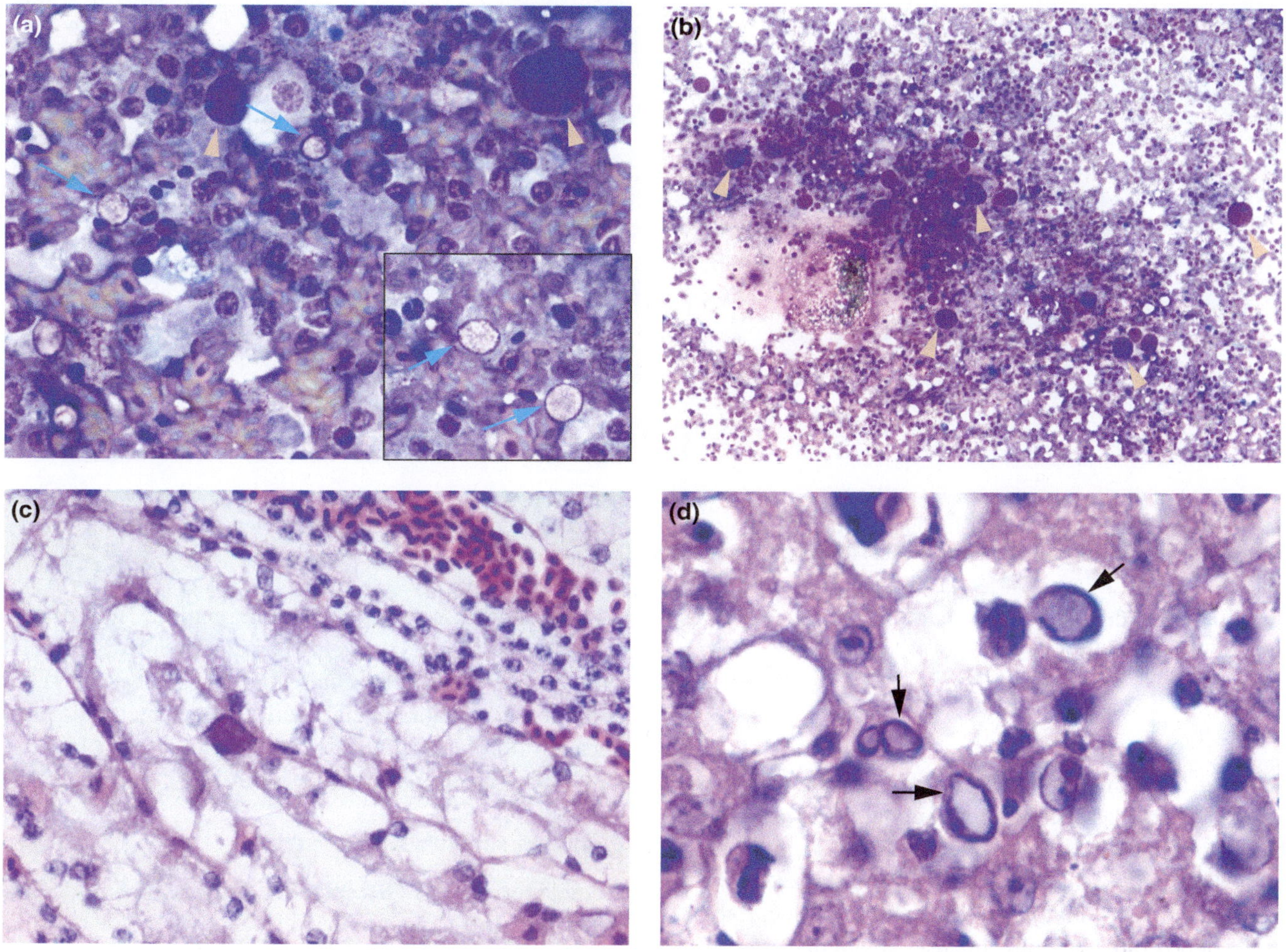

Figure 61.9 Concurrent infection with polyomavirus and adenovirus in a canary (*Serinus canaria*) that was confirmed by PCR. (a) A squash preparation of the kidney illustrates both polyomavirus (arrows) and adenovirus (arrowheads) IBs, which are more distinct with cytology when compared with histopathology (c and d). Inset: Polyomavirus inclusions (Wright–Giemsa, 400×). (b) Large intranuclear adenoviral inclusions (arrowheads) at low magnification demonstrate their size (Wright–Giemsa, 100×). (c) One adenoviral inclusion (center left) is observed (hematoxylin & eosin, 400×). (d) Intranuclear polyomavirus inclusions (arrows) are observed in the center (hematoxylin & eosin, 1000×).

margination results in a delicate, deep basophilic rim around the translucent, lightly colored INIB, giving the nucleus a characteristic hollow-glassy appearance. Like adenoviruses, polyomaviruses can produce multiple small inclusions within a single nucleus.

Other Infectious Agents

Fungal organisms can be observed as contaminants in cytology samples from skin, GIT, or upper respiratory tracts of healthy animals. However, infections with pathogenic fungi are quite common in reptiles and birds.[4,23,24,50–52] Parasites identified in reptilian and avian cytology samples include various hemoparasites in hemodiluted specimens, protozoans, and eggs or larvae of metazoans.[4,23,24,53–55] Further details on protozoan species as recognized by cytology are given in the sections under "Organ Systems."

Hemorrhage

Hemorrhage can be observed in reptiles and birds, often in association with hematoma, inflammation, or neoplasia. Cytologic features of hemorrhage are similar to mammals, including phagocytosis of erythrocytes (acute hemorrhage), intracellular or extracellular blue-black globular hemosiderin (chronic hemorrhage) (Figure 61.11), and golden rhomboid hematoidin crystals (chronic hemorrhage) (Figure 61.4b).

Cysts

Cyst formation is uncommon in reptiles and birds. In birds, epidermal cysts can form in association with feather follicles (Figure 61.12). Cytologic features are similar to epidermal inclusion cysts in mammals and include the presence of well-differentiated squamous epithelial cells, amorphous

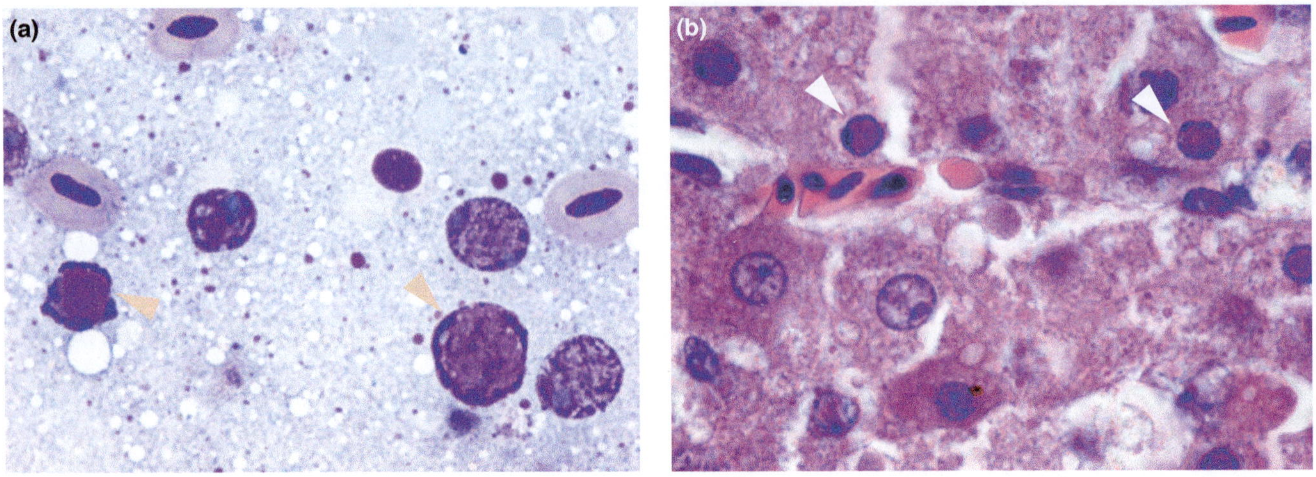

Figure 61.10 (a) Herpesvirus intranuclear inclusion bodies (arrowheads) in a liver squash preparation from a pigeon (*Columba livia*). Infection was confirmed by PCR (Diff-Quik, 1000×). (b) Corresponding histology section from the pigeon demonstrates intranuclear inclusion bodies of herpesvirus (arrowheads) (hematoxylin & eosin, 1000×).

keratinaceous debris, keratin bars, cholesterol crystals, and/or inflammation.

Necrosis

Necrosis is a common result or cause of inflammation or sequela of neoplasia similar to mammals. It is readily visible at low magnification as faded, low to acellular areas with a variably dense pink to basophilic proteinaceous background. The mixture of amorphous nucleoproteinaceous debris often contains nuclear fragments and results in a disorganized, amorphous cytologic appearance, which is infrequently associated with inflammation. Thus, careful scanning for infectious agents is recommended, although their absence does not exclude infection and requires confirmation via additional diagnostics as indicated. The presence of fibroblasts indicates chronicity of the process. Cholesterol crystals also can be observed.

Pigments, Amyloid, and Crystals

Hemosiderin and hematoidin suggest hemorrhage. Prussian blue can enhance visualization and confirm iron in cytologic preparations (Figure 61.4b). In addition to hemorrhagic lesions mentioned above, abundant iron can occur in liver imprints from bird species with

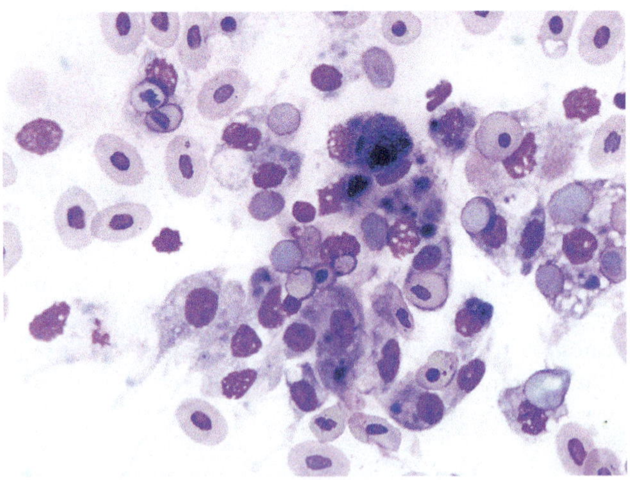

Figure 61.11 Direct smear of coelomic fluid from a yellow rat snake (*Pantherophis alleghaniensis*) is characterized by marked histiocytic coelomitis with acute and chronic hemorrhage, observed as erythrophagia and intracytoplasmic greenish-black globular pigment consistent with hemosiderin. PCV of the fluid was 6% (Wright–Giemsa, 1000×).

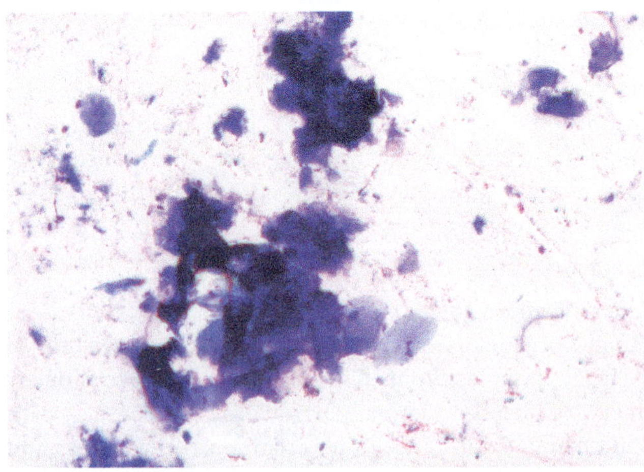

Figure 61.12 Fine-needle aspirate of a small mass closely associated with a feather on the neck of a black swan (*Cygnus atratus*). Numerous well-differentiated squamous epithelial cells are most consistent with a feather cyst (Wright–Giemsa, 1000×).

suspected iron storage disorders, most commonly birds of paradise, quetzals, mynahs, and starlings (Figure 61.13). This has been assumed to result from excess dietary iron absorption in birds, but the pathophysiologic mechanism remains undetermined.[23,56]

Melanin pigment is observed as melanomacrophages in reptiles and melanosis in birds. Melanomacrophages are specialized melanin-synthesizing macrophages that function as effective free radical scavengers and are mainly observed in the liver and, less frequently, in spleen, kidney, and inflammatory lesions.[13] Although variable numbers can be observed in cytology samples, the diagnosis of melanomacrophage hyperplasia is based on histopathology and is nonspecific (e.g. biologic variations, stress, various inflammatory conditions).[13] In certain bird species, deposition of melanin pigment occurs as physiologic melanosis in some organs such as gonads. Cytologic detail can be poor in samples from melanotic proliferations if large numbers of melanin granules are present. Melanomas/melanophoromas are rare and usually malignant in reptiles and birds (Figure 61.14).[23,57–60] Similar to mammals, melanomas grossly present as variably pigmented tissue proliferations. Cytologically, nuclear features of malignancy and variable numbers of melanin pigment granules are characteristic; melanin granule color can be very variable in birds.[61] In contrast to melanomas, melanosis is consistent with an abnormal or excessive melanin pigment production in otherwise normal tissue.[62]

Amyloid in Romanowsky-type stained samples is cytologically similar to other species. It manifests as deposition of amorphous pale eosinophilic or basophilic material, typically in fibrillary strands.[63] Congo red stain is frequently used on histologic sections to help visualize amyloid under polarized light, and it can be applied to cytology samples.[64] Amyloid deposition has been documented to cause renal disease in reptiles.[4] In avian species, amyloidosis most frequently develops as a nonspecific sequela of continuous production of acute phase proteins and formation of alpha-amyloid in the course of chronic granulomatous inflammation, such as in aspergillosis, mycobacteriosis, or pododermatitis. Spleen, liver, and kidneys are frequently affected, and there appears to be a species prevalence for waterfowl, shore birds, passerines, and *Falconiformes* (especially *Falco rusticolus*).[18,65]

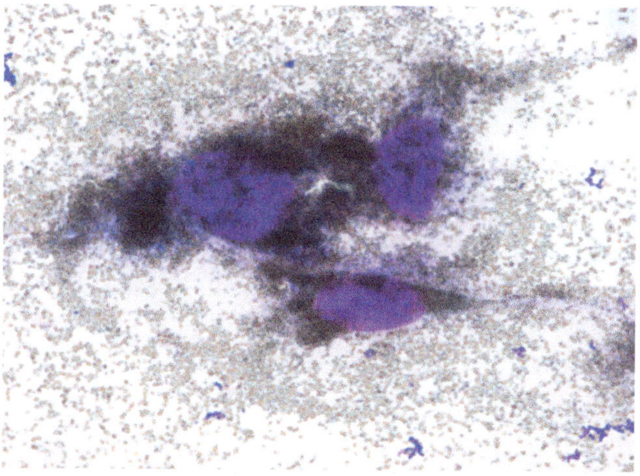

Figure 61.14 Fine-needle aspirate of a black, jelly-like lump over the spine of a Mexican beaded lizard (*Heloderma horridum*). Atypical melanocytes with abundant golden-brown melanin pigment are most consistent with cutaneous melanophoroma. There was no recurrence after surgical removal (Wright–Giemsa, 1000×).

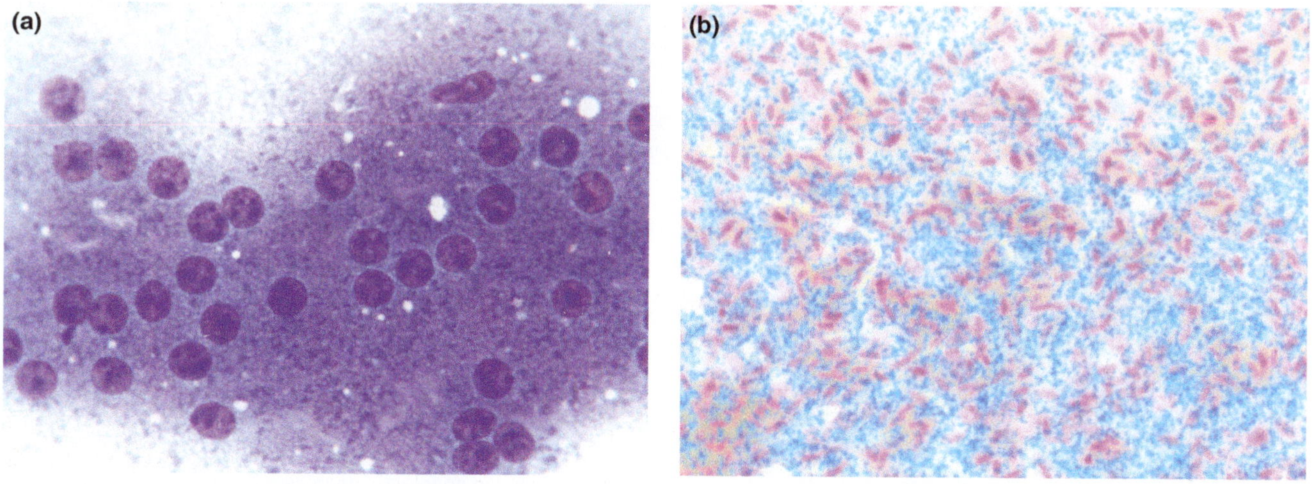

Figure 61.13 Liver tissue imprint from a golden mynah (*Mino anais*). (a) Intracytoplasmic globular pale to medium basophilic material indicative of intracytoplasmic pigment. Given the prevalence of iron storage disorder in this species, pigment accumulation in hepatocytes suggests the presence of hemosiderin (Wright–Giemsa, 1000×). (b) Iron accumulation is confirmed by Prussian blue stain (200×).

Gout is diagnosed cytologically by the identification of characteristic urate crystals. Differentiation from other crystalline material is discussed in sections "Musculoskeletal" and "Urinary Tract."

In birds, cholesterol crystals within foamy macrophages and/or in the background of the sample can reflect impaired systemic lipid metabolism. Such disorders are often associated with hyperlipidemia and manifest as xanthomatosis (see section "Skin and Subcutis" for further information).

Neoplasia

When evaluating tissue cells in a cytology sample, it is important to determine if the cells are normally expected for the tissue of origin and if cellular atypia is present, in order to further differentiate between normal tissue, hyperplasia, or benign or malignant neoplasia.[7,9,66] Although there is need to interpret the degree of atypia in a tissue-specific context, similar to other species, malignant neoplasia in birds and reptiles is suspected if three or more criteria of malignancy are observed, especially in the absence of inflammation (Figure 61.15).

Mixed Cell Populations

Mixed cell populations are defined as a mixture of leukocytes and tissue cells. These lesions often require histopathology for final diagnosis, since cytologic evaluation reveals inflammatory cells admixed with tissue cells infrequently exhibiting atypical features. Considerations for lesions containing inflammatory and atypical tissue cells include an inflamed tumor or an inflammatory lesion in which reactive changes were provoked in tissue cells in response to the inflammation (Figure 61.16). Knowledge of the location and gross appearance of the lesion, clinical history, and prevalence of certain tumors in a particular species can support prioritization of differential diagnoses.

Organ Systems

The following sections address common cytologically evaluated lesions in reptiles and birds and provide a practical general guide since an exhaustive review is beyond the scope of a single chapter. Skin, airways, and GIT are frequently sampled organ systems in reptiles and birds and thus are discussed in more detail than other organ systems.

Skin and Subcutis

Reptile: Normal Structure and Cytology

Reptile skin is composed of two layers: the epidermis with a thick *stratum corneum* that is separated from the underlying dermis by a basement membrane, with scales representing epidermal folds and scutes of chelonians being specialized epidermal hard parts.[67] The dermis contains various pigment-producing cells, which determine an animal's color and pattern based on their arrangement. Melanophores produce melanin, erythrophores and xanthophores contain pteridines and carotenoids, and the light microscopic polarizing iridophores produce purines.[67] Cytology samples of normal reptile skin are composed of polygonal keratinized squamous epithelial

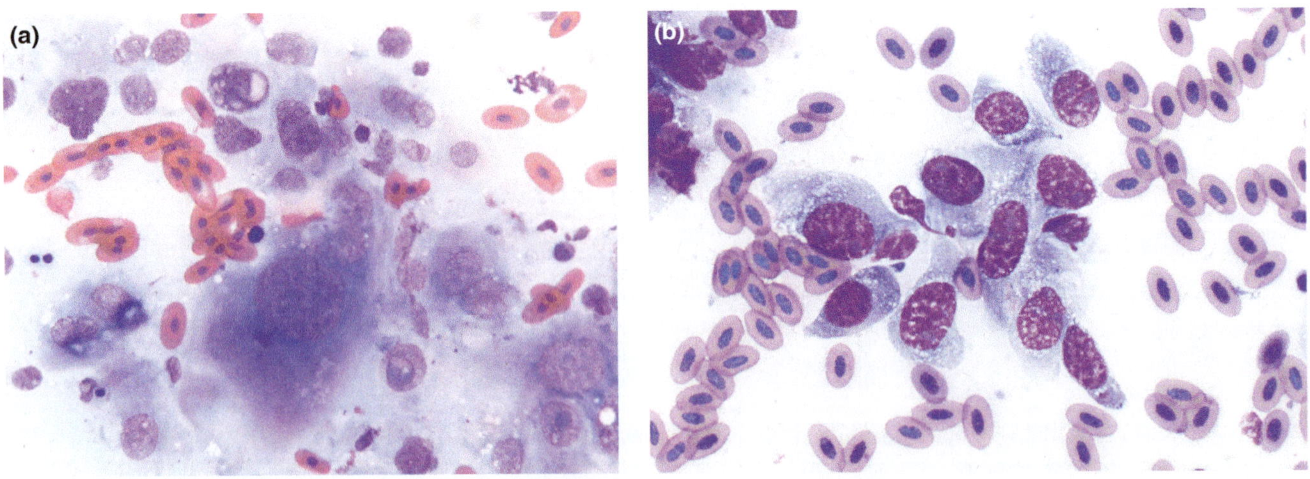

Figure 61.15 (a) Intracoelomic mass diagnosed cytologically and histologically as an anaplastic neoplasm in a pine snake (*Pituophis melanoleucus*). The tissue of origin could not be determined by histopathology (Wright–Giemsa, 1000×). (b) Aggregates of atypical mesenchymal cells from a histopathologically confirmed spindle cell sarcoma of the pectoral muscle from a Northern Saw-whet owl (*Aegolius acadicus*) (Wright–Giemsa, 1000×. *Source:* Image courtesy of Leslie Sharkey).

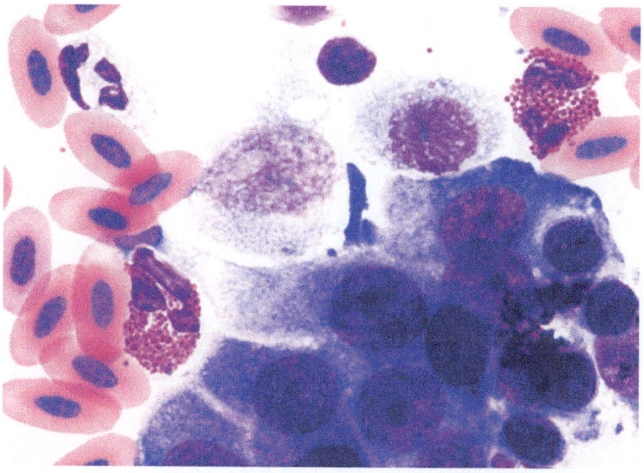

Figure 61.16 Tracheal wash from a Harris' hawk (*Parabuteo unicinctus*). One heterophil (upper left corner) is either degranulated or has poorly staining granules. Two eosinophils are next to a sheet of moderately atypical respiratory epithelial cells that are most consistent with respiratory epithelial hyperplasia in response to the inflammation (Wright–Giemsa, 1000×).

cells with or without variable numbers of melanin pigment and keratinaceous debris. In skin scrapings, immature basal epithelial cells representing deeper layers of the epidermis are infrequently seen. Variable numbers of mixed rod-shaped bacteria compose the normal flora of reptile skin. Environmental contaminants can be observed, such as plant material, fungal elements (i.e. mold), and algae and diatoms in aquatic reptiles.

Avian: Normal Structure and Cytology

The histologic composition of avian skin varies with anatomic location. Apart from non-feathered areas, the epidermis is extremely thin consisting of only a few cell layers per stratum. The *stratum germinativum* consists of a basal, intermediate, and transitional layer, which correspond to the *stratum cylindricum*, *spinosum*, and *granulosum/lucidum* in mammals, respectively. The outer cornified layer, the *stratum corneum*, undergoes permanent desquamation.[23,68,69] Thickened corneal and transitional layers are present in the scaled skin of legs and feet and skin appendages such as combs, wattles, spurs, beak, and claws. In the latter three, multiple layers of strongly keratinized squames are condensed to a keratinized plate fixed onto a keratinized or bony basis. The strong rigidity results from calcium salts incorporated into the keratinized plate.[14] The dermis or *corium* is divided into superficial and deep layers. The *stratum superficiale* is composed of a network of interconnecting ridges of collagen and elastic bundles. It contains feather follicles as well as striated skin musculature (*false skin muscles*) to support the voluntary movement of skin and flight feathers. The flat network of vessels increases in density around the feather follicles and papillae. Seasonally increased vascularization is seen in bald brood patches on chest and abdomen of certain species. A true papillary body providing rigid mechanical attachment of the epidermis is present in areas of increased mechanical strain such as the foot pads. The *stratum profundum* consists of interwoven collagen and elastic tissue bundles containing vessels and non-striated, sympathetically innervated feather muscles, whose elastic tendons extend into the feather follicles of the covering feathers. In contrast to mammals, the avian skin lacks sweat glands, and only few sebaceous glands such as the *glandulae ceruminosae* around the outer ear and the preen gland (*glandula uropygii*) exist as true anatomical structures in most but not all bird species.[68] Instead, lipogenesis takes place in the epidermis, which functions as a holocrine sebaceous gland.[69] The uropygial gland is a bilobed subcutaneous gland located over the dorsal aspect of the tail. Its size and form varies with species and season.[68,70] It acts as holocrine tubular gland, secreting oily contents into a cisterna through a collecting duct, which opens to the outer surface in a single pointed papilla. From there, fat-containing secretions with microbicidal activity are dispersed via the beak onto the plumage during preening.[68] The well-developed subcutis allows for easy movement of the feathers necessary for flight. It contains physiologic fat reservoirs (*Panniculus adiposus*), which can be especially prominent in aquatic birds and obese individuals. Adipose cushions of the digital pads are well developed regardless of the nutritional status.[68] Depending on the anatomical location of sampling, cytologic samples from normal avian skin consist of epithelial cells in various stages of maturation, including basal cells, oval to round intermediate cells, polygonal keratinized squamous epithelial cells with or without melanin pigment, feather fragments, and possibly a few bacteria representing normal microflora. Squash preparations from pulps of growing feathers contain various amounts of blood, globular keratin, and well-differentiated mesenchymal cells (i.e. fibrocytes) (Figure 61.17).

Inflammatory Conditions

Injury to reptile and avian skin typically does not provoke prominent tissue reactions. Consequently, various types of insults lead to a similar gross presentation including erythema, swelling, hemorrhage, necrosis, and/or crusts with or without scale injury or feather dystrophy/loss. Cytologically, such lesions are often composed of necrotic and/or keratinaceous debris, hemorrhage, and variable degrees of inflammation. If ulcerated, opportunistic microbes can be observed, and the initial insult may not be evident. A detailed clinical description of location, size, consistency, color, etc. of

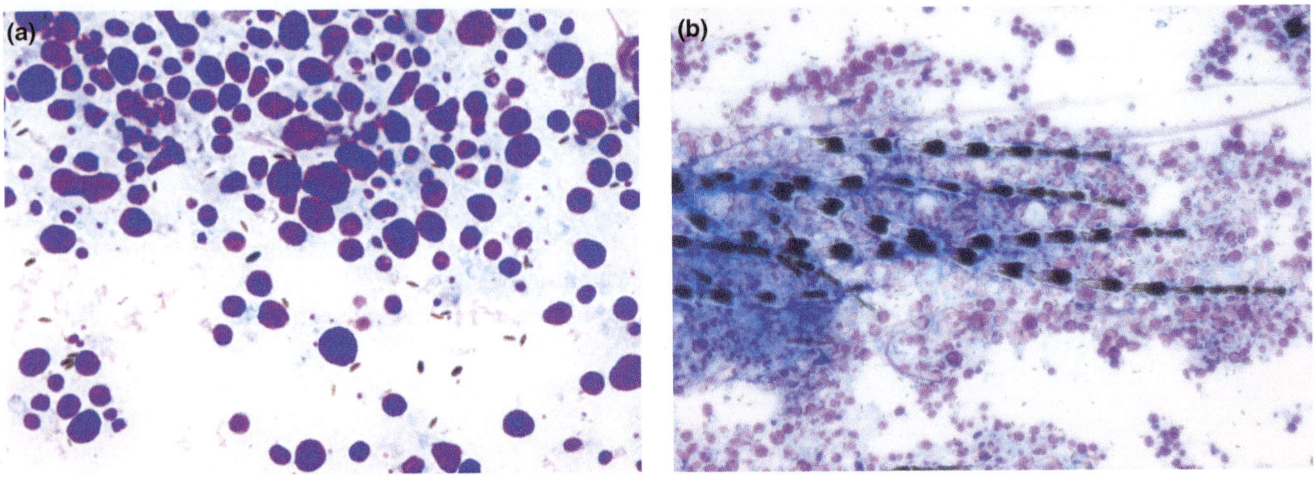

Figure 61.17 Feather squash preparation from a turquoise parrot (*Neophema pulchella*) with normal cytologic findings. (a) Variably sized free globular keratin material and melanin pigment granules (Wright–Giemsa, 1000×). (b) Large feather fragments and variably sized free globular keratin material (Wright–Giemsa, 400×)

the lesion will provide the interpretative context for the cytologic findings.

Noninfectious Inflammatory Conditions

Any condition interfering with normal feather growth such as trauma, inflammation, or genetic predisposition (e.g. Norwich crested canaries [*Serinus canaria domesticus*]) can result in the development of feather cysts that appear as oval to elongated swellings of the affected follicle.[23] Cytologically, the grossly yellowish, layered, dry material is composed of keratinaceous debris, keratinized squamous epithelium in various stages of maturation, and infrequently also feather fragments (Figure 61.12). Epidermal cysts have not been documented in reptiles.

Cutaneous xanthomatosis of birds is a granulomatous inflammatory condition occurring in response to hyperlipidemic blood in tissue. This condition is uncommon in reptiles, but an association with renal disease, diet, and reproductive disorders (e.g. yolk coelomitis) in females is suspected.[4] Cytologically, cutaneous xanthomas consist of foamy macrophages, cholesterol crystals, multinucleated giant cells, extracellular lipid material, and/or necrotic cell debris (Figure 61.18). In birds, cutaneous xanthomas are most commonly seen in areas of mechanical irritation such as blunt or pointed trauma (e.g. bruises, hemorrhages, surgical incisions) or areas of chronic inflammation. Hyperlipidemia caused by high-fat diets, endocrine and kidney imbalances, and genetic predisposition likely contribute to the development of xanthomas.[7,71]

Vitamin A deficiency, a common problem in pet psittacines fed an all seed diet, or captive reptiles on an inappropriate diet clinically presents with scaly skin, poor feather quality, and hyperkeratosis especially of the distal non-feathered areas of the hind limbs in birds. It can be accompanied by various degrees of squamous metaplasia. In birds, the secretory duct of the uropygial gland can become blocked with yellow caseous material. Cytologically, lesions associated with hypovitaminosis A are composed of a large number of uniform squamous epithelial cells and a variable amount of keratinaceous debris. Although the cytologic composition is similar to that observed in feather cysts, the clinical presentation of a feather cyst is focal and localized, whereas hypovitaminosis A often presents with more extensive and systemic lesions, for instance, with nasal discharge, palpebral swelling with discharge, dermatitis, and/or aural abscess formation.

Drug reactions are rare in reptiles and have been empirically suspected to cause hypersensitivity reactions, as reported for injectable cephalosporins, enrofloxacin, or orally administered potentiated sulfa drugs.[4] In birds, dermal hypersensitivity reactions occur but are not fully understood and have been suspected in cases with histologically diagnosed hyperkeratosis, epithelial hyperplasia, and perivascular lymphoplasmacytic cuffing.[23] Heterophilic inflammation due to automutilation and secondary microbial infection can be superimposed. Cytologically, such lesions present with nonspecific findings such as hyperplastic squamous epithelial cells, variable amounts of keratinaceous debris, hemorrhage, necrotic debris, and variable numbers of granulocytes, which, as discussed above, may not be further differentiable.

Feather loss without concurrent evidence of trauma accompanied by increased amounts of mucin has been reported in chicken as primary or secondary cutaneous mucinosis of unknown etiology.[72] Myxedema associated with hypothyroidism has been described in thyroidectomized chickens.[73] Excessive subcutaneous fat deposits and changes in feather quality often accompany mucin

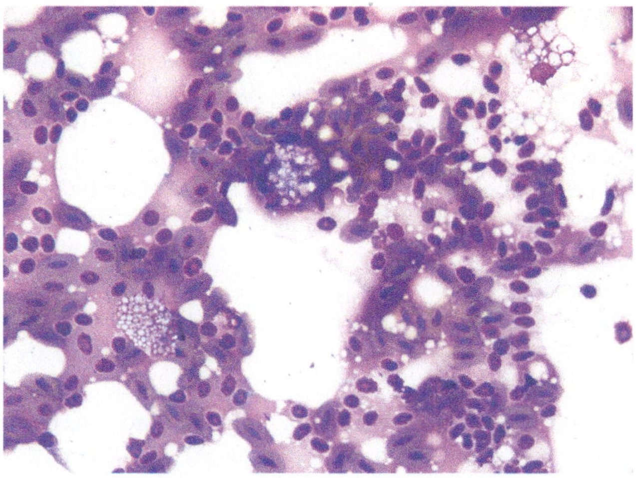

Figure 61.18 Fine-needle aspirate of a soft tissue mass on the body wall of a grey parrot (*Psittacus erithacus*) with hypertriglyceridemia (1600 mg/dL). Large amounts of extracellular lipid material and three highly vacuolated macrophages are most consistent with xanthomatosis. There are free nuclei of lysed erythrocytes and thrombocytes in the background (Wright–Giemsa, 500×).

accumulation. The contour feathers especially of the dorsal, femoral, and crural areas are fringed and elongated with loss of barbules giving them a silky appearance.[74]

Infectious Conditions

A few bacteria are commonly present in skin cytology samples, typically normal microflora composed of variable numbers of pleomorphic bacteria. Cytodiagnosis of bacterial infection, whether primary or secondary, is based on the identification of intracellular bacteria, usually in heterophils, and/or the presence of a monomorphic bacterial population. Similar to mammalian neutrophilic inflammation, heterophils exhibiting hydropic degeneration with swollen nuclei suggest a possible bacterial etiology, even in the absence of phagocytosis of organisms. Cytologic samples of chronic inflammation in reptiles and birds are characterized by necrotic cell debris and histiocytic inflammation with giant cell formation. Microorganisms are often scarce and difficult to find in these advanced-stage inflammatory lesions, and culture is strongly recommended. Ulcerative pododermatitis (bumble foot) is a common example of this type of lesion. *Staphylococcus aureus* and *Escherichia coli* are among the most frequently isolated bacteria. Mycobacterial infections of the skin can be a focal lesion or part of a systemic infection. These lesions appear grossly nodular to diffuse. Cytology samples contain predominantly macrophages with variable numbers of clear nonstaining rod-shaped structures in the cytoplasm and background, which may be difficult to recognize against a pale background. *Mycobacterium* sp. is frequently present in the environment, especially of reptiles. Pathogenic species in reptiles include *Mycobacterium marinum*, *Mycobacterium chelonae*, and *Mycobacterium thamnopheos*. In birds, *Mycobacterium avium* is the most common isolate followed by *Mycobacterium genavense* and, very rarely, *Mycobacterium tuberculosis* (Figure 61.19).[4,23]

A number of viruses can affect the skin of birds, specifically circovirus, poxvirus (Figure 61.20), herpesvirus, and polyomavirus, which can form cytologically detectable IBs (see section "Infectious Agents" and Table 61.2).

Fungal organisms without clinical relevance are frequently observed in skin or shell samples from reptiles and in lubricated or soiled feathers of waterfowl.[14] These specimens contain septate fungal hyphae admixed with numerous mixed bacilli and variable numbers of keratinized squamous epithelial cells. If associated with a gross lesion and cytologic observation of inflammation, cultures and/or molecular diagnostics should be pursued to differentiate pathogenic fungi from environmental contaminants. Dermatomycoses detected in reptile cytology samples include *Acremonium* sp., *Trichosporon* sp., *Fusarium* sp. with its characteristic crescent-shaped microconidia and macroconidia (Figure 61.21), snake fungal disease associated with *Ophidiomyces* (formerly *Chrysosporium*) *ophiodiicola* that is mainly observed in free-ranging snakes in North America, and yellow fungus disease caused by the *Chrysosporium*-related fungus *Nannizziopsis guarroi* which requires specific culture conditions for growth.[4,75] *Cryptococcus neoformans* has been isolated from a skin lesion in a lizard.[50] Fungal infections observed in birds frequently involve species of the genera *Trichophyton* sp., *Microsporum* sp., *Aspergillus* sp., *Mucor* sp., *Rhizopus* sp., *Penicillium* sp., *Candida* sp., *Malassezia/Pityrosporum* sp., and *C. neoformans*. Detection of fungal structures is simplified by dissolution of hyperkeratotic

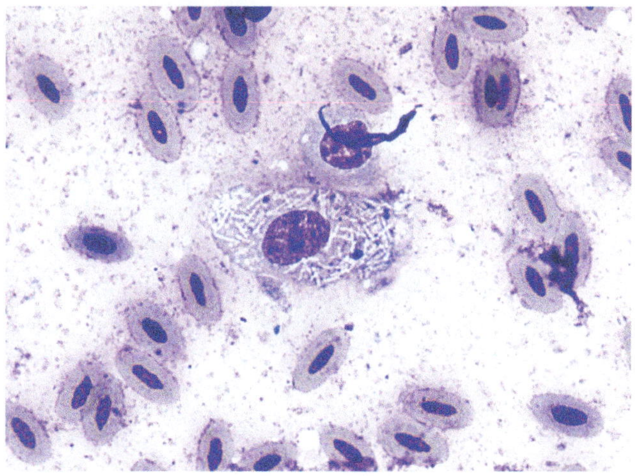

Figure 61.19 Fine-needle aspirate of a subcutaneous mass in a gyrfalcon (*Falco rusticolus*). Negative-staining, phagocytized bacilli are most consistent with *Mycobacterium* sp. in a macrophage (Diff-Quik, 1000×).

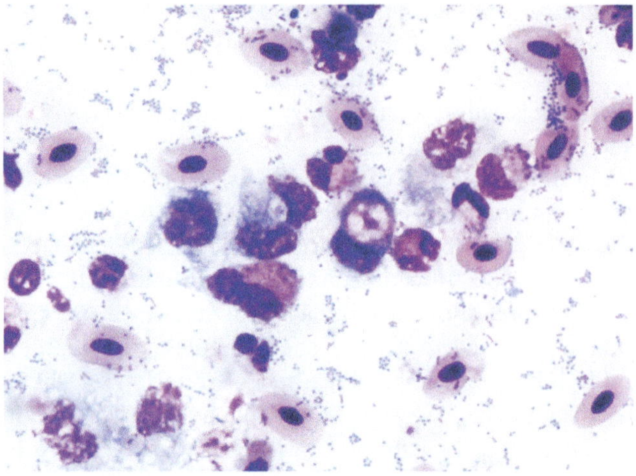

Figure 61.20 Intracytoplasmic poxvirus inclusion in an epithelial cell (center), mixed inflammation (heterophils, histiocytes), and numerous cocci in a skin scraping from a MacQueen's bustard (*Chlamydotis macqueenii*) (Diff-Quik, 500×).

material in potassium hydroxide (KOH) prior to examination.[14] Fungal folliculitis has been reported in avian species but occurs less frequently than in mammals. Fungal infections of the hard cornified plates of beak and claws are rare and most commonly associated with predisposing immunosuppression.[23]

The burrowing activity of female skin mites such as *Knemidocoptes* sp. causes thickening, roughening, and proliferation of the keratinized epidermis. In exotic pet bird species, budgerigars and canaries are most commonly affected. Hyperkeratotic changes are most prominent in the beak and the feet and can result in malformation in severe cases. Diagnosis is made by detection of mites in crusts and deep skin scrapings. Boiling or overnight storage of the sample material in 10% KOH prior to examination will dissolve keratin and cellular debris and simplify recognition of the parasite in a wet mount. Other mite species may be detected in squashes from feather shafts or, rarely, in samples from the subcutis.[55,76–78]

Neoplasia

Neoplasia of the skin has been reported in various reptile species, most frequently in snakes, followed by lizards, chelonians, and crocodilians. Frequent tumors include soft tissue sarcoma including fibrosarcoma, lymphoma, melanomas (chromatophoromas), and lipomas.[57] Cytologic diagnosis of a cutaneous melanophoroma in a green iguana (*Iguana iguana*) revealed predominantly spindloid to stellate melanocytes with fewer round forms and numerous intracellular and extracellular melanin granules.[60] Nuclei were round to oval with small single to multiple nucleoli; anisocytosis and anisokaryosis were mild. Another chromatophoroma, specifically an iridophoroma, was diagnosed cytologically based on the presence of stellate-shaped cells containing pale grey pigment that was birefringent using polarized light.[79] The most commonly encountered skin neoplasms in birds include lipomas, xanthoma, spindle cell tumors (Figure 61.15b), lymphoid neoplasia, and squamous cell carcinoma.[29] Dermal lymphoma in birds occurs both as nodular or diffuse proliferations and can be associated with feather loss. In macaws, facial cutaneous pseudolymphoma, a benign lymphocytic proliferation containing a heterogeneous lymphoid population with lymphoblasts, can mimic lymphoma and requires further

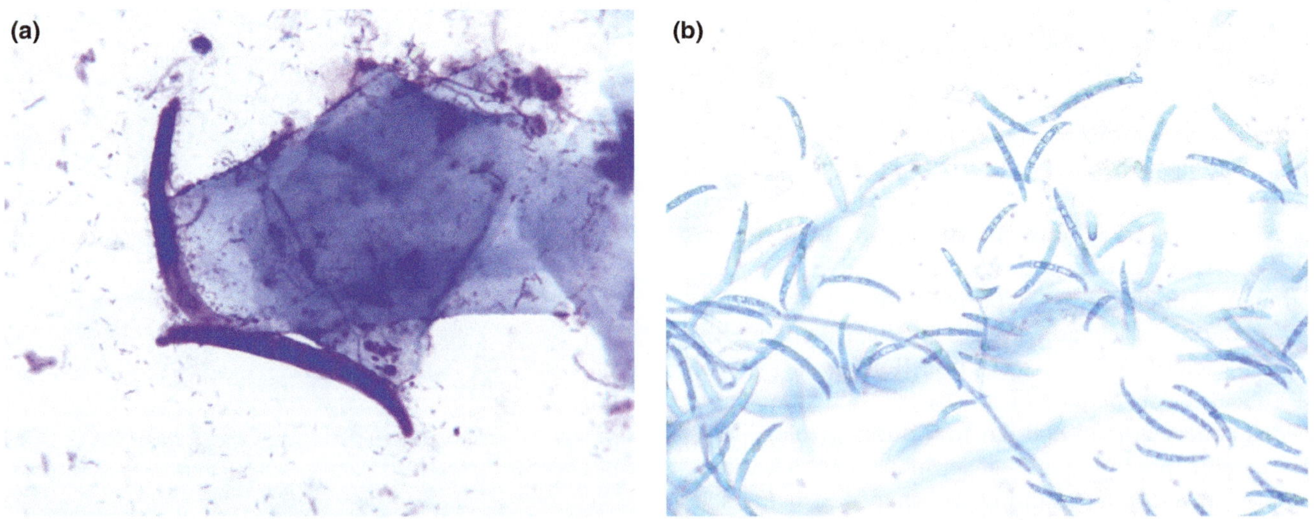

Figure 61.21 Shell scraping from a 2 × 2"shell lesion in a green turtle (*Chelonia mydas*). (a) Characteristic crescent-shaped macroconidia of *Fusarium* sp. are next to anucleated squamous epithelial cells. *Fusarium* sp. was confirmed by culture and PCR (Wright–Giemsa, 500×). (b) *Fusarium* morphology in a culture sample (Lactophenol blue, 100×).

diagnostic means for clear differentiation of these two entities.[80] In contrast to mammalian and human oncology, further differentiation of avian lymphomas beyond the B- and T-cell level is hampered by the lack of diagnostic tools for cellular subtypes applicable for exotic bird species.[81] Mast cell tumors are rare in birds and reptiles and have been described as discrete nodules on the head of a white leghorn chicken (*Gallus callus domesticus*) and a great horned owl (*Bubo virginianus*), a neck mass in a black-masked lovebird (*Agapornis personatus*), a firm mass in skin and skeletal muscle of an eastern king snake (*Lampropeltis getulus getulus*), and pedunculated skin mass in a Galapagos tortoise (*Chelone nigra vicina*); systemic spread was documented in the lovebird.[82–84] Tissue imprints are often diagnostic, provided the granules of the mast cells take up the dye.[23,85] Cutaneous melanomas/melanophoromas have been reported both in reptiles and birds and are malignant in the majority of cases (Figure 61.14).[23,57,58] In psittacines, the facial skin appears to be predisposed.[23]

Ear and Eye

Otitis externa is frequently encountered in some freshwater turtle species and is of fungal (Figure 61.22) and/or bacterial etiology. Exudative otitis externa in birds is often bacterial with possible fungal coinfection. Otitis media is less common in birds and other reptile species and is caused by reactions to infectious agents (bacterial, fungal, parasitic) (Figure 61.23) or foreign material.

Eye lesions in reptiles and birds are often caused by infection (Figure 61.4c) or trauma. *Mycoplasma* sp. is a common infectious cause of upper respiratory tract disease in tortoises, often presenting as conjunctivitis and/or nasal discharge. Since the organism is difficult to reliably identify by cytology, PCR is necessary for diagnosis in suspected cases. Other causes of conjunctivitis in reptiles include bacteria such as *Proteus vulgaris* and *Citrobacter intermedium*, viruses (e.g. ICIBs with iridovirus infections), and exposure to organochlorine pesticides that are used in agriculture and for mosquito control.[4] Infectious agents of various types elicit similar inflammatory responses in the conjunctiva of birds, and cytologic evaluation of swabs helps to narrow potential differential diagnoses. Certain infectious agents, such as *Mycoplasma* sp., *Chlamydia* sp., *Cryptosporidium* sp., poxvirus, cytomegalovirus, and *Encephalitozoon hellem*, can be identified based on characteristic cytologic features, although sensitivity is low.[29,86]

Hypovitaminosis A is cytologically characterized by the presence of numerous squamous epithelial cells at various degrees of keratinization admixed with normal conjunctival cellular components, including conjunctival epithelial cells and goblet cells. This condition can lead to keratoconjunctivitis sicca in reptiles.[4]

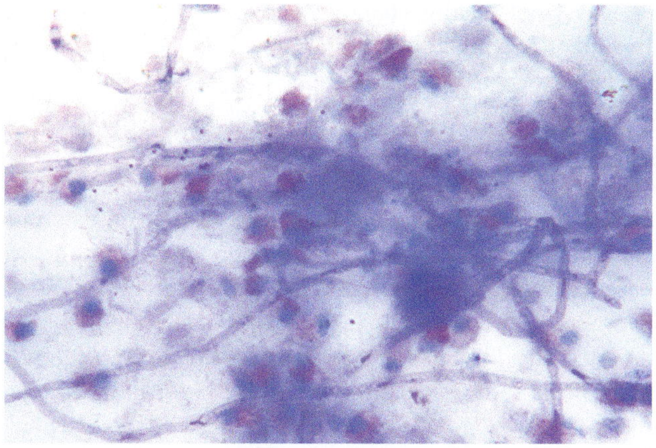

Figure 61.22 Direct smear of surgically removed material from the ear of a red-footed tortoise (*Chelonoidis carbonaria*). Sample consists predominantly of heterophilic inflammation with septate, branching fungal hyphae, and few melanin pigment granules. Cultures identified *Fusarium* sp. (conidia were absent on cytology) and α-hemolytic *Streptococcus* sp., consistent with fungal and bacterial otitis externa (Wright–Giemsa, 500×).

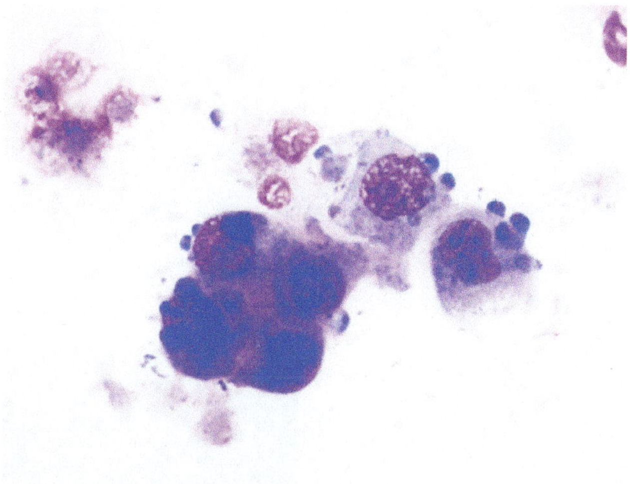

Figure 61.23 *Cryptosporidium baylei* developmental stages attached to epithelial cells from a swab of the pharyngeal opening of the *Tubae auditivae* in a gyrfalcon (*Falco rusticolus*). Heterophilic inflammation and few extracellular bacteria are noted (Diff-Quik, 500×).

Few reports on neoplastic lesions of ears and eyes in birds and reptiles exist. Dacryops (orbital lacrimal cyst) was diagnosed in a red-eared slider (*Chrysemys scripta elegans*) after sonographic examination. Cytologic evaluation of the cyst fluid revealed erythrocytes, cyst-lining macrophages, and degenerated cells on an eosinophilic background; the histopathologic diagnosis was interstitial dacryoadenitis.[87] Retrobulbar adenocarcinoma in a 27-year-old Amazon parrot (*Amazona autumnalis*) with exophthalmos and head tilt was cytologically characterized by occasional acinar clusters of cuboidal to columnar epithelial cells with high nuclear to cytoplasmic ratio (N:C), scant basophilic cytoplasm, central round nuclei, and mild to moderate anisocytosis and anisokaryosis.[88] Aural adenocarcinoma in a grey parrot (*Psittacus erithacus*) with an osteolytic left hemimandibular mass and soft tissue mass in the left external auditory meatus was cytologically diagnosed based on the presence of cohesive sheets of polygonal cells with a moderate amount of basophilic cytoplasm that was sometimes vacuolated.[89] In addition, there were acinar structures, moderate anisocytosis and anisokaryosis, high N:C ratio, and scattered well-differentiated osteoblasts.[89] Diagnosis of periorbital lymphoma in a blue and gold Macaw (*Ara ararauna*) with a 2 cm mass at the dorsomedial aspect of the right eye that displaced the globe was made cytologically with the detection of a homogeneous population of large lymphocytes accompanied by heterophils.[90]

Musculoskeletal

Synovial fluid in reptiles and birds can only be aspirated if there is a significant increase in the amount of fluid present in a diseased joint. Although reference intervals for nucleated cell counts and total protein in synovial fluid of these species are unavailable, general principles of cytologic evaluation apply, i.e. expected presence of a low number of mononuclear cells (synoviocytes and/or macrophages), mucinous background, and windrowing of cells in normal synovial fluid (Chapters 54 and 55). The

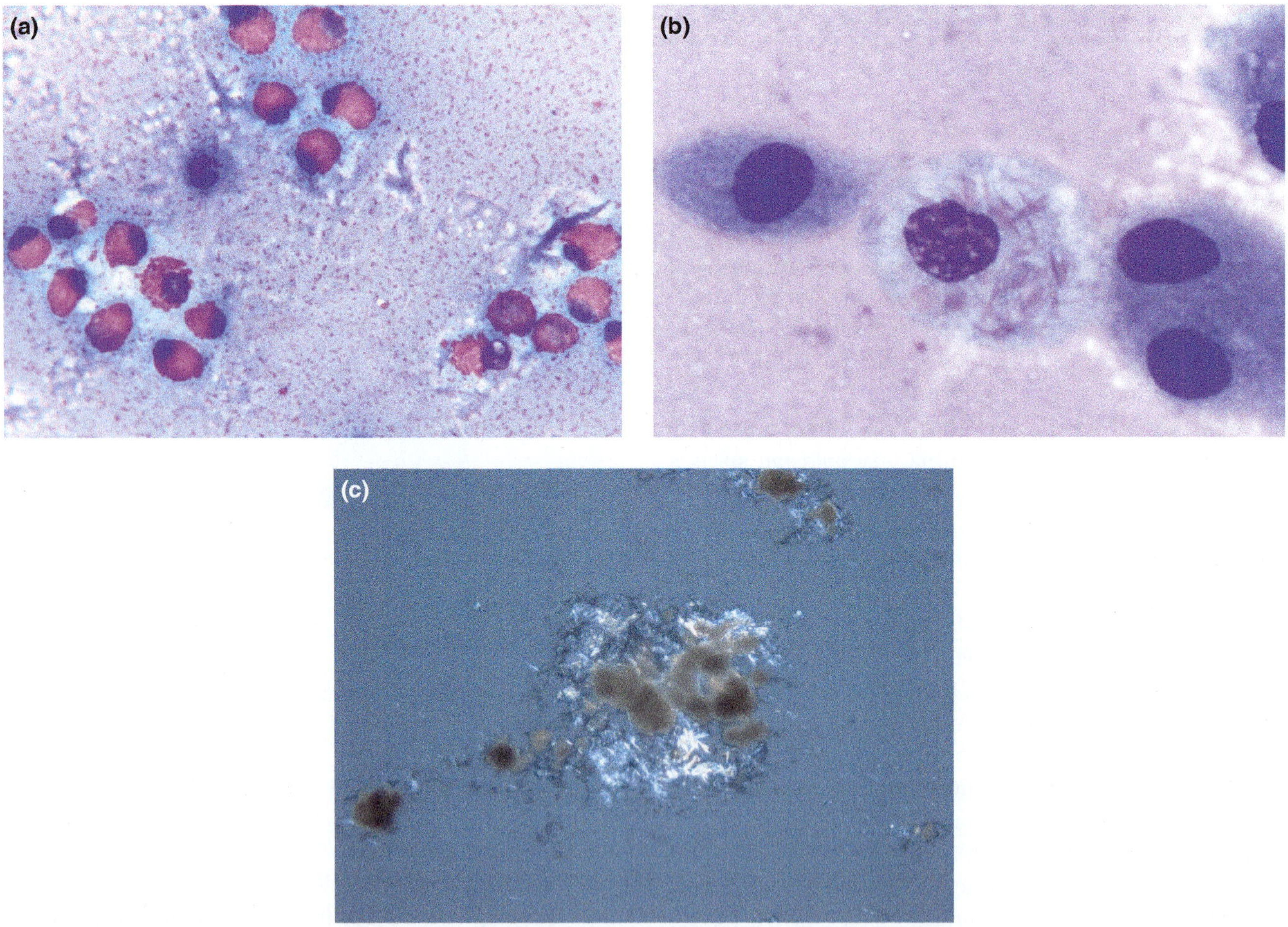

Figure 61.24 (a) Synovial fluid aspirate with mucinous background demonstrating heterophilic synovitis in a Kemp's ridley sea turtle (*Lepidochelys kempii*). No microorganisms were observed cytologically. Synovial fluid and blood culture both were positive for *Serratia marcescens* (Wright–Giemsa, 500×). (b) Synovial fluid with mononuclear phagocytes and intracytoplasmic needle-shaped crystals in an Aracari bird (*Pteroglossus* sp.). The crystals did not polarize and thus were presumed to be variants of the original monosodium urate crystal form. The cytodiagnosis was gout and histiocytic synovitis (Wright–Giemsa, 1000×). (c) Polarizing monosodium urate crystals in a squash preparation of whitish, creamy contents sampled from bilateral swellings of carpus and digits in a giant leaf-tailed gecko (*Uroplatus fimbriatus*). Considerations for the non-polarizing material include proteinaceous and/or degenerated cellular material (unstained fluid wet mount, 100×).

most commonly diagnosed conditions resulting in synovial effusions from reptiles and birds are bacterial synovitis (Figure 61.24a) or gout (Figure 61.24b and c), with pseudogout being less frequent. Gout is cytologically characterized by the presence of mixed or mainly histiocytic inflammation with free or phagocytized, needle-shaped golden-brown or colorless, refractile monosodium urate crystals that are typically birefringent under polarized light (Figure 61.24c). These brittle crystals have a high tendency for aggregation and epitaxial growth, with variable morphology depending on chronicity, surrounding chemical and physical conditions (i.e., supersaturation of uric acid in synovial fluid, temperature), mechanical wear (movements of the joint), and/or fixation of tissue samples.[91] A murexide test can further confirm the presence of urates and differentiate from calcium salts.[7] Briefly, nitric acid is added to fresh synovial fluid on an unstained slide and slowly dried by flame. After addition of ammonia, a red or purple color will occur if urates are present.[92] Pseudogout in reptiles is characterized by calcium deposits (e.g. calcium hydroxyapatite) observed as irregular pleomorphic refractile crystalloid material surrounded by reactive histiocytes. These deposits must be differentiated from calcium carbonate, which can originate from the shell in reptiles (i.e. as part of a cytology sample) or as a sample contaminant. Both gout and pseudogout can result from diet imbalance, some drugs, renal disease, and/or aging.[4,93] A case of renal failure associated gout in an African spur-thighed tortoise (*Geochelone sulcata*) illustrates this entity.[94]

Skeletal muscle lesions are rarely sampled cytologically (Chapter 22). Various microbial and parasitic agents can be detected cytologically and are frequently associated with systemic disease.[23] In birds, apart from sarcocystosis, both cardiac and skeletal muscular involvement is described for *Hemoproteus* sp. and *Leucocytozoon* sp., two commonly occurring avian hemoparasites.[95,96] The exoerythrocytic stages can also occur in organs such as lung, liver, and spleen, sometimes causing severe disease, especially in nonadapted avian hosts.[97,98]

Necrosis, macrophagic inflammation, fibroplasia, and dystrophic calcium deposition are features of exertional rhabdomyolysis and/or capture myopathy in birds (Figure 61.25). Von Kossa stain stains any calcium-containing mineral brown-black in cytologic and histologic samples, suggesting tissue injury from mineralization (Figure 61.25d).

Tumors of musculoskeletal origin reported in reptiles and birds include osteosarcoma, chondrosarcoma, rhabdomyosarcoma, leiomyoma, and leiomyosarcoma.[57,58] Chapters 22 and 23 contain more detailed discussion of such lesions, which are characterized cytologically as for other species. A rhabdomyosarcoma in a free-ranging yellow-headed caracara (*Milvago chimachima*) presented as a 3 cm mass in the muscle around the proximal left humerus and was cytologically composed of pleomorphic elongated spindloid cells with oval nuclei and one or more prominent nucleoli; cross striations were identified in some cells.[99] A benign peripheral nerve sheath tumor associated with the pectoral muscle in a wild toco toucan (*Ramphastos toco*) was cytologically characterized by low numbers of minimally atypical spindloid cells.[100] Cytology of a 3 cm diameter adherent mass 25 cm caudal to the ramus of the mandible in a black rat snake (*Pantherophis obsoletus*) consisted of numerous large clusters of round to polygonal cells with single large round nuclei, single prominent nucleolus, and abundant eosinophilic cytoplasm embedded in homogeneous magenta material, resulting in a diagnosis of chondrosarcoma that was confirmed histologically.[101] Osteosarcoma of the left leg of a kestrel (*Falco tinnunculus*) was presumptively diagnosed based on the presence of lytic bone lesions and cytologic observation of small numbers of atypical spindle cells mixed with multinucleated giant cells; the diagnosis was confirmed histologically.[102]

Respiratory

Disorders of the respiratory tract are quite common in reptiles and birds, and cytology offers a rapid adjunct diagnostic tool that is particularly valuable for this organ system. Although anatomically divergent, the cytologic composition of respiratory tissues of reptiles and birds is similar and even shares features with mammalian samples. The avian air sacs are translucent extensions of the respiratory tract that fill every available space in the avian coelom, surrounding all internal organs with invaginations between muscles and extending into bones. Air sacs are lined by a single layer of flat squamous epithelium, that transitions to ciliated epithelium near the ostia. Normal air sac cytology samples are frequently poorly cellular and composed of squamous or ciliated cuboidal or columnar epithelial cells. Cytospin preparations can be helpful to concentrate the cellular material. A study of methods for processing air sac lavage fluid in turkeys reported that anticoagulant does not influence cell quality.[103] This study proposed optimal concentration speeds and concluded that preparation within an hour of collection and storage at low temperatures resulted in best sample quality.[103] A procedure for bronchoscopy and tracheal wash evaluation in subadult alligators has been published.[104]

Normal findings from the nares to the level of the glottis include keratinized squamous cells, ciliated columnar respiratory epithelial cells, goblet cells, mucus, and variable

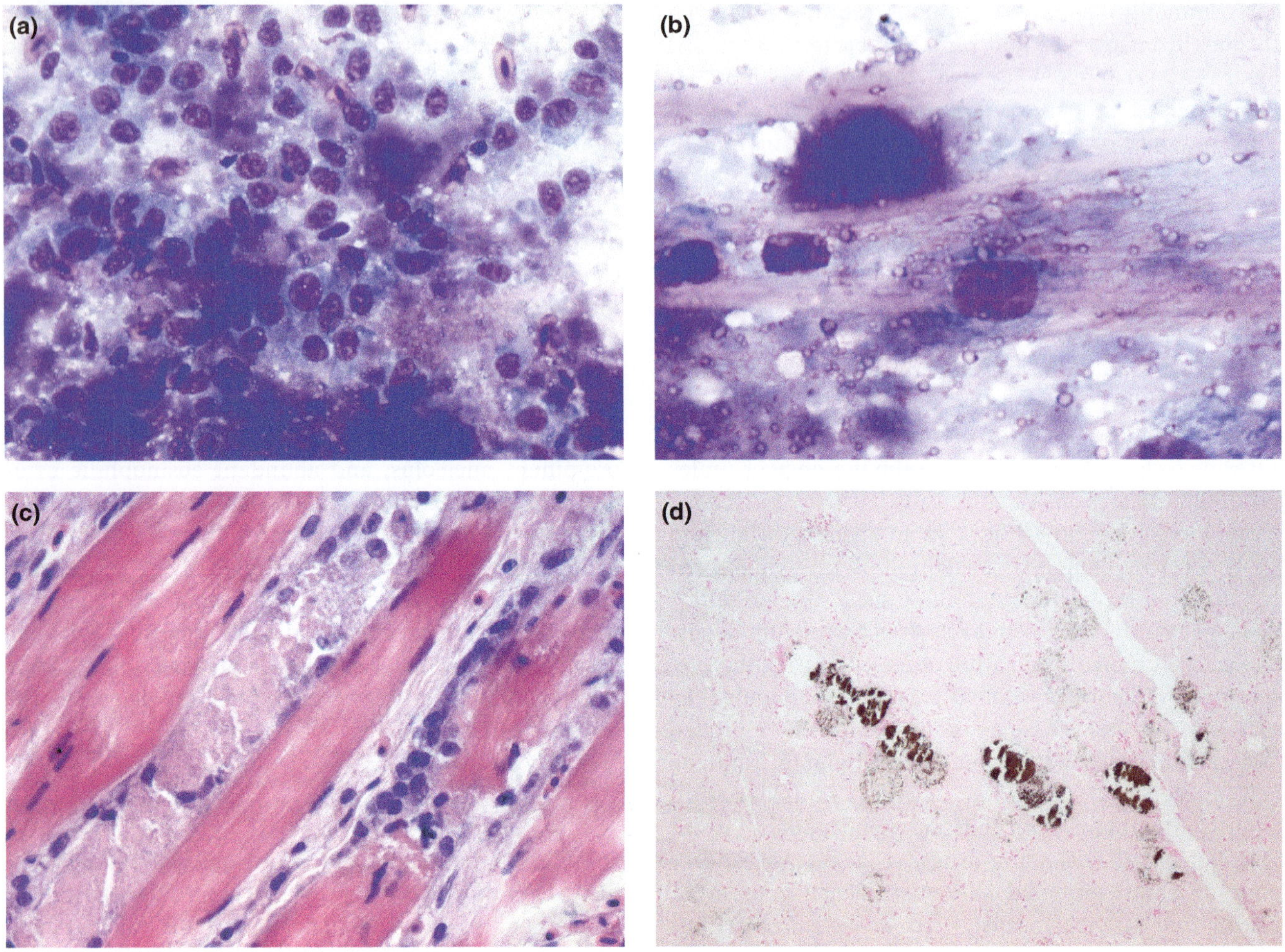

Figure 61.25 Squash preparation of skeletal muscle from a gyrfalcon (*Falco rusticolus*) with exertional myopathy and rhabdomyolysis. (a) Amorphous basophilic to purple necrotic debris, atypical mesenchymal cells most consistent with reactive fibroplasia, and frequent small refractile colorless crystalloid granules are seen.(Diff-Quik, 400×). (b) Fibroblast, lytic myofibers, necrotic cell debris, amorphous crystals (Diff-Quik, 1000×). (c) Corresponding histologic section illustrating fragmentation, swelling, and necrosis of myofibers (rhabdomyolysis) with loss of cross striation. Macrophage infiltration and reactive fibroplasia is seen (hematoxylin & eosin, 400×). (d) Dystrophic calcification of necrotic muscle tissue (Von Kossa stain, 100×).

numbers of a mixed population of bacteria representing normal microflora. Occasionally, some plant material and rare resident inflammatory cells are also present. In samples from areas with respiratory epithelium, cilia are often traumatically detached from apices of epithelial cells and are visible free in the background. These should not be mistaken for thin bacteria. Entire apical segments of ciliated epithelial cells can be traumatically dislodged during sampling and may appear as ciliated bodies lacking nuclei, i.e. "ciliary tufts," also known as ciliocytophthoria, as described in normal and pathologic cytology samples from tissues lined by ciliated epithelium.[105] Normal samples from the trachea are often poorly cellular and mainly composed of columnar respiratory epithelial cells (Figure 61.26), mucus, free cilia, goblet cells, and few inflammatory cells.[104] In swab preparations, rupture of epithelial cells is common, but concentrated tracheal wash samples can provide sufficient intact cells for evaluation. If samples from the trachea or bronchi sampled during bronchoscopy contain squamous epithelial cells with adhered mixed bacteria, oropharyngeal contamination or squamous metaplasia with secondary infection (see below) needs to be considered, depending on the clinical presentation.

Inflammation

Noninfectious Conditions

Gross differential diagnoses for caseous plaques in birds and reptiles in the oropharynx include hypovitaminosis A, bacterial and fungal infections, trichomoniasis (birds), and other parasitic or viral infections.[7] Vitamin A deficiency can be associated with caseous plaques composed of debris from squamous metaplasia that can get secondarily infected.

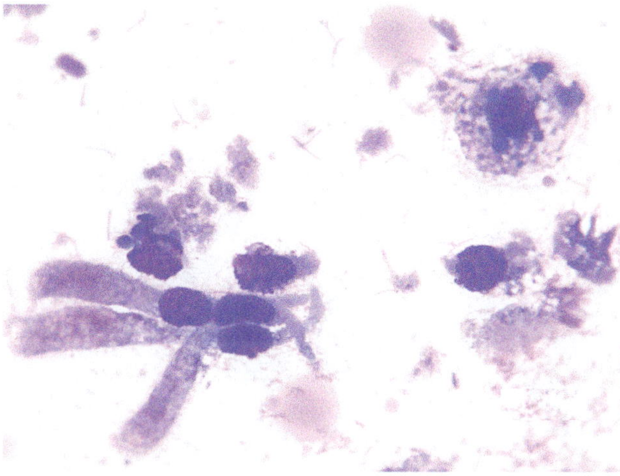

Figure 61.26 Direct smear of mucus from the endotracheal tube in a Kemp's Ridley sea turtle (*Lepidochelys kempii*) illustrate normal cytologic findings: well-differentiated ciliated respiratory epithelial cells, a vacuolated histiocyte with basophilic phagocytized material suggestive of mucus (upper right), and free cilia from respiratory epithelial cells in the background. Free cilia should not be misinterpreted as bacteria (Wright–Giemsa, 1000×).

Infectious Conditions

The nasal cavity and sinuses of birds are frequently affected by bacterial and fungal infections. Various bacteria associated with respiratory infections in reptiles and/or birds include *Salmonella* sp., *E. coli, Klebsiella* sp., *Pasteurella* sp., *Riemerella* sp., *Ornithobacterium* sp., *Bordetella* sp., *Avibacterium* sp., *Mycoplasma* sp., *Staphylococcus* sp., *Enterococcus* sp., *Streptococcus* sp., *Mycobacterium* sp., *Chlamydia* sp., *Campylobacter* sp., and *Pseudomonas* sp. The diagnosis of bacterial infection can be tentatively made by the presence of monomorphic bacterial population and/or bacterial phagocytosis by heterophils and macrophages. Culture and/or PCR are necessary for further differentiation.

Bacteria Chlamydiosis is a common problem in reptiles and birds with potential zoonotic significance. Due to their very small size, chlamydial elements can be easily missed during cytologic evaluation and need to be differentiated from nonspecific granular cellular debris, especially when present free in the background. Chlamydiae form intracellular aggregates of elementary, intermediate, and/or reticular bodies, which are referred to as microcolonies or inclusions (Figure 61.27a). They vary from small to large vacuole-like structures filled with chlamydial organisms. These structures appear as small (0.2–2 μm), round, basophilic granules resembling "poppy seeds," typically much smaller than most cocci. Few elongated structures resembling coccobacilli or very small rods may also be found among typical round bodies. Chlamydial organisms stain in various shades of blue with Romanowsky-type stains and microcolonies are recognized as aggregates of basophilic dots. Special stains for chlamydial inclusions such as Macchiavello, Gimenez, or Stamp will stain organisms red on a blue background. The inclusions are difficult to visualize on Gram stain since they are Gram-negative. Microcolonies are observed most often within macrophages and epithelial cells but also can be found in heterophils. Macrophagic inflammation with foamy/epithelioid macrophages, other leukocytes, and respiratory epithelial cell hyperplasia are often present concurrently. Chlamydiosis in birds can be associated with other bacterial infections of the respiratory tract such as *Salmonella* sp. or *Pseudomonas* sp.; therefore, it is advisable to closely review inflammatory lesions from the avian respiratory tract for bacterial and chlamydial organisms, respectively.

Mycoplasmosis is another bacterial disease that can be difficult to diagnose cytologically, primarily due to small size (typically <1 μm) of the organism. Mycoplasmas are coccobacilli that are typically recognized extracellularly by cytology and are often vertically attached to the surface of epithelial cells where they appear as tiny dark basophilic attachments on the apical surface. Mycoplasmas often cause marked heterophilic to mixed inflammation, typically with more lymphocytes and plasma cells rather than macrophages (Figure 61.27b and c). Acute infections are more likely to be apparent cytologically, whereas few to no organisms are present in chronic infections. Secondary bacterial infections with heterophilic and/or histiocytic components can become predominant in chronic lesions, presenting an additional diagnostic challenge. Whenever suspected clinically, PCR is considered the gold standard for diagnosis.

Similar to mammals, mycobacterial infections of the respiratory tract in reptiles and birds often produce granulomatous inflammation with multinucleated giant cells, foamy/epithelioid macrophages, and other inflammatory cell components. The key diagnostic feature in mycobacterial infections is the presence of negative-staining bacterial rods (Figure 61.28) that stain positive (magenta) with acid-fast stain. These must be distinguished from an artifact in which heterophils have nonstaining granules that can be confused with macrophages containing negative-staining bacilli. The presence of multinucleated giant cells alone is not diagnostic for mycobacterial infections, but should prompt consideration of acid-fast staining. Most pathogenic mycobacteria in birds and reptiles are not considered highly communicable to immunocompetent people. Regardless, *M. tuberculosis* has been reported in reptiles and birds, and speciation of any mycobacteriosis is recommended to assess zoonotic potential.

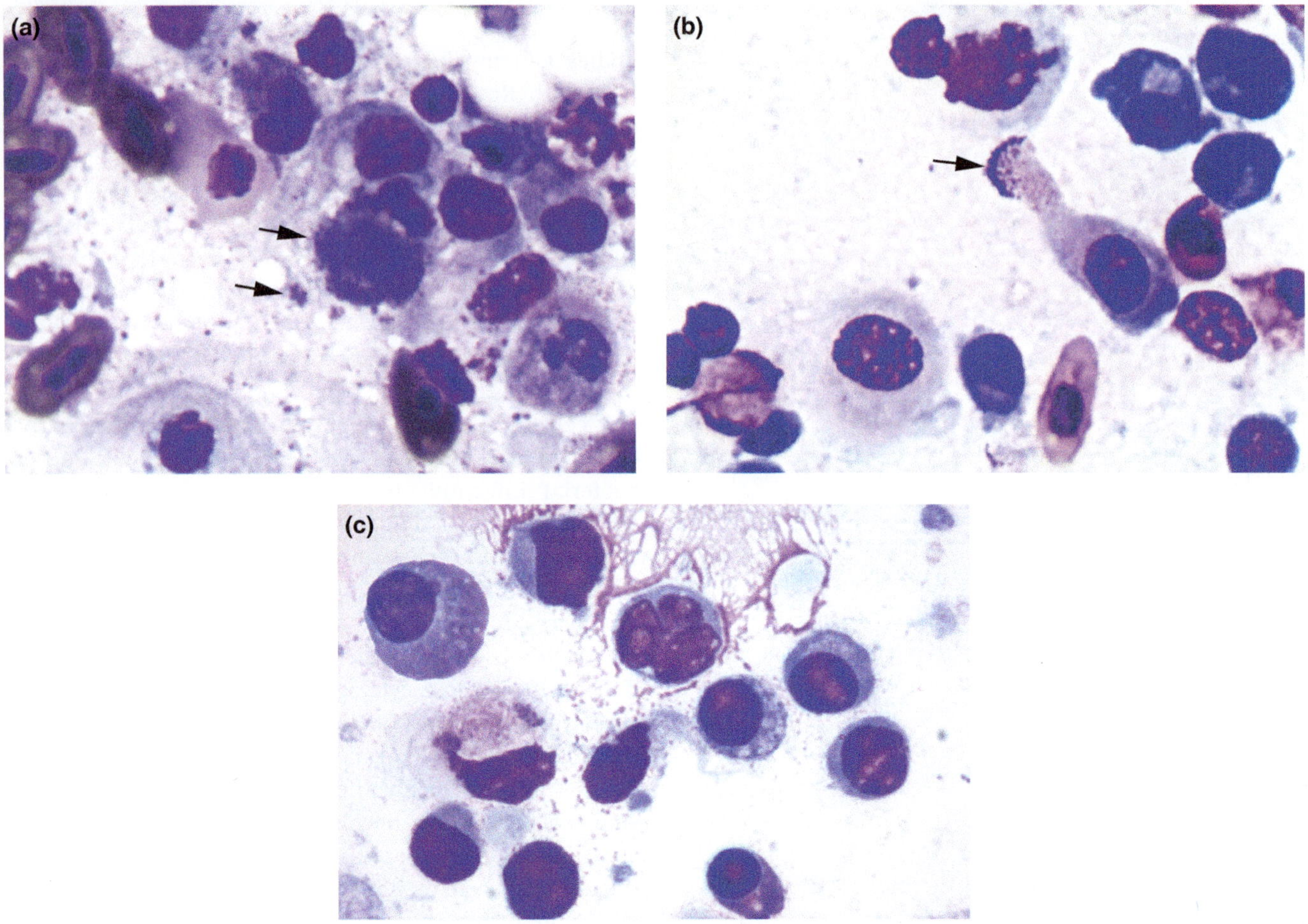

Figure 61.27 (a) Air sac swab from a domestic pigeon (*Columba livia*) showing focal poppy seed-like aggregates most consistent with *Chlamydia* sp. stages in a macrophage and extracellularly (arrows). Intracellular or extracellular granular debris should not be misidentified as chlamydial organisms (Diff-Quik, 1000×). (b) Mycoplasmosis in a conjunctival swab from a domestic chicken showing small coccobacilli attached to the apical surface of a respiratory epithelial cell (arrow). There is mixed inflammation with plasma cells (upper right and position 6) (Diff-Quik, 1000×). (c) Nasal discharge from a gopher tortoise (*Gopherus polyphemus*) with lymphoplasmacytic rhinitis. Although no microorganisms were observed cytologically, this type of inflammation raises suspicion of *Mycoplasma* sp. infection in this species. PCR from nasal discharge confirmed *Mycoplasma aggassizii* (Diff-Quik, 1000×).

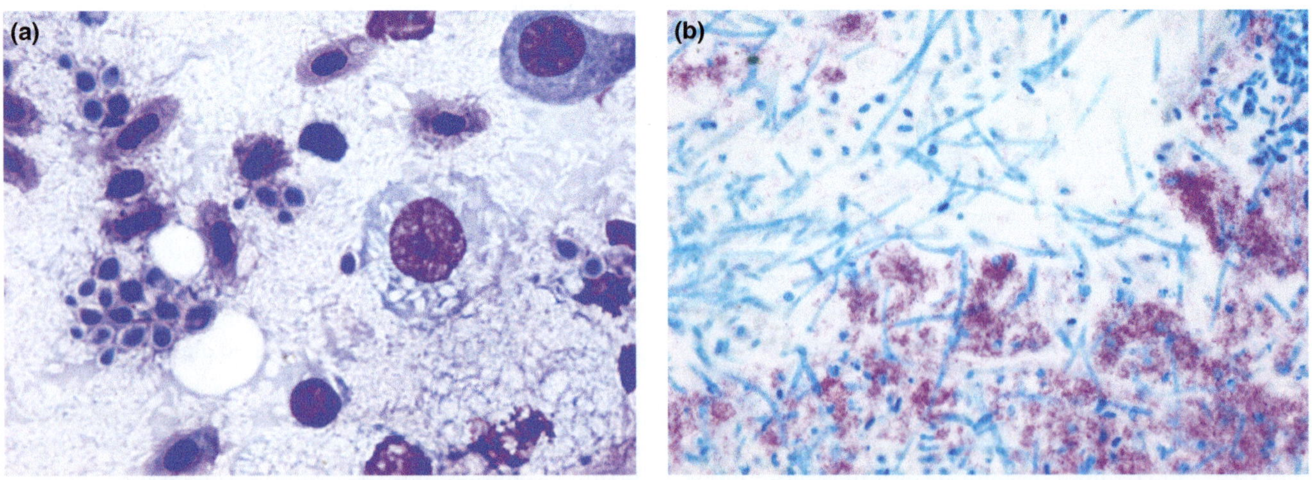

Figure 61.28 (a) Lung imprint from an azure tit (*Cyanistes cyanus*) with granulomatous inflammation and numerous free and phagocytized negative-staining rod-shaped bacilli suggestive of mycobacteriosis and yeast morphologically most consistent with *Candida* sp. (Diff-Quik, 1000×). (b) Corresponding histology section of lung tissue with numerous pink acid-fast positive bacilli and turquoise pseudohyphae (Fite's acid fast stain, 1000×).

Viruses Only a small fraction of viral infections of the respiratory tract cause characteristic cytomorphologic changes with formation of IBs such as poxvirus, adenovirus, herpesvirus, and polyomavirus in birds. For further details, the reader is referred to section "Infectious Agents" and Table 61.2. In reptiles, no specific viral inclusions from respiratory tissue have been described to date, but viral inclusions can be observed in leukocytes originating from peripheral blood in hemodiluted samples.

Fungi Fungal infections of the respiratory tissues are common, including *Aspergillus* sp., *Penicillium* sp., *and* several species of zygomycetes (e.g. *Mucor* sp.). Exposure occurs primarily via inhalation of conidia (spores). Due to their diminutive size (2–3 μm in diameter), conidia can be deposited in the most distal compartments of the respiratory tract such as the intermuscular or intraosseous diverticula of avian air sacs. Key predisposing factors to clinical disease are immunosuppression caused by various stressors, poor ventilation, and the number of inhaled spores. Cytology frequently reveals mixed or granulomatous inflammation. Identification of fungal elements such as septate, branching fungal hyphae and/or conidia is necessary to establish a diagnosis, but structures can be easily missed if present in low number. Visualization of fungal elements can be facilitated by special stains such as Gomori methenamine silver or periodic acid Schiff. Concurrent bacterial and fungal infections are common. Dissolution of sampled material in KOH prior to examination can facilitate detection of fungal structures.[14] Culture and/or PCR are often necessary to differentiate environmental from pathogenic fungal organisms.

Candidiasis is a common disease in immunocompromised animals, especially secondary to primary viral or bacterial infections (e.g. mycobacteriosis) (Figure 61.28) and/or associated with antimicrobial therapy.[106] Other causes include impaired local immunity, altered composition of microflora, discontinuity of the natural epithelial barrier in nasal infections, seeding of the lower respiratory tract with yeast through aspiration of regurgitated food, particularly in avian neonates or sick reptiles, or hematogenous spread. Cytology reveals round to oval, narrow-based budding yeast organisms (3–6 μm in diameter) with both septate mycelium with parallel cell walls and pseudomycelium with constrictions near cell junctions. Inflammation can be subtle, since *Candida* sp. often elicits minimal inflammatory responses. Intraoperative cytologic diagnosis of pulmonary candidiasis was accomplished in a sun conure (*Aratinga solstitialis*) from tissue imprints of a biopsy sample from an endoscopically identified granuloma.[107] Smears consisted of well-differentiated epithelial cells with short segmented fungal hyphae or pseudohyphae and globose spore-like structures accompanied by mixed inflammation.

Respiratory *Cryptococcus* sp. infection has been documented in birds, sometimes in association with sinusitis and potential spread to the lower respiratory tract and central nervous system. Cytology reveals round to oval yeast organisms with narrow-based budding and thick nonstaining capsules of up to 30 μm in diameter along with mixed inflammation, as described in mammals.

Parasites Several respiratory parasitic infections need to be considered in birds and reptiles. Atoxoplasmosis is an important infectious disease of passerine birds, mostly canaries, finches, starlings, and thrushes, which is caused by a coccidian parasite of the genus *Atoxoplasma*. It can cause high mortality in nestlings and older immature birds. The cytologic diagnosis requires the presence of characteristic intracytoplasmic merozoites or meronts in mononuclear cells. Cytologic evaluation of lung tissue is especially rewarding because of typical high organism load compared with other tissues such as liver and spleen. Merozoites appear as elongated whitish, intracytoplasmic, ovoid inclusions with a small eosinophilic center, often displacing the nucleus of the host cell. One or more inclusions can be observed within mononuclear leukocytes.[78]

Toxoplasma sp. causes severe pneumonia in birds, whereas it has been associated with meningoencephalitis in reptiles.[4] Characteristic crescent-shaped tachyzoites are observed individually or in doublets, either free in background or intracellularly, and often with prominent histiocytic inflammation. Variably sized round tissue cysts filled with bradyzoites can also be present. *Sarcocystis* sp. can cause acute rapidly progressive pneumonia, respiratory hemorrhage, and mortality in susceptible hosts. Cytologically, meronts, possibly in rosette formation, are found along with free banana- or cigar-shaped merozoites (Figure 61.29). The inflammation can be lymphoplasmacytic, which is nonspecific and associated with many other conditions. *Sarcocystis* sp. merozoites and *Toxoplasma* sp. tachyzoites appear very similar cytologically; therefore PCR on cytology and/or IHC on tissue sections are recommended for definitive diagnosis.

Cryptosporidium sp. causes respiratory infections ranging from asymptomatic to fatal in birds; however, it is a GIT pathogen in reptiles. Cytologic diagnosis requires identification of the organism, which can be present in several forms, i.e. mature sporulated oocysts, thin-walled oocysts, immature oocysts, several types of budding developmental forms (various types of meronts), or few types of small and

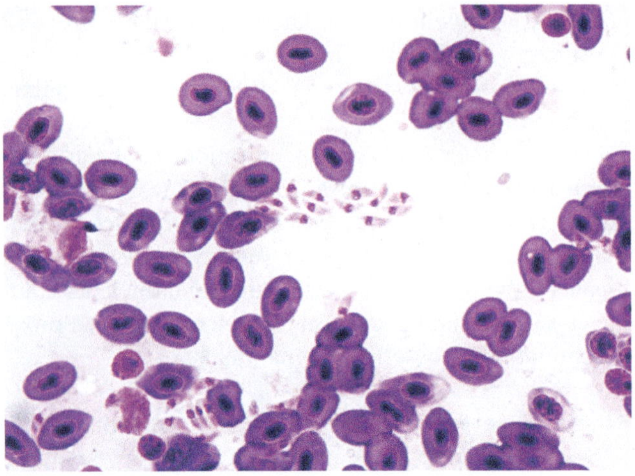

Figure 61.29 Lung imprint from a canary (*Serinus canaria*) with with organisms most consistent with *Toxoplasma gondii* tachyzoites. Nucleated erythrocytes are present in the background (Wright–Giemsa, 400×).

slender merozoites.[108] Mature intact fully sporulated oocysts do not typically take up much stain in Romanowsky-type stained air-dried films and remain as small (5–6 × 4.5 μm) oval ghost structures, which stain positive with acid-fast stain. In contrast, all other developmental stages stain with quick stains but not with acid-fast stains. Meronts can often be observed as small (smaller than oocysts) round structures budding from the apical surface of the parasitized cell. The inflammatory response is mixed, and PCR is necessary for species identification. A technique for rapid cytologic diagnosis of respiratory cryptosporidiosis using Diff-Quik and modified Kinyoun acid-fast staining has been described.[109]

Several nematode species can cause air sac infestation in birds with *Serratospiculum* sp. being most commonly reported.[110,111] They are found frequently in wild or wild-caught captive raptors used for falconry, especially in the Middle East. Infestation often does not cause any obvious evidence of clinical disease; however, it is frequently recognized endoscopically or by presence of parasite ova in crop and fecal samples. In immunocompetent hosts, the reaction to the parasite is often minimal to absent. Severe infestations may cause granulomatous inflammation (Figure 61.30), with presence of multinucleated giant cells. The nematodes are often removed endoscopically. Low-grade infections can be self-limiting. With appropriate treatment, the residual eggs remain within the air sacs without causing any overt tissue reaction.

Neoplasia

Rare reports of primary respiratory neoplasia exist in birds (Figure 61.31), including a bronchial carcinoma.[58] A carcinoma associated with a branchial cyst was described in an umbrella cockatoo (*Cacatua alba*). Cytologic evaluation of the fluid revealed only macrophages and lining epithelial cells, and histopathology was required to identify the carcinoma.[112] Metastasis from other tumors to the lungs has been reported in reptiles and birds.[4,58]

Lymphoid Tissues, Thymus, Spleen

Since reptiles do not have lymph nodes, lymphoid aggregates are well developed in various tissues, especially in the GIT.[13] While lymph nodes are reported in some waterfowl species such as ducks and geese, other birds have

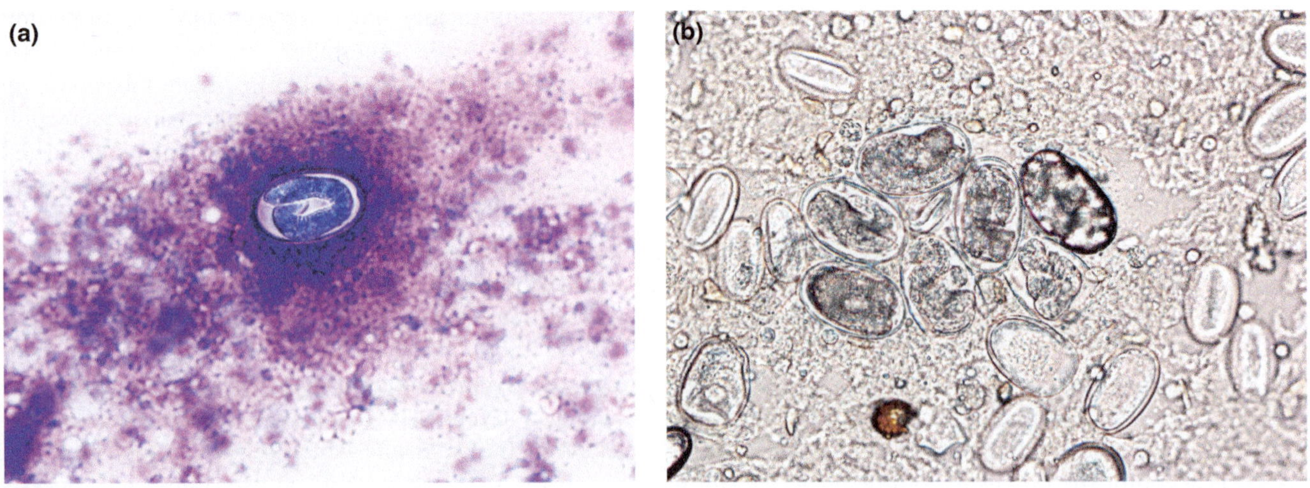

Figure 61.30 (a) Air sac biopsy imprint from a saker falcon (*Falco cherrug*) with *Serratospiculum* sp. larvated ova (Wright–Giemsa, 400×). (b) Unstained wet mount (400×).

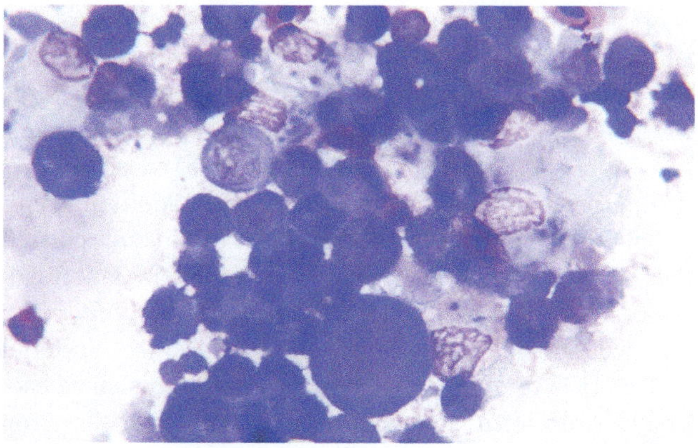

Figure 61.31 Fine-needle aspirate of fluid from a 2 cm soft subcutaneous swelling associated with the right sinuses in a nanday conure (*Aratinga nenday*). Poorly cohesive, atypical epithelial cells are suggestive of adenocarcinoma, which was confirmed by histopathology (Wright–Giemsa, 500×).

functionally similar structures, and mucosal-associated lymphoid tissue is prominent in gastrointestinal and respiratory tracts.[18] Spleen, thymus, and the bursa of Fabricius are the main avian lymphoid organs but are rarely sampled in live animals. Only the spleen is discussed, since samples for cytologic evaluation can be collected by laparoscopy, during necropsy (squash preparation or tissue imprint), or in birds by ultrasound-guided fine-needle aspirate.

Cytologic preparations of normal splenic tissue are highly cellular and consist mainly of mixed lymphocytes with small cell predominance and erythrocytes in various stages of maturation. Lesser numbers of macrophages, plasma cells, granulocytes, and low numbers of immature granulocyte stages, well-differentiated mesenchymal cells, and endothelial cells also can be present. Because the spleen removes senescent erythrocytes, cell debris, erythrophagocytosis, and hemosiderin are also expected. Apart from its function as embryonal hematopoietic, adult lymphopoietic, and erythrocyte processing organ, the spleen serves as major site for mounting and regulating immune responses after antigen exposure.[113] Accurate differentiation of physiologic reactivity from pathologic changes is challenging and not always possible. Careful interpretation in context of peripheral blood leukocyte counts is necessary to differentiate extramedullary hematopoiesis, peripheral leukocytosis, and splenitis. True inflammation is sometimes characterized by heterophil degeneration, necrosis (lympholysis), and phagocytosis of leukocytes or microorganisms by macrophages.

As in other species, any antigenic stimulation can cause reactive lymphoid hyperplasia. Septicemia will result in similar cytologic findings, including variable components of heterophilic and macrophagic inflammation and necrosis. In some cases, infectious organisms can be identified. In reptiles, systemic infections with bacteria and fungi appear to be the most frequent microorganisms observed in the spleen (authors' observation). In birds, bacteria (including mycobacteria), *Chlamydia* sp., and viral INIBs of adenovirus, herpesvirus, and polyomavirus are microbial structures found on a regular basis. Atoxoplasmosis is a coccidian infection mostly seen in passerine birds. It is known as "black spot disease," which refers to the massively congested liver as a black spot visible through the abdominal wall distal to the sternum in juvenile birds. Apart from the intestinal epithelium, merogony occurs in the MPS, most commonly in the liver, spleen, and lung. Cytology is superior to histopathology for detecting the intracytoplasmic 3–5 μm pale pink organisms that indent the host nucleus to a marginal crescent.[23] Developmental stages of *Plasmodium* sp., *Hemoproteus* sp., and *Leucocytozoon* sp. are occasionally detected in splenic samples. As in reptiles, the presence of fungal hyphae typically is associated with systemic mycosis.

Various pigments and crystals may be observed in certain pathologic conditions involving the spleen. Although variable amounts of hemosiderin are expected in normal spleen, increased hemosiderin can occur with hemolysis, splenic hemorrhage, or decreased iron turnover as with anemia of chronic disease.[114] Common causes for hemorrhage and hemolysis include septicemia (bacterial or viral), and heavy metal or rodenticide poisoning.[23,115] Hemosiderin is irregular blackish-blue to blackish-green, globular or granular material within macrophages or in the background of Romanowsky-type stains; it stains bright blue or turquoise with Prussian blue. In *Plasmodium* sp. infections, both Prussian blue-positive hemosiderin granules and Prussian blue-negative hemozoin granules can occur in extra-erythrocytic schizonts phagocytized by macrophages. Prominent accumulation of iron metabolites can be present in infected birds of prey, accompanied by a markedly enlarged spleen with brownish black discoloration. Amyloid can be detected in samples (i.e. liver, spleen, kidney) from patients with chronic granulomatous inflammatory conditions and can be confirmed using polarized light in a Congo red stained preparation. Needle-shaped urate crystals are occasionally detected in splenic tissue in cases of systemic visceral gout. Advanced stages can result in a foreign body inflammatory reaction with macrophages and multinucleated giant cells.[115]

Lymphoproliferative and myeloproliferative malignancies have been reported in reptiles and birds, with frequent splenic involvement.[23,57,116] Prominent erythroid regenerative responses recognized by blood film evaluation in reptiles with concurrent extramedullary hematopoiesis in spleen and liver should not be misinterpreted as erythroleukemia, a condition not recognized in reptiles to date.

Differentiation of hyperplasia (reactive or extramedullary hematopoiesis) from neoplasia often requires histopathology because invasion and disruption of tissue architecture are key diagnostic criteria. Even in histopathology samples, immunohistochemical stains can be necessary for the identification of the affected cell lineage, depending upon availability of validated antibodies. Fibrosarcomas, hemangiomas, hemangiosarcomas, and gastric metastatic carcinomas have been reported to affect the spleen in birds but occur infrequently.[23]

Gastrointestinal Tract, Liver, and Pancreas

Normal Structure and Cytology

Upper GIT

In reptiles and birds, the oropharynx is lined with stratified squamous epithelium, which is keratinized on papillae and in areas of heavy wear such as the tongue. The cytologic evaluation of the upper GIT in birds, i.e. oropharynx or crop, is ideally performed with a dry mount cytology and a concurrent freshly prepared direct wet mount. Wet mounts are particularly useful for the detection of motile organisms in the crop, including *Trichomonas* sp. in pigeons and budgerigars or spirochetes in lovebirds and cockatiels. The latter show very characteristic morphology and movement.[78,117]

Cytology of the normal oropharynx consists of uniform flat, polygonal, nucleated, and anucleated squamous epithelial cells. Superficial squames are large and polygonal with light basophilic cytoplasm. Variable numbers of keratohyalin and melanin granules can be observed in some cells. They exfoliate individually or in loose sheets, often having various surface and contour patterns due to folding. Intermediate squames have comparatively darker basophilic cytoplasm and less angular margins. Basal and parabasal cells as well as salivary gland epithelial cells are rarely present in oropharyngeal swabs of healthy reptiles and birds unless sample collection is traumatic. Cytologic specimens from esophagus and crop (i.e. lavage or swab) consist mainly of superficial and intermediate squames. In addition to epithelial cells, samples from the upper GIT can include ciliated respiratory epithelial cells, pleomorphic food or plant material, oral commensals (*Simonsiella* sp. or *Alysiella filiformis*), and occasional yeast. In healthy animals, the bacterial microflora is composed of abundant mixed rod-shaped bacteria that are often closely adhered to epithelial cells. Crop samples can include calcium carbonate crystals of dietary origin or urate crystals in coprophagous birds.[7] Many passerines, especially granivorous species, i.e. canaries and finches, reportedly have an almost sterile gastrointestinal flora, including oral cavity and crop. In contrast, oropharyngeal samples from clinically healthy and well-performing pigeons contain a mixture of rod-shaped bacteria and possibly occasional *Candida* sp. Trichomonads can be present in their crops without concurrent inflammation (Figure 61.32).[118] During the breeding season, both male and female *Columbiformes* produce a specialized holocrine secretion of desquamated lipid-laden epithelial cells called crop milk to feed their squabs. Grossly, crop milk is yellowish white with curd-like grains originating from the lateral diverticula of the crop. Epithelial cells of crop milk are small polygonal squamous epithelial cells containing variably sized lipid vacuoles and nuclei that are easier to evaluate in wet mounts than in dry mount cytologies.

The avian proventriculus is characterized cytologically by secretory cuboidal and/or columnar epithelial cells and possibly dense mucus. The secretory epithelial cells often

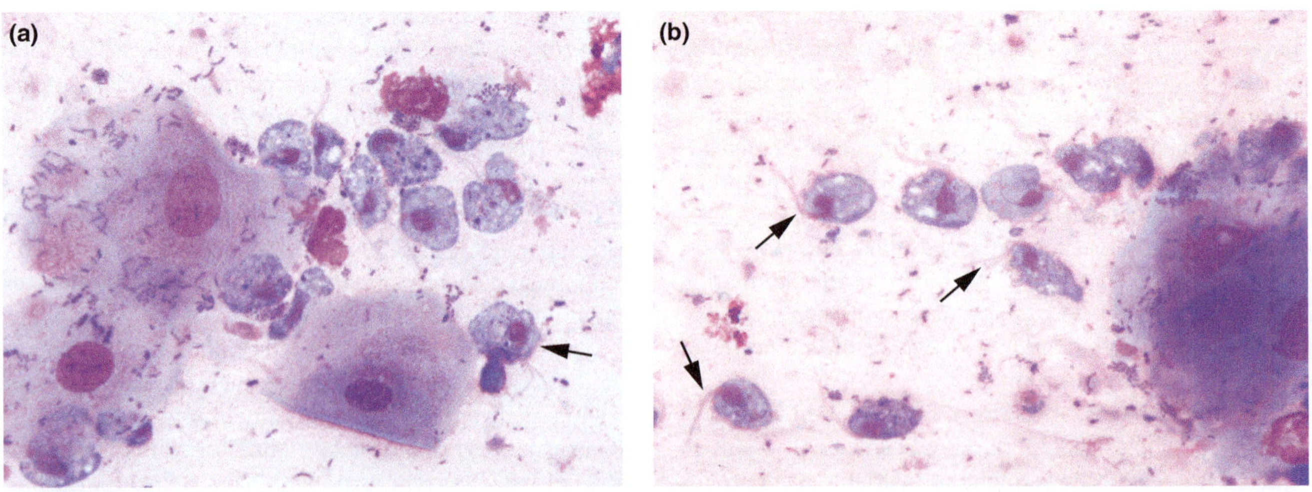

Figure 61.32 *Trichomonas* sp. in a crop swab from a rock dove (*Columba livia*). (a, b) Note anterior flagella (arrows), single nucleus, vacuolated cytoplasm, and an axostyle. There are squamous epithelial cells with adhered mixed bacilli (Diff-Quik, 1000×).

exfoliate poorly and appear as tightly cohesive sheets of orderly honeycomb-like (plane view) or palisade-like (side view) arrangements. They vary from cuboidal to columnar and lack apical cilia. Basal nuclei are round to oval with clumped chromatin and infrequently display one or multiple indistinct small nucleoli. The cytoplasm is granular, pale basophilic, and contains variable numbers of secretory granules. Parietal cells are rarely sampled, but sometimes exfoliate if the mucosa is ulcerated. They resemble exocrine pancreatic epithelial cells with distinct secretory granules and a single round nucleus with clumped chromatin and a small round indistinct nucleolus. The mucosa of the avian ventriculus and reptilian stomach consists of dark-staining, small, columnar epithelial cells. Firm scraping during necropsy examinations is necessary to obtain individual cells or small clusters. The cytoplasm is granular and deeply basophilic. The basally located nucleus contains a single small round indistinct nucleolus. The supranuclear portion of the cytoplasm is packed with deep eosinophilic secretory granules, which produce the koilin layer in birds.

Lower GIT

Small intestinal cytology samples of healthy reptiles and birds reveal striated border epithelial cells, possibly goblet cells, and rarely globular leukocytes. Other cell types such as Paneth cells and enterochromaffin cells require histology and special methods of staining for identification.[119] Additional components of small intestinal samples from clinically healthy reptiles and birds include mucus, food particles, mixed rod-shaped bacteria, low numbers of yeast (incidental and/or *Candida* sp.), and possibly rare parasite ova. Avian caeca vary enormously in form and development among different bird families and are often classified into four types: intestinal, glandular, lymphoid, and vestigial. Cytology of the first two forms closely resembles the small intestine, whereas scrapings from the latter two contain more lymphocytes from the more developed submucosal lymphoid aggregates.

Rectal samples of reptiles and birds are composed of striated border epithelial cells, goblet cells, variable amounts of mucus, and bacterial microflora. The cloaca of reptiles and birds are composed of the coprodeum (intestinal tract opening), urodeum (urinary and reproductive opening), and proctodeum (common opening of coprodeum and urodeum) opening into the vent.[120] These three compartments are not always clearly separated from each other. As a primary lymphoid organ, the bursa of Fabricius of growing birds opens into the dorsum of the proctodeum. The mucosa of the three compartments varies from cuboidal to stratified squamous epithelium, and cytology samples are often composed of both. Mucus, urate crystals, food particles, and spermatozoa also can be present.

Fecal cytology can be performed as a wet mount or dry mount fecal smear; using both methods concurrently is preferred to obtain the most diagnostic information. A wet mount preparation represents diagnostic material in its most original composition and optimizes the observation of motile organisms such as certain protozoans and bacteria. As the sample ages and cools, some microorganisms lose motility, and morphology is altered, hindering identification. An optimal wet mount is prepared by mixing a very small amount of feces, preferably the urate-free portion, with a drop of water (e.g. sterile saline, tap water, or distilled water), and cover-slipping without air bubbles. Room temperature water is acceptable; however, warmed diluent and slides will promote motility. Brownian movement should not be misinterpreted as motility. Diff-Quik® provides excellent staining quality for dry mount fecal cytology samples. A separate staining set designated for fecal sample staining prevents other cytology samples from contamination during staining.

Infectious Disease of the GIT

The emphasis in the following sections is focused on the GIT; however, because many diseases affect multiple organs, particularly the liver, discussion of multiple tissues is included below.

Bacteria

Normal gastrointestinal microflora in most species is typically composed of abundant mixed rod-shaped bacteria of variable size and thickness, possibly with very low numbers of cocci. An overgrown homogeneous population of a monomorphic bacterium is considered abnormal. It can be observed with antimicrobial administration or with bacterial infections, which are often associated with increased mucus, sloughed epithelium, necrotic debris, and inflammation. Abnormal microflora may include spirilliform bacteria (e.g. *Campylobacter* sp. as in certain finches.) and spore formers (i.e., in parrots). Spirilliform bacteria require specialized growth medium, which should be requested at the microbiology laboratory. Spore formers are Gram-positive, and the spores stain bright turquoise with malachite green stain; however, anaerobic culture and toxin enzyme-linked immunosorbent assays can be useful for confirmation. Cytology of an enteric swab was used to diagnose a disseminated mycobacterial infection in a juvenile leatherback sea turtle, demonstrating heterophilic and histiocytic enteritis with characteristic negative staining intrahistiocytic bacteria that were positive with acid-fast stain.[121]

Viruses

In birds, gastrointestinal lesions with cytologically detectable IB formation are most commonly seen with poxvirus, adenovirus, herpesvirus, and polyomavirus infections.

Visualization of IBs is often hampered by concurrent necrosis, inflammation, and secondary opportunistic infections. Deep layer sampling is recommended, especially in lesions of the upper GIT, which are commonly altered by hemorrhage, ulceration, and bacterial superinfections. Nodular to diffuse diphtheroid oropharyngeal lesions are caused by the wet form of poxvirus and need to be differentiated from grossly similar looking lesions caused by hypovitaminosis A, trichomoniasis, capillariasis, candidiasis, *Pseudomonas* sp., and herpes- or circoviral infections. Concurrent infections of all these agents do occur. Adenovirus infections can produce very large basophilic INIBs in enterocytes, hepatocytes, and pancreatic cells. Herpesvirus INIBs can be seen in epithelial cells of oropharynx, crop, intestines, liver, and pancreas. Concurrent presence of syncytia is strongly suggestive of herpesvirus infection. Polyomavirus INIBs are most commonly found in hepatocytes, Kupffer cells, epithelial cells, and leukocytes from samples of the upper GIT and pancreas. An overview of cytologically detectable viral infections in birds is given in section "Infectious Agents" and Table 61.2. In reptiles, the cytodiagnosis of viral infections in the GIT is theoretically possible, e.g. adenoviral INIBs in lizard species, but, to the authors' knowledge, this has not been documented to date.

Fungi

The cytologic finding of *Candida* sp. with characteristic pseudohyphae is interpreted as for other species (Figure 61.33). Low numbers in the GIT in the absence of inflammation are typically not of clinical concern, whereas yeast overgrowth, i.e. candidiasis, with or without inflammation, is consistent with infection as described for the respiratory tract. *Macrorhabdus ornithogaster* (formerly *Megabacterium* sp.) organisms are commonly present in proventricular samples from clinically healthy passerines, parrots, and backyard poultry. In wet mounts, this organism is large (2 × 20–80 μm) and rod shaped with rounded ends and vacuole-like internal structures, infrequently exhibiting dichotomous branching (Figure 61.34). In dry mount cytology, they appear variably blue and can exhibit pink staining vacuole-like structures. Numerous *Macrorhabdus ornithogaster* organisms are consistent with infection, often

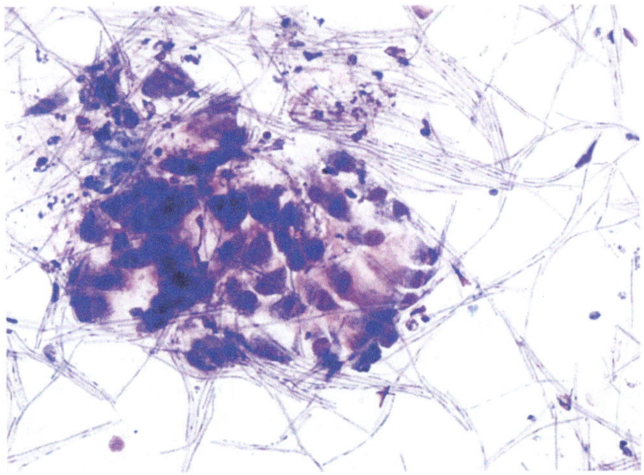

Figure 61.34 Proventriculus scraping from a Gouldian finch (*Erythrura gouldiae*). Well-differentiated secretory columnar epithelial cells are associated with numerous large rod-shaped organisms with rounded ends and vacuole-like internal structures that are consistent with *Macrorhabdus ornithogaster* (Diff-Quik, 500×).

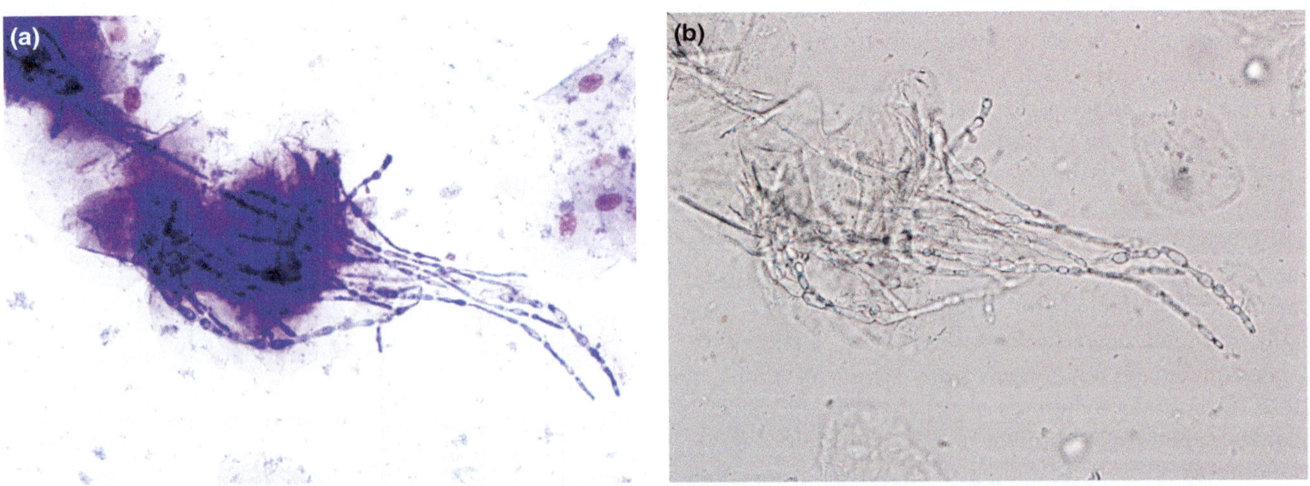

Figure 61.33 (a) Crop swab from a peregrine falcon (*Falco peregrinus*). Budding yeast exhibit pseudohyphae in close association with anucleated squamous epithelial cells. This yeast morphology is characteristic for *Candida* sp. (Diff-Quik, 200×). (b) Unstained wet mount (200×).

accompanied by inflammation and increased mucus. Other fungal organisms observed in GIT samples include fragments of greenish-basophilic fungal structures that often represent mold passing through the GIT and possible infections of septate branching hyphae or nonstaining zygomycetes.

Parasites

Various parasites can be observed cytologically in the GIT of reptiles and birds. Although some of these organisms exhibit a distinct morphology, parasitologic evaluation, special stains, and/or PCR can be necessary for confirmation or identification. Amebiasis is an important diagnosis in various reptile species. Amebic trophozoites and cysts exhibit a similar morphology as those observed in mammalian species (Figure 61.35). Coccidians often pass through the GIT in many reptiles but are of clinical importance in many avian species. In birds, *Eimeria* sp., *Caryospora* sp., and *Isospora* sp. can be present in various segments of the GIT, often exhibiting species-specific localization along the intestines and sometimes pathognomonic gross lesions (especially certain *Eimeria* sp. in chickens). Oocysts are not necessarily present in birds with clinical disease, but identification of different developmental stages of coccidia in significant numbers is necessary to establish the cytologic diagnosis. The developmental stages include meronts, merozoites, macro- and microgametocytes, microgametes, and immature and mature non-sporulated oocysts (Figure 61.36). In active infections, cytology can also contain increased mucus, leukocytes, erythrocytes, and variably degenerate sloughed enterocytes.

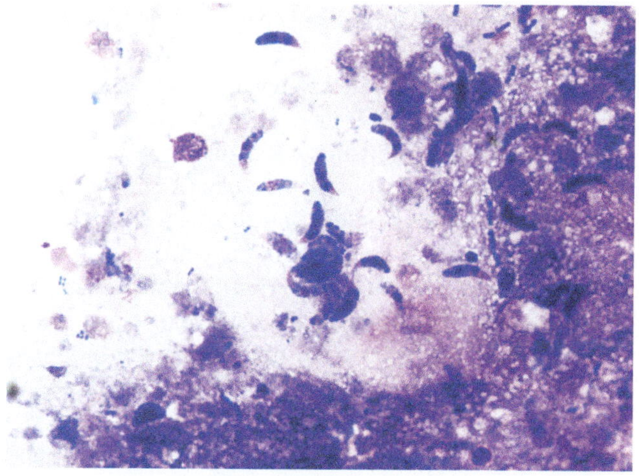

Figure 61.36 Fecal direct smear from a saker falcon (*Falco cherrug*). The crescent-shaped protozoal merozoites and small nucleus are suggestive of *Caryospora* sp., given the host species (Diff-Quik, 1000×).

Disseminated visceral coccidiosis in cranes is caused by *Eimeria gruis* and *Eimeria reichenowi*. Cytologic findings include gametocytes, oocysts, and possibly intracellular asexual stages in macrophages and endothelial cells. Cytologic specimens of granulomatous liver lesions reveal mixed inflammation, necrosis, schizonts, and mononuclear cells with intracytoplasmic coccidial stages. Cytodiagnosis of atoxoplasmosis requires the identification of gametocytes and/or oocysts (usually very few, non-sporulated) in intestinal scrapings and asexual stages of the parasite (merozoites and meronts in

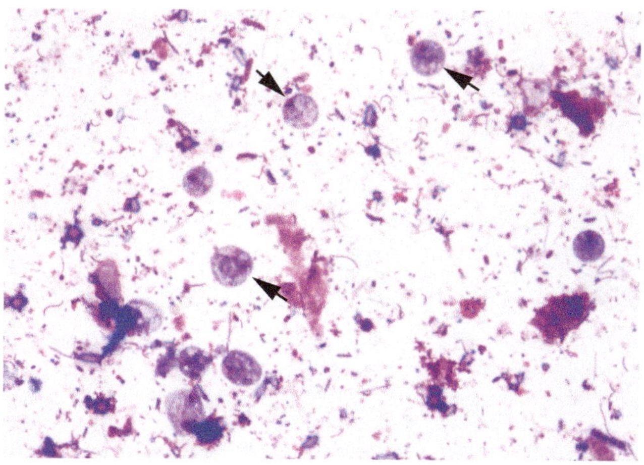

Figure 61.35 Fecal direct smear from a pancake tortoise (*Malacochersus tornieri*). Protozoal cysts (arrows) exhibit central vacuole and eccentrically placed nucleus, suggestive of ameba. There is a background of numerous mixed bacteria. PCR identified *Entamoeba invadens* and was negative for *Blastocystis* sp. (Diff-Quik, 500×).

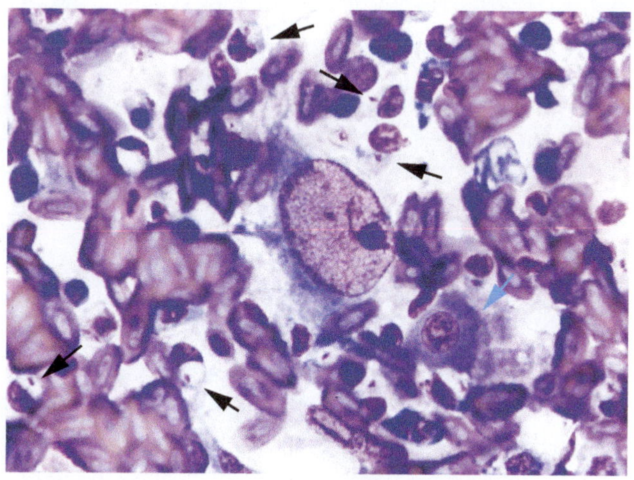

Figure 61.37 Liver squash preparation from a goldfinch (*Carduelis carduelis*). Merozoites of *Atoxoplasma* sp. are found extracellularly or within mononuclear cells (black arrows). A single large intranuclear polyomavirus inclusion (center) is seen in a presumed hepatocyte. One well-differentiated hepatocyte is indicated by the blue arrow. Numerous erythrocytes are present in the background (Diff-Quik, 1000×).

mononuclear cells). Mixed infections with *Atoxoplasma* sp. and other enteric coccidia are not uncommon. Cytology of lung, liver, and spleen can also reveal various stages of this organism (Figure 61.37). Almost every mononuclear cell in these organs will display one or multiple *Atoxoplasma* sp. merozoites.[78] *Sarcocystis* sp. in reptiles and birds is unique in its life cycle during which infective sporulated oocysts are produced in the definitive host, and therefore environmental sporulation is unnecessary. The oocyst wall of the sporulated oocysts is very fragile, which results in release of sporocysts; thus very few or no intact oocysts are present cytologically. Sporocysts are arranged individually or in characteristic doublets. Sporocysts appear similar to *Cryptosporidium* sp. oocysts, are also infective, and contain four well-visible sporozoites. In intermediate hosts, liver cytology can show necrosis and schizonts; however, asymptomatic infections are common in which *Sarcocystis* sp. organisms are very difficult to find. Enteric infections with *Cryptosporidium* sp. may cause clinical disease and mortality (Figure 61.38). In snakes, oocysts of infected rodents can transit the GIT but are of no clinical significance. Thus, PCR (e.g. from gastric lavage, gastric tissue obtained by biopsy) is recommended for species identification. In infections, developmental stages (meronts and gametocytes) and immature oocysts are observed as "budding" from the apical surface of epithelial cells. Mature and immature oocysts can be attached to the epithelium or free in the background. Phagocytosis by inflammatory cells can be observed. *Toxoplasma gondii* infection can result in enteritis with fatal outcome in birds. Cytologically, necrosis, inflammation, sloughing enterocytes, and variable numbers of crescent to oval

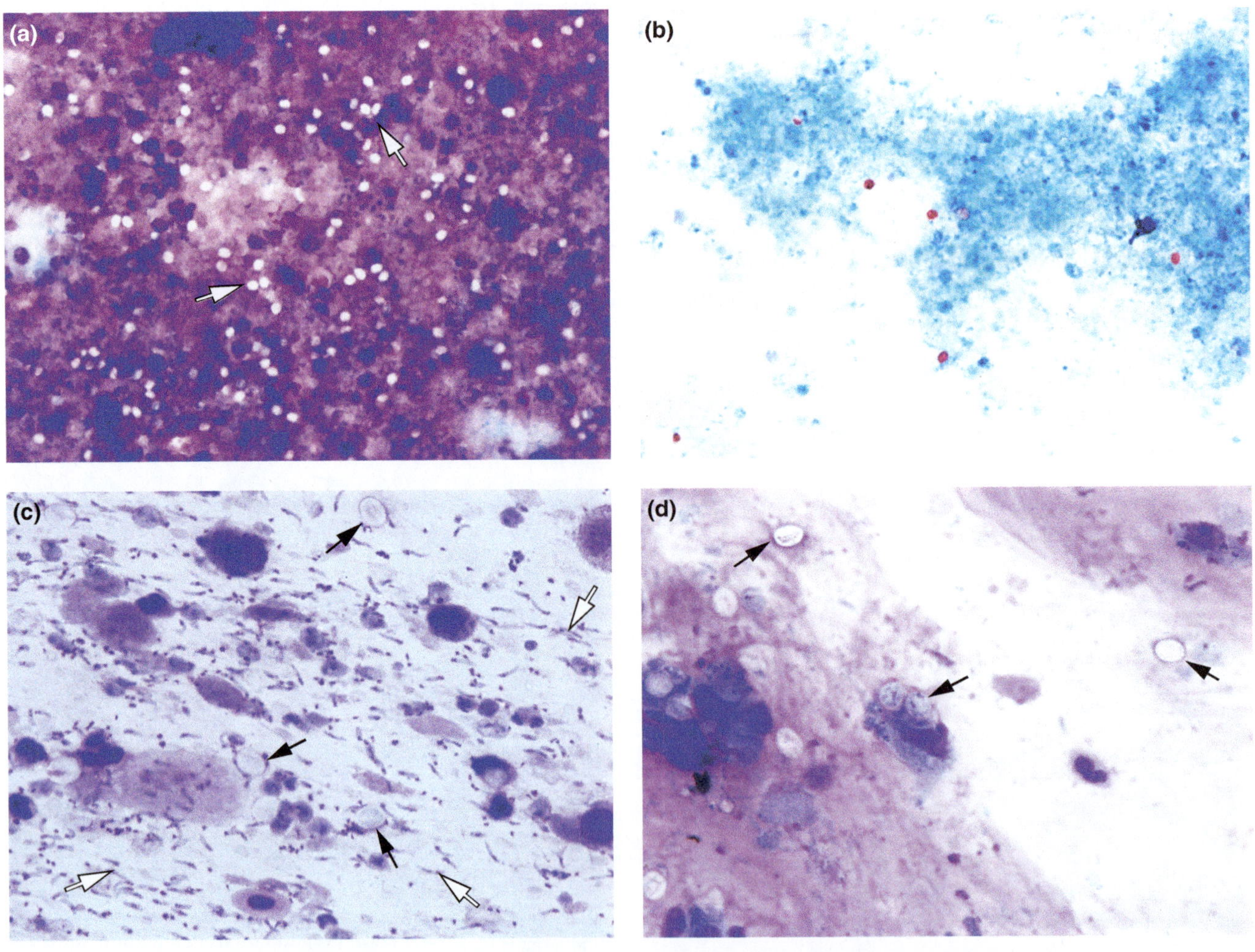

Figure 61.38 (a) *Cryptosporidium baylei* oocysts (arrows) from a swab of the pharyngeal opening of the tubae auditivae in a gyrfalcon (*Falco rusticolus*) (Diff-Quik, 200×). (b) Mature intact *Cryptosporidium* sp. oocysts stain positive with acid fast stain (Ziehl Neelsen stain, 200×). (c and d) Abundant *Cryptosporidium* sp. organisms of different life stages in a choanal swab from a gyrfalcon (*Falco rusticolus*), including oocysts (black arrows) and zoites (white arrows) (Wright stain, (c) 500×, (d) 1000×. *Source:* Images courtesy of Helen Michaels).

tachyzoites of *T. gondii* can be present. IHC of biopsies and/or PCR should be utilized for species identification. Trichomonads can be observed in any samples from the GIT in birds. Organisms are best visualized in fresh wet mounts as active pear- or drop-shaped flagellates with anterior flagella and an undulating membrane of varying size (5–20 µm).[78] In dry mount samples, the organism has pale blue cytoplasm with or without vacuoles, a single small pink anterior nucleus, and, depending on the specimen, an axostyle, anterior flagella, and an undulating membrane. Necrotic debris, inflammation, mixed bacteria, and yeast are often concurrently present. *Giardia* sp., with their characteristic morphology, can be observed in wet mounts and dry cytology GIT samples from reptiles and birds. Although infrequently a clinical problem in bird species, disease has not been documented in reptiles so far. *Hexamita/Spironucleus* sp. organisms are small (3–10 µm in length), very fast moving slender flagellates. Due to their size and varying fast darting motion, they can be easily missed in wet mounts from intestinal samples or fresh feces. Trophozoites appear as slender pear- to comma-shaped organisms with two anterior located pink nuclei (often seen as one bilobed anterior nucleus), multiple long flagella, and pale blue to colorless cytoplasm. Cysts are very similar to *Giardia* cysts but much smaller (usually 2 × 4 µm) and with a single large pink nuclear region. Microsporidiosis can be missed by cytology because of the diminutive size of the spores (~1.5–2 × 1–1.5 µm) and possible confusion with other infectious agents (Figure 61.39). Cytologically, the spores appear nonstaining to barely staining when mature (this stage is also acid-fast positive); however,

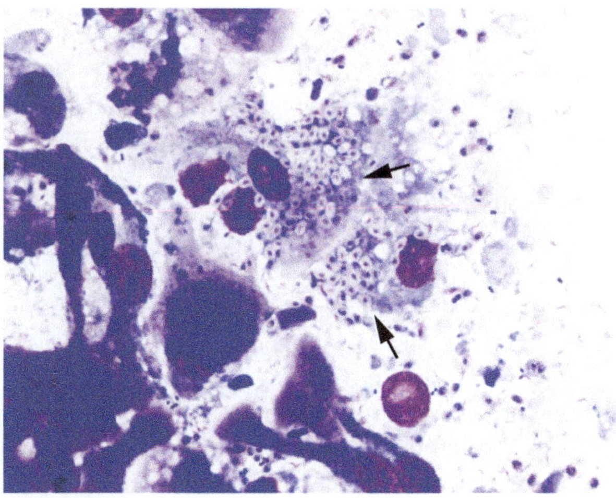

Figure 61.39 Scraping from the rectum of a Gouldian finch (*Erythrura gouldiae*). Microsporidial spores (arrows) are found within two cells, presumably enterocytes (Diff-Quik, 1000×).

immature stages are readily visualized using Romanowsky-type stains. Microsporidia (e.g. *Encephalitozoon* sp. and *Enterocytozoon* sp. in birds, *Pleistophora* sp. in reptiles) are obligate intracellular organisms developing in the cytoplasm of many organs in systemic infections, including the intestine and liver. Clusters of minute organisms (resembling clostridial spores), both staining and nonstaining, can be identified within the cytoplasm of affected cells and free in the background. Inflammation can be observed. Microsporidiosis has been documented in many reptile and bird species.[122] Other parasites include nematode and trematode ova, but the morphology on dry mount preparations does not allow for species identification, and further parasitology testing (e.g. sedimentation) is required.

Liver, Biliary System, and Pancreas

Cytology samples of the pancreas, liver, and biliary epithelium can be collected as tissue imprints of biopsy material taken antemortem or during necropsy examinations. Samples are composed of similar cellular components as described in other species. Liver cytology samples from laying females and newly hatched reptiles and chicks frequently contain extracellular lipid and prominent distinct cytoplasmic hepatocellular vacuolation, consistent with lipid accumulation. In addition to kidney and spleen, the liver is a site of extramedullary hematopoiesis in growing reptiles and chicks. The duration of physiologic hepatic lipidosis and extramedullary hematopoiesis is species-dependent and poorly characterized. Data from psittacines shows cessation of hepatic granulopoiesis/lipidosis at post-hatching day 7–8 for small-sized species and day 9–10 for large-sized species.[123] Despite physiologic cessation at young age, this hematopoietic potential of the liver is maintained throughout life and may be reactivated in adult animals in response to increased peripheral demand from anemia or inflammation. Other cells in liver samples include clumps of thrombocytes from hemodilution, Kupffer cells, endothelial cells, mesothelial cells, and possibly air sac epithelial cells in birds.

Urinary Tract

Cytology of normal kidney tissue is composed of renal tubular epithelial cells accompanied by free nuclei, cytoplasmic debris, and blood. Intact tubular segments or fragments and possibly entire glomeruli can be observed (Figure 61.40). The nuclei of renal tubular epithelial cells are round with clumped chromatin and one or multiple

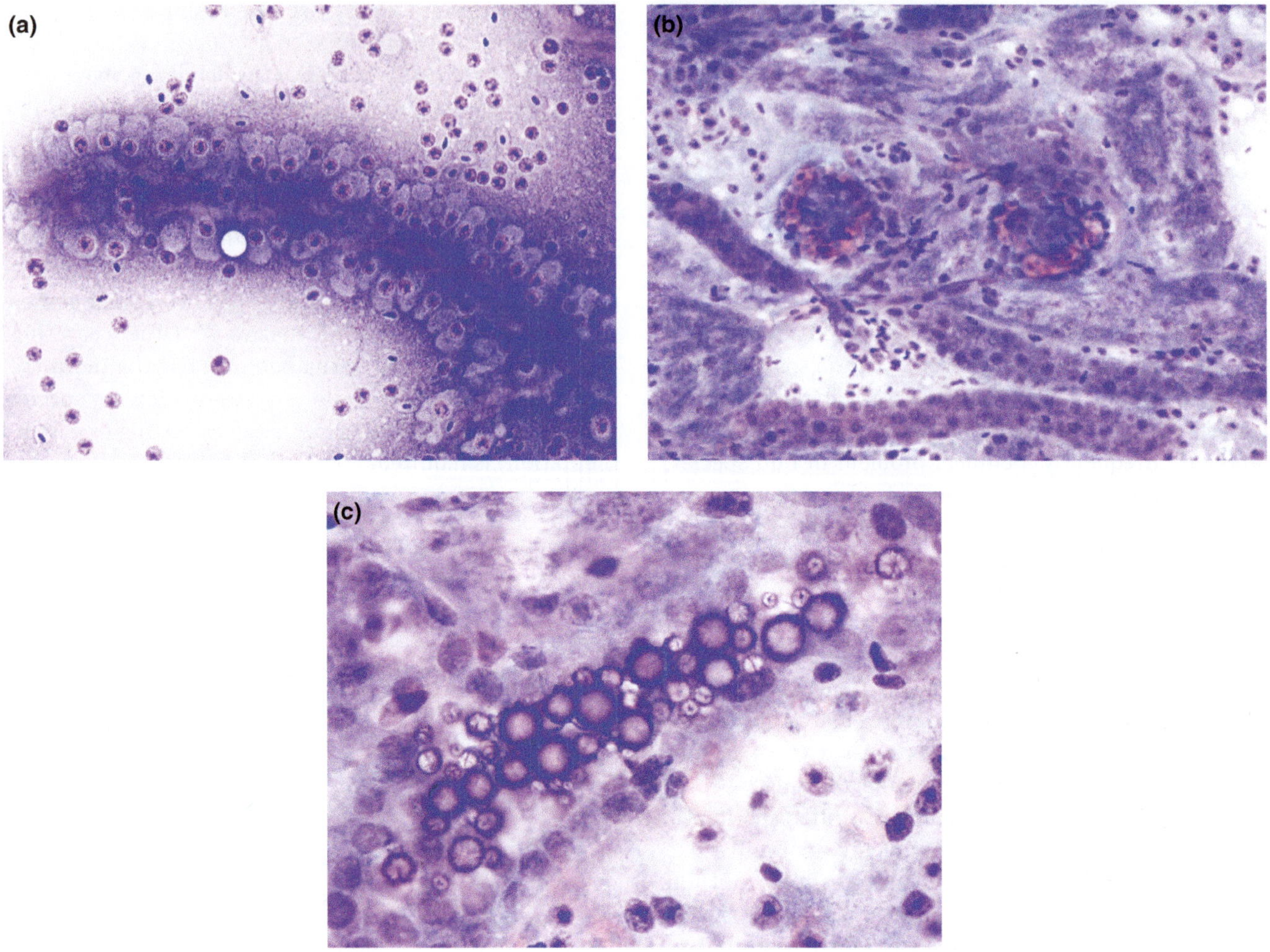

Figure 61.40 Squash preparation of renal tissue from a common quail (*Coturnix coturnix*). (a) Uniform renal tubular epithelium. (b) Glomeruli, renal tubules, and capillaries. (c) Urate crystals within tubular epithelium (Diff-Quik, 500×).

small, round and distinct nucleoli that appear similar in morphology to hepatocyte nuclei. The cytoplasm is abundant, pale to moderately basophilic, and granular. It can contain scant greenish to dark blue amorphous material, which is suspected to be proteinaceous. Urate crystals appear as variably sized round crystalline structures with a dense cartwheel pattern (Figure 61.40c), representing spherical aggregates of monosodium urate crystals that occur under supersaturated conditions.[91] While most bird species excrete uric acid, the nitrogenous waste of reptiles varies in the proportions of uric acid, urea, and ammonia depending on husbandry.[4,7] Uric acid crystals can also be visualized by polarized light (Figure 61.24c). Well-differentiated fibrocytes and endothelial cells can also be observed. Extramedullary granulopoiesis is normal in kidneys of young birds and can reoccur in adult birds with increased peripheral demand for granulocytes.

Urine can provide valuable diagnostic information in reptiles and birds; however, the urinary, genital, and intestinal tracts empty into the cloaca and cloacal samples can contain cellular material from any of these systems. Most urine samples are collected voided from a clean surface, and the fluid component in birds can be aspirated into a syringe. Only chelonians and some lizard species have a urinary bladder, while the posterior cloaca stores urine in snakes and crocodilians. Cystocentesis has been reported in tortoises by experienced clinicians.[4] Catheterization is challenging and sometimes requires anesthesia; thus it is an uncommon technique for urine sampling.[4,124] Green discoloration of urine, i.e., biliverdinuria, in reptiles and birds has been associated with starvation, hepatic disease, and hemolytic anemia.[4,124] Since reptiles do not concentrate their urine, specific gravity measurement is not useful; however birds do have that capacity with reported ranges from 1.005 to 1.020. Urine dipstick analysis for glucose, ketones, blood, and protein can be used, keeping in mind the limitations of cloacal and lower urinary tract contamination.[4,124] If fluid is available, urinalysis follows standard procedures, including wet and dry mount cytology of direct and/or sediment preparations. Normal voided urine is composed of uric acid crystals, amorphous urates, squamous epithelial cells, variable numbers of mixed rod-shaped bacteria from fecal contamination, spermatozoa, and/or possibly a few leukocytes and rarely erythrocytes. Abnormalities of the colonic microflora and parasites can be observed as discussed for fecal cytology. Crystals other than uric acid crystals or urates in reptiles have been documented in sick tortoises and should be carefully evaluated in any species based on clinical history (e.g. dietary imbalances), pH, and type of crystals. Urinalysis is not helpful in the diagnosis of urolithiasis in birds and reptiles, since urate crystals are a physiologic component. The gold standard for diagnosis of urolithiasis is diagnostic imaging. The etiology of calculi in birds and reptiles is thought to be multifactorial and includes diet, dehydration, and possible infection.[4,125,126]

Urinalysis and renal cytology specimens are useful to detect inflammation and some infectious agents in reptiles and birds. The presence of heterophilic inflammation, necrosis, and/or bacteria suggests infection, and culture is recommended. Renal samples from postmortem specimens are easily contaminated by bacteria from the intestines and the cloaca based on anatomic proximity. Viral infections, especially by adenovirus and polyomavirus, can be diagnosed by cytologic observation of characteristic IBs in avian renal samples (Figure 61.9). Glomerular changes associated with viral infections are usually undetectable because of the inconsistent presence of glomeruli in cytologic specimens. Certain strains of pigeon paramyxovirus-1 with renal tropism cause easily identifiable but nonspecific lymphoplasmacytic nephritis. Other infectious agents affecting the avian kidneys include some coccidia, cryptosporidia, and microsporidia. Renal coccidia most commonly affect young waterfowl, especially ducks and geese.[127] Coccidial and microsporidial cytology is detailed in the relevant sections "Respiratory Tract" and "Gastrointestinal Tract, Liver, and Pancreas." Fungal infections of the kidneys result from hematogenous spread (esp. *Candida* sp.) or, in birds, by extension of an air sac infection.

Diagnosis of gout requires finding needle-shaped empty spaces remaining after dissolution of urate crystals during staining, since uric acid is water soluble. Tophus lesions are characterized by the presence of washed out empty urate "needles," often accompanied by multinucleated giant cells, macrophages, and variable numbers of heterophils, lymphocytes, and/or fibrocytes. Renal amyloidosis is characterized by the presence of amorphous pink hyaline to fibrillary material interspersed between cells. If extensive, a minimal cellular component will be entrapped and compressed in dense pink foci of amyloid matrix.

Renal tumors have been documented in various reptile species, including adenocarcinomas (frequently in snakes but less commonly in lizards and chelonians), renal adenomas (in snakes and iguanas), and one case of a malignant nephroblastoma in a leopard gecko.[57]

Reproductive

Cytology samples from the reproductive tract are uncommon in reptiles and birds and can be collected as a fine-needle aspirate of an intracoelomic mass suspected to be associated with the reproductive tract. Physiological melanin deposition, or melanosis, is a common observation in the reproductive tract in certain avian taxa. Cloacal swabs represent excretions from the intestinal and urinary tract; however, unusual discharge from the cloaca can provide useful diagnostic information for the diagnosis of inflammatory conditions. Spermatozoa can be visible in cloacal swabs of males and females in many reptile and bird species, even in females without recent contact with a male, since viable spermatozoa in some reptiles can be stored for up to six years (Figure 61.41).[4] Testicular cytology has been evaluated as an alternative or adjunct to gross and histologic assessment of reproductive status in male

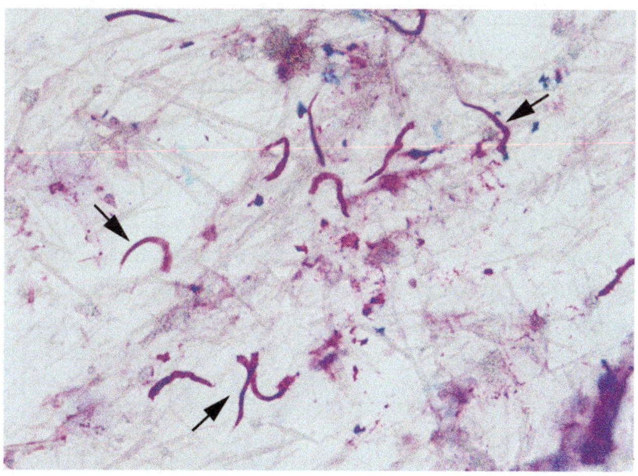

Figure 61.41 Needle-like urate crystals and spermatozoa (arrows) in a direct smear of the white portion of urine from a desert tortoise (*Gopherus agassizii*) (Diff-Quik, 1000×).

budgerigars and psittacines.[128,129] Sample quality was generally high, and results correlated reasonably well with histology with more rapid turnaround.

The most commonly encountered condition of the reproductive tract in reptile and bird patients is associated with folliculogenesis and disorders of egg laying in females, including egg retention, dystocia, and egg or follicle rupture. The latter can result in yolk coelomitis with characteristic gross and cytologic features. Reproductive tumors are common in lizards and snakes and include ovarian adenocarcinoma with or without metastasis, adenocarcinoma of the oviduct, a luteoma with concurrent adenocarcinoma in a green iguana (*Iguana iguana*), and granulosa cell tumors in snakes.[57] An adult spayed female green iguana (*Iguana iguana*) presenting with a history of distended coelom and weight loss had a palpable abdominal mass that was characterized cytologically by markedly pleomorphic oval to polygonal cells occurring in sheets with occasional acinar structures.[130] Concurrent mixed inflammation was noted. An epithelial neoplasm was diagnosed, with consideration given to ovarian origin because of the location, cytology, and concurrent hypercalcemia despite the history of ovarian salpingectomy. Exploratory celiotomy revealed a large mass arising from the area of the left ovary and a normal right ovary; histopathology was consistent with a malignant granulosa cell tumor. An undifferentiated tumor of the ovary in an intact female adult corn snake (*Elaphe guttata guttata*) presenting with anorexia and an abdominal mass was cytologically characterized by a highly pleomorphic population of spindloid to round to polygonal cells with marked anisocytosis and anisokaryosis.[131] Rare multinucleated cells and bizarre mitotic figures were also seen. Histologically, the neoplasm was considered a poorly differentiated ovarian neoplasm, and IHC was most consistent with epithelial origin. Seminomas have been reported in crocodiles, snakes, and lizards; interstitial cell tumors (Leydig cell) in snakes, lizards, and tortoises; and teratomas in lizards, snakes, and turtles.[57] A seminoma presented in a rock dove (*Columba livia*) as a coelomic mass that was cytologically characterized by many pleomorphic round to polygonal cells in dense clusters.[132] Cells contained variable amounts of basophilic vacuolated cytoplasm and a central round to oval nucleus with single large prominent nucleoli. Anisocytosis and anisokaryosis were moderate to marked.

Central Nervous System

Cerebrospinal fluid in reptiles and birds is rarely collected in a clinical setting but has been applied in research.[133] Inflammatory changes and infectious agents are readily detectable in histologic sections. Examples include polyomavirus inclusions in birds, IBD inclusions in boids, acanthamebiasis in snakes, and toxoplasmosis both in birds in reptiles.[4,23]

Body Cavity Fluids

Coelomic fluid of healthy reptiles and birds is scant and often impossible to collect. Coelomic washes are infrequently performed in reptiles. In birds, coelomocentesis can be indicated as part of the emergency treatment in patients with dyspnea. In contrast to most reptiles with one coelomic cavity containing the pericardium as the only separate compartment, birds reportedly have five compartments that are separated by several septae (post-hepatic septum, dorsal mesentery, oblique septum, parietal peritoneum).[3] A single median intestino-peritoneal cavity is flanked bilaterally and cranially by two large ventral hepato-peritoneal cavities and two small dorsal hepato-peritoneal cavities. Depending on the location of the lesion, effusions are confined to one or several of these compartments.

Coelomic fluid is evaluated as described for other species, including color, transparency, total solids, and cytologic evaluation of direct and concentrated smears with a leukocyte estimate and differential, morphologic evaluation of cellular detail, and screening for infectious agents especially in the presence of inflammation. Reference intervals for classification of effusions similar to mammals have not been reported for reptiles and birds.[134] Thus, results from effusion analysis (e.g. leukocyte count, total protein) from reptiles and birds should not be applied as in mammals in order to classify an effusion; however, careful comparisons may be appropriate, i.e. differentiation into low-protein transudate versus high-protein/high-cellularity effusions.[7]

Normal coelomic fluid is colorless or straw colored, clear, and of low cellularity, containing mononuclear phagocytes (macrophages, mesothelial cells) and possibly squamous or ciliated cuboidal or columnar epithelial cells from the air sacs in birds.[135] Low-protein transudates and high-protein/high-cellularity effusions appear to be most frequent in reptiles and birds.[7] Possible etiologies for low-protein transudates include conditions resulting in peripheral hypoalbuminemia such as renal or gastrointestinal protein loss. Protein-rich transudates can result from portal hypertension or right-sided heart failure in association with liver disease. Exudates can be associated with local or systemic infection. Careful evaluation for infectious agents is crucial. Hemorrhagic effusions have been associated with trauma, coagulopathies, or neoplasia (Figures 61.11 and 61.42).

Variably sized, pale to moderately basophilic yolk droplets can result from a pathologic condition in actively

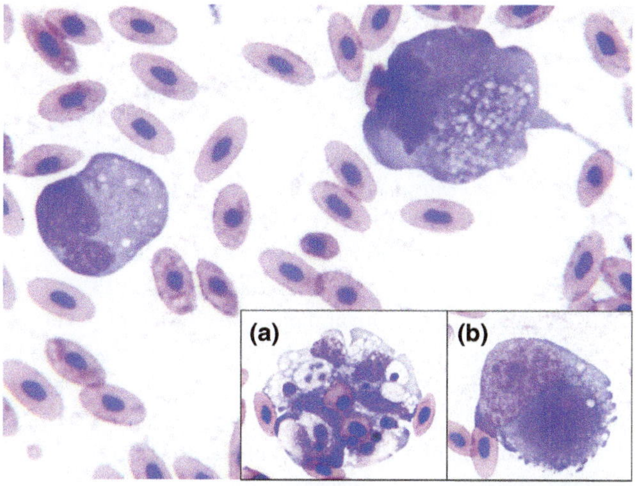

Figure 61.42 Direct smear of a peritoneal effusion in a helmeted guinea fowl (*Numida meleagris*) with mesothelioma that was confirmed by histopathology. The effusion had a PCV of 7% and was consistent with a hemoperitoneum. Cytologically, markedly atypical epithelial cells and mitotic figures were observed (Wright–Giemsa, 1000×). Insets (a) Macrophage with phagocytized erythrocytes and dark blue-black globular pigment suggestive of hemosiderin. (b) Markedly atypical mesothelial cell.

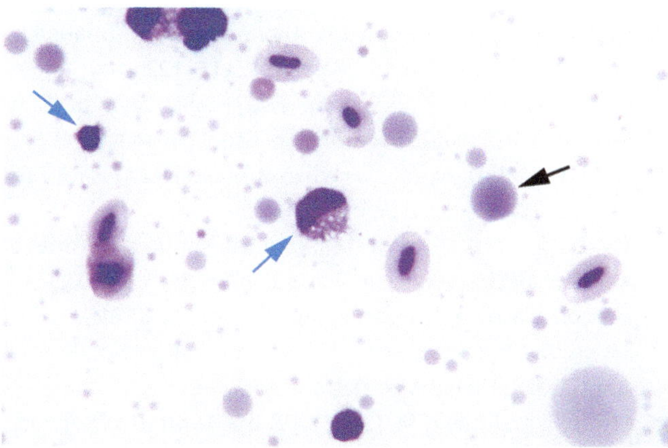

Figure 61.43 Direct smear of a peritoneal effusion in a cockatiel (*Nymphicus hollandicus*). Globular proteinaceous material (black arrows) and dense leukocytes (blue arrows) are consistent with yolk peritonitis (Wright–Giemsa, 500×).

reproductive female reptiles and birds during folliculogenesis. The inflammatory response depends on additional predisposing factors and is usually histiocytic with multinucleated giant cells, possibly heterophils, and variable amounts of globular yolk and lipid.[136] In birds, yolk coelomitis is confined to the intestino-peritoneal cavity (Figure 61.43). Careful evaluation for ascending bacterial infection from the cloaca through the oviduct is indicated and should be confirmed by culture.

Polyomavirus infection frequently results in increased vascular permeability, affecting mainly the pericardial and coelomic cavities. Peracute hemorrhage can especially affect pre-weaned neonates, resulting in various effects on the liver, kidney, central nervous system, and skin. Additionally, hydropericardium with serofibrinous polyserositis can be a sequela of adenovirus infection in *Galliformes*, *Columbiformes*, *Falconiformes*, *Psittaciformes*, and *Passeriformes*. As in mammals, differentiation of mesothelial hyperplasia and carcinoma often requires histopathology.

Conclusion

Cytology has evolved into a valuable diagnostic tool in reptile and bird medicine and is most helpful in the identification of various infectious agents and certain metabolic conditions unique to these species. Since cost effectiveness is often critical, cytology can provide guidance in the strategic selection of additional diagnostic testing such as special stains, culture techniques, targeted plasma chemistry, and/or molecular diagnostics. It is important to be familiar with the unique morphology of various leukocytes in these species to be able to accurately characterize inflammatory lesions in cytology samples. Given the increasing use of laparoscopy in reptile and bird patients, it is expected that cytology will become more and more common practice in clinical and research settings.

References

1 Shedlock, A.M., Botka, C.W., Zhao, S. et al. (2007). Phylogenomics of nonavian reptiles and the structure of the ancestral amniote genome. *Proc Natl Acad Sci U S A* 104: 2767–2772.

2 Campbell, T.W. (ed.) (2015). Cytology sampling techniques and evaluation. In: *Exotic Animal Hematology and Cytology*, 4e, 345–353. Ames, IA: Wiley.

3 Taylor, W.M. (2016). Pleura, pericardium, and peritoneum: the coelomic cavities of birds and their relationship to the lung-air sac system. In: *Current Veterinary Therapy in Avian Medicine*, 1e (ed. B.L. Speer), 345–362. St. Louis: Elsevier.

4 Divers, S.J. and Mader, D.R. (2005). *Reptile Medicine and Surgery*. Philadelphia: Saunders Elsevier.

5 Pendl, H., Wencel, P., and Beaufrère, H. (in press). Cytology. In: *Exotic Animal Emergency* (eds. J. Gladden and J. Graham). Hoboken, NJ: Wiley-Blackwell.

6 Campbell, T.W. (2007). Basics of cytology and fluid cytology. *Vet Clin North Am Exot Anim Pract* 10: 1–24, v.

7 Campbell, T.W. (2015). *Exotic Animal Hematology and Cytology*, 4e. Ames: Wiley.

8 Harmon, B.G. (1998). Avian heterophils in inflammation and disease resistance. *Poult Sci* 77: 972–977.

9 Mischke, R. (2005). *Zytologisches Praktikum für die Veterinärmedizin*. Hannover: Schlütersche Verlagsgesellschaft mbH & Co. KG.

10 Strik, N.I., Alleman, R., and Harr, K.E. (2007). Circulating inflammatory cells. In: *Infectious Diseases and Pathology of Reptiles*, 1e (ed. E.R. Jacobson), 167–218. Boca Raton: CRC Press.

11 Alleman, A.R., Jacobson, E.R., and Raskin, R.E. (1999). Morphologic, cytochemical staining, and ultrastructural characteristics of blood cells from eastern diamondback rattle snakes (*Crotalus adamanteus*). *Am J Vet Res* 60: 507–514.

12 Heard, D., Harr, K.E., and Wellehan, J.F. (2004). Diagnostic sampling and laboratory tests. In: *BSAVA Manual of Reptiles* (eds. S.J. Girling and P. Raiti), 71–86. Gloucester: British Small Animal Veterinary Association Ltd.

13 Stacy, B.A. and Pessier, A.P. (2007). Host response to infectious agents and identification of pathogens in tissue sections. In: *Infectious Diseases and Pathology of Reptiles: Color Atlas and Text* (ed. E.R. Jacobson), 257–297. Boca Raton: CRC Press.

14 Pass, D.A. (1989). The pathology of the avian integument: a review. *Avian Pathol* 18: 1–72.

15 Montali, R.J. (1988). Comparative pathology of inflammation in the higher vertebrates (reptiles, birds and mammals). *J Comp Pathol* 99: 1–26.

16 Stacy, N. and Pendl, H. (2016). Cytology. In: *Current Veterinary Therapy in Avian Medicine*, 1e (ed. B.L. Speer), 501–522. St. Louis, MO: Elsevier.

17 Allison, R.W. and Velguth, K.E. (2010). Appearance of granulated cells in blood films stained by automated aqueous versus methanolic Romanowsky methods. *Vet Clin Pathol* 39: 99–104.

18 Pendl, H. and Tizard, I. (2016). Immunology. In: *Current Veterinary Therapy in Avian Medicine and Surgery*, 1e (ed. B.L. Speer), 400–432. St. Louis, MO: Elsevier.

19 Maxwell, M.H. (1987). The avian eosinophil – a review. *World's Poult Sci J* 43: 190–207.

20 Fudge, A.M. and Joseph, V. (2000). Disorders of avian leukocytes. In: *Laboratory Medicine Avian and Exotic Pets* (ed. A.M. Fudge), 19–27. Philadelphia, PA: W.B. Saunders.

21 Seliger, C., Schaerer, B., Kohn, M. et al. (2012). A rapid high-precision flow cytometry based technique for total white blood cell counting in chickens. *Vet Immunol Immunopathol* 145: 86–99.

22 Mader, D.R., Conzelman, G.M. Jr., and Baggot, J.D. (1985). Effects of ambient temperature on the half-life and dosage regimen of amikacin in the gopher snake. *J Am Vet Med Assoc* 187: 1134–1136.

23 Schmidt, R.E., Reavill, D.R., and Phalen, D.N. (2015). *Pathology of Pet and Aviary Birds*, 2e. Ames: Wiley.

24 Jacobson, E.R. (2007). *Infectious Diseases and Pathology of Reptiles: Color Atlas and Text*. Boca Raton: CRC Press.

25 Hetzel, U., Sironen, T., Laurinmaki, P. et al. (2013). Isolation, identification, and characterization of novel arenaviruses, the etiological agents of boid inclusion body disease. *J Virol* 87: 10918–10935.

26 Gunn, R.G., Wamsley, H.L., and Alleman, A.R. (2007). Tissue imprint of a 10 year old female Hog Island Boa Constrictor (*Boa constrictor imperator*). *ASVCP Conference*, Savannah (10–14 November 2007), pp. 156–164.

27 Allender, M.C., Fry, M.M., Irizarry, A.R. et al. (2006). Intracytoplasmic inclusions in circulating leukocytes from an eastern box turtle (*Terrapene carolina carolina*) with iridoviral infection. *J Wildl Dis* 42: 677–684.

28 Wellehan, J.F. Jr., Strik, N.I., Stacy, B.A. et al. (2008). Characterization of an erythrocytic virus in the family Iridoviridae from a peninsula ribbon snake (*Thamnophis sauritus sackenii*). *Vet Microbiol* 131: 115–122.

29 Latimer, K.S. and Rakich, P.M. (2007). Avian cytology. *Vet Clin North Am Exot Anim Pract* 10: 131–154, vi.

30 Todd, D. (2004). Avian circovirus diseases: lessons for the study of PMWS. *Vet Microbiol* 98: 169–174.

31 Todd, D. (2000). Circoviruses: immunosuppressive threats to avian species: a review. *Avian Pathol* 29: 373–394.

32 Harcourt-Brown, N.H. and Chitty, J. (2005). *BSAVA Manual of Psittacine Birds*. Gloucester: British Small Animal Veterinary Association Ltd.

33 Chitty, J. and Lierz, M. (2008). *BSAVA Manual of Raptors, Pigeons and Passerine Birds*. Gloucester: British Small Animal Veterinary Association Ltd.

34 Beynon, P.H., Forbes, N.A., and Harcourt-Brown, N.H. (1996). *BSAVA Manual of Raptors, Pigeons and Waterfowl*. Gloucester: British Small Animal Veterinary Association Ltd.

35 Vereecken, M., de Herdt, P., and Ducatelle, R. (1998). Adenovirus infections in pigeons: a review. *Avian Pathol* 27: 333–338.

36 Tomaszewski, E.K. and Phalen, D.N. (2007). Falcon adenovirus in an American kestrel (*Falco sparverius*). *J Avian Med Surg* 21: 135–139.

37 Dean, J., Latimer, K.S., Oaks, J.L. et al. (2006). Falcon adenovirus infection in breeding Taita falcons (*Falco fasciinucha*). *J Vet Diagn Invest* 18: 282–286.

38 Hess, M. (2000). Detection and differentiation of avian adenoviruses: a review. *Avian Pathol* 29: 195–206.

39 Oaks, J.L., Schrenzel, M., Rideout, B., and Sandfort, C. (2005). Isolation and epidemiology of falcon adenovirus. *J Clin Microbiol* 43: 3414–3420.

40 Lazic, T., Ackermann, M.R., Drahos, J.M. et al. (2008). Respiratory herpesvirus infection in two Indian Ringneck parakeets. *J Vet Diagn Invest* 20: 235–238.

41 Shivaprasad, H.L. and Phalen, D.N. (2012). A novel herpesvirus associated with respiratory disease in Bourke's parrots (*Neopsephotus bourkii*). *Avian Pathol* 41: 531–539.

42 Wellehan, J.F., Gagea, M., Smith, D.A. et al. (2003). Characterization of a herpesvirus associated with tracheitis in Gouldian finches (*Erythrura [Chloebia] gouldiae*). *J Clin Microbiol* 41: 4054–4057.

43 Barao Da Cunha, M., Correia, J.J., Fagulha, T. et al. (2007). Pacheco's parrot disease in macaws of the Lisbon's Zoological Garden. Description of an outbreak, diagnosis and management, including vaccination. *Dtsch Tierarztl Wochenschr* 114: 423–428.

44 Magnino, S., Conzo, G., Fioretti, A. et al. (1996). An outbreak of Pacheco's parrot disease in psittacine birds recently imported to Campania, Italy: isolation of psittacid herpesvirus 2. *Zentralbl Veterinarmed B* 43: 631–637.

45 Sandhu, T.S. and Shawky, S.A. (2003). Duck virus enteritis (duck plague). In: *Diseases of Poultry*, 11e (ed. Y.M. Saif), 354–363. Ames: Iowa State Press Blackwell.

46 Paulman, A., Lichtensteiger, C.A., and Kohrt, L.J. (2006). Outbreak of herpesviral conjunctivitis and respiratory disease in gouldian finches. *Vet Pathol* 43: 963–970.

47 Heenemann, K., Sieg, M., Rueckner, A. et al. (2015). Complete genome sequence of a novel avian polyomavirus isolated from Gouldian finch. *Genome Announc* 3: e01001-15.

48 Johne, R. and Muller, H. (2007). Polyomaviruses of birds: etiologic agents of inflammatory diseases in a tumor virus family. *J Virol* 81: 11554–11559.

49 Varsani, A., Porzig, E.L., Jennings, S. et al. (2015). Identification of an avian polyomavirus associated with Adelie penguins (*Pygoscelis adeliae*). *J Gen Virol* 96: 851–857.

50 Jacobson, E.R., Cheatwood, J.L., and Maxwell, L.K. (2000). Mycotic diseases of reptiles. *Semin Avian Exotic Pet Med* 9: 94–101.

51 Mycoses, B.L. (1994). *Avian Medicine: Principles and Application*. Lake Worth, FL: Wingers.

52 Flammer, K. and Orosz, S. (2008). Avian mycoses: managing these difficult diseases. *Proceedings of the 29th Annual Conference & Expo of the Association of the Avian Veterinarians*, Savannah, GA (11–14 August 2008).

53 Valkiunas, G. (2004). *Avian Malaria Parasites and Other Haemosporidia*. CRC press.

54 Gardiner, C.H., Fayer, R., and Dubey, J.P. (1988). *An Atlas of Protozoan Parasites in Animal Tissues*, 83. Washington, DC: U.S. Department of Agriculture.

55 Greiner, E.C. and Ritchie, B.W. (1994). Parasites. In: *Avian Medicine: Principles and Application* (eds. B.W. Ritchie, G.J. Harrison and L.R. Harrison), 1007–1029. Lake Worth, FL: Wingers.

56 Gosselin, S.J. and Kramer, L.W. (1983). Pathophysiology of excessive iron storage in mynah birds. *J Am Vet Med Assoc* 183: 1238–1240.

57 Garner, M.M., Hernandez-Divers, S.M., and Raymond, J.T. (2004). Reptile neoplasia: a retrospective study of case submissions to a specialty diagnostic service. *Vet Clin North Am Exot Anim Pract* 7: 653–671.

58 Zehnder, A., Graham, J., Reavill, D.R., and Reavill, D.R. (2016). Neoplastic diseases in avian species. In: *Current Veterinary Therapy in Avian Medicine and Surgery*, 1e (ed. B.L. Speer), 107–142. St. Louis, MO: Elsevier.

59 Heckers, K.O., Aupperle, H., Schmidt, V., and Pees, M. (2012). Melanophoromas and iridophoromas in reptiles. *J Comp Pathol* 146: 258–268.

60 Irizarry-Rovira, A.R., Wolf, A., and Ramos-Vara, J.A. (2006). Cutaneous melanophoroma in a green iguana (*Iguana iguana*). *Vet Clin Pathol* 35: 101–105.

61 Irizarry-Rovira, A.R., Lennox, A.M., and Ramos-Vara, J.A. (2007). Malignant melanoma in a zebra finch (*Taeniopygia guttata*): cytologic, histologic, and ultrastructural characteristics. *Vet Clin Pathol* 36: 297–301.

62 Goldberg, S. (1919). The differential features between melanosis and melanosarcoma. Part I. *J Am Vet Med Assoc* 56: 140–153.

63 Leissinger, M.K., McCauley, C., Fowlkes, N., and Grasperge, B.J. (2017). What is your diagnosis? Nasal lesion in a horse. *Vet Clin Pathol* 46: 361–362.

64 Raskin, R.E. and Meyer, D. (2015). *Canine and Feline Cytology: A Color Atlas and Interpretation Guide*. St Louis, MO: Elsevier Health Sciences.

65 Bennett, P.C., Schmidt, L., Lawen, A. et al. (2002). Cyclosporin A, FK506 and rapamycin produce multiple, temporally distinct, effects on memory following single-trial, passive avoidance training in the chick. *Brain Res* 927: 180–194.

66 Cowell, T.W., Tyler, D.R., Meinkoth, J.H. et al. (2008). *Diagnostic Cytology and Hematology of the Dog and the Cat*, 3e. St. Louis, MO: Mosby Elsevier.

67 Jacobson, E.R. (ed.) (2007). Overview of reptile biology, anatomy, and histology. In: *Infectious Diseases and Pathology of Reptiles: Color Atlas and Text*, 1–130. Boca Raton: CRC Press.

68 Nickel, R., Schummer, A., and Seiferle, E. (1977). *Anatomy of the Domestic Birds*. Berlin, Hamburg: Verlag Paul Parey.

69 Lucas, A.M. and Stettenheim, P.R. (1972). *Avian Anatomy: Integument*, vol. 2. Washington, DC: U.S. Agricultural Research Service.

70 Salibian, A. and Montalti, D. (2009). Physiological and biochemical aspects of the avian uropygial gland. *Braz J Biol* 69: 437–446.

71 Monks, D.J., Zsivanovits, H.P., Cooper, J.E., and Forbes, N.A. (2006). Successful treatment of tracheal xanthogranulomatosis in a red-tailed hawk (*Buteo jamaicensis*) by tracheal resection and anastomosis. *J Avian Med Surg* 20: 247–252.

72 Palmieri, C., Anthenill, L., and Shivaprasad, H.L. (2015). Cutaneous mucinosis in a strain of brown-egg laying chickens. *Vet Pathol* 52: 351–355.

73 Pontes de Carvalho, L.C., Templeman, J., Wick, G., and Roitt, I.M. (1982). The role of self-antigen in the development of autoimmunity in obese strain chickens with spontaneous autoallergic thyroiditis. *J Exp Med* 155: 1255–1266.

74 Cole, R.K., Kite, J.H. Jr., Wick, G., and Witebsky, E. (1970). Recent advances in avian endocrinology. 2. Inherited autoimmune thyroiditis in the fowl. *Poult Sci* 49: 839–848.

75 Le Donne, V., Crossland, N., Brandao, J. et al. (2016). *Nannizziopsis guarroi* infection in 2 inland bearded dragons (*Pogona vitticeps*): clinical, cytologic, histologic, and ultrastructural aspects. *Vet Clin Pathol* 45: 368–375.

76 Burgmann, P.M. (1995). Common psittacine dermatologic diseases. *Semin Avian Exotic Pet Med* 4: 169–183.

77 Doneley, R.J. (2009). Bacterial and parasitic diseases of parrots. *Vet Clin North Am Exot Anim Pract* 12: 417–432.

78 Coutteel, P. and Wencel, P. (2016). Parasitic diseases. In: *Avian Medicine*, 3e (ed. J. Samour), 507–521. St. Louis: Elsevier.

79 Rousselet, E., De Mello Souza, C.H., Wellehan, J.F. et al. (2017). Cutaneous iridophoroma in a Green iguana (Iguana iguana). *Vet Clin Pathol* 46: 625–628.

80 Kollias, G.V., Homer, B., and Thompson, J.P. (1992). Cutaneous pseudolymphoma in a juvenile blue and gold macaw (*Ara ararauna*). *J Zoo Wildl Med* 23: 235–240.

81 Rivera, S., McClearen, J.R., and Reavill, D.R. (2009). Treatment of nonepitheliotropic cutaneous B-cell lymphoma in an umbrella cockatoo (*Cacatua alba*). *J Avian Med Surg* 23: 294–302.

82 Dallwig, R.K., Whittington, J.K., Terio, K., and Barger, A. (2012). Cutaneous mast cell tumor and mastocytosis in a black-masked lovebird (*Agapornis personata*). *J Avian Med Surg* 26: 29–35.

83 Santoro, M., Stacy, B.A., Morales, J.A. et al. (2008). Mast cell tumour in a giant Galapagos tortoise (*Geochelone nigra vicina*). *J Comp Pathol* 138: 156–159.

84 Schumacher, J., Bennett, R.A., Fox, L.E. et al. (1998). Mast cell tumor in an eastern kingsnake (*Lampropeltis getulus getulus*). *J Vet Diagn Invest* 10: 101–104.

85 Swayne, D.E. and Weisbrode, S.E. (1990). Cutaneous mast cell tumor in a great horned owl (*Bubo virginianus*). *Vet Pathol* 27: 124–126.

86 Phalen, D.N., Logan, K.S., and Snowden, K.F. (2006). *Encephalitozoon hellem* infection as the cause of a unilateral chronic keratoconjunctivitis in an umbrella cockatoo (*Cacatua alba*). *Vet Opthalmol* 9: 59–63.

87 Allgoewer, I., Gobel, T., Stockhaus, C., and Schaeffer, E.H. (2002). Dacryops in a red-eared slider (*Chrysemys scripta elegans*): case report. *Vet Ophthalmol* 5: 231–234.

88 Watson, V.E., Murdock, J.H., Cazzini, P. et al. (2013). Retrobulbar adenocarcinoma in an Amazon parrot (*Amazona autumnalis*). *J Vet Diagn Invest* 25: 273–276.

89 Houck, E.L., Keller, K.A., Hawkins, M.G. et al. (2016). Bilateral aural adenocarcinoma in a Congo African grey parrot (*Psittacus erithacus erithacus*). *J Avian Med Surg* 30: 257–262.

90 Alexander, A.B., Griffin, L., and Johnston, M.S. (2016). Radiation therapy of periorbital lymphoma in a Blue-and-Gold Macaw (*Ara ararauna*). *J Avian Med Surg* 31: 39–46.

91 Fiddis, R.W., Vlachos, N., and Calvert, P.D. (1983). Studies of urate crystallisation in relation to gout. *Ann Rheum Dis* 42 (Suppl 1): 12–15.

92 Speer, B.L. (1997). *Diseases of the Urogenital System. Avian Medicine and Surgery*, 625–644. Philadelphia: W.B. Saunders.

93 Alleman, A.R. and Kupprion, E.K. (2007). Cytologic diagnosis of diseases in reptiles. *Vet Clin North Am Exot Anim Pract* 10: 155–186.

94 Casimire-Etzioni, A.L., Wellehan, J.F., Embury, J.E. et al. (2004). Synovial fluid from an African spur-thighed tortoise (*Geochelone sulcata*). *Vet Clin Pathol* 33: 43–46.

95 Olias, P., Gruber, A.D., Kohls, A. et al. (2010). Sarcocystis species lethal for domestic pigeons. *Emerg Infect Dis* 16: 497–499.

96 Page, C.D., Schmidt, R.E., English, J.H. et al. (1992). Antemortem diagnosis and treatment of sarcocystosis in two species of psittacines. *J Zoo Wildl Med* 23: 77–85.

97 Olias, P., Wegelin, M., Zenker, W. et al. (2011). Avian malaria deaths in parrots, Europe. *Emerg Infect Dis* 17: 950–952.

98 Valkiunas, G. and Iezhova, T.A. (2017). Exo-erythrocytic development of avian malaria and related haemosporidian parasites. *Malar J* 16: 101.

99 Maluenda, A.C., Casagrande, R.A., Kanamura, C.T. et al. (2010). Rhabdomyosarcoma in a yellow-headed caracara (*Milvago chimachima*). *Avian Dis* 54: 951–954.

100 Carvalho, M.P., Fernandes, N.C., Nemer, V.C. et al. (2016). Benign peripheral nerve sheath tumor in a wild Toco Toucan (*Ramphastos toco*). *J Avian Med Surg* 30: 280–285.

101 Webb, K.L., Grindem, C., and Dombrowski, D.S. (2015). What is your diagnosis? A soft tissue mass in a Black Rat Snake. *Vet Clin Pathol* 44: 611–612.

102 De Luca Bossa, L.M., Mennonna, G., Meomartino, L. et al. (2015). Polyostotic chondroblastic osteosarcoma in a kestrel (*Falco tinnunculus*). *J Avian Med Surg* 29: 336–339.

103 Crespo, R., Stirtzinger, T., and Hunter, D.B. (1998). Evaluation of different procedures for processing avian air sac lavage fluid. *Avian Dis* 42: 20–27.

104 Lafortune, M., Gobel, T., Jacobson, E. et al. (2005). Respiratory bronchoscopy of subadult American alligators (*Alligator mississippiensis*) and tracheal wash evaluation. *J Zoo Wildl Med* 36: 12–20.

105 DeMay, R.M. (2012). *The Art and Science of Cytopathology*, 211. Chicago: ASCP Press.

106 Donnelly, K., Wellehan, J., and Quesenberry, K.E. (2017). *Gastrointestinal Disease Associated with Non-Albicans Candida Species in Birds*. Dallas, TX: AAZV.

107 Proenca, L.M., Mayer, J., Schnellbacher, R. et al. (2014). Antemortem diagnosis and successful treatment of pulmonary candidiasis in a sun conure (*Aratinga solstitialis*). *J Avian Med Surg* 28: 316–321.

108 Michael, H.T., Willette, M., and Sharkey, L. (2010). What is your diagnosis? Choanal swab from a young Gyrfalcon. *Vet Clin Pathol* 39: 511–512.

109 Latimer, K.S., Goodwin, M.A., and Davis, M.K. (1988). Rapid cytologic diagnosis of respiratory cryptosporidiosis in chickens. *Avian Dis* 32: 826–830.

110 Bigland, C.H., Liu, S.-K., and Perry, M.L. (1964). Five cases of Serratospiculum amaculata (*Nematoda*: Filarioidea) infection in prairie falcons (*Falco mexicanus*). *Avian Dis* 8: 412–419.

111 Ackerman, N., Isaza, R., Greiner, E. et al. (1992). Pneumocoelom associated with Serratospiculum amaculata in a bald eagle. *Vet Rad Ultras* 33: 351–355.

112 Baine, K., Nobrega-Lee, M., Jones, M.P. et al. (2014). Branchial cyst with carcinoma in an umbrella cockatoo (*Cacatua alba*). *J Avian Med Surg* 28: 232–239.

113 Olah, I., Nagy, N., and Vervelde, L. (2014). Structure of the avian lymphoid system. In: *Avian Immunology* (eds. K. Schat, B. Kaspers and P. Kaiser), 11–44. Boston, MA: Academic Press.

114 König, H.E. and Liebich, H.G. (2001). *Anatomie und Propädeutik des Geflügels: Lehrbuch und Farbatlas für Studium und Praxis*. Stuttgart: Schattauer.

115 Randall, C. and Reece, R.L. (1996). *Color Atlas of Avian Histopathology*. Baltimore, MD: Mosby-Wolfe.

116 Löliger, H.C. (1992). Aviäre Onkovirosen. In: *Krankheiten des Wirtschaftsgeflügels Ein Handbuch für Wissenschaft und Praxis Band 1: Allgemeiner Teil und spezieller Teil 1. 1* (eds. G. Heider, M. Gerhard and M. Janos), 742–743. Jena, Stuttgart: Fischer.

117 Evans, E.E., Wade, L.L., and Flammer, K. (2008). Administration of doxycycline in drinking water for treatment of spiral bacterial infection in cockatiels. *J Am Vet Med Assoc* 232: 389–393.

118 Tudor, D.C. (1991). *Pigeon Health and Disease*, 189. Ames, IA: Iowa State University Press.

119 Wang, L., Li, J., Li, J. Jr. et al. (2016). Identification of the Paneth cells in chicken small intestine. *Poult Sci* 95: 1631–1635.

120 Sedacca, C.D., Campbell, T.W., Bright, J.M. et al. (2009). Chronic cor pulmonale secondary to pulmonary atherosclerosis in an African Grey parrot. *J Am Vet Med Assoc* 234: 1055–1059.

121 Donnelly, K., Waltzek, T.B., Wellehan, J.F. Jr. et al. (2016). Mycobacterium haemophilum infection in a juvenile leatherback sea turtle (*Dermochelys coriacea*). *J Vet Diagn Invest* 28: 718–721.

122 Jacobson, E.R., Green, D.E., Undeen, A.H. et al. (1998). Systemic microsporidiosis in inland bearded dragons (*Pogona vitticeps*). *J Zoo Wildl Med* 29: 315–323.

123 Ollé, R.D. (2006). The glycogen body in neonate birds of the order psittaciformes and its role in neonate mortality. Doctoral thesis. Justus-Liebig-Universität Giessen.

124 Harr, K.E. (2002). Clinical chemistry of companion avian species: a review. *Vet Clin Pathol* 31: 140–151.

125 Gonçalves, G.A.M. and Salgado, B.S. (2012). Post-mortem lesions of urolithiasis in a lesser seed finch (*Sporophila angolensis*). *Acta Vet Bras* 6: 52–55.

126 Styles, D.K. and Phalen, D.N. (1998). Clinical avian urology. *Semin Avian Exotic Pet Med* 7: 104–113.

127 Gajadhar, A.A., Wobeser, G., and Stockdale, P.H.G. (1983). Coccidia of domestic and wild waterfowl (*Anseriformes*). *Can J Zool* 61: 1–24.

128 Hanse, M., Krautwald-Junghanns, M.E., Reitemeier, S. et al. (2013). Testicular biopsy in psittacine birds (*Psittaciformes*): comparative evaluation of testicular reproductive status by endoscopic, histologic, and cytologic examination. *J Avian Med Surg* 27: 247–257.

129 Hanse, M., Schmidt, V., Schneider, S. et al. (2008). Comparative examination of testicular biopsy samples and influence on semen characteristics in budgerigars

(*Melopsittacus undulatus*). *J Avian Med Surg* 22: 300–309.

130 Cardona, J.A.C., Conley, K.J., Wellehan, J.F. Jr. et al. (2011). Incomplete ovariosalpingectomy and subsequent malignant granulosa cell tumor in a female green iguana (*Iguana iguana*). *J Am Vet Med Assoc* 239: 237–242.

131 Petterino, C., Bedin, M., Podesta, G. et al. (2006). Undifferentiated tumor in the ovary of a corn snake (*Elaphe guttata guttata*). *Vet Clin Pathol* 35: 95–100.

132 Bedard, C., Lair, S., and Langlois, I. (2007). What is your diagnosis? Coelomic mass in a rock dove (*Columba livia*). *Vet Clin Pathol* 36: 303–305.

133 Anderson, D.K. and Hazelwood, R.L. (1969). Chicken cerebrospinal fluid: normal composition and response to insulin administration. *J Physiol* 202: 83–95.

134 Baker, R. and Lumsden, J.H. (2000). *Color Atlas of Cytology of the Dog and Cat*. St. Louis, MO: Mosby.

135 Rush, E.M., Wernick, M., Beaufrère, H. et al. (2016). Advances in clinical pathology and diagnostic medicine. In: *Current Therapy in Avian Medicine and Surgery* (ed. B.L. Speer), 461–530. St. Louis, MO: Elsevier.

136 Caruso, K., Cowell, R., Meinkoth, J. et al. (2002). Abdominal effusion in a bird [egg yolk peritonitis]. *Vet Clin Pathol* 31: 127–128.

62

Amphibians

Allan P. Pessier

Introduction and Clinical Settings

The amphibians are a diverse vertebrate class with over 7500 described species divided into the orders Anura (frogs and toads), Caudata (newts and salamanders), and Gymniophona (caecilians). The Anura are the largest group and the most likely to be encountered by veterinarians, followed by the caudates. The caecilians are a limbless and mostly fossorial (underground-dwelling) group of animals that are rarely maintained in captivity. Amphibians such as the African clawed frogs (*Xenopus laevis* and *Xenopus tropicalis*) and axolotls (*Ambystoma mexicanum*) are common laboratory animals for studies in embryology, genomics, neurobiology, limb regeneration, and other biological investigations. Other amphibians are found in zoos for education and conservation breeding. Drastic population declines of wild amphibians termed the "Amphibian Extinction Crisis" have increased demand for veterinary involvement in field conservation programs. Other amphibians such as the poison dart frogs (usually *Dendrobates* sp.), White's tree frogs (*Litoria caerulea*), and dwarf African clawed frogs (*Hymenochirus* sp.) are common in the pet trade. Finally, the American bullfrog (*Lithobates catesbeianus*) is farmed for use as a specialty food animal.

Applications of Cytology and Collection Methods

The most common clinical samples from amphibian patients relate to the integumentary system and include skin scrapings, impression smears of ulcers, and aspirates of cutaneous masses. Subcutaneous edema and coelomic cavitary effusions are common clinical problems and another frequent source of diagnostic submissions. Less frequent samples include aspirates and impression smears of visceral organs obtained clinically or at necropsy and review of peripheral blood smears. Comprehensive reviews of amphibian hematology and clinical pathology contain information that will facilitate evaluation of cytology samples and contextual interpretation.[1] In contrast to reptiles (Chapter 61), amphibians have myeloperoxidase-positive neutrophils with multilobed nuclei and fine to indistinct cytoplasmic granules in blood smears and cytologic preparations. Amphibian eosinophils, basophils, lymphocytes, and thrombocytes are morphologically similar to other species. Erythrocytes are usually nucleated, but varying numbers of anucleate cells are seen in plethodontid (lungless) salamanders.

Methods for obtaining samples of cutaneous lesions are similar to those for other species (Chapter 1).[2] Wet-mount examination of skin scrapings such as those used commonly in fish medicine (Chapter 63) is useful for rapid detection of cutaneous parasites and some fungal infections.[3,4] Sheets of shedding skin collected from the animal or the environment are helpful samples for screening for cutaneous fungal infections such as chytridiomycosis (Figure 62.1). The samples are flattened onto glass slides and examined as wet mounts or air-dried prior to routine cytologic staining.[4]

Systems

Skin and Subcutis

Unlike other vertebrates, the skin of amphibians is important for water absorption, electrolyte balance, and, in some species, respiration.[5] Therefore, cutaneous injury and responses to injury (e.g. epidermal hyperplasia) that would have minimal physiologic importance to a mammal or reptile are often very significant to amphibians, especially in terms of osmoregulation.[6] Structurally, the epidermis is thin with minimal keratinization and lacks protective

Veterinary Cytology, First Edition. Edited by Leslie C. Sharkey, M. Judith Radin, and Davis Seelig.

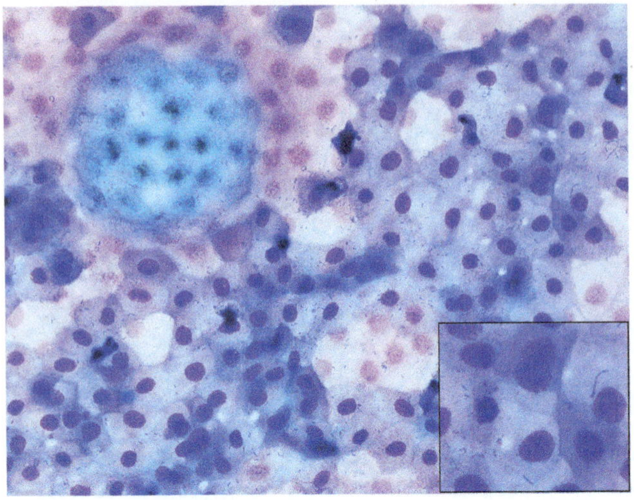

Figure 62.1 A sheet of normal shedding skin from a mountain yellow-legged frog. There are numerous polygonal keratinocytes with variably staining nuclei (Diff-Quik, 200×). Inset: Higher magnification shows bacteria admixed with keratinocytes (Diff-Quik, 1000×).

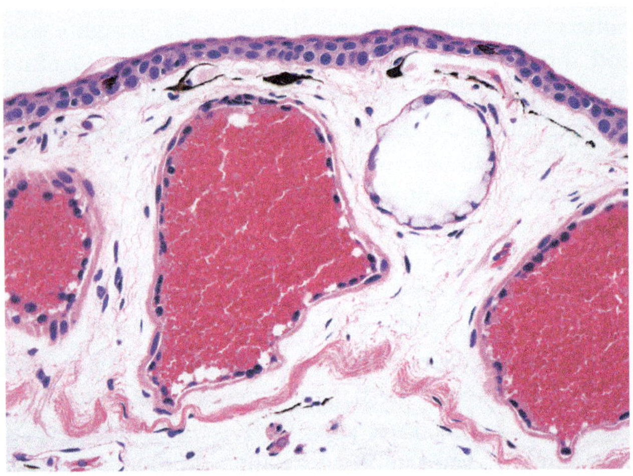

Figure 62.2 A histologic section of normal skin from a White's tree frog. The epidermis (top) is thin with a single, almost imperceptible, keratinized layer. The dermis contains superficial pigmented melanophores, large granular glands with myriad eosinophilic granules, and smaller mucous glands (Hematoxylin & Eosin, 100×).

structures such as hair or scales (Figure 62.2). Within the dermis there are mucous glands that protect against excessive evaporative water loss and granular glands that secrete antimicrobial peptides. In anurans the skin is separated from the underlying body by large subcutaneous lymphatic sacs that have functions related to fluid homeostasis.

Infectious and Inflammatory Conditions

The skin of amphibians hosts diverse bacterial populations that, under normal conditions and proportions, function as part of the innate immune system.[7] As a result, small numbers of mixed and predominantly Gram-negative bacteria are commonly observed in the background of integumentary cytology samples (Figure 62.1 inset). Cutaneous ulcers resulting from trauma, cutaneous fungal infections, viral infections (e.g. ranaviriosis), systemic bacterial infections ("red leg syndrome"), or parasitism are frequently sampled by clinicians. Cytologic findings include neutrophilic and histiocytic inflammation with intracellular bacteria. It can be difficult to distinguish between primary and secondary bacterial infections because many common bacterial isolates are ubiquitous in aquatic environments and readily colonize ulcers or systemically infect animals debilitated by other conditions. For instance, *Aeromonas hydrophila*, classically associated with bacterial "red leg syndrome" in amphibians, is often isolated in pure culture from frogs with ranaviriosis.[8–10] Cutaneous abscesses caused by "atypical" *Brucella* sp. infections such as *Brucella inopinata* are increasingly recognized in anurans, and small Gram-negative coccobacilli are observed cytologically in the exudate of some cases.[11]

Mycobacteriosis associated with *Mycobacterium marinum*, *Mycobacterium chelonae*, *Mycobacterium fortuitum*, and *Mycobacterium liflandii*, among others, is a frequent cause of cutaneous granulomas, abscesses, and cellulitis in captive amphibians.[4,12,13] In stained aspirates and impression smears, there are abundant macrophages with variable numbers of neutrophils and eosinophils. Multinucleated giant cells and epithelioid macrophages are rare, and these infections have been mistaken for round cell neoplasms.[13] Negative staining of intracytoplasmic and extracellular bacilli in routinely stained slides can suggest the diagnosis in cases that have high numbers of organisms (Figure 62.3). Organisms are variably Gram-positive and acid-fast stain

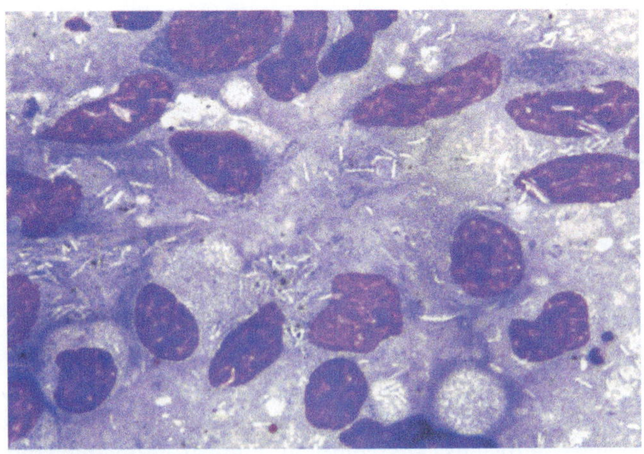

Figure 62.3 Mycobacteriosis. Impression smear from a cutaneous nodule in a Houston toad. There are macrophages with intracytoplasmic negative-staining bacilli. *M. chelonae* was isolated from this lesion (Wright-Giemsa, 1000×).

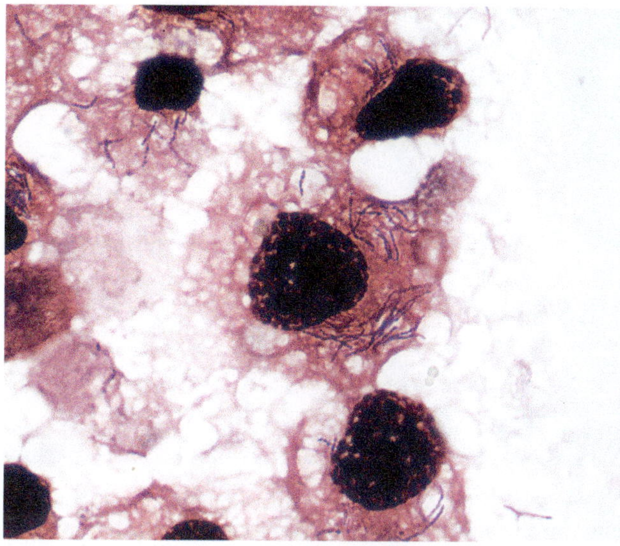

Figure 62.4 Mycobacteriosis. Coelomic fluid from a San Marcos salamander (*Eurycea nana*). Macrophages contain numerous beaded and filamentous Gram-positive bacilli (Gram stain, 1000×).

positive with morphology that ranges from short bacilli to long beaded filamentous bacilli (Figure 62.4).

Fungal and water mold infections of the skin are common in captive amphibians as secondary opportunistic pathogens associated with skin trauma or suboptimal husbandry (e.g. problems with water quality such as elevated environmental ammonia).[4,6] Oomycete water molds, usually from the genus *Saprolegnia,* appear clinically as white, gray, or brown tufts of cottony mycelia on skin surfaces or tadpole mouthparts. On wet-mount or cytologic examination, hyphae are thin walled and infrequently branching with rounded ends (Figure 62.5). Associated inflammatory cells are rare even with infections known to be present for several days. Infections with pigmented (dematiaceous) fungi like *Cladosporium*, *Phialophora*, and *Fonsecaea* cause ulcerative or nodular skin lesions of chromomycosis and phaeohyphomycosis.[6,14] Touch preparations and aspirates contain granulomatous inflammation, often with prominent multinucleated giant cells and fewer neutrophils, eosinophils, and lymphoid cells. Fungal elements are pigmented light brown to blue-green. In cases of chromomycosis, there are distinctive, 10–15 µm in diameter, spherical to oval, internally septate sclerotic bodies that can appear with or without septate hyphae. In phaeohyphomycosis, only hyphae are present. Mucormycosis caused by *Mucor amphibiorum* is associated with granulomatous inflammation similar to that observed with the dematiaceous fungi, but lesions contain 5–40 µm in diameter endosporulating spherules that vaguely resemble *Coccidioides immitis* or algae such as *Prototheca* sp.[15] Infections with other non-pigmented and non-endosporulating fungi in genera such as *Mucor*, *Rhizopus*, and *Fusarium*, among others, can be observed as hyphae in cytologic preparations (Figure 62.6).

Cutaneous chytridiomycosis caused by the zoosporic fungi *Batrachochytrium dendrobatidis* (Bd) or *Batrachochytrium salamandrivorans* (Bsal) is an emerging infectious disease implicated in catastrophic population declines of free-ranging amphibians and mortality events in captive animals. Infections with Bd are proliferative with epidermal hyperplasia and hyperkeratosis, whereas lesions associated with Bsal are necrotizing and ulcerative.[16] Wet mounts or traditional cytologic examination of shed skin fragments or skin scrapings is useful for rapid diagnosis of chytridiomycosis by identification of single or multiple spherical thalli within

Figure 62.5 Saprolegniasis. Skin scraping from a Kaiser newt. There is a dense mat of thin-walled hyphae with rounded ends typical of oomycete water molds (Wet mount stained with new methylene blue, 1000×).

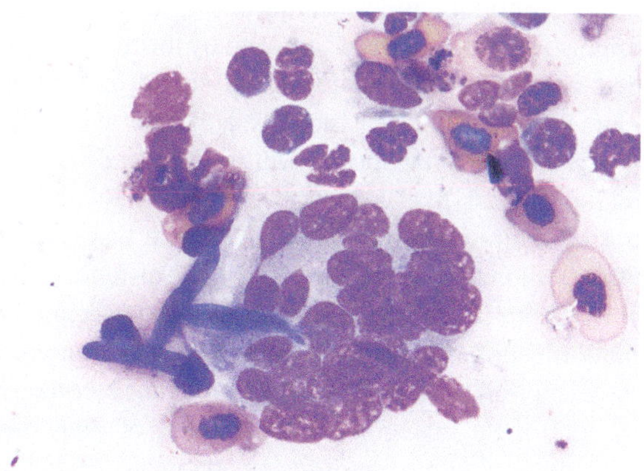

Figure 62.6 Unidentified cutaneous fungal infection. Skin scraping from a Wyoming toad. A multinucleated giant cell partially surrounds branching septate fungal hyphae (Wright-Giemsa, 1000×).

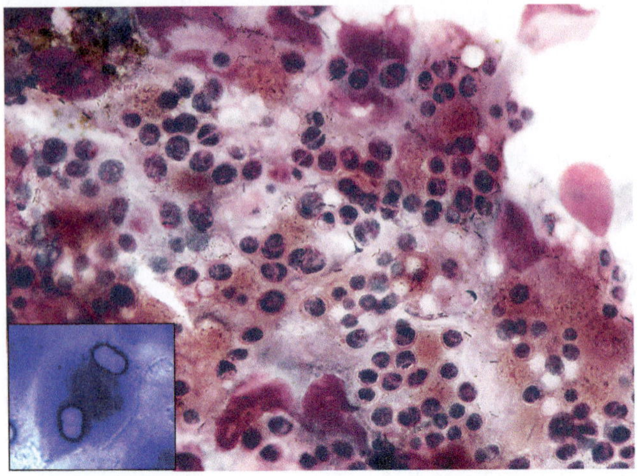

Figure 62.7 Chytridiomycosis caused by *B. dendrobatidis*. A sheet of shedding skin from a mountain yellow-legged frog (compare to Figure 62.1). Keratinocytes have spherical intracytoplasmic fungal thalli. Many thalli have evidence of fine internal septation (colonial thalli) characteristic of *Batrachochytrium* spp. fungi (Diff-Quik, 1000×). Inset: two colonial thalli within the cytoplasm of a keratinocyte in a spotted newt. These are empty thalli that have previously discharged zoospores (new methylene blue stain, 1000×).

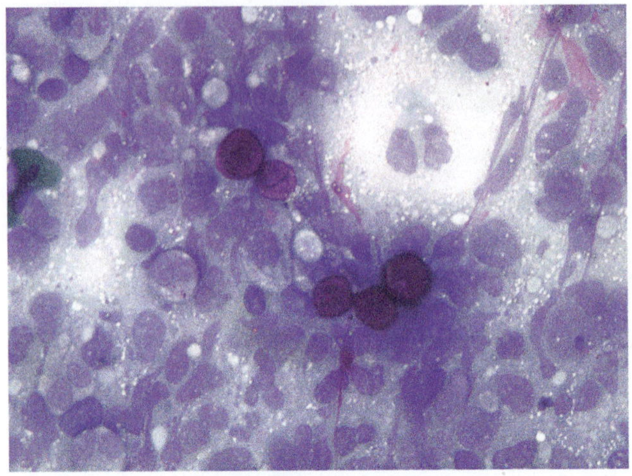

Figure 62.8 Infection with *Amphibiocystidium* spp. Aspirate of a cutaneous nodule in a marine toad. Macrophages and fewer neutrophils surround spherical endospores (Diff-Quik, 1000×).

keratinocyte cytoplasm (Figure 62.7). Extracellular thalli occur in poorly preserved samples or samples from necrotizing lesions of Bsal chytridiomycosis. Staining of wet-mount preparations with new methylene blue, lactophenol cotton blue, or Congo red is helpful in discerning fine details in thalli.[17–19] Multiple developmental stages of thalli are observed, ranging from small 3 to 5 μm wide bodies with thin lightly staining walls to mature zoosporangia up to 20 μm wide that contain discrete 1–2 μm basophilic zoospores. Empty thalli that have previously discharged zoospores are very common in clinical samples.[20,21] Chytrid thalli are distinguished from yeasts or protozoa by forms (colonial thalli) that are internally subdivided by single or multiple thin septa (Figure 62.7). Occasionally, a discharge tube that exits the keratinocyte cytoplasm will be observed that gives the thallus a "flask-like" appearance. Thalli of Bd and Bsal cannot be definitively differentiated on the basis of cytologic examination; however, the thalli of Bsal tend to be larger with greater numbers of colonial thalli. Associated inflammation is not a prominent feature of chytridiomycosis with the exception of cases that have significant secondary bacterial or fungal infections. Confirmation of diagnoses from examination of wet mounts or cytologic preparations is commonly obtained by real-time polymerase chain reaction assays for Bd or Bsal, which is also used to distinguish between these chytrid fungal species.

Infections with mesomycetozoal organisms at the animal–fungal divergence in the genera *Amphibiocystidium*, *Amphibiothecum*, and *Rhinosporidium* cause cutaneous nodules in free-ranging frogs and salamanders.[22,23] Lesions are composed of thick-walled intradermal cysts containing myriad spherical 2–10 μm in diameter endospores observed on wet-mount or cytologic examination (Figure 62.8). An *Ichthyophonus* sp.-like mesomycetozoan causes granulomatous myositis and subcutaneous nodules.

The aphasmid nematode *Pseudocapillaroides xenopi* is an important cause of skin disease in laboratory African clawed frogs (*X. laevis*).[24] These worms inhabit tunnels within the epidermis, and characteristic bioperculate eggs or adult worms can be identified in wet mounts of skin scrapings or shed skin. Other commonly encountered cutaneous or subcutaneous metazoan parasites in amphibians include encysted cercaria of digenetic trematodes (e.g. *Clinostomum* sp.), fish lice (*Argulus* sp.), and trombiculid mites.[4,25] Opportunistic environmental organisms are also occasionally identified in skin samples from amphibians as illustrated by recovery of *Rhizoglyphus* sp. mites from laboratory *X. laevis*.[26] Completely aquatic amphibians are susceptible to some of the same ciliate and dinoflagellate protozoa that affect freshwater fish such as *Trichodina*, *Piscinoodinium*, and *Tetrahymena* spp.[4]

Hyperplasia and Neoplasia

Cutaneous neoplasms including mast cell tumors (morphologically similar to other species; see Chapter 13), cutaneous glandular adenomas and carcinomas, squamous cell carcinomas, sarcomas, and pigment cell neoplasms (chromatophoromas) are reported in amphibians; however, there are few published cytologic descriptions.[27] Chromatophoromas are subclassified by the predominant pigment type (e.g. melanin = melanophoroma). Iridophores contain anisotropic crystalline purines that are easily identified when examined with polarized light. However, melanophore or iridophore hyperplasia occurs at sites of cutaneous injury with resultant black or yellow-white skin discoloration, respectively, and can be difficult to distinguish cytologically from well-differentiated chromatophoromas.[4,27] Ulcerated mass-like lesions on the rostral nose and maxillary oral cavity occur following repeated self-trauma ("nose rub"). Histologically, these lesions can resemble myxomas or myxosarcomas.[27] Nodular hyperplasia of mucous glands is another differential for cutaneous nodules.[28]

Body Cavities and Fluid Analysis

Edema syndromes characterized by fluid accumulation in the coelomic cavity (hydrocoelom) or within the subcutaneous lymphatic sacs of anurans (lymphedema) are a common clinical presentation.[29,30] There is no standardized information on the classification of amphibian effusions using cell counts or total protein levels, and little information has been included in clinical reports. Empirically, guidelines for interpretation of fluid analysis results in mammals have been used, but the results can be misleading. For instance, fluid from an African clawed frog (*X. laevis*) with mycobacterial coelomitis had a low nucleated cell count (40 cells/μL) and low total protein concentration (1.2 g/dL), but macrophages with intracytoplasmic acid-fast bacilli were identified on cytologic examination.[12] In most cases, qualitative estimates of cellularity are used in cytologic evaluation of direct fluid smears and cytospin preparations combined with screening for infectious agents or neoplastic cells. Low numbers of mesothelial cells and macrophages and fewer neutrophils, eosinophils, and lymphocytes are common components of most effusions. Some noninfectious effusions will have very few nucleated cells even in cytospin preparations. Occasionally melanomacrophages and ciliated mesothelial cells are observed.[4,31]

The differential diagnoses for effusions in amphibians are similar to other groups of animals. Common noninfectious causes of effusion are renal disease, hypocalcemia (secondary to dietary calcium deficiency with resulting lymph heart failure), housing in water with low solute levels, hypoproteinemia, heart failure, lymph heart failure, liver disease, and gastrointestinal disease. In the African clawed frog (*X. laevis*), an acellular effusion was associated with a suspected ovarian hyperstimulation syndrome in animals treated with human chorionic gonadotropin.[32] Infectious causes of effusion include bacterial infections that have moderate to high cellularity and intracellular bacteria within neutrophils or macrophages. Effusion associated with mycobacteriosis can show negative-staining bacilli within the cytoplasm of macrophages.[12] Finally, generalized edema is observed secondary to endothelial cell injury with systemic *Ranavirus* infections in anurans and caudates.[8]

Respiratory

Samples obtained from the respiratory tract of amphibians are uncommon. Tracheal washes have been suggested as a means to diagnose infections with the common rhabditiform nematode *Rhabdias* sp. (amphibian lungworm). Larvated eggs, larvae, and occasionally adult worms can be recovered in wash fluid.[33] More commonly these infections are tentatively diagnosed by identification of eggs and larvae in fecal samples; however, differentiation from stages of other nematodes resident in the gastrointestinal tract is sometimes problematic.

Hemolymphatic

Extramedullary hematopoiesis (EMH), especially of granulocytic cell lines, is common in the liver and kidney and is a differential for inflammatory lesions or myeloproliferative disease in cytologic preparations.[27] EMH is especially prominent in tadpoles and recently metamorphosed juvenile animals. Lymphoma and lymphoid leukemia are sporadically observed in amphibians, but as previously noted, lesions of amphibian mycobacteriosis can be confused with round cell neoplasms.[13] Routine acid-fast staining of samples from suspected hematopoietic neoplasms is helpful to avoid this error. Infections with rickettsial organisms previously attributed to the genus *Aegyptianella* result in spherical intracytoplasmic inclusions with clear centers in erythrocytes of anurans and caudates.[34] There is no known clinical significance. Erythrocytic iridoviruses similar to those described in reptiles (Chapter 61) are associated with intracytoplasmic acidophilic to basophilic intracytoplasmic inclusions in erythrocytes of anurans. These inclusions were previously considered to be protozoal (e.g. *Pirhemocyton* or *Toddia* sp.) and are usually incidental findings; however, anemia was reported in heavily infected bullfrogs.[35–36] Iridoviruses in the genus *Ranavirus* cause systemic disease in many amphibians and pink-red intracytoplasmic inclusions can be observed in leukocytes.[37] A variety of hemoparasites are found in peripheral blood and tissue impression smears including *Hepatozoon* sp. (erythrocytes), *Lankesterella* sp. (erythrocytes, leukocytes, melanomacrophages, and hepatocytes), trypanosomes, and microfilaria.[4,38] In most instances these are incidental findings.

Gastrointestinal Tract and Liver

Aggregates of pigmented resident phagocytic cells (melanomacrophages) are normal components of the liver,

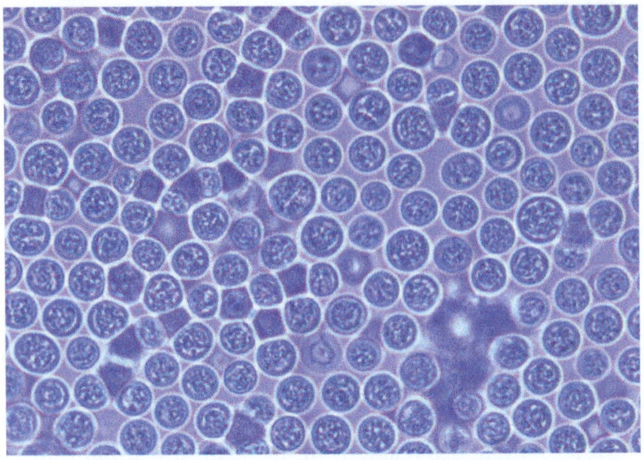

Figure 62.9 Infection with an unnamed alveolate protozoan in a southern leopard frog. An unstained tissue wet mount shows myriad thick-walled spherical spores (400×).

spleen, and kidney.[4,39] Melanomacrophages are observed in impression smears or aspirates of these organs, in effusions, and occasionally at sites of chronic inflammation.[4] Glycogen-type vacuolation of hepatocytes is a common physiologic change that does not have clinical significance.[4,40]

Infection with a pathogenic lineage of alveolate protozoa in the phylum Perkinsea is the cause of mortality events in wild ranid frog tadpoles in the United States.[41,42] Organisms diffusely infiltrate organs such as the liver, kidney, and spleen without significant inflammatory cell infiltrates. Diagnosis is by observation of approximately 6 μm in diameter spherical organisms in impression or squash preparations of affected organs (Figure 62.9).

Several species of opalinid, ciliate, and flagellate protozoa are expected commensal organisms within the intestinal tract.[43] Overgrowth of these organisms in debilitated animals with very high numbers observed on fecal wet mounts is sometimes considered to be clinically significant

Conclusion

Cytology is a valuable component of amphibian diagnostic medicine and its applications are similar to those of domestic animals. Compared with other vertebrates, the skin has exceptional physiologic importance in amphibians, and diagnosis of cutaneous disease forms a large proportion of amphibian cytologic submissions. Edema syndromes (hydrocoelom and lymphedema) are a common presentation in captive amphibians with infectious and noninfectious etiologies. Analysis and classification of these effusions is hampered by a lack of well-documented reference ranges for fluid cell counts and protein levels in relation to etiologic diagnoses.

References

1 Forzan, M.J., Heatley, J., Russell, K.E. et al. (2017). Clinical pathology of amphibians: a review. *Vet Clin Pathol* 46: 11–33.

2 Whitaker, B.R. and Wright, K.M. (2001). Clinical techniques. In: *Amphibian Medicine and Captive Husbandry* (eds. K.M. Wright and B.R. Whitaker), 89–110. Malabar, FL: Krieger Publishing.

3 Reavill, D. and Roberts, H. (2007). Diagnostic cytology of fish. *Vet Clin North Am Exot Anim Pract* 10: 207–234.

4 Pessier, A.P. (2007). Cytologic diagnosis of disease in amphibians. *Vet Clin North Am Exot Anim Pract* 10: 187–206.

5 Campbell, C.R., Voyles, J., Cook, D.I. et al. (2012). Frog skin epithelium: electrolyte transport and chytridiomycosis. *Int J Biochem Cell Biol* 44: 431–434.

6 Pessier, A.P. (2002). An overview of amphibian skin disease. *Sem Avian Exot Pet Med* 11: 162–174.

7 Walke, J.B. and Belden, L.K. (2016). Harnessing the microbiome to prevent fungal infections: lessons from amphibians. *PLoS Pathog* 12: e1005796.

8 Miller, D.L., Pessier, A.P., Hick, P. et al. (2015). Comparative pathology of ranaviruses and diagnostic techniques. In: *Ranaviruses, Lethal Pathogens of Ectothermic Vertebrates* (eds. M.J. Gray and V.G. Chinchar), 171–208. New York, NY: Springer.

9 Schadich, E. and Cole, A.L.J. (2010). Pathogenicity of *Aeromonas hydrophila*, *Klebsiella pneumoniae*, and *Proteus mirabilis* to brown tree frogs (*Litoria ewingii*). *Comp Med* 60: 114–117.

10 Mauel, M.J., Miller, D.L., Frazier, K.S. et al. (2002). Bacterial pathogens isolated from cultured bullfrogs (*Rana catesbeina*). *J Vet Diagn Invest* 14: 431–433.

11 Fischer, D., Lorenz, N., Heuser, W. et al. (2012). Abscesses associated with a *Brucella inopinata*-like bacterium in a big-eyed tree frog (*Leptopelis vermiculatus*). *J Zoo Wildl Med* 43: 625–628.

12 Tarigo, J., Linder, K., Neel, J. et al. (2006). Reluctant to dive: coelomic effusion in a frog. *Vet Clin Pathol* 35: 341–343.

13 Asfari, M. (1988). *Mycobacterium*-induced infectious granuloma in *Xenopus*: histopathology and transmissibility. *Cancer Res J* 48: 958–963.

14 Juopperi, T., Karli, K., DeVoe, R. et al. (2002). Granulomatous dermatitis in a spadefoot toad (*Scaphiopus holbrooki*). *Vet Clin Pathol* 31: 137–139.

15 Creeper, J.H., Main, D.C., Berger, L. et al. (1998). An outbreak of mucormycosis in slender tree frogs (*Litoria adelensis*) and white-lipped tree frogs (*Litoria infrafrenata*). *Aust Vet J* 76: 761–762.

16 White, C.L., Forzan, M.J., Pessier, A.P. et al. (2016). A case definition for *Batrachochytrium salamandrivorans* chytridiomycosis. *Herpetol Rev* 47: 207–209.

17 Briggs, C. and Burgin, S. (2004). Congo red, an effective stain for revealing the chytrid fungus *Batrachochytrium dendrobatidis* in epidermal skin scrapings from frogs. *Mycology* 18: 98–103.

18 Longcore, J.R., Longcore, J.E., Pessier, A.P. et al. (2007). Chytridiomycosis widespread in anurans of northeastern United States. *J Wildl Manag* 71: 435–444.

19 Hyatt, A. (2017). *Infection with Batrachochytrium dendrobatidis Manual of Diagnostic Tests for Aquatic Animals*. Paris, France: World Organization for Animal Health (OIE).

20 Nichols, D.K., Lamirande, E.W., Pessier, A.P. et al. (2001). Experimental transmission of cutaneous chytridiomycosis in dendrobatid frogs. *J Wildl Dis* 37: 1–11.

21 Dusick, A., Flatland, B., Craig, L. et al. (2017). What is your diagnosis? Skin scraping from a hellbender. *Vet Clin Pathol* 46: 183–184.

22 Raffel, T.R., Bommarito, T., Barry, D.S. et al. (2008). Widespread infection of the eastern red spotted newt (*Notophthalmus viridescens*) by a new species of *Amphibiocystidium*, a genus of fungal-like mesomycetozoan parasites not previously reported in North America. *J Parasitol* 135: 203–215.

23 Scheid, P., Balczun, C., Dehling, J.M. et al. (2015). Rhinosporidiosis in African reed frogs *Hyperolius* spp. caused by a new species of *Rhinosporidium*. *Dis Aquat Org* 115: 111–120.

24 Feldman, S.H. and Ramirez, M.P. (2014). Molecular phylogeny of *Pseudocapillaroides xenopi* (Moravec et Cosgrove 1982) and development of a quantitative PCR assay for its detection in aquarium sediment. *J Am Assoc Lab Anim Sci* 53: 668–674.

25 Sladky, K.K., Norton, T.M., and Loomis, M.R. (2000). Trombiculid mites (*Hannemania* sp.) in canyon tree frogs (*Hyla arenacolor*). *J Zoo Wildl Med* 31: 570–575.

26 Ford, T.R., Dillehay, D.L., and Mook, D.M. (2004). Cutaneous acariasis in the African clawed frog (*Xenopus laevis*). *Comp Med* 54: 713–717.

27 Stacy, B.A. and Parker, J.M. (2004). Amphibian oncology. *Vet Clin North Am Exot Anim Pract* 7: 673–695.

28 Shaw, S.D., Berger, L., Harvey, C. et al. (2017). Adenomatous hyperplasia of the mucous glands in captive Archey's frogs (*Leiopelma archeyi*). *N Z Vet J* 65: 140–146.

29 Pessier, A.P. (2009). Edematous frogs, urinary tract disease, and disorders of fluid balance in amphibians. *J Exot Pet Med* 18: 4–13.

30 Clancy, M.M., Clayton, L.A., and Hadfield, C.A. (2015). Hydrocoelom and lymphedema in dendrobatid frogs at National Aquarium, Baltimore: 2003–2011. *J Zoo Wildl Med* 46: 18–26.

31 Green, I.M. (1897). The peritoneal epithelium of some Ithaca amphibians. *Trans Am Microsc Soc* 18: 76–106.

32 Green, S.L., Parker, J., Davis, C. et al. (2007). Ovarian hyperstimulation syndrome in gonadotropin-treated laboratory South African clawed frogs (*Xenopus laevis*). *J Am Assoc Lab Anim Sci* 46: 64–67.

33 Nichols, D.K. (2000). Amphibian respiratory diseases. *Vet Clin North Am Exot Anim Pract* 3: 551–554.

34 Davis, A.K. and Cecala, K. (2010). Intraerythrocytic rickettsial inclusions in Ocoee salamanders (*Desmognathus ocoee*): prevalence, morphology, and comparisons with inclusions of *Plethodon cinereus*. *Parasitol Res* 107: 363–367.

35 Gruia-Gray, J. and Desser, S.S. (1992). Cytopathological observations and epizootiology of frog erythrocytic virus in bullfrogs. *J Wildl Dis* 28: 34–41.

36 Grosset, C., Wellehan, J.F., Owens, S.D. et al. (2014). Intraerythrocytic iridovirus in central bearded dragons (*Pagona vitticeps*). *J Vet Diagn Invest* 26: 354–364.

37 Forzan, M.J., Smith, T.G., Vanderstichel, R.V. et al. (2016). Hematologic reference values for *Rana sylvatica* (*Lithobates sylvaticus*) and effect of infection with Frog Virus 3 (*Ranavirus* sp., Iridoviridae). *Vet Clin Pathol* 45: 430–443.

38 Gericota, B., Garner, M.M., Barr, B. et al. (2010). Morphologic, immunohistochemical and molecular characterization of a novel *Lankesterella* protozoan in two White's tree frogs. *J Zoo Wildl Med* 41: 242–248.

39 Agius, C. and Roberts, R.J. (2003). Melano-macrophage centers and their role in fish pathology. *J Fish Dis* 26: 499–509.

40 Baic, D., Ladewski, B.G., and Frye, B.E. (1979). Quantitative ultrastructural studies of hepatocytes from fed and starved frogs. *J Exp Zool* 210: 381–406.

41 Davis, A.K., Yabsley, M.J., Keel, M.K. et al. (2007). Discovery of a novel alveolate pathogen affecting southern leopard frogs in Georgia: description of the disease and host effects. *EcoHealth* 4: 310–317.

42 Isidoro-Ayza, M., Lorch, J.M., Grear, D.A. et al. (2017). Pathogenic lineage of Perkinsea associated with mass mortality of frogs across the United States. *Sci Rep* 7: 10288.

43 Poynton, S.L. and Whitaker, B.R. (1994). Protozoa in poison dart frogs (Dendrobatidae): clinical assessment and identification. *J Zoo Wildl Med* 25: 29–39.

63

Fish

Charlotte Hollinger and Alisa L. Newton

Introduction

Fish include more species than any other vertebrate group. The extant fish classes comprise bony fish (osteichthyes, e.g. teleosts), cartilaginous fish (chondrichthyes, e.g. sharks and rays), and jawless fish (agnatha, e.g. hagfish and lampreys). Fish inhabit a multitude of different environments worldwide and contribute to healthy ecosystems, economic stability, human nutrition, biomedical and industrial research, recreation and leisure. Cytology is a rapid, nonlethal, inexpensive clinical examination technique and can also be applied during postmortem evaluation to provide diagnostic information for individual patients and to inform group health in aquaculture and laboratory settings, mixed species exhibits, or wildlife environments. This chapter provides a general overview of common fish-focused cytologic techniques and findings, coupled with a brief review of general anatomy and systems pathology. Additional resources are referenced for interested readers.[1–5]

Application of Cytology Techniques in Fish

Cytology in fish is often performed as point-of-care testing and postmortem in "herd health" situations. Wet-mount preparations are utilized most commonly to detect inflammation, infection, and ectoparasitism. Routine air-dried cytologic preparations can characterize and preserve inflammatory and infectious lesions and evaluate neoplasms. Fish health relies heavily on the condition of their skin and gills, and these are frequently sampled. Sampling of internal organs is generally limited to postmortem exams or to antemortem samples collected by veterinarians specialized in fish medicine.

Collection Procedures

Routine collection methods are applicable to fish cytology. Sample site preparation is limited and often not performed to avoid disrupting the external mucus layer, which provides a critical immunological and biological barrier to pathogens and the environment.

External Samples: Skin Scrapes, Fin Clips, and Gill Clips

Skin scrapes, fin clips, and gill clips are useful to screen for infections and detect environmental disturbances such as gas supersaturation (gas bubble disease). These are performed in living and deceased fish.[1,6] Antemortem skin scrapings and fin clips can be performed under manual restraint in some species. Sedation or anesthesia is recommended for gill clips. No site preparation is needed or recommended. All handling and medical management should be performed by experienced personnel.

Skin scrapes are acquired with a dulled blade, coverslip, or other blunt-edged instrument by gently scraping along the body in the direction of the scales. Only limited pressure is needed, and especially antemortem, care should be taken to minimize scale loss and skin damage, as wounds are prone to opportunistic infection. Because secondary agents can overrun established lesions, the leading edge of lesions is the best diagnostic target. Scrapings should include protected sites, such as behind or adjacent to the dorsal and pelvic fins as these may harbor increased numbers of ectoparasites. Proper skin scrapes yield mucus and epithelial cells with only few scales and minimal blood (Figure 63.1). Material is immediately mixed with a drop of fluid on a glass slide, covered with a glass or plastic coverslip, and examined. The fluid media used for the wet mount (saltwater, freshwater, or saline) is guided by the animal's natural environment to prevent cell desiccation and permit survival of bacteria

Veterinary Cytology, First Edition. Edited by Leslie C. Sharkey, M. Judith Radin, and Davis Seelig.

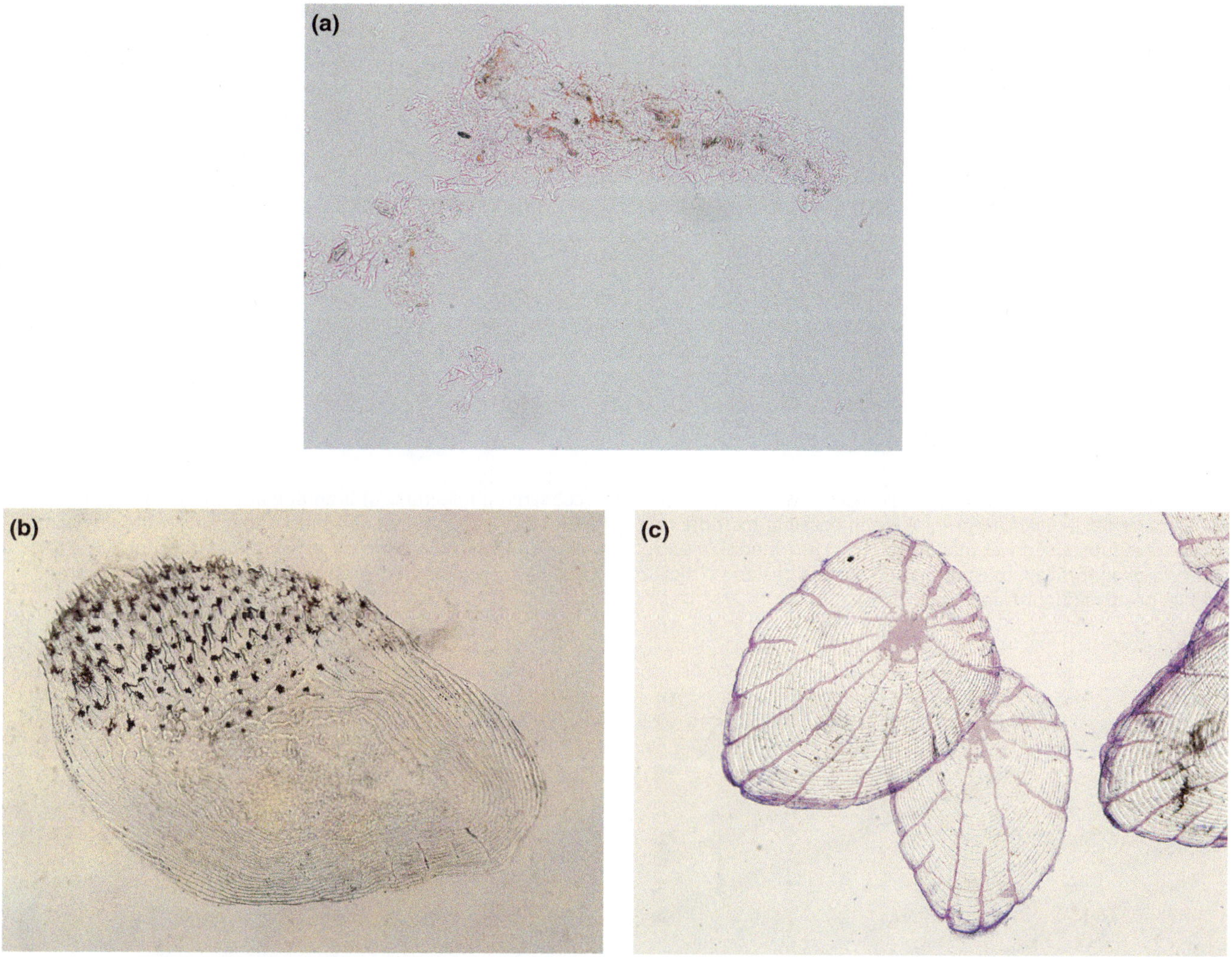

Figure 63.1 (a) Normal skin scrape from a flame hawkfish (*Neocirrhitus armatus*) consisting of mucus and epithelial cells with no scales and minimal erythrocytes (unstained wet mount 100×). (b) Example of scales (unstained wet mount, 100×). (c) Examples of scales air-dried and stained (modified Wright's, 100×).

and ectoparasites in the sample. Evaluation of organism movement in addition to morphology is critical to pathogen identification in many diseases. The condenser is lowered for wet-mount examination to provide appropriate contrast. Contrast can be augmented by addition of a drop of Lugol's iodine to the margin of the coverslip to facilitate identification of bacterial pathogens. Following wet-mount evaluation, the cover slip can be removed, the sample spread thin and air-dried for routine and/or special staining (e.g. modified Wright's stain, Gram stain, acid-fast stain) (Figure 63.2).

Fin clips include evaluation of skin, bone, and local vasculature (Figure 63.3). Samples consist of a small segment (often 1–3 mm, depending on the size of the fish) cut with scissors from the distal margin of one of the fins. As with scrapes, the sample is placed in fluid, cover-slipped, and immediately examined as a wet-mount preparation. Fin choice depends on lesions, species, and personal preference; caudal fins are common. The presence of thick, bony fin rays can create preparations too thick to coverslip and examine. In those cases, only the webbing between the rays is collected and evaluated.

Gill clips are acquired by cutting the tips of a few primary lamellae and transferring the single-layer cut sections to a glass slide with a small amount of fluid for wet mounts (Figure 63.4). Ideally, the second or third gill arches are evaluated as these are protected sites and can harbor ectoparasites. Antemortem gill clips can cause significant bleeding, and adequate hemostasis is required. In most fish, this is accomplished using a small hemostat to clamp the filaments to be sampled proximal to the site of dissection. Rapid autolysis limits the utility of delayed

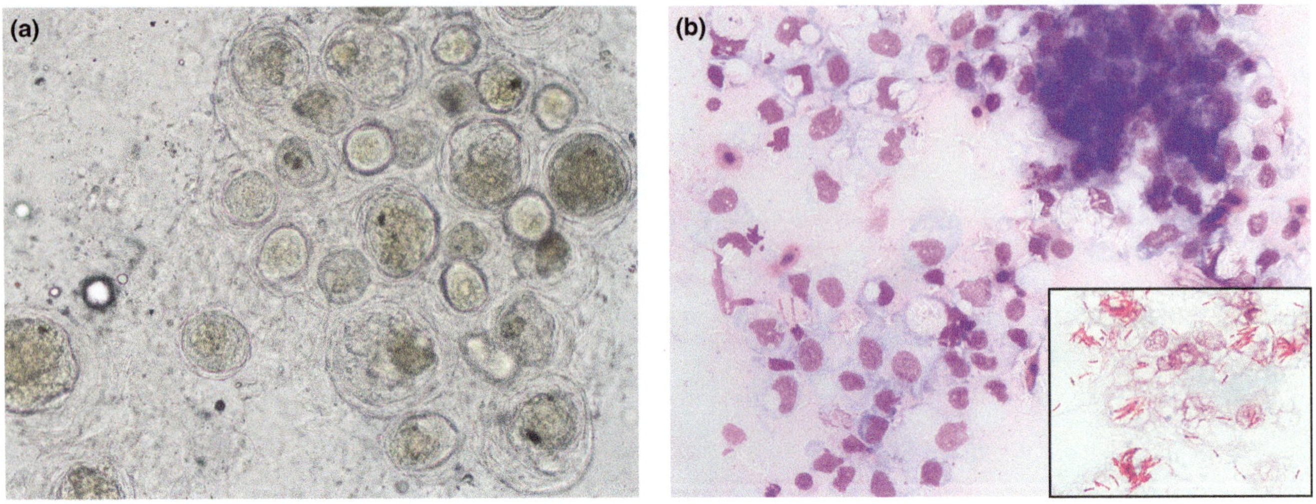

Figure 63.2 Skin scrape cytology from ulcerative lesions caused by mycobacterial infection. (a) Granulomatous inflammation in a blue emperor tetra (*Inpaichthys kerri*) is composed of multiple round granulomas with lamellar periphery and granular brown necrotic central cores (unstained wet mount, 400×). (b) Air-dried skin scraping from a killifish (*Pachypanchax* sp.) shows extracellular and few histiocyte-phagocytized nonstaining rod-shaped bacteria typical of mycobacteriosis (modified Wright's, 1000×) Inset: Bacteria are acid-fast positive (Ziehl-Neelsen, 1000×).

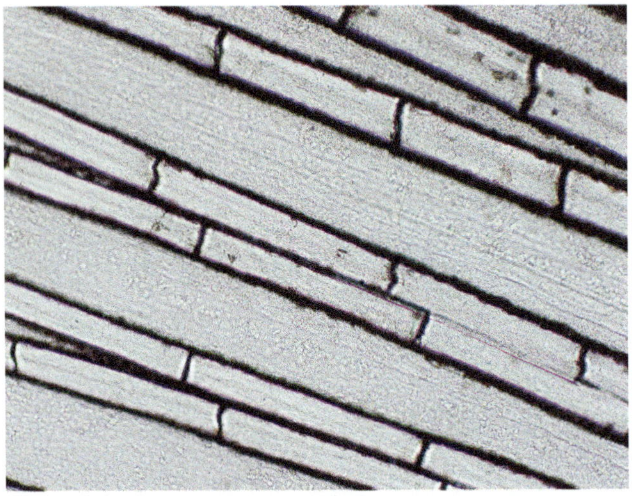

Figure 63.3 Normal fin clip from a longnose butterflyfish (*Forcipiger flavissimus*) consists of bony fin rays and intervening skin with parallel-arrayed small blood vessels (unstained wet mount, 200×).

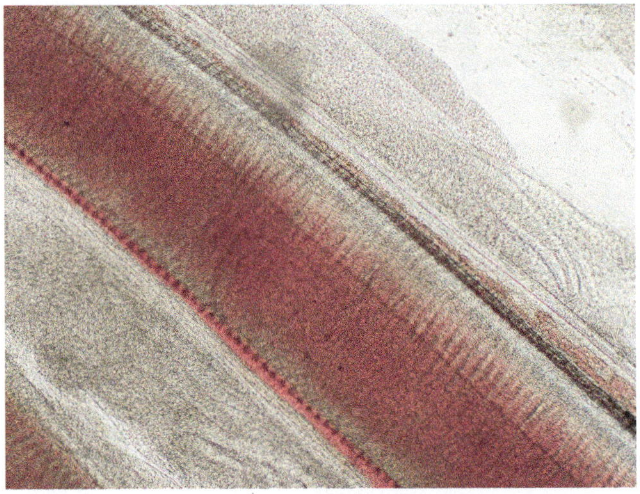

Figure 63.4 Normal gill clip from a lookdown (*Selene vomer*) shows highly vascularized primary lamella (diagonal from upper left to lower right) lined by fine, perpendicularly-oriented and regularly-arrayed secondary lamellae, and overlying amorphous, pale, mucus (unstained wet mount, 200×).

postmortem gill clip samples to predominantly ectoparasite screening.

Assessment of proliferative external lesions (e.g. skin masses) is performed in fish as in other species. Often, fine-needle biopsy with or without aspiration and subsequent air-dried smears are utilized. To diminish contamination and reduce the risk of secondary infection, preparation of antemortem sampling sites can involve rinsing with sterile saline or placing sterile ophthalmic antibiotic drops at the site of aspiration.

Internal Samples: Coelomic Cavity and Organ Samples

Depending on the lesion (e.g. nodule, mass, fluid) and means of clinical assessment (e.g. radiography, ultrasonography, endoscopy), many of the same cytologic techniques used in other taxa are applicable to fish. These include swabs and roll preparations, fecal floats and smears, and fine-needle biopsy or fluid preparations, as described in standard cytology texts.

The coelomic cavity, swim bladder, and internal organs can be aspirated percutaneously with or without ultrasound guidance. Potential complications of internal sampling include hemorrhage and secondary infection. Sampling of the swim bladder can lead to gas leakage into the coelom. Pathologic mechanisms of fluid accumulation are similar to other taxa. Transudates reflect altered hydrostatic or oncotic pressures, and inflammatory exudates can contain microorganisms identified cytologically. Exfoliative neoplastic effusions are uncommon in fish. Hemorrhage occurs secondary to trauma or other processes (e.g. coagulopathy, neoplasia). Unique to some species of elasmobranchs are bilateral pores in the margins of the cloaca (abdominal pores), which communicate directly with the coelomic cavity. A small amount of fluid is common in the coelom of elasmobranchs even in health. Catheter cannulation of the pores allows abnormal fluid to be recovered, or for sterile saline to be introduced and removed, thereby flushing the coelom to sample for infectious agents. The latter is a common method of detecting coelomic coccidial infection in cow-nosed rays. Another common procedure in syngnathids is flushing of the brood pouch of males to treat buoyancy problems and/or recover fluid for diagnosis of luminal protozoal and bacterial infections (Figure 63.5)

Fluid and solid tissue specimens are processed for cytology as in other taxa. Fluid assessment in fish can include measurement of refractometric protein concentration. However, refractometers are not calibrated for fish, results are subject to the effects of other dissolved solutes, and values are often erroneously high. Comparison with findings in health or over time can be diagnostically useful to narrow the diagnostic algorithm of protein-rich vs. protein-poor effusions.

Postmortem organ cytology is used frequently in fish population health assessment as a rapid diagnostic method. Tissue imprints enable assessment of cell and organism features and are performed as in other species (Chapters 1 and 5). Squash preparations include a larger area of tissue screened and assessment of tissue architecture. They are prepared by removing a small (2–4mm diameter) tissue fragment from the target organ, placing it in a small amount of fluid (e.g. water, saline), and compressing the tissue into a thin layer beneath a coverslip or a second glass slide. Commonly sampled organs include liver, anterior kidney, posterior kidney, spleen, stomach, intestine, and any lesions. These preparations typically are used to detect structural changes such as inflammatory foci (granulomas) or necrosis within organs and allow rapid identification of parasites, systemic bacterial or fungal infections, and occasionally metabolic conditions such as nephrocalcinosis. In very small fish (<3cm total length), all of the coelomic viscera can be squashed from a subset of individuals to allow assessment of all organ systems and the interior of the gastrointestinal tract. This can facilitate diagnosis prior to the availability of histology results from other individuals.

Interpretive Considerations and General Disease Responses in Fish

Interpretation of fish cytology samples follows routine diagnostic approaches (Chapter 5). Blood contamination is common, and an understanding of piscine hematology, which is reviewed elsewhere, is needed.[4,7,8] Briefly, major cellular constituents include erythrocytes, leukocytes, and thrombocytes. With few exceptions (e.g. Gonostomidae family), most

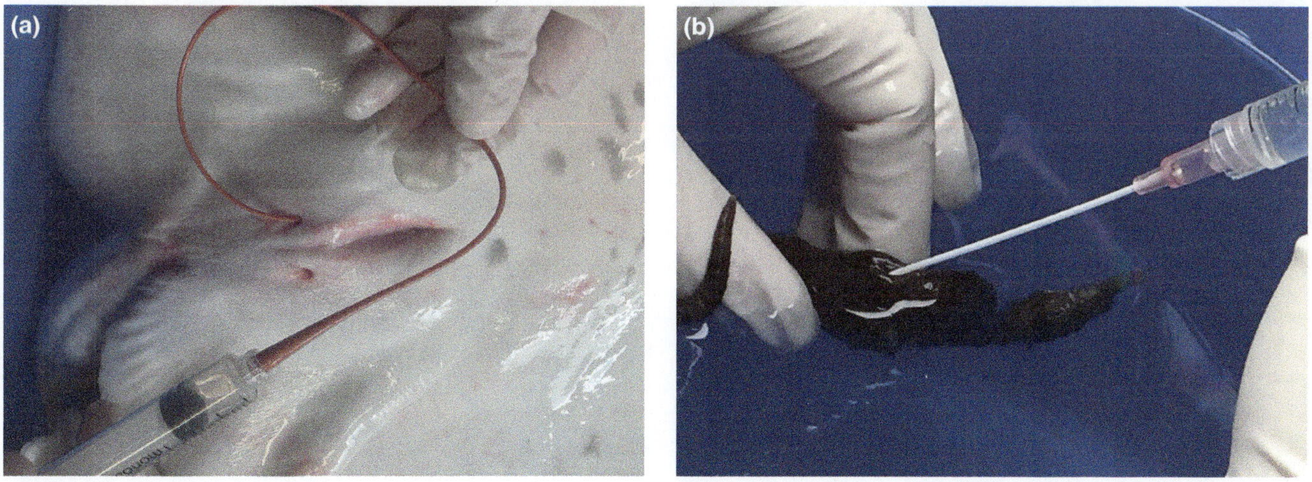

Figure 63.5 (a) Diagnostic coelomic pore fluid collection in a Honeycomb stingray (*Himantura uarnak*) (*Source:* Image courtesy of Natalie Mylniczenko). (b) Therapeutic catheter insertion into the brood pouch of a seahorse allowing fluid installation to relieve abnormal buoyancy.

fish have nucleated erythrocytes. Low numbers of immature erythrocytes (approximately 1%) are found in circulation in health. Immature erythrocytes are smaller, rounder, and polychromatophilic to basophilic, with higher nuclear to cytoplasmic ratio and rare mitotic forms. Leukocytes of fish include lymphocytes, monocytes, and granulocytes. The nomenclature of piscine granulocytes is variable, and conventions generally follow morphologic appearance in other taxa. In teleosts, the terms neutrophil, eosinophil, and basophil are commonly utilized based on microscopic, cytochemical, and ultrastructural evidence. Some teleost neutrophils have been termed heterophils due to eosinophilic cytoplasmic granules on light microscopy. In elasmobranchs, described granulocytes include those with neutral staining granules (neutrophils or G2 cells), fine eosinophilic granules (fine eosinophilic granulocytes, heterophils, or G1 cells), coarse eosinophilic granules (coarse eosinophilic granulocytes, eosinophils, or G3 cells), and purple granules (basophils). The nuclear morphology of piscine granulocytes varies between species from round to indented or lobulated. In most teleosts, the nuclear shape of neutrophils is rounded, whereas that of most elasmobranchs is segmented. Thrombocytes in fish are round to ovoid with usually clear cytoplasm. Elasmobranchs additionally can have granular thrombocytes with dense fine eosinophilic cytoplasmic granules. As in bird and reptiles, thrombocytes must be differentiated from similarly sized lymphocytes in blood and cytologic preparations.

Inflammation

Inflammatory responses in fish are relatively non-insult specific in comparison with other vertebrates.[9] Fish exhibit typical signs of inflammation, including redness, swelling, pain, and loss of function. Heat (calor) is not generally recognized in ectotherms. While granulocytes play a role in the initial stages of inflammation, monocytes/macrophages (histiocytes) from blood or local tissue are generally the predominant inflammatory cell type in fish.[10,11] With chronicity and cell-mediated responses, lymphocytes, multinucleated giant cells, and granulation tissue progressing to mature fibrosis commonly develop. Histologically, chronic granulomas are composed of a central core of necrotic, sometimes mineralized, material surrounded by epithelioid macrophages and more peripheral fibrosis and lymphocytes. Common cytologic findings on air-dried smears include macrophages, fewer lymphocytes, and amorphous debris. Infectious agents may be identified on routine smears or with special staining. To further identify bacteria and define antibiotic sensitivity, culture samples should be submitted promptly (within 24–48 hours). Due to unique growth requirements of some fish pathogens, employing a laboratory experienced with piscine samples is recommended. Advanced techniques, including molecular testing and electron microscopy, can also aid in characterizing infectious agents.

Cell Death

Fish experience typical apoptosis and necrosis.[12] Apoptosis is classically associated with shrinkage, condensation, and fragmentation of individual cells without significant inflammation, while necrotic cells undergo cellular and nuclear swelling and/or lysis, triggering an inflammatory response. On wet-mount preparations, necrosis is apparent as acute loss of architecture, or more chronic foci of cellular debris with variable mineralization and surrounding inflammation or fibrosis (Figure 63.6). Cytologic features

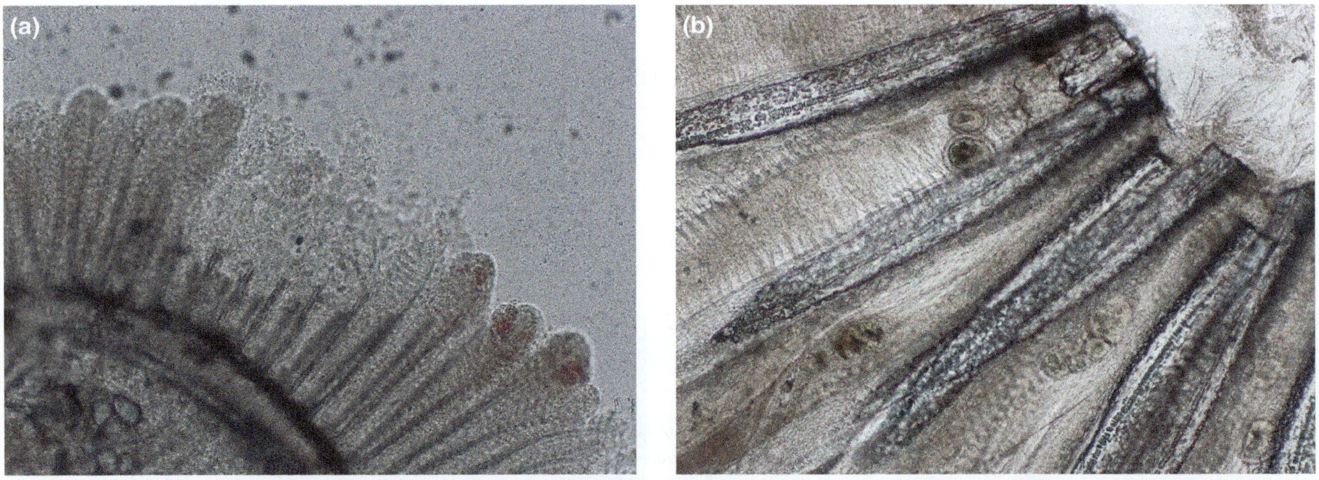

Figure 63.6 Gill clips demonstrating acute necrosis and chronic inflammation. (a) Gill from a northern pipefish (*Syngnathus fuscus*) with focally extensive necrosis characterized by loss of lamellar architecture (center) (unstained wet mount, 100×). (b) Gill from a spotfin butterflyfish (*Chaetodon ocellatus*) demonstrating multifocal chronic granulomas effacing and distorting secondary lamellae (unstained wet mount, 200×).

of necrosis on dry mounts are typical, including faded, indistinct, basophilic cells with diffuse proteinaceous background material and cellular debris. Mineralization is generally not apparent. Necrotic features must be cautiously differentiated from autolytic changes that are especially rapid in aquatic habitats.

Cell Proliferation

Cellular proliferation in fish is particularly influenced by environmental exposures (e.g. carcinogenic and irritant chemicals, infectious agents).[13] As always, cytologic findings must be correlated with clinical and macroscopic findings and results of other diagnostics for optimal interpretation. In some cases, cellular features are sufficient to indicate likelihood of a malignancy. Generally, three or more nuclear features of atypia are expected in cell populations fulfilling morphologic criteria of malignancy (Chapter 5). However, some malignant populations lack apparent pleomorphism, and some nonneoplastic reactive populations exhibit significant atypia. Interpretation of a proliferative lesion in conjunction with inflammation can be particularly challenging due to reactive tissue changes.

Systems

The following sections review body system anatomy and pathology of fish, with an emphasis on relevant cytologic features. Pathologic conditions are divided into infectious/inflammatory and hyperplastic/neoplastic with supporting examples. Entities were selected to demonstrate conditions that are common and/or have significant impact on global captive or wild fish species. For body systems in which multiple infectious agents are important, organisms are subdivided taxonomically to aid organization. Some hyperplastic lesions have an infectious etiology but are grouped under hyperplasia due to the patterns of clinical expression. Other etiologies including metabolic, nutritional, degenerative, vascular, toxic, traumatic, developmental, anomalous, or idiopathic are included only if cytologically important or unique in fish.

Skin and Subcutis

The skin of fish is a critical barrier to the environment and key to osmotic regulation. It is also the most commonly sampled tissue for cytology. Teleost skin consists of a glycocalyx (cuticle), epidermis, basement membrane, dermis, and hypodermis. The epidermis is composed of non-cornified stratified squamous epithelium, which varies in thickness by species, age, site, and reproductive status. All layers of keratinocytes in the teleost epidermis are capable of mitotic division. Other cells variably present in the epidermis include mucus goblet cells, club cells (including Shreckstoffenzellen), granule cells, lymphocytes, and macrophages.[11,14] Club (alarm) cells are associated with defensive function. Eosinophilic granule cells are considered akin to mammalian mast cells and are not often recognized in cytology samples, likely due to low numbers and cell distortion. The superficial dermis is composed of loose collagen and reticulin fibers with interspersed chromatophores (pigment cells), eosinophilic granule cells, and scales. The deeper dermis consists of dense collagen. The described chromatophores of fishes include cyanophores, erythrophores, iridophores, leucophores, melanophores, xanthophores, and dichromatic chromatophores.[15] Scales of teleost fish reside within scale pockets and consist of collagen fibers interspersed with calcified crystals.[14] Elasmobranch fishes have unique surface structures termed placoid scales or dermal denticles, which demonstrate the same histologic structure as teeth.

Scrapes and swabs of skin are used in conjunction with wet-mount preparations for erosive or ulcerative lesions, and fine-needle biopsies are used for expansile nodules or masses. Cytologic findings in healthy fish skin include mucus, squamous epithelial cells, and occasional scales with or without pigment (Figure 63.1). In postmortem samples, bacteria reflect overgrowth or infection. A monomorphic population of bacteria, inflammation, and scale damage support pathogenicity. Low numbers of some parasites may be found incidentally as commensals, as discussed below. Lesions of fish skin typically result from injurious stimuli leading to cellular degeneration, erosion and/or ulceration, or proliferative stimuli causing hyperplasia. The initiating factors can be masked by secondary opportunistic infections including oomycete algae (e.g. *Saprolegnia* sp.) or bacteria (e.g. *Flavobacteria* sp.).

Infection and Inflammation

Infectious agents affecting fish skin span a wide spectrum of microbial agents. Some organisms cause primary infections, while many are secondary opportunists with a range of underlying inciting injuries including inadequate husbandry. Due to the scope of infectious agents relevant to the skin of fish, etiologies are subdivided taxonomically, and examples highlight common and/or significant disease agents. Because many infectious agents also affect deeper tissues, subsequent body system sections refer to some cytologic descriptions in the section "Skin and Subcutis."

Bacteria

Common bacterial infections of fish skin are summarized in Table 63.1. These include Gram-negative bacteria such as *Aeromonas*, *Pseudomonas*, and *Vibrio* species. Many bacteria

Table 63.1 Common bacterial pathogens of fish with characteristic features and selected disease examples.

Bacterial group	Features	Selected examples with disease names
Aeromonads	Gram-negative bacilli Facultative anaerobic Some motile by polar flagella	*Aeromonas salmonicida*: Furunculosis *Aeromonas hydrophila*: Septicemia
Vibrios	Gram-negative, straight or curved bacilli Facultative anaerobic Motile by polar flagella	*Vibrio anguillarum*: vibriosis *Vibrio salmonicida*: cold-water vibriosis
Pseudomonads	Gram-negative bacilli Aerobic Motile by polar flagella	*Pseudomonas fluorescens*: Septicemia *Pseudomonas anguilliseptica*: Red spot
Flavobacteria (formerly Flexibacteria)	Gram-negative, long thin bacilli Aerobic Some motile in gliding motion	*Flavobacterium columnare*: Columnaris disease *Flavobacterium branchiophilum*: Bacterial gill disease, Fin rot
Enterobacteria	Gram-negative bacilli Facultative anaerobic Some motile by flagella	*Edwardsiella tarda*: Edwardsiella septicemia *Yersinia ruckeri*: Enteric red-mouth
Renibacteria	Gram-positive bacilli Aerobic Nonmotile	*Renibacterium salmoninarum*: Bacterial kidney disease
Streptococci	Gram-positive cocci Aerobic Nonmotile	*Streptococcus iniae*: Septicemia *Streptococcus agalactiae*: Septicemia
Mycobacteria	± Beaded, weakly Gram-positive bacilli Acid fast Aerobic Nonmotile	*Mycobacterium marinum*, *Mycobacterium fortuitum*, *Mycobacterium chelonae*: Mycobacteriosis
Nocardia	Gram-positive, pleomorphic to filamentous and branching Acid fast Aerobic Nonmotile	*Nocardia asteroids*: Nocardiosis
Chlamydiaceae	Gram-negative Obligate intracellular Developmental stages: Elementary body (infectious) Reticulate body (noninfectious, reproductive)	*Chlamydia*-like organism: Epitheliocystis

Source: Modified from Roberts,[3] pp. 341–342.

are commensals with opportunistic infections precipitated by factors causing physiologic stress or breakdown in host barriers (e.g. water quality, temperature, nutrition, overcrowding, concurrent disease). The less common obligate pathogens of fish often can survive in the environment and exist on subclinically infected carrier fish, causing morbidity and mortality in times of stress. Many bacterial infections have similar clinical presentations as darkened skin, erosions, or ulcers, leading to sepsis. Antemortem, septic fish can develop prominent erythema and deterioration of the fin margins as well as exophthalmos and coelomic distention with elevation of scales. Postmortem, sepsis commonly presents as enlargement of the anterior kidneys and spleen and/or nodular white foci disseminated throughout multiple organs (Figure 63.7).

Flavobacterium sp. are opportunistic and primary pathogens. *F. columnare* (formerly *Flexibacter columnaris*) causes columnaris disease in captive and wild freshwater, often tropical, fish. Lesions include characteristic areas of pallor near the dorsal fin (saddle lesions), skin ulcers, fin

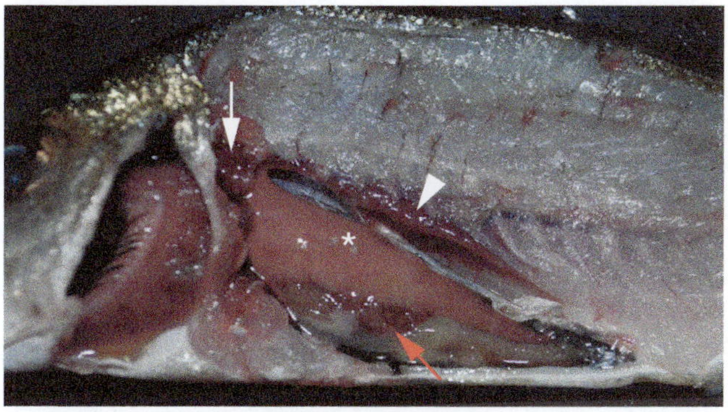

Figure 63.7 Gross necropsy findings in a yellow spot croaker (*Leiostomus xanthurus*) with bacterial sepsis. The anterior kidneys are enlarged and bulging (white arrow), and there are multifocal white nodular foci in the spleen (red arrow), with few in the liver (asterisk) and posterior kidney (arrowhead).

erosion (fin rot), and gill necrosis. Cytologically, long thin bacterial rods (4–10 μm in length) form characteristic aggregates (haystacks) and have gliding motion. Organisms are highlighted by counterstaining with Lugol's iodine (Figure 63.8).[16] A similar organism *Tenacibaculum maritimum* causes ulcerative disease of marine fish manifesting as ulcerative or necrotizing lesions of skin, gills, fins, and oral surfaces. It attaches to external skin and mucosa; infection often originates within gingival pockets of the denticles in the oral cavity.[17]

Mycobacteriosis (piscine tuberculosis) is an important and common cause of localized and systemic lesions in fish. Lesions include skin ulcers or nodules, chronic wasting over months to years with internal granulomas, or chronic spinal deformities. Common pathogenic isolates include *Mycobacterium marinum*, *M. fortuitum*, and *M. chelonea*. Transmission is direct through skin injuries and external parasites, as well as by consumption of contaminated feed including cannibalism.[18] Organisms survive and replicate in macrophages. Granulomas can be visible in wet-mount scrapes and squash preparations. Dry mounts contain macrophages and necrotic debris. Bacteria are identified as extracellular or phagocytized linear nonstaining bacilli with routine staining and are acid-fast positive (Figure 63.2). All fish (freshwater and marine) are susceptible to mycobacteriosis, and the agents are zoonotic causing "fish handler's disease," most common in fish handlers and aquarium hobbyists through skin injuries.[18,19]

Epitheliocystis is caused by chlamydia-like organisms infecting the skin and gills in a variety of freshwater and marine species with variable pathogenicity. Molecular analysis has identified multiple distinct organisms (*Candidatus Piscichlamydia salmonis*, *Candidatus Clavochlamydia salmonicola*, etc.).[20] The intracellular bacteria cause marked hypertrophy of infected host cells that appear as massively enlarged globoid cells filled by granular basophilic inclusion material (organisms) and surrounded by a variably distinct capsule. Peripheral displacement of the host cell nucleus is characteristic. The gills, epidermis, and lining of orobranchial cavities are often involved. Epithelial cells are commonly infected, but infection has also been reported in chloride, mucus, and pillar cells and in macrophages. Developmental forms progress through typical chlamydial development, including a small infectious rigid form (elementary body), large pleomorphic noninfectious form (reticulate

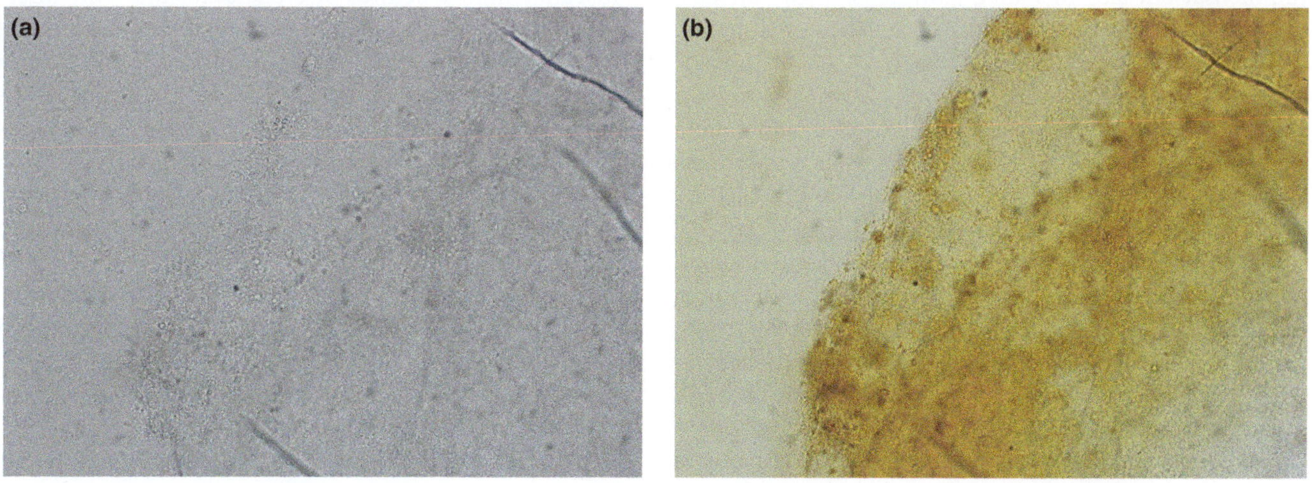

Figure 63.8 Area of skin pallor near the dorsal fin (saddle lesion) in a cardinal tetra (*Paracheirodon axelrodi*) with *Flavobacterium* sp. infection. (a) Skin scrape shows a monomorphic population of filamentous bacteria forming "haystacks" (unstained wet mount, 400×). (b) Bacteria are highlighted by counterstaining (Lugol's iodine, 400×).

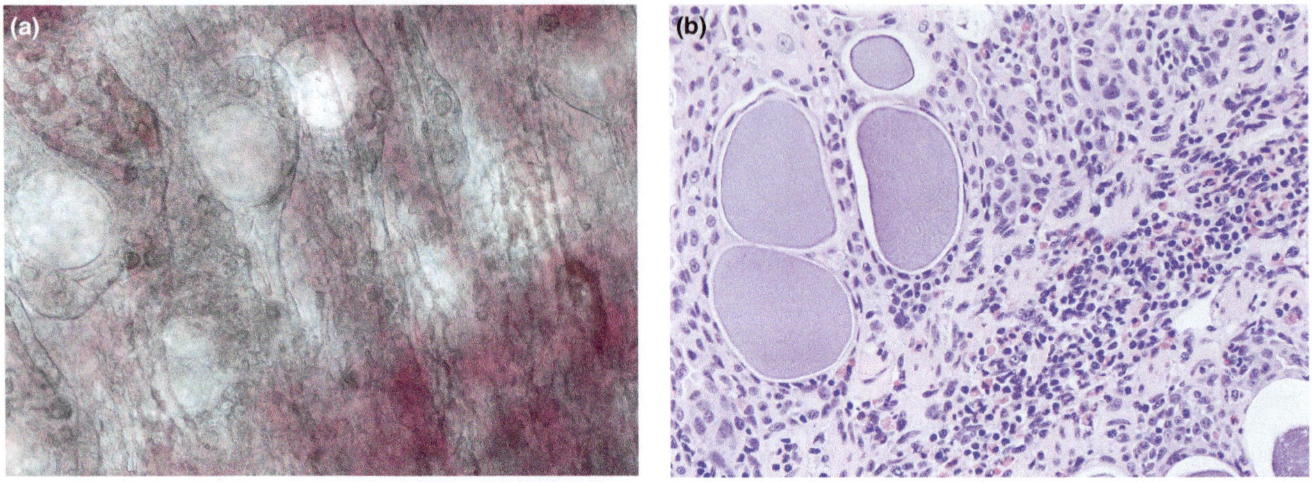

Figure 63.9 Epitheliocystis disease in the gills of a spotted eagle ray (*Aetobatus narinari*). (a) Gill clip shows intraepithelial inclusions as cyst-like structures with a thin limiting capsule and little discernable internal structure (unstained wet mount, 400×. *Source:* Image courtesy of Alexa Delaune). (b) Histology shows multifocal distortion of secondary lamellae by enlarged epithelial cells containing large, finely granular, pale basophilic cytoplasmic inclusions. The primary gill filament is infiltrated by small numbers of lymphocytes and granulocytes (hematoxylin and eosin, 400×. *Source:* Image courtesy of Alvin Camus).

body), and intermediate body. The disease is typically diagnosed histologically but can be seen on skin or gill wet-mount preparations as markedly enlarged cells with amorphous or finely granular content (Figure 63.9).[21]

Parasites

Cytology is commonly used to screen for parasitic infections, which provide a route of entry for secondary invaders. Common ectoparasites and cytologic features are summarized in Table 63.2.

Protozoa

Ciliated protozoa are frequent ectoparasites of fish, often commensal but also including pathogens. These include holotrich ciliates, peritrich ciliates, and free-swimming opportunists causing various degrees of pathology (Table 63.2). Some feed on fish, others use fish only as substrate for attachment, and the degree of irritation and damage depends on extent of infection. Heavy infections are promoted by stressors and poor water quality, such as from high organic loads or high stocking density.

The holotrich ciliate *I. multifiliis* is the causative agent of "white spot disease" or "Ich," which is a clinically important, relatively nonhost-specific disease of freshwater fishes. The counterpart in marine fishes is *Cryptocaryon* spp. *C. irritans* causes rapid fulminant infection across taxa in infected systems, while other *Cryptocaryon* spp. cause low level intermittent disease in debilitated animals. These organisms have a direct life cycle with the trophont stage feeding extensively within the epidermis of the skin and gills. This stage is large, up to 1 mm diameter, and presents as small white spots on the skin and gill surface. On wet mounts, the trophonts are ciliated with slow rotating motion and variably apparent horseshoe-shaped macronucleus (Figure 63.10). After maturation, trophonts exit the epidermis into the water, causing regional skin damage and osmoregulatory failure. Mature trophonts encyst on substrate and divide into numerous ciliated theronts that progress to find new hosts. Epizootics are more common at higher temperatures because trophont maturation accelerates.[22,24]

Peritrich ciliates include sessile and motile organisms. Stalked ciliates, such as *Epistylis* sp., usually attach to environmental structures or crustaceans and only infect fish in high organic environments, especially in bottom dwellers and goldfish.[22] *Epistylis* sp. are colonial, form white tuft-like aggregates, and have a terminal bell-shaped structure (zooid), which retracts and extends (Figure 63.11a).[25] Heavy infections of motile peritrich ciliates, such as *Trichodina* sp., cause clinical disease characterized by increased mucus production, erosions, and eventual systemic effects including reduced food intake and weight loss. Trichodinid ciliates are characterized cytologically by an internal ring of radially arranged denticles (Figure 63.11b).

Free-swimming ciliates such as *Tetrahymena* sp. in freshwater fish and Scuticociliates in marine fish (*Uronema* sp., *Philasterides* sp., etc.) typically feed on decaying organic matter and invade fish with suboptimal conditions including high water temperatures, stress, and high organic loads. These ciliates can become highly invasive opportunists

Table 63.2 Selected common fish parasites with associated lesions and cytologic features.[1,4,22,23]

Parasite (freshwater or marine)	Disease/location	Cytologic features
Protozoa		
Ciliates, holotrich		
Ichthyophthirius multifiliis (freshwater) *Cryptocaryon irritans* (marine)	White spot disease (Ich) Trophonts encyst in epidermis and break out to complete life cycle	Trophonts up to 1 mm diameter with peripheral cilia (holotrich ciliated) Horseshoe-shaped macronucleus (macronucleus of Cryptocaryon may be obscured by granular cytoplasm) Motile in slow rotating/rolling motion
Chilodonella sp. (freshwater) *Brooklynella* sp. (marine)	Feed on epithelial cells causing erosion and hyperplasia	Flattened ovoid shape up to 80 μm long Rows of cilia (holotrich ciliated) Motile in slow gliding motion
Ciliates, Peritrich		
Sessile: *Ambiphyra* (*Scyphidia*) sp., *Glossatella* (*Apiosoma*) sp. Stalked: *Epistylis* sp., *Vorticella* sp., *Heteropolaria* sp. (freshwater, marine)	Often commensal Heavy infections may cause irritation through attachment	Flask-/bell-shaped up to 100 μm long Spiral cilia surrounding buccal cavity (peritrich ciliated) Unipolar adhesive disc ± stalk Nonmotile
Trichodina, Trichodinella, Tripartiella spp. (freshwater, marine)	Irritation with heavier infections Increased mucus production and epithelial erosion	Circular Ring of internal cytoskeletal denticles Spiral cilia surrounding buccal cavity (peritrich ciliated) Motile
Ciliates, Free swimming		
Tetrahymena sp. (freshwater), *Uronema marinum* (marine), *Miamiensis avidus* (marine)	Scuticociliatosis Facultative parasites Can cause ulcerative and invasive lesions into deep tissues and organs	Pyriform, approximately 60 × 100 μm Poorly defined internal vacuoles Free swimming and actively motile in a haphazardly undulating spiral motion ("drunken football spiral")
Flagellates		
Ichthyobodo sp. (freshwater, marine)	Costiasis Epithelial damage, hyperplasia, and mucus production	Oval, approximately 10–15 μm long (similar to fish erythrocytes) Free-swimming with paired flagella of unequal length in groove along body Motile in jerky spiral resembling a flickering flame
Myxozoa		
Myxobolus sp. (freshwater, marine)	Many tissues susceptible	Rounded, ovoid, or pyriform spores, approximately 8–25 μm Refractile wall Two pyriform polar capsules[a]
Henneguya sp. (freshwater, marine)	Gill preferentially affected	Ovoid to fusiform spores, approximately 10 μm Refractile wall Two anterior polar capsules[a] Two tapering elongate caudal tail appendages

(*Continued*)

Table 63.2 (Continued)

Parasite (freshwater or marine)	Disease/location	Cytologic features
Metazoa		
Platyhelminths, Monogenean		
Gyrodactylus sp. (freshwater, brackish, marine)	Mainly at skin Feeding of parasites causes increased mucus, epithelial erosion and ulcers, and gill damage with heavy infections	Small worms (0.3–1 mm) One pair of anchoring hooks, and 16 marginal hooklets Motile in a stretch-and-recoil motion Viviparous with potential to contain multiple generations of internal embryo with hooklets Do not have eyespots
Dactylogyrid (multiple genera) (primarily freshwater; rarely brackish and marine)	Mainly at gills Attachment and feeding causes damage	Small worms (up to 2 mm) Four eyespots (two pairs) One pair of anchoring hooks, ± small marginal hooks (12–14) Oviparous Motile in a stretch-and-recoil motion
Ancyrocephalid (multiple genera) (freshwater, brackish, marine)	Mainly at gills Attachment and feeding causes damage	Resemble dactylogrids (four eyespots, marginal hooks, oviparous) Two pair of terminal anchoring hooks
Capsalid (multiple genera) (brackish, marine)	Skin and gills Damage via suction adhesion	Large (up to 1–2 cm), flattened shape Anterior adhesive/suction discs, posterior haptor with hooks, marginal small hooklets Eyespots present but obscure
Platyhelminths, Digenean		
Multiple genera (freshwater, brackish, marine)	Often incidental Heavy or deep infections may be clinically relevant	Encysted, round to oval metacercariae approximately 0.2–1 mm in various tissues Thin walled with internal larva May see larva move within metacercarial wall
Crustaceans (arthropods)		
Branchiuran crustacean: *Argulus* sp. (freshwater, marine)	Fish lice Attachment and feeding causes hemorrhage and ulcers	Large, can be macroscopic, approximately 0.5–1 cm Dorsoventrally flattened with carapace Proboscis spine, suckers, and hooks
Copepod crustacean: Lernaeid, Ergasilid, Caligidae families (multiple genera) (freshwater, marine)	Anchor worms Damage from attachment ± feeding, causing ulceration	Variably sized, <2 mm up to 1–2 cm, and variably shaped *Lernaea* sp. females are Y-shaped with extruded paired egg sacs
Oomycetes		
Multiple genera (freshwater, marine)	Often opportunistic superficial skin infection, can invade	Pleomorphic Often long, branching, aseptate, nonpigmented hyphae (approximately 7–30 μm) ± terminal zoosporangia and/or zoospores (approximately 5–10 μm)
Microsporidia		
Multiple genera (*Glugea*, *Loma*, *Pleistophora* spp., etc.) (freshwater, marine)	Many tissues susceptible	Oval to pyriform, refractile, spores, approximately 2–10 μm diameter One posterior vacuole

[a] The polar capsules of myxozoan spores each contain a coiled polar filament involved in parasitic adhesion or penetration. This filament is commonly not visualized on cytology but may occasionally be extruded, especially with air-dried preparations, in which it is seen as a long linear strand extending from each polar capsule at the anterior of the spore.

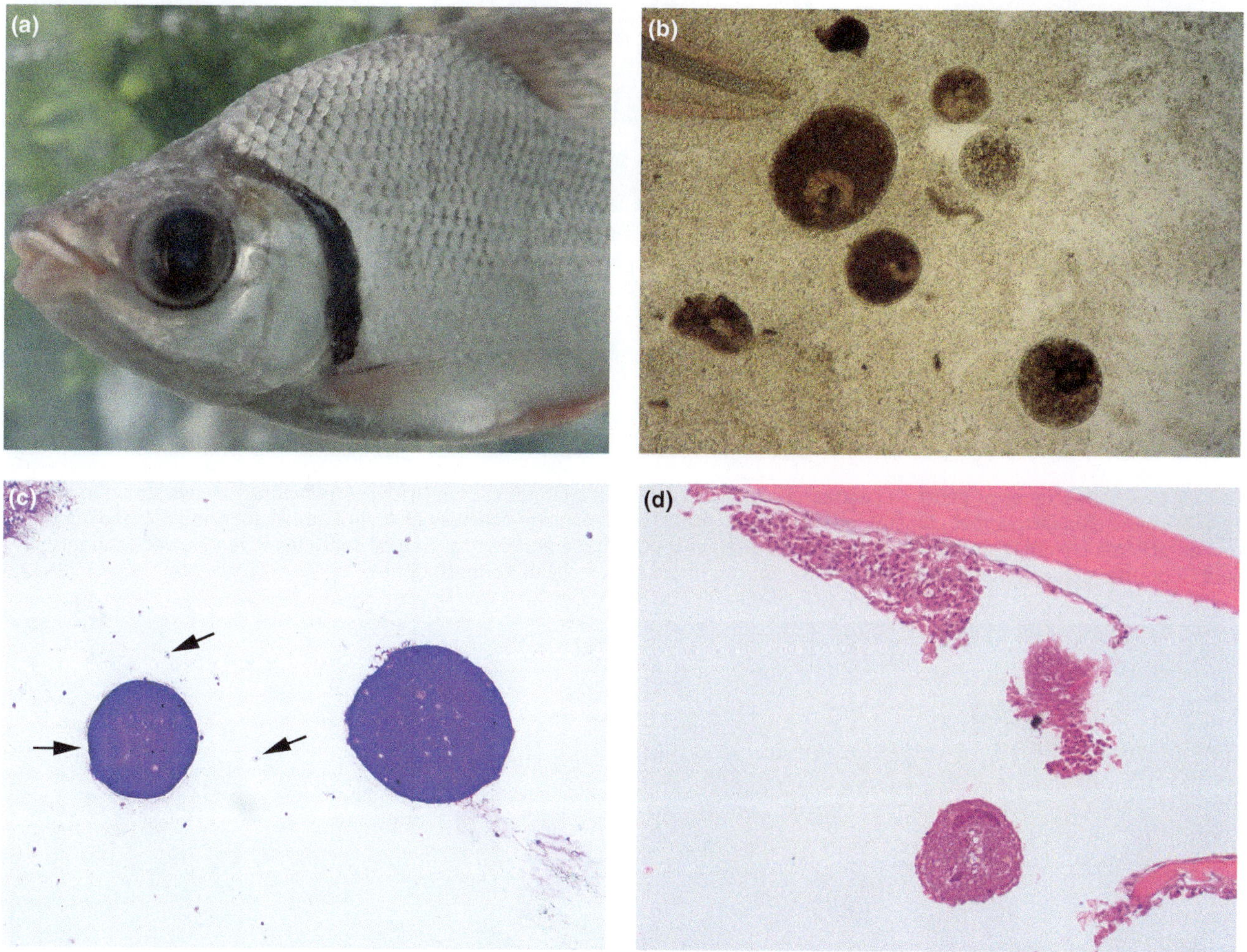

Figure 63.10 Infection by holotrich ciliates. (a) A classic clinical presentation of encysted *Ichthiophthirius multifiliis* organisms in the skin of a redfin prochilodus (*Semaprochilodus taeniurus*) is characterized by pinpoint to 1 mm-diameter white foci across the head and face (*Source:* Image courtesy of Angela Perry). (b) Cytology of *I. multifiliis* trophonts on the gill of a clown loach (*Chromobotia macracanthus*) illustrates the large size and variably apparent C-shaped macronucleus (unstained wet mount, 200×). (c) Air-dried cytology of I. multifiliis organisms from the skin of a paratilapia (Paratilapia polleni). The ciliate organisms are thick and deeply staining. The peripheral cilia give a "fuzzy" appearance. A C-shaped macronucleus is indistinctly discernable in the left organism (black arrow). Poorly stained erythrocytes are present in the background (black arrows), indicating large organism size (modified Wright's, 200×). (d) Histology of *Cryptocaryon* sp. affecting the skin of a pearlscale butterflyfish (*Chaetodon xanthurus*). Morphology is similar, including large size and C-shaped macronucleus (hematoxylin and eosin, 400×).

resulting in muscular and visceral necrotizing to inflammatory lesions in a wide range of fish. Cytologic features include pyriform shape and haphazardly undulating spiraling motion on wet-mount cytology (Figure 63.12).[26,27]

Significant flagellated protozoa on the skin and gills of marine and freshwater fishes include *Cryptobia* sp., which are variably reported to cause pathology, and *Ichthyobodo* sp. such as *Ichthyobodo necatrix* (*Costia necator*), which causes costiasis. Cytologically, free-swimming and early-attached *Ichthyobodo* sp. are oval with fine flagella of unequal length and a quick jerky motion on wet mount (Table 63.2, Figure 63.13). The attached trophont stage lacks apparent flagella and penetrates epithelial cells of the skin and gills using a cytostome complex causing epithelial damage, hyperplasia, and mucus production.[22,28]

Myxozoa

Myxozoans infect many tissues and, as a class, are characterized by multicellular, variably shaped spores containing a sporoplasm and one or multiple polar capsules (commonly two), each with an internal coiled filament. Some common spore morphologies are nicely diagramed elsewhere.[1] Spores develop within multicellular plasmodia (cysts). Cytology is helpful to identify myxozoa and to distinguish spore features that differentiate agents (Table 63.2). Molecular techniques can be used to further characterize

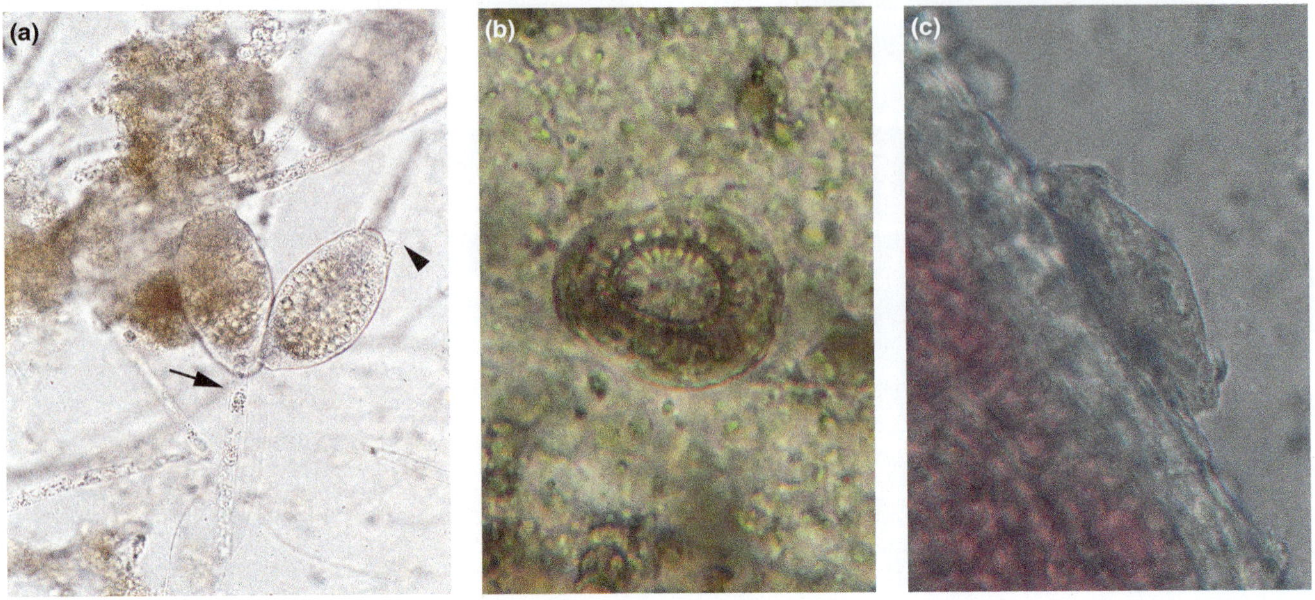

Figure 63.11 Skin scrapes of peritrich ciliates. (a) *Epistylis* sp. from a channel catfish (*Ictalurus punctatus*) shows stalk (arrow) and peritrichous cilia (arrowhead) (unstained wet mount, 400×. *Source:* Image courtesy of Alvin Camus). (b) and (c) *Trichodina* sp. from a paratilapia cichlid (*Paratilapia polleni*) shows distinct round shape and central ring of denticles when viewed straight on (b) and in profile (c) (unstained wet mounts, 400×. *Source:* Images courtesy of Kenneth Conley).

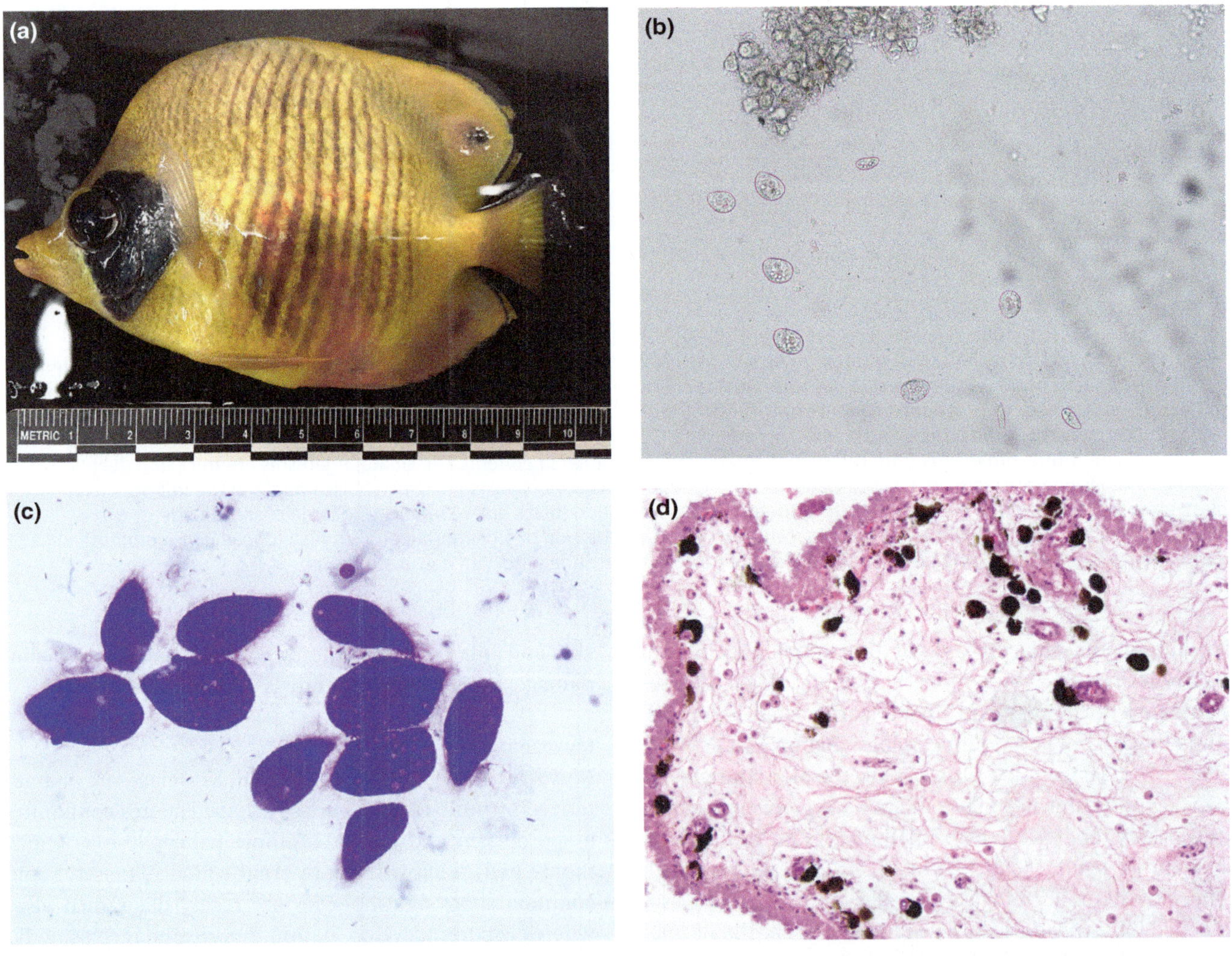

Figure 63.12 Infection by free-swimming ciliates. (a) Golden butterflyfish (*Chaetodon semilarvatus*) has multiple confluent areas of red discoloration, scale elevation, and abnormal gray-discolored mucus coat along the body wall (cm scale). (b) The skin/pouch of a northern seahorse (*Hippocampus erectus*) shows numerous scuticociliates with characteristic pyriform shape and diffuse cilia (unstained wet mount, 400×). (c) Skin scrape from archerfish (*Toxotes jaculatrix*) shows numerous scuticociliates that are deeply staining with cytoplasmic vacuolation, poorly discerned nuclei, and circumferential frill-like cilia (air-dried cytology, modified Wright's, 1000×). (d) Northern seahorse (*H. erectus*) with invasive scuticociliatosis (hematoxylin and eosin, 600×).

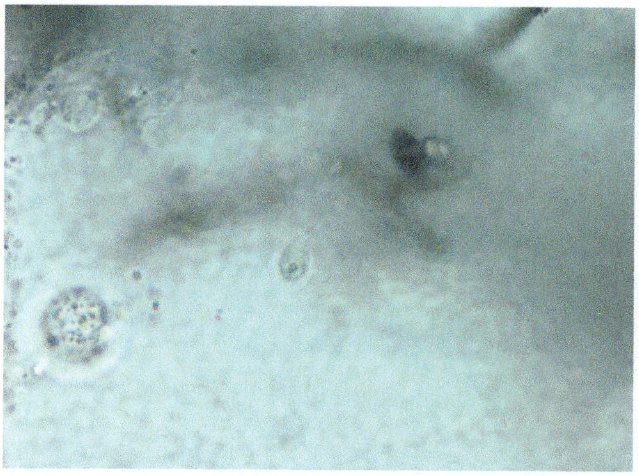

Figure 63.13 Skin from a leopard bushfish (*Leopard ctenopoma*) showing an *Ichthyobodo* sp. flagellate (center) (unstained wet mount, 400×. *Source:* Image courtesy of Kenneth Conley).

specific organisms. Myxozoan parasites affecting the skin include *Myxobolus* sp., *Thelohanellus* sp., and *Henneguya* sp.; however, clinical disease is more frequent in the gills and musculoskeletal system.

Metazoa

Common parasitic metazoans of the skin diagnosed cytologically include monogenean and digenean platyhelminths (flatworms). These parasites are commonly found on wild fish but typically cause disease in captivity, where crowding and environmental factors increase parasite loads.

Monogeneans have direct life cycles and include numerous species within more than 10 families. Major monogenean families diagnosed cytologically are Gyrodactylidae, Dactylogyridae, Ancyrocephalidae, and Capsalidae. Gyrodactylids comprise hundreds of species, most of which are host specific. They are common ectoparasites in freshwater and marine fishes. Many gyrodactylids are viviparous and can reproduce rapidly, with epizootics often linked to poor environmental conditions and stress. Adults can carry fully developed embryos, which in turn can carry embryos (hyperviviparity, akin to "Russian nesting dolls"). Morphologically, gyrodactylids also are characterized by hooks, suckers, and a lack of eyespots (Figure 63.14a). They are transmitted from fish to fish as well as through water. Parasite feeding on blood and tissue in heavy infections causes increased mucus production, frayed fins, skin ulcers, and damaged gills.[23,29] Dactylogyrids include multiple genera (*Dactylogyrus*, *Haliotrema*) and predominantly parasitize the gills, especially in freshwater cyprinids. These organisms are oviparous, and egg development is affected by environmental conditions.[22] Dactylogyrids have hooks and two pairs of distinctive eyespots (Figure 63.14b). Ancyrocephalids also include multiple genera and are closely related and morphologically similar to dactylogyrids, but with two rather than one pair of terminal anchors (Figure 63.14c). Ancyrocephalids are relatively nonhost specific and affect both freshwater and saltwater species.[23] Capsalids, including *Neobenedenia* sp. and *Benedenia* sp., also are considerably less host specific and predominantly parasitize marine fish at the skin and gills, causing damage via suction attachment to the host. These organisms are large and flattened with anterior adhesive suction discs, marginal hooklets, and a posterior haptor with hooks (Figure 63.14d). Masses of brown, triangular, capsalid eggs can also be identified cytologically (Figure 63.14d inset).

Digenean metacercariae of various species have an indirect life cycle and encyst in the skin, fins, and other tissues in freshwater and marine fishes. The encysted metacercariae are round to oval and thin walled with an internal larva that can sometimes be seen to move on wet-mount preparations (Figure 63.15). Encysted metacercariae can cause macroscopic pigment deposition ("black spot"). These parasites usually are not clinically significant unless infesting young fish, causing heavy infections, or penetrating into deep tissues. Examples include *Posthodiplostomum cuticola* in cyprinids and *Cryptocotyle lingua* in marine fish, whose main definitive hosts are fish-eating birds.[22] *Nanophyetus salmincola* in salmonids has carnivores as definitive hosts and is usually incidental except when carrying *Neorickettsia helminthoeca*, the causative agent of salmon poisoning seen most commonly in dogs of the Pacific Northwest.

The skin is also a possible location for nematode infection. One example is infection by *Huffmanela* sp., which is reported to cause grossly apparent, black, serpiginous tracts due to egg deposition in sandbar sharks and rockfish.[30] Eggs are histologically embedded in the epidermis and are seen cytologically (e.g. skin scrape wet mount) as oval, approximately 50–80 μm-long and 20–50 μm-wide structures with a variably dark brown and rugose shell, bipolar plugs, and occasional enclosed coiled larva.[31,32]

Other ectoparasites of fish include crustacean arthropods and less commonly other metazoans (e.g. leeches, mollusks). These parasites are often identified grossly and cytologically. Crustacean parasites affect the skin and gills of freshwater and marine fish, causing pathology due to parasite attachment and feeding. The most common of these parasites are *Argulus* sp., also known as fish lice, which cause pathology by attachment of suckers, hooks, or a spine and subsequent feeding, resulting in ulceration and potential secondary infections. The life cycle is direct, and heavy infections cause skin and gill damage. Copepod crustaceans

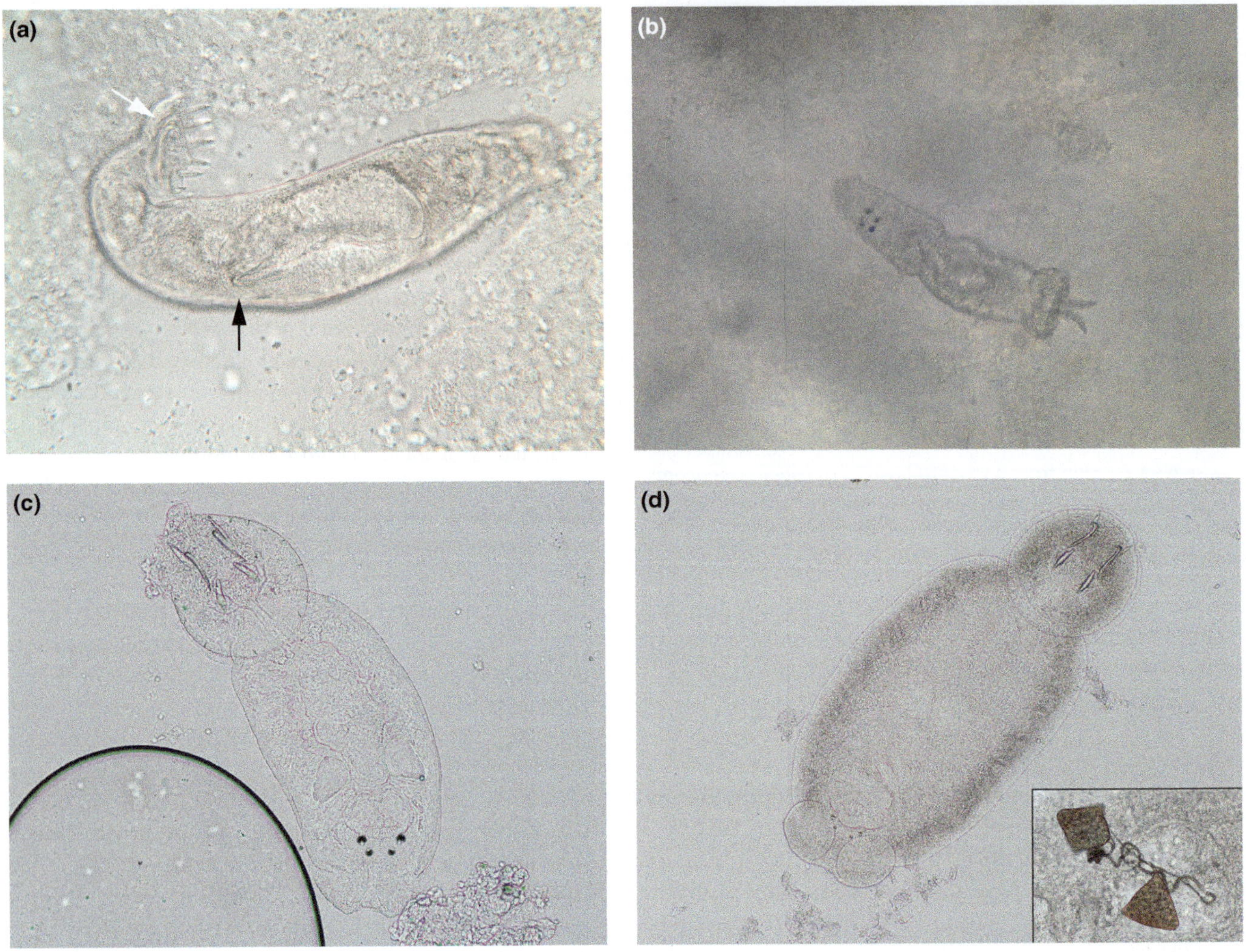

Figure 63.14 Monogenean platyhelminths from the skin and gills. (a) Gyrodactylid from a goldfish (*Carassius auratus*) showing anchoring hooks (white arrow), adjacent marginal hooks, and embryo with hooklets (black arrow). Note the lack of eyespots (unstained wet mount, 200×. *Source:* Image courtesy of Rodman Getchell). (b) Dactylogyrid from a butterfly koi (*Cyprinus carpio*) shows two pairs of eyespots and one pair of anchoring hooks (unstained wet mount, 100×). (c) Ancyrocephalid from a schooling coachman (*Heniochus diphreutes*) showing eyespots and two pairs of terminal anchoring hooks (unstained wet mount, 200×). (d) Capsalid from a longnose hawkfish (*Oxycirrhites typus*) showing anterior suction discs and posterior haptor with hooks (unstained wet mount, 100×). Inset: Typical capsalid-type eggs having long threads used for attachment (unstained wet mount, 200×).

include Lernaeid, Ergasilid, and Caligidae families. Usually, the mature female copepod is parasitic and embeds in the dermis, causing ulceration and extruding posterior egg sacs (Figure 63.16). These infections occasionally penetrate the musculature and coelom, especially in small fish. *Lernaea cyprinacea* is the "anchor worm" of freshwater fish, and causes morbidity and mortality mainly in young fish or with heavy infections of the skin and gills.[22]

Fungi and Fungal-Like Organisms

Oomycete and fungal infections in the skin of fish are usually opportunistic and associated with concurrent skin damage, immunosuppression, and environmental factors. Oomycetes are water molds classed with diatoms and algae. The most common oomycetes are of the Saprolegniales order, including *Saprolegnia*, *Achlya*, and *Aphanomyces* species.[33] Oomycete overgrowth appears grossly as white fuzzy growths on submerged fish and as collapsed, gelatinous, clear to white plaques out of the water. The infections are superficial but can invade the body wall, often with little inflammation. Cytologically, the organisms are pleomorphic between species but generally include long, branching, aseptate, nonpigmented hyphae (approximately 7–30 μm) (Figure 63.17). Reproductive structures such as zoosporangia and zoospores are sometimes present.[25,33] Oomycete infections are not commonly

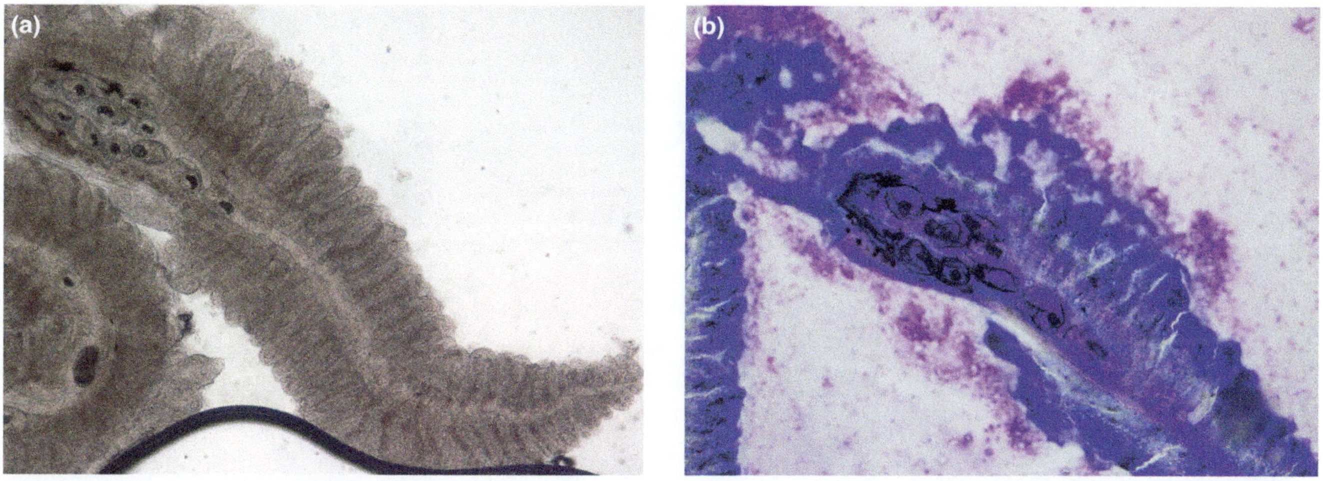

Figure 63.15 Gill clip from an Atlantic mudskipper (*Periophthalmus barbarus*) with encysted digenean platyhelminth metacercariae in the base of the primary gill filament. (a) The encysted metacercariae are rounded to oval with a thin wall within which larvae can be occasionally seen to move (unstained wet mount, 40×). (b) The air-dried cytology loses cellular details but retains larval outlines (modified Wright's, 100×).

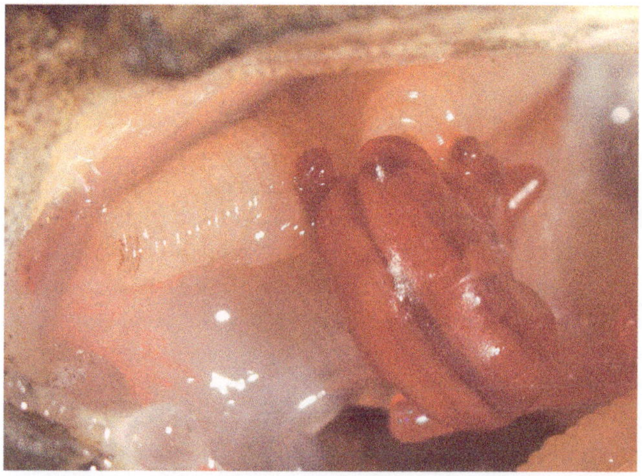

Figure 63.16 Gills and opercular cavity from a Pacific spiny lumpsucker (*Eumicrotremus orbis*) with severe copepod infection. Attached to the gill are multiple large Lernaeid-type crustaceans characterized by a deep red body and elongate yellow spiral egg casings.

speciated by ancillary diagnostics as treatment is usually empirical.

Unlike other oomycetes, *Aphanomyces invadans* is a true primary pathogen causing "epizootic ulcerative syndrome", which since the 1970s has progressed to a worldwide pandemic in freshwater and brackish water fish, causing huge economic losses.[33,34] The infection is acquired by attachment of the free-swimming zoospore to the skin, which goes on to develop vegetative hyphae that invade host tissues. External lesions typically consist of ulcerative lesions and penetrating myopathy with mycotic granulomas. In most, but not all species, infection is enabled by initial skin injury. In addition to skin and muscle, the oomycete can spread extensively in visceral tissues.[35]

Like terrestrial vertebrates, fish are susceptible to true fungal infections including *Aspergillus* sp., *Fusarium* sp., and various zygomycetes. Fungal morphology is consistent with findings in other animals. *Fusarium* infections have been particularly reported in marine species, including angelfish and sharks. Infections by dematiaceous *Exophiala* sp. fungi are reported in various freshwater and marine teleosts, seahorses, and elasmobranchs (Figure 63.18).[30,34,36,37] Mycotic lesions vary from necrotizing to granulomatous and cutaneous to systemic. Underlying husbandry factors or injury are likely involved in establishing infections.

Microsporidians were once considered protists but are now recognized as spore-forming unicellular fungi. Various microsporidia including *Glugea* sp. and *Pleistophora* sp. can cause skin and gill lesions but are more frequently found internally.

Algae

Algal dermatitis caused by nonfilamentous algae has been reported in fish. In a report of cichlids with green to ulcerated skin lesions and cutaneous to disseminated granulomatous inflammation, algae were identified on wet-mount preparations of skin scrapings and tissue squash preparations as variably green, oval cells, morphologically resembling algal infections described in terrestrial vertebrates (e.g. chlorellosis, protothecosis). The organisms in the fish were identified as *Chlorochytrium* sp. and *Scenedesmus* sp., which belong to the Chlorococcales order, along with

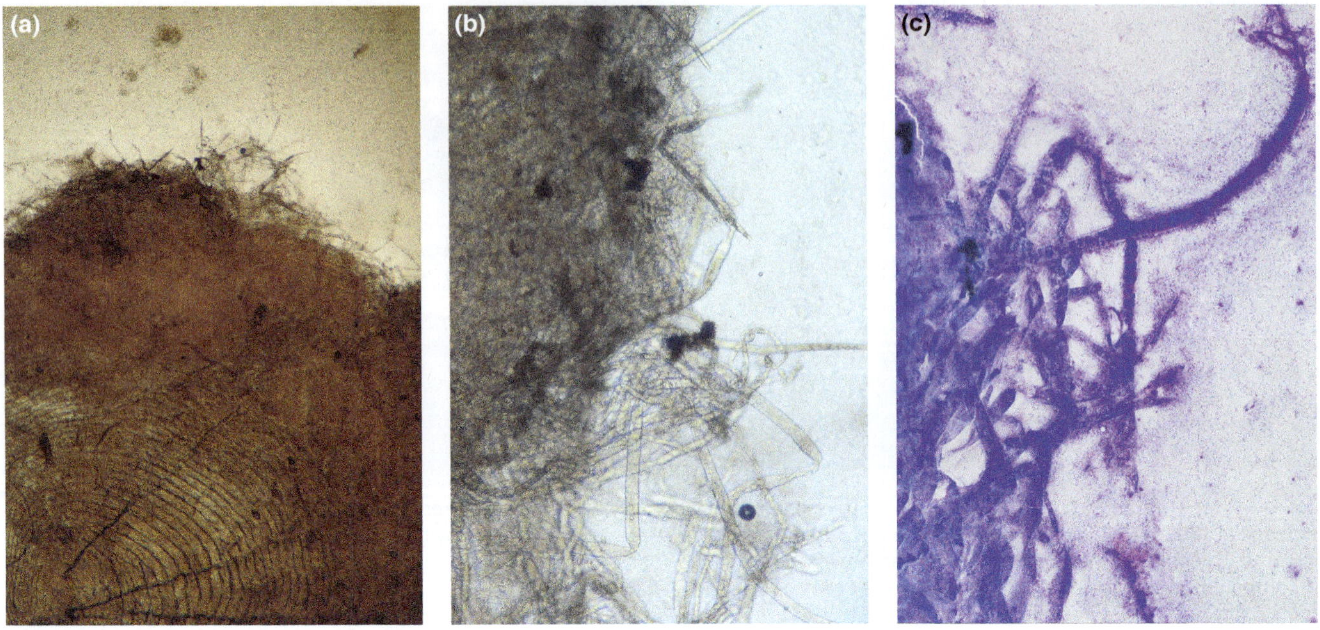

Figure 63.17 Skin scrape from a common shiner (*Luxilus cornutus*) with cutaneous oomycete overgrowth. (a) Dense mats of oomycete hyphae surround the margin of a scale (unstained wet mount, 100×). (b-c) Higher magnification of the scale margin on unstained wet mount (b) and modified Wright's stained preparations (c). Hyphae are branching, nonseptate, and nonpigmented (200×).

Chlorella sp.[38] Dinoflagellates, which are flagellated protists variably grouped with algae, also can parasitize the skin. "Velvet disease" is discussed further under the respiratory system.

Mesomycetozoea

Mesomycetozoea include organisms previous classified under various other orders (e.g. fungi, protozoa) but now recognized as a distinct class including the orders Dermocystida and Ichthyophonida. Infections by *Dermocystidium* sp. affect a variety of freshwater fish, causing skin, gill, and visceral lesions. This organism was previously classified as a fungus but is now under mesomycetozoea (nonanimal, non-fungal eukaryotes). It forms large elongate cysts (approximately 1 mm diameter) containing numerous round spores (5–8 µm diameter) with an eccentric nucleus and vacuole. Cysts and abundant spores are seen on wet-mount preparations, and the vacuolar inclusions appear refractile (refractile body) (Figure 63.19). Host inflammatory and fibrotic responses contribute to pathogenesis, especially in gill infections.[33,39] *Ichthyophonus* sp. infection tends to affect deeper tissues and is discussed below.

Viruses

Viral lesions of the skin are less commonly diagnosed cytologically. Those causing hyperplastic and neoplastic lesions are discussed below. Nodular skin lesions are caused by lymphocystivirus (lymphocystis disease virus 1), an iridovirus, in freshwater and marine fishes. The lesions can be seen cytologically on wet-mount preparations as markedly hypertrophied infected dermal fibroblasts, expanding up to 1–2 mm diameter (Figure 63.20). Histologically, cells exhibit variable karyomegaly and nuclear degeneration, basophilic intracytoplasmic viral inclusion material, and development of a hyaline capsule. While epitheliocystis infection also causes microscopically observable enlarged cells (more often at the gills), the cellular expansion is due to proliferation of chlamydial-like organisms, without karyomegaly or viral inclusion material. The hypertrophied cells in lymphocystis infection occur individually or in clusters, sometimes appearing macroscopically as spots or exophytic tumors.[5,25] Many other viruses affect fish, but cytologic findings are not well characterized overall.[40]

Hyperplasia and Neoplasia

The skin is the most common location of proliferative lesions in fish, and a wide variety of hyperplasic to neoplastic lesions are reported, including epithelial, spindle cell (mesenchymal), and round (discrete) cell lesions.[13,41] Histology is most often required for definitive diagnosis. Ancillary testing can identify underlying infectious causes. Some lesions are promoted by environmental exposures to carcinogens and other toxins. The pathologic

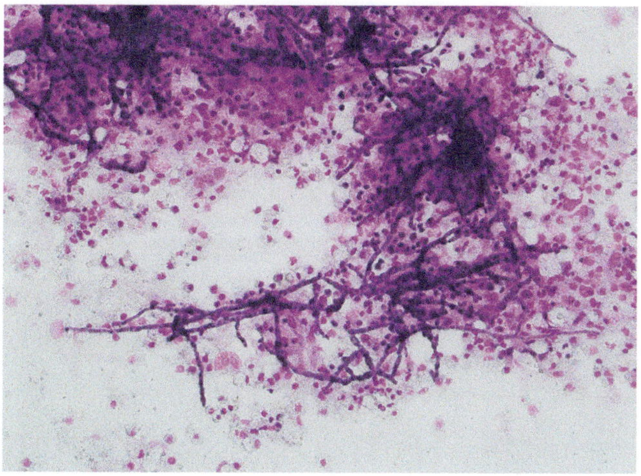

Figure 63.18 Superficial eye and skin scrape from sargassum fish (*Histrio histrio*) with *Exophiala* sp. infection. Pigmented, branching, fungal hyphae are present amid abundant macrophagic inflammation (modified Wright's, 400×).

classification of proliferative lesions in fish extrapolates from schemes used for other taxa. Anatomic and cytologic features of lesions are largely consistent with other vertebrates. Underlying viral etiology is documented or suspected for some entities based on viral isolation, ultrastructure, and/or experimental transmission, but is not cytologically apparent in most cases.

Hyperplastic and neoplastic epithelial lesions of fish are characterized predominantly by non-keratinizing epithelial cells with variable degrees of atypia. Papillomas, which are among the most common cutaneous proliferations in fish, can develop with repeated trauma or irritation, chemical exposures, or viral infection.[13] They are generally raised and papillary to plaque-like. Examples include (i) papillomas of the skin of koi and carp induced by cyprinid herpesvirus 1 (carp pox) with spontaneous resolution and rare transformation to squamous cell carcinoma,[5] (ii) seasonal papillomatosis of Atlantic salmon associated ultrastructurally with retroviral particles,[41,42] and (iii) papillomatous lesions in sharks and rays, with spontaneous resolution and variable evidence for viral underpinnings.[30,43] Histologically, these lesions are predominantly characterized by proliferative non-keratinizing epithelial cells with variably observed viral inclusions (intracytoplasmic or intranuclear). Cytology is rarely reported, but descriptions of increased epithelial cellularity with cohesively clustered cells, increased cytoplasmic basophilia, and mild to moderate pleomorphism (anisocytosis, anisokaryosis) are in the literature. In a guitarfish, intranuclear viral particles were cytologically observed but no definitive virus was isolated.[5,43] Numerous other virus-associated epidermal proliferative lesions of fish are described (e.g. discrete epidermal hyperplasia and diffuse epidermal hyperplasia of walleye, and smooth-type and granular-type epidermal hyperplasia of northern pike, each with retroviral or herpesviral association),[41,44–46] and more are likely to be identified. These conditions vary in gross appearance (multifocal or coalescing, smooth or granular, discrete or diffuse) and histology (e.g. basilar vs. panepidermal hyperplasia, with occasional unique findings such as megalocytic cells in the granular-type lesions of northern pike). However, characteristic cytologic findings are not yet reported.

Squamous cell carcinoma is less common in fish than other vertebrates, reported mainly in individual captive or wild fish. The cranial region might be more commonly involved. Lesions can ulcerate and are locally invasive.[13] Cytology is characterized by non-keratinized squamous

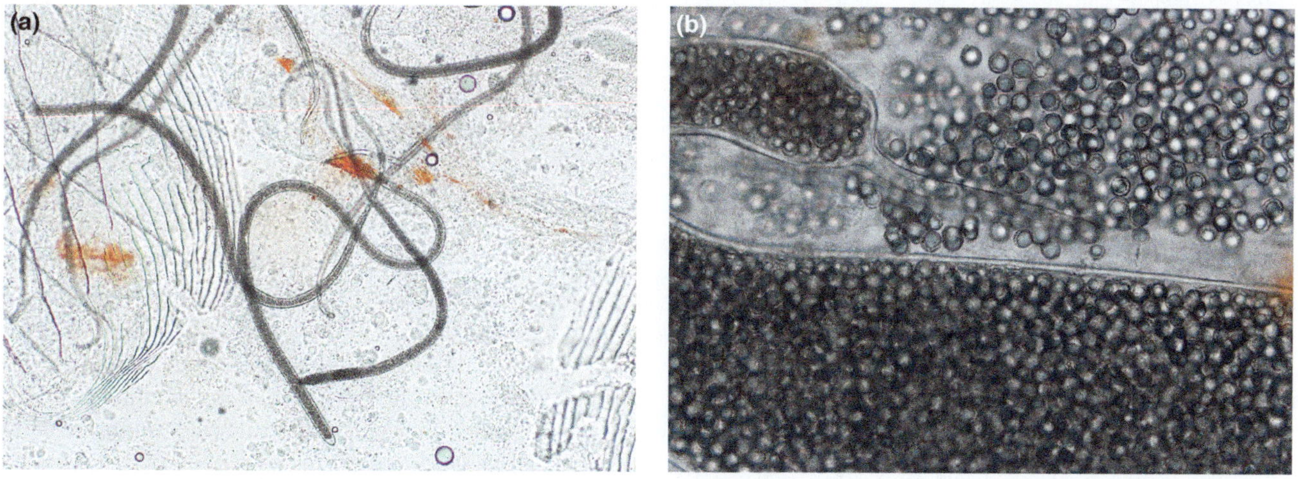

Figure 63.19 Skin scrapes from a cardinal tetra (*P. axelrodi*) with dermocystidium infection. (a) Elongate cysts amid scales and cellular debris. (b) Cysts contain myriad refractile spores (unstained wet mounts, (a) 100×, (b) 400×).

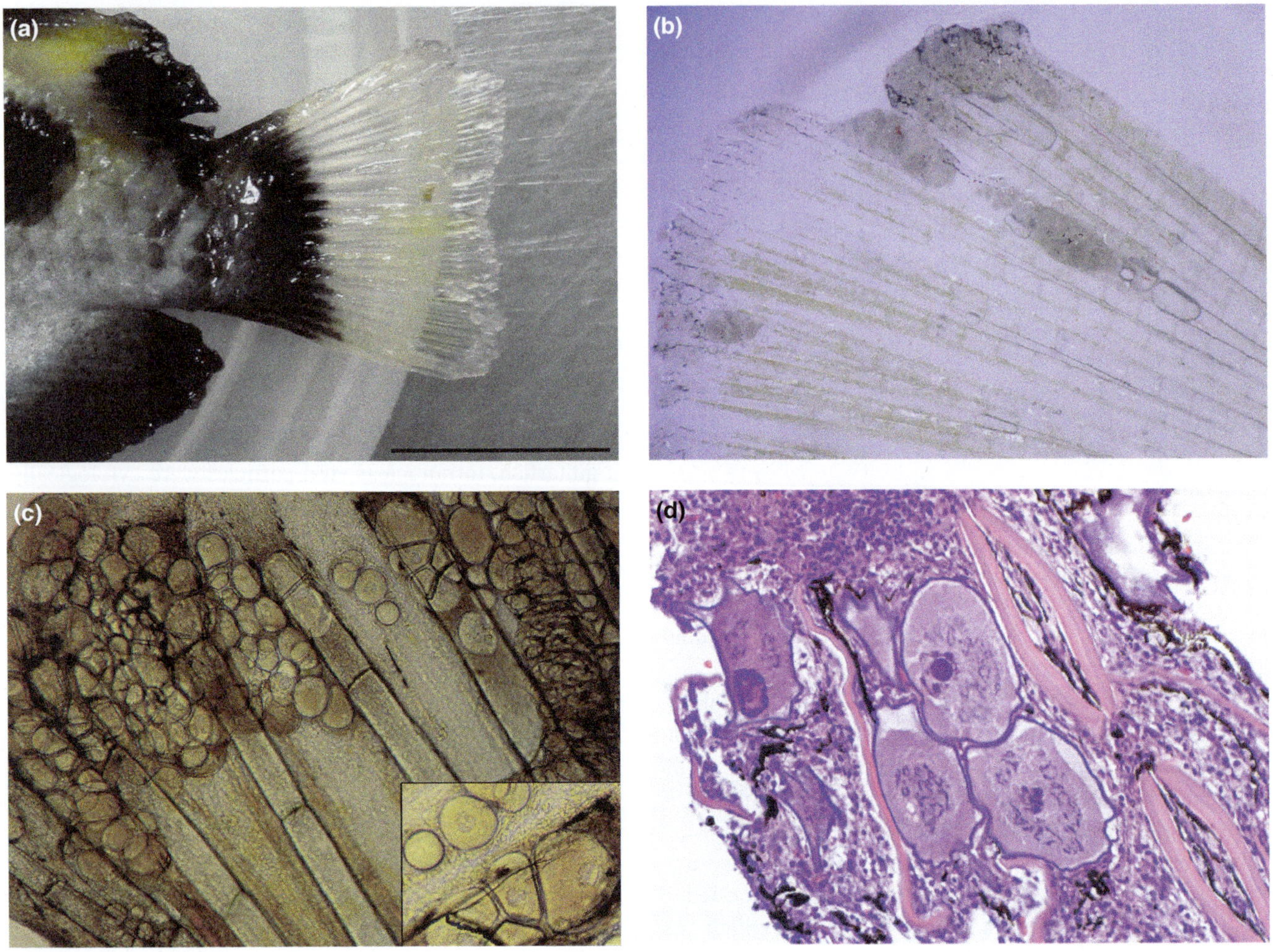

Figure 63.20 Archerfish (*T. jaculatrix*) with lymphocystis disease viral infection. (a) There are multifocal to coalescing 0.1–0.5 mm-diameter nodules along the tips of the fins (Bar = 1 cm). (b) Fin clip shows clusters of hypertrophied dermal fibroblasts corresponding to gross lesions (unstained wet mount, 20×). (c) The distinct hypertrophied and rounded fibroblasts have cytoplasmic and nuclear expansion due to accumulation of poorly discerned viral particles. Inset: Subtle cytoplasmic hazy viral aggregates and irregular degenerating nuclear margins (unstained wet mount, 100×, Inset: 200×). (d) The fin shows hypertrophied infected fibroblasts expanding the dermis, characterized by enlarged degenerate nuclei, finely granular basophilic viral cytoplasmic inclusion material, and hyaline walls. The surrounding dermis is moderately inflamed (hematoxylin and eosin, 600×. *Source:* Images courtesy of Joseph Malatos).

epithelial cells with increased cellular pleomorphism. Due to lack of keratinization, differentiation from carcinomas of other cell lineages can be challenging and often relies on histologic tissue architecture.

Spindle cell neoplasms of fish, including fibromas, schwannomas, neurofibromas, and their malignant counterparts (fibrosarcomas, malignant schwannomas, neurofibrosarcomas) are characterized by spindloid cells arranged in variably dense aggregates with a spectrum of pleomorphism. Cytologic interpretation relies upon identification of routine criteria of malignancy (Chapter 5). Distinguishing neoplastic from nonneoplastic lesions is more difficult in the presence of inflammation, when cellular atypia can reflect reactive rather than neoplastic changes. Cytologic and histologic features are typically insufficient to reach a definitive cell origin identification. Due to limited availability and efficacy of immunohistochemical markers in fish, ultrastructure is often utilized.

The biological behavior of mesenchymal masses ranges from locally expansile to regionally infiltrative and less commonly metastatic. Although not cytologically distinctive, notable spindle cell proliferative lesions in fish include dermal sarcomas of walleye and neurofibromatosis-like disease of bicolor damselfish. In walleye, dermal sarcomas are associated with retrovirus infection causing dome-shaped, multifocal to coalescing, dermal nodules composed of variably pleomorphic spindle cells and collagenous matrix with histologic evidence of osseous metaplasia in some.[41,47] The proliferation can surround a central scale in the dermal scale bed, but invasive tumors are rare. The proliferations are seasonal, and regression is characterized by mononuclear cell infiltration, epidermal ulceration, tumor necrosis, and involution, which can be tolerated or cause secondary systemic compromise depending on the degree of invasion and other factors.[41,47] The well-documented neurofibromatosis-like disease of bicolor damselfish is characterized by multicentric tumors along skin, spinal, cranial, or visceral nerves that are identified as neurofibromas, malignant peripheral nerve sheath tumors, and chromatophoromas. The masses can be plaque-like, pigmented, and locally invasive epidermal lesions or can progress to dermal to subcutaneous masses that are highly invasive internally and externally. The lesions have been reproduced experimentally, but an etiology has not been definitively determined; a "damselfish virus-like agent" is postulated.[41,48,49]

Round cell tumors are less common in fish than in domestic species, and cytology is rare. Lesions described as cutaneous lymphoma are reported in muskellunge and northern pike in association with retrovirus infection, which has been reproduced experimentally. The disease is seasonal and progressive (malignant) with postulated horizontal transmission. Lesions are soft, pale tan, coalescing infiltrative plaques composed of atypical round cells in the dermis and epidermis, and variably extending into deeper tissues. The round cells have moderate eosinophilic cytoplasm, rounded to occasionally reniform nuclei, fine chromatin, and common mitoses. Small lymphocytes are interspersed. Limited immunohistochemical and ultrastructural studies indicate uncertainty as to definitive cellular lineage, with possibilities including T lymphocytic or histiocytic/monocytic origin.[41,50,51]

Other neoplasms reported in the skin of fish include pigmented tumors (melanocytic neoplasms, chromatophoromas, chromatoblastomas), for which the embryologic origin (e.g. neural crest lineage) is not uniformly elucidated.[5] Single and multiple erythrophoromas are reported in goldfish and carp, while melanomas are more common in other fish.[13] Spontaneous melanomas of platyfish × swordtail hybrids were one of the earliest models of genetically regulated neoplastic disease, based on a sex-linked oncogene *Xmrk*.[13] Limited published cytology of these neoplasms is consistent with expected findings of pigment tumors in other taxa, with rounded to polygonal cells variably filled with pigment granules ranging in color and texture. In a chromatophoroma of a crevice kelpfish, neoplastic cells had numerous round, reddish brown, intracytoplasmic granules (Figure 63.21).[52] Cytologic findings in iridophore proliferations include intracellular crystals that are birefringent with polarized light.

Musculoskeletal

Teleosts and elasmobranchs have red and white muscle based on vascular and metabolic differences. Myodegeneration, necrosis, and regenerative changes are similar to other taxa. Inflammation is usually monocytic/macrophagic and less commonly granulocytic. Skeletal muscle diseases are of particular economic impact to the sale of fish meat. The skeletal system of teleosts generally lacks a marrow cavity and haversian systems, reducing the incidence of osteomyelitis except by extension.[10] The entire endoskeleton of sharks, chimaeras and rays is cartilaginous and composed of chondrocytes in an extracellular matrix (ECM) surrounded by a fibrous perichondrium. The ECM is mineralized to varying degrees with crystals of calcium phosphate hydroxyapatite; the extent of mineralization depends on endoskeletal location. Cytologic assessment of the musculoskeletal system in fish is performed primarily for macroscopically apparent lesions, such as those characterized by localized discoloration, alteration in texture, or nodular expansion. These lesions can be noted antemortem but are generally identified and assessed postmortem.

Infection and Inflammation

Many infectious agents affecting the skin and subcutis of fish are capable of involving the musculoskeletal system. The following sections make note of similarities and highlight particular agents of concern for the musculoskeletal system.

Bacteria

Superficial bacterial infections of the skin in fish often extend to involve skeletal muscles and less commonly cartilage and bone. As in the skin, Gram-negative bacteria are common, and numerous other bacteria, including *Mycobacteria* sp., are reported (Table 63.1). The classic lesion of *A. salmonicida* infection is the "furuncle," a localized infection extending from the skin and dermis into the skeletal muscle. Such bacterial infections often cause necrotizing myositis with a central core of necrotic debris, bacterial colonies, and granulocyte infiltration followed by macrophages. With time, inflammatory lesions develop granulation tissue, fibrosis, and usually minimal myoregeneration. Chronic granulomas are common with *Mycobacteria* sp., *Nocardia* sp., and *R. salmoninarum*, creating nodular expansions that are apparent externally in

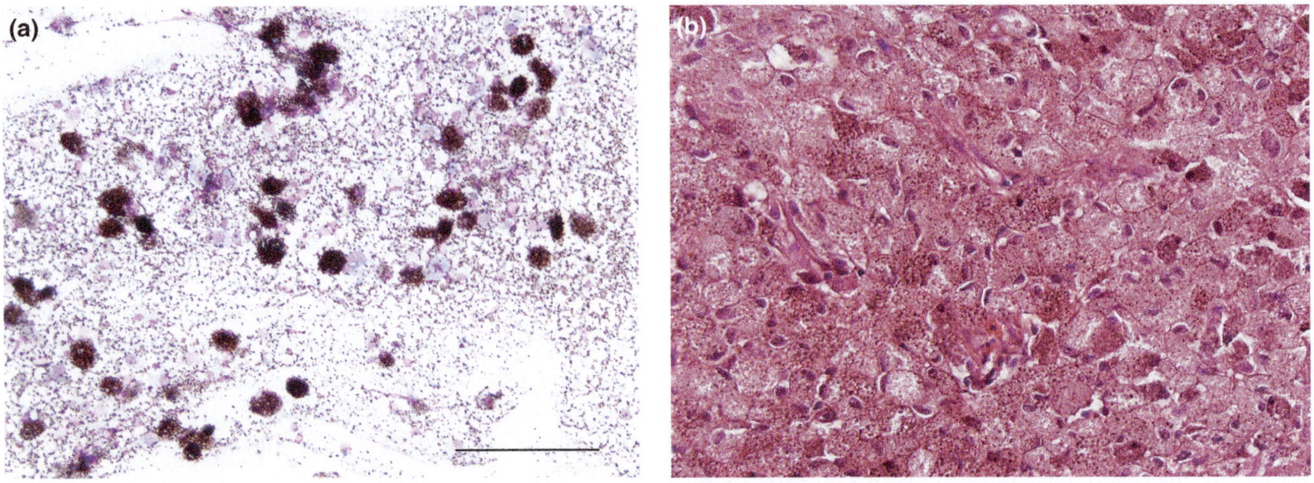

Figure 63.21 Chromatophoroma from a crevice kelpfish (*Gibbonsia montereyensis*). (a) There is a monotypic population of highly pigmented and mildly pleomorphic round cells with abundant free red-brown pigment granules (modified Wright's, bar = 50 μm). (b) Histology shows sheets of round to polygonal cells with fine red-brown cytoplasmic granules (hematoxylin and eosin, 400×. *Source:* Images courtesy of Alvin Camus).

some cases. On cut section, the lesions have caseous centers that form craterous lesions in the muscle. Cytologically, a mixture of cell debris, inflammatory cells, and bacteria are seen. Increased numbers of phagocytized bacteria support pathogenicity, and acid-fast staining is helpful for mycobacteriosis.

Protozoa

Parasitic infections of the musculoskeletal system cause variable tissue damage and include many of the agents affecting the skin and subcutis. Most ciliated protozoa tend to remain on the skin surface but under the right conditions can invade the body wall and viscera. Ciliates more commonly found in deep infections include free-swimming scuticociliates such as *Tetrahymena* and *Uronema* spp. (Figure 63.12). The key cytologic findings in these lesions are identification of organisms (Table 63.2); evidence of tissue degeneration or inflammation can also be noted. Flagellate protozoa, such as *Spironucleus* sp., can also cause myositis and are discussed under the gastrointestinal system.

Myxozoa

Cytologic findings of myxozoans in skeletal muscle and deeper tissues are comparable with other tissues, with spore morphology varying by organism (Table 63.2). Multiple Myxozoa including *Myxobolus*, *Kudoa*, *Henneguya*, and *Ceratomyxa* spp. form parasitic cysts containing spores in skin, muscle, and skeletal tissues; these lesions can be macroscopically visible and spoil meat for sale. Some myxozoan spores are contained within a cyst wall, and others secrete enzymes leading to myocellular injury.[10] An example of this type of infection is *Henneguya salminicola*, which causes salmon "tapioca disease" so named due to grossly apparent small white intramuscular cysts. Cytology of material from *Henneguya* sp. lesions shows oval to fusiform spores with paired polar capsules and caudal appendages (Table 63.2, Figure 63.22).

Myxobolus cerebralis is a well-known myxozoan infecting the skeletal system and causing whirling disease of salmonids. The infective actinospores develop in and are released from environmental tubificids (tubifex worm invertebrates), penetrate the fish, and migrate to cartilaginous tissues of the developing skeleton, especially around the brain, spine, and gill arches. Trophozoites develop in cartilage and form large spore-filled plasmodial cysts causing cartilage destruction, which is identified clinically but usually sampled postmortem. Clinical signs occur due to skeletal and associated nervous system damage causing abnormal swimming (whirling), spinal malformation, and skin discoloration. The infection is variably associated with tissue necrosis and granulomatous inflammation. Cytologically and histologically, *Myxobolus* sp. spores are rounded to pyriform with a sporoplasm and two internal polar capsules containing coiled filaments (Table 63.2). Susceptibility to infection decreases as skeletal maturation progresses and cartilage is ossified.[22] A related agent, *Myxobolus albi*, has been reported to cause cartilage lesions in wild common goby (*Pomatoschistus microps*) and captive lumpfish (*Cyclopterus lumpus*). Cytologic findings were typical of *Myxobolus* sp. spores, and molecular sequencing was used to identify the parasite species (Figure 63.23).[53,54]

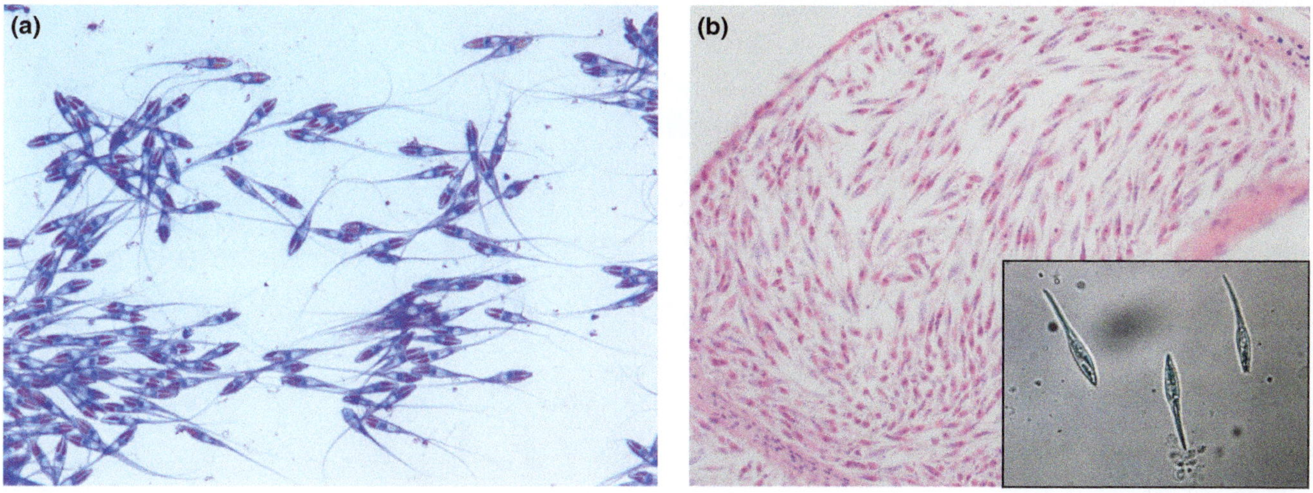

Figure 63.22 *Henneguya* sp. infection (a) Skin scrape from a white catfish (*Ameiurus catus*) shows numerous fusiform spores with two anterior polar capsules, an oval sporoplasm, and paired elongate caudal appendages (modified Wright's, 1000×. *Source:* Image courtesy of Anne Barger, presented at 1999 ASVCP mystery case session). (b) A subepithelial myxozoan cyst containing numerous *Henneguya* sp. spores from a marbled hatchetfish (*Carnegiella strigata*) (hematoxylin and eosin, 500×). Inset: On the wet mount from the same animal, polar capsules, sporoplasm, and caudal processes of the spores are less distinct than on dry mount (unstained wet mount, 1000×).

Metazoa

Metazoan parasites detailed in the section "Skin and Subcutis" occasionally affect deeper tissues including the musculoskeletal system, and cytologic findings are comparable (Table 63.2). Examples include encysted digenean platyhelminths or extension of crustacean arthropods. Depending on the extent of invasion and associated tissue damage, metazoan parasites can predispose to secondary infections.

Fungi and Fungal-Like Organisms

Infections by fungi and fungal-like organisms in the musculoskeletal system generally involve extension from other sites. However, microsporidian parasites, including *Glugea* sp., *Spraguea* sp., and others, cause targeted intramuscular lesions in fish. Microsporidians are obligate intracellular parasites previously considered protists but now classified as spore-forming unicellular fungi. Many microsporidians form large cysts (xenomas) containing numerous spores that markedly hypertrophy host connective tissue cells in a xenoparasitic complex.[55] Xenomas generally consist of the hypertrophied host cell with or without a thick hyaline wall and replacement of part or all of the cytoplasm by the proliferating parasitic spores. These are typically identified histologically but can be seen on wet-mount or dry-mount squash preparations. The microsporidian spores are smaller than myxozoan spores (often <7 μm diameter) and are refractile and oval to pyriform with a single posterior vacuole (Table 63.2).[25] The host response to xenomas is variable but usually involves chronic inflammation and fibrosis.

Pleistophoran microsporidia are notable because they do not form classical xenomas but undergo merogony and sporogony, forming "parasite clusters," that eventually replace the cytoplasm of infected cells with spores and lead to cell rupture and associated host reponse.[22,56] These parasites can extend from primary sites of infection such as myofibers into other tissues and body cavities. *Pleistophora* sp. cause important systemic disease of freshwater fish including research colonies.[57] *Pleistophora hyphessobryconis* causes significant muscular lesions ("neon tetra disease") in neon tetra and laboratory zebrafish.[58] *Pseudoloma neurophilia* is the most commonly detected pathogen of zebrafish, affecting primarily the nervous system and skeletal muscle to a lesser degree. Pyriform refractile spores of *P. hyphessobryconis* are approximately 4×6–7 μm and those of *P. neurophilia* 3×5 μm, each with a posterior vacuole.[57] Spores are variably positive with Luna, Gram, acid-fast, and periodic acid-Schiff stains (Figure 63.24).[59] Specific organism identification by morphology or molecular techniques is mainly performed for biosecurity considerations; infections are handled through colony management rather than treatment of clinical cases. Spores can be harbored by subclinically infected fish and transmitted by multiple routes including ingestion, cohabitation, and reproductive passage.

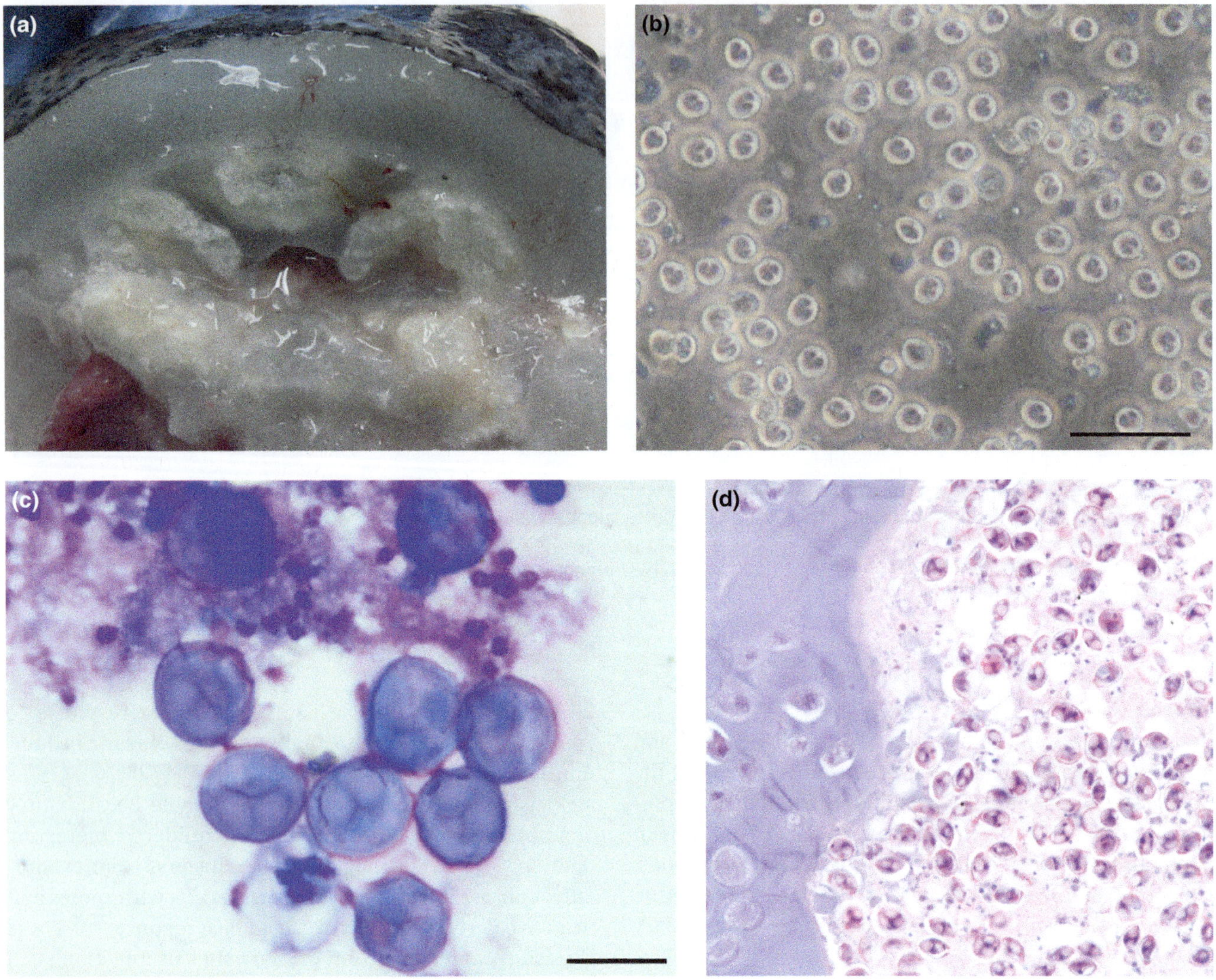

Figure 63.23 *M. albi* infection from lumpfish (*C. lumpus*). (a) Myxozoan infection within cartilage of the cranial calvarium (*Source:* Image courtesy of Julie Cavin). (b) Abundant round refractile myxozoan spores have two pyriform polar capsules (unstained wet mount, bar = 50 µm. *Source:* Image courtesy of Shedd Aquarium). (c) Round myxozoan spores have variably discernable paired polar capsules (modified Wright's, bar = 10 µm. *Source:* Image courtesy of Julie Cavin). (d) Myxozoan cyst in cartilage contains numerous spores (hematoxylin and eosin, 1000×. *Source:* Image courtesy of Sal Frasca Jr.).

Mesomycetozoea

A notable mesomycetozoean infection targeting skeletal muscle is *Ichthyophonus hoferi*, causing disease in marine and freshwater fish. Previously classified as a fungus, infection is thought to be through ingestion and subsequent hematogenous dissemination. Presentation can mimic mycobacteriosis and is characterized by white to tan nodules in muscles and other visceral organs. Squash preparations of infected tissues can show spherical resting spores with broad size variation (10–250 µm) surrounded by a thick chitinous wall that is periodic acid-Schiff positive.[33] Organisms are surrounded by granulomatous inflammation. Germination of spores is helpful in distinguishing *Ichthyophonus* from other infections, and spores are more commonly seen in postmortem samples, likely due to environmental changes (i.e. increasing CO_2) that promote germination.[60,61] Cytologic features of the germinating spores include branching germination tubes (nonseptate hyphae) of up to 40 µm diameter that extend from the spores. Spherical bodies representing new spores (hyphal bodies) can be present at the tips of the hyphae.[33,34]

Hyperplasia and Neoplasia

Musculoskeletal neoplasms are uncommon in fish, though various other neoplasms, especially from skin and

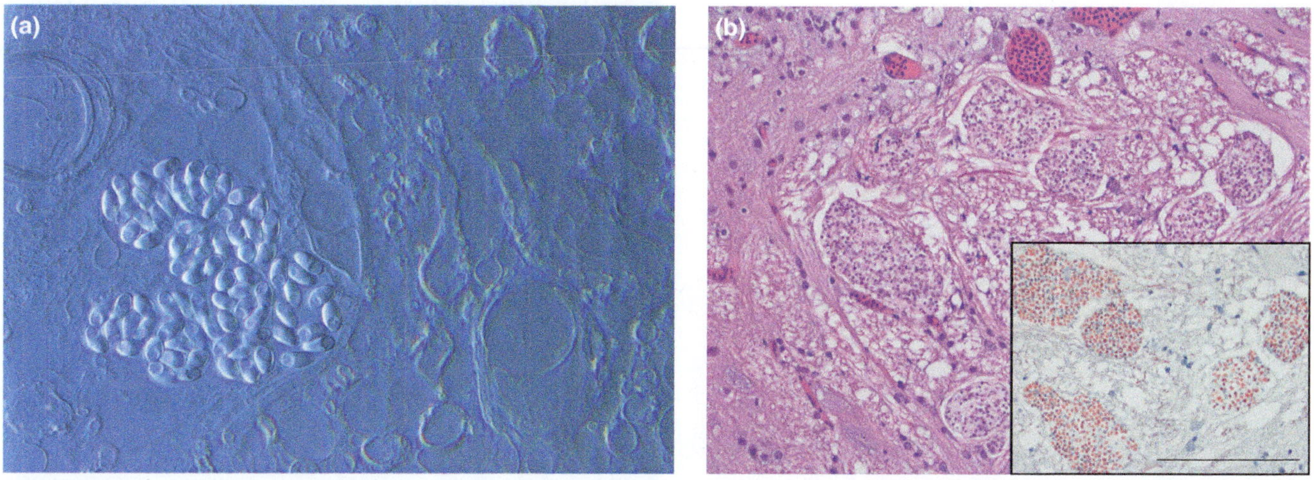

Figure 63.24 *P. neurophilia* infection in laboratory zebrafish (*Danio rerio*). (a) Squash preparation of spinal cord under differential interference contrast highlights clustered oval microsporidial spores (unstained, 1000×. *Source:* Image courtesy of Michael Kent). (b) Multiple microsporidian parasite clusters are within the neuropil (hematoxylin and eosin). Inset: Spores are highlighted by Luna staining (bar = 100 μm. *Source:* Images courtesy of Julie White).

subcutaneous sites, can infiltrate skeletal muscles and bone. Occasional skeletal muscle (rhabdomyoma, rhabdomyosarcoma) and skeletal system (chondromas, chondrosarcomas, osteomas, osteosarcomas) neoplasms are reported spontaneously and in chemically exposed fish.[13] Cytologic findings are expected to be comparable with other vertebrates.

Respiratory

A unique feature of fish is the presence of and reliance (in most species) on gills for respiration. Other key functions of gills include participation in excretion of nitrogenous wastes, electrolyte regulation, and fluid balance. The surface area of the gill epithelium is equal to or greater than the surface area of the body skin in many fish.[14]

The gill arches are supported by a bony skeleton and give rise to macroscopically apparent primary lamellae, which are lined by microscopic secondary lamellae on the dorsal and ventral surfaces. Secondary lamellae are the sites of gas exchange. Deoxygenated blood enters by afferent arteries and flows opposite to the direction of water flow across the gills, allowing countercurrent exchange. Oxygenated blood exits by efferent arteries flowing to the aorta.[14] Secondary lamellae are lined by a single layer of epithelial cells supported by pillar cells, which internally abut the afferent and efferent arteries.[14] Chloride cells, which function in ion exchange, lie along the primary lamellae. The gill arch is covered by slightly larger epithelial cells with interspersed mucus cells at the base of the primary lamellae. Lymphocytes, eosinophilic granular cells, and macrophages are present generally in low numbers within the subepithelial stroma.

Healthy intact gill filaments appear on wet-mount preparations as tapering, smooth-surfaced primary lamellae lined by narrow, perpendicularly oriented, secondary lamellae with approximately equivalent interlamellar spaces (Figure 63.4). Abnormalities of gill structure identifiable on wet-mount cytology include increased mucus production, thickened epithelium (hyperplasia and hypertrophy), lamellar fusion, telangiectasia, necrosis, and inflammation (Figure 63.25). With extensive damage, necrosis can progress to involve secondary lamellae, primarily lamellae, and the cartilage skeleton, causing anatomic distortion. Hyperplastic cells often migrate distally to the leading edge of secondary lamellae resulting in the appearance of "clubbing" of lamellae.[10] The gills have few cellular components and a limited range of responses (inflammation, structural distortion, hyperplasia). However, even slight disturbances to gill function can cause both respiratory and osmoregulatory compromise. Gills are particularly susceptible to infectious agents and environmental exposures including poor water quality (e.g. pH shifts, ammonia or chloride excess) and toxicities (e.g. chemicals, pollutants). Telangiectasia, characterized by dilation of lamellar capillaries, is a nonspecific observation.[25]

Infection and Inflammation

Many infections of the skin also affect the gills and vice versa. The following sections make note of similarities and highlight particular agents of concern for the respiratory system.

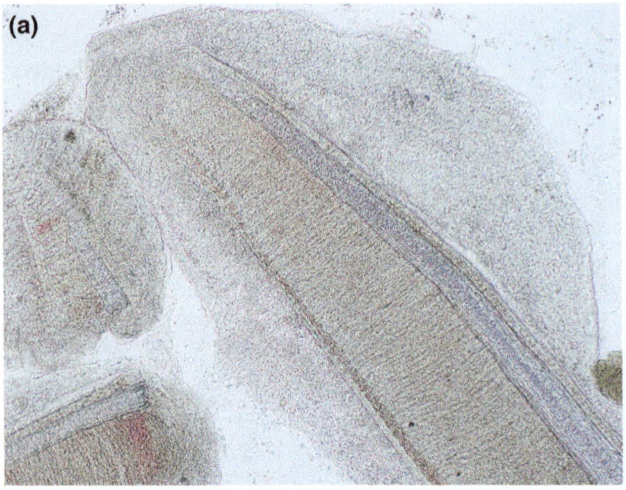

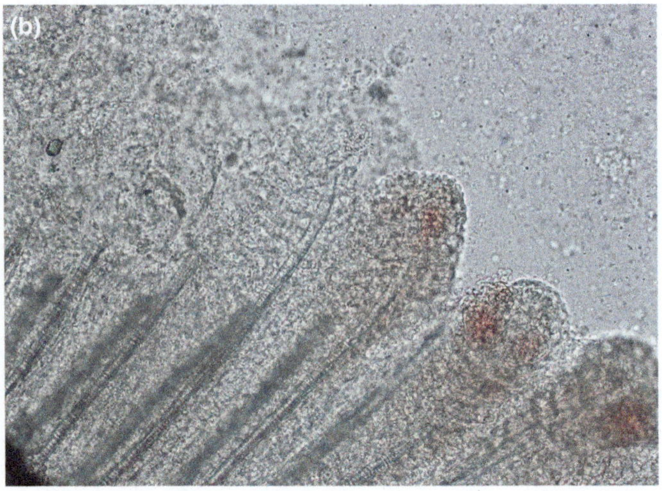

Figure 63.25 Examples of gill pathology. (a) Increased mucus production is seen as thick amorphous material surrounding the primary filaments (unstained wet mount, 100×). (b) Necrosis is evidenced as loss of distal primary filaments and associated secondary filaments (left). Mild telangiectasia is seen as dilation of distal capillaries (right) (unstained wet mount, 200×).

Bacteria

Bacterial infections of the gill are comparable with those of skin (Table 63.1). Although primary infections can occur, many are promoted by adverse husbandry conditions (e.g. crowding, water quality deficiencies), toxin exposures, or other infections (e.g. parasites).

Protozoa

Cytologically identifiable protozoa affecting the gills include many of the organisms discussed above (Table 63.2). Of particular importance for gills is the holotrich ciliate *I. multifiliis* and its marine counterpart *C. irritans*, which in addition to skin disease ("white spot," "Ich"), can cause clinically relevant branchitis in heavy infections (Figure 63.10). Flagellate *Ichthyobodo* sp. protozoa also affect the gills, with cytologic features comparable to findings in skin (Table 63.2).

Myxozoa

Many species of myxozoan parasite also affect the gills and have cytologic features as described in other body systems with variably shaped spores, a refractile wall, and anterior polar capsules (often two) (Table 63.2). *Myxobolus* sp. are common in cyprinid fish; *Myxobolus cyprini* is the agent of "pernicious anemia of carp" that causes gill damage, hemorrhage, and anemia. Spore morphology is similar to other *Myxobolus* sp. (Table 63.2, Figure 63.23). *Henneguya* sp. infect the gill of freshwater and marine fish, forming cysts in the gill arches containing numerous spores. *Henneguya ictaluri* is the causative agent of "proliferative gill disease" ("hamburger gill disease") of catfish, a significant problem of farmed catfish. Infective stages of *H. ictaluri* cause large cysts (plasmodia), granulomatous inflammation, telangiectasia, and hemorrhage in parasitized gills.[22,62] The spore morphology of *Henneguya* sp. includes paired anterior polar capsules and paired tapering caudal tail appendages (Table 63.2, Figure 63.22).

Metazoa

Metazoan parasites of the skin also commonly affect the gills (Table 63.2). The monogenean dactylogrid platyhelminths more commonly parasitize gills than skin, and cause gill filament damage, epithelial hyperplasia, and hypoxia. These organisms are oviparous, and egg development is affected by environmental conditions.[22] As described for the skin, characteristic features of organisms on wet-mount preparations include one pair of anchoring hooks and four eyespots (Table 63.2, Figure 63.14b). Gill damage can be apparent on wet mounts in the form of increased mucus and filament distortion.

Encysted digenean platyhelminth metacercariae are found in the gills, particularly along the arches, and in the cartilaginous support of the primary lamellae (Figure 63.15). While generally nonpathogenic, in large numbers, they can cause respiratory compromise or reduce the resilience of infected fish to environmental stressors. On wet-mount preparations, living larvae can be identified moving within the metacercarial wall.

Arthropods parasitizing the gills include crustacean copepods such as *Lernaeocera branchialis* in marine and *Ergasilus* sp. in freshwater and brackish water species. Females are parasitic, and damage occurs by feeding activity. Cytologic findings are comparable to infections in the skin, with unique organism features including

Y-shaped paired posterior egg sacs in *Lernaea* sp. females (Figure 63.16). Other arthropods are uncommon but include incidental mites that typically reflect aquarium acarofauna rather than true parasites (Figure 63.26).[63]

Fungi and Fungal-Like Organisms

The gills are susceptible to oomycete and fungal infections, which are typically opportunistic and promoted by predisposing factors including crowding, suboptimal water quality, and warmer temperatures. Cytologic findings are comparable to those described for the skin. However, the effects of opportunistic infections, including oomycetes such as *Saprolegnia* sp., are generally more serious in the gill than skin.[10]

"Gill rot", branchiomycosis, is caused by oomycetes *Branchiomyces sanguinis* and *Branchiomyces demigrans* with tropism for vasculature of the gill. These lesions are common in cyprinid fish, but similar findings have been identified in other species including eels and plecostomus.[34] Lesions are characterized by necrosis and infarction of the gill. Typical of oomycetes (Table 63.2, Figure 63.17), hyphae are branched, nonseptate, and 8–30 µm diameter with sometimes observable 5–9 µm-diameter zoospores.[33] Besides the infectious agents, wet-mount preparations can show cellular infiltrate (inflammation) and architectural distortion (necrosis) in the gill. Dry-mount cytology is uncommon but could demonstrate cell debris or inflammation.

Gills are also susceptible to microsporidian infections. For example, *Loma salmonae* infects the gills of salmonids causing formation of xenomas with concurrent necrosis, hemorrhage, hyperplasia, thrombosis, and systemic infection.[22] Like other microsporidians, key cytologic findings are refractile pyriform spores with a single posterior vacuole.

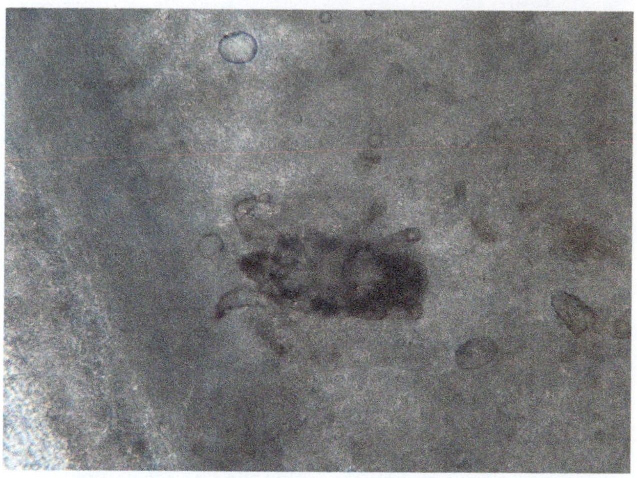

Figure 63.26 Arthropod mite on gill clip from a butterfly koi (*C. carpio*) is considered an incidental finding (unstained wet mount, 200×).

Algae

Amoebic gill disease is described in marine fish and impacts the salmonid industry. Although several species of amoeba have been implicated, disease has been only consistently associated and reproduced by infection with *Neoparamoeba perurans*. This agent is a free-living facultative ectoparasite. Infection causes gill damage including epithelial hyperplasia and lamellar fusion, leading to respiratory distress. Amoeba can be seen on wet mounts, but disease is more commonly diagnosed histologically. Cytologically, the organisms are 15–40 µm in diameter, rounded to amoeboid, with pseudopodia, a nucleus-like structure, and one or more endosymbiont parasomes.[1] Much of the biology of the amoeba organisms and factors contributing to infection are not yet defined.[10,64]

Dinoflagellates are flagellated protists variably grouped with algae that parasitize the skin and gills. The dinoflagellate *Amyloodinium ocellatum* is a free-living dinospore that attaches to the gills and, to a lesser extent, the skin, causing "marine velvet" or "oodiniosis." The developing trophont feeding stage penetrates cells by a rhizoid, causing pathology through attachment and feeding. The other two life stages occur off the host. Tomonts are found in substrate, and dinospores are free swimming and infectious. *Amyloodinium* is a major parasite of the gills of marine fish, causing epithelial hyperplasia and fusion of secondary lamellae. It is one of few fish parasites infecting both teleosts and elasmobranchs.[65] On wet mounts, organisms are seen as dark brown, variably sized (50–350 µm), ovoid to oblong, nonmotile trophonts in the gills; the rhizoid is not usually visible.[1] *Piscinoodinium pillulare* is the freshwater counterpart and contains chlorophyll, creating "velvet disease" or "rust disease" of tropical pet fish.[25]

Viruses

The gills are host to viral infections, most of which lack distinct cytologic features (e.g. lamellar necrosis with koi herpesvirus [Cyprinid herpesvirus 3]). Lymphocystis disease virus and epitheliocystis are both associated with markedly enlarged cells and must be differentiated from one another. Of the two, epitheliocystis is more common in the gill; this chlamydia-like agent fills and enlarges cells, displacing the host cell components (Figure 63.9). In contrast, lymphocystis disease virus-infected cells are hypertrophied with karyomegaly and viral cytoplasmic inclusions (Figure 63.20).

Hyperplasia and Neoplasia

Respiratory neoplasia is uncommon in fish. In the gill, branchioblastomas and branchial lamellar lesions have been reported in salmonids and koi, as well as experimentally with chemical exposure.[13,66] Histologically, branchioblastomas are primitive with possible differentiation toward epithelial, mesenchymal, and blastemal components; cytology is not specifically described. Other reported neoplasms of the gill include epithelial and mesenchymal proliferations (papillomas, carcinomas, osteosarcoma, osteochondroma, chondroma), mainly as individual cases and presumably having similar cytologic features to other vertebrate species.[13]

Supersaturation Disease

Another key noninfectious condition of the teleost gill that is recognized cytologically is gas supersaturation causing intravascular gas emboli ("gas bubble disease"). In severe cases, these lesions also can be seen macroscopically in the fins and eyes. Wet-mount cytology shows well-defined gas emboli within small blood vessels of the gills or fins (Figure 63.27). The condition results from increased total dissolved gas pressure, related to rapid changes in temperature, pump malfunction, and other factors.

Swim Bladder

In fish having swim bladders, the organ arises from the digestive system embryonically and often plays a major role in buoyancy. A pneumatic duct is present in some species (physostomes) and absent or closed in others (physoclistous). In those species lacking a water–air interface, gas release occurs by arterial blood flow through a gas gland and reabsorption through a separate capillary rete (the oval or oval sphincter).[14] Other functions include reception or production of sound in some species.[14] Swim bladder anatomy is highly variable, and the organ can have multiple interconnected chambers. It is generally lined by two layers. The tunica interna consists of cuboidal epithelium and underlying adventitia, and the tunica externa consists of a fibrous layer with variable elastic and muscular components and an outer serosa. Pathology of the swim bladder is usually manifested as buoyancy problems. Many pathologic conditions (infectious and noninfectious) lead to secondary bloating and fluid accumulation. The fluid can be transudative, mucoid, or exudative.

Infection and Inflammation

Inflammatory lesions of the swim bladder (aerocystitis, pneumocystitis) can be organ specific or part of a systemic process. Infectious agents include bacterial, protozoal, myxozoan, metazoan, fungal, algal, mesomycetozoean, and viral agents. The following are particular organ-specific or common agents.

Sphaerospora renicola is a myxozoan parasite causing "swim bladder inflammation" in carp, which manifests as swim bladder thickening. Developing spores also localize to the kidney causing renal degeneration ("kidney enlargement disease"). Organisms can be identified in blood or impression smears of the swim bladder and kidney. As for other myxozoa (Table 63.2), spores are extracellular and refractile with polar capsules and sporoplasm. Mature

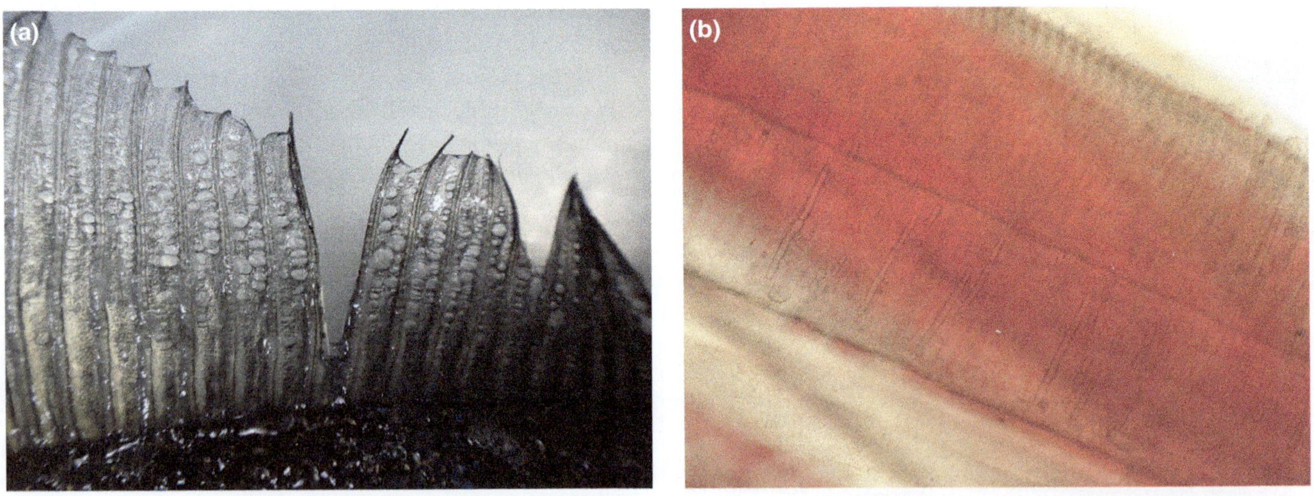

Figure 63.27 Examples of supersaturation (gas bubble disease). (a) Numerous small gas emboli are within the fin vasculature between fin rays. (b) Elongated intravascular gas bubbles are within the vasculature of secondary lamellae in the gill of a cottonwick grunt (*Haemulon melanurum*) (unstained wet mount, 200×).

spores of *S. renicola* are rounded and approximately 7 μm diameter with two polar capsules.[67,68]

Metazoans such as nematodes can be found in the swim bladder on squash preparations often without apparent disease. Cytologically, these larvae are characterized by a round worm-shaped body, cuticle, variable cuticular ornamentations, and sometimes apparent digestive structures. In adults, reproductive structures can be seen. In eels, the fourth stage larval development and adults of the nematode *Anguillicola crassus* occur in the swim bladder, and adults feed on blood. Introduction of this organism from Japanese eels to European eels through aquaculture is thought to have contributed to declines in the European eel population.[69]

Hyperplasia and Neoplasia

Neoplasms of the swim bladder include sporadic benign or malignant proliferations of local or surrounding tissues (epithelial, mesenchymal) or involvement in systemic round cell neoplasms. Uniquely, retroviral related leiomyosarcomas of the swim bladder have been reported in Atlantic salmon.[70] Multinodular masses composed of moderately pleomorphic spindle cells arise from the swim bladder wall, extending into the lumen. Immunohistochemical findings support smooth muscle origin.[71] Other swim bladder tumors include epithelial papilloma, adenoma, and adenocarcinoma in a variety of fish species with and without chemical exposures.[13] Cytology is rarely performed but expected to be consistent with other vertebrates based on histologic similarities.

Hemolymphatic

Fish have an extensive system of lymph drainage but no lymph nodes. The primary hematopoietic tissue of teleosts is the anterior kidney, with minor contributions from spleen, liver, and thymus. The bones of most teleosts lack medullary spaces and bone marrow. Hematopoietic tissues of elasmobranchs include the epigonal organ (adjacent to the gonads), the organ of Leydig (located in the esophageal wall), spleen, and thymus (lymphoid only).[72] The splenic pulp of teleosts is heavily lymphopoietic, with interspersed ellipsoidal capillaries surrounded by erythrocytes and phagocytic cells and scattered melanomacrophage centers. The thymus is paired and located in the dorsal aspect of the operculum, with variable growth and regression across teleost species. In addition to lymphoid tissue, the thymus includes epithelial nests, similar to Hassall's corpuscles.[14] Fish possess an extensive reticuloendothelial system of phagocytic cells, thought to be composed of promonocytes, monocytes, and free and stationary macrophages.[14] Depots of tissue-fixed macrophages are present in the spleen, kidney, and atrial lining of the heart, but unlike mammals, functional hepatic Kupffer cells are absent.[73]

Infection and Inflammation

Hemolymphatic tissues, especially the spleen and kidney, are frequently involved in systemic infections and are particularly prone to bacterial colonization. Common bacterial agents include various Gram-negative bacteria, *Mycobacteria* sp., *Nocardia* sp., *R. salmoninarum*, etc. (Table 63.1). Cytology and histology of acute septicemic lesions often show bacteria with variable necrosis and little inflammation. Wet-mount squash preparations of established lesions demonstrate granulomas composed of a rim of cells surrounding central dark necrotic cores (Figure 63.28). Invasive colonization by other organisms such as protozoa, myxozoa, metazoa, fungi, algae, mesomycetozoea, and viruses also occurs. The cytologic features are largely generic across tissues, as discussed in prior sections.

Notably, some microsporidial agents infecting fish proliferate characteristically in the nucleus of infected cells with or without intracytoplasmic stages (e.g. *Nucleospora salmonis*, *Nucleospora cyclopteri*, *Enterospora nucleophila*). The cellular targets are variable but commonly include lymphocytes, hematopoietic precursors, or rodlet cells. Proliferation of infected cells occurs in diverse body sites, such as kidney, spleen, intestine, and disseminated connective tissues. Infections range from subclinical to pathologic and can resemble leukemia in some cases.[74–76] Microsporidial spores can be seen in cytologic preparations of blood, coelomic fluid, and tissues as developing (merogonial) to maturing oval microsporidial spores within nuclei. The spores are generally more apparent cytologically than histologically and can be highlighted by Luna staining.

Some viral infections, such as piscine iridovirus, causing viral erythrocytic necrosis, can be identified as round basophilic to amphophilic inclusions within the cytoplasm of erythrocytes on blood or tissue cytology. However, in others, such as infectious hematopoietic necrosis virus of salmonids, there is nonspecific necrosis, and no etiology is apparent on cytology.

Hyperplasia and Neoplasia

Neoplasms arising from the hemolymphatic system are most often of round, hemic cell origin, including many reports of lymphoid neoplasia. Progression to leukemia can occur.[13] Neoplastic cells are comparable with lymphocytes in other species. Some reports suggest underlying viral infection. As in cutaneous lymphosarcoma of esocids,

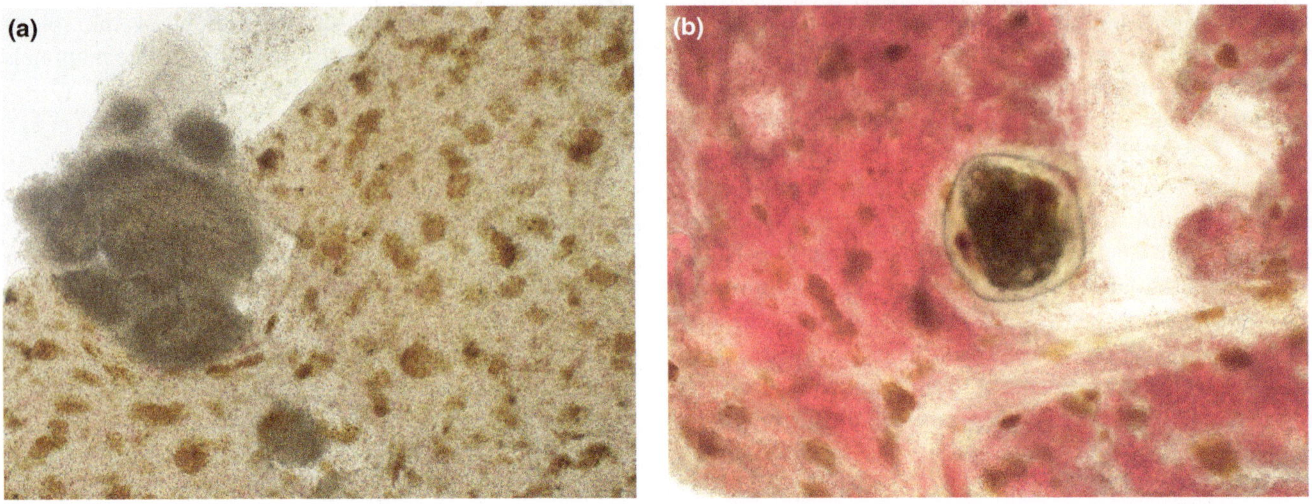

Figure 63.28 Squash preparations of spleen from two yellow spot croakers (*L. xanthurus*) from a group with nocardial sepsis. (a) Acute necrosis and inflammation (b) a chronic granuloma (unstained wet mounts, (a) 100×, (b) 400×).

definitive cell lineage identification has not been completely elucidated by ancillary testing.

Plasmacytoid leukemia is reported in Chinook salmon associated with retroviral infection by salmon leukemia virus, possibly promoted by other infectious cofactors. Also known as "marine anemia," it occurs in fresh- and saltwater salmonids. Cellular infiltrates affect many organs, but enlargement of the spleen and kidneys predominates. Tissue imprints and histology show discrete round to ovoid, plasmacytoid cells with moderate amounts of finely granular cytoplasm, eccentric round to indented nuclei, perinuclear clearing, and many mitoses.[41,77] Epizootic "lympholeukemia" arising from the spleen and infiltrating numerous organs has been reported in Japanese red sea bream, with marked peripheral lymphocytosis, organ infiltration, and adenovirus-like particles seen ultrastructurally in neoplastic cells.[78]

Gastrointestinal

The basic structure of the piscine alimentary tract is similar to other taxa, with adaptations such as in dentition. Generally, the digestive tract of herbivores is longer than carnivores.[14] The oral cavity is lined by stratified epithelium with mucus cells. The esophageal mucosa is commonly folded and lined by cuboidal to columnar and variably ciliated epithelium with interspersed mucus cells. The esophageal muscle is striated, while that of the stomach and aboral alimentary tract is smooth. The stomach is lined by fundic and pyloric glands. Extensions of the stomach, pyloric caeca, are present in many fish and are comparable with intestinal segments histologically. Some fish, including cyprinids (e.g. goldfish, zebrafish, carp), lack a true stomach. The intestine of fish is generally uniform diameter throughout and is lined by simple columnar epithelium with interspersed mucus cells and underlying layers of muscularis mucosae, submucosa, tunica muscularis, and serosa. Mucus cells are increased in the rectum. The ileum of elasmobranchs, lungfishes, and some teleosts is regionally expanded to form the spiral intestine. The mucosa of this region consists of complex convoluted folds, referred to as the spiral valve, which are believed to increased nutrient absorption. In teleosts, eosinophilic granule cells, akin to mammalian mast cells, are common in the lamina propria and submucosa of the digestive tract. Rodlet cells, which may be a form of granular leukocyte, are common in the intestinal lining; these cells are thought to play a role in immune/inflammatory function and contribute to host defense.[11,14]

Infection and Inflammation

Pathology of the alimentary tract is similar to other taxa, including infections linked to bacterial, protozoal, myxozoan, metazoan, and occasionally fungal or algal organisms. Cytologically, protozoan and metazoan infections are among the more commonly identified.

Bacteria

Bacterial infections of the alimentary system can arise from within the tract or by extension. Bacterial agents span those commonly seen in other organ systems (Table 63.1). Interpretation of bacteria seen cytologically relies on typical criteria such as clinical presentation, sample type, concurrent inflammation, etc.

Protozoa

Protozoan alimentary parasites of fish include ciliate, flagellate, and coccidial organisms. Many are common commensal inhabitants of the piscine alimentary tract but also can cause disease. Ciliates affecting the intestinal tract of fish include *Balantidium* sp., as found in mammals. Although often incidental, they can cause enteritis in heavy infections. Cytologic interpretation of the significance of organisms must be based on other clinical or pathologic findings and relative numbers.

Flagellate protozoal infections of the alimentary tract include *Cryptobia* and *Spironucleus* species. *Cryptobia iubulans* is a common infection of cichlids. On wet-mount squash preparations of the gastric wall, characteristic granulomatous inflammation in the submucosa is apparent. Intralesional flagellated protozoa are often very difficult to discern both cytologically and histologically (Figure 63.29). The majority of other *Cryptobia* sp. in fish are hemoparasites closely related to or within the *Trypanoplasma* genus.[79]

The diplomonad flagellate protozoa *Spironucleus* sp. (some formerly classed as *Hexamita* sp.) affect a wide spectrum of freshwater and marine fish. *Spironucleus* flagellates are considered intestinal commensals but have opportunistic invasive potential in conditions of stress.[80] Fish in aquaculture appear to be more susceptible to disease than wild counterparts, likely related to husbandry factors. Disease is intestinal or systemic. Intestinal spironucleosis generally presents as enteritis, emaciation, and ascites with high parasite loads. Systemic spironucleosis occurs when trophozoites invade host tissues and can be identified in blood (Figure 63.30). An example of systemic infection by spironucleus organisms is "hole-in-the-head" disease of cichlids (angelfish, discus) putatively caused by *Spironucleus vortens* infection.[81] Necrotic lesions occur on the head, skeletal muscle, lateral line, and internal organs. The motile trophozoite form is identified cytologically in feces and other tissues as a round to pyriform structure (approximately 10–20 μm long and 5–10 μm wide) with six anteriorly located and two posteriorly located flagella and paired anterior nuclei. The posterior flagella are longer than the anterior (approximately 2 and 1.5 times body length, respectively), and the anterior flagella are arranged in two groups of three.[25,80]

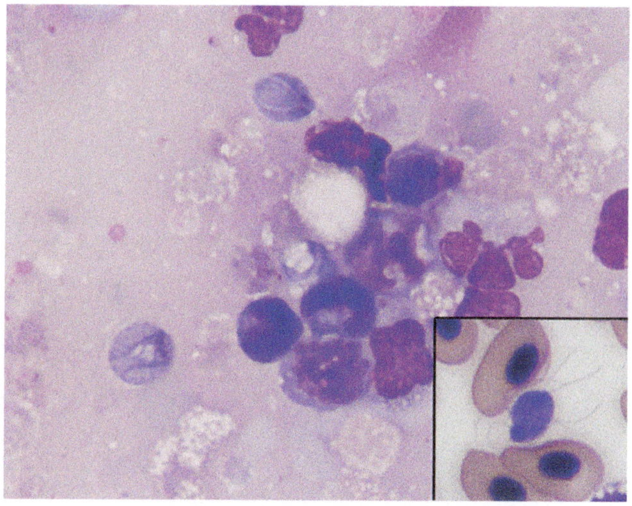

Figure 63.30 Fluid from a cystic cavitary lesion in the musculature of a Chinook salmon (*Oncorhynchus tshawytscha*) shows mixed inflammatory cells with few rounded *Spironucleus* sp. trophozoites. Anterior and posterior flagella are poorly discerned. Inset: In blood from the same animal, multiple thin flagella (six anterior and two posterior) are visible (modified Wright-Giemsa, 1000×. *Source:* Image photographed by Tracy French and provided by Tracy Stokol and Amy Warren from a glass slide presented at the 2006 ASVCP case review session).

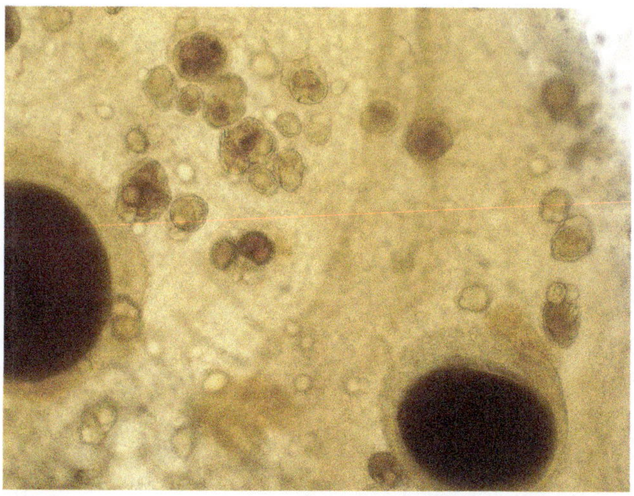

Figure 63.29 Squash preparation of gastric wall from a cichlid with *Crytobia* sp. infection demonstrating multifocal granulomas (unstained wet mount, 200×).

Coccidia (including *Eimeria*, *Caryospora*, and other genera) are found intra- and extraintestinally in fish, including in the liver, swim bladder, and reproductive organs. Although most coccidia do not cause clinical disease, some are significant pathogens (e.g. *Goussia subepithelialis*, *Goussia carpelli*, and *Eimeria carpelli* in cultured carp).[22] Sporulated oocysts can be found cytologically and are consistent with coccidian oocyst morphology seen in other vertebrate taxa (Figure 63.31). In cow-nosed rays, *Eimeria* sp. (*Eimeria southwelli*) cause emaciation, coelomic distention, and mortality; the oocysts can be found in cytology of coelomic fluid.[82]

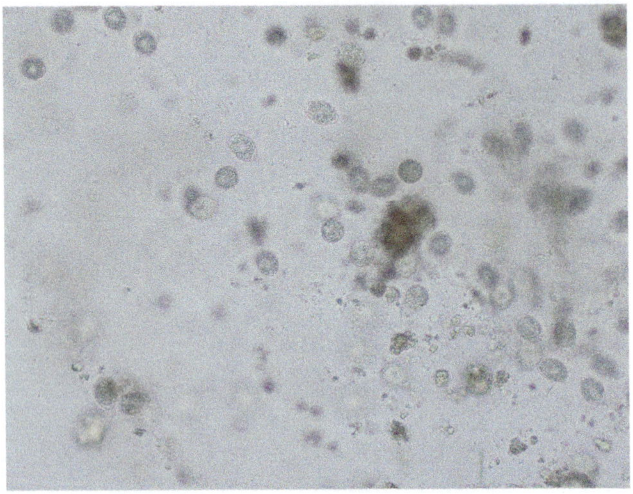

Figure 63.31 Coccidia found in a fecal sample taken as part of quarantine screening from a freshwater stingray (*Potamotrygon jabuti*). This animal was not demonstrating clinical illness (unstained wet mount, 400×).

Cryptosporidia are described in freshwater and marine fish along gastric and intestinal surfaces. Transmission is thought to occur by water, but feeding of brine shrimp has also been implicated along with cannibalism and recirculation systems. Most infections are subclinical, but abdominal swelling, ascites, and abnormal feces are reported in heavy infections of some species (e.g. *Cryptosporidium molnari*).[83] Cryptosporidial morphology is similar to that found in terrestrial vertebrates (Chapter 61).

Myxozoa

Myxozoans of the gastrointestinal tract also range from incidental to pathologic depending on specific agents, organism load, and concurrent pathologic states. *Enteromyxum leei* causes emaciation, enteritis, and mortality (enteromyxosis) in sea bream and a range of other marine and freshwater species.[22] Similarly, the myxozoan parasite *Ceratomyxa shasta* causes ceratomyxosis in salmonids with associated intestinal necrosis and hemorrhage. While often diagnosed histologically, the developing sporoblasts and mature spores can be identified in wet-mount preparations of intestinal squash samples and mucosal scrapings.[84,85] Like other myxozoans, spores of *E. leei* and *C. shasta* have a refractile wall and polar capsules. However, the shape of these mature spores is characteristically arcuated (bent, curved), ranging from approximately 15–20 μm long and 5–10 μm wide. The ends of mature *Enteromyxum* spores are irregularly pointed, and those of *Ceratomyxa* spores are rounded (roughly "boomerang shaped") (Figure 63.32).

Metazoa

Metazoan parasites of the fish alimentary tract include nematodes, cestodes, trematodes, and acanthocephalans. A complete list of parasites is beyond the scope of this chapter, but identification into general parasite group is performed based on body structure (e.g. segmentation, presence or absence of digestive tract) and unique structures (e.g. calcareous corpuscles, glands, hooks, and suckers).[86] Identification of metazoan parasites in fish is often by examination of feces or intestinal content. At necropsy, intestinal squash preparations are often employed.

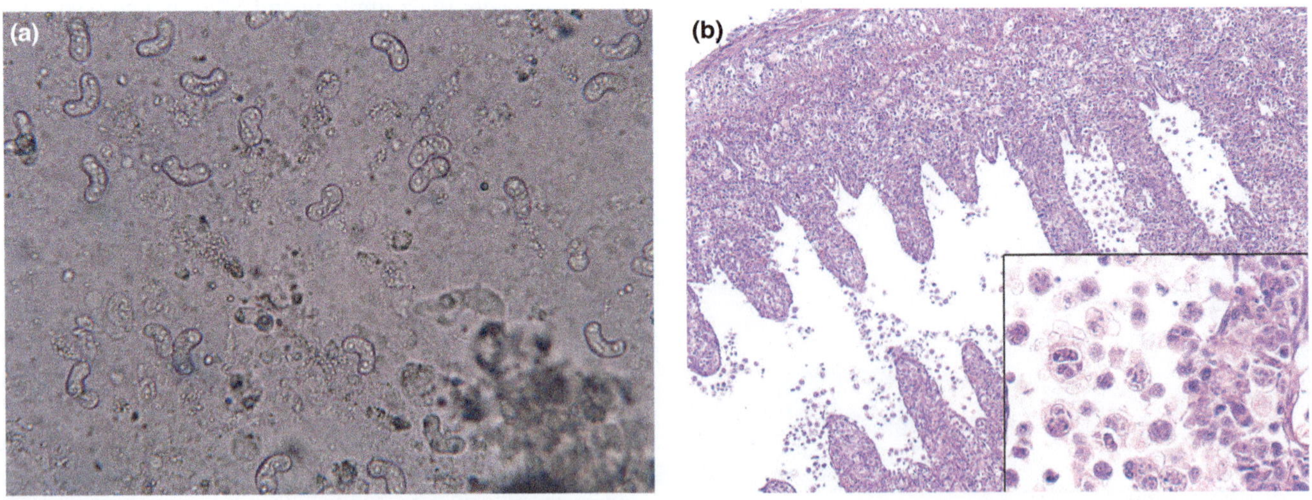

Figure 63.32 *C. shasta* infection in a rainbow trout (*Oncorhynchus mykiss*). (a) intestinal scraping shows numerous characteristic curved spores, each with two polar capsules (unstained wet mount, 1000×). (b) Histology of the posterior intestine shows enteritis with numerous intralesional parasite stages and developing spores sloughed into the lumen (hematoxylin and eosin, (b): 100×. Inset: 400×. *Source:* Images courtesy of Jerri Bartholomew).

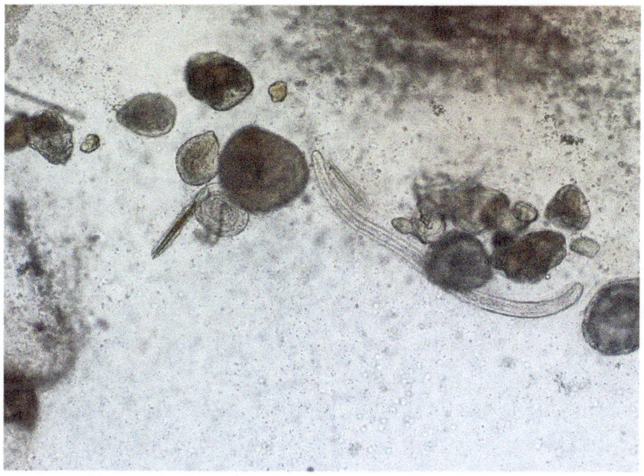

Figure 63.33 Squash preparation of coelomic viscera from a cardinal tetra (*P. axelrodi*). Two free intracoelomic nematode larvae (*Pseudoproleptus* sp.) and multiple granulomas (mycobacterial) are embedded in the thin coelomic connective tissue (unstained wet mount, 200×).

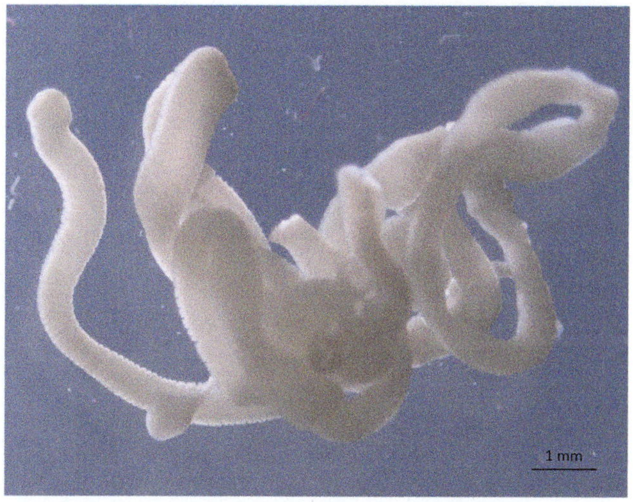

Figure 63.34 Cestode adult *B. acheilognathi* from the intestine of a damba cichlid (*Paretroplus maculatus*) with enteritis. Numerous proglottid body segments and a "heart-shaped" scolex (left) are visible (unstained, 10×. *Source:* Image courtesy of Heather Stockdale Walden).

Metazoan organisms reside in the gastrointestinal lumen, encyst in or around the intestinal wall, or traverse to reside in the coelom or other tissues. Unless heavily infected, many metazoans do not cause significant clinical disease.

Nematode larvae are often found incidentally in body cavity squash preparations (Figure 63.33). Cytologically, larvae are comparable with nematodes in terrestrial vertebrates. Morphologic speciation requires parasitology expertise, and sometimes adults or both male and female organisms are needed. Many fish nematodes have indirect life cycles, and fish serve as intermediate hosts for several nematode genera (*Anisakis*, *Contracaecum*, *Eustrongylides* sp.). The larvae are found in the coelom or viscera, generally causing little disease except in young or heavily infected fish. Definitive hosts, mammals (including humans) and birds, become infected upon consumption. *Pseudocapillaria* sp. are among the less common but clinically significant nematodes of fish. They infect a broad host range and are important parasites of the intestinal tract of zebrafish in laboratory colonies. An association with intestinal neoplasms is reported.[87]

Cestodes are the most clinically significant metazoan infections of the gastrointestinal tract of fish. The Asian fish tapeworm, *Bothriocephalus acheilognathi* (*Schyzocotyl acheilognathi*), is an invasive parasite of freshwater species and is the most important pathogenic cestode of cyprinids.[88] Fish are the definitive host, and tapeworm adults develop in the intestine. They are found on wet mounts as strobila with segmented proglottids and a uniterminal scolex (Figure 63.34). Fish also serve as intermediate hosts in cestode life cycles, during which large metacestodes can sometimes distort viscera or accumulate to cause disease (Figure 63.35). The plerocercoids of *Diphyllobothrium* sp. occur in a wide variety of freshwater fish, most often in skeletal muscle, but also in body cavities and organs. Known as the "broad fish tapeworm," this organism infects humans consuming raw or undercooked fish that carry infective metacestodes.[89]

Digenean platyhelminth metacercariae encyst in viscera and muscle of fish intermediate hosts, generally causing little harm (Figure 63.15). Somewhat more pathologic exceptions include *Clinostomum marginatum*, in which heavy infections of the metacercariae can

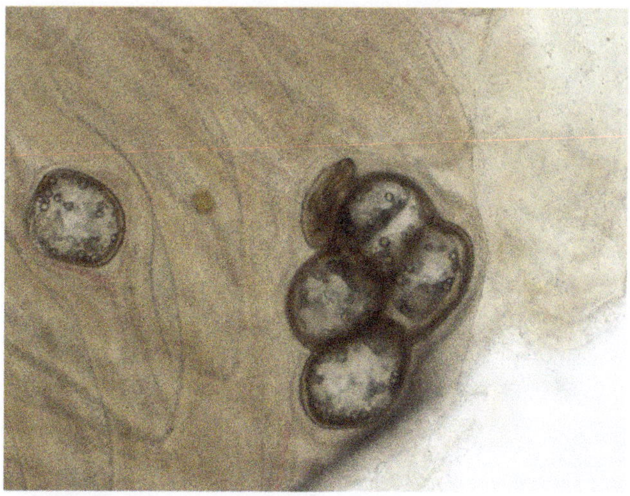

Figure 63.35 Encysted cestode larvae are embedded in the intestinal wall of a silver insignis (*S. taeniurus*) (unstained wet mount, 200×).

cause muscular and visceral damage in many fish species in North America ("yellow grub"). Piscivorous birds are common final hosts.[22]

Fungi and Fungal-Like Organisms

Fungal and oomycete infections are often opportunistic pathogens (see section "Skin and Subcutis"). Microsporidian xenomas (e.g. *Glugea* sp., *Loma* sp.) can occur in the gastrointestinal tract and visceral organs or extend into the coelomic cavity. Heavy infections of the intestinal wall can compromise cells and lead to spread of infection to other organs by extension. Disease manifests when organ function is impaired. Cytologic features are comparable with findings in other organ systems (described more under musculoskeletal) with small, refractile, oval spores containing a single posterior vacuole (Table 63.2).

Hyperplasia and Neoplasia

Gastrointestinal neoplasms are uncommon in fish, with few case reports of epithelial and mesenchymal proliferations largely histologically comparable with other taxa. Notable examples include fibromas on the lips of angelfish associated with retroviruses based on identification of ultrastructural particles[13]; ameloblastomas in chinook salmon[90]; chemical-induced esophageal, gastric, and intestinal adenomas and adenocarcinomas in various fish[13]; and carcinomas and mixed malignant tumors in laboratory zebrafish associated with *Pseudocapillaria tomentosa* infection.[87] Cytology is rarely performed, but extrapolation from histology suggests similarities to the mammalian counterparts.

Hepatobiliary and Pancreas

Normal hepatic color and texture varies from light brown to mahogany-color in teleosts or is pale tan in species with physiologic hepatic lipid storage including sharks and rays. Liver anatomy varies from localized in the cranial coelom to elongated processes extending along the coelomic viscera. The hepatic cords and lobules of fish are less defined than other species. Typically arranged portal tracts and functional Kupffer cells are absent.[14] Hepatocyte morphology is the same as other vertebrates. Melanomacrophage centers are often prominent in the liver, as well as in the spleen and kidney, and are less frequent in gonads and other tissues. Major pigment components of melanomacrophages include lipofuscin, melanin, and hemosiderin. These centers are recognized cytologically on wet mounts as dark brown to black granular nodules, and increased number and/or size of melanomacrophage centers (hyperplasia and hypertrophy) is a nonspecific tissue response (Figure 63.36).[91] The biliary system of fish is comparable with other taxa.

The exocrine pancreatic tissue of fish is anatomically variable and is commonly dispersed in the mesentery and within liver (hepatopancreas). Acinar exocrine cell morphology and function are comparable with other taxa.[14,92] The endocrine pancreas is discussed with the endocrine system.

Infection and Inflammation

The liver is a common site of systemic infectious diseases including bacterial (e.g. mycobacteriosis, nocardiosis),

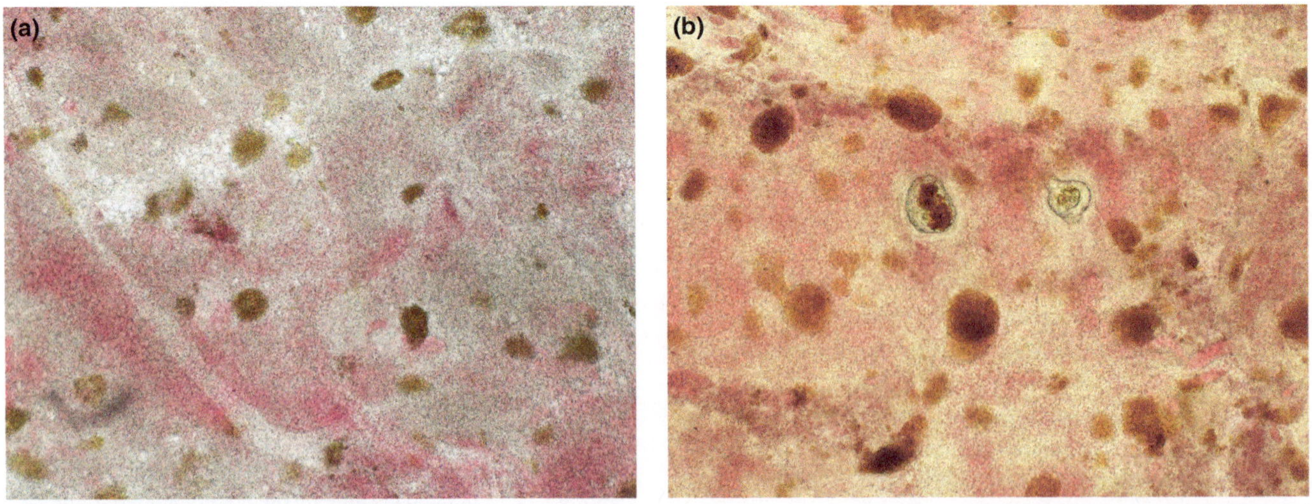

Figure 63.36 (a) Liver from a redbelly yellowtail fusilier (*Caesio cuning*) demonstrates normal melanomacrophage centers (unstained wet mount, 100×). (b) Liver from a yellow spot croaker (*L. xanthurus*) exhibits increased melanomacrophage centers and two granulomatous foci (unstained wet mount, 200×).

protozoal (e.g. invasive scuticociliates), metazoan (e.g. nematodes, trematodes), fungal, mesomycetozoean, and viral agents. These commonly spread hematogenously and/or by direct extension.

The gall bladder is rarely sampled. Protozoa such as *Hexamita* sp. and various myxozoan infections are described but can be present without associated pathology.[10,93] Interpretation of the significance of infectious agents (e.g. bacteria, protozoa, myxozoa) cytologically identified in bile requires consideration of other clinical findings such as imaging, gross lesions, or presence of concurrent inflammation.

The pancreas can also be involved in systemic infections. With the exception of relatively few viral agents (e.g. infectious pancreatic necrosis virus), pancreatic exocrine tissue is rarely a specific target of infectious disease. Cytologic sampling is hindered by low diagnostic yield and the dispersed distribution of exocrine pancreatic tissue.

Hyperplasia and Neoplasia

The hepatobiliary system is one of the more common locations for proliferative lesions in fish, especially in those living in polluted environments or used in laboratory studies of chemically induced tumors. Hepatobiliary neoplasms in rainbow trout associated with aflatoxin exposure are well characterized. The increased incidence after transition to dry feed formulations led to recognition of aflatoxin B1 as a primary carcinogen in fish and humans. Rainbow trout are recognized as a model for environmental carcinogenesis including a wide range of substances (e.g. polycyclic aromatic hydrocarbons, direct chemical carcinonogens) and exposure routes (e.g. dietary, embryonic, microinjection).[94] Lesions range from hyperplastic, to benign neoplastic, to malignant and include nodular atypical hyperplastic foci (basophilic or eosinophilic histologically), hepatic adenomas, cholangiomas, hepatocellular carcinomas, cholangiocarcinomas, and mixed hepatocellular/biliary neoplasms. Carcinomas are invasive and metastatic; ascites is common.[13] Fish livers might be particularly susceptible to chemical damage because of factors such as slow blood and bile flow, high activities of some cytochromes, lack of glutathione S-transferase, and continual growth throughout life vs. mammalian quiescence.[10,94,95] Hepatic tumors in other species of fish are less common but include hepatoblastoma in mummichogs caused by exposure to polycyclic hydrocarbon-contaminated water, and various spontaneous and induced hepatobiliary neoplasms of research zebrafish.[95,96] Cytology of hepatobiliary lesions is uncommon. Histologically, neoplasms resemble mammalian counterparts and are presumed to be cytologically similar. Cytologic features of hyperplasia, benign neoplasia, and well-differentiated carcinomas overlap and require caution in interpretation.

Neoplasms of the exocrine pancreas are rare in fish. Reports include acinar cell adenomas, adenocarcinomas, and cystadenomas, some of which link to fish exposed to environmental chemicals.[13] Histologic morphology is comparable with other vertebrates, and cytology is extrapolated but not sufficiently described.

Hepatocellular Deposits

Fish hepatocytes are prone to pigment (e.g. lipofuscin, hemosiderin) and storage material accumulation. Hepatic glycogen and fat accumulation occur physiologically and pathologically. Excess lipid storage results from over-conditioning, high-fat diets, or negative energy balance. In elasmobranchs, hepatic lipid is a sign of good condition. Hepatic lipidosis cytologically is classical; hepatocytes contain distinct clear cytoplasmic vacuoles, and free lipid occurs in the background. Prolonged starvation can cause hepatocellular atrophy and accumulation of ceroid pigment.[14]

Urinary

The kidneys consist of excretory, hematopoietic, reticuloendothelial, and endocrine components.[14] The anterior kidney (head kidney) of teleost fish is located along the dorsal coelomic cavity, caudal to the gill arches, and is a primary site of hematopoiesis. The posterior kidney (tail kidney) is located in the retroperitoneal position, dorsal to the swim bladder in the mid to caudal coelomic cavity, and is primarily excretory. The kidneys are variably paired to fused in different species, and ureters (archinephric ducts) also variably fuse, forming a bladder in some species, prior to termination at urinary ducts caudal to the anus.[14] Although generally composed of glomeruli, tubular segments, and collecting ducts, nephron structure varies across fishes. Compared with freshwater fish, marine species have shorter nephrons with diminished intermediate and distal segments, and some fish lack glomeruli entirely.[14,97]

Common inflammatory findings on wet-mount squash preparations of anterior and posterior kidney include variably defined granulomas seen as nodules with opaque granular cores and peripheral layers of macrophages and fibrosis. On wet mounts of posterior kidney, tubular lesions present as cellular or granular debris within renal tubules reflecting degenerative or necrotic epithelium or inflammation, or as mineralized concretions signaling nephrocalcinosis (Figure 63.37). Predisposing factors for nephrocalcinosis include high concentrations of CO_2 in water, acid–base shifts, and dietary factors including levels of calcium and magnesium.[98] Cytology is insensitive for evaluating glomerular pathology.

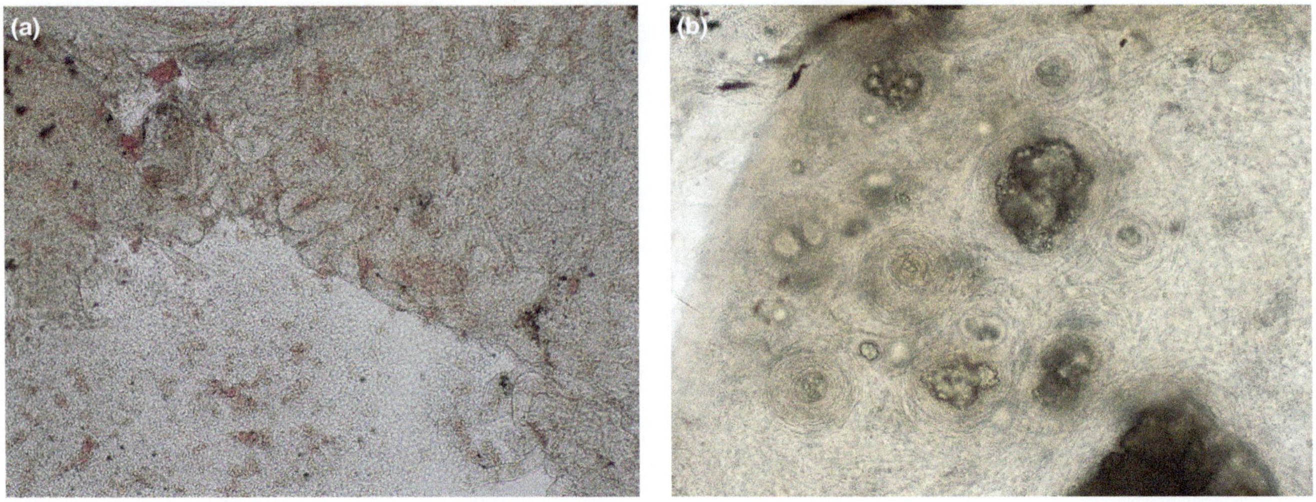

Figure 63.37 Postmortem cytology of normal posterior kidney from a smooth-head unicorn fish (*Naso literatus*) and posterior kidney with nephrocalcinosis from a white finned bedotia (*Bedotia leucopteron*). (a) Normal kidney is largely composed of numerous rows of convoluted, similarly sized renal tubules (unstained wet mount, 400×). (b) With nephrocalcinosis, tubules are multifocally dilated and effaced by large irregular intratubular aggregates of crystalline material that is surrounded by laminated layers, consistent with granulomatous inflammation and fibrosis (unstained wet mount, 200×).

Infection and Inflammation

Fish kidneys are susceptible to systemic infectious diseases as reviewed in other body systems. A few notable nephrotropic diseases are highlighted.

Bacteria

Bacterial infections often localize to the kidneys, and renal samples are the organ of choice for isolation of systemic bacterial infections.[5] *R. salmoninarum* causes "bacterial kidney disease" affecting freshwater and marine salmonids. This agent causes systemic infection with cutaneous and muscle involvement ("spawning rash") in some cases, as well as infection of visceral organs. The kidney is prototypically affected and is enlarged due to inflammation. *Renibacterium* is a facultative intracellular Gram-positive bacillus commonly found in pairs. Granulomatous inflammation is discernable in renal squash preparations, and extra- and intracellular bacilli can be identified within macrophages on air-dried Wright-stained smears. While Gram-positive staining supports the diagnosis, definitive diagnosis is by culture and/or molecular diagnostics. Immunofluorescence staining also can be performed on cytologic preparations.

Myxozoa

"Proliferative kidney disease" of salmonids is caused by the myxozoan *Tetracapsuloides bryosalmonae,* resulting in renal enlargement with chronic interstitial nephritis, granulomatous inflammation, hematopoietic interstitial cell proliferation, and vasculitis. Infection is acquired through the gills and skin, becomes disseminated, and primarily targets the kidney. Proliferation of organisms occurs in the renal interstitium and tubules, and spores are excreted by the urinary system.[99] Mature spores are uncommon, and cytologic diagnosis is accomplished by identification of developing stages on wet-mounts or stained dry-mount imprints. These appear as round to amoeboid, 5–20 μm-diameter primary (mother) cells with 1–7 internal secondary (daughter) cells.[1]

"Polycystic kidney disease" in fish is a generic macroscopic term that encompasses infectious and noninfectious causes. Marked cystic renal enlargement often externally expands the coelom. Cysts arise from both tubules and glomeruli, and the exact etiology, particularly of noninfectious forms (e.g. developmental, inherited), is often unknown. Both genetic predisposition and environmental exposures have been suggested.[100,101] In goldfish, the myxozoan parasite *Hoeferellus carassii* (*Mitraspora cyprini*) causes "kidney bloater disease," characterized by marked hyperplasia and cystic ectasia of renal tubules. Mature spores are often low in number but can be found cytologically as miter-like, approximately 10 × 5 μm, refractile structures with long bristles on the posterior end and two anterior polar capsules. Cystic fluid is typically low in protein and cellularity, and hemorrhage can be present.[5] Myxozoanosis, attributed to *Sinuolinea phyllopteryxa*, in weedy sea dragons also affects the kidneys. Cytologically, spores are round, approximately 15 μm diameter, with two rounded polar capsules and binucleate sporoplasm.[36,102]

Sphaerospora renicola is a myxozoan parasite that can localize to the kidney as well as the swim bladder, causing renal degeneration ("kidney enlargement disease").

Mature spores of *S. renicola* are rounded and approximately 7 μm diameter with two polar capsules[67,68]

Fungi and Fungal-Like Organisms

Microsporidial infections affecting the kidneys include *Nucleospora* species discussed with the hematopoietic system. In addition to distinctive proliferation of hemic/hematopoietic cells, varying degrees of renal tubular and hematopoietic degeneration and necrosis also occur.

Hyperplasia and Neoplasia

Primary renal neoplasms are uncommon in fish, although nephroblastomas, adenomas, and carcinomas are reported. Case series describe nephroblastomas in Japanese eel and tubular epithelial neoplasms in oscars.[103,104] Histology of renal neoplasms is comparable with other taxa, and cytology is poorly characterized. Genetic or toxic factors likely contribute in some cases. Because the kidney is hematopoietic, hemic neoplasms (lymphoma/leukemia) often manifest in the kidneys. Epithelial neoplasms of the renal collecting ducts and urinary bladder have been documented in a few individual reports with limited morphologic description.[105]

Reproductive

Reproductive anatomy of fish is more variable than in other taxa. Although generally divided into male and female sexes, both simultaneous and sequential hermaphroditism occur and are associated with factors including natural history, genetics, environment, and other external cues.[106] Generally, testes are paired, white to pale tan, variably thick streak-shaped organs located adjacent to the swim bladder in the dorsal coelom. The vas deferens collects and transitions sperm and fluid to an excretory meatus at the urinary papilla.[14] The testes consist of seminiferous tubules lined by spermatogenic epithelium and sertoli cells and separated by stromal bands containing interstitial cells responsible for testosterone production.[14] The female genital tract of many teleost fish consists mainly of clustered ovarian follicles, representing more than half of total body weight in mature, reproductively active fish. Depending on the species, ova are released directly into the coelom or into an oviduct.[14] Developing oogonia are progressively surrounded by granulosa cells, and many different stages of development are often present concurrently. Some species of fish, including elasmobranchs, have more developed mesonephric duct systems with variable uterine, cervical, and vaginal structures allowing for internal embryonic development. These structures are generally lined by tunica mucosa, muscularis, and adventitia as in other taxa; the mucosal epithelium is cuboidal to columnar with cilia or microvilli.[14,107] The egg capsules of oviparous sharks and rays are morphologically diverse.

Infection and Inflammation

The reproductive tract of fish is not generally a primary target of infectious agents but can be involved in systemic infections of all kinds. Bacterial infections are most common. Granulomatous inflammation typically results, seen cytologically on wet or dry mounts with or without apparent associated infectious agents. A few highlighted specific infections of reproductive tissues include myxozoan and microsporidian agents.

The myxozoan parasite *Sphaerospora testicularis* is reported to infect sea bass, causing testicular hemorrhage, necrosis, granulomatous inflammation, degeneration, fibrosis, and atrophy.[108] Spores can be identified on cytologic preparations, including seminal fluid. *Sphaerospora* spores are rounded and approximately 10–15 μm diameter with a sporoplasm and two polar capsules.

The microsporidian *Pleistophora ovariae* has been reported to infect ovarian tissues of golden shiner and other minnows. The developing spores infect ova and cause variable degeneration, macrophagic infiltration, fibrosis, and eventual atresia and infertility.[109] The spore morphology is comparable with microsporidia at other sites (Table 63.2).

Fish are susceptible to noninfectious inflammation of ovarian tissue, variably termed "egg binding," and associated with pre- or postovulatory stasis. Histologically, lesions are characterized by follicular degeneration, variable macrophagic inflammation, fibrosis, hemorrhage, and melanomacrophage centers. Degenerate follicles, yolk material, and/or inflammation can be identified cytologically on wet or dry mount, but other means of diagnosis are generally employed (i.e. ultrasound, endoscopy, histology). Underlying infectious conditions must be excluded. Pathogenesis is likely multifactorial, including environmental, nutritional, and hormonal factors.

Hyperplasia and Neoplasia

Reproductive neoplasms are occasionally encountered, especially in some ornamental fish. Testicular neoplasms are relatively common, including seminomas, sertoli cell tumors, and interstitial cell tumors (Figure 63.38).[13] Gonadal neoplasms are reported commonly in koi and carp, sometimes markedly expanding the coelom and even causing body wall herniation. Many of these expansive coelomic neoplasms have been classified as sex cord-stromal tumors, most often arising from the ovary of females, with fewer arising from testes, or rarely from ovotestis or

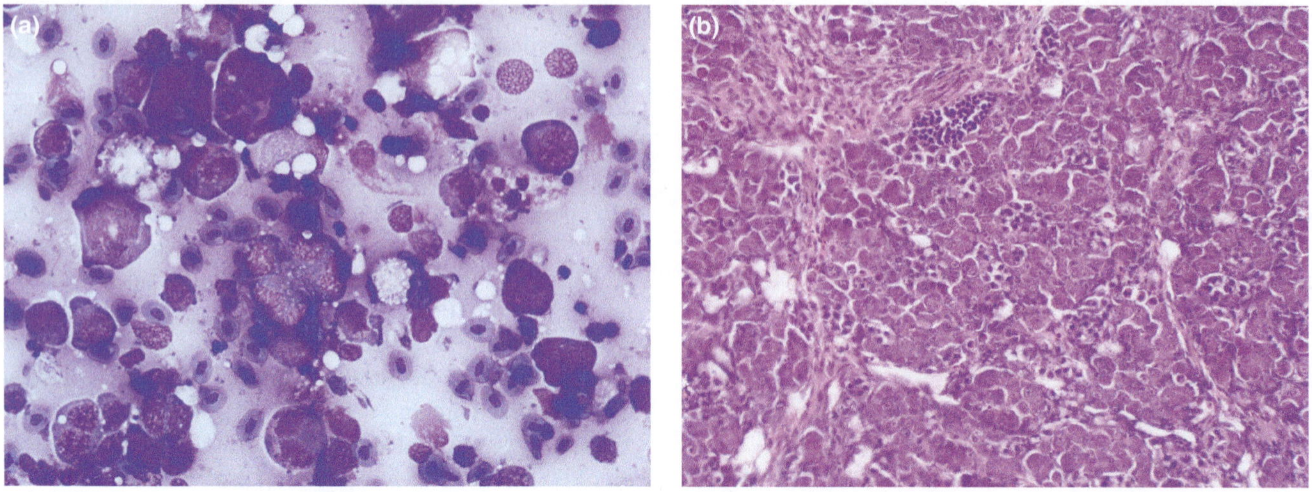

Figure 63.38 Postmortem samples from a gonadal neoplasm (seminoma) in a pachax (*Pachypanchax sakaramyi*). (a) Cytology shows numerous individual round cells with moderate anisocytosis and anisokaryosis, multinucleation, and coarse chromatin. There is mild background blood. Cellular deterioration is consistent with postmortem autolysis (modified Wright's, 1000×). (b) Histology shows sheets of large round cells in a fine fibrovascular stroma with abundant eosinophilic cytoplasm and large open-faced nuclei with a coarse chromatin pattern. Throughout the background are islands of small basophilic cells consistent with spermatids (hematoxylin and eosin, 400×).

unidentified gonads.[110] Other reproductive neoplasms include uncommon cases of smooth muscle neoplasms, mesothelioma, and other systemic or infiltrative lesions. Histologic features and cytologic features are consistent with other vertebrates. Cytology can be used to help differentiate inflammatory from proliferative lesions and, in some cases, to support a specific neoplastic diagnosis.

Nervous System

The basic structure of central and peripheral nervous systems in fish include neurons, neuroglia, white matter, and gray matter, which are similar to other taxa. Fish have a single layer of meninges, the primitive meninx.[14] Eosinophilic granule cells are common around the roots of spinal and cranial nerves.

The central nervous system is not commonly sampled antemortem. A moderate amount of cerebrospinal fluid surrounds the brain in elasmobranchs with a significant accumulation typically present anterior to the telencephalon (Figure 63.39). This can be accessed percutaneously either with ultrasound guidance or through palpation of a small v-shaped notch in the anterior skull. Insertion of a small gauge needle anterior to this site (22 G or smaller) on an appropriate (e.g. 1–5 mL) syringe will permit collection of cerebrospinal fluid for evaluation. Caution should be used in unfamiliar species. In the authors' experience, such samples generally show very low cellularity, but pleocytosis and infectious agents can be identified in disease.

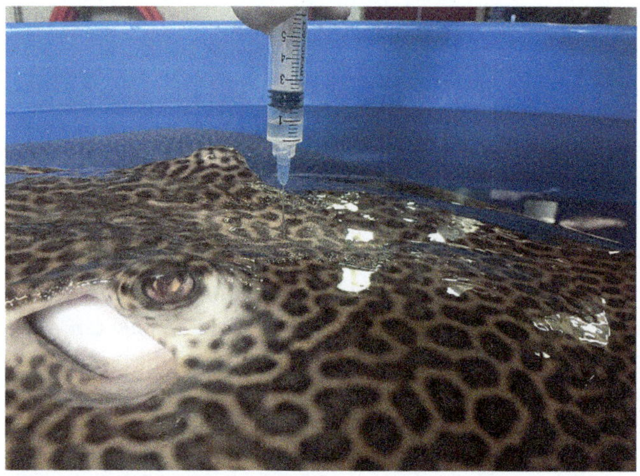

Figure 63.39 Cerebral spinal fluid collection from a honeycomb stingray (*H. uarnak*) (*Source:* Image courtesy of Natalie Mylniczenko).

Infection and Inflammation

Bacteria

Bacteria are the most common cause of meningitis in fish, typically by extension of external infections to or through the dura or by local or systemic spread of internal infections to the meninges. Bacterial agents include *Aeromonas*, *Vibrio*, *Pseudomonas* spp., and others (Table 63.1). The inflammatory response in bacterial meningitis is typically fibrinous and cellular exudate, with monocytes predominating.

Edwardsiella ictaluri causes "hole-in-the-head disease" or "enteric septicemia of catfish" and is occasionally recognized in other fish, such as research zebrafish.[111] In catfish, erosion of the skin and muscle of the head can lead to brain exposure. Necrosis and inflammation of meninges and brain occur, particularly along olfactory and forebrain regions. In established systemic infections, chronic inflammation is also found in coelomic organs.[111,112] Cytologically, evidence of necrosis with macrophages and intracellular rod-shaped bacteria is expected; ancillary testing is required for definitive diagnosis.

Streptococcus iniae is a recognized pathogen of cultured and wild fish causing meningoencephalitis and systemic bacterial sepsis. Fibrinous meningitis with intralesional diplococci can be present, as well as fibrinous, granulocytic, and granulomatous inflammation affecting the pericardium, coelom, systemic blood vessels, and other organs.[113]

Protozoa

Scuticociliate associated meningoencephalitis due to *Miamiensis* sp. is an emerging disease of in situ and ex situ elasmobranch populations. In managed care settings, animals may present with a brief period of lethargy, abnormal behavior, or loss of orientation; many animals die without premonitory signs.[27] In the wild, large scale mortality events associated with infection have been observed.[114,115] Cerebrospinal fluid analysis (antemortem or post mortem) or post mortem brain cytology through direct and stained methods are a sensitive diagnostic tool in these cases and provide an easy, rapid diagnosis. The fluid may demonstrate xanthochromia grossly and moderate mixed pleocytosis with scuticociliates (Figure 63.40). Brain cytology similarly documents inflammatory infiltrates and intralesional protozoa.[27, 114, 115]

Myxozoa

The classic myxozoan agent, *Myxobolus cerebralis*, causes "whirling disease" (see the musculoskeletal system) by targeting the developing skeleton and causing secondary neurological effects. Multiple other myxozoans directly infect the nervous system in a variety of fish species, including *Myxobolus arcticus*, *Myxobolus neurophilus*, and others. Spores can be identified in wet- and dry-mount cytologic preparations (often postmortem touch or squash impressions) and are characterized by a refractile wall, sporoplasm, and polar capsules (Table 63.2). Spore morphology of *Myxobolus* sp. is rounded to pyriform with two polar capsules.[116]

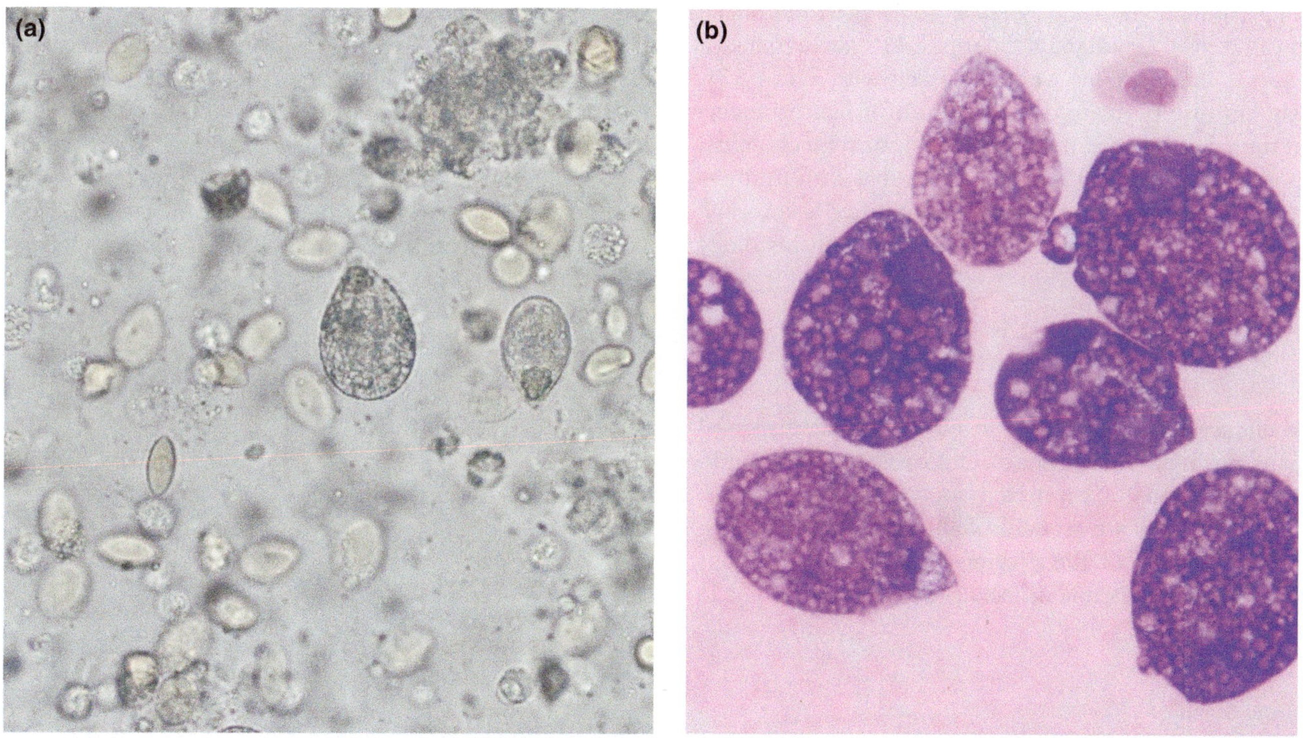

Figure 63.40 (a) Wet mount cytology of a post mortem cerebrospinal fluid sample from a smooth dogfish (Mustelus canis) containing pyriform scuticociliate protozoa amid increased erythrocytes and granulocytes (400×). (b) Wright-Giemsa stained air-dried cytology of cerebrospinal fluid from a smooth dogfish demonstrating 30-50 μm long, 20 μm wide scuticociliates with a eccentric macronucleus and eosinophilic cytoplasmic phagocytic vacuoles (1000×).

Fungi and Fungal-Like Organisms

Fungal infections of the nervous system are uncommon but include oomycetes such as aphanomycosis and true fungi such as exophialiosis. Microsporidians are particularly important infectious agents of the nervous system of fish, including laboratory colonies. *P. neurophilia* is the most common pathogen identified in laboratory zebrafish, affecting the nervous system primarily and skeletal muscle to a lesser degree. Disease is subclinical or characterized by emaciation and spinal deformities.[57] The organisms often localize to spinal cord, nerve roots, and posterior brain.[56] Like *Pleistophora* sp. (see musculoskeletal system), *P. neurophilia* replicate in host cells and can cause cell rupture and host inflammatory response. Like other microsporidia, cytologic features are typified by small refractile oval to pyriform spores with a posterior vacuole (Table 63.2), reported as $3 \times 5\,\mu m$ for *P. neurophila* (Figure 63.24). Other microsporidia infecting the nervous system include *Spraguea* sp. which can form large, macroscopically visible xenomas in the brain, vagus, and spinal nerves. Microsporidian spores are detectable on wet- or dry-mount cytologic preparations of infected tissues.

Hyperplasia and Neoplasia

Most nervous system neoplasms of fish originate from the peripheral nervous system (e.g. neurofibromas, schwannomas, malignant peripheral nerve sheath tumors). These lesions were discussed with skin previously but also occur internally. Primitive neuroectodermal tumors rarely occur spontaneously or with chemical exposures. Cytology is largely comparable with findings in terrestrial vertebrates. However, definitive lesion classification to cellular origin can require not only histology but also ultrastructure.

Endocrine

The endocrine system of fish involves multiple dispersed organs. As in other vertebrates, endocrine tissues are intimately functionally connected to other body systems. Endocrine organs are generally well vascularized and susceptible to many of the previously discussed infectious agents through systemic or localized spread, as well as to toxic exposures.

Thyroid Gland

Thyroid gland microanatomy and function are similar to higher vertebrates, with follicles lined by low cuboidal epithelium and filled with colloid. However, the thyroid gland of fish is widespread and variably distributed, occurring around the pharynx, head, liver, kidney, and other locations. Thyroid proliferations commonly present as nodular swellings at the base of the gills in the ventral opercular cavity and can invade surrounding tissue including gill arches. Hyperplasia (goiter) is often related to husbandry including iodine deficiency, ozone use in managed care, or exposure to other goitrogenic factors.

Thyroid hyperplasia and neoplasia are reported in freshwater and lesser marine fish, both as spontaneous and chemically induced lesions.[13] The proliferations vary from well-differentiated follicles with or without colloid to anaplastic and infiltrative masses including adenomas and adenocarcinomas, but most are benign. Thyroid gland is uncommonly sampled in fish but reported to be comparable with other species and is composed of clusters of epithelial cells and grayish purple staining colloidal material, though many samples are poorly cellular.[5] Cytology can help to differentiate inflammation from tissue proliferation; however, differentiation of hyperplasia vs. neoplasia and benign vs. malignant neoplasms is better performed histologically. Criteria for histologic diagnosis of proliferative thyroid lesions in bony fish are described.[117]

Endocrine Pancreas

Islets of Langerhans are variably dispersed or, in some species, grouped into a single large islet (Brockman body). Islet hormones include insulin (beta cells) and glucagon (alpha cells). The Brockman body should not be mistaken for a proliferative lesion. Although a diabetes syndrome in carp is reported, endocrine pancreatic pathology is not well recognized in fish and specific cytologically diagnostic features are not reported.

Interrenal Gland (Adrenal Function)

Most teleost fish possess interrenal tissue akin to adrenal cortical tissue, which is located in the anterior kidney and produces glucocorticoids and mineralocorticoids. While fish possess mineralocorticoid receptors, most fish do not produce aldosterone (the exception being lungfish) and evidence shows that cortisol plays a greater osmoregulatory role in fish than do other endogenous mineralocorticoids (e.g., 11-deoxycoticosterone).[118] Chromaffin tissue, comparable with adrenal medullary cells, is sometimes located with the interrenal tissue or elsewhere around the anterior kidney or sympathetic ganglia.[14] Although affected by systemic or regionally extensive diseases, particularly from the kidney, specific cytologic lesions of fish interrenal tissue are not described.

Ultimobranchial Gland and Corpuscles of Stannius (Parathyroid Function)

Fish lack parathyroid glands but have functional equivalents involving ultimobranchial glands and corpuscles of Stannius. The ultimobranchial glands are composed of eosinophilic polygonal cells ventral to the esophagus. The corpuscles of Stannius are paired structures in the kidneys and are composed of cords of large polygonal to clear cells that produce piscine calcitonin (teleocalcin).[14] Specific cytologic lesions affecting these tissues are not yet reported.

Pituitary Gland

The pituitary gland of fish is comparable with other vertebrates. Endocrine products include thyroid, adrenal, and gonadal stimulating hormones. Effects on pigmentation, osmoregulation, and growth are described.[14] The pituitary gland can be affected by regional or systemic lesions extending to involve the neuroanatomic region, but cytologic features of organ-specific lesions are not yet reported.

Other Endocrine Structures

Other piscine anatomic structures with possible endocrine function include the pseudobranch in some teleosts and the urophysis in some teleosts and sharks. The pseudobranch is composed of blood capillaries with connections to the choroid of the eye. It is susceptible to toxic and microbial lesions. Pseudobranch tumors are reported in wild cod and other gadoid fish; the histologic features include poorly defined large pale "X-cells," and cytology is not reported.[13,119] The urophysis is present at the posterior spinal cord and consists of neurosecretory cells with hormonal impacts including osmoregulation.[14] Cytology is not reported.

Special Sense Organs

Eye

The eye of teleost fish is similar to other vertebrates. The teleost lens is commonly spherical, enabling a large "fish-eye" field of view and focal depth. The degree of accommodation is less than in other taxa, and muscles of the iris are not well developed. The choroidal vessels are associated with a large gland-like network of capillaries, the choroidal gland (choroidal rete). In contrast, elasmobranch eyes show greater pupillary responsiveness, have less dense and more variably shaped lenses, and no choroidal rete. Retinal morphology in all fish is largely consistent with other vertebrates, although some components (e.g., cone cells, rhodopsin visual pigments) differ across species, environmental conditions, water depth, etc.[14] Unlike mammals, the neural components of the fish retina retain the ability to regenerate throughout life.[120]

Ocular pathology in fish is similar to other vertebrates with the cornea being most vulnerable to trauma and secondary infections, including both bacterial and fungal agents. Like other small vascular beds, the choroidal rete is a common site of secondary involvement in systemic infections. Some parasitic infections of the skin also extend to infect the eye, for example, *Cryptocotyle lingua*, which can be seen as digenean metacercariae encysted in the cornea. A common cause of cataract in fish is parasitic infection by trematode metacercaria of *Diplostomum* sp. (the "eye fluke"). Cytologic sampling of the cornea can be conducted antemortem with anesthesia or postmortem. To examine the lens and other structures, the entire eye (enucleated or postmortem) can be made into a squash preparation. One of the most frequent ocular lesions in fish is gas bubble disease, but cytology is typically performed on the gill.

Fish eyes are infrequently affected by neoplasia. Reported lesions include corneal or intraocular pigment cell tumors (e.g. erythrophoroma, melanoma), mesenchymal tumors, and lymphoma.[13] Spontaneous retinoblastomas are also reported in several fish species; in one series of neuronal embryonal tumors in fish, lesions involved the eyes and less frequently the skin.[121] Most of these ocular neoplasms were consistent with retinoblastoma, and one appeared to be a medulloepithelioma.[121] Rosette formation is a typical histologic feature of these primitive ectodermal neoplasms, which can also be appreciated cytologically, although cytology of ocular neoplasms in fish is rarely reported.

Lateral Line and Labyrinth (Ear)

The lateral line consists of a groove along the trunk of fish, replete in mechanoreceptors, supported by bone, and covered by skin with intermittent pores. In some species, these are contiguous with head canals. The mechanoreceptors are highly sensitive to motion in the water system, including prey movements and wavelengths of sound.[14] The labyrinth is an organ developing from the lateral line, consisting of semicircular canals, chambers, and in teleosts, otolith organs. Movement of endolymphatic fluid results in stimulation of sensory tissue involved in equilibrium and sound perception.[14]

The lateral line can be affected by skin infections and is a common site of *Flavobacterium* sp. infection at low temperatures in marine fish and *Fusarium* sp. infection in elasmobranchs.[10] As in skin, cytologic features of *Flavobacterium* sp. include bacterial aggregates with gliding motion (Table 63.1, Figure 63.8). An epizootic of neoplasia affecting the lateral line was reported in lake trout and presented as soft, white, variably ulcerated, and cerebriform masses. Most were identified histologically as spindle cell sarcomas, but others included benign and malignant peripheral nerve sheath tumors, carcinomas, epitheliomas, astrocytomas, amelanotic melanoma, and others. Causative factors were not identified, but a viral etiology appeared unlikely.[122] Cytologic findings of the labyrinth are not specifically described.

Other Body Systems

Besides collection of blood for hematologic assessment, the cardiovascular system of fish is not typically sampled for cytology. Few disease conditions specifically target the circulatory system. Parasites of the cardiovascular system include flagellates, haemogregarines, rickettsia, and others. Cardiovascular neoplasms include spontaneous or induced hemangiomas and related tumors, often in the dermis and subcutis.[13] Spontaneous hemangiosarcomas are rarely reported.[123]

Conclusion

Cytology has long been used in fish medicine and is particularly effective as a rapid diagnostic technique for individual and group morbidity and mortality situations in relation to infectious disease. As fish continue to grow in companion animal, conservation, aquaculture, and research realms, cytology offers practical, nonfatal, cost-effective benefits to guide diagnostic efforts, management, and intervention. As fish possess unique anatomy, physiology, and pathology, developing familiarity with the species and lesions is helpful and is an ongoing challenge as more is continually learned about these diverse vertebrates.

References

1 Noga, E.J. (2010). *Fish Disease: Diagnosis and Treatment*, 2e. Ames, IA: Wiley-Blackwell.
2 Ferguson, H.W. (2006). *Systemic Pathology of Fish: A Text and Atlas of Comparative Tissue Responses in Diseases of Teleosts*, 2e. London: Scotian Press.
3 Roberts, R.J. (2012). *Fish Pathology*, 4e. Ames, IA: Wiley-Blackwell.
4 Campbell, T.W. (2015). *Exotic Animal Hematology and Cytology*, 4e. Ames, IA: Wiley-Blackwell.
5 Reavill, D. and Roberts, H. (2007). Diagnostic cytology of fish. *Vet Clin North Am Exot Anim Pract* 10: 207–234.
6 Campbell, T.W. (ed.) (2015). Wet-mount sampling techniques in fish. In: *Exotic Animal Hematology and Cytology*, 4e, 373–376. Ames, IA: Wiley-Blackwell.
7 Grant, K.R. (2015). Fish hematology and associated disorders. *Clin Lab Med* 35: 681–701.
8 Arnold, J.E. (2005). Hematology of the sandbar shark, *Carcharhinus plumbeus*: standardization of complete blood count techniques for elasmobranchs. *Vet Clin Pathol* 34: 115–123.
9 Zou, J. and Secombes, C. (2016). The function of fish cytokines. *Biology (Basel)* 5: E23.
10 Roberts, R.J. and Rodger, H. (2012). The pathophysiology and systemic pathology of teleosts. In: *Fish Pathology*, 4e (ed. R.J. Roberts), 62–143. Ames, IA: Wiley-Blackwell.
11 Reite, O.B. and Evensen, Ø. (2006). Inflammatory cells of teleostean fish: a review focusing on mast cells/ eosinophilic granule cells and rodlet cells. *Fish Shellfish Immunol* 20: 192–208.
12 AnvariFar, H., Amirkolaie, A.K., Miandare, H.K. et al. (2017). Apoptosis in fish: environmental factors and programmed cell death. *Cell Tissue Res* 368: 425–439.
13 Groff, J.M. (2004). Neoplasia in fishes. *Vet Clin North Am Exot Anim Pract* 7: 705–756.
14 Roberts, R.J. and Ellis, E.A. (2012). The anatomy and physiology of teleosts. In: *Fish Pathology*, 4e (ed. R.J. Roberts), 17–61. Ames, IA: Wiley-Blackwell.
15 Sköld, H.N., Aspengren, S., Cheney, K.L., and Wallin, M. (2016). Fish chromatophores: from molecular motors to animal behavior. *Int Rev Cell Mol Biol* 321: 171–219.
16 Declercq, A.M., Haesebrouck, F., Van Den Broeck, W. et al. (2013). Columnaris disease in fish: a review with emphasis on bacterium-host interactions. *Vet Res* 44: 1–17.
17 Avendaño-Herrera, R., Toranzo, A.E., and Magariños, B. (2006). Tenacibaculosis infection in marine fish caused by *Tenacibaculum maritimum*: a review. *Dis Aquat Org* 71: 255–266.
18 Decostere, A., Hermans, K., and Haesebrouck, F. (2004). *Piscine mycobacteriosis*: a literature review covering the agent and the disease it causes in fish and humans. *Vet Microbiol* 99: 159–166.
19 Jernigan, J.A. and Farr, B.M. (2000). Incubation period and sources of exposure for cutaneous *Mycobacterium marinum* infection: case report and review of the literature. *Clin Infect Dis* 31: 439–443.
20 Pawlikowska-Warych, M. and Deptuła, W. (2016). Characteristics of chlamydia-like organisms pathogenic to fish. *J Appl Genet* 57: 135–141.
21 Nowak, B.F. and LaPatra, S.E. (2006). Epitheliocystis in fish. *J Fish Dis* 29: 573–588.

22 Wootten, R. (2012). The parasitology of teleosts. In: *Fish Pathology*, 4e (ed. R.J. Roberts), 292–338. Ames, IA: Wiley-Blackwell.

23 Reed, P., Francis-Floyd, R., Klinger, R., and Petty, D. (2009). *Monogenean Parasites of Fish*, 1–4. University of Florida IFAS Extension FA28.

24 Dickerson, H.W. and Findly, R.C. (2014). Immunity to Ichthyophthirius infections in fish: a synopsis. *Dev Comp Immunol* 43: 290–299.

25 Campbell, T.W. (ed.) (2015). Wet mount microscopy in fish. In: *Exotic Animal Hematology and Cytology*, 4e, 357–372. Ames, IA: Wiley-Blackwell.

26 Rossteuscher, S., Wenker, C., Jermann, T. et al. (2008). Severe scuticociliate (*Philasterides dicentrarchi*) infection in a population of sea dragons (*Phycodurus eques* and *Phyllopteryx taeniolatus*). *Vet Pathol* 45: 546–550.

27 Stidworthy, M.F., Garner, M.M., Bradway, D.S. et al. (2014). Systemic scuticociliatosis (*Philasterides dicentrarchi*) in sharks. *Vet Pathol* 51: 628–632.

28 Callahan, H.A., Litaker, R.W., and Noga, E.J. (2005). Genetic relationships among members of the Ichthyobodo necator complex: implications for the management of aquaculture stocks. *J Fish Dis* 28: 111–118.

29 Bakke, T.A., Cable, J., and Harris, P.D. (2007). The biology of gyrodactylid monogeneans: the "Russian-doll killers". *Adv Parasitol* 64: 161–367.

30 Garner, M.M. (2013). A retrospective study of disease in elasmobranchs. *Vet Pathol* 50: 377–389.

31 Conboy, G.A. and Speare, D.J. (2002). Dermal nematodosis in commercially captured rockfish (*Sebastes* spp.) from coastal British Columbia, Canada. *J Comp Pathol* 127: 211–213.

32 MacLean, R.A., Fatzinger, M.H., Woolard, K.D., and Harms, C.A. (2006). Clearance of a dermal *Huffmanela* sp. in a sandbar shark (*Carcharhinus plumbeus*) using levamisole. *Dis Aquat Org* 73: 83–88.

33 Roberts, R.J. (ed.) (2012). The mycology of teleosts. In: *Fish Pathology*, 4e. Ames, IA: Wiley-Blackwell.

34 Yanong, R.P.E. (2003). Fungal diseases of fish. *Vet Clin North Am Exot Anim Pract* 6: 377–400.

35 Oidtmann, B. (2012). Review of biological factors relevant to import risk assessments for epizootic ulcerative syndrome (*Aphanomyces invadans*). *Transbound Emerg Dis* 59: 26–39.

36 Bonar, C.J., Garner, M.M., Weber, E.S. et al. (2013). Pathologic findings in weedy (*Phyllopteryx taeniolatus*) and leafy (*Phycodurus eques*) seadragons. *Vet Pathol* 50: 368–376.

37 Marancik, D.P., Berliner, A.L., Cavin, J.M. et al. (2011). Disseminated fungal infection in two species of captive sharks. *J Zoo Wildl Med* 42: 686–693.

38 Yanong, R.P.E., Francis-Floyd, R., Curtis, E. et al. (2002). Algal dermatitis in cichlids. *J Am Vet Med Assoc* 220: 1353–1358, 1314.

39 Langenmayer, M.C., Lewisch, E., Gotesman, M. et al. (2015). Cutaneous infection with *Dermocystidium salmonis* in cardinal tetra, *Paracheirodon axelrodi* (Schultz, 1956). *J Fish Dis* 38: 503–506.

40 Weber, E.P.S. (2013). Itchy fish and viral dermatopathies. Sampling, diagnosis, and management of common viral diseases. *Vet Clin North Am Exot Anim Pract* 16: 687–703.

41 Coffee, L.L., Casey, J.W., and Bowser, P.R. (2013). Pathology of tumors in fish associated with retroviruses. *Vet Pathol* 50: 390–403.

42 Carlisle, J.C. and Roberts, R.J. (1977). Epidermal papilloma of the Atlantic salmon I: epizootiology, pathology and immunology. *J Wildl Dis* 13: 230–234.

43 Camus, A., Dill, J., McDermott, A. et al. (2016). Virus-associated papillomatous skin lesions in a giant guitarfish *Rhynchobatus djiddensis*: a case report. *Dis Aquat Org* 117: 253–258.

44 Bowser, P.R., Earnest Koons, K.A., Wooster, G.A. et al. (1998). Experimental transmission of discrete epidermal hyperplasia in walleyes. *J Aquat Anim Health* 10: 282–286.

45 Kelly, R.K., Nielsen, O., Mitchell, S.C., and Yamamoto, T. (1983). Characterization of *Herpes virus vitreum* isolated from hyperplastic epidermal tissue of walleye, *Stizostedion vitreum vitreum* (Mitchill). *J Fish Dis* 6: 249–260.

46 Freitas, J.T., Subramaniam, K., Kelley, K.L. et al. (2016). Genetic characterization of esocid herpesvirus 1 (EsHV1). *Dis Aquat Org* 122: 1–11.

47 Martineau, D., Bowser, P.R., Wooster, G., and Forney, J.L. (1990). Histologic and ultrastructural studies of dermal sarcoma of walleye (Pisces: *Stizostedion vitreum*). *Vet Pathol* 27: 340–346.

48 Schmale, M.C. (1995). Experimental induction of neurofibromatosis in bicolor damselfish. *Dis Aquat Org* 23: 201–212.

49 Schmale, M.C., Gibbs, P.D.L., and Campbell, C.E. (2002). A virus-like agent associated with neurofibromatosis in damselfish. *Dis Aquat Org* 49: 107–115.

50 Thompson, J. and Kostiala, A. (1986). Immunological classification of a pike lymphoma. *Vet Immunol Immunopathol* 12: 421–430.

51 Thompson, J.S. and Kostiala, A.A.I. (1990). Immunological and ultrastructural characterization of true histiocytic lymphoma in the northern pike, *Esox lucius* L. *Cancer Res* 50 (Suppl. 17): 5668–5671.

52 Camus, M.S., Hyatt, M.W., Clauss, T.M. et al. (2011). Chromatophoroma in a crevice kelpfish (*Gibbonsia montereyensis*). *Vet Clin Pathol* 40: 549–552.

53 Cavin, J.M., Donahoe, S.L., Frasca, S. et al. (2012). *Myxobolus albi* infection in cartilage of captive lumpfish (*Cyclopterus lumpus*). *J Vet Diagn Invest* 24: 516–524.

54 Picon-Camacho, S.M., Holzer, A.S., Freeman, M.A. et al. (2009). *Myxobolus albi* n. sp. (Myxozoa) from the gills of the common goby pomatoschistus microps krøyer (Teleostei: Gobiidae). *J Eukaryot Microbiol* 56: 421–427.

55 Lom, J. and Dyková, I. (2005). Microsporidian xenomas in fish seen in wider perspective. *Folia Parasitol (Praha)* 52: 69–81.

56 Spagnoli, S.T., Xue, L., Murray, K.N. et al. (2015). *Pseudoloma neurophilia*: a retrospective and descriptive study of nervous system and muscle infections, with new implications for pathogenesis and behavioral phenotypes. *Zebrafish* 12: 189–201.

57 Sanders, J.L., Watral, V., and Kent, M.L. (2012). Microsporidiosis in zebrafish research facilities. *ILAR J* 53: 106–113.

58 Sanders, J.L., Lawrence, C., Nichols, D.K. et al. (2010). *Pleistophora hyphessobryconis* (Microsporidia) infecting zebrafish *Danio rerio* in research facilities. *Dis Aquat Org* 91: 47–56.

59 Peterson, T.S., Spitsbergen, J.M., Feist, S.W., and Kent, M.L. (2011). Luna stain, an improved selective stain for detection of microsporidian spores in histologic sections. *Dis Aquat Org* 95: 175–180.

60 Spanggaard, B. and Huss, H.H. (1996). Growth of the fish parasite *Ichthyophonus hoferi* under food relevant conditions. *Int J Food Sci Technol* 31: 427–432.

61 Spanggaard, B., Huss, H., and Bresciani, J. (1995). Morphology of *Ichthyophonus hoferi* assessed by light and scanning electron microscopy. *J Fish Dis* 18: 567–577.

62 Bahri, S., Marton, S., Marques, A., and Eszterbauer, E. (2010). *Henneguya tunisiensis* n. sp. (Myxosporea: Bivalvulida), a new gill parasite of *Symphodus tinca* (L.) (Teleostei: Labridae) off Tunisia. *Syst Parasitol* 76: 93–101.

63 Fain, A. and Lambrechts, L. (1987). Observations on the acarofauna of fish aquariums. *Bull Ann Soc R D'Entomol Belg* 123: 103–118.

64 Oldham, T., Rodger, H., and Nowak, B.F. (2016). Incidence and distribution of amoebic gill disease (AGD): an epidemiological review. *Aquaculture* 457: 35–42.

65 Lawler, A.R. (1980). Studies on *Amyloodinium ocellatum* (Dinoflagellata) in Mississippi sound: natural and experimental hosts. *Gulf Res Rep* 6: 403–413.

66 Knüsel, R., Brandes, K., Lechleiter, S., and Schmidt-Posthaus, H. (2007). Two independent cases of spontaneously occurring branchioblastomas in koi carp (*Cyprinus carpio*). *Vet Pathol* 44: 237–239.

67 Dykova, I., Lom, J., and Korting, W. (1990). Light and electron microscopic observations on the swimbladder stages of *Sphaerospora renicola*, a parasite of carp (*Cyprinus carpio*). *Parasitol Res* 76: 228–237.

68 Dykova, I. and Lom, J. (1982). *Sphaerospora renicola* n.sp., a Myxosporean from carp kidney, and its pathogenicity. *Z Parasitenkd* 68: 259–268.

69 Knopf, K. (2006). The swimbladder nematode *Anguillicola crassus* in the European eel *Anguilla anguilla* and the Japanese eel *Anguilla japonica*: differences in susceptibility and immunity between a recently colonized host and the original host. *J Helminthol* 80: 129–136.

70 Paul, T., Quackenbush, S.L., Sutton, C. et al. (2006). Identification and characterization of an exogenous retrovirus from Atlantic salmon swim bladder sarcomas. *J Virol* 80: 2941–2948.

71 Bowser, P.R., Casey, J.W., Casey, R.N. et al. (2012). Swimbladder leiomyosarcoma in Atlantic salmon (*Salmo salar*) in North America. *J Wildl Dis* 48: 795–798.

72 Fänge, R. (1977). Size relations of lymphomyeloid organs in some cartilaginous fish. *Acta Zool* 58: 125–128.

73 Ferguson, H.W. (1975). Phagocytosis by the endocardial lining cells of the atrium of plaice (*Pleuronectes platessa*). *J Comp Pathol* 85: 561–569.

74 Freeman, M., Kasper, J., and Kristmundsson, A. (2013). *Nucleospora cyclopteri* n. sp., an intranuclear microsporidian infecting wild lumpfish, (*Cyclopterus lumpus* L.), in Icelandic waters. *Parasit Vectors* 6: 49.

75 Palenzuela, O., Redondo, M.J., Cali, A. et al. (2014). A new intranuclear microsporidium, *Enterospora nucleophila* n. sp., causing an emaciative syndrome in a piscine host (*Sparus aurata*), prompts the redescription of the family Enterocytozoonidae. *Int J Parasitol* 44: 189–203.

76 Hedrick, R., Groff, J., McDowell, T. et al. (1990). Hematopoietic intranuclear microsporidian infections with features of leukemia in Chinook salmon *Oncorhynchus tshawytscha*. *Dis Aquat Org* 8: 189–197.

77 Kent, M.L., Groff, J.M., Traxler, G.S. et al. (1990). Plasmacytoid leukemia in seawater reared Chinook salmon *Oncorhynchus tshawytscha*. *Dis Aquat Org* 8: 199–209.

78 Miyazaki, T., Asai, Y., Kobayashi, T., and Miyata, M. (2000). Lympholeukemia in madai Pagrus major in Japan. *Dis Aquat Org* 40: 147–155.

79 Woo, P.T.K. (2003). Cryptobia (Trypanoplasma) salmositica and salmonid cryptobiosis. *J Fish Dis* 26: 627–646.

80 Williams, C.F., Lloyd, D., Poynton, S.L. et al. (2011). Spironucleus species: economically-important fish pathogens and enigmatic single-celled eukaryotes. *J Aquac Res Development* S2: 002.

81 Paull, G.C. and Matthews, R.A. (2001). *Spironucleus vortens*, a possible cause of hole-in-the-head disease in cichlids. *Dis Aquat Org* 45: 197–202.

82 Stamper, M.A., Lewbart, G.A., Barrington, P.R. et al. (1998). Eimeria southwelli infection associated with high mortality of cownose rays. *J Aquat Anim Health* 10: 264–270.

83 Ryan, U. (2010). Cryptosporidium in birds, fish and amphibians. *Exp Parasitol* 124: 113–120.

84 Katharios, P., Kokkari, C., Sterioti, A. et al. (2014). *Enteromyxum leei* infection in parrotfish, *Sparisoma cretense*: histopathological, morphological and molecular study. *Vet Parasitol* 199: 136–143.

85 Diamant, A., Ram, S., and Paperna, I. (2006). Experimental transmission of *Enteromyxum leei* to freshwater fish. *Dis Aquat Org* 72: 171–178.

86 Gardiner, C. and Poynton, S. (2006). *An Atlas of Metazoan Parasites in Animal Tissues*. Washington, DC: Armed Forces Institute of Pathology.

87 Kent, M.L., Bishop-Stewart, J.K., Matthews, J.L., and Spitsbergen, J.M. (2002). *Pseudocapillaria tomentosa*, a nematode pathogen, and associated neoplasms of zebrafish (*Danio rerio*) kept in research colonies. *Comp Med* 52: 354–358.

88 Pérez-Ponce de León, G., Lagunas-Calvo, O., García-Prieto, L. et al. (2018). Update on the distribution of the co-invasive *Schyzocotyle acheilognathi* (= *Bothriocephalus acheilognathi*), the Asian fish tapeworm, in freshwater fishes of Mexico. *J Helminthol* 92: 279–290.

89 Scholz, T. and Kuchta, R. (2016). Fish-borne, zoonotic cestodes (Diphyllobothrium and relatives) in cold climates: a never-ending story of neglected and (re)-emergent parasites. *Food Waterborne Parasitol* 4: 23–38.

90 Grim, K.C., Wolfe, M.J., Edwards, M. et al. (2009). Epizootic ameloblastomas in Chinook salmon (*Oncorhynchus tshawytscha*) of the northwestern United States. *Vet Pathol* 46: 622–635.

91 Agius, C. and Roberts, R.J. (2003). Melano-macrophage centres and their role in fish pathology. *J Fish Dis* 26: 499–509.

92 Mokhtar, D.M. (2015). Histological, histochemical and ultrastructural characterization of the pancreas of the grass carp (*Ctenopharyngodon idella*). *Eur J Anat* 19: 145–153.

93 Hallett, S.L., Atkinson, S.D., Holt, R.A. et al. (2006). A new myxozoan from feral goldfish (*Carassius auratus*). *J Parasitol* 92: 357–363.

94 Bailey, G.S., Williams, D.E., and Hendricks, J.D. (1996). Fish models for environmental carcinogenesis: the rainbow trout. *Environ Health Perspect* 104 (Suppl. 1): 5–12.

95 Spitsbergen, J.M., Buhler, D.R., and Peterson, T.S. (2012). Neoplasia and neoplasm-associated lesions in laboratory colonies of zebrafish emphasizing key influences of diet and aquaculture system design. *ILAR J* 53: 114–125.

96 Vogelbein, W.K., Fournie, J.W., Cooper, P.S., and Van Veld, P.A. (1999). Hepatoblastomas in the mummichog, *Fundulus heteroclitus* (L.), from a creosote-contaminated environment: a histologic, ultrastructural and immunohistochemical study. *J Fish Dis* 22: 419–431.

97 Ozaka, C., Yamamoto, N., and Somiya, H. (2009). Theaglomerular kidney of the deep-sea fish, *Ateleopus japonicus* (Ateleopodiformes: Ateleopodidae): evidence of wider occurrence of the aglomerular condition in teleostei. *Copeia* 3: 609–617.

98 Smart, G.R., Knox, D., Harrison, J.G. et al. (1979). Nephrocalcinosis in rainbow trout Salmo gairdneri Richardson; the effect of exposure to elevated CO_2 concentrations. *J Fish Dis* 2: 279–289.

99 Schmidt-Posthaus, H., Hirschi, R., and Schneider, E. (2015). Proliferative kidney disease in brown trout: infection level, pathology and mortality under field conditions. *Dis Aquat Org* 114: 139–146.

100 Rahmati holasoo, H., Masoudifard, M., Ebrahimzadeh Mousavi, H. et al. (2015). Cystic lesions in the kidney of flower horn fish, hybrid cichlid. *J Fish Dis* 38: 833–838.

101 Munkittrick, K.R., Moccia, R.D., and Leatherland, J.F. (1985). Polycystic kidney disease in goldfish (*Carassius auratus*) from Hamilton Harbour, Lake Ontario, Canada. *Vet Pathol* 22: 232–237.

102 Garner, M.M., Atkinson, S.D., Hallett, S.L. et al. (2008). Renal myxozoanosis in weedy sea dragons, *Phyllopteryx taeniolatus* (Lacepède), caused by *Sinuolinea phyllopteryxa* n. sp. *J Fish Dis* 31: 27–35.

103 Hochwartner, O., Loupal, G., Wildgoose, W.H., and Schmidt-Posthaus, H. (2010). Occurrence of spontaneous tumours of the renal proximal tubules in oscars *Astronotus ocellatus*. *Dis Aquat Org* 89: 185–189.

104 Masahito, P., Ishikawa, T., Okamoto, N., and Sugano, H. (1992). Nephroblastomas in the Japanese eel, *Anguilla japonica* Temminck and Schlegel. *Cancer Res* 52: 2575–2579.

105 Lombardini, E.D., Hard, G.C., and Harshbarger, J.C. (2014). Neoplasms of the urinary tract in fish. *Vet Pathol* 51: 1000–1012.

106 Desjardins, J.K. and Fernald, R.D. (2009). Fish sex: why so diverse? *Curr Opin Neurobiol* 19: 648–653.

107 McMillan, D.B. (2007). *Fish Histology: Female Reproductive Systems*, 1–65. Dordrecht: Springer.

108 Sitja-Bobadilla, A. and Alvarez-Pellitero, P. (1990). *Sphaerospora testicularis* sp. nov. (Myxosporea: Sphaerosporidae) in wild and cultured sea bass, *Dicentrarchus labrax* (L.), from the Spanish Mediterranean area. *J Fish Dis* 13: 193–203.

109 Nagel, M.L. and Hoffman, G.L. (1977). A new host for *Pleistophora ovariae* (Microsporida). *J Parasitol* 63: 160–162.

110 Ott Knüsel, F., Knüsel, R., Doherr, M.G., and Schmidt-Posthaus, H. (2016). Frequency and histologic characterization of coelomatic neoplasms in koi *Cyprinus carpio* koi. *Dis Aquat Org* 119: 219–229.

111 Hawke, J.P., Kent, M., Rogge, M. et al. (2013). Edwardsiellosis caused by *Edwardsiella ictaluri* in laboratory populations of zebrafish *Danio rerio*. *J Aquat Anim Health* 25: 171–183.

112 Shotts, E.B., Blazer, V.S., and Waltman, W.D. (1986). Pathogenesis of experimental *Edwardsiella ictaluri* infections in channel catfish (*Ictalurus punctatus*). *Can J Fish Aquat Sci* 43: 36–42.

113 Keirstead, N.D., Brake, J.W., Griffin, M.J. et al. (2014). Fatal septicemia caused by the zoonotic bacterium *Streptococcus iniae* during an outbreak in *Caribbean reef* fish. *Vet Pathol* 51: 1035–1041.

114 Retallack, H., Okihiro, M.S., Britton, E., Van Sommeran, S., and DeRisi, J.L. In Press. Metagenomic next-generation sequencing reveals Miamiensis avidus (Ciliophora: Scuticociliatida) in the 2017 epizootic of leopard sharks (Triakis semifasciata) in San Francisco Bay, California, USA. *J Wildl Dis* 55(2): 375–386.

115 Newton, A.L., Hyatt, M.W., Malatos, J.M., Ksepka, S.P., and Bullard, S.A. Scuticociliate (Miamiensis sp.) associated meningoencephalitis in wild Northwest Atlantic smooth dogfish (Mustelus canis). American Elasmobranch Society, Snowbird, UT, 2019.

116 Khoo, L., Rommel, F.A., Smith, S.A. et al. (2010). *Myxobolus neurophilus*: morphologic, histopathologic and molecular characterization. *Dis Aquat Org* 89: 51–61.

117 Fournie, J.W., Wolfe, M.J., Wolf, J.C. et al. (2005). Diagnostic criteria for proliferative thyroid lesions in bony fishes. *Toxicol Pathol* 33: 540–551.

118 Takahashi, H., and Sakamoto, T. (2013). The role of 'mineralocorticoids' in teleost fish: relative importance of glucocorticoid signaling in the osmoregulation and 'central' actions of mineralocorticoid receptor. *Gen Comp Endocrinol* 181:223–228.

119 Alpers, C.E., Cain, B.B., Myers, M. et al. (1977). Pathologic anatomy of pseudobranch tumors in Pacific cod, *Gadus macrocephalus*. *J Natl Cancer Inst* 59: 377–398.

120 Sherpa, T., Fimbel, S., Mallory, D. et al. (2008). Ganglion cell regeneration following whole: retina destruction in zebrafish. *Dev Neurobiol* 68: 166–181.

121 Kagan, R., Pinkerton, M.E., and Kinsel, M.J. (2010). Neuronal embryonal tumors in fish. *Vet Pathol* 47: 553–559.

122 Spitsbergen, J.M., Frattini, S.A., Bowser, P.R. et al. (2013). Epizootic neoplasia of the lateral line system of lake trout (*Salvelinus namaycush*) in New York's Finger Lakes. *Vet Pathol* 50: 418–433.

123 Hyatt, M., Clauss, T., Dennison, S., and Camus, A.C. (2013). Retroperitoneal hemangiosarcoma in a common carp *Cyprinus carpio*: a case report. *Dis Aquat Org* 107: 151–160.

64

Invertebrates

Charlotte Hollinger and Nicole I. Stacy

Introduction

Invertebrates comprise the largest animal group on the planet and include a wide variety of morphologically and physiologically different creatures that inhabit extremely diverse habitats. They are roughly grouped across taxa by the absence of a vertebral column and include insects, arachnids, crustaceans, corals, mollusks, echinoderms, jellyfish, sponges, worms, and more. Most invertebrates have a body composed of differentiated tissues, but structure and function are extremely varied, and complex body system organization into distinct organs and/or body cavities (e.g. coelomates) is not present in all phyla (e.g. sponges, corals). These animals are studied for medical, industrial, and agricultural contributions, are key players in ecosystems and economies, and are also growing in popularity as pets (e.g. tarantulas, scorpions, aquatic species in home aquariums). However, despite their abundance and importance, invertebrates are uncommonly presented for medical assessment and receive relatively little mainstream veterinary attention. Increasing awareness of the role of physiologic stress and diseases in threatened "high profile" invertebrates such as honey bees and corals has brought augmented attention to the impact of diagnostic assessment and application of pathologic techniques in invertebrate health assessment.[1,2] Cytology serves as a low-cost, timely, animal-side diagnostic to guide individual or group health management. This chapter is meant as an introduction to basic cytologic methods used with invertebrates. Invertebrate hematology is reviewed as it is inextricably linked to cytology and not covered in routine veterinary hematology references.

Application of Cytology Techniques in Invertebrates

Cytologic techniques in invertebrates include all of the methods employed with vertebrates. As in other animals, methods are selected based on sample site and composition. Methods of sample collection are reviewed in detail elsewhere (Chapter 1).[3,4] Sedation or anesthesia is utilized in some, as appropriate based on restraint needs, and species-specific nociceptive sensation. For internal samples (e.g. hemolymph), the collection site is often cleaned and disinfected prior to sampling. Resulting wounds in hard-shelled invertebrates can be closed with appropriate adhesive material.[5] For superficial samples (e.g. tape preparations or scrapes), cleaning is generally not indicated due to potential effects on the sample.

Interpretive Considerations and General Disease Responses in Invertebrates

As in other taxa, the quality of cytology interpretation is dependent on sample quality and handling. Cellular morphology is subject to rapid deterioration, and smears should be made as soon as possible after collection.

Invertebrates possess innate, nonadaptive, immune mechanisms functioning through phagocytosis, agglutination, and synthesis of antimicrobial proteins. The phagocytic response (macrophage-like) is the most ancient component of the immune system.[6] The general inflammatory response of invertebrates is cytologically characterized by increased concentrations of responding cells (i.e. hemocytes, coelomocytes) and trafficking of

Veterinary Cytology, First Edition. Edited by Leslie C. Sharkey, M. Judith Radin, and Davis Seelig.

these cells to diseased tissues. The composition and nomenclature of invertebrate cells varies greatly among taxa (discussed in more detail below). Inflammation is often accompanied by evidence of necrosis including cellular fragmentation and dissolution, as in vertebrates. However, the most apparent finding cytologically is typically increased inflammatory cells, with or without infectious agents.

Hemolymph and Coelomic Fluid

Hemolymph is the most common sample collected for cytology across invertebrates. It flows through an open circulatory system in many species. The amount of hemolymph that can be safely withdrawn needs to be carefully considered.[4] Hemolymph assessment includes macroscopic evaluation (color, consistency) and evaluation of hemocytes. In health, the hemolymph of many species is clear or pale blue and clots readily. Changes in color and turbidity (often becoming white and cloudy) and diminished clotting are common nonspecific responses of hemolymph to disease.[4,7] Variably red turbid discoloration of hemolymph in lobsters has been associated with disease, including excretory calcinosis, paramoebiasis, and *Aerococcus viridans* infection (also referred to as "gaffkemia").[4,7,8] Hemocyte concentrations are low in health in some species, requiring concentrated preparations (e.g. cytocentrifugation) in addition to direct smears for cytologic evaluation. Hemocytes are involved in host immune defense, similar to vertebrate leukocytes, and also play a role in coagulation.[4] While hemocytometer and morphologic assessment of undiluted, non-anticoagulated hemolymph has been reported in some species,[9] hemolymph collection and evaluation often utilize processing methods to prevent clotting and osmotic changes, such as the use of endotoxin-free anticoagulant, isosmotic diluent, or use of preservatives (e.g. 10% formalin) to immediately fix the cells.[4] Whatever method is used should be familiar and consistent. Other parameters such as clotting times, refractive index, and fluid chemistry can also be assessed. Ancillary testing (e.g. cultures, electron microscopy, molecular testing) is more often utilized in research settings.

Cytologic assessment of hemolymph is focused on hemocyte quantification by manual hemocytometer counts, morphologic evaluation by slide review, and identification of infectious agents. Inconsistencies in published accounts of cell morphology and lack of understanding about cellular responses pose challenges in interpretation and clinical application of cytologic findings. However, comparative application of cytologic and scientific principles allows for rational interpretation in many cases and contributes to conscientious growth of the body of information on invertebrate hemolymph and other cytologic specimens.

Given the lack of reference intervals for hemocyte cytologic evaluation across taxa of invertebrates, it is recommended to evaluate hemolymph from sick in comparison to representative, apparently healthy individuals of the same species under similar conditions and using consistent sample collection, processing, and evaluation techniques.[4] Cellular composition (numbers and types) can change under seasonal, physiologic, environmental, and other influences. Changes in hemocyte proportions and mitotic hemocytes are reported in circulation during severe inflammatory disease and other causes of hematopoietic stimulation.[10,11] Table 64.1 provides an overview on hemocyte nomenclature across some common invertebrate taxa, and Figures 64.1–64.3 show examples of hemocytes in various species. With the diversity of species and cells, ancillary methods (e.g. special stains, electron microscopy) can be necessary to confirm specific cell identification. For diagnostic samples, utilization of a more simplified classification scheme to differentiate granular versus nongranular/agranular cells offers an alternative to capture shifts in cell patterns without risking cellular misidentification and confused interpretation.

Coelomic fluid sampling is also employed as a research tool and health monitoring system in coelomate and pseudocoelomate invertebrates. Sampling techniques, including anesthetic considerations and reported optimal preservatives for various species based on their environment, i.e. fresh versus saltwater in aquatic invertebrates, are described, with sea stars especially well represented.[3,19]

Cells within the body cavity fluid are generally termed coelomocytes (vs hemocytes in hemolymph), but nomenclature is highly variable between organisms (e.g. coelomocytes, pseudocoelomocytes, phagocytes, hemocytes, amoebocytes, elaeocytes, athrocytes, leucocytes) and based largely on sample type and cell morphology or function.[6] Coelomic cells are described as arising primarily from the coelomic lining.[6,20] Morphology varies between organisms, including round, ovoid, cuboidal, spindle-shaped, or stellate cells.[6] The predominant function of coelomocytes is phagocytosis and encapsulation of foreign agents. Coelomocytes of echinoderms (e.g. sea urchin and sea star) are among the most well studied and, in health, consist of predominantly phagocytes (reported approximately 70–95% of cell counts) with fewer other cells depending on invertebrate species (e.g. amoebocytes, hemocytes) (Figure 64.4).[6,19] Coelomocytes proliferate and accumulate with injury, such as after traumatic arm amputation in sea stars.[19]

Table 64.1 Brief summary of hemocytes found in selected invertebrates.[4,12–18,a]

Taxa	Reported cell types	Comments on morphology +/− function
Arachnids and insects	*Cells are variably reported and classified; organisms do not possess all types* • Prohemocyte • Plasmatocyte • Granulocyte (granular hemocyte) • Cyanocyte • Adipohemocyte • Lebridiocyte • Spherulocyte (spherule cell) • Oenocytoid • Coagulocyte (cystocyte) • Thrombocytoid *With only routine cytology (Wright's stained smears) and without ancillary techniques (e.g. special stains, electron microscopy), simple classification as* *granulocytes* *and* *agranulocytes* *(non-granulocytes) is an alternative and may be more appropriate depending on species and the known level of confidence*	• Prohemocyte: small, rounded cell with round nucleus, condensed chromatin, high N:C, scant cytoplasm • Plasmatocyte: pleomorphic (round, oval, spindle-shaped) cells with oval to indented nucleus; non-granulated or containing fine cytoplasmic granules or vacuoles; role in phagocytosis, encapsulation • Granulocyte: round to oval to pleomorphic cell containing dense round to rod-shaped eosinophilic or basophilic cytoplasmic granules; granules may be in varied stages and can obscure the nucleus; role in engulfment, coagulation *Less uniformly described/reported:* • Cyanocyte: large rounded cell, contains hemocyanin seen as crystalline form in cytoplasm; may be unique to spiders (not yet identified in other arachnids, e.g.scorpions, mites, ticks) • Adipohemocyte: contains globules/lipid inclusions • Lebridiocyte: contains a single large secretory vacuole • Spherulocyte: contains large cytoplasmic inclusions (spherules) • Oenocytoid: rare cell that is large with low N:C • Coagulocyte: may be degranulated granulocyte or plasmatocyte; role in hemolymph clotting • Thrombocytoid: described only in dipteran species, gives off cytoplasmic fragments
Bivalves and gastropods	• Agranulocyte/hyalinocyte (small and large) • Granulocyte (basophilic and eosinophilic)	• Agranulocyte: round with high N:C and thin rim of cytoplasm (lymphocyte-like) • Granulocyte: larger, rounded, oblong to pleomorphic with cytoplasmic granules
Cephalopods	• Large granulocyte • Small granulocyte	*Two morphological hemocyte types only recently recognized (previously only one described); whether the two morphologies could be developmental stages rather than different cell types is uncertain*[12] • Large granulocyte: larger cell with low N:C, indented to U-shaped nucleus, small basophilic cytoplasmic inclusions; more phagocytic activity than small granulocytes • Small granulocyte: smaller cell with high N:C and round to ovoid nucleus
Crustaceans	• Hyalinocyte (amebocyte) • Granular cell (large granule cell) • Semigranular cell (small granule cell)	*It is uncertain whether these represent different cell types or different stages of the same cell type* • Agranular hemocyte (hyalinocyte): smallest hemocyte, high N:C, variably few small cytoplasmic granules; reported functions in some species include coagulation, cuticle tanning, phagocytosis • Granular hemocyte (large granule hemocyte): largest hemocyte, prominent intracytoplasmic granules (>1 μm diameter size, filling cytoplasm), eccentric nucleus; reported functions in some species include phagocytosis • Semigranular cell (small granule hemocyte): fewer, variably sized intracytoplasmic granules (<1 μm diameter in size); reported functions in some species include coagulation, phagocytosis

[a] Reported cell classification and nomenclature schemes are inconsistent within and across taxa. When assessing diagnostic samples, review of literature for the specific species of interest is recommended.

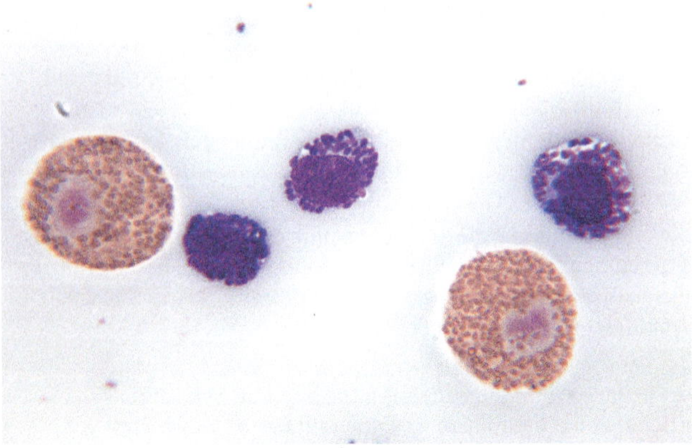

Figure 64.1 Hemolymph direct smear from an apparently healthy Emperor scorpion (*Pandinus imperator*) showing various granulocytes (Wright-Giemsa, 1000×).

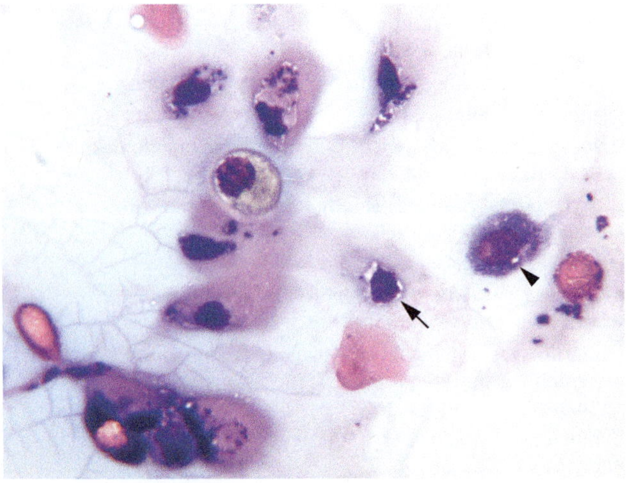

Figure 64.2 Hemolymph direct smears from an apparently healthy rose hair tarantula (*Grammostola rosea*) showing various granulocytes, presumed prohemocyte (arrow), and oenocytoid (arrowhead) (Wright-Giemsa, 500×).

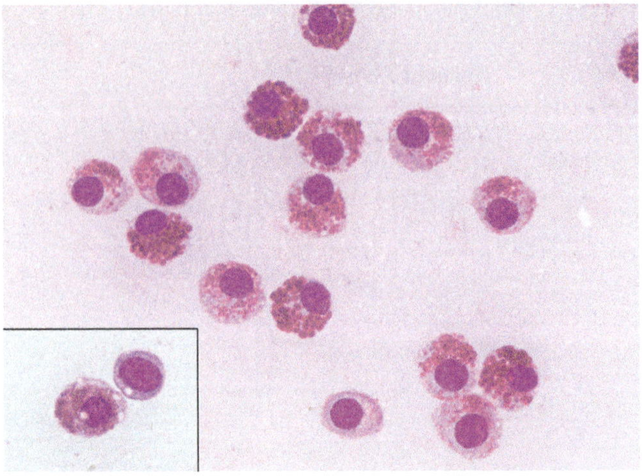

Figure 64.3 Hemolymph direct smear from a nautilus (*Nautilus pompilius*) with histologic evidence of granulocytic enteritis. The hemolymph cellularity is increased compared with healthy conspecifics and consists of approximately 90% granulocytic cells with rare agranulocytes (Inset, right cell) (Wright-Giemsa, 500×. *Source:* Image photographed by author from glass slide provided by Freeland Dunker and Drury Reavill).

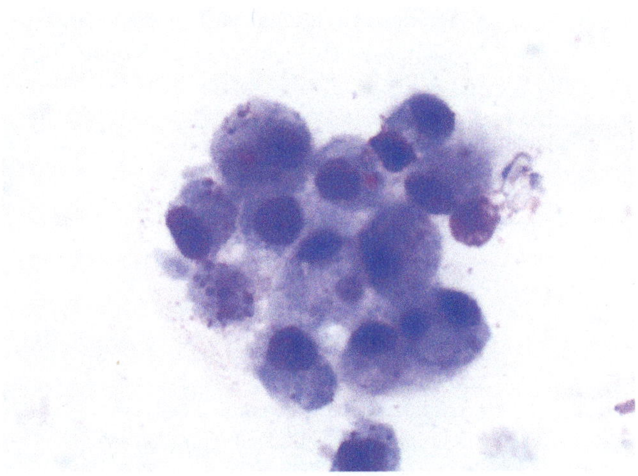

Figure 64.4 Coelomic fluid sediment smear in an apparently healthy purple sea star (*Pisaster ochraceus*) showing an aggregate of phagocytes (Wright-Giemsa, 1000×).

Solid Tissue Samples

Superficial samples such as clips and scrapes are collected and examined similar to vertebrates and include wet mounts in appropriate fluid media (Chapter 63 contains more information on wet mounts). A knowledge of normal anatomy and handling is critical as some invertebrates pose risk to human handlers (e.g. sting or bite). Likewise, diagnosticians unfamiliar with the species can cause inadvertent damage or death of the invertebrate (e.g. skin scrape of tarantulas leading to fatal rupture of the cuticle).[21] Internal lesion and organ samples can utilize needle biopsy, squash, or tissue imprints that are examined directly on wet-mount or as air-dried and stained preparations. As in other animals, the diagnostic value depends on appropriate sampling, sample handling, and skilled evaluation. Parameters for bacterial culture and other tests may need to be optimized to reflect host parameters. Cytology can yield identification of infectious agents, inflammation, and even neoplasia. Some infectious agents are discernable even when tissues are unfamiliar or poorly discerned due to disease or decay. Cytologic interpretation requires judicious consideration of correlated findings including clinical data, gross pathology, and other pertinent data.

Fecal direct smears can be collected as voluntary samples during handling, as observed samples in tank or enclosure (especially when fresh), or via cloacal swabs in species with cloaca. In aquatic species, various diatoms are a common incidental finding (Figure 64.5).

Infection and Inflammation

Infectious agents affecting invertebrates encompass the spectrum of microbes infecting terrestrial and aquatic vertebrates and cytologic features are largely comparable. Since some invertebrates carry commensal and symbiotic organisms (e.g. *Wolbachia* sp. bacteria in nematodes such as the canine heartworm, *Dirofilaria immitis*), knowledge of findings in health are key to understanding disease. The presence of true infection is supported cytologically by increased numbers of hemocytes or coelomocytes and/or phagocytized microorganisms.

Bacterial agents include those common in terrestrial and aquatic environments in other vertebrates (e.g. *Pseudomonas* sp., *Bacillus* sp., *Vibrio* sp., *Aeromonas* sp.) and others that may be unfamiliar to most veterinarians

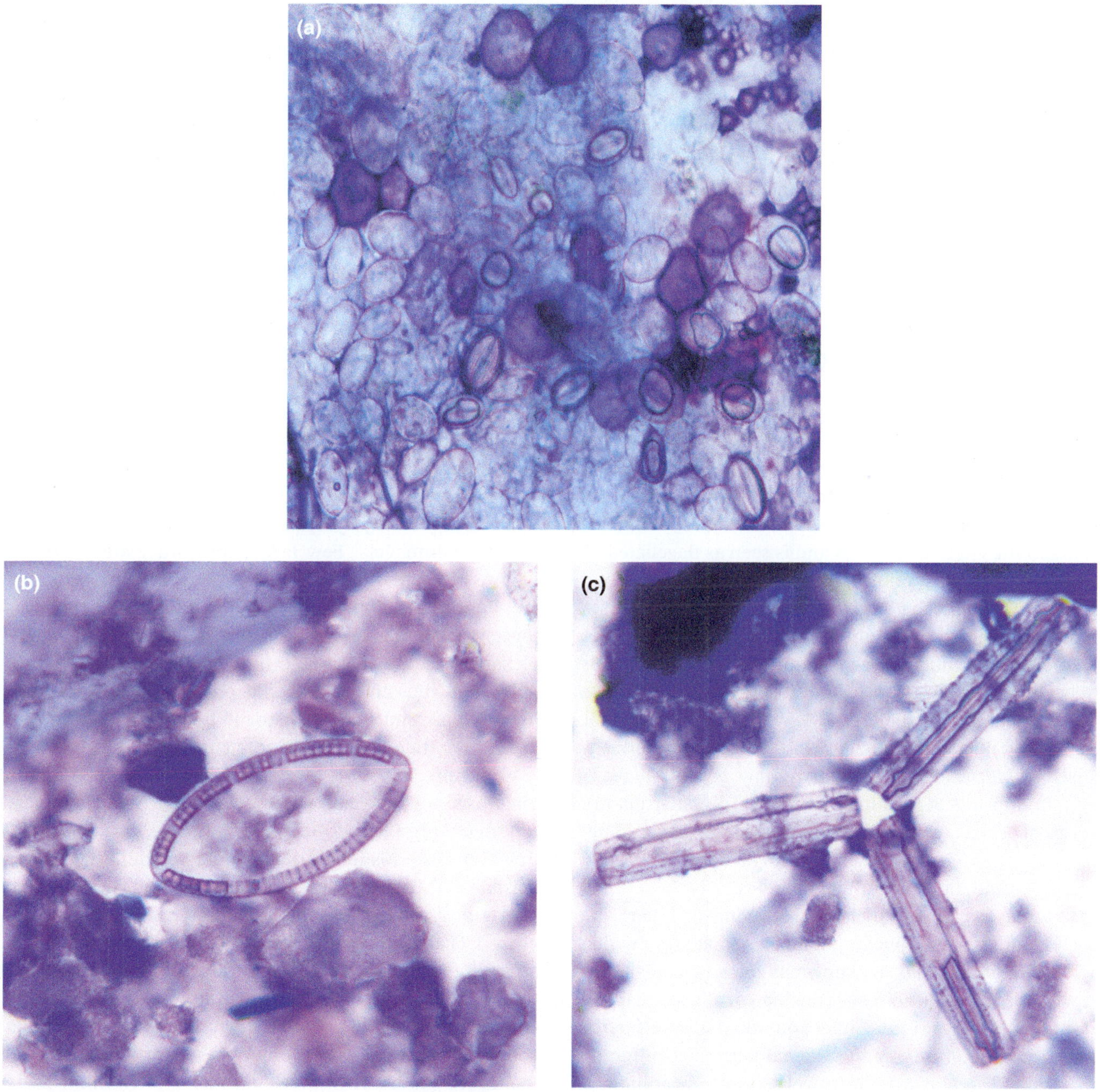

Figure 64.5 (a) Direct fecal smear from an apparently healthy long-spined sea urchin (*Diadema antillarum*) containing diatoms as an incidental finding. (b) and (c) Two commonly observed diatom morphologies (Diff-Quik, (a) 500×, (b) and (c) 1000×).

(e.g. *Beneckia chitinovora* causing "ulcerative shell disease" of hermit crabs, *Serratia marcescens* causing septicemia in larval insects).[22,23] Organisms with a chitinous exoskeleton are susceptible to shell disease caused by chitinolytic bacteria (e.g. "epizootic shell disease" of American lobsters).[22] From a perspective of comparative pathology, the cytologic presentation of bacterial infection (i.e. presence, quantity, and uniformity of bacteria, often with inflammation and phagocytized agents) is largely similar across species. With septicemia, bacteria can be seen in hemolymph preparations.

Other infectious agents include protozoa, myxozoa, metazoa, fungi, and viruses. Some parasites of invertebrates are asymptomatic intermediate stages of parasite life cycles that cause disease in vertebrate hosts. An example is *Myxobolus cerebralis*, for which tubifex worms are intermediate hosts, and infection of fish causes "whirling disease" (Chapter 63).

Infective protozoa of invertebrates include ciliates, coccidia, amoebae, trypanosomes, and others. Cytologic features are comparable to findings in other taxa. Pathogenicity must be assessed in conjunction with knowledge of normal flora, health status, and correlative findings. The following are a few examples of protozoal diseases of invertebrates. *Trichodina* sp. infections of oysters appear cytologically as saucer-shaped ciliates with an internal ring of denticles and cause gill erosions in heavy infections. The scuticociliate *Anophyroides haemophilia* causes "bumper-car disease" of lobsters, with organisms seen as ovoid to pyriform ciliates (approximately 25–40 µm) having internal vacuoles and surface cilia. The trypanosome, *Crithidia mellificae*, occurs in the gut of honeybees and is seen as flagellated or amastigote (rounded, nonflagellated) form (ranging from 5 to 30 µm). The amoeba, *Malpighamoeba mellificae*, causes amoebiasis within the Malpighian tubules of honeybees and presents as amoebic cysts (5–8 µm).[2,22,24–27] Marteiliosis (Aber disease, "digestive gland disease") is an Office International des Epizooties (OIE, World Organization for Animal Health) reportable disease of bivalve mollusks caused by *Marteilia* sp. (*Marteilia refringens*, *Marteilia sydneyi*). In imprints of the alimentary tract (digestive gland), protozoal primary cells and polynucleated sporangia (ranging from 5 to 40 µm) are seen; sporangia contain variably brightly eosinophilic or refringent bodies.[28,29]

Metazoan organisms include free-living and parasitic species and stages. Panagrolaimidae nematodes (which include *Halicephalobus* sp., known as zoonotic parasites of horses) are important disease-causing parasites in captive tarantulas leading to fatal infections of the mouthparts. White material (the mat of nematodes) is commonly observed at the oral region. In wet-mount preparation of this material or fluid from flushing the oral region, motile nematodes less than 2 mm long are seen.[21]

Microsporidia also are important parasites of various invertebrates such as insects. In honeybees, *Nosema* sp. infections (e.g. *Nosema apis*, *Nosema ceranae*, *Nosema bombi*) have been well studied. These microsporidia invade epithelial cells of the gut and can produce millions of spores. The role of *Nosema* sp. infections in bee losses is multifactorial in conjunction with environment, health, genetic, and other factors. Microsporidia can be identified on wet-mount squash preparations of body tissues (e.g. ventriculus, Malpighian tubules, fat) as immature to mature, oval spores (approximately 5–7 µm long) with a refractile wall and little visible internal content.[30,31]

Fungi include both opportunistic and primary pathogens. Depending on the agent, vegetative or reproductive stages can be observed cytologically with similar morphology as in other species, but culture is often needed for definitive diagnosis.

Mites of invertebrates include true parasites and commensals or saprophytes. Even the commensals in high numbers can cause disease. Some predatory mites are also sold commercially (e.g. *Stratiolaelaps scimitus*, formerly *Hypoaspis miles*) for control of pest invertebrates (e.g. thrips).

The dinoflagellate parasite, *Hematodinium* sp., is an important pathogen of crab species and causes high mortality infections of blue crab, Alaska tanner crab, Norway lobster, snow crab, and others. Organisms can be seen on wet-mount or air-dried stained smears of hemolymph or organ impressions as numerous nonmotile trophonts. The trophonts appear as uni- or multinucleated cells, approximately the size of hemocytes, with dense nuclei, and variably frothy cytoplasm. The organisms vastly outnumber hemocytes. Few larger multinucleated plasmodia are also present in some infections.[32,33] *Perkinsus* spp. are important dinoflagellate-like pathogens of bivalves (oysters, clams) and were previously classified as apicomplexans. Disease is variable but includes white cysts on gills, foot, digestive gland, and other tissues. Smears of hemolymph can show spherical bodies (approximately 2–15 µm) with a large eccentric vacuole (signet-ring).[27]

Viral infections of invertebrates are not commonly diagnosed cytologically. However, viral inclusions are reported within hemocytes and tissue cells in various viral infections, so histologic and cytologic identification is feasible.[4,27] One example of documented hemolymph alterations caused by viral infection is *Panulirus argus* virus 1 (PaV1) in the Caribbean spiny lobster, in which affected moribund lobsters had milky white and nonclotting hemolymph. The infected hyalinocytes and semigranulocytes were enlarged with hypertrophied nuclei that contained marginated chromatin and intranuclear viral inclusions in heavily infected cells. The findings were reported cytologically, but histology proved better for diagnosis. Granulocytes were not infected.[34]

Hyperplasia and Neoplasia

Proliferative lesions are less common and generally less well characterized in invertebrates compared with other species. Notable exceptions are neoplasms occurring in species under research such as fruit flies, cockroaches, and beetles, as well as neoplasms in species of economic importance, such as marine bivalve mollusks. Some invertebrates have greater rates of description of neoplasia (e.g. mollusks), while no or only rare cases have been reported in others (e.g. crustaceans, spiders, cephalopods).[35] The Registry of Tumors in Lower Animals (1966–2007) includes cases of benign and malignant lesions spanning the classic categories of epithelial, mesenchymal, and discrete cell lineages.[36] Cytologic features are described for only few naturally occurring neoplasms. In those described, criteria of malignancy are assessed similar to vertebrates, and definitive diagnosis often requires histopathology.

Disseminated neoplasia (hemic neoplasia, hemopoietic sarcoma, hemocytic leukemia) and gonadal neoplasia (germinoma) are the two most commonly identified tumors of invertebrates (occurring in multiple bivalves, shrimp, fruit flies, etc.). In disseminated neoplasia, neoplastic cells suspected to be hemocytes in origin circulate and infiltrate into body tissues. The cells are large (two to four times the diameter of a normal hemocyte) and anaplastic with high N:C ratio, round to pleomorphic nuclei, prominent nucleoli, and frequent mitoses.[35–38] Flow cytometry has been utilized to diagnose hemic neoplasia based on aneuploidy compared with hemocytes in health.[39] The gonadal neoplasms are classified into three histotypes (stroma, germ cell, and combination). The most common are germ cell origin (germinomas). These are characterized by proliferation of small undifferentiated basophilic cells with clumped chromatin and indistinct nucleoli. Neoplasms arise from the germinal epithelium of the gonadal follicles, progress to invade adjacent tissue, and can metastasize.[36,38] Causal factors are known for only few neoplastic entities, such as gene mutations linked to the disseminated (hemic) neoplasia of *Drosophila*. Other proposed contributing factors to neoplasms of invertebrates include environmental pollutants, biotoxins, viruses, and stress.[35]

Conclusion

Invertebrates are critical to the health of virtually every environment on the planet but are impacted by pathogens, stressors from human activities, interactions with environmental factors, and general misunderstanding of their value in global biodiversity. The cumulative load of these pressures threatens the conservation of many of these species. Although much is still to be learned about these diverse animals, cytology is a practical and potentially rewarding component of the diagnostic algorithm that should not be overlooked and deserves further study.

References

1 Work, T. and Meteyer, C. (2014). To understand coral disease, look at coral cells. *EcoHealth* 11: 610–618.

2 Evans, J.D. and Schwarz, R.S. (2011). Bees brought to their knees: microbes affecting honey bee health. *Trends Microbiol* 19: 614–620.

3 Lewbart, G. (2012). *Invertebrate Medicine*, 2e. Ames, IA: Wiley-Blackwell.

4 Van Wettere, A. and Lewbart, G.A. (2007). Cytologic diagnosis of diseases of invertebrates. *Vet Clin North Am Exot Anim Pract* 10: 235–254.

5 Pizzi, R. (2006). Spiders. In: *Invertebrate Medicine*, 2e (ed. G.A. Lewbart), 187–222. Ames, IA: Wiley-Blackwell.

6 Tahseen, Q. (2009). Coelomocytes: biology and possible immune functions in invertebrates with special remarks on nematodes. *Int J Zool* 2009: Article ID 218197.

7 Mullen, T., Russel, S., Tucker, M. et al. (2004). Paramoebiasis associated with mass mortality of American Lobster *Homarus americanus* in Long Island Sound, USA. *J Aquat Anim Health* 16: 29–38.

8 Dove, A.D.M., LoBue, C., Bowser, P., and Powell, M. (2004). Excretory calcinosis: a new fatal disease of wild American lobsters *Homarus americanus*. *Dis Aquat Org* 58: 215–221.

9 Barracco, M., Steil, A., and Gargioni, R. (1993). Morphological characterization of the hemocytes of the pulmonate snail *Biomphalaria tenagophila*. *Mem Inst Oswaldo Cruz* 88: 73–83.

10 Battison, A., Cawthorn, R., and Horney, B. (2003). Classification of *Homarus americanus* hemocytes and the use of differential hemocyte counts in lobsters infected with *Aerococcus viridans* var. homari (Gaffkemia). *J Invertebr Pathol* 84: 177–197.

11 Van De Braak, C.B.T., Botterblom, M.H.A., Liu, W. et al. (2002). The role of the haematopoietic tissue in haemocyte production and maturation in the black tiger shrimp (*Penaeus monodon*). *Fish Shellfish Immunol* 12: 253–272.

12 Castellanos-Martínez, S., Prado-Alvarez, M., Lobo-da-Cunha, A. et al. (2014). Morphologic, cytometric and

functional characterization of the common octopus (*Octopus vulgaris*) hemocytes. *Dev Comp Immunol* 44: 50–58.

13 Tame, A., Yoshida, T., Ohishi, K., and Maruyama, T. (2015). Phagocytic activities of hemocytes from the deep-sea symbiotic mussels *Bathymodiolus japonicus*, *B. platifrons*, and B. *septemdierum*. *Fish Shellfish Immunol* 45: 146–156.

14 Brehelin, M. and Zachary, D. (1986). Insect haemocytes: a new classification to rule out the controversy. In: *Immunity in Invertebrates* (ed. M. Brehélin), 36–48. Berlin: Springer-Verlag.

15 Kuhn-Nentwig, L., Kopp, L.S., Nentwig, W. et al. (2014). Functional differentiation of spider hemocytes by light and transmission electron microscopy, and MALDI-MS-imaging. *Dev Comp Immunol* 43: 59–67.

16 Ravindranath, M.H. (1974). The hemocytes of a scorpion *Palamnaeus swammerdami*. *J Morphol* 144: 1–9.

17 Soares, T., Cavalcanti, M.G., Ferreira, F.R.B. et al. (2013). Ultrastructural characterization of the hemocytes of *Lasiodora* sp. (Koch, 1850) (Araneae: Theraphosidae). *Micron* 48: 11–16.

18 Mahilini, H.M. and Rajendran, A. (2008). Categorization of hemocytes of three gastropod species *Trachea vittata* (Muller), *Pila globosa* (Swainson) and *Indoplanorbis exustus* (Dehays). *J Invertebr Pathol* 97: 20–26.

19 Pinsino, A., Thorndyke, M.C., and Matranga, V. (2007). Coelomocytes and post-traumatic response in the common sea star *Asterias rubens*. *Cell Stress Chaperones* 12: 331–341.

20 Bossche, J.P.V. and Jangoux, M. (1976). Epithelial origin of starfish coelomocytes. *Nature* 261: 227–228.

21 Pizzi, R. (2009). Parasites of tarantulas (Theraphosidae). *J Exotic Pet Med* 18: 283–288.

22 Klaphake, E. (2009). Bacterial and parasitic diseases of selected invertebrates. *Vet Clin North Am Exot Anim Pract* 12: 639–648.

23 Podgwaite, J.D. and Cosenza, B.J. (1976). A strain of *Serratia marcescens* pathogenic for larvae of *Lymantria dispar*: characterization. *J Invertebr Pathol* 27: 185–190.

24 Shimanuki, H. and Knox, D.A. (2000). *Diagnosis of Honey Bee Diseases*, Agriculture Handbook, vol. 690. Washington, DC: US Department of Agriculture.

25 Langridge, D. and McGhee, R.B. (1967). *Crithidia mellificae* n. sp. an acidophilic trypanosomatid of the honey bee *Apis mellifera*. *J Protozool* 14: 485–487.

26 Cawthorn, R.J., Lynn, D.H., Despres, B. et al. (1996). Description of *Anophryoides haemophila* n. sp. (Scuticociliatida: Orchitophryidae), a pathogen of American lobsters *Homarus americanus*. *Dis Aquat Org* 24: 143–148.

27 Bower, S.M., McGladdery, S.E., and Price, I.M. (1994). Synopsis of infectious diseases and parasites of commercially exploited shellfish. *Annu Rev Fish Dis* 4: 1–199.

28 Carella, F., Aceto, S., Maiolino, P., and De Vico, G. (2011). What is your diagnosis? Pale yellowish digestive gland and watery tissues in Mediterranean mussels. *Vet Clin Pathol* 40: 273–274.

29 Levine, J., Law, M., and Corsin, F. (2012). Bivalves. In: *Invertebrate Medicine*, 2e (ed. G.A. Lewbart), 127–152. Ames, IA: Wiley-Blackwell.

30 Fries, I. (2018). Nosemosis of honey bees. In: *Manual of Diagnostic Tests and Vaccines for Terrestrial Animals* (ed. OIE), 744–749. Paris: OIE.

31 Larsson, J.I.R. (2007). Cytological variation and pathogenicity of the bumble bee parasite *Nosema bombi* (Microspora, Nosematidae). *J Invertebr Pathol* 94: 1–11.

32 Noga, E., Hancock, A., and Bullis, R. (2012). Crustaceans. In: *Invertebrate Medicine*, 2e (ed. G.A. Lewbart), 235–254. Ames, IA: Wiley-Blackwell.

33 Bower, S. (2013). Synopsis of infectious diseases and parasites of commercially exploited shellfish: *Hematodinium* sp. (bitter crab disease). Fisheries and Oceans Canada. http://www.dfo-mpo.gc.ca/science/aah-saa/diseases-maladies/hematcb-eng.html (accessed 8 May 2018).

34 Shields, J.D. and Behringer, D.C. (2004). A new pathogenic virus in the Caribbean spiny lobster *Panulirus argus* from the Florida keys. *Dis Aquat Org* 59: 109–118.

35 Newton, A.L. and Lewbart, G.A. (2017). Invertebrate oncology: diseases, diagnostics, and treatment. *Vet Clin North Am Exot Anim Pract* 20: 1–19.

36 Peters, E., Smolowitz, R., and Reynolds, T. (2012). Neoplasia. In: *Invertebrate Medicine*, 2e (ed. G.A. Lewbart), 431–439. Ames, IA: Wiley-Blackwell.

37 Cooper, K.R., Brown, R.S., and Chang, P.W. (1982). Accuracy of blood cytological screening techniques for the diagnosis of a possible hematopoietic neoplasm in the bivalve mollusc, *Mya arenaria*. *J Invertebr Pathol* 39: 281–289.

38 Carballal, M.J., Barber, B.J., Iglesias, D., and Villalba, A. (2015). Neoplastic diseases of marine bivalves. *J Invertebr Pathol* 131: 83–106.

39 Vassilenko, E. and Baldwin, S.A. (2014). Using flow cytometry to detect haemic neoplasia in mussels (*Mytilus trossulus*) from the Pacific coast of Southern British Columbia, Canada. *J Invertebr Pathol* 117: 68–72.

65

Sheep and Goats

Emma Hooijberg, Thomas Jenei, and Leslie C. Sharkey

Introduction

Sheep and goats are versatile livestock that can produce meat, dairy, and fiber products. These animals are also popular as hobby farm or companion animals, and increasingly, goats have economic value in landscape management in urban and suburban areas. They adapt to a variety of environments, but husbandry decisions can be a factor in health and disease in these species. Individual animal and herd health issues are diverse, and use of a variety of diagnostic techniques is required for successful management.

Applications of Cytology and Collection Methods

The diagnostic application of cytology in sheep and goats is similar to other large animal livestock species. Solid tissue cytology of readily accessible lesions of superficial sites such as the skin, ears, and eyes is performed along with fluid analysis of respiratory and body cavity fluids. Evaluation of reproductive tissues is also described. Although veterinarians feel economic pressure to forego diagnostics in favor of empirical treatment, the value of cytological examination should not be underestimated due to the number of diseases transmissible to herdmates or humans.

Body Fluid Samples

Peritoneal fluid can be collected using a 1.5 in., 20 G needle in a standing animal. Two collection sites, which should be clipped and aseptically prepared, have been described: (i) the center of the inguinal area to the left or right of the udder or (ii) 5 cm on either side of the midline at 5 cm caudal to the xiphoid.[1,2] In the Author's experience, sampling to the right of the midline will decrease the risk of inadvertently performing a rumenocentesis. In addition, a teat cannula can be used to minimize the risk of penetrating the gastrointestinal tract.

Cerebrospinal fluid (CSF) is collected from animals in sternal recumbency from the lumbar site. After local lidocaine anesthesia, a 1 cm skin incision made between lumbar vertebrae 3 and 4 in goats and between the last lumbar vertebra and the sacrum in sheep.[3,4] Synovial fluid collection is of variable difficulty depending on the site, and sedation may be required. Site preparation is similar to other species.

Respiratory Washes

Two methods are described for the collection of bronchoalveolar lavage fluid (BALF). The first method can be performed in a standing animal. An area on the ventral neck about 5 cm distal to the larynx is aseptically prepared and infiltrated with lidocaine. A 21 G venous catheter is inserted into the trachea between two tracheal rings. The needle is removed and the stylet advanced until firmly in place. A size five French catheter is then advanced through the stylet down to the lungs until resistance is felt, after which 30 mL of physiological saline is instilled down the tube and re-aspirated after 5 seconds.[5] The second method involves the collection of BALF from a sedated sheep in sternal recumbency. A 30–40 cm long PVC tube with an internal diameter of 0.8 cm is passed into the trachea, and a 100 cm long, 0.25 cm diameter feeding tube is fed through the PVC tube until the end becomes lodged in a bronchus. Four 25 mL aliquots of physiological saline are instilled through the feeding tube and recovered. The sample material is placed into EDTA for cytological processing.[6] A 200-cell differential count is performed.

Veterinary Cytology, First Edition. Edited by Leslie C. Sharkey, M. Judith Radin, and Davis Seelig.

Solid Tissues

Sampling of cutaneous lesions, masses, and lymph nodes is similar to other species. Specific concerns will be outlined in each system.

Systems

Skin, Subcutis, and Ears

Ectoparasites

Ectoparasites identified using skin scrapes include biting and sucking lice (*Bovicola* spp. and *Linognathus* spp.) and mites (*Chorioptes bovis*, *Demodex* spp., *Psorobia* spp., *Psoroptes* spp., *Sarcoptes scabiei*).[7] A 2-month-old Lacaune ewe lamb presenting for alopecia, hypotrichosis, erythema, and crusting skin lesions underwent skin scraping that revealed particles of *S. scabiei* mites. Cytology of otic exudate revealed more dead mites, keratinocytes, and cocci; bilateral ear hematomas were also noted.[8]

Bacterial and Fungal Skin Disease

Dermatophilus congolensis causes exudative dermatitis and scabbing in many animal species, including sheep and goats. Bacteria are visualized as branching filaments consisting of cocci arranged in parallel rows on Giemsa-stained smears (Chapters 3 and 11). Smears are prepared directly from the underside of crusts or from scabs crushed with water.[9–11] *Staphylococcus* spp. causes crusting and scaling, folliculitis, and/or furunculosis in goats and sheep. Staphylococcal skin infections are often secondary to other skin diseases in goats, like *Malassezia*, parapox, mange, or nutritional deficiencies. Cytological samples made from exudate or pustules reveal neutrophilic inflammation and the presence of intracellular cocci. Culture is necessary for a definitive diagnosis.[12]

Malassezia spp. are an uncommon cause of dermatitis in goats. The organism appears as a round, oval, or boot-shaped yeast using sticky-tape samples (Chapters 3, 11, and 17). The underlying histopathological lesion is a seborrheic dermatitis that is sometimes accompanied by hyperkeratosis.[13,14] *Cryptococcus gattii* was diagnosed by cytology (no further description provided) and culture from a dairy goat with a postsurgical abdominal wound infection.[15]

Neoplasia

Squamous cell carcinoma (SCC) is a common skin tumor in sheep and goats.[16] SCCs occur as enzootic outbreaks in sheep and goats in arid or hot areas, probably due to a combination of high ultraviolet light exposure and the presence of poorly pigmented skin (as with tail docking, for example).[17,18] Papillomavirus also might play a role. Common sites in both species are the ears, perianal area, vulva, muzzle, and eyelids.[17,18] SCC lesions are characterized by erythema, ulcerated nodules, and hyperkeratosis.[17] Cytologic features are sparsely reported in sheep and goats, with one goat in a case series having a pedunculated ulcerated lesion dorsal to the rectum. Skin scrapings contained sheets of vacuolated epithelial cells characterized by anisokaryosis and bacteria.[18] Otherwise, cytologic features should be similar to other species (Chapters 12 and 21). Lymphoid metastasis of SCC can be identified cytologically.[18]

Although uncommon, malignant melanoma has been reported in goats in sites such as the horn base, coronary band, and perineal region.[19–21] Metastasis to regional lymph nodes is common.[21] Although cytology is not reported, polygonal or spindle-shaped cells with varying amounts of melanin pigment and frequent mitoses are seen on histopathology.[21] Other skin-associated tumors that have been reported in sheep and goats, albeit without cytological descriptions, include lymphoma, cutaneous histiocytoma, mast cell tumor, hemangioma, hemangiosarcoma, fibroma, fibrosarcoma, lipoma, papilloma, sebaceous gland tumor, and apocrine sweat gland tumor.[16,19,22,23]

Eye

Eye diseases including infectious keratoconjunctivitis, foreign bodies, and trauma can affect small ruminants. Pain can reduce weight gain and have economic impact on herds. Infectious keratoconjunctivitis can be related to *Chlamydia* spp. infection, which can be transmitted between sheep and goats. *Mycoplasma* spp. is another implicated agent that can cause disease in combination with other bacteria such as *Escherichia coli* and *Staphylococcus aureus* in goats.[24]

The most common microflora of sheep include *Bacillus*, *Enterococcus*, *Corynebacterium*, *Staphylococcus* spp., *E. coli*, and *Alcaligenes faecalis*.[25] *Mycoplasma conjunctivae* has been identified in normal conjunctival samples.[26] Fungi, including *Mucor*, *Aspergillus*, and *Penicillium* spp. have also been cultured from healthy ovine conjunctivae.[25] Smears made from scrapes of the palpebral conjunctivae in healthy sheep contained epithelial cells from both deep and superficial layers, low numbers of goblet cells, and occasional lymphocytes. Melanin pigment can occur in epithelial cells. Scrapes from sheep with keratoconjunctivitis caused by *M. conjunctivae* had an increased number of goblet cells, high numbers of neutrophils, and variable numbers of plasma cells. Mycoplasms were visualized as clumps of bilobed or triangular structures, often attached to epithelial cells.[26]

Cytocentrifuge preparations, prepared from fixative fluid in which conjunctival cytobrushes have been placed, are useful for diagnosing keratoconjunctivitis in goats.[27] The normal flora of goat conjunctiva has been described and includes *Staphylococcus* spp., *Streptococcus* spp., *Moraxella bovis*, and *Mycoplasma* spp.[24] Samples from caprine eyes with keratoconjunctivitis had a mixed population of variably dysplastic epithelial cells, which included basal cells, goblet cells, columnar cells, and non-keratinizing squamous epithelial cells. An inflammatory cell component was also present, dominated by neutrophils, with lower numbers of macrophages and lymphocytes. Bacteria can present intracellularly or extracellularly, and common pathogens include *S. aureus, Pseudomonas aeruginosa,* and *E. coli.*[27]

The cytology of ocular neoplasia in sheep and goats is not well described, although periocular tissues are predisposed to SCC in sheep, and ocular involvement of multicentric lymphoma in a ewe was described.[16,28]

Musculoskeletal

Reports detailing cytological findings in normal ovine or caprine joint fluid appear rarely in the primary literature, although fluids are expected to be of low nucleated cellularity and viscous as in other species. Sheep with chronic septic arthritis do not show distention of affected joints, and attempts to collect synovial fluid are usually not successful.[4,29] A goat kid with polyarthritis caused by *Mycoplasma mycoides* subspecies *mycoides* had carpal synovial fluid with a total nucleated cell count (TNCC) of 12 000/μL and total protein (TP) of 50 g/L. Neutrophils predominated (85%) with 11% large mononuclear cells and 4% lymphocytes. Small basophilic ring-shaped or linear *Mycoplasma* organisms were seen in the background.[30]

Respiratory

A variety of respiratory diseases occur in small ruminants in both the upper and lower respiratory tract. A thorough clinical examination of an animal will often help to localize the cause of the respiratory signs, but due to the varied causes, a definitive diagnosis often is elusive without clinicopathological testing. Pneumonia is a relatively common cause of lower airway disease, and etiologies include bacterial, mycoplasmal, parasitic, and fungal organisms. With the aid of appropriate diagnostics, targeted rather than empirical, therapy can be instituted. When respiratory disease is encountered, housing of the small ruminant should be assessed for contributing factors such as poor ventilation or overcrowding.

Bronchoalveolar Lavage

BALF from healthy sheep contains mostly alveolar macrophages. BAL fluid collected postmortem from healthy ovine lungs contained 52–92% macrophages, 1–16% lymphocytes, 0–21% neutrophils, 0–19% eosinophils, and 0–3% mast cells.[31] Mean percentage cell counts (± standard deviation) described for BALF in living sheep were 84 ± 5% macrophages, 10 ± 3% lymphocytes, 7 ± 2% neutrophils, and 1 ± 1% eosinophils.[6] Postmortem caprine BALF samples from healthy goats have a primarily mononuclear composition as well, with approximately 5% neutrophils in one study.[32]

A mild increase in lymphocytes occurs in maedi-visna virus infections, with an increase above 13.5% correctly predicting maedi-visna infection in 91% of cases and a value below 13.5% correctly predicting healthy sheep in 90% of cases.[6,31] However, this study did not include sheep with other lung diseases.[6] Neutrophils can increase up to 49% in pulmonary adenomatosis.[31] An increase in eosinophils of up to 50% and mast cells of up to 7% is a good indicator for parasitic lung infections (e.g. *Muellerius capillaris*), but these changes are not consistently seen.[31]

A large Nigerian study of postmortem BALF findings in goats with various types of pneumonia revealed increased numbers of neutrophils, macrophages, lymphocytes, and eosinophils, typically with increased neutrophil to macrophage ratios compared with goats that did not have pneumonia.[32] Various infectious agents such as bacteria, fungi, and larval helminths were observed in washings.

Although the neoplastic lesions of pulmonary adenomatosis are present in the alveoli and bronchi, descriptions of the frequency and appearance of tumor cells in ovine BALF fluid do not appear to exist in the English-language published literature. Sediment smears made of the fluid nasal discharge can contain clusters or spheres of rounded, swollen respiratory epithelial cells, with occasional regular mitoses, and high numbers of neutrophils.[33] The use of polymerase chain reaction assays for detection of Jaagsiekte sheep retrovirus (the causative agent of pulmonary adenomatosis) in ovine BALF samples has a reported sensitivity of 89% and specificity of 93% and may be useful for the detection of infected animals not yet showing clinical signs.[34]

Enzootic Nasal Adenocarcinoma

These tumors are unilateral or bilateral, originating from the ethmoid turbinates, and are caused by a betaretrovirus, enzootic nasal tumor virus-1 (ENTV-1) in sheep and ENTV-2 in goats.[35] Fine-needle aspirates (FNA) of these tumors contain numerous round, cuboidal, or polygonal epithelial cells arranged in clusters. Cells have a moderate to high nuclear to cytoplasmic ratio (N:C), with medium blue cytoplasm and a central round nucleus with a coarse chromatin pattern and one to two nucleoli. Binucleation may be present.[35,36] This cytological appearance is not specific to the enzootic nasal adenocarcinoma and could be characteristic of hyperplasia or other nasal epithelial tumors.

Lymphatic

The Gram-positive bacterium *Corynebacterium pseudotuberculosis* is the causative agent of caseous lymphadenitis and causes lymphadenomegaly and abscessation of both superficial and visceral lymph nodes in sheep and goats. Histology findings include pyogranulomatous inflammation, which presumably would be observed cytologically as mixed inflammation with pleomorphic bacteria with coccoid to filamentous forms within macrophages.[37,38] Definitive diagnosis requires culture and isolation of the organism, as other bacteria like *S. aureus* and *Actinomyces pyogenes* can also cause a septic pyogranulomatous lymphadenitis.[37]

Lymphoma is one of the most common neoplasms in goats, typically with a multicentric presentation.[19] Both large and small cell subtypes have been reported. A recent histopathologic study found that 11 out of 15 goats with lymphoma had T-cell neoplasms, often with involvement of the thoracic cavity or cervical area.[39] Cytological reports of caprine lymphoma are rare. One case involving a multicentric large B-cell lymphoma described a monomorphic population of large lymphoid cells with a high N:C, which is consistent with that found in other species.[40]

Gastrointestinal

Rumen Fluid

Like other ruminants, sheep and goats are at risk for rumen dysbiosis due to disruption of the normal bacterial and protozoal populations of their rumen.[41–43] An orogastric tube can be passed to collect a sample of rumen fluid from these species. Alternatively, direct percutaneous rumenocentesis has been described in cows (Chapter 58) and likely could be adapted to sheep and goats to avoid contamination of the sample with saliva, which could alter the pH and bicarbonate levels.[44]

Peritoneal Fluid Cytology

The volume of peritoneal fluid collected for analysis in healthy sheep is around 2 mL of pale yellow and clear fluid. TNCC ranges from 0.2 to 3.9×10^9/L with a cell population generally dominated by macrophages (3–93%) and lymphocytes (0–86%) with low proportions of neutrophils (0–16%) and eosinophils (0–7%).[1] TP ranges from 5 to 32 g/L.[1] TP in normal peritoneal fluid from goats should be less than 27 g/L and TNCC less than 0.4×10^9/L with a majority of lymphocytes and/or macrophages (0–62%) and up to 32% neutrophils.[2,45,46] Increases in TNCC of up to 1.2×10^9/L and TP of 37 g/L can occur in goats after rumenotomy, exploratory laparotomy, and enterectomy.[2,45,46] Neutrophils can increase up to 84% after uncomplicated abdominal surgery.[2,46]

Peritoneal effusions can occur associated with underlying neoplasia. Examples of such tumors include gastric carcinoma, intestinal adenocarcinoma, ovarian adenocarcinoma, and mesothelioma.[47–51] When reported, fluid characteristics are that of a transudate, with low cellularity (TNCC 0.2–0.6×10^9/L) and TP of 20–36 g/L.[47,49,51] Neoplastic cells were either not seen or not reported in these cases. The mechanism of fluid formation is thought to be due to the presence of neoplastic emboli in the lymphatics.[49]

Central Nervous System

The most common cytologic tool for evaluation of the central nervous system (CNS) in sheep and goats is assessment of CSF. Many of the underlying diseases manifesting as central depression are infectious. However, it can be difficult to clinically differentiate infectious diseases and conditions such as polioencephalomalacia without the use of CSF analysis.

Normal CSF Cytology

Normal caprine CSF is clear and colorless, with TNCC of 2–5/μL with the cell population consisting mostly of small lymphocytes.[3] Protein concentration is less than 14 mg/dL.[3] Normal ovine CSF has TNCC of <10/μL, also with lymphocytes predominating, and protein concentration of <40 mg/dL.[4]

CSF in Disease

A mild to marked neutrophilic pleocytosis (TNCC 13–1300/μL) and protein concentrations ranging from normal to markedly elevated (20–250 mg/dL) are reported in sheep with brain abscesses.[52,53] Bacterial meningoencephalitis in lambs and listeriosis in adult sheep can cause a marked neutrophilic pleocytosis (TNCC > 120/μL) with protein concentration >100 mg/dL.[52–55] Bacteria can be visualized microscopically in the CSF in cases of neonatal meningoencephalitis.[56]

Eosinophilic pleocytosis can indicate parasitic CNS disease, but this finding is not consistent.[52] CSF from a goat with cerebrospinal nematodiasis caused by *Parelaphostrongylus tenuis* had a TNCC of 33 000/μL, with 17% eosinophils.[57] Eosinophils (ranging from 0.5 to 29.9%) were found in the CSF of 16/24 sheep with chronic coenurosis, caused by *Coenurus cerebralis*, the larval stage of *Taenia multiceps*.[58] Concurrent changes included a mixed mononuclear or lymphocytic pleocytosis (18/24) and/or increased TP (7/24). Four animals had normal CSF.[58] The absence of CSF eosinophilia does not exclude the presence of coenurosis.

Sarcocystis ovicanis is the causative agent of ovine protozoal myeloencephalitis, causing non-suppurative encephalomyelitis.[59] Two of the sheep with coenurosis from the study mentioned above were also found to have *S. ovicanis* in their CSF samples; the significance of this organism in these cases was unclear.[60] One of these sheep had a mild mononuclear pleocytosis (TNCC 33/μL) and the other a mild increase in TP (58 mg/dL); these changes were thought to be due to the coenurosis rather than the *Sarcocystis*.[60] *Sarcocystis capricanis*, which cycles through goats, has been identified in the CSF of two sheep with neurological signs.[61] One of these animals had a mixed cell pleocytosis and the other a predominance of foamy macrophages (TNCC not reported).[61] The organisms were oval, slightly curved, 4–7 μm in width and 12–17 μm in length, with a granular blue cytoplasm containing a clear area toward one pole and a pink-staining structure close to the other pole.[61]

A severe mixed cell pleocytosis was found in a goat with *Cryptococcus neoformans* meningitis, but no organisms were identified in the CSF.[62] In summary, a mixed or mononuclear cell pleocytosis can indicate infection with *C. cerebralis* or *Sarcocystis* spp. in sheep and *Cryptococcus* in goats. Increased CSF protein with normal TNCC has been reported in sheep with neurological lentivirus infection (maedi-visna), where protein can range from 20 to 190 mg/dL.[52] In a sheep with neurological signs localized to one of the limbs, an increase in CSF protein (range 55–692 mg/dL) without pleocytosis indicates a spinal lesion such as localized spinal cord swelling, neoplasia, or vertebral or epidural abscessation.[53,54,56,63] There are no significant changes in ovine CSF with metabolic diseases, scrapie and polioencephalomalacia, which may aid discrimination of these diseases from other CNS infections.[52,53]

Choroid Plexus Cytology

Wright-Giemsa-stained impression smears of the choroid plexus from a healthy sheep revealed the presence of choroid plexus epithelial cells with two distinct morphologies. One cell type was round to polygonal, 15–20 μm in diameter, with a granular, dark blue cytoplasm and a small round nucleus. The second type was larger (17–25 μm), with a pale gray or pink cytoplasm containing a slightly larger nucleus with fine chromatin and a small visible nucleolus. Whether these two cell types represent a mature and immature population of a single type or two functionally different cell lines was not determined.[64]

Urinary Tract

While it may be possible to identify urinary tract infection, inflammation, or, rarely, neoplasia by examination of urine sediment sample, collection can be challenging. Although a voided sample is most readily obtained, a "free catch" specimen is at risk for contamination leading to a misdiagnosis. The smaller size of sheep and goats can make catheterization of the females difficult compared with cows. In the case of bucks and rams, catheterization is generally impossible due to the urethral recess, although limited success has been reported with angiographic catheters.[65] Cystocentesis can be considered when a sterile sample is required although due to the size of the animals ultrasonographic guidance may be required.

Reproductive

Breeding soundness examination in production animals can include cytology. Assessment of the reproductive tract would utilize similar methodology as in other farm species. Due to the smaller size of these patients, palpation per rectum is typically not appropriate, although transrectal ultrasound is valuable in the assessment of reproductive concerns of breeding females.

Vaginal Cytology

Exfoliative vaginal cytology findings during various phases of the estrus cycle in sheep and goats can be summarized as follows[66–69]:

Anestrus: Low numbers of parabasal cells, very high numbers of intermediate cells, very low numbers of superficial cells.

Proestrus: Moderate numbers of parabasal, intermediate, and superficial cells, low numbers of keratinized squames, very low numbers of neutrophils.

Estrus: No parabasal cells, very few intermediate cells, very high numbers of superficial cells, moderate numbers of keratinized squames, very low numbers of neutrophils.

Metestrus: Very low numbers of parabasal cells, few intermediate cells, moderate numbers of superficial cells, moderate to high numbers of keratinized squames, moderate to high numbers of neutrophils, many bacteria.

Diestrus: Very low numbers of parabasal cells, very few intermediate cells, low numbers of superficial cells, high numbers of keratinized squames, high numbers of neutrophils, many bacteria.

Testicle

Transscrotal ultrasonography combined with FNA of the testicle has been shown to provide useful information about breeding soundness in rams.[70] FNA is performed using a 21 G butterfly needle connected to a 20 mL syringe. The needle is placed into a stabilized testicle and redirected several times while aspirating. A 200-cell count is performed on the resulting smears and encompasses identification and enumeration of spermatogonia, primary and secondary spermatocytes, early and later spermatids, spermatozoa, and Sertoli cells. The spermatic index, defined as the percentage of spermatozoa of all spermatogenic cells (spermatogonia, spermatocytes, and spermatids), was found to correlate positively with semen quality.[70] Social stress can cause leukocytospermia and increased sperm anomalies.[71]

Conclusion

Due to a multitude of diseases manifesting with similar clinical presentations, a multimodal diagnostic approach is necessary in the small ruminant. Unfortunately, for some of these conditions, there remains limited clinicopathological data from goats or sheep for comparison. However, their similarity in many respects to larger ruminants such as cows should aid in the interpretation of cytology and fluid samples.

References

1. Al-Rukibat, R.K., Ismail, Z.B., Al-Majali, A.M., and Al-Zghoul, M.B. (2006). Peritoneal fluid analysis in adult, nonpregnant Awassi sheep. *Vet Clin Pathol* 35: 215–218.
2. Nazifi, S., Dehghani, S., and Barzegar, M.R. (2000). Evaluation of cellular and biochemical parameters of blood and peritoneal fluid following enterectomy in the goat. *Small Rumin Res* 37: 65–71.
3. Mozaffari, A.A., Shahriarzadeh, M.H., and Ja'fari, H. (2011). Analysis of serum and cerebrospinal fluid in clinically normal adult Iranian Cashmere (Rayeni) goats. *Comp Clin Pathol* 20: 85–88.
4. Scott, P.R. (2013). Analysis of samples of cerebrospinal fluid, thoracic ultrasonography and arthrocentesis/radiography of joints as ancillary aids to clinical diagnosis and treatment in small ruminant practice. *Small Rumin Res* 110: 82–87.
5. Sheehan, M., Markey, B., Cassidy, J. et al. (2005). New transtracheal bronchoalveolar lavage technique for the diagnosis of respiratory disease in sheep. *Vet Rec* 157: 309.
6. Katsoulos, P.D., Christodoulopoulos, G., Kontopidis, G. et al. (2009). Leukocyte counts in bronchoalveolar lavage fluid obtained from normal and Maedi-Visna-infected sheep. *Vet Clin Pathol* 38: 397–402.
7. Cortinas, R. and Jones, C.J. (2006). Ectoparasites of cattle and small ruminants. *Vet Clin North Am Food Anim Pract* 22: 673–693.
8. Tsioli, V., Farmaki, R., Papastefanou, A. et al. (2013). A case of bilateral auricular haematoma in a ewe-lamb with sarcoptic mange. *Small Rumin Res* 110: 145–149.
9. Chitra, M.A., Jayalakshmi, K., Ponnusamy, P. et al. (2017). *Dermatophilus congolensis* infection in sheep and goats in Delta region of Tamil Nadu. *Vet World* 10: 1314–1318.
10. Yeruham, I., Elad, D., and Perl, S. (2003). Dermatophilosis in goats in the Judean foothills. *Rev Med Vet Toulouse* 154: 785–788.
11. Awad, W.S., Nadra-Elwgoud, M.I., and El-Sayed, A.A. (2008). Diagnosis and treatment of bovine, ovine and equine dermatophilosis. *J Appl Sci Res* 4: 367–374.
12. Foster, A.P. (2012). Staphylococcal skin disease in livestock. *Vet Dermatol* 23: 342–363.
13. Pin, D. (2004). Seborrhoeic dermatitis in a goat due to *Malassezia pachydermatis*. *Vet Dermatol* 15: 53–56.
14. Eguchi-Coe, Y., Valentine, B.A., Gorman, E., and Villarroel, A. (2011). Putative *Malassezia dermatitis* in six goats. *Vet Dermatol* 22: 497–501.
15. Villarroel, A. and Maggiulli, T.R. (2012). Rare *Cryptococus gattii* infection in an immunocompetent dairy goat following a cesarean section. *Med Mycol Case Reports* 1: 91–94.
16. Ahmed, A.F. and Hassanein, K.M.A. (2012). Ovine and caprine cutaneous and ocular neoplasms. *Small Rumin Res* 106: 189–200.
17. Mendez, A., Perez, J., Ruiz-Villamor, E. et al. (1997). Clinicopathological study of an outbreak of squamous cell carcinoma in sheep. *Vet Rec* 141: 597–600.
18. Gibbons, P.M., Lamb, L., and Mansell, J. (2015). Presentation, treatment, and outcome of squamous cell carcinoma in the perineal region of 9 goats. *Can Vet J* 56: 1043–1047.
19. Lohr, C.V. (2013). One hundred two tumors in 100 goats (1987–2011). *Vet Pathol* 50: 668–675.
20. Mavangira, V., Hughes, J.M., Middleton, J.R. et al. (2008). Malignant melanoma of the horn base in a Pygora goat. *J Vet Diagn Invest* 20: 104–107.

21 Ramadan, R.O., el Hassan, A.M., and Taj el Deen, M.H. (1988). Malignant melanoma in goats: a clinico-pathological study. *J Comp Pathol* 98: 237–246.

22 Scott, P.R., Rhind, S., and Dun, K. (1997). Cutaneous lymphoma in a Scottish blackface ram. *Vet Rec* 141: 473–474.

23 Cordes, D.O. and Shortridge, E.H. (1971). Neoplasms of sheep: a survey of 256 cases recorded at Ruakura animal health laboratory. *N Z Vet J* 19: 55–64.

24 Meekins, J.M., Apley, M.D., Lubbers, B. et al. (2017). Evaluation of conjunctival bacterial flora in a herd of goats in the Midwestern United States. *Vet Ophthalmol* 20: 40–45.

25 Bonelli, F., Barsotti, G., Attili, A.R. et al. (2014). Conjunctival bacterial and fungal flora in clinically normal sheep. *Vet Rec Open* 1: e000017.

26 Dagnall, G.J. (1994). Use of exfoliative cytology in the diagnosis of ovine keratoconjunctivitis. *Vet Rec* 135: 127–130.

27 Cakir, L., Gümüşsoy, K.S., Kutsal, O., and Tunç, A.S. (2014). Evaluation of brush cytology (cytospin technique) and cultural results in the diagnosis of keratoconjunctivitis in a goat herd. *Ankara Üniv Vet Fak Derg* 61: 35–41.

28 Rushton, J.O., Thaller, D., and Krametter-Froetscher, R. (2017). Ocular involvement of multicentric malignant B-cell lymphoma in a ewe. A case report. *Tierarztl Prax G N* 45: 182–186.

29 Scott, P.R. and Sargison, N.D. (2012). Diagnosis and treatment of joint infections in 39 adult sheep. *Small Rumin Res* 106: 16–20.

30 Alleman, A.R., Henson, K.L., Polkes, A. et al. (1999). Synovial fluid from a kid with polyarthritis. *Vet Clin Pathol* 28: 64.

31 Dawson, S., Else, R.W., Rhind, S.M., and Collie, D.D. (2005). Diagnostic value of cytology of bronchoalveolar fluid for lung diseases of sheep. *Vet Rec* 157: 433–436.

32 Jarikre, T.A., Emikpe, B.O., Ohore, O.G. et al. (2016). Bronchoalveolar lavage fluid cellular and haematological changes in different types of caprine pneumonia. *Niger J Physiol Sci* 31: 31–36.

33 Nobel, T.A., Neumann, F., and Klopfer, U. (1970). Clinico-pathological investigations in sheep pulmonary adenomatosis (Jaagsiekte). I. Exfoliative cytology. *entralbl Veterinarmed B* 17: 958–962.

34 Voigt, K., Brugmann, M., Huber, K. et al. (2007). PCR examination of bronchoalveolar lavage samples is a useful tool in pre-clinical diagnosis of ovine pulmonary adenocarcinoma (Jaagsiekte). *Res Vet Sci* 83: 419–427.

35 Stowe, D.M., Anderson, K.L., Guy, J.S. et al. (2012). A case of enzootic nasal adenocarcinoma in a ewe. *Case Report Vet Med* 2012: 4.

36 Ajayi, O., Oyewusi, I.K., Olaniyi, M.O. et al. (2013). Enzootic nasal adenocarcinoma: cytological and clinicopathological observations in a West African dwarf goat. *Bull Anim Health Prod Afr* 61: 231–336.

37 de Sá Guimarães, A., do Carmo, F.B., Pauletti, R.B. et al. (2011). Caseous lymphadenitis: epidemiology, diagnosis, and control. *IIOAB J* 2: 33–43.

38 Ribeiro, M.G., Dias Junior, J.G., Barbosa, P.G. et al. (2001). Punção aspirativa com agulha fina no diagnóstico do *Corynebacterium pseudotuberculosis* na linfadenite caseosa caprina. *Arq Inst Biol* 68: 23–28.

39 Kiser, P.K. and Lohr, C.V. (2017). Lymphoma classification in goats. *Vet Pathol* 54: 611–619.

40 Versnaeyen, H., Kolkman, I., Van Aert, M. et al. (2016). Multicentric B-cell lymphoma in a pygmy goat. *Vlaams Diergeneeskundig Tijdschrift* 85: 291–295.

41 Dehority, B.A. and Grubb, J.A. (1977). Characterization of the predominant bacteria occurring in the rumen of goats (*Capra hircus*). *Appl Environ Microbiol* 33: 1030–1036.

42 Wang, L., Xu, Q., Kong, F. et al. (2016). Exploring the goat rumen microbiome from seven days to two years. *PLoS One* 11: e0154354.

43 Franzolin, R. and Dehority, B.A. (1996). Effect of prolonged high-concentrate feeding on ruminal protozoa concentrations. *J Anim Sci* 74: 2803–2809.

44 Duffield, T., Plaizier, J.C., Fairfield, A. et al. (2004). Comparison of techniques for measurement of rumen pH in lactating dairy cows. *J Dairy Sci* 87: 59–66.

45 Adamu, S.S., Egwu, G.O., and Malgwi, J.T. (1991). Biochemical changes in the peritoneal fluid following rumenotomy in goats. *Vet Res Commun* 15: 363–367.

46 Dehghani, S., Nazifi, S., and Barzegar, M.R. (2000). Evaluation of cellular and biochemical parameters of blood and peritoneal fluid following exploratory laparotomy in the goat. *J Vet Med A Physiol Pathol Clin Med* 47: 143–148.

47 Haibel, G.K. (1990). Intestinal adenocarcinoma in a goat. *J Am Vet Med Assoc* 196: 326–328.

48 Krametter, R., Bago, Z., Floeck, M. et al. (2004). Abdominal mesothelioma in a goat. *N Z Vet J* 52: 293–296.

49 Stern, A.W., Stewart, J.L., Chu, C., and Garrett, E. (2015). Signet-ring cell carcinoma in a goat. *Vet Q* 35: 111–115.

50 Perez, V., Corpa, J.M., and Garcia Marin, J.F. (1998). Adenocarcinoma of the small intestine in a goat. *J Comp Pathol* 119: 311–316.

51 Memon, M.A., Schelling, S.H., and Sherman, D.M. (1995). Mucinous adenocarcinoma of the ovary as a cause of ascites in a goat. *J Am Vet Med Assoc* 206: 362–364.

52 Scott, P.R. (2010). Cerebrospinal fluid collection and analysis in suspected sheep neurological disease. *Small Rumin Res* 92: 96–103.

53 Scott, P.R. (1992). Analysis of cerebrospinal fluid from field cases of some common ovine neurological diseases. *Br Vet J* 148: 15–22.

54 Scott, P. (1994). Cerebrospinal fluid analysis in the differential diagnosis of spinal cord lesions in ruminants. *In Pract* 16: 298–301.

55 Scott, P.R. (1993). A field study of ovine listerial meningo-encephalitis with particular reference to cerebrospinal fluid analysis as an aid to diagnosis and prognosis. *Br Vet J* 2: 165–170.

56 Scott, P.R. (1995). The collection and analysis of cerebrospinal fluid as an aid to diagnosis in ruminant neurological disease. *Br Vet J* 151: 603–614.

57 Kopcha, M., Marteniuk, J.V., Sills, R. et al. (1989). Cerebrospinal nematodiasis in a goat herd. *J Am Vet Med Assoc* 194: 1439–1442.

58 Zobba, R., Manunta, M.L., Evangelisti, M.A. et al. (2014). Cisternal cerebrospinal fluid analysis in 24 sheep with chronic coenurosis. *Vet Ital* 50: 57–63.

59 Caldow, G.L., Gidlow, J.R., and Schock, A. (2000). Clinical, pathological and epidemiological findings in three outbreaks of ovine protozoan myeloencephalitis. *Vet Rec* 146: 7–10.

60 Zobba, R., Alberti, A., Manunta, M.L. et al. (2014). What is your diagnosis? Cerebrospinal fluid from a sheep. *Vet Clin Pathol* 43: 467–468.

61 Formisano, P., Aldridge, B., Alony, Y. et al. (2013). Identification of *Sarcocystis capracanis* in cerebrospinal fluid from sheep with neurological disease. *Vet Parasitol* 193: 252–255.

62 Stilwell, G. and Pissarra, H. (2014). Cryptococcal meningitis in a goat: a case report. *BMC Vet Res* 10: 84–84.

63 Scott, P.R. and Will, R.G. (1991). A report of Froin's syndrome in five ovine thoracolumbar epidural abscess cases. *Br Vet J* 147: 582–584.

64 Garma-Aviña, A. (2004). Cytology of the normal and abnormal choroid plexi in selected domestic mammals, wildlife species, and man. *J Vet Diagn Invest* 16: 283–292.

65 Reppert, E.J., Streeter, R.N., Simpson, K.M., and Taylor, J.D. (2016). Retrograde catheterization of the urinary bladder in healthy male goats by use of angiographic catheters. *Am J Vet Res* 77: 1295–1299.

66 Zohara, F., Azizunnesa, A., Faruk, M. et al. (2014). Exfoliative vaginal cytology and serum progesterone during the estrous cycle of indigenous ewes in Bangladesh. *J Embryol Trans* 29: 183–188.

67 Ola, S.I., Sanni, W.A., and Egbunike, G. (2006). Exfoliative vaginal cytology during the oestrous cycle of West African dwarf goats. *Reprod Nutr Dev* 46: 87–95.

68 Pérez-Martínez, M., Mendoza, M.E., and Romano, M.C. (1999). Exfoliative vaginal cytology and plasma levels of estrone and estradiol-17beta in young and adult goats. *Small Rumin Res* 33: 153–158.

69 Sanger, V.L., Engle, P.H., and Bell, D.S. (1958). The vaginal cytology of the ewe during the estrous cycle. *Am J Vet Res* 19: 283–287.

70 Vencato, J., Romagnoli, S., and Stelletta, C. (2014). Trans-scrotal ultrasonography and testicular fine-needle aspiration cytology in the evaluation of ram sperm production. *Small Rumin Res* 120: 112–115.

71 Garrido-Fariña, G.I., Castillo-Hernández, G., Gutiérrez-Hernández, J.L. et al. (2016). Stress-induced leokocytospermia in rams with healthy reproductive tract. *Small Rumin Res* 137: 34–39.

Part XVI

Applications of Cytology in Industry

66

Cytological Evaluation in Biomedical Research and Toxicity Studies

Florence Poitout-Belissent, Michelle Cora, and Angela Wilcox

Introduction

Laboratory animal species, including rats, mice, dogs, and nonhuman primates (NHP) are often utilized in biomedical research and toxicity studies. These include basic and applied research studies, studies investigating substances as potential human health hazards, and studies conducted during drug development. Drug development requires compound efficacy and safety (preclinical or toxicity) studies. Efficacy studies evaluate the effects of candidate compounds on animal models, while preclinical studies evaluate the toxicity of compounds in laboratory animals before their utilization in clinical human studies and are regulated by government agencies. Cytological evaluation of biological samples can be a valuable endpoint for evaluation.

Agencies responsible for investigation of the safety and efficacy of health products – the US Food and Drug Administration (FDA), European Agency for Evaluation of Medicinal Products (EMEA), and Japan's Ministry of Health, Labor and Welfare (MHLW) – have published guidance documents for preclinical toxicology studies with recommendations for clinical pathology evaluation.[1–3] These documents contain similar information, largely based on a position paper from the Joint Scientific Committee for International Harmonization of Clinical Pathology,[4] although a more recent position report has been published by the American Society for Veterinary Clinical Pathology (ASVCP) Regulatory Affairs Committee.[5] While cytological endpoints are rarely mentioned in the guidance documents, regulatory agencies recommend a flexible approach depending on the species and the observed or expected effect of a substance, explicitly stating that additional testing and endpoints may be necessary to identify toxic effects attributable to test material.

In toxicological studies, evaluation of thoracic or peritoneal fluid is uncommon because these fluids rarely form during short-term studies. Fluid cytological evaluation is sometimes an important endpoint for certain biomedical and toxicity studies, often from lavages performed at the end of compound efficacy studies. Fluid cytological evaluation may be utilized in the following: (i) bronchoalveolar lavage fluid (BALF) evaluation in inhalation studies or asthma and chronic obstructive pulmonary disease (COPD) models, (ii) abdominal lavage fluid evaluation in peritoneal inflammation model studies, (iii) cerebrospinal fluid (CSF) evaluation to estimate direct compound effects on the central nervous system (CNS), and (iv) synovial fluid evaluation in studies involving joints.

Another type of toxicity study evaluates the effects of a compound on the mammalian reproductive system to identify potential risk to human fertility or embryo/fetal development. Such studies evaluate all stages of development from conception to sexual maturity and are known as developmental and reproductive toxicology (DART) studies. DART studies undertaken for drug development are regulated and are usually conducted in one species, most often the rat, but occasionally use NHP. Embryotoxicity studies require an additional mammalian species, usually rabbits.[6,7] Direct assessment of male and female reproductive systems may be added to chronic or subchronic general toxicity studies. Evaluation of vaginal cytology preparations assesses sexual maturity and longitudinal menstrual or estrous cyclicity. Sperm evaluation assesses compound effects on spermatogenesis and sperm maturation. Additionally, the results of sperm evaluation can be used to corroborate histopathological lesions related to defective spermatogenesis or to further characterize compound effects.[8] Vaginal cytology and sperm evaluations are also performed in pre-study screenings for confirmation of sexual maturity.[8]

The FDA Redbook[2] and Weingand et al.[4] both recommend that urinalysis includes measurements of urine volume, specific gravity, pH, glucose, and protein. Urine

Veterinary Cytology, First Edition. Edited by Leslie C. Sharkey, M. Judith Radin, and Davis Seelig.

sediment microscopy should be considered when the toxicology and pharmacology suggest urinary tract changes. Because of high potential for compounds to affect the renal system, urine sediment evaluation is commonly done. Collection of urine samples is easy in NHP, dogs, minipigs, rabbits and rats, but not in mice due to the limited amounts of urine produced.

Bone marrow cytological evaluation is not discussed in this chapter. Regulatory agencies do not always provide recommendations on bone marrow cytology, but a few agencies recommend preparation of bone marrow smears from each animal for subchronic toxicity studies with evaluation only being performed if effects on the hematopoietic system were noted during the bone marrow histological and hematological evaluations.[2] Best practices for bone marrow evaluation are included in a recent paper produced by the Bone Marrow Working Group of the ACVP/Society of Toxicologic Pathology (STP).[9]

Fluid Cytology

Bronchoalveolar Lavage Evaluation in Drug Efficacy and Inhalation Studies

Bronchoalveolar lavage (BAL) samples cells and fluid within the lower airways. The first surface encountered by inhaled materials is the epithelium of the respiratory tract, which is coated by a fluid that can be sampled via saline wash. BALF collected from animals acutely exposed to various test materials by inhalation or instillation can be used as a standard method to evaluate lung changes. BALF evaluation may detect early lung changes, which either precede or confirm histomorphological changes.

Early in development, compounds can be tested on rodents to screen for efficacy, and BALF evaluation assesses the efficacy of anti-inflammatory drugs in the resolution of induced lung changes. For such studies, neutrophilic inflammation is induced by intratracheal administration or inhalation of lipopolysaccharides, reproducing COPD.[10] Alternatively, animals are sensitized by intraperitoneal ovalbumin administration and then challenged by a second exposure to ovalbumin via aerosol administration, inducing pulmonary eosinophilia and replicating asthma.[11–13] In either approach, animals are subsequently treated with the test compound, and BALF is collected at 6, 24, 48, and/or 72 hours post-exposure.

Other studies evaluate the development of primary or secondary lung changes in animals directly exposed to a compound by inhalation.[14] In these types of studies, BALF evaluation aids in the detection of early lung effects.

Collection

Specimens should be collected using consistent and reproducible methods. Many pre-analytical variables – including age, sex, source of the animals, randomization, time of collection, anesthesia, diet, housing, sample handling, collection site, method of collection, means of restraint, and experience of handler and/or collector – should be considered prior to study start, with efforts made to minimize variation to ensure robust cytological data.

To collect a BALF sample in dogs and NHP, the animals undergo general anesthesia, and saline is instilled into a bronchus via a bronchoscope. The fluid is then aspirated and placed in the appropriate tube(s) (see section "Laboratory Methods"). In rodents, BALF is collected at necropsy, after suppression of the respiratory function of an anesthetized animal.[15] The trachea is then surgically exposed for catheterization and instillation of saline in the bronchus (approximately 3 mL in rats). Once the lung is adequately washed, the saline is aspirated and placed into the appropriate tube(s). This procedure can be repeated once or twice. Approximately 60% of the instilled fluid will be recovered. Large volumes can be collected with repeated lavages, even in rats. Some authors suggest gently massaging the lungs prior to removal of each lavage; however, this method is controversial as it will increase the number of macrophages and epithelial cells released into the fluid and potentially lead to increased variability between samples.

Laboratory Methods

Cell Counts

Standard BALF analysis includes enumeration of the total nucleated cell count (TNCC) and a differential cell count. The differential cell count is essential and considered a reliable parameter because the proportion of the different cell populations is independent of the volume of fluid collected. BALF TNCC should be interpreted with caution as the number of cells present depends on the amount of fluid collected. TNCC can still be informative if the collection method is consistent.

A common practice is to pool all fluids collected from a single animal into one tube, perform the TNCC and differential counts, centrifuge the remaining fluid, and then collect the supernatant for biochemical analysis.[5] Alternatively, the fluid collected from the first instillation can be reserved for biochemistry or cytokine analyses, as analytes tend to be more concentrated in the first wash. After a short low speed centrifugation (6 minutes at 700g), the supernatant is placed on ice or refrigerated and used for analysis of biochemical parameters and cytokines. The cell pellet can be washed and mixed with the other instillations for cell count evaluation. In these cases, the first wash should be collected in a plain tube without anticoagulant for biochemical and cytokine analysis, and subsequent washes collected in ethylenediaminetetraacetic acid (EDTA)-coated tubes for TNCC and differential counts. Cells are better individualized in EDTA (K2 or K3), although BALF cells collected into plain tubes rarely clump if lung massage is avoided.[5]

When small volumes of BALF are collected (<2 mL), for example, in mice, a direct measurement of TNCC is recommended. When large volumes of fluid are collected from one animal, concentration of the cells by centrifugation of the EDTA preserved fluid is advised. The supernatant is discarded, and cells are resuspended in a smaller volume of saline or a buffer (e.g. HEPES buffered medium). This method is useful when measuring TNCC using an automated analyzer because it elevates the cell count above the minimum threshold for detection. Initial cell concentrations can be calculated based on the concentration procedure. BALF collected under anesthesia often contains more mucus, which can be separated by washing. The fluid is centrifuged, the cell pellet is resuspended in saline and then centrifuged again; and the cell pellet is resuspended once more in a determined amount of saline.

Based on our experience, the stability of cells in BALF is approximately 3 hours at room temperature and 24 hours at 4 °C (refrigerated). The reference method or the most common procedure for measuring TNCC in body fluids is manual counting using a counting chamber (hemocytometer). While considered accurate, it is time consuming and prone to errors. Accurate results have been reported using automated hematology analyzers in humans.[16] Hematology analyzers equipped with multi-species software should be validated to perform BALF TNCC in animals.[17,18] The Sysmex® 2000iV analyzer (Sysmex Europe GmbH, Norderstedt, Germany) was suitable for the calculation of the total leukocyte count (i.e. TNCC) in BALF from various animal species[19] and was reliable in differentiating neutrophils and eosinophils in rats and mice.[20] Software developed for BALF analysis of rats and mice on the Advia® analyzer (Siemens Healthcare Diagnostics, Tarrytown, NY, USA) generated adequate results.[21]

Red blood cells (RBCs) in BALF are usually blood associated, and counts offer little information beyond the microscopic observation of blood contamination considered sufficient for most studies. Epithelial cells can be observed, often in cohesive sheets that are subjectively described rather than enumerated.

Slide Preparation

Microscopic evaluation of BALF for differential cell counts and assessment of cell morphology is performed using cytospin slide preparations of the resuspended EDTA BALF. After air drying, slides are stained with a Romanowsky-type stain (e.g. Wright-Giemsa, May-Grünwald-Giemsa). Mast cell granules typically stain well with alcohol based Romanowsky-type stains in rodents and dogs (e.g. Wright-Giemsa), but variably stain with aqueous Romanowsky-type stains (e.g. Diff-Quik).[22] Mast cell granules do not stain well with either type of Romanowsky stain in NHP; staining with 0.5% toluidine blue at an acidic pH is necessary in these species.[23]

Cytological Evaluation

Cell Types

In all species, alveolar macrophages are the predominant cell, with low numbers of small lymphocytes and occasional neutrophils, eosinophils, and mast cells. Ciliated and non-ciliated columnar and cuboidal epithelial cells are commonly observed in sheets or individually in BALF. Macrophages and lymphocytes tend to have a similar morphology across species, but cytologic differences are observed in other cell types (Figure 66.1a and c). For example, neutrophil segmentation and the morphology of eosinophil and mast cell granules vary between different laboratory species.[24] Two hundred cell differentials are performed enumerating the absolute concentrations and percentages of alveolar macrophages, neutrophils, monocytes, eosinophils, lymphocytes, and mast cells. Automated cell differential is feasible with hematology analyzers adapted and gated for this type of sample.[20,21] However automated differentiation of only three or four different cell types is possible, and microscopic screening for verification of the results remains essential. Phenotyping of lymphocytes in BALF expression can be assessed by flow cytometry.[25]

Inflammation

Post-challenge (e.g. lipopolysaccharides or ovalbumin), BALF cell composition varies significantly over time; thus the timing of samples is essential. Based on our experience, sampling 12–24 hours after stimulation is often optimal.[25] After challenge with ovalbumin in brown rats, fluids contain up to 2000 cells/μL, mostly neutrophils and few macrophages. With betamethasone treatment, the proportion of neutrophils decreases rapidly within 4–24 hours, and the proportion of macrophages increases significantly. A predominance of eosinophils and neutrophils was seen in BALF after administration of ovalbumin to mice.[13,25]

At the end of inhalation studies, TNCC in BALF collected from untreated control laboratory animals is usually <500 cells/μL (counts depend on the lavage method), composed mostly of macrophages with low numbers of

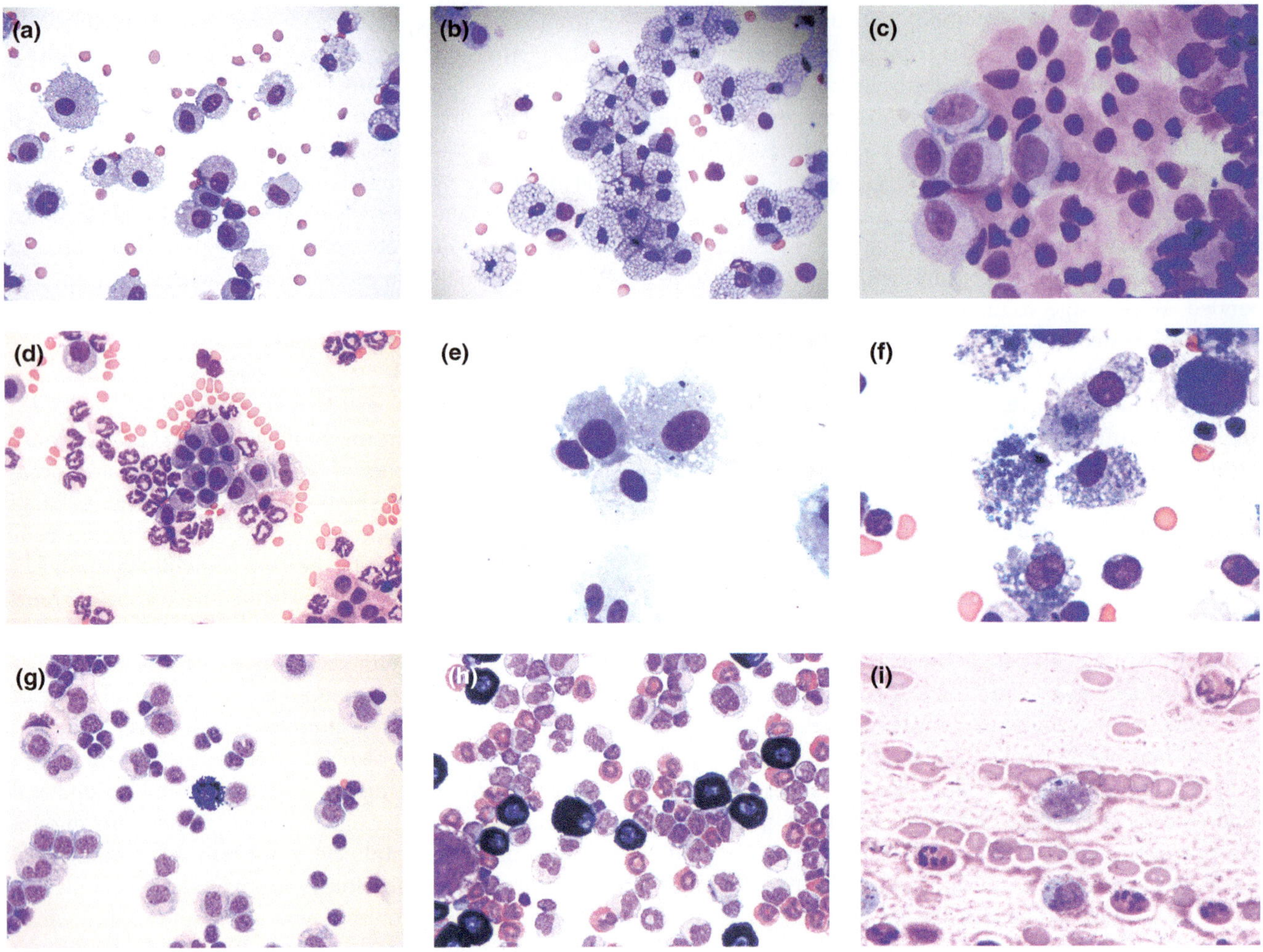

Figure 66.1 Body fluids. (a) BAL from a healthy control rat. Macrophages are predominant (Thiazin-eosin, 500×). (b) BAL from a rat receiving compound by inhalation. The numerous small vacuoles present within the macrophages represent an accumulation of the compound or its metabolites (Thiazin-eosin, 500×). (c) BAL from a healthy control mouse is characterized by macrophages and ciliated epithelial cells (Thiazin-eosin, 1000×). (d) BAL from a mouse treated with lipopolysaccharides, resulting in increased numbers of neutrophils and macrophages (Thiazin-eosin, 200×). (e) BAL from a healthy control NHP with several macrophages, one mast cell with unstained granules (center), and a small lymphocyte (Thiazin-eosin, 1000× oil). (f) BAL from a NHP receiving a compound by inhalation. The pigmented material present within the macrophages is consistent with hemosiderin (Thiazin-eosin, 1000×). (g) Peritoneal fluid from a mouse receiving thioglycollate by intraperitoneal injection (a model of peritoneal inflammation). Increased numbers of macrophages and small lymphocytes are seen. There is one mast cell (center) (Thiazin-eosin, 200×). (h) Peritoneal fluid from a rat receiving thioglycollate by intraperitoneal injection. There are increased numbers of eosinophils, neutrophils, mast cells, and macrophages (Thiazin-eosin, 200×). (i) Joint fluid from a rabbit following an intra-articular treatment is characterized by increased numbers of neutrophils and a few macrophages (Wright-Giemsa, 500×).

lymphocytes. Neutrophils are rare under normal conditions; increased numbers are consistent with an inflammatory response. Eosinophilia is indicative of hypersensitivity/allergic reactions (Figure 66.1d and e).

Compound Accumulation

Compound material can be observed in alveolar macrophages, appearing as cytoplasmic vacuoles containing the compound or its derivatives (Figure 66.1b). This is considered a major finding because compound should not accumulate in the lungs.

Biochemistry, Cytokines, and Immunological Evaluation

Changes in BALF biochemical parameters can be observed early in a study, possibly signifying later morphological changes. With inflammation, total protein concentration increases due to increased permeability of the air–blood barrier and leakage of albumin. Because BALF albumin concentrations are usually below the limit of quantification for automated chemistry analyzers, protein electrophoresis has been used to measure BALF albumin.[26] Total lactate dehydrogenase activity is a useful marker of cell damage or inflammation.[27–29] In primates, C-reactive protein levels can be analyzed with appropriately sensitive methodology.[30]

Other immunomodulatory soluble factors measureable in BALF include secretory products of macrophages and epithelial cells, such as tumor necrosis factor-alpha, fibronectin, interleukins (IL), chemotactic factors, growth factors, proteases, and antiproteases. IL-1, IL-2, IL-4, IL-5, IL-6, IL-8, IL-10, IL-13, IL-12/23, IL-17, granulocyte colony-stimulating factor, granulocyte-monocyte colony-stimulating factor, interferon-γ, RANTES, eotaxin, histamine, monocyte chemoattractant protein-1, and IgE have all been measured in BALF.[31]

Peritoneal Fluid

Ascites formation is uncommon in toxicological studies, but when present, it can be evaluated as described (Chapter 50). There are no reference values for abdominal fluids of rodents and NHP, but values are expected to be close to the published values from other domestic animals. Most peritoneal fluid evaluation in toxicological studies is performed in rodents using lavage samples.

Peritoneal lavages are used to evaluate the anti-inflammatory properties of compounds in rodents. For example, intraperitoneal injection of thioglycollate in mice stimulates the rapid migration of macrophages and neutrophils into the peritoneal cavity. Peritoneal lavage fluid analysis is employed to assess the ability of a candidate compound to reduce inflammatory cell recruitment.[32,33] After thioglycollate administration, there is a typical pattern of cell migration into the peritoneal cavity: neutrophils first influx 4–24 hours post-injection and large number of monocytes influx between 24 and 72 hours.[34,35] The candidate compound plus thioglycollate is usually compared to a commercialized anti-inflammatory drug (e.g. dexamethasone plus thioglycollate) and to controls receiving thioglycollate only.

Collection

Similar to BALF collection, peritoneal lavage is performed on rodents receiving inhalant (usually isoflurane) anesthesia before euthanasia. A solution of saline containing EDTA (approximately 2 mL for mice and 10 mL for rats) is injected into the abdominal cavity followed by re-aspiration and collection into a plain tube. The same procedure is repeated once or twice more. The TNCC and differential cell count of the fluid are determined. The fluid can also be used for cytokine analysis.

Sample Processing and Cell Counts

TNCC can be determined using a hemocytometer or an automated hematology analyzer.[19,35] Cell clumping, cell fragments, and noncellular debris can cause counting errors with both techniques. There is no reference range for cell counts as they strongly depend on the collection method; however, most control animal cell counts obtained in our laboratory are below 500 cells/μL after instillations of 5 mL in rats and 2 mL in mice (authors' observations). It is standard to compare study animals with controls to assess compound effects.

Lavage fluid from control animals consists mainly of macrophages with low numbers of lymphocytes and rare neutrophils, eosinophils, and mast cells. RBCs in peritoneal lavage fluid indicate blood contamination, cavity hemorrhage, or increased capillary permeability with diapedesis of RBCs. RBC counts offer little information over visual assessment. Cellularity of the lavage varies with the nature of the compound administered. Macrophages and neutrophils remain the hallmark of inflammation, while eosinophils increase with hypersensitivity (Figure 66.1g and h). Flat sheets of quiescent mesothelial cells can be observed. Reactive individual mesothelial cells are not observed in lavages.

Cerebrospinal Fluid

CSF evaluation is most often used to monitor neurotropic drugs and includes cytological, biochemical, immunologic, or pharmacokinetic analyses. Most compounds do not cross the blood–brain barrier after intravenous administration. Direct central neural axis neuromodulation has become a viable means to treat chronic neurologic disease; thus compounds are being developed for direct delivery to the CNS. Intrathecal drug administration by catheterization of the subarachnoid space is commonly done.[36] Other modes of administration include intra-cerebroventricular catheterization or direct injection, direct or continuous injection into the parenchyma, or use of vectors that gain access to the brain/spinal cord following systemic administration.[36] Evaluation of potential toxicity of such compounds requires CSF evaluation during preclinical studies.

Collection

CSF collection has been performed in NHP,[34] dogs,[37] swine, and rats[38] during studies or as a terminal procedure. CSF is collected under anesthesia via cerebromedullary (cisterna magna) or lumbosacral dural needle puncture or via an indwelling catheter surgically implanted for infusion of the compound and repeated punctures. CSF should be placed in EDTA tubes for cytological evaluation, while tubes without anticoagulant are preferred for biochemistry.[38]

Chronic intrathecal infusion studies in NHP and swine use an indwelling catheter, and a baseline CSF sample is collected prior to the administration of the first dose of the test compound as an in-study reference. Sample collection is repeated one to four hours post-dose depending on the distribution and absorption of the compound in the CNS compartment.[39] While indwelling catheters with a subcutaneous access port can theoretically be left in place for up to 6–9 months, obstruction is reported at a rate of 40% after 40 days[40] to 3 months.[39] Catheters are generally well tolerated, with no remarkable changes in neurological, physical, or ophthalmologic examinations; however, transient increases in CSF cellularity with increased numbers of neutrophils can occur.[36] Complications including encephalitis, osteitis, blockage of cannulas with fibrous connective tissue, and longer collection times have been reported.[36] Studies using implanted catheters in rats have been reported but remain anecdotal.[41]

In rats, CSF may be collected under isoflurane anesthesia or immediately after carbon dioxide asphyxiation. A 27 G winged infusion set connected to a syringe is passed through the dura mater into the cistern magna. Gentle negative pressure is applied in the syringe, and approximately 50–70 μL[38] to 120 μL[42] of CSF is drawn into the tubing and placed in a collection tube. Without negative pressure, up to 25 μL can be acquired with minimal blood contamination. In NHP and dogs, larger volumes of up to 250 μL/kg can be collected and replaced with artificial CSF.

Cell Counts

CSF samples placed in an EDTA tube for cell counting should be evaluated within two to three hours of sample collection. Manual determination of white blood cell (WBC) and RBC concentrations are performed using a hemocytometer. Software for CSF cell counting and differential cell determination has been developed for the Advia automated hematology analyzer and was found to generate accurate CSF cell counts in humans[43] and correlate well with manual WBC and RBC counts in dogs.[43,44] Most healthy dogs have a CSF WBC count of 0–2 cells/μL and RBCs are not present in normal CSF.[45] However, CSF collected after chronic intrathecal catheterization was reported to contain a mean of 6–10 WBC/μL and 0–7 RBC/μL.[37] RBCs most likely represent blood contamination.

In a rat study collecting CSF immediately after CO_2 asphyxiation, the mean CSF RBC count from untreated rats was $6.2 \pm 1.2 \times 10^3/\mu L$ after exclusion of samples with visual evidence of blood contamination (discolored samples); the mean WBC count was $2.3 \pm 4.9/\mu L$ (mean ± SEM).[38] In NHP with indwelling intrathecal catheters, the total mean WBC count was $61 \pm 136/\mu L$, as cell numbers tend to increase with device implantation.[39]

Cytological Evaluation

Cytospin slide preparations are used to evaluate cells and perform a differential cell count. As with other fluids, slides are stained with a Romanowsky-type stain (e.g. Wright-Giemsa, May-Grünwald-Giemsa). Normal CSF in rats is composed predominantly of lymphocytes (~60%), with the remaining cells being macrophages (~34%) and neutrophils (~6%).[38] However, cell classification may vary, with some investigators classifying cells as small lymphocytes, small mononuclear cells, large mononuclear cells, or large foamy macrophages (Chapter 48). In preclinical intrathecal studies in NHP, CSF leukocytosis with increased neutrophils is commonly observed in vehicle control and treated groups after intrathecal catheter placement; increased albumin values and lower glucose levels are also seen.[39]

Biochemical Evaluation

For biochemical and other non-cytological evaluations, CSF is placed in a tube without anticoagulant. CSF has a low total protein concentration, usually less than 45 mg/dL, and albumin accounts for 80–95% of total protein in normal CSF.[46] The concentration of proteins will increase with inflammation and alterations of the blood–brain barrier. Blood contamination (as indicated by >30 RBC/μL) can also increase the total protein concentration. Refractometry or chemical methods used for serum protein measurements are inappropriate for the evaluation of CSF protein concentration due to the low concentrations. However, ultrasensitive assays designed for measuring urine protein may be used; Coomassie blue spectrophotometric or benzethonium chloride turbidometric methods can be assayed on an automated chemistry analyzer.[47] Protein electrophoresis can be performed on CSF to evaluate albumin or gamma-globulin concentrations.

Proteins are more stable than cells; therefore, samples may reliably be held refrigerated up to 48 hours (author's laboratory validation) before protein concentration is determined. CSF protein concentration is collection site dependent. The total protein concentration of CSF in rats obtained by percutaneous aspiration of the cistern magna was 17.1 ± 2.7 mg/dL.[38] The total protein concentration was 76 ± 228 mg/dL in NHP when collected from an indwelling intrathecal catheter.[39]

Glucose is commonly measured in CSF. In cases of inflammation, glucose tends to decrease from inflammatory cell utilization.[39] In untreated NHP with indwelling catheters, glucose concentrations averaged 46 ± 6 mg/dL.[39]

Monitoring of changes in CSF cellularity and protein and glucose concentration correlate with morphological changes noted in histopathological evaluation for intrathecal compounds.[39]

Synovial Fluid

Animal models of synovial disease can evaluate early effects of drugs on inflammatory markers. For example, collagen-induced arthritis in rodents is a well-established disease model for rheumatoid arthritis.[48,49] Repeated sampling of synovial fluid by the perfusion methods described below allows for serial monitoring instead of needing to rely on a single study endpoint histologic result.[50]

Collection

The synovium is lavaged because joints are rarely swollen. Lavage is aseptically performed on a stifle joint under general anesthesia or at necropsy. The needle is inserted approximately 2–3 mm above the tibia head and laterally behind the patellar ligament. Recommended needles vary between species: 29.5 G for rats and 25 G for dogs and NHP. Sterile saline is injected until resistance to articulation is noted (approximately 1–1.5 mL in large animals, 0.2 mL in small animals). The syringe is removed and the limb is gently flexcd and extended several times before collecting the synovial fluid. The needle is then reinserted in the area of the injection for rodents and medially at an angle of 90° in large species. In rats, it is possible to perfuse a joint by inserting two needles on two opposite sides and collect the fluid passing through the joint.[50] Synovial lavages for cytologic analysis should be promptly placed in EDTA tubes and refrigerated if not analyzed immediately. Samples for biochemical and cytokines evaluation are placed in tubes without anticoagulant.

Cell Counts and Analysis

TNCC are performed on a hemocytometer or an automated analyzer.[18] Prior to analysis, undiluted synovial fluid should be treated with hyaluronidase to decrease viscosity and improve the accuracy and precision of total and differential cell counts.[51] Target final concentration of hyaluronidase concentration in synovial fluid is 0.01 mg/mL.[51] However, synovial lavages usually have a lower viscosity and can be evaluated by an automated analyzer without the addition of hyaluronidase.

After addition of hyaluronidase, cytospin slides can be prepared and provide an adequate concentration of synovial cells allowing a good visualization of the cells. Normal synovial fluid is composed of few cells, and the numbers vary with infusion technique and the volume utilized; therefore counts are only reliable if the method is highly standardized. Normal synovial fluid contains mononuclear cells, predominantly macrophages with low numbers of lymphocytes. Neutrophil counts increase with inflammation (Figure 66.1i). Eosinophils are rarely observed with compound administration but reflect a hypersensitivity reaction. With serial collections, neutrophilic inflammation is common and will limit the evaluation.

Synovial fluid is often collected for the measurement of cytokines, including matrix metalloproteinase activity, IL-6, IL-17, and tumor necrosis factor-alpha, which are interesting inflammatory markers in experimental-induced arthritis studies.[48] Indicators of cartilage degradation (COMP and CTX-II) or bone damage (CTX-I) are also reliable markers when measured in synovial fluid and plasma.[48,49]

Vaginal Cytology

Rats and Mice

Assessment of the estrous cycle is used both as a principal determinant of reproductive cyclicity and as an ancillary test in reproductive toxicity studies.[52] The relative changes in the cell types directly reflect circulating levels of estrogen and progesterone from the ovaries. Conventionally, the estrous cycle has four stages: proestrus, estrus, metestrus, and diestrus. Some investigators divide it into as few as three stages (proestrus, estrus, diestrus),[52] while others have subcategorized the 4 stages into as many as 13 stages.[53] This section will describe the four classic stages.

Methodology

To assess estrous cycles, vaginal cytology samples are collected over at least 14 consecutive days, but 21 is ideal.[54] Collection of samples can be done at any time of the day, but typically in the morning after the lights are turned on. Regardless of timing, collection should be consistent to reduce variability. Lavage is preferred because it yields better cellularity samples, but moistened swabs can be used. Lavage is performed using a pipette or eyedropper with smooth tapered ends, preferably a new one for each animal, although thorough rinsing can prevent carryover of cells. Normal or phosphate-buffered saline is preferred over water to reduce cell distortion and rupture. Approximately 0.1 mL (mice) or 0.2 mL (rats) of saline is drawn into the pipette, and the tip is gently inserted into the vaginal orifice 1–2 mm in mice and 5–10 mm in rats. The saline is then flushed in and back out of the vagina two to three times. It is critical to avoid inserting the tip too deeply into the canal because cervical stimulation can cause pseudopregnancy.[52] Pseudopregnancies present as a persistent diestrus for up to 14 days. Details regarding vaginal lavage technique and collection using cotton swabs are available.[55,56]

A drop of sample is placed evenly in a thin layer on a glass slide and read immediately as a direct wet mount. Alternatively, or after wet-mount evaluation, smears can be dry fixed for later staining and evaluation. For archiving, six to eight consecutive days' samples from one animal can be placed on a 1×3 in. glass slide with a labeled box grid of six to eight cells drawn with a solvent resistant marker; glass slides with pre-drawn grids are also available. Wet mounts allow for immediate identification of the stage. However, stained smears are easier to evaluate, facilitate serial evaluation in individual animals to document cycling, and can be archived.

Romanowsky-type stains (e.g. Wright-Giemsa, Diff-Quik™) and toluidine blue are recommended. Papanicolaou stain has also been used for better visualization of chromatin and degree of keratinization, but this is not usually needed to assess rodent estrous cycles. For Papanicolaou staining, fixation of the slide is required before drying (i.e. wet fixation) with the use of a fixative such as Spray-Cyte® (Becton, Dickinson & Co., Franklin Lakes, NJ, USA).

Slide Evaluation

Training is critical for accurate interpretation. Important considerations include inherent variations in the appearance of the stages such as relative proportions of cells, recognition of artifactual changes in cells, and an appreciation that smears represent a snapshot of a dynamic process.[57] Use of practice sets following animals over time helps build proficiency. It is important to limit the number of individuals evaluating vaginal smears in a lab or study and to make a concerted effort to standardize criteria for classification of stages to ensure consistent results. Most smears can be evaluated with a 10× objective, but use of a 20× or 40× objective can verify the presence of neutrophils. Evaluating the whole smear using low magnification is important because cell types and numbers can vary regionally.

Cells and Stages of the Estrous Cycle

In rats and mice, the estrous cycle averages four to five days, but six-day cycles are occasionally encountered.[52,58–63] There are many factors that influence cycle length including light: dark cycle, age, noise, stress, social interactions, and the presence of males.[52,58,64–67] The length of the four stages varies between 6 and 72 hours depending on the stage and individual rodent, so shorter stages can be missed in a 24 hour sample interval. In some individual rodents, only estrus and diestrus might be detected over the course of the collection window.

Cells of the Estrous Cycle

Neutrophils During processing neutrophils can condense or "ball up," appearing as small dark round dots on lower power. Neutrophils can partially rupture during collection or processing, and it is important to recognize condensed or ruptured neutrophils for accurate interpretation of vaginal smears.

Small Nucleated Epithelial Cells These cells are small, round to oval with a round nucleus and blue cytoplasm. They are nonkeratinized and have a higher nuclear to cytoplasmic ratio (N:C) than large nucleated epithelial cells. They can stain very dark, precluding visualization of the nucleus. Small epithelial cells of proestrus may contain small cytoplasmic vacuoles.

Large Nucleated Epithelial Cells These cells are round to polygonal and have smooth, jagged, or irregular borders with moderate or abundant amounts of blue, variably keratinized cytoplasm and a lower N:C than small epithelial cells. Nuclei may be intact, degenerate, or pyknotic.

Anucleated Keratinized Epithelial Cells Anucleated epithelial cells are aged cells with abundant blue to sky blue cytoplasm and jagged or angular edges. As the name infers, they lack nuclei but can contain a pale round area where a nucleus once existed (ghost nuclei).

Stages of the Estrous Cycle

The stages of the estrous cycle are identified by the absence, presence, or proportion of cell types (Table 66.1). Cell density and the arrangement of the cells in the smear also aid identification of stage.

Proestrus Proestrus is a short stage averaging 14 hours in rats and less than 24 hours in mice.[61,68–70] It is characterized by small nucleated epithelial cells of relatively uniform size and appearance (Figure 66.2a). They sometimes stain deeply basophilic or can have a delicate or wispy appearance, especially in low cellularity smears. The small epithelial cells can form cohesive clusters (so-called "grape" clusters), sheets, or strands; however, these patterns are not prerequisite in the determination of proestrus since they may be absent, especially in low cellularity samples. Neutrophils are uncommon, but can be found in low numbers in early proestrus, during the transition out of diestrus. Few large nucleated and anucleated epithelial cells also can be seen throughout proestrus. As estrus approaches, anucleated keratinized cells will become more abundant. Low numbers of neutrophils, large epithelial cells, or anucleated epithelial cells do not preclude a proestrus stage when the predominating feature of the smear is high numbers of small epithelial cells.

Estrus Estrus averages between 24 and 48 hours in rats and 12 and 48 hours in mice.[59,61,68–70] Keratinized anucleated epithelial cells predominate during estrus. Numerous bacteria can be seen epicellularly or throughout the background of the smear. Low numbers of nucleated epithelial cells can be present. Neutrophils are absent, although rare to occasional neutrophils appear toward the end of estrus,

Table 66.1 Classification of the stages of estrous cycle based on types and relative numbers of cells in vaginal smears in rats and mice.

Stage	Neutrophils	Small nucleated epithelial cells	Large nucleated epithelial cells	Anucleated keratinized epithelial cells	Relative cell density
Proestrus	0 to +	++ to +++	0 to +	0 to +	Low to moderate
Estrus					
Rat	0 to +	0 to ++	0 to ++	++ to +++	Moderate to high
Mouse	0 to +	0 to +	0 to +	++ to +++	Moderate to high
Metestrus					
Rat	+ to +++	+ to ++	+ to ++	+ to +++	Moderate to high
Mouse	+ to +++	0 to +	0 to +	++ to +++	Moderate to high
Diestrus	++ to +++	+ to ++	+ to ++	0 to +	Low to moderate

0, none; +, few; ++, moderate; +++, high.

during the transition to metestrus. While consisting mostly of anucleated epithelial cells, the first and second halves or phases of estrus differ in their cellular appearance and also differ between rats and mice.[57]

When two consecutive days of estrus are observed in mice, two distinct phases are usually appreciated.[57] Initially, the anucleated cells are smaller and usually arranged in loose clusters or sheets reminiscent of proestrus. As estrus progresses, anucleated cells become larger, more evenly distributed, and cell numbers generally increase (Figure 66.2b). Cells can form stacks or layers.

In rats, the short late estrus phase is distinctly different in appearance from the rest of the stage, but is not always observed[57] (Figure 66.2c). Late estrus is characterized by the emergence of numerous small and large nucleated epithelial cells interspersed among the anucleated cells. The nucleated cells are smooth to irregular and can be round, oval, or spindle shaped and sometimes stain deeply basophilic. The large oval nucleated cells of late estrus called "pavement cells" indicate that metestrus is rapidly approaching.[71] Late estrus should not be mistaken for proestrus. Evaluating the previous day's smear should help avoid confusion. Additionally, the nucleated cells of proestrus are generally more uniform in appearance and have a higher N:C compared with late estrus.

Metestrus Metestrus is a short stage in rats, lasting between six and eight hours.[59,61,69] In mice it can be as long as 24 hours and infrequently can be two days.[57,68,70] Metestrus is characterized by a combination of anucleated epithelial cells and neutrophils. In mice, rare to occasional nucleated epithelial cells can be observed. In rats, the nucleated epithelial cells of late estrus are present in moderate numbers throughout the stage.

In early metestrus, neutrophils are scattered among the epithelial cells and are sometimes found in clumps or tightly packed around the epithelial cells. At this point, the epithelial cells predominate or are equal in number to the neutrophils. As metestrus progresses, neutrophil numbers increase, exceeding epithelial cells up to 10-fold, resulting in a highly cellular smear (Figure 66.2d and e).[72]

Numbers of neutrophils and epithelial cells fall during the transition to diestrus. While early and mid-metestrus are easily identified, distinguishing between late metestrus and early diestrus can be challenging because they are defined by the same cell types. If there is uncertainty whether a smear is late metestrus or early diestrus, best practice is to "err" on the side of diestrus. There is little value in overly scrutinizing a late metestrus/early diestrus smear.[57]

Diestrus Diestrus is the longest stage, averaging 48–72 hours in rats and mice.[59,61,68–70] There is a substantial decrease in, but not necessarily an absence of, anucleated epithelial cells. Cellularity is moderate to low consisting of small and large epithelial cells, neutrophils, and low numbers of anucleated epithelial cells (Figure 66.2f). Neutrophils usually exceed epithelial cells with some smears containing only neutrophils. Diestrus smears can have very low cellularity with just a scattering of cells, especially on days 2 and 3. Toward the end of diestrus, epithelial cells can occur in small clumps indicating impending proestrus, but neutrophils remain the predominant feature of the smear.

Transitional Smears Transitional smears will invariably be encountered and can be classified based on the predominating feature(s). For example, during transition from proestrus to estrus, if the majority (>50%) of the cells are small nucleated epithelial cells, the stage should be classified as proestrus. Alternatively, the data could be recorded as P(e), where the capital letter indicates that proestrus is the predominant stage and the lowercase "e" denotes that many anucleated cells were also present, suggesting transition to estrus. The method of documentation depends on the purpose for monitoring the estrous cycle.

Nonhuman Primates

The need to predict ovulation and reproductive or ovarian cyclicity in monkeys is essential for many developmental and reproductive toxicity studies. Breeding seasons and ovarian cycle lengths vary widely among different monkey species. Old World primates, such as cynomolgus monkeys (*Macaca fascicularis*) and rhesus monkeys (*Macaca mulatta*), have a menstrual cycle, while New World and prosimian primates, such as marmosets (*Callithrix jacchus*), have an estrous cycle. Both the menstrual and estrous cycles consist of follicular, periovulatory, and luteal phases. Monkeys with a menstrual cycle will have menstruation or menses following the luteal phase, although many mature monkeys have irregular or anovulatory cycles due to stress and hierarchical status.[73]

Vaginal Cytology of the Menstrual Cycle

Monitoring ovarian cyclicity in Old World monkeys is easily accomplished by the detection of overt menses through

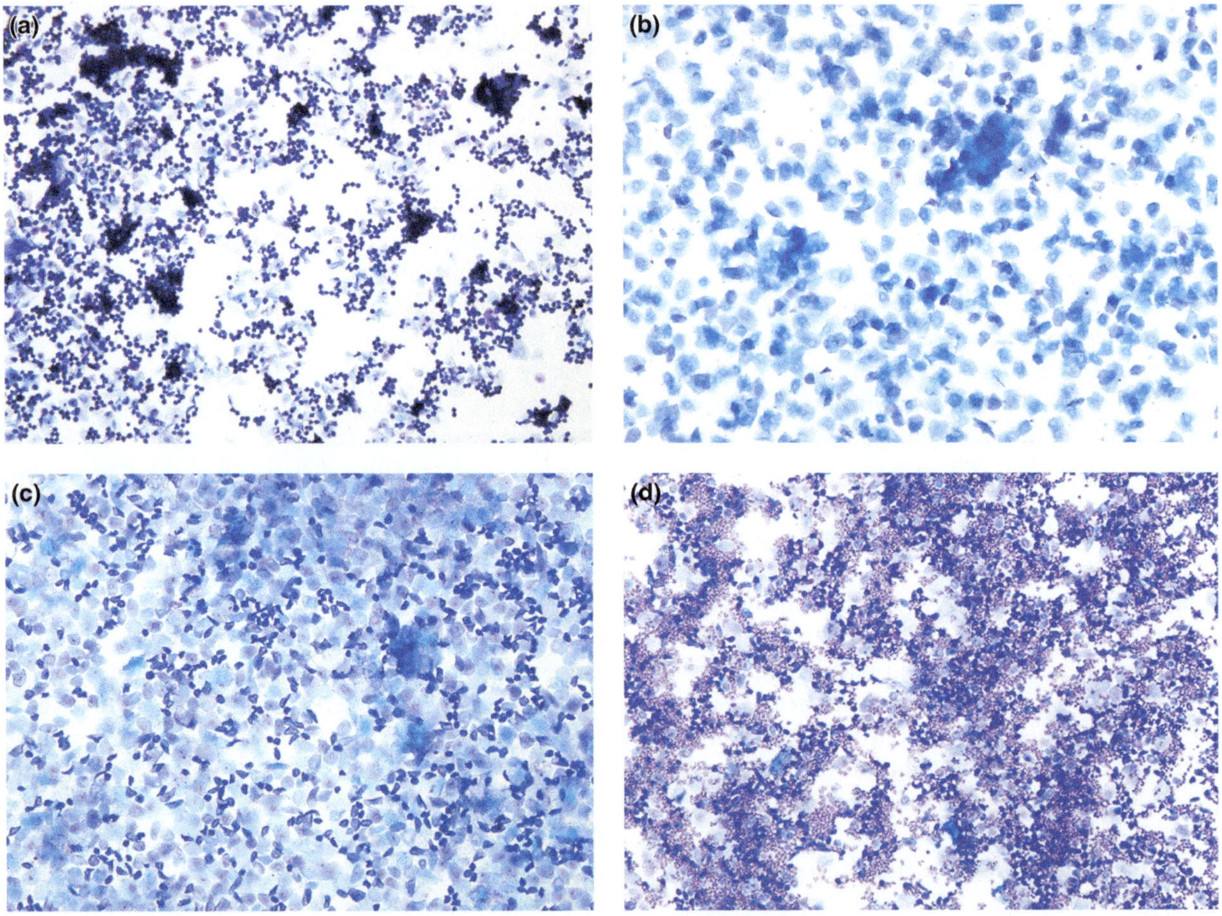

Figure 66.2 Vaginal cytology. (a) Proestrus in a rat. Small nucleated epithelial cells, sometimes in clumps, predominate. It is not unusual for small epithelial cells to stain darkly. No neutrophils are present. Proestrus appears similar in mice (Toluidine blue, 100×). (b) Estrus in a mouse. This smear represents the so-called second phase of estrus in mice. Anucleated epithelial cells predominate. Estrus appears similar in rats with the exception of late estrus (Figure 66.2c) (modified Wright-Giemsa, 100×. *Source:* Reprinted with permission from Cora et al.[57]). (c) Late estrus in a rat. The late estrus phase in a rat is characterized by the emergence of round, oval, or spindle-shaped nucleated epithelial cells interspersed among the anucleated cells. This phase should not be confused with proestrus (Toluidine blue, 100×). (d) Metestrus in a rat. Neutrophils are interspersed among the anucleated and nucleated epithelial cells of late estrus. At the peak of metestrus, the cell density is high, and neutrophils are present in substantial numbers (Toluidine blue, 100×. *Source:* Reprinted with permission from Cora et al.[57]). (e) Metestrus in a mouse. Neutrophils, present in very high numbers, and anucleated cells characterize the peak of metestrus in mice (Toluidine blue, 100×). (f) Diestrus in a mouse. Diestrus is characterized by smears of moderate to low cellularity with neutrophil numbers usually higher relative to the epithelial cell numbers. Diestrus appears the same in rats (Toluidine blue, 100×). (g) Follicular stage in a NHP. Superficial epithelial cells are predominant, and numerous bacteria are present (Wright-Giemsa, 500×). (h) Peri-ovulatory stage in a NHP. Superficial epithelial cells with abundant cytoplasm and small pyknotic nuclei are predominant. Numerous bacteria are present (Wright-Giemsa, 200×). (i) Luteal stage in a NHP. Intermediate cells are predominant (Wright-Giemsa, 500×).

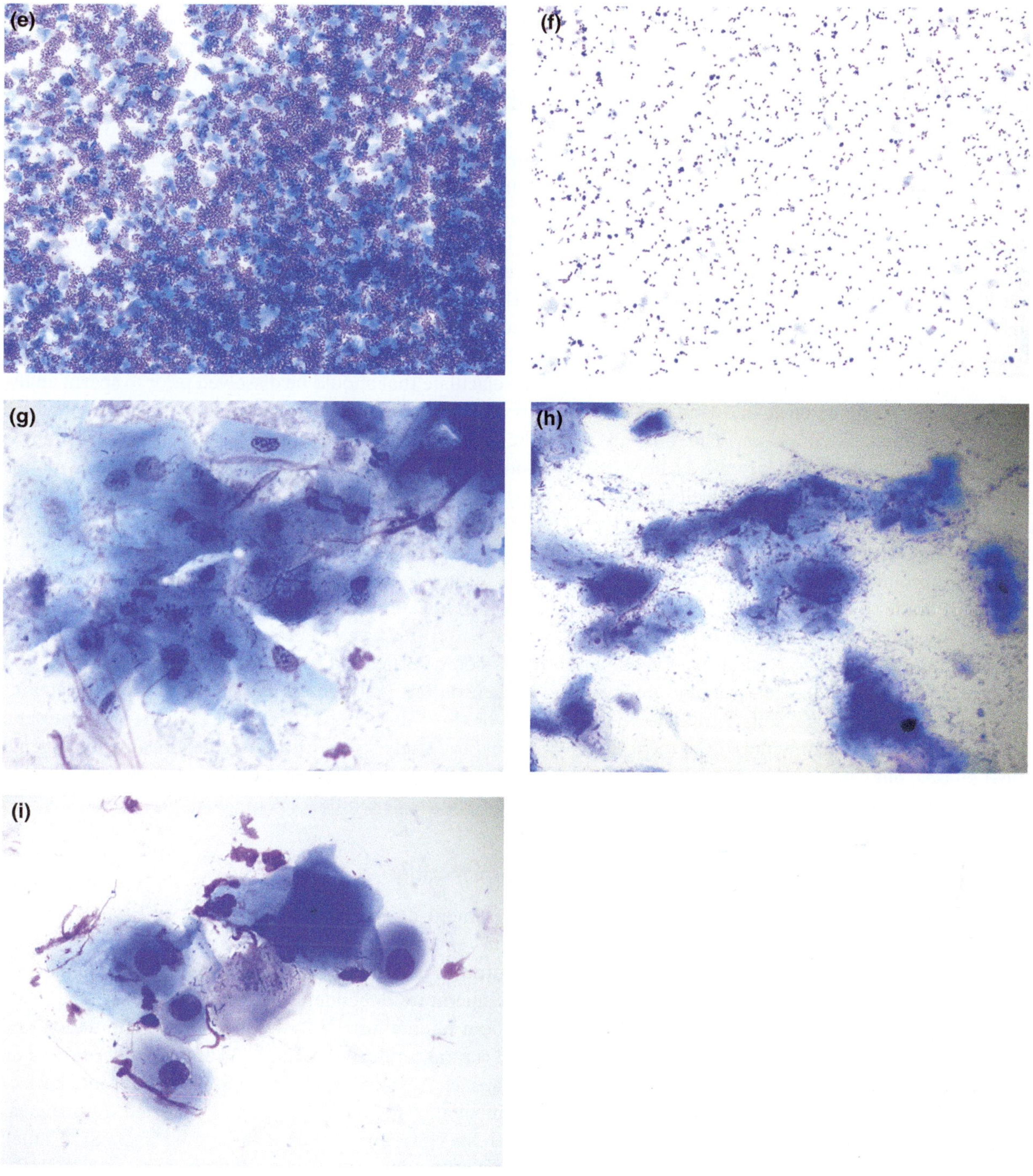

Figure 66.2 (Continued)

daily vaginal smear evaluation. Hormone levels can be monitored but can be impracticable. In cynomolgus and rhesus monkeys, a normal ovarian cycle is 28–32 days.[73] To evaluate for menses, the monkey is first conditioned to "present" for vaginal swabbing. A cotton-tipped applicator is moistened with water or saline, placed in the peri-vaginal area and gently rotated and then visually examined for blood. Results can be recorded as a negative or positive, or a subjective grading scale can be used, including observation of no menses, or slight, heavy, or very heavy (visible) bleeding.[74]

Vaginal Cytology of the Estrous Cycle

Cytologic evaluation of the estrous cycle in New World monkeys and prosimians to monitor ovarian cyclicity is more challenging because the cyclic changes are not as apparent as in rodents. Thus, daily vaginal cytology is not commonly performed; however it has been evaluated with mixed results.[75–80] Appropriate training and expertise, routine practice, and knowledge of the normal range of variation in epithelial cell types throughout the cycle are required for accurate vaginal cytology staging. More commonly, ovarian cyclicity in New World monkeys is monitored by endocrinological evaluations.

Vaginal Cytology Evaluation

To make a vaginal smear for microscopic evaluation, after collection, gently roll the swab onto a glass slide and stain with a Romanowsky-type or Papanicolaou stain. The stages of the estrous cycle are recognized by evaluating the relative numbers of parabasal, intermediate, and superficial vaginal epithelial cells (Figure 66.2g–h). Parabasal cells have moderate amounts of cytoplasm. The nucleus is round to oval with fine chromatin and usually is more than one third of the cell diameter. Intermediate cells are larger than parabasal cells with abundant cytoplasm that typically stains light blue with Papanicolaou stain. The nucleus is round with fine chromatin. Superficial cells have irregular or jagged cell borders and abundant cytoplasm that typically stains pink with Papanicolaou stain. The nucleus is smaller and pyknotic. In general, superficial cells will predominate in the follicular stage, peaking midcycle (periovulatory), and intermediate cells dominate in the luteal phase. Neutrophils are mainly present in the follicular and luteal phases, but can occasionally be seen during the periovulatory phase of the estrous cycle.[75,77,79,80]

Calculation of the karyopyknotic index (KPI) can be a useful way to determine if ovulation has occurred.[75,78,81] KPI is the ratio of superficial epithelial cells to intermediate epithelial cells. In normally cycling monkeys, the KPI will fluctuate during the cycle, peaking at or around the time of ovulation. Non-cycling monkeys will have little variation. To calculate the KPI, stained vaginal smears are collected regularly throughout the cycle, and between 100 and 300 epithelial cells are categorized as intermediate or superficial cells.[78] For example, if 178 epithelial cells were classified as superficial cells and 22 were classified as intermediate, the KPI ratio would be 8.

Semen Evaluation

There is increasing concern about potential compound-related effects on male reproduction. These are generally subtle and can be induced by direct germ cell toxicity or indirectly through hormonal disturbance. Mating success is the most common method for detecting effects on spermatogenesis. Because of excess sperm production in rodents, use of this endpoint for the detection of pathology lacks sensitivity and is questionably reflective of effects on human sperm production.[82] Histopathology of the testis is the most sensitive method for the detection of effects on spermatogenesis. Sperm evaluation can complement histopathology and confirm histopathological lesions related to spermatogenesis or detect alterations in sperm maturation. Semen evaluation includes sperm counts, sperm motility, and sperm morphology.

In rats and mice, semen is obtained at necropsy from the vas deferens or the cauda epididymis. Ejaculate evaluation in large animals (e.g. dogs, NHP) requires sexually mature animals carefully selected prior to study initiation.[73,83] In NHP, rabbits, and dogs, the semen is obtained by induced or electroejaculation, and the semen is immediately mixed with a buffer for evaluation. In NHP, there is a gel plug in the ejaculate that should be dissolved prior to sperm analysis. In dogs, the ejaculate occurs in three fractions, of which the first two are used for analysis: the first is a small volume containing few sperm, the second contains most of the sperm, and the third is clear prostatic fluid (Chapter 41).[82]

One advantage of rabbit, dog, and NHP studies is the ability to conduct longitudinal studies in which baseline data serves individual animal pretreatment controls. In rabbits, collection is recommended once or twice a week for at least three weeks, because evaluating multiple ejaculates compensates for variability in sperm numbers and concentrations.[82,84] In dogs and NHP, multiple collections two or three days apart should be evaluated prior to and during the study, as they are more genetically heterogeneous with more variable sperm morphology and motility than rodents or rabbits.[82]

Sperm Motility

Assessment of sperm motility should be performed in a warm environment (media, instruments, etc.) within 30 minutes of collection because the spermatozoa motility is temperature dependent. Sperm collection is conducted at room temperature.[82] Post collection, manipulation and analysis are conducted between 34 and 38 °C depending on the species, using a slide warmer and a warm water bath or an incubator. In rodents, semen is collected from the vas deferens (rat) and cauda epididymis (mouse).[60] Small pieces of the vas deferens or a sample from a notch in the cauda epididymis are placed in a warm petri dish containing warm phosphate-buffered saline mixed with bovine serum albumin. The sperm is allowed to diffuse in the media for an incubation period of approximately five minutes; the turbidity of the suspension can be adjusted. An aliquot is then taken directly from the semen sample in the petri dish to fill the two chambers of a sperm counting chamber (e.g. Cell-Vu®, Millennium Inc., New York, NY, USA) or of an automated counter using a computer-assisted sperm motion analysis (CASA) system. In NHP, dogs, and rabbits, a sample is taken directly from the ejaculate and put in a warm media prior to sperm motility analysis.

Sperm motility of all species can be evaluated by a CASA system. Such systems determine the number of motile and nonmotile sperm for each field of vision. The motility is generally assessed using a single 200 spermatozoa count. CASA systems have revolutionized the assessment of sperm motion parameters by offering a practical method for measuring sperm motility and velocity and by permitting analysis of spermatozoa swimming freely in deep chambers. Appropriate sample preparation is essential to avoid artifactual changes.[85] Laboratories without such systems can perform manual microscopic assessment of motility, although this is time consuming and more prone to analytical variation.

Semen Collection for Sperm Counts

While temperature is critical for accurate motility assessment, sperm count analysis can be performed at room temperature. To calculate sperm counts in rodents, the cauda epididymis is transected at the junction with the corpus. Once weighed, the cauda epididymis is placed in a petri dish containing a known quantity of Triton solution. The tissue is then homogenized or minced to make a homogeneous sample. In dogs and rabbits, the amount of sperm ejaculate is directly calculated and then diluted in a 10% buffered formalin and saline solution.[82] In NHP, the gel plug should be dissolved with Triton for several hours prior to the evaluation and then placed in 10% buffered formalin. Further dilution with known amounts of solutions (as applicable for each species) may be required. Sperm count analysis can be performed manually using a hemocytometer or with a CASA system.[85] Sperm concentration results are expressed in sperm/g of cauda epididymis for rodents and rabbits or expressed in sperm/mL or sperm/ejaculate for NHP, rabbits, and dogs.[82,84]

Sperm Morphology

Typically, aliquots of the sperm suspension prepared for evaluation of counts are used for assessing morphology. For rats, dry-fixed slide preparations are made by placing a drop of sperm suspension on a slide, letting it air dry, and staining it with eosin.[82] The sample can be stained prior to application to the slide. Head and tail abnormalities can be induced by air-drying preparations made with unfixed semen.[82]

A preferred method for evaluating sperm morphology in rabbit, dog, and NHP is to prepare a wet smear by spreading a defined volume of sperm suspension (10–200 μL depending on the dilution) on a slide and covering it with a coverslip to avoid artifacts. Evaluation is performed on unstained preparations using a contrast-phase microscope. The key factor is evaluation of a minimum of 200 spermatozoa.

The following morphological features are assessed: head, acrosome, midpiece or tail abnormalities, and sperm agglutination. A simplified system is used in rodents (Tables 66.2 and 66.3).[86] In dogs and NHP, defects are classified as primary or major and secondary or minor.[87] Rat and mouse spermatozoa have a typical head in the shape of a hook, while it is oval in NHPs, rabbits, and dogs (Figure 66.3).[88]

Table 66.2 Abnormal spermatozoa morphology in the rat.

Normally shaped head separated from flagellum
Normally shaped head with abnormal flagellum
Misshapen head with normal flagellum
Misshapen head separated from flagellum
Misshapen head with abnormal flagellum

Table 66.3 Abnormal spermatozoa morphology in the mouse.

Head abnormalities	Lack of usual hook
Tail abnormalities	Banana-like shape
	Amorphous
	Folded
	Two tails
	Others

Urine Sediment Analysis

Species-Specific Methods of Urine Collection

A variety of urine collection methods for laboratory animals include overnight collection, metabolism cages, morning cage pan collection, cystocentesis, catheterization, and manual stimulation. Timed urine collections (approximately 16 hours) are recommended but are more susceptible to bacterial, fecal, or food contamination because of housing conditions. To preserve the urine sediment and reduce bacterial growth, urine samples can be collected on ice overnight by the attachment of tubing to the cage pan that transfers urine into a conical tube immersed in ice within a collection container. Urine collection should be standardized during the study, and procedural-related effects should be considered during interpretation of the urinalysis data. For example, urine volume and specific gravity differ greatly between urine from a 12 to 16 hour metabolic cage collection and catheterization, which collects only the urine accumulated in the bladder.[89] Urine collected from NHP by cystocentesis can have increased RBCs and protein because of the collection technique. All data from treated animals are compared with control animals to distinguish test article-related changes from procedure-related findings.

Food is withheld during overnight collections to limit contamination of urine. Urine collection in mice is limited

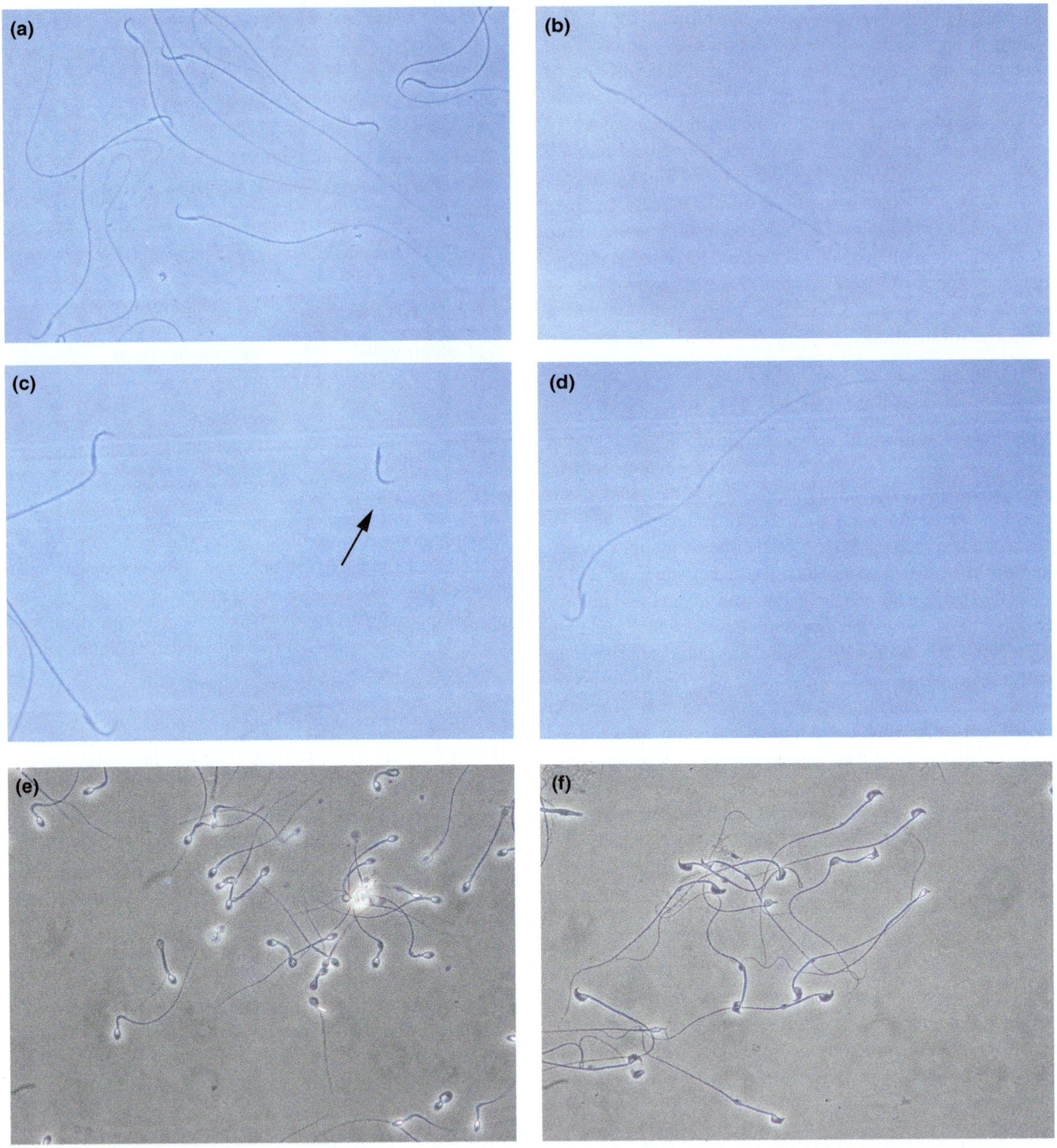

Figure 66.3 Sperm evaluation using unstained wet preparations and phase-contrast microscopy. (a) Untreated rat. Spermatozoa have normal morphology with typical thin hooked heads (400×). (b) Rat. Spermatozoa with a misshapened, extended head and normal flagellum (400×). (c) Rat. Normal detached spermatozoa head (arrow) (400×). (d) Rat. Spermatozoa has a normal head but with a misshapen flagellum (400×). (e) NHP. Spermatozoa with normal morphology. A few have coiled tails and broken heads (100×). (f) Mouse. Spermatozoa exhibit normal morphology (hook head) (200×).

to three to five hours with no food because of the rapid development of hypoglycemia. Water is provided and is particularly important because of the risk of renal toxicity, but contamination of the sample by water can be difficult to avoid when animals play with the water delivery systems. Water access is separated from the living area of rats, and in dogs and monkeys, it is possible to place water catchers below the water access to limit water contamination.

Nonhuman Primates

While NHP are routinely housed in pairs or small groups (European caging), they should be singly housed for urine collection to ensure accurate results. Urine is typically collected in concert with other clinical pathology endpoints necessitating overnight fasting, which prevents urine contamination by food. Overnight urine samples can be obtained from the cage pan and a collection container placed below a hole in the pan. Alternatively, urine can be obtained from a morning cage pan placed in the animal housing cage prior to turning on room lighting at the end of the dark cycle. Once the lights are turned on, the natural inclination of NHP is to urinate, and most monkeys will provide urine within 15 minutes of lights on, providing a quick and relatively contaminant-free sample. Additional collection methods done under sedation or at necropsy include cystocentesis, catheterization, and manual expression.

Minipigs

Urine can be collected using a metabolism cage, via cystocentesis at necropsy, or by catheterization under sedation.[90] Females are easily catheterized, and this method is commonly used; however, catheterization of male minipigs is difficult due to the preputial diverticulum, corkscrew-shaped tip of the penis, and sigmoid flexure of the penis. If a metabolism cage is used, an acclimation period is required to reduce the stress of singly housed animals.

Rats

The most common collection technique for rats uses commercially available plastic or stainless steel metabolism cages constructed to separate urine and feces. Food is withheld overnight, and urine is collected in the morning. It is also possible to collect urine by cystocentesis at necropsy. Less frequent techniques include stimulation or massage by gentle transabdominal pressure and catheterization under anesthesia with the animal restrained in a supine position. In females, a catheter is carefully inserted into the external urethral ostium and advanced parallel to the spinal cord approximately 10 mm to ensure bladder access.[91] In males, compression next to the base of the foreskin causes the tip of the penis to extrude, and a catheter can be inserted.[92]

Mice

For urine collection, mice are usually placed in metabolic cage for a few hours (a maximum of five hours) with no food. The quantities obtained are often insufficient for standard urinalysis, and sediment is rarely evaluated. Kurien and Scofield[92] describe a urine collection method whereby clear plastic wrap is placed upon a sheet of white paper. A mouse is then placed on the plastic wrap and kept there until it urinates. It was possible to obtain volumes of 10–250 μL in a relatively short period of time (as quickly as 12 seconds) with this method. Mice also can be placed on a hydrophobic sand (Labsand®, Coastline Global Inc., Palo Alto, CA, USA) that keeps the animal urine on top, making sample collection easy by aspiration of the urine droplets. It allows collection of a sufficient quantity of urine for urinalysis and does not interfere with the enzymatic reactions of the urine strips (authors' observations).

Dogs

Urine collection in dogs is most often performed with the use of metabolism cages but can also be done via cystocentesis (restrained or at necropsy) or catheterization. With the use of metabolism cages, food is withheld, but animals have access to water; however, samples can be compromised by fecal contamination. The collection trays of metabolism cages are constructed to allow urine to drain through tubing into a collection container. A porous metal screen is used to cover the tray in order to reduce fecal contamination. Cystocentesis provides the highest quality sample; however, it is a more labor intensive procedure and may be prohibitive in large toxicology studies.

Rabbits

Voided rabbit urine is thick and cloudy because of large amounts of mucus, numerous calcium carbonate crystals, and lesser numbers of triple phosphates.[93] Like horses, rabbits have relatively high total serum calcium concentrations and increased renal calcium excretion.[94] Thus, urine requires centrifugation prior to evaluation because of the abundance of crystals.[95] Urine collection in rabbits is best performed using cystocentesis in dorsal recumbency under sedation or at necropsy. Collection in newborn rabbits (2–10 days old) by manual stimulation is recommended.[92] This method can be used in adults, but it takes longer for urine to be released, and animals are more prone to injury during restraint. Urine can be collected from a pan placed under the wire grid floor of the cage; however, metabolism cages enhance separation of urine from feces. The physical properties of rabbit urine and crystalluria make microscopic sediment examination difficult, and therefore, it is not recommended as part of routine clinical pathology evaluation in this species.[95]

Urine Storage and Processing

Urine at room temperature should be evaluated within a few hours of collection. When prompt evaluation is not feasible, specimens can be refrigerated for up to 24 hours. If urine was collected on ice, it should be maintained on ice or stored in a refrigerator set at 4 °C until analysis. For evaluation of urine sediment, samples from adult rats and large animal species should be mixed gently by inversion and a sufficient volume of urine (1–5 mL) placed in a conical tube for centrifugation at 700g for 5 minutes. The supernatant is decanted, leaving approximately 0.5 mL for resuspension of the sediment pellet. The resuspended sample is maintained at ambient temperature for the sediment evaluation. In mice and juvenile rats, urine sediment can be prepared with urine volumes of less than 1.0 mL. In a recent study comparing urine sediments prepared with urine volumes as low as 30 µL with no centrifugation to sediments prepared with large urine volumes (5 mL) after centrifugation, it was found that results were more reproducible with lower urine volume than with large volumes.[96]

Urine Color and Clarity

Urine can be a variety of colors and is most often shades of yellow ranging from very pale or colorless to very dark or amber. Urine color changes with the degree of urine concentration or dilution. Red or brown colored urine may be a sign of hematuria and should be confirmed with examination of urine sediment. Reddish coloration in the urine of rabbits may be associated with excretion of dietary porphyrin pigment and is often incorrectly identified as hematuria.[97,98] Normal urine in laboratory animals is generally clear to slightly cloudy. Increased turbidity can be associated with the presence of blood, inflammation, crystals, mucus, and/or debris in the urine.

Microscopic Sediment Exam

Urine sediment evaluation involves semiquantitative microscopic analysis of WBCs, RBCs, casts, crystals, bacteria, and other routine elements. A urine sediment stain (i.e. Sedi-Stain™, BD Worldwide, Franklin Lakes, NJ, USA) and/or polarized light can be used to further enhance identification. A small drop of resuspended urine sediment is placed on a glass microscope slide using a pipette, and a coverslip is applied. When evaluating multiple animals on a toxicology study, KOVA Glasstic® Slides (KOVA International, Garden Grove, CA, USA) allow for preparation of 10 specimens at a time for faster evaluation. When a large amount of sediment prevents identification of microscopic elements, the sediment is diluted with isotonic saline at 1 : 1 or greater, if needed. Microscopic evaluation of urine in toxicological studies should adhere to rigid preparation techniques, and the same method should be used for all urine samples of a study. Low microscopic lighting is helpful in highlighting elements of an unstained preparation. The entire chamber or coverslipped area should be examined with a 10× objective (low magnification) for the presence of casts. Five to ten microscopic fields of the sediment should be examined with the 40× objective (high power field, HPF) for cells, crystals, and bacteria. Depending on the species, elements such as spermatozoa, epithelial cells, mucus, yeast, and amorphous crystals are of limited toxicological significance and are generally not reported. Prolonged exposure of cells and casts to urine leads to degenerative changes or cell lysis, which can become a problem with prolonged, timed urine collections. If changes in urine sediment are a consideration, an alternative method of urine collection should be used.

Cells

Leukocytes Neutrophils, eosinophils, lymphocytes, monocytes, or macrophages can rapidly lyse in alkaline or dilute urine samples. Neutrophils are the cells most commonly present in urine, and observing an average of 0–5 cells per HPF is considered normal.[99] Increased numbers of neutrophils indicate inflammation due to a urinary tract infection, urolithiasis, or prostatitis. Lymphocytes, plasma cells, and macrophages can be present with chronic inflammatory disease.[100]

Erythrocytes RBCs are small, measuring ~6–7 µm, and lack internal structures. In diluted or alkaline urine, they can appear colorless and swollen and can lyse. Prolonged time in urine causes RBCs to crenate, making them easier to distinguish from lipid droplets, yeast, WBCs, or amorphous urate crystals.[101] To aid examination, acetic acid can be added to a portion the sediment to lyse the RBCs, leaving other elements intact.[102] Normal urine can contain 0–5 RBCs per HPF, while higher numbers characterize the urine of female monkeys during menses and dogs during proestrus. Larger numbers can indicate hemorrhage, inflammation, or necrosis.

Epithelial Cells Low numbers of epithelial cells including squamous, transitional, and renal are considered normal in urine. However, large numbers may be pathological, and histopathologic evaluation of the kidneys and bladder is warranted. Large, thin squamous epithelial cells can be observed in the sediment of healthy animals and originate from the urethra, vulva, or vagina.[100]

Casts

Casts are cylindrical-shaped concretions of fluid and/or cells that form in the loops of Henle, distal tubules, and collecting ducts.[101] Casts are primarily composed of Tamm–Horsfall mucoprotein secreted by epithelial cells and can accumulate disintegrated material, WBCs, RBCs, or epithelial cells. They are generally categorized as cellular, hyaline, granular, waxy, broad, or mixed. Hyaline and granular casts are occasionally observed in low numbers

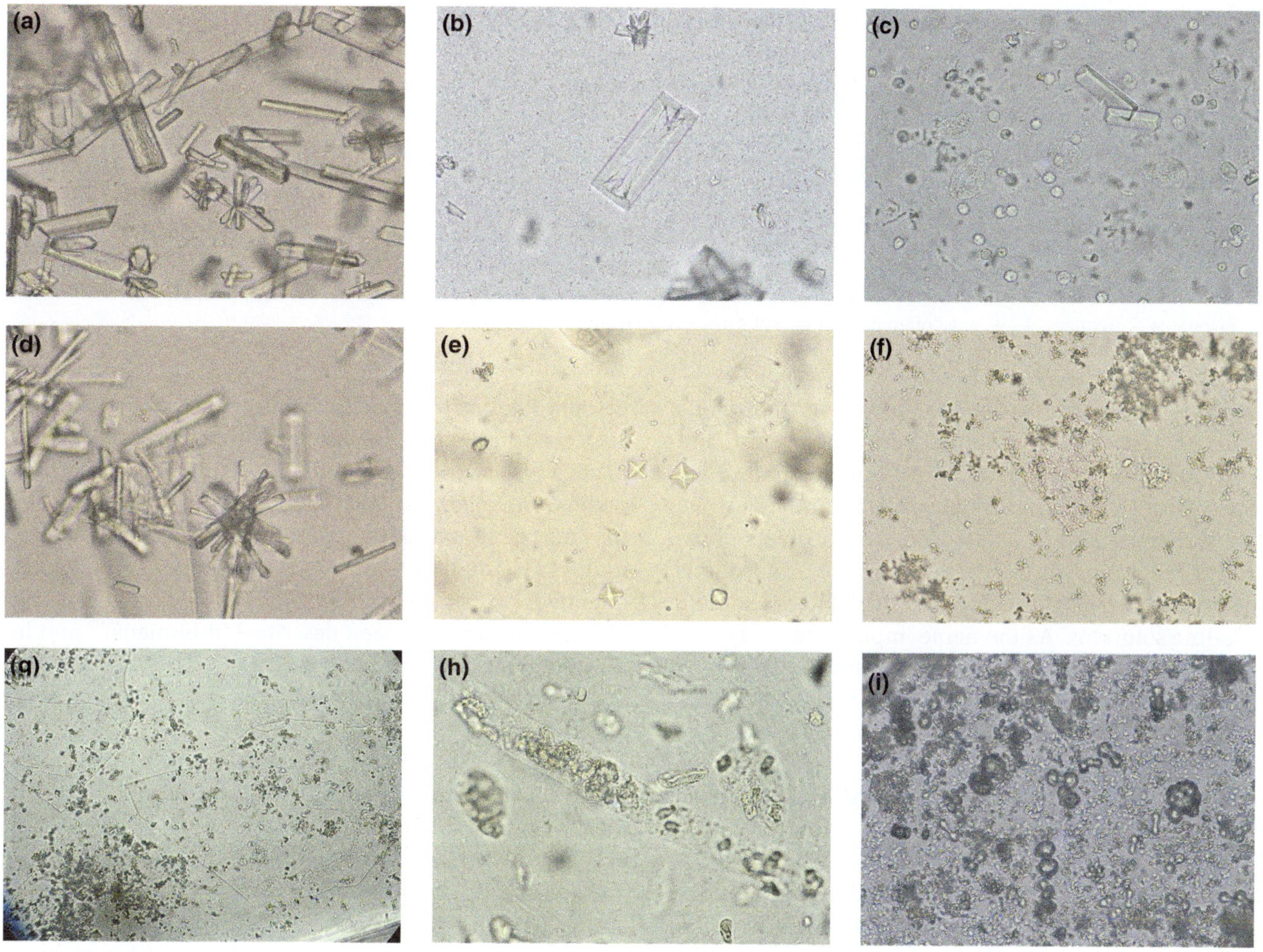

Figure 66.4 Unstained urine sediment. (a) Rat. Numerous triple phosphate crystals are common in this species (400×). (b) Rat. There are a few triple phosphate crystals and numerous bacteria. Bacterial contamination of samples is common with overnight cage pan collections (400×). (c) Dog. This sample contains a few epithelial cells, RBCs, occasional leukocytes, occasional bacteria, and several triple phosphate crystals (100×). (d) Dog. Calcium phosphate crystals (brushites) in alkaline urine (400×). (e) NHP. Calcium oxalate dihydrate crystals are common in this species (100×). (f and g) Overnight cage pan collection from a NHP. Calcium phosphate plates and amorphous phosphates (100×). (h) NHP. Example of a hyaline cast and epithelial cells, with occasional leukocytes and RBCs (400×). (i) Rabbit. Calcium carbonate crystals with a "dumbbell" form and amorphous phosphates are common in this species (100×).

in urine from healthy animals (Figure 66.4g).[95,100] Cellular casts (RBC, WBC, epithelial) degenerate to become granular casts, which then become waxy casts, all of which indicate injury to the renal tubules and/or urine stasis. Waxy casts are rarely observed in toxicological studies. The observation of cellular casts usually correlates with the histopathological findings of casts within the renal tubules.

Crystals

Urinary crystals are commonly observed in healthy laboratory animals, and their formation is dependent upon the pH, temperature, food, and test article.[101,103] Crystals commonly observed in the urine of laboratory animals include amorphous, calcium oxalate, triple phosphate, calcium phosphate, and calcium carbonate (Table 66.4). These can be observed in low numbers in control animals with no renal lesions, but their concentrations can increase with pathological conditions. Test articles can induce crystalluria by modifying the pH or renal excretion of minerals such as calcium and phosphorus. Test articles and metabolites excreted by the kidney can form urinary crystals or droplets. Pathological crystals include bilirubin, sodium urates, cholesterol, uric acid, and ammonium urates. The formation of cystine or leucine crystals is unlikely in preclinical studies.[104]

Table 66.4 Common urinary crystals and casts in laboratory animal species.

	Amorphous crystals	Calcium oxalate crystals	Triple phosphate crystals	Calcium phosphate	Calcium carbonate	Hyaline cast	Granular cast
Rat	++	+	+++	Rare	Rare	Rare	Rare
Dog	+	+++	++	+ (brushites)	–	+	+
NHP	+	+	+	+ (plates)	+	+	+
Rabbit	+++	Rare	+	–	+++	–	–

+, occasional; ++, frequent; +++, most often present; –, not expected; NHP, nonhuman primate.

Amorphous Phosphate and Urate Crystals Amorphous crystals consist of sodium, potassium, magnesium, and calcium urates or phosphates.[101] Amorphous phosphate crystals form in alkaline urine, while amorphous urate crystals are observed in acidic urine. Amorphous phosphate crystals are soluble in acetic acid. Amorphous urate crystals are insoluble in acetic acid, but are soluble in alkaline solutions. As the name implies, these crystals have no definite shape, and visual distinction between the two crystals type is not possible. As such, classification is usually based on the pH of the urine. These crystals are frequently observed in the urine of all laboratory animal species, but are usually not recorded, as they have no known significance.

Calcium Oxalate Calcium oxalate dihydrate crystals are usually colorless and have a distinctive dipyramidal, octahedral, or envelope shape (Figure 66.4e). They most often form in urine with an acidic or neutral pH and are soluble in hypochloric acid, but insoluble in acetic acid. Dihydrate calcium oxalate crystals are frequently observed in the urine of dogs and can also be observed in the urine of rats and NHP. In general, these crystals have no clinical significance; however, increased numbers can be seen with increased urinary excretion of calcium. Calcium oxalate monohydrate crystals are unusual and are observed in pathological conditions. They vary in size and can have a spindle, oval, or dumbbell appearance.

Triple Phosphate Triple phosphate (magnesium ammonium phosphate or struvite) crystals may be seen in abundant numbers in rats and are commonly observed in dogs, monkeys, and rabbits (Figure 66.4a and b). In low numbers, they have no clinical significance, but their concentration increases with dehydration and urinary tract lesions. These crystals are easily identified in urine, appearing as colorless prisms referred to as "coffin lids" with three to six sides and oblique ends. They form in neutral and alkaline urine and are soluble in acetic acid.

Calcium Phosphate Calcium phosphate crystals form in alkaline urine and are soluble in acetic acid. Calcium phosphate crystals can be observed as long, thin, colorless prisms with a pointed end that may resemble a rosette, or they may be spherical in shape, and referred to as brushites in dogs (Figure 66.4d). In the urine of monkeys, they frequently form large asymmetrical plates (Figure 66.4f and g). These plates have been described in humans[105] and in no other species other than NHP. In NHP, they are frequently observed in urine collected overnight (authors' observations).

Calcium Carbonate Calcium carbonate crystals form in alkaline or neutral urine and are soluble when mixed with acetic acid. They are colorless to yellow-brown crystals that are dumbbell to oval in shape but are also seen as large spheroids with radial striations. They can be found individually or in large granular masses. Calcium carbonate crystals are larger than amorphous crystals and, when observed in clumps, can have a dark color. These crystals are abundant in rabbit urine and are usually present with large amounts of amorphous phosphates, precluding visualization of other urine elements (Figure 66.4i). These crystals are also considered a normal finding in guinea pig urine.

Bilirubin (Crystals and/or Pigment) Bilirubin crystals are an uncommon finding in urine sediment. They form in acidic urine with the presence of soluble conjugated bilirubin and appear as orange-reddish needles or orange-yellow-brown granules. Bilirubin crystals can be found in low numbers in healthy dogs but are considered abnormal in other laboratory animal species. Their presence may be an indication of hepatic toxicity or biliary obstruction, and should be correlated to hepatic or gastrointestinal lesions and the presence of bilirubin in urine.

Cholesterol Crystals Cholesterol crystals are infrequently observed. They form in acidic urine and are soluble in chloroform. They are large, flat, colorless plates with notched corners and are occasionally observed in normal dogs,

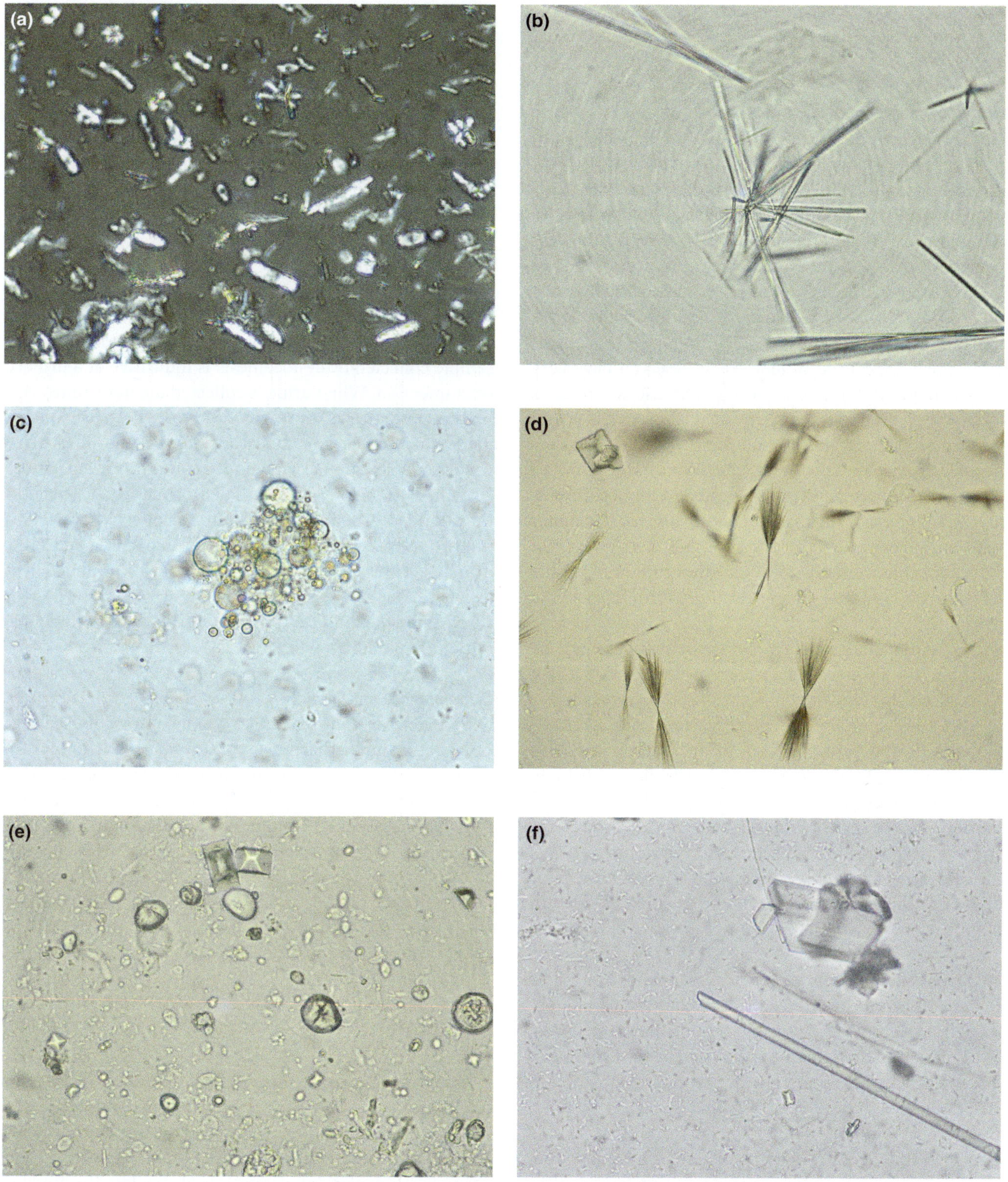

Figure 66.5 Examples of compound-induced urine crystals or material and contaminants in unstained urine sediments. (a) Rat. Compound-induced crystals (Refractive light, 100×). (b) NHP. Thin compound-induced crystals (400×). (c) Rat. Compound-induced droplets (400×). (d) Dog. Tyrosine-like compound-induced crystals and a few calcium oxalate dihydrate crystals (400×). (e) Rat. Food contamination in urine from an overnight collection in a cage pan. The large round crystal-like forms are food debris. Numerous bacteria and a few triple phosphate crystals are present in the background (100×). (f) Rat. Contamination of urine with cage bedding material appears as long thin crystal-like debris. Numerous bacteria and a few triple phosphate crystals are present in the background (400×).

although rarely in toxicological studies. The finding of large numbers of cholesterol crystals may indicate renal disease.[101]

Uric Acid, Ammonium Urate, and Sodium Urate Crystals Uric acid crystals are not expected in most mammalian species with the exception of humans and great apes (e.g. chimpanzee and gorilla). This is because humans and great apes lack the enzyme uricase that, in other mammalian species including those used in research studies, catalyzes the degradation of uric acid into allantoin in the liver.[106,107] The allantoin is then excreted by the kidneys. Because humans and great apes lack uricase, they excrete uric acid instead of allantoin in the urine. Cynomolgus monkeys (not classified as great apes) used in biomedical research have very low to barely detectable concentrations of uric acid in their blood.[108] However, in rabbits, uric acid is present in serum and may be elevated with renal toxicity.[94] Although rarely affected in toxicological studies, alterations in the elimination of uric acid are regularly suspected. With hepatic toxicity and decreased uricase function, uric acid urinary excretion will occur. Uric acid crystals have a yellow-brown color and characteristic form of diamond or rhombic plates, which may contain rosettes. They form in an acidic environment.

Ammonium urate crystals are uncommon but can be present in normal dogs and also form with hepatic toxicity and reduced ammonia metabolism.[101] It is therefore possible to observe such crystals during a toxicological study. Ammonium urate crystals form in an acid environment and appear as yellow-brown spherical bodies with long, irregular protrusions. Among the amorphous urates, described earlier, sodium urate crystals can be observed for the same reasons and have been observed in normal dogs and rats (Authors' observations). They are colorless or yellowish needles, are present in clusters, and dissolve in alkaline urine.

Compound-Related Crystals Test compounds or their metabolites can form urine crystals if they are eliminated through the kidneys and precipitate in urine. For example, the formation of sulfonamide crystals in the urine has been well described and is due to the low solubility of sulfonamides; the solubility of sulfonamides has now been improved.[100] Similarly, ampicillin and xanthine crystals have been described in dogs.[101] Urine crystals are rarely observed and are not expected to form during toxicological studies. Thus, when observed, they are considered an important finding. Compound-related crystals have been observed in various forms (Figure 66.5) including rosette, needles, circular, and oval shapes (authors' observations). They have not been observed in animals receiving vehicle controls, and their concentration tends to depend on the dose of compound administered. The crystalloid nature can be verified by the evaluation of urine sediment with a contrast-phase microscope, as crystals tend to refract the light (Figure 66.5a). Further characterization of such crystals can be done by liquid chromatography and mass spectrometry.[101]

Bacteria

Pleomorphic populations of bacteria are frequently observed in urine samples collected via cage pan or metabolism cage, but should not be observed in samples collected via cystocentesis. The presence of bacteria and WBCs in a sample collected by cystocentesis is indicative of a urinary tract infection. When urine is collected during a timed collection period (e.g. overnight), the presence of contaminants such as feces or food can increase the number of bacteria; collection of urine on ice can minimize bacterial growth.[109] Hence, evaluation for a urinary tract bacterial infection is not reliable with samples collected overnight, unless there is a significant difference in bacteria and WBC numbers between the treated and control animals. Test article-related decreases in numbers of bacteria are more easily evaluated and can occur if a drug or its metabolites inhibits bacterial growth.[104]

Contaminants and Normal Elements

Other elements that are unlikely to be of toxicological significance include urine mucus, protozoa (i.e. Trichomonas), parasite ova, sperm, lipid droplets, and amorphous crystals. These generally represent incidental background findings and may indicate contamination. Fecal contamination of samples is not unusual and may lead to the observation of trophozoites, such as *Balantidium coli*, in the urine.[110] Food and cage material can contaminate the urine and are easily confused with crystals (Figure 66.4e and f), but are not dissolved with acetic acid or alkali.

Conclusions

Cytology is an important endpoint for many studies in biomedical research and toxicology. In this particular context, evaluation of cytological samples uses methods similar to those in diagnostic laboratories for companion animals. However, interpretation of cytology findings is different within such studies, as it is necessary to take into consideration the peculiarities of laboratory animal species and the differences in methods of sample collection. Comparisons to reference intervals are of limited use for study interpretation because of the complexity and variable conditions of each study. Comparisons with control groups are essential in distinguishing compound-related findings from analytical and biological variations. The cytopathologist has an essential role to play in such studies, as the understanding of animal physiology and laboratory methods remain essential for study interpretation.

References

1 EMEA (2010). *Guideline on Repeated Dose Toxicity*. CPMP/SWP/1042/99 Rev 1 Corr*. London: European Medicines Agency.

2 FDA (2003). *Guidance for Industry and Other Stakeholders. Toxicological Principles for the Safety Assessment of Food Ingredients. Redbook 2000: IV.B.1 General Guidelines for Designing and Conducting Toxicity Studies*. College Park, MD: U.S. Department of Health and Human Services.

3 EMA (2009). ICH guideline M3(R2) on non-clinical safety studies for the conduct of human clinical trials and marketing authorization for pharmaceuticals, EMA/CPMP/ICH/286/1995.

4 Weingand, K., Brown, G., Hall, R. et al. (1996). Harmonization of animal clinical pathology testing in toxicity and safety studies. *Fundam Appl Toxicol* 29: 198–201.

5 Tomlinson, L., Boone, L.I., Ramaiah, L. et al. (2013). Best practices for veterinary toxicologic clinical pathology, with emphasis on the pharmaceutical and biotechnology industries. *Vet Clin Pathol* 42: 252–269.

6 International Conference on Harmonization. (2005). Detection of toxicity to reproduction for medicinal products & toxicity to male fertility S5(R2). http://www.ich.org/products/guidelines/safety/safety-single/article/detection-of-toxicity-to-reproduction-for-medicinal-products-toxicity-to-male-fertility.html (accessed 5 December 2019).

7 International Conference on Harmonization (2009). S6(R1) Preclinical safety evaluation of biotechnology-derived pharmaceuticals. http://www.ich.org/products/guidelines/safety/safety-single/article/preclinical-safety-evaluation-of-biotechnology-derived-pharmaceuticals.html (accessed 5 December 2019).

8 Halpern, W.G., Ameri, M., Bowman, C.J. et al. (2016). Scientific and regulatory policy committee points to consider review: inclusion of reproductive and pathology end points for assessment of reproductive and developmental toxicity in pharmaceutical drug development. *Toxicol Pathol* 44: 789–809.

9 Reagan, W.J., Irizarry-Rovira, A., Poitout-Belissent, F. et al. (2011). Best practices for evaluation of bone marrow in nonclinical toxicity studies. *Toxicol Pathol* 39: 435–448.

10 Wright, J.L., Cosio, M., and Churg, A. (2008). Animal models of chronic obstructive pulmonary disease. *Am J Physiol Lung Cell Mol Physiol* 295: L1–L15.

11 Hannon, J.P., Tigani, B., Williams, I. et al. (2001). Mechanism of airway hyperresponsiveness to adenosine induced by allergen challenge in actively sensitized Brown Norway rats. *Br J Pharmacol* 132: 1509–1523.

12 Lapa e Silva, J.R., Ruffie, C., Lefort, J. et al. (1997). Role of eosinophilic airway inflammation in models of asthma. *Mem Inst Oswaldo Cruz* 92 (Suppl. 2): 223–226.

13 Nials, A.T. and Uddin, S. (2008). Mouse models of allergic asthma: acute and chronic allergen challenge. *Dis Model Mech* 1: 213–220.

14 Dorato, M.A. (1990). Overview of inhalation toxicology. *Environ Health Perspect* 85: 163–170.

15 Porter, D.W., Hubbs, A.F., Baron, P.A. et al. (2007). Pulmonary toxicity of Expancel microspheres in the rat. *Toxicol Pathol* 35: 702–714.

16 Harris, N., Kunicka, J., and Kratz, A. (2005). The ADVIA 2120 hematology system: flow cytometry-based analysis of blood and body fluids in the routine hematology laboratory. *Lab Hematol* 11: 47–61.

17 Gorman, M.E., Villarroel, A., Tornquist, S.J. et al. (2009). Comparison between manual and automated total nucleated cell counts using the ADVIA 120 for pleural and peritoneal fluid samples from dogs, cats, horses, and alpacas. *Vet Clin Pathol* 38: 388–391.

18 Brudvig, J.M. and Swenson, C.L. (2015). Total nucleated cell and leukocyte differential counts in canine pleural and peritoneal fluid and equine synovial fluid samples: comparison of automated and manual methods. *Vet Clin Pathol* 44: 570–579.

19 Pinto da Cunha, N., Giordano, A., Caniatti, M., and Paltrinieri, S. (2009). Analytical validation of the Sysmex XT-2000iV for cell counts in canine and feline effusions and concordance with cytologic diagnosis. *Vet Clin Pathol* 38: 230–241.

20 Hatzelmann, A., Haefner, D., Beume, R., and Schudt, C. (1996). Automatic leukocyte differentiation in bronchoalveolar lavage fluids of guinea pigs and brown-Norway rats. *J Pharmacol Toxicol Methods* 35: 91–99.

21 Natiello, M., Kelly, G., Lamca, J. et al. (2009). Manual and automated leukocyte differentiation in bronchoalveolar lavage fluids from rodent models of pulmonary inflammation. *Comp Clin Pathol* 18: 101–111.

22 Allison, R.W. and Velguth, K.E. (2010). Appearance of granulated cells in blood films stained by automated aqueous versus methanolic Romanowsky methods. *Vet Clin Pathol* 39: 99–104.

23 Haley, P.J., Muggenburg, B.A., Rebar, A.H. et al. (1989). Bronchoalveolar lavage cytology in cynomolgus monkeys and identification of cytologic alterations following sequential saline lavage. *Vet Pathol* 26: 265–273.

24 Raskin, R.E. and Wardrop, K.J. (2010). Species specific hematology. In: *Schalm's Veterinary Hematology* (eds. D.J. Weiss and K.J. Wardrop), 797–1018. Ames, IA: Wiley-Blackwell.

25 Fiscus, L.C., Van Herpen, J., Steeber, D.A. et al. (2001). L-Selectin is required for the development of airway hyperresponsiveness but not airway inflammation in a murine model of asthma. *J Allergy Clin Immunol* 107: 1019–1024.

26 Ito, M., Takeuchi, N., Masuno, T. et al. (1975). Lung damage caused by phospholipase C and the changes in phospholipids in the rat lung. *Jpn J Exp Med* 45: 479–488.

27 Drent, M., Cobben, N.A., Henderson, R.F. et al. (1996). Usefulness of lactate dehydrogenase and its isoenzymes as indicators of lung damage or inflammation. *Eur Respir J* 9: 1736–1742.

28 DeNicola, D.B., Rebar, A.H., and Henderson, R.F. (1981). Early damage indicators in the lung. V. Biochemical and cytological response to NO_2 inhalation. *Toxicol Appl Pharmacol* 60: 301–312.

29 Beck, B.D., Gerson, B., Feldman, H.A., and Brain, J.D. (1983). Lactate dehydrogenase isoenzymes in hamster lung lavage fluid after lung injury. *Toxicol Appl Pharmacol* 71: 59–71.

30 Dahl, M. and Nordestgaard, B.G. (2009). Markers of early disease and prognosis in COPD. *Int J Chron Obstruct Pulmon Dis* 4: 157–167.

31 Henderson, R.F. (2005). Use of bronchoalveolar lavage to detect respiratory tract toxicity of inhaled material. *Exp Toxicol Pathol* 57 (Suppl 1): 155–159.

32 Keul, P., Lucke, S., von Wnuck Lipinski, K. et al. (2011). Sphingosine-1-phosphate receptor 3 promotes recruitment of monocyte/macrophages in inflammation and atherosclerosis. *Circ Res* 108: 314–323.

33 Segal, B.H., Kuhns, D.B., Ding, L. et al. (2002). Thioglycollate peritonitis in mice lacking C5, 5-lipoxygenase, or p47(phox): complement, leukotrienes, and reactive oxidants in acute inflammation. *J Leukoc Biol* 71: 410–416.

34 Smith, S.R., Denhardt, G., and Terminelli, C. (2001). The anti-inflammatory activities of cannabinoid receptor ligands in mouse peritonitis models. *Eur J Pharmacol* 432: 107–119.

35 Lefebvre, E., Moyle, G., Reshef, R. et al. (2016). Antifibrotic effects of the dual CCR2/CCR5 antagonist cenicriviroc in animal models of liver and kidney fibrosis. *PLoS One* 11: e0158156.

36 Butt, M.T. (2011). Morphologic changes associated with intrathecal catheters for direct delivery to the central nervous system in preclinical studies. *Toxicol Pathol* 39: 213–219.

37 West, W., Ehrmann, J., and Johnson, W. (2014). Chronic lumbar intrathecal catheterization for the collection of cerebrospinal fluid in the canine. *J Investig Surg* 27: 226–233.

38 Sharma, A.K., Schultze, A.E., Cooper, D.M. et al. (2006). Development of a percutaneous cerebrospinal fluid collection technique in F-344 rats and evaluation of cell counts and total protein concentrations. *Toxicol Pathol* 34: 393–395.

39 Felice, B.R., Wright, T.L., Boyd, R.B. et al. (2011). Safety evaluation of chronic intrathecal administration of idursulfase-IT in cynomolgus monkeys. *Toxicol Pathol* 39: 879–892.

40 Perron, J., Trude, Y., Emond, F. et al. (2008). Collection of cerebrospinal fluid by direct puncture or by surgically implanted ports in monkeys. *Proceedings of the Society of Toxicology*, Seattle, WA (16–20 March 2008).

41 Consiglio, A.R. and Lucion, A.B. (2000). Technique for collecting cerebrospinal fluid in the cisterna magna of non-anesthetized rats. *Brain Res Brain Res Protoc* 5: 109–114.

42 Nirogi, R., Kandikere, V., Mudigonda, K. et al. (2009). A simple and rapid method to collect the cerebrospinal fluid of rats and its application for the assessment of drug penetration into the central nervous system. *J Neurosci Methods* 178: 116–119.

43 Aune, M.W., Becker, J.L., Brugnara, C. et al. (2004). Automated flow cytometric analysis of blood cells in cerebrospinal fluid: analytic performance. *Am J Clin Pathol* 121: 690–700.

44 Ruotsalo, K., Poma, R., da Costa, R.C., and Bienzle, D. (2008). Evaluation of the ADVIA 120 for analysis of canine cerebrospinal fluid. *Vet Clin Pathol* 37: 242–248.

45 Cowell, R.L., Tyler, R.D., and Meinkoth, J.H. (1998). Cerebrospinal fluid analysis. In: *Diagnostic Cytology and Hematology of the Dog and Cat*, 2e (eds. R.L. Cowell, R.D. Tyler and J.H. Meinkoth), 125–141. St Louis, MO: Mosby, Inc.

46 De Lorenzi, D. and Mandara, M.T. (2009). The central nervous system. In: *Canine and Feline Cytology: A Color

Atlas and Interpretation Guide, 2e (eds. R.E. Raskin and D.J. Meyer), 325–365. St Louis, MO: Elsevier.

47 Stokol, T., Divers, T.J., Arrigan, J.W., and SP, M.D. (2009). Cerebrospinal fluid findings in cattle with central nervous system disorders: a retrospective study of 102 cases (1990–2008). *Vet Clin Pathol* 38: 103–112.

48 Seeuws, S., Jacques, P., Van Praet, J. et al. (2010). A multiparameter approach to monitor disease activity in collagen-induced arthritis. *Arthritis Res Ther* 12: R160.

49 Oestergaard, S., Chouinard, L., Doyle, N. et al. (2006). The utility of measuring C-terminal telopeptides of collagen type II (CTX-II) in serum and synovial fluid samples for estimation of articular cartilage status in experimental models of destructive joint diseases. *Osteoarthr Cartil* 14: 670–679.

50 Barton, N.J., Stevens, D.A., Hughes, J.P. et al. (2007). Demonstration of a novel technique to quantitatively assess inflammatory mediators and cells in rat knee joints. *J Inflamm* 4: 13.

51 Ekmann, A., Rigdal, M.L., and Grondahl, G. (2010). Automated counting of nucleated cells in equine synovial fluid without and with hyaluronidase pretreatment. *Vet Clin Pathol* 39: 83–89.

52 Goldman, J.M., Murr, A.S., and Cooper, R.L. (2007). The rodent estrous cycle: characterization of vaginal cytology and its utility in toxicological studies. *Birth Defects Res B Dev Reprod Toxicol* 80: 84–97.

53 Boot, L.M., Muhlbock, O., and Thung, P.J. (1956). Senile changes in the oestrous cycle and in ovarian structure in some inbred strains of mice. *Acta Endocrinol* 23: 8–32.

54 Cooper, R.L. and Goldman, J.M. (1999). Vaginal cytology. In: *An Evaluation and Interpretation of Reproductive Endpoints for Human Health Risk Assessment* (eds. G.P. Daston and C.A. Kimmel), 42–56. Washington, DC: ILSI Press.

55 Byers, S.L., Wiles, M.V., Dunn, S.L., and Taft, R.A. (2012). Mouse estrous cycle identification tool and images. *PLoS One* 7: e35538.

56 OECD. Organisation for the Economic Co-operation and Development (n.d.). Part 5: Preparation, Reading and Reporting of Vaginal Smears. April 1, 2014. http://www.oecd.org/chemicalsafety/testing/40581357.pdf (accessed 5 December 2019).

57 Cora, M.C., Kooistra, L., and Travlos, G. (2015). Vaginal cytology of the laboratory rat and mouse: review and criteria for the staging of the estrous cycle using stained vaginal smears. *Toxicol Pathol* 43: 776–793.

58 Nelson, J.F., Felicio, L.S., Randall, P.K. et al. (1982). A longitudinal study of estrous cyclicity in aging C57BL/6J mice. I. Cycle frequency, length and vaginal cytology. *Biol Reprod* 27: 327–339.

59 Mandl, A.M. (1951). The phases of the oestrous cycle in the adult white rat. *J Exp Biol* 28: 576–584.

60 Morrissey, R.E., Schwetz, B.A., Lamb, J.C. et al. (1988). Evaluation of rodent sperm, vaginal cytology, and reproductive organ weight data from National Toxicology Program 13-week studies. *Fundam Appl Toxicol* 11: 343–358.

61 Long, J.A. and Evans, H.M. (1922). *The Oestrous Cycle in the Rat and its Associated Phenomena*, Memoirs of the University of California, 1–148. University of California.

62 Parkes, A.S. (1928). The length of the oestrous cycle in the unmated normal mouse: records of one thousand cycles. *J Exp Biol* 5: 371–377.

63 Blandau, R.J., Boling, J.L., and Young, W.C. (1941). The length of heat in the albino rat as determined by copulatory response. *Anat Rec* 79: 453–463.

64 Li, S. and Davis, B. (2007). Evaluating rodent vaginal and uterine histology in toxicity studies. *Birth Defects Res B Dev Reprod Toxicol* 80: 246–252.

65 Campbell, C.S., Ryan, K.D., and Schwartz, N.B. (1976). Estrous cycles in the mouse: relative influence of continuous light and the presence of a male. *Biol Reprod* 14: 292–299.

66 Campbell, C.S. and Schwartz, N.B. (1980). The impact of constant light on the estrous cycle of the rat. *J Endocrinol* 106: 1230–1238.

67 Whitten, W.K. (1956). Modification of the oestrous cycle of the mouse by external stimuli associated with the male. *J Endocrinol* 13: 399–404.

68 Allen, E.W. (1922). The oestrous cycle in the mouse. *Am J Anat* 30: 297–371.

69 Astwood, E.B. (1939). Changes in the weight and water content of the uterus of the normal adult rat. *Am J Phys* 261: 162–170.

70 Grasso, P., Rozhavskaya, M., and Reichert, L.E. Jr. (1998). In vivo effects of human follicle-stimulating hormone-related synthetic peptide hFSH-beta-(81–95) and its subdomain hFSH-beta-(90–95) on the mouse estrous cycle. *Biol Reprod* 58: 821–825.

71 Young, W.C., Boling, J.L., and Blandau, R.J. (1941). The vaginal smear picture, sexual receptivity and time of ovulation in the albino rat. *Anat Rec* 80: 37–45.

72 Hubscher, C.H., Brooks, D.L., and Johnson, J.R. (2005). A quantitative method for assessing stages of the rat estrous cycle. *Biotech Histochem* 80: 79–87.

73 Weinbauer, G.F., Niehoff, M., Niehaus, M. et al. (2008). Physiology and endocrinology of the ovarian cycle in macaques. *Toxicol Pathol* 36: 7S–23S.

74 Bussiere, J.L., Moffat, G., Zhou, L., and Tarlo, K.S. (2013). Assessment of menstrual cycle length in cynomolgus monkeys as a female fertility endpoint of a biopharmaceutical in a 6 month toxicity study. *Regul Toxicol Pharmacol* 66: 269–278.

75 Travis, J.C. and Holmes, W.N. (1974). Some physiological and behavioural changes associated with oestrus and pregnancy in the squirrel monkey (*Saimiri sciureus*). *J Zool* 174: 41–66.

76 Tarif, S., Carville, A., Elmore, D. et al. (2012). Reproduction and breeding of nonhuman primates. In: *Nonhuman Primates in Biomedical Research*, 2e (eds. C.R. Abee, K. Mansfield, S. Tardif and T. Morris), 197–249. Waltham, MA: Elsevier.

77 Hernandez-Lopez, L., Mayagoitia, L., Esquivel-Lacroix, C. et al. (1998). The menstrual cycle of the spider monkey (*Ateles geoffroyi*). *Am J Primatol* 44: 183–195.

78 Gluckman, T.L., Walz, S.E., Schultz-Darken, N., and Bolton, I.D. (2004). Cytologic assessment of the vaginal epithelium in the common marmoset (*Callithrix jacchus*): a preliminary new approach to reproductive screening. *Contemp Top Lab Anim Sci* 43: 28–31.

79 Izard, M.K. and Rasmussen, D.T. (1985). Reproduction in the slender Loris (*Loris tardigradus malabaricus*). *Am J Primatol* 8: 153–165.

80 Dukelow, W.R. (1983). The squirrel monkey. In: *Reproduction in New World Primates* (ed. J. Hearn), 151–179. Hingham, MA: MTP Press.

81 Mehta, R.R., Jenco, J.M., Gaynor, L.V., and Chatterton, R.T. Jr. (1986). Relationships between ovarian morphology, vaginal cytology, serum progesterone, and urinary immunoreactive pregnanediol during the menstrual cycle of the cynomolgus monkey. *Biol Reprod* 35: 981–986.

82 Seed, J., Chapin, R.E., Clegg, E.D. et al. (1996). Methods for assessing sperm motility, morphology, and counts in the rat, rabbit, and dog: a consensus report. ILSI Risk Science Institute Expert Working Group on Sperm Evaluation. *Reprod Toxicol* 10: 237–244.

83 Luetjens, C.M. and Weinbauer, G.F. (2012). Functional assessment of sexual maturity in male macaques (*Macaca fascicularis*). *Regul Toxicol Pharmacol* 63: 391–400.

84 Williams, J., Gladen, B.C., Schrader, S.M. et al. (1990). Semen analysis and fertility assessment in rabbits: statistical power and design considerations for toxicology studies. *Fundam Appl Toxicol* 15: 651–665.

85 Slott, V.L. and Perreault, S. (1993). *Computer-Assisted Sperm Analysis of Rodent Epididymal Sperm Motility Using the Hamilton-Thorn Motility Analyzer. Methods in Toxicology*, 319–333. San Diego, CA: Academic Press.

86 Filler, R. (1993). Sperm morphology evaluation. In: *Methods in Toxicology* (eds. G. Jolles and A. Cordier), 334–343. San Diego, CA: Academic Press.

87 Oettle, E.E. (1993). Sperm morphology and fertility in the dog. *J Reprod Fertil Suppl* 47: 257–260.

88 Paufler, S.K. and Foote, R.H. (1968). Morphology, motility and fertility of spermatozoa recovered from different areas of ligated rabbit epididymides. *J Reprod Fertil* 17: 125–137.

89 Patience, J.F., Friend, D.W., Hartin, K.E., and Wolynetz, M.S. (1987). A comparison of two urine collection methods for female swine. *Can J Anim Sci* 67: 859–863.

90 Preube, C. and Skaanild, M.T. (2012). Minipigs in absorption, distribution, metabolism, and excretion (ADME) studies. In: *The Minipig in Biomedical Research*, vol. 155 (eds. P.A. McAnulty, A.D. Dayan, N.-C. Ganderup and K.L. Hastings). Boca Raton, FL: CRC Press.

91 Reis, L.O., Sopena, J.M., Favaro, W.J. et al. (2011). Anatomical features of the urethra and urinary bladder catheterization in female mice and rats. An essential translational tool. *Acta Cir Bras* 26 (Suppl 2): 106–110.

92 Kurien, B.T., Everds, N.E., and Scofield, R.H. (2004). Experimental animal urine collection: a review. *Lab Anim* 38: 333–361.

93 Flatt, R.E. and Carpenter, A.B. (1971). Identification of crystalline material in urine of rabbits. *Am J Vet Res* 32: 655–658.

94 Loeb, W.F. and Quimby, F.W. (1999). The rabbit. In: *The Clinical Chemistry of Laboratory Animals*, 2e (eds. W.F. Loeb and F.W. Quimby), 70–81. Philadelphia, PA: Taylor & Francis.

95 Hall, R.L. (2007). Clinical pathology of laboratory animals. In: *Animal Models in Toxicology* (ed. S.C. Gad), 787–830. Boca Raton, FL: CRC Press/Taylor & Francis.

96 Chase, J., Hammond, J., Bilbrough, G. et al. (2015). Examination of imprecision and effectiveness of different centrifugation and uncentrifugation methods for urine sediment microscopic evaluation. *Proceedings: ACVP-STP*, Minneapolis, MN (17–21 October 2015).

97 Rosenthal, K.L. (2008). Small mammals. In: *Rapid Review of Exotic Animal Medicine and Husbandry* (eds. K.L. Rosenthal, N. Forbes, F.L. Frye and G.A. Lewbart), 19. Boca Raton, FL: CRC Press.

98 Hillyer, E.V. and Quesenberry, K.E. (1997). Rabbits: reproductive and urogenital disorders. In: *Ferrets, Rabbits, and Rodents Clinical Medicine and Surgery* (eds. E.V. Hillyer and K.E. Quesenberry), 202–211. Philadelphia, PA: W.B. Saunders.

99 Haber, M.H. and PCJ, W. (2002). Urine. In: *Clinical Laboratory Medicine* (ed. K.D. McClatchey), 519–551. Philadelphia, PA: Lippincott Williams and Wilkins.

100 Loeb, W.F. and Quimby, F.W. (1999). *The Clinical Chemistry of Laboratory Animals*. Philadelphia, PA: Taylor & Francis.

101 Osborne, C.A. and Stevens, J.B. (eds.) (1999). Urine sediment. In: *Urinalysis: A Clinical Guide to Compassionate Patient Care*, 132–141. Shawnee Mission, KS: Bayer Corporation.

102 Strasinger, S.K. and Di Lorenzo, M.S. (eds.) (2014). Urine sediment constituents. In: *Urinalysis and Body Fluids*, 111. Philadelphia, PA: F.A. Davis.

103 Hall, R.L. and Everds, N.E. (2014). Principles of clinical pathology for toxicology studies. In: *Principles and Methods of Toxicology*, 5e (eds. A.W. Hayes and C.L. Kruger), 1336. Boca Raton, FL: CRC Press.

104 Hall, R.L. (2013). Principles of clinical pathology. In: *Toxicologic Pathology: Nonclinical Safety Assessment*, 1e, vol. 166 (eds. J.A. Popp, P.S. Sahota and J.F. Hardisty). Boca Raton, FL: CRC Press.

105 Graff, S. (1983). *A Handbook of Routine Urinalysis*. Philadelphia, PA: J.B. Lippincott.

106 Motojima, K. and Goto, S. (1990). Organization of rat uricase chromosomal gene differs greatly from that of the corresponding plant gene. *FEBS Lett* 264 (1): 156–158.

107 Roch-Ramel, F. and Peters, G. (1978). Urinary excretion of uric acid in nonhuman mammalian species. In: *Handbook of Experimental Pharmacology (Continuation of Handbuch der Experimentellen Pharmakologie)*, vol. 51 (eds. W.N. Kelley and I.M. Weiner), 211–255. Berlin, Heidelberg: Springer.

108 Chen, Y., Qin, S., Ding, Y. et al. (2009). Reference values of clinical chemistry and hematology parameters in rhesus monkeys (*Macaca mulatta*). *Xenotransplantation* 16: 496–501.

109 Denny, K.H. and Stewart, C.W. (2013). Acute, sub-acute, sub-chronic, and chronic general toxicity testing for preclinical development. In: *A Comprehensive Guide to Toxicology in Preclinical Drug Development*, vol. 103 (ed. A.S. Faqi). Waltham, MA: Academic Press.

110 Parrula, M.C. and Pandya, D. (2015). What is your diagnosis? Urine from a cynomolgus monkey. *Vet Clin Pathol* 44: 169–170.

Index

Page locators in **bold** indicate tables. Page locators in *italics* indicate figures. This index uses letter-by-letter alphabetization.

a

Veterinary Cytology, First Edition. Edited by Leslie C. Sharkey, M. Judith Radin, and Davis Seelig.

C